Pediatric Lower Limb Deformities

Sanjeev Sabharwal • Christopher A. Iobst
Editors

Pediatric Lower Limb Deformities

Principles and Techniques of Management

Second Edition

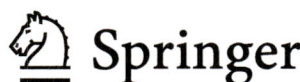

Editors
Sanjeev Sabharwal
Department of Orthopedics
UCSF Benioff Children's Hospital
Oakland, CA, USA

Christopher A. Iobst
Department of Orthopedics
Nationwide Children's Hospital
Columbus, OH, USA

ISBN 978-3-031-55766-8   ISBN 978-3-031-55767-5 (eBook)
https://doi.org/10.1007/978-3-031-55767-5

© The Editor(s) (if applicable) and The Author(s), under exclusive license to Springer Nature Switzerland AG 2016, 2024

This work is subject to copyright. All rights are solely and exclusively licensed by the Publisher, whether the whole or part of the material is concerned, specifically the rights of translation, reprinting, reuse of illustrations, recitation, broadcasting, reproduction on microfilms or in any other physical way, and transmission or information storage and retrieval, electronic adaptation, computer software, or by similar or dissimilar methodology now known or hereafter developed.

The use of general descriptive names, registered names, trademarks, service marks, etc. in this publication does not imply, even in the absence of a specific statement, that such names are exempt from the relevant protective laws and regulations and therefore free for general use.

The publisher, the authors, and the editors are safe to assume that the advice and information in this book are believed to be true and accurate at the date of publication. Neither the publisher nor the authors or the editors give a warranty, expressed or implied, with respect to the material contained herein or for any errors or omissions that may have been made. The publisher remains neutral with regard to jurisdictional claims in published maps and institutional affiliations.

This Springer imprint is published by the registered company Springer Nature Switzerland AG
The registered company address is: Gewerbestrasse 11, 6330 Cham, Switzerland

If disposing of this product, please recycle the paper.

Preface

Welcome to the second edition of *Pediatric Lower Limb Deformities: Principles and Techniques of Management*. In line with the goals of the previous edition, this updated textbook comprehensively covers all aspects of pediatric lower limb deformity from the hip to the toes. The author of each chapter was carefully chosen as an international expert for the assigned topic and was asked to provide current, state-of-the-art management principles for the reader to use in their day-to-day clinical practice. This up-to-date treatise is presented in a format that not only provides valuable fundamental information for the young surgeon but also covers nuances, including practical tips and tricks that will be relevant to the advanced limb deformity surgeon as well.

There are two special features of this second edition that are worth highlighting. First, besides updating the content of each chapter, ten entirely new chapters have been added including those highlighting Patient Reported Outcome Measures (PROMs) in limb lengthening and deformity correction; how to set up a limb deformity practice; pin site care and management of bone defects. The second update involves supplementing the content of each of the 40 chapters with an invited commentary from another authority in the field. In this way, the reader gets the benefit of at least two different perspectives on the topic as well as additional pearls and insights from experts in the field.

Finally, on reviewing the Table of Contents for the list of contributors, you will notice that this unique textbook has a decidedly international flavor. In order to make this work relevant to a broad audience of limb reconstruction surgeons and trainees, we have made a concerted effort to include perspectives from surgeons practicing in regions with varying degrees of resource availability and unique clinical pathology. Thus, we purposely invited contributions from a diverse group of professionals who were not only content experts in the assigned topic but also practiced in different clinical settings. Our goal was to tap into the incredible pediatric limb reconstruction work being done around the globe and to share this amazing repository of resources with you, the reader. We both have thoroughly enjoyed preparing this second edition and have learned an enormous amount from our colleagues and hope that you will too.

Oakland, CA, USA Sanjeev Sabharwal
Columbus, OH, USA Christopher A. Iobst

Acknowledgments

Acknowledgement by Sanjeev Sabharwal, MD, MPH (Director, Limb Lengthening and Complex Reconstruction Center, UCSF Benioff Children's Hospital, Oakland, CA, USA)

This second edition would not have been possible without the professional relationships and friendships that were developed over the years with members of the Limb Lengthening and Reconstruction Society (LLRS), Pediatric Orthopaedic Society of North America (POSNA), and Paediatric Orthopaedic Society of India (POSI). I am thankful to the residents, staff, and faculty of the Department of Orthopaedics at the University of California, San Francisco, who have taught me the value of patience and persistence. I have been lucky to have the institutional and academic infrastructure and an awesome team, here at UCSF Benioff Children's Hospital in Oakland, California.

The constant support of my dear friend and co-editor, Chris Iobst and the Springer publishing team, especially Kristopher Spring was vital in making this second edition a reality.

I am extremely grateful to my parents, grandparents, mentors, and students for helping me recognize the importance of integrity and hard work. Thanks to my dearest wife, Ranjit, who for the past 35 years took care of essentially everything so that I could pursue an academic career in pediatric orthopedics and limb reconstruction. I appreciate our three lovely children, Samir, Simran, and Sabhyta and their growing families for keeping me honest and grounded.

Acknowledgement by Christopher A. Iobst, MD (Director, Center for Limb Lengthening and Reconstruction, Nationwide Children's Hospital, Columbus, OH, USA)

I would like to reiterate Sanjeev's message of appreciation and gratitude to the entire international limb lengthening and reconstruction community. I am eternally indebted to the generosity and kindness of my mentors and countless colleagues who have guided and educated me along the way. I am constantly impressed by the spirit of kindness and willingness to help displayed throughout the entire limb reconstruction field. This second edition is an example of that collaborative power and sharing of knowledge. We hope it will continue to provide valuable reference and education to surgeons both young and old.

Personally, I must thank the Center for Limb Lengthening and Reconstruction team at Nationwide Children's Hospital for their hard work and dedication to taking care of patients with limb deformities. We have been able to make our dream of establishing a Center that provides comprehensive care for patients and their families become a reality. As we recently celebrated our eighth birthday, I would especially like to thank Danielle, Ashley, Cheri, and Jessica who have been critical, invaluable team members from the start.

Finally, I would like to thank my family. My parents, for their lifelong support and for teaching me the value of hard work and education. I could never have been able to follow this path without them. To my wife, Sybil, for providing the peaceful atmosphere, understanding and love necessary to complete the time-consuming process of editing a reference textbook.

Contents

Part I General Principles and Techniques

1. **Etiology of Lower Limb Deformity** 3
   Allyson Zakrzewski and Viral V. Jain

2. **Clinical Evaluation Including Imaging** 19
   Raymond W. Liu

3. **Decision-Making in Lower Extremity Deformity Correction** 39
   J. Eric Gordon

4. **Outcome Measures in Limb Lengthening and Deformity Correction** 59
   Harpreet Chhina and Anthony Cooper

5. **Keys to Building a Successful Pediatric Limb Reconstruction Program** 69
   Christopher A. Iobst and Anirejuoritse Bafor

6. **Growth Modulation for Angular and Length Correction** 83
   Peter M. Stevens

7. **Physeal Bar Excision** 103
   David A. Podeszwa, Anthony I. Riccio, and Karl E. Rathjen

8. **Acute Deformity Correction Using an Osteotomy** 117
   Vrisha Madhuri and Jonathan Reddy

9. **Gradual Deformity Correction in Children and Adolescents** 151
   Mark Eidelman, Pavel Kotlarsky, and John E. Herzenberg

10. **Pin Site Care** 173
    Nando Ferreira and William D. Harrison

11. **Fixator Assisted Nailing and Plating** 189
    Chang-Wug Oh

12. **Hybrid Techniques for Limb Length and Deformity Correction** 211
    Mark T. Dahl, Andrew G. Georgiadis, and Stewart G. Morrison

13. **Motorized Intramedullary Lengthening of the Femur: Antegrade and Retrograde** ... 227
    Søren Kold and Christopher A. Iobst

14. **Motorized Intramedullary Lengthening of the Tibia** 281
    Austin T. Fragomen

Part II Related Concepts and Management Options

15 **Biomechanically Based Clinical Decision Making in Pediatric Foot and Ankle Surgery**... 295
Jon R. Davids

16 **Congenital Foot Deformities** 307
Mitzi L. Williams and Matthew B. Dobbs

17 **Management of Pediatric Foot and Ankle Deformities: Gradual Correction** 337
Bradley M. Lamm

18 **Pediatric Joint Contractures** 353
Aaron J. Huser and David S. Feldman

19 **Physical Therapy During Limb Lengthening and Deformity Correction: Principles and Techniques** 363
Anil Bhave, Erin Baker, and Mary Campbell

20 **Amputation and Prosthetic Management: Amputation as a Reconstructive Option** 383
John A. Herring

21 **Working in Resource-Challenged Environments** 405
Scott C. Nelson and Philip K. McClure

Part III Underlying Conditions

22 **Metabolic Disorders** 429
Ali Bas, Mehmet Kocaoglu, Levent Eralp, and F. Erkal Bilen

23 **Osteogenesis Imperfecta** 457
Reggie C. Hamdy, Yousef Marwan, Frank Rauch, Kathleen Montpetit, and François R. Fassier

24 **Lower Limb Deformity in Neuromuscular Disorders: Pathophysiology, Assessment, Goals, and Principles of Management** 479
Unni G. Narayanan

25 **Arthrogryposis** 517
Reggie C. Hamdy, Yousef Marwan, Khaled Abu Dalu, and Noémi Dahan-Oliel

26 **Limb Lengthening and Deformity Correction in Patients with Skeletal Dysplasias** 537
Mihir M. Thacker, Colleen Ditro, W. G. Stuart Mackenzie, and William G. Mackenzie

27 **Lower Extremity Benign Bone Lesions and Related Conditions** 561
Lori Karol and Daniel E. Prince

28 **Management of Juxtaphyseal Malignant Bone Tumors Around the Knee Joint: New Concepts in Limb-Sparing Surgery** 581
Hidenori Matsubara and Hiroyuki Tsuchiya

Part IV Congenital and Developmental Disorders

29 Congenital Femoral Deficiency Reconstruction and Lengthening Surgery 595
Dror Paley and Claire E. Shannon

30 Fibular Hemimelia in the Pediatric Patient 713
Philip K. McClure, John E. Herzenberg, and Shawn C. Standard

31 Tibial Hemimelia 747
Dror Paley, Katherine Miller, and David Y. Chong

32 Treatment of Congenital Pseudarthrosis of the Tibia 791
Claire E. Shannon and Dror Paley

33 Congenital Posteromedial Bowing of the Tibia 831
Benjamin Joseph, Hitesh Shah, and N. D. Siddesh

34 Controversies in Blount's Disease 843
David A. Podeszwa and John G. Birch

Part V Sequelae and Complications

35 Methods to Enhance Bone Formation in Distraction Osteogenesis 863
Hae-Ryong Song, Dong-Hoon Lee, Young-Hwan Park, and Ashok Kumar Ramanathan

36 Residual Deformities of the Hip 883
Shawn C. Standard and Daniel K. Ruggles

37 Posttraumatic Lower Limb Deformities in Children 927
Ashok N. Johari, Sandeep A. Patwardhan, and Taral Vishanji Nagda

38 Postinfectious Deformities of the Lower Limb 959
In Ho Choi and Chang Ho Shin

39 Bone Defects 977
Abdullah Addar, Reggie C. Hamdy, and Mitchell Bernstein

40 Iatrogenic Deformities 993
Austin T. Fragomen and Robert Rozbruch

Index 1017

Contributors and Commentators

Contributors

Abdullah Addar Department of Orthopaedics, King Saud University, Riyadh, Saudi Arabia

Anirejuoritse Bafor Department of Orthopedic Surgery, Nationwide Children's Hospital, Columbus, OH, USA

Erin Baker OrthoNY, Albany, NY, USA

Ali Bas Department of Orthopedics and Traumatology, Koç University Hospital, Istanbul, Turkey

Mitchell Bernstein Shriners Hospital for Children-Canada, Montreal, QC, Canada
Department of Surgery and Pediatric Surgery, McGill University, Montreal, QC, Canada
Montreal Children's Hospital, Montreal, QC, Canada
Montreal General Hospital, Montreal, QC, Canada

Anil Bhave Rubin Institute for Advanced Orthopedics, Sinai Hospital, Baltimore, MD, USA

F. Erkal Bilen Macka EMAR Medical Center, Istanbul, Turkey

John G. Birch Department of Orthopedics, Scottish Rite for Children, Dallas, TX, USA

Mary Campbell Baltimore, MD, USA

Harpreet Chhina Department of Orthopaedic Surgery, BC Children's Hospital, Vancouver, BC, Canada

Department of Orthopaedics, University of British Columbia, Vancouver, BC, Canada

In Ho Choi Division of Pediatric Orthopedics, Seoul National University Children's Hospital, Seoul, Republic of Korea
Department of Orthopedic Surgery, Chung-Ang University Hospital, Seoul, South Korea

David Y. Chong Department of Orthopedic Surgery, University of Oklahoma Health Sciences Center, Oklahoma City, OK, USA

Anthony Cooper Department of Orthopaedics, University of British Columbia, Vancouver, BC, Canada

Noémi Dahan-Oliel Clinical Research/Rehabilitation, Shriners Hospital for Children, Montreal, QC, Canada

Mark T. Dahl Limb Lengthening Service, Minneapolis, MN, USA
Department of Orthopaedics, Gillettte Children's Hospital, St. Paul, MN, USA
Orthopedic Surgery, University of Minnesota, Minneapolis, MN, USA

Khaled Abu Dalu Division of Pediatric Orthopedics, Department of Orthopedics, Shriners Hospital for Children, McGill University, Montreal, QC, Canada

Jon R. Davids Shriners Children's Northern California, Sacramento, CA, USA

Department of Orthopaedic Surgery, University of California Davis, Sacramento, CA, USA

Colleen Ditro Department of Orthopedic Surgery, Nemours Children's Hospital, Delaware, Wilmington, DE, USA

Matthew B. Dobbs Dobbs Clubfoot Center, Paley Institute, West Palm Beach, FL, USA

Clinical Orthopaedics and Related Research, Park Ridge, IL, USA

United States Bone and Joint Initiative, Warrenville, IL, USA

Association of Bone and Joint Surgeons, Park Ridge, IL, USA

International Federation of Pediatric Orthopaedic Societies, St. Louis, MO, USA

Mark Eidelman Pediatric Orthopedics, Ruth Rappoport Children's Hospital, Rambam Health Care Campus, Haifa, Israel

Levent Eralp Istanbul Faculty of Medicine, Istanbul University, Istanbul, Turkey

François R. Fassier Shriners Hospital for Children – Canada and McGill University Health Centre, Montreal, QC, Canada

David S. Feldman Paley Orthopedic and Spine Institute, West Palm Beach, FL, USA

Nando Ferreira Division of Orthopaedic Surgery, Department of Surgical Sciences, Faculty of Medicine and Health Sciences, Stellenbosch University, Cape Town, South Africa

Austin T. Fragomen Limb Lengthening & Complex Reconstruction Service, Hospital for Special Surgery, New York, NY, USA

Department of Orthopedics, Hospital for Special Surgery, New York, NY, USA

Andrew G. Georgiadis Department of Orthopaedics, Gillettte Children's Hospital, St. Paul, MN, USA

Orthopedic Surgery, University of Minnesota, Minneapolis, MN, USA

J. Eric Gordon St. Louis Children's Hospital, St Louis, MO, USA

Department of Orthopaedic Surgery, Washington University School of Medicine, St. Louis, MO, USA

St. Louis Shriner's Hospital for Children, St. Louis, MO, USA

Reggie C. Hamdy Shriners Hospital for Children – Canada and McGill University Health Centre, Montreal, QC, Canada

Department of Pediatric Surgery, McGill University Health Center, Quebec, Canada

Division of Pediatric Orthopedics, Department of Orthopedics, Shriners Hospital for Children, McGill University, Montreal, QC, Canada

William D. Harrison Limb Reconstruction Service, Liverpool University Hospitals, Liverpool, UK

John A. Herring Department of Orthopedic Surgery, Scottish Rite for Children, University of Texas Southwestern Medical School, Dallas, TX, USA

John E. Herzenberg International Center for Limb Lengthening, Rubin Institute for Advanced Orthopedics, Sinai Hospital of Baltimore, Baltimore, MD, USA

Aaron J. Huser Paley Orthopedic and Spine Institute, West Palm Beach, FL, USA

Christopher A. Iobst Department of Orthopedic Surgery, Nationwide Children's Hospital, Columbus, OH, USA

Center for Limb Lengthening and Reconstruction, Orthopaedic Surgery, Nationwide Children's Hospital, Columbus, OH, USA

Viral V. Jain Division of Orthopedic Surgery—MLC# 2017, Cincinnati Children's Hospital Medical Center, Cincinnati, OH, USA

Ashok N. Johari Department of Paediatric Orthopaedics, Children's Orthopaedic Centre, Mumbai, Maharashtra, India

Benjamin Joseph Kasturba Medical College, Manipal, Karnataka, India

Lori Karol Department of Orthopedic Surgery, Texas Scottish Rite Hospital, Dallas, TX, USA

Mehmet Kocaoglu Istanbul Faculty of Medicine, Unimed Center, Istanbul, Turkey

Søren Kold Limb Lengthening and Reconstruction, Department of Orthopaedics, Aalborg University Hospital, Aalborg, Denmark

Pavel Kotlarsky Pediatric Orthopedics, Ruth Rappoport Children's Hospital, Rambam Health Care Campus, Haifa, Israel

Bradley M. Lamm Foot and Ankle Surgery at St. Mary's Medical Center & Palm Beach Children's Hospital, West Palm Beach, FL, USA

Foot and Ankle Deformity Correction Center and Fellowship, Paley Orthopedic and Spine Institute, West Palm Beach, FL, USA

Dong-Hoon Lee Department of Orthopedic Surgery, Severance Children's Hospital, Seoul, Republic of Korea

Raymond W. Liu Rainbow Babies and Children's Hospital, Cleveland, OH, USA

W. G. Stuart Mackenzie Department of Orthopedic Surgery, Nemours Children's Hospital, Delaware, Wilmington, DE, USA

William G. Mackenzie Department of Orthopedic Surgery, Nemours Children's Hospital, Delaware, Wilmington, DE, USA

Vrisha Madhuri Department of Paediatric Orthopaedics, Amara hospital, Tirupati, India

Department of Paediatric Orthopaedics, Christian Medical College and Hospital, Vellore, Tamil Nadu, India

Yousef Marwan Shriners Hospital for Children – Canada and McGill University Health Centre, Montreal, QC, Canada

Division of Pediatric Orthopedics, Department of Orthopedics, Shriners Hospital for Children, McGill University, Montreal, QC, Canada

Hidenori Matsubara Department of Orthopedic Surgery, Kanazawa University Hospital, Kanazawa, Ishikawa, Japan

Philip K. McClure International Center for Limb Lengthening, Rubin Institute for Advanced Orthopedics, Sinai Hospital of Baltimore, Baltimore, MD, USA

Katherine Miller St. Mary's Medical Center, Paley Orthopedic and Spine Institute, West Palm Beach, FL, USA

Kathleen Montpetit Shriners Hospital for Children – Canada and McGill University Health Centre, Montreal, QC, Canada

Stewart G. Morrison The Royal Children's Hospital—Melbourne, Parkville, VIC, Australia

Victorian Orthoapedic Centre, Melbourne, VIC, Australia

The Bob Dickens Pediatric Orthopaedic Research Fellowship, Melbourne, VIC, Australia

Taral Vishanji Nagda Department of Pediatric Orthopedics, SRCC Children's Hospital Mumbai, Mumbai, Maharashtra, India

Unni G. Narayanan Department of Surgery and Rehabilitation Sciences Institute, University of Toronto, Toronto, ON, Canada

Division of Orthopaedic Surgery and Child Health Evaluative Sciences Program, The Hospital for Sick Children, Toronto, ON, Canada

Scott C. Nelson Department of Orthopaedic Surgery, Loma Linda University School of Medicine, Loma Linda, CA, USA

Chang-Wug Oh Department of Orthopedic Surgery, School of Medicine, Kyungpook National University, Kyungpook National University Hospital, Daegu, Republic of Korea

Dror Paley Paley Orthopedic and Spine Institute, West Palm Beach, FL, USA

St. Mary's Medical Center, Paley Orthopedic and Spine Institute, West Palm Beach, FL, USA

Young-Hwan Park Department of Orthopedic Surgery, Korea University Medical Center, Guro Hospital, Seoul, Republic of Korea

Sandeep A. Patwardhan Department of Pediatric Orthopedics, Sancheti Institute for Orthopedics and Rehabilitation, Pune, Maharashtra, India

David A. Podeszwa, MD Department of Orthopedics, Scottish Rite for Children, Dallas, TX, USA

Daniel E. Prince Division of Orthopaedic Oncology, Department of Surgery, Memorial Sloan Kettering Cancer Center, New York, NY, USA

Ashok Kumar Ramanathan Department of Orthopedic Surgery, Madurai Medical College, Madurai, Tamil Nadu, India

Karl E. Rathjen, MD Department of Orthopedic Surgery, Scottish Rite for Children, Dallas, TX, USA

Frank Rauch Shriners Hospital for Children – Canada and McGill University Health Centre, Montreal, QC, Canada

Jonathan Reddy Department of Paediatric Orthopaedics, Christian Medical College and Hospital, Vellore, Tamil Nadu, India

Anthony I. Riccio, MD Department of Orthopedic Surgery, Scottish Rite for Children, Dallas, TX, USA

Robert Rozbruch Department of Orthopedics, Hospital for Special Surgery, New York, NY, USA

Weill Cornell Medical College, Cornell University, New York, NY, USA

Daniel K. Ruggles Department of Orthopedic Surgery, Nicklaus Children's Hospital, Miami, FL, USA

Hitesh Shah Department of Paediatric Orthopedics, Kasturba Medical College, Kasturba Hospital, Manipal Academy of Higher Education, Manipal, Karnataka, India

Claire E. Shannon Paley Orthopedic and Spine Institute, West Palm Beach, FL, USA

Chang Ho Shin Division of Pediatric Orthopedics, Seoul National University Children's Hospital, Seoul, Republic of Korea

N. D. Siddesh Department of Orthopaedics, Dubai Hospital, Dubai Health Authority, Dubai, United Arab Emirates

Hae-Ryong Song Department of Orthopedic Surgery, Korea University Medical Center, Guro Hospital, Seoul, Republic of Korea

Shawn C. Standard International Center for Limb Lengthening, Rubin Institute for Advanced Orthopedics, Sinai Hospital of Baltimore, Baltimore, MD, USA

Peter M. Stevens Department of Orthopedics, University of Utah School of Medicine, Salt Lake City, UT, USA

Mihir M. Thacker Department of Orthopedic Surgery, Nemours Children's Hospital, Delaware, Wilmington, DE, USA

Hiroyuki Tsuchiya Department of Orthopedic Surgery, Kanazawa University Hospital, Kanazawa, Ishikawa, Japan

Mitzi L. Williams Kaiser San Francisco Bay Area Foot and Ankle Residency Program, Department of Orthopedics and Podiatric Surgery, Kaiser Permanente, Oakland, CA, USA

Allyson Zakrzewski SUNY Upstate, Syracuse, NY, USA

Commentators

Alexandre Arkader Pediatric Orthopedics & Orthopedic Oncology, Perelman School of Medicine at University of Pennsylvania, The Children's Hospital of Philadelphia, Philadelphia, PA, USA

Anirejuoritse Bafor Department of Orthopedic Surgery, Nationwide Children's Hospital, Columbus, OH, USA

Oliver Birke The Children's Hospital at Westmead, Sydney, NSW, Australia

University of Sydney, Sydney, NSW, Australia

Franz Birkholtz Institute of Orthopaedics and Rheumatology, Mediclinic Winelands Orthopaedic Hospital, Stellenbosch, South Africa

Peter Calder The Royal National Orthopaedic Hospital, Stanmore, London, UK

Milind Chaudhary Centre for Ilizarov Techniques in India, Chaudhary Hospital, Akola, Maharashtra, India

In-Ho Choi Department of Orthopedic Surgery, Chung-Ang University Hospital, Seoul, South Korea

Janet D. Conway Head of Bone and Joint Infection, International Center for Limb Lengthening, Rubin Institute for Advanced Orthopedics, Sinai Hospital of Baltimore, Baltimore, MD, USA

Mark T. Dahl Department of Orthopedic Surgery, University of Minnesota, Minneapolis, MN, USA

Limb Lengthening and Deformity Correction, Gillette Children's Specialty Healthcare, St. Paul, MN, USA

Mark Eidelman Department of Pediatric Orthopedics, Ruth Children's Hospital, Haifa, Israel

Jill C. Flanagan Department of Orthopedic Surgery, Children's Healthcare of Atlanta, Atlanta, GA, USA

David B. Frumberg Yale School of Medicine, New Haven, CT, USA

J. Eric Gordon St. Louis Children's Hospital, St Louis, MO, USA

Fran Guardo Paley Orthopedic and Spine Institute, West Palm Beach, FL, USA

Reggie C. Hamdy McGill University Health Centre, The Montreal Children's Hospital, Shriners Hospital for Children-Canada, Montreal, QC, Canada

Philip K. McClure Sinai Hospital of Baltimore, Baltimore, MD, USA

Mindaugas Mikužis, MD Limb Lengthening and Reconstruction, Department of Orthopedics, Aalborg University Hospital, Aalborg, Denmark

Fergal Monsell Department of Paediatric Orthopaedic Surgery, Bristol Royal Hospital for Children, Bristol, UK

Unni G. Narayanan Departments of Surgery & Rehabilitation Sciences Institute, Division of Orthopaedic Surgery, University of Toronto, Toronto, ON, Canada

Child Health Evaluative Sciences Program, The Hospital for Sick Children, Toronto, ON, Canada

Stephen M. Quinnan Department of Orthopaedic Surgery, Florida Atlantic University, Boca Raton, FL, USA

Department of Orthopaedic Trauma and Amputee Reconstruction, Paley Orthopedic and Spine Institute, St. Mary's Medical Center, West Palm Beach, FL, USA

J. Spence Reid Penn State Bone and Joint Institute, Hershey, PA, USA

Craig Robbins Paley Orthopedic and Spine Institute, West Palm Beach, FL, USA

Jan Duedal Rölfing Children's Orthopaedics and Reconstruction, Aarhus University Hospital, Aarhus, Denmark

R. E. Christopher Rose Division of Orthopaedics, University Hospital of the West Indies, Kingston, Jamaica, West Indies

Tom Scharschmidt Department of Orthopedics, Nationwide Children's Hospital, Columbus, OH, USA

Hemant K. Sharma Hull York Medical School, Hull Limb Reconstruction and Bone Infection Unit, University of Hull, Hull University Teaching Hospitals, Hull, UK

Noman A. Siddiqui International Center for Limb Lengthening, Rubin Institute Advanced Orthopedics, Sinai Hospital of Baltimore, Baltimore, MD, USA

David A. Spiegel Department of Orthopaedic Surgery, Children's Hospital of Philadelphia, Perelman School of Medicine at the University of Pennsylvania, Philadelphia, PA, USA

Louis-Nicolas Veilleux Montreal General Hospital, Montreal, QC, Canada

Bjoern Vogt Pediatric Orthopedics, Deformity Reconstruction and Foot Surgery, Muenster University Hospital, Muenster, Germany

Hugh G. Watts Department of Orthopedics, University of California at Los Angeles, Shriners Hospitals for Children, Pasadena, CA, USA

Klane K. White Department of Pediatric Orthopedics, The Rose Brown Endowed Chair of Pediatric Orthopedic Surgery, Children's Hospital Colorado, Aurora, CO, USA

Department of Orthopedics, University of Colorado School of Medicine, Aurora, CO, USA

University of Colorado Anschutz Medical Campus, Aurora, CO, USA

Part I
General Principles and Techniques

Etiology of Lower Limb Deformity

Allyson Zakrzewski and Viral V. Jain

Etiologies of lower extremity deformity include conditions that result in limb length inequality, angular deformity, and/or asymmetric girth. There are many different conditions that can result in deformity in children. Despite some overlap, categorizing them can help simplify diagnosis and treatment. Pediatric limb deformities can be classified into four main etiologic groups: (1) underlying conditions, (2) congenital, (3) developmental, and (4) acquired. Table 1.1 demonstrates the wide variety of etiologies that contributed to limb length inequality, deformity, and asymmetric girth.

Table 1.1 General categorization of lower limb deformity in children

Underlying conditions with examples	
Metabolic	Rickets
	Renal osteodystrophy
	Endocrinopathies (hypothyroidism, growth hormone deficiency)
Genetic conditions	Osteogenesis imperfecta
	Neurofibromatosis
	Skeletal dysplasia's
	Arthrogryposis
	Larsen Syndrome
Tumor and tumor-related conditions	Benign tumors
	Malignant tumors
	Fibrous dysplasia
	Ollier's syndrome
	Multiple hereditary exostosis
Inflammatory conditions	Juvenile idiopathic arthritis
	Hemophilic arthropathy
Congenital	
Limb deficiencies	Congenital femoral deficiency (proximal focal femoral deficiency)
	Congenital fibular deficiency (fibular hemimelia)
	Congenital tibial deficiency (tibial hemimelia)
Tibial bowing	Posteromedial bowing
	Anteromedial bowing
	Anterolateral bowing (congenital pseudarthrosis)
Others	Coxa vara
	Congenital knee dislocation
	Congenital patella dislocation
	Hemihypertrophy
Developmental	
Genu varum	Physiologic varus
	Blount's disease—Infantile, adolescent
	Focal fibrocartilaginous dysplasia
Genu valgum	Physiologic valgus
	Idiopathic genu valgum
Acquired	
Residual deformity	Slipped capital femoral epiphysis
	Legg-calve perthes disease
	Developmental dysplasia of the hip
	Avascular necrosis
Post-traumatic	Physeal arrest from fracture involving the growth plate
	Fracture malunion
	Cozen's phenomenon
	Femoral overgrowth
Post-infectious	Physeal arrest from osteomyelitis
	Physeal arrest from septic arthritis
	Physeal bar equivalent
	Meningococcal septicemia
Iatrogenic	Repetitive and aggressive physeal fracture reduction
	Contracture manipulation
	Surgery at or around the physis
	Physeal injury following ligamentous reconstruction

A. Zakrzewski
SUNY Upstate, Syracuse, NY, USA
e-mail: zakrzewA@upstate.edu

V. V. Jain (✉)
Division of Orthopedic Surgery - MLC# 2017, Cincinnati Children's Hospital Medical Center, Cincinnati, OH, USA
e-mail: Viral.Jain@cchmc.org

Underlying Medical Conditions

Metabolic Disorders

Endocrinopathies and metabolic disorders can affect normal regulatory signals necessary for chondrocyte maturation and new bone formation. Disorders such as hypothyroidism and growth hormone deficiency have been shown to weaken the physis and can result in conditions such as slipped capital femoral epiphysis (SCFE) [1]. Compressive forces across these weakened growth plates can lead to the development of angular deformities.

Rickets

Rickets is a clinical manifestation of defective mineralization of the physis secondary to disruption of calcium/phosphate homeostasis. This can be related to genetic as well as nutritional causes. Hypophosphatemic rickets is a Vitamin D resistant form that is caused by the inability of renal tubules to absorb phosphate. While this can be inherited in an autosomal dominant and autosomal recessive fashion, the most common form has an X-linked dominant inheritance. This group of disorders results from a mutation in the phosphate-regulating endopeptidase X-linked gene (PHEX), which is expressed in osteocytes. Mutation in this gene leads to increased levels of fibroblast growth factor 23 (FGF 23), leading to decreased renal phosphate absorption and suppression of (25)-OH-1α hydroxylase activity [2]. Vitamin D-dependent rickets is less common and is related to mutations of (25)-OH-1α hydroxylase.

Nutritional causes are important to consider as well (Fig. 1.1). Risk factors that predispose children to rickets and Vitamin D deficiency include poor nutritional intake, premature birth, dark skin, living in higher latitudes with limited sun exposure, obesity, and malabsorption syndromes (celiac disease, pancreatic insufficiency, and biliary obstruction). Exclusive breast-feeding particularly in non-white children has also been associated with the development of nutritional rickets [3]. The different forms of rickets have similar skeletal manifestations often presenting with lower extremity angular deformity and decreased longitudinal growth with radiographic findings including widened irregular physis and cupped or flared metaphysis.

Renal Osteodystrophy

Renal osteodystrophy occurs secondary to end-stage renal disease and results from the kidney's inability to produce adequate amounts of 1, 25 dihydroxyvitamin D3 as well as phosphate retention. The elevated phosphate levels lead to hyperparathyroidism, which can result in brown tumors and

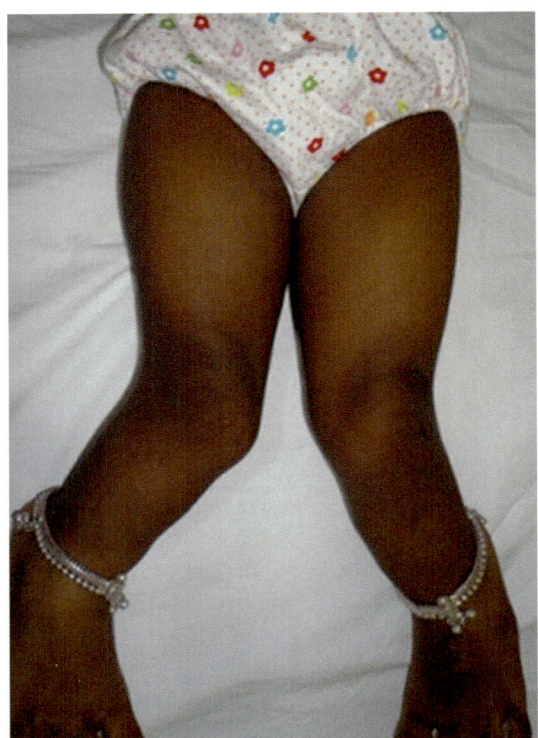

Fig. 1.1 Genu valgum in a 7-year-old female secondary to nutritional rickets

subperiosteal erosions. In children, renal osteodystrophy can lead to growth retardation as well as angular deformities. In addition to the development of valgus or varus lower extremity alignment (typically at the knee but also at the ankle), children with renal osteodystrophy are also at risk for the development of SCFE. The severity of skeletal deformity does not correlate with the degree of control of the renal disease [4].

Genetic Disorders

Osteogenesis Imperfecta

Osteogenesis imperfecta is broadly used to describe a group of genetic disorders that result in increased bone fragility and low bone mass. The most common mutations are in COL1A1 and COL1A2, which encode alpha chains of type I collagen. Clinical presentation varies but patients frequently present to an orthopedic surgeon with lower extremity fragility fractures. The underlying disorder results in poor remodeling potential during healing, and multiple fractures can result in deformity of long bones, which can be in a single plane or multiple planes. Additionally, these children typically have short stature and coxa vara. Bisphosphonates are often used for treatment to increase bone mineral density with the goal of reducing overall fracture rates [5].

Neurofibromatosis

Neurofibromatosis (NF) is a group of genetic disorders involving products of all three germ lines: neuroectoderm, mesoderm, and endoderm. The most orthopedically relevant disorder in this group is Neurofibromatosis Type 1, which previously had been known as von Recklinghausen disease. This is an autosomal dominant disorder with a prevalence rate of 1:4000. It occurs equally in all ethnic groups and 50% are a result of new genetic mutations. The clinical presentation itself is variable with some patients having subclinical to severe manifestations. The associated gene is located on chromosome 17 (17q) and affects neurofibromin, which acts as a tumor suppressor gene [6].

Diagnosis of neurofibromatosis is made by several distinguishing clinical features (Table 1.2). Orthopedic clinical manifestations include tibial dysplasia and hemihypertrophy, which can lead to limb length discrepancies and limb deformities. Both are discussed in greater detail later in the chapter. In addition to lower extremity deformity, spinal deformities are commonly seen in children with neurofibromatosis. Spinal deformities remain the most common orthopedic manifestation with rates of incidence reported around 30% [6]. All patients with neurofibromatosis should be screened for scoliosis during orthopedic evaluation.

Neuromuscular Conditions

Cerebral Palsy

Cerebral palsy is a static encephalopathy that results secondary to an injury to the premature brain. This results in cognitive and musculoskeletal manifestations. From an orthopedic perspective, the presentation of children with cerebral palsy is varied and is based on the presence, distribution, and severity of underlying spasticity. Tone imbalances can lead to the development of deformities of the lower extremity including rotational and angular deformities along with joint contractures.

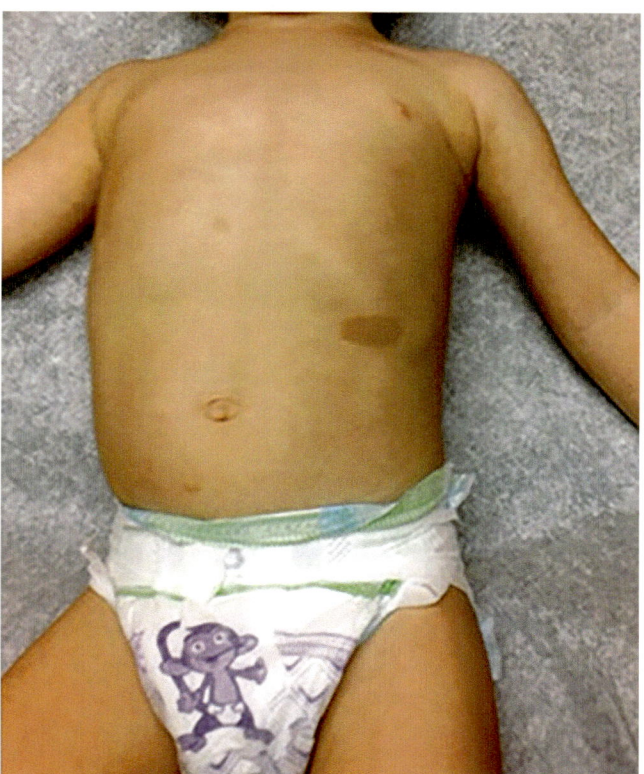

Fig. 1.2 Three-year-old female with neurofibromatosis type 1 (NF1). Café au lait spots are seen on the abdomen

Charcot Marie Tooth

Charcot Maire Tooth disease (CMT) is the most common hereditary motor and sensory neuropathy. There are many described subtypes with the most common subtype being a duplication of the peripheral myelin protein 22 gene (PMP 22) on chromosome 17, which is inherited in an autosomal dominant fashion. Demyelination of peripheral nerves and dorsal root ganglia is progressive and leads to muscle atrophy as well as loss of proprioception and deep tendon reflexes. Weakness in the peroneus brevis, tibialis anterior, as well as intrinsic muscles of the foot results in the most common presentation of a cavovarus foot with claw toes (Fig. 1.3). Other musculoskeletal manifestations include calf atrophy, scoliosis, hip dysplasia, as well as upper extremity intrinsic wasting, resulting in weak pinch and grasp [7].

Arthrogryposis and Related Syndromes

Arthrogryposis multiplex congenital is a heterogeneous group of conditions that present as nonprogressive contractures involving at least two joints at more than two different areas of the body at the time of birth. While not well understood, arthrogryposis is thought to be a genetically mediated syndrome that is related to decreased fetal movement during in-utero development. Hips are commonly involved with typical flexion and abduction contractures with hip

Table 1.2 Diagnostic criteria of neurofibromatosis

Diagnostic Criteria of Neurofibromatosis Type 1 (> 2 criteria for diagnosis)
Six or more café au lait spots measuring at least 15 mm in adults and 5 mm in prepubertal individuals (Fig. 1.2)
Two or more neurofibromas of any type or one plexiform neurofibroma
Freckling in the axillary or inguinal region
Optic Glioma
Two or more Lisch nodules (iris Hamartomas)
A distinctive bony lesion (sphenoid wing dysplasia, thinning of long bone cortex, anterolateral bowing of the tibia, or pseudoarthrosis of a long bone)
A first-degree relative with NF1

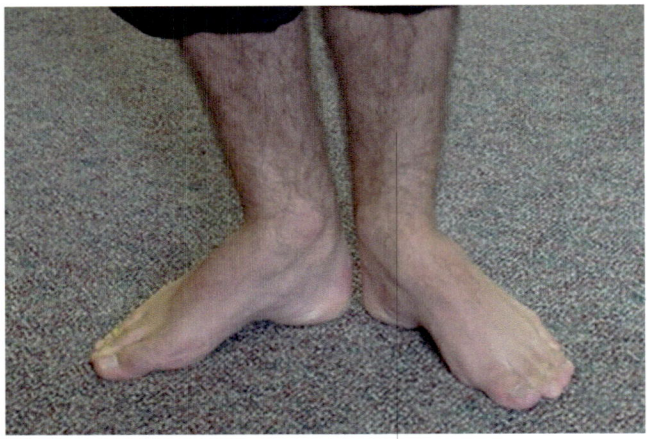

Fig. 1.3 Seventeen-year-old patient with Charcot Marie Tooth Disease (CMT). Cavus deformity of the foot is seen bilaterally

dislocation noted in 15–30% of cases. Involvement of the knees can be with either flexion or extension contractures, although flexion contractures are more common. Foot deformities are frequent with 80–90% of children with arthrogryposis having a clubfoot or congenital vertical talus [8].

Larsen syndrome is a rare disorder that is characterized by multiple joint dislocations that are noted at birth. Mutation has been noted in the FLNB gene, which encodes for filamin B, a cytoskeletal binder that helps chondrocytes differentiate and proliferate [9]. Dislocations of the hips, knees, and cervical spine abnormalities are commonly seen. Clubfoot deformities are rigid and can be difficult to treat [10].

Multiple Pterygium syndrome is a spectrum of disorders, resulting in skin webbing of joints, commonly the elbows and knees. Most cases involve a mutation in the CHRNG gene, which encodes for the gamma subunit of the fetal acetylcholine receptor protein important in neuromuscular signaling. As the adult acetylcholine receptor gene predominates after 33 weeks gestation, joint contractures without concomitant muscle weakness are the typical presentation [11].

Skeletal Dysplasia

Osteochondral dysplasias are disorders of growth and development of cartilage and bone. There are numerous conditions included in the category of skeletal dysplasias with most variations resulting in short stature and angular deformities of the lower extremity. Relevant skeletal dysplasia, underlying genetic findings, lower extremity findings, as well as other orthopedic findings are shown in Table 1.3.

Bone Tumors

Benign bone tumors and tumor-like lesions can result in lower extremity deformity. This is related to pathologic fracture, proximity of the tumor to the physis, or as a result of treatment. Therapeutic curettage or injection can also result in damage to the adjacent growth plate. Additionally, radiation therapy can inhibit the growth of the physis by altering chondroblast activity [14]. The overall risk is related to the amount of radiation delivered, the size of the field, and the patient's overall growth potential. Malignant tumors frequently require wide resection often including the nearby physis, which can lead to an increasing limb length discrepancy with growth.

Polyostotic diseases can result in severe limb deformities. Multiple hereditary exostosis (MHE) is a condition that results secondary to the loss of function of EXT1 and EXT2 proteins, resulting in multiple osteochondromas. These patients typically have short stature and can develop valgus alignment of the hip, knee, and ankle. Fibrous dysplasia is a developmental abnormality that is caused by a mutation in the GS-α protein that leads to failure of the production of normal lamellar bone. While any bone can be involved, the proximal femur is the most common and leads to the characteristic Shepard's crook deformity. Additionally, progressive bowing deformities of the long bones are seen with fibrous dysplasia, and 60% of patients with polyostotic fibrous dysplasia have a reported limb length discrepancy. Ollier's disease is a form of multiple enchondromatosis, which produces islands of cartilage in the diaphyseal and metaphyseal regions of long bones. These lesions often encroach on the physis and can result in inhibition of growth. Typically, this involves one limb more than the other and, as such, can lead to both angular deformities and significant limb length discrepancy [15].

Inflammatory Conditions

Juvenile idiopathic arthritis is a group of conditions that is characterized by chronic joint inflammation of unknown etiology that lasts longer than 6 weeks in a child under the age of 16. This was previously referred to as juvenile rheumatoid arthritis but few children were found to be rheumatoid factor positive. Etiology is multifactorial and likely due to several environmental and genetic factors [16]. Contractures can develop from chronic inflammation and may need to be released. Overgrowth has been reported and is associated with younger age at the time of presentation [16].

1 Etiology of Lower Limb Deformity

Table 1.3 Relevant skeletal dysplasia's and orthopedic manifestations [12, 13]

Condition	Typical inheritance	Involved protein	Common lower extremity deformities	Other orthopedic manifestations
Achondroplasia	Autosomal dominant	Gain of function FGFR3	Rhizomelic dwarfism Genu varum	Lumbar stenosis Thoracolumbar kyphosis Foramen magnum stenosis Trident hand
Pseudoachondroplasia	Autosomal dominant	COMP	Hip dysplasia Genu valgum Genu varum Wind-swept deformity	Cervical instability Kyphoscoliosis Platyspondyly
Hypochondroplasia	Autosomal dominant	FGFR3	Mild short stature Rhizomelic dwarfism Genu varum	Spinal stenosis
Diastrophic Dysplasia	Autosomal recessive	SLC6A2 (sulfate transporter)	Joint contractures Genu valgum Patella dislocation Equinovarus feet	Hitchhiker's thumbs Cervical kyphosis Thoracic kyphosis
Kniest Syndrome	Autosomal dominant	COL2A1	Large stiff joints Equinovarus foot	Odontoid hypoplasia Kyphoscoliosis
Spondyloepiphyseal dysplasia congenita	Autosomal dominant	COL2A1	Short stature Coxa vara Genu valgum Equinovarus foot	C1–C2 instability Scoliosis Platyspondyly
Spondyloepiphyseal dysplasia tarda	X linked	COL2A1	Short stature	Platyspondyly
Multiple epiphyseal Dysplasia	Autosomal dominant	COMP, type IX collagen	Coxa vara Valgus deformity Joint contractures	Normal spine
MPS Type 1 (hurler)	Autosomal recessive	α-l-Iduronidase	Hip dysplasia Genu valgum	Kyphoscoliosis Carpal tunnel syndrome Gibbus deformity
MPS Type IV (Morquio)	Autosomal recessive	Keratin sulfate	Ligamentous laxity Genu valgum Progressive acetabular dysplasia	Odontoid hypoplasia C1–C2 instability Platyspondyly Carpal tunnel

Hemophilic arthropathy results in repeated intra-articular bleeding, leading to synovitis, joint contractures, and joint destruction. Recurrent hemarthrosis can result in lasting changes to chondrocyte activity and cartilage matrix integrity, leading to abnormalities in epiphyseal growth. Asymmetrical growth can result leading to angular deformities. Limb Length discrepancy can also result in related hyperemia [17].

Congenital Etiology

Hemihypertrophy and Hemiatrophy

Hemihypertrophy and hemiatophy are conditions that result in abnormal growth of the affected extremity. These conditions can be idiopathic or related to an underlying syndrome but, in general, lead to significant differences in limb girth and limb length equality. Figure 1.4 demonstrates the limb length discrepancy and asymmetrical girth seen in idiopathic hemihypertrophy. Overgrowth and undergrowth syndromes are detailed in Table 1.4.

Both syndromic and idiopathic hemihypertrophy have been associated with embryonal tumors, such as Wilm's tumor, adrenal cell carcinoma, and hepatoblastoma [18]. Genetic evaluation is important to identify subgroups of patients in which this risk is increased. Beckwith–Wiedemann syndrome has an incidence of embryonal tumors of 8.8%, and serial abdominal exams and ultrasounds are recommended every 3–4 months in this population until age 7 [19].

Congenital Femoral Deficiency

Congenital femoral deficiency is a spectrum of disorders that involve abnormalities in the femur. Proximal focal femoral deficiency (PFFD) is a distinct subset in which the defect is within the primary ossification center of the proximal femur. Variable deficiencies are noted with the mildest form, resulting in a short femur to more severe forms in which the proximal femur is absent and the distal femoral shaft creates a pseudo articulation at the hip. Patients with PFFD present with a short thigh with the hip in a flexed, abducted, and externally rotated position (Fig. 1.5). Additionally, knee contractures are common, and this condition is also associated with ACL deficiency.

In most cases, the underlying genetic link is unknown although there is a form associated with abnormal facies (femoral hypoplasia—unusual facies syndrome), which is inherited in an autosomal dominant fashion [21].

Congenital Fibular Deficiency

This condition, also known as fibular hemimelia, consists of shortening or absence of the fibula along with variable involvement of the lateral bones of the lower extremity. This is the most common long-bone deficiency with an incidence between 7.4 and 20 cases per million live births [22]. The exact etiology is unknown and cases are typically sporadic. Graham et al. suggested that exogenous vascular or mechanical disruption of limb bud function on the apical ectodermal ridge may lead to fibular hemimelia [23]. Angiographic abnormalities have been identified as well [24].

Typically, patients with fibular hemimelia present with a short tibia, anteromedial bowing, and marked equinovalgus deformity of the ankle. Additional abnormalities associated with the condition are hypoplastic lateral femoral condyle, cruciate ligament deficiency, coxa vara, ball and socket ankle joint, tarsal coalitions, and absent lateral rays of the foot. Femoral deficiencies are often seen in conjunction with fibular hemimelia. While the magnitude of femoral shortening is variable, it often contributes to the overall limb shortening. In addition to limb length discrepancy, valgus alignment of the lower extremity often develops from the dysplastic lateral condyle, seen in 93% of children with fibular hemimelia [25].

Congenital Tibia Deficiency

Congenital tibia deficiency (Tibia Hemimelia) is a partial to complete absence of the tibia at birth. It is one of the rare congenital lower limb deformities. While most cases have an unknown etiology, there are some associated syndromes that have autosomal dominant inheritance patterns. Four different autosomal dominant syndromes have been identified and include Warner Syndrome (Tibia Hemimelia-foot polydactly–tripahlangeal thumb syndrome), Tibia hemimeliala–micromelia–trigonobrachycephaly syndrome, Tibial hemimelia diplopodia syndrome, and Tibial hemimelia split hand and foot syndrome. In syndromic forms of tibia deficiency, defects in the sonic hedgehog pathway have been identified [26, 27]. Inherited forms of tibial hemimelia are typically bilateral and are associated with other congenital anomalies. In a review, 79% of patients had associated abnormalities of the hip, hand, or spine occurring alone or in various combinations [28]. Unlike other longitudinal deficiencies, tibial hemimelia is associated with visceral involvement typically of the cardiac,

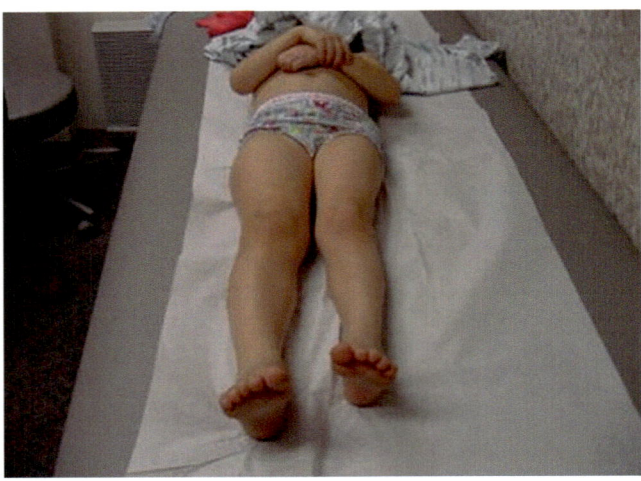

Fig. 1.4 Limb length discrepancy and asymmetrical girth in idiopathic hemihypertrophy

Table 1.4 Common overgrowth and undergrowth syndromes [20]

Syndrome	Genetic association	Common clinical features
Common overgrowth syndrome		
Beckwith–Wiedemann syndrome	Mutation of 11p15 leading to overactivity of the IGF-2 gene	Macroglossia, macrosomia, midline abdominal wall defects, neonatal hypoglycemia, and hemihypertrophy
Proteus syndrome	Somatic activating mutation in AKT1 kinase	Progressive macrodactyly, hemihypertrophy, thickening of the skin, lipomas, subcutaneous tumors, epidermal nevus, and macrocephaly
Neurofibromatosis type 1	Mutation of the NF1 gene located on chromosome 17 results in disruption of Ras signaling controlled by neurofibromin	Café-au-lait spots, cutaneous neurofibromas, axillary freckling, optic glioma, Lisch nodules, vertebral scalloping, tibial dysplasia, and plexiform neurofibroma
Klippel–Trenaunay syndrome	In some patients—angiogenic factor VG5Q, translocation (5:11, 8:14)	Nevus Flammeus (port-wine stain), venous and lymphatic malformations, soft tissue and bony hypertrophy
Common undergrowth syndrome		
Syndrome	Genetic association	Common clinical features
Russel–silver Syndrome	Loss of methylation on chromosome 11p15 (30–60%) Maternal uniparental disomy on chromosome 7 (10% of patients)	Short stature, small triangular faces, disproportionately normal head circumference, and clinodactyly
Cutis marmorata telangiectatica congenita	Unknown	Generalized or localized reticulated cutaneous vascular mottling, macrocephaly, glaucoma, hemiatrophy, vascular anomalies

Fig. 1.5 (a and b) Clinical and radiographic findings of proximal focal femoral deficiency. Eighteen-month-old male with proximal focal femoral deficiency. Note the short femur and absence of the proximal femur on the left side

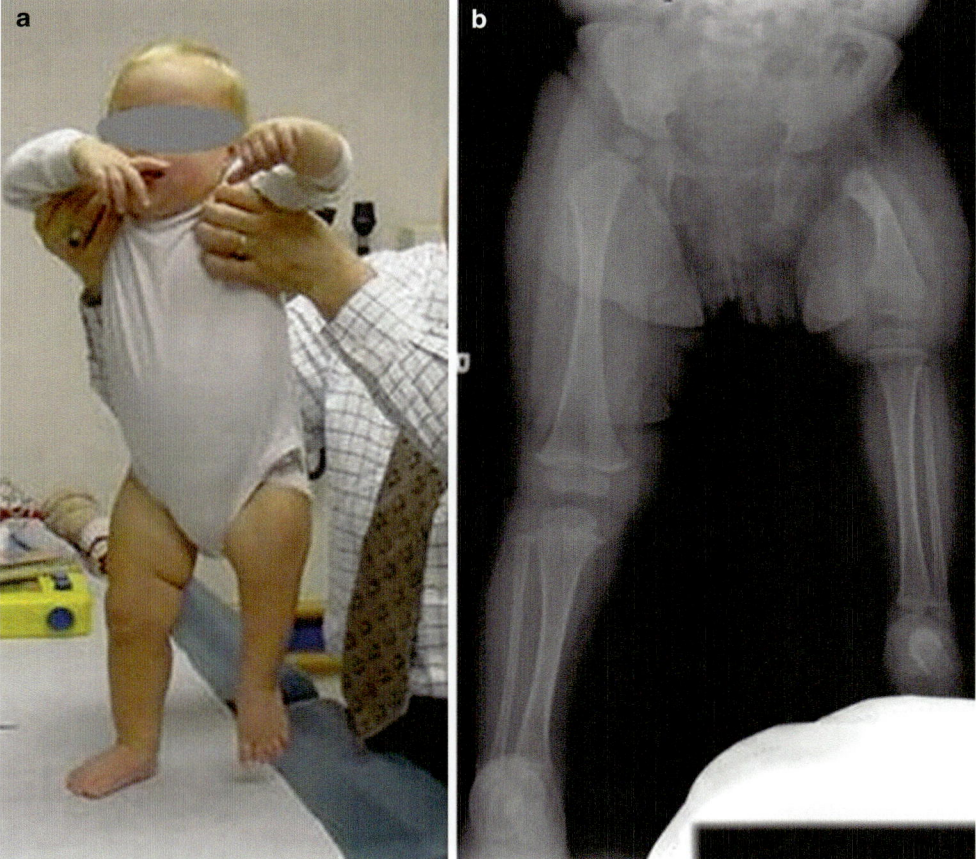

gastrointestinal, and genitourinary systems [28]. Presentation typically includes anterolateral bowing of the tibia, flexion contracture of the knee, and rigid equinovarus and supination deformity of the foot. Most children will have hamstring function, but presence of quadricep function is variable and related to the degree of absence of tibia.

Congenital Knee Dislocation

Congenital knee dislocation is the most severe form of congenital knee hyperextension. The overall incidence of congenital knee dislocation has an incidence of 1 per 100,000 [29]. It is readily identifiable at birth as there is marked hyperextension at the knee with the foot typically pointing toward the infant's mouth or shoulder (Fig. 1.6). This condition is thought to be secondary to abnormal fetal positioning. Once in an abnormal position, limited movement related to an underlying neuromuscular condition or hyperlaxity results in persistent hyperextension, which leads to quadriceps atrophy and fibrosis. Others have postulated that the absence of the cruciate ligaments is a key factor in the development of congenital knee dislocation [30].

Bilateral congenital knee dislocation is almost always syndromic in nature and has been associated with hyperlaxity syndromes (such as Larsen Syndrome, Beal's Syndrome, and Ehlers–Danlos syndrome) as well as underlying neuromuscular conditions (such as arthrogryposis, myelomeningocele). It is also important to assess for additional orthopedic manifestations including ipsilateral hip dislocation and club foot that are commonly seen in infants with congenital knee dislocation [30, 31].

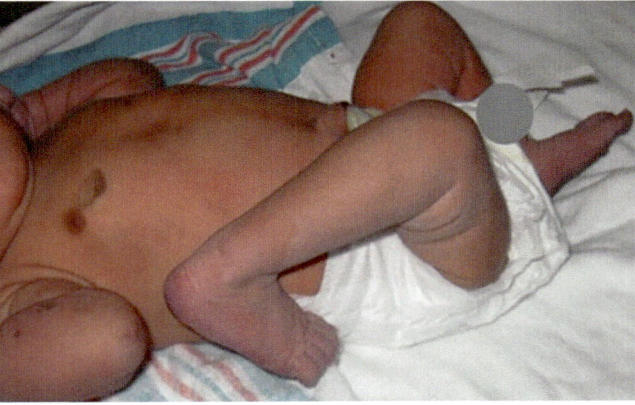

Fig. 1.6 Clinical presentation of congenital knee dislocation. Newborn with congenital knee dislocation. Initially treated with serial casting and eventually required quadricep release

Congenital Patella Dislocation

This is a relatively rare condition that presents with a laterally displaced and hypoplastic patella. This is present at birth and has a spectrum of severity. The most severe forms result in knee flexion contracture and are diagnosed in infancy while milder forms may not present until the child is older when functional problems related to quadricep weakness are noted. These children are typically present with genu valgum with significant external rotation of the tibia noted on exam. The patella is small and is often difficult to palpate in its lateral location [32].

Congenital patella dislocation is thought to be secondary to an embryologic cause. Normally, the quadriceps rotates from a lateral to an anterior position during fetal development. In children with a congenital patella dislocation, the quadriceps is short and found to be more lateral and a thickened iliotibial band is often present. This may prevent the normal rotation of the quadriceps during development and result in a dislocated patella at birth. Others have reported a possible hereditary link. Congenital patella dislocation has been associated with a variety of conditions including diastrophic dysplasia, arthrogryposis, Rubinstein-Taybi Syndrome, nail-patella syndrome, and Ellis van Creveld Syndrome [32, 33].

Coxa Vara

Congenital coxa vara is a developmental abnormality of the proximal femur that is characterized by a cartilaginous defect in the femoral neck. This leads to an abnormal decrease in the femoral neck-shaft angle, shortening of the femoral neck, relative overgrowth of the greater trochanter, and shortening of the affected limb. Overall the incidence is rare with 1 in 25,000 live births being affected [34]. While not all patients have progression, worsening of coxa vara is thought to occur secondary to excessive biomechanical stress on the abnormally positioned proximal femoral physis.

Presentation typically occurs after walking age and even into adolescence. Children with unilateral involvement typically present with easy fatigability or aching pain in the gluteal musculature, a Trendelenburg gait pattern, or mild limb length discrepancy. Bilateral involvement typically presents with a waddling gait with or without fatigue or muscular pain. Bilateral cases are associated with underlying conditions or skeletal dysplasias including Cleidocranial dysostosis, spondylometaphyseal dysplasia, and metaphyseal dysostosis (Jansen type). Coxa vara is thought to have a genetic component, as well as it can occur in families and twins [35].

In addition to congenital coxa vara, other causes include coxa vara secondary to congenital femoral deficiency and acquired coxa vara. These are considered separate entities as different radiographic and clinical findings are seen. Some causes of acquired coxa vara include slipped capital femoral epiphysis, sequelae of avascular necrosis from Legg–Calve–Perthes Disease, femoral neck fracture or traumatic dislocation, and septic necrosis. Additionally, coxa vara can be seen in underlying bone disorders including osteogenesis imperfecta, fibrous dysplasia, osteopetrosis, and renal osteodystrophy.

Congenital Bowing of the Tibia

Anterolateral bowing of the tibia is a condition seen at birth with an apical prominence of the lateral tibia. It is most frequently associated with tibial dysplasia or congenital pseudarthrosis. The pseudarthrosis is typically not present at birth but develops due to underlying disease process and deformation, resulting in a fracture that often progresses to a nonunion. Overall, this is a rare condition with an incidence of 1: 140,000—190,000. Anterolateral bowing and congenital pseudarthrosis have been associated with underlying conditions. Neurofibromatosis Type 1 is frequently associated with both conditions. While 5.7% of patients with neurofibromatosis have this tibial deformity, 55% of cases of anterolateral bowing and pseudarthrosis are associated with neurofibromatosis [36]. Additionally, fibrous dysplasia can be seen in 15% of children with anterolateral tibial bowing [36]. While rare, amniotic band syndrome can result in local constriction leading to the development of pseudarthrosis [37].

Posteromedial bowing of the tibia is a deformity that is present at birth and is typically seen in combination with calcaneovalgus foot, although they can occur independently (Fig. 1.7). The underlying cause is thought to be secondary to intrauterine malposition [38]. Typically, there is spontaneous but incomplete correction of bowing within the first 4 years of life. The most common sequelae of posteromedial bowing is a limb length discrepancy, and children should be followed until skeletal maturity [38, 39].

Anteromedial bowing is most commonly seen in association with congenital fibular deficiency as noted in the previous section.

Developmental

Physiologic Genu Varum

Most newborns are born with 10–15 degrees of varus angulation of the lower extremities. As the child stands and walks, this deformity can appear more prominent. Internal tibial torsion, which is also a common finding in this age group, can also exacerbate the deformity. Parental concern over the

1 Etiology of Lower Limb Deformity

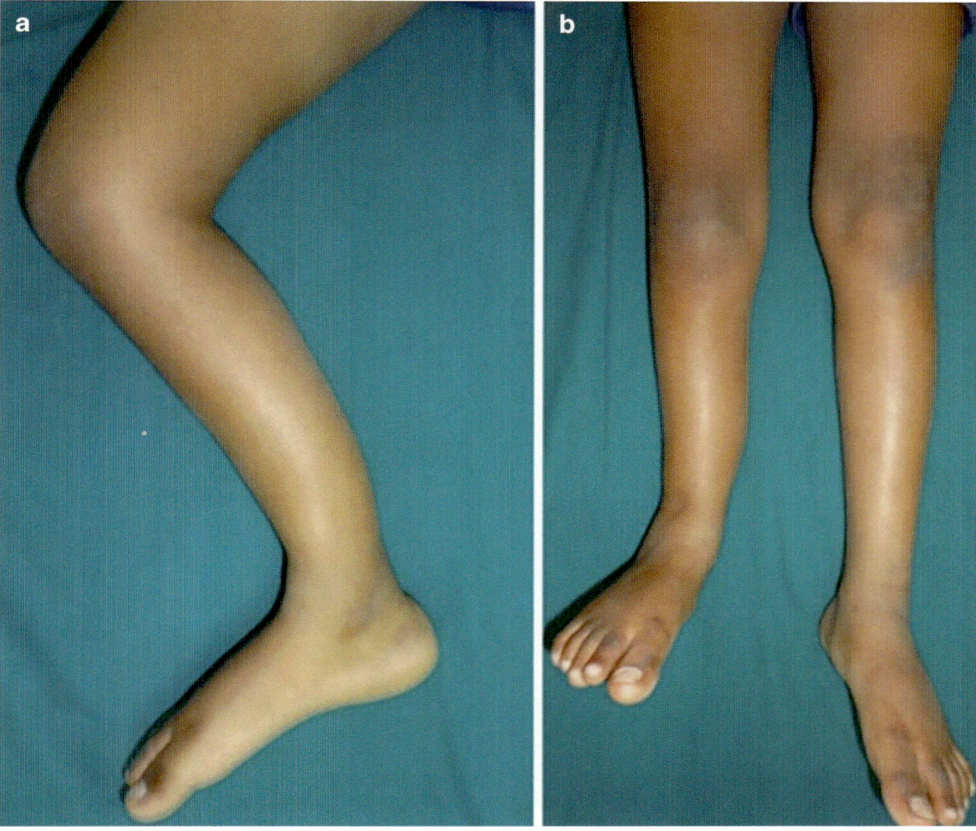

Fig. 1.7 (**a** and **b**) Posteromedial bowing. Nine-year old with right-sided posteromedial bowing and limb shortening. No significant calcaneus deformity noted

appearance of the lower extremities as the child begins to stand and walk is what typically prompts evaluation. Cases are often bilateral and are noted to improve with time. Spontaneous resolution is common by 18–24 months. Typically, alignment through childhood progresses to maximum valgus between ages 3 and 4 before gradual correction to adult alignment by the age of 7 years. While usually, this condition self-corrects, if varus alignment is persistent past 24 months or if significant clinical progression is noted, radiographs should be obtained to evaluate for underlying disorders [40].

Blount's Disease

Tibia vara, often referred to as Blount's disease, is characterized by abrupt varus deformity of the proximal tibia. In Blount's description in 1937, he described an irregular physeal line of the proximal medial tibia and a wedge-shaped epiphysis with medial metaphyseal beaking [41]. In contrast to physiologic genu varum, this is a progressive deformity. Two main forms exist and are classified based on time of onset—infantile (<4 years old) and adolescent (>10 years old).

While there may be a positive family history, infantile Blount's disease is considered a developmental disorder as radiographic features are typically not seen in children younger than 1 year (Fig. 1.8). Typically, children with Blount's disease are early walkers and are often obese. Finite element modeling has shown that compressive forces sufficient to retard physeal growth can be produced on the medial tibial plateau in a 2-year-old in the 90th percentile for body weight and with a 20-degree deformity [42]. Additionally, higher BMIs have been associated with greater overall varus alignment in children with infantile tibia vara [43].

Adolescent Blount's disease is a distinct form of tibia vara that presents later in childhood. The underlying etiology of adolescent Blount's disease is multifactorial and is not fully understood [44]. It is thought that progressive varus deformity results from repetitive trauma to the posteromedial proximal tibial physis due to increased body weight. While some have postulated that residual static varus alignment influences the development of adolescent Blount's disease, Davids et al. demonstrated that increased thigh girth and the resulting "fat-thigh gait" has been shown to lead to dynamic loading of the medial proximal tibial physis that can lead to compressive forces capable of inhibiting physeal growth [45]. The role of Vitamin D deficiency in the development of Blount's Disease continues to be investigated. Race has also been shown to be a factor, with adolescent Blount's disease being more common in African American populations, although it is seen in all races and ethnicities [44].

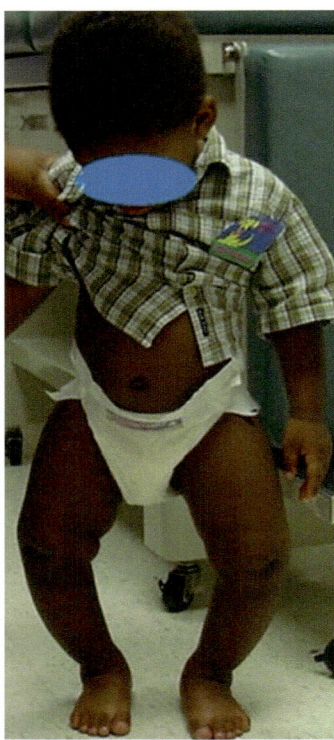

Fig. 1.8 Infantile blounts. Four-year-old male with Infantile Blount's disease. This is more common in African American populations

Proximal Focal Fibrocartilaginous Dysplasia

This is a rare idiopathic benign condition that can cause tibia vara. This typically presents as an abrupt varus deformity distal to the joint line of the knee and corresponds to cortical sclerosis at the metaphyseal–diaphyseal junction of the proximal tibia (at the insertion of the pes anserine). Abnormal fibrocartilage has been identified at the tendon insertion and the concept of this acting as a fibrous tether has been proposed. This deformity has the potential to correct spontaneously even with large varus deformities [46].

Genu Valgum

Physiologic valgus first becomes apparent around age 2 and reaches a maximum between ages 3 and 4. The valgus alignment of the lower extremity typically decreases over the next couple of years until adult alignment (5–7 degrees of valgus) is achieved at around age 7. Worsening genu valgum after age 7 is often pathologic. Common causes of genu valgum are shown in Table 1.5. In addition to underlying causes or injuries to the physis of the distal femur or proximal tibia, genu valgum can be idiopathic in nature. A recent study showed that 71% of children with idiopathic genu valgum were obese, which was significantly higher than in the normal population [47].

Table 1.5 Common causes of genu valgum

Unilateral presentation	Bilateral presentation
Post traumatic physeal injury	Physiologic
Proximal tibial metaphyseal fracture (Cozen's phenomenon)	Rickets
Osteochondroma	Idiopathic
Focal Fibrocartilaginous dysplasia	Pseudoachondroplasia
Fibrous Dysplasia	Morquio's (MPS IV)
Encondromatosis	Chondroectodermal dysplasia (Ellis van Creveld)
Fibular hemimelia	Multiple Hereditary exostosis
	Spondyloeiphyseal dysplasia

Acquired

Residual Hip Deformity

Outcomes of pediatric hip disorders (such as developmental hip dysplasia, SCFE, and Perthes Disease) are largely dependent on the congruency of the hip joint and avoidance of complications including avascular necrosis. It is important to consider the effect that these disorders, and their treatment, have on lower extremity limb length and alignment. Complete physeal arrest, either from the condition itself or as a result of treatment, can lead to limb length discrepancy. Children may present with an abductor lurch secondary to the corresponding greater trochanteric "overgrowth." Partial arrest can lead to the development of coxa vara or coxa valga. Additionally, studies evaluating coronal lower extremity alignment after Legg Calve Perthes Disease and SCFE have shown the development of valgus lower extremity alignment over time [48, 49].

Physeal Fractures

Injuries that are juxtaphyseal or ones that involve the physis can cause direct injury to the chondrocytes and interrupt normal growth of the extremity. This can lead to complete arrest with no further growth or partial arrest which can lead to angular deformity or slowing of growth. The risk of development of a physeal arrest is related to the Salter-Harris Classification, mechanism of injury, and degree of initial displacement. Reduction should be carefully attempted as repeated reductions may increase the risk of premature physeal closure [50]. Significant clinical deformity or limb length discrepancy can develop and is based on the age of the patient and the amount of growth remaining.

Physeal injuries of the distal femur are the most clinically relevant, given the magnitude of potential growth and the undulating nature of the physis. This undulation leaves the physis vulnerable to arrest as a fracture line can potentially cross multiple zones of the physis encouraging the potential of bony bar formation.

Salter-Harris Classification and initial displacement of the fracture correlate with complications [51]. The incidence of physeal arrest has been shown to be as high as 50% [51, 52]. Leg length discrepancies or angular deformity can develop and often necessitate additional intervention.

Femoral neck fractures occur typically as part of high-energy polytrauma. While avascular necrosis remains a significant and devastating complication of these fractures, premature physeal arrest can occur in up to 22% of cases [53]. This can be related to the injury at the time of fracture or secondary to implant placement. Limb length discrepancy tends to be minimal given the robust nature of the distal femoral physis. The angular deformity can occur from partial arrest resulting in coxa valga or coxa vara.

Distal tibia fractures have an overall rate of premature physeal closure of 13% with a reported range between 0.2% and 42%. Salter Harris IV fractures are most likely to develop arrest followed by Salter-Harris II fractures [54]. Mechanism of injury also plays a role as supination-external rotation injuries have a premature arrest rate of 35% in comparison to the 54% seen in children with pronation abduction-type injuries [55]. An important criterion for the development of physeal arrest in these injuries is displacement following reduction [53, 54]. Angular deformity is more common in pronation external rotation injuries [56].

Nonphyseal Fractures

Fractures of the lower extremities can result in angular deformity and limb length discrepancy even if the growth plate is not directly involved. Fracture malunion can result in long bone deformity. In younger children, this may remodel over time but as the child ages and approaches skeletal maturity, little remodeling will occur.

Femoral overgrowth is a well-documented phenomenon after femoral shaft fracture. This is related to increased vascular perfusion of the femoral physis during fracture healing. Typically, this measures about 1 cm and rarely exceeds 2 cm [57]. Femoral overgrowth has been reported, irrespective of the treatment methods. Given the anticipation of overgrowth, 1 cm of shortening is acceptable in young children when treating femoral shaft fractures with hip spica casting.

Progressive valgus angulation has been documented after a nondisplaced or minimally displaced fracture of the proximal tibia metaphysis. Known as Cozen's phenomenon, after healing of the fracture, a valgus deformity develops, which can be alarming in appearance (Fig. 1.9). There are many theories in regard to the mechanism of the phenomenon including soft tissue interposition, stimulation of the medial physis or tethering of the lateral physis by the intact fibula. The reported incidence of Cozen's Phenomenon varies between 50 and 90% with multiple studies noting the resolution of this deformity with time with few having clinically significant genu valgum requiring intervention [58, 59].

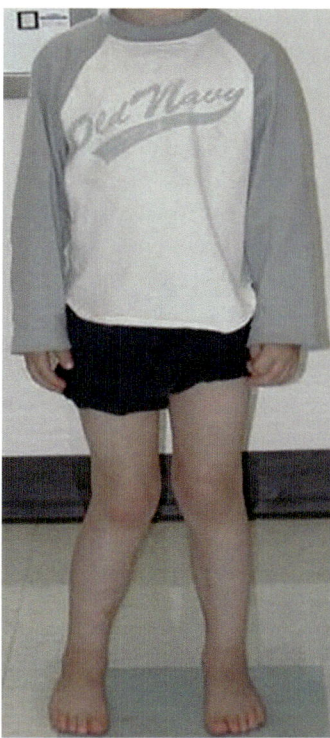

Fig. 1.9 Cozen's phenomenon after proximal tibia metaphyseal fracture. Six-year-old male, 1-year-post-proximal tibia metaphyseal fracture that developed genu valgum. He was observed serially and noted to completely remodel the valgus deformity

Post-Infectious

Both osteomyelitis and septic arthritis can lead to growth arrest or disturbance. Chondrocytes can be damaged by the infection itself or by the surgical debridement required to treat it, resulting in a bony bar formation. Even with the infection being successfully treated, the clinical effect may not be apparent for several years.

The infectious process can result in physeal cell death, which can produce similar tethering properties without osseous bar formation. Physeal bar equivalent has been reported early in life after infection near the distal femur physis [60]. Additionally, meningococcal septicemia can lead to a vascular occlusive process, resulting in damage to multiple growth plates and ultimately may present years later as limb length discrepancy or angular deformity [61].

Iatrogenic

Physeal damage leading to growth arrest can be from iatrogenic causes. Reduction of physeal fractures should be done carefully as repeated or overaggressive reduction attempts can lead to physeal damage and arrest. Additionally, manipulation after partial healing can also lead to physeal injury. Closed manipulation of a lower extremity contracture should be done carefully as physeal separations can occur with excessive force.

Surgical procedures near the physis also have the potential to cause iatrogenic injury to the physis, and careful dissection is important to avoid injury to the perichondral ring. Additionally, transphyseal hardware, improperly placed intramedullary nails, or instrumentation for guided growth can result in premature physeal growth arrest.

Ligament reconstruction around the knee often requires drilling tunnels that are near or across the distal femoral or proximal tibial physis. Both the cross-sectional area of the drilled tunnel and the angulation of the tunnel are thought to contribute to the development of both angular deformity and limb length discrepancy after anterior cruciate ligament (ACL) reconstruction with animal studies demonstrating that disruption of 7% of cross-sectional area leads to growth disturbance [62]. Growth abnormalities have been seen with both transphyseal and all epiphyseal ACL reconstruction. The most common deformities are genu valgum, recurvatum, and overgrowth. Overgrowth is seen in 62% of cases of limb length discrepancy after ACL reconstruction [63]. Growth disturbances have also been reported after Medial patellofemoral ligament (MPFL) reconstruction secondary to variability in tunnel placement [64].

Summary

The purpose of this chapter is to introduce the vast array of etiologies of lower limb deformities in the pediatric population. These deformities can be classified into underlying, congenital, developmental, or acquired conditions. The remaining chapters in this book will further discuss the diagnosis, classification, and management of specific disorders.

Commentary

Craig Robbins
crobbins@paleyinstitute.org

Limb deformities in children may result from innumerable causes, and the severity and functional impairment of a deformity can vary widely between patients. Drs. Zakrzewski and Jain have done a commendable job broadly categorizing these myriad causes into congenital, acquired, developmental, and those associated with underlying conditions. As they aptly say, "despite some overlap, categorizing them can help simplify diagnosis and treatment." Identifying the etiology of a limb deformity may uncover associated orthopedic and non-orthopedic problems. In appropriate patients, genetic counseling is an important consideration; a genetic counselor can help decide if and what testing may be germane and can provide useful information about future family planning [65, 66]. Testing may confirm or refute a diagnosis, guide treatment, and help access services and research trials. Advanced imaging such as MRI may provide useful information such as the presence of unossified cartilage and define neurovascular and soft tissue anatomy. The accumulated information from a thorough evaluation and work-up allows the family and clinical team to understand the natural history and prognosis of the deformity and develop a comprehensive treatment plan, and in some cases a "life plan."

Treatment options for pediatric limb deformities are almost as varied as the deformities themselves. They depend on patient, family, and surgeon/clinical team factors. These factors include, but are not limited to diagnosis, prognosis, comorbidities, cultural, religious, social, family economics, surgeon/clinical team experience, and medical care access. After a diagnosis is established, treatment goals need to be clearly defined and a personalized reconstructive plan created. Regardless of the particular cause, treatment goals may include any or several of the following: prevent deformity progression, decrease disability, decrease pain, improve function, correct deformity, stabilize joints, normalize limb alignment, equalize limb lengths, and prevent deformity recurrence.

The orthopedic surgeon must be part of the comprehensive treatment team. Prior, during, and after orthopedic interventions, associated conditions, comorbidities, and abnormalities may need to be treated or optimized by the appropriate specialist. Examples include metabolic (e.g., rickets), hematologic (e.g., TAR syndrome), and structural (e.g., Arnold-Chiari) abnormalities. The surgical treatment plan must include pre-operative, intra-operative, and post-operative considerations for associated problems. Examples include screening for spinal stenosis, taking precautions for malignant hyperthermia and latex allergies, and monitoring platelet counts. Understanding potential problems, obstacles, and complications for a particular deformity allow the surgeon and treatment team to optimize their reconstructive plan and minimize sub-optimal outcomes [67].

The reconstructive plan for limb deformity may include operative and/or non-operative options. Non-operative treatment for limb length discrepancies and deformities includes the use of shoe lifts (for lower extremity), orthoses, and prostheses depending on the etiology, amount, and underlying shape and function of the extremity [68]. Surgical options depend on the defined goals of treatment and include combinations of acute and gradual correction with internal and external fixation in single or multiple stages. The reconstructive plan may evolve over time based on outcomes, response to previous treatments, changes in goals, and advances in medical and surgical treatments.

Limb deformities in pediatric patients may progress with time and future growth. Complete and partial growth arrest results in axial and angular deformities. Progressive limb length discrepancy, for most conditions, can be accurately predicted which helps guide the reconstructive plan [69, 70]. Predicted discrepancies above a certain threshold may alter a surgeon's treatment plan (e.g., prosthetic fitting–with or without amputation–in lieu of multiple staged lengthenings, or combining contralateral shortening by growth arrest with ipsilateral lengthening. Patients should be followed through skeletal maturity with discrepancy calculations repeated throughout growth. If the predicted discrepancy or reconstructive complexity exceeds the surgeon's capabilities, experience, or comfort level, they have the opportunity to refer.

Treatment options for pediatric limb deformities continually evolve and mature. Advances in orthotics, alongside prosthetics design and manufacturing, have improved their use and functionality. Surgical advances have come from modifications of existing procedures, advent of new reconstructive procedures, introduction of new hardware and software, and repurposing existing hardware in innovative ways. Examples of these advances include percutaneous osteotomy and fixation, cross-union technique for congenital pseudarthrosis of the tibia [71], femoral shortening with posterior knee soft-tissue lengthening and capsulotomy for arthrogryposis [72, 73], computer-dependent hexapod fixators that can accommodate more complex deformities, and extra-medullary placement of lengthening rods in younger and smaller patients [74, 75].

Generalizations for limb deformity surgeons:

- Understand the pathoanatomy
- Formulate an individualized reconstructive plan
- Optimize patients prior to surgery
- Plan to obtain and then maintain deformity correction
- Consider how a deformity may change over time
- Anticipate and prevent complications but be prepared to treat them
- Remember that limb function is more important than limb length

References

1. Loder RT, Wittenberg B, DeSilva G. Slipped capital femoral epiphysis associated with endocrine disorders. J Pediatr Orthop. 1995;15(3):349–56.
2. Bitzan M, Goodyer PR. Hypophosphatemic rickets. Pediatr Clin N Am. 2019;66(1):179–207.
3. Misra M, Pacaud D, Petryk A, et al. Vitamin D deficiency in children and its management: review of current knowledge and recommendations. Pediatrics. 2008;122(2):398–417.
4. Barrett IR, Papadimitriou DG. Skeletal disorders in children with renal failure. J Pediatr Orthop. 1996;16(2):264–72.
5. Dwan K, Phillipi CA, Steiner RD, et al. Bisphosphonate therapy for osteogenesis imperfecta. Cochrane Database Syst Rev. 2016;10(10):Cd005088.
6. Crawford AH, Schorry EK. Neurofibromatosis update. J Pediatr Orthop. 2006;26(3):413–23.
7. Jani-Acsadi A, Ounpuu S, Pierz K, et al. Pediatric Charcot-Marie-Tooth disease. Pediatr Clin N Am. 2015;62(3):767–86.
8. van Bosse HJP, Pontén E, Wada A, et al. Treatment of the lower extremity contracture/deformities. J Pediatr Orthop. 2017;37(Suppl 1):S16–s23.
9. Dobbs MB, Boehm S, Grange DK, et al. Case report: congenital knee dislocation in a patient with larsen syndrome and a novel filamin B mutation. Clin Orthop Relat Res. 2008;466(6):1503–9.
10. Larsen LJ, Schottstaedt ER, Bost FC. Multiple congenital dislocations associated with characteristic facial abnormality. J Pediatr. 1950;37(4):574–81.
11. Carrera-García L, Natera-de Benito D, Dieterich K, et al. CHRNG-related nonlethal multiple pterygium syndrome: muscle imaging pattern and clinical, histopathological, and molecular genetic findings. Am J Med Genet A. 2019;179(6):915–26.
12. Baitner AC, Maurer SG, Gruen MB, et al. The genetic basis of the osteochondrodysplasias. J Pediatr Orthop. 2000;20(5):594–605.
13. White KK, Sousa T. Mucopolysaccharide disorders in orthopaedic surgery. J Am Acad Orthop Surg. 2013;21(1):12–22.
14. Goldwein JW. Effects of radiation therapy on skeletal growth in childhood. Clin Orthop Relat Res. 1991;262:101–7.
15. Reif TJ, Matthias J, Fragomen AT, et al. Limb length discrepancy and angular deformity due to benign bone tumors and tumor-like lesions. J Am Acad Orthop Surg Glob Res Rev. 2021;5(3):e00214.
16. Bovid KM, Moore MD. Juvenile idiopathic arthritis for the pediatric orthopedic surgeon. Orthop Clin North Am. 2019;50(4):471–88.
17. Rodriguez-Merchan EC. Prevention of the musculoskeletal complications of hemophilia. Adv Prev Med. 2012;2012:201271.
18. Dempsey-Robertson M, Wilkes D, Stall A, et al. Incidence of abdominal tumors in syndromic and idiopathic hemihypertrophy/isolated hemihyperplasia. J Pediatr Orthop. 2012;32(3):322–6.
19. Brioude F, Kalish JM, Mussa A, et al. Expert consensus document: clinical and molecular diagnosis, screening and management of Beckwith-Wiedemann syndrome: an international consensus statement. Nat Rev Endocrinol. 2018;14(4):229–49.
20. Ballock RT, Wiesner GL, Myers MT, et al. Hemihypertrophy. Concepts and controversies. J Bone Joint Surg Am. 1997;79(11):1731–8.
21. Burn J, Winter RM, Baraitser M, et al. The femoral hypoplasia-unusual facies syndrome. J Med Genet. 1984;21(5):331–40.
22. Crawford DA, Tompkins BJ, Baird GO, et al. The long-term function of the knee in patients with fibular hemimelia and anterior cruciate ligament deficiency. J Bone Joint Surg Br. 2012;94(3):328–33.
23. Graham JM Jr. Limb anomalies as a consequence of spatially-restricting uterine environments. Prog Clin Biol Res. 1983;110(Pt A):413–22.

24. Hootnick DR, Levinsohn EM, Randall PA, et al. Vascular dysgenesis associated with skeletal dysplasia of the lower limb. J Bone Joint Surg Am. 1980;62(7):1123–9.
25. Rodriguez-Ramirez A, Thacker MM, Becerra LC, et al. Limb length discrepancy and congenital limb anomalies in fibular hemimelia. J Pediatr Orthop B. 2010;19(5):436–40.
26. Cho TJ, Baek GH, Lee HR, et al. Tibial hemimelia-polydactyly-five-fingered hand syndrome associated with a 404 G>a mutation in a distant sonic hedgehog cis-regulator (ZRS): a case report. J Pediatr Orthop B. 2013;22(3):219–21.
27. Deimling S, Sotiropoulos C, Lau K, et al. Tibial hemimelia associated with GLI3 truncation. J Hum Genet. 2016;61(5):443–6.
28. Clinton R, Birch JG. Congenital tibial deficiency: a 37-year experience at 1 institution. J Pediatr Orthop. 2015;35(4):385–90.
29. Jacobsen K, Vopalecky F. Congenital dislocation of the knee. Acta Orthop Scand. 1985;56(1):1–7.
30. Katz MP, Grogono BJ, Soper KC. The etiology and treatment of congenital dislocation of the knee. J Bone Joint Surg Br. 1967;49(1):112–20.
31. Curtis BH, Fisher RL. Congenital hyperextension with anterior subluxation of the knee. Surgical treatment and long-term observations. J Bone Joint Surg Am. 1969;51(2):255–69.
32. Wada A, Fujii T, Takamura K, et al. Congenital dislocation of the patella. J Child Orthop. 2008;2(2):119–23.
33. Ghanem I, Wattincourt L, Seringe R. Congenital dislocation of the patella. Part I: pathologic anatomy. J Pediatr Orthop. 2000;20(6):812–6.
34. Johanning K, Coxa vara infantum. I. Clinical appearance and aetiological problems. Acta Orthop Scand. 1951;21(4):273–99.
35. Duncan GA. Congenital coxa vara occurring in identical twins. Am J Surg. 1937;37(1):112–5.
36. Hefti F, Bollini G, Dungl P, et al. Congenital pseudarthrosis of the tibia: history, etiology, classification, and epidemiologic data. J Pediatr Orthop B. 2000;9(1):11–5.
37. Tanguy AF, Dalens BJ, Boisgard S. Congenital constricting band with pseudarthrosis of the tibia and fibula. A case report. J Bone Joint Surg Am. 1995;77(8):1251–4.
38. Hofmann A, Wenger DR. Posteromedial bowing of the tibia. Progression of discrepancy in leg lengths. JBJS. 1981;63(3):384.
39. Wright J, Hill RA, Eastwood DM, et al. Posteromedial bowing of the tibia: a benign condition or a case for limb reconstruction? J Child Orthop. 2018;12(2):187–96.
40. Salenius P, Vankka E. The development of the tibiofemoral angle in children. J Bone Joint Surg Am. 1975;57(2):259–61.
41. Blount WP. TIBIA VARA: osteochondrosis deformans tibiae. JBJS. 1937;19:1.
42. Cook SD, Lavernia CJ, Burke SW, et al. A biomechanical analysis of the etiology of tibia vara. J Pediatr Orthop. 1983;3(4):449–54.
43. Sabharwal S, Zhao C, McClemens E. Correlation of body mass index and radiographic deformities in children with Blount disease. J Bone Joint Surg Am. 2007;89(6):1275–83.
44. Banwarie RR, Hollman F, Meijs N, et al. Insight into the possible aetiologies of Blount's disease: a systematic review of the literature. J Pediatr Orthop B. 2020;29(4):323–36.
45. Davids JR, Huskamp M, Bagley AM. A dynamic biomechanical analysis of the etiology of adolescent tibia vara. J Pediatr Orthop. 1996;16(4):461–8.
46. Jouve JL, Kohler R, Mubarak SJ, et al. Focal fibrocartilaginous dysplasia ("fibrous periosteal inclusion"): an additional series of eleven cases and literature review. J Pediatr Orthop. 2007;27(1):75–84.
47. Walker JL, Hosseinzadeh P, White H, et al. Idiopathic genu valgum and its association with obesity in children and adolescents. J Pediatr Orthop. 2019;39(7):347–52.
48. Tercier S, Shah H, Siddesh ND, et al. Does proximal femoral varus osteotomy in Legg-Calvé-Perthes disease predispose to angular mal-alignment of the knee? A clinical and radiographic study at skeletal maturity. J Child Orthop. 2013;7(3):205–11.
49. Ucpunar H, Tas SK, Camurcu Y, et al. The effects of residual hip deformity on coronal alignment of the lower extremity in patients with unilateral slipped capital femoral epiphysis. J Child Orthop. 2018;12(6):599–605.
50. Leary JT, Handling M, Talerico M, et al. Physeal fractures of the distal tibia: predictive factors of premature physeal closure and growth arrest. J Pediatr Orthop. 2009;29(4):256–61.
51. Basener CJ, Mehlman CT, DiPasquale TG. Growth disturbance after distal femoral growth plate fractures in children: a meta-analysis. J Orthop Trauma. 2009;23(9):663–7.
52. Bellamy JT, Ward LA, Fletcher ND. Evaluation of pediatric distal femoral physeal fractures and the factors impacting poor outcome requiring further corrective surgery. J Pediatr Orthop B. 2021;30(1):6–12.
53. Yeranosian M, Horneff JG, Baldwin K, et al. Factors affecting the outcome of fractures of the femoral neck in children and adolescents: a systematic review. Bone Joint J. 2013;95-b(1):135–42.
54. Jalkanen J, Sinikumpu JJ, Puhakka J, et al. Physeal fractures of distal tibia: a systematic review and meta-analysis. J Pediatr Orthop. 2021;41:e506.
55. Rohmiller MT, Gaynor TP, Pawelek J, et al. Salter-Harris I and II fractures of the distal tibia: does mechanism of injury relate to premature physeal closure? J Pediatr Orthop. 2006;26(3):322–8.
56. Binkley A, Mehlman CT, Freeh E. Salter-Harris II ankle fractures in children: does fracture pattern matter? J Orthop Trauma. 2019;33(5):e190–e95.
57. Hougaard K. Femoral shaft fractures in children: a prospective study of the overgrowth phenomenon. Injury. 1989;20(3):170–2.
58. Yang BW, Shore BJ, Rademacher E, et al. Prevalence of Cozen's phenomenon of the proximal tibia. J Pediatr Orthop. 2019;39(6):e417–e21.
59. Nenopoulos S, Vrettakos A, Chaftikis N, et al. The effect of proximal tibial fractures on the limb axis in children. Acta Orthop Belg. 2007;73(3):345–53.
60. Peterson HA, Shaughnessy WJ, Stans AA. Physeal bar equivalent. J Pediatr Orthop B. 2017;26(6):507–14.
61. Park DH, Bradish CF. The management of the orthopaedic sequelae of meningococcal septicaemia: patients treated to skeletal maturity. J Bone Joint Surg Br. 2011;93(7):984–9.
62. Mäkelä EA, Vainionpää S, Vihtonen K, et al. The effect of trauma to the lower femoral epiphysis plate. An experimental study in rabbits. J Bone Joint Surg Br. 1988;70(2):187–91.
63. Collins MJ, Arns TA, Leroux T, et al. Growth abnormalities following anterior cruciate ligament reconstruction in the skeletally immature patient: a systematic review. Arthroscopy. 2016;32(8):1714–23.
64. Seitlinger G, Moroder P, Fink C, et al. Acquired femoral flexion deformity due to physeal injury during medial patellofemoral ligament reconstruction. Knee. 2017;24(3):680–5.
65. Aicale R, Tarantino D, Maccauro G, Peretti G, Maffulli N. Genetics in orthopaedic practice. J Biol Regul Homeos Agents. 2019;33:103–17.
66. Zelzer E, Olsen BR. The genetic basis for skeletal diseases. Nature. 2003;423(6937):343–8. https://doi.org/10.1038/nature01659.
67. Paley D, Chong DY, Prince DE. Congenital femoral deficiency reconstruction and lengthening surgery. In: Pediatric lower limb deformities: principles and techniques of management; 2015. p. 361.
68. Paley D. Problems, obstacles, and complications of limb lengthening by the Ilizarov technique. Clin Orthop Relat Res. 1990;250:81–104.
69. Anderson M, Green WT, Messner MB. Growth and predictions of growth in the lower extremities. J Bone Joint Surg Am. 1963;45-A:1–14.

70. Paley J, Talor J, Levin A, Bhave A, Paley D, Herzenberg JE. The multiplier method for prediction of adult height. J Pediatr Orthop. 2004;24(6):732–7.
71. Paley D. Paley cross-union protocol for treatment of congenital pseudarthrosis of the Tibia. Oper Tech Orthop. 2021;31:100881. https://doi.org/10.1016/j.oto.2021.100881.
72. Feldman D, Rand T, Huser A. Novel approach to improving knee range of motion in arthrogryposis with a new working classification. Children. 2021;8:546. https://doi.org/10.3390/children8070546.
73. Paley D. Shortening: the orthopedic theory of relativity. J Limb Lengthening Reconstr. 2020;6:1. https://doi.org/10.4103/2455-3719.288573.
74. Shannon C, Paley D. Extramedullary internal limb lengthening. Tech Orthop. 2020;35(3):195–200.
75. Dahl MT, Morrison SG, Laine JC, Novotny SA, Georgiadis AG. Extramedullary motorized lengthening of the femur in young children. J Pediatr Orthop. 2020;40(10):e978–83.

Clinical Evaluation Including Imaging

Raymond W. Liu

Introduction

The majority of pediatric lower extremity deformities presenting for evaluation are normal physiologic angular and/or rotational conditions that improve spontaneously and do not need imaging studies. However, limb length discrepancy and asymmetric and/or severe limb deformities often require imaging and eventual treatment. The focus of this chapter is on patients who present with deformities that will likely warrant treatment.

History

The chief complaint is very important for deformity assessment. Knowing whether the child has symptoms such as excessive tripping, difficulty with gait, or pain is helpful. For complaints of pain, associated activities should be elicited. Oftentimes, parents have brought their child because of recommendations from other family members, friends, or physician referrals rather than the presence of any symptoms and are seeking reassurance. Sometimes, they present because physicians prescribed treatment in the past to family members of previous generations [1]. In many of these situations, the physician can explain to the parents that treatment has subsequently not been found to improve upon natural history, and further testing is not indicated [2].

The clinician should determine at what age the deformity was first noticed. For example, in-toeing from femoral anteversion, which does not appear until approximately age 2 years, is usually due to the resolution of the physiologic external rotation contracture of the infant's hip, unmasking femoral anteversion. If the family is expressing concerns that do not fit the normal developmental pattern, then further investigation may be warranted.

Asking whether the deformity seems to be getting better, worse, or remaining the same is important. For example, bowing of the lower extremities is a normal consequence of the in utero position and will resolve spontaneously; the gradual improvement in the bowing helps establish the diagnosis and rules out Blount disease or metabolic bone disease, two conditions that require a more extensive work-up and treatment.

One should inquire whether there is any history of fractures, lower extremity injuries, bone or soft-tissue infections, or previous surgery. The development of an angular deformity or leg length discrepancy following a fracture or infection may indicate a partial or complete injury to the growth plate.

Determining whether the child is firstborn, had a breech presentation, or had any family history of hip issues can help screen for hip dysplasia. If the child was premature or had delayed motor milestones, a neuromuscular etiology could be considered.

Family history is also important, particularly any family history of orthopedic, neuromuscular, renal, or endocrine disorders.

Physical Examination

Although many children who present for evaluation have an obvious diagnosis, one should consider a comprehensive evaluation including an assessment of body mass index (BMI), upper extremities, spine and trunk, neurological, gait, and lower extremities. Many of these can be performed rapidly.

R. W. Liu (✉)
Victor M. Goldberg Professor of Orthopaedics, Rainbow Babies and Children's Hospital, Cleveland, OH, USA
e-mail: raymond.liu@uhhospitals.org

Body Mass Index

Height and weight should be measured at the office visit instead of asking the family to furnish this information because parents often are quite inaccurate with their child's stated height and weight [3]. BMI percentiles can be determined from charts available from the Centers for Disease Control (http://www.cdc.gov/growthcharts/clinical_charts.htm). Very large age-related Z scores may indicate a condition associated with obesity such as Blount disease or Prader–Willi syndrome. Very low Z scores may indicate malnutrition, malabsorption, chronic metabolic disease, or skeletal dysplasia.

Upper Extremity

An abnormal carrying angle of the elbow, especially if symmetric, may indicate a skeletal dysplasia. Joint laxity with excessive motion, such as hyperextension of the elbows or fingers, may indicate a connective tissue disorder. Palpable metaphyseal enlargements may indicate a rachitic disorder or multiple hereditary exostoses.

Spine and Trunk

The rib cage can be palpated for a rachitic rosary: swellings at the costochondral junction are indicative of a rachitic disorder. Screening for scoliosis is performed by checking for thoracic and/or lumbar asymmetry with forward bending. If there is any concern for a possible leg length discrepancy, always examine the spine in the sitting position. This will eliminate the compensatory curve of the spine caused by standing with a tilted pelvis that is often confused for scoliosis.

Neurologic

A quick but quite sensitive screening battery for the detection of neurological disease affecting the lower extremity can be done in walking-age children by having them walk on their heels in dorsiflexion, on their toes in equinus, and hop on one leg at a time. To perform these maneuvers, the child utilizes quadriceps (L2, L3, L4), hip extensors (L5, S1, S2), hip abductors (L5, S1), ankle plantar flexors (L5, S1, S2), and ankle dorsiflexors (L4, L5). If there is a high level of suspicion for the presence of a neurological abnormality, a more detailed exam must be done, including searching for pathologic primitive reflexes.

Gait

The examiner should watch the child walk. Sometimes children walk in a certain pattern as instructed by their parents when aware that the physician is watching. Thus, it is helpful to watch the child walk from the waiting area to the exam room or on their way to get a radiograph when he or she is unaware of being examined. Alternatively, try to distract the child with conversation or games as they walk or instruct them to walk faster while being observed. One can watch the child walk both with shoes and barefoot to better observe the dynamic movements of the foot. Try to observe the gait pattern as they walk away from you, toward you, and from the side to get a complete picture of the gait.

Foot Progression Angle

The foot progression angle is the angle between the axis of the foot and the line of progression, with in-toeing expressed as negative values and out-toeing expressed as positive values [4, 5]. A study of gait in 160 children (up to 14 years of age) concluded that the normal angle of gait was approximately 10° external at all ages with a slight decrease after age 7 [6] (Fig. 2.1). Etiologies contributing to an internal rotation gait include excessive acetabular anteversion, excessive femoral anteversion, internal tibial torsion, and metatarsus adducts (MTA). Etiologies contributing to an external rotation gait include acetabular retroversion, physiologic external rotation contracture of the hips, femoral retroversion, external tibial torsion, and flat foot. These conditions may be additive or may compensate for each other [7].

Short Leg Gait

A child with a limb length inequality will most commonly walk with the foot and ankle in equinus or with an abductor lurch on the short side during the stance phase of gait. Other compensatory mechanisms for a short lower extremity include flexing the contralateral knee and/or dropping the ipsilateral hemipelvis.

Equinus

Unilateral equinus is often seen in patients with hemiparetic cerebral palsy, some unilateral foot deformities, and limb length inequality. Bilateral equinus may indicate idiopathic toe walking or neuromuscular disease, such as cerebral palsy or muscular dystrophy.

Trendelenburg Sign

The child stands on one foot while the clinician observes the pelvis dropping toward the opposite side. Normally, the child should not allow the pelvis to drop for at least 15 s. A positive sign with the pelvis dropping indicates abnormal ipsilateral femoral pelvis anatomy (such as acetabular dysplasia, dislocated or subluxated femoral head, and proximal femoral deformity) or abductor weakness. Although not initially described by trendelenburg, tilting of the hemipelvis over the leg in stance during gait is commonly described as a tredelenburg gait.

Knee Thrust

It is important to assess for any dynamic increase in deformity when the foot strikes the ground. A varus thrust suggests lateral collateral ligament laxity and can be seen in multiple conditions including Blount disease and achondroplasia (Fig. 2.2). This finding typically indicates surgery and should be factored into the treatment plan. A valgus thrust is less common but indicates a lack of medial collateral ligament function.

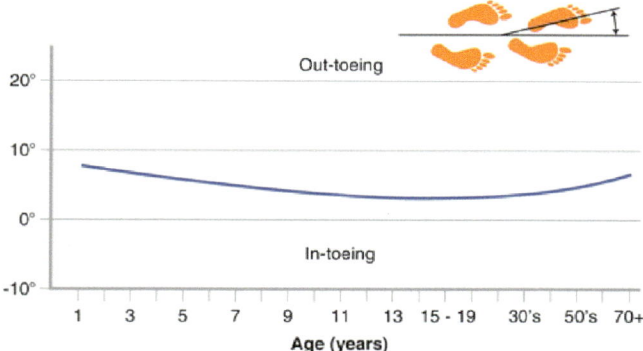

Fig. 2.1 Foot progression angle changes with age. The normal range is very broad. Adapted from [2]

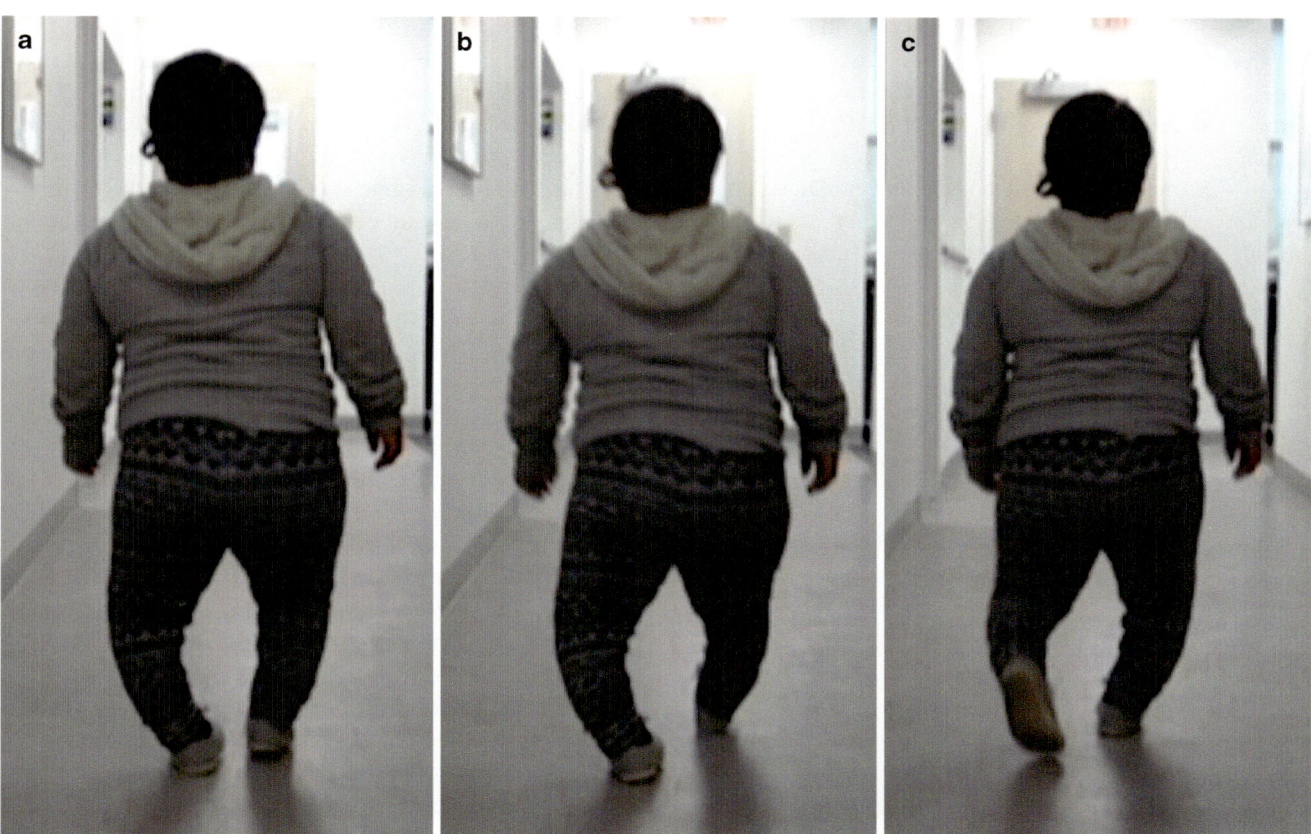

Fig. 2.2 An adolescent female with achondroplasia demonstrates a lateral thrust. (**a**) Right leg is in swing, and the right knee has mild varus. (**b**) Right foot just begins a heel strike. (**c**) Right foot has just started a single-leg stance and demonstrates maximal varus as the lax lateral collateral ligament is fully stretched

Lower Extremities

Supine Exam

A general assessment of the lower extremities in the supine position on the exam table includes evaluation of the limb lengths, as seen by the levels of the heels of both feet after assuring that the pelvis is level. Any asymmetry of thigh circumference, leg circumference, or foot length should also be noted. Size discrepancies are seen in hemihypertrophy, neurological disease, and vascular disease.

Hip abduction in flexion is typically at least 60°, and tightness may indicate hip dysplasia. Abduction and adduction range of motion should be assessed, and any contracture noted. Hip flexion contracture can be assessed with the Thomas test by placing the contralateral hip in maximal flexion to neutralize the lumbar spine and then noting any lack of full extension of the ipsilateral hip.

Knee laxity in the anterior/posterior and medial/lateral directions should be assessed, with increased laxity common in limb deficiencies and many syndromic conditions. Maximal knee extension should be assessed for potential hyper-extension or knee flexion contracture (Fig. 2.3), and maximal knee flexion can also be assessed. Patellar tracking as well as any pain or laxity with patellofemoral motion should be assessed if the child has pain in this region.

Ankle exam should include an assessment of maximal dorsiflexion with the midfoot supinated to lock the midfoot and measured with both knee flexion and extension, with the decreased amount of dorsiflexion in extension representing tightness from the gastrocnemius. Subtalar inversion and eversion can be assessed. This is particularly important in fibular hemimelia as this can help guide whether the ankle should be tilted into varus to compensate for the lack of the fibular buttress. Anterior/posterior laxity can be assessed as well.

Standing Exam

If a discrepancy in limb lengths is noted, children who can stand adequately should be examined with blocks underneath the short leg to determine how much of a lift is necessary to level the pelvis. This method has been shown to be the most reliable clinical measurement for leg length discrepancy, although the studies were done in adults [8, 9]. Older children and adolescents should be asked to report what amount of elevation for the short extremity makes them feel level and well-corrected. Patients with long-standing limb length discrepancies usually report that they feel well-corrected when the blocks under the foot undercompensate for the discrepancy because they have become partially accustomed to the discrepancy. Standing on blocks is more accurate (greater reliability) and also incorporates the foot and pelvis, unlike tape measure techniques [10].

The lower extremity may appear shorter if an ipsilateral hip or knee flexion contracture or an adduction contracture of the hip is present while standing; likewise, the extremity may appear longer if an ipsilateral hip abduction or equinus contracture is present.

To determine if a discrepancy is due to a femoral or tibial difference, the child can sit on the exam table with the hips and knees flexed 90°, the patellas forward, and feet unsupported. If there is a femoral discrepancy, the knees will appear to be at a different level when viewed from above; if a tibial discrepancy is present, the feet will be at different levels when viewed from the front. In many cases, there is a discrepancy in both segments.

Examination of the feet in stance includes assessment of pes planus. The child can stand on their tiptoes to confirm flexibility. The position of the heel compared to the tibia can be assessed from the posterior and normally is in slight valgus. With a high-arched foot and a varus heel, a Coleman block test can be performed where the child stands on a lift with the first ray free, to see if the hindfoot is flexible and can correct into the valgus. If it is flexible, no calcaneal osteotomy is generally necessary.

Prone Exam

The prone exam allows excellent qualitative assessment of rotational conditions affecting the lower extremity and can also assess limb length discrepancy.

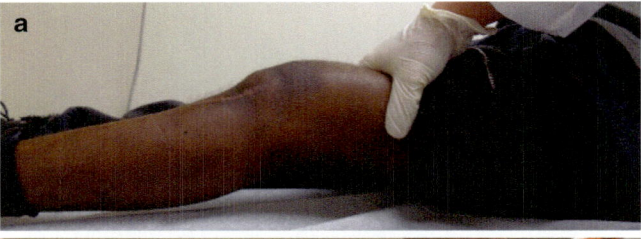
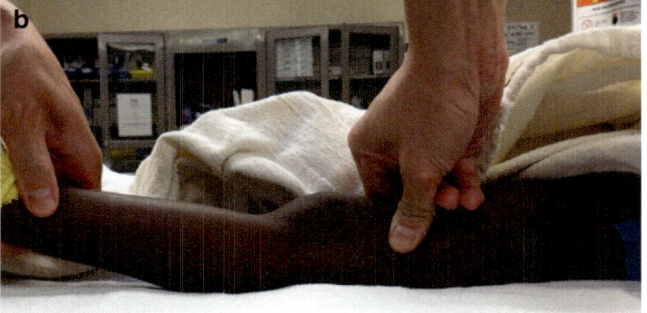

Fig. 2.3 Knee extension can be tested with the patient supine with the hip extended relaxing the hamstrings. (**a**) With a knee flexion contracture, it is not possible to push the popliteal fossa into the examination table. (**b**) With knee hyperextension, the popliteal fossa is pushed into the table and the lower leg is extended

Femoral Version

Hip rotation in the prone position is the net result of soft-tissue rotation contracture, acetabular version, and femoral version. Hip rotation should be evaluated with the child prone and the hip extended because the hip functions largely in extension during normal gait. Moreover, hip flexion in the supine position relaxes the anterior hip capsule, causing an inaccurate assessment of rotation [11]. The child should be positioned prone, the pelvis leveled, and the knees flexed at 90°. The leg serves as an indicator of rotation, measuring its angulation from vertical [5] (Fig. 2.4). Abduction of the hip should be avoided; otherwise, measurement of external rotation will be inflated. The normal hip arc of motion, or sum of internal and external rotations, is approximately 80–100° [5, 12], and typically, there is a little more internal than external rotation, while a large imbalance suggests anteversion or retroversion.

Etiologies of excessive external rotation include acetabular retroversion, as seen in Down syndrome [13], and femoral retroversion, as seen in slipped capital femoral epiphysis (SCFE), coxa vara, and congenital femoral deficiency.

A severe valgus deformity of the proximal tibia will cause an apparent increase in internal rotation and decrease in external rotation without affecting the total rotational arc, whereas a severe varus deformity will cause an apparent increase in external rotation and decrease in internal rotation (Fig. 2.5) [15].

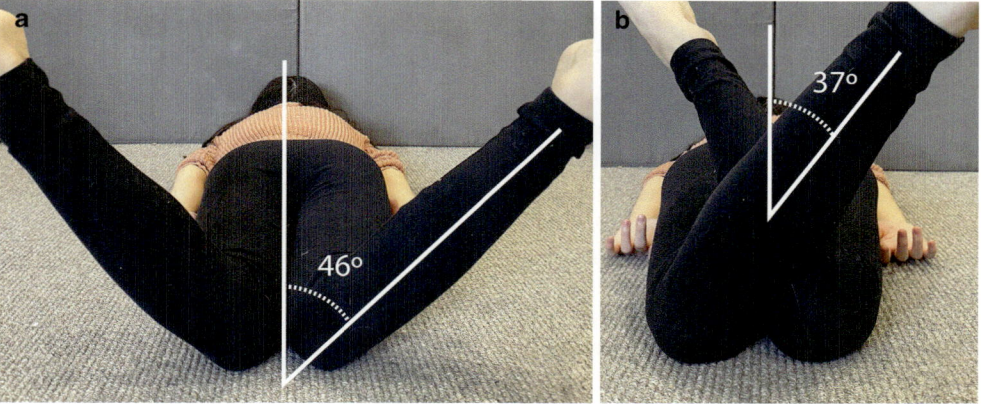

Fig. 2.4 Hip internal and external rotation is commonly assessed in the prone position, with the pelvis level and the knees touching. (**a**) Hip internal rotation is assessed as the axial angle between a line orthogonal to the pelvis and a line along the lower leg with both legs maximal internally rotated. (**b**) Hip external rotation is assessed as the axial angle between a line orthogonal to the pelvis and a line along the lower leg with both legs maximal external rotated. Sometimes it is advantageous to example external rotation in each side separately, if the position of the legs is interfering with the ability to assess rotation without inadvertently abduction the hips

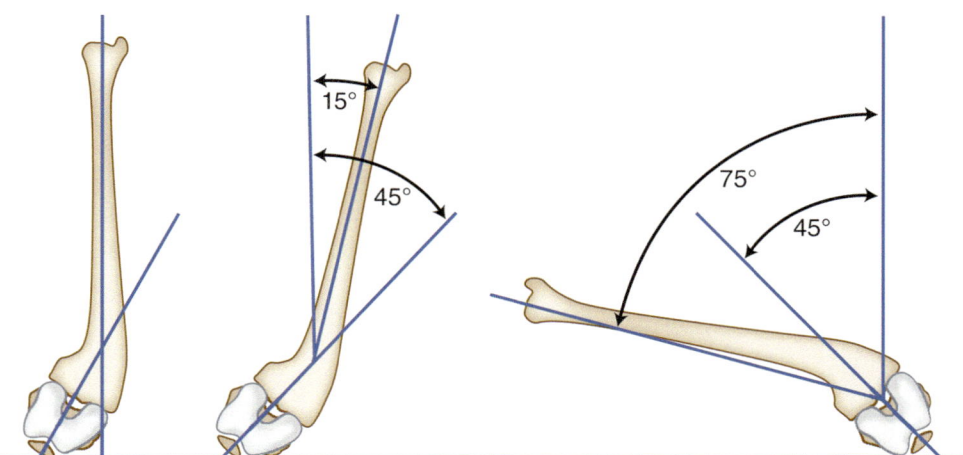

Fig. 2.5 Left lower extremity in the prone position viewed from the caudal–cranial is depicted. A 30° valgus deformity of the proximal tibia results in an incorrect assessment of 75° internal rotation (instead of 45°) and 15° external rotation (instead of 45°). Adapted with permission from Lippincott Williams and Wilkins/Wolters Kluwer Health; Jacquemier M, Jouve JL, Bollini G, Panuel M, Migliani R. Acetabular anteversion in children. J Pediatr Orthop. 1992;12(3): 373–5 [14]

In most cases, a qualitative clinical examination, based on comparing hip internal and external rotations, is sufficient without a quantitative imaging study. Imaging to quantify the femoral version is considered if hip rotation is significantly asymmetrical, operative correction is planned, or the version must be measured to determine the cause of failure of prior surgical procedure around the hip [2]. Most authors conclude that femoral anteversion is not harmful [7, 11, 16, 17], although it may benefit from surgical correction when associated with excessive external tibial torsion [2, 12], abnormal acetabular version [12, 18], neuromuscular disease [19], developmental dysplasia of the hip (DDH) [18, 19], or when associated with significant lower extremity pain or functional issues.

Tibial Torsion

The thigh–foot angle (TFA) is the angle formed by the longitudinal axis of the thigh with the longitudinal axis of the hindfoot. The TFA is measured in the prone position with the hip in neutral rotation, the knee in 90° flexion, and the ankle and foot in neutral dorsiflexion (Fig. 2.6). One needs to be cautious about knee joint laxity and foot deformity, which can alter this value. Although assessment of the TFA and many other parameters is commonly done visually, a goniometer may be used for quantifying this angle and to compare on subsequent exams. A positive value is in the external direction, while a negative value is in the internal direction.

The TFA averages 5° internal (range − 30° to +20°) in infants and averages 10° external (range −5° to +30°) by the age of 8 years [7]. Katz reported internal tibial torsion on the left side more frequently than the right in a series of 54 females and 45 males [20].

Tibial torsion can also be diagnosed and quantified by determining the transmalleolar axis (TMA). Measurement can also be done in the prone position by locating the transmalleolar axis, drawing a line perpendicular to this axis, and then measuring the angle this line forms with the long axis of the thigh. The result obtained by the TMA method yields a value more external than the TFA method, with TMA preferable with foot deformities that make TFA difficult to measure.

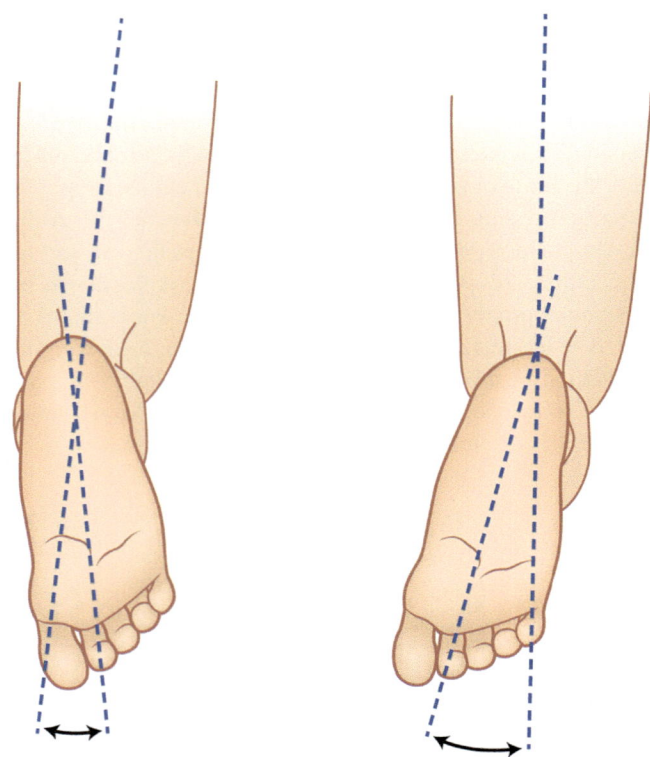

Fig. 2.6 Thigh–foot angle (TFA) assesses tibial torsion. The left image demonstrates external tibial torsion, while the right side demonstrates internal tibial torsion. Adapted with kind permission from Springer Science+Business Media: Paley D. Principles of deformity correction. Berlin, Heidelberg; 2002 [15]

Axial Foot Deformities

The alignment of the foot as a possible cause of in-toeing or out-toeing can also be assessed with the child in the prone position [21]. The examiner should note whether the medial and lateral borders of the foot are straight (Fig. 2.7). The heel bisector line, a line through the midline axis of the hindfoot and forefoot, passes through the second web space in a normal foot. If the heel bisector line passes lateral to the second web space, then there is metatarsus adductus (MTA). If the line passes medial to the second web space, valgus is present. A concave medial border of the midfoot also indicates MTA. If MTA is present, the hindfoot can then be held with one hand while the examiner's other hand abducts the forefoot to

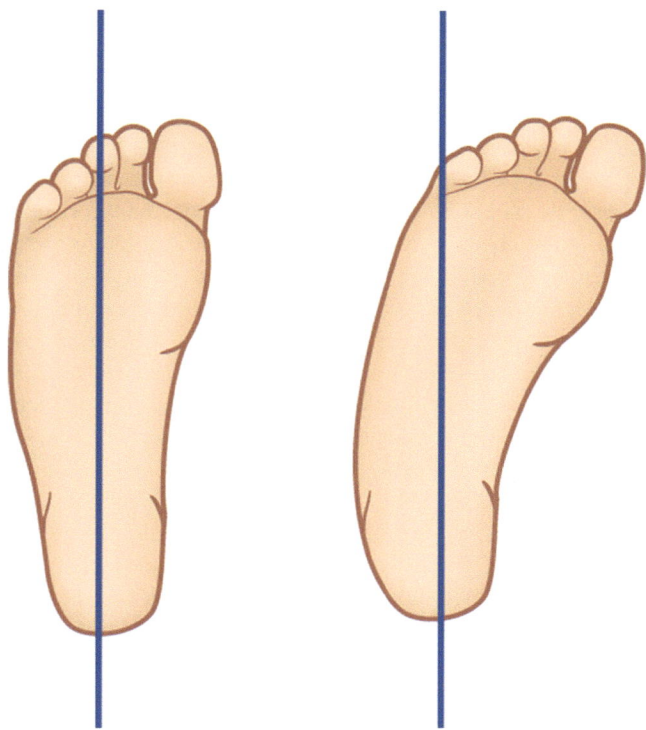

Fig. 2.7 Heel bisector line passes through the second web space in the normal foot and lateral to the second web space in the metatarsus adductus. Adapted with permission from Smith JT, Bleck EE, Gamble JG, Rinsky LA, Pena T. Simple method of documenting metatarsus adductus. J Pediatr Orthop. 1991;11(5):679–80 [21]

determine whether the MTA is rigid or supple. A normal foot should be flexible and exhibit slight forefoot abduction with gentle manipulation.

Limb Length Discrepancy

With the child prone, the pelvis is leveled and the knees bent to 90°. The position of the knees when viewed from posterior quantifies femur length discrepancy. The height of the heels quantifies the tibia and foot length discrepancy.

Physical Exam Summary

The physical exam is critical in the assessment of the limb deformity patient. There are multiple examination findings that influence surgical treatment but may be difficult to assess on imaging, summarized in Table 2.1.

Table 2.1 Key physical exam tests

Exam maneuver	Relevant conditions	Implications
Gait: Knee thrust	Genu varum and valgum	Generally indicates surgery, and the plan should consider the ligament laxity
Gait: Tredelenburg	Hip pathology, abductor weakness	Significant hip pathology, need for rehabilitation in postop patients
Gait: Foot progression angle	Torsional abnormalities	When deciding on which rotational components to correct the overall foot progression angle should be considered
Leveling pelvis with blocks	Limb length discrepancy	Determines the appropriate size lift to use when imaging
Hip/knee/ankle contractures	Multiple	These all can influence the limb length discrepancy seen clinically and on imaging
Coleman block test	Cavus foot	Determines whether a calcaneal osteotomy should be included
Knee/ankle laxity	Multiple including limb deficiency and syndromic	Joints with laxity need to be protected particularly with lengthening procedures
Maximal knee extension	Knee pathology	Knee hyperextension and flexion contracture should be considered when planning correction, and a maximal extension lateral radiograph is very helpful with either finding
Ankle dorsiflexion	Ankle/foot pathology	Surgical release or preoperative casting should be considered with tightness
Subtalar inversion and eversion	Fibular hemimelia	The distal tibia can be purposely tilted into varus to allow these parameters to match the regular side or normal parameters
Prone hip rotation	Femoral version	Imbalance suggests an aberrant femoral version, although one should always consider the contribution from the acetabular side
Thigh foot angle and transmalleolar Axis	Tibial torsion	Assess for internal or external tibial torsion

Diagnostic Imaging

Although many common deformities in younger children can be managed without imaging, most limb length discrepancy, asymmetric angular deformity, or angulation outside the range of normal for age merits radiographic evaluation.

Guidelines for performing imaging studies for rotational conditions are less clear.

Assessment of Limb Length

Several techniques have been developed for the measurement of limb length discrepancies, including orthoroentgenograms [22], standing teleroentgenograms [15, 23], scanograms [24], computerized tomography (CT) scanogram [25], and low-dose biplanar radiographs with the EOS machine. The ideal method should be accurate, readily available in the physician's office, technically easy, have reasonable cost and radiation dosage, and be reproducible. Scanograms are seldom used due to potential issues with positioning and movement, lack of assessment of foot height, as well as the inability to assess angular deformity or potential lesions in the diaphyses. A single-exposure standing teleroentgenogram taken with the patella straight forward with a distance of 10 ft. between the beam source and the film offers the benefits of an easy-to-perform and complete image in a weight-bearing position (Fig. 2.8). The main downside is the parallax from a single image, although this can be partially mitigated with the long distance. In severely obese children or in the presence of severe angular deformity, it may be necessary to perform separate AP radiographs of the two lower extremities. A magnification standard, such as a 25 mm ball bearing, can be affixed to the extremity at the main site of interest or at the knee when assessing leg length. The ball bearing should be positioned the same distance from the cassette as the bone. Placing a ruler with radiopaque graduations on the cassette may not accurately quantify magnification because the ruler is closer to the film than the bone.

Standing orthoroentgenography is a radiographic technique of performing three exposures of the lower extremity on a long cassette and is a common option for assessing limb deformity. Similar to the scanogram, the beam for each exposure is centered over the hip, knee, and ankle to minimize magnification and parallax. By using rectangular collimation, the three exposures can be performed to obtain a full-length image from the hip to the ankle [22]. Direct measurement and deformity analysis on the image can be performed. However, the patient needs to avoid any movement while the three exposures are made. Higher radiation dose is also an issue.

CT scanograms exhibit reasonable accuracy and reliability [10] but are not available in most clinicians' office settings. Lateral CT scanograms have low radiation exposure compared to other radiographic methods and can be performed in the presence of flexion contractures. Magnification error is not an issue. However, since the scan is usually performed in a nonweight-bearing position, it is impossible to measure the contribution of the foot to the leg length discrepancy.

Low-dose biplanar radiographs using EOS are becoming more common, with low radiation dosage and theoretically no axial plane magnification. A study compared EOS, orthoroentgenogram, and teleoroentgenogram on a 70 cm radiodense phantom and found EOS and orethoroentgenogram to both be more accurate than teleoroentgenogram [26]. A clinical study comparing EOS to CT scanogram found near-perfect correlation and high

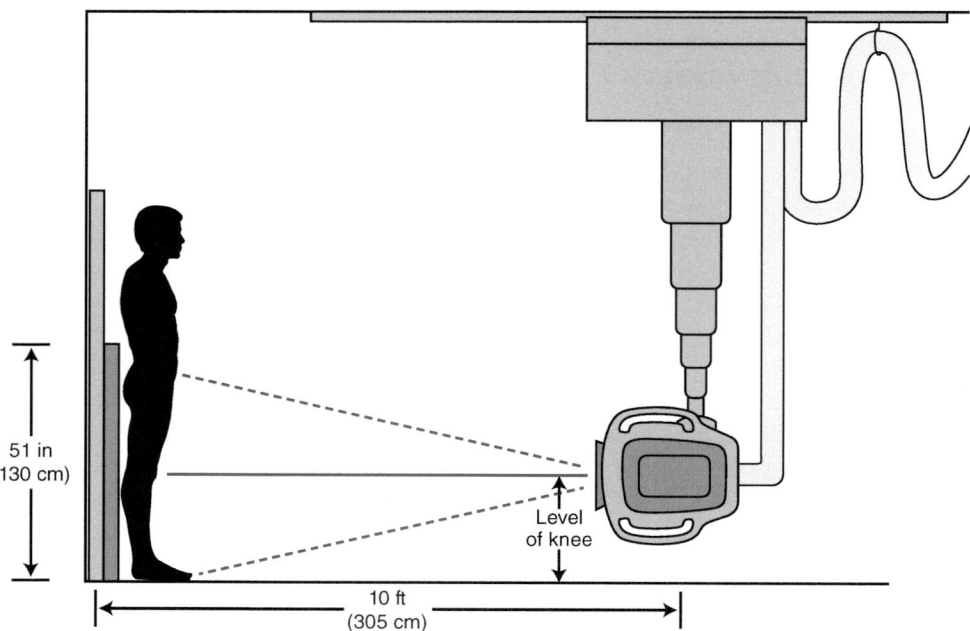

Fig. 2.8 Single-exposure standing full-length radiograph with patella forward is used to evaluate limb length and deformity. Adapted with kind permission from Springer Science+Business Media: Paley D. Principles of deformity correction. Berlin, Heidelberg, 2002 [15]

reliability [27]. Of note, while EOS offers scanning of the AP and lateral images at the same time, the overlap of the limbs on the lateral necessitates either some deviation from normal positioning or separate images. In addition, the child needs to be able to stand still during the scanning process.

For all standing views, the limb is classically positioned with the patella centered on the distal femur, although one should recognize that when a knee is positioned with the femoral condyles overlapped and an orthogonal image is taken, the patella is naturally situated lateral from center [28, 29]. It is important to avoid inadvertent correction of deformity, which occurs most often in genu valgum when the patient is positioned with the feet nearly touching, pushing the knee joints into varus.

Lateral imaging of the entire lower extremity should be performed with the knee in maximal extension, which allows one to separately assess distal femoral deformity, proximal tibial deformity, and soft tissue contracture components of deformity.

Version Diagnostic Imaging

Abnormal femoral version is usually apparent from the physical exam based on a mismatch between hip internal and external rotation. If the diagnosis is in doubt, or if corrective surgery is being planned, imaging for diagnosis and quantification may be indicated to confirm the suspected femoral version and investigate for potential acetabular version abnormalities. MRI and CT with limited slices taken at the hips, knees, and ankles are an option, while low-dose biplanar imaging is being investigated as a more convenient alternative.

Acetabular Version

Computerized tomography measurements show that the normal acetabulum is anteverted approximately 13° in children from ages 1 to 15 years, with a large range of normal between ages 1 and 2 years [13, 14]. Visser et al. reported a mean acetabular anteversion of 6.5° in a newborn and 16.5° in adults [30]. Excessive acetabular anteversion is often seen in children with DDH, and acetabular retroversion has been reported in children with Down syndrome [13]. McKibbin developed an "instability index" based on the sum of the acetabular version angle and the femoral anteversion angle. Values less than 20° or greater than 58° were associated with hip instability. He hypothesized that the version of the femur and acetabulum must develop in a coordinated manner [18]. Tönnis and Heinecke reported increasing pain and osteoarthritis in adult hips with a McKibbin instability index at the upper and lower limits of normal [12].

Femoral Version

The femoral version is the angle formed by the axis of the femoral neck with the tangent of the posterior aspect of the femoral condyles (Fig. 2.9). The normal femur is mildly anteverted, with the neck extending anteriorly from the coronal plane. Normal values for infants and children have been published, with an average value of 30–40° at birth, declining to 8° in adult men and 14° in adult women [2, 4, 5, 12, 19].

Computerized tomography is currently the most accurate method of quantifying the femoral version [31]. The equipment is less easily available in the clinic and exposes children to ionizing radiation. The morphologies of the femoral neck and greater trochanter sometimes make measurement

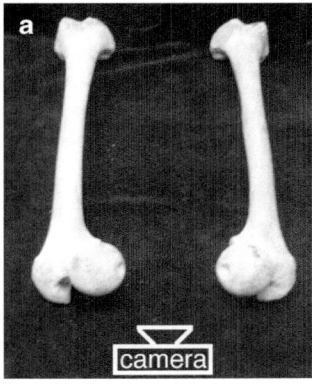
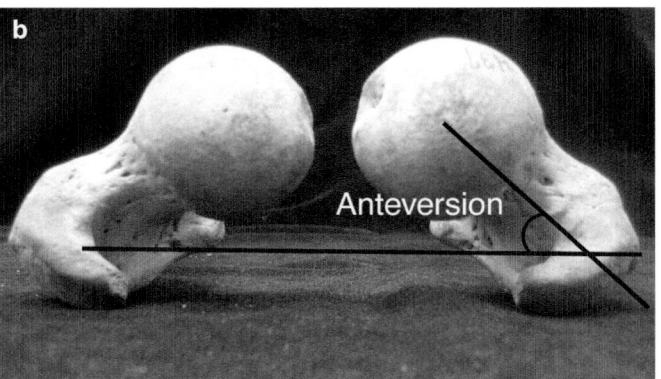

Fig. 2.9 Cadaveric femora illustrating measurement of femoral version. (**a**) Femora are positioned resting on the posterior aspect of the greater trochanter and the posterior aspects of the femoral condyles. A camera icon representing the viewpoint for panel **b**. (**b**) When viewed from cranial to caudal, the femoral version is measured as the angle between the femoral neck and a line representing the posterior aspects of the femoral condyles. (Adapted with kind permission from Wolters Kluwer Health Inc.: Liu RW, Toogood P, Hart DE, Davy DT, Cooperman DR. The effect of varus and valgus osteotomies on femoral version. J Pediatr Orthop. 2009 Oct-Nov;29(7):666–75)

difficult [32]. Various other radiographic techniques have been used, including biplanar radiography (RyderCrane [32] and Magilligan [33] techniques), fluoroscopy [34], ultrasound [35, 36], and MRI.

Low-dose biplanar radiographs with the EOS system offer a low dose and quick option for institutions with this machine and has been found to be comparable to CT scans for measuring femoral version and tibial torsion in patients preoperative for total hip replacements [37]. However, patient positioning can be an issue. One study of 53 patients, 37 with cerebral palsy, found large variations in the femoral version in serial EOS images of patients not treated with surgery, and lower amounts of correction in both the femoral version and tibial torsion than expected in those who underwent surgery; these differences were attributed to patient positioning issues [38]. Another study purposely rotated patients by 15° in the machine and found acceptable femoral version measurements with acceptable correlation to CT scan data but decreased inter-observer reliability and decreased correction with CT scan data when measuring tibial torsion [39]. A recent study compared EOS to CT versus MRI in patients with abnormal rotational parameters and found that the femoral version measured with EOS was significantly lower than CT/MRI, while tibial torsion measurements were comparable [40]. Overall, the utility of EOS for measuring rotational profiles shows some promise but needs additional research.

Intraoperative assessment of the femoral version can be challenging. Clinical examination can be limited by patient positioning and instability of provisional fixation. Intraoperative CT scanning is an option but requires special equipment and adds operative time. Biplanar radiographs traditionally are limited by the need to get two orthogonal views and then refer to a calculation table, with the added issue that most systems mathematically neglect the anterior bow leading to additional error [41]. A modified Ogata approach consists of obtaining a lateral view with the femoral condyles aligned, laying a linear radiodense object at the posterior aspect of the femoral condyles, and then obtaining a lateral at the hip with the same object at the posterior aspect of the greater trochanter (Fig. 2.10). If the angle between the femoral neck and the radiodense object is 5°, then the femoral version is between 2° and 11°, assuming the neck-shaft angle is between 115° and 155° [41].

Tibial Torsion

Tibial torsion less commonly requires imaging for diagnosis or quantification since unlike the femur, it can be assessed on examination both in the clinic and the operating room. Computerized tomography has been described to measure tibial torsion as the angle formed by a line through the proximal tibial juxtaarticular area and the distal bimalleolar axis or distal articular surface [42], and the use of EOS is discussed in the femoral version section above.

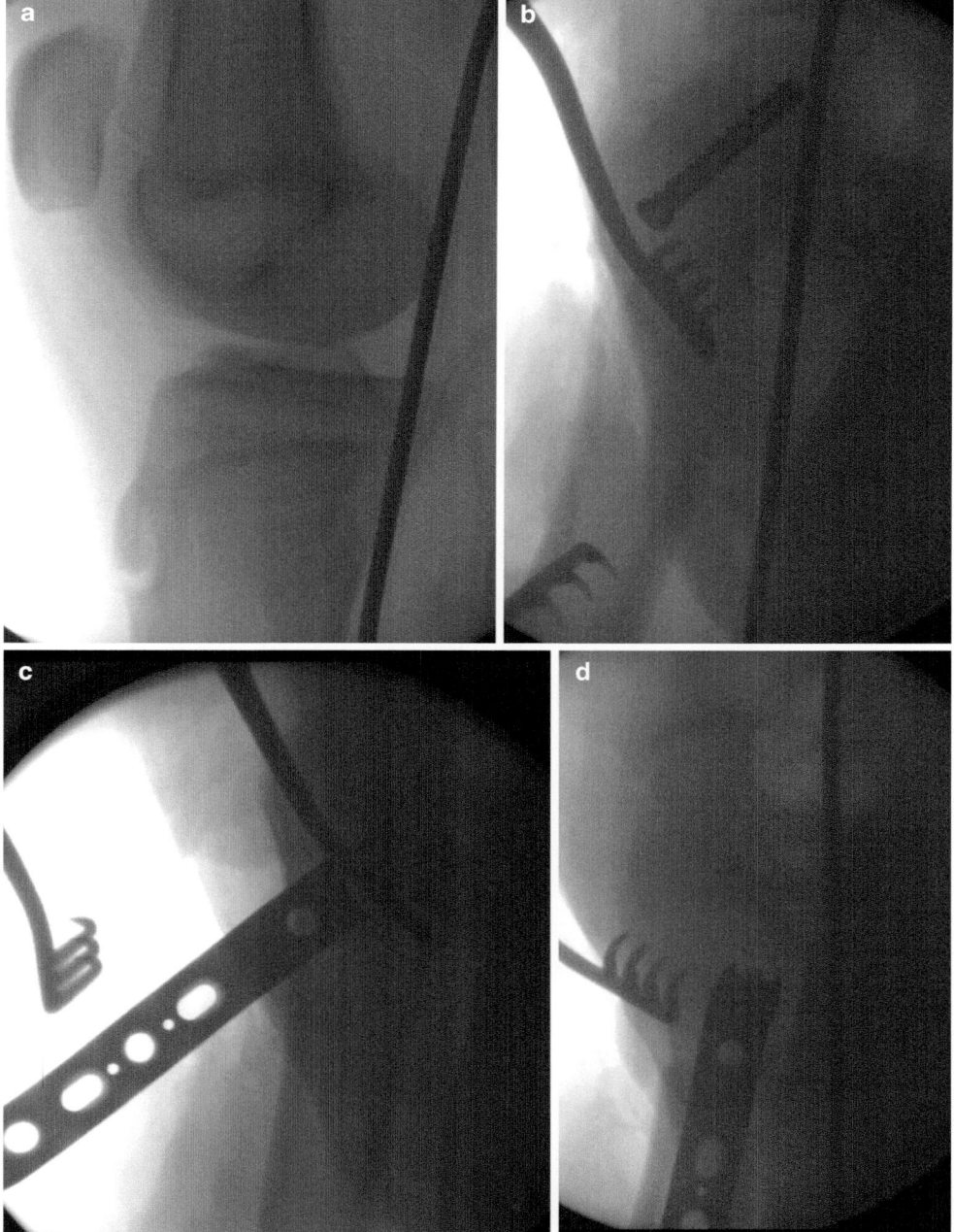

Fig. 2.10 Modified Ogata method is useful when the femoral version cannot be directly measured and with experience relatively quick to do intraoperatively. This patient with deformity secondary to slipped capital femoral epiphysis was treated with a proximal femur flexion osteotomy. Since the flexion osteotomy will significantly change the femoral version, the Ogata method was utilized. Before surgical preparation, both the hip and knee are bumped since direct lateral views are necessary, and overlap from the contralateral extremity can obscure the images. (**a**) Using a direct lateral view the knee is positioned such that the femoral condyles are overlapped, and a radiodense wire is positioned such that it projects on the posterior aspect of the femoral condyles. The wire is held at this position at the knee by the surgeon. (**b**) A direct lateral hip image is then obtained, and the wire is pivoted by an assistant until the wire projects over the posterior aspect of the greater trochanter. The angle between femoral neck and the wire here is significantly downsloping (negative), indicating severe retroversion before the osteotomy. (**c**) The position of the blade chisel demonstrates the planned flexion osteotomy. (**d**) The osteotomy is performed with the plate clamped to the shaft. The first step is repeated at the knee to position the leg and then the wire. The hip view now demonstrates mild downsloping, indicating improved but persistent retroversion after the flexion osteotomy. The femur can now be rotated at the osteotomy and the imaging rechecked until the femoral version is acceptable, with the goal to see the femoral neck upsloping approximately 5°

Quantitative Deformity Analysis

It is important to perform deformity analysis in a systematic fashion, and while basic concepts with a focus on the knee are presented, additional detail and assessment of other sites can be found [15, 43].

In the coronal plane, the mechanical axis is drawn from the center of the femoral head to the center of the talus and normally passes through the medial tibia spine at the level of the knee. Mechanical axis deviation (MAD) is the distance from the center of the knee to the mechanical axis line and is typically between 0 and 15 mm (Fig. 2.11a). After one has determined an overall varus versus valgus alignment, angles can be drawn to look for deformity in the distal femur, proximal tibia, or joint. Occasionally, the MAD is normal but there is substantial obliquity to the joint line. If so, measuring specific angles again is the proper next step.

Angles are typically defined by whether they are mechanical or anatomic, whether they are measured medial or lateral (or anterior or posterior), whether they are proximal or distal, and whether they are of the femur or tibia. Mechanical lateral distal femoral angle (mLDFA) is the lateral angle between a line from the center of the hip to the center of the knee, and a line defined by the distal ends of the femoral condyles (Fig 2.11b). mLDFA is normally 88° (range 85–90°), and values outside this range define distal femoral deformity.

Tibial angles typically forgo the mechanical versus anatomic specification since these two lines are very similar. Medial proximal tibial angle (MPTA) is the medial angle between a line connecting the tibial plateaus, and a line from the center of the knee to the center of the talus (Fig 2.11c). If there is no visible joint line deformity, the line from the distal femoral condyles can be shifted distally to serve as the proximal tibial line. MPTA is normally 87° (range 85–90°), and values outside this range define proximal tibial deformity.

mLDFA and MPTA do vary in younger children. Sabharwal et al. demonstrated that mLDFA is higher (more varus) as younger ages and decreases with time, while MPTA stays more constant, with all parameters within adult normative ranges by age 7 years [44]. Asymmetric cartilage thickness should also be considered in younger children, with the medial distal femur thicker than lateral, resulting in more distal femur valgus than is appreciated on plain radiographs. This effect also resolves by age 7 years based on a MRI-based study, and in younger children with circumstances where mild changes in angulation may change surgical management, an intraoperative arthrogram can be considered [45].

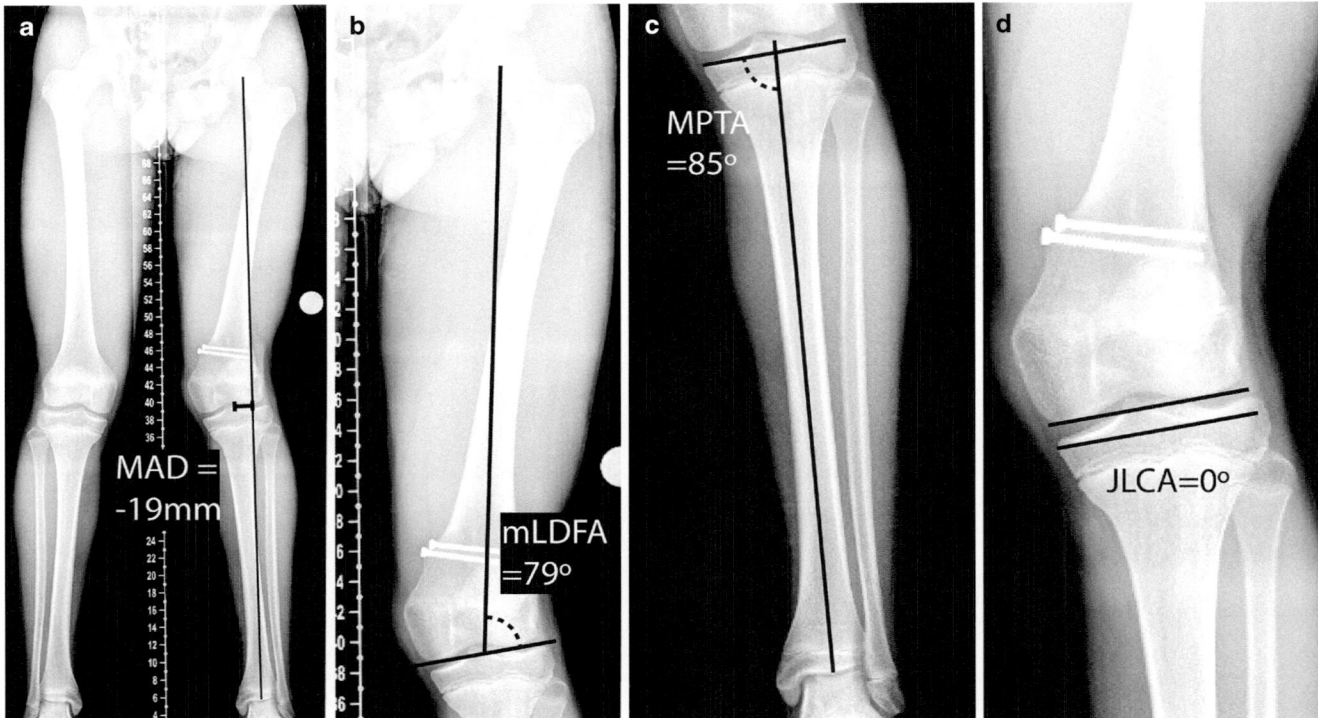

Fig. 2.11 Standing orthoroentgenogram of a 15-year-old male with a partial growth arrest of his left distal femur. (**a**) Mechanical axis line is first drawn from the center of the femoral head to the center of the talus. The MAD is the orthogonal distance from the center of the knee to this line and is −19 mm in this case, indicating valgus knee deformity. (**b**) mLDFA is the lateral angle between a line from the center of the femoral head to the center of the knee versus a line along the distal femoral condyles. It is 79° in this case, indicating distal femur valgus. (**c**) MPTA is the medial angle between a line from the center of the knee to the center of the talus versus a line along the proximal tibial plateaus. It is 85° in this case, which is within the normal range, indicating no coronal proximal tibial deformity. (**d**) JLCA is the angle between lines along the distal femoral condyles and along the proximal tibial plateaus. These lines are parallel so the angle is 0°, which is within the normal range indicating no intraarticular deformity

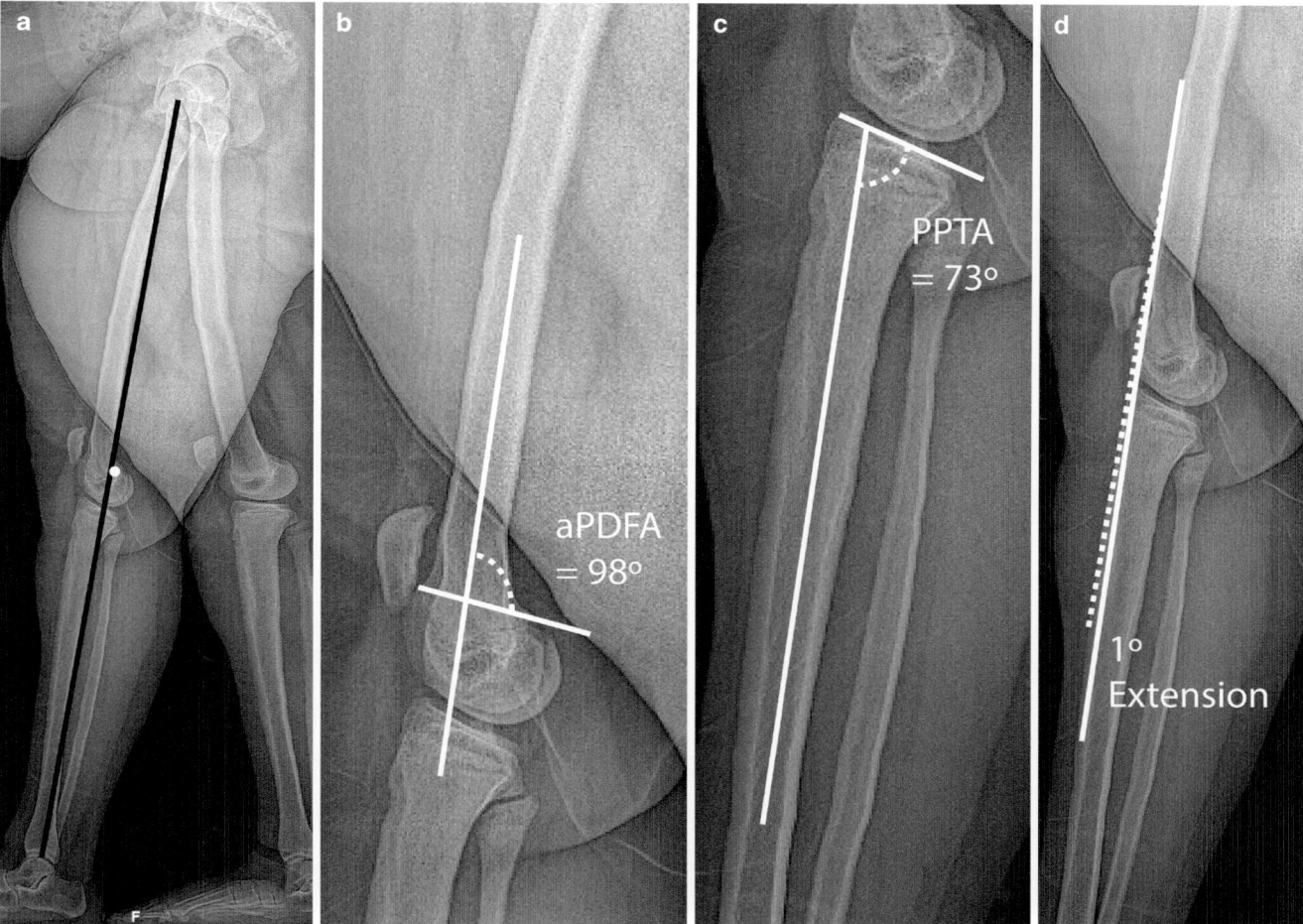

Fig. 2.12 Lateral EOS view of a 13-year-old female with adolescent Blount's disease. The right knee is anterior and maximally extended. (**a**) Mechanical axis line is drawn from the center of the femoral head to the center of the talus and is just barely anterior to the rotational axis of the knee, marked with a white circle. Deformity planning should take care to avoid adding any procurvatum to this patient, which could take away her ability to lock her knee into an extension. (**b**) aPDFA is the posterior angle between a line along the center of the distal femoral shaft and a line across the physis and is 98°, indicating recurvatum of the distal femur. (**c**) PPTA is the posterior angle between a line along the tibial plateau and a line along the center of the proximal tibial shaft and is 73°, indicating procurvatum of the proximal tibia. (**d**) Solid line along the anterior distal femoral shaft and a dotted line along the anterior proximal tibial shaft form an overall 1° extension deformity. Based on 15° of recurvatum at the distal femur and 8° of procurvatum at the proximal tibia, there should be a 6° of flexion contracture in the joint ($-15 + 8 + 6 = -1$)

The joint line congruence angle (JLCA) is the angle between the lines defined by the distal ends of the femoral condyles and the proximal tibial plateaus (Fig. 2.11d). JLCA is normally 0–2°, and values outside this range define joint deformity, such as lateral collateral ligament laxity in Blount disease.

For the sagittal plane, it is ideal to have a full-length image from the hips to ankles with the knee in maximal extension. A normal mechanical axis typically passes through the anterior third of the femur and the anterior fifth of the tibia. It is important for the mechanical axis to be anterior to the center of rotation of the knee, which is located at the junction of a line extending down the posterior femoral cortex and the growth plate (Fig 2.12a). If the mechanical axis is posterior to this point, then the knee cannot lock in extension and the energy requirement of stance and gait is greatly increased.

Anatomic posterior distal femoral angle (aPDFA) is the posterior angle between a line along the distal femoral shaft versus a line between the anterior and posterior physis and is normally 83° (range 79–87°) (Fig 2.12b). Posterior proximal tibial angle (PPTA) is the posterior angle between a line starting one-fifth of the way from the anterior aspect of the proximal tibia extending to the middle of the ankle and a line along the tibia plateau and is normally 81° (range 77–84°) (Fig. 2.12c). Anatomical lines along the anterior cortices of the distal femur and proximal tibia should be parallel, and the angle between them defines the overall knee deformity (Fig. 2.12d). If this overall deformity does not match the amount of deformity from the distal femur and proximal tibia, then there is an additional soft tissue component that makes up the difference.

The hip in the coronal plane is typically assessed with mechanical lateral proximal femoral angle (mLPFA), which is the lateral angle between a line from the superior tip of the greater trochanter to the center of the femoral head versus a line from the center of the femoral head to the center of the knee, normally 90° (range 85–95°). The ankle in the coronal plane is assessed with lateral distal tibial angle (LDTA), which is the lateral angle between a line from the center of the knee to the center of the talus versus a line along the superior talus, normally 89° (range 86–92°). The ankle in the sagittal plane is assessed with anterior distal tibial angle (ADTA), which is the anterior angle between a line from the center of the knee to the center of the talus versus a line between the anterior and posterior aspects of the distal tibial, normally 80° (range 78–82°).

The location and magnitude of the deformity should be quantified in the coronal, sagittal, and axial planes. In the coronal plane, the femoral deformity can be determined using either anatomic or mechanical methods. For the anatomic method, the proximal line is drawn from the piriformis fossa extending along the femoral shaft, while the distal line is drawn forming a lateral angle between it and a line along the distal femoral condyles that matches the other normal side versus using the normative angle of 81° if the other side is abnormal. The intersection of these lines determines the location and magnitude of the deformity (Fig. 2.13a).

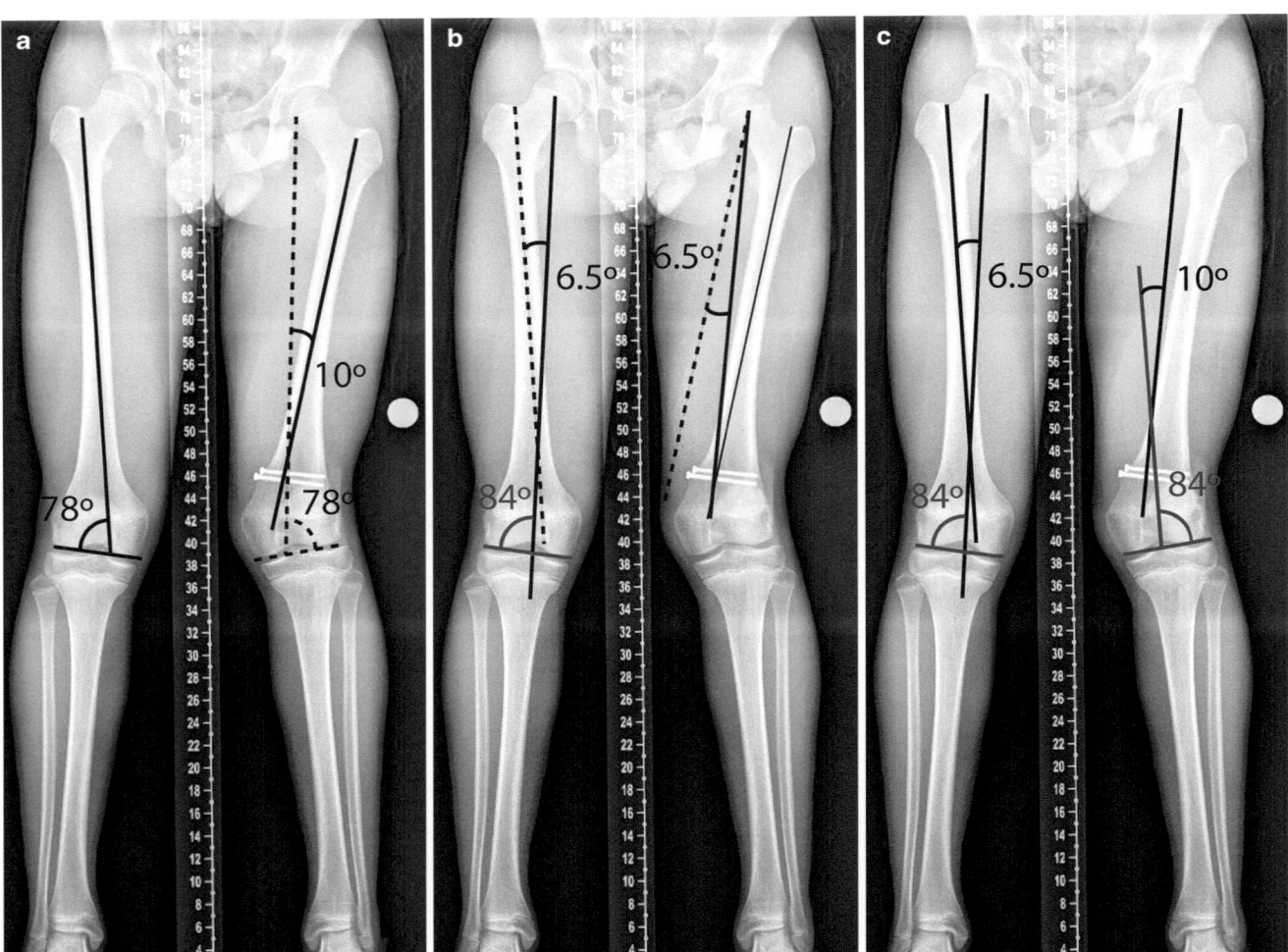

Fig. 2.13 Same patient from Fig. 2.11 is used here to demonstrate how to determine the location and magnitude of the femoral deformity. (**a**) To perform anatomical planning, an anatomical line is drawn on the right side, and its angle versus a line across the joint is measured at 78°. An equal 78° angle is then drawn on the left side using the distal femoral condyle line as a guide (dashed line), with careful attention to have the line extending proximally meet the femoral condyle similarly to the right side. An anatomical line (solid line) is then drawn from proximal, and the intersection of these lines is the level of the deformity, with a magnitude of 10° here. (**b**) To perform mechanical planning, a mechanical axis line is first drawn on the right side (solid line). The angle between this line and a line within the proximal femur shaft (dashed line) is measured at 6.5° here, and the angle between the mechanical axis line and the distal femoral condyles (purple line) is measured at 84°. On the left side, a line is first drawn within the proximal shaft (thin black line). A parallel line to this is drawn originating at the femoral head (dashed line), and then, a line 6.5° angled to the dashed line is drawn representing the proximal mechanical line (solid line). (**c**) With the proximal mechanical line maintained, a second line is drawn distally oriented 84° from a line along the distal femoral condyles (purple line), to represent the distal mechanical axis. The intersection of the two mechanical lines identifies the level of the deformity with again a magnitude of 10°. Note that the level of deformity with mechanical planning is slightly different from the level with anatomical planning, which is typical. Also, note that one could draw a distal mechanical line originating from the center of the talus and passing through the medial tibial spine since the tibia does not have coronal plane deformity

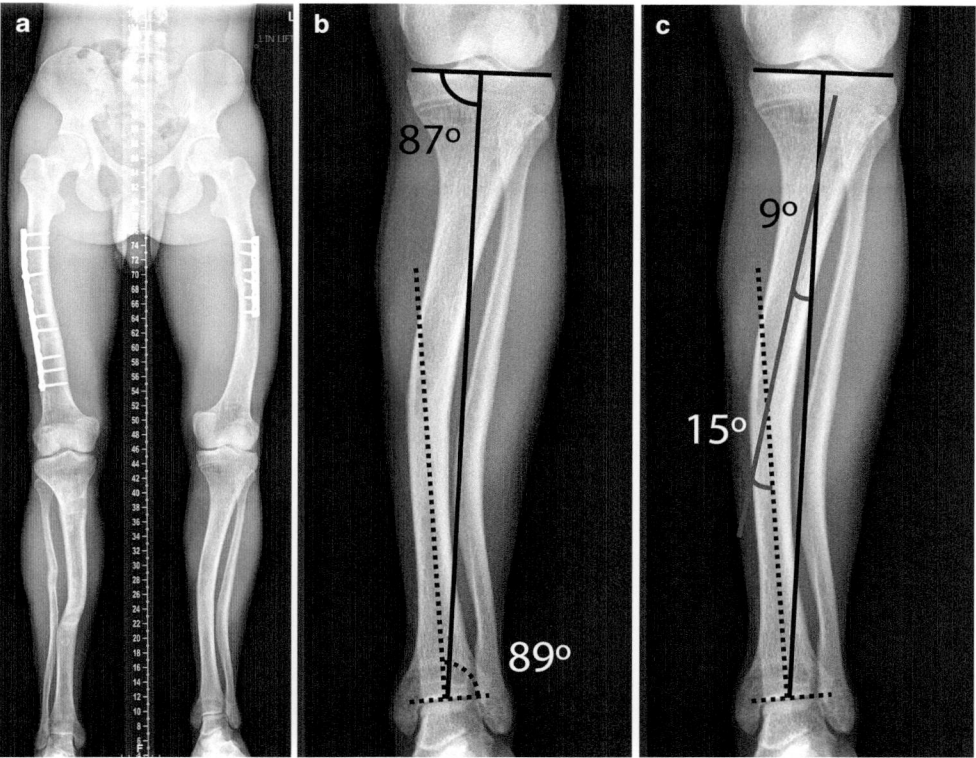

Fig. 2.14 Twenty-one-year-old male with x-linked hypophosphatemic rickets, status post multiple previous surgeries. (**a**) Although all four bones have deformities, the focus for this example is the left tibia. (**b**) Without a normal femur or contralateral tibia, planning is instead done using normative angles of 87° proximally (solid line) and 89° distally (dashed line). The lines intersect at the ankle, despite obvious deformities at other levels, suggesting multi-level deformity. (**c**) Anatomical line is drawn in the middle segment (purple line), identifying the levels of the two deformities and their magnitude

Whenever two lines are drawn to define any deformity, if they do not meet at the visible deformity, then at least two deformities are likely to present, and a third line should be drawn along the anatomical axis of the middle segment and its intersections with the first two lines defines the two deformities.

The femoral deformity can also be determined using a mechanical line. The angle between a line along the anatomical proximal femoral shaft versus a line from the center of the femoral head to the center of the knee can be first measured on the opposite normal side, and then, the same angle is drawn between the shaft and a line originating from the femoral head on the deformity side. If the opposite side is abnormal, a normative angle of 6° can be used. A distal line can be drawn based on measuring the mLDFA on the opposite normal side and then drawing a line originating from the center of the knee that forms an equal lateral angle versus a line connecting the distal femoral condyles. Alternatively, a normative 88° line can be drawn. The intersection of the line is then used to determine the level and magnitude of the deformity (Fig. 2.13b-c).

In the tibia in the coronal plane, the proximal line can be drawn extending from the center of the hip through the medial tibial spine and extending distally if the femur is normal or if femoral deformity will not be corrected. Otherwise, a line can be drawn with a medial angle to a line along the tibial plateaus equal to the opposite normal side versus at a 87° normative angle. The distal angle can be based on a line through the center of the talus extending up the tibial shaft. Alternatively, one can draw a line originating from the center of the talus and forming a lateral angle to a line along the talus equal to the opposite side versus at a 89° normative angle. Once again, the intersection of the line is then used to determine the level and magnitude of the deformity, and if the deformity is not at this point then a double-level deformity should be suspected (Fig. 2.14).

For the sagittal plane in the tibia, the proximal line can similarly be drawn from the femoral head through the anterior fifth of the joint, or a line can be drawn with respect to the proximal tibial using an approach similar to the coronal plane. If the level of the deformity on the lateral view is different than the level on the AP view, then a translational deformity also exists, which is generally the case. The distance between the proximal and distal lines at the level of the deformity is the translational deformity (Fig. 2.15). As noted above, there may also be a soft tissue component to the deformity in the sagittal plane, and in general, one should be cautious about fully correcting the bony deformity if it accentuates a soft tissue deformity. For example in a child with 10° of tibial procurvatum and 10° of knee hyperextension with femoral deformity, there is a 20° soft tissue extension deformity and one might choose to leave the tibial procurvatum minimally corrected or uncorrected.

Axial plane deformity is composed of limb length discrepancy (LLD) and rotational deformity. Rotational deformity can be assessed as noted above with the physical exam and imaging if deemed necessary. Direct LLD is calculated based on the difference between the combined femur and tibial lengths, measured from the acetabulum or proximal femur proximally and the talus distally. Direct LLD does

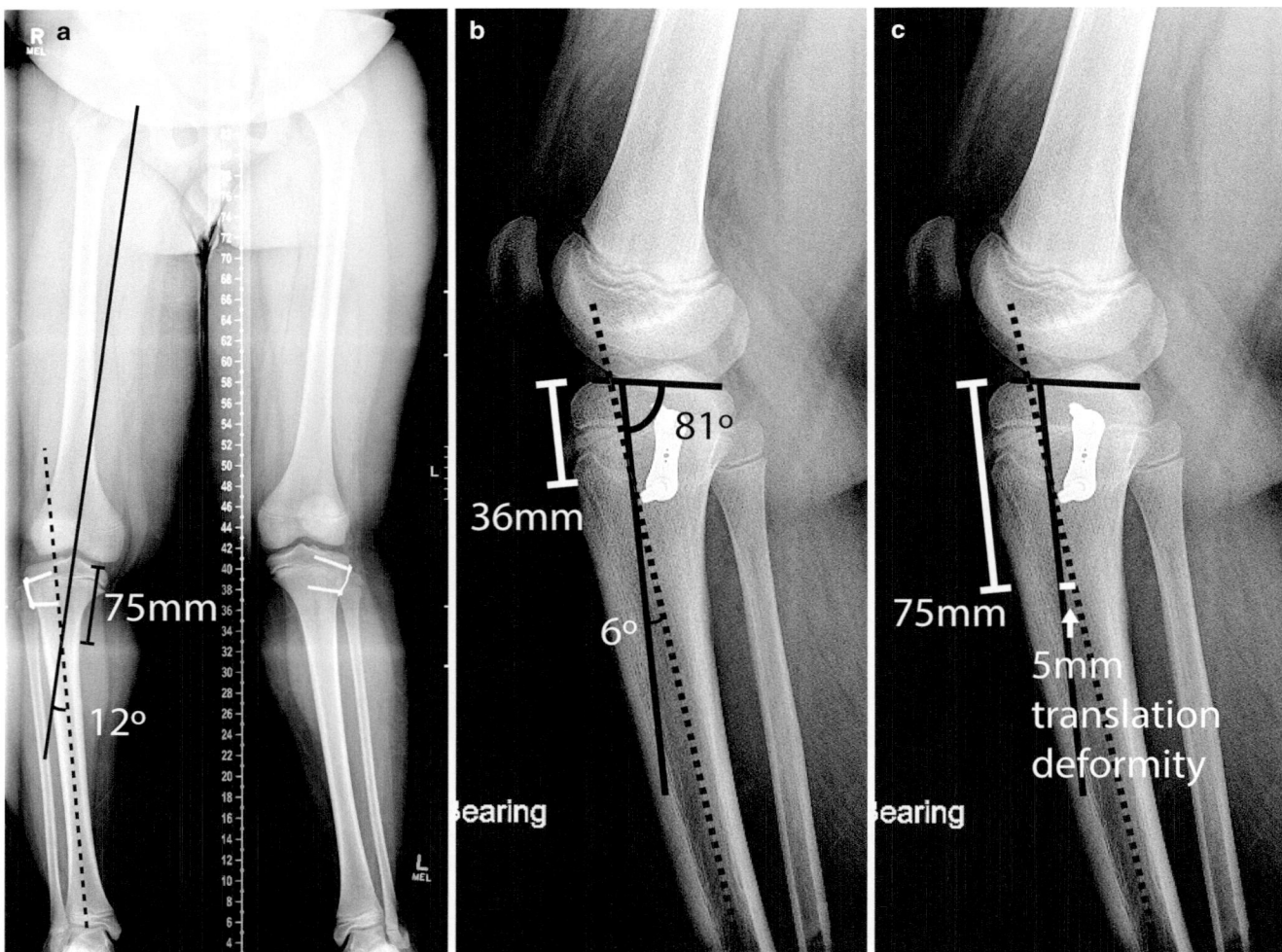

Fig. 2.15 Eleven-year-male with bilateral Blount's disease. He was lost to follow-up after bilateral guided growth plates and developed overcorrection on the left but no correction on the right. Planning is focused on the right side. (**a**) His right femur is within normal limits, and so the proximal mechanical axis line is drawn from the center of the hip through the medial tibial spine (solid line). A distal line is drawn through the center of the tibial shaft (dotted line). The lines intersect demonstrating a 12° varus deformity located 75 mm from the joint. (**b**) In the sagittal plane, an 81° proximal line is drawn off the tibial plateau (solid line), and a distal line is drawn through the center of the tibial shaft (dotted line). These intersect to create a 6° procurvatum deformity 36 mm distal to the joint line. (**c**) Since this bone will be corrected at only one level, there must be some translation deformity component. If one decides to set the level of the correction at the level of deformity in the coronal plane (75 mm from the joint), then the amount of translational deformity in the sagittal plane can be calculated by measuring the distance between the lines 75 mm from the joint. Thus, the deformity in the sagittal plane is 6° procurvatum and 5 mm of posterior translation of the distal fragment versus the proximal fragment. Note that the level of the correction can be at any level, and the translational deformity in both planes is determined with this same approach

not account for foot deformity. Indirect LLD is calculated based on the difference in distances from the acetabulum or proximal femur to the top of the image on the two sides, while also accounting for the lift size. Thus, indirect LLD includes femur, tibia, and foot discrepancy, and the difference between direct LLD and indirect LLD is the foot height discrepancy, assuming no hip, knee, or ankle contractures. Individual femur and tibia differences can be directly measured as well.

After all three components of the deformity are assessed, correction can proceed. Please see the chapters on acute and gradual correction for details on correction options.

Oblique Plane Deformities

A deformity seen in both the AP and lateral views is an oblique plane deformity. Biplanar deformity is a misnomer because the deformity is only in a single plane (the plane of maximum deformity), located between the AP and lateral planes (Fig. 2.16). Historically, the exact calculation of the Olique plane deformity was important to determine the placement of the hinge in the Ilizarov correction technique. Nevertheless, it is still important to understand the concept of an oblique plane deformity.

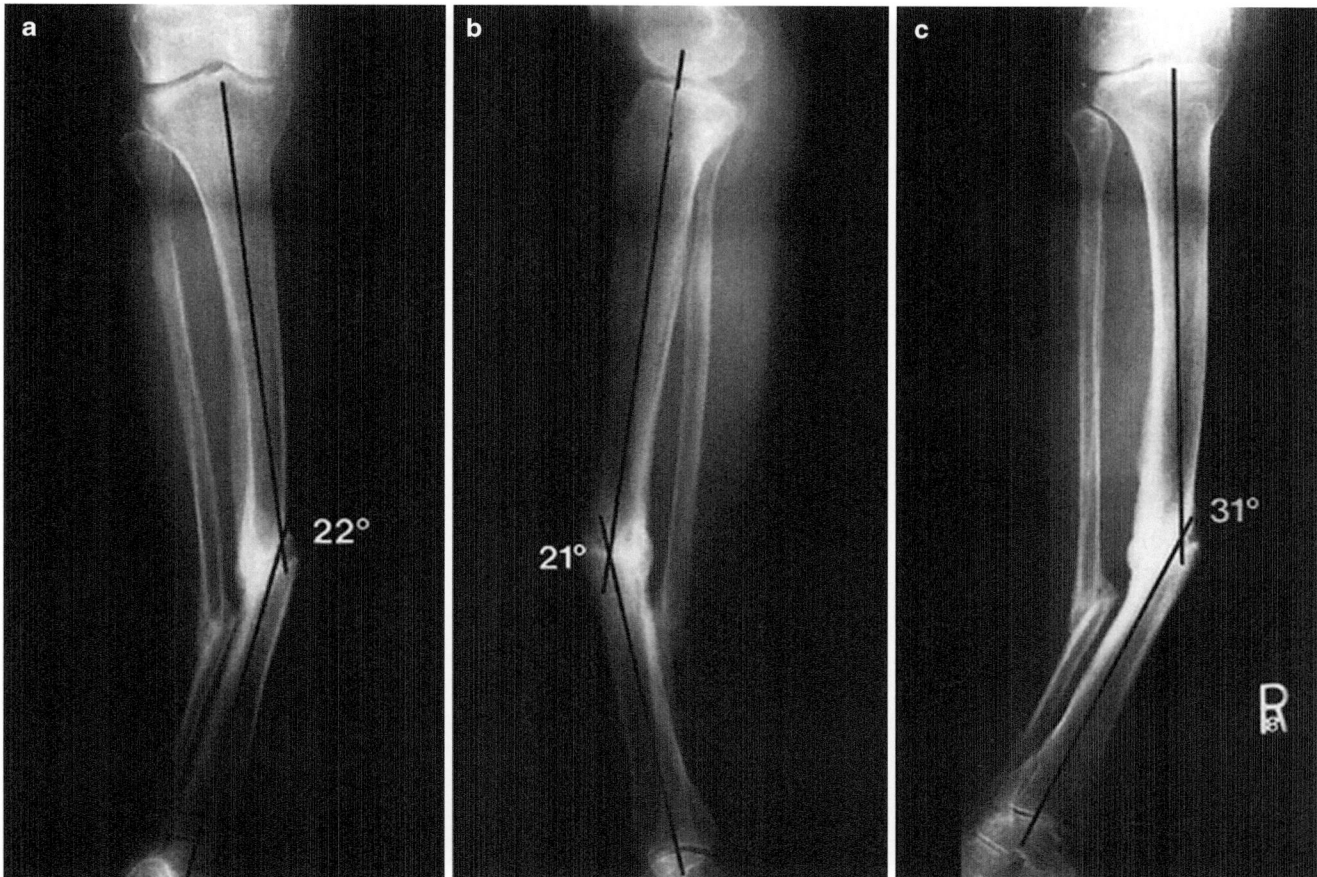

Fig. 2.16 (a, b) Oblique plane angular deformity of the tibia. Radiographs show angulation on the AP (22°) and LAT (21°) projections of magnitude. This is not a biplanar deformity but rather a single plane of angulation where the true plane of angulation lies between the frontal and sagittal planes. (c) An oblique radiograph obtained perpendicular to the plane of angulation shows the maximum angulation (31°). With kind permission from Springer Science+Business Media: Paley D. Principles of deformity correction. Berlin, Heidelberg; 2002 [15]

Conclusions

In summary, many children present to a pediatric orthopedic surgeon to assess limb deformity. While most are treated with reassurance, some need a more thorough history to help determine whether there is a need for correction and to identify any related conditions. A careful physical examination provides important data that might not otherwise be available on imaging. Radiographic analysis should be approached with a systemic assessment to identify the location and magnitude of the deformity in the coronal and sagittal planes, and limb length discrepancy in the axial plane. With this information, a surgeon can then develop a comprehensive plan to address the unique deformity characteristics of each patient.

Commentary

Jan Duedal Rölfing
jan.rolfing@rm.dk and Bjoern Vogt
bjoern.vogt@ukmuenster.de

In recent years, technological advances such as planning software, 3D-printed guides, and patient-specific implants have revolutionized limb deformity surgery and vastly improved its accuracy. However, history-taking and clinical examination remain fundamental medical skills that must be mastered in order to determine if radiological investigations are needed and when surgery should be considered. Reassurance of children and their parents that certain deformities are self-limiting or likely to correct as the child grows older requires profound knowledge of the physiological development of alignment and benign deformities. Knowledge of which conditions require surgical intervention and which do not is just as important as clinical experience when deciding if patients are suitable to undergo surgery at all.

Calibrated long-standing radiographs are the mainstay of limb deformity correction and indispensable for evaluation and planning of reconstruction of limb length and angular deformities. On the other hand, radiological evaluation of torsion, in particular of the lower leg, is rarely indicated, and children can thus be protected from unnecessary radiation. However, if osteotomies for rotational malalignment are scheduled or the examiner is uncertain, radiological assessment with MRI or low-dose CT is appropriate for examining the version of the acetabulum, femur, and lower leg.

Clinical evaluation of joint stability and contractures is crucial—not only before surgery but also during gradual limb deformity correction. If clinical instability of the adjacent joints is evident, stabilizing procedures are most often needed if lengthening has been considered. Moreover, varus thrust of the knee during gait is not necessarily apparent on long-standing radiographs, but the underlying laxity of the collateral ligament may warrant surgery. In the sagittal plane, radiographs should be taken with maximum knee extension. Importantly, clinical examination outweighs the radiological measurements in the sagittal plane. For instance, if an excessive tibial slope is measured and the knee can be completely extended, one should refrain from correction in order to prevent hyperextension.

During limb lengthening, the motion range of adjacent joints should be monitored closely. In particular, the lack of full extension of the knee should warrant caution and intensive physiotherapy in order to prevent rotational subluxation, dislocation, and permanent sequelae. Most often, it is neither the lack of new bone formation, nor the capacity of the implant, but soft tissue conditions that cause failure to achieve a particular treatment goal. In addition, during gradual limb reconstruction, the patient should be examined for changes in sensibility as nerves are structures at risk of temporary and permanent damage.

The goal of realigning the limb may not necessarily translate into complete equalization of limb length discrepancy as measured on long-standing radiographs. The functional discrepancy may be either more or less pronounced than indicated by the radiological values. Furthermore, many patients preoperatively feel most at ease with a slight under-correction of limb length when standing on blocks in the outpatient clinic. Likewise, patients may request a temporary shoe raise in order to adapt after complete equalization of limb length.

In conclusion, history taking and physical examination are essential from the first meeting with the patient and throughout the reconstructive journey.

References

1. Driano AN, Staheli L, Staheli LT. Psychosocial development and corrective shoe wear use in childhood. J Pediatr Orthop. 1998;18(3):346–9.
2. Staheli LT. Rotational problems in children. J Bone Joint Surg Am. 1993;75(6):939–49.
3. O'Connor DP, Gugenheim JJ. Comparison of measured and parents' reported height and weight in children and adolescents. Obesity. 2011;19(5):1040–6.
4. Staheli LT, Corbett M, Wyss C, King H. Lower-extremity rotational problems in children. Normal values to guide management. J Bone Joint Surg Am. 1985;67(1):39–47.

5. Staheli LT. Torsional deformity. Pediatr Clin N Am. 1977;24(4):799–811.
6. Engel GM, Staheli LT. The natural history of torsion and other factors influencing gait in childhood. A study of the angle of gait, tibial torsion, knee angle, hip rotation, and development of the arch in normal children. Clin Orthop Relat Res. 1974;99:12–7.
7. Lincoln TL, Suen PW. Common rotational variations in children. J Am Acad Orthop Surg. 2003;11(5):312–20.
8. Jonson SR, Gross MT. Intraexaminer reliability, interexaminer reliability, and mean values for nine lower extremity skeletal measures in healthy naval midshipmen. J Orthop Sports Phys Ther. 1997;25(4):253–63.
9. Woerman AL, Binder-Macleod SA. Leg length discrepancy assessment: accuracy and precision in five clinical methods of evaluation*. J Orthop Sports Phys Ther. 1984;5(5):230–9.
10. Sabharwal S, Kumar A. Methods for assessing leg length discrepancy. Clin Orthop Relat Res. 2008;466(12):2910–22.
11. Kling TF Jr, Hensinger RN. Angular and torsional deformities of the lower limbs in children. Clin Orthop Relat Res. 1983;176:136–47.
12. Tönnis D, Heinecke A. Current concepts review. Acetabular and femoral anteversion: relationship with osteoarthritis of the hip. J Bone Joint Surg Am. 1999;81(12):1747–70.
13. Sankar WN, Schoenecker JG, Mayfield ME, Kim YJ, Millis MB. Acetabular retroversion in down syndrome. J Pediatr Orthop. 2012;32(3):277–81.
14. Jacquemier M, Jouve JL, Bollini G, Panuel M, Migliani R. Acetabular anteversion in children. J Pediatr Orthop. 1992;12(3):373–5.
15. Paley D. Principles of deformity correction. Heidelberg: Springer; 2002.
16. Hubbard DD, Staheli LT, Chew DE, Mosca VS. Medial femoral torsion and osteoarthritis. J Pediatr Orthop. 1988;8(5):540–2.
17. Weinberg DS, Park PJ, Morris WZ, Liu RW. Femoral version and tibial torsion are not associated with hip or knee arthritis in a large osteological collection. J Pediatr Orthop. 2017;37(2):e120–8.
18. McKibbin B. Anatomical factors in the stability of the hip joint in the newborn. J Bone Joint Surg. 1970;52(1):148–59.
19. Fabry G, MacEwen GD, Shands AR Jr. Torsion of the femur. A follow-up study in normal and abnormal conditions. J Bone Joint Surg Am. 1973;55(8):1726–38.
20. Katz JF. Behavior of internal tibial torsion in infancy. Mt Sinai J Med. 1982;49(1):7–12.
21. Smith JT, Bleck EE, Gamble JG, Rinsky LA, Pena T. Simple method of documenting metatarsus adductus. J Pediatr Orthop. 1991;11(5):679–80.
22. Green WT, Wyatt GM, Anderson M. Orthoroentgenography as a method of measuring the bones of the lower extremities. J Bone Joint Surg Am. 1946;28:60–5.
23. Sabharwal S, Zhao C, McKeon JJ, McClemens E, Edgar M, Behrens F. Computed radiographic measurement of limb-length discrepancy. Full-length standing anteroposterior radiograph compared with scanogram. J Bone Joint Surg Am. 2006;88(10):2243–51.
24. Sabharwal S, Zhao C, McKeon J, Melaghari T, Blacksin M, Wenekor C. Reliability analysis for radiographic measurement of limb length discrepancy: full-length standing anteroposterior radiograph versus scanogram. J Pediatr Orthop. 2007;27(1):46–50.
25. Poutawera V, Stott NS. The reliability of computed tomography scanograms in the measurement of limb length discrepancy. J Pediatr Orthop B. 2010;19(1):42–6.
26. Asma A, Nichols LR, Ulusaloglu AC, Kazmi F, Rogers KJ, Drozdowski B, Bowen JR. Applications and error ratios of calibration techniques in EOS, orthoroentgenogram, and teleoroentgenogram for length measurement: a comparative study. J Pediatr Orthop. 2022;42(1):e21–6.
27. Garner MR, Dow M, Bixby E, Mintz DN, Widmann RF, Dodwell ER. Evaluating length: the use of low-dose biplanar radiography (EOS) and tantalum bead implantation. J Pediatr Orthop. 2016;36(1):e6–9.
28. Kyriakedes JC, Liu RW. An anatomic study on whether the immature patella is centered on an anteroposterior radiograph. J Pediatr Orthop. 2017;37(2):138–43.
29. Ajuwon AA, Desai R, Farhang K, Lasko CE, Liu RW. An anatomic study on whether the patella is centered in an ideal anteroposterior radiograph of the knee. HSS J. 2015;11(2):117–22.
30. Visser JD, Jonkers A, Hillen B. Hip joint measurements with computerized tomography. J Pediatr Orthop. 1982;2(2):143–6.
31. Delialioglu MO, Tasbas BA, Bayrakci K, Daglar B, Kurt M, Agar M, et al. Alternative reliable techniques in femoral torsion measurement. J Pediatr Orthop B. 2006;15(1):28–33.
32. Ryder CT, Crane L. Measuring femoral anteversion; the problem and a method. J Bone Joint Surg Am. 1953;35-A(2):321–8.
33. Magilligan DJ. Calculation of the angle of anteversion by means of horizontal lateral roentgenography. J Bone Joint Surg Am. 1956;38-A(6):1231–46.
34. Ruwe PA, Gage JR, Ozonoff MB, DeLuca PA. Clinical determination of femoral anteversion. A comparison with established techniques. J Bone Joint Surg Am. 1992;74(6):820–30.
35. Phillips HO, Greene WB, Guilford WB, Mittelstaedt CA, Gaisie G, Vincent LM, et al. Measurement of femoral torsion: comparison of standard roentgenographic techniques with ultrasound. J Pediatr Orthop. 1985;5(5):546–9.
36. Terjesen T, Anda S, Svenningsen S. Femoral anteversion in adolescents and adults measured by ultrasound. Clin Orthop Relat Res. 1990;256:274–9.
37. Folinais D, Thelen P, Delin C, Radier C, Catonne Y, Lazennec JY. Measuring femoral and rotational alignment: EOS system versus computed tomography. Orthop Traumatol Surg Res. 2013;99(5):509–16. https://doi.org/10.1016/j.otsr.2012.12.023.
38. Westberry DE, Carpenter AM. 3D modeling of lower extremities with biplanar radiographs: reliability of measures on subsequent examinations. J Pediatr Orthop. 2019;39(10):521–6. https://doi.org/10.1097/BPO.0000000000001046.
39. Cho BW, Lee TH, Kim S, Choi CH, Jung M, Lee KY, Kim SH. Evaluation of the reliability of lower extremity alignment measurements using EOS imaging system while standing in an even weight-bearing posture. Sci Rep. 2021;11(1):22039.
40. Brooks JT, Bomar JD, Jeffords ME, Farnsworth CL, Pennock AT, Upasani VV. Reliability of low-dose biplanar radiography in assessing pediatric torsional pathology. J Pediatr Orthop. 2021;41(1):33–9. https://doi.org/10.1097/BPO.0000000000001700.
41. Morris WZ, Henry H, Liu RW, Streit JJ, Grant RE, Cooperman DR. A modified ogata-goldsand technique for simplified intraoperative measurement of femoral version. J Pediatr Orthop. 2015;35(6):593–9.
42. Jakob RP, Haertel M, Stussi E. Tibial torsion calculated by computerised tomography and compared to other methods of measurement. J Bone Joint Surg (Br). 1980;62-B(2):238–42.
43. Herzenberg JE, Standard SC, Conway JD, Lamm BM, Siddiqui NA. The art of limb alignment. Baltimore: Sinai Hospital of Baltimore; 2013.
44. Sabharwal S, Zhao C, Edgar M. Lower limb alignment in children: reference values based on a full-length standing radiograph. J Pediatr Orthop. 2008;28(7):740–6.
45. Bigach SD, Carender CN, Liu RW. Is bony knee alignment representative of the true joint surface in skeletally immature patients? A magnetic resonance imaging study. Strategies Trauma Limb Reconstr. 2020;15(2):79–83.

Decision-Making in Lower Extremity Deformity Correction

J. Eric Gordon

Introduction

Comprehensive preoperative planning is essential for effective lower extremity reconstruction in children. These plans should consider a number of factors including an analysis of the deformity, the biology of the problem, and the family and patient's perception of the problem. This planning can and should take two different forms. Firstly, there is global planning that should occur when a patient is initially evaluated; this can take the form of a discussion with the family regarding general approaches and goals, outlining potential treatment approaches and potential results and complications. Secondly, treatment episodes should be planned thoroughly and in detail, addressing alternative techniques, issues, and potential complications. Lower extremity deformities can vary widely with regard to their etiology, magnitude, the integrity of the soft tissue envelope, and natural history. Because of this variation, it is impossible to create a formulaic method of approaching a patient with a lower limb deformity. This difficulty is compounded by differences in the patient's environment, the surgeon's skills, the resources available to treat the patient, and the ability of the patient or family to comply with a treatment program. Because of these differences, it is important to assess how each of these factors may influence the treatment method that is ultimately chosen and to follow a consistent approach in analyzing the deformity and planning the surgical correction. The nature and location of the deformity should guide the surgeon's choice of implant and technique, not vice versa.

When considering both global and episodic planning, a deformity analysis is crucial in understanding the deformity and making treatment choices. In addition to an analysis of the child's deformity, the biology of the problem is important to assess as the treatment options appropriate to different diagnoses vary greatly. Appropriate treatment of a congenital pseudarthrosis of the tibia, a rigid post-traumatic pseudarthrosis, and a developmental deformity such as tibia vara differ significantly. Finally, the family's perception of the problem should also be explored in depth as the family's perception of the problem may be very different from the surgeon's perception. The family of a young child with tibia vara may be so focused on the rotational abnormality that they minimize the bowing which may be the surgeon's primary focus. A comprehensive preoperative discussion should lead to an understanding by the family of the surgeon's concerns as well as an understanding by the surgeon of the family's concerns.

Global planning should include an assessment of the child's deformity and the natural history of the deformity as the child grows and develops. This should account for the child's projected limb length discrepancy, angulatory and rotational deformities, joint instability and stiffness, and the ultimate function of the limb. The surgeon should be prepared to outline to the family, the expected results and function of different treatment regimens. It is often helpful to summarize these factors in a problem list.

Episodic planning involves a focused evaluation of the child at a single point within the global plan. There should be clear goals that are communicated to the family and there should be an understanding of where a specific episode fits into the global plan. It is important also to communicate to the family the commitment that would be required in terms of visit frequency, the need for other services such as physical or occupational therapy, the long- and short-term financial burden for the family, and the potential complications with the impact of those complications on the chosen treat-

---

J. E. Gordon (✉)
Department of Orthopaedic Surgery, Washington University School of Medicine, St. Louis, MO, USA

St. Louis Children's Hospital, St. Louis, MO, USA

St. Louis Shriner's Hospital for Children, St. Louis, MO, USA
e-mail: Gordone@wustl.edu

ment regimen. The formation of a problem list is helpful in summarizing the issues, deformity, and potential pitfalls in episodic planning.

The problem list is helpful in summarizing the issues associated with the correction of a limb deformity. This problem list may be quite short and unwritten in treating simple issues such as mild familial genu valgum. In other situations, however, these lists can be quite complex, combining multiple deformities in different planes and locations, soft tissue issues, joint instability and psychological, and family issues that can be extremely challenging. A written problem list is quite helpful as deformities become more complex and are often quite long when treating difficult issues such as large congenital limb length discrepancies. The problem list should include issues with regard to the deformity and pathology being treated and factors such as joint stability and motion that may affect the frequency of complications.

It is important to remember that even with a consistent approach to decision-making, it is not uncommon that multiple approaches to similar clinical deformities and symptoms may be appropriate and that there may not be a single "best" approach. Although there can be suboptimal approaches, seldom is there only a single correct treatment approach. Surgeon skills as well as patient and caretaker preferences can often influence the final decision-making in these situations and it is important that the surgeon discusses the various options and potential complications with the patient and family prior to making a final decision.

Clinical Evaluation

When evaluating a patient, there is a temptation for surgeons to consider radiographs of the patient and make decisions regarding the ultimate treatment without taking into account other factors. Like other areas of medicine, it is important for the surgeon to obtain a history of the problem, perform a careful physical examination and obtain appropriate laboratory studies and imaging prior to making a diagnosis and developing a treatment plan.

When obtaining a history, it is important to elicit from the patient or family a chronologic account of the development of the deformity as well as the current symptoms of pain, instability, and functional limitations. The surgeon should understand the limitations that the patient and their caretakers perceive as well as their expectations of treatment. The presence of joint instability, the limitation of motion, pain, neurologic symptoms, signs of infection, and previous treatment are crucial to elicit from the patient or family. Past medical histories, such as coagulopathy or bleeding issues, compromised immune system and chronic medical conditions, can also influence decision-making.

Examination of the patient generally starts with the observation of the individual's stance and gait. Factors that contribute to the ultimate plan include general conditioning (for instance, is the patient obese?). The examination should also include an assessment of motion and stability of the major lower extremity joints. Limitations of joint motion or instability can have a direct impact on both the etiology and the treatment of deformities. For example, a hip adduction contracture can lead to the development of knee valgus in patients, and attempts to correct the knee valgus without addressing the hip adduction contracture can lead to postoperative recurrence and gait problems. Children with congenital limb length discrepancies frequently have hip, knee, and/or ankle instability of the shorter extremity, which can have a substantial impact on subsequent limb lengthening. Additionally, the rotational profile should be assessed by physical examination, documenting femoral version and tibial torsion clinically.

Imaging studies provide information about the static deformity in both the anteroposterior and lateral planes. It is crucial when evaluating the radiographs that the surgeon ascertains not only the presence of malalignment, but also the location of one or more deformities. This can be best accomplished by either mechanical axis planning or anatomic axis planning utilizing full-length radiographs of the entire lower extremity including the hip, knee, and ankle. This portion of the evaluation has been addressed in the previous chapter. Components of the deformity can include angulation, translation, length, and rotation. Of these components, angulation, translation, and length can be largely described from the radiographs. Rotation is often adequately ascertained by examining the patient, although specialized rotational studies such as CT scans and MRI can complement the physical examination in selected situations [1].

One must elucidate why the patient and/or family are seeking medical care for their deformity. Is the patient concerned by the appearance of the extremity; is the patient having functional difficulties or is the primary concern pain? Often families seek care for growing children because of concerns not about the current state of the limb but because of concerns that the deformity will worsen or that pain or disability will result at a later time. It is important to engage the patient and caretaker regarding the natural history of the deformity and counsel them as to how the surgical correction may or may not address their concerns. Occasionally, the patient or caretaker may be seeking care for a complaint that is only minimally or not related to the patient's deformity.

The surgeon must also evaluate the social situation of both the patient and the psychological issues and family dynamics when planning correction of a deformity. In particular, the surgeon should consider the ability of the patient and family to comply with a proposed treatment regimen. For example, the gradual correction of deformities utilizing a circular external fixation system in a patient with autism might be ill-advised. The ability of patients and families to comply with postoperative protocols should be evaluated prior to finalizing a surgical plan and prearrangements for the anticipated need for physical therapy and follow-up visits may be necessary in certain situations. The surgeon's skill set and available medical resources should also be taken into account when developing a plan. The institution of a complex reconstruction while traveling internationally might be ill-advised if appropriate follow-up cannot be arranged. Finally, relevant cultural norms should also be considered and may dictate pursuing reconstructive options that might otherwise be contraindicated and lead the surgeon and patient to accept perhaps less function in order to be more culturally acceptable. For example, in some parts of the world there is a strong cultural bias against accepting amputation as part of what otherwise might be a preferred treatment.

The Problem List

The history, physical examination, imaging studies, and patient and family perceptions of the problem and dynamics of the situation should be brought together by the surgeon to form a problem list (see Table 3.1). This list should summarize the deformities, the pertinent pathology, co-morbidities as they impact the treatment of the deformity, the patient's perceptions of the problem, and the potential obstacles to treatment whether they are related to the patient or the environment in which treatment is occurring. It is important to remember that the problem list is a problem list and not necessarily a surgical agenda and that a complete problem list often includes potential problems.

After a problem list has been developed, the anatomy and biology of the underlying deformity must be considered. In particular, the surgeon should decide whether the location of the deformity is more amenable to acute or gradual correction based on the anatomy of the neurovascular structures and postoperative or post-traumatic scarring. Are the physes open, leaving the option of growth modulation to correct the deformity? The presence of active or prior infection is another important factor to be considered, as are factors such as the presence of pseudarthrosis.

When considering the problem list in conjunction with the anatomy and biology of the problem, the surgeon should be able to outline options for an appropriate treatment agenda for addressing the deformity comprehensively over time. Some of these plans may be relatively simple comprising an acute correction of a uniapical deformity. Other cases may require a much more complex plan, including a series of interventions over a number of years such as for an infant with proximal femoral focal deficiency.

Surgical Indications: General

The decision about whether to correct a given deformity or not can be quite individual for each patient and there are no absolute rules. Relative indications for surgical correction of a deformity include the presence of pain or a deformity with a natural history of substantial progression (see Table 3.2). In general, the current or anticipated limb length discrepancies greater than 2 cm should be addressed although in certain patients discrepancies smaller than this may be important [2].

Table 3.1 Important elements of a problem list to describe in planning a lower extremity deformity correction

Elements of a problem list
The site(s) of the deformity
Coronal, sagittal, and rotational parameters of each deformity
Soft tissue envelope/vascularity of bone
Relevant joint stability issues
The biology of the problem
Patient/caretaker perception of a problem
Patient co-morbidities
Prior treatment successes and challenges
Potential complications and problems
Family limitations
Cultural limitations

Table 3.2 Relative indications for surgical correction of lower extremity deformity

Surgical indications for deformity correction
Persistent pain
Mechanical axis in zone 2 with symptoms
Mechanical Axis in zone 3 or greater with or without symptoms
Uncompensated hindfoot deformity
Sagittal plane deformities impeding gait and function

Surgical Indications: The Knee

Angulatory deformities about the knee should generally be corrected if the mechanical axis falls within zone 2 and the patient is symptomatic and should be corrected if the mechanical axis is beyond zone 2 (Fig. 3.1) even if the patient is asymptomatic. When the deformity of the knee requires correction, the joint orientation angles such as the lateral distal femur angle (LDFA), the medial proximal tibial angle (MPTA), and the joint line congruency angle (JLCA) should be measured. If the JLCA is more than 5° in conjunction with a bony deformity, then we prefer to address the ligamentous laxity as well. If the deformity of the knee involves only the femur or the tibia and the other bone is normal, then correction should nearly always occur within the affected bone. If both bones are abnormal but the majority of the deformity is within one of the bones, then there may be some consideration to correcting only the bone with the majority of the deformity if less than 5° of abnormality is present in either the LDFA or MPTA. If greater than 5° of abnormality is noted in both the LDFA and MPTA, then we prefer to address the deformity at both sites.

For sagittal plane deformities about the knee, one must consider both the bony deformity within the distal femur and proximal tibia as well as the soft tissue constraints about the knee joint. The goal of treatment of sagittal deformity in the knee is a functional range of motion in both extension and flexion. My preference is to develop a surgical plan that achieves knee extension within 5° of full extension and without hyperextension of greater than 5° as well as knee flexion of at least 90°. For patients with limited extension, one must consider concomitant hamstring, iliotibial band, or posterior capsule releases while correcting the bony sagittal deformity. Likewise, one can consider quadriceps lengthening to augment a deformity correction in a patient with limited knee flexion.

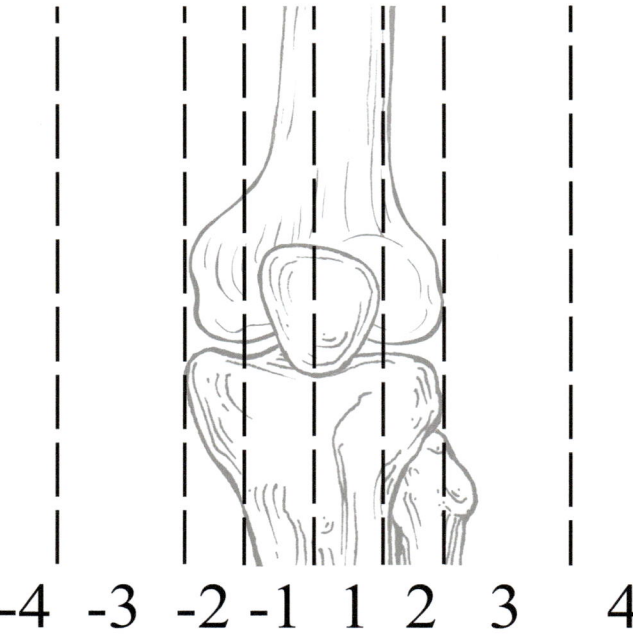

Fig. 3.1 Depiction of the zone of a mechanical axis deviation at the knee. Zone 1 is within the tibial spine. Zone 2 is within the tibial condyles. Zone 3 is within the knee joint width away from the center of the knee joint. Zone 4 is greater than one knee joint width from the center of knee joint [3]

Surgical Indications: The Ankle

The decision to correct ankle alignment must be made in conjunction with a careful examination of the hindfoot. Patients with substantial deformity of the ankle may be clinically well aligned with a compensatory hindfoot deformity (Fig. 3.2). Patients with such well-compensated deformity and with limited subtalar motion may not be well served by a decision to correct the ankle and thus "create" a more visible deformity by uncovering the fixed hindfoot abnormality.

Fig. 3.2 (**a** and **b**) Radiographs (**a**) and clinical images (**b**) of a patient with distal tibial valgus and compensatory hindfoot varus. Note the radiographic valgus of the left ankle and the apparent normal clinical alignment of the left hindfoot

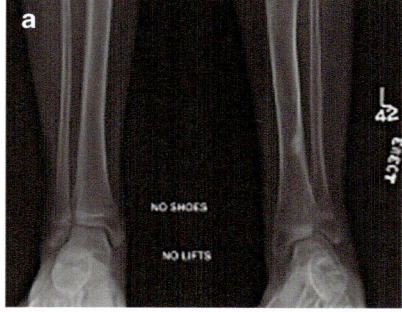
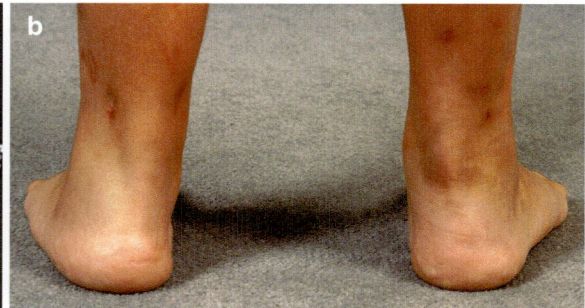

Relative Contraindications

Contraindications to surgery are necessarily somewhat vague and include a number of patient-related factors including unrealistic expectations on the part of the patient and caretakers, their inability to follow through with the necessary outpatient components of both a treatment program and situations where the risks of surgical intervention outweigh the potential benefits to the patient (see Table 3.3). For instance, patients with severe mental illness or with limited ability to comprehend the treatment plan may not have the ability to comply with more complex treatment protocols including gradual correction using external fixation. Although more complex treatment protocols may be contraindicated in these patients, simplified alternatives may represent better choices. For example, for some patients, the difficulties involved in complying with instructions and a physical therapy program associated with a limb lengthening may be able to comply easily with the less strenuous instructions and therapy associated with a closed femoral shortening (Fig. 3.3).

Table 3.3 Relative surgical contraindications to performing lower extremity deformity correction

Surgical contraindications
Natural history of the deformity is benign
Unrealistic patient/family expectations
Patient/family unable to comply with postoperative protocol
Potential complications of treatment outweigh the benefits to patient

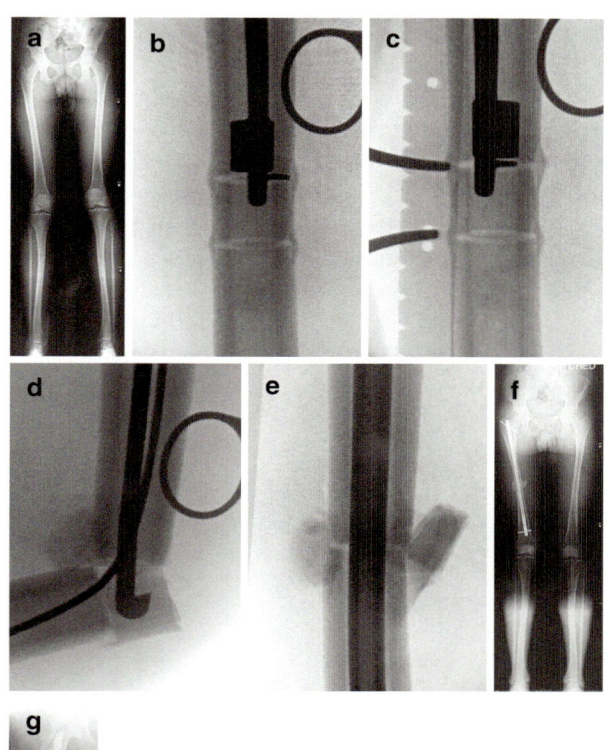

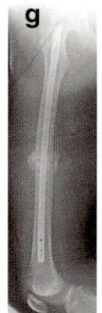

Fig. 3.3 (a–g) Femoral shortening case study. (a) Preoperative standing AP of both lower extremities with a 2.5-cm block under the left foot of a 19-year-old male with a 2.5-cm right greater than left limb length discrepancy due to the right hemihypertrophy. (b) Intramedullary saw completing the more proximal cut within the femur. (c) Intramedullary saw in place completing the proximal cut with a ruler in place confirming 2.5 cm of shortening. (d) Intramedullary chisel splitting the intercalary segment. (e) The final intraoperative image showing the intramedullary nail crossing the shortening site with the intercalary fragment split and adjacent to the osteotomy. (f) Standing AP of both lower extremities 6 weeks postoperatively showing equal leg lengths and a healing osteotomy. At this point, the patient is walking with a mild abductor lurch without crutches. (g) Lateral radiograph of the right femur 6 weeks postoperatively showing the healing closed femoral shortening

Surgical Options

The plan for each deformity may comprise several different techniques that might be applicable in a given situation (see Table 3.4). There is no reason to avoid combining techniques when clinically applicable. General categories that should be considered include soft tissue surgery, physeal bar resection, growth modulation, acute correction with internal or external fixation, or gradual correction (including lengthening) with internal or external fixation. A brief description of the techniques follows with a general description of indications and contraindications.

Table 3.4 Available techniques to perform deformity correction

Surgical options
Soft tissue modification
Physeal modulation or ablation
Osteotomy with acute correction
Osteotomy with gradual correction

Soft Tissue Modification

Soft tissue surgery can be effective either as a solitary procedure or in conjunction with bony surgery. Modification of the soft tissues is not only limited to procedures that directly approach the soft tissues themselves but also can be an intended consequence of bony procedures. Tightening of the lateral collateral ligament at the knee can be performed by translating the fibular head distally either with a fibular osteotomy or gradual bone transport with an external fixator or in cases of adolescent tibia vara utilizing a circular external fixator. In these cases, tibial osteotomy can be performed while leaving the fibula intact and securing it distally to the tibia. The angulatory deformity is then corrected while lengthening gradually, thus transporting the fibula distally in relation to the proximal tibia resulting in tightening of the lateral collateral ligament (Fig. 3.4). Correction of present or antici-

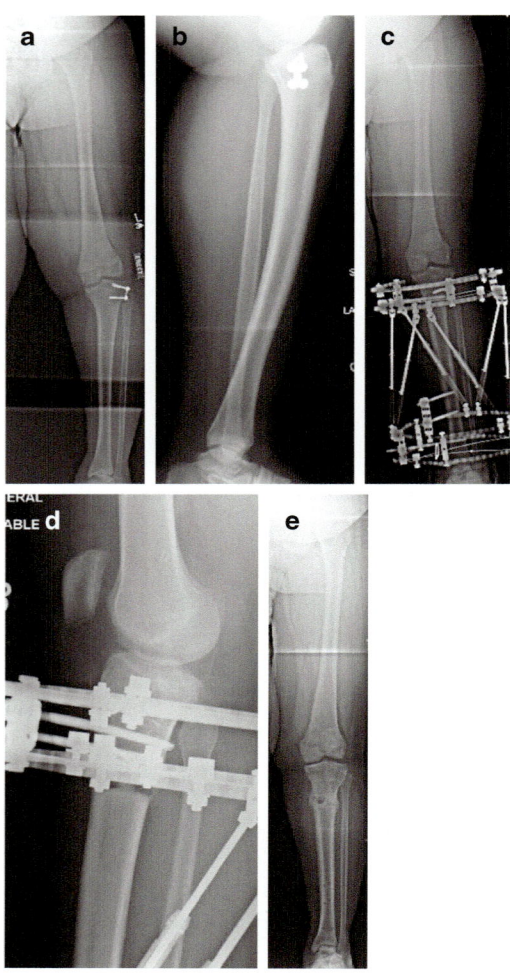

Fig. 3.4 (a–e) Case example of adolescent tibia vara treated with circular external fixator and tightening of the lateral collateral ligament. (a, b) AP and lateral preoperative radiographs of a 12-year-old male with tibia vara. (c, d) Immediate postoperative radiographs depicting a ring circular external fixator with fixation of the fibula distally into the tibia and no proximal transfibular fixation. (e) Postoperative radiographs after fixator removal showing distal transport of the fibula relative to the proximal tibia, thus tightening the lateral collateral ligament

pated contractures via soft tissue release (such as the iliotibial band during lengthening of a congenitally short femur) or by gradual stretching with an external fixator is also effective and can be incorporated into a treatment plan.

Physeal Modulation or Ablation

Physeal modulation can take many forms. Physeal bar resection following traumatic or developmental partial arrest can be performed successfully in situations where a partial arrest of the physis, as documented by progressive deformity, is present that involves less than 50% of the physis with more than 2.5 cm of growth remaining at the involved physis and more than 2 years of growth are expected [4, 5]. Advantages of physeal bar resection include the relative simplicity involved in postoperative care and relatively rapid patient recovery and return to activity (Fig. 3.5). Disadvantages of physeal bar resection include a high failure rate and frequent late closure of the physis necessitating close follow-up and further surgical treatment.

Complete epiphyseodesis by either percutaneous drilling or, more commonly, utilizing either plates or staples can be performed in skeletally immature individuals who have adequate growth remaining to contribute to the correction of a limb length discrepancy [6]. The technique, however, can be utilized in limb length discrepancies as part of a comprehensive treatment plan or as an isolated procedure depending on the projected limb length discrepancy and the growth remaining. Temporary hemiepiphyseodesis using medial and lateral staples or plates has been reported [7] but needs close follow-up to skeletal maturity due to concerns about permanent physeal closure and the possibility of rebound growth following implant removal.

Hemiepiphyseodesis by plate, screw, drilling, or Blount's staples should be considered in patients who are skeletally immature and who have adequate growth available to reasonably expect correction of an angulatory deformity [8]. These deformities can be in the coronal, sagittal, or oblique planes (Fig. 3.6). Physeal modification can be utilized even in situations where the physis is abnormal [9] such as chronic renal failure and hypophosphatemic rickets. Deformities such as proximal tibial valgus following a Cozen's type fracture which tend to recur following osteotomy correction are particularly amenable to treatment with plate hemiepiphyseodesis. Following correction of the deformity in a patient who has substantial growth remaining, the metaphyseal screw can be removed percutaneously, and the plate and epiphyseal screw can be left in place allowing continued growth (Fig. 3.7). If the deformity recurs, then the metaphyseal screw can be replaced percutaneously resulting in re-hemiepiphyseodesis and repeat correction. Keshet et al. have advocated against this technique because of the risk of late physeal bar formation and the frequency of the plate position necessitating removal and repositioning of the plate at the time of re-hemiepiphyseodesis [10].

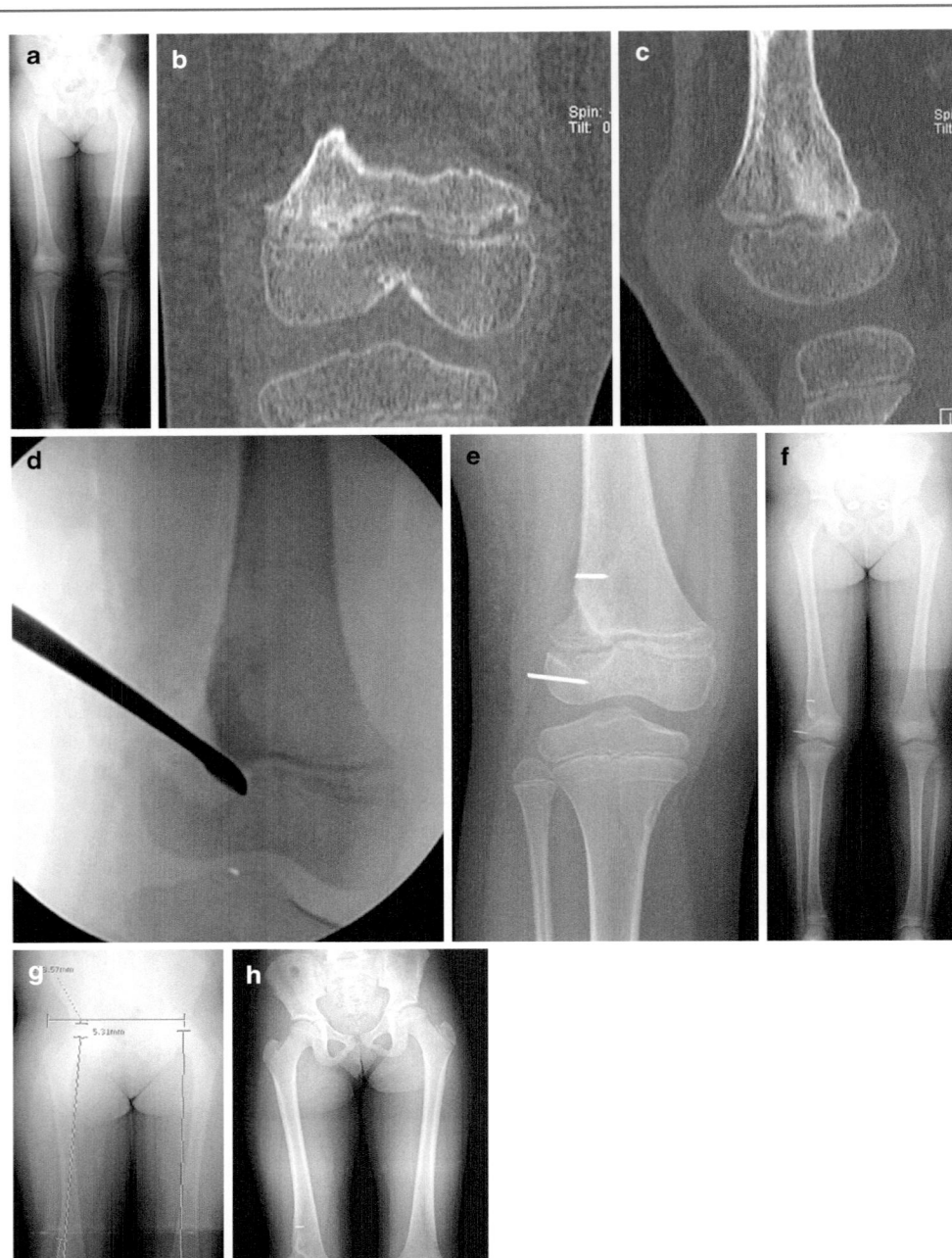

Fig. 3.5 (a–h) Case example of a 9-year-old female with a post-traumatic physeal bar formation in the right distal femur. (a) Standing AP demonstrating the right distal femur physeal bar. (b, c) coronal and sagittal slice of a CT scan showing lateral distal femoral bar with less than 20% of physis involvement. (d) Fluoroscopic image showing curettage of physeal bar. (e) Postoperative AP after physeal bar resection. K-wires are placed in order to follow eventual growth, radiolucent cranioplast is placed on the epiphyseal side to limit the reformation of a bar. (f) Immediate postoperative standing AP. (g) Standing radiographs demonstrating growth within the distal femoral physis 2 years postoperatively. (h) Standing anteroposterior radiograph demonstrating continued growth with a migration of the cranioplast proximal to the physis with a resultant recurrence of the physeal bar associated with a limb length discrepancy and valgus deformity 3 years postoperatively

Fig. 3.6 (a–f) Oblique plane deformity of the right distal femur in a 6-year-old male with arthrogryposis. (**a**) Standing AP demonstrating the right distal femoral valgus. (**b**) Lateral of the right knee in less than maximal extension showing a knee flexion contracture of approximately25°. (**c, d**) AP and lateral of the knee showing hemiepiphyseodesis of the anteromedial distal femur, promoting distal femoral varus and procurvatum. (**e, f**) Standing AP and maximal extension lateral views 18 months postoperative with a resultant correction of deformity. The patient had a full knee extension

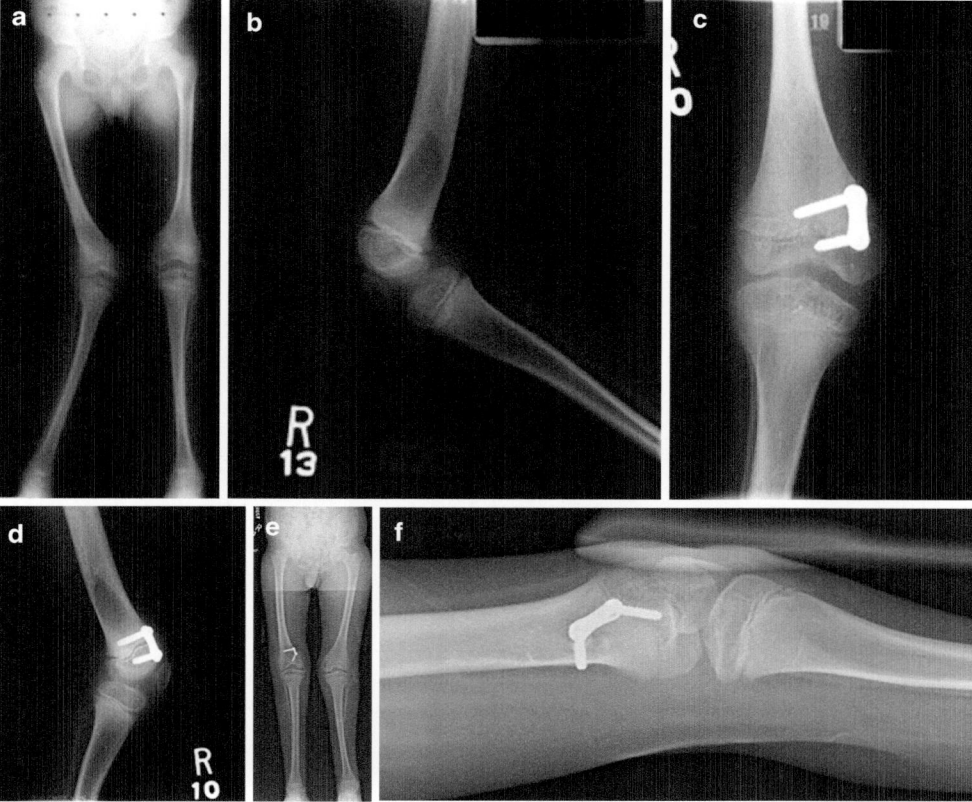

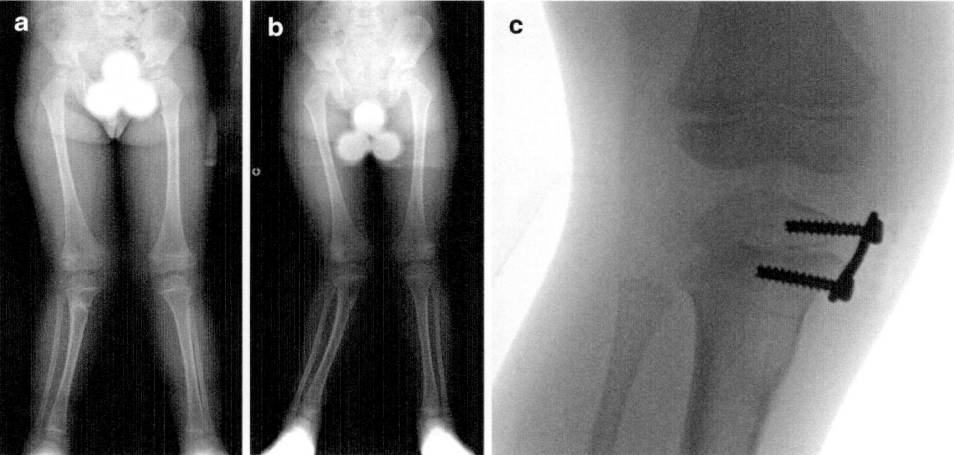

Fig. 3.7 (a–f) Four-year-old male with a proximal tibial valgus deformity after proximal tibia fracture (Cozen's fracture). (**a**) Standing AP after cast treatment for the right proximal tibia fracture. (**b**) 6-Month postinjury film demonstration proximal tibial valgus deformity. (**c**) Fluoroscopic image showing the placement of hemiepiphyseodesis plate medially. (**d**) Immediate postoperative standing AP. (**e**) 9-Month postoperative radiographs showing normal mechanical axis. (**f**) Metaphyseal screw is removed after deformity correction in order to facilitate replacement of hemiepiphyseodesis if deformity recurs

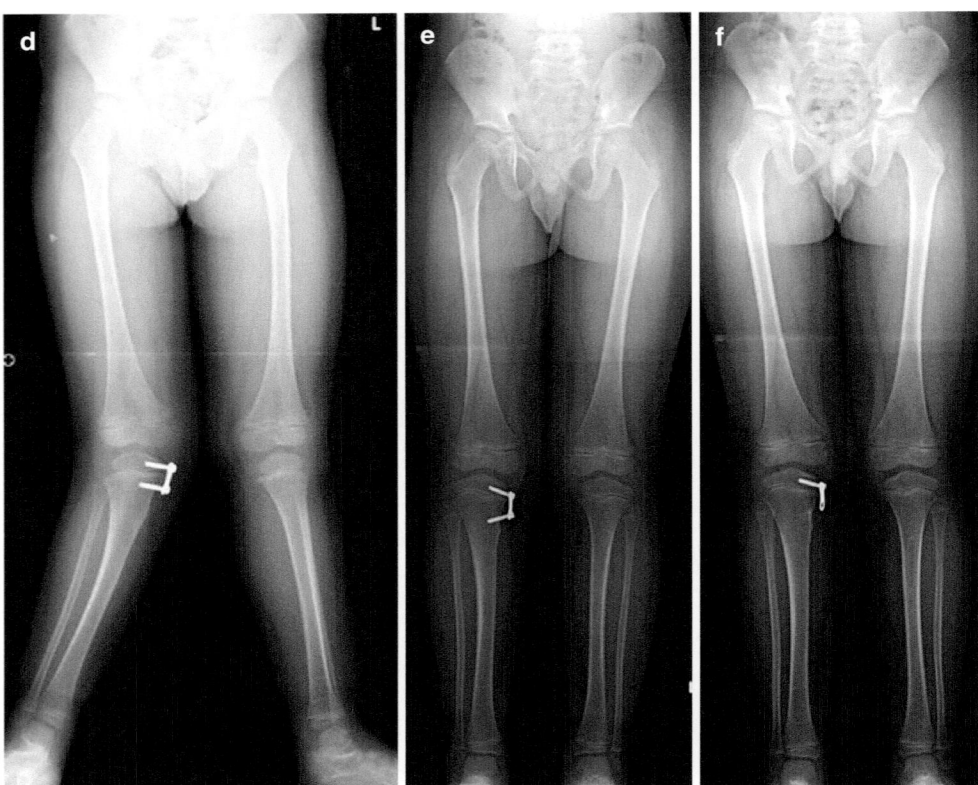

Fig. 3.7 (continued)

Acute Correction with Osteotomy

Osteotomies with acute correction are particularly indicated in angulatory deformities in patients with minimal limb length discrepancies allowing correction of the deformity without placing undue stress on the neurovascular structures. Most often the acute correction is combined with a rigid internal fixation although it can be utilized in conjunction with an external fixation or Kirschner wire fixation and cast immobilization. The choice of implants is determined by the site of the osteotomy and can potentially include intramedullary fixation, screw fixation, locking, or non-locking plates or external fixation.

Intramedullary fixation can be helpful when combined with percutaneous diaphyseal osteotomy techniques such as in patients with an isolated femoral rotational deformity [11, 12]. Intramedullary stabilization can also be helpful when angulatory deformities exist in the diaphyseal region after either traumatic malunion or in cases of hypophosphatemic rickets with a residual femoral lateral bow (Fig. 3.8). In these cases, often the percutaneous osteotomy can correct both the apparent genu varum deformity and correcting the coxa vara that can produce a significant abductor lurch during gait. The disadvantage of intramedullary fixation is the limitation in the magnitude of the correction that can be obtained. Intramedullary stabilization results in a comparatively straight diaphyseal segment when combined with a diaphyseal osteotomy. Intramedullary stabilization can also be utilized with blocking screws in conjunction with acute correction of a supracondylar distal femoral or proximal tibial osteotomy with or without the intraoperative assistance of external fixation. Contraindications to intramedullary fixation include open physes with substantial remaining growth in the proximal tibia or distal femur and the inability to pass an intramedullary nail through an obstructed intramedullary canal. In addition, intramedullary nailing should be generally avoided in the presence of active infection.

Screw fixation provides the surgeon with the ability to stabilize osteotomies with some inherent bony stability while achieving rigid correction of the deformity. Cannulated screws are particularly helpful when performing osteotomies in the epiphyseal region that requires rigid control of the osteotomy. One specialized use of these screws is to stabilize intraarticular osteotomies in the proximal tibia. This can be performed in cases of medial tibial plateau depression due to delayed treatment of early onset tibia vara with a resulting "pagoda" deformity [13]. These tibial plateau osteotomies can be effectively stabilized after an acute correction using cannulated screws with an incomplete osteotomy and allograft cortical bone as a structural graft (Fig. 3.9).

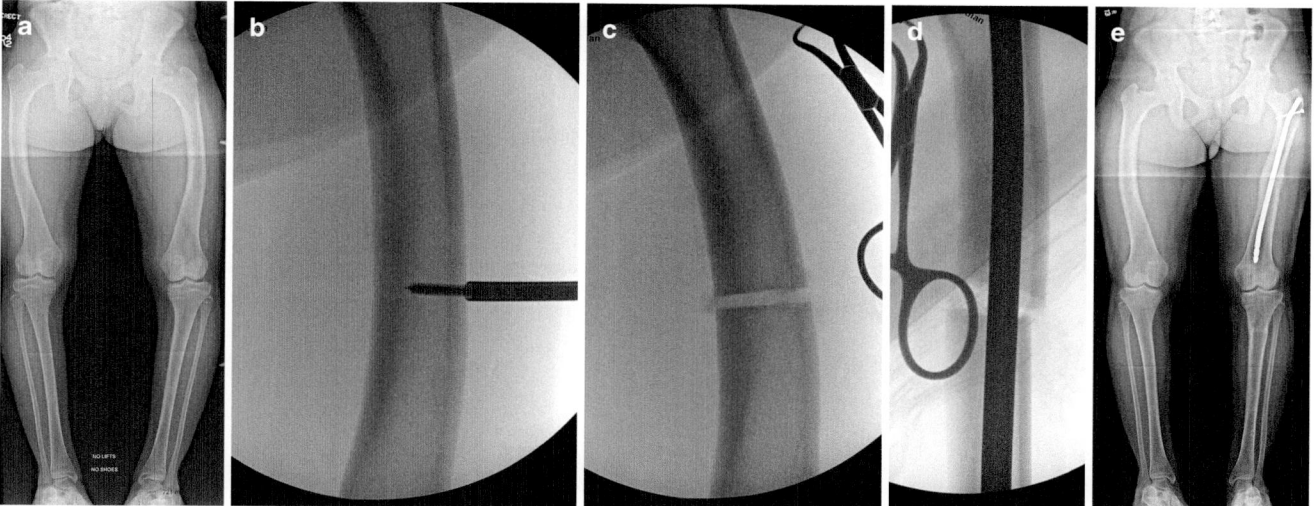

Fig. 3.8 (a–e) Use of intramedullary nail for deformity correction. (a) Standing AP of a 12-year-old female with X-linked hypophosphatemic rickets and midshaft bowing of both femurs at the isthmus. (b) Fluoroscopy demonstrating percutaneous diaphyseal femoral osteotomy using drill. (c) Completion of diaphyseal femoral osteotomy. (d) Insertion of pediatric femoral nail. As the osteotomy was performed at the isthmus and deformity, this results in an opening wedge osteotomy medially. (e) Postoperative standing AP demonstration correction of the right femoral deformity

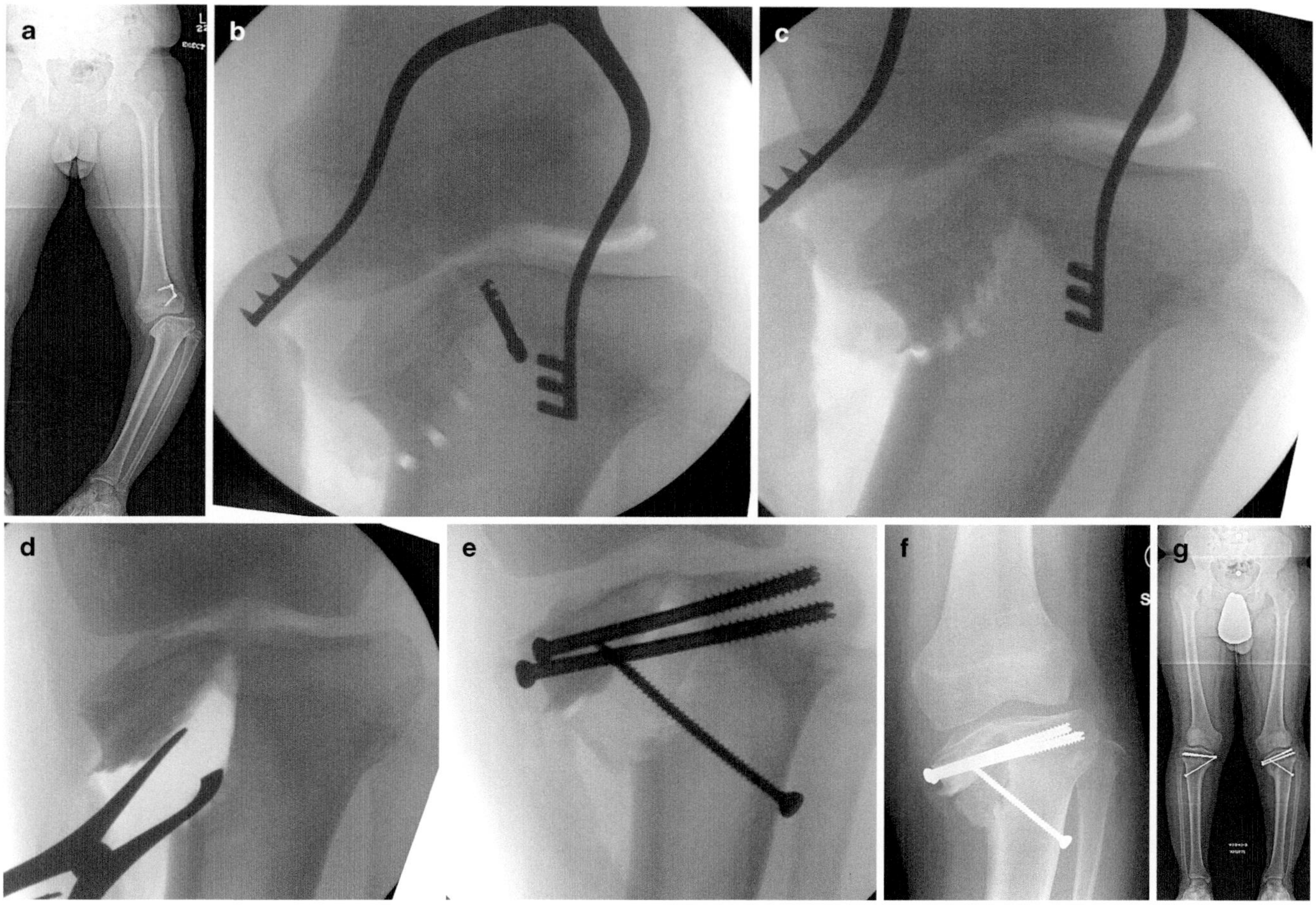

Fig. 3.9 (a–g) Twelve-year-old male with Blount disease and proximal tibia intra-articular deformity. (a) Standing AP demonstrating intra-articular proximal tibial deformity and medial growth arrest (Langenskiold Type VI). (b, c) Fluoroscopy demonstrating drill holes along the path of intra-articular osteotomy for tibial plateau elevation, the completion of osteotomy with an osteotome. (d) Laminar spreader simulating correction of intra-articular deformity. (e, f) Intraoperative fluoroscopy and postoperative radiographs demonstrating fixation with large fragment screws after structural bone graft placement. (g) Healed osteotomy sites with persistent proximal tibial varus. Tibial plateau elevation corrects intra-articular deformity but often does not correct overall varus deformity completely

Plates provide a rigid method of stabilizing osteotomies following an acute correction. They are particularly useful in stabilizing metaphyseal osteotomies after correction of either angulatory or rotational deformities. Plates utilized can be conventional plates, locking plates, or blade plates [14]. In particular, blade plates and locking plates (Fig. 3.10) can be used to stabilize osteotomies that have little or no inherent stability, and locking plates can be utilized with a submuscular technique that may minimize soft tissue dissection. Advantages of their use include the ability to begin early motion at adjacent joints, rigid fixation, and immediate correction of the deformity (Fig. 3.11). Disadvantages to the use of conventional plates are the relatively larger amount of soft tissue dissection that is necessary, the lack of ability to adjust

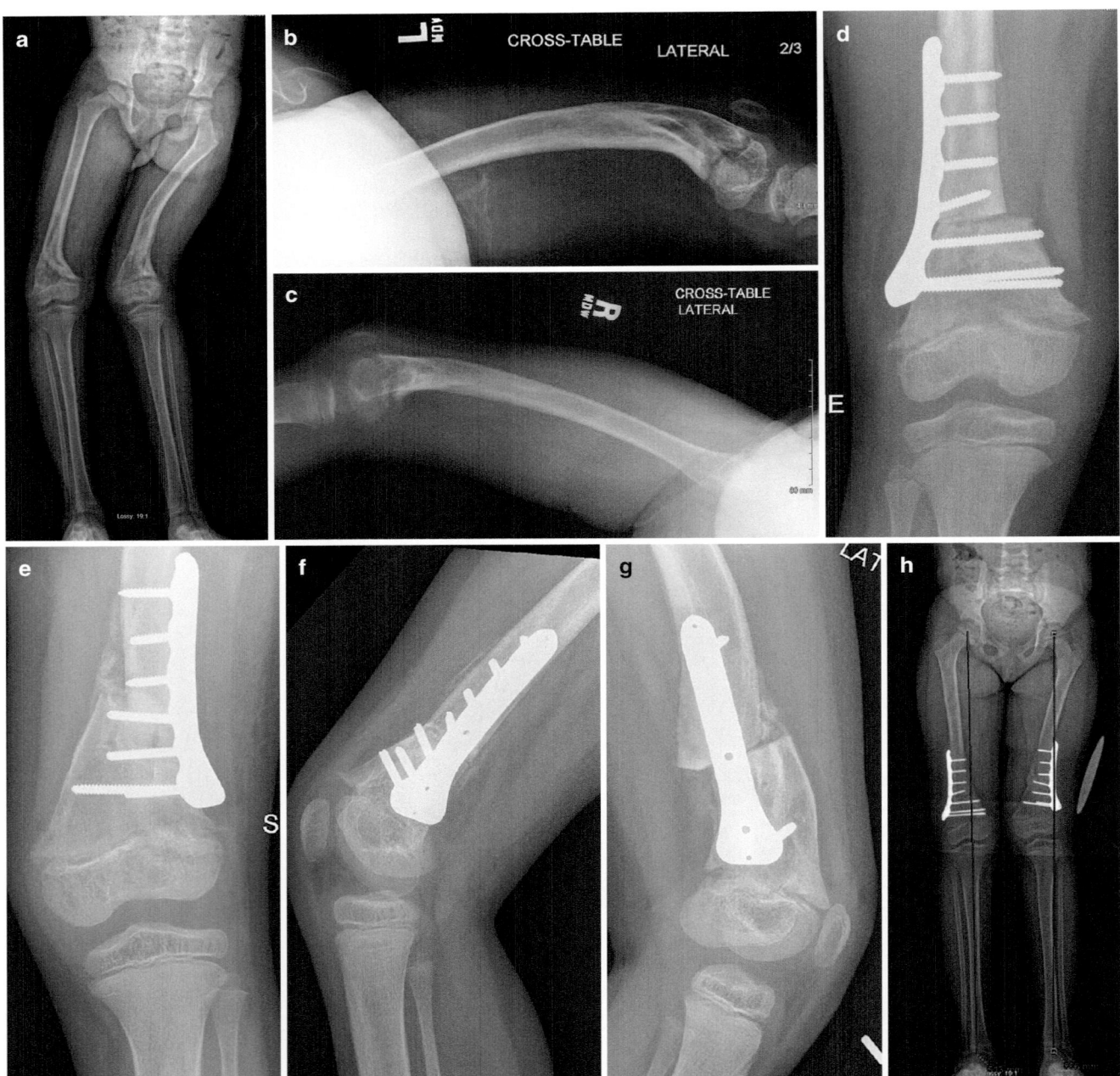

Fig. 3.10 (a–h) 6-Year-old female from West Africa with a history of SC hemoglobinopathy. (a–c) Standing AP demonstrating the right distal femoral varus-procurvatum oblique plane deformity and left distal femoral valgus-procurvatum oblique plane deformity. (b) Lateral radiograph of the right femur demonstrating a procurvatum. (d–g) AP and lateral radiographs 3 weeks postoperatively showing acute correction of the oblique plane deformities with stabilization using locking plates. (h) Standing AP radiograph of both lower extremities showing healing osteotomies of the distal femur showing near normal alignment

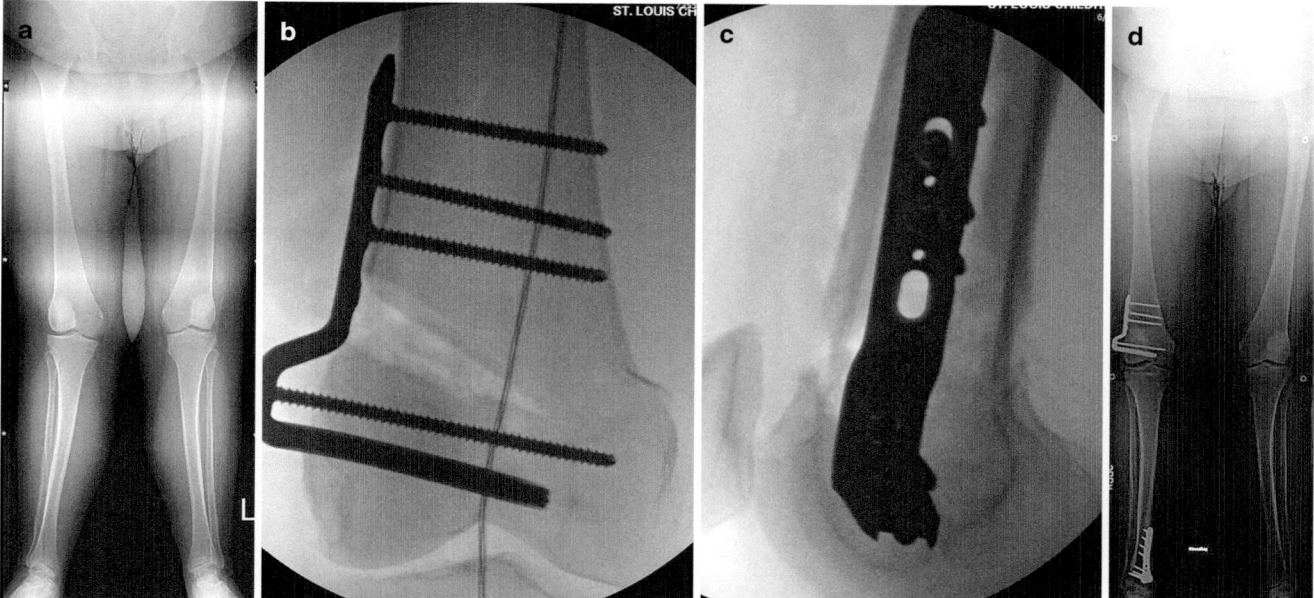

Fig. 3.11 (a–d) Sixteen-year-old female with distal femoral valgus deformity. (a) Standing AP demonstrating distal femoral valgus deformity. (b, c) AP and lateral fluoroscopic images showing distal femoral osteotomy with blade plate correction of deformity. (d) Postoperative radiographs demonstrating the restoration of the mechanical axis. Of note, the patient had a concomitant derotational distal tibial osteotomy for excessive external tibial torsion

the correction postoperatively, and the difficulties associated with soft tissue coverage in areas with little overlying soft tissue resulting in issues with infection.

Gradual Correction with Osteotomy

The workhorse of complex deformity correction is gradual correction. Gradual correction is effective in treating deformities with components of angulation, rotation, translation, and/or length. Gradual correction can be achieved with monolateral external fixation; circular external fixation utilizing the classic Ilizarov-type hinges and distractors, or computer-controlled six-strut circular external fixation. Most recently, motorized nails have combined some of the advantages of gradual correction with an internal fixation [15]. Motorized nails, however, provide no ability to correct angulatory deformities gradually but do allow for an acute correction of angulatory deformities followed by gradual lengthening. Advantages of gradual correction include minimal soft tissue dissection and early weight bearing with the ability to deal with problems that arise during the postoperative period and the ability to "fine tune" the correction to optimize the final alignment [16–19]. Disadvantages of gradual correction include complex postoperative care requiring substantial compliance with a physical therapy protocol and rigid adherence to a follow-up schedule by the patient and family with the possibility of damaging adjacent joints by the injudicious use of distraction at an osteotomy site. In addition, external fixation systems tend to be less well tolerated by patients, and issues with pain and pin tract problems are often noted [20–24]. As the lower limb deformities become more complex, the degree of required patient compliance and the physician learning curve also increase substantially. The trade-off, however, is the increasing ability to deal with complex three-dimensional deformities and achieve accurate corrections (Figs. 3.12 and 3.13).

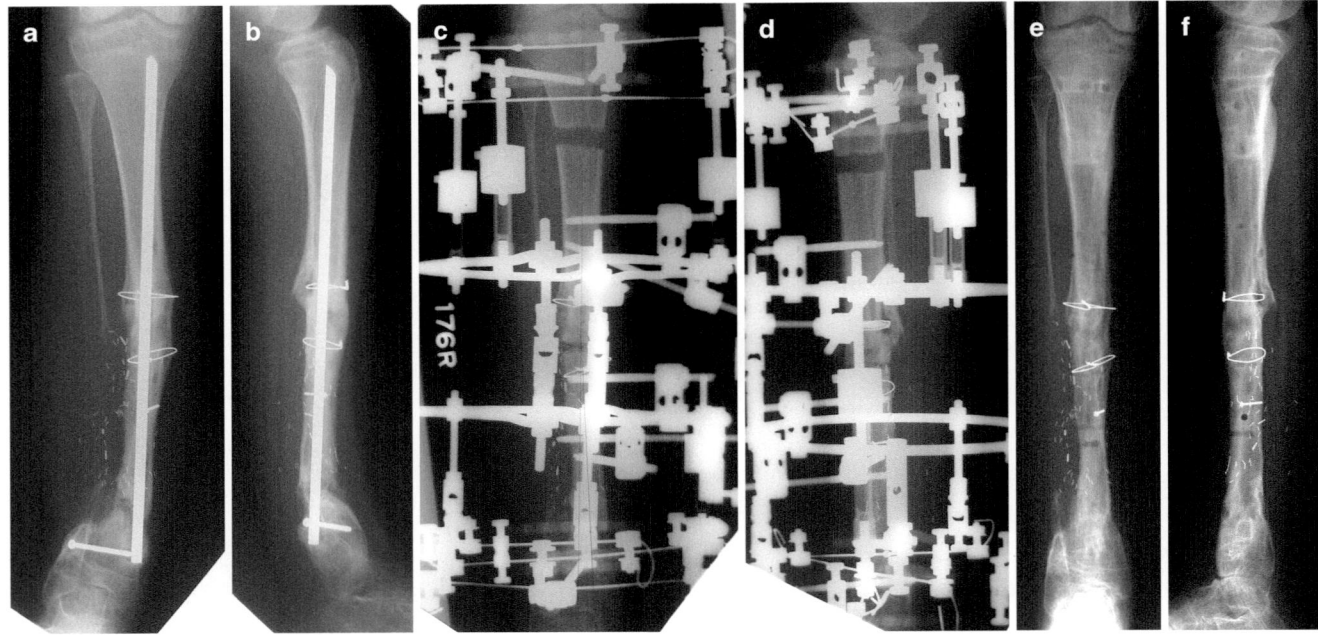

Fig. 3.12 (a–f) Thirteen-year-old female with tibial pseudarthrosis, status postmultiple attempts at correction and healing with Peter Williams rod. (**a, b**) AP and lateral of the right tibia demonstrating deformity and the occurrence of a new distal tibial pseudarthrosis. (**c, d**) AP and lateral views of Ilizarov application with multilevel osteotomy, proximal osteotomy for tibial lengthening and distal tibial osteotomy for deformity correction and bone transport into pseudarthrosis site. (**e, f**) AP and lateral views after frame removal and pseudarthrosis healing

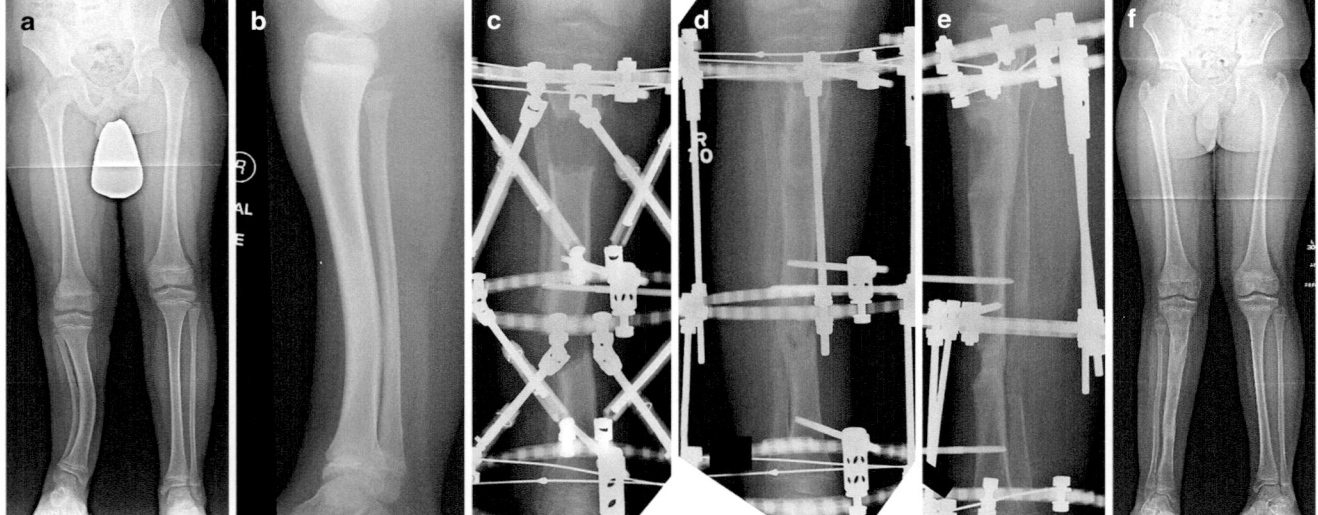

Fig. 3.13 (a–f) Ten-year-old male with posteromedial bowing and limb length discrepancy. (**a, b**) Standing AP and lateral view demonstrating deformity and limb length discrepancy. (**c**) AP radiograph showing the application of a bi-level circular external fixator. A proximal tibial osteotomy was performed for lengthening and a midshaft osteotomy for deformity correction. (**d, e**) AP and lateral views demonstrate healing of regenerate and the correction of deformity. (**f**) Standing AP showing the restoration of the mechanical axis and the correction of leg length discrepancy

Combined Acute and Gradual Correction

The increased availability of motorized intramedullary nails has allowed the increased utilization of intramedullary nails to perform metaphyseal osteotomies with acute deformity correction followed by gradual lengthening to correct a limb length discrepancy. Blocking screws can be used to stabilize the fragments during the acute correction and gradual lengthening then can be performed after an appropriate latency period. This technique increasingly allows more complex

Fig. 3.14 (a–g) 15-year-old male with a history of the left distal femoral physeal arrest. (**a**) Standing AP of both lower extremities showing a 3.1-cm limb length discrepancy and the left distal femoral valgus deformity. (**b, c**) AP and lateral radiographs of the left femur 1 week after a distal femoral osteotomy correcting the valgus deformity stabilized using a retrograde-motorized intramedullary nail and blocking screws. (**d, e**) Standing AP of both lower extremities and lateral of the left femur 6 weeks after surgery following 3.1 cm of lengthening. (**f, g**) Standing AP of both lower extremities and lateral of the left knee 9 months after surgery showing the restoration of the mechanical axis and correction of leg length discrepancy with healing of the distraction site

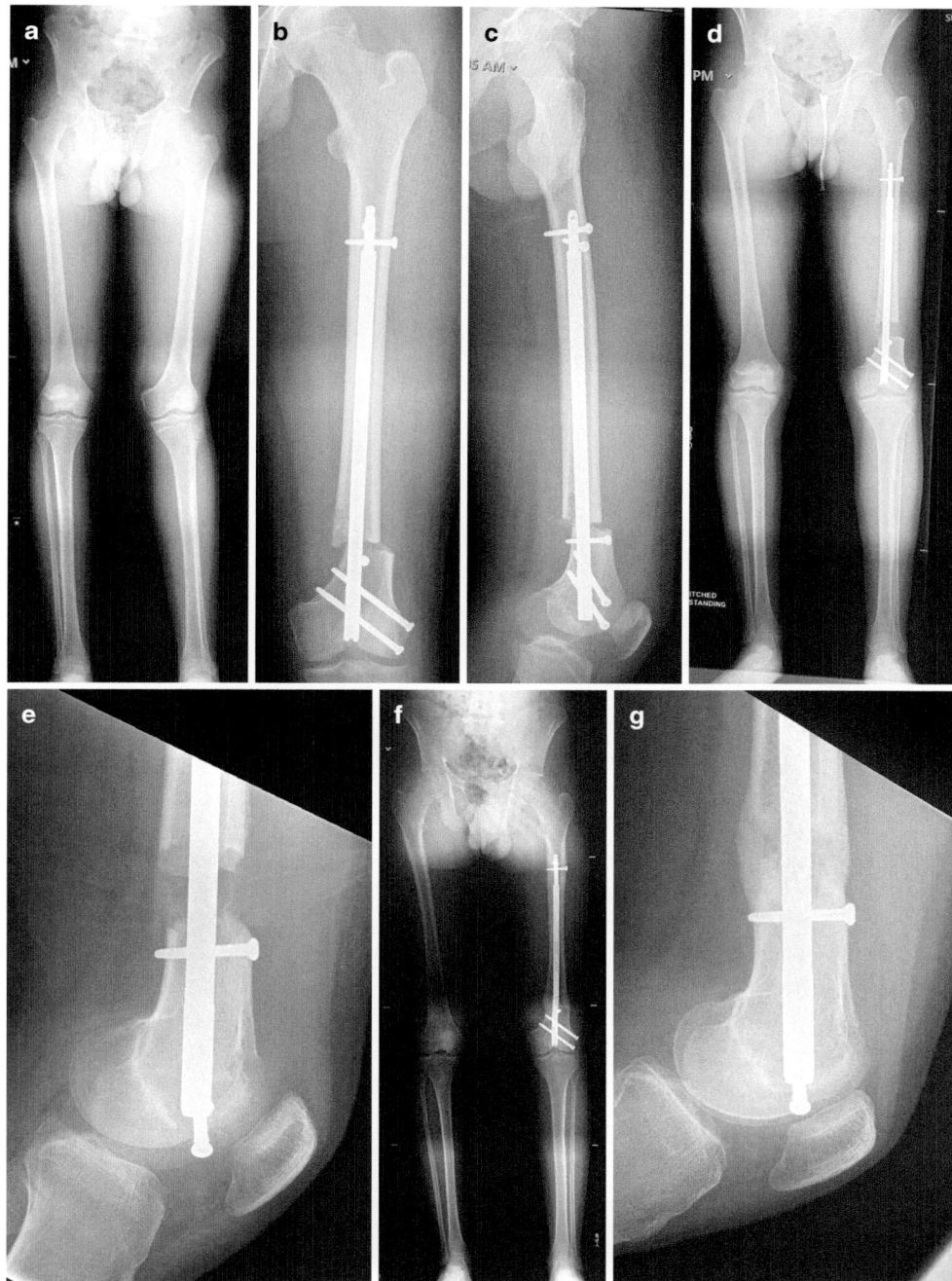

deformities to be treated without the disadvantages of external fixation (Fig. 3.14).

Summary

Decision-making in the lower extremity deformity correction is a necessary, but arduous task. One must develop a complete problem list which addresses the pertinent difficulties associated with the patient's deformity, perceived problem, and ability of the caretaker and patient to implement the plan of care as well as potential likely complications. This problem list then should help guide the location of the correction and select which mode or the combination of modes of deformity correction is optimal, whether it be soft tissue modification, physeal modulation/ablation, or osteotomy through either an acute or a gradual approach. The approach(es) selected then should guide the surgical plan. With advances in technology devices such as motorized nails and computer-controlled six strut circular external fixators,

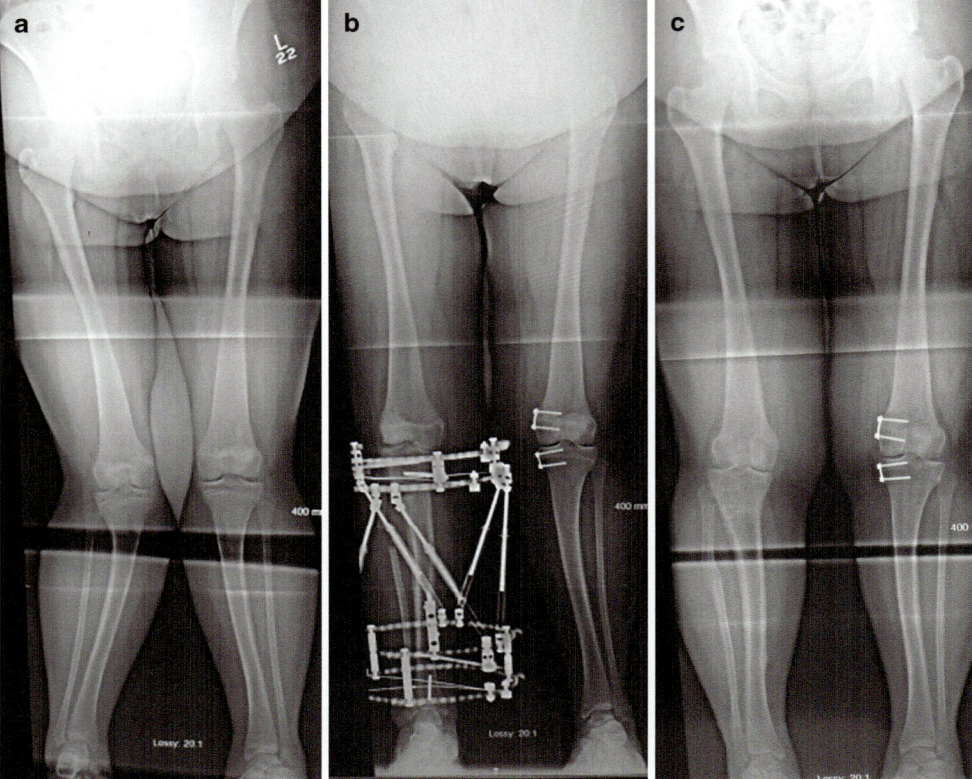

Fig. 3.15 (a–c) 11-year-old female with bilateral valgus deformities and knee pain. (**a**) Standing AP of both lower extremities showing bilateral valgus deformities worse on the right than the left with the right tibial valgus and the left distal femoral and proximal tibial valgus. (**b**) Standing AP of both lower extremities 6 weeks after surgery showing the application of the left tibial circular external fixator with gradual correction through a proximal tibial osteotomy and the left medial distal femoral and proximal tibial plate hemiepiphyseodesis. (**c**) Standing AP of both lower extremities 2 years after surgery showing healing of the right proximal tibial osteotomy 19 months after the removal of the external fixator and correction of the left-sided valgus deformity with closed physes

the complex deformities can safely be addressed in a comprehensive way. It is important to start with a thorough evaluation of each patient, his or her environment and the resources available and apply the principles of deformity correction to develop a customized treatment plan which may incorporate multiple modalities (Fig. 3.15).

Commentary 1

Fergal Monsell
fergal.monsell@uhbw.nhs.uk

Deformity analysis requires an understanding of patient characteristics, deformity characteristics, and surgeon characteristics. Patient characteristics include an appreciation of the natural history of the index condition and an understanding of the biology of correction. This mandates a cautious approach to surgery, particularly in rare conditions or common conditions presenting in an unusual way.

An understanding between patient, caregiver, and physician is also a requirement of any form of treatment and is particularly relevant in complex limb reconstruction, which may be difficult and protracted. A key consideration is optimization of the overall limb function and this has many facets and includes axis realignment, improvement in appearance, and the modification of symptoms.

It is important to carefully document a full medical history. Chronic medical conditions, such as obesity and diabetes, are becoming more prevalent and can have an impact on how a patient contends with deformity correction, particularly if this is conducted over a protracted period. Seemingly unconnected episodes of the previous illness may also be important and should be discussed. This is particularly relevant to apparently uncomplicated sepsis in the neonatal and early infantile period, which may cause subtle growth arrest that results in substantial deformity many years later. The effect of the previous treatment, regardless of whether this has been successful or unsuccessful, should also be discussed. This will have an impact on the patient's perception of their surgical journey and it is useful to understand this at an early stage.

Part of the evaluation of the ability of a patient to comply with the proposed treatment involves identifying additional assistance that may be required. This may take the form of equipment including wheelchairs and crutches, modifications of the home environment involving ramps and hoists, or modifications to the employment or educational environment. It is difficult to reactively organize the provision of equipment if surgery occurs at short notice.

The patient's perception of their individual problem is also key to offering advice and is important to ensure that their expectations and the ability of the surgeon are aligned. Issues that are important to the surgeon may not intuitively coincide with those of the patient and their family and failure is often the result of unrealistic expectations by either surgeon, patient or both. It is necessary to clearly explain that anatomical perfection may not be possible and that the goal is to produce improvement within defined parameters to achieve a useful enhancement of function.

Sufficient time is required for good communication and attempting to have a complicated and often difficult discussion with a patient or family in the context of a busy clinic is suboptimal. Important conversations ideally should be separated from a general clinic, with adequate time for a full and frank appraisal of the details of a planned procedure, the potential alternatives, the complication profile and the requirements for follow-up.

Goals should be expressed in a language that is understood by the patients and caregivers and misunderstanding or miscommunication about the fundamental aim of treatment may result in an unsatisfactory outcome, regardless of the technical success of the procedure. In addition to a written problem list, it is instructive to provide patients with an explanatory letter, expressed in lay terms, particularly if the clinical correspondence contains complicated medical jargon.

The surgeon should be able to give an honest appraisal of their personal experience in addition to the published literature on any given subject. It is easy to be overambitious about what is possible, particularly when the outcome may not be clearly defined for a considerable period. Whilst the surgeon may forget the promises that are made in the early stages of treatment, the patient and family will not, and will judge the outcome against these initial claims.

A further opinion may be requested in complex conditions and those that do not have a recognized treatment algorithm. The benefit of an additional perspective should not be underestimated and should be facilitated as a part of the ongoing management responsibility. If the opinions are identical, this is reassuring, if there is a conflict between opinions, then the treating surgeon has a responsibility to reconcile these in a way that the patient is comfortable with. Ongoing disagreement is destructive and it is unfair to expect, even a well-informed patient, to arbitrate on disparate medical opinions.

There are several components to an individual deformity and each must be properly evaluated. These are usually described in terms of the plane (frontal, sagittal, and axial) and type (angulation and translation). Frontal plane angulation can either be apex lateral or medial, and translation in this plane is either medial or lateral. Lateral plane angulation can be either apex anterior or posterior and translation can be either anterior or posterior. Axial plane angulation can either be internal or external torsion and translation in this plane can be short or long. It is generally accepted that torsion describes a pathological angular deformity in the axial plane, version describes a normal geometry and rotation refers to the movement of a joint.

Lengthening in congenital deformity, irrespective of the type of device, should be performed cautiously because of the inherent joint stability associated with these conditions. Joint stability is a prerequisite and if this is not present, then the risk of subluxation is prohibitively high. This is particularly relevant in congenital femoral shortening and it often requires pre-emptive joint stabilization, prior to surgical lengthening. Correction of femoral length or angular deformity should include routine division of the iliotibial band as this structure is unyielding, resists tensile forces, and introduces considerable resistance to deformity correction.

Correction of diaphyseal deformity can be undertaken using an intramedullary device. This, however, may not be possible in the presence of a multiapical deformity. Whilst this can be reduced to a single apex, the diaphysis does not align in a manner that permits passage of an intramedullary nail and this may require an alternative surgical strategy including a locking plate. Complex multilevel correction in three axes is technically difficult. This can be conducted using an external fixator as a temporary, intraoperative device to produce stable diaphyseal correction, suitable for intramedullary stabilization. Implant-based fixation should be approached cautiously in the presence of previous infection and if there is evidence of active infection, there should be a very specific reason to conduct implant-based surgery and an external fixator is often a safer alternative.

Growth plate modulation has become a popular method of correcting angular deformities in the growing limb. This, however, should not occur at the expense of creating an additional deformity, which may complicate the subsequent re-alignment surgery. This is illustrated by axis correction using hemiepiphyseal stapling in the X-linked rickets. This improves overall alignment but does not address the common multiapical diaphyseal deformity, which often becomes painful in adolescence and requires surgical correction. If this has been prefaced by a growth modulation, then there is an additional periphyseal deformity, which requires an additional level of correction. This technique should also be used cautiously in the presence of a "sick physis." This is particularly relevant after generalized infection, in which growth appears to be viable on plain radiology, but occurs at an unpredictably slow rate, making it difficult to predict axial and angular correction.

Commentary 2

Reggie C. Hamdy
rhamdy@shriners.mcgill.ca and

Louis-Nicolas Veilleux
ln.veilleux@mcgill.ca

Knee height asymmetry (KHA) is defined clinically as any difference in the level of both knees in the standing, sitting, or supine positions and is measured radiologically on an AP view of the whole lower limbs standing with the pelvis level (1). It may or may not be associated with limb length discrepancy (LLD). Although it is a largely ignored deformity and rarely discussed, this topic was presented at the POSNA meeting in 2023 and, surprisingly, elicited an unexpected and intense discussion between all participants that raised more questions than answers. There are several reasons for this interest in KHA:

Firstly, KHA is not a well-known deformity and is very poorly described in the most standard textbooks on limb deformities. It is not part of the standard analysis of any long bone deformity—that includes angular, rotational, transverse, and length deformities. In most pediatric hospitals, there is an LLD clinic but there is no KHA clinic and there is a lack of documentation regarding KHA.

Secondly, very little has been written in the literature regarding KHA. However, the little that has been written is very concerning! Veilleux et al. [25] in one of the rare papers published on KHA, retrospectively reviewed a series of 55 consecutive patients followed in the LLD clinic and who were surgically operated on to address their LLD. They reported a high incidence of KHA in these patients with more than one-third of them having KHA of more than 2.0 cm. This was the first reported study demonstrating the close relationship between LLD and KHA. However, more concerning than the high incidence of KHA was the fact that following successful surgery for equalization of their LLD, more than half of these patients had an increase in their KHA! While Veilleux et al. studied asymmetry between the knee height of both limbs, Weinberg and Lui [26] studied the effects of asymmetry between the segments of the same lower limb. They analyzed the tibio-femoral ratio in 1152 cadaveric tibiae and femorae and reported that any increase in the tibio-femoral ratio of 0.80/1.00 predisposed to knee osteoarthritis. They were the first ones to demonstrate that any asymmetry between the segments of the same limb (which automatically leads to a KHA) has negative effects on the knee joint. Veilleux et al. [27] reported the results of gait assessment on two patients with KHA (of 2.0 cm and 4.00 cm, respectively) and LLD and demonstrated the presence of abnormal gait parameters, whereas self-perception and pain assessment were negatively affected. In a further analysis of one patient with no LLD but significant KHA (unpublished data), functional impairment was present, specifically during squatting activities and driving a car. Although these are only anecdotal reports, they do, however, raise the concern that KHA may have a significant impact on gait and function.

There are still too many unanswered questions regarding the true impact of KHA on gait, function, and psychosocial aspects and how much KHA is safe and acceptable. We hope that this debate at the last POSNA meeting (2023) will not only lead to an increased awareness of KHA as a potentially significant deformity that should not be ignored but will also lead to the development of well-designed longitudinal and multi-centric studies in order to be able to answer the question: *'Knee Height Asymmetry: Does it Matter?'*

References

1. Davids JR, Benfanti P, Blackhurst DW, et al. Assessment of femoral anteversion in children with cerebral palsy: accuracy of the trochanteric prominence angle test. J Pediatr Orthop. 2002;22:173–8.
2. Gordon JE, Davis LE. Leg length discrepancy: the natural history (and what do we really know). J Pediatr Orthop. 2019;39:S10–3.
3. Park SS, Gordon JE, Luhmann SJ, et al. Outcome of hemiepiphyseal stapling for late-onset tibia vara. J Bone Joint Surg Am. 2005;87:2259–66.
4. Kasser JR. Physeal bar resections after growth arrest about the knee. Clin Orthop Relat Res. 1990;255:68–74.
5. Langenskiold A. Surgical treatment of partial closure of the growth plate. J Pediatr Orthop. 1981;1:3–11.
6. Gabriel KR, Crawford AH, Roy DR, et al. Percutaneous epiphyseodesis. J Pediatr Orthop. 1994;14:358–62.
7. Skytta ET, Savolainen HA, Kautiainen HJ, et al. Long-term results of leg length discrepancy treated with temporary epiphyseal stapling in children with juvenile chronic arthritis. Clin Exp Rheumatol. 2003;21:669–71.
8. Mielke CH, Stevens PM. Hemiepiphyseal stapling for knee deformities in children younger than 10 years: a preliminary report. J Pediatr Orthop. 1996;16:423–9.
9. Stevens PM, Klatt JB. Guided growth for pathological physes: radiographic improvement during realignment. J Pediatr Orthop. 2008;28:632–9.
10. Keshet D, Katzman A, Zaidman M, et al. Removal of metaphyseal screw only after hemiepiphysiodesis correction of coronal plane deformities around the knee joint: is this a safe and advisable strategy? J Pediatr Orthop. 2019;39:e236–9.
11. Chapman MW, Dwellius PW, Bray TJ, et al. Closed intramedullary femoral osteotomy: shortening and derotation procedures. Clin Orthop. 1993;287:245–51.
12. Gordon JE, Pappademos PC, Schoenecker PL, et al. Diaphyseal derotational osteotomy with intramedullary fixation for correction of excessive femoral anteversion in children. J Pediatr Orthop. 2004;25(4):548–53.
13. Schoenecker PL, Johnston R, Rich MM, et al. Elevation of the medical plateau of the tibia in the treatment of Blount disease. J Bone Joint Surg Am. 1992;74:351–8.
14. Gordon JE, Heidenreich FP, Carpenter CJ, et al. Comprehensive treatment of late-onset tibia vara. J Bone Joint Surg Am. 2005;87:1561–70.
15. Schiedel FM, Vogt B, Tretow HL, et al. How precise is the PRECICE compared to the ISKD in intramedullary limb lengthening? Acta Orthop. 2014;85:293.
16. Feldman DS, Madan SS, Ruchelsman DE, et al. Accuracy of correction of tibia vara: acute versus gradual correction. J Pediatr Orthop. 2006;26:794–8.
17. Feldman DS, Madan SS, Koval KJ, et al. Correction of tibia vara with six-axis deformity analysis and the Taylor Spatial Frame. J Pediatr Orthop. 2003;23:387–91.
18. Feldman DS, Shin SS, Madan S, et al. Correction of tibial malunion and nonunion with six-axis analysis deformity correction using the Taylor Spatial Frame. J Orthop Trauma. 2003;17:549–54.
19. Gordon JE, Jani M, Dobbs M, et al. Treatment of rigid hypertrophic posttraumatic pseudarthrosis of the tibia in children using distraction osteogenesis. J Pediatr Orthop. 2002;22:419–23.
20. Camathias C, Valderrabano V, Oberli H. Routine pin tract care in external fixation is unnecessary: a randomised, prospective, blinded controlled study. Injury. 2012;43:1969–73.
21. Dayton P, Prins DB, Hensley N, et al. A user-friendly method of pin site management for external fixators. Foot Ankle Spec. 2011;4:370–2.
22. Gordon JE, Kelly-Hahn J, Carpenter CJ, et al. Pin site care during external fixation in children: results of a nihilistic approach. J Pediatr Orthop. 2000;20:163–5.
23. Jennison T, McNally M, Pandit H. Prevention of infection in external fixator pin sites. Acta Biomater. 2014;10:595–603.
24. Lee CK, Chua YP, Saw A. Antimicrobial gauze as a dressing reduces pin site infection: a randomized controlled trial. Clin Orthop Relat Res. 2012;470:610–5.
25. Veilleux LN, et al. Incidence of knee height asymmetry in a paediatric population of corrected leg length discrepancy: a retrospective chart review study. Int Ortho. 2018;42(8):1979–85.
26. Weinberg & Lui. J Paediatric Ortho, 2017.
27. Veilleux LN. September 2016, Gait & Posture 49, Conference Abstract.

Outcome Measures in Limb Lengthening and Deformity Correction

Harpreet Chhina and Anthony Cooper

Introduction

The measures used to assess the impact of treatments on a patient are called outcome measures. Apart from mortality, the most commonly measured outcomes in healthcare include function, pain, and health-related quality of life (HRQL). These outcome measures could be patient reported (patient-reported outcome measures or PROMs) or proxy reports from a clinician or a parent. Outcome measures can further be classified into generic outcome measures and condition-specific outcome measures. For example, generic questionnaires, such as Short Form Health Survey (SF-36), Pediatric Quality of Life Inventory (PedsQL) and Child Health Questionnaire (CHQ), measure common HRQL concerns that apply to any condition or disease or to healthy individuals [1–3]. As generic questionnaires are meant to cover any health condition and can be used to compare patient groups with each other and with the general population, they often fail to ask about issues that matter most to patients with a specific health condition. As a result, generic questionnaires tend to be less sensitive to detecting clinical changes as a result of an intervention [4]. Condition-specific outcome measures are designed for a particular group of patients that may have unique problems. Such instruments tend to have higher content validity than generic outcome measures and are thus considered more appropriate for measuring specific concerns of a target patient group. These tools are especially useful in the measurement of change in a patient's function, pain, and HRQL after an intervention.

Outcome Assessment in Lower Limb Deformities

Outcome assessment in lower limb deformities has been complicated due to the lack of a universally accepted classification system for assessing lower limb deformities. However, the classification system developed by the Limb Lengthening and Reconstruction Society (LLRS-AIM classification) was introduced to address this deficiency [5]. The use of PROMs in general has increased considerably in last two decades to assess the effect of interventions, quality of care, and evaluate policies to inform health economics [6]. Overall, there has also been an increase in the use of PROMs in the field of pediatric orthopedics but limited utilization of PROMs specifically validated for the pediatric population [7]. The field of limb lengthening and deformity correction has observed some progress in the use of PROMs [8, 9] and hence the development of new measures specific to limb lengthening and deformity correction has also increased [10–13]. These outcome measures, specific to limb lengthening and deformity correction, include the Limb Deformity-Scoliosis Research Society (LD-SRS) score for adults, the Stanmore Limb Reconstruction Score (SLRS) for adults and patient-reported outcome measure for lower limb reconstruction (PROLLIT). Fabricant et al. introduced the LD-SRS score for adults with lower limb deformities [12]. LD-SRS score is a modification of the Scoliosis Research Society (SRS) outcome instrument [12, 14]. The modifications included are removing the joint and arthritis-specific scales and replacing the words 'back' and 'trunk' with 'limb'. The validation study included adult patients between the ages of 18 and 70 years with a diagnosis of congenital or acquired lower limb deformity and/or angular deformity.

H. Chhina (✉)
Department of Orthopaedic Surgery, BC Children's Hospital, Vancouver, BC, Canada

Department of Orthopaedics, University of British Columbia, Vancouver, BC, Canada
e-mail: hchhina@cw.bc.ca

A. Cooper
Department of Orthopaedics, University of British Columbia, Vancouver, BC, Canada
e-mail: anthony.cooper@cw.bc.ca

The LD-SRS score has since been used in a few studies in adults undergoing limb lengthening and reconstruction [15, 16]. SLRS was developed based on the interviews with the adult patients undergoing limb reconstruction surgery followed by interviews with limb reconstruction surgeons, clinical nurse specialists, and therapists [9]. It has been shown to have face validity in a recent pilot study [13]. A protocol paper published for PROLLIT indicates that it is a PROM specific to lower limb reconstruction [11]. However, no further information about the development of this new PROM has been published to date. The aforementioned new PROMs are specifically being developed for an adult population undergoing limb lengthening and reconstruction procedures. There has also been some progress specifically in the PROMs developed for children undergoing limb lengthening and reconstruction procedures.

PROMS in Children

A systematic review published by Chhina et al. in 2017 indicated the lack of a validated condition-specific PROM for children with lower limb deformities [8]. In the absence of a condition-specific PROM, the studies included in this systematic review had used 24 different measurement instruments. The most commonly used instruments were the American Academy of Orthopaedic Surgeons (AAOS) Lower Limb Outcomes Questionnaire, Pediatric Quality of Life Inventory (PedsQL), Pediatric Outcomes Data Collection Instrument (PODCI), and Short-Form Health Survey (SF-36). There were only two lower limb specific questionnaires identified from this systematic review. These were the AAOS Lower Limb Outcomes Questionnaire [17] and a lower limb questionnaire [18]. However, the AAOS Lower Limb Outcomes Questionnaire was not designed specifically for children and included items around the function of the lower limb. The lower limb questionnaire was an in-house questionnaire focused on parental satisfaction with their child's leg length discrepancy.

Since the publication of this systematic review in 2017, more recent studies have identified other lower limb specific instruments such as an in-house limb deficiencies questionnaire developed by Johansen et al. [19], Limb Lengthening Satisfaction Questionnaire (LLSQ), Childhood Amputee Prosthetics Project-Prosthetics Satisfaction Inventory (CAPP-PSI) [2, 19–25], and Gait Outcomes Assessment List—Lower Limb Differences (GOAL-LD) [26]. The in-house limb deficiencies questionnaire was developed by input from organizations representing this diagnosis, parents of children with limb deficiencies, and adults particularly with limb deficiencies. This questionnaire was completed only by the parents of children with limb deficiencies [19]. The LLSQ is a 5-item questionnaire that uses a 10-cm visual analog scale to assess a child's satisfaction with their limb lengthening. The LLSQ was first developed as a parent-reported questionnaire to assess the parental satisfaction with their child's limb lengthening procedure and the parental report of their child's satisfaction with the limb lengthening procedure. The parental version of the LLSQ was adapted from the parent version of CAPP-PSI [25]. There is no further information available on the validation of the LLSQ. Childhood Amputee Prosthetics Project-Functional Status Inventory (CAPP-FSI) is a standardized measure of the parent-reported functional status of children ages 3–17 years with upper and lower limb deficiencies exclusively. The content was developed based on a literature review and input from the clinicians. There was no involvement of children with limb deficiencies in any phase of content development.

GOAL-LD is a new questionnaire developed for gait outcome assessment for children with lower limb differences [26]. It is the first outcome assessment questionnaire that has been developed specifically for children with lower limb differences. GOAL-LD has been developed by modifying the Gait Outcomes Assessment List (GOAL), which is an assessment tool for children with cerebral palsy. The development and initial validation studies for GOAL-LD were conducted in the United States, Australia, and Canada. At the time of writing this chapter, the validity and reliability of this new questionnaire in other countries and languages have not yet been published.

The Patient-Reported Outcome Measurement Information System (PROMIS) includes a number of person-centered measures to evaluate and monitor physical, mental, and social health in adults and children [27]. Self-report measures for children between the ages 8 and 17 years are available. PROMIS measures are psychometrically sound and when needed can be used as complementary generic measures along with condition-specific measurement instruments for patients with lower limb deformities. However, it is important to remember when using generic measurement instruments such as PROMIS that they may not have adequate content validity (i.e. may not have items most relevant to this patient population) for patients with lower limb deformities.

A recent review from high-impact pediatric orthopedic journals over a 2-year period has identified and assessed the most commonly used PROMs in pediatric limb deformity [28]. PROMs were used and reported in 23 studies involving children, in which 10 studies used PROMs that have been validated in children and 13 studies used adult PROMs that have not been validated in children. PROMs validated in children included 2 generic PROMs (EuroQol-5and Rosenberg self-esteem scale) and 8 condition-specific PROMs (PODCI for musculoskeletal conditions, PedsQL-CP version, FAQ, CPCHILD, Oxford Foot and Ankle questionnaire, Kujala score for anterior knee pain, Non-communicating Children's Pain Checklist Postoperative Version for pain in severe intellectual disabilities, and Barnhoft questionnaire for Hip). This review has once again confirmed the findings from a previous systematic review from 2017 [8] by demonstrating that there is no consensus on the use of PROMs in the field of pediatric limb deformity. This is due to the lack of availability of a condition-specific PROM for this patient population. The lack of a condition-specific PROM and consensus on the use of PROMs make it challenging to compare results across studies. The findings from these two reviews [8, 28] also align with the results from two other reviews which also demonstrated the variability in the use of PROMs in pediatric orthopedics in general and the use of adult PROMs in pediatric population [7, 29]. Hence, there is a clear need for education for clinicians and researchers about the use of appropriate PROMs in pediatric orthopedics in addition to the development of condition-specific PROMs following the appropriate methodology [28, 30].

How to Choose an Appropriate PROM?

- How to select a PROM from the plethora of available instruments can be a daunting task. There are certain key considerations to be made while selecting a PROM for use. Below we present a summary of these key considerations based on recommendations from various sources including the US Food and Drug Administration (FDA) [31], European Medicine Agency (EMA), The International Society for Pharmacoeconomics and Outcomes Research (ISPOR), International Society for Quality of Life Research (ISOQOL), and COnsensus-based Standards for the selection of health Measurement INstruments (COSMIN).

  1. *What Is the Context of the Use of PROM?*
     Prior to selecting a PROM for use, it is important to understand the purpose of using PROMs for a specific context. PROMs can be used in multiple ways to inform the patients, clinicians, and policymakers. In a clinical context, PROMs can specifically be used for several purposes including looking at the effectiveness of interventions, measuring the change in a specific PRO such as HRQL or function or pain over time and comparing specific patient population with the general population.
  2. *What Is Your Target Patient Population?*
     Once the context of use is defined and a target patient population has been selected, it can be decided further whether to use a condition-specific PROM or a generic PROM or both. They both have advantages and disadvantages as discussed in the previous sections.
  3. *What Is the Concept of Interest?*
     It is important to understand, what is it that you want to measure. For example, in the context of limb reconstruction, are you interested in measuring HRQL or just function or appearance-related concerns of patients?
  4. *What PROMs Are Available for Use?*
     Once the concepts of interest are identified, there are multiple ways to identify available PROMs that exist already and could be potentially used. While formal literature searches and systematic reviews are the correct way to have a list of available PROMs, this is time consuming and not always practical. There are a few key resources to refer to when looking for a PROM to use. These include the Q-portfolio website, PROQOLID and Patient-Reported Outcomes Measurement Information System (PROMIS), and International Consortium for Health Outcomes Measurement (ICHOM).

     The Q-portfolio website provides a list of available PROMs to be used in various conditions in children and adults. These PROMs were developed by experts in PROM development by using modern psychometric approaches with the aim to measure what matters most to patients with a specific health condition. PROQOLID™ is an online database created by the Mapi Research Trust that provides a comprehensive list of measurement instruments to be used for clinical outcome assessments. For the instruments listed in this database, there is information available on the basic description (authors, copyright, use, therapeutic area of use, therapeutic indication, languages available, contact information, and conditions of use) and descriptive information (concepts of interest it is measuring, number of items, mode of administration, recall period, time for completion, population for intended use, population age range, domains covered by the questionnaire, scoring details, documentation of measurement properties of the instrument, ability to detect change, minimally important difference, and relevant references and websites) [32]. Another relevant resource is PROMIS, an initiative that has developed and validated a set of outcome measures to evaluate and monitor physical, mental, and social health across various chronic conditions and health statuses [27]. International Consortium for Health Outcomes Measurement (ICHOM) is a nonprofit organization promoting the measurement of outcomes that matter most to patients. ICHOM sets of patient-centered outcome measures are standardized outcomes, measurement tools, and time points and risk adjustment factors for a given condition. ICHOM standard sets are developed by a consortium of patient representatives, healthcare professionals, and researchers in a specific field. ICHOM uses International Society for Quality of Life Research (ISOQOL) minimum standards to guide their PROM research. Though ICHOM currently doesn't have a standard set for lower limb conditions, it is a valuable resource to check before deciding on a PROM for use. They have currently published 40 sets of patient-centered outcome measures for different conditions and specific patient populations [33]. However, it should be noted that there is no single resource that provides a list of outcome measures dedicated to orthopedic surgery.

5. *Is the PROM Validated for Use in Your Specific Patient Population?*

    Once there is a list of PROMs of interest, before looking into any evidence for the development or psychometric properties of the PROM, it is important to ascertain whether the PROM has been validated for use in your specific patient population. Instruments validated in one population will not necessarily perform well among patients with different medical conditions. To validate a measurement instrument in a specific patient population, the measurement properties of that instrument need to be assessed in that specific patient population.

6. *Does the PROM Meet the Minimum Standards for Use in Patient-Centered Outcomes and Comparative Effectiveness Research?*

    Once a list of PROMs that can be potentially used in your target population has been identified, they need to be evaluated to determine whether they meet the minimum standards for PROMs [31, 34, 35]. Below is a summary based on ISOQOL's recommendation for minimum standards for PROMs used in patient-centered research [34].

(a) Documentation of conceptual and measurement model: For a particular PROM, there should be documentation of what concepts are being measured, what is the target population for its use, what is the measurement model, how items are related to concepts being measured and what is the relationship between the concepts being measured.

(b) Documentation of psychometric properties of a PROM document: Below is a list of key psychometric properties of a PROM that should be documented. However, it is important to note that the psychometric evaluation of a measurement instrument is an ongoing process. Data accumulated from multiple studies and samples overtime are required to strengthen the confidence in the performance of a PROM [36].

Content validity: Content validity is the empiric evidence that demonstrates that the items and scales of an instrument are appropriate and comprehensive relative to its intended measurement concept, population, and use [31, 37]. For example, when looking at a PROM for children with lower limb differences, it needs to be ensured that the PROM covers a wide range of items under a particular concept, items are understandable by children with lower limb differences, and the items are also clinically relevant. The US FDA and European Medicines Agency have both highlighted the importance of establishing content validity for PROMs [38, 39]. The COSMIN group states that content validity is the most important psychometric property among various measurement properties of a PROM including reliability, validity, and responsiveness [40]. Both ISPOR and COSMIN group provides detailed guidance on establishing and reporting the content validity of PROMs [40–42]. COSMIN group provides detailed recommendations for evaluating the content validity of PROMs, how to perform a systematic review on content validity of PROMs, and how to establish the content validity of new PROMs [43]. In terms of developing PROMs for use in pediatrics, qualitative methods have been strongly recommended to include children in the concept elicitation and content validation phases as opposed to only including the parents [44]. Levels of agreement between child self-reports and parent proxy reports have been well documented in general and specifically in pediatric orthopedic population. The agreement between the child's self-report and the parents' proxy report of the child's quality of life is higher for commonly observable domains (e.g., physical functioning) than for less observable (e.g., emotional domain) [45]. Several psychological factors have been related to discrepancies in a child's self-reports and parents' proxy reports including projection of the parents' feelings and assumptions [46, 47]. A study specifically looking at agreement between child and parent reports in the pediatric orthopedic population found low levels of agreement on physical function, general health, and mental health domains as measured by Child Health Questionnaire and expectations domain in PODCI [48]. Children reported higher levels of Physical Function while lower levels for General Health and Mental Health as compared to their parents.

Construct validity: This is the degree to which scores from a PROM are consistent with hypotheses based on the assumption that the PROM is measuring the construct it is supposed to measure. Three aspects of construct validity include structural validity (internal relationships), hypotheses testing, and cross-cultural validity. Both hypothesis testing and cross-cultural validity are about the relationships to scores of other instruments or differences between relevant groups [35, 49]. Hypotheses testing is about whether the direction and magnitude of a correlation or difference are similar to what could be expected based on the construct(s) that are being measured. For example, to establish the structural validity of a new PROM assessing the HRQL in children, this new PROM may be administered alongside the PedsQL, a generic HRQL instrument measuring physical, social, emotional, and school function. Scores from the new instrument that is measuring similar domains to the generic PedsQL instrument will be expected to correlate more strongly than domains measuring dissimilar constructs.

Responsiveness: Responsiveness, also referred to as sensitivity to changes, is the ability of a PROM to measure the clinically meaningful change in scores over time. Anchor-based and distribution-based approaches have been recommended to assess the responsiveness of a PROM [50–53]. The responsiveness of a PROM can be compromised if the items included in the PROM are not relevant to a specific patient population. In other words, a lack of content validity can affect the responsiveness of a PROM.

Reliability: This is the degree to which the scores from a PROM are free from measurement error. Measurement error is the systematic and random error of a score that is not due to the true change in the construct being measured. Evidence for the reliability of a PROM can be obtained using various methods including internal consistency reliability and test–retest reliability. Internal consistency reliability is the degree to which the items of a PROM are consistent with each other. Test—retest reliability is the degree to which a person's responses to items for a measurement instrument are consistent between two separate administrations of the same instrument provided that the construct being measured remains unchanged between the two time intervals. It is worth mentioning that due to the rigorous and resource-intensive methodology required to establish measurement properties such as content validity and responsiveness, reliability is one of the most commonly reported measurement properties for PROMs.

(c) Interpretability of scores: There should be documentation of the details for the interpretation of scores for a PROM. For example, does a high score on a PROM mean better HRQL?

(d) Availability of the PROM in your language: Is the PROM available in the language you are planning to implement it? International collaborative research using PROMs would require a PROM to be available for use in multiple languages. In such cases, it is important to know the methods used for the translation and cultural adaptation (TCA) of a specific PROM as this will ensure the quality of the translation. There are standardized guidelines available from various resources to perform TCA including WHO, FDA, ISOQOL, and ISPOR. The most frequently used recommendations are from the ISPOR patient-reported outcomes translation and linguistic validation good research practice task force report [54, 55]. Evidence of cross-cultural validity should be assessed for PROMs that are translated and used in different languages. The degree to which the items on a translated PROM are an adequate reflection of the performance of items of the original version of the PROM.

(e) Clinician/researcher and the patient burden is also an important consideration to be made while choosing a PROM for use in a clinical or research setting. In terms of burden, the length of the PROM, frequency of use, and mode of administration are to be considered.

(f) The literacy level of the patient population and the appropriate reading level of the items included in the PROM also require to be considered before selecting a PROM. A PROM should have documentation on the reading level of the items which can be taken into consideration by the users.

(g) Pilot testing the PROM in your target population could be considered before implementing it in a large multicenter study. These small-scale pilot testing studies can be useful to determine the logistics of implementing a new PROM in a particular clinical setting, test the platforms used to implement the PROM such as Research Electronic Data Capture (REDCap) and perform a preliminary analysis of the data collected.

How Are PROMs Developed?

Guidelines for the development of new PROMs, translation and cultural adaptation, and establishing the measurement properties of PROMs are available from World Health Organisation (WHO), Food and Drug Administration (FDA) [31], European Medicine Agency (EMA), The International Society for Pharmacoeconomics and Outcomes Research (ISPOR), International Society for Quality of Life Research (ISOQOL) and COnsensus-based Standards for the selection of health Measurement INstruments (COSMIN).

There are three main phases in the development of any PROM [56]. These phases generally involve an interactive mixed methods approach with an *exploratory sequential design* 'QUAL-quant' where the qualitative phase is followed by a quantitative phase [57]. This approach is particularly useful for developing new instruments or revising existing instruments. Below we present three iterative and interactive phases involved in the development of a new PROM using the development of an HRQL PROM as an example.

1. Item generation: This phase starts with the development of a conceptual framework of HRQL for the target patient population followed by item generation and scale development. Development of the conceptual framework further involves multiple steps including a systematic review of literature, developing a preliminary conceptual framework based on the literature, and finally revising this conceptual framework based on a qualitative study involving the target patient population. A rigorous qualitative study is crucial in the development of a new PROM [44, 58]. Qualitative interviews with the target patient population can provide a deeper understanding of what is important to the patients and are the first step toward establishing the instrument's content validity [41, 42]. If the aim is to develop a PROM that is applicable to an international patient population, it is important to include patients from a wide range of countries to ensure that the final conceptual framework captures the concepts of interest from a heterogeneous patient population. The final conceptual framework developed based on the systematic review and the qualitative study is used to create an exhaustive item pool that is used to inform a set of preliminary scales for the new PROM.

   Once the items are developed and scales are formed, the next step is to establish the content validity of the new PROM. ISPOR and COSMIN groups provide detailed guidance to establish the content validity of a PROM [37, 41, 42, 59]. This involves conducting cognitive debriefing interviews with the target patient population and getting input from experts involved in the care of that patient population. Items and scales are revised based on the cognitive debriefing interviews and expert input.

2. Item reduction: This phase involves conducting a field-test study to perform item reduction, further refining the scales, and examining their psychometric properties. If the PROM is being developed for use in an international patient population, an international field test is conducted which involves collecting data using new the PROM from a large sample of the target patient population. To perform item reduction using modern psychometric approaches such as Rasch Measurement Theory (RMT), a minimum sample size of 150 patients per country is usually required [60]. RMT is a modern psychometric approach that uses the 1 parameter item-response theory model [61, 62]. Modern psychometric methods such as Rasch are increasingly used to develop scales that form clinical hierarchies and have interval-level measurement properties. Such scales allow for meaningful and interpretable measurement of change in patient status, which is difficult for scales developed using the traditional psychometric approaches [63].

   Before collecting field test data from various sites internationally, the new PROM will need to be translated and culturally adapted for use in each of the countries involved. Translation and cultural adaptation (TCA) can be performed using the available guidelines [54, 55, 64]. It is important to perform TCA and include data from different countries to establish the cross-cultural validity of the new PROM. This method provides an opportunity to perform differential item functioning with the field test data from different countries. The items that differ in performance across different countries can be dropped to ensure cross-cultural validity.

   Data from the field test are analyzed using a number of tests and criteria to examine the item and scale performance [62, 65]. The statistical tests indicating the item performance along with the clinical relevance of items guide the item reduction process. RMT analysis also provides a scoring system for the scale. Analysis of the field test data helps to establish some psychometric properties of the PROM based on the field test data including construct validity, test re-test reliability, and internal consistency reliability.

3. Psychometric evaluation: This phase involves further evaluation of measurement properties that have not been evaluated in the prior steps including reliability, validity, and responsiveness (discussed in previous sections).

Integrating into Clinical Practice/Implementation Science

Despite the widespread acknowledgment of the importance of patient-centered healthcare and the potential of PROMs to influence the care of patients, PROMs are still not widely used in clinical practice. The studies examining the challenges and barriers to incorporate PROMs in clinical practice state the length of the PROM as the biggest barrier indicated by the patients and the need for adequate resources to collect PROMs as the main barrier for investigators [66, 67]. There has also been an increased effort in developing frameworks and protocols to facilitate the incorporation of PROMs in clinical practice using technology [68–71]. However, these frameworks can only provide some guidance while individual healthcare systems will need to modify or develop their implementation frameworks based on the available resources.

Some steps to facilitate PROM use in clinical practice include integrating outcome measures within Electronic Medical Records (EMR), providing training to clinicians and healthcare professionals on implementing PROMs, and interpreting and communicating the results of PROMs. To make implementing PROMs in routine clinical practice a success, it has to be easy for patients and families to complete them. Incorporating these into an EMR and having the opportunity to complete PROMs ahead of their clinical visit either at home or at the time of check-in at the clinic are some examples of how this can be made more manageable for the patients. Patients and families will also be more inclined to complete the PROMs if they see a meaningful discussion about the results from their PROMs with their healthcare providers. Individual teams will need to tailor their clinic flows to fit these important discussions around the results of PROMs to review the success of certain treatments or to discuss significant unexpected changes in results. Visuals such as Power BI (Business intelligence) dashboards used to show the change in PROM scores over time is one of the many examples to share data with the clinical teams and patients for more meaningful engagement.

Future Directions

Though clinical data will always take precedence over other outcome measures, it will still be highly important for healthcare systems to implement appropriate frameworks that can support the routine incorporation of validated outcome measures into clinical practice. Improved results from PROMs can be important indicators of the success of procedures. Unexpected changes in scores from PROMs can be used to flag patients and help identify problems that can otherwise remain undetected during routine clinical appointments. The use of PROMs to measure the value and quality of orthopedic surgery, in general, has been well advocated in the past and can be used to estimate the quality-adjusted life-years (QALYs) and provide informed value-based care [72–75]. However, we have yet to see PROMs being used to calculate QALYs and inform value-based care in pediatric limb reconstruction. Lastly, future work also needs to focus on examining how we can incorporate PROMs to optimize surgical decision-making to improve patient-reported outcomes while still aligning with the patient's goals and expectations.

Commentary

Unni G. Narayanan
unni.narayanan@sickkids.ca

The effectiveness of an intervention, or how well it works, is best judged by whether it achieves the goals for which it is intended. The goals are those that arise from the lived experiences of patients (with a particular condition) which influence their concerns, desires, and expectations, collectively labeled as patient priorities [76]. Effectiveness is most meaningfully evaluated using outcome measures that incorporate the priorities and goals of patients, and therefore must be reported by patients themselves. The value of patient-reported outcome measures (PROMs) is increasingly well acknowledged but not as widely applied in pediatric orthopedics [77]. Too often our field has focused on outcomes that are technical [78], such as radiographic measures of length and alignment. These metrics are important to consider as they are direct measures of the immediate objectives of our interventions. However, these are just a means to an end, and cannot be assumed to translate to the outcomes that really matter to patients. In children with lower limb deformities, these might include the domains of appearance, body image and self-esteem, or participation in life activities. The quality of a PROM isn't merely a function of its completion by the patient. What they report on must be relevant and important to them. The content of the PROM must have been derived from direct input of patients with the lived experience, or their parents (proxy perspective), when we are considering pediatric conditions.

In their chapter entitled *"Outcome measures in limb lengthening and deformity correction,"* Chhina and Cooper provide an excellent overview of these concepts and shed light on PROMs in general and the current state of PROMs for pediatric lower limb differences. They introduce the concepts of generic and condition-specific PROMs and make a compelling argument for the latter when it comes to capturing issues that are most relevant to the population of interest. The chapter includes a list of resources and repositories of PROMs and provides an excellent summary of what goes into the development of a PROM. They provide a comprehensive list of criteria to consider when choosing a PROM and judging its merits—based on its content, structure, and psychometric properties. They go further to discuss how to incorporate the use of PROMs within routine clinical practice by incorporating these into the electronic medical record, and how these efforts can facilitate shared decision-making and promote Quality Improvement (QI).

The chapter includes a review of the PROMs that have been used in published studies of lower limb deformity in children and discusses their many limitations. Some are generic measures, whose content is unlikely to be pertinent to the population. Many were developed and intended for adults, while others were adapted from

PROMs developed for another condition. Most were developed without sufficient, if any, input from children with limb deformities or their parents. It would have been helpful if the authors had used their listed criteria to evaluate each of these PROMs to systematically illustrate their deficiencies and provide the justification for a new measure.

The authors surprisingly neglect to mention their own rigorous efforts to develop a PROM following from their published systematic review on the subject. They have followed the guidelines for PROM development, using qualitative methods to engage participants from many countries and cultures to generate the items for a new PROM, the LIMB-Q Kids for this population [79]. Their approach is exemplary, and this ongoing work is proceeding with the next steps to establish the psychometric properties of this PROM.

The authors identify only the condition-specific measure developed specifically for lower limb differences in children, the development, and validation of which was published after their systematic review. The GOAL-LD was created on the model of the GOAL questionnaire, originally developed for children with ambulatory cerebral palsy. Using the Patient Priority Framework [80] to underpin the development of this PROM, children with lower limb deficiencies, deformities, and length differences, their parents were iteratively interviewed to generate the content and structure of GOAL-LD. The content was vetted by an international group of clinician experts, and subsequently tested for its sensibility (face and content validity, including relevance and importance, comprehensiveness comprehensibility, and feasibility) using cognitive interviews of additional patients and parents to establish the final version of the GOAL-LD [81]. It then underwent formal psychometric evaluation of its reliability, construct, and convergent validity in an international multicenter study [82]. Its responsiveness or sensitivity to change has not yet been established. The GOAL-LD is unique in that it asks respondents to report for each item whether making an improvement on that item is an important goal they are seeking. In doing so, the GOAL-LD serves as an instrument to elicit patient and parent goals and to facilitate shared decision-making and informed consent. How the GOAL-LD compares with LIMB-Q Kids will require further study.

In the meantime, clinicians and researchers involved in the care of children with lower limb differences may need to well read this chapter to familiarize themselves with the concepts that can guide their assessments of the effectiveness of their interventions or their research efforts to make these judgments.

References

1. Ware JE Jr, Sherbourne CD. The MOS 36-item short-form health survey (SF-36). I. Conceptual framework and item selection. Med Care. 1992;30(6):473–83.
2. Varni JWP, Seid MP, Kurtin PSMD. PedsQL(TM) 4.0: reliability and validity of the pediatric quality of life inventory(TM) version 4.0 generic core scales in healthy and patient populations. Med Care. 2001;39(8):800–12.
3. Landgraf JM, Maunsell E, Speechley KN, Bullinger M, Campbell S, Abetz L, et al. Canadian-French, German and UK versions of the Child Health Questionnaire: methodology and preliminary item scaling results. Qual Life Res. 1998;7(5):433–45.
4. Patrick DL, Deyo RA. Generic and disease-specific measures in assessing health status and quality of life. Med Care. 1989;27(3 Suppl):217–32.
5. McCarthy J, Iobst C, Rozbruch SR, Sabharwal S, Eismann E. Limb lengthening and reconstruction society AIM index reliably assesses lower limb deformity. Clin Orthop Relat Res. 2013;471(2):621–7.
6. Kluzek S, Dean B, Wartolowska KA. Patient-reported outcome measures (PROMs) as proof of treatment efficacy. BMJ Evid Based Med. 2021:bmjebm-2020-111573. Available from: http://ebm.bmj.com/content/early/2021/06/03/bmjebm-2020-111573.abstract
7. Truong WH, Price MJ, Agarwal KN, Suryavanshi JR, Somasegar S, Thompson M, et al. Utilization of a wide array of nonvalidated outcome scales in pediatric orthopaedic publications: can't we all measure the same thing? J Pediatr Orthop. 2019;39(2):E153–8.
8. Chhina H, Klassen A, Kopec J, Park S, Fortes C, Cooper A. Quality of life of children with lower limb deformities: a systematic review of patient-reported outcomes and developement of a preliminary conceptual framework. J Limb Lengthening Reconstr. 2017;3(1):19–29.
9. Antonios T, Barker A, Ibrahim I, Scarsbrook C, Smitham PJ, David Goodier W, et al. A systematic review of patient-reported outcome measures used in circular frame fixation. Strateg Trauma Limb Reconstr. 2019;14(1):34–44.
10. Sabharwal S. Patient reported outcome measures for lower limb deformities: let's do it. J Limb Lengthening Reconstr. 2017;3(1):30. Available from: https://www.jlimblengthrecon.org/article.asp?issn=2455-3719
11. Leggett H, Scantlebury A, Sharma H, Hewitt C, Harden M, McDaid C. Quality of life following a lower limb reconstructive procedure: a protocol for the development of a conceptual framework. BMJ Open. 2020;10(12):1–7.
12. Fabricant P, Borst E, Green S, Marx R, Fragomen A, Rozbruch S. Validation of a modified Scoliosis Research Society instrument for patients with limb deformity: the limb deformity-Scoliosis Research Society (LD-SRS) score. J Limb Lengthen Reconstr. 2016;2(2):86–93.
13. Wright J, Timms A, Fugazzotto S, Goodier D. Development of a patient-reported outcome measure in limb reconstruction: a pilot study assesing face validity. Bone Joint Open. 2021;2(9):705–9.
14. Haher TR. Results of the scoliosis research society instrument for evaluation of surgical outcome in adolescent idiopathic scoliosis. Spine. 1999;24(14):1435–40.
15. Heath MR, Shin TJ, Mehta R, Principe PS, Rozbruch SR. Patients with lower limb deformity report worse quality of life than control subjects regardless of degree of deformity. J AAOS Glob Res Rev. 2021;5(8):1–6.
16. Galal S, Shin J, Principe P, Khabyeh-Hasbani N, Mehta R, Hamilton A, et al. STRYDE versus PRECICE magnetic internal lengthening nail for femur lengthening. Arch Orthop Trauma Surg. 2021;142:0123456789. https://doi.org/10.1007/s00402-021-03943-8.

17. Johanson NA, Liang MH, Daltroy L, Rudicel S, Richmond J. American Academy of Orthopaedic Surgeons lower limb outcomes assessment instruments. Reliability, validity, and sensitivity to change. J Bone Jt Surg. 2004;86(5):902.
18. Lee KM, Chung CY, Gwon DK, Sung KH, Cho JH, Kim TW, et al. Parental perspectives on leg length discrepancy. J Pediatr Orthop Part B. 2012 Mar;21(2):146–9.
19. Johansen H, Dammann B, Øinæs Andersen L, Andresen IL. Children with congenital limb deficiency in Norway: issues related to school life and health-related quality of life. A cross-sectional study. Disabil Rehabil. 2016;38(18):1803–10.
20. Varni JW, Thompson KL, Hanson V. The Varni/Thompson Pediatric Pain Questionnaire. I. Chronic musculoskeletal pain in juvenile rheumatoid arthritis. Pain. 1987;28(1):27–38.
21. Varni JW, Sherman SA, Burwinkle TM, Dickinson PE, Dixon P. The PedsQL™ family impact module: preliminary reliability and validity. Heal Qual Life Outcomes. 2004;2(55):1–6.
22. Piers E, Harris D, Herzberg D. Piers-Harris 2: Piers-Harris children's self-concept scale. 2nd ed. Los Angeles: Western Psychological Services; 2002.
23. Reynolds C, Kamphaus R. BASC-2: behaviour assessment system for children. 2nd ed. Circle Pines: American Guidance Service; 2004.
24. Birch JG, Paley D, Herzenberg JE, Morton A, Ward S, Riddle R, et al. Amputation versus staged reconstruction for severe fibular hemimelia. JBJS Open Access. 2019;4(2):e0053.
25. Pruitt SD, Varni JW, Seid M, Setoguchi Y. Prosthesis satisfaction outcome measurement in pediatric limb deficiency. Arch Phys Med Rehabil. 1997;78(7):750–4.
26. Griffiths AL, Donnan LT, Iobst CA, Kelley SP, Bouchard M, Narayanan UG. The gait outcomes assessment list for children with lower limb difference (GOAL-LD): assessment of reliability and validity. J Pediatr Orthop. 2021;41(7):450–6.
27. Cella D, Yount S, Rothrock N, Gershon R, Cook K, Reeve B, et al. The patient-reported outcomes measurement information system (PROMIS): progress of an NIH roadmap cooperative group during its first two years. Med Care. 2007;45(5 SUPPL. 1):S3–S11.
28. Amakoutou K, Liu RW. Current use of patient-reported outcomes in pediatric limb deformity surgery. J Pediatr Orthop Part B. 2021;30:399–404.
29. Phillips L, Carsen S, Vasireddi A, Mulpuri K. Use of patient-reported outcome measures in pediatric orthopaedic literature. J Pediatr Orthop. 2018;38(8):393–7.
30. d'Entremont AG, Cooper AP, Johari A, Mulpuri K. What clinimetric evidence exists for using hip-specific patient-reported outcome measures in pediatric hip impingement? Clin Orthop Relat Res. 2015;473(4):1361–7.
31. U.S Food and Drug Administration. U.S Department of Health and Human Services Food and Drug Administration guidance for industry: patient-reported outcome measures: use in medical product development to support labeling claims. [Internet]. Vol. 2014; 2009 [cited 2016 Feb 19]. Available from: http://www.fda.gov/downloads/Drugs/GuidanceComplianceRegulatoryInformation/Guidances/UCM193282.pdf.
32. Emery MP, Lou PL, Acquardo C. Patient-reported outcome and quality of life instruments database (PROQOLID): frequently asked questions. Health Qual Life Outcomes. 2005;3:1–6.
33. ICHOM Connect [Internet]. [cited 2022 Mar 16]. Available from: https://connect.ichom.org/resources/?rcat=overall-paediatric-health
34. Reeve BB, Wyrwich KW, Wu AW, Velikova G, Terwee CB, Snyder CF, et al. ISOQOL recommends minimum standards for patient-reported outcome measures used in patient-centered outcomes and comparative effectiveness research. Qual Life Res. 2013;22(8):1889–905.
35. Mokkink LB, Terwee CB, Patrick DL, Alonso J, Stratford PW, Knol DL, et al. The COSMIN study reached international consensus on taxonomy, terminology, and definitions of measurement properties for health-related patient-reported outcomes. J Clin Epidemiol. 2010 Jul;63(7):737–45.
36. Revicki DA, Osoba D, Fairclough D, Barofsky I, Berzon R, Leidy NK, et al. Recommendations on health-related quality of life research to support labeling and promotional claims in the United States. Qual Life Res. 2000;9(8):887–900.
37. Mokkink LB, Terwee CB, Patrick DL, Alonso J, Stratford PW, Knol DL, et al. The COSMIN checklist for assessing the methodological quality of studies on measurement properties of health status measurement instruments: an international Delphi study. Qual Life Res. 2010 May;19(4):539–49.
38. U.S. Department of Health and Human Services FDA Center for Drug Evaluation and Research. Guidance for industry: patient-reported outcome measures: use in medical product development to support labeling claims: draft guidance. Health Qual Life Outcomes. 2006;4:79.
39. European Medicines Agency. Reflection paper on the regulatory guidance for the use of health-related quality of life (Hrql) measures in the evaluation of medicinal products. Reproduction. 2005;January 2006:1–5.
40. Terwee CB, Prinsen CAC, Chiarotto A, Westerman MJ, Patrick DL, Alonso J, et al. COSMIN methodology for evaluating the content validity of patient-reported outcome measures: a Delphi study, Quality of life research, vol. 27. Springer International Publishing; 2018. p. 1159–70.
41. Patrick DL, Burke LB, Gwaltney CJ, Leidy NK, Martin ML, Molsen E, et al. Content validity—establishing and reporting the evidence in newly developed patient-reported outcomes (PRO) instruments for medical product evaluation: ISPOR PRO good research practices task force report: part 1—eliciting concepts for a new PRO instrument. Value Heal. 2011;14(8):967–77.
42. Patrick DL, Burke LB, Gwaltney CJ, Leidy NK, Martin ML, Molsen E, et al. Content validity - establishing and reporting the evidence in newly developed patient-reported outcomes (PRO) instruments for medical product evaluation: ISPOR PRO good research practices task force report: part 2 - assessing respondent understanding. Value Heal. 2011 Dec;14(8):978–88.
43. Mokkink LB, Terwee CB, Knol DL, Stratford PW, Alonso J, Patrick DL, et al. The COSMIN checklist for evaluating the methodological quality of studies on measurement properties: a clarification of its content. BMC Med Res Methodol. 2010;10:1–8.
44. Arbuckle R, Abetz-Webb L. Not just little adults: qualitative methods to support the development of pediatric patient-reported outcomes. Patient. 2013;6(3):143–59.
45. Eiser C, Morse R. Can parents rate their child's health-related quality of life? Results of a systematic review. Qual Life Res. 2001;10(4):347–57.
46. Tomlinson D, Plenert E, Dadzie G, Loves R, Cook S, Schechter T, et al. Reasons for disagreement between proxy-report and self-report rating of symptoms in children receiving cancer therapies. Support Care Cancer. 2021;29(7):4165–70.
47. Smith LE, Weinman J, Yiend J, Rubin J. Psychosocial factors affecting parental report of symptoms in children: a systematic review. Psychosom Med. 2020;82(2):187–96.
48. Matsumoto H, Vitale MG, Hyman JE, Roye DP. Can parents rate their children's quality of life? Perspectives on pediatric orthopedic outcomes. J Pediatr Orthop Part B. 2011;20(3):184–90.
49. Mokkink LB, Terwee CB, Patrick DL, Alonso J, Stratford W, Knol DL, et al. The COSMIN checklist for assessing the methodological quality of studies on measurement properties of health status measurement instruments: an international Delphi study. Qual Life Res. 2010;19(4):539–49.
50. Revicki D, Hays RD, Cella D, Sloan J. Recommended methods for determining responsiveness and minimally important differences for patient-reported outcomes. J Clin Epidemiol. 2008;61(2):102–9.

51. Guyatt G, Walter S, Norman G. Measuring change over time: assessing the usefulness of evaluative instruments. J Chronic Dis. 1987;40(2):171–8.
52. Sprangers MA, Moinpour CM, Moynihan TJ, Patrick DL, Revicki DA. Assessing meaningful change in quality of life over time: a users' guide for clinicians. Mayo Clin Proc. 2002;77(6):561–71.
53. Hobart JC, Cano SJ, Thompson AJ. Effect sizes can be misleading: is it time to change the way we measure change ? J Neurol Neurosurg Psychiatry. 2010;81(9):1044–8.
54. Wild D, Eremenco S, Mear I, Martin M, Houchin C, Gawlicki M, et al. Multinational trials-recommendations on the translations required, approaches to using the same language in different c. Value Heal. 2009;12(4):430–40.
55. Wild D, Grove A, Martin M, Eremenco S, McElroy S, Verjee-Lorenz A, et al. Principles of good practice for the translation and cultural adaptation process for patient-reported outcomes (PRO) measures: report of the ISPOR task force for translating adaptation. Value Heal. 2005;2(2):94–104.
56. Wong Riff KWY, Tsangaris E, Goodacre T, Forrest CR, Pusic AL, Cano SJ, et al. International multiphase mixed methods study protocol to develop a cross-cultural patient-reported outcome instrument for children and young adults with cleft lip and/or palate (CLEFT-Q). BMJ Open. 2017;7:e015467.
57. Creswell JW, Plano Clark VL, Gutmann M, Hanson W. Advanced mixed methods research designs. In: Tashakkori A, Teddlie C, editors. Handbook of mixed methods in social & behavioral research. Thousand Oaks: Sage; 2003. p. 209–40.
58. Lasch KE, Marquis P, Vigneux M, Abetz L, Arnould B, Bayliss M, et al. PRO development: rigorous qualitative research as the crucial foundation. Qual Life Res. 2010;19(8):1087–96.
59. Terwee CB, Prinsen CA, Chiarotto A, De Vet H, Bouter LM, Marjan JA, et al. COSMIN methodology for assessing the content validity of PROMs User manual version 1.0 [Internet]. Available from: www.cosmin.nl
60. Linacre J. Sample size and item calibration stability. Rasch Meas Trans. 1994;7(28):328.
61. Rasch G. Probabilistic models for some intelligence and attainment tests. Inf Control. 1961;4:382.
62. Andrich D. Rasch models for measurement. Newbury Park: SAGE Publications, Inc; 1988.
63. Hobart J, Cano S. Improving the evaluation of therapeutic interventions in multiple sclerosis: the role of new psychometric methods. In: Health technology assessment, vol. 13; 2009. p. 1–177.
64. World Health Organisation. Process of translation and adaptation of instruments [Internet]. [cited 2017 Jan 19]. Available from: http://www.who.int/substance_abuse/research_tools/translation/en/
65. Wright B. Rating scale analysis: Rasch measurement. Chicago: MESA; 1982.
66. Philpot LM, Barnes SA, Brown RM, Austin JA, James CS, Stanford RH, et al. Barriers and benefits to the use of patient-reported outcome measures in routine clinical care: a qualitative study. Am J Med Qual. 2018;33(4):359–64.
67. Foster A, Croot L, Brazier J, Harris J, O'cathain A. The facilitators and barriers to implementing patient reported outcome measures in organisations delivering health related services: a systematic review of reviews. J Patient Rep Outcomes. 2018;2:1–16.
68. Hsiao CJ, Dymek C, Kim B, Russell B. Advancing the use of patient-reported outcomes in practice: understanding challenges, opportunities, and the potential of health information technology. Qual Life Res. 2019;28(6):1575–83. https://doi.org/10.1007/s11136-019-02112-0.
69. Nguyen H, Butow P, Dhillon H, Sundaresan P. A review of the barriers to using Patient-Reported Outcomes (PROs) and Patient-Reported Outcome Measures (PROMs) in routine cancer care. J Med Radiat Sci. 2021;68(2):186–95.
70. Porter I, Gonçalves-Bradley D, Ricci-Cabello I, Gibbons C, Gangannagaripalli J, Fitzpatrick R, et al. Framework and guidance for implementing patient-reported outcomes in clinical practice: evidence, challenges and opportunities. J Comp Eff Res. 2016;5(5):507–19.
71. Stover AM, Haverman L, van Oers HA, Greenhalgh J, Potter CM, Ahmed S, et al. Using an implementation science approach to implement and evaluate patient-reported outcome measures (PROM) initiatives in routine care settings. Qual Life Res. 2020;30:3015–33.
72. Devlin NJ, Appleby J, Buxton M, Vallance-Owen A. Getting the most out of PROMS. Putting health outcomes at the heart of NHS decision making. Health Econ. 2010;
73. Ayers DC, Zheng H, Franklin PD. Integrating patient-reported outcomes into orthopaedic clinical practice: proof of concept from FORCE-TJR. Clin Orthop Relat Res. 2013;471(11):3419–25.
74. (AAOS) AA of OS. Public Reporting of Provider Performance. 2012.
75. Schilling C, Dowsey MM, Clarke PM, Choong PF. Using patient-reported outcomes for economic evaluation: getting the timing right. Value Heal. 2016;19(8):945–50. https://doi.org/10.1016/j.jval.2016.05.014.
76. Narayanan UG. Concerns, desires and expectations of surgery for adolescent idiopathic scoliosis: a comparison of patients', parents' and surgeons' perspectives. Toronto: Health Policy Management & Evaluation, University of Toronto; 2008. Available from: https://tspace.library.utoronto.ca/bitstream/1807/11155/1/Narayanan_Unni_G_2008June_MSc_thesis.pdf
77. Narayanan UG. Outcomes in pediatric orthopaedics. In: Bhandari M, editor. Evidence-based orthopaedics. 2nd ed. Wiley Blackwell BMJ Books; 2021. Chapter 173. p. 1019–28.
78. Goldberg MJ. Measuring outcomes in cerebral palsy. J Pediatr Orthop. 1991;11(5):682–5.
79. Chhina H, Klassen A, Bade D, Kopec J, Cooper A. Establishing content validity of LIMB-Q Kids: a new patient-reported outcome measure for lower limb deformities. Qual Life Res. 2022;31(9):2805–18.
80. Narayanan UG. The patient priority framework. In: Priority based scales for children's outcomes—research & evaluation (PSCORE) program: https://lab.research.sickkids.ca/pscoreprogram/.
81. Dermott JA, Wright FV, Salbach NM, Narayanan UG. Development of the gait outcomes assessment list for lower-limb differences (GOAL-LD) questionnaire: a child and parent reported outcome measure. Health Qual Life Outcomes. 2021;19(1):139.
82. Griffiths AL, Donnan LT, Iobst CA, Kelley SP, Bouchard M, Narayanan UG. The gait outcomes assessment list for children with lower limb difference (GOAL-LD): Assessment of reliability and validity. J Pediatr Orthop. 2021;41(7):450–6.

Keys to Building a Successful Pediatric Limb Reconstruction Program

Christopher A. Iobst and Anirejuoritse Bafor

Introduction

Over the past 20 years, pediatric orthopedics has gradually become increasingly subspecialized. The increasingly rapid advancement of pediatric orthopedic knowledge and surgical techniques has made it more difficult to remain proficient in all areas of the field. Surgeons have also started to identify and concentrate on personal areas of special interest within pediatric orthopedics. As a result, specific disciplines within pediatric orthopedics, such as spine, sports, hip, and hand, are now recognized as distinct subspecialties.

Pediatric limb reconstruction, however, is not universally recognized as a separate subspecialty. For example, it was not listed as one of the choices of primary clinical interest in the 2017 POSNA member needs assessment. 2023 was the first year that the American Academy of Orthopedic Surgeons gave limb lengthening and limb reconstruction a separate designation for instructional course lectures and scientific presentations. These omissions may be explained by the fact that limb reconstruction appears to overlap with so many different aspects of orthopedics. Nevertheless, developing a distinct limb reconstruction program as part of your institution's orthopedic strategy should be encouraged. The existence of such programs has been shown to have multiple benefits to the entire orthopedic department [1].

The purpose of this chapter is to provide recommendations regarding how to build a dedicated limb reconstruction practice from two vantage points: (1) for surgeons who work in resource-available environments and (2) for surgeons who work in resource-limited environments.

C. A. Iobst (✉) · A. Bafor
Department of Orthopedic Surgery, Nationwide Children's Hospital, Columbus, OH, USA
e-mail: christopher.iobst@nationwidechildrens.org;
Anirejuoritse.Bafor@nationwidechildrens.org

Resource Available Model

Surgeon

The keystone of any limb reconstruction practice is the surgeon. As the supervisor of the entire program, the surgeon must perform many roles. Beyond the expected clinical duties involving patients in the clinic and the operating room, the surgeon must organize and manage a large multi-disciplinary team of providers that support the daily activities of the program. In addition, to this clinical team, the surgeon may desire to develop and coordinate a research team and a marketing team. The required management and promotional skills are not concepts that are usually taught as part of the formal medical school or residency education process. Nevertheless, it is this combination of clinical, surgical, research, leadership, and interpersonal skills that make the limb reconstruction surgeon's job description unique.

Pediatric limb reconstruction is a challenging profession both mentally and physically. Not only does it require surgical dexterity but it demands fastidious attention to detail and the ability to effectively analyze and design solutions to complex problems. To become proficient at limb reconstruction, it is highly recommended that the surgeon fully dedicate himself/herself to the field. Limb reconstruction needs to be the focus of the practice not just an occasional occurrence. The following are suggested items to help prepare the surgeon who may be interested in limb reconstruction:

1. Building an educational foundation

    Before requesting to manage limb reconstruction patients, the surgeon first needs to develop a knowledge base. This foundation is ideally formed by supervised training either through a fellowship(s) or by working with an experienced colleague. While it is possible to try to train yourself in situations where direct supervision is not available, the process takes longer and is not as smooth. The following options provide directed training in limb reconstruction:

(a) Pediatric orthopedic or orthopedic trauma fellowship

Traditional fellowship programs at institutions that also contain a well-established limb reconstruction program provide an opportunity for training. Although the limb reconstruction experience is limited by the time required in the other disciplines of the fellowship specialty, the fellow can still build a solid base if he/she can spend at least 3–6 months with the limb reconstruction team.

(b) Limb reconstruction fellowship

There are several centers in the United States (and internationally) that offer dedicated limb lengthening and reconstruction fellowships. These reconstruction fellowships often incorporate a mixture of pediatric and adult deformity patients and provide a strong foundation for a career in limb reconstruction. Depending on the surgeon's goals, these reconstruction fellowships can be taken in isolation or as a complement to another orthopedic fellowship.

(c) Traveling fellowship

The Limb Lengthening and Reconstruction Society (LLRS) offers a 1 month traveling fellowship that sends participants to four different limb reconstruction centers each for a week at a time. This intensive learning experience is designed for young surgeons to enhance their prior training and gain exposure to current limb reconstruction techniques.

2. Continuing education

Once the fellowship training is over, the real learning begins. As your limb reconstruction experience begins to grow, you will realize that your knowledge base continuously needs to be augmented and expanded. There are several methods to continue the education process:

(a) Educational courses

Educational courses, both CME and non-CME events, provide an avenue for learning either broad topics (i.e., limb deformity analysis) or more specific surgical techniques (i.e., internal lengthening nails). Not only is it recommended to attend these courses but it is often beneficial to repeat them. With each successive exposure to the course material, the surgeon will absorb new information as his/her experience grows. Courses also provide an opportunity for networking with fellow attendees and faculty members. This is an understated but valuable component of the courses. Connecting with colleagues and potential mentors who will become resources for advice is crucial to a young surgeon's development. This networking is also a useful way to develop research partnerships.

(b) Visiting limb reconstruction surgeons

Arrange short private visits to experienced limb reconstruction surgeons. These visits provide the opportunity to shadow one on one with an established limb reconstruction surgeon and observe how he/she manages the clinic team, organizes his/her operating room, and he/she evaluates patients. Some visits may even be sponsored by industry if they are designed to observe and learn a specific skill set. Multiple visits to several different surgeons are recommended because they provide the opportunity to compare and contrast different styles and select the components from each practice that are the most beneficial to you. Repeat visits to the same surgeon provide the opportunity to pick up nuances that you may have missed the first time and strengthen the professional rapport between you and your host.

(c) Find a mentor

Because pediatric limb reconstruction encompasses such a wide array of patient types and surgical procedures, finding a mentor (or mentors) to guide you is extremely important. Joining a group that already has an established limb deformity specialist is the ideal situation for a young surgeon. Working side by side with an experienced surgeon who can provide daily guidance provides the best framework for success. Unfortunately, many pediatric orthopedic departments do not have a dedicated limb deformity specialist on staff. Therefore, young surgeons need to find a trusted and willing mentor. Fortunately, email and video chats allow cases to be discussed almost instantaneously with practically any colleague around the world. Despite these virtual opportunities to interface with an experienced surgeon, finding a local mentor, i.e., someone within easy driving distance, is still recommended. Face-to-face discussions are still the most valuable means to discuss cases/techniques. In addition, a local mentor provides an opportunity to conveniently observe cases, which will increase your knowledge base.

(d) Reading list

There are vast volumes of material written about limb reconstruction. Deciding what are the most valuable resources to read can be confusing. Appendix A provides a suggested core reading list for limb reconstruction surgeons.

(e) Limb reconstruction societies

Most countries have a national limb reconstruction or Association for the Study and Application of the Methods of Ilizarov (ASAMI) society. In North America, the Limb Lengthening and Reconstruction Society (LLRS) hosts an annual scientific meeting. These meetings provide an opportunity to see the latest research and surgical techniques being performed by colleagues around the world. There are usually educational workshops or courses attached to the meeting where you can learn new skills or enhance existing ones. The meeting exhibit hall conveniently assembles all the orthopedic companies related to limb reconstruction in one place, which makes it easy to explore the latest available technology. Volunteering your time on society committees keeps you informed of policies and discussions that may be affecting the field and allows you to contribute to the decision-making.

(f) Teaching

Inviting medical students, residents, or fellows to the clinic/OR provides an opportunity to teach. Instead of focusing on how they may slow you down, consider these two points:

1. There is no better way to develop mastery of a subject than having to teach it to another person. By teaching others, you will benefit by improving your own skills.
2. Create an environment where the students/residents/fellows are encouraged to be curious and ask questions. Answering their questions will keep you intellectually stimulated, and the subsequent discussions may generate a research idea or concept that may not have been apparent to you.

(g) Share your experience

Presenting your work at society meetings and conferences is another valuable method to increase your experience and knowledge base. Direct feedback from colleagues can help to identify strengths and weaknesses in your development. Initially, study what you have available and then gradually expand into multi-center studies or basic science research.

Develop a Limb Reconstruction Team

No limb reconstruction program can achieve success without a well-organized team. While the surgeon may be considered the main element of a limb reconstruction practice, he/she represents just one piece of a much larger interconnected network of care providers. Like other high-performance units, such as Navy SEALs, airline flight crews, or auto racing pit crews, an effective limb reconstruction program requires a cohesive team of people working toward a common goal [3].

1. Clinic co-pilot

After the surgeon, the most indispensable limb reconstruction team member is the designated provider responsible for running the clinic. In many ways, this person is more important than the surgeon since he/she will be interacting with the patients on the front lines every day. The medical background of this team member may be different at different centers (nurse, nurse practitioner, physician assistant, and nonoperative physician) but their role is the same. He/she is the person(s) responsible for knowing the details of every patient and how to manage their care in coordination with the surgeon. Depending on how busy the program is, this may be one person or multiple people, but their role is to function as the surgeon's most trusted assistant. This person must be proficient in many vital (and time-consuming) patient care areas such as educating pin site care, educating limb lengthening protocols, changing dressings, managing pin site infections, performing frame adjustments, and troubleshooting limb lengthening devices. While it requires a substantial investment of time to prepare the "co-pilot" to be comfortable and competent to independently manage the nuances of limb reconstruction patients, the development of this provider is essential to the success of the program. In addition to training the co-pilot yourself, consider sending him/her to educational courses to complement and boost their knowledge base. This provider must be dedicated solely to the limb reconstruction program on a full-time basis and should be the first person the surgeon adds to the team.

2. Additional clinic staff

For the clinic to run efficiently, each surgeon should have a medical assistant, a nurse, and a mid-level provider (physician assistant or nurse practitioner) at a minimum. Residents and fellows will come and go but these providers should be assigned to work with the surgeon on a full-time, daily basis. Because the management of limb reconstruction patients has so many unique components, the effectiveness of the care suffers when there are multiple different, rotating providers rather than the same team at each clinic. In addition to regular clinic duties, this core team will be responsible for handling the daily patient phone calls, emails, paperwork, and unscheduled visits especially when the surgeon is in the operating room or out of the office.

3. Limb reconstruction program administrative assistant or office coordinator

A person dedicated to the scheduling of limb reconstruction patient clinic visits and surgeries is another necessary team member. Many patients will have frequent visits to clinics and/or physical therapy that need to be organized and monitored. The coordinator will be responsible for arranging this process and alerting the team when patients miss scheduled visits. This coordination is especially vital for families that routinely travel long distances or for those that are traveling to your program from out of state or out of the country.

4. Physical therapists

Having physical therapists specifically trained in limb reconstruction rehabilitation is crucial to the success of any program. The physical therapist(s) will be working closely with many of the limb reconstruction patients and provide a central role in the surgical outcomes. Often the therapist will be the first to recognize subtle changes in the range of motion, weight-bearing status, or pain levels in your patients and can alert you to potential trouble. Ideally, the therapist should be on-site to allow direct, real-time communication about each patient. Having a therapist who is dedicated to your clinic is essential for two reasons:

  (a) A therapist assigned to your patients full-time allows the therapist to rapidly develop his/her expertise in limb reconstruction patient rehabilitation. These patients have their own unique therapy needs, and an experienced therapist can often make the difference between a mediocre and a good outcome. If your patients are sent to various therapists at multiple locations around the community, it is virtually impossible to know the level of care quality that your patients are receiving. The designated therapist will also be a resource for communicating with and educating other therapists who will provide ongoing care and guidance within the patient's home community. This is especially important in more rural settings where exposure to limb lengthening and reconstruction will be rare.

  (b) Having a dedicated therapist(s) allows the surgeon to obtain near-instantaneous feedback on the patient's progress and make appropriate decisions based on this information. Offsite therapists can communicate with the surgeon by phone or email, but it is usually hours or days after the session takes place when it is too late to make meaningful changes.

  Once you have identified your primary therapist or team of therapists, send them to visit established limb-lengthening centers. Visiting other centers to exchange ideas and learn new skills is just as important for the therapist as it is for the surgeon.

5. Psychologist

  Pediatric limb reconstruction patients often undergo prolonged, sometimes repeated, treatment regimens over the course of their lifetime. Having a psychologist to help them and their families through these stressful situations is valuable on multiple levels.

  (a) The psychologist can help them navigate the anxiety and depression that are often associated with the reconstruction journey.
  (b) They can also teach pain management strategies to help decrease the need for prescription pain medicine and muscle relaxants.
  (c) The psychologist can screen preoperative patients for warning signs that may indicate the patient or family may not be a good candidate for a limb reconstruction procedure at that time. There are often many co-existing medical, family, or social stressors that the surgeon may not recognize (or have time to recognize) that could negatively influence the postoperative course. The psychologist can analyze these factors and help the surgeon make an informed decision about the best surgical option for each individual patient and family.

6. Physiatrist

  Limb reconstruction patients will often have orthotic and prosthetic needs. Partnering with a physiatrist who has expertise in managing limb deficiency patients can be very helpful. If possible, try to schedule the physiatrist's clinic concurrently with yours so patients can see each of you in the same setting. This also facilitates discussing the patient's management together in real time.

7. Social worker

  An evaluation of the patient and their family's home/social situation prior to surgery is important. Because many patients will need to be seen in the clinic on a weekly or bi-weekly basis (as well as supplemental visits for therapy), reliable transportation must be available. The social worker can determine the family's transportation, medical equipment, and additional support needs. Having this analysis before surgery will minimize any post-surgical logistical problems that may jeopardize the patient's outcome.

8. Radiology team

  A large portion of the decision making in limb reconstruction is based on analyzing radiographs. Obtaining accurate, high-quality pre- and postoperative radiographs on a consistent basis is crucial to the surgeon's success. Because getting proper radiographs of limb reconstruction patients can be challenging, it is important to educate the radiology technicians on how to obtain the proper views. Invest time teaching the technicians who work in your clinic how to correctly position the patient and what pitfalls to avoid. Most importantly, do not hesitate to go with the patient to the X-ray suite and assist the technician with the radiograph. Try to keep the same technicians in your clinic each time to minimize the variability in radiograph quality. Obtaining the radiographs can be a stressful and painful experience for the patient and their family. Having the same technician allows him/her to establish a relationship with the patients that they radiograph each week and learn what makes the process more comfortable for them.

  Although most of the immediate radiographic interpretation will be done by the surgeon in the clinic, having a trusted musculoskeletal radiologist is essential. Rare or unusual cases will benefit from having an additional perspective from the radiologist. In addition, discussing the need for advanced imaging on certain patients and the subsequent interpretation of the obtained studies will be enhanced by an experienced orthopedic radiologist.

Limb Reconstruction Clinic Setting

To maximize the quality and efficiency of the limb reconstruction clinic, the following elements are recommended:

(a) Space

The clinic area needs to be big enough to accommodate patients in wheelchairs, multiple family members, and your team. If the rooms are too cramped, it will be difficult to properly evaluate and manage limb reconstruction patients. In addition, there needs to be an unobstructed area where the patient can walk and run a sufficient distance to observe the gait pattern.

(b) Clinic patient scheduling

It is recommended to have a dedicated limb reconstruction clinic where all limb reconstruction patients are seen at the same time. Rather than sprinkle your patients intermittently through your other clinics, create a half-day/whole day that involves only limb reconstruction patients. This arrangement will utilize your team resources most efficiently, especially in the early stages when your practice is just starting to grow. It also provides an opportunity for patients with similar conditions to meet each other and share experiences. Finally, some patient visits can be lengthy, whether it is discussing the treatment options for leg length discrepancy with a new patient or making frame modifications on a postoperative patient. Plan adequate time for each patient visit into the clinic schedule. A very busy limb reconstruction clinic may only see 20–25 patients in an entire day.

(c) Blocks

Have multiple sets of blocks available to evaluate leg length discrepancy in the clinic area. Make sure each block is labeled to allow an accurate calculation of the total height. The radiology suite should also have a set of blocks to use for your standing radiographs. Instruct the radiology technician to note the size of the blocks used on each standing radiograph so the information is easy to reference.

(d) Equipment room/equipment cart

Patients with external fixators will often require frame maintenance during the clinic. Rather than sending someone to the operating room to get supplies each time, create an organized collection of fixation elements, struts, wrenches, ring sizing templates, pin caps, pin clips, etc., and store them in a safe, convenient place in the clinic. Depending on the size of your collection and the available space in your clinic, this equipment can be housed in an entirely separate room or in a large rolling cart. In addition, to save time, try to have several, smaller portable containers filled with the essential items needed for frame maintenance that can be easily transported into the patient room.

(e) Photo/video space

Documenting your patient's preoperative condition and the postoperative change is important in limb reconstruction. Create a designated space for taking high-quality photographs and gait videos. Although modern smartphones have great embedded cameras, you may not be allowed to use your private phone to capture patient images. Therefore, it is recommended to invest in a high-quality digital camera that can be used to store patient images securely. Train one of your team members or have someone from the hospital media department available to be the designated clinic photographer. This will save time for the surgeon and improve the quality and consistency of your images.

Operating Room (OR) Setting

Consistency is the key to running an efficient operating room. Utilizing the same circulating nurse, scrub technician, and radiology technician (C-arm) every day will maximize the productivity of the surgeon. Working with a trained OR team that is familiar with the equipment and flow of limb reconstruction cases can make the difference between a smooth surgery and a stressful surgery. Limb reconstruction cases often involve a lot of equipment trays, often from multiple different companies, which can be overwhelming for a scrub technician who is not familiar with the process. When the same scrub technician is present every day, he/she will not only know the equipment but also be able to anticipate each step of the procedure and have the appropriate instruments ready for the surgeon. In addition, having the same OR staff allows a relationship with the industry representatives to develop, which helps everyone anticipate equipment needs and troubleshoot potential equipment problems for the surgeon.

If you are in a program that has residents and fellows, then you will most likely have their assistance in the operating room. Because their positions are constantly rotating, they may not be familiar with you or your cases. To increase efficiency, consider having a dedicated assistant in the operating room for each case. This person will know your preferences and can provide meaningful assistance with all aspects of the case. In addition, he/she can keep things moving while you stop to teach the residents/fellows.

Using the same radiology technician or core pair of technicians to operate the fluoroscopy machine (C-arm) in every case is another factor that can make a huge difference in the level of stress in the operating room. A technician who is familiar with your cases and understands the required views to complete the surgery is invaluable. Dealing with a different technician each time can decrease efficiency because each image takes longer to acquire. Increased radiation exposure to everyone in the room also becomes an issue with inexperienced technicians who require multiple attempts to obtain the correct image. Having a laser pointer attached to the C-arm helps to eliminate some of the erroneous images.

While it may not be possible to have the same anesthesia staff every day, it is advisable to communicate your antibiotic, regional anesthesia, and muscle relaxation requirements to them before each case. Establishing a consistent routine and promoting open communication with your anesthesia colleagues will also help them perform more efficiently during your cases.

Patient Volume

Once the care team is in place, the next component to building a successful limb reconstruction program is developing a large, consistent patient volume. Many limb reconstruction patients have relatively rare conditions and gaining management experience requires adequate exposure to them. To truly become successful, a surgeon needs to dedicate his/her practice to limb reconstruction and not just dabble in it. Obtaining true expertise requires repetition [3]. Applying one or two hexapod frames or inserting one or two internal lengthening nails per year will not provide the necessary feedback to improve or even maintain the minimum surgical skills. Moreover, mastering the surgical techniques is only part of the required skill set. Gaining the experience to properly manage these patients through the extended and sometimes complicated postoperative period is arguably an even more critical skill to acquire. The only way to effectively develop this competence is if there is a steady supply of limb reconstruction cases in your practice.

There are multiple factors that contribute to establishing patient volume:

1. Joining a department with an already existing limb reconstruction program and surgeon(s)

    Having a well-established patient referral base is the easiest way to ensure being busy from the outset. Unfortunately, these positions and opportunities are relatively rare.
2. Joining a department without an established limb reconstruction program:

    It is far more common that the surgeon will need to build a program de novo or expand a partially developed one. In these situations, choosing to practice in a heavily populated geographic area is important. Pediatric limb reconstruction cases are not as common as other pediatric conditions, such as sports medicine injuries, and require a large population of patients to achieve a critical mass of cases. Trying to establish a dedicated pediatric limb deformity practice in a rural area will be difficult, especially if your patients are required to drive long distances to see you. Keep in mind that many patients will need to see you on a weekly or bi-weekly basis during the postoperative period. Imagine a catchment area that encompasses a population of potential patients within a reasonable driving distance (2–3 h) from your institution. If less than a million people fit within that imaginary circle, it may be hard to develop a robust limb reconstruction practice.
3. Cooperation from colleagues

    Your primary referral source will be patients seen initially by an orthopedic surgeon in your department or the surrounding orthopedic community. These colleagues need to be willing to refer desired patients to you rather than keeping them for themselves. While this can be a sensitive subject in an "eat what you kill" practice model, establishing an environment of reciprocal patient sharing should be encouraged. Fortunately, the limb reconstruction surgeon can be portrayed as a resource to manage complicated patients that other surgeons do not want rather than as a direct competitor for cases. For example, make yourself available to manage complicated extremity fractures that present when other orthopedic colleagues are on call. In many cases, by demonstrating a readiness to take care of complex patients, more straightforward cases will gradually start to follow. Establish a set of criteria for desired and appropriate patient referrals not only with your partners but also with your scheduling department (i.e., leg length evaluations, knock-knee/bowing, contractures, etc.). Having the congenital deficiency cases funneled to you is usually not difficult to arrange, but the relative paucity of these patients will force you to supplement your practice with other types of patients. Convincing your colleagues that it is worthwhile to send all the guided growth and angular/rotational osteotomy cases is critical since these patients will likely become the bulk of your practice. Providing your services as a "resource" for colleagues rather than a "competitor" is a nuanced skill set that one must learn to navigate as your practice grows.
4. Marketing

    Your hospital should help to market your program to attract new patients. This should be a multi-layered approach including print media and social media. The goal is to increase community awareness of your program. Create brochures and newsletters that highlight patient success stories, explain unique features of your program, and describe the services your limb reconstruction team provides. These should be consistently updated and mailed out repeatedly to all physicians in the region. While having a website is essential, it is even more important to have a motivated marketing team to constantly manage and update the content. The website should be easy to navigate and provide educational information to patients and parents. Emphasizing key internet search terms will help to keep your website relevant. Other forms of social media, such as Facebook pages, blogs, or support groups, can be helpful but are time-consuming. Be sure you are ready to commit the necessary resources to maintain these endeavors before you start them. Find a team member who is interested and willing to dedicate time to maintaining your program's social media presence rather than trying to do it by yourself.

5. Speaking engagements

   Speaking engagements are an understated but valuable commodity. Get in front of as many groups of people as possible to showcase the value of your program. No matter how small the audience is, speaking is the most effective method to spread awareness of your practice in the community. Try to give a grand rounds lecture at every hospital in the area. Speak to every department that may be a potential referral source, such as family medicine, pediatrics, endocrinology, nephrology, and genetics. It always helps to place a face with a name—physicians will be more likely to refer appropriate patients to you if they know who you are and what you do. Limb reconstruction is a very visual medium that lends itself well to presentations. Most audiences aren't aware of the current limb reconstruction capabilities and generally leave the talks very impressed with what is possible.

6. Be available

   If you are affable, available, and able, colleagues will notice and increase their willingness to send patients your way. Word of mouth in your local medical community will spread awareness of your skills (good or bad), which will create opportunities for growth. However, for a limb reconstruction program to be successful, it is vitally important that the surgeon stay in one place for a prolonged period of time. Because these programs take time to build, a surgeon who moves from one location to another every few years will not be able to develop a strong referral pattern or community awareness.

7. Adult patients

   Even in the best circumstances, there may not be enough pediatric limb reconstruction patients to entirely fill your practice. Opening your clinic to adults with limb reconstruction needs has the potential to vastly increase your volume. Although some pediatric hospitals have strict age restriction rules, many centers will allow healthy adult patients to have surgery, especially young adults. If you are in an institution where adult surgery is strictly prohibited, acquiring privileges at a local adult hospital is an alternative. Because managing adult patients involves different issues (medical co-morbidities, drug/alcohol/ cigarette use, DVT prophylaxis, workers compensation, etc.), each surgeon will need to decide for himself/herself whether the access to an increased number of cases is worth the additional responsibilities.

Practice Habits

Being organized and punctual are essential prerequisites to maximizing your potential as a limb reconstruction surgeon. These qualities are not only beneficial to you but also provide a positive role model to everyone working with you. Demanding high standards of yourself will inspire others to do the same. The following suggestions represent some of the fundamental habits to adopt in your limb reconstruction practice.

1. Preoperative planning

   Spend time planning and reviewing each surgical case as thoroughly as possible. Formulating a plan several days or weeks ahead of the surgery date is recommended. Waiting until the night before the case is scheduled is often too late. Last-minute preparation makes it difficult to change or add unanticipated equipment. By analyzing, templating, illustrating, and writing out the surgical plan step-by-step ahead of time, the surgeon will have mentally visualized the surgery prior to entering the operating room. This virtual surgical rehearsal will improve the OR efficiency and allow potential problems to be anticipated and addressed before surgery rather than during surgery. Try to involve your assistants, nurses, and mid-level providers to participate in the preoperative planning. It helps them understand the procedure and postoperative care better. At some point, you may delegate some of the preoperative planning to the other member of the team and let him/her present the planning to you and the team. Bring your plan to the operating room and share it with the staff so everyone is aware of your intentions. Finally, no matter how many times you may have performed the same surgery, always bring your cross-sectional anatomy atlas to the operating room to use as a reference when placing half pins or Ilizarov wires. Post your preoperative plans on the wall, easily seen by all members of the OR staff, and include a brief description of the patient's pathology and your surgical steps at the preoperative "briefing" before initiating the case.

2. Surgical journal

   Keep a journal of your surgical cases. After each case, write down things that went well and any obstacles you encountered. Whenever you are planning a similar case in the future, you can refer to your notes to ensure you do not repeat the same mistakes again. By continually recording the modifications and refinements to each technique, your surgical skill and proficiency will keep improving.

3. Weekly clinic visits

    Any patient who is in the process of lengthening or adjusting an external fixator should be seen on a weekly basis. Because the potential for complications to arise in these patients is so great, a weekly visit is advisable to recognize any subtle changes and intervene before they become more complex problems. As you become more experienced, you may be able to relax on this schedule for certain patients, but for the young surgeon, close and frequent monitoring of your patients is mandatory.

4. Accepting complications

    Complications are going to happen. While we all may strive for perfection, no limb reconstruction surgeon can expect to have a perfect outcome every time. Rather than ignoring a problem, it is crucial that the surgeon recognizes when a patient is having trouble and acts aggressively to solve the issue. Very often serious complications start with insignificant problems, which are not properly addressed. Ignoring a problem will not make it go away—in fact, in most cases, it will only continue to get worse until something is done to correct it. Being open and honest with the patient and the family is always the best policy. Acknowledge the concern with the patient and family and then outline the plans to resolve it. Do not hesitate to seek counsel from a mentor or colleague when you sense an impending complication and take immediate steps to mitigate the problem.

    When a complication does occur, however, do not let it consume you. If you are losing sleep or becoming depressed over a particular incident, then you are preventing yourself from being at your best for all your other patients. It is normal to feel empathy and concern when something goes wrong but try not to let it dominate your thoughts for an extended period of time. If you plan thoroughly, operate carefully, and treat your patient with compassion and respect, then there is not much more you can expect from yourself.

5. Postoperative patient clinic visits

    In the clinic, the mid-level provider can be utilized to see postoperative patients. This allows the surgeon to be available to see all new patients and regular follow-up patients. However, it is still critical that the surgeon visit with all the postoperative patients even if just for a brief period. The patient and family always expect to see the surgeon even when they have a scheduled appointment with the physician extender. Stopping to acknowledge their presence in your clinic shows respect and provides reassurance that you have not forgotten about them. In addition, no matter how talented the mid-level provider may be, the surgeon may pick up on a subtle issue that was missed and address it before the patient leaves the clinic.

6. Pre- and post-clinic huddle

    Because limb reconstruction patients can have so many details to coordinate and monitor, it is important that all team members are regularly updated on any new information or changes in the care plan. Gathering the team members together to look at the day's list before the clinic can ensure that mundane things like X-ray orders are prepared and can help the day go more smoothly. Also, any planned frame adjustments or more time-consuming visits can be adjusted for the best clinic flow. There is no better way to stop a clinic in its tracks than to have simultaneous complex frame cases that need adjustments scheduled back-to-back. The entire team should also meet at the end of the clinic to review each patient seen that day. This provides an opportunity for everyone to share and discuss the findings from the visit. This communication ensures that a consistent message can be delivered to the patient from all team members. It also prepares everyone for the plan of the patient's next visit or surgery.

7. Team meetings

    To keep the team organized and cohesive, schedule regular team meetings involving all the key clinic and OR personnel involved in the limb reconstruction program. The common goal of the meetings should be to identify opportunities to improve patient care and clinic/OR efficiency at every level. Many of the issues identified may not be apparent to everyone (especially the surgeon), and this format helps to keep everyone equally aware. The meetings also provide a forum for expressing opinions and/or concerns to the group and exploring solutions. Acknowledging and implementing other team members' ideas gives everyone a sense of involvement in the success of the group. Cultivating and maintaining relationships between the individual team members will help to boost the overall team morale.

8. Conferences

    A regular schedule of conferences can pique and maintain interest in the program, further enhancing common knowledge and sharing insights by team members. This also provides an opportunity for trainees to learn and become involved in case planning, furthering the input from different members.

9. Branding

    Another method to unify the team is to create a brand for your program. Design a team name, slogan, or emblem that can be displayed on apparel, office supplies, and accessories. These items should be shared among the team members and patients. For example, wearing matching team scrubs or shirts in the clinic not only encourages team unity but it presents a consistent

message to the patients. You may consider investing in t-shirts or small everyday items for patients with your team logo/brand name. Give these items to the patient to mark the achievements and milestones in their treatment process.
10. Customer service

    Like it or not, medicine has become a business. Patients can go online and rate their visit with the provider just like any other purchase or life experience. Negative ratings from patients, warranted or not, attract attention. Successful businesses demand excellent customer service from their employees. Emphasize the concept of treating patients the way you would want to be treated. A few simple points like answering all patient calls and emails in a timely manner, reporting test results immediately, and keeping patient appointments on time will produce positive feedback for the program.

Working with Industry

Limb reconstruction often requires unique equipment from orthopedic device companies to be used during surgery. Because a company representative (rep) is responsible for arranging that the appropriate equipment is available for each case, it is important to develop clear lines of communication with each rep. Establish a list of preferences with each rep and clarify your expectations of his/her role. All reps appreciate surgeons who are organized and order their equipment with as much advanced notice as possible. In most cases, the reps will go out of their way to ensure that you receive excellent service. However, as the customer, do not hesitate to express concerns to the company if the rep is unreliable or unprofessional in their duties.

Hospital Commitment

Developing a dedicated pediatric limb reconstruction program requires commitment and understanding from the hospital administration. Establishing the program will benefit the hospital because it can publicize a unique patient care element that most other institutions do not have. However, a clear conversation with the hospital administration about the resources required to be successful is recommended prior to agreeing to develop the program. The hospital will need to invest substantial resources (as outlined above) in the program from the outset and accept that the return on the investment will take time to materialize. At a minimum, when negotiating with the hospital, make sure that the program will have the appropriate clinic team staffing, available and appropriate clinic and OR space, a thorough marketing plan, and opportunities for expansion. The creation of a program research team that will manage patient databases, administer outcome measures/consent forms, write grants, and submit institutional research board (IRB) protocols, will also be necessary.

In terms of compensation, it is important to communicate that the process of managing limb reconstruction patients is different than other types of pediatric orthopedic patients. Because of their complexity, a smaller number of patients can be seen within a given clinic block compared to colleagues seeing primarily fractures and sports injuries. Many clinic spaces will also be occupied for weeks at a time by postoperative lengthening/fixator patients during the global period when there is no charge for the visit. In addition, many limb reconstruction surgeries do not have recognized current procedural terminology (CPT) codes that accurately characterize the complexity of the cases. Consequently, when negotiating a salary, any portion that is based on the annual relative value units (RVUs) accumulated by the surgeon will need to have realistically low-value expectations. During negotiations, emphasize to the administration that a limb reconstruction program can generate huge downstream revenue for an institution when physical therapy visits, psychology assessments, radiologic imaging, in-patient hospital stays, and regional anesthesia charges from patients are included in the business analysis.

Managing Expectations

Many young surgeons find limb reconstruction to be an attractive subspecialty. However, it is a demanding field that requires dedication, a desire to stay and work in one location, and an unwavering passion for the discipline. While there is tremendous satisfaction in the patient success stories, there can also be devastating disappointments when complications occur. Before you start down this path, honestly analyze yourself and be sure that your personality is wired to handle the tremendous ups and downs of a limb reconstruction practice.

In a world where instant gratification is expected, building a limb reconstruction program takes tremendous patience. Unless you are in the rare situation to join an existing pediatric limb reconstruction practice, it will take years to build up a steady stream of cases and it requires continuous effort to maintain the case referrals. While you may have to supplement your practice with other types of cases in the beginning, do not become frustrated or lose faith in your decision. A career in pediatric limb reconstruction surgery is an extremely rewarding and intellectually stimulating experience that is worth navigating the difficulties that exist when first getting started.

Resource Challenged Environment

One of the most glaring peculiarities of a limb deformity service in a resource-challenged environment is a shortage of practice-specific resources. These deficiencies encompass both human and material resources as well as organizational structure. In many of these settings, a deformity correction practice is an ad-hoc, usually single-individual-driven venture, often embedded within a larger practice, with little to no support from the establishment. Yet, as daunting as some of the challenges are, limb reconstruction surgeons in these environments have devised means of overcoming some of these issues. This requires a combination of improvisation and some level of ingenuity. From modifications to the ideal standard of care procedures to "out of the box" thinking, this section looks at the challenges of setting up a limb deformity practice in a resource-challenged setting [4].

1. *Personnel*—Having adequate staffing is key to the smooth functioning of a limb deformity practice. As pointed out earlier in the chapter, a multi-disciplinary approach to care is ideal for success. This multi-disciplinary team, however, is a luxury in many practice settings in low-income countries (LIC) and lower-middle-income countries (LMIC). Countries in this category have struggled to meet the requirements for an adequate surgeon-to-patient ratio. In a 2015 survey by Spiegel et al., only 3.3% of hospitals in LICs and LMICs had access to full-time surgeons [5]. Nigeria, with a population estimated at 211 million people, has less than 500 practicing orthopedic surgeons, while South Sudan, with a population estimated at nearly 13 million, has only three orthopedic surgeons. Invariably, this means that the practice is not likely to be exclusively dedicated to limb reconstruction where an orthopedic surgeon is present. The inadequacies in personnel numbers also affect other relevant service areas, including physical therapy, the operating room, nursing staff, radiology, clinical administration, etc.

    To overcome these challenges, the surgeon needs to "wear many caps." In some cases, he may be required to double up as the scrub nurse. He may also be responsible for sourcing and organizing the supply of inventory in the operating room. This problem is further compounded by the absence of industry support in a lot of these settings. Consequently, the surgeon is responsible for training the operating room personnel on the technicalities and expectations for surgery. This can be a frustratingly difficult enterprise, especially in situations where the shortage of personnel like a dedicated scrub nurse, leads to a prolongation of the surgery duration. In some larger centers, advocacy for a dedicated team is beginning to yield results in overcoming this challenge.

2. *Training and Education*—The importance of having the right foundation in training and education cannot be overemphasized. Unfortunately, most LICs and LMICs do not have formal post-residency limb reconstruction fellowship programs. Exposure to limb reconstruction surgery is usually limited to time spent during the formal residency training program. When applying for positions that offer hands-on training in formal post-residency fellowships in developed countries, international medical graduates not only have to face stiff competition from locally trained residents in these countries but they also must overcome licensing hurdles, cultural barriers, and sometimes, language difficulties. This adds layers to the difficulty of getting the desired education and hands-on training in this specialty. Furthermore, the general shortage of personnel makes investment in dedicated training in a highly specialized field of orthopedic surgery an undesirable venture for the hospital administration, who would rather have personnel that can function in a multi-specialty capacity. These same challenges also exist for the nursing staff, operating room personnel, physical therapists, etc.

    In addressing some of these challenges, exploring opportunities for a South–South academic partnership (between two LMICs) as opposed to a North–South (between HIC and LMIC) may be more relevant and somewhat easier to establish. Nevertheless, collaborative efforts with peers as well as mentors in developed countries have proved invaluable [6]. These efforts provide crucial training and educational support in this subspecialty area for local surgeons. This has been achieved via formal and informal observerships as well as dedicated fellowships in centers in developed countries. For example, the Limb Lengthening and Reconstruction Society (LLRS) hosts an annual traveling fellowship that is open to surgeons from all over the world, including LICs and LMICs. This is a huge learning resource for surgeons from resource-challenged centers. Other methods include attendance at conferences, courses, and workshops organized by specialty associations like the LLRS, surgical mission trips, and local training workshops with experienced specialist volunteer faculty. Other organizations like the Institute for Global Orthopaedics and Traumatology (IGOT) provide sustainable academic partnerships and opportunities for collaboration and support for pursuing clinical and research activities. Teaming up with peers in LICs and LMICs who have been fortunate enough to get post-residency fellowship training in specialized centers with established programs also helps.

    The idea of a "reverse fellowship" model is an interesting concept and provides a method to gain some specialist training. In this model, faculty from high-income countries (HICs) spend time in resource-challenged settings, training local surgeons. To date, this has only occurred for short periods during mission trips or via training workshops lasting a few days to a week or two. Longer visits, perhaps during a sabbatical, or developing institutional relationships would be more sustainable and give a much-needed boost to the training and education needs of surgeons working in these challenging environments. Most importantly, the reverse fellowship model allows the acquisition of critical hands-on learning.

Repetition is the best way to ensure continuing education, so regularly attending training workshops, observerships, and specialty meetings should be encouraged to maintain education and skill levels. Establishing and cultivating mentor relationships with experienced limb deformity surgeons is very important for surgeons from LICs and LMICs.

3. *Social Media*

The ability to utilize current technology has also been employed as a method to overcome some of these challenges. Training and education can be advanced by utilizing virtual classroom technologies like Zoom, while social media platforms like WhatsApp have been used for case planning and discussion. The use of social media platforms for case discussions is an effective method not only for virtual consultation with experts in the field but also as a form of continuing education. Its popularity is based on the relative ease of use and the potential for real-time feedback from experts and mentors. An example of this is the "SIGN Limb Deformity Network" which, so far, has surgeons from North America and several LMICs. Difficult cases are discussed and opinions regarding decision-making and planning can be obtained from experts in the field using simple social media tools.

4. *Clinic Organization*—In many resource-challenged settings, the practice setup may not be the most ideal. Some of the common obstacles include:

    (a) Clinic space: Securing adequate space might be difficult especially when these limited facilities are shared by several other specialties. Even if space is available, the physical structure is not likely to be designed with limb reconstruction patients in mind. It is likely to be generic in nature without the necessary accommodations required for a limb reconstruction clinic.

    (b) Ancillary services: Services like radiology and physical therapy may not be available in the same location. Patients need to go to a different site in the hospital or a different facility altogether to acquire these services. Consequently, patients may need to be scheduled for a second visit to review radiographs ordered after an initial clinical evaluation. This naturally prolongs the decision-making process, from hours to a waiting period of days to weeks. This is particularly difficult in situations where patients travel long distances to access their care. It also contributes to an increase in the volume of reviews that a surgeon must make during the clinic.

    (c) Patient scheduling: These clinics are unlikely to be homogenous and specific to limb lengthening and reconstruction patients. This makes it difficult for peer support among patients undergoing the same type of treatment. In some facilities, surgeons have tried to overcome this challenge by setting up extra day or half-day specialty clinics. A typical example is the clubfoot clinic, which may be run for an hour or 2 in some settings. Networking to foster a spirit of subspecialty referrals is also helping to provide more homogeneity to the patient population in the clinic setting.

    (d) Cost and Inventory—A robust inventory of equipment and hardware is needed to support an ideal limb deformity practice. In many resource-challenged settings, this is lacking. The reasons for this include funds limitation and competing purchasing interests in the healthcare facility as well as a lack of industry support in many instances. Refurbished equipment and implants manufactured locally or from another LMIC are useful alternatives.

5. *Travel Logistics/Availability of Service*—The paucity of specialists available means that many patients must travel long distances to access this type of care. Compounding this issue are the difficult travel logistics for patients in this setting, which may compromise their ability to maintain scheduled follow-up appointments. This is particularly important in conditions where regular close monitoring is required.

    As an alternative, in some settings, surgeons have utilized social media platforms to connect with patients. Patients can provide feedback to questions about their progress and provide images and/or videos for the surgeon to review. While this method of telemedicine is not always ideal, it at least allows the surgeon to connect with the patient when in-person visits are impossible.

6. *Intraoperative Solutions*: One-way surgeons have overcome these obstacles is by modifying the treatment plans for these cases. Combining acute deformity correction with gradual deformity correction helps to limit or eliminate the need for strut changes when using hexapod devices to manage patients with significant angular deformity.

    The use of cheaper and readily available alternatives also provides a way around some of these problems. Utilizing regular cancellous screws and washers in combination with steel wires oriented in a figure-of-8 fashion has been used to create a flexible construct that offers an

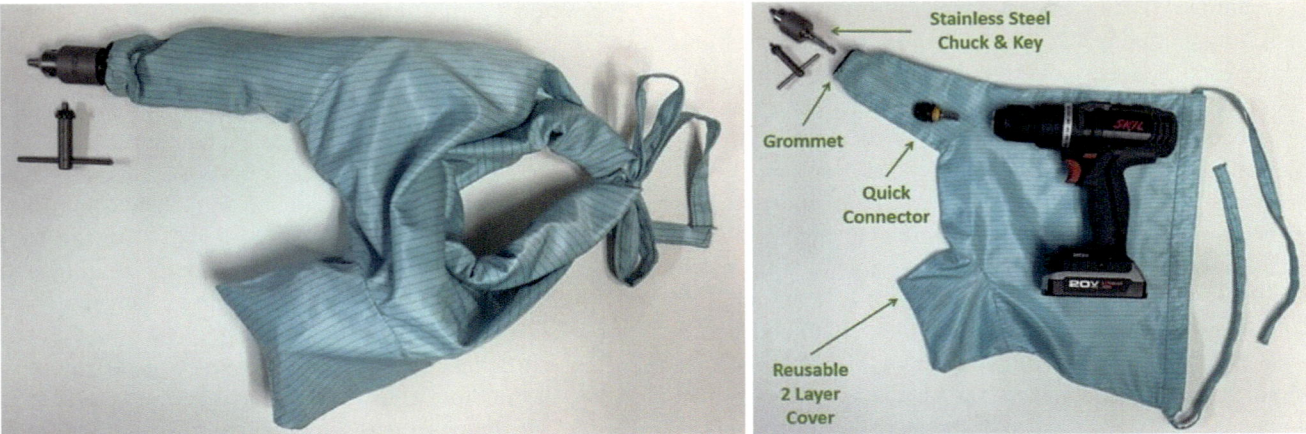

Fig. 5.1 Sterilizable hardware drill cover (courtesy SIGN Fracture Care International)

alternative to the "8-plate" for achieving guided growth in patients with angular deformity [7]. Where possible, donated equipment, implants, and frames provide a useful source of hardware to support treatment options. Utilizing nonmedical equipment like a regular power drill obtained from a hardware store provides improvisations that help to make surgery feasible in these settings. Ingenious and sterilizable drill covers have been created to allow these tools to be used in a hospital setting (Fig. 5.1).

Acknowledgment Mikhail Samchukov MD, Alex Cherkashin MD, John Birch MD, and Mark Dahl MD contributed to the development of this chapter.

Appendix: Reading List

Books

1. Ilizarov, Gavriil. Transosseous Osteosynthesis. Springer-Verlag Berlin Heidelberg, 1992.
2. Paley, Dror. Principles of Deformity Correction. Springer Science & Business Media, 2002.
3. Kirienko, Alexander. Ilizarov Technique for Complex Foot and Ankle Deformities. Taylor and Francis, 2003.
4. Catagni, Maurizio. Atlas for the Insertion of Trans-Osseous Wires and Half Pins. Medi Surgical Video, Milan, 2003.
5. Rozbruch, S. Robert and Ilizarov, Svetlana. Limb Lengthening and Reconstruction Surgery. Taylor and Francis, 2007.
6. Solomin, Leonid. The Basic Principles of External Skeletal Fixation Using the Ilizarov and Other Devices. Springer, 2012.
7. Kocaoglu, Mehmet, Tsuchiya, Hiroyuki, and Eralp, Levent. Advanced Techniques in Limb Reconstruction Surgery. Springer, 2014.
8. Sabharwal, Sanjeev. Pediatric Lower Limb Deformities: Principles and Techniques of Management. Springer, 2015.
9. Rozbruch, S. Robert and Hamdy, Reggie. Limb Lengthening and Reconstruction Surgery Case Atlas. Springer, 2015.
10. Green, Stuart and Dahl, Mark. Intramedullary Limb Lengthening: Principles and Practice. Springer, 2017.
11. Standard, Shawn et al. The Art of Limb Alignment. Independently published, 2019.
12. Herzenberg, John. The Art of Limb Alignment: Taylor Spatial Frame. Independently published, 2019.

Reference Articles

1. Ilizarov GA. The tension-stress effect on the genesis and growth of tissues. Part I. The influence of stability of fixation and soft-tissue preservation. *Clin Orthop Relat Res* 1989;238.
2. Ilizarov GA. The tension-stress effect on the genesis and growth of tissues: Part II. The influence of the rate and frequency of distraction. *Clin Orthop Relat Res* 1989;239.
3. Fleming B et al. A biomechanical analysis of the Ilizarov external fixator. *Clin Orthop Rel Res.* 1989;241.
4. Ilizarov GA. Clinical application of the tension-stress effect for limb lengthening. *Clin Orthop Relat Res* 1990;250.
5. Paley D. Problems, obstacles, and complications of limb lengthening by the Ilizarov technique. *Clin Orthop Relat Res.* 1990;250.

6. Dahl MT, Gulli B, Berg T. Complications of limb lengthening. A learning curve. *Clin Orthop Relat Res* 1994;301:10-18.
7. Ilizarov GA. The principles of the Ilizarov method. 1988. *Bull Hosp Jt Dis*. 1997;56(1).
8. Dahl MT. Preoperative planning in deformity correction and limb lengthening surgery. *Instr Course Lect.* 2000;49.
9. Birch JG and Samchukov ML. Use of the Ilizarov method to correct lower limb deformities in children and adolescents. *J Am Acad Orthop Surg* 2004;12(3).
10. Watson JT. Distraction osteogenesis. *J Am Acad Orthop Surg* 2006;14(10).
11. Baumgart R. The reverse planning method for lengthening of the lower limb using a straight intramedullary nail with or without deformity correction. A new method. *Oper Orthop Traumatol.* 2009;21(2).
12. Sabharwal S. Enhancement of bone formation during distraction osteogenesis: Pediatric applications. *J Am Acad Orthop Surg* 2011;19(2).
13. Makarov MR, Samchukov ML, Birch JG, Cherkashin AM, Sparagana SP, Delgado MR. Somatosensory evoked potential monitoring of peripheral nerves during external fixation for limb lengthening and correction of deformity in children. *J Bone Joint Surg Br*. 2012;94(10).
14. Iobst CA. Advances in Pediatric Limb Lengthening: Part I. *JBJS Reviews* 2015;3(8)
15. Iobst CA. Advances in Pediatric Limb Lengthening: Part II. *JBJS Reviews* 2015;3(9)
16. Paley D. Precice intramedullary limb lengthening system. *Expert Rev Med Devices* 2015;12(3).
17. Paley D. Surgical reconstruction for fibular hemimelia. *J Child Orthop* 2016;10(6).
18. Paley D. Tibial hemimelia: new classification and reconstructive options. *J Child Orthop* 2016;10(6).
19. Paley D. The Paley ulnarization of the carpus with ulnar shortening osteotomy for treatment of radial club hand. *SICOT J* 2017;3.
20. Sheha ED, et al. Leg-Length Discrepancy, Functional Scoliosis, and Low Back Pain. *JBJS Reviews* 2018;6(8).
21. Iobst CA. Intramedullary Limb Lengthening: Lessons Learned. *JBJS Reviews* 2019;7(12).
22. Hubbard EW, Liu RW, Iobst CA. Understanding skeletal growth and predicting limb-length inequality in pediatric patients. *J Am Acad Orthop Surg* 2019;27(9).
23. Paley D. Congenital pseudarthrosis of the tibia: biological and biomechanical considerations to achieve union and prevent fracture. *J Child Orthop* 2019;13(2).
24. Dahl MT, et al. Motorized internal limb lengthening: An updated review. *JPOSNA* 2020;2(1).

Commentary

Milind Chaudhary
milind.chaudhary@gmail.com

It is difficult to find something that has not been covered by Drs Iobst and Bafour in the comprehensively written chapter on how to set up a Pediatric limb reconstruction practice.

The young surgeon is likely to find pearls in each and every line. Especially insights like "Residents and Fellows will come and go but providers and specific clinic staff must be groomed to be available daily and full-time." After 34 years of setting up such a practice, I can unhesitatingly state that these full-time assistants are almost worth their weight in silver and should be remunerated handsomely so that they stay permanently and grow along with you.

I will attempt to add a few bits and pieces and hope they will resonate with someone with a similar cultural and resource background as mine.

For patients who are self-paying and not covered by insurance (such as many with congenital anomalies in our environment), it is prudent to inform them(or parents) at the outset about the need for additional surgery and its costs. In our practice environment, maintaining the trust of the patient and their extended family and community may mean a "partial meter down" or "full meter down" policy, i.e., subsidized billing. For repeat surgeries, we may charge the patient negligible sums or nothing at all if they develop disturbing complications. Recently, we had a child who fractured her femur a few days after frame removal through the osteotomy site. We offered immediate reapplication of the fixator at less than 10–15% of the cost of initial surgery. A clear message is sent that the surgeon and hospital care about a good outcome without having to subject the family to unexpected financial burdens.

Surgeon availability: patients under treatment frequently need doubts to be clarified at all odd hours and insist that the surgeon give them his personal cell phone number. I recommend that junior team members be answerable at specific times to answer calls. Except at the very beginning of practice, surgeons need not be available at the patients' beck and call to retain objectivity.

A big difference between resource-enabled environments and some other cultures, such as in India, patients (nonlimb reconstruction) feel offended if they have to wait days or weeks to see the surgeon. It is culturally inappropriate to turn away a patient who comes to our clinic. This puts time pressure on the surgeon and may take time and attention away from the postoperative care of limb reconstruction patients. I recommend developing flexibility and clinical "triage" to ensure the most time and effort is reserved for the most deserving limb recon patients in follow-up.

One essential piece of furniture in the equipment room that may be lacking in resource-challenged environs are variable height examination couches, which enable our associates and team members to look after the external fixation devices without having to bend over. Bending while working causes fatigue and when unsupervised, can lead to hasty or incomplete actions. If not variable height, they should be higher than normal couches, enabling team members to work for longer durations on these patients without having to bend.

Most patients treated with external fixation repeatedly ask when will the apparatus come off. I have found it useful to perform all communication in follow-up visits in the treatment area (especially, if it is a common treatment area), rather than in the consultation chamber. This does not tax the surgeon's patience in the office. While treatments are being administered, advice and instructions tend to be accepted and understood, giving rise to less friction between patients and the limb recon team, over the long run.

In our practice, certain external fixation parts are reused and help in reducing costs significantly. Rail fixators, rings, hinges, and other undamaged external fixation elements can safely be reused and help reduce the costs for patients.

At the beginning of setting up a limb recon practice, it is a good idea to collaborate with social organizations like Rotary International, etc. to offer surgeries at reduced or modest costs to the underprivileged. The service should maintain the same high standards of follow-up care, despite there being no remuneration for it.

Low-cost accommodation should be arranged for people coming from long distances, to enable frequent follow-ups without expensive travel costs. To enable adequate follow-up care of patients undergoing limb lengthening and deformity correction, we allow as many as three days a week and perform elective surgeries only three days a week. Any changes in the montage of fixators could be done within a few hours, rather than calling in the patient again in a few days.

Any unplanned surgeries (pin exchange, repeat corticotomy for premature consolidation) may be done on the same day under local or regional/ultrasound-guided blocks.

The limb recon surgeon must also be good at applying plaster casts (such as needed for recently healed osteotomies where the apparatus cannot be retained any longer due to loosening). Casts should be well molded, should not come off, or have pressure areas. Applying casts for some patients by the chief surgeon will send the message that there is a master craftsman at work: one who takes pride in using the most sophisticated tools like the TSF fixator or Precice nail as well the simplest ones like the plaster cast. A surgeon works with his head, hands, and his heart, and it should be visible from time to time in a limb recon practice.

References

1. Rozbruch SR, Rozbruch ES, Zonshayn S, Borst EW, Fragomen AT. What is the utility of a limb lengthening and reconstruction service in an academic department of orthopedic surgery? Clin Orthop Relat Res. 2015;473:3124–32.
2. Dahl MT, Gulli B, Berg T. Complications of limb lengthening. A learning curve. Clin Orthop Relat Res. 1994;301:10–8.
3. Gladwell M. Outliers: the story of success. New York: Back Bay Books; 2011.
4. Ferreira N, Sabharwal S, Hosny GA, Sharma H, Johari A, Nandalan VP, Vivas M, Nayagam S, Parihar M, Ferguson D, Rölfing JD. Limb reconstruction in a resource-limited environment. SICOT-J. 2021;7:66.
5. Spiegel DA, Nduaguba A, Cherian MN, Monono M, Kelley ET. Deficiencies in the availability of essential musculoskeletal surgical services at 883 health facilities in 24 low- and lower-middle-income countries. World J Surg. 2015;39(6):1421–32. https://doi.org/10.1007/s00268-015-2971-2.
6. Morshed S, Shearer DW, Coughlin RR. Collaborative partnerships and the future of global orthopaedics. Clin Orthop Relat Res. 2013;471(10):3088–92. https://doi.org/10.1007/s11999-013-3145-x.
7. Bafor A, Ogbemudia AO. Temporary hemiepiphyseodesis for angular deformity of the knee using screws and figure-of-8 wiring. Nigerian J Orthopaedics Trauma. 13(1):40–4.

Growth Modulation for Angular and Length Correction

Peter M. Stevens

Background

As pediatric orthopedists, we are often consulted to evaluate and manage evolving deformities of the lower extremities that, if left untreated, may have lifelong adverse impacts on gait and the spine. Previous management strategies such as "corrective shoes," orthotics, and bracing have yielded to surgical management because the natural history of pathological deformities may be inexorable progression. In 1933, Phemister introduced the concept of open epiphysiodesis for the management of angular deformities and limb length inequality [1]. With the advent of fluoroscopy, this method evolved to the comparatively less invasive percutaneous growth arrest [2–4]. However, the acknowledged drawback of such ablative methods is that they are permanent and hence, irreversible. Therefore, open or percutaneous epiphysiodesis must be delayed until adolescence and perfectly timed in order to avoid over- or under-correction of a given deformity. The vagaries of determining skeletal maturity and parental compliance, including timely follow-up, may make this goal challenging [5]. The same drawbacks pertain to other experimental methods of chemical, electrical, or radiofrequency ablation that are permanent and irreversible.

Given these limitations, many still consider osteotomy to be the "gold standard" for treating progressive angular deformities such as Blount's disease, rickets, and idiopathic genu valgum. Some surgeons also feel compelled to cut bone(s) in order to correct associated torsional deformity. However, the potential disadvantages of any osteotomy include blood loss, neurovascular compromise, immobilization, over- or under-correction, and malunion or nonunion [6]. Comparative cost, cast immobilization, weight-bearing restrictions, unsightly scars, and difficult hardware retrieval must be considered as well.

The appeal of temporary reversible epiphysiodesis is that, in addition to being more cost-effective, it circumvents the above list of iatrogenic problems. Haas was the first to document this using a wire loop initially in dogs and eventually in human subjects [7, 8]. Soon, thereafter, in 1947, Blount introduced his staple for the correction of angular deformities and limb length inequality, and this technique was widely practiced for decades [9]. Because the physis is dynamic and the forces of growth so powerful, there was a propensity for staples to eventually (or precipitously) bend, break, or migrate (Fig. 6.1). The use of multiple staples failed to consistently address these problems. Furthermore, staple removal often proved challenging, sometimes resulting in physeal damage or local bone loss that could compromise the reversibility of this technique. This placed doubt upon the wisdom and necessity of using such rigid implants; their popularity has, therefore, declined.

Frustrated by some of the aforementioned problems associated with stapling, the concept of using an extraperiosteal nonlocking plate serving as a tension band was developed in 2002 and introduced in 2004 [10, 11]. Since then, similar implants have been introduced into the market worldwide (Fig. 6.2). It is not critical which implant one selects; rather it is the tension band principle that counts. The implant construct should be low profile and flexible. However, one should avoid locking plates because the rigid construct will predispose to implant failure.

In disadvantaged regions of the world, the 8-plate or facsimiles may not be available. In such an environment, an option is to take a 1/3 semi-tubular plate or a pelvic reconstruction plate and cut it into 2-hole segments [12–14]. The potential disadvantages of homemade implants relate to the relative bulkiness or stiffness (will not reverse bend) when compared to the real device. Some favor the use of quad

P. M. Stevens (✉)
Department of Orthopedics, University of Utah School of Medicine, Salt Lake City, UT, USA
e-mail: peter.stevens@hsc.utah.edu

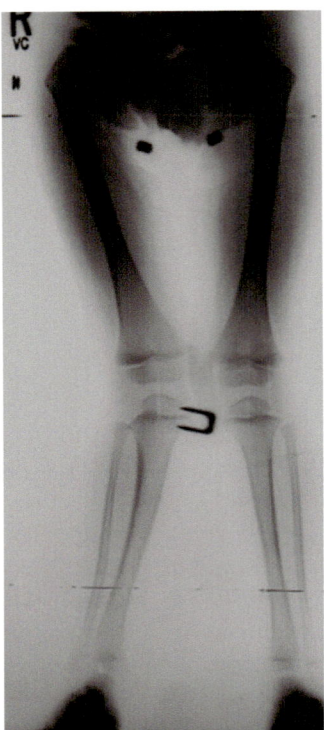

Fig. 6.1 A 4-year-old girl, with post-traumatic tibia valga (Cozen's phenomenon), treated by stapling. Rigid implants are subject to failure through bending, breakage, or migration, as a result of the inexorable forces of physeal growth. Note the extrusion of her single staple; occurring inexplicably, 9 months following implantation

plates (4-hole) in heavy children, particularly those with Blount's disease. Inevitably, a variety of plate shapes have been proposed (step-off, hinge plates, H-plates) and the controversy is unresolved as to whether titanium or stainless steel implants are superior. Unfortunately, there is currently no literature to convincingly support or refute these ideas. Suffice it to say that any device that is flexible and permits differential growth can work.

An alternative strategy, popularized by Metaizeau, involves the insertion of large diameter screws (6.5 or 7.3 mm) cancellous screws across one or both sides of the physis (percutaneous epiphysiodesis using transphyseal screws = P.E.T.S.) [15]. While also minimally invasive and deceptively simple, the theoretical objection is the drawback of having to violate the physis with a large threaded implant. Series reports of P.E.T.S. are largely confined to the adolescent age group; therefore, the reversibility of this technique has not been well documented. It has not been described in younger children or in sagittal or oblique plane deformities. Thus, P.E.T.S. has comparatively narrow ranges of age and applications. Tension band plating has emerged as the most versatile and preeminent form of guided growth [16].

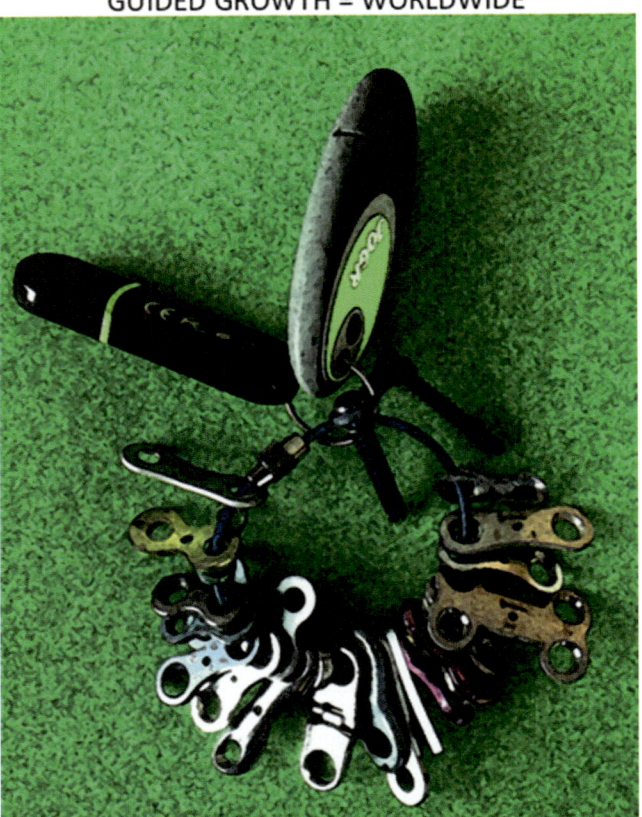

Fig. 6.2 Since the introduction of the 8-plate in 2004, many facsimiles have been produced worldwide and used successfully for guided growth. The common denominators for success are low profile and nonlocking

Deformities of the Lower Extremities

General With the notable exception of physiologic varus and valgus, lower extremity deformities often progress with growth. While angular deformities at the knee are most obvious and perplexing, one must examine the patient for concomitant limb length discrepancy, rotational deformities, and ligamentous laxity that present confounding factors. Also, examine the hip and ankle clinically and, when indicated, radiographically, for coexisting or compensatory angular deformities. If the deformity is unilateral, then the normal leg serves as a comparison. However, oftentimes deformities are bilateral and not necessarily symmetrical. Finally, observe the alteration of gait as a result of limb deformity. Genu valgum is often associated with circumduction and out-toeing. Genu varum may present with a waddling, Trendelenburg gait pattern, in-toeing, and lateral thrust. Unilateral pathology will often be associated with limb length discrepancy.

The age at presentation and history of persistence or progression of deformity are important to consider. If a deformity is thought to be physiologic or borderline in severity, a follow-up visit after 6–12 months may clarify this and affect the timing of intervention. Alternatively, in the age of smartphones and electronic communication, parents may send periodic pictures (see below). For adolescents, one must be cognizant of remaining growth and the predicted natural history of a given problem. It is important to document concomitant deformity of the hip and/or ankle because simultaneous multilevel guided growth may be employed.

Angular: Frontal

Physiologic It is well-recognized that children under the age of two may present with symmetrical and painless bowing of the legs associated with ligamentous laxity and in-toeing. With observation alone, all components of this deformity will spontaneously correct without treatment. While there is no need for intervention, parental education, reassurance, and periodic follow-up as needed are tantamount to success. Likewise, physiologic genu valgum should be managed expectantly without requiring bracing, physical therapy, or shoe modification up until the age of six. These self-limiting conditions are a contraindication to surgical intervention of any kind [17–19]. When in doubt, periodic reexamination of the patient, with or without radiographs, may be employed. An alternative is to have the parents send a picture of the child standing in 6–12 months and decide whether further consultation/radiographs/surgery are indicated.

Pathologic In contradistinction to the above noted problems, the pathologic deformities may be unilateral or bilateral and multilevel. The etiology may be idiopathic, developmental (Blount's), acquired (Cozen's), metabolic (Rickets), genetic (neurofibromatosis, hereditary multiple exostoses, Schmid dysplasia), or dysplastic (fibrous dysplasia, Ollier's) to name a few. Deformities may occur in the frontal, sagittal, or oblique plane compounded by torsion and ligamentous laxity. They are insidious in their progression and refractory to attempts at orthotic management or physical therapy.

Regardless of the underlying etiology, individually and collectively, these deformities constitute the indication for guided growth as the treatment of choice instead of osteotomy (salvage procedure). Clinically, genu valgum is often associated with anterior knee pain and a circumduction gait; patellar instability may ensue. It is documented by measuring the intermalleolar distance when standing and prone. Genu varum may also be seen with knee pain and a waddling Trendelenburg positive gait often in association with in-toeing, ligamentous laxity, and lateral thrust. This is documented clinically using the intercondylar distance. Furthermore, when the deformity is unilateral, progressive relative limb length discrepancy is common.

While knee deformities represent, by far, the most common indication for guided growth, there are specific deformities such as ankle valgus or coxa vara that may also lend themselves to the same principle and technique. Timely guided growth may prevent or forestall the need for distal tibial or proximal femoral osteotomies. In some patients, multilevel guided growth to simultaneously address concomitant deformities is efficient and well-tolerated [20] (Fig. 6.3).

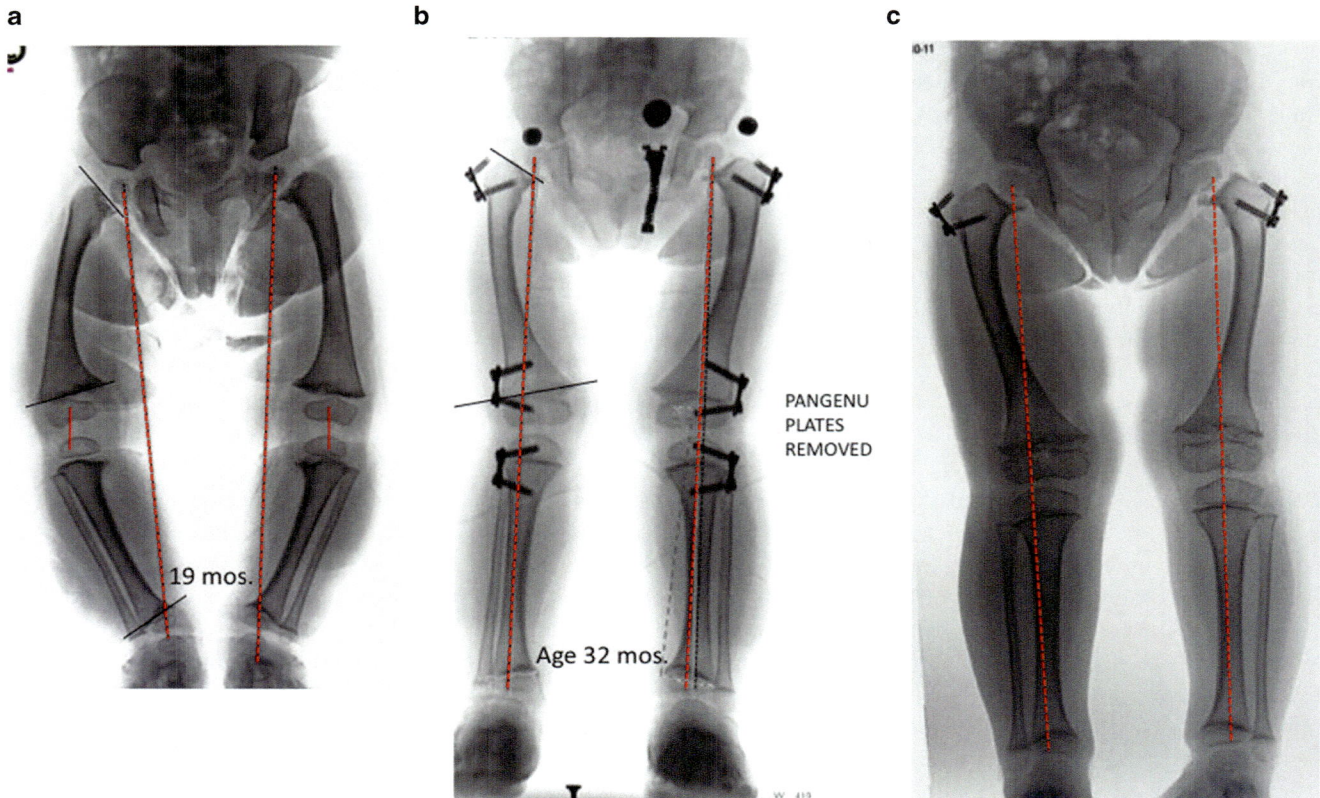

Fig. 6.3 (a) This 19-month-old girl with Schmid-type chondroepiphyseal dysplasia, presented with a waddling gait and hip pain (due to stress fractures of the femoral neck). (b) Thirteen months following bilateral, 3-level guided growth (outpatient/no cast), her mechanical axis neutral; her gait has become normal and hip pain abated. (c) At age 6, she remains asymptomatic, with neutral alignment. Note the indirect resolution of her ankle varus. Her femoral neck fractures remain healed; the plates will be left in situ, pending further growth. Proximal femoral osteotomies was successfully averted

Treatment

Timing/Angular When dealing with progressive angular deformities, the previously preferred method of epiphysiodesis—now largely of historic interest—involved permanent arrest by either open or percutaneous techniques [21, 22]. These required serial scanograms and bone age determinations with calculations using various methods [23–25]. Guided growth with tension band plates is more forgiving in terms of timing and calculations. The Multiplier Method has been used as a way of trying to perfectly time-guided growth [26]. However, this presupposes that the parents will return during the prescribed window in order to achieve the desired outcome. Because guided growth is reversible and may be repeated, timing is rarely an issue. The only caveat is that in adolescents with encroaching maturity, skeletal age determination should document that at least one year of growth remains.

On a standing AP teleoroentgenogram, the relative limb lengths and mechanical axis are documented. The mechanical axis should bisect the horizontal knee at an 87-degree angle or at least fall within the center of two quadrants (zones ± 1) of the knee. When it is in medial or lateral zone 2 or 3, surgical intervention is generally warranted. If two levels of deformity, for example, femur + tibia, are identified, then pan genu-guided growth is indicated in order to preserve a horizontal knee joint line. The other indication for pan genu guided growth is when limited remaining growth is predicted; meaning, time is running short.

In children older than 10, the standard anatomic angles have been codified [27, 28] (Table 6.1). These reference the joint/shaft orientation for the femur and tibia and can be useful to monitor progression following guided growth. The joint congruence angle is typically 0 degrees (parallel lines), indicating ligamentous balance/integrity. There may be concomitant deformity in both the femur and tibia. Depending upon the direction, these may be compounding or compensatory. By envisioning the knee joint horizontally, one can readily detect multilevel deformities. For example, in patients with Blount's disease, there may be concomitant varus or varus deformity of the distal femur that must be taken into account.

6 Growth Modulation for Angular and Length Correction

Table 6.1 Lower extremity anatomic and joint orientation angles

Abbreviation	Angle	Degrees
PMFA	Proximal medial femoral angle	90
LDFA	Lateral distal femoral angle	87
PMTA	Proximal medial tibial angle	87
LDTA	Lateral distal tibial angle	87
PPTA	Posterior proximal tibial angle	81
PDTA	Posterior distal tibial angle	90
JCA	Joint congruence angle	Parallel

To benefit from guided growth, the age of the patient is not critical provided there is at least a year of predicted growth remaining. Guided growth has been safely and successfully utilized in patients ranging from as young as 18 months through late adolescence, which may be delayed in various patients, provided a year of growth remains. For younger patients, with clearly pathologic, progressive, and symptomatic deformity, it is preferable to correct the problem, even if it requires repeated guided growth subsequently, rather than await perfect timing or resort to osteotomy. The risks of delaying surgical realignment include compensatory deformity of the hip, knee, or ankle, ligamentous laxity, patellar instability, and gait disturbance.

Technique/Angular Under tourniquet control, the designated physis is approached through a 3-cm incision. The dissection is deepened through fascial and submuscular planes down to the bone and preserving the periosteum. A Keith needle is inserted into the physis checking its position in the frontal and sagittal planes with the fluoroscope. The plate is then inserted, placing the small center hole over the Keith needle to align it with the physis. The transverse Keith needle will not damage the physis. It is desirable to position the plate mid-sagitally unless an oblique plane deformity is being corrected. For example, a knee flexion/varus deformity may call for a single anterolateral tension band plate. One plate per physis is usually sufficient. The smooth 1.6-mm guide pins are inserted; they need not be parallel but must avoid the physis and joint. It has been demonstrated that the size of the plate, the length of the screws, and the screw orientation at the outset do not affect the outcome [29]. While screw length is arbitrary and sizes may be mixed, the longest practical screw is usually recommended. There is no evidence to mandate that the screw tip must be past the midline of the bone. However, longer screws provide more purchase and are less apt to drag and encroach upon the physis during subsequent growth. At the discretion of the surgeon, each hole is predrilled to a depth of 5 mm in order to facilitate the advancement of the 4.5-mm cannulated screws, without undue torque. Each screw is advanced to be touching the plate. It is then important to remove the guide pins, which may be binding on the screw, and further tighten each screw to countersink within the plate. This should be documented fluoroscopically. Avoid leaving gap between the plate and the metaphysic. This critical maneuver will avoid 3-point bending stresses reported in some patients with Blount's disease, which could produce stress fracture of the screw. This is a potential technical error that may compromise any screw, be it titanium or stainless steel, cannulated or solid. If the plate is not well coapted to the bone, consider removing it and increasing the 10° convex bend so that it contours better with the bone; this is particularly germane for the proximal lateral tibia. Once the hardware is secured, with fluoroscopic confirmation of optimal placement, the wound is closed in layers, and a soft dressing is applied.

Although guided growth is minimally invasive and performed through small incisions, it is not without associated postoperative discomfort. Parents need to be educated in this regard so they know what to anticipate. Full weight-bearing and activities are encouraged, as tolerated. Physical therapy may be helpful for a minority of children who cannot flex their knee to 90° by one month following surgery.

Follow-up Historically, routine follow-up has been recommended every 3 months (for angle) or every 6 months (for length) until correction is achieved (Fig. 6.4). However, this is both costly and impractical for many families. Some parents simply forget and neglect to return at a prescribed time. As a result, significant overcorrection may occur requiring revision surgery. Keeping a separate list of the patients currently undergoing guided growth is helpful to monitor for any missed appointments and ensure timely evaluation to prevent overcorrection.

An excellent alternative is to instruct the parents to take a monthly smartphone picture of their child clad in shorts and with the knees facing forward. The child holds a placard that includes their name, date of birth, date of surgery, and type of surgery (implant inserted or removed). The picture is then shared by the electronic platform of choice and the provider directs the parents to either (1) repeat the picture in a month or (2) return to the clinic/hospital for a comparison standing radiograph (± bone age determination) and insertion, repositioning or removal of implant(s). This smartphone exchange then continues—monitoring for improvement of alignment, rebound deformity, or overcorrection. The obvious benefits to the surgeon include streamlined clinics, fewer extraneous radiographs, enhanced and timely surgical scheduling, and more consistent communication with engaged parents. By obviating routine postoperative office visits every 3 months, the benefits to the family are economical, less time off work and school, and less travel. The aggregate savings of time and cost are obvious. Perhaps, most importantly, rebound deformity is anticipated and overcorrection rarely occurs. This method of monthly documentation mitigates against the "lost to follow-up" risk that has been reported with some

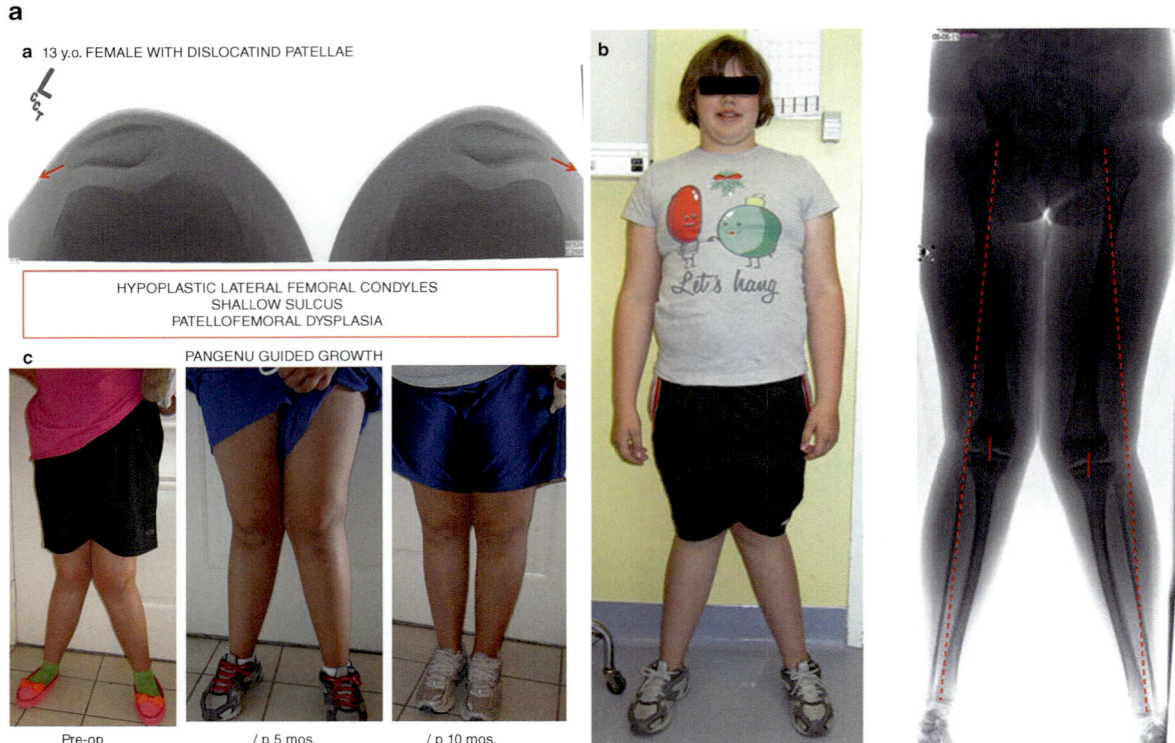

Fig. 6.4 (**a**) This 13-year-old girl presented with "patello-femoral dysplasia" manifest by bilateral patellar instability. (**b**) Clinically, her intermalleolar distance measured 20 cm. Her mechanical axis is lateral zone 3. It was apparent that idiopathic genu valgum (femur + tibia) was the proximate cause of her patellar dislocations and recognized that an MPFL reconstruction or patellar tendon transfer would not suffice to solve her problems. (**c**) Having hit her adolescent growth spurt, her deformities completely corrected within 10 months of pan genu plate application and her patellae stabilized, without direct intervention. (**d**) Radiographic comparison of before vs. 10 months after pan genu guided growth, whereupon the plates were removed. (**e**) "Sunrise" radiographs demonstrating improvement in the patello-femoral sulcus depth, presumably as a consequence of normalizing the mechanical axis and directing the patella in front of the femur

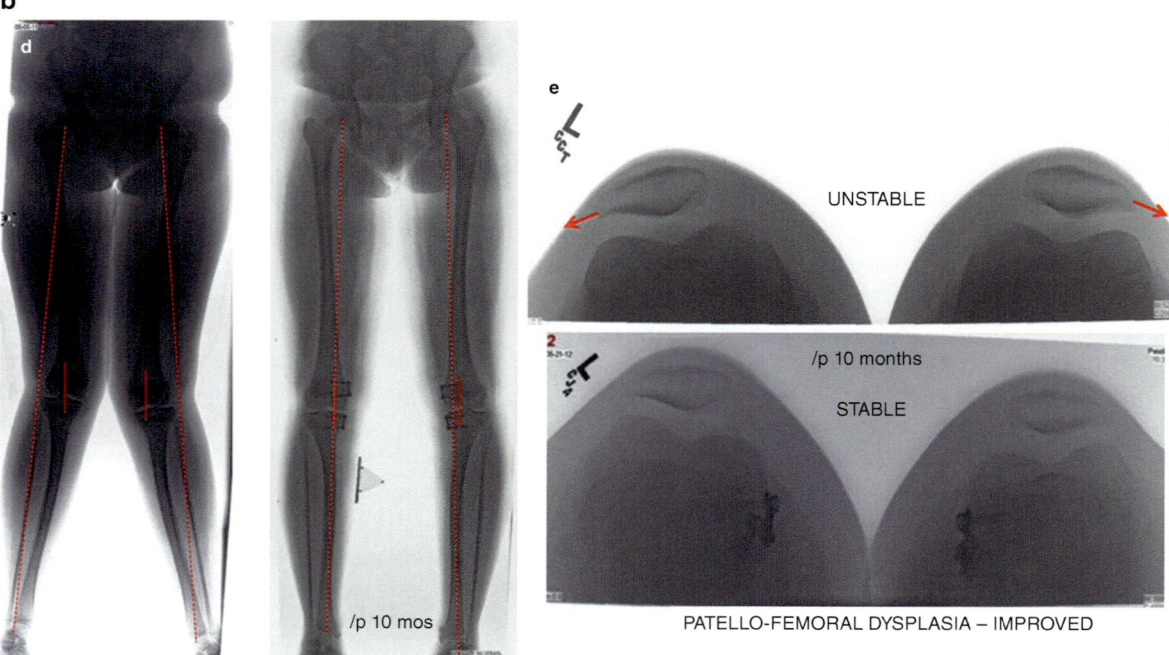

Fig. 6.4 (continued)

patients undergoing guided growth. Revision or repeated guided growth is certainly preferable to resorting to osteotomies, which have more significant associated risks.

Time to Correction For angular correction, most deformities will be resolved within 6–18 months (Fig. 6.4). However, certain syndromes and skeletal dysplasias such as achondroplasia may require more time. There is no proven limit as to how long one can safely restrain one side of the physis. Since continued growth is unabated in the presence of a unilateral flexible tether, premature physeal closure is highly unlikely. Clinical correction is corroborated by a full-length, weight-bearing teleoroentgenogram, noting limb lengths and the mechanical axis. In children younger than 10, or with delay in skeletal maturity, it may be advisable to allow slight overcorrection of the mechanical axis into medial or lateral zone 1. In the event of rebound/recurrent deformity, guided growth may be safely repeated. Once the screws have reached maximum divergence, the narrow waist of the plate accommodates reverse bending of the plate, facilitating further correction. This characteristic is not shared by the more rigid quad plates.

Intermittent Guided Growth It is impossible to determine the perfect timing for correcting a given angular deformity, nor is it possible to predict or prevent rebound deformity after implant removal; meaning that for some patients, repeat tethering of the physis may be indicated. Fortunately, tension band plating is uniformly reversible. Rather than having to remove and reinsert the entire construct when the mechanical axis is restored, a useful technique is to percutaneously remove only the metaphyseal screw providing the plate and epiphyseal screw are in a good position. The smartphone method of follow-up is then employed in order to detect rebound deformity and metaphyseal screws may then be percutaneously reinserted. Likewise, the unlikely event of persistent tethering causing overcorrection of a deformity is readily detected and the plate and epiphyseal screw are removed and/or repositioned. This has proven to be a very economical and well-tolerated method of serial intervention for younger children or adolescents with unanticipated growth spurts.

Angular: Sagittal/Oblique

Knee Fixed knee flexion deformity (FKFD) may be associated with conditions including cerebral palsy, spina bifida, and arthrogryposis. It is important to differentiate between dynamic vs. fixed contracture because the treatment is very different. Both conditions will limit the straight leg raise. With the former, the popliteal angle will change as the hip is flexed in the supine position. In addition to the typical supine straight leg raise, it is helpful to examine the patient prone with the hip extended and relaxing the hamstrings. If the knee remains flexed and the foot does not reach the table, this indicates a fixed, rather than dynamic, knee deformity that will not respond to hamstring recession.

In children with lower limb spasticity, bilateral FKFD causes a progressive crouch gait that is refractory to bracing and physical therapy. The shortened stride length and anterior knee pain, frequently seen with radiographic evidence of patella alta ± avulsion fractures, may preclude sustained ambulation. Supracondylar extension osteotomy of the femur ± patellar advancement has enjoyed recent popularity. However, recurrent knee flexion deformity is common and represents a major drawback. Additionally, because involvement is bilateral, simultaneous osteotomies represent a major undertaking and a daunting recovery.

An alternative approach is to employ guided growth of the distal anterior femur to gradually correct the sagittal or oblique plane deformities [30]. It is important to place the plates medial and/or lateral to the sulcus (intracapsular but nonarticular) in order to avoid irritation of the patella. While the initial postoperative pain and crepitus may exceed the expectations of the parents and physical therapist, these symptoms abate as the legs gradually straighten. In contradistinction to osteotomies or external frames, there is no loss of knee flexion. Postoperative bracing (usually floor reaction) may still be helpful until the crouch deformity fully corrects. Typically, this takes 12–18 months following guided growth treatment. Overcorrection into recurvatum is rare, as is recurrence. In the author's experience, simultaneous or subsequent advancement of the patellar tendon is not required because knee pain typically abates as the knee gains extension and patella alta is rendered unimportant. Symptomatic patella alta can be addressed separately but is rarely warranted.

Furthermore, concomitant hamstring lengthening is also unnecessary. In fact, as the knee straightens, the hamstrings may actually pull upon the ischium, extending the pelvis and mitigating the hip flexion deformity, while preserving hip extensor power. Finally, the apparent equinus is improved indirectly as the knee extends and the heel may reach the floor. Thus, by primarily addressing the FKFD with anterior tension band plates, gradual correction is realized. In contradistinction to supracondylar osteotomy, posterior capsulotomy, or frames, knee flexion is preserved while extension is gained (Fig. 6.5). Perhaps this should be called "single level, multievent surgery" (SLMES).

Surgical Technique Under tourniquet control, with a bolster to support the flexed knee, the fluoroscope is positioned horizontally. The femoral physis is approached, through short incisions that are medial and lateral to the patella. The medial and lateral retinaculum and synovium are opened and the articular surface of the sulcus is visualized. Under fluoroscopic guidance, Keith needles are inserted into the physis. Avoiding the articular surface, medial and lateral tension band plates are inserted over each needle to center each upon the physis, and the two 1.6-mm smooth guide wires are placed. Once the cannulated screws are seated, remove the guide wires and further tighten the screws in order to countersink them into the plate and minimize their prominence. The retinacula and skin are closed in layers.

Postoperative Management No immobilization or weight-bearing precautions are required. If the child was ambulating with AFOs, these may be reapplied and ambulation encouraged. This particular form of guided growth is accompanied by more pain and crepitus than parents and physical therapists typically expect (but certainly far less than distal femoral extension osteotomies). The caretakers need to be reassured that the implants are not beneath the patella and informed that the crepitance is due to the presence of plates beneath the extensor retinaculum. These symptoms will spontaneously abate by three months postoperatively.

Ankle/Coronal Progressive ankle valgus is common and insidious sequelae of a variety of conditions (Table 6.2). The detection of insidious ankle valgus is more challenging than knee deformities because of the relatively short height of the foot. It may be mistaken for an overcorrected clubfoot, planovalgus, or pronated foot. The critical radiographic study is a weight-bearing AP of the ankles. The normal LDTA (lateral distal tibial angle) should be approximately 87–90° [28].

As the deformity progresses, there is often lateral pain around the ankle and hindfoot due to impingement of the distal fibula upon the talus or calcaneus. As the ground reaction force shifts laterally, the distal fibular epiphysis may enlarge in response to the increased weight-bearing load imposed. This situation does not lend itself to correction with orthoses.

Guided growth of the distal tibia inserting a single transphyseal screw in the medial malleolus offers an easy method of correcting ankle valgus [31]. However, a decided drawback is that one is applying a rigid implant across the open and very dynamic physis. This may lead to implant failure or difficult removal. It is preferable to utilize a flexible extraperiosteal tension band that will produce more rapid correction and is simple to remove [32]. In comparison to the knee, the time to correction of the ankle is slower, often taking 18–24 months. It is recommended to overcorrect into slight varus (LDTA of up to 95 degrees) in anticipation of rebound valgus, which is relatively common. The subtalar joint can readily accommodate and compensate for the slight overcorrection. The concerns expressed regarding hardware prominence have not been borne out in practice. However, if the child is wearing an AFO, it is desirable to mold or pad the brace p.r.n. to avoid rubbing.

Ankle/Sagittal At the distal tibia, one may insert an anterior plate for residual fixed equinus or a posterior plate for calcaneus deformity, rather than resort to supramalleolar osteotomy. If the deformity is greater than 15 degrees, however, an osteotomy may be required.

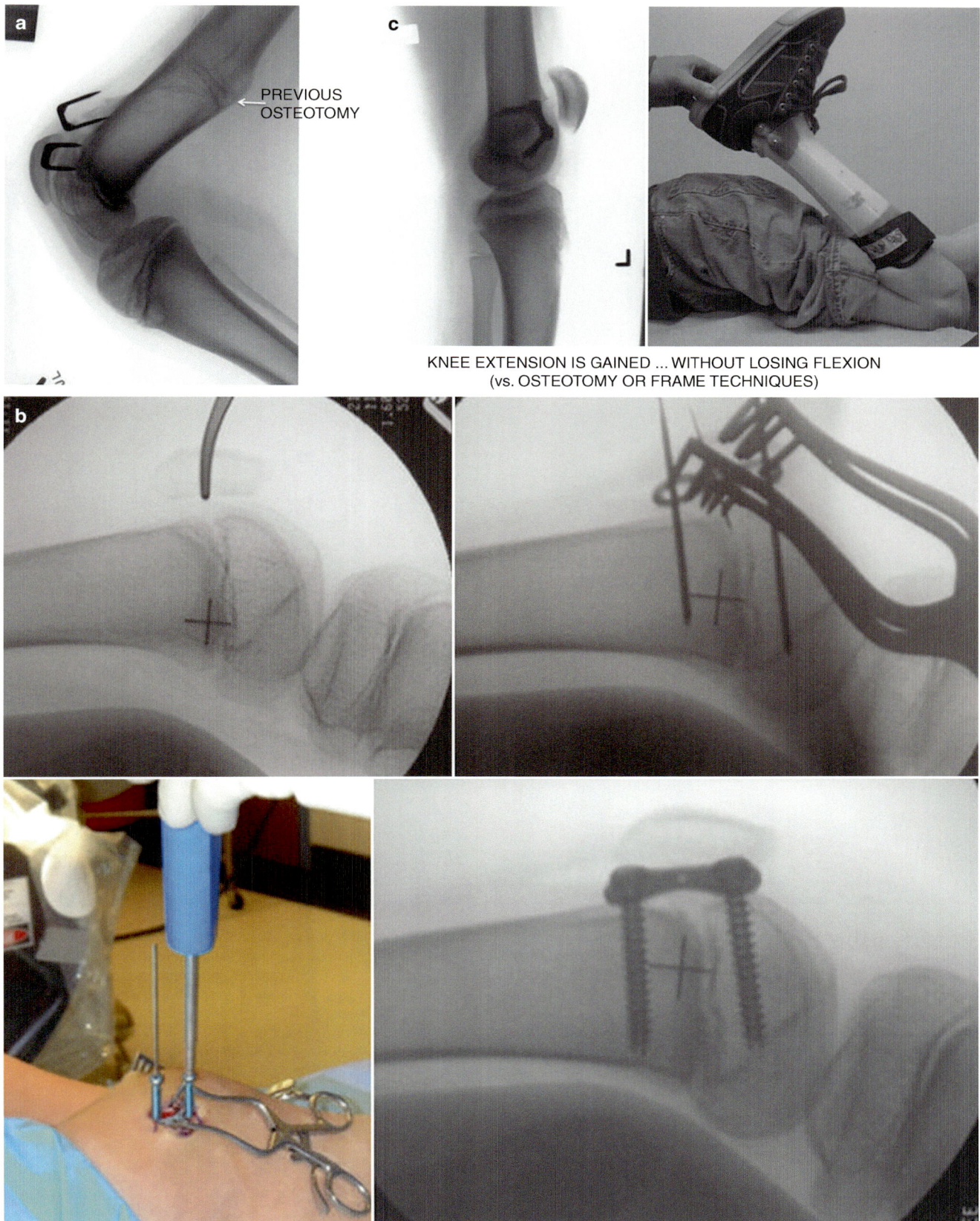

Fig. 6.5 (a) This 7-year-old patient with congenital fixed knee flexion deformity (FKFD), had a previous extension osteotomy (dotted arrow) at age 3, with the inevitable recurrence of her deformity. Anterior femoral staples migrated and had to be removed. (b) Intraoperative images show the technique of sagittal plane correction by applying tension band plates to the anterior distal femur, one on each side of the sulcus. (c) In contradistinction to osteotomy or frame application, knee extension is achieved, without losing correction. Regarding patella alta, if the patient is ambulatory and pain-free, there is no requirement that the patellar tendon be advanced

Table 6.2 Etiology of ankle valgus

Dysplastic	Neuromuscular	Genetic	/P traumatic
Clubfoot	Cerebral palsy	Rickets	Fracture
Postaxial hypoplasia	Spina bifida	Down syndrome	Osteotomy
Tibial pseudarthrosis	Neurofibromatosis	MHE	

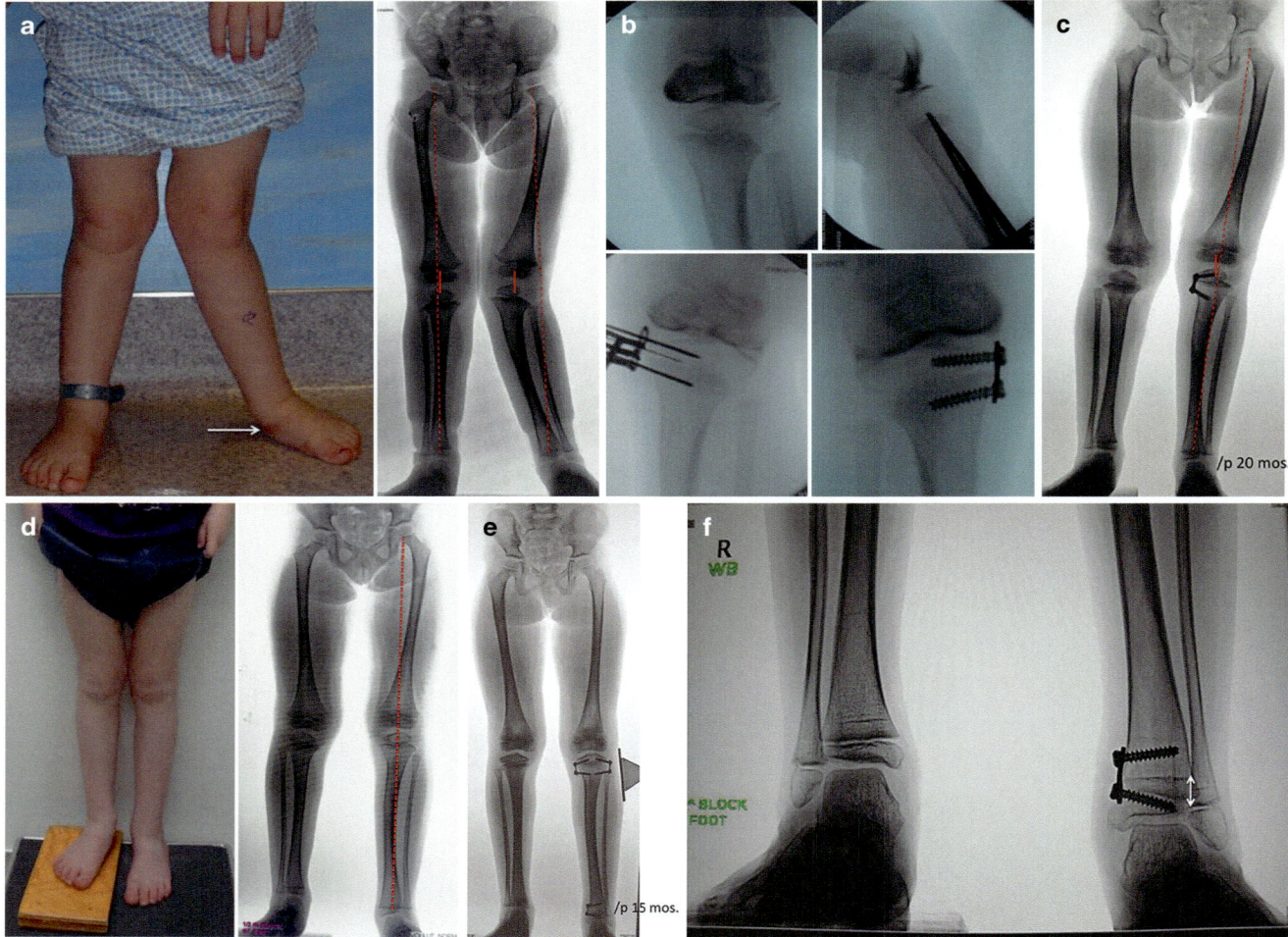

Fig. 6.6 (**a**) A 3-year-old girl with Cozen's post-traumatic genu valgum, presenting 18 months/p proximal tibial fracture. Note the small hemangioma on the instep (arrow). (**b**) An arthrogram was employed to better delineate the chondro-epiphyses and aid in placing the guide wires and cannulated screws. (**c**) Full correction of the angular deformity took 20 months, whereupon the implant was removed. Follow-up continued to monitor for recurrent valgus and LLD. (**d**) At age 7, she is noted to have a 2.5-cm discrepancy and symptomatic ankle valgus. These were attributed to her congenital hemangioma causing growth imbalance. This was managed via bifocal guided growth—proximal tibia for length inhibition and distal medial tibia for valgus. (**e**) Fifteen months later, her length discrepancy measures 1.2 cm and the ankle valgus has resolved. (**f**) Note the asymmetrical growth line in the left distal tibia, with correction of the ankle valgus to neutral. The strategy is to wait for 9 months, allowing slight overcorrection into the ankle varus, then remove the metaphyseal screws from the distal and proximal plates. Following 6 months of reprieve from guided growth, allowing growth to resume, the metaphyseal screws may be reinserted. Follow-up will be continued until maturity, repeating this process of screw removal/reinsertion as indicated

Complications of Guided Growth

Perioperative complications pertaining to tension band plate insertion are decidedly rare, provided the routine precautions are exercised. These include protecting and preserving the periosteum and avoidance of violating the physis or joint with the screws. With respect to the latter, it may be helpful to perform an arthrogram in young children in order to outline the entire chondro-epiphysis (Fig. 6.6). Parents also need to be apprised of the importance of follow-up, be it in person, or via monthly smartphone images, so as to avoid overcorrection.

There have been sporadic reports of *broken screws*. Most commonly this occurs in Blount's disease and involves the metaphyseal screw. While some authors have attributed this to increased BMI, there is no factual corroboration of such. Screw breakage occurs, not at the head/shank junction, but where the exposed screw shank enters the cortex [33]. This may occur regardless of the material (stainless vs. titanium), design (cannulated vs. noncannulated), or size of the screw (Fig. 6.7). This situation is best avoided by anticipation and attention to surgical technique. Steps to avoid screw fatigue failure include: (1) remove the guide pins and alternately tighten the screws to bend the plate in situ or (2) remove the plate and increase its convex bend to better contour to the lateral cortex of the tibia. When encountered, broken screws may be percutaneously exchanged as needed rather than resort to osteotomy. Other proposed but unproven options to consider are the use of dual plates or quad plates and the choice of solid (noncannulated) screws. Without corroborative evidence, these choices reflect surgeon preference.

The issue of *rebound growth* imbalance and recurrent deformity, which is more common under the age of 10, is not a true complication. Rather, it is an educational challenge, requiring the surgeon to establish parental expectations, maintain vigilance, and pursue meticulous follow-up. The rebound deformity phenomenon can generally be detected within 12 months of implant removal. Properly informed, most parents (and patients) would prefer to repeat guided growth to any osteotomy.

Regarding angular correction, some have cited concerns about overcorrection [34]. This is actually not a complication of the tension band technique per se. Rather, it represents a failure of informed consent. Either the surgeon failed to communicate the need for consistent monitoring or the parents failed to comprehend and follow instructions. Perhaps, following minimally invasive surgery, they simply forget to return in a timely manner (as opposed to osteotomy). The simple remedy for this situation is to engage the parents in sending monthly pictures. In this manner, significant overcorrection will be prevented.

Management Weighing the potential for rebound growth causing recurrent deformity (more common under the age of 10), it may be desirable to permit slight overcorrection (of varus into medial zone 1 valgus—or vice versa). This will extend the "mileage" of a given procedure. If the rebound is deemed likely, one option is to remove just the metaphyseal screw and continue observation, reinserting the screw if and when rebound is documented. In other words, the modular nature of reversible guided growth lends itself to handling a myriad of conditions and situations. Frequent minimally invasive, outpatient surgeries may be preferable to major, more invasive techniques.

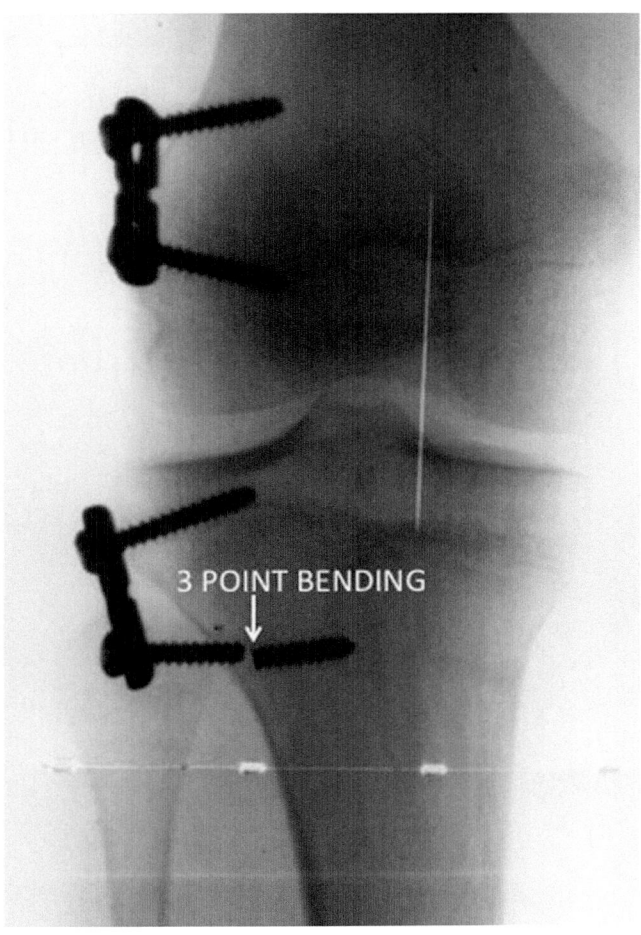

Fig. 6.7 If there is no contact between the plate and tibial metaphysis, the screw be subject to 3-point bending, regardless of the screw size and material. This 4.5-mm solid stainless screw demonstrates such a technical error

Length: Anisomelia

Physiologic According to the literature, it is widely accepted that limb length discrepancy of up to 1.2 cm is well-tolerated by most adults. With few exceptions, surgical treatment is not recommended for children who have a discrepancy that is not predicted to exceed 1.2 cm at maturity. While shoe lifts may be prescribed, they are merely compensatory and few children will consistently wear them.

Pathologic Whether the etiology is congenital, developmental, or acquired, if the predicted discrepancy will exceed 1.2 cm at maturity, then surgical treatment may be warranted. It is important to see the growing child biannually in order to identify the trend (static vs. progressive), educate the parents, anticipate the predicted discrepancy at maturity, and determine the optimal timing of surgical intervention.

The most practical radiograph to obtain is the teleoroentgenogram, which is a full-length weight-bearing AP of the legs [35]. It is helpful to level the pelvis with an appropriate height wooden block under the shorter leg. If one uses a radiographic magnification marker, then relative limb lengths may accurately be measured, along with the mechanical axis [36]. A horizontal line across the top of the iliac crests will reflect the aggregate limb length discrepancy because it includes both the ileum and the foot, as well as the femur and tibia. It is noteworthy that the "entire leg" tab in the Multiplier App includes only the femur + tibia and does not include the pelvis or foot; this may lead to underestimation of the discrepancy. If there is mechanical axis deviation of either (or both) limbs, this needs to be taken into account because angular deformity will cause a disparity between the true and apparent length of the affected long bone(s). Correcting an angular deformity will add length and reconcile this discrepancy.

Treatment: Length

Timing: Adolescent:

The typical application for guided growth inhibition is during adolescence, hoping to achieve limb equalization at skeletal maturity. Several methods of determining skeletal maturity have been published in an attempt to predict the discrepancy at maturity and select the optimum time for epiphysiodesis [22–25, 37, 38]. However, other investigators have cast doubt about the reliability of such methods [39–42]. Clearly, problems inherent in determining skeletal maturity may result in over- or under-correction, especially when using permanent and irreversible techniques

Regardless of the technique and implants chosen (staples, tension band plates, Metaizeau P.E.T.S.), there is a latency effect before longitudinal growth is inhibited. Consequently, many reports of surgical outcomes following epiphysiodesis accept residual discrepancies <1.5 cm as a good result. This latency should be taken into account and epiphysiodesis undertaken 6–12 months in advance of what was formerly deemed "ideal". By using reversible technology, much earlier intervention is permitted because the implants may be removed if a correction occurs before skeletal maturity is reached. If a given child has reached 2 cm of discrepancy and becomes symptomatic, serial tethering may commence, regardless of age.

Some authors still favor permanent epiphysiodesis over reversible instrumented techniques. They cite various ablative methods as being more rapid or "definitive," when compared to tension band plating [43–49]. What they fail to appreciate is the subtle difference between growth arrest, which is permanent and requires accurate prediction, and *growth deceleration* using tension band plates [50]. The speed of correction becomes irrelevant because correction of LLD using tension band plates relies upon the principle of *reversible tethering* and, therefore, does not require precise calculations. The qualifier is that for adolescents, the Menelaus method is useful in determining that, based upon skeletal age, there is at least one year of predicted growth remaining [51, 52]. Respecting these principles, good success can be achieved using tension band plates [53] (Fig. 6.8).

Timing: < age 10 years

A given physis may be restrained for up to 2 years and will resume growing when the implants are removed. This guideline is based upon personal communication between Drs. Phemister and Blount but has never been corroborated in the literature. Nevertheless, it has proven to be reliable in practice. A physis that is relieved of tethering within this window will not close permanently. Because extra-periosteal tethering is reliably reversible, it may be utilized in children less than 10 years old. This is in contradistinction to percutaneous other methods of epiphysiodesis including epiphysiodesis or P.E.T.S. Comparatively, young children with "gigantism" due to specific conditions such as Trevor's

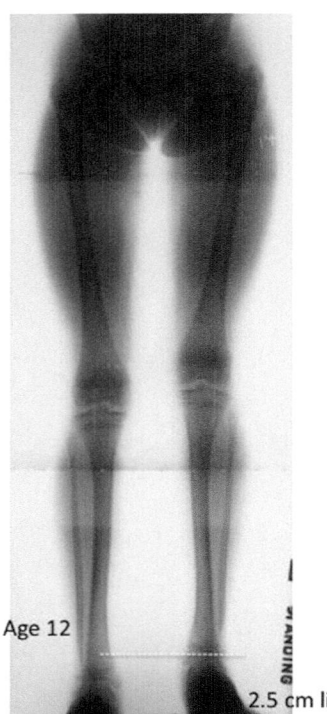
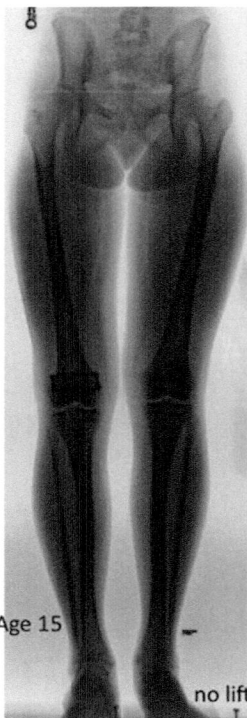

Fig. 6.8 As a sequela of DDH, this 12-year-old girl became symptomatic with a 2.5 cm limb length discrepancy. Three years following guided growth, her limb lengths are equal

Disease, Klippel-Trenaunay-Weber, hemangioma, Beckwith-Wiedemann Syndrome, and neurofibromatosis, may be candidates for intermittent longitudinal restraint of the overgrown limb, via guided growth (Figs. 6.6 and 6.9). Similarly, children with limb dysplasia, such as postaxial hypoplasia, may be considered for serial/intermittent guided growth of the normal longer limb. The goal is to forestall, minimize or perhaps obviate limb lengthening, with all of its associated risks. At the very least, one may forego lengthening with an external fixator in children in favor of an expanding intramedullary rod during adolescence.

In patients undergoing major long bone resection/limb salvage for oncologic disease, intermittent guided growth of the contralateral limb may mitigate some of the problems encountered with expanding implants. When employing this strategy, it is important to respect the 2-year window of opportunity, because, if a given physis is restrained indefinitely, the physis could permanently shut down. Therefore, one strategy is to remove the metaphyseal screws, wait for six months and reinsert them (Fig. 6.10). This may serve as an adjunct to the contralateral lengthening of the shorter limb or circumvent the need for it altogether.

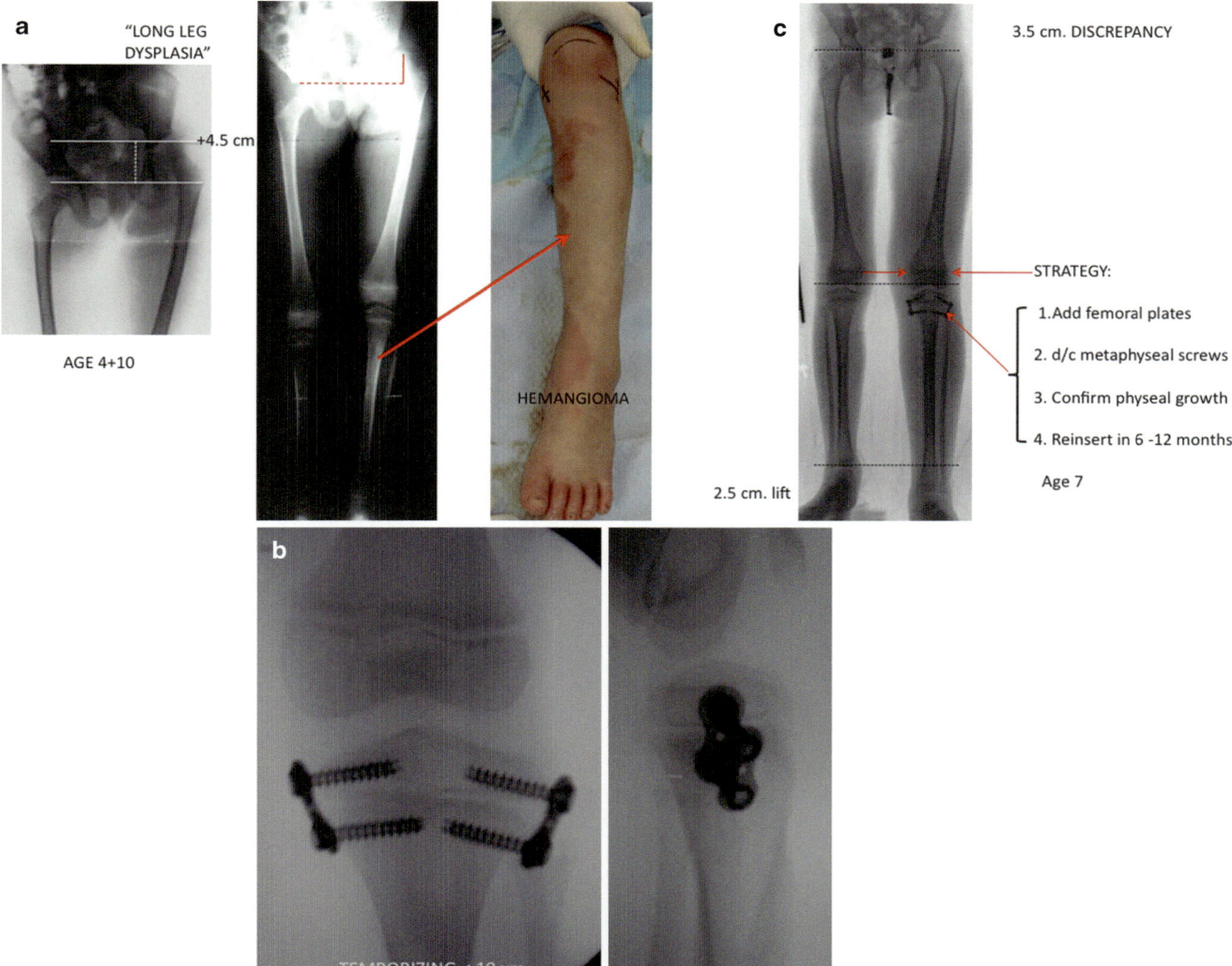

Fig. 6.9 (**a**) This girl presented with hemangioma causing a progressive LLD (4.5 cm), left hip and back pain, and projected 6–7 cm discrepancy (if untreated) at maturity. (**b**) She started at 4 + 10 years with guided growth of the proximal tibia. The fibula was not prominent, and thus was not included. (**c**) Two years later, her discrepancy measured 3.5 cm. The empirical tolerance of physeal restraint is 2 years. (**d**) Therefore, the tibial metaphyseal screws were removed and femoral plates were added. (**e**) Asymptomatic at age 9, with a 2.5-cm discrepancy (would have been 5–6 cm by now). (**f**) At age 10, with a 2-cm discrepancy and varus drift of the mechanical axis into zone -2. This was managed by reinserting the lateral metaphyseal screw in the tibia and percutaneously drilling the proximal fibular physis. When the axis returned to neutral over the ensuing 8 months, medial screws were added. (**g**) A summary of guided growth procedures as of age 11+4, when her limb lengths became equal for the first time in her life. The financial savings and reduced risk, as compared to osteotomy/shortening of the involved leg, or frame/lengthening of the normal right leg, are obvious

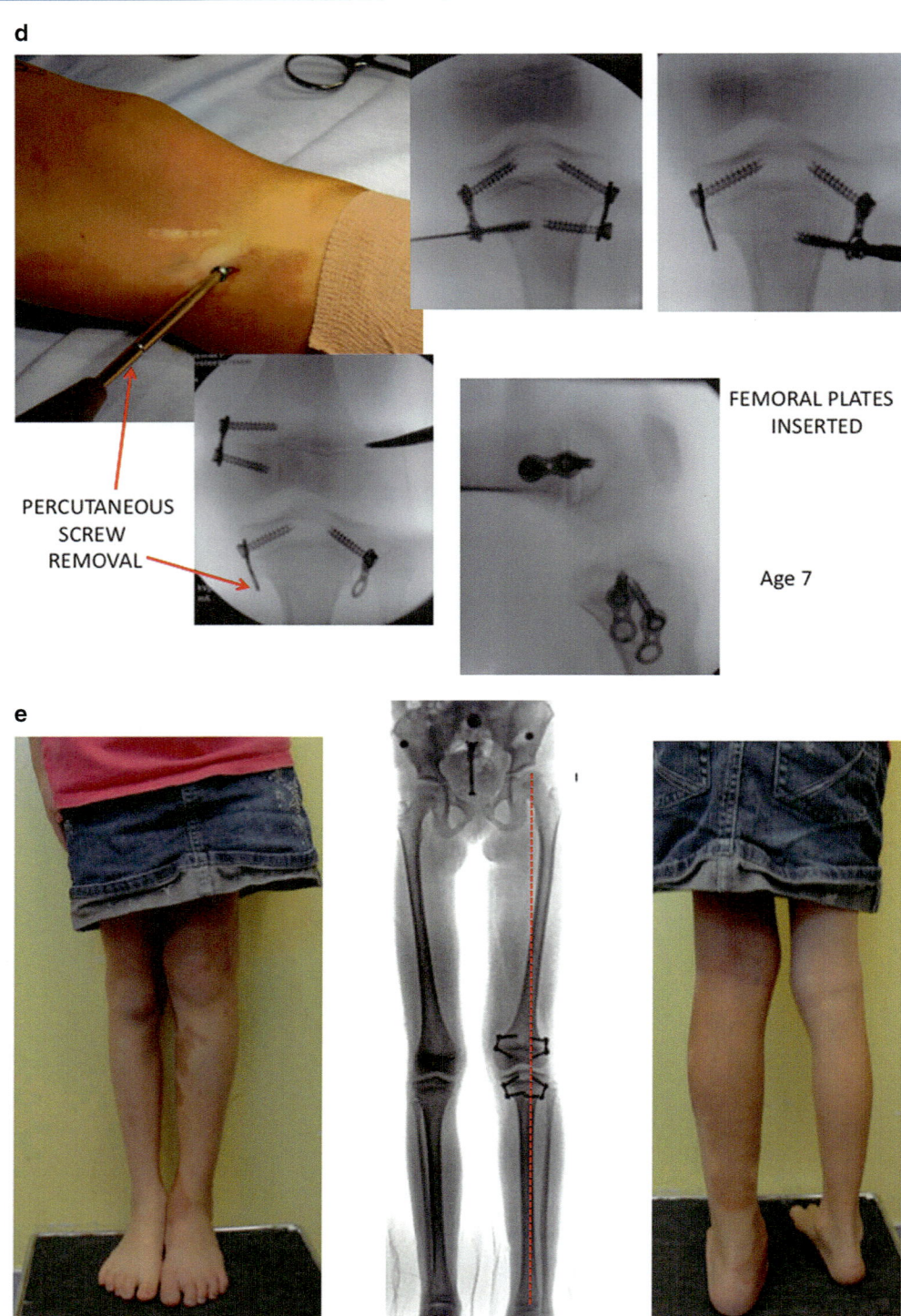

Fig. 6.9 (continued)

f

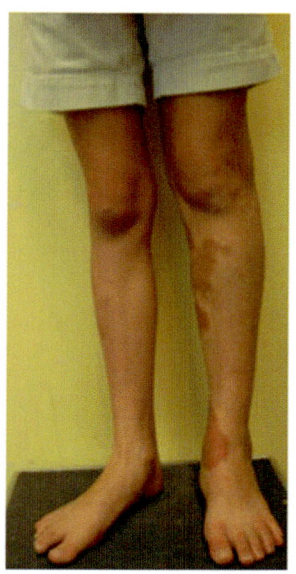
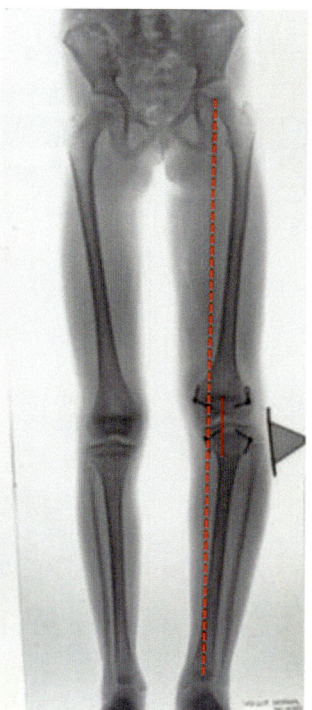
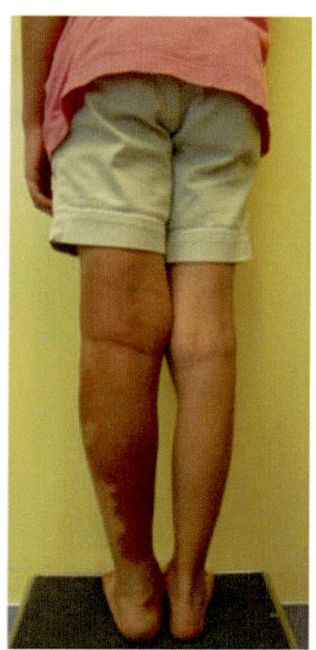

Age 10

g

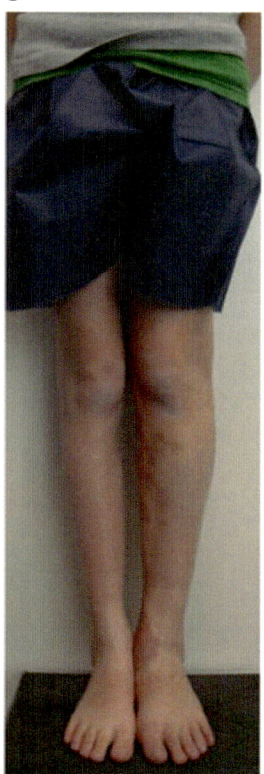

(D.O.B. 8/02 – now 11+4 yrs. old)

6/07 Plates proximal tibia

7/09 d/c metaph screws + plates femur

11/09 reinsert tibial screws

8/11 d/c tibial / femoral screws

9/11 lateral tibial screws / drill fibula (varus)

12/12 reinsert femoral and medial tib. screws

WITHOUT:
shoe lift
hospitalization
cast
osteotomy
frame

EQUAL LENGTHS

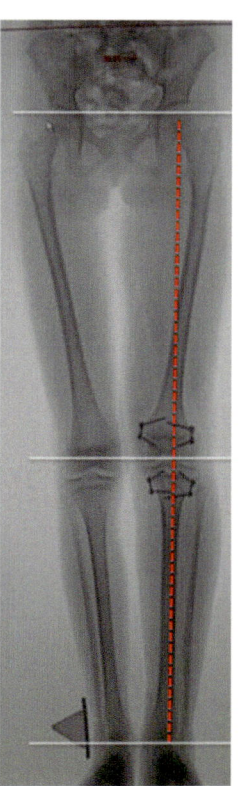

Fig. 6.9 (continued)

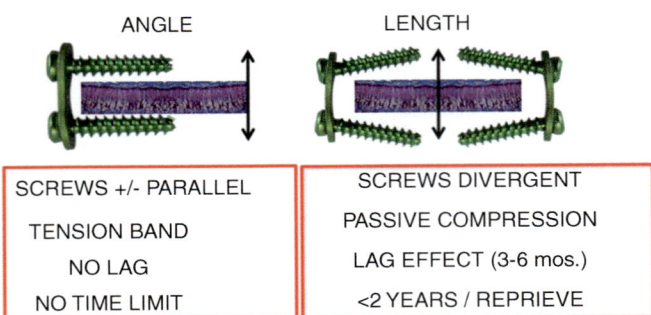

Fig. 6.10 When effecting angular correction, the screws are placed more or less parallel to each other and there is no time limit. Most angular deformities are correct within 12–18 months. When placed for length inhibition, the screws are placed divergent to each other. This may reduce the lag time and avoid screw bending. After 2 years of growth inhibition, one may remove the implant, or just the metaphyseal screw(s), wait 6 months, and repeat the process p.r.n.

Treatment/Length

Despite utilizing the same implants and surgical roaches as for angular guided growth, there are subtle differences in technique. Specifically, for length inhibition, the screws are placed in a *divergent* orientation within the plate (Figs. 6.9 and 6.10). This will mitigate against screws bending and may reduce the aforementioned latency period. It may also prevent intra-artuclar deformity such as the "pagoda tibia" effect reported by some - the consequences of which are unknown.

Complications/Length

Length equalization is slower and, therefore, less apparent than angular correction. Consequently, follow-up every 6 months is recommended for monitoring progress. In the interim, parents should be instructed to send a picture if they detect the development of a bow leg or knock knee deformity in the restrained extremity. This will also allow detection of drift of the mechanical axis and timely intervention. The proximal lateral tibia may pose problems and lead to iatrogenic genu varum. This situation may be encountered whether one uses staples or tension band plates. If such an angular drift is noted, one should remove the medial tibial plate (or metaphyseal screw), allowing gradual normalization of the mechanical axis and reimplant when the alignment is neutral (Fig. 6.9). In some cases, unopposed fibular growth may contribute to the deformity. If this is suspected, or if the fibular head is relatively prominent, it may be desirable to percutaneously drill the proximal fibular physis.

There have been concerns expressed regarding the potential to cause intraarticular deformity of the tibia, secondary to medial and lateral tension band plating [54, 55]. This effect may be prevented by inserting the screws in a divergent pattern from the outset. This will serve to mitigate against central physeal growth in the face of peripheral restraint.

Rotational Guided Growth?

Guided growth has proven to be versatile and in lieu of osteotomies, has become the treatment of choice for the management of most pediatric angular deformities. It is also a useful technique for managing progressive limb length inequality. Consequently, limb lengthening may be deferred or even prevented in some cases. The open question remaining is whether physeal engineering can be employed to correct malrotation.

Commonly, as an angular deformity (such as Blount's disease or Cozen's phenomenon) is corrected with guided growth, the rotational deformity will resolve when the mechanical axis is restored to neutral. This occurs regardless of whether the 8-plate is inserted vertically or in a diagonal orientation. Presumably, the rotational deformity that occurred through the physis is reversible as coronal alignment is corrected.

Now, there is mounting interest in the possibility of guiding the physis to respond to oblique restraint, for the express purpose of correcting malrotation of the femur or tibia. This has been successfully demonstrated in animal models [56–58]. More recently, investigators have reported correction employing various implants including 8-plates, obliquely placed cannulated screws connected with a wire, and modified Pega plate components secured with fiber-wire. The time for modest correction to occur has been reported as approximately 18 months. Upon correcting the rotational deformity, the aforementioned implants should be removed to accommodate continued longitudinal growth. Long term outcomes have not been reported. It is certainly appealing to avert the need for rotational osteotomy through "physeal engineering." The efficacy of such techniques awaits validation in children.

Summary

The classic method of epiphysiodesis, first described by Phemister nine decades ago, has evolved to a more versatile, less invasive, and reversible method, such as employing a low-profile tension band plate. This technique lends itself to the correction of both angular deformities and limb length discrepancy and may safely be applied in very young children without the risk of permanent physeal closure (provided the periosteum is protected). Bilateral and multilevel deformities may be addressed on an outpatient basis. Postoperative complications are rare and readily managed. The treatment costs are very low, compared to osteotomy. This method should be considered the treatment of choice for a wide variety of conditions, reserving osteotomy for salvage situations.

Commentary

Philip K. McClure
pmcclure@lifebridgehealth.org

The technique of growth modulation without question has made tremendous impacts on patient quality of life when undergoing deformity correction. The presence of open growth plates makes most deformity correction decisions fairly straightforward. It is of critical importance to keep in mind that while it is less invasive, risks remain in growth modulation surgery. Given the minimal attention in the literature, it's likely that iatrogenic Sagittal deformity is more prevalent than currently reported, though it may be of debatable short-term clinical significance. Careful deformity analysis is needed in each case, as the generation of a large joint line obliquely is likely a risk factor for degenerative disease in the future.

Various dogmas need up-to-date review—for instance, the mantra of "straight by age 4" when applied to Blount disease. Certainly, some insight into the nuances of this statement is needed, as the decision-making is no longer simply osteotomy vs. observation. Studies have demonstrated favorable responses to growth modulation despite skeletal dysplasia and metabolic bone disease, though clear-minded monitoring is required in order to change plans if needed. The combination of growth modulation and metabolic treatment should be entertained wherever possible for these patients. Growth modulation has recently been shown to improve outcomes for patients affected by tibial dysplasia, potentially decreasing fracture risk and the need for more invasive procedures.

Certainly, there are general preferences for technique of growth modulation, mostly either the PETS or tension band plates, though there are occasions where a simple inexpensive Blount staple remains tempting. The principle of growth modulation remains one of critical importance for deformity correction, and the means of optimal implementation may change depending on patient characteristics. Most surgeons can be categorized as devotees of either PETS or plates, both of which may be generally appropriate. The key to optimal practice is to identify in which category you find yourself and make a special effort to understand the instances in which that option may not be the best fit. Tunnel vision is of limited benefit to patients affected by uncommon problems or constellations of problems.

What follows is a brief (and incomplete) discussion of the relative advantages of each method.

PETS: minimally invasive and soft tissue friendly, rapid recovery, minimal to no need for PT (particularly relevant for medial distal femoral growth modulation in conjunction with intramedullary lengthening). Disadvantages include possible risk to the preadolescent physis. This can be mitigated by using the exacting technique, and only crossing the physis with the guide wire when the final position is optimized, maintaining a steep angle minimizes the cross-sectional area of the compromise to the physis, though it is technically more difficult. Implant prominence has been an issue with TBP's on the anterior distal femur, depending on the clinical series. Similar corrections have been obtained in neuromuscular corrections using PETS screws, with a decreased rate of anterior knee pain. Transphyseal screws may be preferable to tension band plates for patients with limited growth remaining due to faster correction. PETS screws may have application in the spastic hip to prevent proximal femoral valgus.

TBP: less invasive than osteotomy, faster recovery than osteotomy, less PT than osteotomy, truly "physeal sparing." Disadvantages include relatively large implant profiles on areas with minimal soft tissue coverage (medial distal tibia; distal radius) or areas with large amounts of relative motion between bone and overlying structures (medial distal femur).

The prominence is often not an issue, and newer generation implants have aimed for lower profiles. Tension band plates offer a convincing advantage in patients with large amounts of growth remaining

Finally, the inability to fully correct a deformity is not necessarily a contraindication to growth modulation techniques. An adolescent patient with Blount's disease may benefit from growth modulation even if there may not be enough time to fully correct the deformity. In my practice, I refer to this as a "get to know your plate" in which the patient's likely compliance with more rigorous deformity correction techniques can be evaluated without the risks associated with larger procedures. In addition, simplification from an angular deformity with LLD to simple LLD is particularly attractive in the era of intramedullary lengthening. In this setting, however, care must be taken to do a complete deformity analysis: intramedullary lengthening may generate unexpected results if a deformity is corrected away from its apex using growth modulation and then lengthened internally (consider the typical triple-level deformity of postermedial bowing of the tibia).

References

1. Phemister DP. Operative arrestment of longitudinal growth of bones in the treatment of deformities. J Bone Joint Surg Am. 1933;15:1–15.
2. Bowen JR, Leahey JL, Zhang ZH, Macewen GD. Partial epiphysiodesis at the knee to correct angular deformity. Clin Orthop Relat Res. 1985;198:184–90.
3. Canale ST, Russell TA, Holcomb RL. Percutaneous epiphysiodesis: experimental study and preliminary clinical results. J Pediatr Orthop. 1986;6(2):150–6.
4. Ogilvie JW. Epiphysiodesis: evaluation of a new technique. J Pediatr Orthop. 1986;6(2):147–9.
5. Blair VP, Walker SJ, Sheridan JJ, Schoenecker PL. Epiphysiodesis: a problem of timing. J Pediatr Orthop. 1982;2(3):281–4.
6. Steel HH, Sandrow RE, Sullivan PD. Complications of tibial osteotomy in children for genu varum or valgum. Evidence that neurological changes are due to ischemia. J Bone Joint Surg Am. 1971;53(8):1629–35.
7. Haas SL. Retardation of growth by a wire loop. J Bone Joint Surg Am. 1945;27:25–36.
8. Haas SL. Mechanical retardation of bone growth. J Bone Joint Surg Am. 1948;30a(2):506–12.
9. Blount WP, Clarke GR. Control of bone growth by epiphyseal stapling; a preliminary report. J Bone Joint Surg Am. 1949;31a(3):464–78.
10. Pm S. Guided growth: 1933 to the present. Strategies Trauma Limb Reconstr. 2006;1(1):29–35.
11. Stevens PM. Guided growth for angular correction: a preliminary series using a tension band plate. J Pediatr Orthop. 2007;27(3):253–9.
12. Bohm S, Krieg AH, et al. Growth guidance of angular lower limb deformities using a one-third two-hole tubular plate. J Child Orthop. 2013:289–94.
13. Jamil K, Abdul Rashid AH, et al. Guided growth implants for low-income to middle-income countries. J Pediatr Orthop B. 2013;22(6):608.
14. Lin TY, Kao HK, et al. Guided growth by a stainless-steel tubular plate. J Pediatr Orthop B. 2013;22(4):306–10.
15. Métaizeau JP, Wong-Chung J, Bertrand H, Pasquier P. Percutaneous epiphysiodesis using transphyseal screws (pets). J Pediatr Orthop. 1998;18(3):363–9.
16. Masquijo J, Artigas C, De Pablos J. Growth modulation with tension-band plates for the correction of paediatric lower limb angular deformity: current concepts and indications for rational use. Effort Open Rev. 2021;6(8):658–68.
17. Salenius P, Vankka E. The development of the tibiofemoral angle in children. J Bone Joint Surg Am. 1975;57(2):259–61.
18. Heath CH, Staheli LT. Normal limits of knee angle in white children – genu varum and genu valgum. J Pediatr Orthop. 1993;13(2):259–62.
19. Kling TF, Hensinger RN. Angular and torsional deformities of the lower limbs in children. Clin Orthop Relat Res. 1983;176:136–47.
20. Stevens PM, Novais EN. Multilevel guided growth for hip and knee varus secondary to chondrodysplasia. J Pediatr Orthop. 2012;32(6):626–30.
21. Inan M, Chan G, Littleton AG, Kubiak P, Bowen JR. Efficacy and safety of percutaneous epiphysiodesis. J Pediatr Orthop. 2008;28(6):648–51.
22. Bowen JR, Johnson WJ. Percutaneous epiphysiodesis. Clin Orthop Relat Res. 1984;190:170–3.
23. Paley D, Bhave A, Herzenberg JE, Bowen JR. Multiplier method for predicting limb-length discrepancy. J Bone Joint Surg Am. 2000;82-A(10):1432–46.
24. Moseley CF. A straight-line graph for leg-length discrepancies. J Bone Joint Surg Am. 1977;59(2):174–9.
25. Heyworth BE, Osei DA, Fabricant PD, Schneider R, Doyle SM, Green DW, et al. The shorthand bone age assessment: a simpler alternative to current methods. J Pediatr Orthop. 2013;33(5):569–74.
26. Eltayeby H, Gwam C, Frederick M, Herzenberg J. How accurate is the multiplier method in predicting the timing of angular correction after hemiepiphysiodesis? J Pediatr Orthop. 2019;39(2):E91–4.
27. Sabharwal S, Zhao C, Edgar M. Lower limb alignment in children: reference values based on a full-length standing radiograph. J Pediatr Orthop. 2008;28(7):740–6.
28. Paley D. Principles of deformity correction. Berlin: Springer; 2002.
29. Schoenleber S, Iobst C, Baitner A, Standard S. The biomechanics of guided, growth: does screw size, plate size, or screw configuration matter? J Pediatr Orthop B. 2014;23(2):122–5.
30. Klatt J, Stevens PM. Guided growth for fixed knee flexion deformity. J Pediatr Orthop. 2008;28(6):626–31.
31. Stevens PM, Belle RM. Screw epiphysiodesis for ankle valgus. J Pediatr Orthop. 1997;17(1):9–12.
32. Stevens PM, Kennedy JM, Hung M. Guided growth for ankle valgus. J Pediatr Orthop. 2011;31(8):878–83.
33. Stevens PM. The broken screw dilemma. J Pediatr Orthop. 2013;5(1):3.
34. Cheng Y-H, Lee W-C, Tsai Y-F, Kao H-K, Yang W-E. Chang C-H tension band plates have a greater risks of complications in temporary epiphysiodesis. J Child Orthop. 2021;15:106–13.

35. Machen MS, Stevens PM. Should full-length standing anteroposterior radiographs replace the scanogram for the measurement of limb length discrepancy? J Pediatr Orthop B. 2005;14(1):30–7.
36. Stevens PM. Radiographic distortion of bones: a marker study. Orthopedics. 1989;12(11):1457–63.
37. Green W, Anderson M. Skeletal age and the control of bone growth. Instr Lect Am Acad Orthop Surg. 1960;17:199–217.
38. Song H, Eun-Seok C, Seok M, et al. Percutaneous epiphysiodesis using transphyseal screws in the management of leg length discrepancy: optimal operation timing and techniques to avoid complication. J Pediatr Ortho. 2015;35(1):89–93.
39. Lee SC, Shim JS, Seo SW, Lim KS, Ko KR. The accuracy of current methods in determining the timing of epiphysiodesis. J Bone Joint Surg. 1995;7:993–1000.
40. Dimeglio A, Kelly P. Lower-limb growth: how predictable are predictions? J Child Orthop. 2008;2:407–15.
41. Makarov MR, Jackson TJ, Jo CH, Birch JG. Timing of epiphysiodesis to correct leg-length discrepancy: a comparison of prediction methods. J Bone Joint Surg. 2018;100(14):1217–22.
42. Birch JG, Makarov MA, Jackson TJ, Jo CH. Comparison of Anderson-Green graphs and White-Menelaus predictions of growth remaining in the distal femoral and proximal tibial physes. J Bone Joint Surg Am. 2019;101(11):1016–22.
43. Lykissas MG, Jain VV, Manickam V, Nathan S, Eismann EA, Mccarthy JJ. Guided growth for the treatment of limb length discrepancy: a comparative study of the three most commonly used surgical techniques. J Pediatr Orthop B. 2013;22(4):311–7.
44. Stewart D, Cheema A, Szalay EA. Dual 8-plate technique is not as effective as ablation for epiphysiodesis about the knee. J Pediatr Orthop. 2013;33(8):843–6.
45. Lauge-Pedersen H, Hagglund. Eight plate should not be used for leg length discrepancy. J Child Orthop. 2013;7(4):285–837.
46. Bayhan I, Karatas A, Rogers K, et al. Comparing percutaneous epiphysiodesis for the treatment of limb length discrepancy. J Pediatr Orthop. 2017;37(5):323–7.
47. Kaymaz B, Komurcu E. Comment On the article "dual 8-plate technique is not as effective as ablation for epiphysiodesis about the knee" By Stewart, et al. J Pediatr Orthop. 2014;34(8):E67.
48. Borbas P, Agten C, Rosskopf A, et al. Guided growth with tension band plate or definitive epiphysiodesis for treatment of limb length discrepancy? J Orthop Surg Res. 2019;14(1):99.
49. Gaumetou E, Mallet C, Souchet P, et al. Poor efficiency of eight-plates in the treatment of lower limb length discrepancy. J Pediatr Orthop. 2016;37(7):715–9.
50. Stevens PM. Invalid comparison between methods of epiphysiodesis. J Pediatr Ortho. 2018;38(1):e29–30.
51. Menelaus MB. Correction of leg length discrepancy by epiphyseal arrest. J Bone Joint Surg (B). 1966;48(2):336–9.
52. Westh R, Menelaus M. A simple calculation for the timing of epiphyseal arrest: a further report. J Bone Joint Surg. 1981;63(B):117–9.
53. Pendleton A, Stevens PM, Hung M. Guided growth for the treatment of moderate leg-length discrepancy. Orthop. 2013;36(5):e575–80.
54. Ballhause TM, Steil N, Breyer S, Stucker R, Spiro A. Does eight-plate epiphysiodesis of the proximal tibia in treating angular deformity create intraarticular deformity? Bone Joint J. 2020;102-B(10)
55. Sinha R, Weigl E, Mercado T, Becker P, Kedem P, Bar-On E. Eight-plate epiphysiodesis: are we creating an intra-articular deformity? Bone Joint J. 2018;100-B(8)
56. Martel G, Holmes L, Sobrado G, Paley D, Praglia F, Arguello G, Arellano E, Flores G. Rotational-guided growth. J Limb Lengthen Reconstruct. 2019;4(2):97–1056.
57. Arami A, Bar-On E, Herman A, Velkes S, Heller S. Guiding femoral rotational growth in an animal model. J Bone Joint Surg Am. 2013;95(22):2022–7.
58. Moreland MS. Morphological effects of torsion applied to growing bone: an in vivo study in rabbits. Bone Joint J. 1980;62-B(2)

Physeal Bar Excision

David A. Podeszwa, Anthony I. Riccio, and Karl E. Rathjen

Introduction

As with any clinical dilemma in the growing child, the management of a physeal growth disturbance begins with careful consideration of the natural history of the pathologic process. Appropriate treatment of a physeal arrest starts with understanding the patient and disease characteristics that may act in concert to create limb deformity. Knowledge of the nature and characteristics of the arrest, an understanding of normal physeal behavior, and an appreciation of factors influencing future growth allow the clinician to assess the potential for deformity if a physeal arrest was left untreated. Appreciation of these factors is also essential for generating realistic expectations for the restoration of normal growth following surgical intervention. To ensure optimal outcomes, the treatment choice must be tailored to the individual patient and, in many instances, the individual physis.

Etiology

Physeal injury can occur via both direct and indirect mechanisms. While physeal fractures account for the majority of physeal arrests and premature physeal closures, growth disturbance is also reported following osteomyelitis, vascular insult, radiation exposure, as well as neoplastic and tumor-like conditions [1–10]. Infantile Blount's disease is yet another cause of physeal growth disturbance. Unlike other etiologies, physeal arrest in infantile Blount's disease is likely the result of sustained altered physiologic function within the physis itself [3, 11, 12].

Growth disturbance can occur from physical loss of the physis, altered physeal physiology without any loss of the physeal structure, or disruption of normal physeal architecture. Disruption of normal physeal architecture may produce an osseous bridge across the cartilaginous physis, which is termed a physeal bar (Fig. 7.1). However, it is important to realize that physeal growth disturbance may produce deformity without physeal arrest (Fig. 7.2). The etiology of a physeal growth disturbance appears to have some bearing in the successful restoration of growth following the resection of a physeal bar. In the authors' experience, growth arrests associated with fractures and infantile Blount's disease carry a better prognosis for resumption of growth following epiphysiolysis than arrests resulting from infection, radiation, or intraosseous space-occupying lesions. As the treatment strategies can differ based on the etiology of a growth disturbance, an understanding of the nature of the physeal disturbance is essential.

D. A. Podeszwa (✉) · A. I. Riccio · K. E. Rathjen
Department of Orthopedic Surgery, Scottish Rite for Children, Dallas, TX, USA
e-mail: David.podeszwa@tsrh.org; Anthony.riccio@tsrh.org; karl.rathjen@tsrh.org

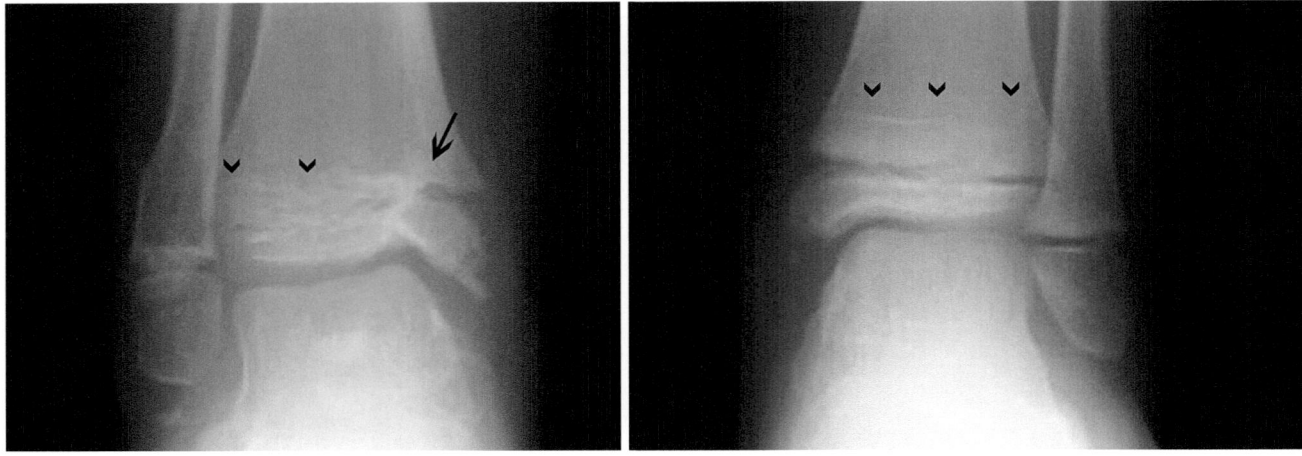

Fig. 7.1 AP radiograph of bilateral ankles. Note the "Harris growth arrest" lines (*arrowheads*) on both sides. On the right ankle, the Harris line is asymmetrical and terminates medially at the area of physeal arrest or "bony bar" (*arrow*)

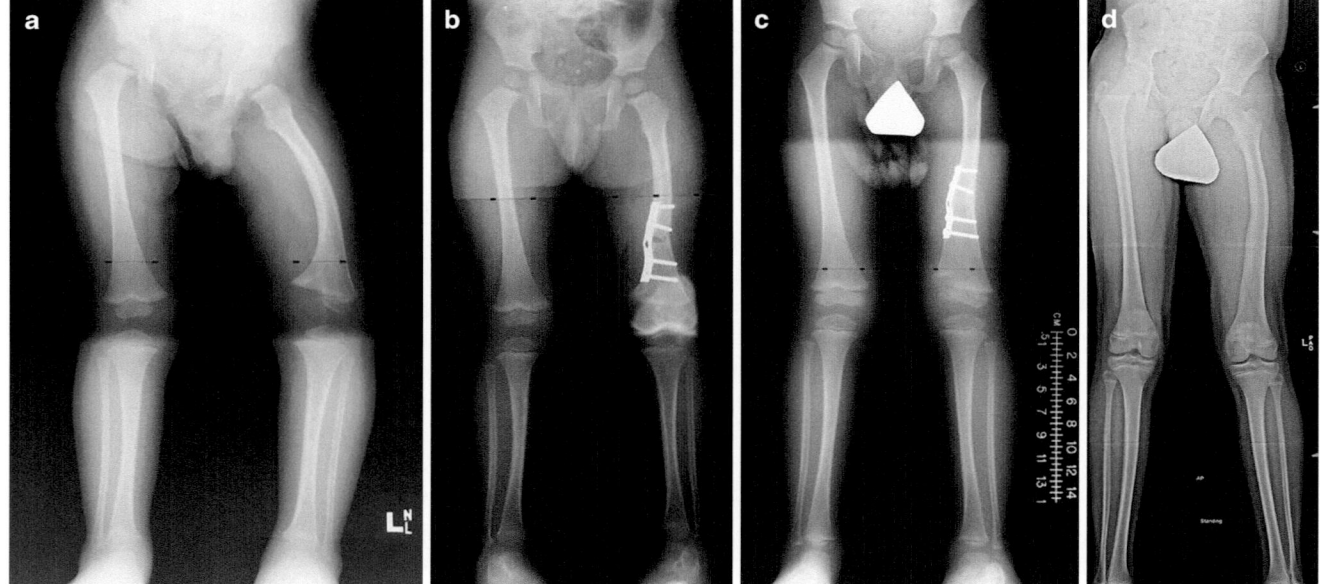

Fig. 7.2 (**a**) A 2-year-old with a history of neonatal sepsis. MRI at this age showed no physeal bar and a relatively normal cartilaginous epiphysis. Despite the significant diaphyseal deformity and appearance of the secondary ossification center, the patient was felt to have mild (albeit long-standing) growth disturbance without physeal arrest. (**b**) Intraoperative radiograph with opening wedge osteotomy and arthrogram which demonstrates normal cartilaginous anatomy of the distal femur. (**c**) With the restoration of normal limb alignment and mechanical forces, the secondary ossification of the distal femur begins to ossify. This is an excellent example of the Heuter–Volkmann principle. (**d**) Nine years postoperatively, there has been relatively normal growth. Note the absence of angular deformity, the pelvic obliquity associated with limb length inequality, and the premature closure of the ipsilateral distal femoral growth plate

Trauma

It is well documented that the physis' cartilaginous nature provides a path of minimal resistance to forces traversing an extremity. The majority of physeal fractures course through the hypertrophic zone of the growth plate, which is mechanically the weakest zone of the physis and therefore the most susceptible to disruption. Physeal fractures that progress from the hypertrophic zone into the adjacent metaphysis (Salter–Harris II fractures) course away from the germinal and proliferative zones and therefore away from the regions of maximal growth and metabolic activity. As a result, these fractures generally have a lower rate of physeal arrests than those that course from the hypertrophic zone, through the germinal and proliferative zone, and toward the epiphysis [13] (Salter–Harris III and IV fractures) [14, 15] (Fig. 7.3).

In addition to the Salter–Harris classification, fracture location can be prognostic for the development of a growth arrest. Fractures involving the distal femoral physis and, to a lesser extent, those involving the medial malleolus are notorious for relatively high rates of growth arrest [15].

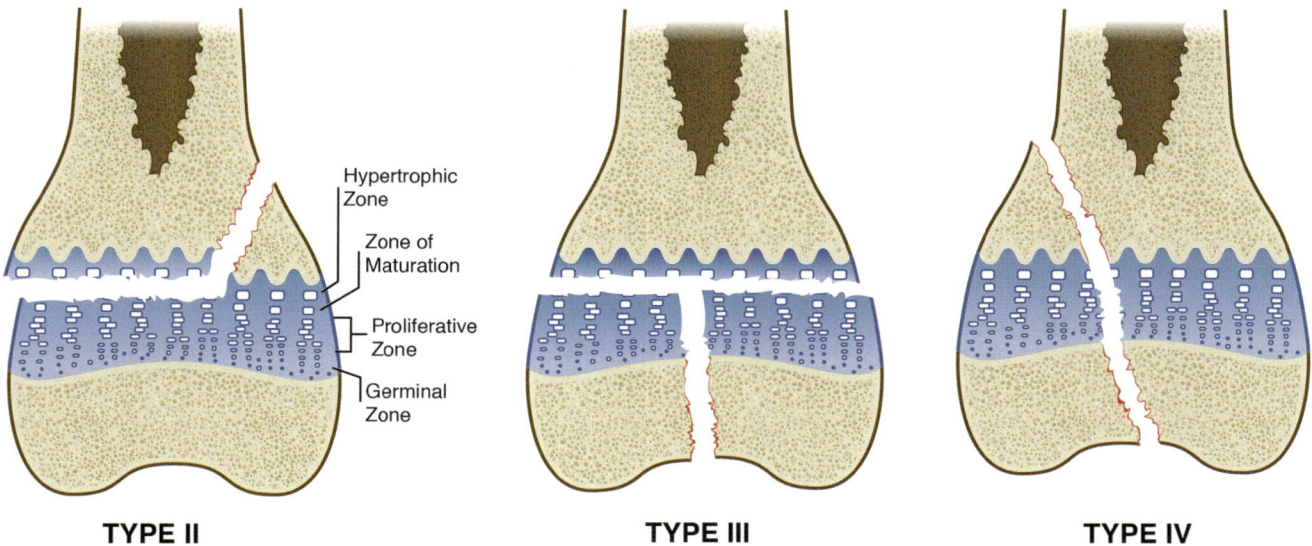

Fig. 7.3 Salter–Harris type II, type III, and type IV injuries. Note that the germinal zone of the physis is disrupted in type III and IV injuries

Infection

Osteomyelitis and septic arthritis can lead to both physeal growth disturbance and growth arrest. As with trauma, physeal destruction from musculoskeletal infection can result in both complete and partial growth disturbance resulting in angular deformities, altered joint morphology, and limb length differences [7]. Widespread systemic neonatal sepsis can result in multifocal physeal arrests and severe deformity (Fig. 7.4).

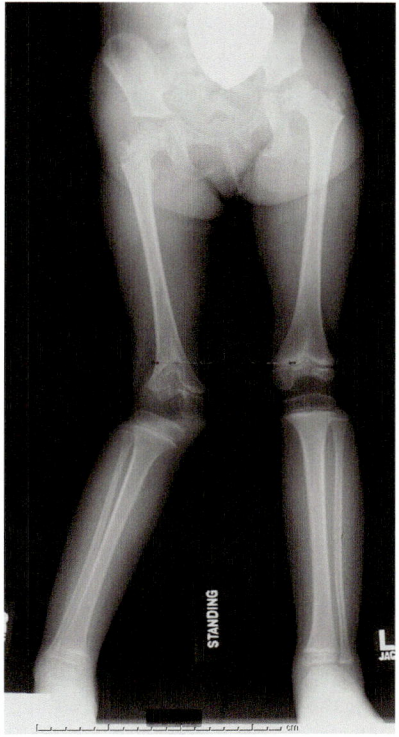

Fig. 7.4 AP bilateral lower extremities of a 4-year-old with a history of neonatal sepsis. Note the shortening and angular deformity of the right leg. Note also that the central growth arrest has created intra-articular abnormality of the right knee. Note the irregularities in the left proximal and distal femoral epiphyses

Neoplasm and Tumor-Like Conditions

Growth disturbance from physeal injury has been reported in the presence of both malignant and benign neoplasms [16, 17].

Physical encroachment of the growth plate by these lesions is the usual mechanism of physeal damage, although additional injury can occur during treatment (surgical or radiation). Growth disturbance resulting from space-occupying lesions can be challenging to treat as it is often difficult to predict the degree of altered growth resulting from irradiation and the behavior of physeal tissue preserved following tumor resection or a limb salvage operation. Small physeal bars are only rarely encountered, usually obviating epiphysiolysis as a surgical option. Completion epiphysiodesis and staged or concurrent deformity correction or limb lengthening procedures are more commonly required.

Vascular Insult

Limb hypoperfusion due to either severe systemic hypotension or local limb ischemia resulting from vascular injury, altered venous outflow, or compartment syndrome can result in altered physeal physiology and growth disturbance [18–20].

This relatively rare cause of abnormal growth plate function has been associated with both partial and complete physeal arrests. A small proportion of growth arrests without an obvious attributable cause may in fact have resulted from unrecognized transient vascular injury insufficiently following local trauma without fracture or injury remote to the area of arrest in the ipsilateral limb.

Other Causes of Physeal Injury

Rare etiologies of growth plate disturbance include burns, frostbite, electrical injury, radiation exposure, and repetitive stress injuries. Growth disturbance due to repetitive stress is commonly encountered in the young athlete. Altered proximal humeral physeal growth is well described in children who engage in extensive overhead throwing activities [21, 22]. Fortunately, the cessation of the offending activity usually results in the restoration of normal physeal function.

Assessment of the Abnormal Physis

Timely identification of a growth disturbance, differentiation between partial and complete physeal arrests, determination of the location and extent of a physeal bar, and an accurate assessment of remaining growth of the involved physis are all necessary for a complete assessment of the abnormal physis and selection of appropriate treatment.

Timely Identification

Early identification of a physeal growth disturbance usually affords the clinician a wider array of management options and can simplify management by allowing for treatment of the growth arrest without the concomitant management of an associated deformity. Careful serial radiographic follow-up of physeal injuries is recommended until the clinician is confident regarding the resumption of normal growth. Even when normal growth ensues, radiographic surveillance until skeletal maturity is advised as physes with a history of injury are known to close prematurely [23]. If the identification of a growth disturbance is delayed and a significant acquired deformity has developed, both the deformity and the growth disturbance usually require treatment.

Partial Versus Complete Physeal Arrest

The effect of a bar (bony, cartilaginous, or fibrous) on the adjacent physeal growth varies with location and size of the arrest. Large bars and those bars associated with extensive injury to surrounding physeal cartilage usually retard growth of the entire physis causing a complete growth arrest (Fig. 7.5). Such bars usually result in a limb length discrep-

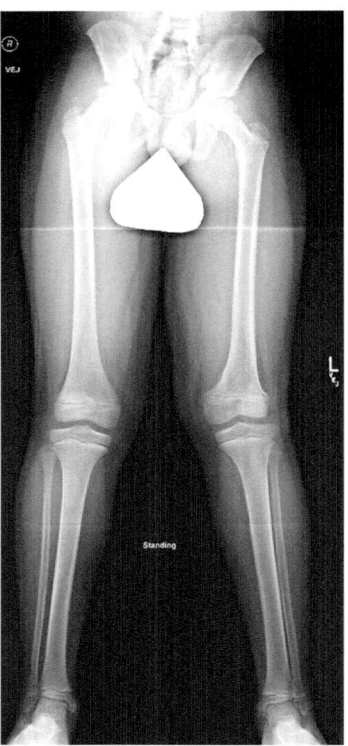

Fig. 7.5 AP bilateral lower extremities of a 9-year-old who sustained a distal femoral physeal fracture 2 years earlier. Note the premature complete closure of the left distal femoral physis and the pelvic obliquity associated with mild limb length inequality

ancy without associated intra-articular or angular deformity. Smaller central bars and those that are more peripherally located usually result in a partial physeal growth disturbance. As the bar causes local restriction of growth in the presence of normal physeal function remote to the bar, angular deformity, limb length difference, tenting of the physis, and intra-articular deformity can ensue (see Fig. 7.4).

Resumption of growth following resection of a physeal bar relies upon the integrity and health of the normal physis surrounding the physeal bar. There is no role for physeal bar resection in the presence of a complete growth arrest of the entire physis, therefore, differentiating between a partial and complete disturbance is the first step in developing a management strategy.

Location of Physeal Arrest

Partial growth arrests are classified based upon their location within the physis. Determination of location of a physeal bar is important, as it is predictive of the potential deformity that might ensue if left untreated. Furthermore, the choice of a surgical approach for a bar resection is largely dependent upon its location.

Physeal bars are generally classified as central or peripheral [10]. Peripheral bars, as the name suggests, involve an outer edge of the growth plate. If left untreated, peripheral bars are likely to create marked angular deformity in a child with considerable growth remaining. We typically classify peripheral bars as Type A arrests (Fig. 7.6). Central bars are subclassified based upon the amount of healthy physis surrounding the arrest. Type B arrests are surrounded circumferentially by normal physeal cartilage. As the normal physis continues to grow around a Type B bar, tenting of the growth plate, and eventually the epiphysis, can develop. This may ultimately result in the distortion of the underlying articular cartilage. A Type C arrest is a variation of a central bar in which the area of arrest traverses the entire growth plate in one direction with healthy physis present on the remaining two sides. This type of arrest is often seen following Salter–Harris III and IV fractures of the medial malleolus in which physeal bars frequently extend from anterior to posterior with normal physis being found medially and laterally (an example is shown in Fig. 7.10).

Resection of a bar while minimizing concomitant damage to the surrounding normal physis is of paramount importance regardless of the type of arrest encountered. The importance of classification lies in the fact that accomplishing this goal in the presence of central bars (Types B and C) may be more challenging than in those located peripherally.

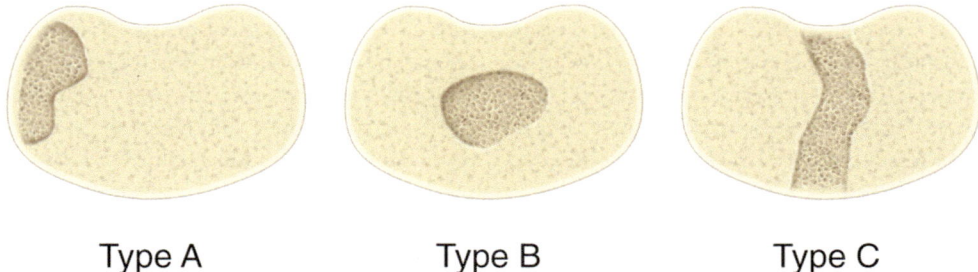

Fig. 7.6 Anatomic classification of physeal arrest. Type A: Peripheral. Type B: Central surrounded by normal physis. Type C: Central traversing the physis completely. Reprinted with permission from Herring JA (ed). Tachdjian's Pediatric Orthopedics: From the Texas Scottish Rite Hospital for Children. 5th ed. Philadelphia: Elsevier; 2013

Extent of Physeal Arrest

Determination of the extent of physeal involvement in a partial growth plate arrest is the next step in developing an appropriate treatment strategy. Size of a physeal bar, typically documented as a percentage of the entire physis, has been shown to correlate with successful outcomes following resection surgery [4, 24, 25]. Successful restoration of growth has been reported to be more likely in bars that comprise less than 25 % of the involved growth plate [25]. While it is important to note that no firm cutoff exists as to a percentage of physeal area beyond which bar resection should not be attempted, the restoration of meaningful growth following excision of arrests that involve greater than 50 % of the growth plate is less likely. Although three-dimensional imaging is now nearly universally used to assess the extent of a physeal arrest, we believe that it is important to understand the process of "mapping" a physeal arrest in two planes and that this exercise can ensure that the surgeon has a comprehensive understanding of the three-dimensional anatomy of the physis [3, 23, 26–29]. This nuanced knowledge will likely aid the surgeon who attempts resection of a physeal arrest.

Plain Radiographs

Standard orthogonal radiographs are an appropriate initial diagnostic study for any patient with a suspected physeal arrest. Though advanced imaging modalities allow for more accurate determination of the presence, extent, and exact location of a physeal arrest, much information can be garnered from plain radiography. Physeal narrowing and areas of bridging can often be seen using plain radiographs prior to the development of deformity (as demonstrated in Figs. 7.1 and 7.5). More readily determined, however, are the presence and orientation of growth arrest lines, which often are the earliest heralds of altered growth [4]. These thin sclerotic lines develop at the growth plate during most physeal insults. If normal growth resumes, this line becomes progressively distant from the physis. If normal symmetric physeal growth resumes, the arrest line will remain parallel to the physis. In the presence of a growth arrest, the line (if the arrest is peripheral) or lines (if the arrest is central) will converge toward the area of abnormal growth. Identification of such convergence should alert the clinician to a likely arrest and will usually prompt additional imaging to assess the extent of the bar (see Fig. 7.1).

Computed Tomography

Computed tomography (CT) is often the imaging modality of choice for assessment of a physeal bar. A CT scan can generally be obtained quickly and without sedation, which is often necessary for magnetic resonance imaging (MRI). Modern image reconstruction and manipulation software usually allow for excellent visualization of both normal and diseased physis, thereby allowing for very accurate determination of the extent and location of a physeal bar (see also Fig. 7.10a) [28]. A preoperative CT scan is helpful if using intraoperative CT scanning for the localization of the physeal bar and confirmation of complete resection.

Magnetic Resonance Imaging

MRI is a highly sensitive test for the detection and delineation of areas of physeal arrest. This study allows for the localization of both normal physeal cartilage and regions of bony bars. Furthermore, the use of three-dimensional MRI utilizing fat-suppressed spoiled gradient-recalled echo sequences allows for the manual reconstruction of the growth plate, thereby allowing the clinician to accurately map an area of growth arrest which can be invaluable in developing a surgical plan for epiphysiolysis (see also Fig. 7.7c) [3, 27, 29, 30]. Accurate mapping of a physeal bar should include localization in relation to known and identifiable anatomic markers which can be useful during surgical resection [31, 32] (Fig. 7.7).

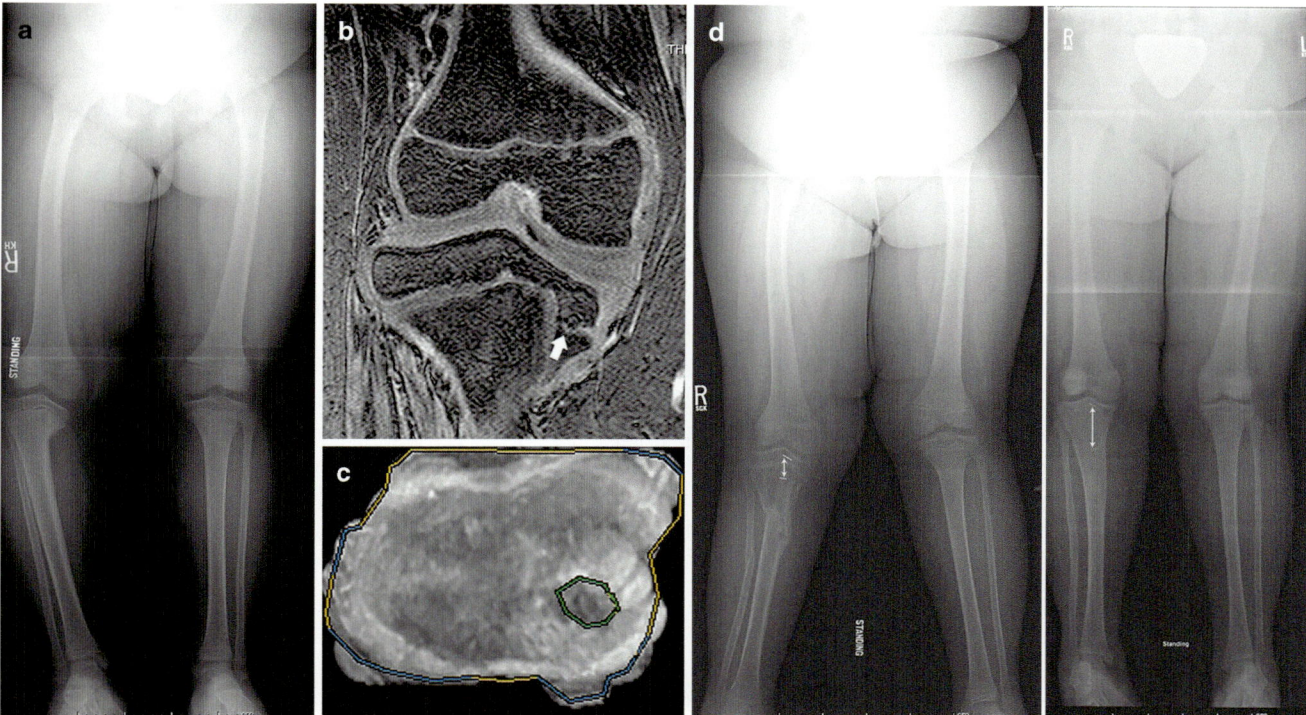

Fig. 7.7 (a) AP bilateral lower extremities of an 8-year-old with infantile Blount's. (b) Coronal MRI demonstrating a small physeal bar in a proximal tibia (*arrow*). (c) Modern software can facilitate the construction of a "map" which defines the area of physeal closure. (d) Early postoperative and final standing radiographs. Note the resumption of growth as demonstrated between the markers (*arrows*)

Growth Remaining

The greater the growth potential in a physis, the more likely it will resume growth following the resection of a physeal bar, and the greater the benefit from the restoration of growth. The amount of growth remaining from a particular physis is determined by which physis is involved and the age of the patient. A number of studies have assessed longitudinal limb growth and allow general estimates of yearly growth from each long bone physis [33–35]. As physiologic or skeletal age may differ significantly from chronological age; the former is important to consider when assessing growth potential. Traditionally, this is most commonly achieved using standards for skeletal age published in atlas format using radiographs of the left hand and wrist [36]. Skeletal age can also be determined using AP and lateral radiographs of the elbow [37, 38]. This information, in conjunction with the knowledge that extremities typically grow until a bone age of 14 in women and 16 in men, can provide estimations of the amount of growth remaining in a particular physis.

Surgical Indications

Traditional indications for physeal bar excision include a growth plate arrest occupying less than 50% of the involved physis in a child with more than 2 years or 2 cm of growth remaining at the involved physis. Interestingly, there is surprisingly little scientific evidence to support this "dogma" [4, 25]. Because of the modest results of physeal bar resection in most modern reports, we believe that physeal bar resection is ideally performed in patients in the first decade of life, and patients closer to skeletal maturity (i.e., only 3 or 4 years of limb growth remaining) may be better treated with completion epiphysiodesis, with or without a contralateral epiphysiodesis to mitigate any limb length difference. Consideration can be given to resection of larger bars in very young children as success might spare the child from multiple subsequent procedures. Lastly, excision of a physeal arrest is ideally performed prior to the development of angular deformity. Once deformity is present, consideration must be given to concomitant corrective osteotomy.

Surgical Technique and Pitfalls

Once the determination has been made to resect a physeal bar, meticulous preoperative planning should address the following considerations: need for concomitant deformity correction, approach for bar resection, interposition material following resection, and radiographic markers in the epiphysis and metaphysis to aid in assessment of future growth.

Role of Osteotomy

The decision to surgically correct any concomitant angular deformity should be the first consideration when planning a physeal bar resection. In our experience, it is unlikely that a successful bar resection will "overgrow" to correct angular deformity. Although growth modulation of an injured physis after bar resection is possible, there is no way to predict which physes may respond to modulation. Therefore, we believe it unwise to plan for "guided growth" via physeal tethering in an injured physis. Thus, osteotomy with acute correction of deformity is often the most attractive option when a physeal bar is associated with clinically unacceptable angular deformity. Acute correction of the angular deformity to restore normal alignment has the added theoretical benefit of eliminating any asymmetrical forces across the physis which may be contributing to abnormal physeal growth via the Heuter–Volkmann principle. If acute angular correction is performed, careful consideration and planning must be given to determine appropriate fixation of the osteotomy. Fortunately, many of these patients are young and can be managed with relatively simple constructs including variations of "pins and plaster" (Fig. 7.11). Obviously, more extensive internal or external fixation will be necessary for larger children and adolescents.

Surgical Approaches (Tips and Tricks)

Once the need for osteotomy to correct angular deformity has been assessed, the determination can be made regarding the best approach to resect the physeal bar. Peripheral bars are the simplest and are approached directly (Fig. 7.8). Central bars can be more challenging and can be addressed in a variety of ways, including through a metaphyseal window or tunnel (perhaps most common) (Fig. 7.9), percutane-

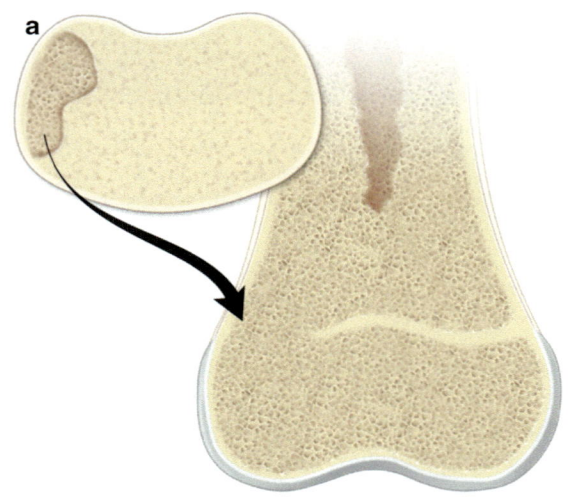
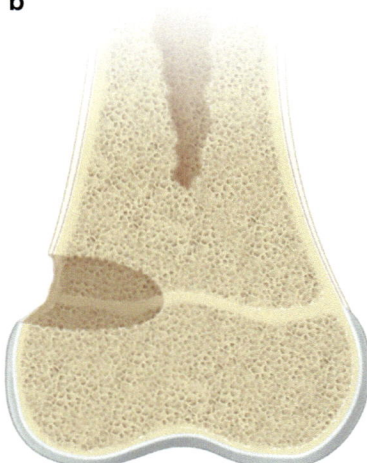

Fig. 7.8 Schematic representation of a peripheral bar resection. (**a**) Peripheral physeal bar of the distal femur. (**b**) The bar can be approached directly and excised with a small amount of the metaphysis and epiphysis using a high-speed burr

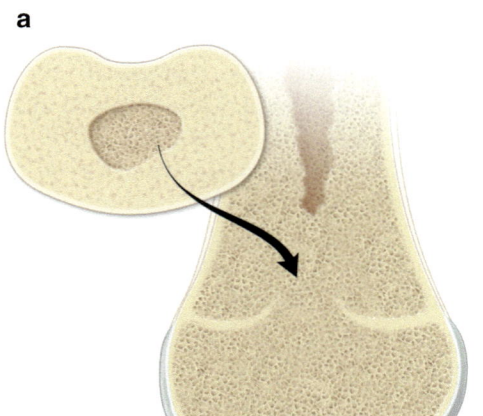
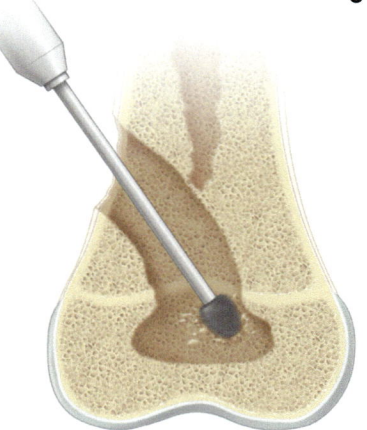
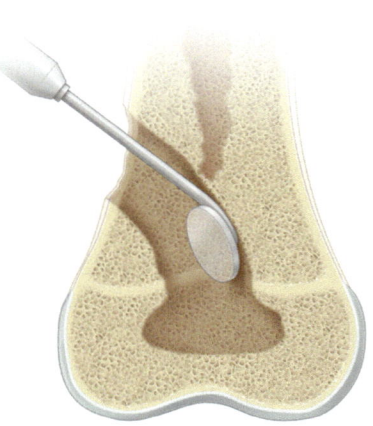

Fig. 7.9 Illustration of central physeal bar resection. (**a**) Central bar of the distal femur. (**b**) A high-speed burr is used to approach the bar through a tunnel in the metaphysis. (**c**) A dental mirror or arthroscopy camera (and fluoroscopic guidance, fiberoptic suction lighting, and small curved currets) can be helpful in assessing the resection. Reprinted with permission from Herring JA (ed). Tachdjian's Pediatric Orthopedics: From the Texas Scottish Rite Hospital for Children. 5th ed. Philadelphia: Elsevier; 2013

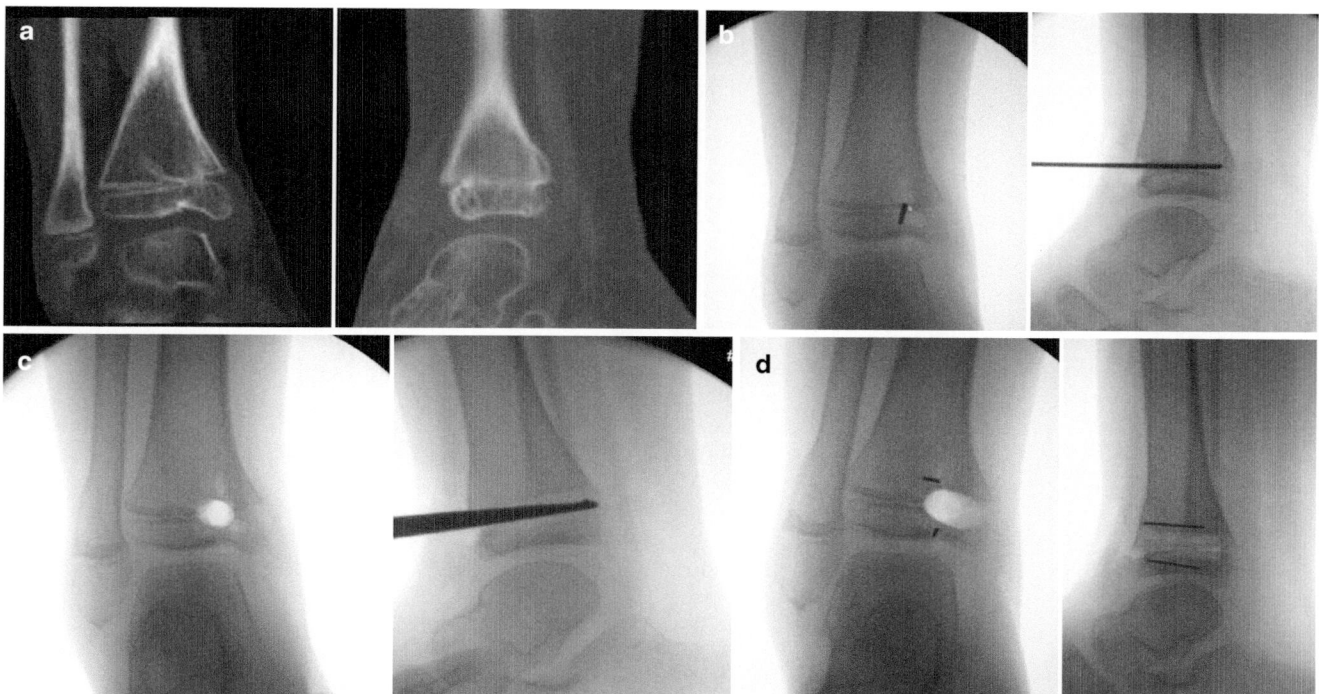

Fig. 7.10 (a) Coronal and sagittal CT scan demonstrating Type C central bar following a Salter–Harris IV fracture of the medial malleolus. (b) Intraoperative fluoroscopy is used to place a guide pin through the area of physeal closure. (c) A cannulated reamer is placed over the guide to resect the bony bar. Resection is confirmed with a curette. (d) Final appearance after radiographic markers are placed to facilitate postoperative assessment

ously (ideal for Type C bars as illustrated in Fig. 7.10), and directly through an osteotomy (most commonly an option when performing concomitant angular deformity correction). Although distraction through the physis prior to bar resection has been reported [39], we have no experience with this technique and have concerns that distraction across the physis may further damage the germinal layer and lead to premature closure. The surgeon should select an approach that will give him or her the confidence that he or she can reach the entire extent of the bar. Most commonly the bony bar is resected by initially reaming over a guide wire and completing the resection with a high-speed burr, taking care to always run the burr perpendicular to the physis. It is paramount that the surgeon visualizes normal physis separating the epiphysis and metaphysis. Again this is relatively straightforward for peripheral bars but can be more challenging for central bars. Fiber-optic lighted suction, dental mirrors, and arthroscopes may aid in confirming a normal physis "360°" around the resection of a central bar. Additionally, radio-opaque dye can be placed in the resection bed to allow fluoroscopic assessment of the extent of the resection (Figs. 7.9 and 7.11).

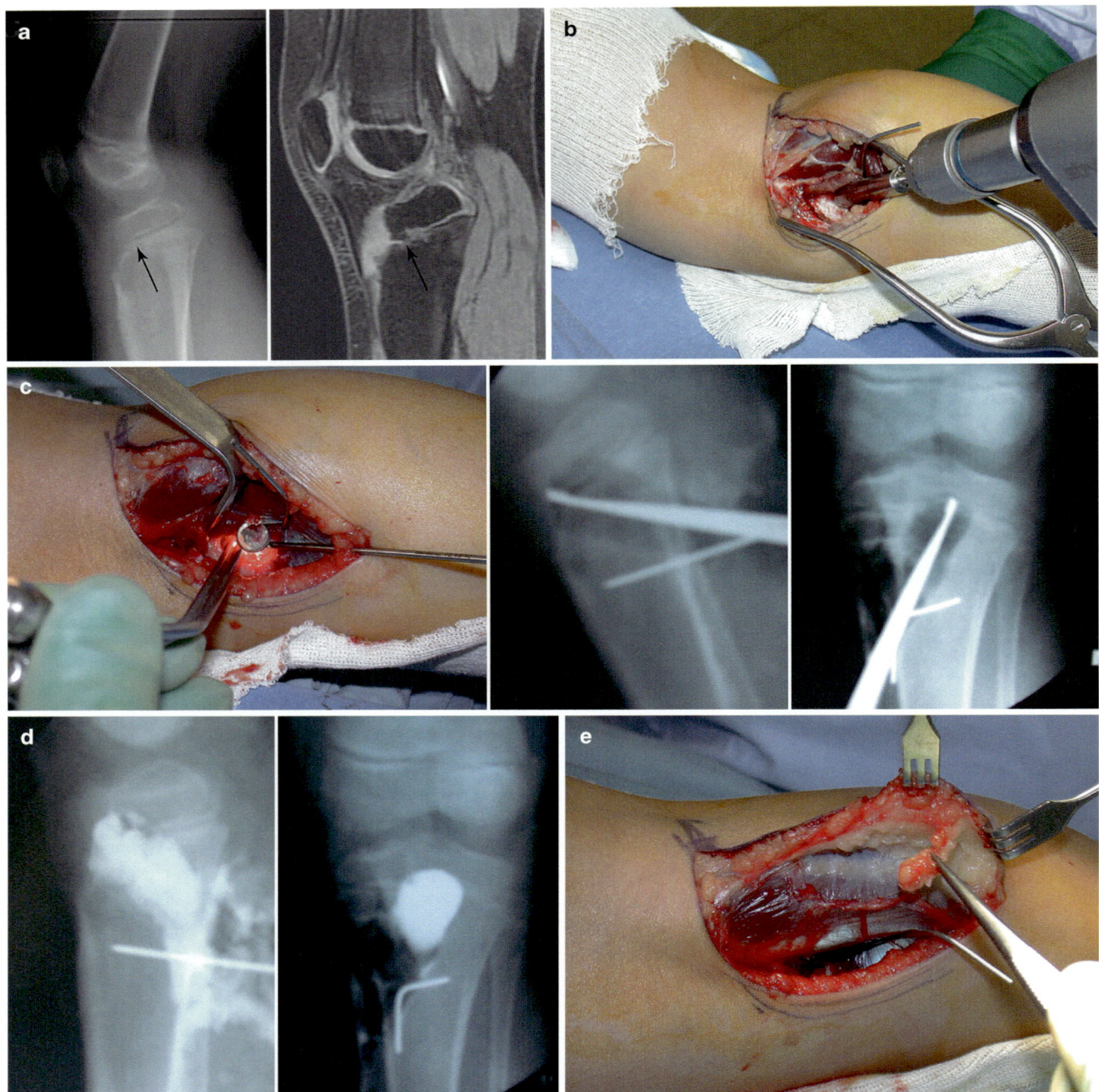

Fig. 7.11 (a) Lateral X-ray and MRI showing a recurvatum deformity and an anterior physeal bar (*arrow*) following a proximal tibial fracture. (b) A cannulated ACL reamer is used to create a tunnel through the posterior tibial metaphysis after placing a guide wire in the physeal bar. (c) Fiber-optic lighted suction, dental mirrors, and fluoroscopy are used to confirm adequate resection of the bar. (d) Radio-opaque dye can be used to document the extent of the resection. (e) Local fat is harvested to use as an interposition material. (f) Lateral radiograph before and after opening wedge osteotomy with allograft (*arrow*) to correct angular deformity. Note the radio-opaque markers in the epiphysis and metaphysis to help with postoperative assessment of subsequent growth

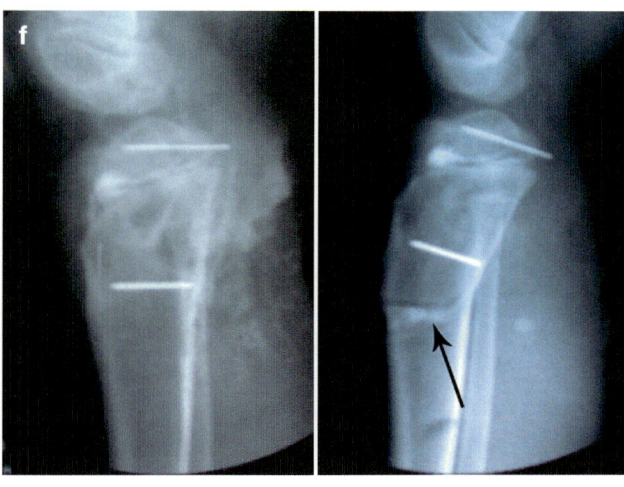

Fig. 7.11 (continued)

Interposition Material

Once the surgeon is satisfied that the bar has been completely excised, interposition material should be placed in an effort to limit recurrence. Interposition materials have included bone wax, fat, silicone, and cranioplast [4, 6, 9, 25]. (Silicone is no longer clinically available.) While a few recent investigations have assessed the possibility of cartilaginous cells as an interposition material, they are, to the best of our knowledge, not yet clinically viable [40–42]. Subsequently, for peripheral bars we ensure that the adjacent periosteum has been widely and sharply excised from the resection area and apply bone wax to the exposed metaphyseal and epiphyseal bone. For central bars we prefer local fat interposition. Cranioplast has the purported advantage of completely and permanently filling the resection void and has been shown to be effective in a large series of bar resections [43]. However, we believe that it has several disadvantages when further reconstructive procedures are required; particularly, it is difficult to remove and leaves a bony deficit post-removal, often exactly at the level of deformity, potentially significantly complicating subsequent procedures.

Radiographic Markers

The surgeon's final intraoperative task is to place small radiographic markers in the epiphysis and metaphysis to serve as markers to make comparison measurements on radiographs over time. We usually use small stainless steel k-wires [44], although some advocate for titanium wires in case MRI evaluation of the physis is needed in the future [43]. Small (0.8 mm) tantalum beads inserted into the cortex above and below the physis may prove to be the most effective method of determining early growth following bar removal of epiphysiodesis [45, 46]. It is imperative that the surgeon communicates to the family the need to follow the child to skeletal maturity. A close follow-up can allow early detection of recurrence and allow completion epiphysiodesis prior to the development of angular deformity. Even with excellent resumption of growth, the surgeon should expect the involved physis to close earlier than the contralateral limb as the patient nears skeletal maturity [25, 43, 44].

Clinical Outcome

The reported results of physeal bar resection are variable. Perhaps the most cited report is Peterson's 1984 report where some growth was noted in 70 of 71 cases. They noted a wide variation in the growth of the operated bone relative to the normal bone (0–200%) with a mean of 84% in patients followed to maturity. Perhaps not completely appreciated, they also noted that in some cases the "normal" bone was treated with an epiphysiodesis which "favorably influences the result expressed as a percentage" [10]. Williamson and Staheli reported "near-normal" longitudinal growth (>93% of the contralateral limb segment) and no progression of angular deformity in 11 of 29 patients [25].

Yuan et al. reported the results of 48 patients who underwent physeal bar resection over a 30 year period by Peterson and followed prospectively until skeletal maturity. The average age at the time of surgery was 9.7 years (range 3.4–14.5 years) and the average bar size was 30% of the physis cross-sectional area (range 10–60%). Cranioplast was used in 86% of cases. Their results demonstrated a frequent initial burst of physeal growth, actually greater than that of the normal contralateral physis. The initial increased growth was most marked in the first 2 years and then receded to equal the uninjured side. Eliminating the effect of young age, there were no factors that were significantly correlated with an increased bone growth rate. Seventy-one percent of patients underwent a concurrent or subsequent surgery, with 24% undergoing 3 or 4 additional surgeries.

The largest series in the literature includes 89 patients, including 26 distal femoral, 49 proximal tibial (40 due to infantile Blount disease), and 14 distal tibial bars [44]. Thirty-seven (42%) had at least 2 years of growth after bar resection and an additional 13 patients (15%) demonstrated at least 6 months but less than 2 years or growth. There was no significant difference in the rate of success based on the physis affected, patient age, bar size, gender, location, bar morphology, or etiology. Fat graft was used in 77 cases and cranioplastic in the remaining cases. There was a statistically significant increase in successful cases using cranioplastic as compared to fat. Only 10 patients (11%) grew to maturity without requiring a secondary procedure. In those patients who resumed growth after bar resection, premature cessation of growth occurred in 28/51 (55%) at an average of 18 months postoperatively. In the infantile Bount disease group, there were 14 (35%) successful resections, 5 (13%) partial successes, and 21 (53%) failures. Thirty-six (90%) infantile Blount patients required a second reconstructive procedure.

Summary

Physeal bar excision is an important tool in the armamentarium in treating children with acquired limb deformity. The surgeon considering physeal bar resection should be familiar with the anatomy and physiology of the normal physis and the etiology and anatomy of the physeal growth arrest and should have an understanding of skeletal maturation. Because of the complexities of the factors involved, the outcome of attempted bar resection can be unpredictable. In spite of a technically adequate bar resection, the failure of resumption of growth or premature cessation of growth is common. As such, the surgeon should educate patients and families the importance of close clinical follow-up as well as the likelihood of needing subsequent procedures. Despite the unpredictable nature of physeal bar resection, it can result in meaningful and gratifying resumption of growth in carefully selected patients.

Commentary

Mindaugas Mikužis
mim@rn.dk

As a result of the fragile nature of the growth plate, special care should be taken when treating physeal fractures to avoid iatrogenic injuries to the physis. Multiple or forced attempts to manipulate the fracture to improve alignment may cause damage to the growth plate. Reduction of physeal fractures is recommended to be done immediately, as prolonged time after trauma increases the risk of growth arrest. In our institute, we aim to treat all physeal fractures within 72 h.

Transfixation through the growth plate with K-wires should be done with as few attempts as possible. Moreover, the perichondrial ring is the especially damage-sensitive zone and can lead to peripheral physeal arrest. Therefore, it must be kept intact and free from implant contact. It is better to perforate the growth plate more centrally, as a small physeal bar (under 7%) can resolve on its own.

Physeal bar excision is a procedure that is cumbersome to perform and has a low success rate. The treatment is divided into bar resection and correction of secondary deformities.

When resecting a physeal bar, it is paramount to fill the defect with stationary and nondegradable material to avoid re-formation of bone in the defect through the physis and thus bar recurrence.

Often a fat graft is applied, however the success rate is unpredictable, which could be due to either degradation or migration of the graft. To avoid migration of the material used to fill the gap, i.e., cement, a K-wire can be used to anchor the cement plug into the epiphysis during axial growth.

The continuous development of technology improves diagnostics with higher quality images and the possibility to obtain computer-assisted 3D mapping of the physeal bar. 3D images with advanced software open various possibilities including virtual bone models, 3D printing for preoperative planning, and production of patient-specific positioning guides that allow the surgeon to determine the exact location of instrumentation access to type B and C physeal bars.

Fortunately, physeal fractures in children tend to occur mostly in the second decade, and higher patient age correlates negatively with an indication for physeal bar resection. As the success rate of physeal bar resection without any required additional interventions is low, our opinion is rather to perform epiphysiodesis based on the following reasons: In the last two decades, limb lengthening with intramedullary lengthening nails has shown advantages due to the improved minimally invasive technique and the optimized nail design which has improved patient comfort. This represents a substantial improvement compared to lengthening with external fixation. Bone length correction with a lengthening nail for small length increments is today a more manageable procedure. In addition, deformity correction can be done at the same time with long-term results demonstrating low risk of recurrence of any pathology. Furthermore, future lengthening plates will provide another treatment method in the toolbox. Lengthening plates do not cross the growth plate and thus allow bone lengthening in patients before skeletal maturity without the need to postpone the lengthening procedure. The treatment scenario would consist of an epiphysiodesis of the "sick" growth plate combined with acute deformity correction and gradual lengthening at the same procedure with the lengthening plate.

However, since a physeal bar resection still represents a "nothing to lose" option, especially in very young children, this would still be considered the first choice of treatment, when it is suitable.

References

1. Birch JG. Surgical technique of physeal bar resection. Instr Course Lect. 1992;41:445–50.
2. Bright RW. Operative correction of partial epiphyseal plate closure by osseous-bridge resection and silicone-rubber implant. An experimental study in dogs. J Bone Joint Surg Am. 1974;56(4):655–64.
3. Craig JG, Cramer KE, Cody DD, Hearshen DO, Ceulemans RY, van Holsbeeck MT, et al. Premature partial closure and other deformities of the growth plate: MR imaging and three-dimensional modeling. Radiology. 1999;210(3):835–43.
4. Kasser JR. Physeal bar resections after growth arrest about the knee. Clin Orthop Relat Res. 1990;255:68–74.
5. Langenskiold A. An operation for partial closure of an epiphysial plate in children, and its experimental basis. J Bone Joint Surg Br. 1975;57(3):325–30.
6. Langenskiold A. Surgical treatment of partial closure of the growth plate. J Pediatr Orthop. 1981;1(1):3–11.
7. Langenskiold A. Growth disturbance after osteomyelitis of femoral condyles in infants. Acta Orthop Scand. 1984;55(1):1–13.
8. Langenskiold A. Partial closure of the epiphyseal plate. Principles of treatment. Clin Orthop Relat Res. 1978;1993(297):4–6.
9. Langenskiold A, Osterman K. Surgical treatment of partial closure of the epiphysial plate. Reconstr Surg Traumatol. 1979;17:48–64.
10. Peterson HA. Partial growth plate arrest and its treatment. J Pediatr Orthop. 1984;4(2):246–58.
11. Langenskiold A. Tibia vara: osteochondrosis deformans tibiae. Blount's disease. Clin Orthop Relat Res. 1981;158:77–82.
12. Beck CL, Burke SW, Roberts JM, Johnston CE 2nd. Physeal bridge resection in infantile Blount disease. J Pediatr Orthop. 1987;7(2):161–3.
13. Salter R, Harris W. Injuries involving the epiphyseal plate. J Bone Joint Surg Am. 1963;45-A:587.
14. Peterson HA. Physeal fractures: Part 3. Classification. J Pediatr Orthop. 1994;14(4):439–48.
15. Salter R. Epiphyseal plate injuries. In: Letts R, editor. Management of pediatric fractures. New York, NY: Churchill LIvingston; 1994. p. 11.
16. Lampasi M, Magnani M, Donzelli O. Aneurysmal bone cysts of the distal fibula in children: long-term results of curettage and resection in nine patients. J Bone Joint Surg Br. 2007;89(10):1356–62.
17. Clayer M, Boatright C, Conrad E. Growth disturbances associated with untreated benign bone cysts. Aust N Z J Surg. 1997;67(12):872–3.
18. Sanpera I Jr, Fixsen JA, Hill RA. Injuries to the physis by extravasation. A rare cause of growth plate arrest. J Bone Joint Surg Br. 1994;76(2):278–80.
19. Bloom JD, Mozersky DJ, Buckley CJ, Hagood CO Jr. Defective limb growth as a complication of catheterization of the femoral artery. Surg Gynecol Obstet. 1974;138(4):524–6.
20. Macnicol MF, Anagnostopoulos J. Arrest of the growth plate after arterial cannulation in infancy. J Bone Joint Surg Br. 2000;82(2):172–5.
21. Barnett LS. Little League shoulder syndrome: proximal humeral epiphyseolysis in adolescent baseball pitchers. A case report. J Bone Joint Surg Am. 1985;67(3):495–6.
22. Sabick MB, Kim YK, Torry MR, Keirns MA, Hawkins RJ. Biomechanics of the shoulder in youth baseball pitchers: implications for the development of proximal humeral epiphysiolysis and humeral retrotorsion. Am J Sports Med. 2005;33(11):1716–22.
23. Birch JG, Herring JA, Wenger DR. Surgical anatomy of selected physes. J Pediatr Orthop. 1984;4(2):224–31.
24. Broughton NS, Dickens DR, Cole WG, Menelaus MB. Epiphyseolysis for partial growth arrest. Results after four years or at maturity. J Bone Joint Surg Br. 1989;71(1):13–6.
25. Williamson RV, Staheli LT. Partial physeal growth arrest: treatment by bridge resection and fat interposition. J Pediatr Orthop. 1990;10(6):769–76.
26. Carlson WO, Wenger DR. A mapping method to prepare for surgical excision of a partial physeal arrest. J Pediatr Orthop. 1984;4(2):232–8.
27. Ecklund K, Jaramillo D. Patterns of premature physeal arrest: MR imaging of 111 children. AJR Am J Roentgenol. 2002;178(4):967–72.
28. Loder RT, Swinford AE, Kuhns LR. The use of helical computed tomographic scan to assess bony physeal bridges. J Pediatr Orthop. 1997;17(3):356–9.
29. Sailhan F, Chotel F, Guibal AL, Gollogly S, Adam P, Berard J, et al. Three-dimensional MR imaging in the assessment of physeal growth arrest. Eur Radiol. 2004;14(9):1600–8.
30. Cheon JE, Kim IO, Choi IH, Kim CJ, Cho TJ, Kim WS, et al. Magnetic resonance imaging of remaining physis in partial physeal resection with graft interposition in a rabbit model: a comparison with physeal resection alone. Invest Radiol. 2005;40(4):235–42.
31. Hasler CC, Foster BK. Secondary tethers after physeal bar resection: a common source of failure? Clin Orthop Relat Res. 2002;405:242–9.
32. Lurie B, Koff MF, Shah P, Feldmann EJ, Amacker N, Downey-Zayas T, et al. Three-dimensional magnetic resonance imaging of physeal injury: reliability and clinical utility. J Pediatr Orthop. 2014;34(3):239–45.
33. Anderson M, Green WT. Lengths of the femur and the tibia; norms derived from orthoroentgenograms of children from 5 years of age until epiphysial closure. Am J Dis Child. 1948;75(3):279–90.
34. Anderson M, Green WT, Messner MB. Growth and predictions of growth in the lower extremities. J Bone Joint Surg Am. 1963;45-A:1–14.
35. Anderson M, Messner MB, Green WT. Distribution of lengths of the normal femur and Tibia in children from one to eighteen years of age. J Bone Joint Surg Am. 1964;46:1197–202.
36. Greulich W, Pyle S. Radiographic atlas of the skeletal development of the hand and wrist. Stanford, CA: Stanford University Press; 1959.
37. Charles YP, Dimeglio A, Canavese F, Daures JP. Skeletal age assessment from the olecranon for idiopathic scoliosis at Risser grade 0. J Bone Joint Surg Am. 2007;89(12):2737–44.
38. Dimeglio A, Charles YP, Daures JP, de Rosa V, Kabore B. Accuracy of the Sauvegrain method in determining skeletal age during puberty. J Bone Joint Surg Am. 2005;87(8):1689–96.
39. Bollini G, Tallet JM, Jacquemier M, Bouyala JM. New procedure to remove a centrally located bone bar. J Pediatr Orthop. 1990;10(5):662–6.
40. Lee KM, Cheng AS, Cheung WH, Lui PP, Ooi V, Fung KP, et al. Bioengineering and characterization of physeal transplant with physeal reconstruction potential. Tissue Eng. 2003;9(4):703–11.
41. Li L, Hui JH, Goh JC, Chen F, Lee EH. Chitin as a scaffold for mesenchymal stem cells transfers in the treatment of partial growth arrest. J Pediatr Orthop. 2004;24(2):205–10.
42. Tobita M, Ochi M, Uchio Y, Mori R, Iwasa J, Katsube K, et al. Treatment of growth plate injury with autogenous chondrocytes: a study in rabbits. Acta Orthop Scand. 2002;73(3):352–8.
43. Yuan BJ, Stans AA, Larson DR, Peterson HA. Excision of physeal bars of the distal femur, proximal and distal tibia followed to maturity. J Pediatr Orthop. 2019;39(6):e422–e9.
44. Manchanda K, Rodgers J, Kanaan Y, Ho C, Podeszwa D, Birch J. Results of lower extremity physeal bar resection. Iranian J Orthopaedic Surg. 2019;17(4):132–41.
45. Lauge-Pedersen H, Hagglund G, Johnsson R. Radiostereometric analysis for monitoring percutaneous physiodesis. A preliminary study. J Bone Joint Surg Br. 2006;88(11):1502–7.
46. Garner MR, Dow M, Bixby E, Mintz DN, Widmann RF, Dodwell ER. Evaluating length: the use of low-dose biplanar radiography (EOS) and tantalum bead implantation. J Pediatr Orthop. 2016;36(1):e6–9.

Acute Deformity Correction Using an Osteotomy

Vrisha Madhuri and Jonathan Reddy

This chapter discusses the indications, principles, specific considerations, choice of hardware, and complications of acute correction of lower limb deformities using an osteotomy.

Principles of Acute Deformity Correction

General Considerations

It is generally preferable to perform an acute correction when the magnitude of angular correction required is small and the deformity is in a single plane. The bone gap created by an opening wedge osteotomy heals well in children due to better healing potential and a thick, biologically active periosteum. The skin overlying the affected area should be healthy as acute correction can cause skin necrosis because of stretch or impaired vascularity. Long-standing deformities are associated with soft-tissue contractures on the concave side of the deformity, which must be considered when planning.

Age Considerations

The outcome of treatment of certain deformities depends on the age at which the corrective osteotomy was performed. It is due to the correction or worsening of the deformity or the underlying bony pathology with increasing age. In some conditions, there is a high prevalence of recurrence when correction is done at an earlier age. For instance, in congenital posteromedial bowing of the tibia, it is wise to defer surgery till at least 3–4 years of age since spontaneous correction of the deformity is noted to a large extent, and the complication rate and chance of recurrence are higher if done at a younger age 1. Softtissue and bony correction of deformities in cerebral palsy tend to fail if performed before 8–10 years of age due to worsening spasticity with growth and persisting muscle imbalance [1].

The magnitude of correction should take into account the possibility of progressive deformity with future growth. Physeal injuries and conditions such as Blount's disease, where only a portion of the growth plate is affected, may require fusion of the healthy (lateral) portion of the open physis or overcorrection of the deformity (Fig. 8.1). In some situations, deformity correction may be combined with treatment of the pathology such as excision of a physeal bar (Fig. 8.2) [2, 3].

V. Madhuri (✉)
Department of Paediatric Orthopaedics, Amara hospital, Tirupati, India

Department of Paediatric Orthopaedics, Christian Medical College and Hospital, Vellore, Tamil Nadu, India

J. Reddy
Department of Paediatric Orthopaedics, Christian Medical College and Hospital, Vellore, Tamil Nadu, India
e-mail: jonathan.reddy@cmcvellore.ac.in

Fig. 8.1 (a) Radiograph of a 7-year-old girl with Blount's disease. The apex of the deformity is seen at the intersection of the two lines (*red lines* indicate the proximal and distal tibial mechanical axes). (b) Overcorrection by Rab's osteotomy. (c) Radiograph at 3-year follow-up shows a good alignment of the mechanical axis of the tibia

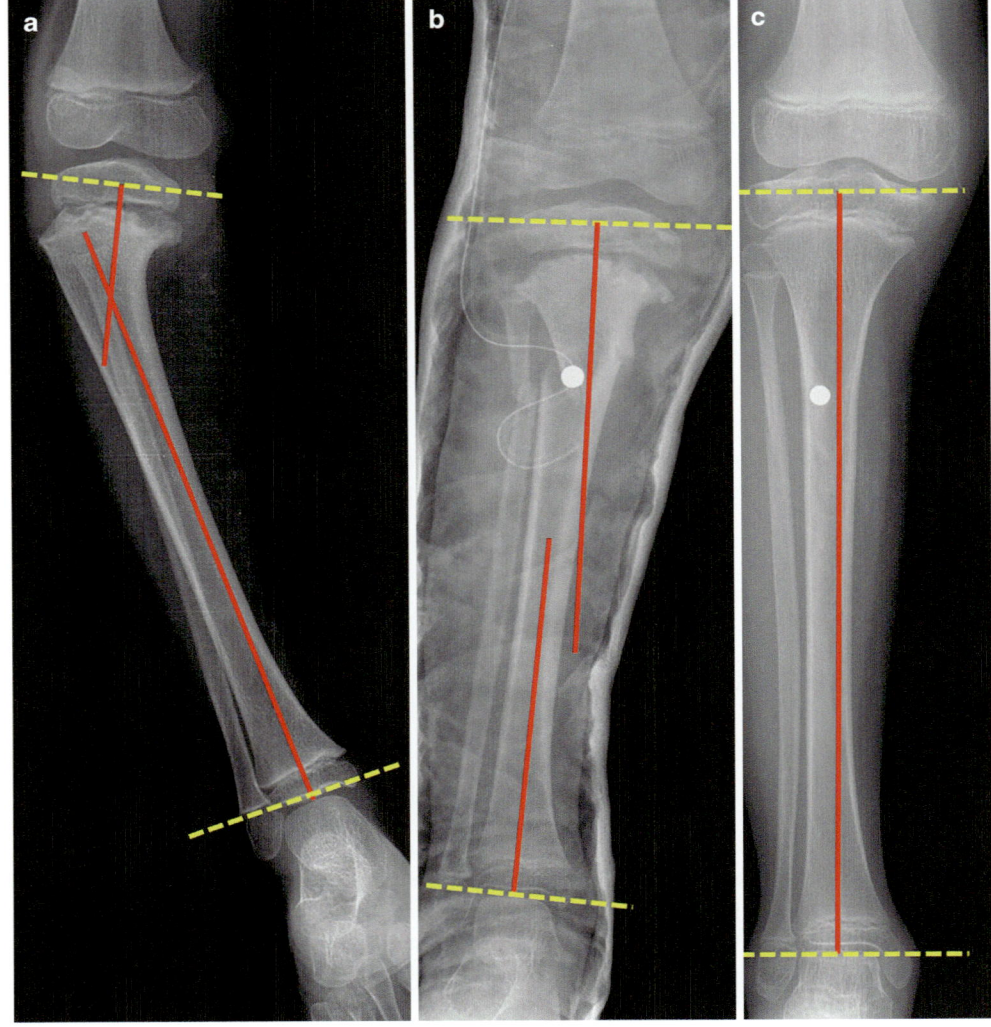

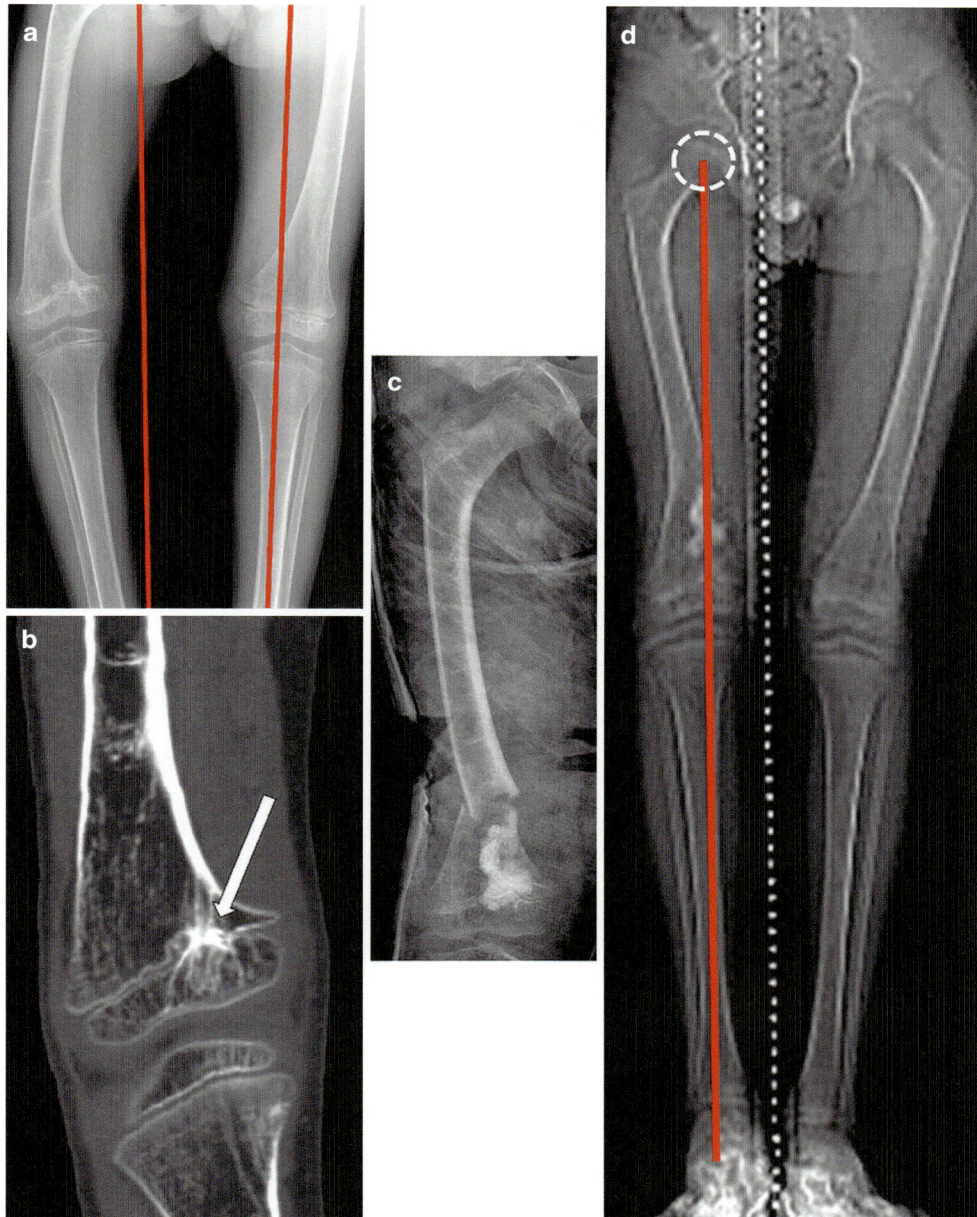

Fig. 8.2 (a) Right-sided genu varum in a 7-year-old boy with the hemi-epiphyseal arrest of the right distal femur (*red lines* represent the mechanical axes of both lower limbs). (b) A CT scan shows a peripheral physeal bar (*white arrow*). (c) Bar resection and cement interposition were performed in addition to corrective osteotomy of the distal femur. (d) CT scanogram (supine) shows restoration of the mechanical axis and proximal migration of cement, indicating restoration of growth at the 18-month follow-up. A supine CT scanogram was taken in this case; however, a full-length standing radiograph is a more accurate measure of alignment and should be preferred

Principles Pertaining to Correction of Lower Limb Alignment

Minor changes in lower limb alignment following corrective osteotomy often remodel in children. Bone remodeling following correction occurs in both sagittal and coronal planes, although such remodeling is greater in the plane of joint movement and when the osteotomy is close to the growing end of the bone. This remodeling occurs at the site of osteotomy in accordance with Wolff's law [4]. This law infers that remodeling will occur on the compression side by laying new bone. Pauwels postulated that malalignment of bone produces a differential growth at the physis, which tends to realign the shaft perpendicular to the major joint reaction forces [5]. This observation is similar to the epiphyseal pressure rule of Heuter-Volkmann (growth is retarded by increased mechanical compression) [6]. Any residual deformity would tend to decrease by remodeling in 4–5 years following surgery [7]. Seventy-five percent of this remodeling occurs at the physis and 25% by bone drift or translation [8, 9]. Thus, a perfect anatomical alignment may not be necessary; however, long-term follow-up is required in children with remaining growth.

Influence of Level of Osteotomy

In children, often, the osteotomies are at a site distant from the apex or center of rotation of angulation (CORA). When planning an osteotomy, one should consider various factors such as the proximity of the CORA to the adjacent physis and/or joint, the presence of pathological bone and neurovascular structures in the vicinity. Overall, metaphyseal osteotomies have a better healing potential than diaphyseal ones. The ease of rotational correction is the same at both levels in the case of the femur, but the proximal shaft is preferable as large corrections at the distal third would be theoretically at the expense of an undesirable alteration in the patella-femoral dynamics [10]. Any corrective osteotomy or lengthening should not be performed at the site of pathological bone to avoid healing problems [11, 12]. The exceptions are where the entire bone is pathologic, like in osteogenesis imperfecta or fibrous dysplasia.

Adjuvant Fibular Osteotomy: When and Where?

The fibula acts as a strut to prevent large angular or rotational tibial corrections. Thus, with opening wedge correction of the tibia, an adjuvant fibular osteotomy is often performed along with tibial osteotomy.

- Fibular osteotomy should be avoided in its proximal third to safeguard the common peroneal nerve [13]. In the middle third, there is a risk of damage to peroneal vessels [14–16].
- The classic recommendation of doing a distal tibial derotation without a fibula osteotomy is for rotational corrections of up to 35° [17]. However, derotational osteotomies of up to 55° internal and 45° external have been reported without fibular osteotomy and neurovascular compromise [18]. We, however, prefer a fibular osteotomy while doing a rotational correction of greater than 30°.
- We tend to perform osteotomy at the proximal and middle third junction in case of proximal tibial angular osteotomy and the close to distal and middle third junction in distal tibial/rotational osteotomies.
- A fibula segment should be resected when the desired angular correction in the tibia is considerable [19]. Fibula osteotomy, if performed at a site far away from CORA, leads to wide displacement of the fibula and may require resection of the projecting portion of the fibula. A distal tibiofibular fusion should be performed to avoid ankle instability when a fibular pseudarthrosis is anticipated following such resections [20].
- At least 10% of the total fibular length should be preserved distal to the osteotomy to avoid ankle instability [21]. Our experience shows that proximal fibular migration occurs if the fibula does not unite, irrespective of the level of the osteotomy.
- A concomitant fibula osteotomy at the apex of deformity is recommended in conditions like posteromedial bowing of the tibia [22], where the fibula is also deformed. It prevents the deformed bone from acting as a tether and causing the recurrence of deformity.

Principles Pertaining to Specific Osteotomies

Opening Wedge Osteotomy

The axis of deformity correction lies on the convex cortex. The overall length of the limb increases following deformity correction. The final length achieved will equal the sum of the lengths of the convex border of the deformity (Fig. 8.3a). If the combined total correction exceeds 2.5–3 cm of lengthening, shortening may be required as a cautionary measure since significant lengthening could compromise the neurovascular status. The nerve stretch in certain circumstances may be further influenced by the direction of rotation, such as the risk of iatrogenic injury being somewhat less in external than internal rotation when performing a proximal tibial osteotomy because of tethering of the peroneal nerve at the proximal fibula [23]. When the axis of correction lies away from the osteotomy site, further lengthening is achieved; for instance, in calcaneal lengthening osteotomy the axis of correction lies away from the calcaneum, i.e., at the talar head [24] (Fig. 8.4).

8 Acute Deformity Correction Using an Osteotomy

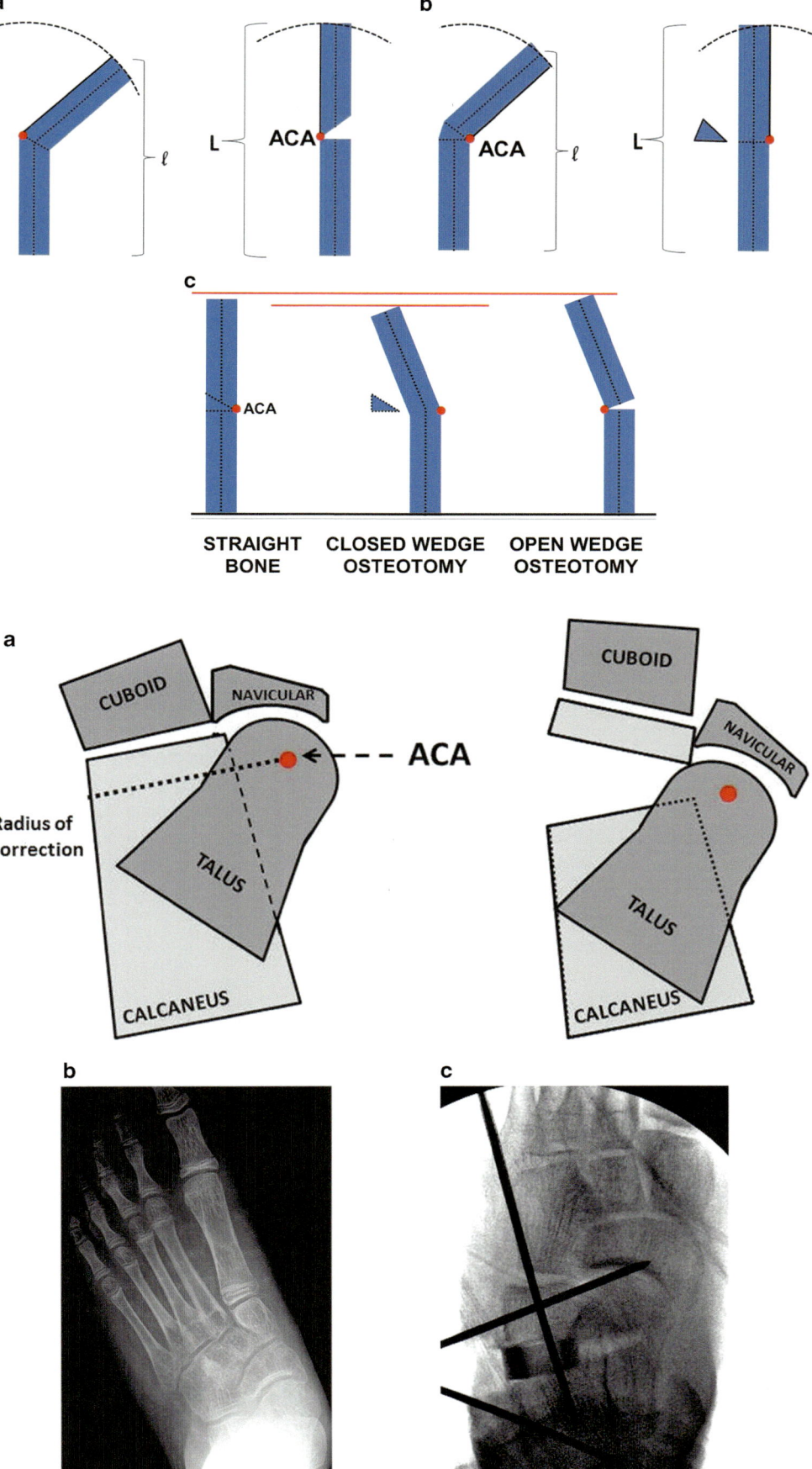

Fig. 8.3 (a) Open wedge osteotomy in a deformed bone of length "l" showing an increase in length of the bone. The final length "L" is the sum of the convex borders of the deformed bone. (b) Closed wedge osteotomy in an angular deformed bone shows an increase in the length of the bone. The final length "L" is the sum of the concave borders of the deformed bone (*ACA* axis of correction of angulation). (c) In a straight bone, an open wedge angular osteotomy causes less shortening than a closed wedge, as shown by the *red lines*. Hence, the former is preferred when minimal lengthening is desired along with corrective osteotomy

Fig. 8.4 (a) Axis of correction of angulation (ACA) is located away from the calcaneum, i.e., at the talar head. The effective lengthening along with open wedge osteotomy can be seen. (b) Preoperative and (c) intraoperative radiographic views of left calcaneal lengthening osteotomy and the increase in talar head coverage brought about by it

Closing Wedge Osteotomy

The axis of deformity correction lies on the concave side of the deformity. The overall length of the limb increases following deformity correction and is equal to the sum of the concave borders of the deformity, as shown in Fig. 8.3b. Generally, a closed wedge osteotomy in a straight bone reduces the limb length, whereas the bone length increases or remains the same with an open wedge osteotomy, for instance, with compensatory osteotomies for the proximal femur in Perthes disease and nonunion of the neck of femur (Fig. 8.3c).

Dome Osteotomy

Dome osteotomy is ideal for deformities with CORA close to the joint line, such as in physeal or metaphyseal injuries near the knee or ankle. The displacement of the osteotomy is directly proportional to the radius of correction. Dome osteotomy causes minimal length alteration as the CORA is usually at or near the site of deformity in the metaphysis. The advantage of such an osteotomy is good bony contact and intrinsic stability. However, this technique is limited by its inability to correct rotational malalignments. In addition, it is technically more demanding than more straightforward open and closed wedge osteotomy and does not allow for translation if the dome's apex is away from CORA.

Angular Correction and Translation

An angular osteotomy involves shifting of the mechanical axis in the direction of correction of the deformity; that is, the mechanical axis shifts medially in the varus and laterally in the valgus osteotomy. Hence, the translation of the distal fragment has been advised to restore the mechanical axis [23]. A valgus proximal femoral osteotomy requires lateralization of the distal fragment. However, when doing an angular correction below the knee, the direction of translation is opposite, i.e., lateral translation for varus and medial translation for a valgus osteotomy. Glard et al. showed that proximal femoral varus osteotomy with medial translation in Perthes disease did not affect the mechanical axis deviation at the knee [25]. Several studies show remodeling of the femoral neck-shaft angle following varus osteotomy with or without translation [25–30]. In a child, do we need to translate the distal fragment when performing angular correction to optimize the mechanical axis? Sanghavi et al. found that after varus derotation osteotomy, the neck-shaft angle tends to revert to normal depending on the age at which the operation was undertaken [26]. Tercier et al. showed that following proximal femoral osteotomy in Perthes, the resulting mechanical axis deviation is usually subtle and clinically insignificant in children [27]. Following varus osteotomy of the proximal femur in cerebral palsy, 60% of the correction is lost after 8 years by remodeling [28]. In pelvic support osteotomy, up to 30° of valgus angulation at the osteotomy site does not cause any significant change in the mechanical axis [31]. Therefore, it is our assumption that translation of the distal fragment during angular correction of proximal femoral deformities is not mandatory in younger children unless the magnitude of the correction is outsized, such as greater than 30°. This observation is also supported by the acceptability of overriding/bayoneting fracture reduction in younger children where after a few years complete restoration of the anatomy occurs [32]. The advantages of not translating are that the periosteal hinge medial or lateral stays intact, and the final lengthening is greater than with translation (Fig. 8.5).

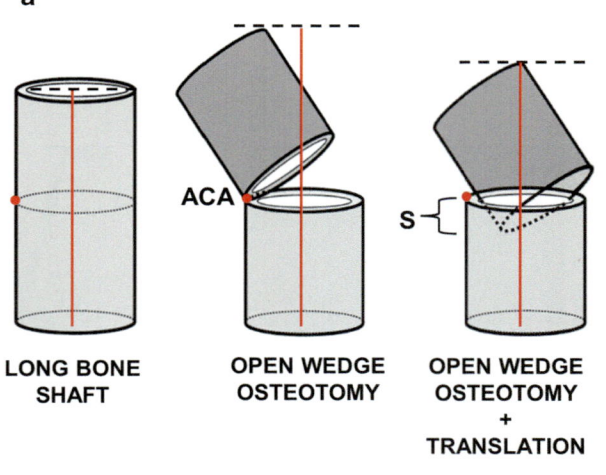
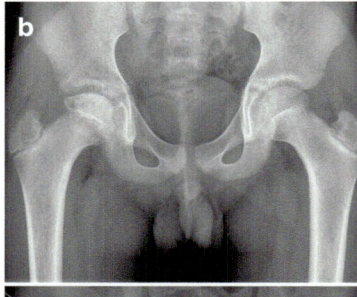
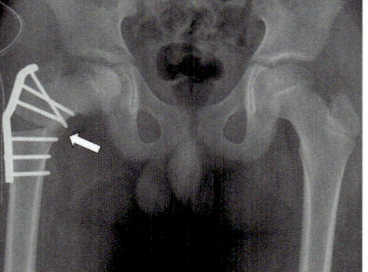

Fig. 8.5 (a) Effect of angular correction on length of a straight bone. *Red solid lines* indicate the length of the straight bone. An increase in length is seen following opening wedge osteotomy without translation. Translation has relatively less effect on the final limb length. "S" is the amount of shortening achieved following translation. *ACA* axis of correction of angulation. (b) *Top*: Radiograph of a child with Perthes disease of the right hip. *Bottom*: A varus derotation osteotomy was performed. The medial intact periosteal hinge is shown (*white arrow*)

Oblique Osteotomy

An oblique osteotomy corrects multiplanar deformities at the same time. Meticulous preoperative planning is essential as it involves correcting deformities in various planes through a single osteotomy. The lesser the obliquity of the plane, the lesser the bony contact after angular correction but the easier and greater the rotational correction, such as in Rab's osteotomy (Fig. 8.6).

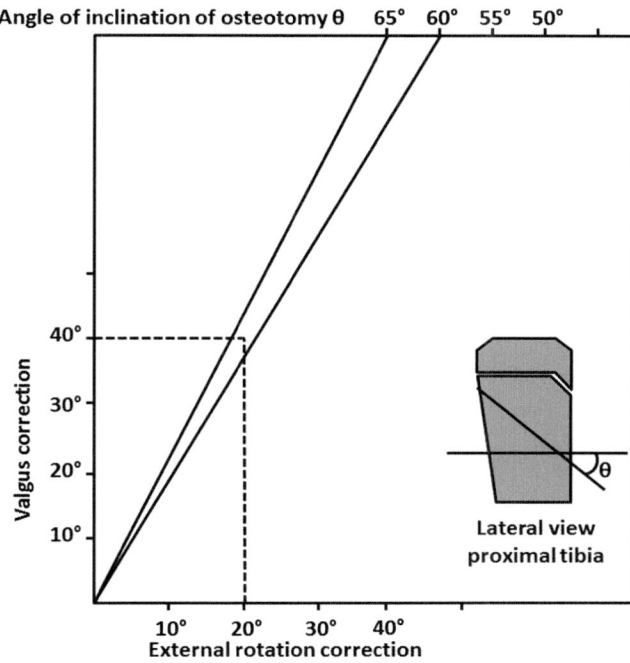

Fig. 8.6 In this example, the amount of desired external rotational (20°) and valgus angular correction (40°) (indicated by *dotted lines*) is plotted on the graph. θ, the angle of inclination of proximal tibial osteotomy with the horizontal lies between 60 and 65°. Adapted from [33]

Lengthening/Shortening Osteotomy

Lengthening osteotomy in a single stage is best achieved either by a step cut/long oblique osteotomy to maintain adequate contact while lengthening at the same time, such as in distal fibula, metatarsals, or proximal ulna. Acute lengthening of 1.7 cm and 3.2 cm for the tibia and femur, respectively, have been performed with minimal complications in adults [34]. Opening wedge angular correction can sometimes offset the shortening caused by varus angulation and gain in length to some extent, for instance, in Perthes disease (see Fig. 8.4a). It is important to keep in mind the change in length ratio as compared to the companion bones in the case of osteotomies of the leg and foot [35]. Acute shortening of up to 3 cm can be performed safely in young adults with open tibial fractures with bone loss [36]. Any further shortening should be gauged based on the clinical assessment of limb vascularity. Fibular shortening osteotomy can be combined with proximal tibia corrective osteotomy in achondroplasia to correct the lateral collateral laxity and fibular overriding [37]. The major shortenings are required in children with plexiform neurofibromas, where the limb may be longer by more than 10 cm, and the child is near maturity. In these conditions, a shortening of up to 5 cm in each segment is well tolerated (Fig. 8.7). The laxity of muscles around the knee and ankle causes significant laxity and affects function when shortened to more than 5 cm [38]. The major disadvantage of lengthening/shortening osteotomy with acute correction is that the amount of correction safely gained is limited. In the case of angular deformity, if the magnitude of the correction is considerable, either a simultaneous shortening osteotomy or gradual distraction osteogenesis is preferred to avoid significant risk to the neurovascular structures and soft-tissue tightness (Fig. 8.8).

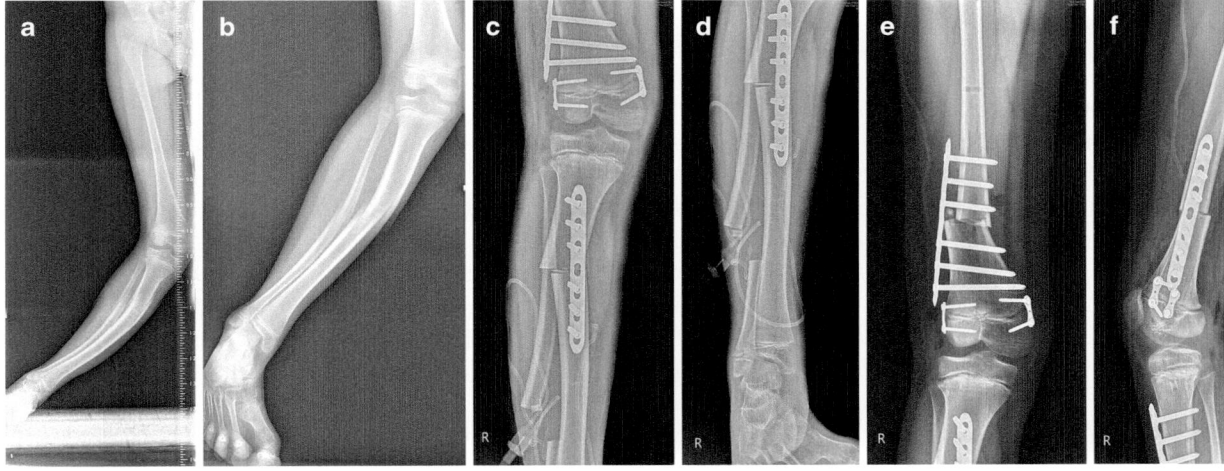

Fig. 8.7 (**a**, **b**) 14 year old boy with 14 cm shortening accommodated by holding the limb in gross valgus and flexion. (**c**, **d**). Five cm diaphyseal segments of femur and tibia were removed along with deformity correction (**e**, **f**). Epiphyseodesis of distal femur was carried out to achieve further gradual shortening in the femur to equalize limb length by maturity

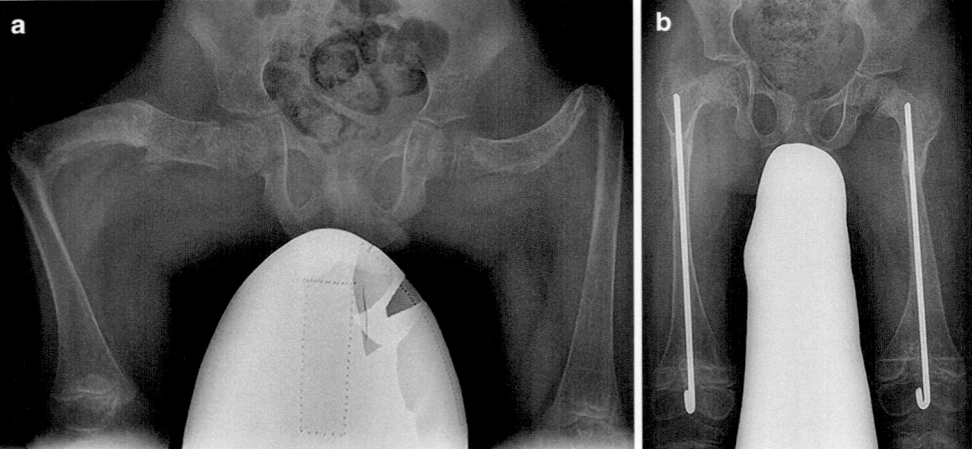

Fig. 8.8 (a) Radiograph of a 10-year-old girl with osteogenesis imperfecta and bowing deformity of both femora. Restoring the length of the femur is limited by the stretch of neurovascular structures and soft tissues. (b) Hence, corrective osteotomies are combined with shortening

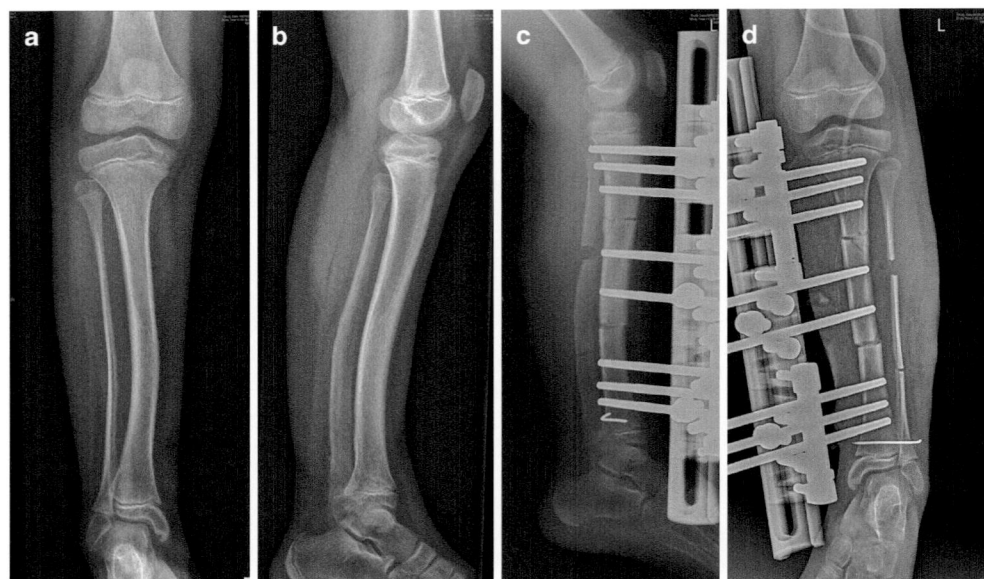

Fig. 8.9 AP and lateral radiographs of a 7-year-old girl with posteromedial bowing deformity (a and b) who underwent bifocal osteotomy with gradual lengthening at proximal end and deformity correction at distal end using an limb reconstruction system (Orthofix, Verona, Italy)

Bifocal Procedures

In bifocal deformities in the same or adjacent bone, overcorrection of one deformity to avoid a second osteotomy can lead to obliquity of the joint surface or abnormal mechanical and anatomical axis, for instance, compensation for a valgus deformity of the tibia by overcorrection at the supracondylar osteotomy for femoral valgus has been shown to cause a shift of the mechanical axis, and arthritic changes with pain in the long term [39]. Many deformities are multiaxial such as in physeal arrests and metabolic bone disease. They require multiple sites of deformity correction. Sometimes a single procedure can be used to achieve correction at two levels; one of which is acute, and the second one is a gradual correction. An excellent example of this is acute deformity correction at the metaphyseal end of the bone and gradual lengthening over a frame at the diaphyseal level. The correction can be achieved using a bifocal procedure on a single frame such as the Orthofix (Fig. 8.9) limb reconstruction system or Ilizarov or a combination of two fixation systems such as an intramedullary device for lengthening combined with a plate [40].

Special Considerations

Deformity Secondary to Physeal Injury

Angular deformity secondary to physeal insult is usually progressive until skeletal maturity. The following strategies can be adopted for such corrections:

- Overcorrection of the deformity to compensate for future progression of the deformity.
- A combination of acute corrective osteotomy is combined with the excision of the physeal bar and interposition.

- Acute corrective osteotomy combined with a growth modulation technique: This would, however, invoke a shortening effect due to arrest of either side of the physis.
- An opening wedge osteotomy would simultaneously address the existing limb length discrepancy.

Mango Slice Effect

In the Indian subcontinent, raw mango slice, a savory seasonal snack for children, is split into multiple radial cuts for better seasoning. It makes a good illustration for osteotomy with multiple open wedges for diaphyseal deformity, as seen following rickets and other metabolic disorders. The concept and execution are explained in the following illustration. Small corrections at two or more CORAs allow lengthening, and deformity correction spreads over the bone length (Fig. 8.10).

Deformity Memory Effect

Pediatric congenital and developmental conditions such as developmental coxa vara, fibular hemimelia, and posteromedial bowing of the tibia have a memory because of associated soft-tissue contractures. Following an osteotomy, either the deformity can recur by bending the callus or slow relapse occurs due to abnormal forces on the growing physis [Heuter-Volkmann]. In these situations, the osteotomies should be combined with soft-tissue lengthening or shortening of the bone (Fig. 8.11).

Cozen's Phenomenon

Certain proximal tibia fractures in a growing child are associated with a proximal tibial valgus deformity. These deformities may correct spontaneously over a few years, and thus an acute corrective surgery for the tibial valgus should be deferred for at least 3–4 years following the fracture [41, 42] (Fig. 8.12).

Box 8.1
- Acute deformity correction is preferred in children, especially when the magnitude of deformity or length discrepancy is relatively small.
- Soft-tissue constraints should be addressed simultaneously where needed, to avoid recurrence.
- Knowledge of the natural history of the underlying pathology is crucial before executing an acute osteotomy.
- Anatomical alignment of the mechanical axis is not mandatory in younger children because of remodeling potential.
- A dome osteotomy can be performed when the CORA is juxta-articular.
- Fibular osteotomy may be necessary for tibial osteotomies for a large correction.

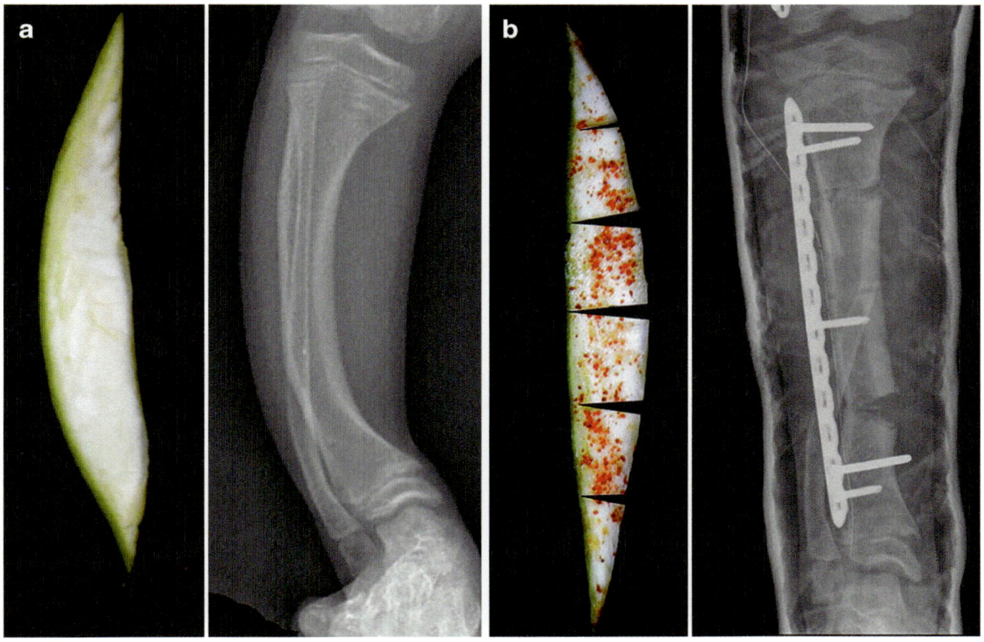

Fig. 8.10 (**a**) An intact mango slice and (**b**) a slit, seasoned one can be compared with multiple opening wedge osteotomies in a bowed tibia

Indications

The indications for acute correction with an osteotomy in children are varied and include correction of certain uniplanar or multiplanar skeletal deformities. The indications include angular and rotational correction as well as treatment of mild length discrepancies.

Site-Specific Osteotomies

Metaphysis

Frontal plane angular deformities around the knee [genu varum or genu valgum] related to conditions such as Blount's disease, metabolic bone disease, physeal arrests, and coxa vara are often treated with acute correction via a metaphyseal osteotomy (Fig. 8.13).

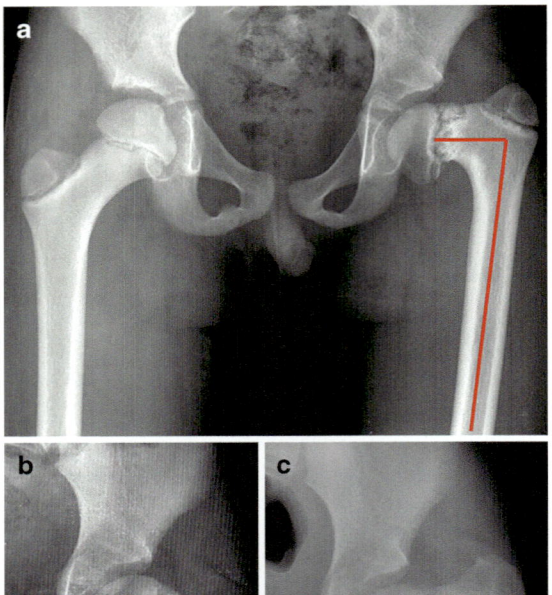

Fig. 8.11 The deformity memory effect. (**a**) Developmental coxa vara in a 15-year-old boy. (**b**) Corrective osteotomy and blade plate fixation. (**c**) Radiograph at 16-month post-op follow-up shows reduction of neck-shaft angle (*red angles*) despite the implant position remaining unchanged

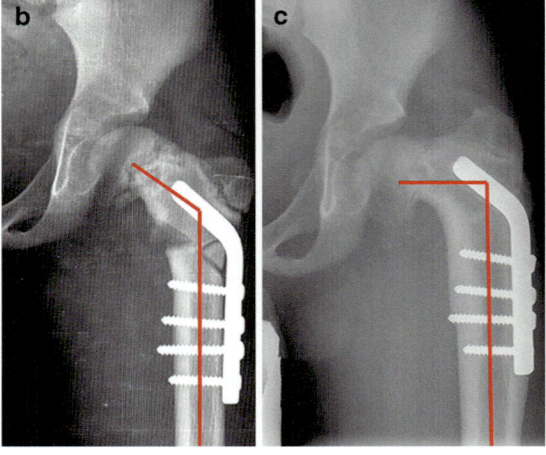

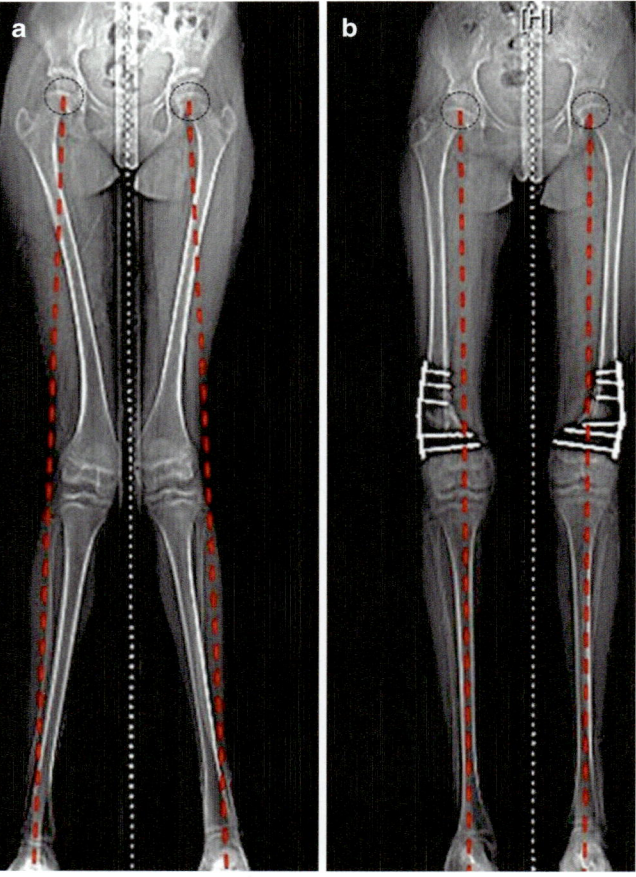

Fig. 8.13 CT scanograms (supine) comparing (**a**) pre-op and (**b**) post-op mechanical axis alignment (*dotted red lines*) in a 14-year-old girl with bilateral genu valgus. She underwent bilateral varus osteotomies of the distal femora and fixation with locked compression plates. A supine CT scanogram was taken in this case. However, a full-length standing radiograph is a more accurate measure of alignment and should be preferred

Fig. 8.12 Cozen's phenomenon. (**a**) Three-year-old boy with proximal tibia fracture. (**b**) Radiograph after 4 years shows tibial valgus deformity

Epiphyseal

Osteotomies may also be performed at the epiphyseal level to accomplish joint elevation, such as medial hemi-plateau elevation (Fig. 8.14) for Blount's disease [43–45]. Such osteotomy also addresses laxity at the adjacent joint.

Juxta-Apophyseal

Re-directional osteotomies of greater trochanter, calcaneal, and tibial tuberosity improve muscle function by optimizing the lever arm dysfunction [46–49] (Fig. 8.12).

Diaphysis

The common indications for diaphyseal osteotomies include metabolic bone disorders such as rickets, osteogenesis imperfecta, renal osteodystrophy, and deformities secondary to traumatic or pathological fractures due to osteomyelitis and cystic lesions of bone. Posteromedial bowing of the tibia and congenital limb deficiency form a particular subset of diaphyseal osteotomies due to their propensity for complications caused by associated soft-tissue inelasticity, requiring special measures to avoid complications. For instance, postponing the deformity correction until the child with posteromedial tibial bowing is older and using a locked plate to prevent fractures or bowing of the regenerate which may cause the recurrence of deformity. Congenital pseudarthrosis of the tibia is another rare disorder where the primary aim of treatment is to achieve union and maintain the normal mechanical axis by deformity correction and limb lengthening (Fig. 8.15).

Metabolic bone disorders often exaggerate the natural curves of shafts of long bones, leading to anterolateral bowing in the femur and tibia. The associated diaphyseal deformities are typically generalized bow and multiapical, requiring multilevel osteotomies for correction. Severe forms of osteogenesis imperfecta often cause grotesque diaphyseal deformities. The osteoporosis of underlying bone warrants an intramedullary device to splint the bone after correction (see Fig. 8.8).

Specific Considerations Based on Location of the Deformity

Proximal Femur

In order to avoid damage to the capital physis, most proximal femoral osteotomies in children are carried out distant from the site (apex) of deformity. Such acute correction reorients the femoral head in valgus or varus, extension or flexion, and rotation and is also used for shortening the femoral segment in some instances of long-standing dislocated dysplastic hips.

Most of these osteotomies cannot be performed at the CORA due to the presence of the pathological bone at the site of deformity as in proximal focal femoral deficiency or because of proximity to the proximal femoral physis and the tenuous blood supply to the femoral head [11, 12]. A common example is Perthes disease, where proximal femoral varus or valgus osteotomies realign the articulation to either

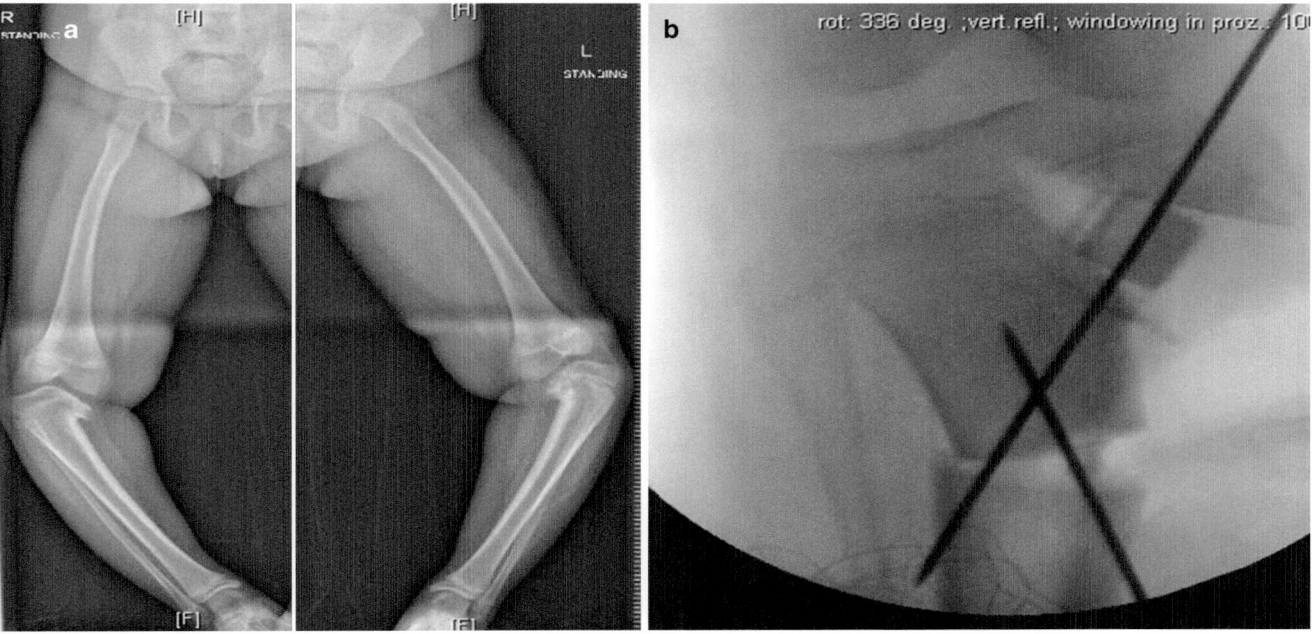

Fig. 8.14 (a) Radiographs of a 6 year old child with Blount's disease. (b) shows epiphyseal osteotomy to elevate medial epiphysis to restore medial height combined with a metaphyseal osteotomy to treat the residual deformity

Fig. 8.15 (a) Anteroposterior and lateral views showing congenital pseudarthrosis of tibia in a 6-year-old boy. (b) Six years following corrective shortening osteotomy, resection of hamartomatous periosteum, bone grafting, and revision intramedullary rodding

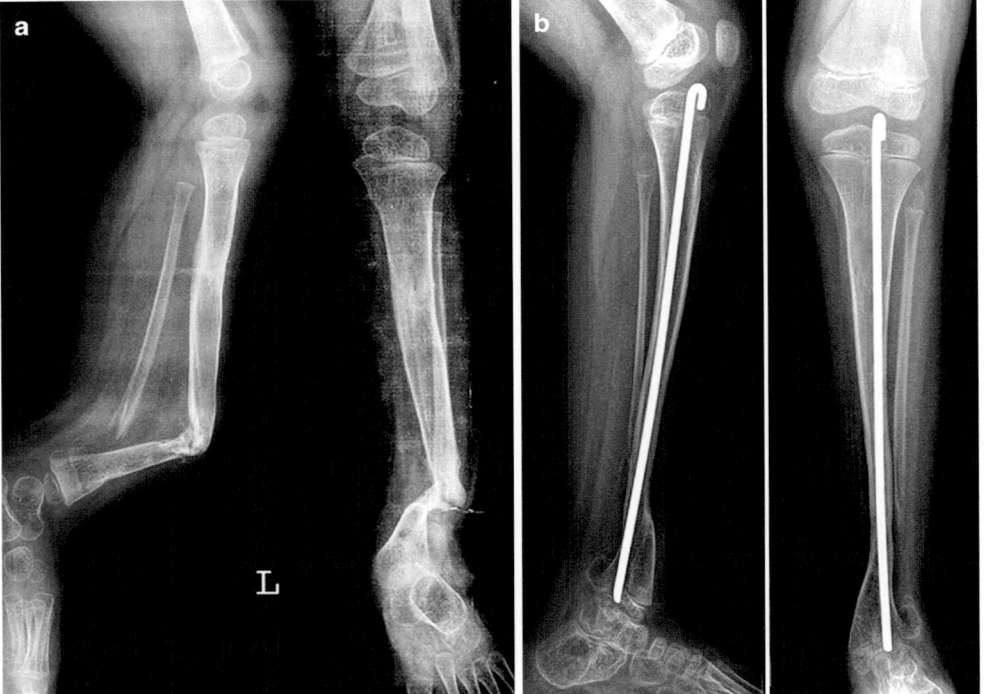

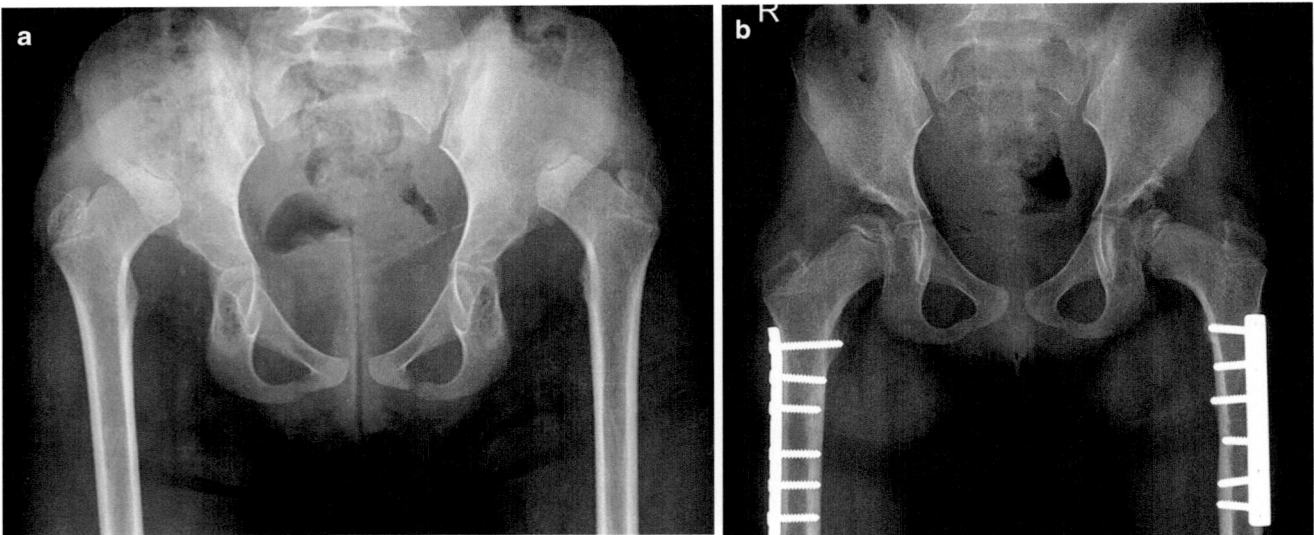

Fig. 8.16 (a) Radiograph of a 6-year-old girl with bilateral dysplastic hips. (b) Open reduction was performed in conjunction with femoral shortening osteotomy to avoid avascular necrosis and derotation to correct anteversion and reduce the hip

increase femoral head coverage or avoid impingement by the deformed head (Figs. 8.16 and 8.17). A combination of angulation, shortening, and rotation is sometimes necessary to achieve optimal reorientation, for instance, a proximal femoral osteotomy in a child with a congenital and neurogenic hip dislocation (Fig. 8.18). In developmental coxa valga, realignment of the physis to a more horizontal position prevents relapse.

Acute osteotomy of the intertrochanteric and subtrochanteric regions of the femur orients the proximal femoral physis more horizontally, thus converting shear forces to compressive forces.

Subcapital realignment osteotomies are an example of correction at the level of deformity (CORA) in slipped capital femoral epiphysis but are rarely done because of the risk of vascular compromise to the femoral head blood supply (Fig. 8.19).

8 Acute Deformity Correction Using an Osteotomy

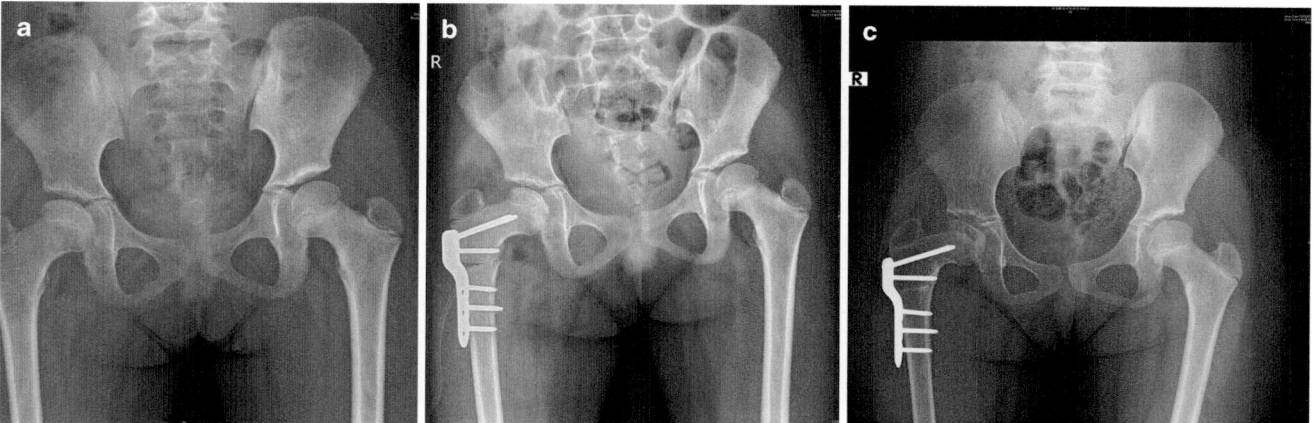

Fig. 8.17 Radiographs shows (**a**) Perthes disease with decrease of femoral epiphyseal height on right. (**b**) images showing proximal femoral varus osteotomies realigning the articulation to increase femoral head containment. (**c**) AP radiograph showing 6 months post op with head contained

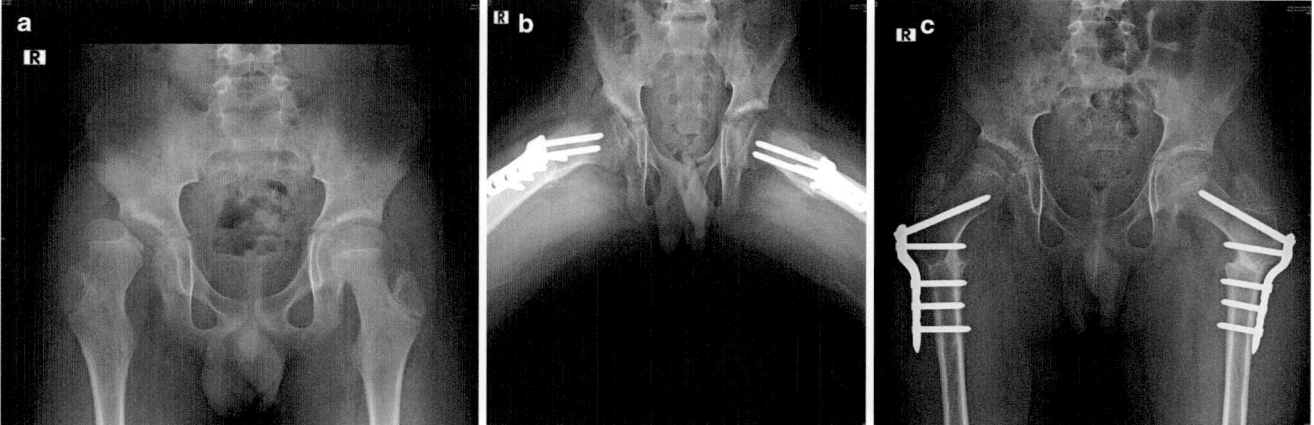

Fig. 8.18 (**a**) AP pelvis radiographs show neurologic dislocation on the right and bilateral coxa valga. (**b** and **c**) Lateral and AP views of the hips following proximal femoral osteotomy fixed with a proximal hip locked plate correcting the anteversion and valgus 6 months after surgery. Hip containment is improved

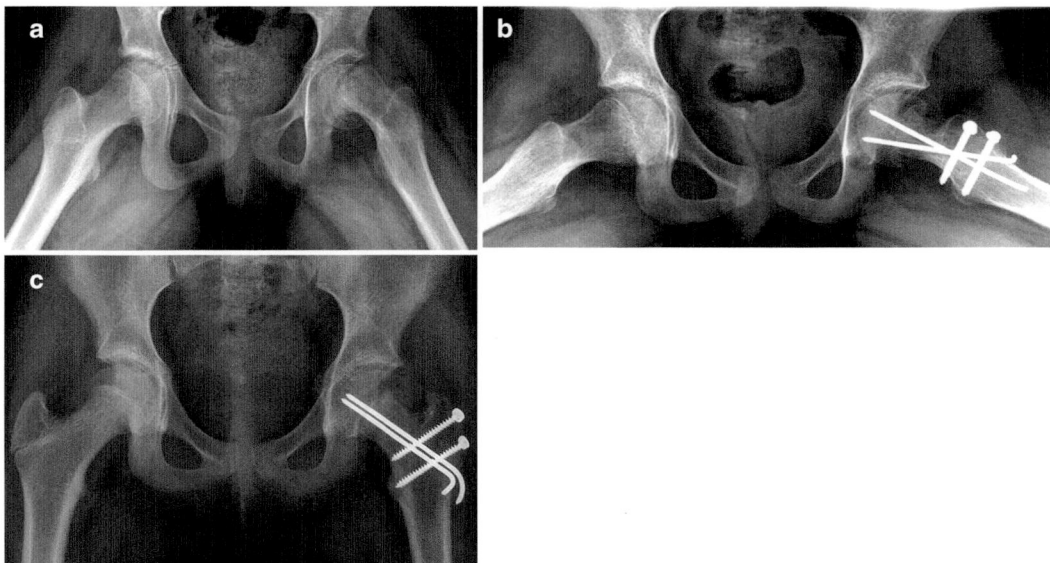

Fig. 8.19 (**a**) Acute on chronic SCFE left hip in a 12-year-old girl. (**b, c**) A modified Dunn's osteotomy was done to realign the head and avoid femoro-acetabular impingement

Osteotomies Around the Knee

Flexion deformity of the knee associated with intractable joint contractures and muscle imbalance such as myelodysplasia, arthrogryposis, cerebral palsy, and poliomyelitis can be corrected by supracondylar extension osteotomy of the femur. Such osteotomies reorient the arc of knee motion allowing full apparent extension and improving the child's gait and function. A distal femur-shortening osteotomy can counter the long-standing flexion contracture without significantly affecting the hip extensor power. Correction of coronal plane angular deformities by closed or open wedge is the commonest indication around the knee. While the growth modulation technique is rapidly replacing this, correction via an osteotomy has a role when the deformity is severe and growth potential is limited or where rapid correction is desirable. Lower limb deformities in children with certain skeletal dysplasias where growth modulation techniques play a limited role can also be treated by acute corrective osteotomy. Correcting deformity around the knee requires consideration of neurological and vascular structures due to their proximity to the osteotomy site (Fig. 8.20). Epiphyseal/physeal osteotomies for severe Blount's in stage IV–VI ()or a physeal osteotomy to correct severe valgus at the knee in adolescents with Morquio's disease are necessary where there is not enough remaining growth potential [50].

Acute Correction of Length Discrepancy

Correction of minor shortening can be obtained by acute lengthening. Brachymetatarsia correction by acute lengthening of up to 15 mm can be performed safely without any neurovascular compromise [35]. *Trans*-iliac osteotomy is a rarely done procedure that achieves lengthening when angular correction is not sought. In relative femoral neck lengthening, displacement osteotomy of the trochanter is combined with the reshaping of the head, neck, and trochanter to eliminate femoro-acetabular impingement and lengthen the lever arm (Fig. 8.21). Another example is the acute lengthening of the distal fibula by a step-cut or long oblique osteotomy [47].

Reorientation Osteotomy of Acetabulum

Ganz, triple, Dega's, and Salter's osteotomy in dysplastic acetabulum augments femoral head coverage and redistributes hip joint force [49, 51].

Osteotomy with Adjuvant Procedures

Sometimes acute correction of the deformity can be combined with another procedure. This can be unifocal such as physeal

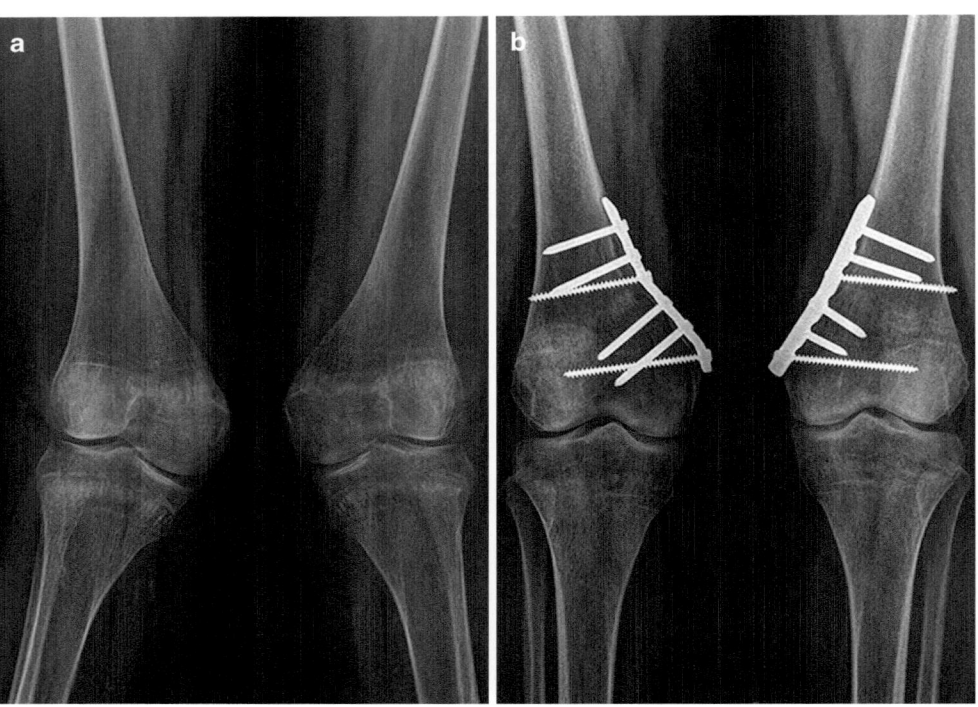

Fig. 8.20 (a) Bilateral genu valgus in a skeletally mature girl. (b) Bilateral closed wedge osteotomies and metaphyseal plate fixation were performed. Closing rather than open wedge osteotomies were performed to avoid common peroneal nerve injury. In femoral valgus deformity corrections greater than 30°, we prefer to decompress the nerve

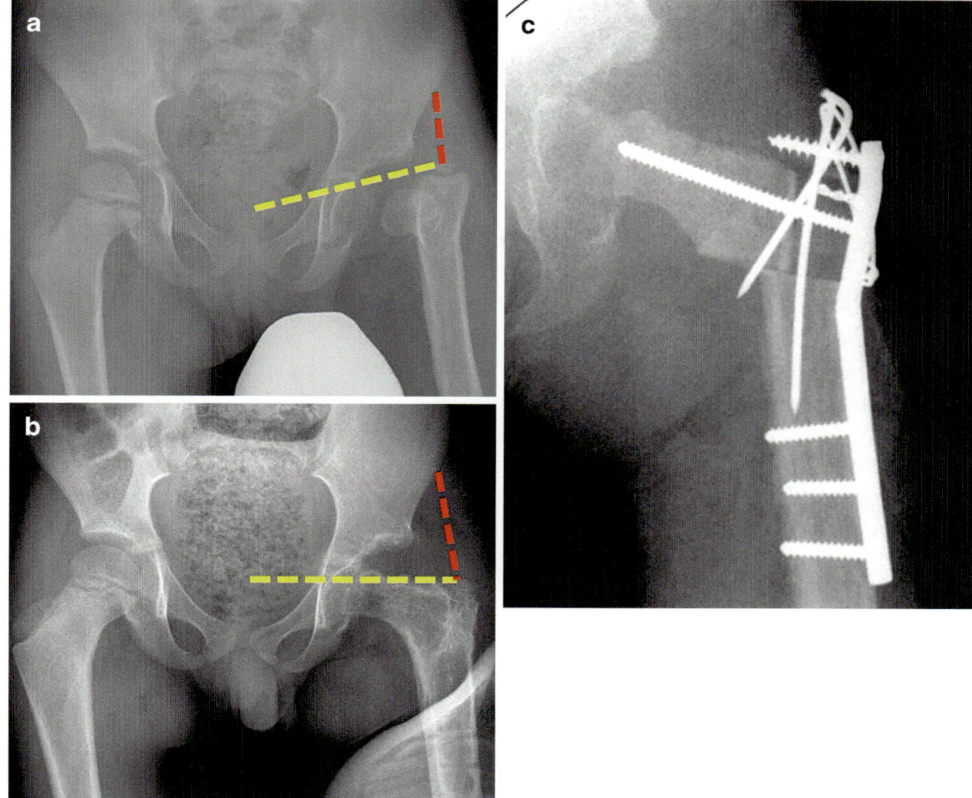

Fig. 8.21 (a) Radiograph of a 6-year-old boy with Choi's type IVa [48] postseptic sequel left hip. (b) A neck-lengthening osteotomy with the distal transfer of the greater trochanter shows optimization of the hip abductor lever arm function. *Red- and yellow-dotted lines* indicate the abductor lever arm and moment arm, respectively. (c) Immediate postoperative radiograph

bar excision with corrective osteotomy in hemiphyseal arrests around the knee (see Fig. 8.2). Alternatively, it could be bifocal, where it is not optimal to do the angular correction at the same site as that of lengthening, for instance, pelvic support osteotomy with distal femoral lengthening [52, 53]. Guided growth procedures can also be performed along with acute osteotomy, e.g., lateral proximal tibial guided growth along with ipsilateral Rab's osteotomy for a child with Blount's disease [54]. In patients with physeal arrests being corrected at maturity, it is possible to do angular and rotation deformity correction acutely and fine-tune the correction by combining it with the gradual angular correction or lengthening by distraction at the osteotomy site by callotasis [55]. The muscle-balancing procedure is combined with a corrective osteotomy to counter the muscle imbalances brought about by cerebral palsy or meningomyelocele and other neuromuscular disorders, thereby avoiding relapse. For example, patellar tendon reefing is done following supracondylar extension osteotomy for fixed flexion deformity of the knee in cerebral palsy and tibialis anterior transfer to the heel is combined with a calcaneal osteotomy in a child with excessive ankle dorsiflexion and weak plantar flexors.

Disease-Specific Indications

In certain conditions like osteogenesis imperfecta, when the child is nonambulatory, the indication for a corrective osteotomy is to aid seating on a wheelchair, better hygiene, and prevent further deformities rather than aligning the mechanical axis. A long-standing dislocated or destroyed painful hip in a child can be managed by a pelvic support osteotomy combined with excision of the femoral head.

Skeletal dysplasia and storage disorders form a specific indication of guided growth because of slower correction [56]. They may require more acute corrections because of lower growth velocity.

> **Box 8.2**
> - Apophyseal reorientation osteotomies (calcaneal, greater trochanter, and tibial tuberosity) lengthen the lever arm for optimal joint function.
> - Metabolic bone disorders usually cause multiapical deformities, often requiring acute multilevel corrective osteotomies.
> - Acute shortening osteotomy may be performed primarily in the proximal femur to avoid avascular necrosis or in conjunction with deformity correction to avoid stretch on neurovascular structures.
> - Various realignment osteotomies of the proximal femur are described to increase joint coverage, reduce impingement, realign capital physis, and increase the arc of motion.

Planning

Rules Governing Osteotomy Planning

Growth considerations have to be kept in mind when planning deformity correction. Hence, osteotomy planning in children is somewhat different from that of adults, where accurate line diagrams and metaphyseal angles are drawn to achieve precise alignment of the knee mechanical axis. While restoring the mechanical axis is important in children, deformity correction involves aligning the proximal and distal physes parallel to each other and perpendicular to the ground rather than merely achieving exact anatomical alignment. However, in older children nearing skeletal maturity, the principles of restoring the mechanical axis used for adults are more applicable. While there are several methods for preoperative planning, we will illustrate our preferred planning methods for acute correction of the tibial and femoral deformities in children.

Planning for Tibial Deformity Correction

Step 1: Finding the CORA

The aim of surgical correction via an osteotomy is to achieve near-normal mechanical alignment and joint orientation of the lower extremity. After obtaining standing radiographs in the orthogonal planes, the joint lines at the knee and ankle are drawn (yellow-dotted lines) as shown in Fig. 8.22b. Red lines form the anticipated mechanical alignment angles of the tibia, with the yellow-dotted lines tangential to the knee joint and talar dome. We consider the talar dome as the reference line for the distal mechanical axis since the epiphysis and physis of the distal tibia are often misshapen in angular deformity in growing children. The mechanical axes intersect at the CORA and the angle [α] thus subtended is the magnitude of correction of the deformity (Fig. 8.22b). When the CORA is located in the bone

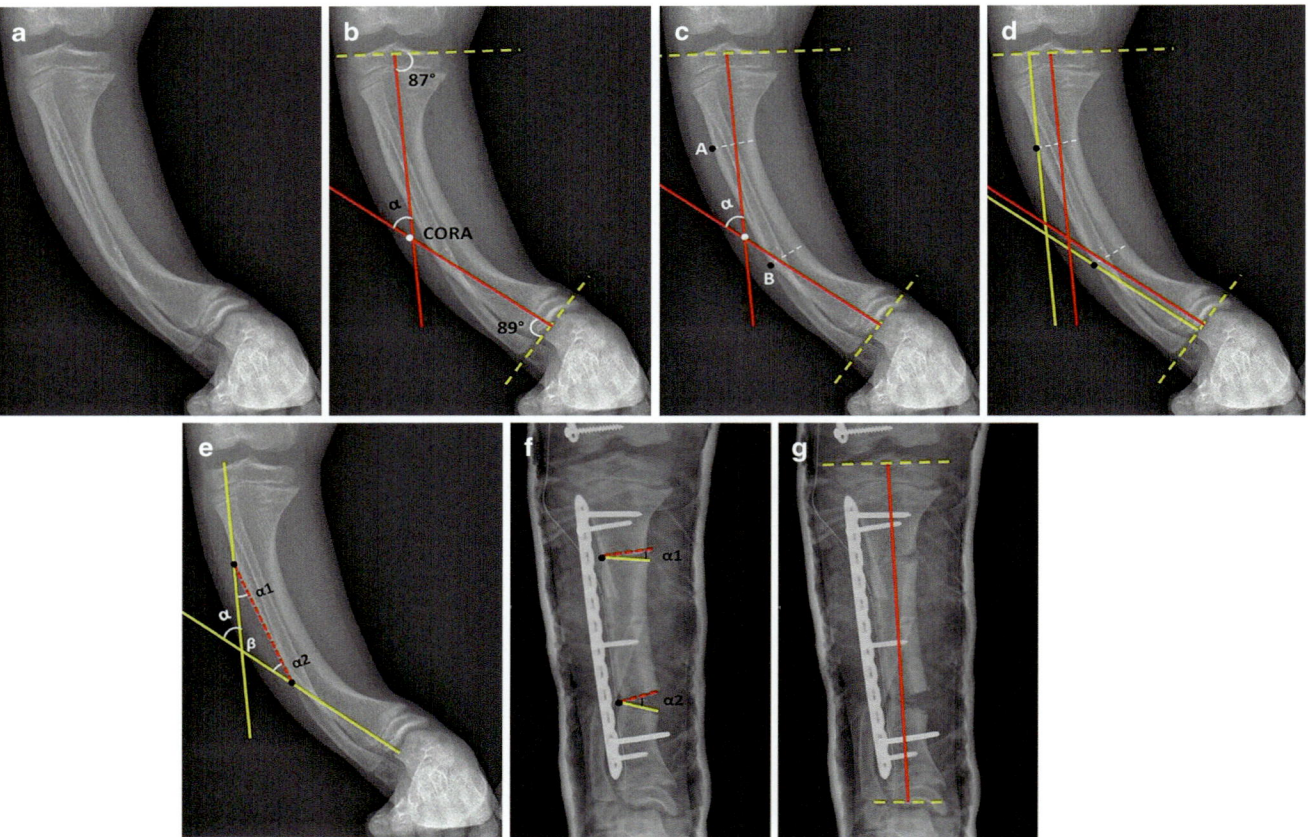

Fig. 8.22 Steps in planning correction of the tibial deformity. (**a**) Bowing deformity of the tibia due to metabolic bone disease. (**b**) *Yellow-dotted lines* drawn tangential to the tibial plateau and talar dome. Mechanical axes [*red dotted*] of the proximal and distal tibia are drawn from the center of the former landmarks. The point of intersection of these lines is the CORA of the deformity and the angle "α" subtended is the magnitude of the correction. (**c**) Two suitable sites for osteotomy, "A" and "B" are plotted on the convex or concave tibial border based on the execution of an open or closed wedge osteotomy, respectively. (**d**) Lines (*yellow solid*) are drawn parallel to the proximal and distal mechanical axes through these points. (**e, f**) The two points are connected by a line (*red dotted*), thus forming a triangle with α1, α2, and β angles. An opening wedge osteotomy of "α1" magnitude proximally and "α2" distally is planned. (**g**) Final radiographs after executing the osteotomies showing the corrected mechanical axis

near the obvious apex of deformity (the area where the deformity visually appears to be maximum), correction can be obtained by a single osteotomy of magnitude "α" at this level.

Step 2: Finding the Axis of Correction for Two CORAs.

In bowing deformities, the CORA could be located away from the obvious apex of deformity, suggesting the presence of two or more CORAs (Fig. 8.22a,b) [23]. In such situations, two points (A and B) are plotted at the desired osteotomy sites on the cortex of the bone (Fig. 8.22c). These points form the center of the arc of correction of the deformity. Lines (yellow) parallel to the mechanical axis of the individual fragments [red] are drawn through the proximal and distal points, respectively (Fig. 8.22d). These points are now connected by a single line (dotted red) (Fig. 8.22e,f,g). The sum of the two acute angles, α1 and α2, subtended in the triangle formed is equal to the total magnitude of correction "α."

Explanation:
The obtuse angle "β" in the triangle = 180° − [α1 + α2] (sum of all angles in a triangle = 180°).
Also, β = 180° − α (angles on a straight line add to 180°).
Hence, α = α1 + α2.

The equation proves that the magnitude of multiple wedge osteotomies at the two desired points should sum up to the magnitude of deformity correction.

The osteotomies can be thus planned at the marked points. It is prudent to confirm the mechanical axis alignment intraoperatively with the Bovie cord method [57]. The electrocautery cord is stretched between the center of the hip and the talar dome following correction. The correction is then fixed using an appropriate fixation device. If desired, the CORAs could be identified on the concave border, and closing wedge osteotomies were carried out.

Contrary to the widespread practice, we do not draw the mid-diaphyseal line as this would produce two fixed apices at sites that may be unacceptable to undergo osteotomy. The advantage of the described technique is that the surgeon can choose the osteotomy sites in consideration of adjacent structures like a neurovascular bundle, physis, pathological bone, or unhealthy skin.

Planning for Femoral Deformity Correction Other than Coxa Vara

The mechanical and anatomical axes for the femur are different. There are no pediatric standards for proximal lateral femoral angle, and the greater trochanter may be incompletely ossified or unossified in young children. This requires alternative planning for femoral deformity correction.

Step 1: Plotting Mechanical Axis for Distal Femur

Standing orthogonal films are obtained in both anteroposterior (Fig. 8.23a) and lateral views. The mechanical lateral distal femoral angle (mLDFA = 88°) is drawn (see Chap. 2). This gives the distal mechanical axis [red line] as shown in Fig. 8.23b.

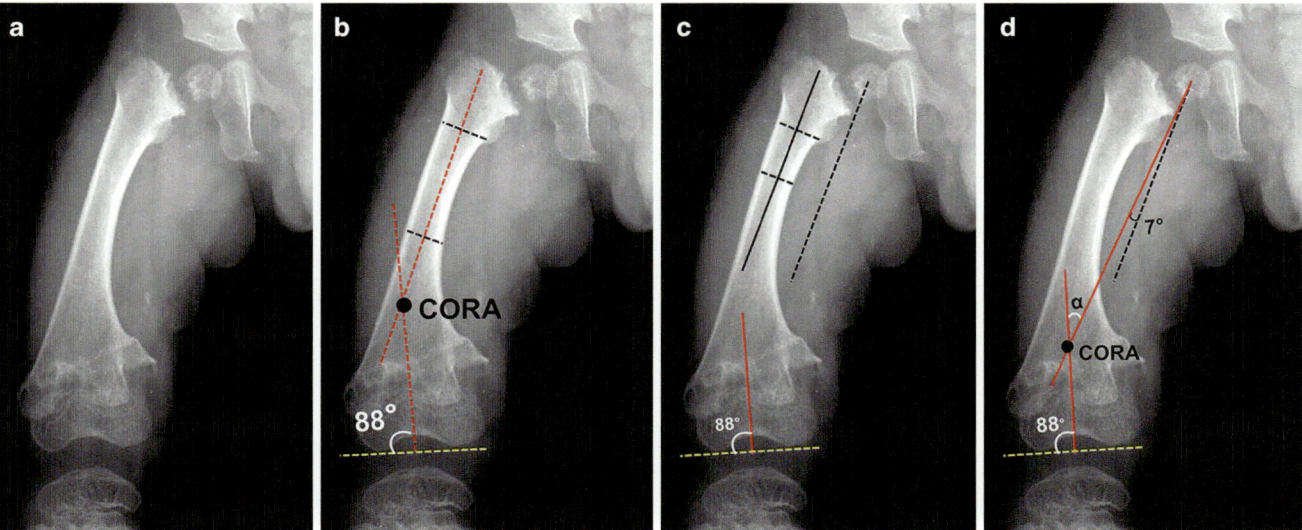

Fig. 8.23 (**a**) A femoral bowing deformity in a 4-year-old boy with unossified greater trochanteric apophysis. (**b**) mLDFA and mid-diaphyseal line for the proximal femur are plotted (*red solid line*, mechanical axis; *black solid line*, anatomical axis). (**c**) The *black-dotted line* is drawn parallel to the anatomical axis from the center of capital femoral ossific nucleus. (**d**) The mechanical axis (*red solid line*) at the proximal femur is drawn from the same point at 7° to the *black-dotted line*. The intersection of the two axes is the CORA and "α" is the magnitude of deformity correction

Step 2: Plotting Proximal Femoral Mechanical Axis

As there are no standards for mLPFA for different age groups in children, we consider plotting the mechanical axis as follows. The mid-diaphyseal line is drawn as shown in Fig. 8.23c. A line parallel to this is drawn from the center of the capital femoral ossific nucleus [black dotted]. The proximal femoral mechanical axis is a line angled 7° lateral to this line (Fig. 8.23d). The point of intersection of these lines is the CORA and the angle subtended gives the magnitude of the correction. The axis of correction should be located in the axial plane of the CORA depending upon whether an open, closed, or neutral wedge osteotomy is desired. In the case of bowing deformity with two or more CORAs, *step 2* shown in Fig. 8.22e for tibial correction can be carried out. In the case of coxa vara, the principle of deformity correction lies in aligning the capital femoral physis as horizontally as possible. In all other cases, we wait for the neck-shaft angle to remodel once the mechanical axis is restored. In adolescents where the trochanter is ossified, mLPFA and mLDFA are plotted as described in Chap. 2.

Planning for Multiple Bony Deformities in the Same Limb

Children with deformities secondary to metabolic disorders or osteogenesis imperfecta often present with multiple bony deformities in the same limb (Fig. 8.24a). When planning such sequential corrections, single or multi-staged, we perform the tibial correction first, which has essentially the same mechanical axis and anatomical axis. For checking the femoral alignment, if the tibial alignment is normal, the Bovie cord is stretched between the hip and ankle. Following correction of the femoral deformity, the cord should pass through the center of the knee if the mechanical axis of the lower extremity is restored. However, when the tibia is also deformed, despite restoring the femoral mechanical axis, the cord may lie on the medial or lateral side of the knee if the tibia has residual varus or valgus deformity, respectively (Fig. 8.24b). There is no such problem when checking the tibia as the Bovie cord can be stretched between the center of the knee and ankle, and if it lies along the axis of the tibia, the tibial deformity correction is confirmed independently of the hip reference point (Fig. 8.24c).

If the femoral deformity is corrected first, the cord has only one reference point, i.e., the center of the femoral head, the distal reference point being outside the corrected mechanical axis, i.e., the center of the talar dome (Fig. 8.24d). On the other hand, the tibial deformity can be corrected without using the limb mechanical axis for reference, as the anatomical and mechanical axes are the same in the case of the tibia. Hence, when ipsilateral femoral and tibial deformities are being addressed with acute osteotomy correction, either at the same sitting or in a staged fashion, we recommend performing the tibial correction first (Fig. 8.25).

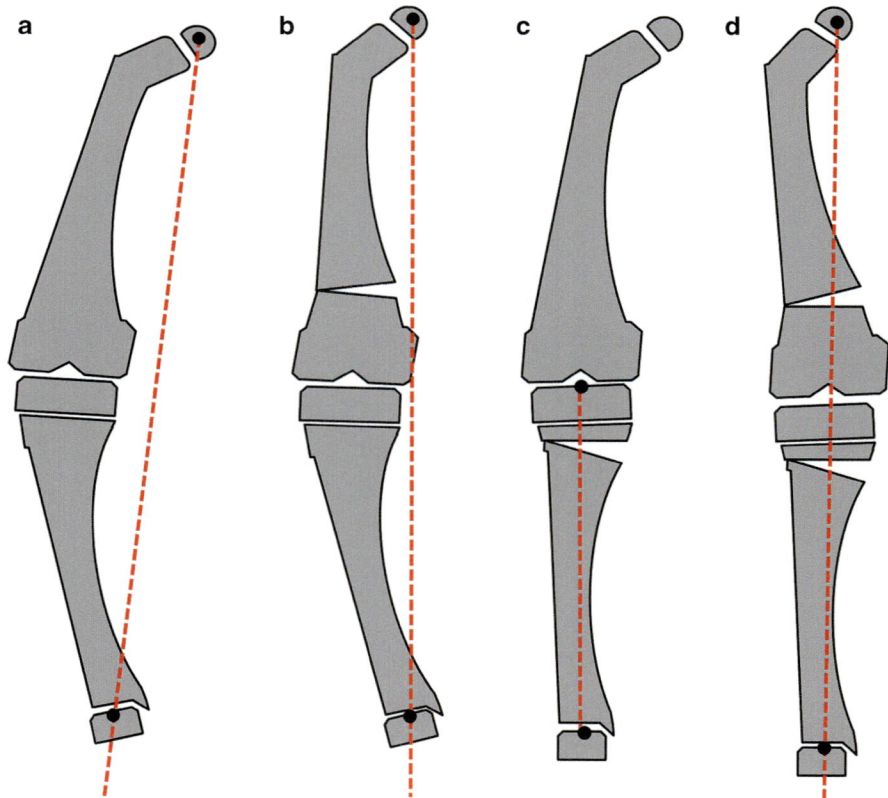

Fig. 8.24 (**a**) Illustration showing mechanical axis deviation (MAD) in a limb with tibial and femoral deformities. (**b**) Distal femoral corrective osteotomy without addressing the tibia deformity. Cross-checking MAD with the Bovie cord between the hip and talar dome as reference points is not possible as the tibial axis is abnormal. (**c**) Cross-checking correction of the tibial deformity is possible with the Bovie cord using the centers of the tibial plateau and talar dome as reference points. (**d**) The corrected tibial mechanical axis allows the mechanical axis of the limb to pass through the center of the knee joint when the femoral head and the talar dome are the reference points

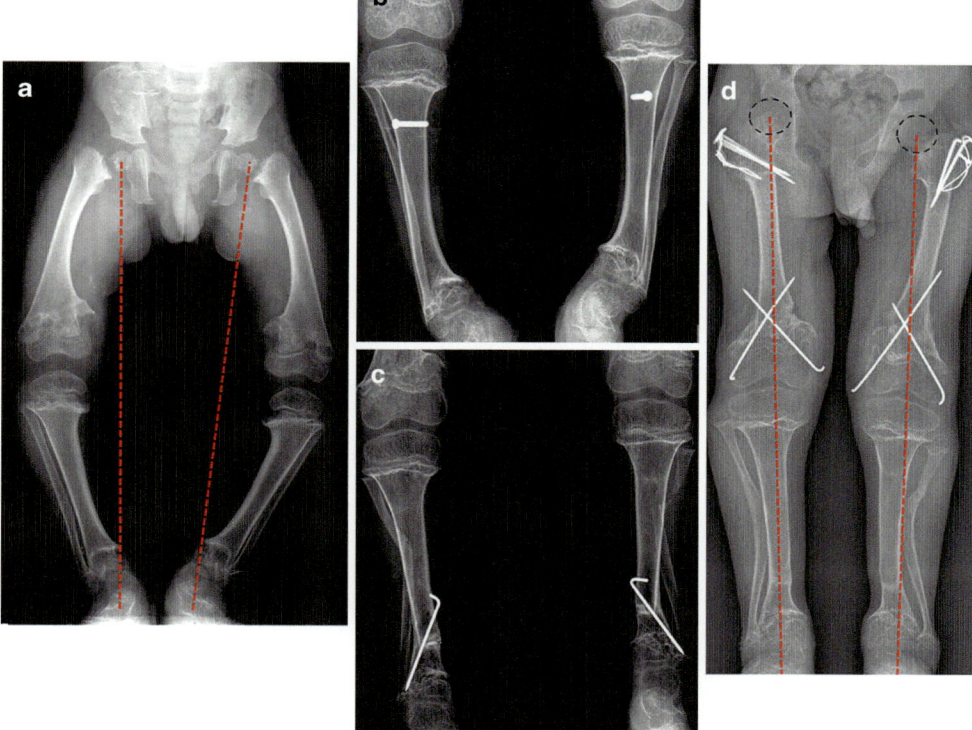

Fig. 8.25 (**a**) Preoperative standing radiograph of a child with spondylometaphyseal dysplasia. He underwent serial corrections of lower limb deformities. (**b**, **c**) The tibial deformity was addressed initially. (**d**) It was followed by the correction of the femoral deformity

Box 8.3
- Judicious preoperative planning with standing radiographs or CT scanograms is essential before executing acute corrective osteotomy.
- Consider the talar dome as a reference line for drawing the mechanical axis of the distal tibia as the distal tibial epiphysis often misshapen in deformities of the tibia.
- Intraoperative confirmation of mechanical axis alignment with a Bovie cord is prudent for accurately correcting deformities.
- When dealing with concomitant deformities of the ipsilateral tibia and femur, it is wise to correct the tibial deformity first to avoid malalignment.

Hardware Considerations

Casts are often used following acute deformity correction in young children. They are often used to maintain deformity correction after no fixation or minimal fixation with screws or wires [57]. The casts need to be well molded to avoid loss of correction in a cast. In the operating room, correction of the deformity in the cast is checked by the electrocautery cord method [58]. A well-done cast wedging allows further fine-tuning of deformity correction (see Fig. 8.26). However, casts must be used with caution in acute correction as postoperative swelling may lead to compartment syndrome.

Kirschner Wires

Smooth Kirschner (K) wires are safe and easy to use, especially in infants and toddlers where plaster casts are often needed. The smooth wires are less traumatic to the physis and allow for fine-tuning of the correction in the postoperative period by wedging of the casts. Their use allows the osteotomies to be placed close to the physis and the CORA of the metaphyseal deformity. They are also used when corrective osteotomies are combined with other procedures such as physeal surgeries in the vicinity and where the anticipated healing times are short, and the forces across the osteotomy site are not excessive. Examples of K wire use are Bowen's technique for tibia vara correction, supramalleolar osteotomy, calcaneal lengthening osteotomy, Salter's innominate osteotomy, and metatarsal osteotomies for hallux valgus correction [17, 59, 60].

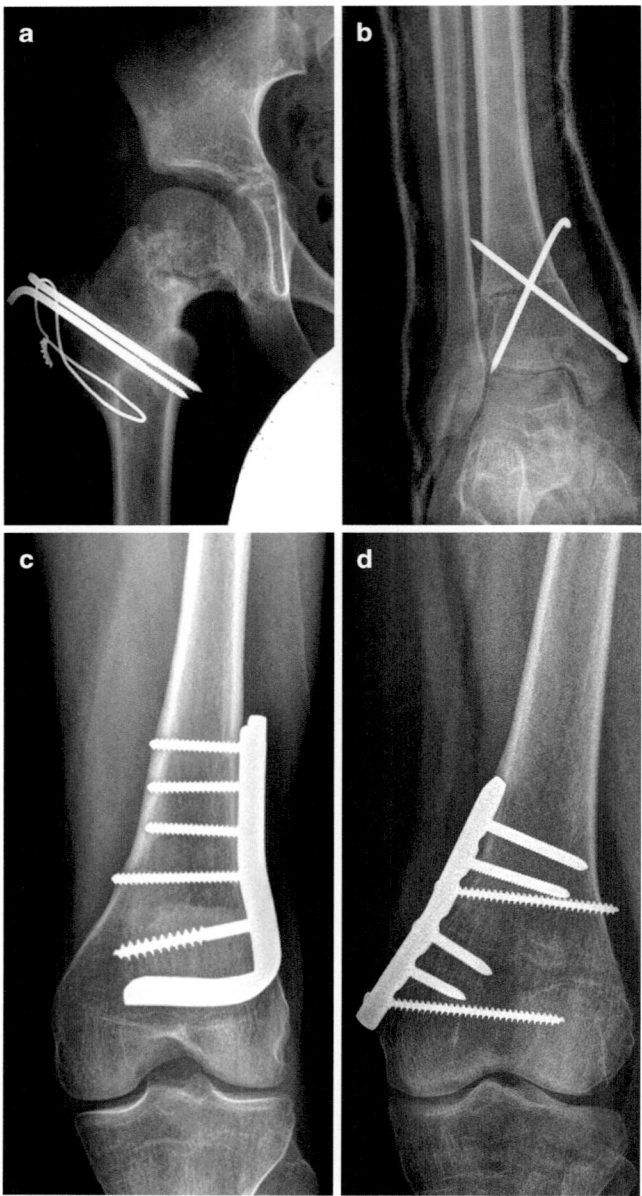

Fig. 8.26 Shows the use of various implants at different sites. (**a**) Distal transfer of the greater trochanter fixed with tension band wiring. (**b**) Use of Kirschner wires and plaster cast for the fixation of supramalleolar corrective osteotomy. (**c**) Lateral closed wedge osteotomy of distal femur and fixation with the blade plate for genu varus deformity. (**d**) Use of the metaphyseal plate for juxta-articular fixation following medial closed wedge osteotomy for correction of genu valgus deformity

Screws

Screws are useful for small fragments and sometimes allow postoperative adjustment in one plane only when a single screw is used, e.g., in Rab's osteotomy (see Fig. 8.1) [61]. They are also used for the fixation of small apophyseal fragments in trochanteric (see Fig. 8.27) and tibial tuberosity reattachments.

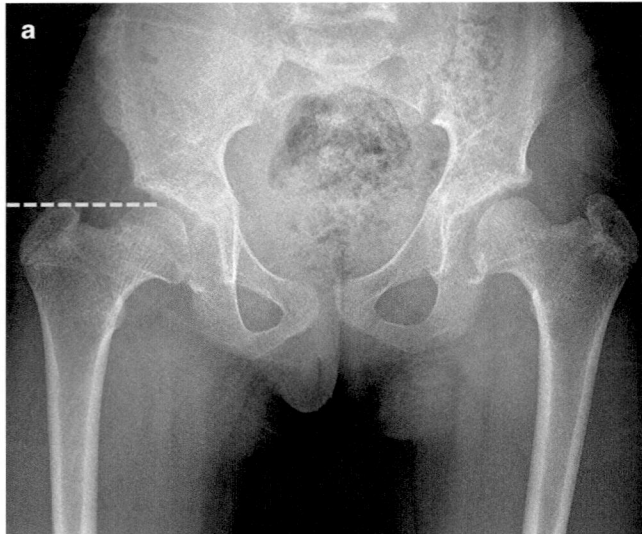

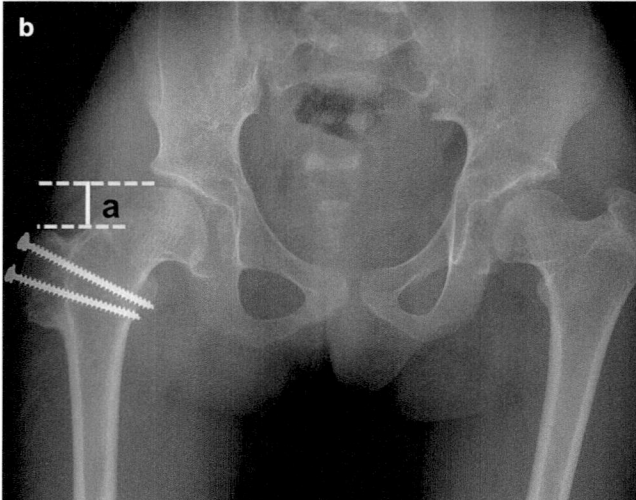

Fig. 8.27 (**a**) A 10-year-old girl with skeletal dysplasia with shortened abductor lever arm and abnormal articulo-trochanteric distance bilaterally. (**b**) Distal and lateral transfers of the right greater trochanter were performed. The increased length of the abductor lever arm following trochanteric transfer improves abductor power and gait, and eliminates trochanteric impingement. a, restored articulo-trochanteric distance

They can cross the growth plate near or after physeal closure, as in osteotomy involving mal-united condyles and malleoli.

Dynamic Compression Plate

A contoured dynamic compression plate (DCP) can hold the angular correction required for small deformities. With such internal fixation devices, a predetermined correction can be achieved by translating the bone fragments to the plate. Rotational correction can be achieved by inserting K wires on either side of the planned osteotomy at the desired angle and making them parallel at the fixation time. This technique is easy for beginners as the proximal or distal fragment can be predrilled and tapped before osteotomy and is controlled during osteotomy and fixation [62].

Tension Band Wiring

Even large fragments such as proximal femur fragments during coxa vara correction can be fixed in children with tension band wiring (Fig. 8.26). It is a useful technique in closing wedge osteotomy. Another example is the distal transfer of the greater trochanter [63]. There is a lesser degree of physeal damage when correction is desired in younger children wherein screws or plates cannot be used.

Blade Plate

Specific osteotomy plates such as condylar blade plates with preset angles can be used for proximal tibial as well as proximal and distal femoral metaphyseal corrections (see Fig. 8.26). Minor adjustment in angular correction is possible by varying the angle of insertions/entry points in condylar plates. Rotational correction can also be achieved by directing the blade in an appropriate anteversion. They have a tendency to cut out in the osteoporotic metaphysis such as in children with cerebral palsy. These devices are less forgiving and require a thorough understanding of the implant design's local anatomy and the constraints. Locked plates have replaced them in metaphyseal osteotomies which have better angular stability and allow appropriate translation.

Locked Plates (LCP)

These are ideal for holding correction in osteoporotic bones and in multiple osteotomies within a single bone. They permit early weight bearing and promote improved bone healing due to reduced plate bone contact. The metaphyseal-locked plate allows better hold in a short fragment near the joint (see Fig. 8.26). Pediatric varus and valgus hip LCP and distal femoral LCP for osteotomies around the hip and lower femur allow multiple locked screw fixations, thus achieving rigid fixation and avoiding early or late joint penetration as can be seen with some of the more conventional plating systems. As each hole provides fixation of two cortices, a shorter plate length is needed.

Angle Stable Devices for Metaphyseal Deformity Correction

These devices are preferred implants for osteoporotic bones and have been devised for deformities involving the neck of the femur, distal femur, and proximal tibia. In children, developmental coxa vara and cerebral palsy with coxa valga and subluxation are ideal candidates for locking compression pediatric hip plates [64]. These low-profile implants are devised to provide angular stability in addition to the measured amounts of displacement at the osteotomy site and thus restore the mechanical axis by providing medial displacement in the varus and lateral displacement in the valgus osteotomy. The rigid compression allows early mobilization.

Intramedullary Devices (Such as Rush Rods and Fassier-Duval Telescoping Rods)

These devices are preferred when the bone quality is poor and cannot be improved completely by medical treatment such as in osteogenesis imperfecta, metabolic disease, resistant forms of rickets, and renal osteodystrophy. The rate of reported complications with telescoping rods has been high [65, 66]. Rush rods can also be used for corrective valgus osteotomy in the proximal femur in proximal femoral focal deficiency (PFFD). Overlapping rush rods accommodate future growth in metabolic bone disorders and osteogenesis imperfecta (Fig. 8.28). The overlapping Rush rods need to be of the same diameter to avoid stress risers. Fassier Duval rod and similar devices provide a telescopic rod with epiphyseal fixation with a screw and a similar arrangement at the entry end. The telescoping rod allows the device to lengthen, allowing for bone growth. The major problems with this are bending the telescopic rod and migration of the anchoring screw into the metaphysis.

Fig. 8.28 (a) An 8-year-old boy with osteogenesis imperfecta presented a month after a trivial fall. The radiograph shows healing fractures of both femora and a broken Rush rod in the right femur. (b) Bilateral double Rush rodding was done to accommodate future growth of bone and fracture beyond the bone was protected by the implant

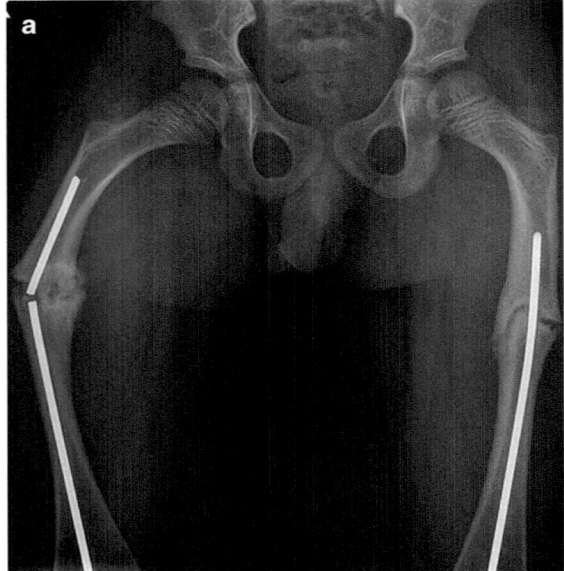
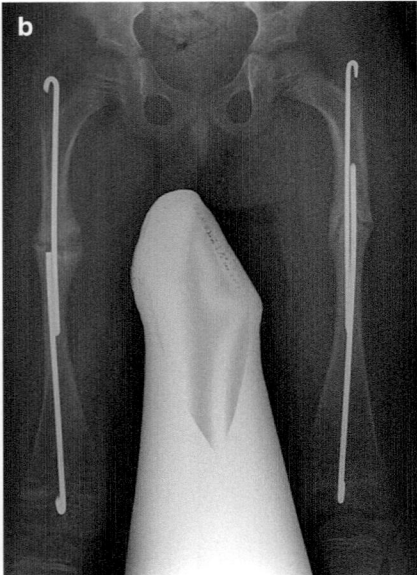

External Fixation and Limb Reconstruction Systems

Acute correction with external fixation offers potential advantages of allowing dynamic compression, distraction following acute correction, permitting minor realignments postoperatively, and having a lower incidence of peroneal nerve palsy and compartment syndrome following a proximal tibial osteotomy in obese or adolescent patients [67]. The stability offered by circular external fixators often allows patients to weight bear as tolerated. The fixator can span the physis till the healing of the osteotomy and then be removed, thereby not significantly affecting growth.

Bone Void Fillers

Autografts, allografts, xenografts, and varied combinations of commercially available synthetic bone substitutes can be used as fillers or scaffolds following an opening wedge osteotomy as promoters of bone healing. Such fillers may also provide structural support in maintaining alignment following an acute correction. Ceramic-based bone graft substitutes include hydroxyapatite, calcium phosphate, tricalcium phosphate, or bioglass. Hydroxyapatite-based scaffolds are the most preferred for bone reconstruction as the natural bone has similar stoichiometry [68]. However, except for autografts, these substitutes do not have osteogenic potential. Synthetic bone graft substitutes are often brittle leading to loss of correction, and cannot be used to fill large defects in long bones [69]. The resorption of hydroxyapatite-based ceramics is faster in young children [70]. In a recent study, Balakumar et al. showed that a hydroxyapatite tricalcium phosphate calcium silicate scaffold (HASi) incorporates faster and can be used safely for metaphyseal defects in children and adolescents [56] (Fig. 8.29). Anatomical locking metal block plates for open wedge proximal tibia osteotomy have been described [71].

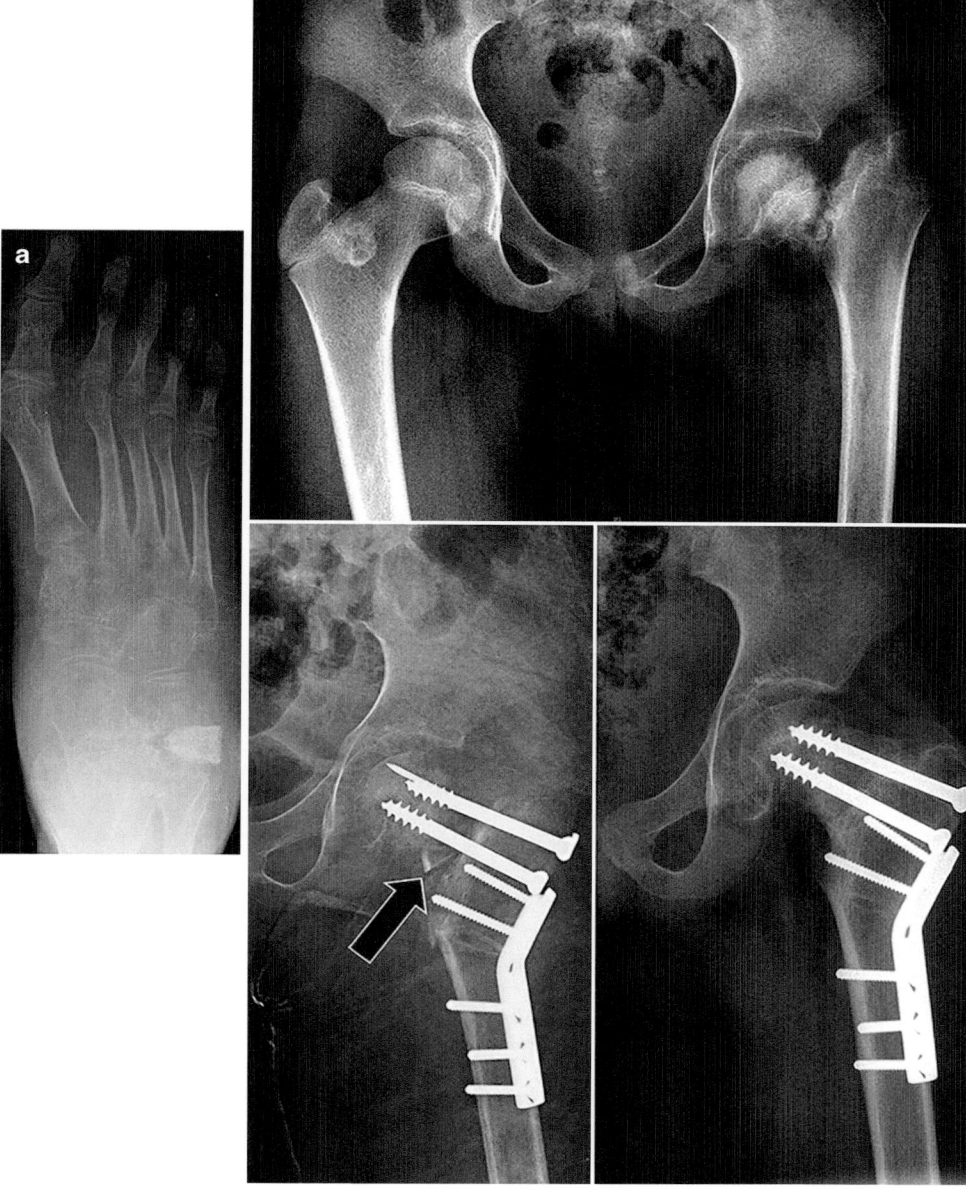

Fig. 8.29 (**a**) Use of hydroxyapatite-tricalcium phosphate-calcium silicate (HASi) scaffold as a wedge to maintain correction in calcaneal lengthening osteotomy. (**b**) Nonunion and resorption of the right femoral neck fracture in an 11-year-old girl who underwent neck reconstruction by autograft (*arrow*) and valgus subtrochanteric osteotomy. A follow-up radiograph shows evidence of union

Adapted Fixation Techniques

Fixator-Assisted Plating

Maintaining accurate alignment can be difficult when using plate fixation following acute deformity correction. The fixator-assisted plating (FAP) technique, as described by Bar-On et al., uses a temporary external fixator to acutely correct the deformity and stabilize it before application of the plate [72, 73]. Fixator-assisted manipulation of osteotomy fragments using either a tubular, rail, or ring fixator allows easy placement of LCP or DCP by using a minimally invasive technique, thus maintaining the biology and decreasing the need for assistance during surgery. Indications for this technique include angular or rotational correction of metaphyseal or diaphyseal and multiplanar and multiapical deformities. Distal femoral valgus deformities treated with fixator-assisted locking plating can be performed precisely by a minimally invasive technique, with minimal morbidity, allowing early weight bearing and early union at 6 weeks [74].

Technique

The technique described by Bar-On et al. involves using a monoplanar external fixator and locked plates [72]. Metaphyseal plates are used for juxta-articular deformities and straight narrow plates for diaphyseal deformities. External fixator pins are introduced beyond the proximal and distal ends of the selected locked plate. When this is not possible, the half-pins can be closer together; however, their placement should avoid the anticipated site of plate fixation. The osteotomy is placed as close to the CORA as possible. Bar-On et al. recommend two locked screws per segment. Rozbruch described a similar technique in adults employing a designated deformity correction frame such as Taylor spatial or multiaxial correction frames [73]. The fixator placement must not impede subsequent internal fixation. The deformity is then incrementally corrected intraoperatively with this fixator.

We slightly modify the above techniques by placing the proximal and distal pins at right angles to the mechanical axis and fixed to the clamps of a monolateral fixator or a two-ring circular fixator. For tibial deformities, one or two half-pins are passed parallel to the proximal and distal joint lines, each under image intensifier in the plane of maximum deformity and preferably on the concave side of the deformity as distraction holds the alignment better. For the femur, the distal pin is inserted parallel to the joint line, and the proximal pin is inserted in the proximal shaft angled 7° caudad to a perpendicular (valgus with respect to the anatomical axis in the anterolateral plane) to the femoral shaft (Fig. 8.30a-g). When rotational correction is required, the pins are aligned at the desired magnitude of rotational alignment in each fragment. In a large epiphysis like the femur, the pins can be passed through the distal femoral epiphysis if necessary. A two-ring Ilizarov frame with two wires in each fragment may be used in corrections close to the ankle (Fig. 8.31).

A hinged monolateral or ring fixator permits fine-tuning of correction before plate insertion. Acute correction by osteotomy is carried out at or near the CORA, and alignment is confirmed in both planes. In the case of multilevel deformity correction or corrective femoral osteotomy, we use the Bovie cord technique to confirm final alignment. The locked plate is introduced by making longitudinal incisions proximally, distally, or through the osteotomy site [72]. One end is fixed with a K wire to achieve plate alignment close to the shaft of the bone following correction and fixed with distal and proximal locking screws. At this stage,

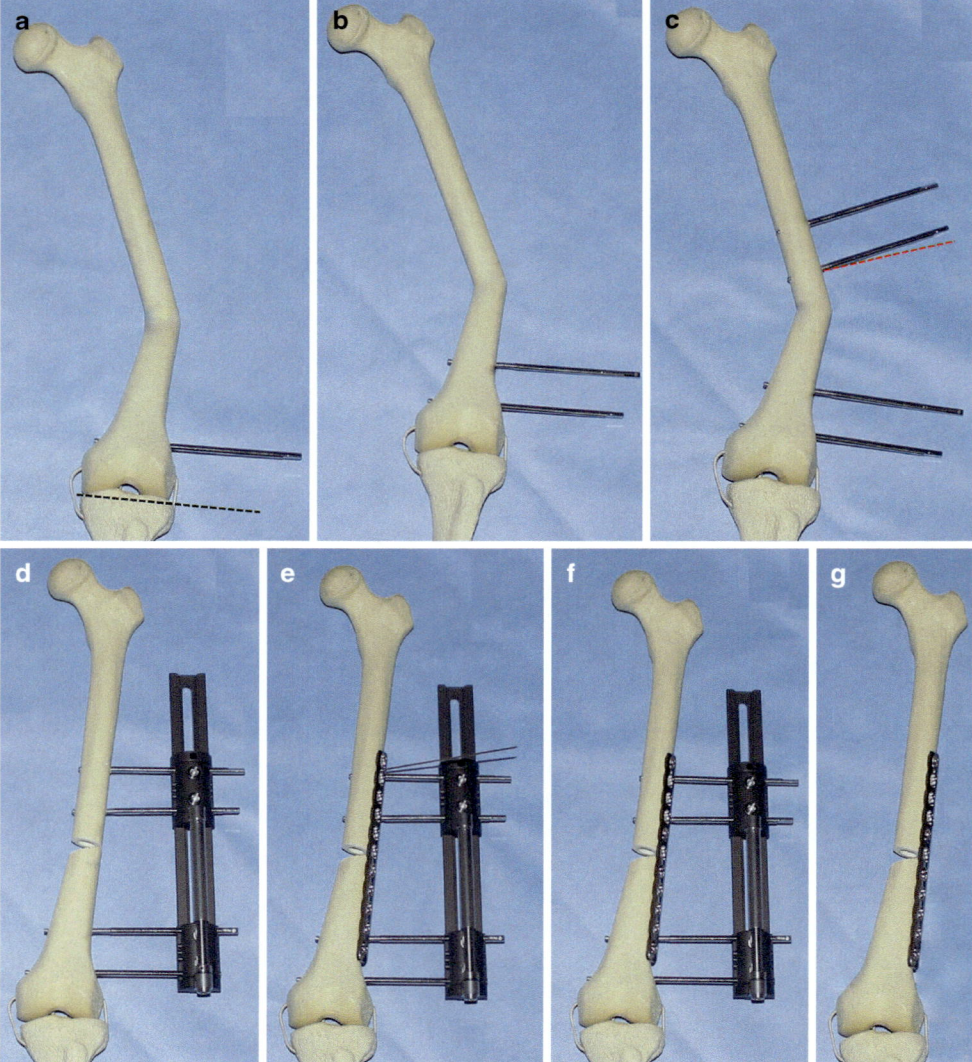

Fig. 8.30 The saw bone model illustrates the technique of deformity correction with limb reconstruction system (LRS) and subsequent plating. (**a**) The distal pin is placed freehand parallel to the knee joint line (*dotted line*). (**b**) The second pin is placed using the LRS pin template. (**c**) The second set of screws is angled 7° caudad perpendicular to the underlying diaphysis (*red-dotted line*). This restores the mechanical axis of the femur which lies at 7° to the anatomical axis of the proximal fragment. (**d**) Osteotomy is carried out at or near the CORA, and deformity is corrected using the monolateral fixator using the compression distraction unit. (**e**) A locked compression plate is aligned parallel to the shaft anterior to the fixator and temporarily stabilized with a K wire proximally and a locked screw distally. (**f**) The remaining two screws proximally and one distally are inserted through the locking holes, and the K wire is removed. (**g**) LRS is removed

8 Acute Deformity Correction Using an Osteotomy

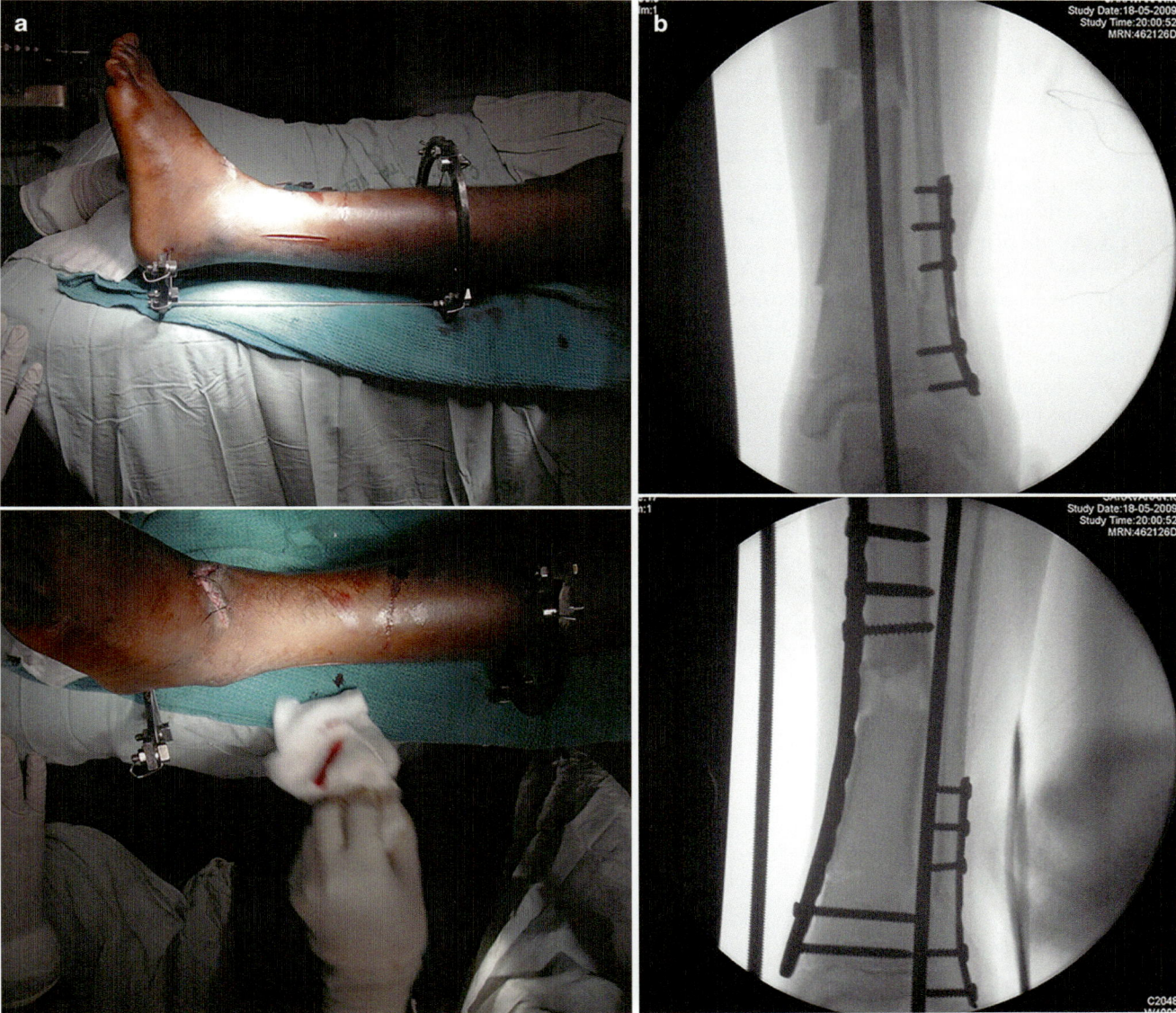

Fig. 8.31 (a) Photographs show the use of the Ilizarov frame in the fixator-assisted technique for reduction and maintaining alignment of fracture fragments in a 17-year-old boy with an open fracture tibia. (b) Intraoperative radiographs show the attainment of alignment and the connecting Ilizarov rods, which are seen overlying the skin

there is the opportunity for minor translation of the underlying bone fragment by adjusting the screw lengths or using a nonlocking cortical screw in the distal or proximal fragment of the plate to achieve the desired displacement of the fragment. The prominence of the plate may be avoided by precontouring the plate. Precontouring the plate with locked screws engaged in the plate is recommended to avoid distortion of the screw holes. Alternatively, a contoured DCP can also be used. Postoperatively, toe touch ambulation is usually permitted.

Fixator-assisted deformity correction offers fine alignment control, eases correction, and requires minimal assistance during the application of internal fixation. The main advantage over conventional techniques of correction is that there is less risk of losing correction. We often use a similar technique when plating at the end of gradual lengthening with a fixator to shorten the time in external fixation.

The technique, however, is challenging to use in smaller children. A difficult exposure or plate introduction due to the presence of a fixator can be avoided by judicious preoperative planning and outlining the plate position with a skin marker [72]. Another problem is that a large pin tract may act as a stress riser. This could be prevented by extending the plate beyond the fixator or providing cast protection for a short period. The technique is also unsuitable for corrections of large magnitude involving bone shortening as actual contact between the two fragments is lost. We have had no pin tack infection thus far when doing locked plate following acute or gradual deformity correction using external fixation, but there is a theoretical risk of deep infection.

Supracutaneous Locked Plating

A supracutaneous plate is an attractive option for acute deformity correction or shortening in the presence of poor skin condition or infection [75–77]. The indications are similar to those for external fixation, except that it allows the fixation of small metaphyseal fragments when a metaphyseal locked plate is used. The additional advantages are its lightweight, low profile, and easy concealment under regular clothing, especially in a small child. We extensively use this technique for open fractures as well [78]. A supracutaneous locked plate can serve as a lightweight external fixator in the presence of or before infection. The usual indications are deformity correction secondary to osteomyelitis sequel, physeal arrest, or pathological fractures. The technique involves initial deformity correction at the non-union/mal-union site. In the presence of a gap, nonunion shortening is affected, and the fragments are held with a conventional or fixator-assisted technique (Fig. 8.32). One centimeter thick folded linen is inserted between the plate and skin to aid screw length measurement. A supracutaneous locked plate holds this position with a minimum of four cortices (two locked screws) on either side. Following this, the fixator is removed. We do not hesitate to put one screw in the epiphysis when the fragment is very small as the plate is removed in a few weeks to months and the effect on growth is negligible. Pin care protocols are followed, and removal is done when all four cortices at the osteotomy site are noted on radiographs.

> **Box 8.4 Fixation Techniques and Implants**
> - Internal fixation with K wire and/or plaster cast allows minor postoperative realignment during molding or by cast wedging.
> - Metaphyseal locking plates offer a better hold of short metaphyseal fragments following corrective osteotomy.
> - Deformity correction in poor bone quality can be stabilized with intramedullary devices, which permit growth and provide internal splinting.
> - An external fixator following corrective osteotomy offers the added advantage of compression, distraction, and minor postoperative realignments.
> - Bone void fillers provide structural support and act as a promoter of bone healing as well.
> - Fixator-assisted plating technique allows deformity correction and stabilization of fragments until plate fixation is done.
> - A locked compression plate can be used as a low-profile and lightweight external fixator following acute osteotomy.

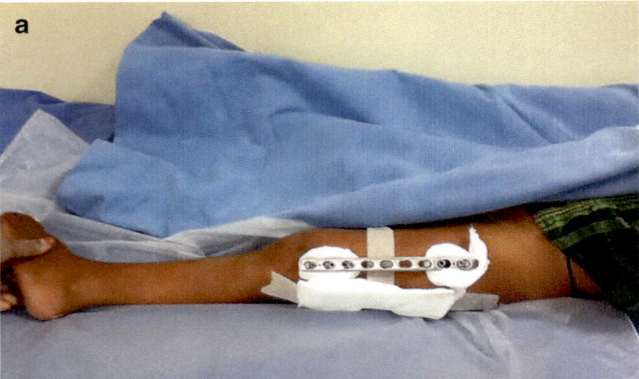

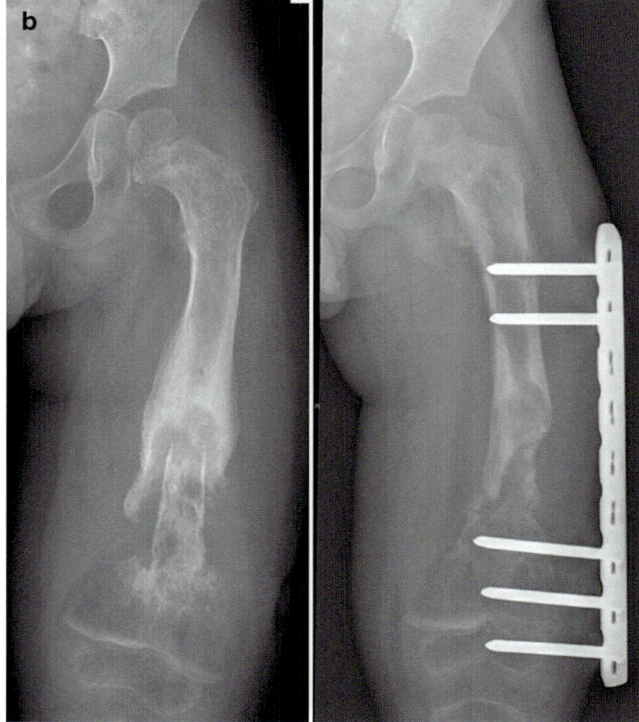

Fig. 8.32 (a) Picture of a 6-year-old boy with chronic osteomyelitis left femur with a supracutaneous locked plate fixation. (b) Pre- and postoperative radiographs show corrective angulation and shortening osteotomy following sequestrectomy

Complications

The complications in acute deformity correction include complications of skin and soft tissues, osteotomies, fixation failure, and lengthening associated with acute deformity correction. The risk of complications may vary with age, the site of deformity, underlying pathology, proximity to physis, and adjacent neurovascular structures. There is no consensus in the literature on the amount of acute deformity correction and the frequency of complications. Angular deformity correction has been noted to have more complications than rotational correction [79].

Acute Complications

Neurological

The rate of neurological complications following acute deformity correction is varied. There is evidence that acute correction of a proximal tibial varus deformity is associated with a greater risk of peroneal nerve palsy than with gradual correction [80]. Some studies have shown no complications, whereas others have reported a variable rate of such injuries ranging from 5 to 20% [79]. The neurological deficit could be due to direct intraoperative injury, ischemia, acute stretch, or fibular osteotomy [79]. Acute correction of a deformity via an osteotomy can potentially stretch the adjacent nerve(s) when the osteotomy and correction result in the lengthening of the limb, especially if the neurovascular bundle lies on the concave side of the deformity. This iatrogenic risk is less with a closing wedge than with an opening wedge osteotomy. The degree of nerve stretch also depends on the mobility of the neurovascular bundle in the surrounding soft tissues and is related to the magnitude of angular correction and its distance from the center of correction (Fig. 8.33). The neurologic risk could further increase when rotational correction is attempted; for instance, acute internal rotational correction in the proximal tibia can often lead to common peroneal nerve palsy. Another cause of peroneal nerve palsy is a fibular osteotomy, especially in the proximal third. The ideal position for fibular osteotomy is closer to the lower and middle third junction as the peroneal nerve is relatively less mobile in the upper third [14]. Judicious use of intraoperative somatosensory evoked potential (SSEP) monitoring and prophylactic nerve decompression, e.g., in genu valgum and in certain high-risk instances, could minimize the risk of iatrogenic nerve injuries [79].

Compartment Syndrome

Concomitant acute lengthening with deformity correction, pressure on vessels, or soft-tissue edema following surgery can lead to a compartment syndrome. When performing a proximal tibial osteotomy with acute correction, it is advisable not to close the deep fascia after deformity correction. Prophylactic anterior compartment fasciotomy and drain insertion have also decreased the chance of compartment syndrome in acute correction for Blount's disease [81]. Opening wedge osteotomy, large displacements, and multiple osteotomies in the same or different segments of the same limb predispose to the development of a postoperative compartment syndrome.

Vascular

Vascular injury may occur secondary to direct injury, instrumentation, or deformity correction. Such iatrogenic injuries may be due to drill/osteotome/oscillating saw/inappropriate retractor placement or implant placements such as screws, external fixator pins, or excessive stretch following open wedge osteotomy. The popliteal artery is at specific risk for osteotomies around the knee joint, e.g., Rab's osteotomy. The peroneal vessels are at risk when doing an adjuvant fibular osteotomy at its middle third [15].

Skin and Wound Problems

When the CORA is away from the site of correction, large bone displacements occur, which could result in a risk to the skin and soft tissue and wound dehiscence. Other causes for skin necrosis are poor skin conditions before surgery, multiple prior surgeries, subcutaneous bones such as the tibia, and hardware prominence, especially in subcutaneous areas such as femoral condyles.

Iatrogenic Fractures

Intraoperative fractures or a longitudinal split can occur, as in osteogenesis imperfecta, while trying to stabilize fragments in excessive soft-tissue tension.

Physeal Injury

Physeal damage can occur when correcting close to the joint or due to multiple penetrations by the fixation devices such as nails or wide Kirschner wires. The use of an intraoperative

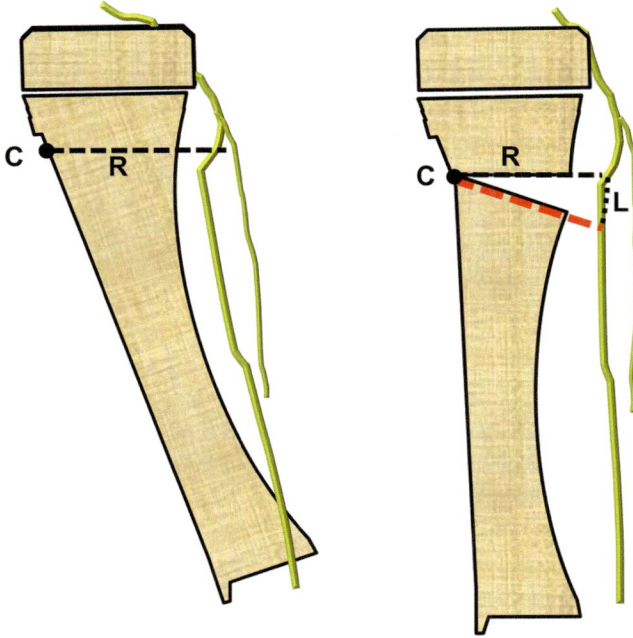

Fig. 8.33 Illustration of valgus deformity of the tibia. The effect of nerve stretch brought about by an opening wedge osteotomy is shown. The amount of stretch affected "L" on the nerve is directly proportional to the magnitude of angular correction "θ," and this can be calculated by the formula $L = 2\pi R \dfrac{\theta}{360°}$ where "R" is the distance of the relatively immobile nerve segment at the level of osteotomy from "C," the center of rotational correction. With kind permission from Springer Science + Business Media: Paley D. Principles of deformity correction. Berlin, Heidelberg; 2002

image intensifier is advised when dealing with juxta-physeal deformity corrections to prevent accidental implant penetration of the physis.

Late Complications

Joint Stiffness

Soft-tissue adhesions following acute osteotomy correction often cause joint stiffness, more so around the knee and the ankle. Tethering of the iliotibial band and the quadriceps may also occur when external fixators are applied to the thigh. Excessive intra-articular pressure following a juxta-articular acute opening wedge osteotomy correction could lead to sequelae such as chondrolysis and stiffness. Chondrolysis and avascular necrosis may be associated with the distal transfer of the greater trochanter.

Vascular

There are reports of delayed presentation of pseudoaneurysms caused by vascular injury related to instruments such as an osteotome or the penetration of vessels by fixator pins, screws, or wires [82]. Once recognized, the treatment options include ligating the involved vessel if insignificant for the vascularity of the limb, embolization, and vascular repair. Following surgery for proximal tibia hemorrhage in the popliteal fossa and the leg, the compartment has been reported to cause a deep vein thrombosis, compartment syndrome, a false aneurysm of the popliteal artery, and an arteriovenous fistula [83].

Recurrent Deformity

Recurrence of the deformity following an osteotomy is likely in the presence of metabolic bone disease, especially if the underlying metabolic disorder is not corrected or controlled. Other causes are residual soft-tissue contractures requiring soft-tissue lengthening or muscle balancing, such as in neuromuscular foot deformity (Fig. 8.34). In coxa vara, the presence of an open physis and failure to appropriately realign the capital physis increase the risk of recurrence. In some of the congenital limb deficiency and posteromedial bowing, there is a deformity memory that causes a recurrence by bowing an immature callus. Another instance is a valgus deformity of the proximal tibia in Cozen's phenomenon, where the deformity tends to recur after acute osteotomy [84]. Lack of planning for further disturbed growth in the affected physis, poor bone quality, and ongoing disease processes such as cystic lesions and fibrous dysplasia are other causes. Recurrence may also be related to the severity of soft-tissue deformity or magnitude of initial deformity, poor choice of implant, or premature weight bearing. Correction or optimizing the underlying metabolic disorder before surgical correction is essential,

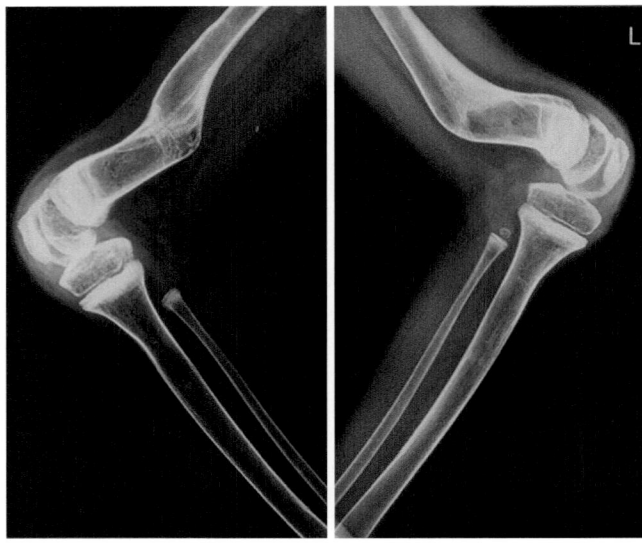

Fig. 8.34 Radiograph of 7-year-old boy referred for recurrence of flexion deformity of both knees 2 years following corrective femoral osteotomy for the same

and supplemental external or internal splinting following osteotomy correction is required in those with impaired metabolic states [57]. However, the level of osteotomy, whether metaphyseal or diaphyseal, may not be related to the risk of recurrence [57, 85]. In children with cerebral palsy, rotational deformities tend to recur if derotation is performed in children less than 10 years of age [1].

Nonunion and Delayed Union

Nonunion and delayed union are rare in children but could occur in excessive motion at the osteotomy site, decreased bone contact, and bone gap associated with large angular corrections and thermal necrosis due to the use of power instruments such as an oscillating saw. It is also more likely when combining acute correction with gradual lengthening. Some of this can be avoided by adding translation and collapse, which increases stability and bone contact and decreases the length gained at the osteotomy site. Poor healing is possible when doing acute corrections of greater than 30° with associated lengthening [86]. Acute lengthening of less than 3 cm is generally well tolerated for neurovascular status. However, the rate of secondary procedures for achieving union is high [87].

Hardware-Related Complications

In children, peri-implant complications are high because of the greater difference in the stiffness of the implant and bone. As the underlying bone is smaller and the overlying soft-tissue envelope less bulky, implant prominence is greater. Intramedullary implants being less elastic, if not perfectly aligned with the longitudinal mechanical axis, tend to cut out or bone bends at the implant–bone junction. The suggested periods for implant removal will vary from 9 months to one and a half years, based on the underlying cause. In some conditions such as osteogenesis imperfecta, these implants are not removed but revised with further growth.

Even after the healing of osteotomy in deformity correction in osteoporotic bone, fractures or bowing can occur at the implant–bone interphase and cause the hardware to fail. The wrong choice of hardware, especially in those with osteopenia, is another cause of implant failure or recurrence of deformity (Fig. 8.35).

Cast-Related Complications

Patients with anesthetic limbs, impaired cognition, and spasticity are predisposed to develop skin and soft-tissue sores related to overlying casts. Bony prominences should be adequately padded to minimize the risk of such cast-related problems, and attempts at gaining further correction by wedging the cast must be avoided, especially in these at-risk children. If cast wedging is done, it should include the removal of a cast wedge on the collapsing side to avoid excessive pressure on the underlying skin and soft tissues. Tight plaster casts should be avoided in the immediate postoperative phase to prevent compartment syndrome.

Muscle Weakness

When performing a closing wedge osteotomy and substantial shortening, there is a relative lengthening of the overlying muscle-tendon unit. For instance, a closing wedge supracondylar extension osteotomy can be associated with quadriceps insufficiency and weak knee extension. In some cases where the weakness persists despite physical therapy, one may require surgical measures such as patellar tendon reefing. Shortening of greater than 3 cm of tibia or femur causes weakness of the thigh and leg muscles and may require temporary use of braces.

> **Box 8.5 Staying out of Trouble when Doing Acute Deformity Correction**
> - Leave the deep fascia open following acute deformity correction to minimize the risk of compartment syndrome.
> - Judicious use of intraoperative SSEP monitoring and nerve decompression in high-risk cases is recommended to avoid iatrogenic nerve palsy.
> - Physeal injury can be avoided by using intraoperative imaging and avoiding multiple penetrations of the physes by nails and wires for juxtaphyseal osteotomies.
> - The bony pathology and associated soft-tissue contracture or muscle imbalance should be addressed during deformity correction to minimize recurrence.
> - Avoid acute correction when poor skin conditions, and multiple prior surgeries with scarring.

Acute Versus Gradual Correction

The complication rates with acute correction are generally higher than those of gradual correction in the tibia [67, 80]. In the postoperative rigid equinus deformity, acute correction in the presence of poor skin condition, neurovascular compromise, and multiple prior surgeries is more likely to lead to complications [88]. On the other hand, gradual correction gives a better outcome when simultaneous length-

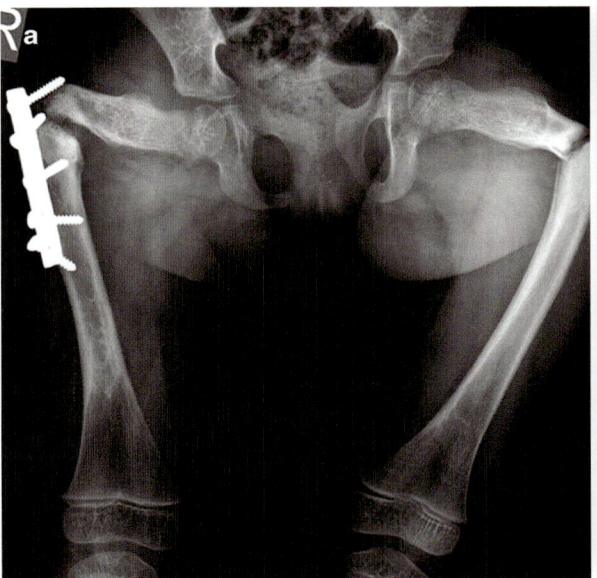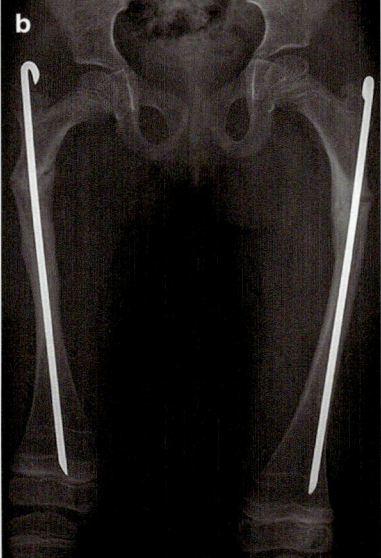

Fig. 8.35 (a) Radiograph of a 10-year-old girl with osteogenesis imperfecta (OI) shows fixation failure due to poor choice of implant and soft bones. (b) The ideal implant for OI would be an intramedullary device

ening is required [89]. Gradual correction of tibia vara has been shown to correct angular deformity more accurately than acute correction [67, 80]. The possible cause could be the flexibility to correct minimal malalignments with gradual correction techniques, especially with computer-assisted technology. However, the acute correction requires less supervision. It is also better for correcting rotational deformities. Before choosing acute or gradual correction for managing a child with a lower limb deformity, the treating surgeon should consider factors such as the patient's growth remaining, the magnitude of current and anticipated deformity and limb length discrepancy, availability of resources, and familiarity with instrumentation and psychosocial issues.

Commentary

Anirejuoritse Bafor
anirejuoritse.bafor@nationwidechildrens.org

Acute correction is a versatile concept in deformity correction surgery with applications in pediatric and adult limb reconstruction. Particularly in low-income countries (LIC) and lower-middle-income countries (LMIC) where resources for gradual correction, like the computerized hexapod systems, are limited or lacking, this is the mainstay of deformity correction and limb reconstruction surgery. Although more easily suited to correcting mild to moderate grade uniplanar deformities, with diligent planning and technique modifications, it may also be useful in severe and multiplanar deformity correction surgery.

Acute deformity correction has several advantages.

1. It shortens treatment duration and, by extension, reduces treatment costs while promoting an earlier return to function. In addition, achieving all the desired corrections in one sitting precludes the need for the sometimes logistically challenging weekly clinic visits during the correction phase for patients managed with a circular fixator.
2. In some instances, it does not require internal or external fixation to maintain the correction achieved. This eliminates potential complications like pin-site infection and discomfort specific to external fixators or the need to return to the operating room for hardware removal.

Some of the disadvantages include

1. Where correction is unsatisfactory, postoperative adjustments to the correction's magnitude are impossible without returning to the operating room. Naturally, this comes at a cost, financial and timewise. These postoperative adjustments are valuable in determining final patient satisfaction with treatment using gradual correction, particularly for rotational deformities.
2. Correction of severe deformities is not advisable without compromise, such as shortening or accepting some residual deformity. These compromises are necessary to help mitigate the risk of complications like neurovascular injury and skin necrosis.

Age considerations—in conditions like Blount's disease, where recurrence of deformity is a consideration, some authorities have argued for overcorrection to shift the mechanical axis of the lower limb to the lateral compartment of the knee, thus unloading the medial compartment and encouraging growth. However, a study by Eamsobhana et al. showed that over-correction by more than 15 degrees did not always prevent the recurrence of deformity in early-stage Blount's disease in children aged 30–40 months [90]. Therefore, it is essential to consider the stage of the disease and the growth remaining when planning treatment. In late-stage Blount's disease, an eccentric fusion of the physis has invariably occurred, and regardless of age, this will be a factor that determines recurrence.

Adjuvant Fibular Osteotomy: When and Where?—Aside from a reduced incidence of common peroneal nerve injury, one of the other advantages of doing a fibular osteotomy in the region of the junction of the middle and distal third when performing a high tibial osteotomy rather than in the proximal third is that correction is "less unstable" and less likely to require hardware to maintain the corrected position of the limb. In addition, when carrying out a fibula resection (fibulectomy), the resected segment can be used as an autograft to hold up a tibial hemiplateau elevation [91].

Bifocal procedures—In situations where deformities affect sites in adjacent bones, such as the distal femur and the proximal tibia, compensatory overcorrection may be permissible if the magnitude is small enough. This allows all the corrections to be limited to one surgical site, saving cost and effectively reducing surgery-related morbidity. Five degrees of overcorrection of the mechanical lateral distal femur angle (mLDFA) have been suggested as being permissible around the knee without compromising the biomechanics of the knee joint [92]. However, a recent cadaveric study by Wang et al. showed that the knee was more tolerant of a laterally oriented joint line obliquity than a medial joint line obliquity in full extension and in 20 degrees of knee flexion [93].

Osteotomy with Adjuvant Procedures—Laxity of the lateral collateral ligament (LCL) may be present in some patients with genu varum. Using external fixators, this laxity of the LCL is generally addressed by a combination of gradual deformity correction and lengthening of the tibia following a high tibial osteotomy without performing a fibular osteotomy. In acute correction of deformity following a high tibial osteotomy, laxity of the lateral collateral ligament may be addressed by reefing the ligament. The resultant shortening of the ligament achieved acutely in this fashion helps to restore its integrity and confer stability to the knee joint.

Other considerations –

1. *Acute correction in multiplane deformities*—Correction of multiplanar deformities can be achieved acutely in conditions like Blount's disease. An anterior–posterior dome or "inverted-U" osteotomy performed in the proximal tibial metaphysis can achieve angulation, rotation, and translation correction at the same sitting. The geometry of the osteotomy confers stability to the correction, thus eliminating the need for internal fixation to hold correction, while the larger surface area involved is ideal for healing [94]. We have found this technique useful even in addressing severe deformities by incorporating a laterally based closing wedge osteotomy at the dome osteotomy site. This reduces the potential complications that may arise from acutely stretching adjacent soft tissue structures.
2. *Combining acute correction with gradual correction*—The goal here is to reduce the magnitude of the deformity before frame application while protecting the adjacent soft tissues from the effects of acute stretching. This shortens treatment time and, in many cases, eliminates the need for strut changes when using hexapod frames. It also allows fine-tuning the magnitude of correction postoperatively. We have found this protocol useful for severe angular deformities. Because acute correction is achieved through an open osteotomy rather than the minimally invasive procedures used with gradual correction, we advocate a longer latency period prior to the commencement of distraction.
3. *Reverse planning method and acute correction using IM nails*—Using motorized lengthening nails is now considered the gold standard for managing significant limb length discrepancy. In femoral length discrepancy correction, intramedullary lengthening results in a lateral shift of the mechanical axis of the lower limb because lengthening occurs along the anatomical axis rather than the mechanical axis of the femur. The reverse planning method was designed to address this problem and maintain a normal mechanical axis during lengthening of the femur or tibia [95]. In combination with acute deformity correction, this technique has been used to restore length with good effect in patients with shortening and concomitant deformity. Iobst et al. demonstrated their technique using intraoperative temporary external fixation to achieve acute correction [96]. Modifications to this technique now mean that using external fixators intraoperatively is no longer necessary or required, with deformity correction now achieved intraoperatively using rigid reamers and appropriately placed blocking screws.

References

1. Kim H, Aiona M, Sussman M. Recurrence after femoral derotational osteotomy in cerebral palsy. J Pediatr Orthop. 2005;25(6):739–43.
2. Williamson RV, Staheli LT. Partial physeal growth arrest: treatment by bridge resection and fat interposition. J Pediatr Orthop. 1990;10(6):769–76.
3. Lalonde K-A, Letts M. Traumatic growth arrest of the distal tibia: a clinical and radiographic review. Can J Surg. 2005;48(2):143.
4. Boyle C, Kim IY. Three-dimensional micro-level computational study of Wolff's law via trabecular bone remodeling in the human proximal femur using design space topology optimization. J Biomech. 2011;44(5):935–42.
5. Pauwels F. Biomechanics of the locomotor apparatus. Berlin, Heidelberg: Springer; 1980. Translated by Maquet P, Furlong R
6. Bries AD, Weiner DS, Jacquet R, Adamczyk MJ, Morscher MA, Lowder E, et al. A study in vivo of the effects of a static compressive load on the proximal tibial physis in rabbits. J Bone Joint Surg Am. 2012;94(15):e1111–0.
7. Wallace ME, Hoffman EB. Remodelling of angular deformity after femoral shaft fractures in children. J Bone Joint Surg (Br). 1992;74(5):765–9.
8. Murray DW, Wilson-MacDonald J, Morscher E, Rahn BA, Käslin M. Bone growth and remodelling after fracture. J Bone Joint Surg (Br). 1996;78:42–50.
9. Karaharju EO, Ryoppy SA, Makinen RJ. Remodelling by asymmetrical epiphyseal growth: an experimental study in dogs. J Bone Joint Surg (Br). 1976;58-B:122–6.
10. Feller JA, Amis AA, Andrish JT, Arendt EA, Erasmus PJ, Powers CM. Surgical biomechanics of the patellofemoral joint. Arthroscopy. 2007;23(5):542–53.

11. Rozbruch SR, Ilizarov S. Limb lengthening and reconstruction surgery. Boca Raton, FL: CRC; 2013.
12. Shah HH, Doddabasappa SN, Joseph B. Congenital posteromedial bowing of the tibia: a retrospective analysis of growth abnormalities in the leg. J Pediatr Orthop B. 2009;18(3):120–8.
13. Curley P, Eyres K, Brezinova V, Allen M, Chan R, Barnes M. Common peroneal nerve dysfunction after high tibial osteotomy. J Bone Joint Surg (Br). 1990;72(3):405–8.
14. Mont MA, Dellon AL, Chen F, Hungerford MW, Krackow KA, Hungerford DS. The operative treatment of peroneal nerve palsy. J Bone Joint Surg. 1996;78(6):863–9.
15. Rupp RE, Podeszwa D, Ebraheim NA. Danger zones associated with fibular osteotomy. J Orthop Trauma. 1994;8:54–8.
16. Ogbemudia AO, Umebese PFA, Bafor A, Igbinovia E, Ogbemudia PE. The level of fibula osteotomy and incidence of peroneal nerve palsy in proximal tibial osteotomy. J Surg Tech Case Rep. 2010;2(1):17–9.
17. Inan M, Ferri-de Baros F, Chan G, Dabney K, Miller F. Correction of rotational deformity of the tibia in cerebral palsy by percutaneous supramalleolar osteotomy. J Bone Joint Surg (Br). 2005;87(10):1411–5.
18. Aydoğdu S, Yercan H, Saylam C, Sur H. Peroneal nerve dysfunction after high tibial osteotomy. An anatomical cadaver study. Acta Orthop Belg. 1996;62(3):156–60.
19. Pacelli LL, Gillard J, McLoughlin SW, Buehler MJ. A biomechanical analysis of donor-site ankle instability following free fibular graft harvest. J Bone Joint Surg. 2003;85(4):597–603.
20. Ryan DD, Rethlefsen SA, Skaggs DL, Kay RM. Results of tibial rotational osteotomy without concomitant fibular osteotomy in children with cerebral palsy. J Pediatr Orthop. 2005;25(1):84–8.
21. Kang SH, Rhee SK, Song SW, Chung JW, Kim YC, Suhl KH. Ankle deformity secondary to acquired fibular segmental defect in children. Clin Orthop Surg. 2010;2(3):179.
22. Johari AN, Dhawale AA, Salaskar A, Aroojis AJ. Congenital posteromedial bowing of the tibia and fibula: is early surgery worthwhile? J Pediatr Orthop B. 2010;19(6):479–86.
23. Paley D. Principles of deformity correction. Heidelberg: Springer; 2002.
24. Mosca VS. Flexible flatfoot in children and adolescents. J Child Orthop. 2010;4(2):107–21.
25. Glard Y, Katchburian MV, Jacquemier M, Guillaume J-M, Bollini G. Genu valgum in Legg-Calvé-Perthes disease treated with femoral varus osteotomy. Clin Orthop Relat Res. 2009;467(6):1587–90.
26. Sangavi SM, Szöke G, Murray DW, Benson MKD. Femoral remodelling after subtrochanteric osteotomy for developmental dysplasia of the hip. J Bone Joint Surg (Br). 1996;78(6):917–23.
27. Tercier S, Shah H, Siddesh ND, Joseph B. Does proximal femoral varus osteotomy in Legg–Calvé–Perthes disease predispose to angular mal-alignment of the knee? A clinical and radiographic study at skeletal maturity. J Child Orthop. 2013;7(3):205–11.
28. Mazur JM, Danko AM, Standard SC, Loveless EA, Cummings RJ. Remodeling of the proximal femur after varus osteotomy in children with cerebral palsy. Dev Med Child Neurol. 2004;46(06):412–5.
29. Herceg MB, Cutright MT, Weiner DS. Remodeling of the proximal femur after upper femoral varus osteotomy for the treatment of Legg-Calvé-Perthes disease. J Pediatr Orthop. 2004;24(6):654–7.
30. Talkhani IS, Moore DP, Dow-Ling FE, Fogarty EE. Neck-shaft angle remodelling after derotation varus osteotomy for severe Perthes disease. Acta Orthop Belg. 2001;67(3):248–51.
31. Milch H. The "pelvic support" osteotomy. 1941. Clin Orthop Relat Res. 1989;249:4–11.
32. Beaty JH, Kasser JR. Rockwood and Wilkins' fractures in children. 7th ed. Philadelphia, PA: Lippincott Williams & Wilkins; 2010.
33. Rab GT. Oblique tibial osteotomy for Blount's disease (tibia vara). J Pediatr Orthop. 1988;8(6):715–20.
34. Johnson E. Acute lengthening of shortened lower extremities after malunion or non-union of a fracture. J Bone Joint Surg. 1994;76(3):379–89.
35. Kim HT, Lee SH, Yoo CI, Kang JH, Suh JT. The management of brachymetatarsia. J Bone Joint Surg (Br). 2003;85(5):683–90.
36. Sen C, Kocaoglu M, Eralp L, Gulsen M, Cinar M. Bifocal compression-distraction in the acute treatment of grade III open tibia fractures with bone and soft-tissue loss: a report of 24 cases. J Orthop Trauma. 2004;18(3):150–7.
37. Beals RK, Stanley G. Surgical correction of bowlegs in achondroplasia. J Pediatr Orthop B. 2005;14(4):245–9.
38. El-Rosasy MA. Acute shortening and re-lengthening in the management of bone and soft-tissue loss in complicated fractures of the tibia. J Bone Joint Surg Br. 2007;89(1):80–8. https://doi.org/10.1302/0301-620X.89B1.17595.
39. Nizaj N, Sukesh AN, Jacob B, George B, Kandathil JC, Theruvil B. Double level osteotomy in an overcorrected distal femoral Varisation osteotomy: a case report. JBJS case. Connect. 2022;12(1) Published 2022 Mar 23 https://doi.org/10.2106/JBJS.CC.21.00771.
40. Jardaly A, Gilbert SR. Combined antegrade femur lengthening and distal deformity correction: a case series. J Orthop Surg Res. 2021;16(1):60. https://doi.org/10.1186/s13018-020-02168-6.
41. Brougham DI, Nicol RO. Valgus deformity after proximal tibial fractures in children. J Bone Joint Surg (Br). 1987;69(3):482.
42. Robert M, Khouri N, Carlioz H, Alain JL. Fractures of the proximal tibial metaphysis in children: review of a series of 25 cases. J Pediatr Orthop. 1987;7(4):444–9.
43. Hefny H, Shalaby H, El-kawy S, Thakeb M, Elmoatasem E. A new double elevating osteotomy in management of severe neglected infantile tibia vara using the Ilizarov technique. J Pediatr Orthop. 2006;26(2):233–7.
44. McCarthy JJ, MacIntyre NR 3rd, Hooks B, Davidson RS. Double osteotomy for the treatment of severe Blount disease. J Pediatr Orthop. 2009;29(2):115–9.
45. Van Huyssteen AL, Hastings CJ, Olesak M, Hoffman EB. Double-elevating osteotomy for late-presenting infantile Blount's disease. The importance of concomitant lateral epiphysiodesis. J Bone Joint Surg B. 2005;87(5):710–5.
46. Schneidmueller D, Carstens C, Thomsen M. Surgical treatment of overgrowth of the greater trochanter in children and adolescents. J Pediatr Orthop. 2006;26(4):486–90.
47. Iliadis AD, Jaiswal PK, Khan W, Johnstone D. The operative management of patella malalignment. Open Orthop J. 2012;6(Suppl 2):327.
48. Choi I, Pizzutillo P, Bowen J, Dragann R, Malhis T. Sequelae and reconstruction after septic arthritis of the hip in infants. J Bone Joint Surg. 1990;72(8):1150–65.
49. Mitchell GP. Posterior displacement osteotomy of the calcaneus. J Bone Joint Surg (Br). 1977;59(2):233–5.
50. Colmenares-Bonilla D, Vasconcelos-Martinez M, Guerra-Jasso J, Ocampo-Perez L. Guided growth may not be the best option for knee valgus deformity in adolescent patients with Morquio-a. Musculoskelet Surg. 2017;101(2):113–8. https://doi.org/10.1007/s12306-016-0441-0.
51. Brown DE, Alexander AH, Lichtman DM. The Elmslie-Trillat procedure: evaluation in patellar dislocation and subluxation. Am J Sports Med. 1984;12(2):104–9.
52. Mahran MA, ElGebeily MA, Ghaly NAM, Thakeb MF, Hefny HM. Pelvic support osteotomy by Ilizarov's concept: is it a valuable option in managing neglected hip problems in adolescents and young adults? Strategies Trauma Limb Reconstr. 2011;6(1):13–20.
53. Gursu S. An effective treatment for hip instabilities: pelvic support osteotomy and femoral lengthening. Acta Orthop Traumatol Turc. 2011;45(6):437–45.

54. Abdelgawad AA. Combined distal tibial rotational osteotomy and proximal growth plate modulation for treatment of infantile Blount's disease. World J Orthop. 2013;4(2):90.
55. Sabharwal S. Blount disease. J Bone Joint Surg Am. 2009;91(7):1758–76. https://doi.org/10.2106/JBJS.H.01348.
56. Balakumar B, Babu S, Varma HK, Madhuri V. Triphasic ceramic scaffold in paediatric and adolescent bone defects. J Pediatr Orthop B. 2013;23(2):187–95.
57. Petje G, Meizer R, Radler C, Aigner N, Grill F. Deformity correction in children with hereditary hypophosphatemic rickets. Clin Orthop Relat Res. 2008;466(12):3078–85.
58. Sabharwal S, Kumar A. Methods for assessing leg length discrepancy. Clin Orthop Relat Res. 2008;466(12):2910–22. https://doi.org/10.1007/s11999-008-0524-9.
59. Ferriter P, Shapiro F. Infantile tibia vara: factors affecting outcome following proximal tibial osteotomy. J Pediatr Orthop. 1987;7(1):1–7.
60. Lee K-B, Seo C-Y, Hur C-I, Moon E-S, Lee J-J. Outcome of proximal chevron osteotomy for hallux valgus with and without transverse Kirschner wire fixation. Foot Ankle Int. 2008;29(11):1101–6.
61. Rab GT. Oblique tibial osteotomy revisited. J Child Orthop. 2009;4(2):169–72.
62. Joseph B, Srinivas G, Thomas R. Management of Perthes' disease of late onset in southern India. J Bone Joint Surg (Br). 1996;78:625–30.
63. Cordes S, Dickens DR, Cole WG. Correction of coxa vara in childhood. The use of Pauwels' Y-shaped osteotomy. J Bone Joint Surg Br. 1991;73(1):3–6.
64. Ziebarth K, Slongo T. Osteotomien am proximalen femur mit der winkelstabilen kindlichen Hüftplatte (LCP): Valgusosteotomie [proximal femoral osteotomies with the paediatric hip plate (LCP): valgus osteotomy]. Oper Orthop Traumatol. 2015;27(3):210–20. https://doi.org/10.1007/s00064-015-0402-z.
65. Birke O, Davies N, Latimer M, Little DG, Bellemore M. Experience with the Fassier-Duval telescopic rod: first 24 consecutive cases with a minimum of 1-year follow-up. J Pediatr Orthop. 2011;31(4):458–64.
66. Wright DM, Sampath J, Nayagam SN, Bass A. Experience and complications associated with the Fassier-Duval telescoping nailing system. J Bone Joint Surg Br. 2012;94-B(SUPP XXIV):6.
67. Feldman DS, Madan SS, Ruchelsman DE, Sala DA, Lehman WB. Accuracy of correction of tibia vara: acute versus gradual correction. J Pediatr Orthop. 2006;26(6):794–8.
68. Giannoudis PV, Dinopoulos H, Tsiridis E. Bone substitutes: an update. Injury. 2005;36(Suppl 3):S20–7.
69. Dorozhkin S. Calcium orthophosphate-based bioceramics. Materials. 2013;6(9):3840–942.
70. Matsumine A, Myoui A, Kusuzaki K, Araki N, Seto M, Yoshikawa H, et al. Calcium hydroxyapatite ceramic implants in bone tumour surgery. A long-term follow-up study. J Bone Joint Surg Br. 2004;86(5):719–25.
71. Han S-B, et al. Biomechanical properties of a new anatomical locking metal block plate for opening wedge high tibial osteotomy: Uniplane osteotomy. Knee Surg Related Res. 2014;26:155–61.
72. Bar-On E, Becker T, Katz K, Velkes S, Salai M, Weigl DM. Corrective lower limb osteotomies in children using temporary external fixation and percutaneous locking plates. J Child Orthop. 2009;3(2):137–43.
73. Rozbruch SR. Fixator-assisted plating of limb deformities. Oper Tech Orthop. 2011;21(2):174–9.
74. Eidelman M, Keren Y, Norman D. Correction of distal femoral valgus deformities in adolescents and young adults using minimally invasive fixator-assisted locking plating (FALP). J Pediatr Orthop B. 2012;21(6):558–62. https://doi.org/10.1097/BPB.0b013e328358f884.
75. Woon CY, Wong M-K, Howe T-S. LCP external fixation-external application of an internal fixator: two cases and a review of the literature. J Orthop Surg Res. 2010;20(5):19.
76. Gupta SKV, Parimala SP. Supracutaneous locking compression plate for Grade I &; II compound fracture distal tibia—a case series. Open J Orthop. 2013;03(02):106–9.
77. Tulner SAF, Strackee SD, Kloen P. Metaphyseal locking compression plate as an external fixator for the distal tibia. Int Orthop. 2012;36(9):1923–7.
78. Radhakrishna VN, Madhuri V. Management of pediatric open tibia fractures with supracutaneous locked plates. J Pediatr Orthop B. 2018;27(1):13–6. https://doi.org/10.1097/BPB.0000000000000425.
79. Makarov MR, Samchukov ML, Birch JG, Johnston CE, Delgado MR, Rampy PL, et al. Acute deformity correction of lower extremities under SSEP-monitoring control. J Pediatr Orthop. 2003;23(4):470–7.
80. Gilbody J, Thomas G, Ho K. Acute versus gradual correction of idiopathic tibia vara in children: a systematic review. J Pediatr Orthop. 2009;29(2):110–4.
81. Sabharwal S. Blount disease. J Bone Joint Surg Am. 2009;91(7):18.
82. Rickman M, Saleh M, Gaines PA, Eyres K. Vascular complications of osteotomies in limb reconstruction. J Bone Joint Surg (Br). 1999;81(5):890–2.
83. Franke L, Gossé F. Angiologische Komplikationen nach valgisierender Tibiakopfkorrekturosteotomie–eine Fallbeschreibung [Angiological complications following high tibial head correcting osteotomy–a case report]. Z Orthop Ihre Grenzgeb. 1997;135(1):76–8. https://doi.org/10.1055/s-2008-1039559.
84. Jackson DW, Cozen L. Genu valgum as a complication of proximal tibial metaphyseal fractures in children. JBJS. 1971;53(8):1571–8.
85. Song HR, Soma Raju VV, Kumar S, Lee SH, Suh SW, Kim JR, Hong JS. Deformity correction by external fixation and/or intramedullary nailing in hypophosphatemic rickets. Acta Orthop. 2006;77:307–14.
86. Donnan LT, Saleh M, Rigby AS. Acute correction of lower limb deformity and simultaneous lengthening with a monolateral fixator. J Bone Joint Surg (Br). 2003;85(2):254–60.
87. Johnson EE. Acute lengthening of shortened lower extremities after malunion or non-union of a fracture. J Bone Joint Surg Am. 1994;76(3):379–89. https://doi.org/10.2106/00004623-199403000-00008.
88. Fuentes P, Cuchacovich N, Gutierrez P, Hube M, Bastías GF. Treatment of severe rigid posttraumatic Equinus deformity with gradual deformity correction and arthroscopic ankle arthrodesis. Foot Ankle Int. 2021;42(12):1525–35. https://doi.org/10.1177/10711007211018201.
89. Matsubara H, Tsuchiya H, Sakurakichi K, Watanabe K, Tomita K. Deformity correction and lengthening of lower legs with an external fixator. Int Orthop. 2006;30(6):550–4. https://doi.org/10.1007/s00264-006-0133-8.
90. Eamsobhana P, Kaewpornsawan K, Yusuwan K. Do we need to do overcorrection in Blount's disease? Int Orthop. 2014;38(8):1661–4. https://doi.org/10.1007/s00264-014-2365-3.
91. Ogbemudia AO, Bafor A, Ogbemudia EJ, Edomwonyi E. Combined Antero-Posterior inverted-U Metaphyseal and open-wedge medial-epiphyseal osteotomy for advanced blount disease. Surg Sci. 2015;6:162–9. https://doi.org/10.4236/ss.2015.64026.
92. Miller ML, Gordon JE. Decision making in lower extremity deformity correction. In: Sabharwal S, editor. Pediatric lower limb deformities: principles and techniques of management. Switzerland: Springer International Publishing; 2016. p. 37–50. https://doi.org/10.1007/978-3-319-17,097-8.
93. Wang D, Willinger L, Athwal KK, Williams A, Amis AA. Knee joint line obliquity causes tibiofemoral subluxation that alters contact

94. Ogbemudia AO, Bafor A, Ogbemudia PE. Anterior-posterior inverted-U' osteotomy for tibia vara: technique and early results. Arch Orthop Trauma Surg. 2011;131(4):437–42. https://doi.org/10.1007/s00402-010-1139-7.
95. Baumgart R. The reverse planning method for lengthening of the lower limb using a straight intramedullary nail with or without deformity correction. Oper Orthop Traumatol. 2009;21(2):221–33. https://doi.org/10.1007/s00064-009-1709-4.
96. Iobst CA, Rozbruch SR, Nelson S, Fragomen A. Simultaneous acute femoral deformity correction and gradual limb lengthening using a retrograde femoral nail: technique and clinical results. J Am Acad Orthop Surg. 2018;26(7):241–50. https://doi.org/10.5435/JAAOS-D-16-00573.

Gradual Deformity Correction in Children and Adolescents

Mark Eidelman, Pavel Kotlarsky, and John E. Herzenberg

Introduction

Pediatric limb deformities may be congenital or acquired, and simple or complex. Subsequently, multiple methods of correction are available: acute, gradual, or a combination of the approaches. Several factors must be considered when outlining a pediatric deformity correction plan. The open physis of an immature patient is an important factor that must be taken into account. Iatrogenic damage to a normal open growth plate must be avoided. Another challenge in pediatric cases is the "sick" physis that may be sequela of premature growth arrest (GA) due to various reasons (e.g., metabolic conditions, Blount disease, Ollier disease, posttraumatic injury, postinfection, and tumor-induced growth arrest). An abnormal physis may cause a recurrence of deformity and persistent limb shortening when not addressed (Fig. 9.1).

Acute correction of deformity offers the advantage of immediate results, usually with a shorter period of healing and rehabilitation when compared to gradual correction. However, acute correction has the disadvantage of being unforgiving. An error in acute correction often cannot be adjusted postoperatively without another surgical intervention. Acute correction may create adverse effects that are less likely when a correction is performed gradually. For example, compartment syndrome is rare in patients with Blount disease who have undergone gradual correction. However, compartment syndrome is commonly described in children undergoing tibial osteotomy with acute correction, often due to kinking of the tibialis anterior artery that subsequently contributes to the syndrome [1, 2].

Gradual correction techniques not only assess the deformity but also allow simultaneous limb lengthening in cases where there is substantial shortening. Gradual correction is preferred with lengthening of affected bones in congenital short femur, congenital leg deformity, and all conditions related to premature growth arrest when a deformity exists with shortening. The most common method of gradual deformity correction for children with open physes is guided growth, also referred to as temporary hemiepiphysiodesis. In this chapter, we will focus on pediatric gradual correction and bone lengthening using external and internal devices.

M. Eidelman (✉) · P. Kotlarsky
Pediatric Orthopedics, Ruth Rappoport Children's Hospital, Rambam Health Care Campus, Haifa, Israel
e-mail: m_eidelman@rmc.gov.il; p_kotlarsky@rmc.gov.il

J. E. Herzenberg
The Rubin Institute for Advanced Orthopedics, Sinai Hospital of Baltimore, Baltimore, USA
e-mail: jherzenb@lifebridgehealth.org

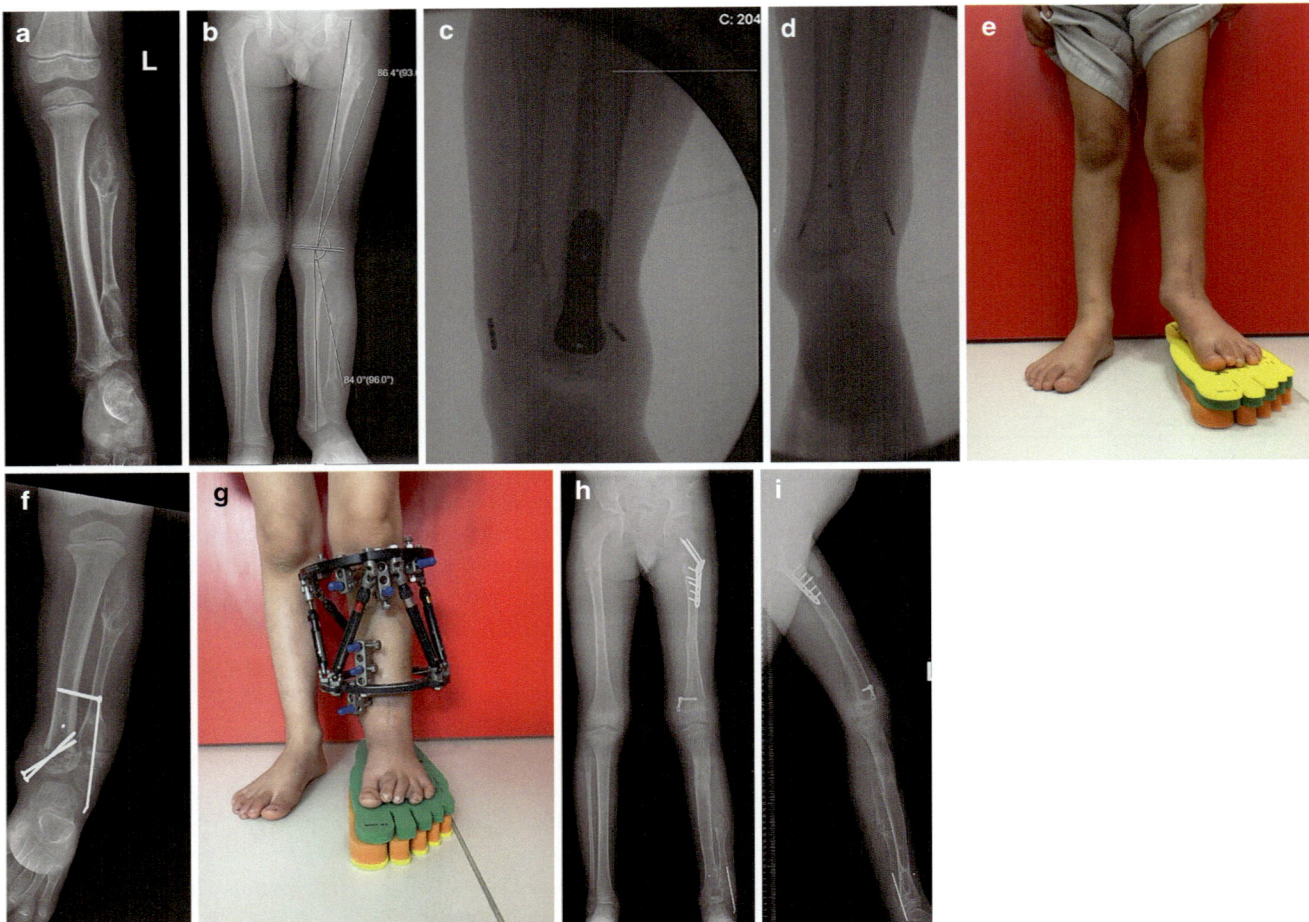

Fig. 9.1 (**a, b**) x-rays of 4-year-old child with Ollier disease before correction, (**c**) correction of deformities (without closure of the epiphysis of the distal tibia), (**d**) recurrence of deformities, (**e**) clinical appearance of the leg after recurrence, (**f**) epiphysiodesis of the sick physis and closing wedge osteotomy, (**g**) leg appearance before tibial lengthening, and (**h-i**) x-rays after two tibial lengthening procedures 9 years later

Gradual Correction Using External Fixation

Modern deformity correction and bone lengthening can be attributed to Gavriil Abramovich Ilizarov [3, 4]. Attempts to perform bone lengthening which predate Ilizarov [5, 6] were either acute lengthening or employed a relatively rapid distraction rate with filling of the distraction gap with bone graft and internal fixation with a plate [7, 8]. Before Ilizarov, bone lengthening was prone to numerous complications [7–9]. Prior to Ilizarov, correction and lengthening usually were performed by relatively high-speed correction without special respect to the periosteum and soft tissues around bones, which led to poor bone formation after osteotomy. Although circular external fixators were developed before Ilizarov [10], his method of gradual correction and lengthening by distraction for new bone formation was revolutionary. From Ilizarov's contributions, a latency period of 5–7 days before distraction was adopted, as well as a standard of 1 mm daily lengthening, divided into 3–4 steps throughout the day. This rate of lengthening does not damage vascular supply or nerves and is optimal for the formation of bone regeneration. Lengthening >1.5 mm daily can cause nonunion and neurovascular damage, whereas lengthening <0.75 mm/day may cause premature bone consolidation.

External fixators come in two main types: monolateral and circular. De Bastiani and colleagues [11] designed a useful monolateral external fixatorr and described the corticotomy method of bone osteotomy through a minimal skin incision, limited periosteal stripping, multiple drill holes, and completion of the osteotomy by osteotome [8, 11, 12]. They also coined the term *callotasis* (lengthening of the callus) to describe the formation of the regenerate during lengthening. While monolateral fixation has some advantages (e.g., it is less bulky and easier to apply), it also has several disadvantages. It is less stable, and it is difficult to perform a correction with the apex of the deformity near a joint. Moreover, it is practically impossible to perform a gradual correction of rotational deformities with a monoliteral fixator. For these reasons, the device is less useful for gradual correction [13–15]. Most modern monoliteral applications are limited to the femur in straight-lengthening situations.

The circular external fixator—specifically the classic Ilizarov frame—in our opinion is still the most useful reconstructive external fixation system. The circular frame uses hinges and other devices to allow the correction of all possible deformities. The Ilizarov frame's main disadvantage is its learning curve. To be a master of correcting severe deformities, one requires significant experience using this circular frame. Correction of rotation with the frame is possible, but difficult even for experts to achieve [13–15]. Replacing hinges and making modifications for multiplanar deformities are other obstacles that contribute to the rather steep learning curve [14].

The Taylor Spatial Frame™ was the first hexapod frame, an advancement that further enhanced surgeon ability and opened new doors [13–16]. Currently, there are numerous hexapods on the market, all of which allow for the simultaneous correction of six-axis deformities using virtual hinges. Six axis refers to varus/valgus, procurvatum/recurvatum, translation (anterior/posterior; medial/lateral; length), and rotation. The greatest advantage of hexapod systems is their elimination of the need for frame adjustments (other than strut changes) because all deformities, from simple to the most complex, are treated with essentially the same frame that consists of two rings and six struts. Accurate deformity analysis can be done with the aid of a hexapod system's software program. Hexapods have become the treatment of choice for gradual correction of multiplanar skeletal deformities, especially those with rotational components [13–16].

Basic Principles of Gradual Correction Using External Fixation

Accurate deformity analysis is crucial before beginning treatment. Multiple factors should be taken into account. Is it a simple or multilevel deformity? Is rotational deformity present? What is the proximity of the deformity apex to the growth plate? Both the current and the projected limb length discrepancy (LLD) must be analyzed to not only correct the deformity but also the length of the affected limb.

Numerous factors affect the planning of gradual correction using external fixation. The surgeon must decide the apex of the deformity, level of the osteotomy, type of frame, and diameter of each ring. If the deformity is close to the ankle joint, a decision will need to be made about whether the foot will be incorporated into the frame for increased stability. Multilevel deformities will require even more complex technical considerations.

Let us turn our attention to a relatively simple example of growth arrest of the proximal tibia in an adolescent close to maturity (Fig. 9.2).

Before correction, one must decide the patient's projected LLD at maturity. An easy method of prediction is the use of the Multiplier method which is available for free as an iPad, iPhone, and Android applications [17–19]. Multiplier apps save time and can prove invaluable in pediatric orthopedics. Knowledge of the projected LLD is important for the surgeon to restore length and even perform pre-emptive lengthening to equalize limbs at maturity. The Multiplier method can also project height at maturity. For example, in patients with a projected height of <170 cm, surgeons will likely opt to perform gradual correction and lengthening, instead of correction with epiphysiodesis of the longer limb.

Partial GA should be addressed first. A partially open physis will lead to the recurrence of deformity. The options are to resect the bar or to complete the closure of the remaining intact physis (completion of epiphysiodesis). The are several ways to achieve complete epiphysiodesis; the authors recommend percutaneous drilling and curettage of the physis under fluoroscopy (Fig. 9.3a–b). From the authors' experience, this option is the simplest, cheapest, and most predictable. An alternative to drilling and curettage is to insert a staple or other implant on the convex side of the deformity, straddling the physis. To prevent the overgrowth of the proximal physis, closure of the proximal fibula (Fig. 9.3c) should be performed in patients with >2 years of remaining growth [20]. Proximal fibular closure can be achieved by either inserting a 5.5 mm longitudinal fully threaded cannulated screw from the top of the fibular, crossing the growth plate, or by simply curetting the physis.

Following proper physeal closure, the treatment can be planned, depending on the LLD and specific deformity. In most cases, deformity and shortening of the affected limb can be addressed by osteotomy, external fixator application, and gradual correction with lengthening (Fig. 9.2).

The tibia and fibula are typical sites for gradual correction of deformity. Common examples include tibia vara, post-traumatic malunions, and congenital leg deformities such as fibular and tibial hemimelia and congenital pseudarthrosis of the tibia.

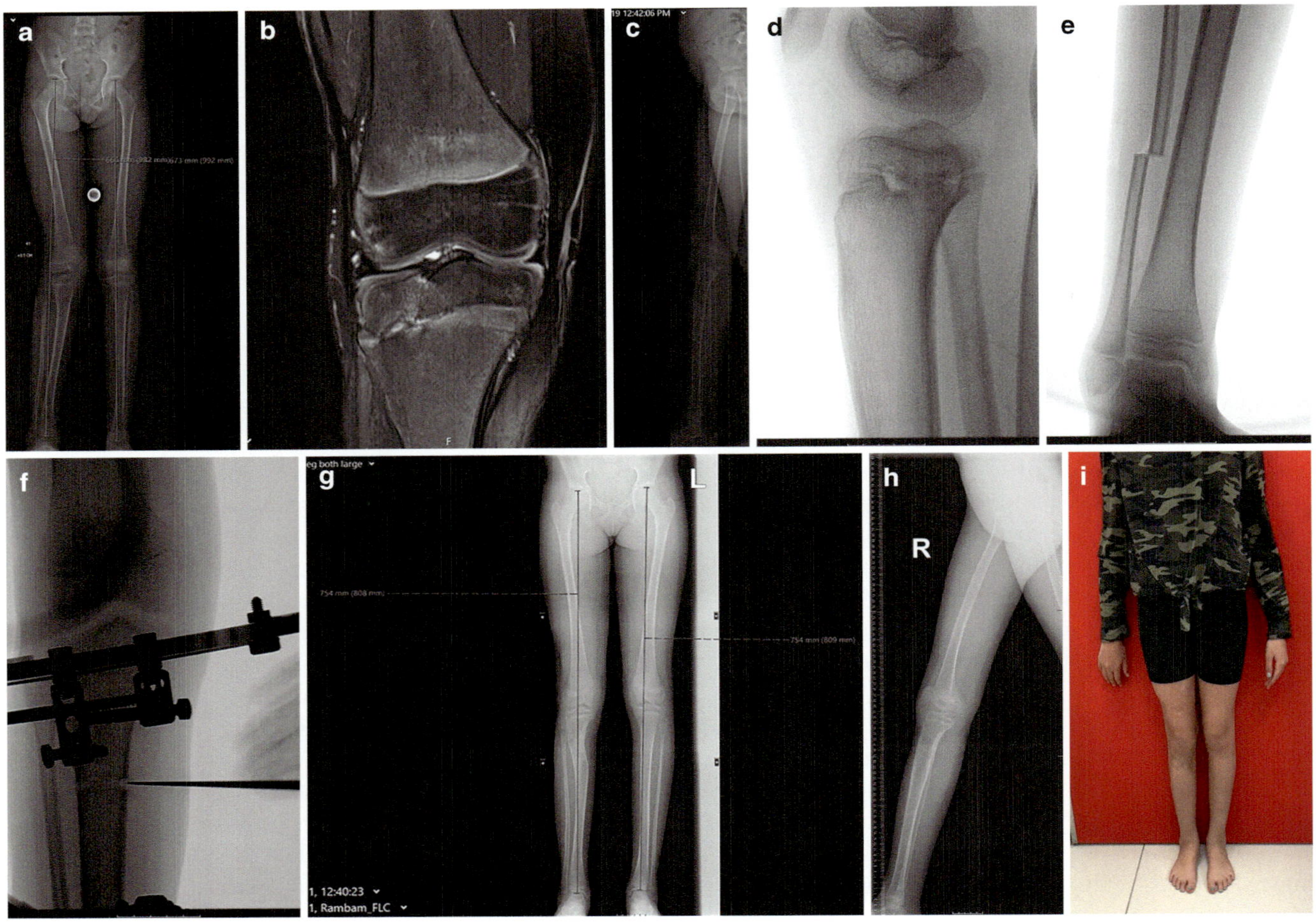

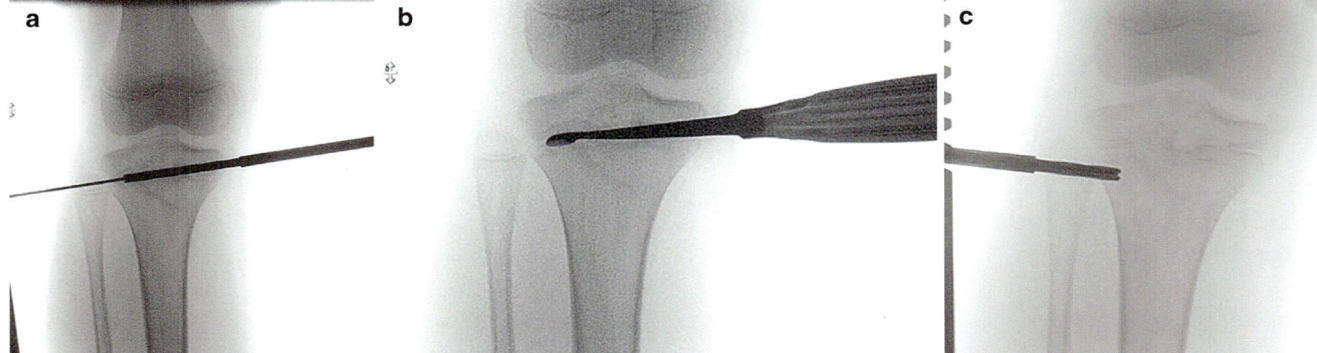

Fig. 9.2 (a-c) 10-year-old girl, 2 years after post-traumatic growth arrest of the right lateral proximal tibial physis with subsequent shortening, valgus and procurvarum, (d) percutaneous epiphysiodesis of the proximal tibia and fibula, (e) osteotomy of the fibula between distal and mid diaphysis, (f) percutaneous proximal tibial osteotomy just below the tibial tubercle, (g-h) x-rays 2 years after correction and contralateral proximal tibia epiphysiodesis, and i. clinical appearance 3 years after correction

Fig. 9.3 (a, b) Completion of the epiphysiodesis of the proximal tibia using cannulated technique and curettage and (c) percutaneous epiphysiodesis of the proximal tibia

The femur is another good location for gradual correction. GA after trauma or infection and congenital short femur are typical indications for correction. External fixation remains a valuable option for the femur, but there are also newer methods using internal lengthening nails which patients may find more comfortable, and which may be applicable down to school age children.

The upper limb is a less common site for gradual correction; acute correction is often all that a patient requires. Furthermore, LLDs in the arms—even when they are several centimeters—are not as crucial as in lower limbs where the asymmetry causes limping and issues with gait. Cubitus varus can be treated accurately with hexapods and yields predictable results. GA of the humerus with subsequent deformity and shortening can also be treated gradually. However, the forearm's narrow indication and complex anatomy restrict the wide use of external fixation, and most of its deformities are corrected acutely.

Gradual Correction of Femoral Deformities Using External Fixation

In recent years, external fixation for the gradual correction of femoral deformity is becoming a less attractive option to many surgeons as more internal lengthening devices become available. However, external fixation remains a practical and effective method of correction—and may be the only technique available in many scenarios.

The thigh's anatomy, as well as the motion of the knee and hip, should be taken into consideration before application of the frame. Knee flexion can be preserved by leaving the distal ring open posteriorly. The inner thigh portion of the fixator is left relatively unencumbered when a mid-thigh ring is applied laterally and with the open side medially (Fig. 9.4). In most femoral lengthenings, the surgeon should consider releasing the iliotibial band under sterile tourniquet before application of the frame (the iliotibial band restricts knee motion). This is best done distally, at the superior pole of the patella, to avoid muscle herniation. Prophylactic release of the peroneal nerve may be important when significant acute valgus correction with lengthening is planned (Fig. 9.5).

The femur's unique anatomy will dictate the pin and wire insertion. Wire placement through the thigh muscles can be problematic and restricting. Transmuscular penetration with

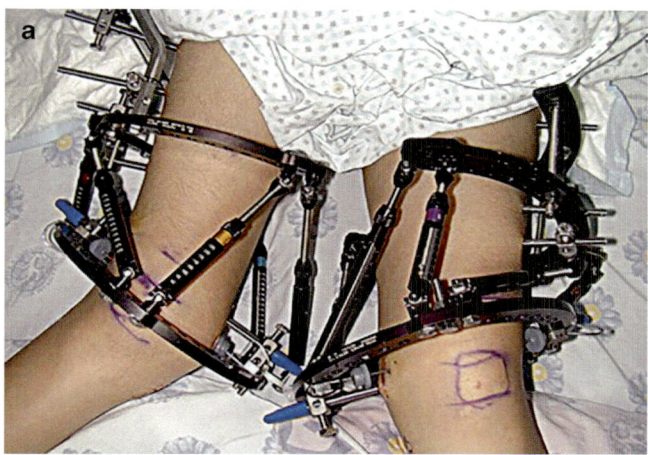
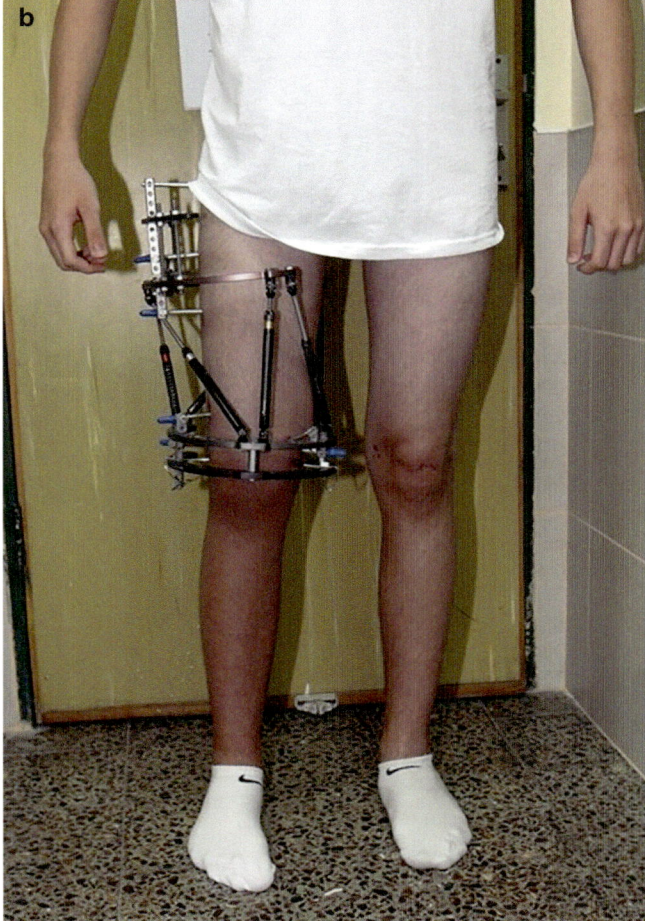

Fig. 9.4 (a, b) Application of a hexapod external fixation system on the femur

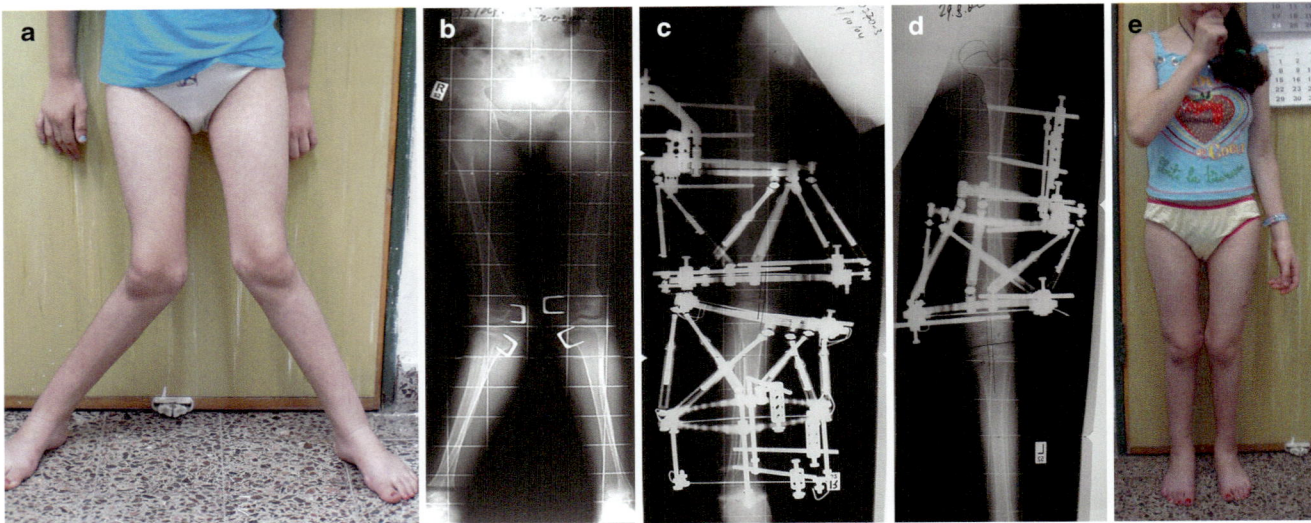

Fig. 9.5 (**a**) Severe bilateral genu valgum in a 14-year-old girl, (**b**) x-rays before gradual correction, (**c, d**) after correction and preventive peroneal nerve release, and (**e**) clinical picture after frame removal

a wire may lead to joint stiffness, infection, and loss of function [16]. Careful placement of each half-pin is crucially important to prevent complications during the correction process.

Another challenge is the creation of the stable distal block fixation. Usually, the apex of deformity is close to the knee joint, requiring a very distal femoral osteotomy to prevent significant translation. Posterolateral and posteromedial 6 mm half-pins ("Mercedes style") typically provide sufficient stability for fixation (Fig. 9.6).

Knee stability must be considered, particularly in children with congenital deformities. Spanning of the knee joint with hinges at the functional knee axis point should be performed in any case where knee stability is questionable (Fig. 9.7).

Finally, the osteotomy technique is a pivotal factor for success. The authors prefer to perform femoral osteotomy at any level percutaneously using multiple drills and the osteotome technique.

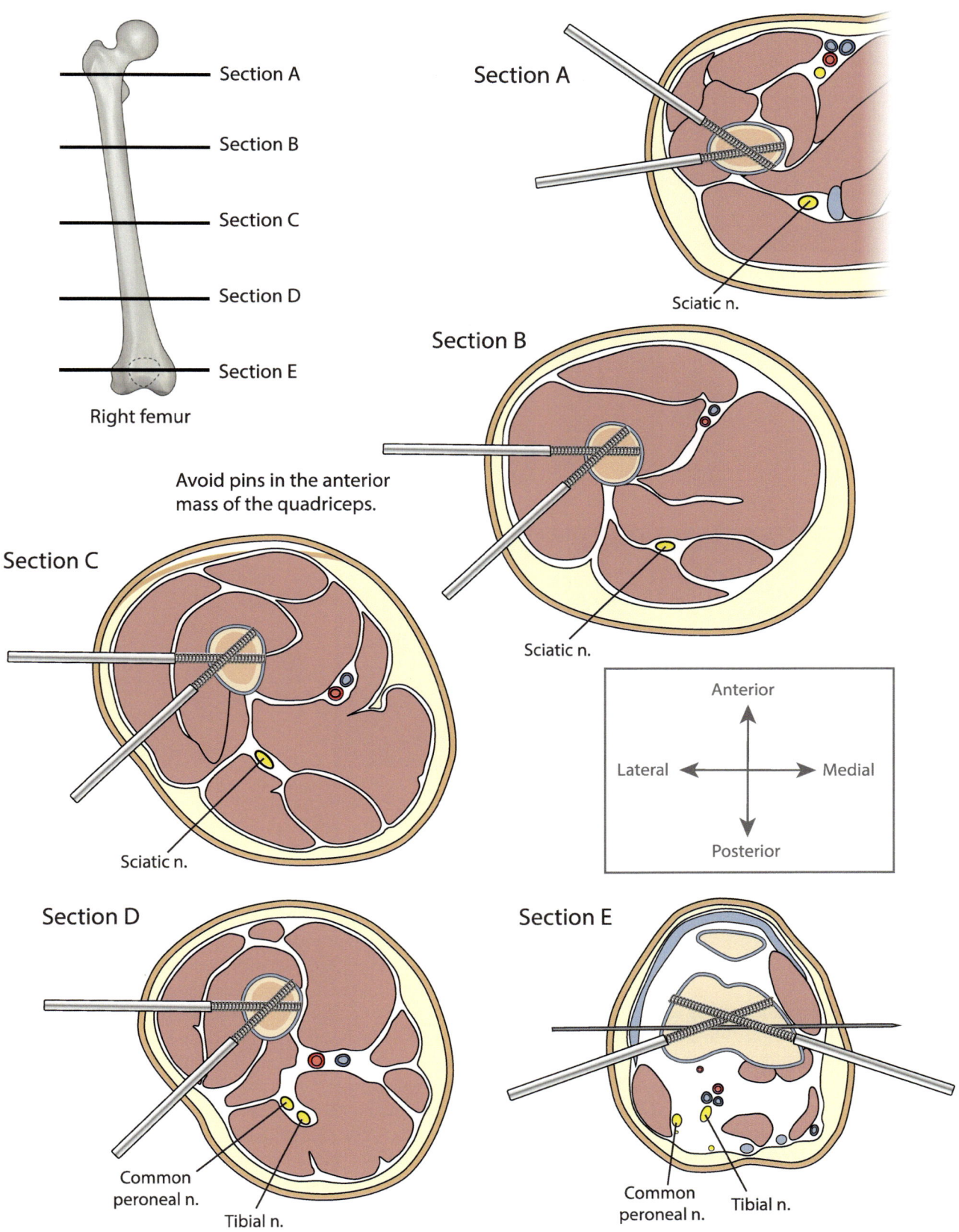

Fig. 9.6 External Fixation patterns for femur. Note the position of the 6 mm diameter pins at level E: posteromedial and posterolateral, avoiding the major muscle groups. The transverse wire at level E is typically placed as an initial reference wire for distal ring mounting, but removed at the end of the surgery, as it impedes the knee range of motion. In the more proximal levels, pin placement avoids transfixing the bulk of the quadriceps. (reproduced with permission, Rubin Institute for Advanced Orthopedics, Sinai Hospital of Baltimore)

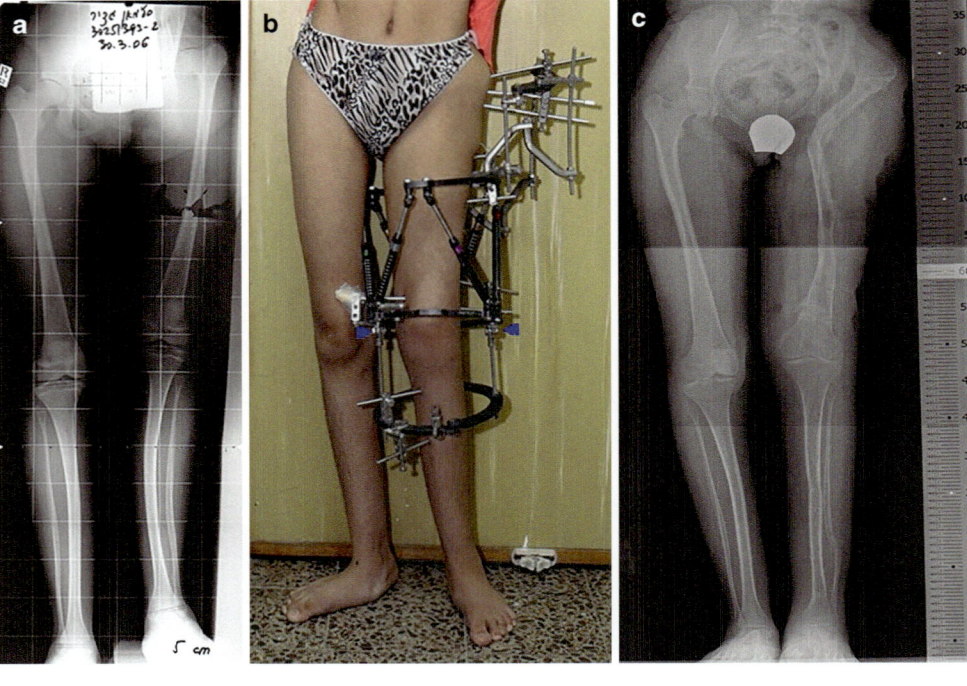

Fig. 9.7 (**a**) A 16-year-old girl with neglected hip dislocation and 11 cm leg length discrepancy. (**b**) clinical picture during correction and application of hinges (marked with blue arrows) to prevent knee instability. (**c**) x-rays after pelvic support osteotomy and gradual correction of femoral and double level tibial deformities with lengthening of 9 cm. Note that new mechanical axis goes through the sacroiliac joint to the ankle and cross the knee joint exactly in the middle

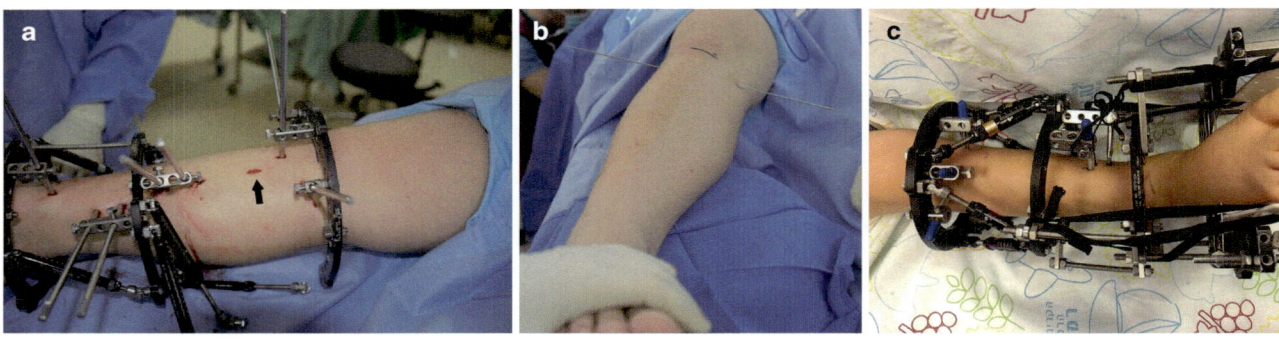

Fig. 9.8 (**a**) Incision for proximal tibial osteotomy (marked with a black arrow), (**b**) insertion of reference Ilizarov wire parallel to the joint, and (**c**) insertion of 3 half-pins above the tibial tubercle

Gradual Correction of Tibial Deformities Using External Fixation

Tibial Osteotomy

The osteotomy level and technique will vary for each specific case, yet some principles are universal. It is imperative to deal with periosteum delicately for successful callotasis and regenerate growth because most of blood supply for new bone formation comes from the periosteal vessels. The authors prefer to perform osteotomy through a percutaneous incision using multiple drill holes and osteotome with minimal periosteum rupture. The osteotomy incision width is slightly greater than the width of the 10 mm osteotome (Fig. 9.8a).

Proximal tibial osteotomy is common for deformities around the knee joint (e.g., tibia vara or any deformity that involves physis of the proximal tibia). The apex of the deformity is usually near the joint, however, an osteotomy above the tibial tubercle is technically difficult, allows little real estate for fixation, and therefore should be avoided. Typically, osteotomy is performed just below the level of the tibial tubercle. This site allows for correction of the deformity with minimal translation. Osteotomy at this level provides a relatively limited space for fixation in children with open physes. Space available for proximal fixation is from the level below the physis to the level of the osteotomy.

The authors prefer beginning with a wire parallel to the joint line (Fig. 9.8b). If space is limited, the ring should be attached above the wire. Even in smaller children there is often enough space to allow insertion of 3 half-pins (Fig. 9.8c). The first half-pin is inserted through the one-hole cube, and then the second half-pin through the two-hole cube. Finally, the third half-pin is inserted through the three-hole cube (or, if space is limited, by two-hole cube) with extension using a thick washer. Therefore, the proximal block of fixation consists of 3 half-pins and one Ilizarov wire. This wire may cause pain, infection, irritation to soft tissue surrounding the knee joint, and restrict knee motion. If any of these occur and the wire is removed in clinic, the 3 half-pins provide sufficient stability. Additionally, the authors assert the importance of frequent pauses during drilling to prevent heating the bone at the osteotomy site and during insertion of half-pins. Infection is a rare occurrence when half-pins are inserted properly.

Osteotomy Technique

A small (maximum 15 mm) longitudinal periosteal incision is made just below the tibial tubercle. Pediatric periosteal elevators are used gently to elevate the periosteum on the lateral side, and to a lesser extent medially, to create space for drilling of the bone. Several holes are then created in the bone using a solid 4.8- or 3.8-mm drill through a drill sleeve. After several (3–6) pathways being created, the authors recommend fluoroscopy to determine where drilling was not performed (Fig. 9.9). Next, the osteotomy is completed with use of an osteotome.

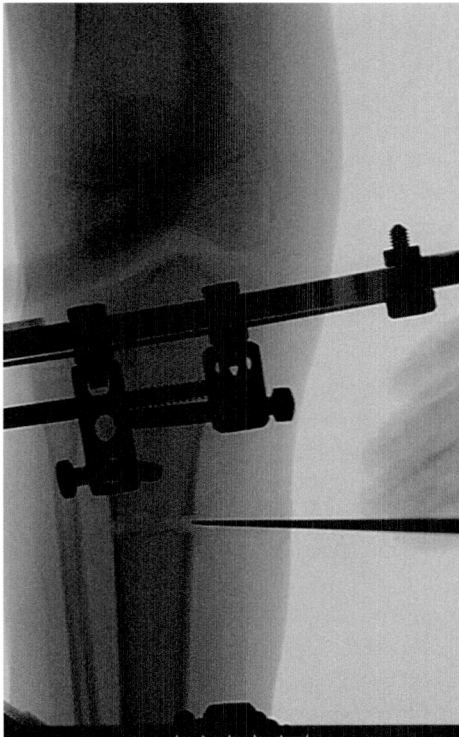

Fig. 9.9 Fluoroscopy shows that drilling is done properly, and osteotomy is safely performed

Another useful osteotomy method is by means of a Gigli saw [21–23]. Gigli saw osteotomy is always complete, and complications are minimal when done properly. It is similar to the drill and osteotome technique for immature patients with wide periosteum bone formation. The Gigli saw always makes a complete cut, with no comminution, so half-pins can be inserted within a few mm above the osteotomy site. The disadvantages of the Gigli saw technique are a longer learning curve, technical difficulties, and, in some cases, delayed union. It is relatively contraindicated for use in diaphyseal bone, as the Gigli may cause thermal necrosis around the osteotomy with subsequent delayed union or even nonunion. Therefore, Gigli saw use is primarily restricted to metaphyseal bone. Common indications for Gigli saw osteotomies are proximal tibial osteotomy, supramalleolar osteotomy, and osteotomy through the tarsal bones of the foot [23].

Deformities surrounding the ankle joint are usually corrected acutely. However, in instances when length is important, an effective solution may be supramalleolar osteotomy and circular external fixator application for simultaneous deformity correction and lengthening [22].

Supramalleolar osteotomy can be performed via separate incisions for the distal tibia and fibula using drill and osteotome. The authors contend that supramalleolar osteotomy by using the Gigli saw is a superior option. Because supramalleolar osteotomy occurs in the metaphyseal area, healing of the regenerate is excellent, provided the osteotomy is made within 1.5–2.0 cm from the joint. Additional advantages are completeness of the osteotomy, lack of comminution (makes translation easier), pin and wire application very close to the level of osteotomy, and easier correction of rotational osteotomy when done at this level. Disadvantages are the necessary learning curve and potential damage to structures around the osteotomy if it is performed incorrectly. Several structures are at risk. Anteriorly, there are the tibialis anterior tendon and anterior neurovascular bundle. Laterally are the peroneal tendons. Medially are the tibialis posterior tendon and posterior neurovascular bundle.

This osteotomy is completely subperiosteal and performed approximately 20–25 mm above the ankle joint. At this level, there is no space between tibia and fibula, so the bones are osteotomized simultaneously. Success and safety of this osteotomy are dependent on the precise execution of several steps. First, a small anteromedial transverse incision is performed just medial to the tibialis anterior tendon. Next, the periosteum is elevated with pediatric elevators all the way to the fibula on the lateral aspect of the ankle. Second, a lateral fibular longitudinal skin cut is made over the tip of the periosteal elevator. This incision is approximately 15 mm. Using a hemostat, a stout suture is passed subperiosteally to the medial aspect of the ankle for later attachment of the Gigli saw. The periosteum is elevated circumferentially all the way around the ankle joint. Next, a third incision is made posteromedial, and must be done just anterior to the tibialis posterior tendon that passes over the posterior slope of the distal tibia. Probe the slope with wire to find the correct point of the incision, a transverse posteromedial incision made just anterior to the wire. Last, pass the saw attached to the suture around the ankle. Before osteotomy, ensure that peroneal tendons are not entrapped within the saw (Fig. 9.10).

A tip for this procedure is that it is more convenient to activate the Gigli saw to make an osteotomy three-fourth of the way from lateral to medial, apply the external fixator, and then complete the osteotomy so that the fixator keeps the tibia stable. Another advantage of this osteotomy is that only two antero-medial struts need to be removed, contrary to the standard technique that requires removing every strut to ensure completion of the osteotomy.

Gradual Correction of Foot Deformities

Most children who need gradual correction of foot deformities are clubfoot and clubfoot-like cases (e.g., forefoot adduction, cavus, and rotational deformities) and nearly all have equinus. The conservative Ponseti method of clubfoot treatment involving a heelcord tenotomy has dramatically decreased the need for extensive surgical procedures for children with clubfoot deformities. However, relapsed and recurrent clubfeet are still common, especially in cases of noncompliance with braces and deviation from Ponseti's principles of treatment.

Relapses are defined as recurrent deformities in previously well-corrected feet, and residual deformities are persistent deformities of incompletely corrected feet. Many relapses might be treated conservatively with Ponseti principles, but some will need operative correction [24]. The majority of relapses in children aged <2.5 years (early relapse group) can be treated by using the casting technique. Older children aged between 2.5 and 8 years (late relapse group) might benefit from casting followed by tibialis anterior transfer and a second tenotomy of the Achilles tendon or gastrocsoleus recession (majority of relapses have equinus). The goal of treatment in this age is to obtain proper correction using casting and then maintain correction with the tendon transfer [24]. The authors prefer to avoid extensive traditional soft tissue release because of problems related to deep scarring, muscle weakness, and subsequent permanent foot stiffness.

Ilizarov principles of correcting foot deformities in children are based on soft tissue distraction in children aged <8 years and osteotomies (hindfoot/tarsal/supramalleolar) in older children [24–27]. While any correction is possible with the classic circular Ilizarov frame for soft tissue distraction, the authors prefer to use a computer-guided hexapod frame.

The "Ponse-Taylor"method of correction for clubfeet is so named in dual homage to Drs. Ponseti (sequential method of clubfoot correction) and Taylor (hexapod fixator).

The Ponse-Taylor method is a specific soft tissue distraction method that attempts to present the Ponseti principle sequence in two stages. The first stage includes correction of the internal tibial torsion and hindfoot varus. A talar neck olive wire is inserted laterally, bent outside the skin, and attached as a stirrup wire to the proximal ring. Some lengthening through the subtalar joint must be programmed to allow derotation and varus correction through it. The second stage is the equivalent of a Ponseti tenotomy to gain foot dorsiflexion. This procedure is typically done in the operating room. The talar neck wire should be disconnected from the proximal tibial ring, straightened, and attached to the foot ring, so the talus can dorsiflex with the entire foot [24, 26]. Overcorrection is advised, due to the tendency of recurrence of equinus (Fig. 9.11).

Gradual Correction of Upper Limb Deformities

Gradually correcting deformities of the upper extremities is not a common practice. Because length is less important of a factor than in lower limbs, most deformities of the arm can be successfully treated with acute correction. However, several conditions might be treated using gradual correction methods, particularly elbow deformities: cubitus varus and cubitus valgus.

Cubitus varus is often a complex three-dimensional deformity including not only coronal but also sagittal and rotational plane deformities. Failure to recognize the complexity of deformity in the past had led to a relatively high complication rate after acute correction [16, 28]. Herzenberg introduced a method of insertion half-pins in the distal humerus to avoid the disturbance of the open growth plate in children and minimize injury to the radial nerve [16] (Fig. 9.12c-d).

The method begins with the insertion of an Ilizarov wire in the distal humerus under fluoroscopic control. When the wire is verified on both views to be in the correct position, a cannulated drill is inserted over the wire. The authors use 4.5 mm half-pins on young children and 6 mm half-pins on adolescents. The pins attach to the 2/3 ring open anteriorly for free elbow movements, with an additional 2 half-pins inserted into the humerus above the deltoid tuberosity and attached to the 2/3 ring, open medially. After completion of fixation and spreading the struts, percutaneous osteotomy is performed just above the upper half-pin placed distally (Fig. 9.12).

Gradual correction of humeral deformities typically begins with a daily distraction of 0.75 mm starting post-op day seven, with passive and active elbow motions as soon as possible (can start post-op day one). Children tend to tolerate

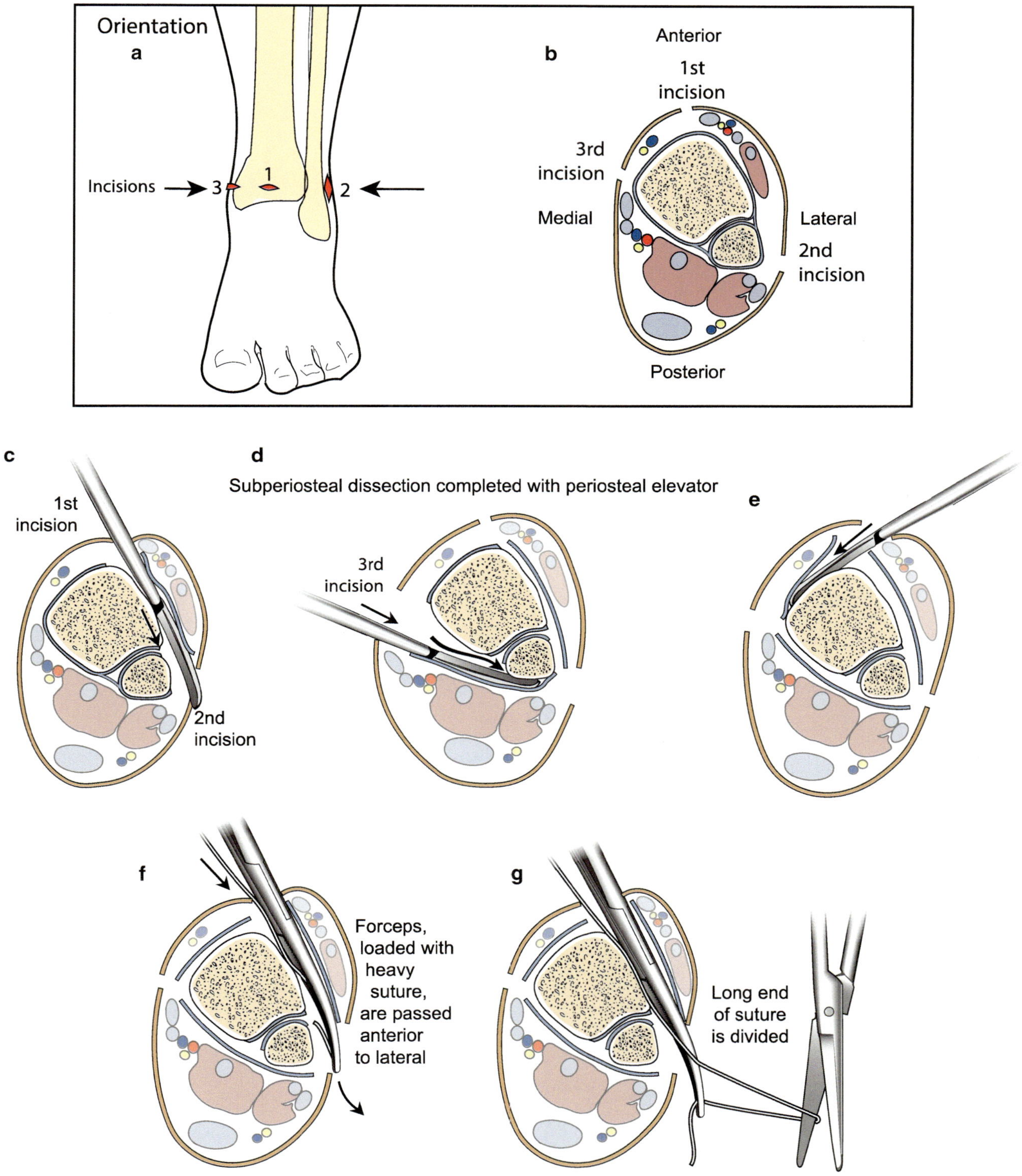

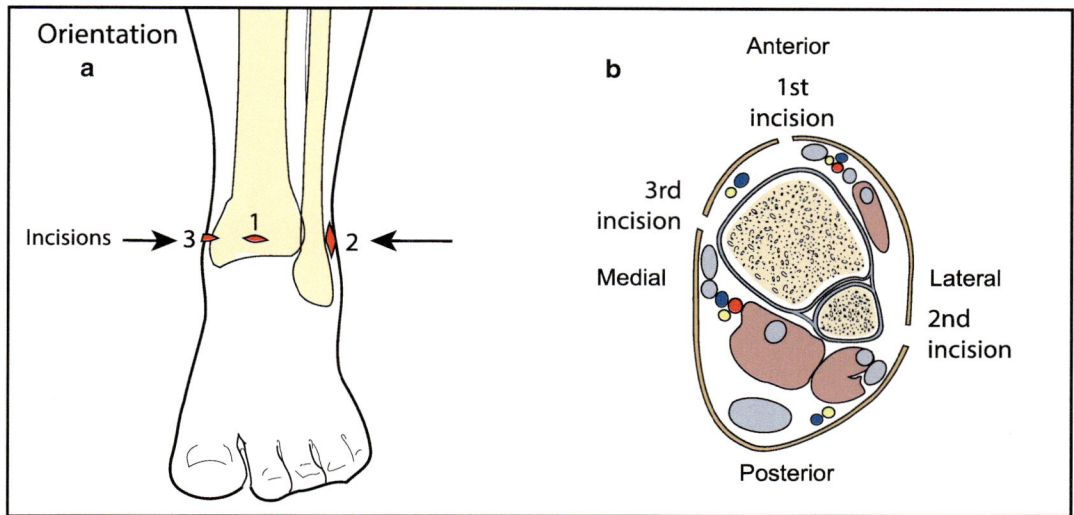

Fig. 9.10 Percutaneous supramalleolar Gigli saw osteotomy—step by step. (**a**) three incisions, (**b**) cross-sectional view, (**c**) elevation of anterior periosteum, (**d**) elevation of posterior periosteum, (**e**) elevation of medial periosteum, (**f**) suture passage anteriorly, (**g**) suture divided, (**h**) forceps withdrawn, (**i**) Gigli tied to suture, (**j**) Gigli passed medial to lateral, (**k**) forceps with suture passed posteriorly, (**l**) suture divided, (**m**) forceps withdrawn, (**n**) suture tied to Gigli, (**o**) Gigli pulled back inside posteriorly from lateral to medial, (**p**) Gigli activated, hugging the bone, (**q**) before exiting medially, elevator inserted to protect medial periosteum, (**r**) osteotomy completed, and (**s**) Gigli cut and extracted. (reproduced with permission, Rubin Institute for Advanced Orthopedics, Sinai Hospital of Baltimore)

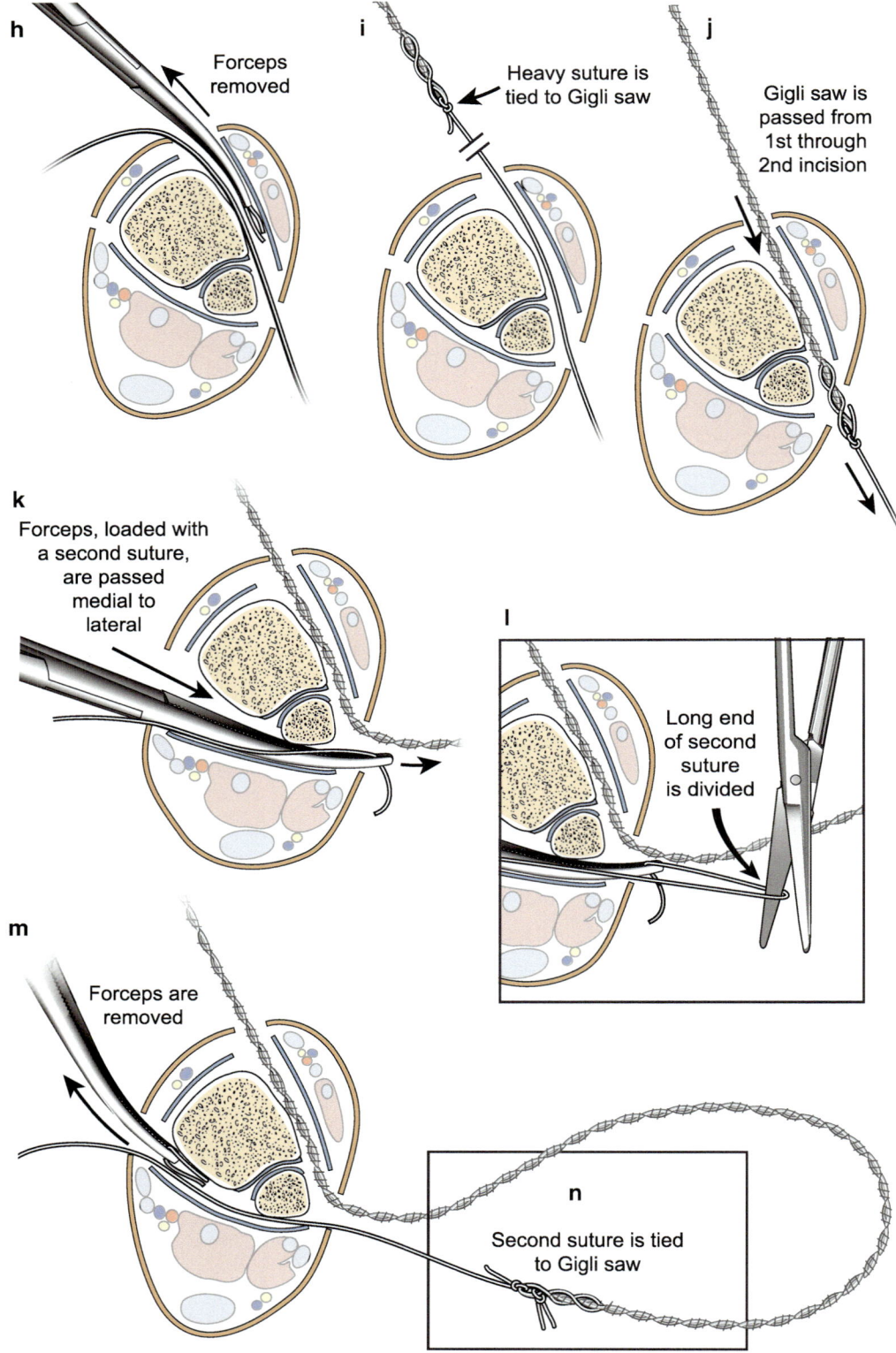

Fig. 9.10 (continued)

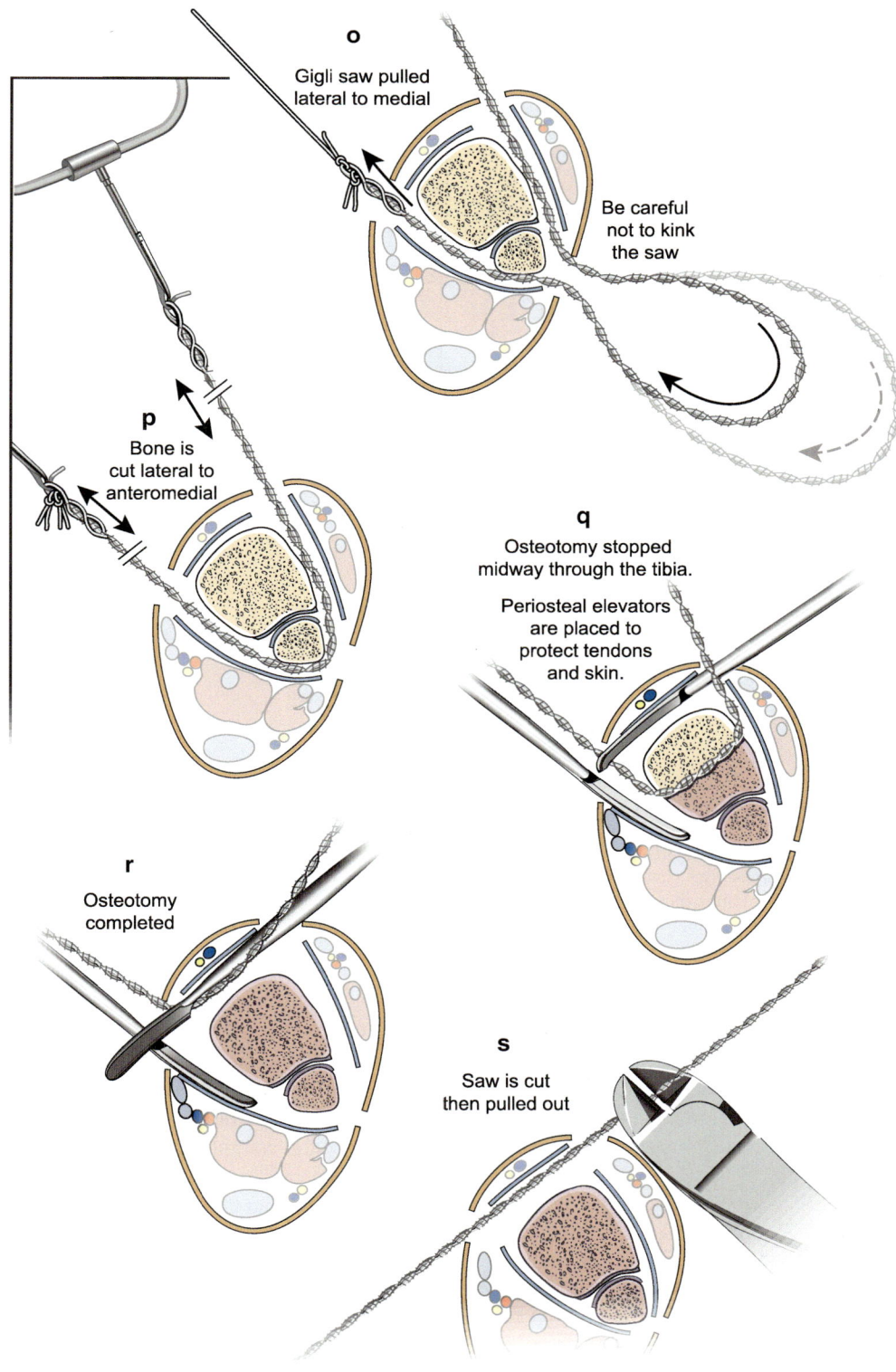

Fig. 9.10 (continued)

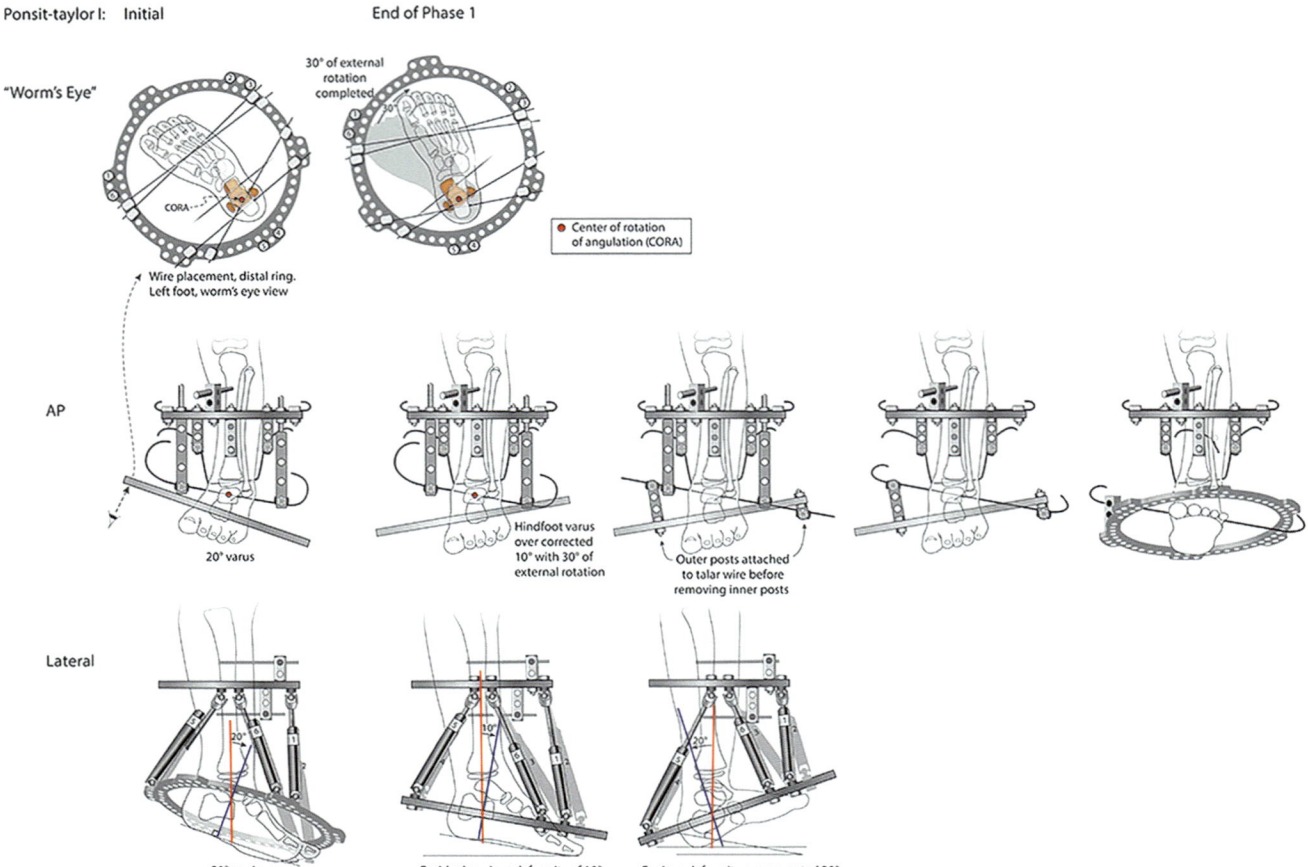

Fig. 9.11 Ponse–Taylor sequence for clubfoot correction. The initial program is for external rotation (30 degrees) of the foot through the subtalar joint, shown in the worm's eye views of the distal ring. Overcorrection is intentional, due to some expected rebound after frame removal. The AP views show the initial program also correcting varus and distracting the subtalar joint. Also depicted the transfer of the talar neck wire from the tibia ring to the foot ring, done at the end of the initial sequence. The lateral views show the correction in the second stage, from equinus to dorsiflexion. Overcorrection is recommended due to expected rebound after frame removal. (reproduced with permission, Rubin Institute for Advanced Orthopedics, Sinai Hospital of Baltimore)

the simple frame well and achieve a full range of elbow motions without problems. Mature regenerate usually becomes visible at the end of second month after correction. It is suggested to dynamize the frame one week before removal using partial strut removal to see the consolidation more clearly.

Acute Correction of Deformities Using Internal Lengthening Nail

Recently, internal lengthening has become part of a popular practice within deformity surgery, particularly in the West [29–31]. Unlike external fixation, there is no chronic pin/wire transfixion of soft tissue with internal lengthening. Hence, patients tend to regain motion quicker, with less pain and fewer instances of infection. Insertion of the nail is a relatively simple procedure technically; most surgeons can perform the correction after a short learning curve. However, there are also some disadvantages, particularly that full weight bearing cannot commence until at least substantial regenerate consolidation. The short lived Stryde™ Biodur nail allowed full weight bearing but turned out to be plagued with corrosion at the male female junction, creating osteolysis, which prompted its withdrawal from the market [32, 33]. Gradual correction in patients who previously underwent external fixation may have an increased risk of deep tract infections, and the high cost of nails (nonreusable as opposed to external fixators) restricts their use worldwide.

Perhaps acute correction using internal lengthening nails is the best example of the combined method of correction (Fig. 9.13). Femoral nails can be inserted antegrade or retrograde. Normal open physis of the distal femur restricts the use of retrograde nails, but it could be the preferred option for patients with a closed distal femoral or proximal tibial physis and with an apex of deformity close to the

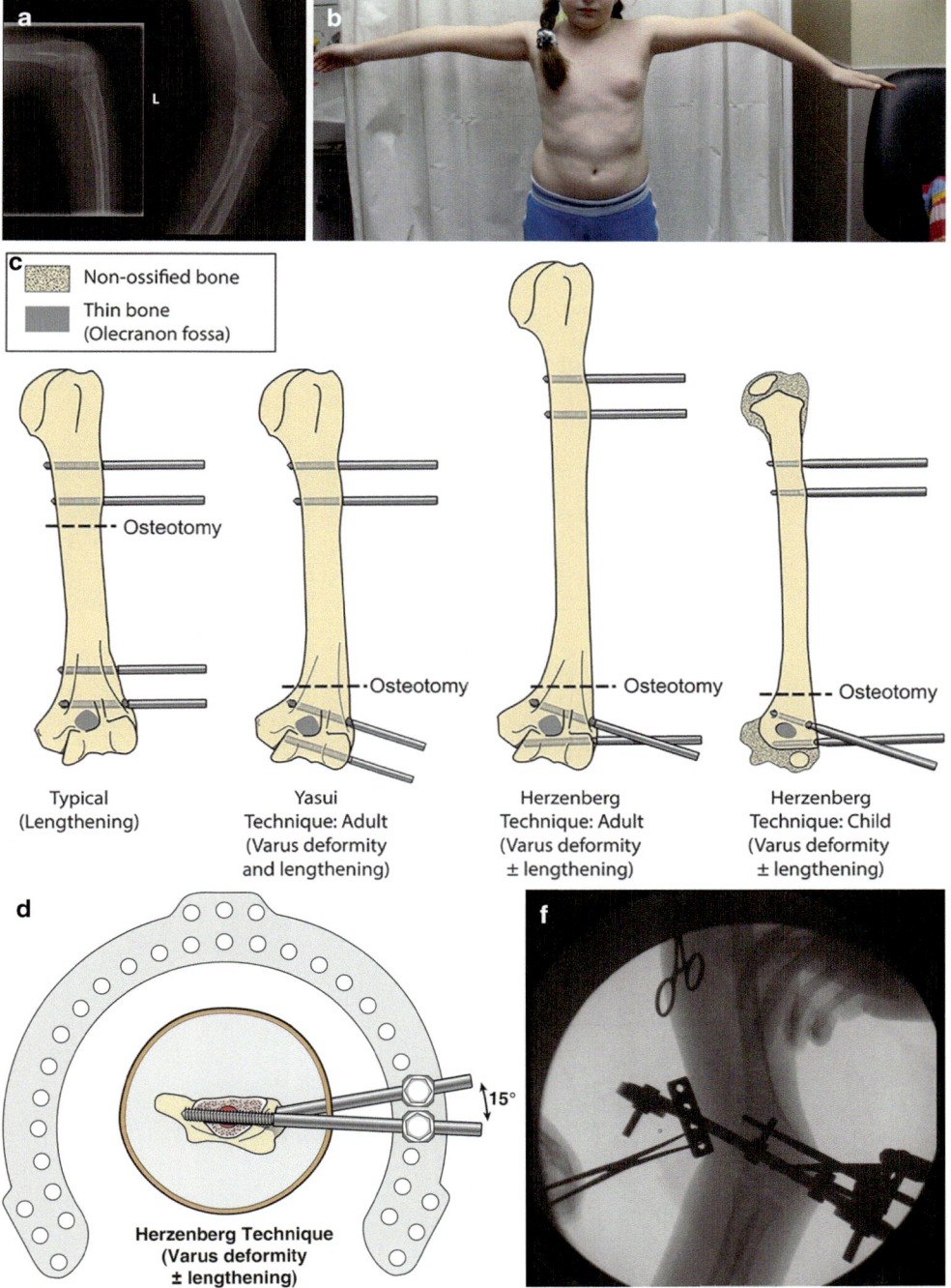

Fig. 9.12 (**a**) A 7 year-old girl with severe left distal humeral varus deformity after supracondylar fracture (40 degrees of varus, 30 degrees of flexion contracture, and 10 degrees of internal rotation), (**b**) clinical photo demonstrating "gun stock" deformity, and (**c**, **d**) the Herzenberg method of half-pin placement allowed fixation of the distal humerus without risk of growth plate penetration. Shown here in comparison with other options. The cross-sectional diagram shows the delta con- figuration of the two pins, giving added stability. Reproduced with permission, Rubin Institute for Advanced Orthopedics, Sinai Hospital of Baltimore. (**e**) Cannulated technique of half-pin placement, (**f**, **g**) x-rays and clinical picture of half-pin insertion, (**h**, **i**) x-rays after correction, (**j**, **k**) clinical picture before hexapod removal, and l. clinical photo 10 years after correction

knee joint. Fixator-assisted acute correction of distal femoral deformity and insertion of retrograde nails with blocking screws to ensure proper nail position, with acute deformity correction and subsequent bone lengthening, is an excellent choice for combined acute deformity and gradual length correction. Antegrade nailing might be through

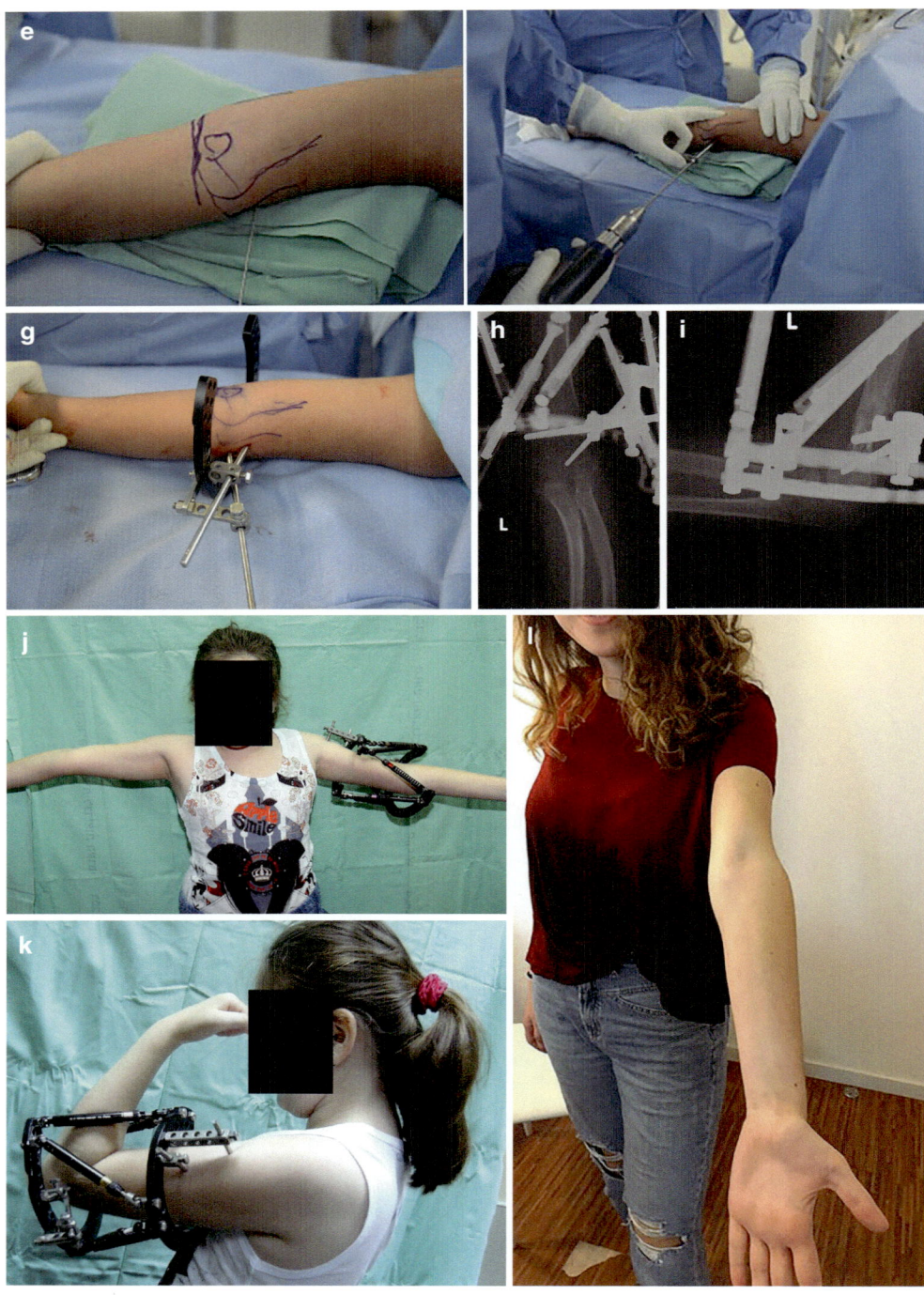

Fig. 9.12 (continued)

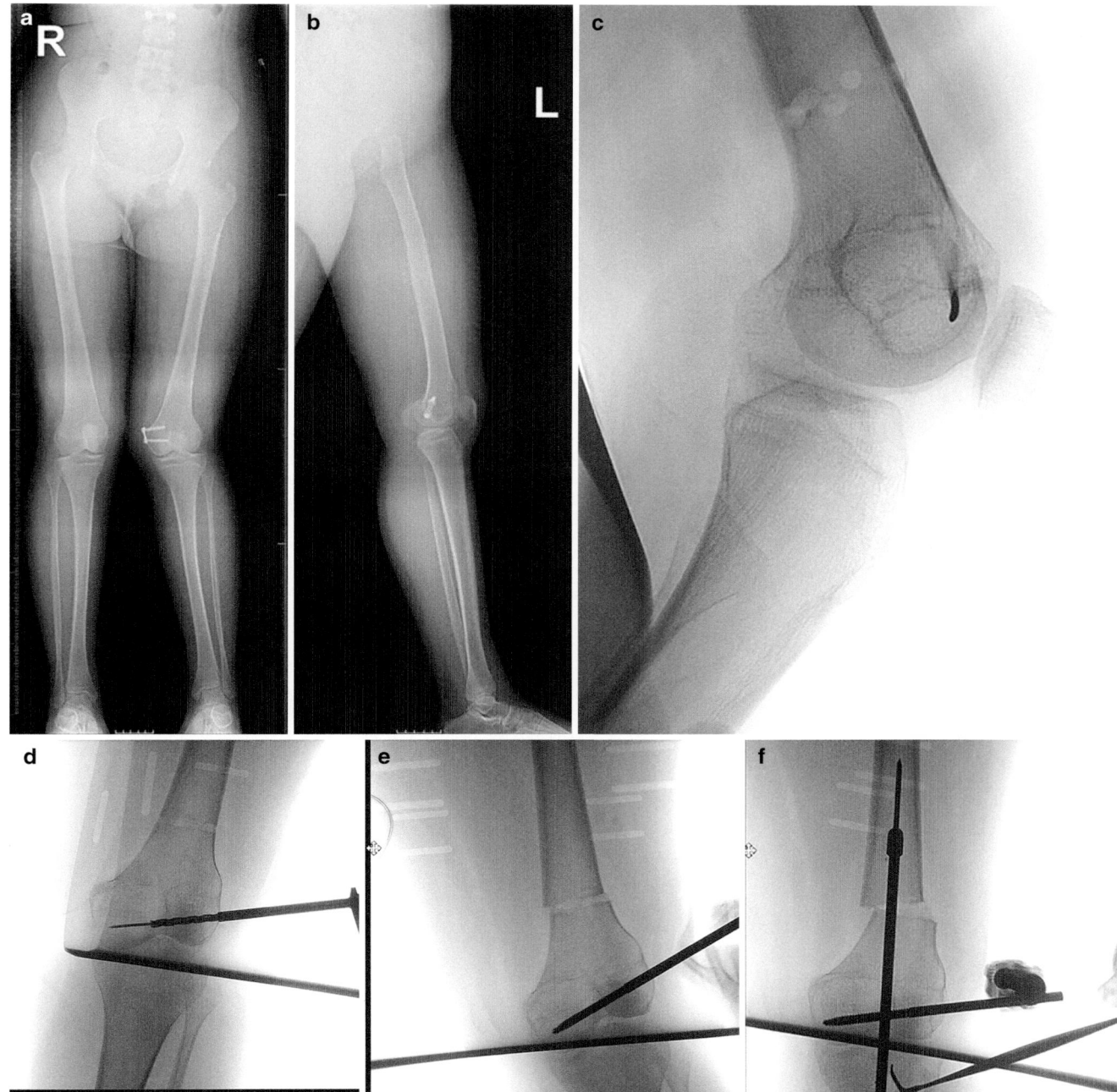

Fig. 9.13 (**a, b**) x-rays of 14 years-old girl with valgus deformity of left distal femur and 4 cm shortening, (**c, d**) after predrilling of the osteotomy, wire was inserted anteriorly and parallel to the knee joint, (**e**) osteotomy performed near the apex of femoral deformity, (**f**) acute correction of valgus using an external fixator and retrograde reaming of the distal femur before nail insertion, (**g**) insertion of retrograde femoral nail (note that bowie cord transects knee joint slightly medial), (**h**) insertion of blocking screws to prevent loss of correction, (**i, j**) x-rays after correction, and (**k, l**) standing X-rays 1 year after correction

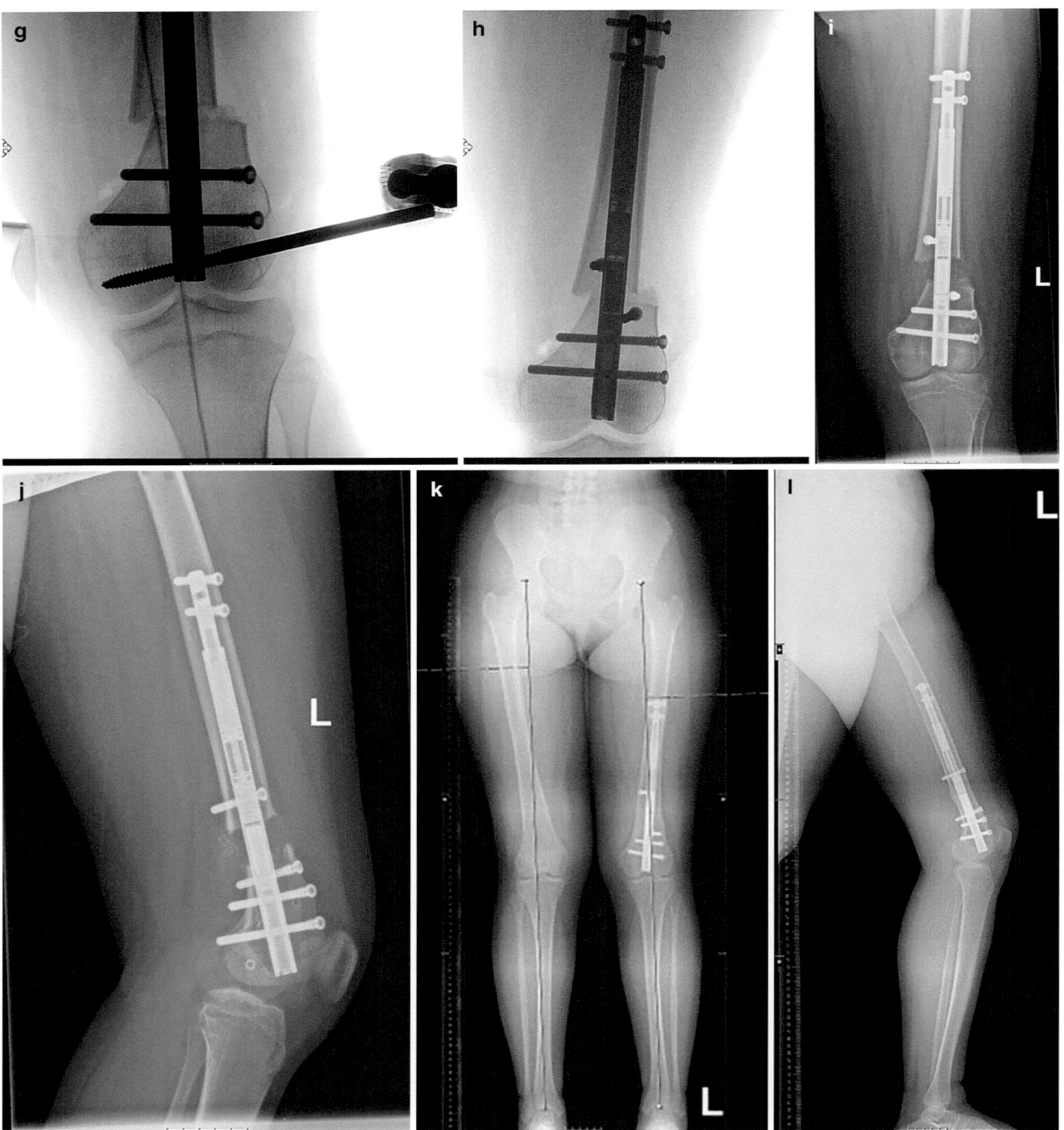

Fig. 9.13 (continued)

piriformis fossa in skeletally mature patients with closed physes or trochanteric entry in immature patients with open physes. Insertion of a trochanteric nail may cause mid proximal femoral varus, therefore in patients with valgus deformities it could potentially improve the limb's mechanical axis. For patients with closed physis, a straight nail through piriformis fossa is the preferred option because this entry does not acutely change limb alignment. Lengthening along the anatomic axis may, however, induce some valgus mechanical axis deviation.

Internal lengthening using a tibial nail is another powerful alternative to external fixation (Fig. 9.14). This is less commonly used in children, as the growth plate is typically open, except in cases of premature GA. Options for nail insertion include infrapatellar or suprapatellar approaches. The infrapatellar approach assumes that the knee is capable of full flexion. Both methods may result in long-term anterior knee pain that might not resolve with hardware removal. Given these problems, it seems much easier and safer to apply external fixation to the tibia.

The past decade has brought a shift from external fixation for lengthening and deformity correction toward more use of acute deformity correction with internal fixation and internal lengthening nails for LLD. Despite this change, there will be, at least for the foreseeable future, an important role for external fixation, underscoring the importance of mastering the techniques described in this chapter.

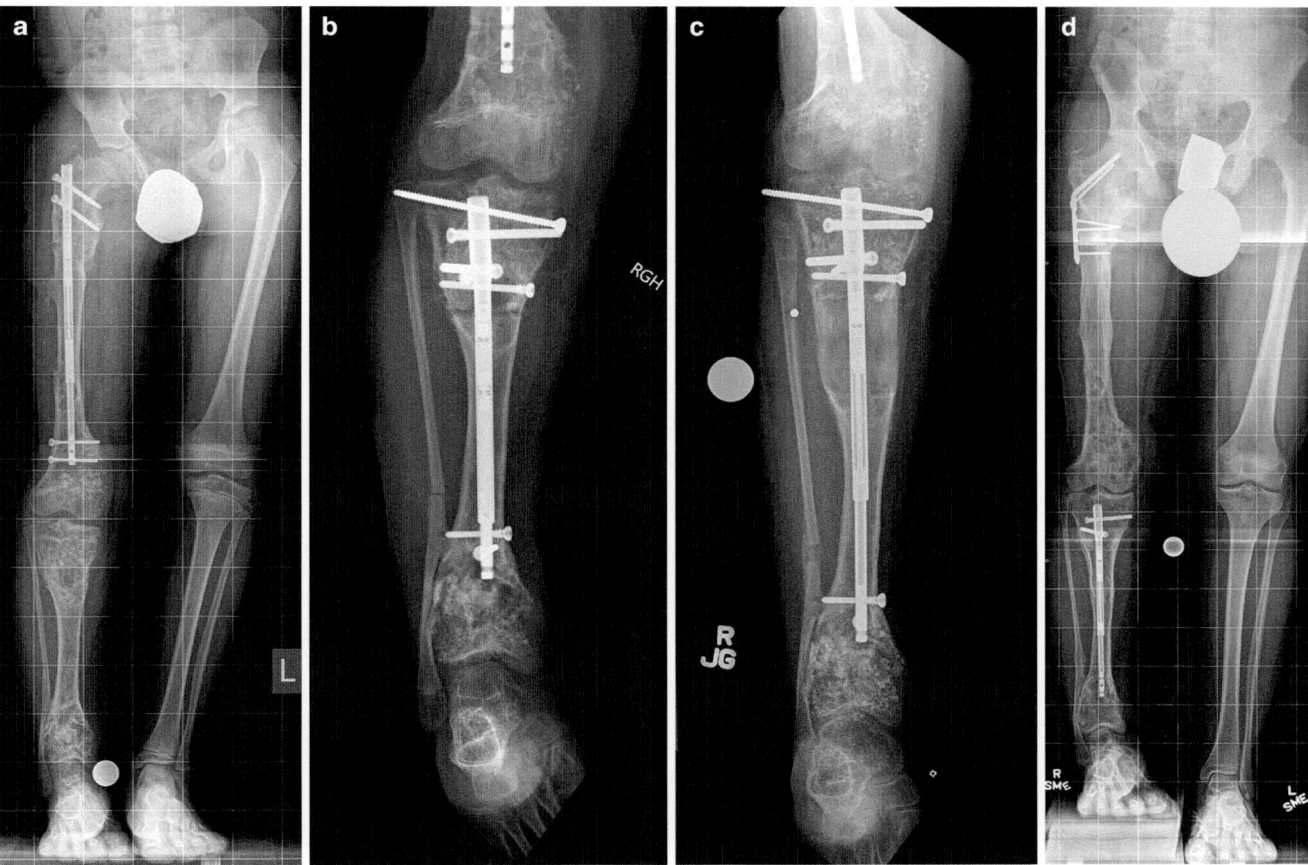

Fig. 9.14 PRECICE tibial nail lengthening in a 10-year-old boy with Ollier disease. The proximal tibial growth plate is functionally closed due to the massive involvement of the enchondromatosis (reproduced with permission, Rubin Institute for Advanced Orthopedics, Sinai Hospital of Baltimore). (**a**) Preop erect legs film shows the destruction of the growth plates at the right knee and ankle. The patient had a prior PRECICE nail lengthening of the right femur. (**b**) Immediate post-op film shows the PRECICE nail in place with the corticotomy through the wide, meta-diaphyseal segment. Note the blocking screws to prevent malalignment. (**c**) Three months post op, there is 5 cm wide, healthy regenerate bone, consolidating appropriately. Note that there was premature consolidation of the distal fibular osteotomy. This led to descent of the proximal fibula, despite it being initially transfixed with a cortical bone screw in the head of the fibula. (**d**) Five years post op. In the interval, the femur was re-lengthened with another PRECICE nail, and the coxa vara was corrected with a cannulated blade plate. The distal locking screws were removed for dynamization purposes. Despite the varus inclination of the ankle joint, the foot is plantigrade, so no correction of the increased LDTA is indicated

Commentary

Franz Birkholtz
fbirkholtz@ior.health

This well written chapter on Gradual Deformity Correction in Children and Adolescents by prominent authors in the field needs very little commentary or addition. Nevertheless, it may be worthwhile to share a few ideas on the topic from the perspective of a surgeon practicing in the "developing world", henceforth referred as "low and middle-income countries". The dichotomy of dealing with advanced, often neglected pathologies on the one hand and being situated in a resource constrained environment on the other, leads to some interesting challenges when employing gradual correction strategies.

It is not unusual to have patients present very late with untreated and advanced pathologies. The reason for this ranges from cultural perceptions of disease, religious considerations and indeed access (or the lack thereof) to appropriate healthcare. Untreated clubfoot or Blount's deformities that present at a later age are a common sight in the clinics in the region.

Limited resources in terms of the patient or family means that patients travel long distances to hospitals and cannot necessarily follow up regularly, if at all. Access to clean running water, electricity and proper nutrition remain problems for a significant section of this patient population. Limited resources in the healthcare system means an overloaded system with a low specialist-to-patient ratio and simply not enough time to have the luxury of multiple trips to the operating room. External fixators are often removed in the clinic, even in younger patients. The re-use of external fixation components is near-standard practice. Because of the limited ability to get people for multiple complex surgical procedures at different times, I have coined the term "Simple Single Surgery", as this is often the only shot that these patients have at improvement. Treatment goals are pragmatically also chunked down to more basic goals like simple axis deviation correction or limb equalization instead of complex multi-level staged corrections.

Gradual Correction as described in this chapter does not include guided growth (which is covered in Chap. 6). In this context it is then an iteration of the purest form of limb reconstruction: distraction osteogenesis after the creation of a very special type of osteotomy. Gradual correction strategies can then serve to restore length, alignment or compensate for future length or alignment issues that may still develop as a result of the growing skeleton. The Ilizarov Method was born in an environment very much like that of low and middle-income countries today: relatively complex pathologies attached to patients with limited resources and significant logistic challenges. The extreme modularity of the Ilizarov external fixation system, coupled to the relatively simple operation of a 'nut-driven-correction-machine' make it a tried and tested method to manage complex pathologies in these circumstances. Although the learning curve is steep, the volume and nature of the pathologies mean that a dedicated surgeons practicing in low and middle-income countries can climb the curve in a relatively short time.

Of course, the hexapod fixators have revolutionized the way that we move rings in relation to each other, giving us some very elegant ways to correct very complex three-dimensional deformities with reasonably simple frames. They are however dependent on software and, in the vast majority of cases needs a stable internet connection. Additionally, a basic level of patient literacy is needed to understand and read the prescription used to adjust the struts. Nonetheless, the hexapod fixators have become workhorses in multiplanar deformities like Blount's Disease, and have been adapted with some modifications by surgeons practicing in low and middle-income countries.

Monolateral rail fixators offer a relatively (often)cheap, simple and robust alternative for longitudinal gradual corrections like lengthenings and segmental bone transport. Although, often being replaced in favor of its circular cousins, monolateral rail fixators still are workhorses in limb reconstruction in the low and middle-income countries.

To deploy gradual deformity corrections efficiently and accurately, meticulous and systematic deformity analysis is necessary. This includes the current deformity as well as the projected future deformity. Of course, this is contingent on radiographic views that reproduce the patient's patho-anatomy accurately. Unfortunately, this remains a weak point in a lot of hospitals around the world. The limb reconstruction surgeon who spends extra time in the radiology suite to ensure an improvement in the quality of the x-rays taken in their hospital, will certainly reap the benefits in improved patient outcomes.

Femoral gradual correction with external fixation is problematic in terms of the transfixing of soft tissues as well as the discomfort related to prolonged external fixation. Although internal lengthening nails have become a gold standard in many instances around the world, their high price tag and limited availability in some countries still limit their use somewhat. Other concerns regarding open growth plates, bone length and canal diameter may limit the use of an internal lengthening nail.

The move to try and shorten (and even eliminate) time spent in a femoral external fixator has led to the development of a number of interesting techniques where external and internal fixation are combined to provide gradual correction. Typically, an acute deformity correction would be performed, followed by gradual lengthening and then finally internal fixation to allow for consolidation without an external fixator. Examples of these techniques are: Lengthening Over a Nail (LON); Lengthening Over a Plate (LOP); Lengthening And Then Nailing (LATN); Lengthening And then Plating (LATP).

'The quality of your osteotomy determines your quality as a limb reconstruction surgeon'. This is my favorite lesson to teach when someone embarks on the journey to become a limb reconstruction surgeon. Performing a low energy, biologically sound, complete osteotomy without destabilizing the fixation elements will determine the quality and speed of the lengthening regenerate, the frame time and ultimately the complication rate. A well-executed predrilled osteotomy (corticotomy) remains the technique of choice in the majority of cases.

Gigli saw osteotomies, especially in the foot, benefit from guiding Ilizarov wires to prevent the Gigli form deviating from the intended course. An Ilizarov wire is placed parallel to and on either side of, the intended osteotomy path. This prevents the Gigli from deviating too far from the intended osteotomy plane. If the guiding wires are still stable in the frame after the osteotomy, they could be incorporated into the frame through a bent wire (stirrup wire) technique.

The Ponse-Taylor or Ponse-Hex technique is not only useful in the younger patient, but can be used in adolescent or adult patients with untreated clubfoot. An interesting variation is to prepare the joints for a triple arthrodesis in situ and then apply a Ponse-Hex frame to the deformed foot. After a lag period, the staged correction sequence is followed to spin the foot out into a better shape and then bring it out of equinus. The frame then holds the triple arthrodesis in the corrected position until union.

Gradual correction is limb reconstruction in the purest form. Regardless of the hardware device used to perform the correction, the underlying principles of pre-operative planning, biomechanics, distraction osteogenesis and functional rehabilitation remain the main components of a successful outcome.

References

1. Ferriter P, Shapiro F. Infantile tibia vara: factors affecting outcome following proximal tibial osteotomy. J Pediatr Orthop. 1987;7:1–7.
2. McCarthy JJ, Mark AK, Davidson RS. Treatment of angular deformities of the tibia in children: acute versus gradual correction. J Surg Orthop Adv. 2007;16(3):118–22.
3. Ilizarov GA. Trans Osseous osteosynthesis: theoretical and clinical regeneration of the regeneration and growth of tissue. Berlin, Germany: Springer-Verlag; 1992.
4. Ilizarov GA. Clinical application of the tension-stress effect for limb lengthening. Clin Orthop Relat Res. 1990;250:8–26.
5. Codivilla A. On the means of lengthening in the lower limbs, the muscles and tissues which are shortened through deformity. J Bone Joint Surg Am. 1905;2:353–69.
6. Putti V. The operative lengthening of the femur. 1921. Clin Orthop Relat Res. 1990;250:4–7.
7. Wagner H. Operative lengthening of the femur. Clin Orthop Relat Res. 1978;136:125–42.
8. Birch JG. A brief history of limb lengthening. J Pediatr Orthop. 2017;37:S1–8.
9. Abbot LC, Saunders JB. The operative lengthening of the tibia and fibula: a preliminary report on the further development of the principles and technic. Ann Surg. 1939;110:961–91.
10. Paley D. The Ilizarov technology revolution. J Limb Lengthen Reconstr. 2018;4:115–28.
11. De Bastiani G, Aldegheri R, Renzi-Brivo L, Trivella G. Limb lengthening by callus distraction (callotasis). J Pediatr Orthop. 1987;7:129–34.
12. Paley D. Principles of deformity correction. Heidelberg: Spinger-Verlag; 2002.
13. Eidelman M, Bialik V, Katzman A. Correction of deformities in children using the Taylor spatial frame. J Pediatr Orthop B. 2006;15:387–95.
14. Keshet D, Eidelman M. Clinical utility of the Taylor spatial frame for limb deformities. Orthop Res Rev. 2017;9:51–61.
15. Binski JC. Taylor spatial frame in acute fracture care. Techniques Orthop. 2002;17:173–1849.
16. Herzenberg JE. The art of limb alignment: taylor spatial frame. 1st ed. Baltimore: The Rubin Institute for Advanced Orthopedics (RIAO), Sinai Hospital of Baltimore; 2018.
17. Paley D, Bhave A, Herzenberg JE, Bowen JR. Multiplier method for predicting limb-length discrepancy. J Bone Joint Surg Am. 2000;82:1432–46.
18. The Multiplier–phone application (iPhone and Android). Herzenberg JE, Bhave A, Standard SC. Rubin Institute for Advanced Orthopaedics, Sinai Hospital of Baltimore; 2019.
19. Paley Growth—phone application (iPhone and Ipad). Paley Institute, West Palm Beach, FL; 2018.
20. Boyle J, Makarov MR, Podeszwa DA, Rodgers JA, Jo CH, Birch JG. Is proximal fibula epiphysiodesis necessary when performing a proximal tibial epiphysiodesis? J Pediatr Orthop. 2020;40(10):e984–9.

21. Paktiss AS, Gross RH. Afgan percutaneous osteotomy. Pediatric Orthop. 1993;13:531–3.
22. Eidelman M, Katsman A, Zaidman M, Keren Y. Deformity correction using supramalleolar gigli saw osteotomy and Taylor spatial frame: how to perform this osteotomy safely? J Pediatr Orthop B. 2011;20:318–22.
23. Eidelman M, Katsman A, Keren Y. Correction of residual clubfoot deformities in older children using the Taylor spatial butt frame and midfoot gigli saw osteotomy. J Pediatr Orthop. 2012;32:527–33.
24. Eidelman M, Kotlarsky P, Herzenberg JE. Treatment of relapsed, residual and neglected clubfoot: adjunctive surgery. J Child Orthop. 2019;13:293–303.
25. Jauregui JJ, Zamani S, Abawi HH, Herzenberg JE. Ankle range of motion after posterior subtalar and ankle capsulotomy for relapsed equinus in idiopathic clubfoot. J Pediatr Orthop. 2017;37:199–203.
26. Eidelman M, Katzman A. Treatment of complex foot deformities in children with Taylor spatial frame. Orthopedics. 2008;31:1–5.
27. Kirienko A, Villa A, Calhoun JH. Ilizarov technique for complex foot and ankle deformities. Philadelphia PA: Taylor & Francis; 2004.
28. Belthur MV, Iobst CA, Bor N, Segev E, Eidelman M, Standard SC, Herzenberg JE. Correction of cubitus varus after pediatric supracondylar elbow fracture: alternative method using the Taylor spatial frame. J Pediatr Orthop. 2016;36:608–17.
29. Rozbruch SR, Birch JG, Dahl MT, Herzenberg JE. Motorized intramedullary nail for treatment of limb length discrepancy. J Am Acad Orthop Surgeons. 2014;22:403–9.
30. Makarewich CA, Herzenberg JE, McClure PK. Latest advances in limb lengthening using magnetically controlled intramedullary lengthening nails. Surg Technol Int. 2020;36:4040–411.
31. Radler C, Mindler GT, Stauffer A, Weiß C, Ganger R. Limb lengthening with Precice intramedullary lengthening nails in children and adolescents. J Pediatr Orthop. 2022;42(2):e192–200.
32. Iliadis AD, Wright J, Stoddart MT, Goodier WD, Calder P. Early results from a single centre's experience with STRYDE nail: a cause for concern? Bone Joint J. 2021;103–B(6):1168–72.
33. Sax OC, Molavi DW, Herzenberg JE, Standard SC, McClure PK. Biopsy proven focal osteolysis in a stainless-steel limb-lengthening device: a report of three cases. J Am Acad Orthop Surg Glob Res Rev. 2021;5:1–6.

Pin Site Care

Nando Ferreira and William D. Harrison

Introduction

The success of any external fixator-assisted reconstructive surgery relies on the bone–pin interface surviving the duration of the process. Loss of this crucial interface threatens the stability of the construct and may necessitate its revision through the exchange of pins or wires or abandonment of the fixator.

With pin site infection being an almost universal finding in limb reconstruction with external fixation, with incidences of up to 100% reported in the literature, a conscious effort is required to prevent infection and manage it when it occurs [1–9]. The discrepancy in reported infection rates results from inconsistent definitions used for pin site infection, variation in the description of infection frequency, the use of different pins, wires and devices, and different pathologies being treated [10–12]. A 2016 systematic review found a 27% cumulative pin site infection rate [13].

In most instances, these infections are not severe and adequately treated by local pin site care and oral antistaphylococcal antibiotics [1, 9, 14, 15]. Severe infections, however, threaten the longevity of the fixator and may necessitate the treatment to be abandoned.

Multiple variables that potentially influence the integrity and longevity of the bone–pin interface have been identified and researched, and in most instances, have failed to provide concrete proof to guide practice. The fact that these variables each contribute a relatively small influence on the overall risk of developing pin site infection and the lack of sufficiently powered, high-quality research on the subject makes the identification of robust evidence-based treatment protocols challenging.

It is, however, essential to note that the lack of proof does not mean a lack of effect, and a nihilistic approach to pin insertion and pin site care should be discouraged. Current practice is generally guided by expert opinion and consensus statements based on the best available evidence.

Preoperative Preparation

Davies et al. emphasize that any strategy that aims to reduce pin site complications begins in the operating theatre [12]. There is definite merit in the statement, but we contend that the optimal strategy to limit pin sites complications would include preoperative considerations.

When discussing the considerations before external fixator application, a distinction between the elective and emergency scenario is acknowledged. Elective reconstruction affords the opportunity to optimize modifiable host factors, which the acute trauma setting does not [15]. This opportunity should be used effectively to address all factors influencing pin site longevity.

Potential systemic factors that may predispose to pin site complications include diabetes mellitus, Human Immunodeficiency virus (HIV) infection, smoking, and systemic steroid use [16, 17].

In a comparative study, Wukich et al. found people with diabetes to have a sevenfold increased risk for wire site complications [18]. The contributing factors are poor neutrophil function, glycosylation of tissues, compromised vascular supply, poor bone quality, instability from bone lysis, and excessive weight-bearing in neuropathic individuals. Finkler et al. provided further insight by showing that patients with elevated haemoglobin A1C levels specifically had higher

---

N. Ferreira (✉)
Division of Orthopaedic Surgery, Department of Surgical Sciences, Faculty of Medicine and Health Sciences, Stellenbosch University, Cape Town, South Africa
e-mail: nferreira@sun.ac.za

W. D. Harrison
Limb Reconstruction Service, Liverpool University Hospitals, Liverpool, UK
e-mail: William.Harrison2@liverpoolft.nhs.uk

rates of pin site infection, potentially indicating that glucose control could counter the increased risk that diabetes poses [9]. This theory is supported by Wukich et al., who found that well-controlled diabetics did not have an increased risk for surgical site complications during foot and ankle surgery [19].

Studying the effect of HIV on pin site infection, Norrish et al. found a higher incidence of patients who required pin removal in HIV positive patients. The study was conducted on patients who sustained open fractures and were exclusively managed in monolateral external fixators. The cohort was also mostly anti-retroviral treatment-naive [20]. Ferreira and Marais failed to show any difference in HIV-positive patients when using circular fixators to manage tibial non-unions [15]. The interpretation of these results shows that HIV may potentially influence pin site complications, but that host optimization and fixator choice might negate these risks.

Preoperative smoking has been shown to negatively affect wound healing and predispose to wound breakdown and infection [21]. Both Hussein et al. and Sharma et al. showed a statistically significant increased rate of pin site infection in smokers [17, 22]. Extrapolating the preventative effects of smoking cessation on infection rates in hip and knee arthroplasty, it is feasible to predict similar outcomes for pin site infection [21].

The preoperative preparation period is also an extremely valuable time to discuss potential pin site problems with the patient and their family and start the information sharing and education process. Sources of information can be from clinicians, dedicated limb reconstruction specialist nurses, written hand-outs, or increasingly online videos, meeting other patients, or joining support groups. The role of prehabilitation and meeting other patients in physiotherapy or support groups is also incredibly important. [23]

Intra-Operative Considerations

Fixator Stability Principles

Before surgery, careful consideration is given to the appropriate fixator for the task at hand, as fixator-bone stability and pin site infection are bi-directionally related. Consequently, it is not surprising that different fixator types show different incidences of pin site infection, with monolateral and hybrid fixators showing a higher incidence of pin site infections than ring fixators [3, 24]. As pin site infection and loosening can result in loss of fixator stability, so can an unstable fixator cause additional pin site stresses that can result in instability and infection. The chosen design and the application of an external fixator is, therefore, a vital step in limiting pin site complications.

How fixation elements are arranged is also crucial in limiting additional stresses on the pin–bone interface, and a thorough understanding of external fixator mechanics is paramount. Half pin biomechanics exert cantilever stresses on the bone–pin interface, and fixation elements are positioned in such a manner as to reduce the effect of the cantilever bending. For example, a monolateral rail is brought closer to the bone to reduce the moment arm of the half-pin cantilever effect. Also, the inter-connecting rods in a circular fixator should be circumferential around the limb to mitigate asymmetrical cantilever forces between rings. Thiart et al. showed how the arrangement of inter-connecting rods could influence overall stability, where the bone should ideally be placed within the constructed "area of support" [25] (Fig. 10.1).

External fixators are, however, not always required to only withstand axial loading during ambulation and rehabilitation. Where these devices are required to perform additional "work" such as during gradual deformity correction, bone transport or limb lengthening, added demand is placed on the bone–pin interface. In these instances, the fixator might also be expected to be in situ for longer than in the acute trauma scenario. Dynamic frames that allow active joint motion also place added demand on the pin sites compared to static frames [26, 27]. In these instances, it is critical to ensure that fixation elements are chosen in such a way as to counteract the expected forces acting on the frame and bone.

Skin Prep and Decolonization

In vivo, the literature favours chlorhexidine-alcohol solutions for skin preparation to cover the common skin commensals [28]. A review article of ten randomized control trials has also demonstrated that chlorhexidine-isopropyl alcohol has superior protection against surgical site infection and that alcohol-based skin preparation had a 98% probability of having better protection than aqueous-based preparations. [29]

Revision of Frame: How to Clean the Frame

Revision of a frame can be necessary for several reasons, including broken wires, loose half pins or as part of the management of an actively infected pin site. Due to the large surface area and inaccessible recesses within a circular fixator, it can be challenging to achieve sufficient sterility of the frame.

Once the patient is anaesthetized, all dressings should be removed, and a general wash with soapy water should be undertaken. The frame should be dried to allow the subse-

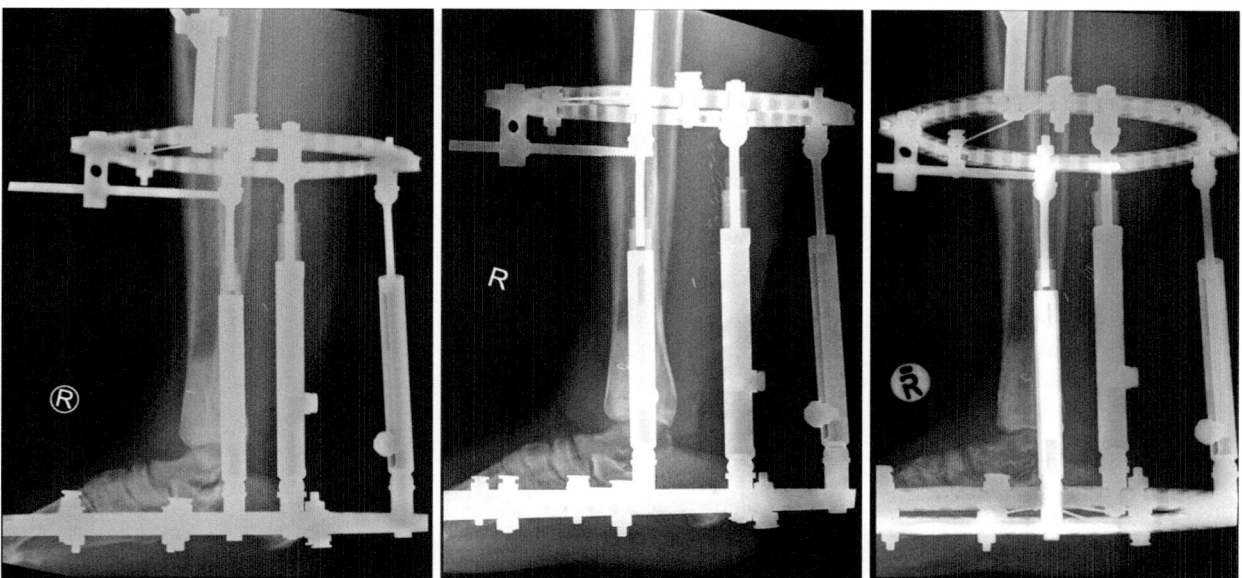

Fig. 10.1 Ankle spanning circular external fixator shows the tibia and ankle outside the constructed "area of support" and progressive lysis around the anterior half-pin, subjected to excessive cantilever loading

quent alcohol-based skin preparation. Chlorhexidine-alcohol solutions can then be liberally sprayed over the frame, with attention to cover difficult to access areas. If the frame needs to be partly dissembled, this is done in such a way as to avoid contamination of other instruments and gloves and drapes should be changed before any open procedure. The frame is then secondarily cleaned through a skin paint technique at the time of the formal limb preparation and draping. Large gauze wound packs can be soaked in alcoholic chlorhexidine, squeezed dry and then wrapped around areas of the frame that do not require access for revision. The aim is to have a minimal amount of the frame surface area exposed to the operative field. These swabs are then secured to one another by surgical clips or sutures.

Fixation Elements: Wire and Pin Design

- Pin diameter has not been specifically linked to pin site infection. However, larger diameter pins afford greater stability of the pin–bone interface [30].
- Half pins are designed with a graduated conical diameter. This is to produce radial preload, which in essence disperses forces symmetrically around the pin–bone interface. The opposite of this is axial preload, which causes focal stress on the pin–bone interface and, therefore, focal osteolysis [30].
- Fine wires vary in tip geometry. The tip aims to drill through bone effectively and with a minimal amount of thermal heat generation. A three-edged bayonet-shaped eccentric tip is the most commonly used design.
- Olive wires intrinsically have more stability than smooth wires and translational stability is not solely reliant on wire crossing angles. Where smooth wires are used, crossing angles of greater than 60° are required to limit translational instability.

Half Pin/Wire Coating

Several studies have shown that HA-coating protects against deterioration of pin fixation [31–34]. Although the HA-coating does not have any inherent anti-microbial properties, their ability to create a more stable bone–pin interface may secondarily help prevent pin site infections. Despite coated pins generally being preferred for long-term fixators, a recent meta-analysis failed to show any clinical evidence of their use to decrease pin site infection [10]. A 2016 systematic review, however, showed that HA-coating reduces loosening in patients undergoing prolonged fixation procedures but again failed to show an influence on infection rates [35].

Magyar et al. showed that HA-coating significantly improved extraction torque forces of half pins in both the metaphysis and diaphysis compared to uncoated pins [31]. Toksvig-Larsen et al. examined the performance of bisphosphonate-coated pins and showed similar extraction torque to HA-coated pins in metaphyseal bone and uncoated pins in diaphyseal bone [33].

In summary, coated pins probably impart clinical benefit, although their effect on pin site infection might not be as evident. It is, therefore, probably prudent to use coated pins in the metaphyseal and poor-quality bone, while uncoated pins could be used in good-quality diaphyseal bone.

Insertion Technique: Soft Tissue Considerations

- Fixation elements should not place tension on the skin–pin interface. If tension does occur on one side of the pin/wire, then consider releasing the skin.
- To prevent transfixing muscles in a shortened position, muscles should be placed in maximal stretch (lengthened position) when traversing them with a pin or half pin.
- To limit heat generation and iatrogenic soft tissue trauma, wires are pushed onto the near cortex, then drill through the bone and advanced through the far side tissues with a mallet (Fig. 10.2).
- If wires do not sit flush with the ring on the axial plane, then washers or blocks must "build the frame to the wire" rather than bending the wire onto the ring. This reduces skin tension, improves wire biomechanics, and reduces the risks of broken wires.
- When using olive wires, a small skin cut using a 15 blade scalpel will decrease iatrogenic soft-tissue trauma when seating the olive onto the bone.
- Avoiding transfixion of unnecessary muscle groups. This is particularly relevant to the medial head of the gastrocnemius, which is a common focus of irritation.
- Close adjacent open wounds before passing wires/half pins as this can make wound closure difficult and put tension on the skin–pin interface.
- Common pin site irritation areas (painful but not necessarily infection hotspots) include the medial proximal gastrocnemius, calcaneus, midfoot, and wires close to tendons. To minimize the effect of soft tissue irritation, various authors have identified ideal corridors for pin and wire placement [36–38].

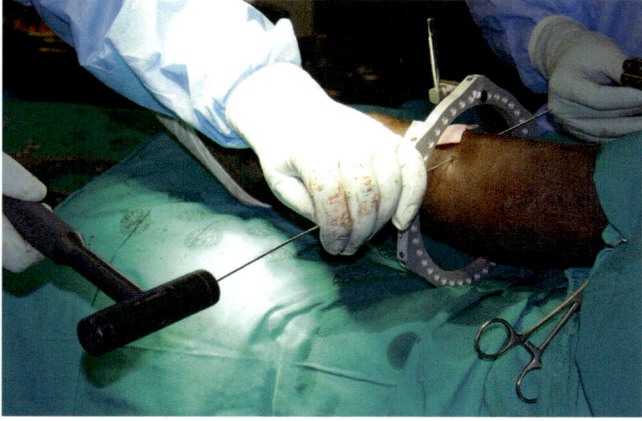

Fig. 10.2 Wire advanced using a mallet

Insertion Technique: Bone Considerations

- Wire or pin fixation should ideally have a bi-cortical fixation, as this forms a simple supported beam that promotes the best mechanical environment. Wires and pins that pass through areas of thick cortical bone, such as the anterior tibial crest, are at significant risk of inducing thermal necrosis during insertion. Unicortical pins and wires also produce a poorer mechanical hold than bi-cortical fixation.
- Half pins should be attached to the ring without tension. Bending a half pin to the fixator attachment produces preload that may result in focal osteolysis on the near cortex and the subsequent instability and infection.
- In the same vein, fine wires should be fixed to the ring in the line in which they pass through the bone. If the wire is brought to the ring by force, then the wire is at increased risk of breaking, and the bone is also at risk of focal osteolysis.
- It can occasionally be challenging to pass a fine wire through diaphyseal bone. This is more relevant in adults but is also essential for paediatric osteopetrosis, melorheostosis, or linear scleroderma of bone. During difficult wire passage, check that the wire tip has not blunted as this could lead to excessive heat generation. If the wire tip has blunted, then have a low threshold for using a new wire.
- Although it is less relevant to the paediatric population, neuropathic patients are highly prone to experience wire breakages, and therefore, additional fixation is recommended. Neuropathic patients should be warned preoperatively of their increased risk of requiring unscheduled returns to theatre.

Multiple studies have shown the mechanical superiority of self-drilling pins over predrilled pins [39, 40]. Oliphant et al., in a biomechanical study, found that predrilling had no effect on pin pull-out strength and that the near cortex showed no stripping with self-drilling pins [41].

It is important to note that mechanical superiority doesn't necessarily translate to better clinical results, especially if that mechanical advantage comes at the expense of local biology. Hutchinson et al. recorded significantly elevated temperatures with the direct pin drilling technique [42]. When considering that immediate thermal osteonecrosis occurs when temperatures exceed 60 °C, and after 30 s when the temperature exceeds 50 °C, it is prudent to consider heat generation during pin and wire insertion [43–45]. As such, to avoid excessive heat generation, predrilling half-pin sites is recommended [12, 46].

Heat generation during bone drilling is a factor of friction and time. Variables to consider regarding heat generation during drilling are drill speed, feed rate, and pressure [47].

Drill speed is directly proportional to heat generation, while feed rate is inversely proportional to heat generation. However, low speed and fast advancement do not produce good clinical results. This is because low drill speed with a high feed rate would require increased drill pressure which again increases heat generation and causes cortical bone fragmentation [48]. Brisman et al. further showed that low speed and minimal pressure produced similar temperature increases as the high speed with high pressure because of more efficient cutting by the drill flutes and decreased drilling times [49].

Several drilling techniques have been advocated to prevent heat generation, varying from intermittent/pulsatile drilling to fast drill speed with slow feed rate to slow drill speed and fast feed rate. Nam et al. concluded that using either low speed and high pressure or high speed and low pressure to be the optimal strategy for maintaining bone temperatures below the critical 50 °C [50]. We prefer high drill speed and low pressure, allowing the "drill to do the work". In addition to its effects on heat generation, high drill speed and low pressure also have a spin-stabilizing effect on fine wires being passed through bone, helping to improve wire trajectory accuracy.

After drilling, we advocate irrigation of the drill tract before pin insertion. This removes any bone swarf left in the tract, which might act as sequestra and impede osseointegration of the pin. A simple feeding tube or rubber catheter connected to a 20 cc syringe allows for an easy and inexpensive method [12, 46].

In addition to predrilling, other techniques to reduce heat generation include the use of clean, sharp drill bits, a drill sleeve to protect the soft tissue envelope and saline lavage of the drill and drill site and to clean the drill flutes after every use (Fig. 10.3). Cold saline lavage is effective in reducing heat generation below critical values [51, 52]. Room temperature saline lavage is satisfactory, as long as intermittent drilling is being used.

Intra-Operative Pin Site Dressing

Pin site dressings in theatre usually mirror the same process used in the postoperative setting. Pin site dressings are more extensively discussed in the next section. The authors prefer to use slotted 2 cm × 2 cm gauze swabs soaked in a chlorhexidine-alcohol solution (Fig. 10.4). The gauze is squeezed dry before application and placed flat on the skin to avoid excessive chlorhexidine that may cause skin irritation. Using chlorhexidine provides a local antiseptic environment and makes the gauze less likely to adhere to the skin. Dry dressings at the early postoperative phase are painful to exchange and can cause local skin trauma during removal.

Pin site dressings are placed immediately after the wire or pin is passed. The early application of dressings and gentle compression (using stoppers or bungs) stop any bleeding around the pin site and prevent the formation of a small haematoma [12]. Dressings are placed flat on the skin and not bunched to prevent local areas of increased pressure that can predispose to tissue necrosis [12].

The ideal bung reduces the risk of needlestick injury, is a cheap, pliable material that can be easily inserted onto the wire, maintains friction on the wire to exert gentle compression, has a flat underside to uniformly compress the dressing, and has minimal dead space to allow accumulation of debris.

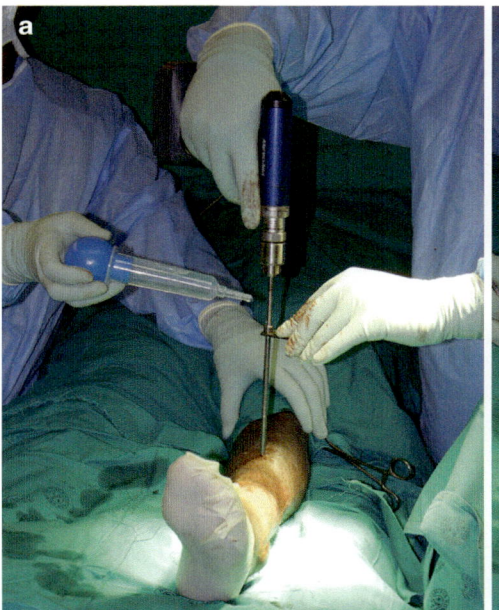 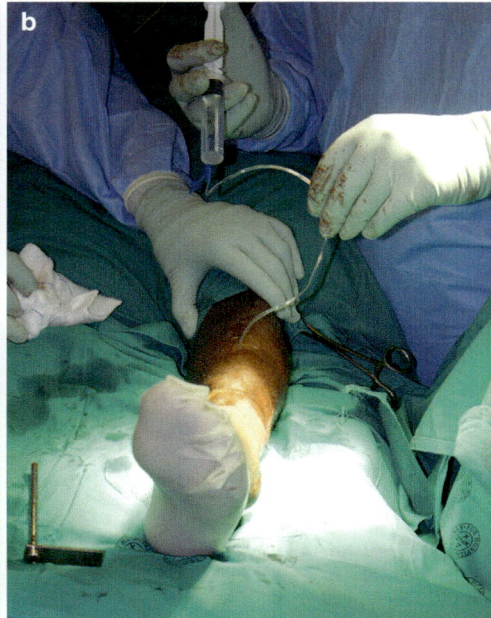

Fig. 10.3 (a) Half-pin site predrilling using a sharp drill bit, drill sleeve, and cold saline irrigation. (b) Drill hole irrigation to remove the swarf from the cavity

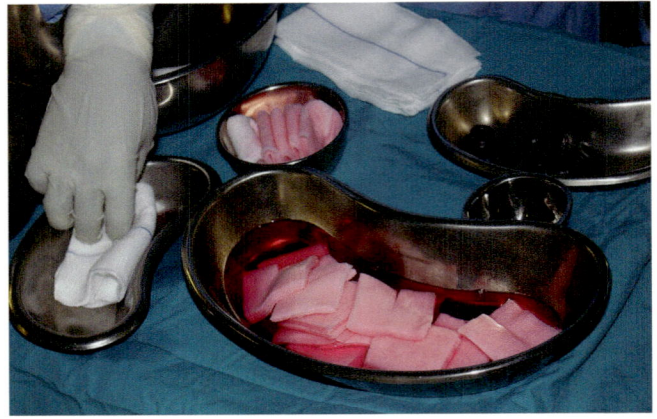

Fig. 10.4 Slotted 2×2 gauze dressings soaked in a chlorhexidine-alcohol solution

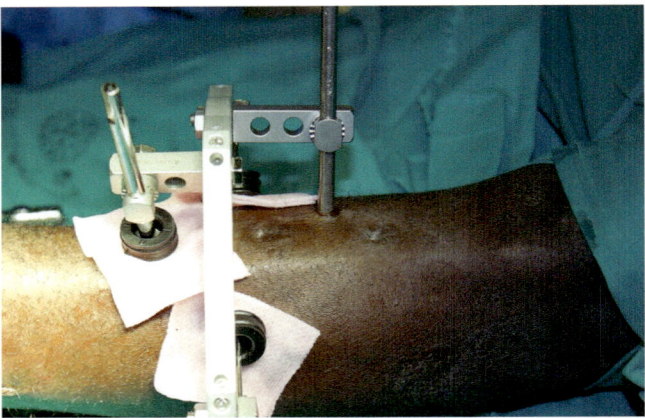

Fig. 10.5 Pin site dressings are held in place by syringe rubbers

Bespoke stoppers may be provided by the fixator manufacturer or custom made using materials readily available in the operating room. Two options include the use of a 20 ml syringe rubber or a 2 cm section of sterile airway tubing (Macaroni). Both the syringe rubber and the macaroni need to be incised with a scalpel before passing onto the wire. The scalpel incision should be small enough to allow easy passage of the wire; however, it should maintain enough friction to exert gentle compression to the dressing (Fig. 10.5).

At the completion of the procedure, all blood-soaked dressings are exchanged for fresh dressings.

Considerable variation exists for dressing the external fixator, with many authors preferring not to dress it at all. It is unknown if dressing the external fixator (sometimes called a sympathy bandage) has a placebo effect, a clinical effect on pain, or no effect at all. The authors use fluffed large gauze packs (a nest) placed inside the rings and then over-wrapped with a bandage. This theoretically helps stabilize the soft tissues and provides additional soft tissue compression to limit bleeding. If using this technique, care must be taken to remove the radio-opaque markers inside the gauze material.

Some surgeons bandage the contralateral leg to prevent collision with the frame in the early postoperative recovery (Fig. 10.6).

Stabilizing the foot, if not already incorporated into the frame, has the benefit of avoiding equinus contractures and reduces irritation and bleeding around the pin-sites from the motion of adjacent muscles and tendons. This can be achieved with a flat bottom "post-op shoe" attached to the frame or a bandage/therapy band pulling the forefoot up towards the frame (Fig. 10.7). This can be removed during mobilization and rehabilitation but should ideally be replaced when patients are sedentary and sleeping.

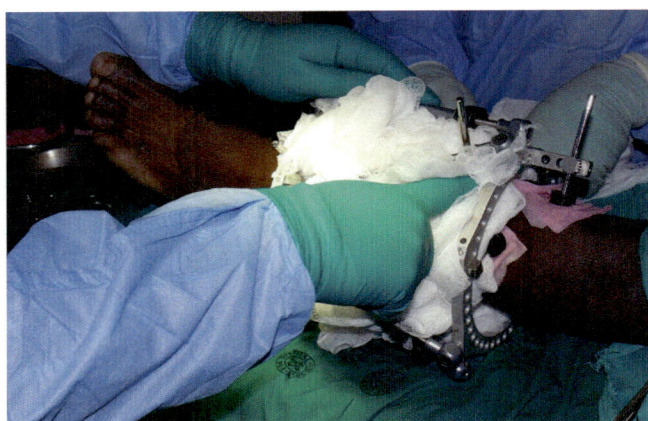

Fig. 10.6 External fixator "sympathy bandage" wrap

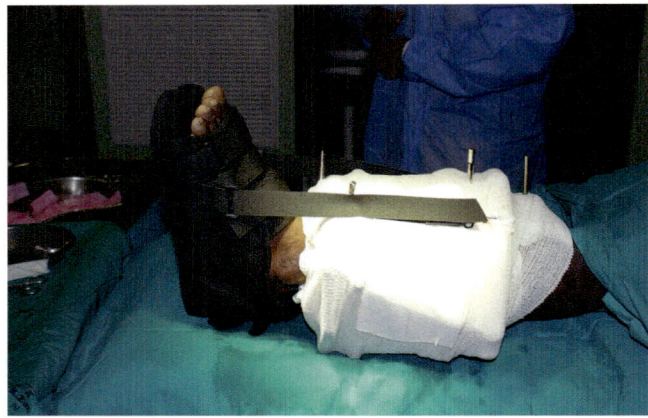

Fig. 10.7 Post-op frame shoe that prevents ankle equinus and excessive soft tissue movement

Postoperative Pin Site Care

Recovery

Limb elevation is a simple method to reduce the initial swelling and bleeding from surgical wounds and pin sites. When the patient is transferred to the recovery area, they experience increased mean arterial blood pressure and start moving in their bed. This translates to bleeding around wounds and soiled dressings. Occasionally, dressings will need to be changed in recovery, and bleeding pin sites usually respond to gentle compression bandages and elevation. Dressing changes should be done in a sterile fashion. The principle of limb elevation is to make sure the foot is higher than the knee, and the knee is higher than the hip. The limb should be roughly level with the heart. The knee should be supported while avoiding a flexed knee position which can be challenging to overcome without early physiotherapy intervention.

On the Ward

Mobilization in the early postoperative period should be encouraged. Surgeons often want to demonstrate to patients that the frame is suitable for early full weight-bearing, but the condition of the soft tissues needs to be appreciated. In the early phase, mobilization can lead to painful pin sites and bleeding. Later, excessive mobilization can lead to irritation or infection of pin sites and broken wires. Patients who excessively weight bear, such as neuropathic individuals or those with mental health problems, may encounter significant problems [53]. Other patients at risk of pin site problems during the early phases are those who are undergoing:

- Femoral external fixation due to large group muscle transfixation and soft tissue shear around the pin from exaggerated cantilever effects.
- Deformity correction (including lengthening).
- Bone transport.

Prophylactic Antibiotics

Routine prophylactic antibiotics for external fixation, beyond normal post-operative prophylaxis, have historically been recommended with some evidence of reduced pin site infection rates within the first 10–14 days [54]. However, a more recent study specifically assessing infection rates postoperatively of 106 patients demonstrated no benefit of prophylactic postoperative antibiotics during external fixation [55]. Consensus among the limb reconstruction community is not to use routine prophylactic antibiotics after frame application.

Timing of the First Dressing Change

Pin site materials and protocols are a source of continued investigation, and there is a significant variation in practice among clinicians. Pin site protocols internationally have primarily developed as a result of consensus, habit, or individual preference [12]. Efforts have been taken to create an international consensus amongst the limb reconstruction community to find ways to drive best practices.

In 2005, Davies et al. performed a case-controlled study of two different protocols (the authors' local protocol vs the "Russian protocol") and demonstrated superior results with the Russian protocol of daily dressing changes for the first 3 days than compared to undisturbed dressings for the first 48 h [12]. There were, however, confounding factors as they used chlorhexidine dressings and compression bandages in the daily dressing group, whereas they used dry gauze for the other.

A cohort study of 101 patients demonstrated that undisturbed dressings in the first postoperative week conferred a clinical advantage, with less requirement for antibiotics ($p < 0.0001$) [56]. One criticism of this article is that all pin sites infections were defined by having positive swab cultures rather than clinical infections. All pin sites were swabbed, irrespective of their clinical appearance, which may have been a confounding factor. The authors suggest that dressings should be changed early in the situation of heavy pin site leakage that does not respond to reinforced compressive dressings. [56]

Pin Site Care

Dressings materials and frequency of changes vary significantly between protocols and in terms of cost. It should be recognized that a patient with a frame will have many hundreds of individual pin site dressings throughout their treatment. Clinicians should consider the cost-effectiveness of dressings and appraise whether expensive dressings confer any clinically significant benefit. The ideal protocol and dressing material will also allow self-pin-site care without the need for frequent health facility or caregiver visits. The cheapest, easiest protocol with the least complications should be adopted for each clinical environment.

Dahl et al. failed to show any difference between daily and weekly pin site care in terms of infection, pain, or the use of antibiotics [57]. Dry adhesive dressings are not recommended, especially in the early pin site care. The use of chlorhexidine dressings has become the most widely accepted cleaning solution. W-Dahl et al. demonstrated that chlorhexidine solution is superior to sodium chloride, with 8.5% vs. 14% of pins site infections [58]. The chlorhexidine group also used significantly fewer antibiotics and had lower pain scores at weeks six and ten. When compared to antibiotic ointment dressings, chlorhexidine dressings also showed superior results [59].

A well-conducted but potentially underpowered randomized controlled trial compared chlorhexidine solution and

Dermol 500 (an emollient solution) for pin site dressings [60]. They demonstrated no significant differences in pin site infection rates or other secondary outcomes. Chlorhexidine had four adverse skin reactions (6.7%), whereas the Dermol group had none. The patients who had chlorhexidine-related skin reactions were crossed over to the Dermol group and had no further problems.

Patient and Caregiver Education

The maturation of the pin site will impact the timing of whether a bath or shower is appropriate. For the first two weeks after surgery, the leg should not be submerged. Thereafter, if the pin sites are healthy and the patient can carry out self-care, they can be permitted to bathe or shower on the understanding that the frame is rinsed with fresh water immediately afterwards, and they are to avoid irritant products such as bubble-bath. The same is true of swimming in pools or the sea. However, this is only permitted after a minimum of six weeks in the frame. The patient should apply fresh pin site dressings after a wash or a swim.

Pin Site Infection

The diagnosis of pin site infection is usually apparent, although no formal diagnostic criteria have been proposed or accepted. Consensus must also be reached on the exact distinction between an irritated, inflamed, or colonized and infected pin site. Regardless of this, the diagnosis is evident from an inflamed, painful, and weeping pin site in most instances. None of the available classifications has been validated, and there is considerable inter-observer bias in their interpretation [11].

Multiple classifications have been proposed. Each classification has a slightly different take on the interpretation of subjective clinical findings. Holmes et al. (2005) describe clinical features that differentiate between normal healing of a pin site (reaction), an inflamed (colonized) pin site, and a frankly infected one [61]. Ward classification (1998) separates simple pin site infections that respond to simple dressing changes and systemic antibiotics and more severe infections that require surgical management [62].

The "Good, Bad and Ugly" grading by Clint and Eastwood and the "Clam, Irritated and Infected" system from Santy et al. attempt to simplify the classification of pin site infections [63, 64]. They also incorporate symptoms and various stages of the inflammatory response into the interpretation of clinical findings. Checketts and Otterburn (2000) remain the most popular classification as it provides a graduated six clinical stages with guidance for the management of the infection [65] (Table 10.1). The modified Oppenheim wound score [66], Saleh and Scott [67], and Dahl [58] classifications do not differ significantly from Checketts and Otterburn.

Table 10.1 Checketts and Otterburn classification [65] of pin site infections

Grade	Characteristics	Treatment
Minor infection		
1	Slight redness, little discharge	Local pin site care
2	Redness of the skin, discharge, pain, and tenderness in the soft tissue	Local pin site care plus oral antibiotics
3	Grade 2 but no improvement with oral antibiotics	Affected pins must be removed
Major infection		
4	Severe soft tissue infection involving several pins, sometimes with associated loosening of the pin	External fixation must be abandoned
5	Grade 4 but radiographic changes	External fixation must be abandoned
6	Infection after fixator removal. Pin track heals initially but subsequently break down and discharge. Radiographs may show sequestrum	Curettage of the pin tract

Once diagnosed, the location of the infection should be documented and classified, the patient educated and treatment initiated with an early plan for follow-up. It is helpful to have a template letter for general practitioners to guide pin site infection prescriptions to fast track the getting of antibiotics to patients in peripheral areas.

Bacteriology and Antibiogram Properties

The most common organisms are *Staphylococcus aureus* and *Staphylococcus epidermidis* [24, 68, 69]. *Staphylococcus aureus* has been cultured in as high as 80% of pin site infections [70]. Other organisms from a different study include *Staph. epidermidis* (22%) and *Strep. viridans* (17%) [14]. Other less commonly reported organisms include *Pseudomonas, Strep. milleri, coagulase-negative staphylococcus,* and *Enterobacter* sp. [56].

A biofilm analysis of in vivo Kirschner wire sites and control pins demonstrates that staphylococcal bacteria most commonly colonized wires, but no bacterial biofilm was formed at six weeks [66]. The presence of a biofilm makes antibiotic penetration more difficult, which is inevitable with a pin site present for long periods. The development of crusts on a pin site undoubtedly represents an established biofilm. Once crusts become actively infected they should be removed. [53]

Treatment Principles

Early identification through patient education should form part of the pre-habilitation. This, along with the need for committed physiotherapy, constitutes a significant reason for intensive postoperative follow-up and often input from general practitioners in peripheral areas.

Swabbing of the pin site is intuitive to clinicians but does not alter the empirical management of inflamed or infected pin sites. The swab is unlikely to differentiate between inflammation and infection, as the pin site is colonized with skin flora from a very early stage. There is no correlation between positive swabs culturing skin commensals and active infection [58]. The swab culture can be helpful for clinically infected pin-sites that are refractory to first-line empirical antibiotics to target specific microbes or identify antibiotic resistance.

Occasionally, small abscesses can form at the pin site, and these need early attention as they can rapidly lead to cellulitis and develop deeper infections. The authors' preference is to use an antiseptic freeze spray as means of analgesia and gently lance the fluctuant swelling with an 11 or 15 blade scalpel. Small children may require light sedation or anaesthesia for significant collections.

Skin crusts naturally form at the pin-site as a process of normal exudates, regardless of dressing protocols. Crusting is more exaggerated during active infection. Beneath the crust, it is possible for a potential dead space, or reservoir, to form, which can lead to secondary infection [71, 72]. The function of the crusts and clinicians' response to them has been a source of controversy. The crusts are formed of exudates and sloughed skin and are heavily colonized with bacteria. They have no blood supply and therefore no access to systemic antibiotics. Adherent crusts are protective of pin site infection and arguably form a biological seal of natural skin commensals with protective flora that prevent pathological bacterial infection [53]. Routine removal of skin crusts can be a source of pain and anxiety in children. However, the work from Britten et al. demonstrates that once a pin site gets infected, the crusts should be removed [53].

Antimicrobials should be targeted towards the most commonly encountered causative organisms; *S. aureus and S. epidermidis* [24, 68, 69]. The cause for the infection is the presence of foreign material (a pin or wire) in the skin and cannot be easily removed. The role of antibiotics in pin site infection is to treat the soft tissue infection aggressively and avoid recurrent infection. Most pin site infections can be managed with a single agent, high-dose anti-staphylococcal with good soft tissue penetration [1, 9, 14, 46]. Flucloxacillin at a higher dose for two weeks has a very high rate of success. Patients with risk factors for infection such as the immunocompromised, those with recurrent infections or infections that have failed to respond to the first-line antibiotics should have a second-line empirical antibiotic given concurrently. Clindamycin or ciprofloxacin are good second-line antibiotics or alternative first-line options for penicillin-allergic patients. Both clindamycin and ciprofloxacin induce gastrointestinal side effects, which can be intolerable to some patients.

According to the Checketts and Otterburn classification, a pin site that does not respond to antibiotics may require removal [65]. It is prudent at that stage to get a radiograph to look for bony changes suggestive of osteomyelitis or a broken wire. A pin site swab is also recommended at the stage of an infection that has not responded to the first-line antibiotics.

The culture result is likely to confirm that empirical antibiotics have been appropriately selected. If the antibiotics are well tolerated, then they should continue for the entire two-week course. If a decision to start dual antimicrobial therapy has been made, then this should also continue (unless there are significant side effects to one or both antibiotics). If there is an unusual finding of an atypical antimicrobial infection or a resistance to empirical antibiotics, then antibiotics should be adjusted and targeted appropriately. It may be prudent to ask for microbiology consult in those rare situations.

It is important to note that not all inflamed pin sites are the result of infection. Both contact dermatitis allergic reactions to the stainless steel pins and the chlorhexidine cleaning solution have been observed by the senior author and reported in the literature [73–78]. In these cases, every pin site is inflamed, may have a slight serous discharge, and does not respond to a course of oral antibiotics. Cessation of chlorhexidine pin site cleaning will resolve contact dermatitis, but pin removal is necessary to treat metal allergy to pins and wires. The use of an alternative solution, such as Dermol 500, is recommended in that scenario [60].

Surgical Management of Pin Site Infections

If there is a decision to revise a wire, then all wires should be critically appraised in the clinic. If wires are causing irritation or could be adjusted to ease discomfort, then this should be addressed at the time of surgery. Occasionally, additional surgical procedures may be incorporated into the unscheduled wire exchange, such as grafting a docking site or soft tissue release to avoid contracture. The aim is to minimize the number of scheduled or unscheduled operations for the patient.

The same rationale should be applied to a revision of the entire frame. A revision of the frame is rarely required for a refractory pin site infection. If there are ongoing pin site problems, then it may be because there are issues with frame stability. A critical assessment of the frame biomechanics needs to be made in conjunction with understanding the mechanobiology of the fracture/regenerate site/docking site, etc. If the mechanobiology or limb alignment can be significantly improved through a complete revision of the frame, then this should be seriously considered. The "time in frame" can be reduced by revising to a frame with better biomechanics or exchanging to internal fixation. Pin site infections should be entirely quiescent before committing to the secondary internal fixation. If internal fixation is not an option and the patient has exhausted their frame time, an alternative is to provide a "frame holiday" before returning to complete treatment. This is a difficult judgement call and needs to be made with an experienced clinician in conjunction with the patient and carers.

Checketts and Otterburn VI pin site infections pose a unique situation where the pin site fails to heal, even after removing the offending pin (Fig. 10.8). Localized osteitis of the pin tract is usually the cause, and sequestrum can often be seen in the tract. Proposed treatment options for these scenarios include endoscopic debridement and the use of the Versajet Hydrosurgery system (Smith & Nephew, Memphis, Tennessee) [6, 79, 80] (Fig. 10.9). Formal bone debridement is rarely required. The same principles of type II and III Cierny and Mader chronic osteomyelitis prevail. Host status should be optimized. The extent and cause of infection are determined. Dead bone is debrided with dead space management and empirical local and systemic antibiotics followed by targeted systemic antibiotics.

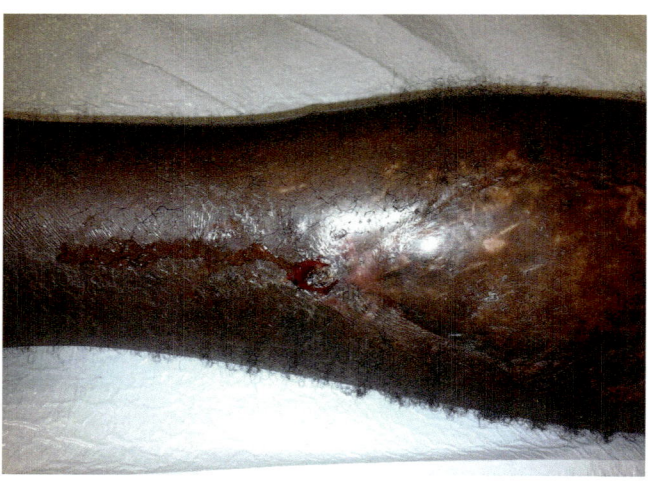

Fig. 10.8 Non-healing pin site, two weeks after external fixator removal

End of Treatment Considerations

At the completion of treatment, consideration for the removal of the external fixator is required. In most instances of paediatric reconstruction cases, this is done in the operating room under sedation or general anaesthetic. If the patient is awake during fixator removal, then generally try to remove the most accessible pins that will cause the least amount of pain first. Leave the olive wires, half pins, and those with inflamed skin until last. Before removal, the fixator is cleaned as previously described and then dismantled. All pin sites are cleaned and any crust or detritus is removed.

Wire Removal

It is important to differentiate between olive and smooth wires before removal. Some manufacturers place laser-etched markings on the olive side of the wire to assist with identification. If this is not the case, or the markings have been removed, then the radiographs should be studied to identify the location of the olives.

During removal, the far side of the wire is cut close to the skin and cleaned with chlorhexidine-alcohol before being pulled through the limb. This is to avoid pulling excessive contaminated material through the bone unnecessarily.

Half Pin Removal

Half pins are more difficult and more painful to remove than fine wires, especially half pins that are coated. As osseointegrated pins may shear during removal one should loosen the bone–pin interface before placing an extraction force on the pin. A ¼ clockwise turn would loosen adhesions while placing a compressive force on the pin after which the pin can be removed without fear of breakage. Where trans-osseous pins were used, thorough cleaning of the far side of the pin is

Fig. 10.9 Intra-operative images of Checketts and Otterburn VI pin site infection treated by Versajet hydrosurgical debridement

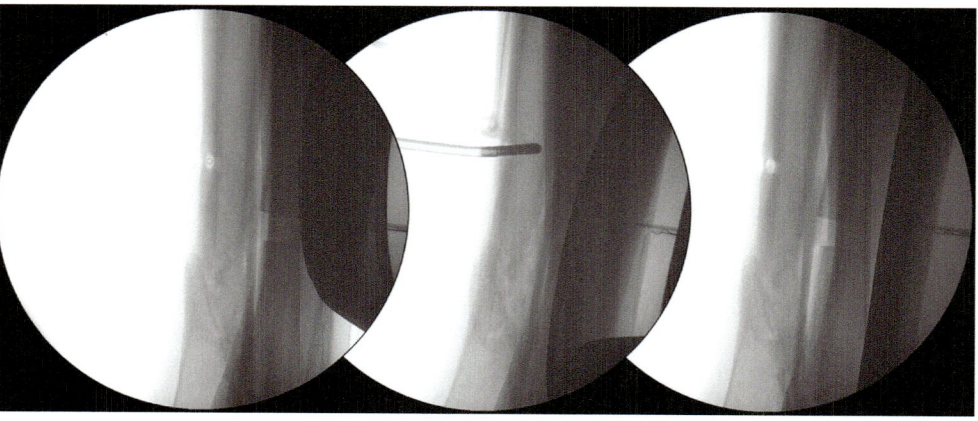

required to avoid pulling excessive contaminated material through the bone.

Following pin removal, the pin site is curetted and irrigated with normal saline. Chemical debridement with peroxide is also advocated by some surgeons. This step is omitted when the fixator is removed in the outpatient clinic. The pin sites are dressed without the routine skin closure. Bleeding and haematoma formation are unavoidable and addressed with compressive dry dressings. Unless pins are removed for the reason of infection, no post-removal antibiotics are required.

Conclusion

The success of every external fixator-assisted reconstructive procedure hinges on the survival of the bone–pin interface until the treatment goal is reached. Despite the lack of high-quality, evidence-based guidelines, all aspects of treatment should be aimed at protecting this crucial part of the fixator–patient interface. Care should be taken to control as many factors implicated in the development of pin site infection to decrease the risk or severity of pin site infections.

Commentary

Hemant K. Sharma
hemant.sharma5@nhs.net

The external fixator is a commonly used, extremely versatile device; however, it has the constant drawback of discomfort and pin site infections. Ferriera and Harrison have written a comprehensive chapter which would be useful for all practicing limb reconstruction surgeons. Despite being a common problem, this subject historically is under-researched, which is surprising considering that it is such a common problem. Because of the relatively large volume of available patients, finding volunteers to recruit into research study trials should not be a problem. Pin site research, however, has several core issues including a lack of consensus on simple things like "what defines a pin site infection" as there are no validated classification systems for pin site infection.

Current evidence on pin site infections is very heterogeneous [81, 82] (systematic reviews published by Lobst and Rozbruch), which happens to be the basis of current pin site literature across the globe. There are no high-quality trials to answer common questions. In the absence of robust evidence, rational and logical practice seems to be the right way forward. Clinical experience in pin site infections is a potent weapon.

Hydroxy-apatite coated pins are not anti-microbial and therefore do not reduce pin site infections directly. These coated pins decrease the incidence of loosening and thereby prevent frame instability which decreases return trips to the operating room [82, 83]. Therefore, despite the higher initial cost than standard titanium pins, they should be cost-effective, although there is no evidence in the literature to confirm it. In practices where resources are limited, surgeons commonly use titanium (cheaper) pins for trauma and HA-coated pins for elective/long duration frames. Several other coatings and nano-technology are currently being tested with encouraging results, which in the future, may help reduce the pin site problems.

Clinical experience suggests metaphyseal half pins tend to loosen more frequently compared to diaphyseal pins although true evidence is lacking. Therefore, wires are often used in the metaphysis rather than half pins.

Pre-tensioning of half pins may lead to cantilever loading resulting in stress concentration on the pin–bone junction resulting in pin loosening. Therefore, tightening the fixation element like a cube/rancho to the ring prior to drilling ensures a centralized pin in the fixation element which prevents deflection stress concentration (Fig. 10.10 and 10.11).

Pin site infection consequences can vary from minor inconvenience to osteomyelitis. Peri-articular pins are more prone for discomfort and infection. The risk of developing a deep infection is reported around 4% (Ting et al.). A recent study [84] suggested that peri-articular wires in close proximity to internal fixation are more prone to develop a deep infection. The same study also reported no deep infections in the elective frames but the number of the elective frames in the study was small.

Proximal and distal tibio-fibular joints can be stabilized with half pins instead of fine wires, which may be more tolerable for the patients. To do this, start by drilling a wire from the fibula that exits on the medial side of the tibia. A cannulated drill is then used over the wire from medial to lateral allowing the wire to be replaced by a half pin. This technique is easier to perform in elective situations than trauma.

Another under-recognized consequence of pin site infection (and sometimes with loss of wire tension) is instability of the frame, which can lead to delayed/nonunion/delayed consolidation of the regenerate. There is no objective way of checking wire tension. Recurrent infections/discharge from a wire should alert the surgeon for a potentially loose wire. In the absence of any available objective testing method, subjective methods are commonly used. Hitting the wire with the spanner and listening to sound (varies with wire tension) is totally unscientific and relies more on experience. However, lucent lines across the wires and half pins, along with the clinical picture is a better and more reliable way of identifying the loosening.

Cooling of wires and half pins during drilling with alcohol is common practice although some units use cool water as Prof Ferreira has eluded to in the chapter. Alcohol evaporates at a much faster rate than water. Therefore, for a given amount of time, alcohol, transfers more heat and, therefore, will have a better cooling effect.

There is a wide variation in pin site dressings [81–83, 85]: type of dressing/no dressings, weekly/daily dressings, etc. Due to the lack of robust evidence, current practice is anecdotal and based on personal experiences. Therefore, it is safe to say that pin site care and dressings (or no dressings) should be based on the available resources, the local cultural practices, and frame and patient factors. For example, a hot equatorial climate is perhaps more suited for daily showering and therefore open pin site (no dressing) care.

The reported incidence of pin site infection is also under debate. Should all pin site infections be pooled for the patient? Should recurrence be counted as a separate infection? Should incidence be reported as per patient or percentage of pins infected? Ting et al.'s study [86] reported a 4.6% deep pin site infection rate. If this is reported differently, then from 871 half pins 1 half pin had deep infection and 12 wires from 1385 wires had deep infection. This results in 0.11% and 0.86% deep infection for half pins and wires, respectively.

International pin site consensus group [87] (ASAMI 2019, Liverpool), utilizing modified Delphi's approach have identified nine top research questions in pin site infections according to surgeons across the world. The answers to these nine questions in the form of a systematic review were published in a special issue of the *Journal of Limb Lengthening and* Reconstruction [84]. Editorial [88] in this issue suggests that this priority setting exercise will hopefully inform future research and identify solutions for this very common problem.

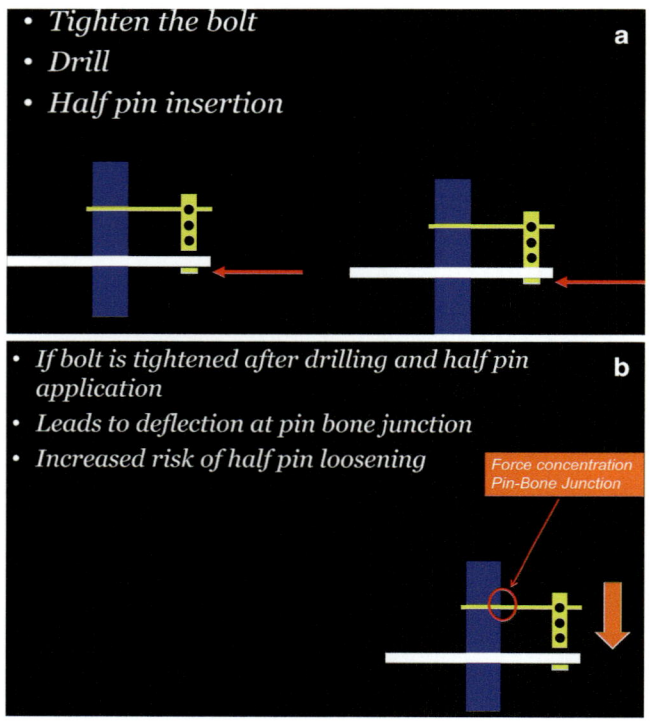

Figs. 10.10 and 10.11 Copyright H K Sharma, Image used with permission

References

1. Ferreira N, Marais LC. Pin tract sepsis: incidence with the use of circular fixators in a limb reconstruction unit. SA Orthop J. 2012;11(1):10–8.
2. Sims M, Saleh M. External fixation–the incidence of pin site infection: a prospective audit. J Orthop Nurs [Internet]. 2000;4(2):59–63. Available from: https://linkinghub.elsevier.com/retrieve/pii/S1361311100900670
3. Parameswaran AD, Roberts CS, Seligson D, Voor M. Pin tract infection with contemporary external fixation: how much of a problem? J Orthop Trauma [Internet]. 2003;17(7):503–7. Available from: http://www.ncbi.nlm.nih.gov/pubmed/12902788
4. Cavusoglu AT, Er MS, Inal S, Ozsoy MH, Dincel VE, Sakaogullari A. Pin site care during circular external fixation using two different protocols. J Orthop Trauma [Internet]. 2009;23(10):724–30. Available from: http://www.ncbi.nlm.nih.gov/pubmed/19858981
5. Lee CK, Chua YP, Saw A. Antimicrobial gauze as a dressing reduces pin site infection: A randomized controlled trial. Clin Orthop Relat Res [Internet]. 2012;470(2):610–5. Available from: https://pubmed.ncbi.nlm.nih.gov/21842299/
6. Bibbo C, Brueggeman J. Prevention and management of complications arising from external fixation pin sites. J Foot Ankle Surg [Internet]. 2010;49(1):87–92. Available from: http://www.ncbi.nlm.nih.gov/pubmed/20123298
7. Patterson MM. Multicenter pin care study. Orthop Nurs [Internet]. 2005;24(5):349–60. Available from: https://pubmed.ncbi.nlm.nih.gov/16272914/

8. Pizà G, Caja VL, González-Viejo MA, Navarro A. Hydroxyapatite-coated external-fixation pins. J Bone Joint Surg Br [Internet]. 2004;86-B(6):892–897. Available from: https://pubmed.ncbi.nlm.nih.gov/15330032/.
9. Finkler ES, Kasia C, Kroin E, Davidson-Bell V, Schiff AP, Pinzur MS. Pin tract infection following correction of Charcot foot with static circular fixation. Foot ankle Int [Internet]. 2015;36(11):1310–5. Available from: https://pubmed.ncbi.nlm.nih.gov/26223236/
10. Stoffel C, Eltz B, Salles MJ. Role of coatings and materials of external fixation pins on the rates of pin tract infection: A systematic review and meta-analysis. World J Orthop [Internet]. 2021;12(11):920–30. Available from: https://www.wjgnet.com/2218-5836/abstract/v12/i11/920.htm
11. Santy J. A review of pin site wound infection assessment criteria. Int J Orthop Trauma Nurs [Internet]. 2010;14(3):125–31. Available from: https://linkinghub.elsevier.com/retrieve/pii/S1878124109002482
12. Davies R, Holt N, Nayagam S. The care of pin sites with external fixation. J Bone Joint Surg Br [Internet]. 2005;87-B(5):716–9. Available from: https://online.boneandjoint.org.uk/doi/10.1302/0301-620X.87B5.15623
13. Iobst C, Liu R. A systematic review of incidence of pin track infections associated with external fixation. J Limb Lengthening Reconstr [Internet]. 2016;2(1):6. Available from: https://www.jlimblengthrecon.org/article.asp?issn=2455-3719;year=2016;volume=2;issue=1;spage=6;epage=16;aulast=Iobst
14. Schalamon J, Petnehazy T, Ainoedhofer H, Zwick EB, Singer G, Hoellwarth ME. Pin tract infection with external fixation of pediatric fractures. J Pediatr Surg [Internet]. 2007;42(9):1584–7. Available from: http://www.jpedsurg.org/article/S0022346807002874/fulltext
15. Ferreira N, Marais LC. The effect of HIV infection on the incidence and severity of circular external fixator pin track sepsis: a retrospective comparative study of 229 patients. Strateg Trauma Limb Reconstr [Internet]. 2014;9(2):111–5. Available from: https://www.stlrjournal.com/doi/10.1007/s11751-014-0194-y
16. Egol KA, Paksima N, Puopolo S, Klugman J, Hiebert R, Koval KJ. Treatment of external fixation pins about the wrist: a prospective, randomized trial. J Bone Joint Surg Am [Internet]. 2006 Feb;88(2):349–354. Available from: https://pubmed.ncbi.nlm.nih.gov/16452747/.
17. Hussein IM, Wang L, Yu B. Treatment options for pin site infection during Kirschner wires in elective forefoot surgery. Open J Orthop [Internet]. 2021;11(02):47–66. Available from: http://www.scirp.org/journal/PaperInformation.aspx?PaperID=107441
18. Wukich DK, Belczyk RJ, Burns PR, Frykberg RG. Complications encountered with circular ring fixation in persons with diabetes mellitus. Foot Ankle Int [Internet]. 2008;29(10):994–1000. Available from: https://journals.sagepub.com/doi/10.3113/FAI.2008.0994
19. Wukich DK, Crim BE, Frykberg RG, Rosario BL. Neuropathy and poorly controlled diabetes increase the rate of surgical site infection after foot and ankle surgery. J Bone Jt Surg [Internet]. 2014;96(10):832–9. Available from: /pmc/articles/PMC4018772/
20. Norrish AR, Lewis CP, Harrison WJ. Pin-track infection in HIV-positive and HIV-negative patients with open fractures treated by external fixation: a prospective, blinded, case-controlled study. J Bone Jt Surg Br [Internet]. 2007;89(6):790–3. Available from: http://www.ncbi.nlm.nih.gov/pubmed/17613506
21. Møller AM, Villebro N, Pedersen T, Tønnesen H. Effect of preoperative smoking intervention on postoperative complications: a randomised clinical trial. Lancet (London, England) [Internet]. 2002 Jan 12 [cited 2021 Nov 23];359(9301):114–7. Available from: https://pubmed.ncbi.nlm.nih.gov/11809253/
22. Sharma SK, Vati J, Wali I, Sen R. The effect of smoking on pin site infection rate among patients with external skeletal fixation. Nurs Midwifery Res Journal, [Internet]. 2008 Apr 6 [cited 2021 Nov 23]; Available from: https://nrfninechd.com/the-effect-of-smoking-on-pin-site-infection-rate-among-patients-with-external-skeletal-fixation/
23. Ede MPN, Malik MHA, Prudhoe L, Miller C, Khan SA, Wilkes RA. Supporting Limb Reconstruction Patients: A Fine-Wire Circular Fixator Support Group. Ann R Coll Surg Engl [Internet]. 2009 Jan [cited 2021 Nov 30];91(1):63. Available from: /pmc/articles/PMC2752247/.
24. Antoci V, Ono CM, Antoci V, Raney EM. Pin-tract infection during limb lengthening using external fixation. Am J Orthop (Belle Mead NJ) [Internet]. 2008 Sep 1 [cited 2021 Nov 21];37(9):E150–4. Available from: https://europepmc.org/article/med/18982187
25. Thiart G, Herbert C, Sivarasu S, Gasant S, Laubscher M. Influence of different connecting rod configurations on the stability of the Ilizarov/TSF frame: A biomechanical study. Strateg Trauma Limb Reconstr [Internet]. 2020 Oct 15 [cited 2021 Aug 10];15(1):23–27. Available from: https://creativecommons.
26. Hove LM, Krukhaug Y, Revheim K, Helland P, Finsen V. Dynamic compared with static external fixation of unstable fractures of the distal part of the radius: a prospective, randomized multicenter study. J Bone Joint Surg Am [Internet] 2010 Jul 21 [cited 2021 Nov 24];92(8):1687–1696. Available from: https://pubmed.ncbi.nlm.nih.gov/20660231/
27. Sommerkamp TG, Seeman M, Silliman J, Jones A, Patterson S, Walker J, et al. Dynamic external fixation of unstable fractures of the distal part of the radius. A prospective, randomized comparison with static external fixation. undefined. 1994;76(8):1149–61.
28. Miller HJ, Awad SS, Crosby CT, Mosier MC, Ph D, Alsharif A, et al. Chlorhexidine–Alcohol versus Povidone–Iodine for Surgical-Site Antisepsis. 2010;18–26.
29. Sidhwa F, Itani KMF. Skin preparation before surgery: options and evidence. Surg Infect. 2015;16(1):14–23.
30. Giotakis N, Narayan B. Stability with unilateral external fixation in the tibia. Strateg Trauma Limb Reconstr. 2007;2(1):13–20.
31. Magyar G, Toksvig-Larsen S, Moroni A. Hydroxyapatite coating of threaded pins enhances fixation. J Bone Joint Surg Br [Internet]. 1997 May [cited 2021 Nov 21];79(3):487–489. Available from: https://pubmed.ncbi.nlm.nih.gov/9180334/
32. Moroni A, Toksvig-Larsen S, Maltarello MC, Orienti L, Stea S, Giannini S. A Comparison of Hydroxyapatite-Coated, Titanium-Coated, and Uncoated Tapered External-Fixation Pins. An in Vivo Study in Sheep*. J Bone Jt Surg [Internet]. 1998 Apr;80(4):547–54. Available from: http://journals.lww.com/00004623-199804000-00011
33. Toksvig-Larsen S, Aspenberg P. Bisphosphonate-coated external fixation pins appear similar to hydroxyapatite-coated pins in the tibial metaphysis and to uncoated pins in the shaft. Acta Orthop [Internet] 2013 Jun 28 [cited 2021 Nov 21];84(3):314–318. Available from: https://pubmed.ncbi.nlm.nih.gov/23621808/
34. Moroni A, Pegreffi F, Cadossi M, Hoang-Kim A, Lio V, Giannini S. Hydroxyapatite-coated external fixation pins. Expert Rev Med Devices [Internet] 2005 Jul 9 [cited 2021 Nov 21];2(4):465–471. Available from: https://pubmed.ncbi.nlm.nih.gov/16293085/
35. Patel A, Ghai A, Anand A. Clinical benefit of hydroxyapatite-coated versus uncoated external fixation: A systematic review. Int J Orthop [Internet] 2016 Jun 28 [cited 2021 Nov 21];3(3):581–590. Available from: http://www.ghrnet.org/index.php/ijo/article/view/1627/2056
36. Nayagam S. Safe corridors in external fixation: the lower leg (tibia, fibula, hindfoot and forefoot). Strateg Trauma Limb Reconstr [Internet]. 2007 Dec [cited 2021 Dec 2];2(2):105. Available from: /pmc/articles/PMC2322836/.
37. Kishan S, Sabharwal S, Behrens F, Reilly M, Sirkin M. External fixation of the femur: basic concepts. Tech Orthop. 2002 Jun;17(2):239–44.

38. Safe zones in the tibia for pin insertion [Internet]. [cited 2021 Dec 2]. Available from: https://surgeryreference.aofoundation.org/orthopedic-trauma/adult-trauma/tibial-shaft/approach/safe-zones-of-the-tibia-for-pin-insertion
39. Pei Chee L, Bin Daud R, Bin FK, Mohamad Khan S, Alia Md Zain N, Abdullah S, Bajuri Y. Pre-drilling and self-drilling pins screw-bone fixation stress interaction analysis induced by uniaxial compression loading. undefined. 2019 Feb 4;15(1):99–108.
40. Arango D, Tiedeken N, Clippinger B, Samuel SP, Saldanha V, Shaffer G. Biomechanical analysis of four external fixation pin insertion techniques. Orthop Rev (Pavia) [Internet] 2017 Oct 3 [cited 2021 Nov 21];9(3):68–70. Available from: /pmc/articles/PMC5646427/.
41. Oliphant BW, Kim H, Osgood GM, Golden RD, Hawks MA, Hsieh AH, et al. Predrilling does not improve the pullout strength of external fixator pins: a biomechanical study. J Orthop Trauma [Internet]. 2013 [cited 2021 Nov 21];27(2):e25–e30. Available from: https://pubmed.ncbi.nlm.nih.gov/22495530/
42. Hutchinson DT, Bachus KN, Higgenbotham T. External fixation of the distal radius: to predrill or not to predrill. J Hand Surg Am [Internet] 2000 [cited 2021 Nov 21];25(6):1064–1068. Available from: https://pubmed.ncbi.nlm.nih.gov/11119664/
43. Li S, Chien S, Brånemark PI. Heat shock-induced necrosis and apoptosis in osteoblasts. J Orthop Res [Internet] 1999 [cited 2021 Nov 21];17(6):891–899. Available from: https://pubmed.ncbi.nlm.nih.gov/10632456/
44. Boner V, Kuhn P, Mendel T, Gisep A. Temperature evaluation during PMMA screw augmentation in osteoporotic bone-an in vitro study about the risk of thermal necrosis in human femoral heads. J Biomed Mater Res Part B Appl Biomater [Internet] 2009 Aug [cited 2021 Nov 21];90B(2):842–848. Available from: https://onlinelibrary.wiley.com/doi/10.1002/jbm.b.31353
45. Eriksson AR, Albrektsson T. Temperature threshold levels for heat-induced bone tissue injury: A vital-microscopic study in the rabbit. J Prosthet Dent [Internet] 1983 Jul [cited 2021 Nov 21];50(1):101–107. Available from: https://pubmed.ncbi.nlm.nih.gov/6576145/
46. Ferreira N, Marais LC. Prevention and management of external fixator pin track sepsis. Strateg Trauma Limb Reconstr [Internet]. 2012 Aug 31 [cited 2021 Nov 21];7(2):67–72. Available from: /pmc/articles/PMC3535127/.
47. Timon C, Keady C. Thermal osteonecrosis caused by bone Drilling in Orthopedic Surgery: A literature review. Cureus [Internet] 2019 Jul 24 [cited 2021 Nov 24];11(7). Available from: /pmc/articles/PMC6759003/.
48. Thompson HC. Effect of drilling into bone. J Oral Surg (Chic) [Internet]. 1958;16(1):22–30. Available from: http://www.ncbi.nlm.nih.gov/pubmed/13492103
49. Brisman DL. The effect of speed, pressure, and time on bone temperature during the drilling of implant sites. Int J Oral Maxillofac Implants. 1996;11(1):35–7.
50. Nam O, Yu W, Choi MY, Kyung HM. Monitoring of Bone Temperature during Osseous Preparation for Orthodontic Micro-Screw Implants: Effect of Motor Speed and Ressure. Key Eng Mater [Internet]. 2006 Oct [cited 2021 Nov 24];321–323:1044–7. Available from: https://www.scientific.net/KEM.321-323.1044
51. Augustin G, Davila S, Mihoci K, Udiljak T, Vedrina DS, Antabak A. Thermal osteonecrosis and bone drilling parameters revisited. Arch Orthop Trauma Surg [Internet]. 2008 Jan [cited 2021 Nov 24];128(1):71–77. Available from: https://pubmed.ncbi.nlm.nih.gov/17762937/
52. Effatparvar MR, Jamshidi N, Mosavar A. Appraising efficiency of OpSite as coolant in drilling of bone. J Orthop Surg Res 2020 151 [Internet]. 2020 May 29 [cited 2021 Nov 24];15(1):1–5. Available from: https://josr-online.biomedcentral.com/articles/10.1186/s13018-020-01710-w
53. Britten S, Ghoz A, Duffield B, Giannoudis PV. Ilizarov fixator pin site care: the role of crusts in the prevention of infection. Injury [Internet]. 2013;44(10):1275–8. Available from: https://linkinghub.elsevier.com/retrieve/pii/S0020138313003082
54. Magyar G, Ahl TL, Vibe P, Toksvig-Larsen AL. Open-wedge osteotomy by hemicallotasis or the closed-wedge technique for osteoarthritis of the knee. J Bone Joint Surg Br. 1999:81-B(3).
55. W-Dahl A, Toksvig-Larsen S. Infection prophylaxis: A prospective study in 106 patients operated on by tibial osteotomy using the hemicallotasis technique. Arch Orthop Trauma Surg. 2006;126(7):441–7.
56. W-Dahl A, Toksvig-Larsen S. Undisturbed theatre dressing during the first postoperative week. A benefit in the treatment by external fixation: A cohort study. Strateg Trauma Limb Reconstr. 2009;4(1):7–12.
57. W-Dahl A, Toksvig-Larsen S, Lindstrand A. No difference between daily and weekly pin site careA randomized study of 50 patients with external fixation. Acta Orthop Scand [Internet]. 2003;74(6):704–8. Available from: http://www.tandfonline.com/doi/full/10.1080/00016470310018234
58. W-Dahl A, Toksvig-Larsen S. Pin site care in external fixation sodium chloride or chlorhexidine solution as a cleansing agent. Arch Orthop Trauma Surg [Internet] 2004 Oct [cited 2021 Nov 21];124(8):555–558. Available from: https://pubmed.ncbi.nlm.nih.gov/15338244/
59. Wu SC, Crews RT, Zelen C, Wrobel JS, Armstrong DG. Use of chlorhexidine-impregnated patch at pin site to reduce local morbidity: the ChIPPS pilot trial. Int Wound J [Internet] 2008 Jun [cited 2021 Nov 21];5(3):416–422. Available from: /pmc/articles/PMC7951341/.
60. Roth F, Cagienard F, Link BC, Hodel S, Lehnick D, Babst R, et al. Primary or secondary wound healing of the pin sites after removal of the external fixator: study protocol for a prospective, randomized controlled, monocenter trial. Trials [Internet] 2020 Feb 19;21(1):205. Available from: http://www.ncbi.nlm.nih.gov/pubmed/32075685
61. Holmes SB, Brown SJ. Skeletal pin site care: national association of orthopaedic nurses guidelines for orthopaedic nursing. Orthop Nurs. 2005;24(2):99–107.
62. Ward P. Care of skeletal pins: a literature review. Nurs Stand [Internet] 1998 [cited 2021 Nov 21];12(39):34–38. Available from: https://pubmed.ncbi.nlm.nih.gov/9776884/
63. Clint SA, Eastwood DM, Chasseaud M, Calder PR, Marsh DR. The "good, bad and ugly" pin site grading system. Injury [Internet]. 2010;41(2):147–50. Available from: https://linkinghub.elsevier.com/retrieve/pii/S0020138309003350
64. Santy-Tomlinson J, Jomeen J, Ersser SJ. Patient-reported symptoms of 'calm', 'irritated' and 'infected' skeletal external fixator pin site wound states; a cross-sectional study. Int J Orthop Trauma Nurs [Internet]. 2019;33:44–51. Available from: https://linkinghub.elsevier.com/retrieve/pii/S1878124118301035
65. Checketts RG, MacEachem AG, Otterburn M. Pin track infection and the principles of pin site care. Orthofix Extern Fixat Trauma Orthop. 2001:97–103.
66. Hargreaves D, Pajkos A, Vickery K, Filan S., Tonkin M. The role of biofilm formation in percutaneous Kirschner-wire fixation of radial fractures. J Hand Surg Am 2002;27 B(4):365–8.
67. Saleh M, Scott BW. The Complications of Leg Lengthening. In: Orthofix External Fixation in Trauma and Orthopaedics [Internet]. London: Springer London; 2000 [cited 2021 Nov 21]. p. 496–510. Available from: https://link.springer.com/chapter/10.1007/978-1-4471-0691-3_47
68. Jennison T, McNally M, Pandit H. Prevention of infection in external fixator pin sites. Acta Biomater [Internet] 2014 [cited 2021 Nov 21];10(2):595–603. Available from: https://pubmed.ncbi.nlm.nih.gov/24076071/

69. Charville GW, Hetrick EM, Geer CB, Schoenfisch MH. Reduced bacterial adhesion to fibrinogen-coated substrates via nitric oxide release. Biomaterials [Internet] 2008 Oct [cited 2021 Nov 21];29(30):4039–4044. Available from: https://pubmed.ncbi.nlm.nih.gov/18657857/
70. Lerner A, Chezar A, Haddad M, Kaufman H, Rozen N, Stein H. Complications encountered while using thin-wire-hybrid-external fixation modular frames for fracture fixation: A retrospective clinical analysis and possible support for "damage control orthopaedic surgery". Injury. 2005;36(5):590–8.
71. Clasper JC, Cannon LB, Stapley SA, Taylor VM, Watkins PE. Fluid accumulation and the rapid spread of bacteria in the pathogenesis of external fixator pin track infection. Injury. 2001;32(5):377–81.
72. Santy J, Newton-Triggs L. A survey of current practice in skeletal pin site management. J Orthop Nurs. 2006;10(4):198–205.
73. Qi Y, Ding Y, Liu B, Xu Y. TCM treatment of allergy induced by stainless steel implants for tibiofibular fracture: A case report. Allergol Sel [Internet] 2019 Jan 1 [cited 2021 Nov 21];3(01):15–21. Available from: https://www.dustri.com/article_response_page.html?artId=186279&doi=10.5414/ALX02095E&L=0
74. Chiewchalermsri C, Sompornrattanaphan M, Wongsa C, Thongngarm T. Chlorhexidine Allergy: Current Challenges and Future Prospects. J Asthma Allergy [Internet]. 2020 Mar [cited 2021 Nov 21];Volume 13:127–33. Available from: /pmc/articles/PMC7069565/.
75. Wittczak T, Dudek W, Walusiak-Skorupa J, Swierczynska-Machura D, Palczynski C. Chlorhexidine–still an underestimated allergic hazard for health care professionals. Occup Med (Chic Ill) [Internet]. 2013 Jun 1 [cited 2021 Nov 21];63(4):301–5. Available from: https://academic.oup.com/occmed/article/63/4/301/1430007
76. Rose MA, Garcez T, Savic S, Garvey LH. Chlorhexidine allergy in the perioperative setting: a narrative review. Br J Anaesth [Internet] 2019 Jul 1 [cited 2021 Nov 21];123(1):e95–103. Available from: https://linkinghub.elsevier.com/retrieve/pii/S0007091219300807
77. Bhardwaj P, Bekeny JC, Zolper EG, Nigam M, Sher SR. Chlorhexidine hypersensitivity. Plast Reconstr Surg–Glob Open [Internet]. 2020 Aug 14 [cited 2021 Nov 21];Publish Ah. Available from: https://journals.lww.com/prsgo/Fulltext/2020/08000/Chlorhexidine_Hypersensitivity__A_Case_Report_of.10.aspx
78. Sáenz-Jalón M, Sarabia-Cobo CM, Roscales Bartolome E, Santiago Fernández M, Vélez B, Escudero M, et al. A randomized clinical trial on the use of antiseptic solutions for the pin-site Care of External Fixators: chlorhexidine–alcohol versus povidone–iodine. J Trauma Nurs [Internet]. 2020;27(3):146–50. Available from: https://journals.lww.com/10.1097/JTN.0000000000000503
79. Morgan-Jones RL, Burgert S, Richardson JB. Arthroscopic debridement of external fixator pin tracts. Injury [Internet]. 1998 Jan [cited 2021 Nov 23];29(1):41–42. Available from: https://pubmed.ncbi.nlm.nih.gov/9659480/
80. Saini A, Grey J, Venter R, Ferreira N. Hydrosurgical debridement of Grade VI external fixator pin site infection. J Limb Lengthening Reconstr [Internet]. 2022 [cited 2023 Aug 14];8(1):84. Available from: https://journals.lww.com/jllr/fulltext/2022/08010/hydrosurgical_debridement_of_grade_vi_external.14.aspx
81. Iobst CA, Liu RW. A systematic review of incidence of pin track infections associated with external fixation. J Limb Lengthen Reconstr. 2016;2(1):6–16. https://doi.org/10.4103/2455-3719.182570.
82. Kazmers NH, Fragomen AT, Robert Rozbruch S. Prevention of pin site infection in external fixation: a review of the literature. Strat Traum Limb Recon. 2016;11:75–85. https://doi.org/10.1007/s11751-016-0256-4.
83. Iobst CA. Pin-track infections: Past, present, and future. J Limb Lengthen Reconstr. 2017;3(2):78–84. https://doi.org/10.4103/jllr.jllr_17_17.
84. Journal of limb lengthening and reconstruction; special supplement, October 2022, https://www.jlimblengthrecon.org/showBackIssue.asp?issn=2455-3719;year=2022;volume=8;issue=3;month=October;supp=Y
85. Ferguson D, Harwood P, Allgar V, Roy A, Foster P, Taylor M, Moulder E, Sharma H. The PINS Trial: a prospective randomized clinical trial comparing a traditional versus an emollient skincare regimen for the care of pin-sites in patients with circular frames. Bone Joint J. 103-B:2. https://doi.org/10.1302/0301-620X.103B2.BJJ-2020-0680.R1.
86. Ting J, Moulder E, Muir R, Barron E, Hadland Y, Sharma H. The incidence of deep infection following lower leg circular frame fixation with minimum of 1-year follow-up from frame removal. Strategies Trauma Limb Reconstr. 2022;17(2):88–91. https://doi.org/10.5005/jp-journals-10,080-1558.
87. Hemant K Sharma, Nando Ferreira. International pin site consensus; fourth Combined Congress of the ASAMI-BR & ILLRS societies combined ASAMI international, 27–30 Aug 2019, Liverpool.
88. Sharma HK, Ferreira N, McDaid C, McNally M. International Pin Site Consensus: Time to develop common grounds and collaborate? J Limb Lengthen Reconstr. 2022;8:S1–2. https://doi.org/10.4103/jllr.jllr_30_22.

Fixator Assisted Nailing and Plating

Chang-Wug Oh

Introduction

Angular and/or rotational deformities of the lower extremity can be due to congenital, acquired or developmental etiologies and can be seen in patients with fracture malunion, skeletal dysplasia, metabolic disorders, and other clinical entities. Lower limb deformities often affect the axial alignment of the lower extremity and are especially important regarding mechanical forces sustained across articular cartilage of the weight bearing joints during ambulation. Coronal deformities around the knee, such as distal femur or proximal tibia, increase medial and lateral load, which theoretically could lead to osteoarthritis in later life. Therefore, realignment by corrective osteotomy is often required in the deformities of the lower extremities. Restoration of normal mechanical alignment may decrease pain, improve function, and slow or prevent further degeneration of adjacent joints [1].

Either closing or opening wedge osteotomy has been used to achieve an acute correction of angular deformity. These traditional methods are commonly combined with the use of either an intramedullary nail or plate. They usually require extensive surgical exposure with soft-tissue stripping, which may increase the amount of bleeding, the need for bone grafts, the risk of infection, and the healing time of the osteotomy site. These techniques are difficult to use in order to perform precise deformity corrections during an operation. Moreover, it is more technically challenging to perform in the deformities of an oblique plane. Deformity correction often necessitates translation of the bony fragments, which may be very difficult with the opening or closing wedge technique. When intact cortical contact is lost, it may be difficult to maintain stability during internal fixation. Then, the planned correction may not be achieved during the fixation after osteotomy, especially when using a free-hand technique [2]. When an optimal correction is not achieved, additional surgery is inevitable to adjust the further wanted alignment. A high rate of complications has been reported by traditional osteotomy techniques, including nonunion, inaccurate correction of the deformity, implant irritation, loss of correction, and reoperation [3].

External fixation has been used to correct complex deformities in the lower extremities. Either a circular or unilateral external fixator can be chosen to achieve a successful alignment, either acutely or gradually. An external fixator has advantages for controllability until achieving the desired amount of correction and maintaining the segments until satisfactory healing of the osteotomy [4]. Moreover, its benefit of performing distraction osteogenesis simultaneously enables correction of deformity as well as potential lengthening [5]. The recent improvement of hexapod external fixators has given the concept of placement of a virtual hinge and the ability to re-run correction programs, which is an extremely versatile option to achieve an accurate deformity correction [6]. However, until the complete healing of the osteotomy site, it is uncomfortable for patients to wear the bulky external fixator for a considerable time. External fixator pins and wires tether soft tissue and frequently cause pin site irritation and deep infection. Complications are not uncommon, including delayed bone healing, fractures, or recurrence of deformity after frame removal [7].

Recently, hybrid techniques for correcting the deformity have been implemented to use the advantages of both, internal and external fixation techniques, such as fixator-assisted plating (FAP) or fixator-assisted nailing (FAN). As these techniques are performed with a minimally invasive procedure, patients have the advantage of not having to wear an external fixator for a long duration and starting early rehabilitation with less restriction of daily life activities [8].

This hybrid technique is based on the concept that the desired correction is obtained and maintained intraopera-

C.-W. Oh (✉)
Department of Orthopedic Surgery, School of Medicine, Kyungpook National University, Kyungpook National University Hospital, Daegu, Republic of Korea
e-mail: cwoh@knu.ac.kr

tively using an external fixator and stabilized by the internal implants until the bone heals. Temporary external fixation has the role of correcting the deformity as well as maintaining the preoperative planned osteotomy accurately until the end of internal implant fixation. After external fixation, the corrected alignment is confirmed under fluoroscopy without losing the desired reduction.

Internal fixation is important in both the types of implant hardware and the techniques used to place them. From a biomechanical standpoint, intramedullary (IM) nailing is generally recommended due to the benefit of a load-sharing device. Biologically, it has an advantage of promoting bone healing without the need for a bone graft since it can be fixed percutaneously without the violation of surrounding soft tissue and providing local bone graft during intramedullary reaming [2]. However, IM nailing may have potential disadvantages such as violating the growth plates, damaging the articular cartilage, and being of limited value in patients with small-diameter medullary canals [9]. Therefore, the choice of plate is often advantageous in the young pediatric populations. Traditional plate fixation required extensive surgical exposure and periosteal stripping, which may interfere with bone healing biology. Currently, minimally invasive plate osteosynthesis (MIPO) or submuscular plating techniques have become popular in fracture management, which preserves the periosteum and soft tissue around the osteotomy as in the principle of closed IM nailing [10]. It overcomes the complications of the conventional open technique, resulting in a small amount of blood loss, a low infection rate, and a high rate of bone healing. This less invasive method is commonly used for internal fixation after corrective osteotomy. Compared to the conventional nonlocking plate/screw system, the locking plate/screw system provides more stable fixation. Due to the fixed-angle stabilizing mechanism, a locking plate does not have to precisely contact the underlying bone while stabilizing the segments without pulling the bone to the plate. Because of these advantages of the fixation construct, the locking plate is frequently used to correct pediatric limb deformities when the IM nail is not a viable option [8, 9, 11].

Preoperative Planning

Preoperative assessment and planning of deformity are very important. Patients must be evaluated for malalignment and limb length discrepancy with standing orthoroentgenograms in both the frontal and sagittal planes. The center of rotation of angulation (CORA) should be noted in coronal and sagittal angular deformities. Besides a thorough clinical exam, documenting the rotational profile of the lower extremity, a CT scan is an important tool to help confirm and quantify the contribution of the rotational malalignment from the femoral and tibial segments. Either by the use of paper tracing or computer-based tracing methods, the operative procedure should be simulated preoperatively.

The location of the osteotomy should be decided after considering the CORA, the shape of the osteotomy, the placement of the temporary external fixation, the final construct of fixation, and bone healing. The temporary external fixation needs to consider the location of Schanz pins or wires attached to the external fixator, the type of external fixator (mono-planar or circular), the desired location of the internal implant, and the adjacent neuro-vascular structures. The pin location should not disturb the anticipated site of the plate or IM nail. The osteotomy may need to be placed as close to the CORA as possible.

Preoperative planning also includes the choice of an adequate internal implant for definitive fixation, such as an IM nail or plate. Several factors are important to consider, including the age of the patient, the size of the bone, the level of deformity, the status of the growth plate, and the diameter of the intramedullary canal. In pediatric deformities, the open physeal plate should be protected by the damage of an IM nail or screws. Over-reaming of a small medullary canal may disturb the bone healing as well as the fixation with the IM nailing. When the IM nail is selected, the diameter and length of the IM nail to be used should be estimated. The possible use and location of the interference (or poller) screws is to be determined [12]. Mostly, plates are commonly chosen as the final internal implants with pediatric anatomical restrictions. Anatomical plates are well suited for juxta-articular or metaphyseal deformities, while straight plates are optimal for diaphyseal deformities. [13]

Fixator-Assisted Nailing (FAN)

FAN has become one of the more familiar techniques to correct femoral deformities. Retrograde nailing may be an optimal implant in the deformities of the distal femur when the physeal plate is already closed. Antegrade nailing is commonly used for proximal or diaphyseal deformities. (Fig. 11.1) The patient is usually placed supine or laterally on a radiolucent table in order to check the intraoperative alignment from the hip to the ankle using fluoroscopy. If needed to compare with the contralateral side as the guide of normal alignment, both extremities may be draped together.

Prior to performing the osteotomy, it is necessary to locate the optimal sites to insert the pins of the external fixator. One or two pairs of external fixator pins (1 distal and 1 proximal) are inserted from the lateral side. It is important to place the pins away from the path of the intramedullary nail. In particular, the site of nail insertion should have sufficient space in the coronal or sagittal plane. It is preferred to insert these

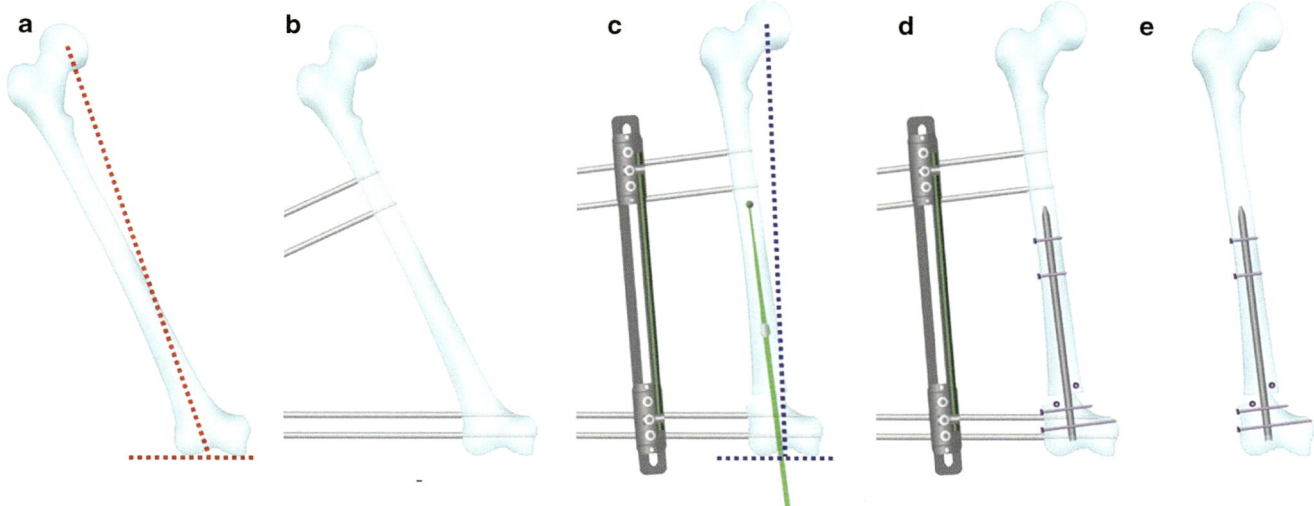

Fig. 11.1 FAN procedure of distal femur deformity
In a valgus deformity of the distal femur (**a**), Schanz pins are fixed at the lateral aspect of the distal condyle and proximal shaft. Then, the osteotomy is made at the distal metaphyseal area (**b**). Then, the desired amount of angular correction is made with the use of the external fixator. Poller screws are often inserted in order to guide the reamer and the IM nail (**c**). The retrograde IM nail is inserted and locked proximally and distally while the external fixator maintains the achieved correction (**d**). Then, the external fixator is removed as the IM nail secures the achieved correction (**e**)

pins in a parallel fashion, which may be advantageous to maintain or correct the rotational alignment.

Then, the osteotomy is performed through a mini incision, preferably by the multiple drill hole technique or with the use of the focal dome drill guide. The medial or lateral edges of the osteotomy are completed with an osteotome. The osteotome can be used to perform the translation, if desired. At the osteotomy, it may work as the leverage to push the cortex. Alternatively, the pins of an external fixator may be used as a joystick to produce the translation manually. The angular and/or rotational correction is then performed either manually or more accurately with the use of the external fixator. The accuracy of the correction may be confirmed under the image intensifier. When the desired correction is achieved, the external fixator is "locked" by tightening all connections and the surgeon can then proceed with the nailing. An interference or blocking screw may be needed to guide the IM nail as well as to prevent loss of the correction [12]. The interference screw may be inserted before or after reaming. When an interference screw is inserted before the reaming, the reamer may collide the pre-existed screw. If the location of the screw is placed away from the desired location, there is a risk of fracture or overcorrection of deformity by impeding of the nail passage. When it is inserted after reaming, the path of the nail is already set and the interference screw may not work to achieve the wanted correction. After confirming the adequate alignment, the nail with the adequate size and length is inserted and locked with proximal and distal interlocking screws. Then, the external fixator is removed at the end of internal fixation. An electrocautery test may be used to confirm the alignment of the lower limb before removing the half-pins of the external fixator. When the proximal physis is closed, FAN can be performed on the tibial deformities similarly using an antegrade nailing technique. In contrast to the femur, the fibula will almost always need to be osteotomized to allow the desired correction of angular deformity. (Fig. 11.2a–f).

When the limb length discrepancy is present, the external fixator remains in place as a distraction device to lengthen the bone, as the process of lengthening over the IM nail [5, 14]. A recent advanced lengthening nail may simultaneously continue the lengthening procedure, after FAN to correct the deformity [15].

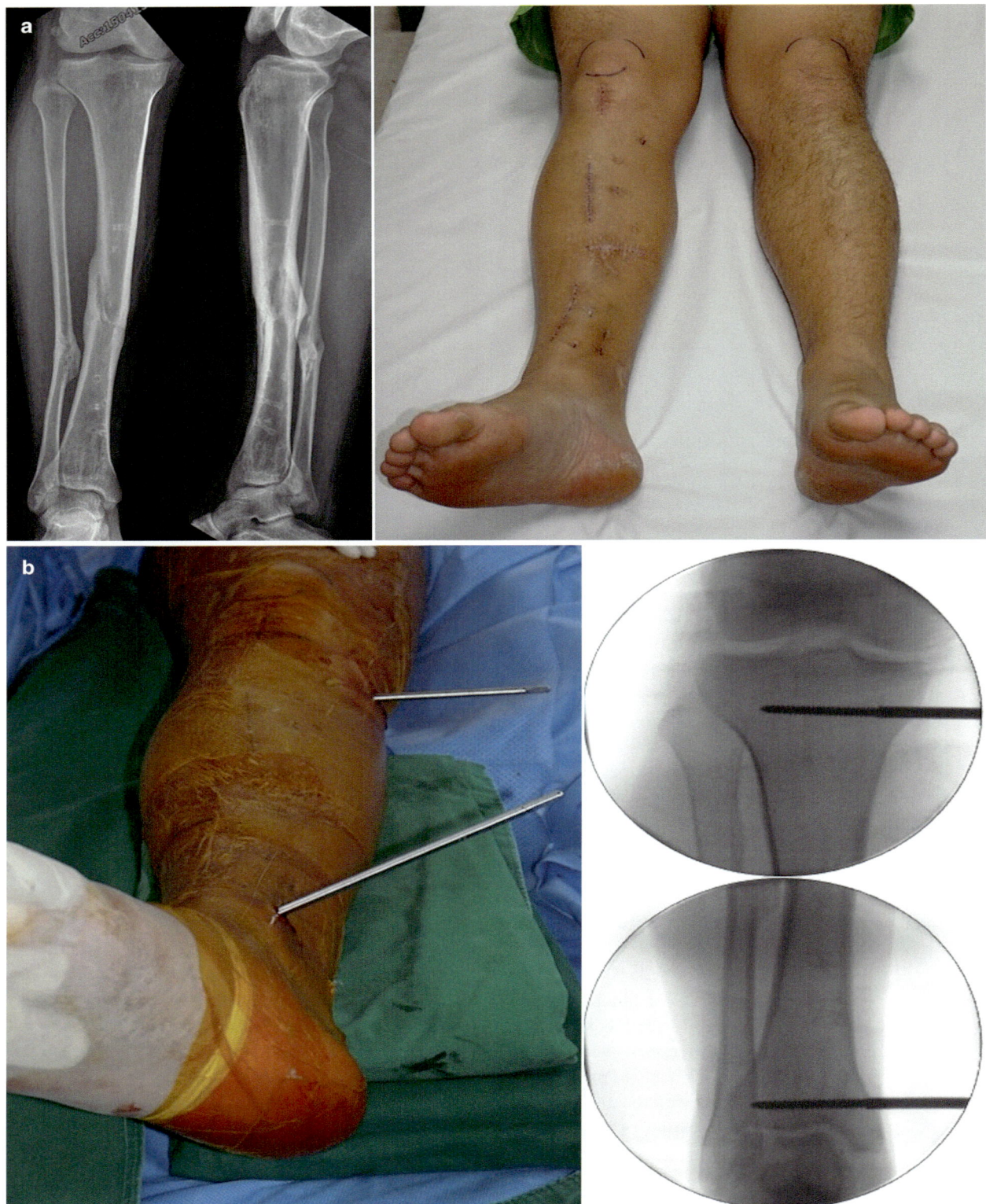

Fig. 11.2 FAN to correct rotational malalignment
A 17-year-old boy had a deformity of external rotation in the right tibia after suffering the fracture. Note the difference in foot position (**a**). Schanz pins were fixed at the medial aspect of the proximal condyle and distal malleolus (**b**). An osteotomy was made at the midshaft, followed by the rotational correction into the desired alignment (**c**). Then, IM nailing was performed while the external fixator maintained the achieved correction. In the sagittal plane, Schanz pins were placed posteriorly to the nail trajectory in order to not conflict with the insertion of the IM nail (**d**). Post-operatively, a satisfactory reduction was gained after fixator-assisted nailing (**e**). Successful healing was achieved, with a similar rotational alignment compared with the non-injured side (**f**)

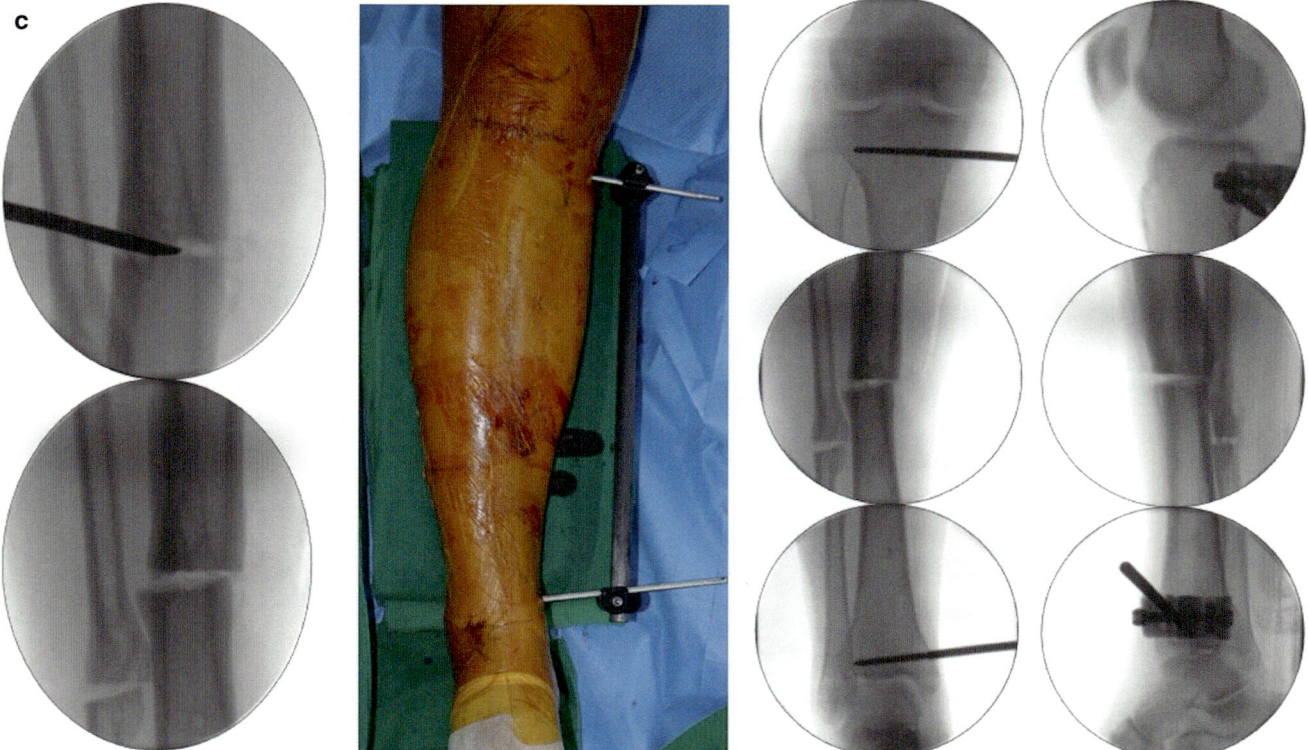

Fig. 11.2 (continued)

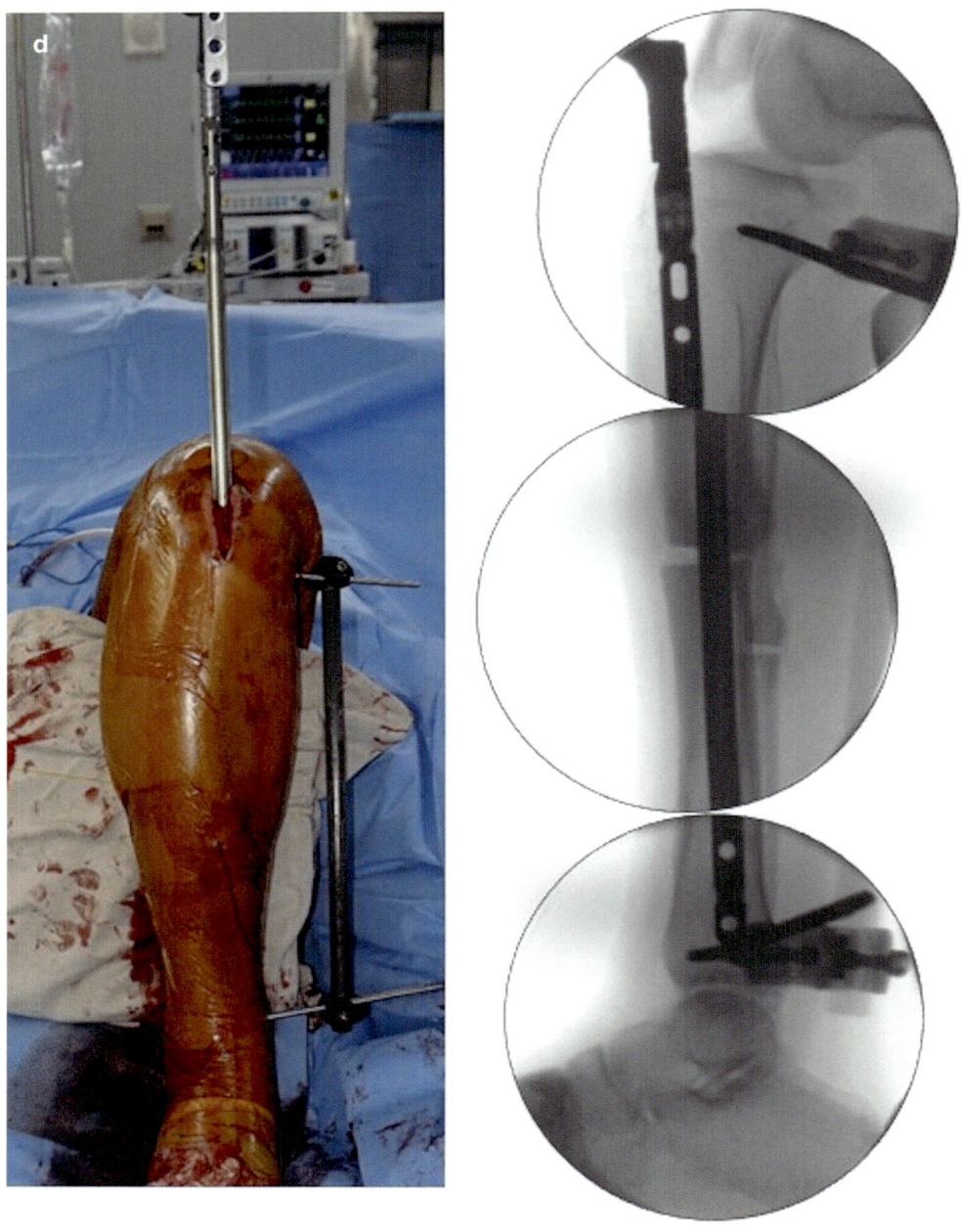

Fig. 11.2 (continued)

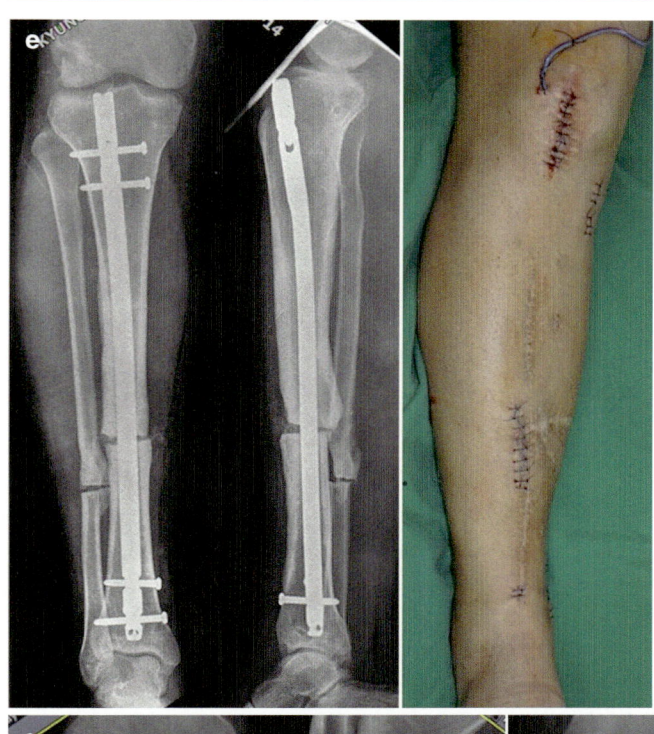
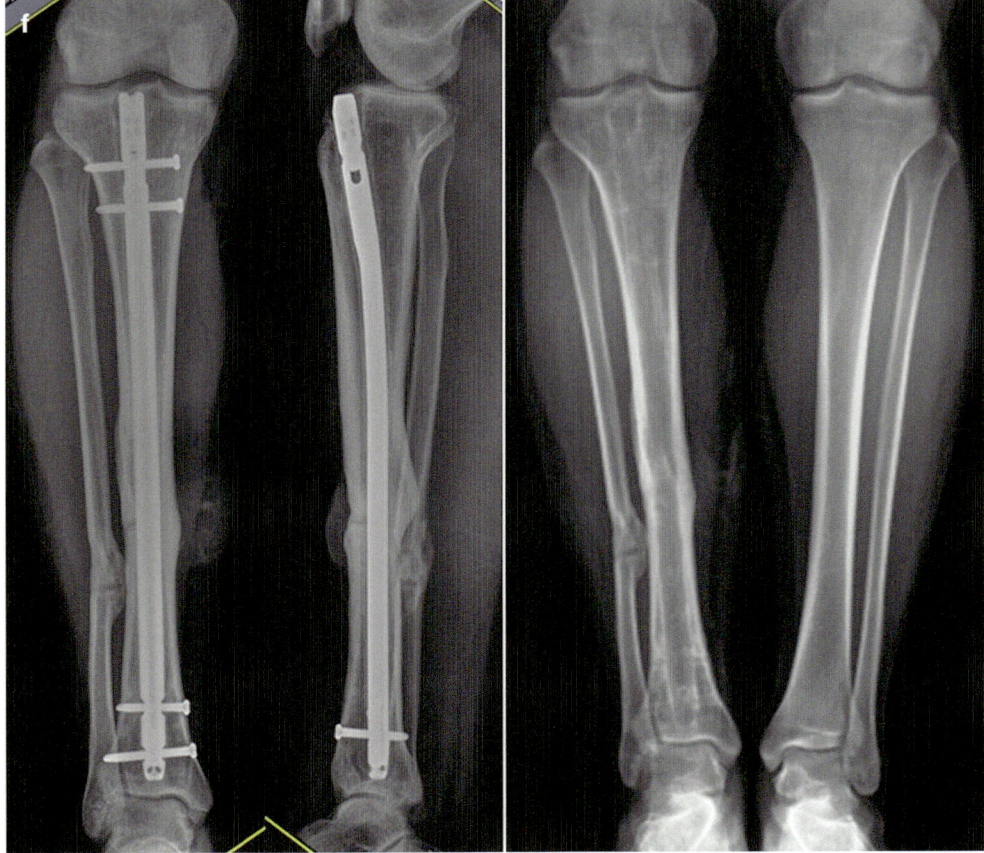

Fig. 11.2 (continued)

Fixator-Assisted Plating (FAP)

Compared with the FAN technique, FAP may have broader indications for correcting pediatric deformities. (Fig. 11.3) When the diameter of the marrow canal is smaller than that of the smallest diameter available IM nail, the plate can be an alternative implant to fix. Also, the growth plate can be preserved by the use of the plate [8, 9, 13].

Surgical preparation is similar to FAN, which should allow the clear C-arm images to define the procedure of osteotomies and correction. It is also important to find adequate locations for the pins of the external fixator before the osteotomy. It is necessary to consider the anticipated location of the plate. In the distal femoral deformities, the author prefers to fix on the medial aspect of the femur as the anatomical locking plate will be fixed on the lateral aspect; one is placed at the medial femoral condyle, perpendicular to the femoral shaft, and the other is placed at the distal diaphysis (about 3–5 cm above the adductor tubercle), with care taken not to damage the femoral vasculature. The descending geniculate artery, a branch from the superficial femoral artery, is a possible bleeding source when pins are inserted without the open incision. The medial pin should be fixed very carefully, around 5 cm above the adductor tubercle, which is the crossing point of the arterial branch at the medial aspect of the distal femur. In cases where rotational correction is required, two pins may be inserted parallel to each other, in order to easily measure the amount of surgical derotation; one at the proximal one-third level and one at the distal one-third level.

Plate fixation is performed in the fashion of the submuscular plating technique. In the distal femur, a lateral parapatellar approach is commonly used. With a 5–6 cm longitudinal skin incision along the lateral border of the patella, the lateral aspect of the femoral condyle was exposed to ensure space for the plate fixation. Through this window, the level of the osteotomy can be chosen mostly at the meta-diaphyseal junction of the distal femur. At the distal part of the plate, it may be necessary to create a distal fragment of sufficient size in order to fix at least 5 or 6 locking screws. With care taken to avoid denuding the soft tissue, the osteotomy is completed. The length of the plate is chosen according to the availability of proximal screw fixation (at least 3 or 4 screws for fixation, alternatively with empty holes in the plate). The proximal window is made at the lateral aspect of the anticipated proximal end of the plate.

After opening the lateral or medial side of the osteotomy, angular correction is achieved manually or by joystick-handling of the medially inserted pins. In the case of rotational correction, the proximal and distal pins are aligned at the desired magnitude of rotational alignment in each fragment. The amount of rotation may be estimated by the angle between two pins. When the desired correction is achieved, the proximal and distal pins are temporarily locked by an external fixator.

Confirming the corrected alignment using fluoroscopic examination, the chosen plate is inserted through the submuscular tunnel, followed by the completion of screw fixation. Thereafter, the external fixator and pre-inserted two medial pins are removed. (Fig. 11.4a–e).

A similar FAP technique is applicable to the tibia deformities [16]. It is preferred to insert external fixator pins at the anterior aspect so that the next step of plate fixation is not disrupted. After the osteotomy, the desired alignment is achieved by using the inserted pins. (Figs. 11.5a–e and

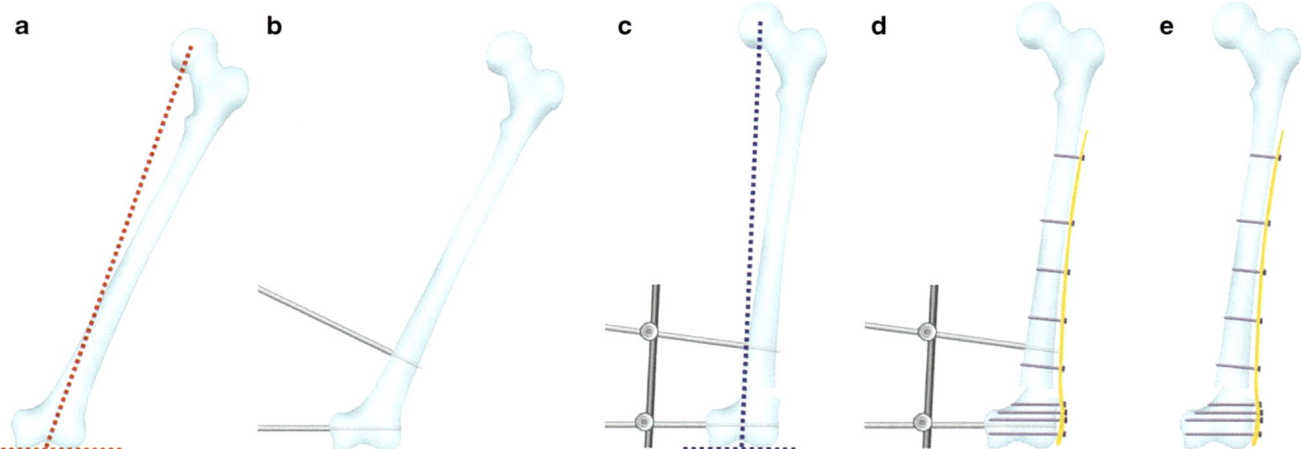

Fig. 11.3 FAP procedure of distal femur deformity
In a valgus deformity of the distal femur (**a**), Schanz pins are fixed at the medial aspect of the distal condyle and distal shaft. Then, the osteotomy is made at the distal metaphyseal area (**b**). With the use of the external fixator, the desired alignment is achieved with angular correction and translation (**c**). While the external fixator maintains the achieved correction, the locking plate is fixed to the lateral aspect of the femur (**d**). Then, the external fixator is removed as the locking plate secures the achieved correction (**e**)

Fig. 11.4 FAP procedure to correct the tibia malunion
An 8-year-old boy suffered a malunion of the right tibia, showing valgus and posterior angulation (**a**). After performing the osteotomy of the previous fracture site, a satisfactory alignment was achieved using the external fixator (**b**). A locking plate was inserted on the medial side of the tibia with the minimally invasive technique, while the alignment was maintained by the external fixator (**c**). Postoperative X-rays showed a satisfactory alignment after FAP (**d**). At 4 months, successful healing was achieved (**e**)

11.6a–d) Accurate alignment is maintained by locking the external fixator to the pins. Then, plate fixation is performed percutaneously on the medial side of the tibia or submuscularly on the lateral side of the tibia, according to the soft tissue condition or the location of the osteotomy [17].

When it is needed, lengthening over the plate procedure may be continued, remaining the external fixator in place as a distraction device to lengthen the bone [18] (Fig. 11.7a–e).

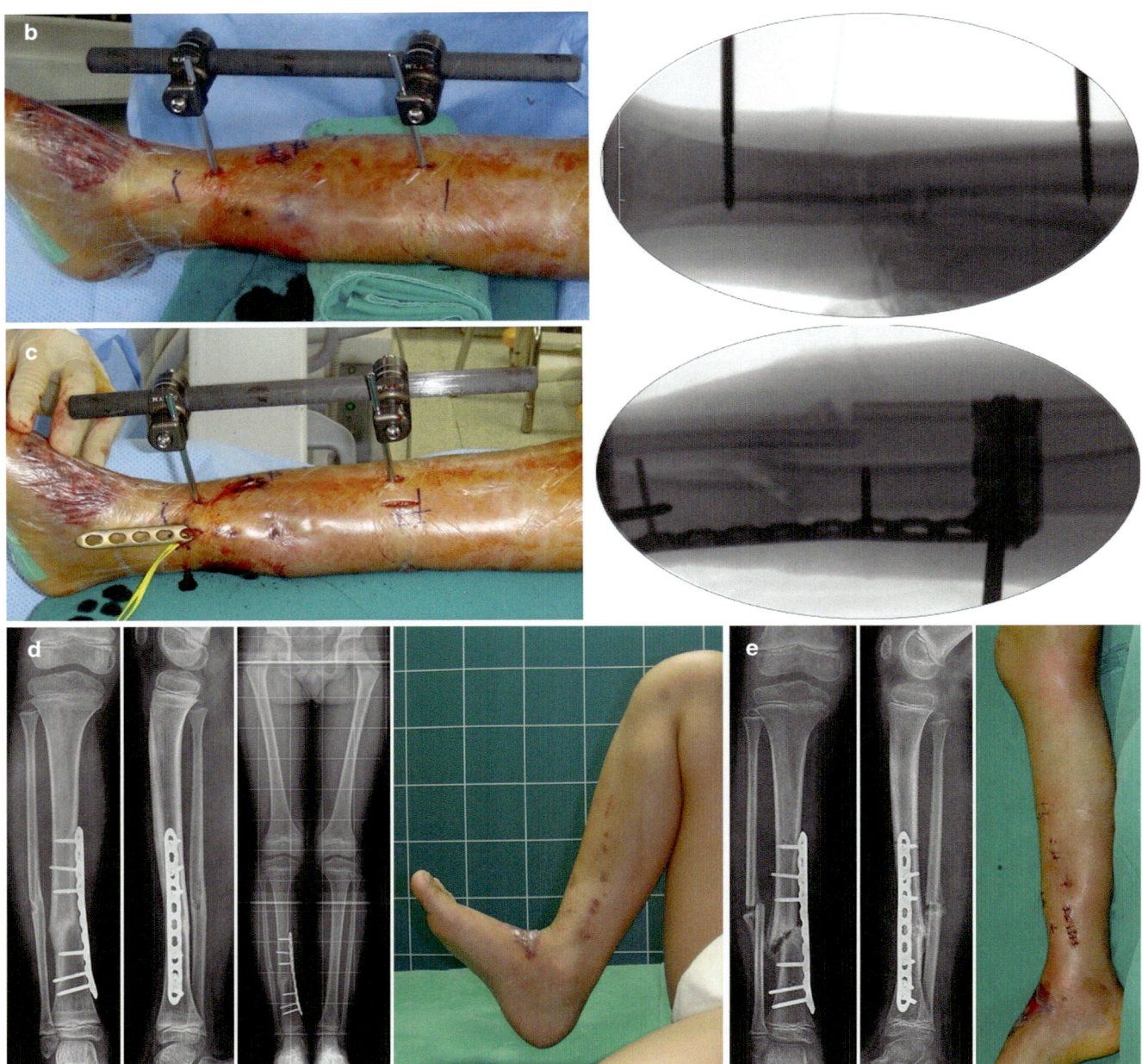

Fig. 11.4 (continued)

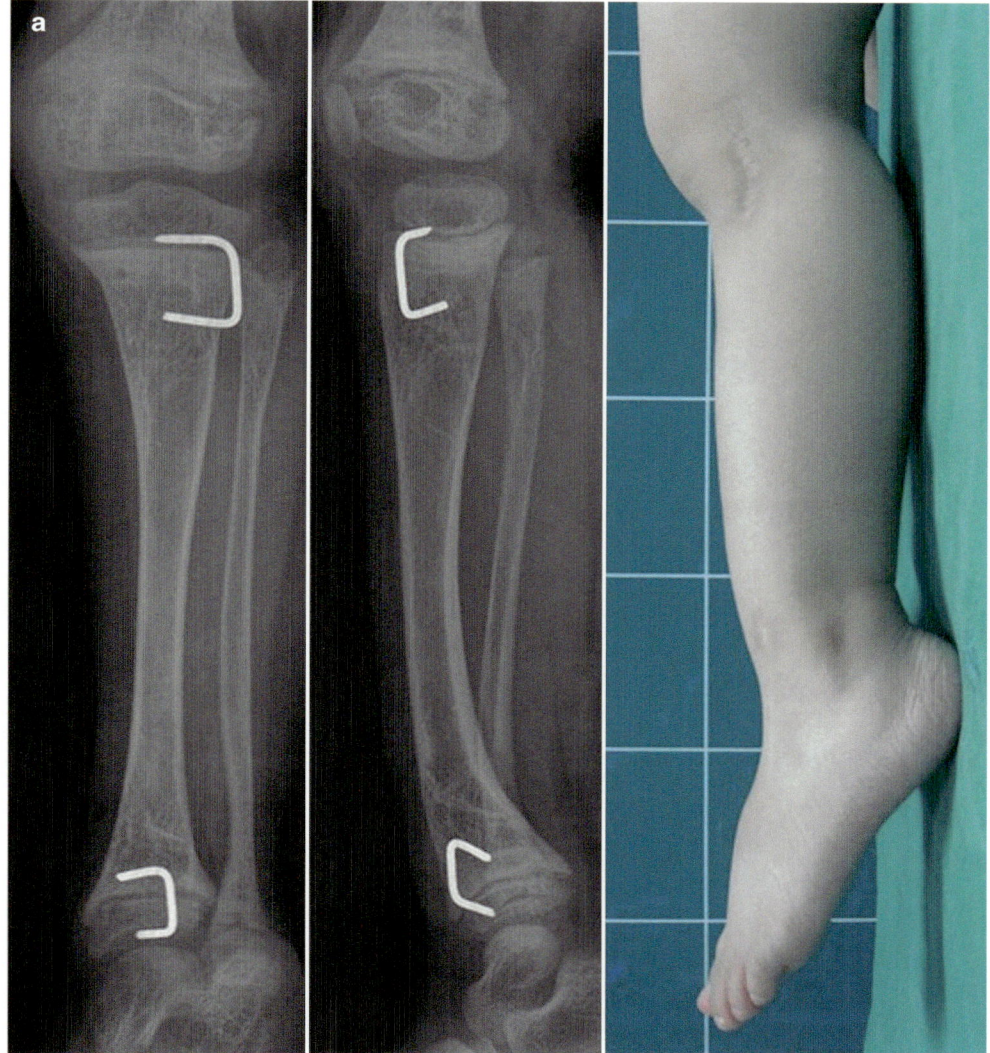

Fig. 11.5 FAP procedure to correct the deformity of tibia
A 6-year-old girl with Vit-D resistant rickets showed a deformity of the tibia, showing internal rotation and anterior angulation (**a**). After the osteotomy at the distal tibia, a satisfactory alignment was gained using the external fixator (**b**). Minimally invasive plating was performed on the medial side of the tibia with the maintenance of alignment by the external fixator (**c**). A satisfactory alignment was achieved after FAP (**d**). At 6 months, successful healing was achieved (**e**)

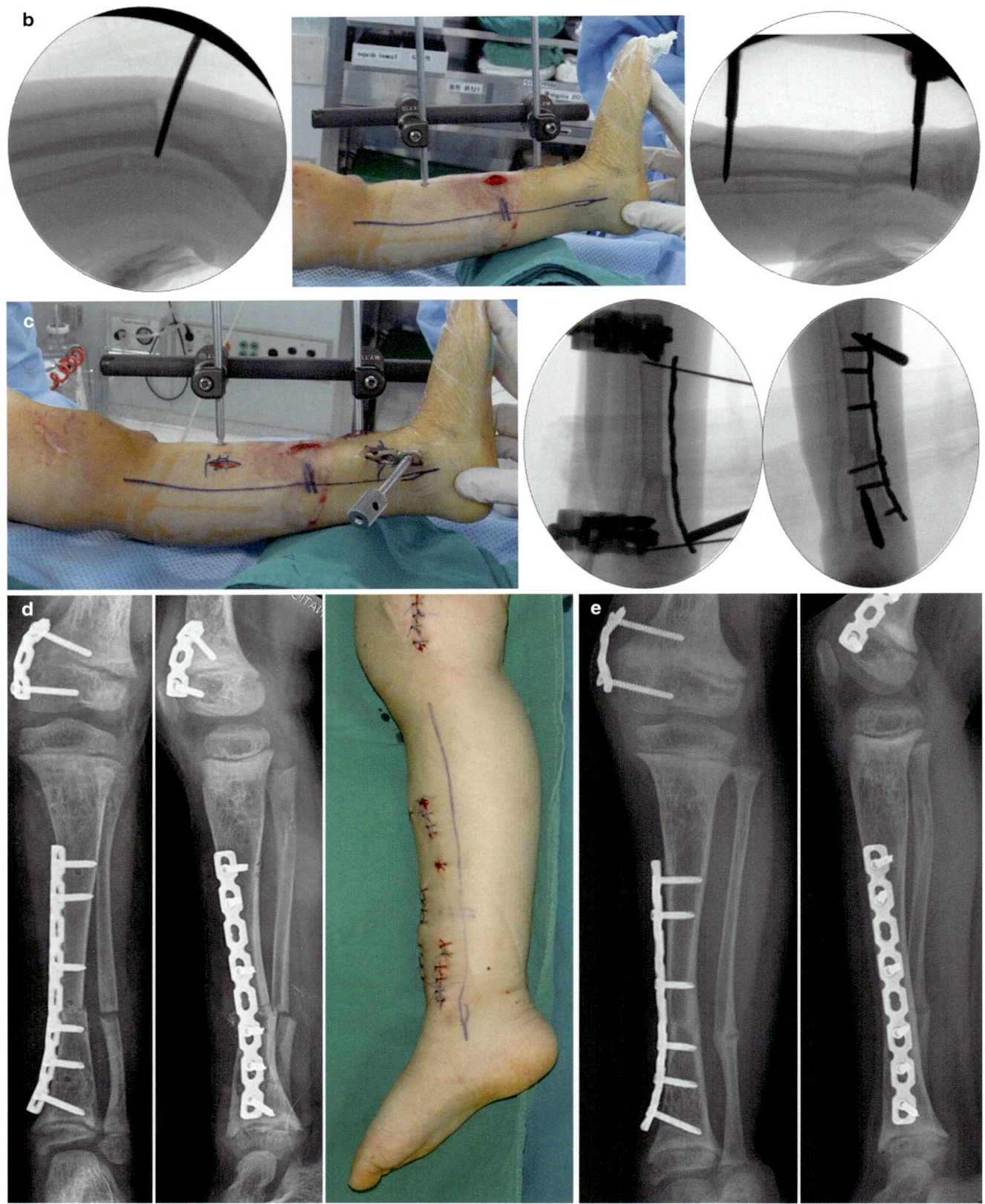

Fig. 11.5 (continued)

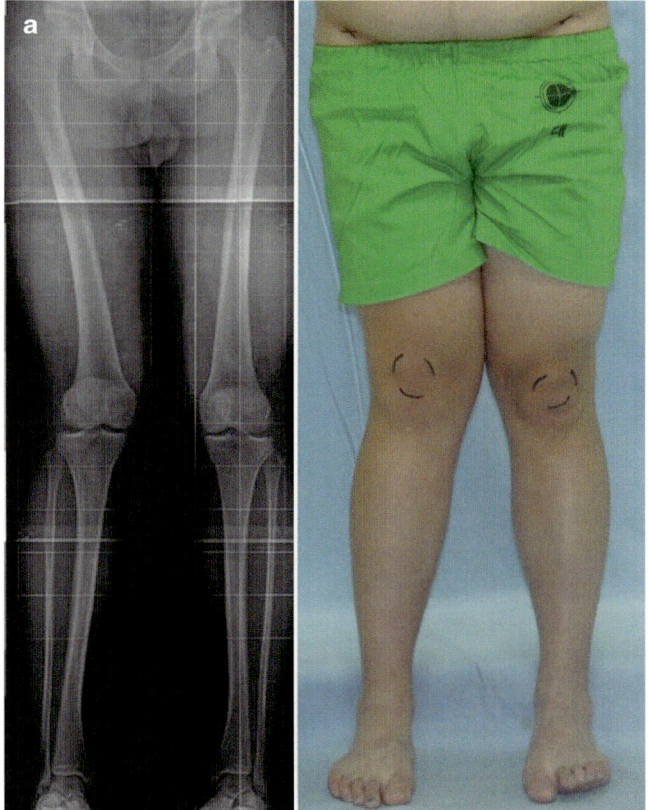

Fig. 11.6 FAP procedure to correct the deformity of distal femur
A 17-year-old boy had a moderate valgus deformity of the distal femur after a previous physeal injury. Note the lateral deviation of the mechanical axis (dotted line), compared with the non-injured limb (**a**). Schanz pins are fixed at the medial aspect of the distal femoral shaft and condyle, respectively. Then, the osteotomy is made at the distal metaphyseal area. After correcting the desired alignment, Schanz pins were locked by an external fixator. Note that an electrocautery cord was positioned at the middle of the intercondylar notch (**b**). A minimally invasive technique was used to insert and fix the anatomical locking plate. A postoperative radiograph showed satisfactory correction of deformity (**c**). At 1 year postoperatively, successful healing was achieved, and the mechanical axis was maintained (**d**)

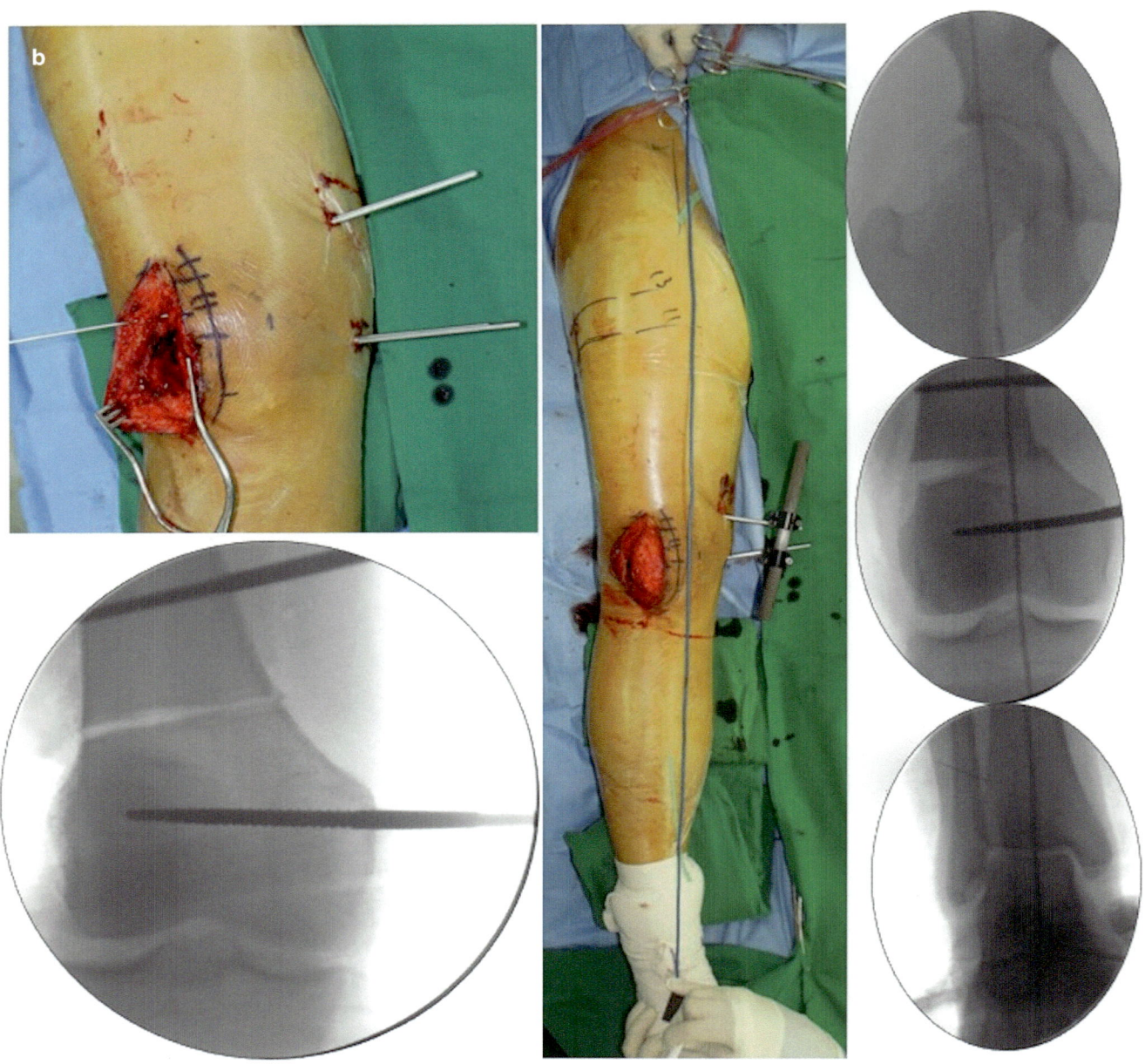

Fig. 11.6 (continued)

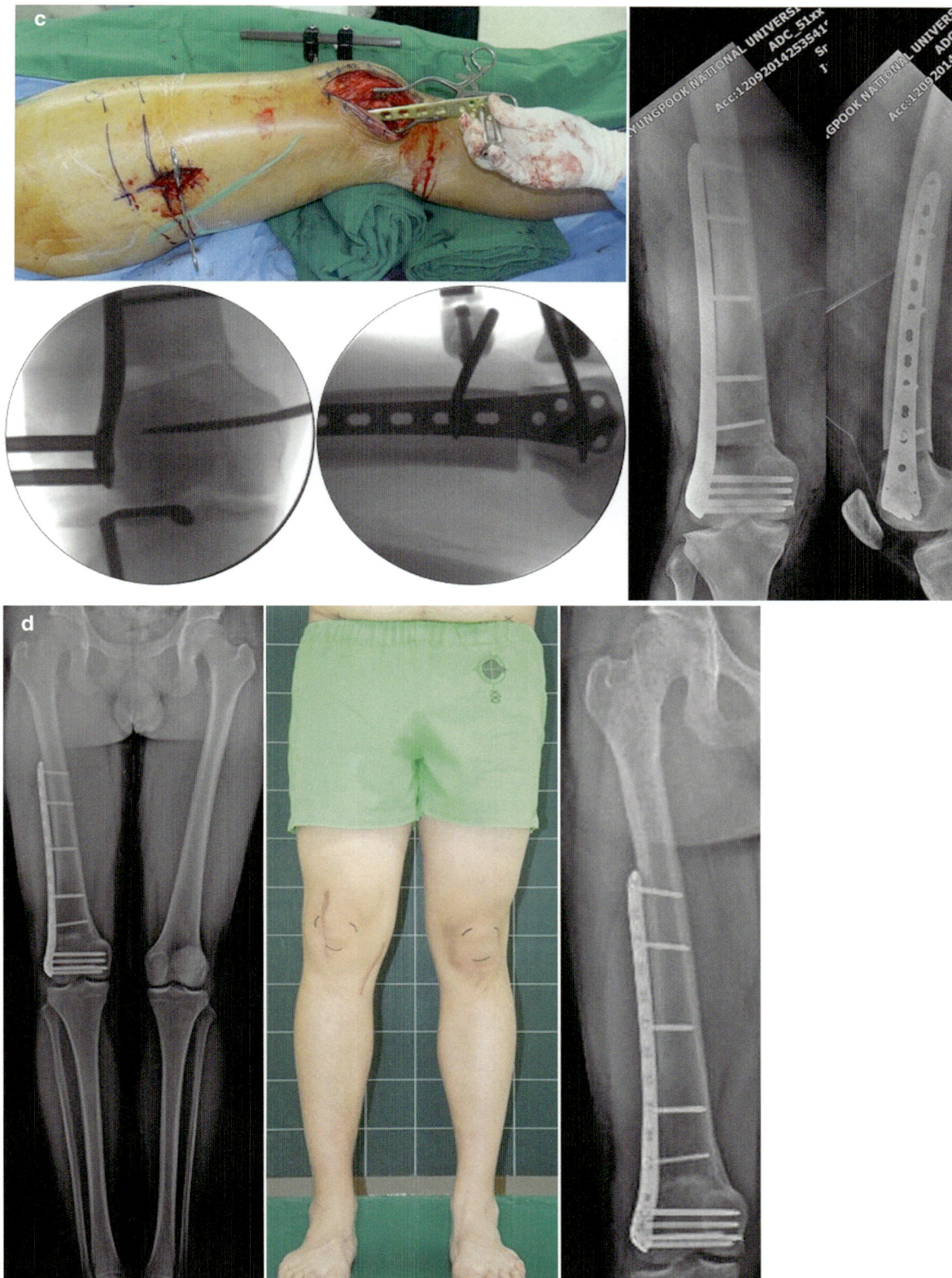

Fig. 11.6 (continued)

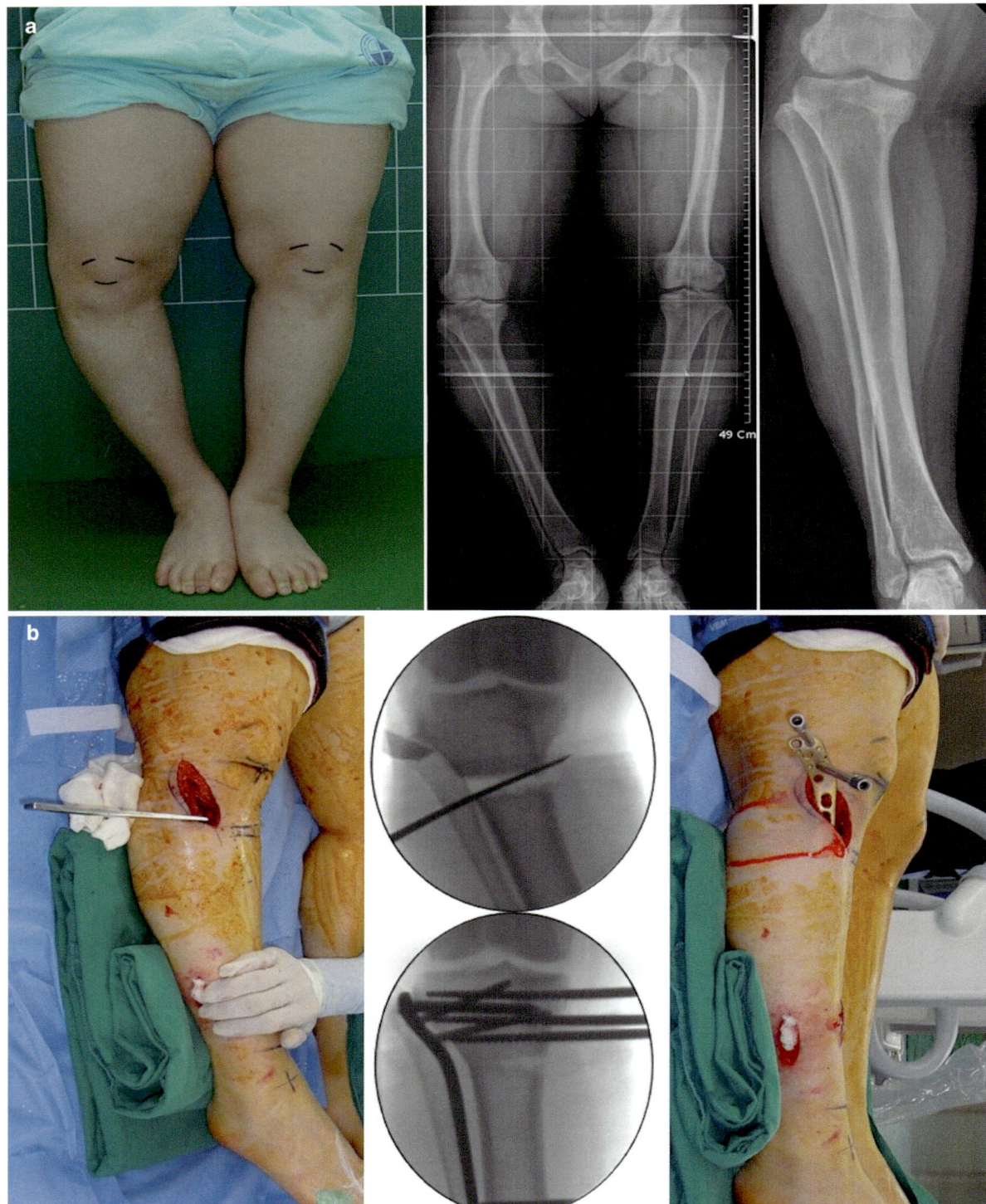

Fig. 11.7 FAP followed by tibia lengthening in the deformity of proximal tibia

A 17-year-old girl suffering from rickets showed a moderate varus deformity of the tibia (**a**). After the osteotomy was made at the proximal tibia, angular correction was achieved by the assistance of an external fixator, followed by the fixation of the locking plate (**b**). Lengthening with the plate procedure was performed, with acute correction of the tibia deformity. Note that the monolateral external fixator was fixed medially to lengthen the tibia (**c**). After achieving the target length of 4.5 cm, screws were placed in the distal segment and the external fixator was removed (**d**). Six months later, the distraction callus had healed with a successful correction of malalignment in both legs (**e**). Note that FAP procedure made a successful healing in both femurs

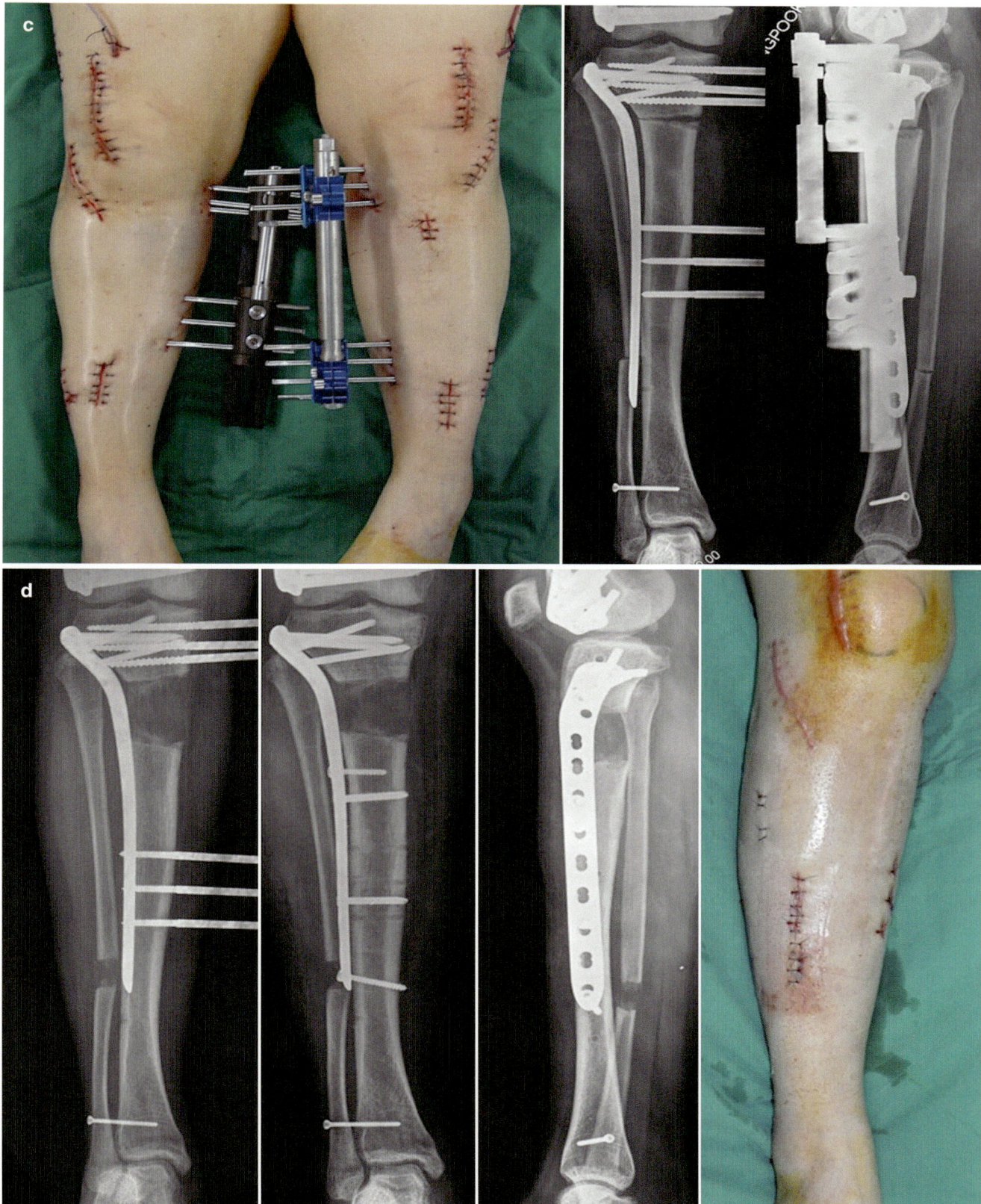

Fig. 11.7 (continued)

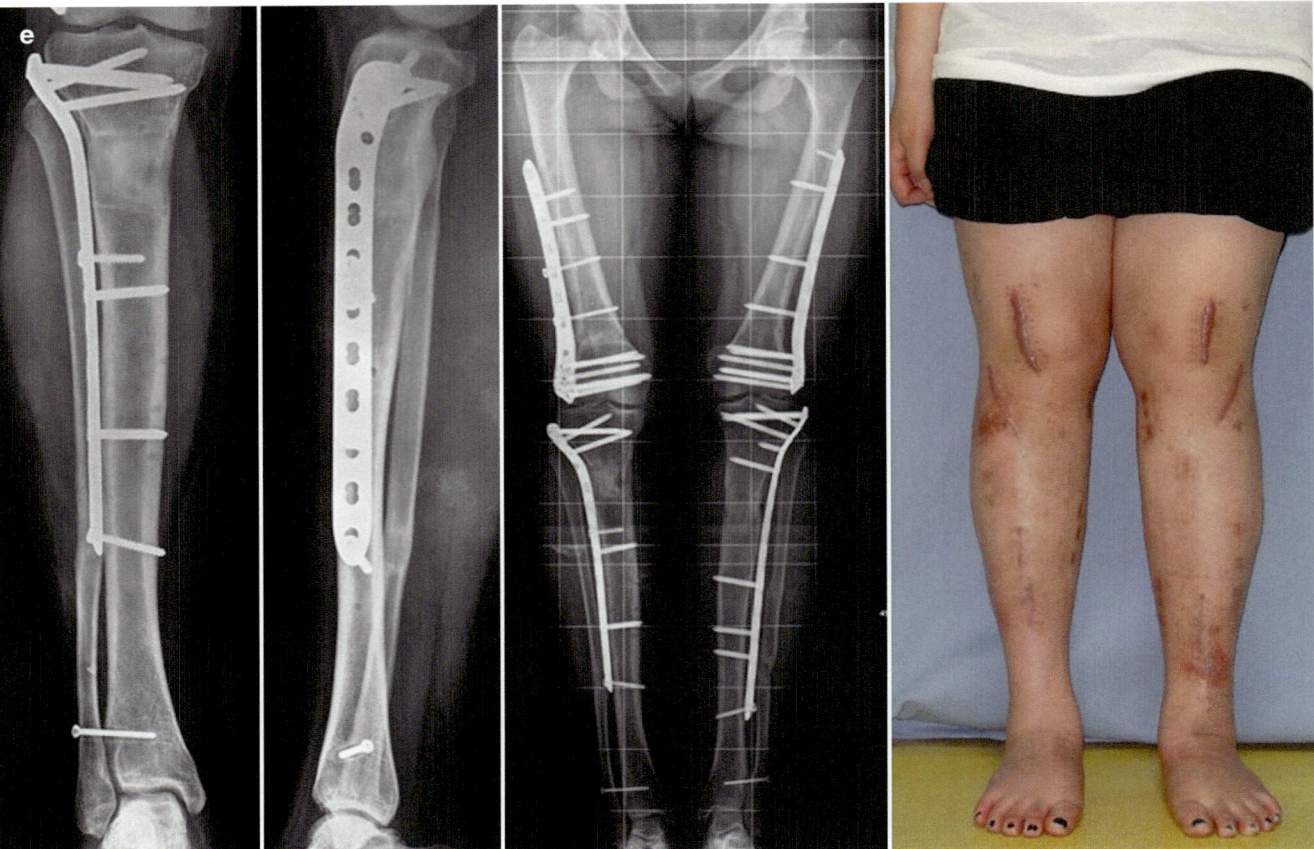

Fig. 11.7 (continued)

Postoperative Management

As long as the IM nailing or locking plate fixation has sufficient stability, external immobilization may not be needed. Postoperative pain should be controlled with either oral or intravenous patient-controlled analgesia. Patients are allowed and encouraged to begin joint motion exercises as soon as possible. Partial weight bearing is also allowed with the use of crutches. If there is adequate radiographic evidence of osseous healing, the transition to full weight bearing is allowed.

Complications

FAN or FAP may have complications related to osteotomy, acute correction of angles, and fixation failure. The risk of complications may vary with age, the site of deformity, underlying pathology, adjacent physis, and surrounding neurovascular structures.

Acute Complications

Neurological Complication

The immediate correction of angular deformities raises concerns regarding neurovascular compromise. An opening wedge osteotomy may have a higher risk than a closing wedge osteotomy. The possibility of nerve stretch may depend on the mobility of the neurovascular bundle in the surrounding soft tissues and the magnitude of angular correction. Furthermore, when rotational correction is combined, the risk may increase even more. There is a particularly high risk of peroneal nerve injury when an acute correction of a valgus knee is performed.

Another cause of peroneal nerve palsy is a fibular osteotomy, when the deformity of the proximal tibia is corrected. As the peroneal nerve is relatively less mobile in the upper third, a fibular osteotomy may be performed at the lower and middle third junction. Its risk may be high in valgus deformities around the knee (proximal tibia or distal femur) which needs to varus correction, or deformities which needs a lengthening procedure simultaneously. In these conditions, prophylactic decompression of the peroneal nerve is recommended in order to prevent this complication. Also, intraoperative SSEP monitoring may minimize the risk of iatrogenic nerve injuries.

Compartment Syndrome

Acute corrective osteotomy may put pressure on adjacent vessels and increase the soft tissue edema after surgery, which may result in unexpected compartment syndrome. It is advised not to close the deep fascia after osteotomy when it is performed for the proximal tibia deformity. Prophylactically, anterior compartment fasciotomy is advocated to decrease the risk of acute correction of Blount's disease or other similar deformities. It can be performed through small incisions, with the minimally invasive surgery technique. Opening wedge osteotomy with a large displacement may predispose to the development of postoperative compartment syndrome.

Vascular Injury

This may occur directly from the surgical procedure of osteotomy and implant fixation, or indirectly with deformity correction. Inappropriate use of drills, osteotome, saw, or implants may cause this iatrogenic injury. Also, excessive stretching with open wedge osteotomy may be another reason. The popliteal vessel is at risk when the osteotomy is performed around the knee joint. Peroneal vessels should be protected when doing a fibular osteotomy.

Soft tissue problems

Healing disturbance of soft tissue may occur when a large displacement of bone occurs after osteotomy. It may increase the pressure on the surrounding soft tissue, resulting in wound dehiscence or skin necrosis. When the poor skin condition is present prior to the surgery, it increases this risk. It is also prudent to keep this risk in mind when performing the procedure at a subcutaneous bone, such as the tibia, due to the prominence of the hardware.

Late Complications

Delayed Union and Nonunion

In children, healing disturbance at the osteotomy is not common, unless excessive motion is present because of unstable fixation. Other potential causes include decreased bone contact and increased gap with a large angular correction. Stability at the osteotomy can be increased by adding translation and bony contact. Excessive acute lengthening at the osteotomy site should be avoided.

Recurrence of Deformity

If the underlying disorder, such as metabolic bone disease, is not corrected or controlled, the deformity may recur following surgical correction. Other reasons include poor bone quality (e.g., fibrous dysplasia) and severe contracture of soft tissue (e.g., cerebral palsy). Controlling or optimizing the underlying disease before and after corrective osteotomy is important to avoid the risk of recurrent deformity.

Peri-implant Complications

The prominence of implants is not uncommon in children because the bone is smaller and the soft tissue envelope is less bulky. It is important to select the appropriate size of internal implant to fix. In some metabolic diseases or osteogenesis imperfecta, fractures or bowing can occur at the interface of bone and implant, even after the healing of an osteotomy. As it may cause hardware failure or the recurrence of deformity, the choice of implant should be carefully decided.

Summary

To correct complex deformities, external fixation has been the standard method to achieve a satisfactory outcome. It has several advantages of controllability to achieve the desired amount of correction and performing the lengthening procedure simultaneously. Hexapod external fixators provide a precise correction in all planes combining gradual distraction principles and deformity analysis conducted by the web-based software. However, the external fixator should maintain the segments until the solid healing of the osteotomy site. It is very uncomfortable for patients to wear the external fixator for a long duration, as it results in inevitable complications such as pin site infection and deep infection. Moreover, delayed complications are not uncommon after the removal of external fixator, including the delayed healing, fractures of osteotomy site, or recurred deformity.

Fixator-assisted plating (FAP) and fixator-assisted nailing (FAN) are recent innovative techniques, combining the advantages of external fixator and internal implants. These techniques need diligent planning and execution to achieve an accurate correction of deformity, and decrease the time in external fixation and the resultant complications. However, it is important to know the tips and pitfalls, in order to reduce the complications from the acute correction, including neurovascular injuries, compartment syndrome, and soft tissue complications.

Commentary

Janet Conway
jconway@lifebridgehealth.org

The technique of fixator assisted nailing and plating has a tremendous value in deformity correction. It combines the accuracy of external fixator correction without the disadvantages of external fixation with its associated prolonged external fixation times and pin site complications. Especially in pediatrics, this technique is much more comfortable for the patients. For the surgeons, however, this technique requires extensive preoperative planning to ensure that the technique is feasible given the deformity. There are some extremely complex or multilevel deformities that may not be amenable to this technique.

There are many considerations during the preoperative planning that Dr. Oh nicely mentions in this chapter. Open growth plates require plates, and closed growth plates can accept intramedullary nails. Acute corrections also need to be accompanied by peroneal nerve decompressions, tarsal tunnel decompressions, or prophylactic fasciotomies depending upon the level and degree of correction. The peroneal nerve should be decompressed in all tibial rotational deformity corrections, knee flexion contractures, and distal femoral and proximal tibial valgus to neutral corrections. The tarsal tunnel should be decompressed with distal tibial derotations and varus to valgus corrections. Anterior fasciotomies are useful with derotational tibial osteotomies. The level of the osteotomy needs to be close to the correction angle because too much translation will not allow for the passage of a nail or stable plate fixation. In addition, fixator pin placement needs to be carefully planned to avoid interfering with nail locking gigs, reamers and plate fixation. The preoperative planning and intraoperative time of surgery will take longer than traditional deformity correction using external fixation but the easy post operative orthopedic care and excellent patient satisfaction are worth it.

For anyone interested in deformity correction, this technique is an essential tool. For the new deformity correction surgeon, starting out with easy, single plane deformities will ensure that they get comfortable with this technique. The figures provide excellent case examples of this technique and show some of the useful places for the temporary external fixator pins.

References

1. Sharma L, Song J, Felson DT, Cahue S, Shamiyeh E, Dunlop DD. The role of knee alignment in disease progression and functional decline in knee osteoarthritis. JAMA. 2001;286(2):188–95.
2. Gugenheim JJ Jr, Brinker MR. Bone realignment with use of temporary external fixation for distal femoral valgus and varus deformities. J Bone Joint Surg Am. 2003;85(7):1229–37.
3. Iobst C, Waseemuddin M, Bafor A. Accuracy and safety of distal femoral valgus correction: a comparison of three techniques. Strategies Trauma Limb Reconstr. 2020;15(1):41–6.
4. Rozbruch SR, Segal K, Ilizarov S, Fragomen AT, Ilizarov G. Does the Taylor spatial frame accurately correct tibial deformities? Clin Orthop Relat Res. 2010;468(5):1352–61.
5. Kocaoglu M, Eralp L, Bilen FE, Balci HI. Fixator-assisted acute femoral deformity correction and consecutive lengthening over an intramedullary nail. J Bone Joint Surg Am. 2009;91(1):152–9.
6. Pesenti S, Iobst CA, Launay F. Evaluation of the external fixator TrueLok Hexapod System for tibial deformity correction in children. Orthop Traumatol Surg Res. 2017;103(5):761–4.
7. Seah KT, Shafi R, Fragomen AT, Rozbruch SR. Distal femoral osteotomy: is internal fixation better than external? Clin Orthop Relat Res. 2011;469(7):2003–11.
8. Park KH, Kim JW, Kim HJ, Kyung HS, Oh JK, Cho TJ, Seo I, Oh CW. Corrective osteotomy of the distal femur with fixator assistance: a novel technique of minimally invasive osteosynthesis. J Orthop Sci. 2017;22(3):474–80.
9. Lee HJ, Oh CW, Song KS, Kim JW, Jung JW, Park BC, Kim JY. Rotational osteotomy with submuscular plating in skeletally immature patients with cerebral palsy. J Orthop Sci. 2013;18(4):557–62.
10. Özcan Ç, Sökücü S, Beng K, Çetinkaya E, Demir B, Kabukçuoğlu YS. Prospective comparative study of two methods for fixation after distal femur corrective osteotomy for valgus deformity; retrograde intramedullary nailing versus less invasive stabilization system plating. Int Orthop. 2016;40(10):2121–6.
11. Oh CW, Song HR, Kim JW, Kyung HS, Lee HJ, Min WK, Park BC. Deformity correction with submuscular plating technique in children. J Pediatr Orthop B. 2010;19(1):47–54.
12. Dabash S, Zhang DT, Rozbruch SR, Fragomen AT. Blocking screw-assisted intramedullary nailing using the reverse-rule-of-thumbs for limb lengthening and deformity correction. Strategies Trauma Limb Reconstr. 2019;14(2):77–84.
13. Bar-On E, Becker T, Katz K, Velkes S, Salai M, Weigl DM. Corrective lower limb osteotomies in children using temporary external fixation and percutaneous locking plates. J Child Orthop. 2009;3(2):137–43.

14. Song HR, Oh CW, Mattoo R, Park BC, Kim SJ, Park IH, Jeon IH, Ihn JC. Femoral lengthening over an intramedullary nail using the external fixator: risk of infection and knee problems in 22 patients with a follow-up of 2 years or more. Acta Orthop. 2005;76(2):245–52.
15. Iobst CA, Rozbruch SR, Nelson S, Fragomen A. Simultaneous acute femoral deformity correction and gradual limb lengthening using a retrograde femoral nail: technique and clinical results. J Am Acad Orthop Surg. 2018;26(7):241–50.
16. Lee DH, Ryu KJ, Kim JH, Soung S, Shin S. Fixator-assisted technique enables less invasive plate osteosynthesis in medial opening-wedge high tibial osteotomy: a novel technique. Clin Orthop Relat Res. 2015;473(10):3133–42.
17. Yusof NM, Oh CW, Oh JK, Kim JW, Min WK, Park IH, Kim HJ. Percutaneous plating in paediatric tibial fractures. Injury. 2009;40(12):1286–91.
18. Oh CW, Song HR, Kim JW, Choi JW, Min WK, Park BC. Limb lengthening with a submuscular locking plate. J Bone Joint Surg Br. 2009;91(10):1394–9.

Hybrid Techniques for Limb Length and Deformity Correction

Mark T. Dahl, Andrew G. Georgiadis, and Stewart G. Morrison

Introduction

Limb lengthening and the correction of severe deformities with external skeletal fixation is known to be a difficult process. While motorized internal devices are used increasingly for both lengthening and even deformity correction in certain situations, many lengthenings and deformity corrections can only be achieved with external fixation. These circumstances may include particular clinical features (large deformity magnitude, anatomic location, younger children), but also austere practice environments, surgeon familiarity, and cost.

This chapter will describe five external fixation lengthening methods supplemented with plates, nails, or screws. Each method adheres to Ilizarov's principles of distraction osteogenesis for limb lengthening [1–4] but utilizes readily available internal fixation devices to protect bone regenerate, shorten the consolidation phase and minimize the burden of prolonged external fixation. Clinical reports indicate more rapid joint motion recovery and less discomfort when adding supplemental internal fixation than when using external fixation alone for lengthening [5].

Preoperative planning is critical to success, with each technique having pitfalls to avoid. Acute intraoperative correction with fixator-assisted techniques may be required and the limits this method will be discussed.

Indications for bone lengthening and deformity correction include limb length discrepancy resulting from congenital conditions such as fibular hemimelia and congenital short femur, or acquired conditions like fracture malunion and premature physeal arrest. Both children and adults are candidates for such treatment, with specific implant and technical considerations, detailed in the chapter below. The overarching principles of distraction osteogenesis (DO) have been successfully used over the last half-century to lengthen and straighten bone [6]. The six essential elements of successful DO by the Ilizarov method are:

1. Preservation of blood supply (endosteal and periosteal)
2. Stable external fixation
3. A delay prior to distraction
4. Slow fractionated distraction (~1 mm/day)
5. A period of stable neutral fixation after lengthening
6. Physiologic use of the elongated limb

Despite tremendous advances in the field of limb lengthening and deformity reconstruction, patients and their families undergo months of pin site maintenance [7] and

Supplementary Information The online version contains supplementary material available at https://doi.org/10.1007/978-3-031-55767-5_12.

M. T. Dahl
Limb Lengthening Service, Minneapolis, MN, USA

Department of Orthopaedics, Gillettte Children's Hospital, St. Paul, MN, USA

Orthopedic Surgery, University of Minnesota, Minneapolis, MN, USA
e-mail: mdahl@gillettechildrens.com

A. G. Georgiadis (✉)
Department of Orthopaedics, Gillettte Children's Hospital, St. Paul, MN, USA

Orthopedic Surgery, University of Minnesota, Minneapolis, MN, USA
e-mail: andrewgeorgiadis@gillettechildrens.com

S. G. Morrison
The Royal Children's Hospital—Melbourne, Parkville, VIC, Australia

Victorian Orthoapedic Centre, Melbourne, VIC, Australia

The Bob Dickens Pediatric Orthopaedic Research Fellowship, Melbourne, VIC, Australia
e-mail: stewart.morrison@rch.org.au

ever-present external fixation. The resulting soft tissue scarring can lead to further contracture and adjacent joint difficulty. Additionally, Ilizarov's methods take years and scores of cases for surgeons to master the techniques [8]. Complications common to any lengthening like joint contracture, subluxation, fracture, residual deformity, and chronic pain are all well documented [8]. Even after years of experience with bone regeneration, surgeons commonly confront yet another new complication arising from the treatment.

While many of the above principles of DO can be achieved with external fixation, they can be further complemented by adjunctive technology. For example, physiologic use of the limb can occur with stable internal fixation that secures lengthening regenerate in proper alignment, thus diminishing time in the external fixator. Hybrid techniques like this have evolved because external fixation has several attendant disadvantages including: pin site infections, pain, soft-tissue tethering, and psychological acceptance. The prolonged treatment of bone lengthening with external fixation can now be shortened by substituting internal fixation for the external fixator during the consolidation phase of lengthening.

A recent meta-analysis assessed all available comparative studies of "integrated limb lengthening" (herein we use the term "hybrid") versus traditional external fixation alone, concluding that the time in frame, "problems", and "sequelae" were all significantly minimized with a hybrid approach [9]. Still, there are potential complications unique to hybrid techniques, which will be discussed below.

Lengthening Over Nail (LON)

Using an intramedullary nail or device in the presence of an external fixator lengthening was first described by Bost and Larsen, who used a smooth pin intended to prevent deformity during lengthening [10]. They describe rod migration as an encountered complication, and to mitigate this mentioned drilling a hole within the rod to obtain cross fixation with another smooth wire.

The term "Lengthening-Over-Nail" (LON) was coined by Paley, Herzenberg, and Bhave who introduced the modern method in 1997 (Fig. 12.1) [5]. Their series described 29 patients treated with femoral corticotomy and simultaneous application of an external fixator and locked intramedullary nail. At the index procedure, the distal interlocking screws were not inserted in the nail. Once the desired length was achieved, the distal interlocking screws could be inserted which then allowed the fixator to be removed well before full consolidation had occurred. They compared the LON group to 31 patients treated previously with external fixators alone, demonstrating a near 50% reduction in the average of external fixation duration, and markedly improved return of knee range of motion. Six fractures occurred in the historical group, compared to none in the LON group, and though one case was complicated by interlocking screw failure, overall complications were reduced by 25%.

Critical to the technique was over-reaming of the intermedullary canal to 2 mm larger than the planned nail diameter, to prevent entrapment of the rod that may prevent lengthening. Such reaming has an acknowledged effect on the endosteal blood supply to the planned lengthening site, but this effect is mitigated by the increased mechanical stability afforded by the nail. The risk of deep infection when internal fixation is placed in a close proximity to external fixation should be considered, and the paper's illustrations highlight the technique of posteriorly located, cortically based external fixation half pins in order to (i) allow passage of the nail, and (ii) avoid direct contact with the intramedullary space. LON can also be used retrograde, as demonstrated by a 2002 case by the senior author in which acute deformity correction and retrograde lengthening was performed concomitantly. This technique anticipates the valgus that will be produced with lengthening along the anatomic axis of the femur (Fig. 12.2).

The technique also has been demonstrated in a pediatric population. Gordon et al. described femoral LON in a preliminary retrospective series of 9 patients in 2002, then in 37 patients in 2013 [11, 12]. In the initial series, nine children (average age 10 years 9 months) were treated with humeral interlocking nails due to size considerations, and in the latter 37 were treated with newer generation, pediatric-specific lateral entry femoral nails. Highlighted is the importance of trochanteric tip, or lateral trochanteric nail entry, with strict avoidance of the piriformis fossa and the circumflex femoral artery. After nail insertion, a monolateral external fixator was applied, and lengthening achieved through a proximal corticotomy. No patients in either series developed femoral head avascular necrosis. Joint instability is discussed, with both hip and knee subluxation being reported as complications. Certainly, a move away from joint-spanning external fixation mandates careful evaluation of joint stability pre-operatively, as well as during lengthening, particularly in patients with congenital limb deficiencies.

> **Box 12.1**
> - When positioning the external fixator pins or wires, contact with the IM nail must be avoided. If possible, pins should be placed unicortical or intra-cortical
> - Over-reaming of the medullary canal by 2 mm is recommended to under-size the diameter of nail and prevent "binding" of the nail during lengthening.

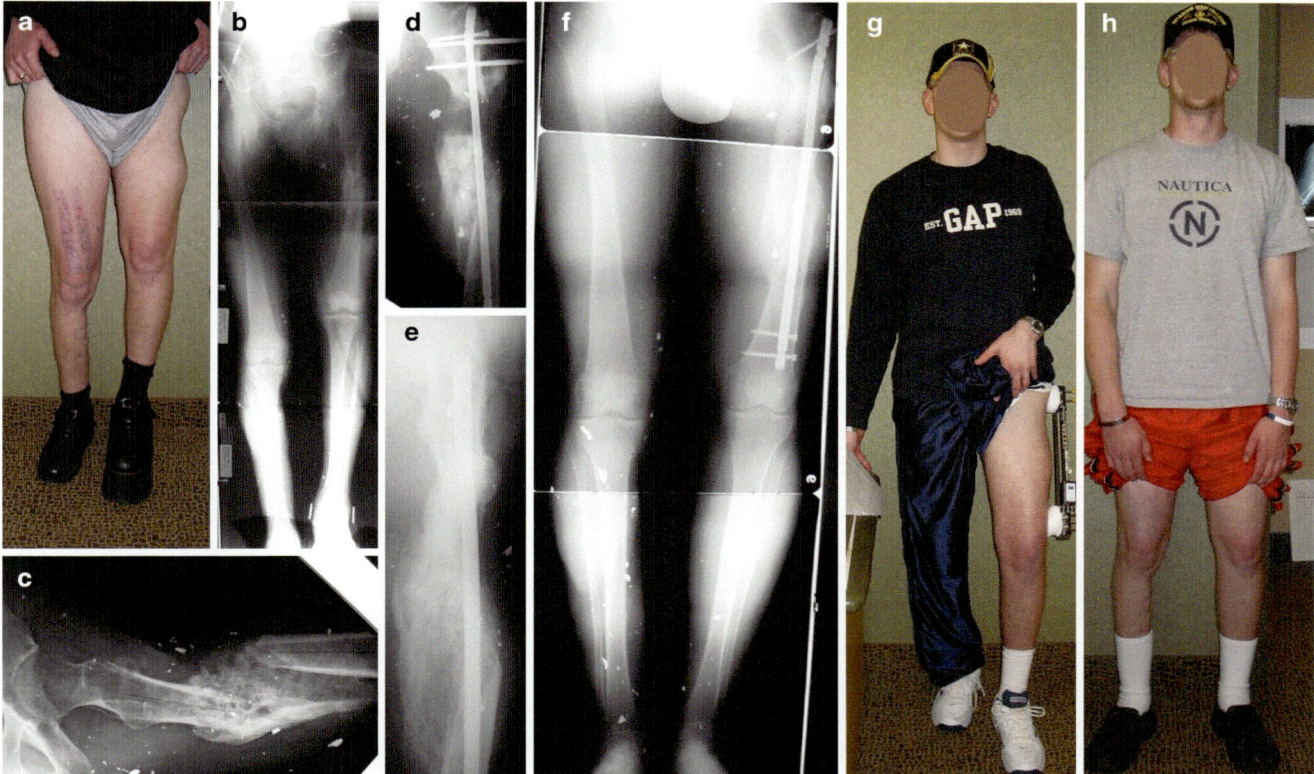

Fig. 12.1 This soldier was struck by an IED (improvised explosive device), causing open brain trauma and open fractures of the left femur and right forearm. A 10-cm leg length discrepancy (LLD) with angulation, rotation, and translation of the femur developed (**a–c**). Acute correction of the angulation, translation, and rotation was followed by lengthening over nail of 10 cm (**d, e**) with final equalization of limb lengths (**f**) and good tolerance of the lengthening (**g**) with final clinical result (**h**)

The use of flexible intramedullary nails to augment external fixation lengthening is also described. Lampasi et al. [13] performed 7 pediatric femoral lengthenings with monolateral fixators after retrograde placement of elastic stable intramedullary nails (ESIN), with fixator duration average 212 days to achieve an average lengthening of 4.8 cm. A comparative study by Popkov et al. [14] included patients, in which this technique was used in both the femur and tibia as well as the upper limb. All nails were removed 3–8 months post external fixator removal, and they concluded that the use of ESIN reduced fixator duration. It must be acknowledged, however, that the ability of flexible nails (without any sort of cross fixation) to maintain length is extremely limited, and their main role is likely in the maintenance of sagittal and coronal alignment. Preliminary studies in an animal model propose an advantage to the use of hydroxyapatite coated intramedullary wires in that they may improve regenerate formation during lengthening, however this has not been demonstrated in a human model [15].

Hybrid techniques to safely correct an extreme tibial torsion ("Deformity correction over a nail") are illustrated in Fig. 12.3. Note an externally rotated foot, similar to a "lateral" ankle radiograph, with an AP knee view, suggestive of external tibial torsion. Subsequently, a hexapod frame and IM nail are applied with a midshaft osteotomy. Internal rotation was performed at 5° per day for a total external fixation time of 8 days. Importantly, over-reaming of 2 mm was performed to prevent "binding" of the derotation. Fixation included a wire and a half pin proximally and 2 half pins distally. The nail was locked in compression and frame removed, allowing her to return to her university studies 2 weeks after the index procedure.

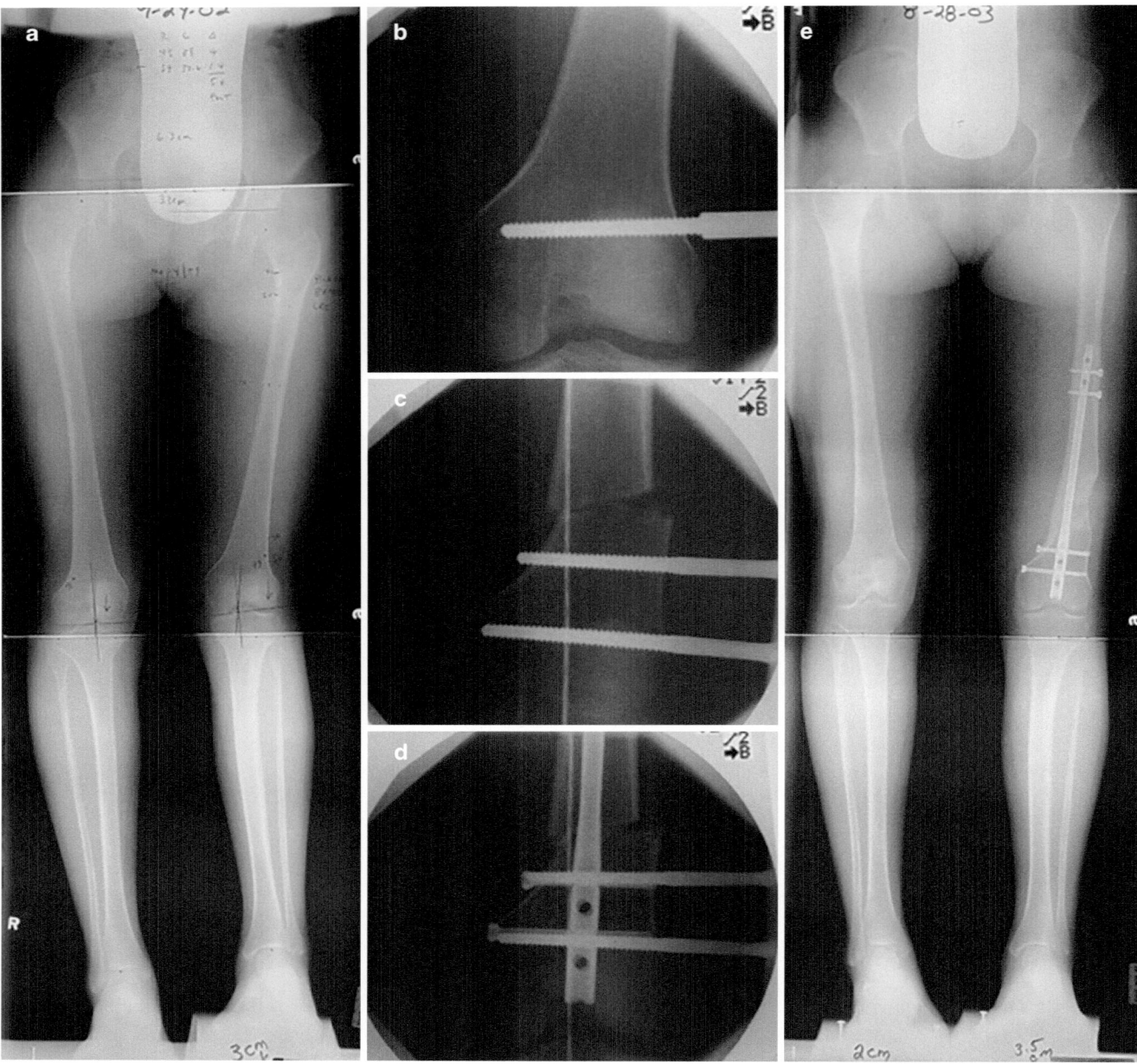

Fig. 12.2 Adult female with fibular hemimelia, distal femoral valgus, and a 6.5 cm discrepancy, left shorter (**a**). Intraoperatively, half-pins were placed parallel to the distal femoral joint line to control the distal fragment (**b**), and a corticotomy was performed with acute deformity correction into local varus and small magnitude overall varus (**c**, **d**). This alignment anticipates the valgus that will develop with lengthening along the anatomic axis of the femur, resulting in a neutral final mechanical axis (**e**)

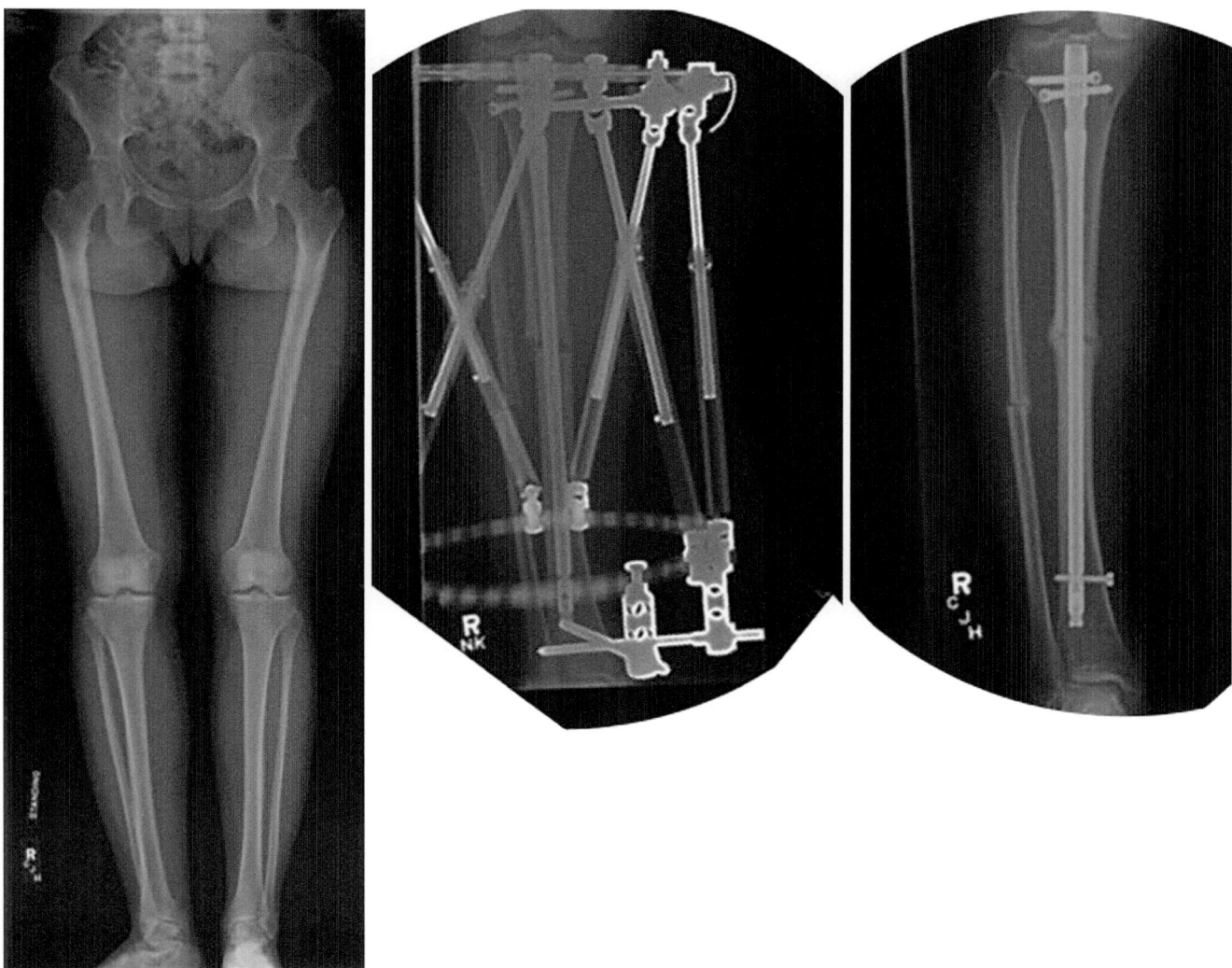

Fig. 12.3 An adult with right external tibial torsion underwent large magnitude (>30°) tibial derotation over a nail, to mitigate the risk of peroneal nerve palsy

Lengthening and Then Nailing (LATN)

This technique was described by Rozbruch in 2008 [16] employing deformity correction and concomitant external fixator lengthening, after which the external fixator is replaced by a locked intramedullary nail at the completion of lengthening. This may reduce (but certainly not eliminate) the risk of deep infection of the medullary cavity or the implant, but has a role primarily in situations where gradual correction of deformity is required (via external fixation) before an intramedullary nail can be implanted. Acute deformity correction, depending on the location, magnitude, and soft tissue considerations, may be difficult or dangerous. The circular fixator gradually corrects deformities, of length, angulation, and/or rotation with a locked nail inserted at the completion of correction. The application of the frame should adhere to the principles of lengthening over a nail, which fixation avoiding the eventual path of the nail whenever possible.

Plate-Assisted Lengthening (PAL)

Iobst and Dahl first introduced PAL in 2007 [17]. The index report was a description of the surgical steps and a retrospective examination of six patients with open physes, using a

Fig. 12.4 Plate assisted lengthening technique employed for a seven-year-old with fibular hemimelia. Notice that a simple three-ring frame has been applied (a foot frame to mitigate equinus during lengthening). Threaded rods are used as the "motor" for lengthening, and these are parallel to the long axis of the tibia on orthogonal views. All points of fixation are planned deliberately to be out of the way of the submuscular plate, and distal fixation will move away from the end of the plate with continued lengthening. It is technically easiest to apply the plate to the medial face of the tibia, but can be applied laterally to try and mitigate predictable valgus deformity of the regenerate

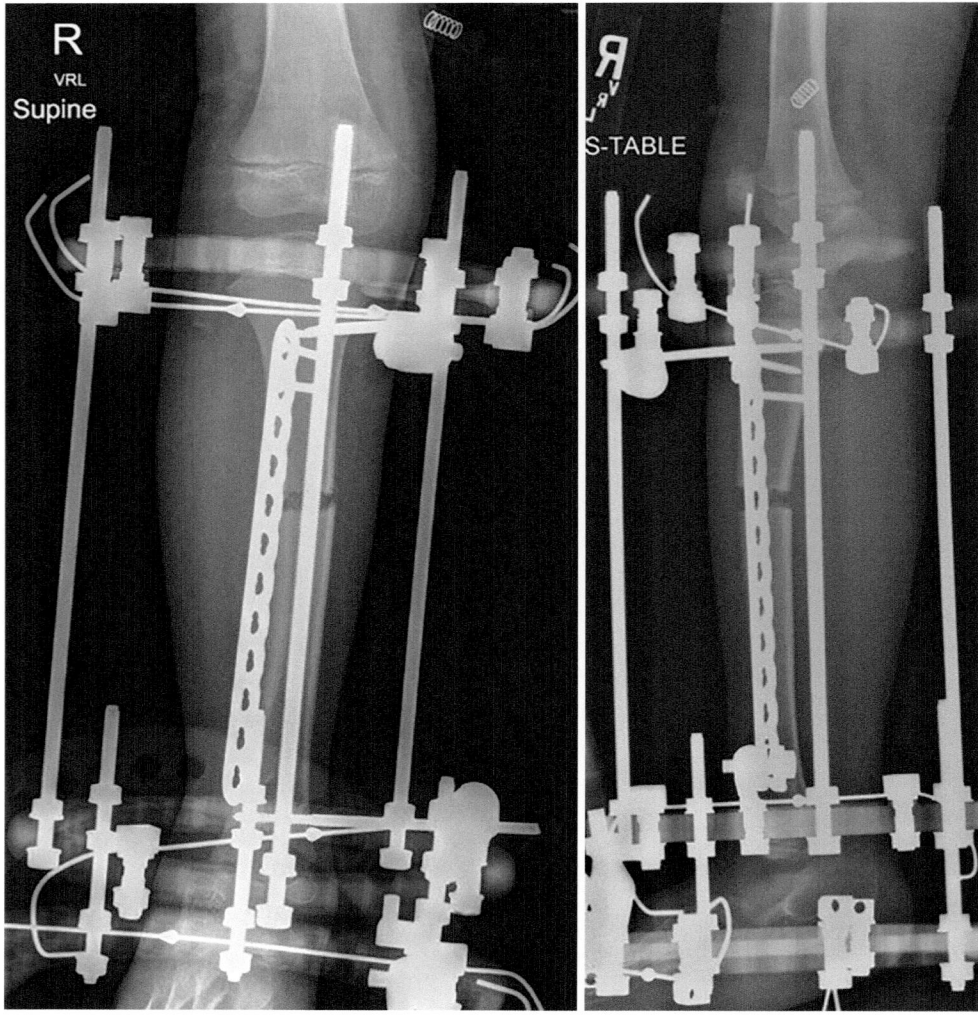

technique intended to shorten time in fixator by application of a percutaneous locking plate at frame application, which is then locked when lengthening is complete. This allows immediate fixator removal and allows consolidation to occur with internal fixation only. The main indication for PAL is instances when intramedullary nail is not a viable option, as in those patients with a narrow medullary canal, bone deformity, open physes, or joint contractures. Generally, patients eligible for this technique have skeletally immature tibiae or any femoral segment in a child <10 years of age. Lengthenings were completed with complication rates comparable to other methods of lengthening, but with a shorter external fixation index. Any deformities that occurred with lengthening (particularly varus and procurvatum of the regenerate) could be corrected at the time of plate locking.

Intraoperatively, a drill corticotomy is performed, maintaining an intact bone segment while the plate and fixator are applied. A percutaneous submuscular plate is applied laterally on the femur or medially on the tibia, and is provisionally secured with one or two screws on one side of the corticotomy. A circular fixator is then applied in a standard fashion, again with fixation points attached to the intact, pre-corticotomized bone segment for ease of application. Care must be taken to keep wires and half pins away from the plate (Fig. 12.4). Finally, the fixator is loosened to allow for interfragmentary motion, and the corticotomy is completed. Acute deformities can be corrected at this time, or gradually corrected with the frame during lengthening. At the time of lengthening completion, the plate is percutaneously locked and the fixator removed, thus almost eliminating the consolidation phase time in the frame.

Half-pin and wire fixation area may be more limited in this technique, because of its application to small bones and the presence of adjacent internal fixation. As a result, axis deviation can occur and can often be adjusted at the time of fixator removal and plate locking. It should be noted that the locking procedure is tedious because the external fixation components block access to the limb, but are critical to maintain until the plate is locked so as to mitigate shortening or deformity (Fig. 12.5).

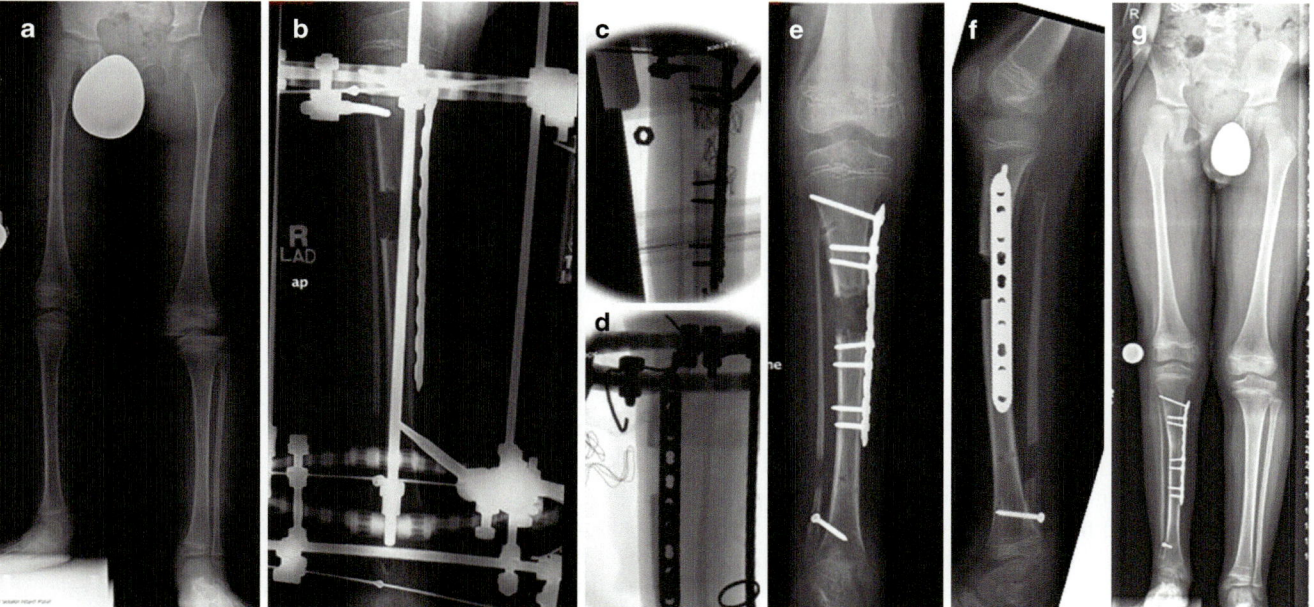

Fig. 12.5 A six-year-old with fibular hemimelia and LLD emanating primarily from the tibial segment (**a**). To minimize fixator time, a PAL technique was applied. Notice fixation points are maximally distanced from the internal fixation, and the plate is on the medial face of the tibia (**b**). After 4 weeks of lengthening, 3.5 cm is achieved and the plate is locked. On intraoperative fluoroscopy, notice that strategic positioning of the threaded rods which allow access for instruments to the medial face of the tibia, facilitating plate locking (**c, d**). Immediately after locking, plain radiographs are taken (**e, f**). Standing films several months after plate locking reveal maturation of the regenerate and improved discrepancy, with maintained coronal alignment (**g**)

A follow-up study from Georgiadis, Dahl and colleagues was performed on 38 patients in 2017 [18]. The goal of shortened fixator time was accomplished with a mean external fixation index of 13.1 ± 4.29 days/cm, with an average fixator time of 48 days while achieving an average 3.8 cm of lengthening. Oh et al. also described a similar technique in older children and adults, using a submuscular locking plate [19, 20]. Submuscular plating has the advantage of providing angular stability and preserving the periosteal and endosteal blood supply, which is beneficial for distraction osteogenesis. The authors continue to use this technique in younger children with particularly short tibia segments, to gently increase the segment length in preparation for later extramedullary or intramedullary lengthening, depending on bone size and age.

Box 12.2
- External fixation half-pins and wires should not contact plate or screws, to avoid cross contamination, which may evolve into deep infection.
- The longest possible plate should be chosen for an individual patient's anatomy, to maximize stability after locking and allow sufficient number of screws on each side of the lengthened segment (remember that a 3–4 cm lengthening will mean 2–3 fewer screw holes between the time of placement and when lengthening is complete).
- Protection from full weight bearing and the use of a protective device (such as a patellar tendon bearing brace in tibia lengthening) is recommended until sufficient consolidation of the distraction callus is achieved.
- When fixing a screw in skeletally immature patients, the adjacent physis should not be violated.
- Insertion of screws in the distal segment at the end of distraction period should be performed prior to removal of the external fixator. This will prevent loss of correction that was gained at the lengthening site.

Lengthening and Then Plating (LAP)

This technique is analogous to plate assisted lengthening, except that the percutaneous plate is inserted at the terminus of lengthening. Rozbruch and Fragomen reported a retrospective case-matched comparison between LAP and traditional Ilizarov techniques alone [21]. The duration of frame use and external fixation index were lower in the LAP group (4.5 vs. 6.2 months and 1.5 vs. 2 months/cm). The rates of angular deformity during lengthening were no different between groups, although varus malalignment and plate breakage did occur in two LAP patients. Pin-tract infection was more common in the classic group (12 vs. 2). No deep infections occurred in the LAP group. These results further emphasize coronal and sagittal deviation as a problem, presumably because the presence of the plate limits the pin positions of the external fixation.

The advantage to plating after lengthening is that the circular fixator is unencumbered to allow a precise alignment correction before plating. As in PAL, care must be taken to leave open access for the plate insertion, so that contaminated pin sites do not later cause infection of the plating site. At the time of plate locking, Uysal et al. [22] recommended removing only the rods or struts that obstruct screw placement, while keeping the remainder of the frame intact, until the plate is locked on both sides of the lengthening.

> **Box 12.3**
> - A LAP technique is advantageous for children who have an open physis or a small intramedullary canal, especially for whom the IM nailing may be difficult to perform.
> - Because this technique does not require exposing the distraction area and soft tissue dissection is kept to the minimum, the risk of deep infection can be minimized.
> - Caution is still needed not to involve pin tracks of the external fixator, which can be a source of delayed infection.
> - Insertion of screws in the distal segment at the end of distraction period should be performed prior to removal of the external fixator. This will prevent loss of correction that was gained at the lengthening site.

Bone Transport with a Plate or Nail Assist

Segmental bone defects can result from trauma, infection, tumor, nonunion, and congenital conditions [23]. The principals of distraction osteogenesis can be utilized for treating such intercalary defects, and this process is commonly known as 'bone transport'. Due to the various complex etiologies of a bone defect, distraction osteogenesis is often complicated by poor local biology, leading to prolonged treatment times. Trifocal (two sites of distraction osteogenesis) and even tetrafocal techniques can be employed to shorten overall treatment time, however even then the duration of external fixation required for bony consolidation is associated with pin tract infection, joint stiffness, and patient discomfort. Premature removal can lead to fracture.

Bone transport over an IM nail has been described, in a similar fashion to lengthening over an IM nail, most extensively by Oh [24]. The IM nail provides stability for the transport segment, potentially reducing the amount of external fixation required. One major disadvantage of using external fixation during transport is the 'dragging' of wires or pins through skin, traveling with pressure necrosis on the leading side and healing by secondary intention on the trailing side. This commonly leads to deeply clefted and elongated scars. If an IM nail can be safely placed early in treatment, once the bone segment transport is complete and docking site healing achieved, the nail can be locked allowing fixator removal. Standard IM nails provide no interlocking fixation points in their mid-section, undesirably allowing the backward migration of the transport segment. A method to prevent this has been developed by Oh et al. They describe securing the docked segment in place under compression by plate and screw fixation, allowing immediate removal of the external fixator. A later publication by Bernstein et al. describes customizing an intramedullary nail by the addition of an extra interlocking screw hole, allowing fixation of the transport segment in the docked position and avoiding the plate altogether [25]. Such customization must be very carefully planned. As with any use of an IM nail, the length of each segment should be considered, if a docking site is in close proximity to a joint (particularly in the distal tibia), an IM nail and its interlocking screw options may be inadequate for the extent of stability required.

Oh et al. in 2013 also introduced "bone transport with a plate," which again affords a shorter period of external fixation [26]. A plate allows more transverse fixation options when compared to a standard intramedullary nail, allowing control of each of the segments of bone as required and optimizing stability and subsequent healing at both distraction and docking sites.

Any existing infection of the bone is, of course, an absolute contraindication to combining internal fixation during transport. Additionally, all techniques involving both internal and external fixation must consider the potential for pin site inoculation of an implant, which could result in deep infection. "Pin site holidays" can be employed, in which the patient returns to the operating room and all pins and wires are removed, new pins and wires inserted, all while planning to avoid obstruction to final fixation (Fig. 12.6). In instances where regenerate is thin, the object of plating can be to protect regenerate indefinitely (Fig. 12.7).

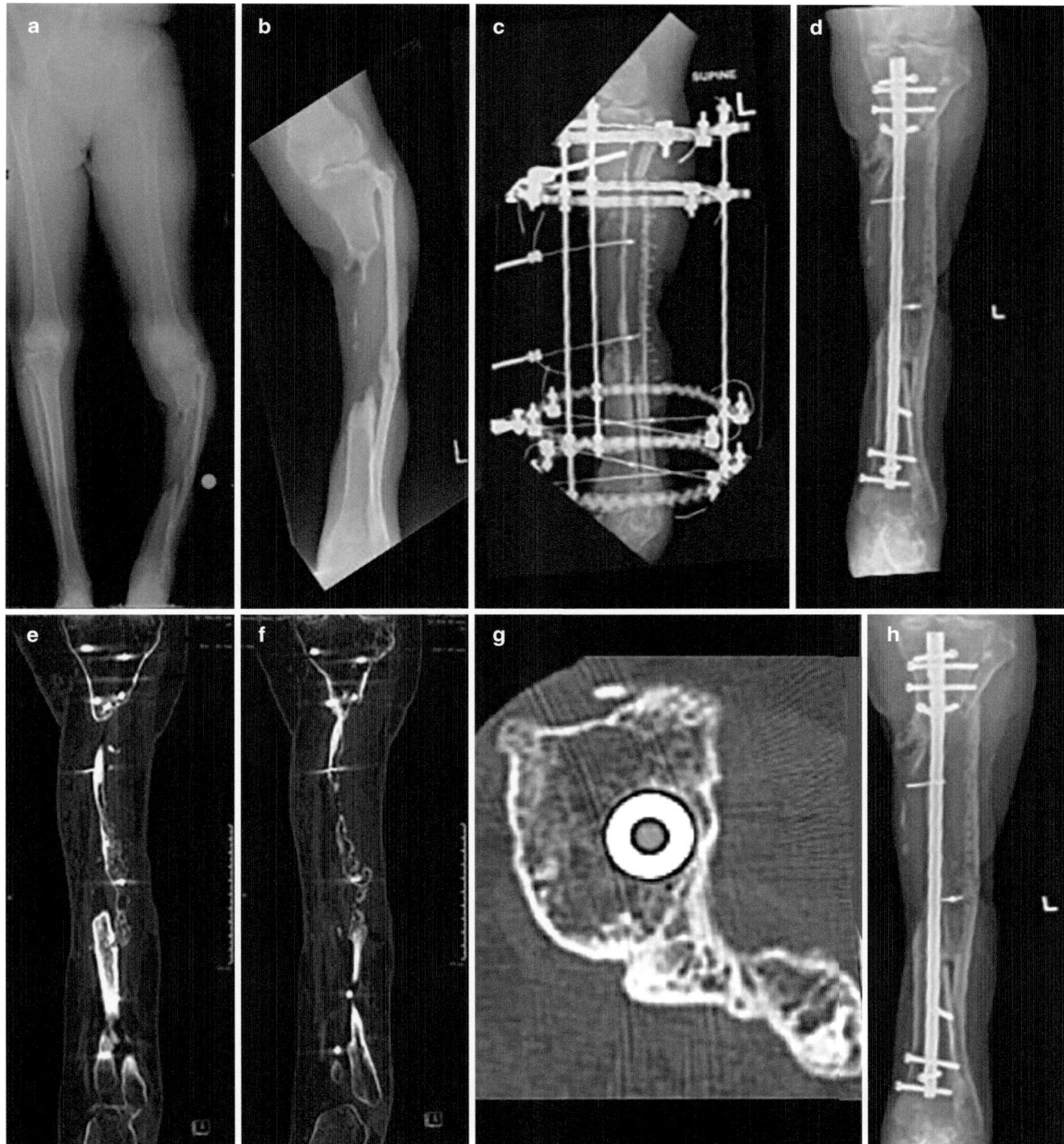

Fig. 12.6 A 23-year-old female presented with a 22 cm tibial defect secondary to open trauma at age eight in East Africa (**a**—standing AP, **b**—AP tibia). Thin and invaginated skin made a conventional longitudinal transport impossible, so a lateral half fibula-to-tibia transport was performed (**c**—mid-transport). Once docking proximally and distally was achieved at 12 weeks, it was elected to insert an intramedullary nail to maintain position while the regenerate bone matured (**d**). As existing pin and wire sites posed the potential threat of infection with a newly inserted IM nail, a "pin site holiday" was achieved by removing all pins and wires and placing a new pair of pins proximally and distally, eccentric to the future nail position for 4 weeks before nail insertion. (**e**) and (**f**) denote bridging consolidation of the fibula-pro-tibia, further denoted in cross sectional CT (**g**) and final AP radiograph (**h**)

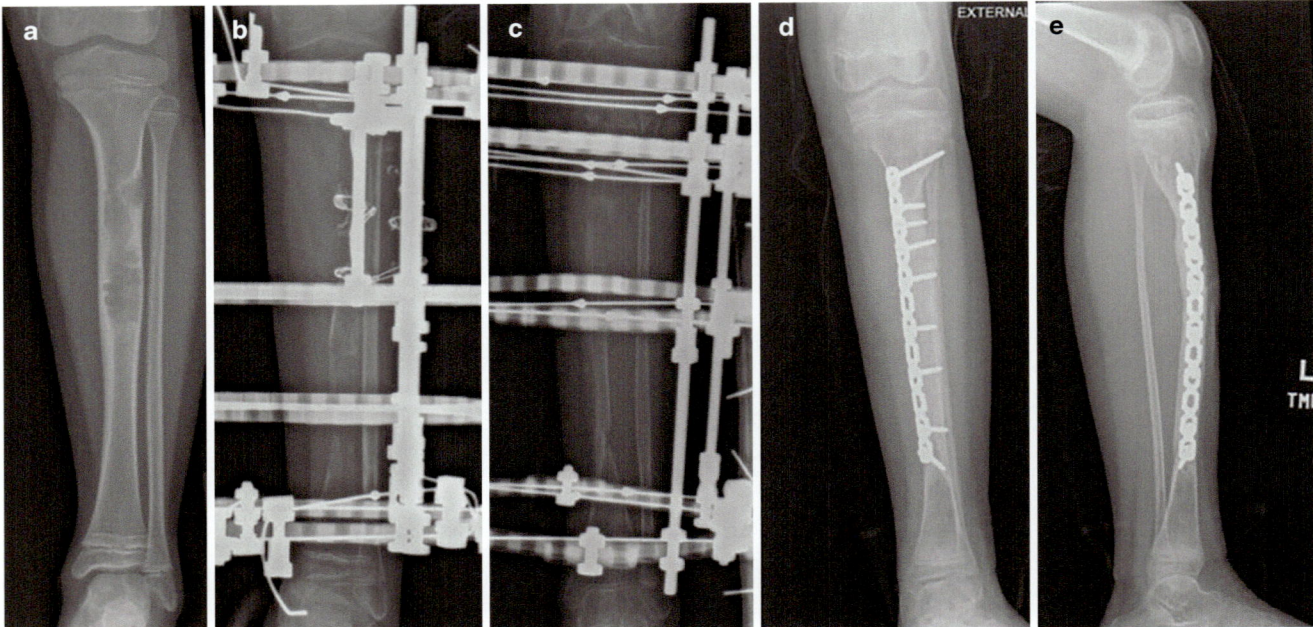

Fig. 12.7 A six-year-old female with adamantinoma (**a**) underwent wide resection and double level retrograde cable assisted transport (**b**, **c**). The docking site is healing (**c**) but thin regenerate requires a prolonged consolidation period in frame. The docking and lengthening sites matured slowly, protected by a percutaneously inserted plate (**d**, **e**), after a "pin site holiday" to minimize the chance of infection

Box 12.4
- Compared to bone transport over a nail, bone transport with a plate may further reduce the external fixation time because the screw fixation at the transported segment adds stability and can eliminate the time required for union at the docking site.
- If the remaining segment is too short for intramedullary fixation, such as in the case of juxta-articular bone defects, the use of transport with a plate is particularly useful.
- In order to minimize the risk of secondary infection, the external fixation pins are inserted sufficiently remotely from the plate or screws.

Lengthening and Then Screw Fixation

Extreme foot deformities must be corrected gradually to stretch the soft tissues and neurovascular structures safely into the corrected position. Conditions such as recalcitrant clubfeet and extreme equinus can be corrected with external fixation, with or without osteotomy. While using external fixation for such corrections, the static phase of external fixation (maintenance of the achieved correction) is usually three times the duration of the correction phase. This prolonged subsequent external fixation protects the regenerate bone and the stretched soft tissues in the corrected position, but often results in foot stiffness and discomfort.

Inserting percutaneous screws, pins, or staples at the time of completion of deformity correction allows for earlier removal of the fixator. This technique has been employed after foot correction to spare patients' months in a foot frame (Figs. 12.8 and 12.9). The percutaneous, fluoroscopic-guided insertion of cannulated screws thus protects the osteotomy sites along with casts or braces.

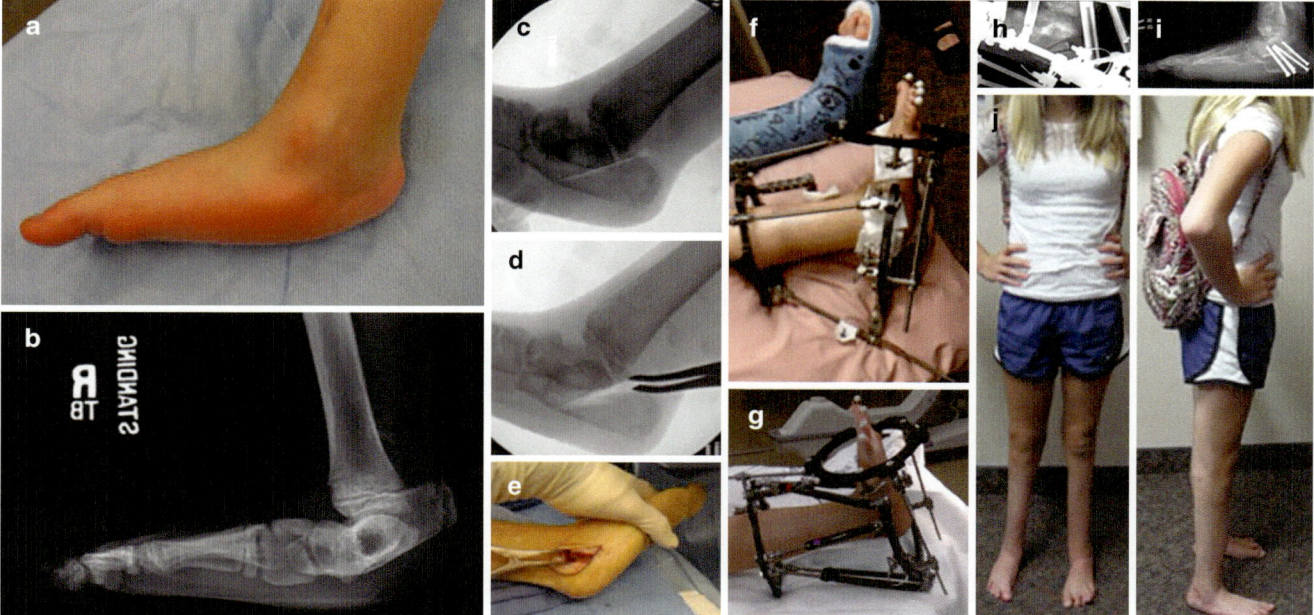

Fig. 12.8 An 11-year-old girl with bilateral fibular hemimelia and severe equinoplanovaglus foot deformity underwent previous unsuccessful R foot surgery. External fixation and then screw fixation was employed. (**a**) and (**b**) denote the preoperative clinical appearance and lateral radiograph of the foot. Intraoperatively, an opening wedge calcaneal osteotomy was performed (**c–e**) with interpositional graft to maintain the acute opening wedge. Gradual equinus and hindfoot valgus correction was performed with an external fixator (**f**, **g**). Once correction was achieved (**h**), Internal fixation was placed (**i**) which reduced time in frame significantly and resulted in a patient with a plantigrade foot that allowed normal shoe-wear (**j**)

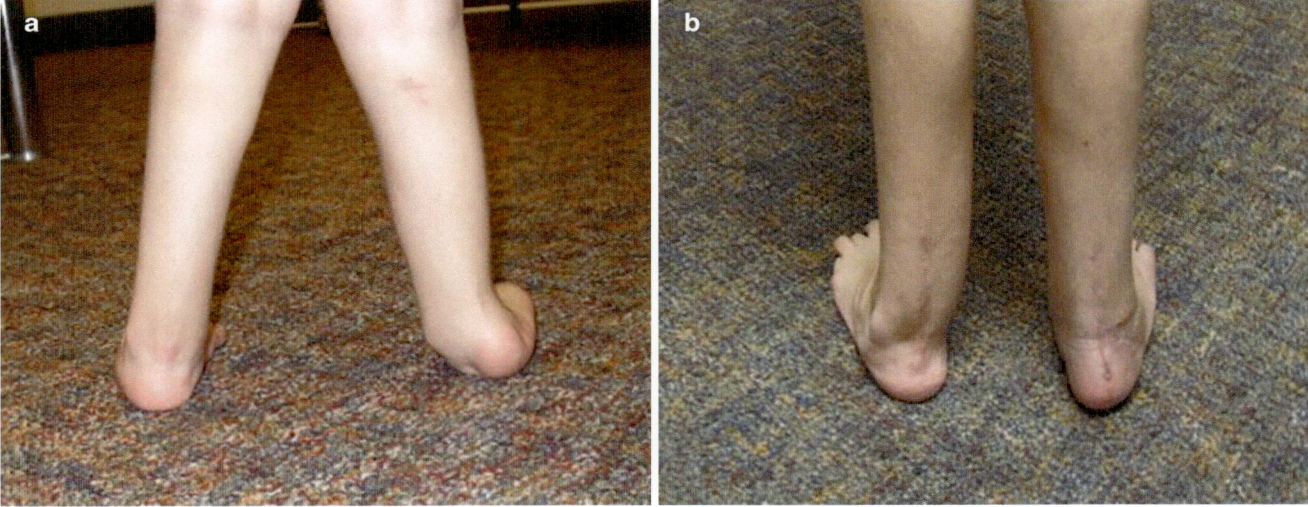

Fig. 12.9 The 11-year-old girl from Fig. 12.4, with pre (**a**) and postoperative (**b**) views of the hindfeet, demonstrating improved plantigrade positioning

Summary

A variety of hybrid techniques have been established to improve the patient experience during limb length and deformity correction by limiting external fixation time to the latency and distraction phases. Each of these techniques shares the requirements of careful preoperative planning, prevention of cross-contamination of external fixator pins, and skill with internal fixation devices.

- Lengthening over nail reduces external fixation time and facilitates early rehabilitation.
- Plate-assisted lengthening in children reduces fixator time.
- Lengthening and then nailing allows for complex deformity correction followed by nailing to shorten fixator time.
- For complex foot correction that must be done gradually, securing the desired correction with screws will hasten fixator removal.

Commentary

Commentary on Hybrid Fixation for Lengthening and Deformity Correction

Milind Chaudary
milind@ilizarov.org

Motorized internal lengthening devices have enabled the surgeon to completely avoid using external fixation. Their ubiquitous use is curtailed by the high cost. They cannot be used in the presence of active or dormant infection. These also cannot be used in bones with narrower canals or in the skeletally immature.

Other drawbacks include the inability to use these in the presence of large and bowing deformities, or to be able to perform two different tasks in the same segment. Many designs and iterations of Motorized Internal Lengthening Nails like the ISKD [27], Albizzia, Fitbone as well as the Precice [28] have had failures, some mildly troublesome and some catastrophic, which make their easy adoption in many geographies impossible.

For many of these drawbacks, hybrid methods of lengthening and deformity correction offer alternative solutions.

The first advantage, of course, is low-cost. These hybrid methods employ routine external fixation devices. The internal fixation devices such as locking nails and plates, are familiar and easily available. Any modifications needed in the devices to enable lengthening and deformity correction are easy and inexpensive to make. The indications for using lengthening over nails and lengthening over plates, are broader, with only acute or dormant infection being true contra indications.

For many adults who have limb shortening and deformities the use of hybrid fixation, methods to reduce fixator duration, can be a great boon and advantage.

Lengthening over nails has the advantage of enabling long lengthenings. In the absence of a deformity, limb lengthening is easiest over an intramedullary nail [29].

Dahl et al. have given a comprehensive outline of hybrid limb lengthening and deformity correction methods. While they have adequately emphasized the role of separating the external fixation pins from the intramedullary nail using C-Arm and the K-wire-&-cannulated-drill technique, other factors need to be recognized too. Excessive reaming to accommodate a large nail size can result in blood loss and infection. Poor hygiene and improper dressing technique, and poor nourishment of the patient also play a role in the development of deep intramedullary infection [29].

Poor soft tissue coverage or poor muscle envelope over the osteotomy site, as in poliomyelitis, may also predispose the patient to infection. Not only excessive reaming, but continuous high-speed reaming generates heat that may be responsible for cell death, in the heat affected zone. Reaming also needs to be slow and in a start stop fashion. Guichet [30] has designed special reamers with large flutings which enable the reamers to come out easily and not generate heat. A simpler alternative could also be to use hand-held reamers and ream slowly. Sharp reamers will reduce heat generation and the chance of infection. Most important of all are rigid reamers, rather than the commonly available flexible ones to allow reaming the canal only 1 mm larger than the nail diameter. A straight nail can easily slide and lengthen with less reaming as compared to a curved trauma nail, which will need a large amount of reaming.

The next scenario is shortening of the limb accompanied by deformity. When lengthening of the segment is planned at the apex of the deformity after its acute correction, the technical difficulties increase significantly in comparison with simple lengthening. Deformity correction is ideally performed using a Dome osteotomy or an angulation translation osteotomy or a closing wedge osteotomy at the deformity site. It is possible to do the former two percutaneously. The aids to correct the deformity are external fixation pins, rings or clamps, the reamer jutting out through the entry portal, the use of an F-Tool, and also the use of poller screws. Poller screws [31, 32] will narrow the canal diameter and guide the reamer and nail in the desired track. Poller screws inserted on either side of the nail using the reverse rule of thumbs will prevent secondary migration of the reamer or nail and help correct an angular deformity. The nail can be passed up to the osteotomy site from the entry portal and after acute correction of the deformity, slid in to the proximal or distal fragment. Poller screws may be passed in either the proximal or distal fragments to prevent secondary translations of the nail. The nail is locked in the short fragment and remains unlocked in the longer one allowing it to slide and lengthen the bone using the external fixation.

Sometimes it is not possible to negotiate a nail due to difficulties in the entry portal especially in the presence of a large deformity that is very close to the joint near the entry portal. Some other concerns include difficulties in reaming the far fragment due to a bowing deformity. This is where eccentric reaming is helpful. For example, the posterior cortex may need more reaming [33] for a procurvatum deformity. This entails exerting downward pressure on the working end of the reamer which will elevates the reamer at the entry point to widen its track. To prevent this problem, a series of steel tubes have been designed by Baumgart & Thaller [34]. These tubes will prevent widening of the canal at the entry point, and enable eccentric reaming, in whichever direction is needed closer to the osteotomy side or beyond. In large lengthening, the nail may be kept protruding outside out of the piriformis fossa, to be allowed to slide inwards as the lengthening progresses.

In tibial lengthenings, there is a tendency for formation of a procurvatum deformity as the nail slides posteriorly in the canal. This can be prevented by passing a poller screw from medial to lateral posterior to the track of the nail, before inserting it. Similarly, the nail tends to migrate lateral in the proximal fragment, causing a valgus deformity. The tendency of valgus and procurvatum is similar, regardless of the hardware used for lengthening. The proper entry point has a big role in the causation of deformity. A lateral entry point in the Femur near the greater trochanter can cause a varus deformity. A medial entry point, more commonly seen in the distal entry portal can cause a valgus deformity. Entry point in the proximal tibia is very important as supra tuberosity entry is very likely to have deviated entry points due to the presence of patellar pressure upon knee flexion >120°. A suprapatellar portal enables central entry while flexing the knee only 30°.

A common problem with lengthening over nails is premature consolidation. This can happen due to the enhanced stability. There is another reason which may not be detected and that is lack of parallelism of the external distraction mechanism, in relation to the intramedullary nail, both in the AP and lateral views or in the sagittal and coronal plane.

Large or full segment or full-length x-ray films will show the bone and the struts of the circular fixator or the rail fixator. Adjustments of strut direction or rail to ensure they become parallel to the nail will enable continued lengthening. Performing a repeat corticotomy is difficult in the presence of a nail. The nail may have to be extracted proximal to the osteotomy, which is then repeated, and the nail slid back in and locked.

Poor regenerate formation is less of a problem with this method, than with external fixation. As soon as the length is achieved, the external device is removed after the nail is locked at the new length. Advancing to full weight-bearing during consolidation occurs quickly and rarely requires augmenting of the region with bone marrow aspirate or bone grafting. Deep intramedullary infection is indeed a problem and can be solved by removing the nail, reaming the canal, inserting an antibiotic-coated nail, retaining the external fixation, and giving parenteral antibiotics as suggested by the culture reports. In this instance, it may or may not be possible to achieve the full length, as originally planned.

With more experience, the limitations of performing the deformity correction and lengthening through a single site becomes evident. It may be necessary to perform a large deformity correction at one level and perform the lengthening at the other end or perform a second task like heal a non-union, or fuse a joint.

Both the tasks can be performed using a single intramedullary nail [35], with custom holes in the center for locking bolts that will isolate the two separate locations. Lengthenings larger than 10–12 cm can be performed by two osteotomies and the nail may be locked in the center, or not. These can be accompanied by deformity correction as well. In all these situations, we can perform a double level fixator assisted nailing (see Video 12.1).

Lengthening over a plate and lengthening and then plating are also good methods that enable early removal of the fixator. There are issues of late migration away from the bone in lengthening over the plate, which is solved by the ingenious method of lengthening over a custom slotted plate [36]. This may enable moderately long lengthening in the femur or tibia. A plate may present difficulties in contouring to match the bone, and may stay away from the bone creating some difficulties in knee ROM. While lengthening the femur, an anatomic plate cannot be used as space is needed to fix the half pins posterior to the plate. Since the plate must be fixed with at least three screws, it may need an osteotomy to be made more proximally, closer to the diaphysis. However, enhanced stability of the fixator and plate could ensure early bone formation. One of the limitations of this technique is the inability to correct large deformities and perform the lengthening, and it possibly may make long lengthenings difficult.

The choice of lengthening over a nail or a plate is individual and depends on the felicity, comfort, and control the surgeon has with the hardware. Lengthening and then nailing enables easier deformity correction using the external fixation. Nailing a straight bone would present less challenges, especially if the external fixator pins have been placed away from the intended track of the nail.

References

1. Ilizarov GA. The principles of the Ilizarov method. Bull Hosp Jt Dis Orthop Inst. 1988;48(1):1.
2. Ilizarov GA. The tension-stress effect on the genesis and growth of tissues: part II. The influence of the rate and frequency of distraction. Clin Orthop Relat Res. 1989;239:263.
3. Ilizarov GA. The tension-stress effect on the genesis and growth of tissues. Part I. The influence of stability of fixation and soft-tissue preservation. Clin Orthop Relat Res. 1989;238:249.
4. Ilizarov GA. Clinical application of the tension-stress effect for limb lengthening. Clin Orthop Relat Res. 1990;250:8.
5. Paley D, Herzenberg JE, Paremain G, Bhave A. Femoral lengthening over an intramedullary nail. A matched-case comparison with Ilizarov femoral lengthening. J Bone Joint Surg Am. 1997;79(10):1464.
6. Green SA. The Ilizarov method: Rancho technique. Orthop Clin North Am. 1991;22(4):677.
7. Antoci V, Ono CM, Antoci V Jr, Raney EM. Pin-tract infection during limb lengthening using external fixation. Am J Orthop. 2008;37(9):E150.
8. Dahl MT, Gulli B, Berg T. Complications of limb lengthening. A learning curve. Clin Orthop Relat Res. 1994;301:10.
9. Sheridan GA, Fragomen AT, Rozbruch SR. Integrated limb lengthening is superior to classical limb lengthening: a systematic review and meta-analysis of the literature. J Am Acad Orthop Surg Glob Res Rev. 2020;4(6)
10. Bost FC, Larsen LJ. Experiences with lengthening of the femur over n intramedullary rod. J Bone Joint Surg Am. 1956;38-A(3):567.
11. Gordon JE, Goldfarb CA, Luhmann SJ, Lyons D, Schoenecker PL. Femoral lengthening over a humeral intramedullary nail in preadolescent children. J Bone Joint Surg Am. 2002;84(6):930.
12. Gordon JE, Manske MC, Lewis TR, O'Donnell JC, Schoenecker PL, Keeler KA. Femoral lengthening over a pediatric femoral nail: results and complications. J Pediatr Orthop. 2013;33(7):730.
13. Lampasi M, Launay F, Jouve JL, Bollini G. Femoral lengthening over elastic stable intramedullary nailing in children using the monolateral external fixator. La Chirurgia degli organi di movimento. 2009;93(2):57.
14. Popkov D, Popkov A, Haumont T, Journeau P, Lascombes P. Flexible intramedullary nail use in limb lengthening. J Pediatr Orthop. 2010;30(8):910.
15. Popkov A, Pietrzak S, Antonov A, Parol T, Lazovic M, Podeszwa D, Popkov D. Limb lengthening for congenital deficiencies using external fixation combined with flexible intramedullary nailing: a multicenter study. J Pediatr Orthop. 2021;41(6):e439.
16. Rozbruch SR, Kleinman D, Fragomen AT, Ilizarov S. Limb lengthening and then insertion of an intramedullary nail: a case-matched comparison. Clin Orthop Relat Res. 2008;466(12):2923.
17. Iobst CA, Dahl MT. Limb lengthening with submuscular plate stabilization: a case series and description of the technique. J Pediatr Orthop. 2007;27(5):504.
18. Georgiadis AG, Rossow JK, Laine JC, Iobst CA, Dahl MT. Plate-assisted lengthening of the femur and tibia in pediatric patients. J Pediatr Orthop. 2017;37(7):473.
19. Oh CW, Kim JW, Baek SG, Kyung HS, Lee HJ. Limb lengthening with a submuscular locking plate. JBJS Essent Surg Tech. 2014;3(4):e24.
20. Oh CW, Song HR, Kim JW, Choi JW, Min WK, Park BC. Limb lengthening with a submuscular locking plate. J Bone Joint Surg Br. 2009;91(10):1394.
21. Harbacheuski R, Fragomen AT, Rozbruch SR. Does lengthening and then plating (LAP) shorten duration of external fixation? Clin Orthop Relat Res. 2012;470(6):1771.
22. Uysal M, Akpinar S, Cesur N, Hersekli MA, Tandogan RN. Plating after lengthening (PAL): technical notes and preliminary clinical experiences. Arch Orthop Trauma Surg. 2007;127(10):889.
23. Dahl MT, Morrison S. Segmental Bone Defects and the History of Bone Transport. J Orthop Trauma. 2021;35(Suppl 4):S1–S7. https://doi.org/10.1097/BOT.0000000000002124. PMID: 34533479.
24. Oh CW, Song HR, Roh JY, Oh JK, Min WK, Kyung HS, Kim JW, Kim PT, Ihn JC. Bone transport over an intramedullary nail for reconstruction of long bone defects in tibia. Arch Orthop Trauma Surg. 2008;128(8):801.
25. Bernstein M, Fragomen A, Rozbruch SR. Tibial bone transport over an intramedullary nail using cable and pulleys. JBJS Essent Surg Tech. 2018;8(1):e9.
26. Oh CW, Apivatthakakul T, Oh JK, Kim JW, Lee HJ, Kyung HS, Baek SG, Jung GH. Bone transport with an external fixator and a locking plate for segmental tibial defects. Bone Joint J. 2013;95-B(12):1667.
27. Medium-term evaluation of leg lengthening by ISKD® intramedullary nail in 28 patients: should we still use this lengthening system? Orthop Traumatol Surg Res. 2020;106(7):1433–40.
28. Thaller PH, Frankenberg F, Degen N, Soo C, Wolf F, Euler E, Fürmetz J. Complications and effectiveness of intramedullary limb lengthening: a matched pair analysis of two different lengthening nails. Strategies Trauma Limb Reconstr. 2020;15(1):7–12.
29. Chaudhary M. Limb lengthening over a nail can safely reduce the duration of external fixation. Indian J Orthop. 2008;42(3):323–9.
30. Guichet J-M. Personal communication. ILLRS Congress Miami; Nov 2015.

31. Ross KA, Steinhaus M, Rozbruch SR, Fragomen AT. Blocking screws for intramedullary nail guidance. J Limb Lengthen Reconstr. 2019;5. 62. 10.4103.
32. Dabash S, Zhang DT, Rozbruch SR, Fragomen AT. Blocking screw-assisted intramedullary nailing using the reverse-rule-of-thumbs for limb lengthening and deformity correction. Strategies Trauma Limb Reconstr. 2019;14(2):77–84.
33. Kucukkaya M, Karakoyun Ö, Erol MF. The importance of reaming the posterior femoral cortex before inserting lengthening nails and calculation of the amount of reaming. J Orthop Surg Res. 2016;11:11.
34. Thaller PH, Furmetz F. Retrograde femur technique for motorized internal limb lengthening. Techn Orthop. 35(3):171–5.
35. Chaudhary MM, Lakhani PH. Double-level fixator-assisted nailing (DL-FAN). Bone Joint J. 2019;101-B(2):178–88.
36. Kulkarni SM, Kulkarni RM. Femoral lengthening using ilizarov ring fixator and slotted plate. J Limb Lengthen Reconstr. 2022;8:110–4.

Motorized Intramedullary Lengthening of the Femur: Antegrade and Retrograde

Søren Kold and Christopher A. Iobst

Evolution

In "A Brief History of Limb Lengthening" from 2017, John G. Birch mentions three major advances in limb lengthening within the last 35 years: (1) distraction osteogenesis with circular frames, (2) the introduction of computer assisted hexapod frames, and (3) the development of motorized intramedullary lengthening nails [1]. Limb lengthening by fully implantable intramedullary lengthening nails builds on the principles of distraction osteogenesis developed by Gavriil Ilizarov [2]. Distraction osteogenesis by external fixation provides solutions for very complex limb deformities. However, there are drawbacks inherent to using an external fixator for limb lengthening such as pin-site infection, patient discomfort and risk of regenerate bending or fracture after removal of the external fixator. By residing within the intramedullary canal and avoiding the need for pins and wires traversing the soft tissue envelope, fully implantable lengthening nails eliminate some of the disadvantages with external fixators. Table 13.1 highlights the pros and cons of motorized lengthening nails and external fixators in limb lengthening. Retrospective studies comparing fully implantable lengthening nails with external fixators for bone lengthening of the femur have suggested that lengthening nails: (a) reduce the overall number of complications, (b) better preserve knee range of motion, (c) result in faster healing of the regenerate, (d) result in less pain, and, (e) result in higher patient satisfaction [3–5].

S. Kold (✉)
Limb Lengthening and Reconstruction, Department of Orthopaedics, Aalborg University Hospital, Aalborg, Denmark
e-mail: sovk@rn.dk

C. A. Iobst
Center for Limb Lengthening and Reconstruction, Orthopaedic Surgery, Nationwide Children's Hospital, Columbus, OH, USA
e-mail: Christopher.iobst@nationwidechildrens.org

Table 13.1 Comparison between internal lengthening nails and external fixation for lower limb lengthening

Internal lengthening nail	External fixation
Advantages • Higher patient comfort • No pin problems **Disadvantages** • Can only distract along the long axis of the nail • Deformity correction must be performed acutely at surgery. The limitations for acute deformity correction regarding risk of neurologic damage or delayed union are not known • Soft-tissue coverage mandatory to prevent infection **Complications** • Less frequent than with external fixation, especially on the femur • However, complications are still frequent	**Advantages** • Can be applied in children with open growth plates • Can be applied in bones with small intramedullary diameter or short length • Gradual correction can be performed in all planes • Less risk of reactivating previous bone infection • An unstable joint can be spanned by the external fixator during lengthening **Disadvantages (especially on the femur)** • Uncomfortable for the patient • Pin problems (infection, pain) • Decreased range of motion of joints due to transfixation of muscles and other soft-tissues • Difficult to assess when to remove the frame with risk of regenerate bending or fracture after frame removal **Complications** • More frequent than with lengthening nails; however, external fixation often used for more complex cases

A Ukrainian surgeon, Alexander Bliskunov, was the first to introduce a mechanical femoral lengthening nail that was attached to the iliac bone [6]. The first generation of intramedullary lengthening nails were fully mechanical using a rachet mechanism to achieve lengthening. Over time, unfor-

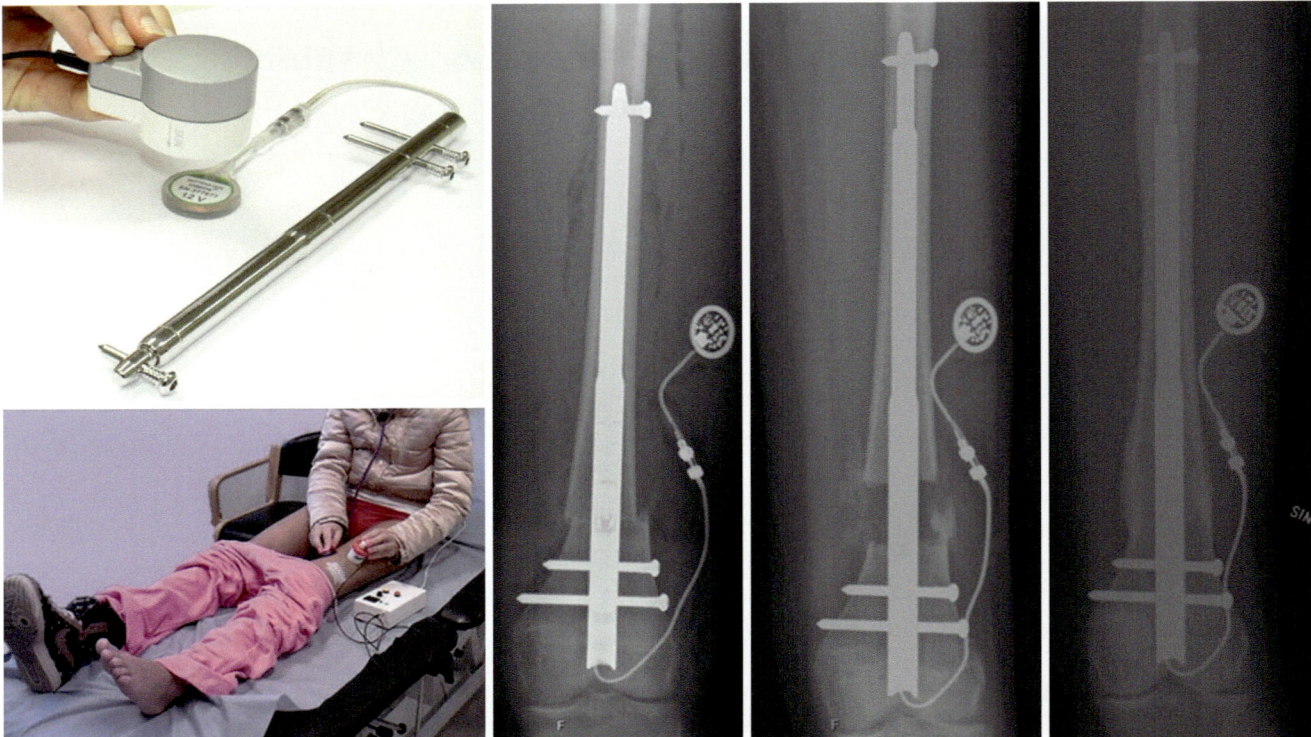

Fig. 13.1 Electric motorized FITBONE™ nail. Energy is transmitted from an external transducer through the skin to an internal receiver. The energy is transmitted from the internal receiver to the motor inside the nail by a connecting cord. The activation of the motor can be heard by a stethoscope placed over the nail

tunately, these types of nails were found to have design flaws that limited their success. Some nails, like the Albizzia™ nail, required the patients to twist their lower limb to activate the nail, which was extremely painful and required a high re-admission rate to the hospital. Other nails, such as the Intramedullary Skeletal Kinetic Distractor (ISKD™) did not allow the surgeon to control the rate of lengthening. This resulted in cases of "runaway" lengthening with subsequent poor regenerate bone formation.

The current generation of lengthening nails contain internal mechanisms that are controlled from outside the limb. Currently, there are two FDA approved motorized lengthening nails: the Fitbone™ and the Precice™ nails. Both nails elongate by use of gearing systems but the powering of the motors differs. The Fitbone™ nail, developed by Rainer Baumgart, contains an electric motor that is powered from the outside as electricity is transmitted through the skin (Fig. 13.1). An induction coil (called the receiver or antenna) underneath the skin is connected to the nail via a cable, and a second induction coil placed outside the body transmits energy through the skin.

The Precice™ nail is controlled by a magnet system (Fig. 13.2). Inside the nail, there is a strong rare earth magnet that can rotate. A handheld device containing two additional magnets is placed on the skin over the nail magnet. As the two magnets in the handheld device rotate, they create a magnetic field that captures and spins the magnet inside the nail. The rotational force of the internal magnet is converted through a series of gears to a longitudinal force enabling expansion or retraction of the nail.

Fig. 13.2 Magnetically powered PRECICE™ nail. A cylindrical magnet inside the nail rotates when an external magnetic field is activated outside the limb. The rotational force is transferred through gearing systems to enable longitudinal elongation (or compression) of the nail. Radiographs showing good regenerate bone after acute deformity correction and immediate bone lengthening through the same osteotomy

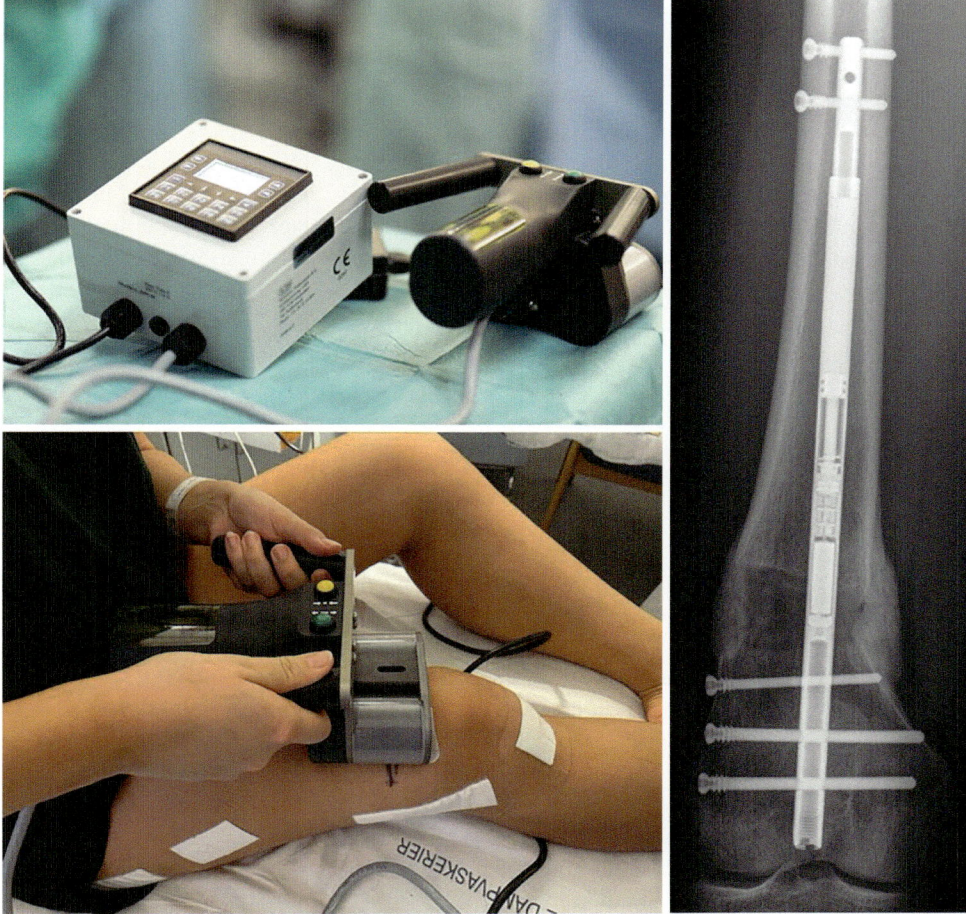

Indications

Whenever limb lengthening is required on the femur, the possibility of treating the patient with an internal lengthening nail should be considered. Particularly on the femur, the external fixator is cumbersome and uncomfortable for the patient. In addition, due to the need for pins and wires to traverse the skin and underlying soft tissues, external fixators often develop pin site infections during the course of treatment. Fractures through pin-holes or the lengthening regenerate can also occur after fixator removal. Since internal lengthening nails do not require transfixion elements through the skin and muscles, there are no pin site infections, there is improved early joint motion and the resulting surgical scars are more cosmetically acceptable.

However, there are some limitations that must be considered when contemplating using an internal lengthening nail. For example, in pediatric patients, the implantation of an internal lengthening nail is limited by the intramedullary diameter and/or the length of the femoral bone. Furthermore, open growth plates and the vascular supply to the femoral head must be considered in skeletally immature patients.

In general, the limitations for using bone lengthening nails on the femur include:

- The physis should ideally be closed.
  - If the proximal physis of the femoral epiphysis is still open, an antegrade insertion through the piriformis fossa should be avoided to prevent iatrogenic injury to the vascular supply to the femoral head resulting in risk of avascular necrosis of the femoral head. A trochanteric entry nail should be considered instead.
  - The age limitation of patients for insertion through the trochanteric apophysis with a trochanteric entry point is not known. Experienced surgeons are routinely placing nails in skeletally immature patients (from 8 years of age) [7, 8]. However, if the surgeon has any concern about the possibility of avascular necrosis of the femoral head, the surgeon should wait until skeletal maturity to place an antegrade femoral nail.

- The age limitation of patients for insertion of a retrograde nail through an open growth plate distally on the femur is not known. If placing a nail through an open distal physis is considered, keeping the nail entry point at the very center of the physis and maintaining the nail across the physis until skeletal maturity may help to prevent growth abnormalities [9, 10]. However, if retrograde nail is to be inserted for rare cases through an open distal femoral epiphysis, it might be safer to perform an epiphysiodesis at the time of nail insertion. Hereby, additional lengthening is required but the introduction of a secondary deformity from an injured growth plate is prevented.
- If the diameter or length of the femur is too small to safely insert the currently available implant sizes, then an alternative to intramedullary lengthening should be investigated.
- When using a retrograde femoral lengthening nail, the osteotomy level should optimally not be closer than 5 cm from the joint line to ensure good purchase of locking screws.
- Since it is not possible to span the adjacent joint such as an unstable knee (or hip) joint with an internal lengthening nail, patients with unstable hip or knee joints will need reconstruction prior to lengthening (preparatory surgery).
- If the intramedullary canal path is obstructed (incarcerated hardware, cement, etc.) then using an internal lengthening nail will not be possible.
- Complicated femoral deformity requiring multiple osteotomy sites to allow insertion of the internal lengthening nail may require a staged approach.
- The size of the thigh is especially important to consider when determining whether to use the magnetically powered internal lengthening nail. If the size of the soft tissue envelope creates a distance that is too large for the magnet inside the nail to communicate with the handheld magnet at the level of the skin, then the nail will not function properly (or at all).
- Intramedullary lengthening nails are relative contraindicated in high-risk patients for deep infection, i.e., previous osteomyelitis [7] or in patients with compromised soft tissue coverage.

Some paediatric patients, such as those with congenital shortening related to congenital femoral deficiency (CFD) and fibular hemimelia have a high risk of joint subluxation or dislocation during lengthening that cannot be prevented by external spanning of the joint when performing fully internal lengthening. Therefore, realignment of joint angles and ligamentous laxity should be addressed prior to internal limb lengthening to reduce the risk of joint subluxation/luxation. Examples are a SuperHip procedure in CFD [11] or guided growth with a hemi-epiphysiodesis for distal valgus deformity. If the patient has a grossly unstable knee examination or lateral radiographs of the knee that demonstrate subluxation of the tibia on the femur prior to embarking on the lengthening, then knee reconstruction is highly recommended before using an internal lengthening nail. Preoperative MRI of the knee can demonstrate patients with lack of cruciate ligaments, which increases the risk of knee subluxation during lengthening. Soft-tissue release of the ilio-tibial band might be performed in high-risk patients distally on the femur to prevent postero-lateral subluxation of the knee joint [12]. Postoperative physiotherapy is mandatory to prevent and treat muscle contractures and lengthening should be as slow as possible without having premature consolidation of the regenerate. Finally, the needed lengthening can be obtained during repeated nail lengthening procedures. Lengthening should be terminated when the risk of joint subluxation/luxation gets too high, and then lengthening can be resumed at a later point, either by using the same nail as previously or applying a new nail. Reusing the same PRECICE™ nail, the so-called "sleeper" concept, appears to be safe if the nail has no signs of bending or breakage and if the nail has not been fully deployed [13].

To date, the following etiologies have been managed with internal lengthening nails to treat limb shortening secondary to various etiologies [7, 14–16]:

- Idiopathic shortening
- Fibular hemimelia
- Congenital femoral deficiency
- Postraumatic deformity
- Ollier's disease
- Congenital clubfoot
- Post-septic growth arrest
- LLD after hip arthroplasty
- Gradual relocation of femoral head in hip dysplasia
- Hemihypertrophy
- Tumor
- Hypochondroplasia/achondroplasia
- Short stature

Preoperative Evaluation

History and Physical Examination

Gait/Alignment/Muscles/Shortening/Rotation

The etiology of shortening must be sought to anticipate any problems with limb lengthening such as knee subluxation in severe fibular hemimelia or infection in patients with a previous history of osteomyelitis.

The surgeon should consider the following when examining a potential femoral internal lengthening nail patient:

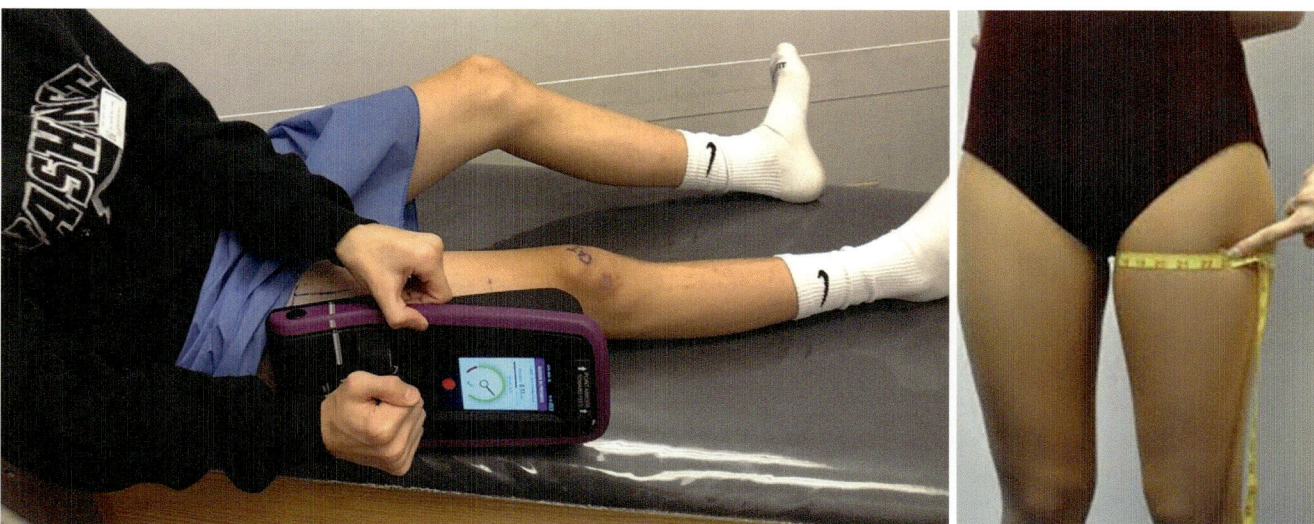

Fig. 13.3 A rough estimate of the distance from the skin to the nail can be obtained clinically to ensure that the external magnet can drive the internal magnet in the Precice™ lengthening nail

Is the gait influenced by the limb shortening? Is the gait pattern corrected to some extent by shoe lift?

Overall limb shortening and contributions of each segment (femur, tibia, foot) to the shortening.

How is the overall mechanical alignment of the lower limbs in frontal and sagittal plane? Some deformities might potentially be corrected through the same lengthening osteotomy. However, deformities leading to unstable joints or larger deformities should be corrected at separate surgery prior to lengthening.

Are there any rotational deformities visible during gait? Analysis of femoral rotation is best examined with the patient prone. For the tibia, this can be assessed either prone (thigh foot angle) or with the patient sitting with 90° of knee flexion and neutral ankle position (malleolar axis).

Overall personality of the muscles in the thigh: Are the muscles long and "ready" for limb lengthening as in hypochondroplasia or are the muscles tight in a small limb as in congenital femoral deficiency? Remember, tight muscles on pre-operative examination will only get tighter during the lengthening process.

Size of the thigh: Any problems when using a magnetic nail? (Fig. 13.3).

Signs of gluteal weakness (Trendelenburg sign) should caution the surgeon to analyze the radiographs for a potentially unstable hip joint. If the hip is stable but the gluteal muscles are weak, it might be better to perform lengthening through a distal femoral osteotomy with retrograde lengthening nail.

Strength of knee extensor muscles. Weak muscles should caution the surgeon when considering a retrograde lengthening.

When weakness of muscles is present, it might be advantageous to perform smaller, but repeated, lengthening procedures. Furthermore, the ultimate lengthening goal might be to leave the weakened limb a little short (0.5–1 cm) compared to the contralateral leg in order to achieve a well-functioning gait.

Joint Stability

Hip Joint

Hip joint stability is assessed from:

- The etiology of the limb shortening
- Physical examination focused on hip range of motion (flexion/extension, abduction/adduction, internal and external rotation). Any contractures identified must be corrected prior to lengthening.
- Pelvic radiographs and hip radiographs in AP and lateral plane. Risk factors for unstable hip are low CE (Center Edge) angle or varus angulation of the femoral neck associated with femoral retroversion and acetabular dysplasia.

Special considerations with unstable hip joint:

- Soft-tissue release of the iliopsoas muscle can be performed prior to lengthening.
- For congenital femoral deficiency, the following are often performed prior to lengthening:
  - Soft tissue releases: iliopsoas, rectus femoris, piriformis, abductors
  - Correction osteotomies: Pelvic osteotomy and femoral valgus and derotation osteotomy

- When lengthening in a patient with previously unstable hip joint, it might be safer to lengthen through a distal femoral osteotomy. This brings the primary forces of lengthening closer to the knee and further away from the hip. The lengthening goal should be small but the lengthening procedure can be repeated. The lengthening rate should be as low as possible without having premature consolidation.

Knee Joint

Knee joint stability is assessed from:

- The etiology of the limb shortening
- Physical examination: Knee range of motion (flexion/extension) and knee laxity.
- AP and lateral radiographs of the knee joint. Radiographic risk factors for unstable knee are: (1) malalignment of knee joint, (2) dysplasia of femoral condyle, (3) lateral subluxation of patella, and (4) absence of tibial spines.
- MRI can be used to help determine the presence of anterior and posterior cruciate ligaments.

Special considerations with unstable knee joint:

- The patient should be capable of fully extending the knee joint prior to lengthening. Soft-tissue release of the iliotibial band at time of lengthening can be performed. Corrective extension osteotomies are best performed at separate surgery prior to lengthening, enabling physiotherapy and gain of full knee extension prior to lengthening.
- When lengthening in a patient with unstable knee joint, it might be safer to lengthen through a proximal femoral osteotomy. The lengthening goal should be small for each lengthening procedure as the lengthening procedure can be repeated. The lengthening rate should be as low as possible without having premature consolidation.
- Static and dynamic external braces can be applied to ensure full knee extension throughout the lengthening.
- Loss of knee extension is a warning sign for subluxation.
- Lateral knee radiographs should be taken to examine for signs of subluxation.

Ankle Joint

Ankle joint motion and the position of the weightbearing foot is examined. If the patient is not capable of weightbearing with a plantigrade foot, additional surgeries might be planned prior to femoral lengthening.

Mental Health Examination

Limb lengthening, even with motorized lengthening nails, requires a high degree of patient collaboration and effort to reach a successful outcome without complications. Even in the best circumstances, the long medical journey required by limb lengthening surgery can provoke feelings of frustration, depression and anxiety in patients. The patient should be screened for: (1) Depression, (2) Anxiety, (3) Chronic pain, (4) Addictions since these may all be exacerbated by the limb lengthening experience. Scheduling behavioral health sessions before surgery and throughout the post-operative recovery period is recommended for any patient but especially for all at-risk patients.

Social Examination

Limb lengthening requires regular follow-up examinations at the outpatient clinic as well as regular physiotherapy. The patient and his/her family will need to have appropriate resources at their disposal to fulfill the postoperative rehabilitation requirements. Transportation to weekly office visits and multiple physical therapy sessions will be needed. The parent or guardian must have time available to care for the child and accompany him/her to each visit. Therefore, a preoperative assessment of the patient's psychosocial situation is recommended before starting the lengthening. Risk factors for a more challenging treatment process have been identified such as living with a single parent, having a preexisting mental health condition, and having a history of previous surgery [17].

Bone Health Examination

Does the patient have any medical co-morbidities that may affect bone healing? Medical conditions (e.g., diabetes) or medications (e.g., nicotine) that inhibit blood flow are particularly important to investigate.

The vitamin-D and endocrinological status should also be evaluated. If the patient has a low vitamin-D level preoperatively, Vitamin D supplementation should be started and monitored before surgery (pre-habilitation).

Does the patient receive antirheumatic treatment (such as methotrexate or other immunosuppressive drugs)?

Does the patient smoke?

Any previous history of infection?

Previous history of external fixator on the femur?

Any sclerotic areas on the radiograph as a warning of previous infection or reduced bone healing capacity?

Femoral Lengthening Along the Long Axis of the Lengthening Nail

Theoretically, lengthening with an internal intramedullary nail results in lengthening along the anatomical axis of the femur. For femoral lengthening, this leads to medialization of the knee joint which shifts the lower limb mechanical axis laterally resulting in a distal femoral valgus deformity. Lengthening along the anatomical femoral axis in a normally aligned limb has been shown to shift the mechanical axis by 1 mm for each 1 cm lengthening [18]. This shift might not be clinically important in small lengthenings. Furthermore, the mechanical axis shift occurring during femoral lengthening may change depending on the osteotomy level. For example, if the nail is not fully filling the intramedullary canal on both sides of the osteotomy and if blocking screws are not applied, the osteotomy will have a tendency to angulate corresponding to the tension forces arising during lengthening. When lengthening through a proximal or mid-diaphyseal osteotomy on the femur, this often leads to a varus angulation and thus reduces the lateral shift of the mechanical axis. When lengthening through a distal osteotomy on the femur, this often leads to a valgus angulation and thus enhances the lateral shift of the mechanical axis. The factors mentioned above, however, are controllable with a detailed preoperative plan. A final consideration is the diameter of the implant itself. Using small diameter nails, such as the 8.5 mm diameter Precice nail™, with a larger lengthening might result in unforeseen angulation of the bone regenerate due to bending of the nail.

Antegrade Versus Retrograde

An antegrade approach is applied for straight forward lengthening without simultaneous deformity correction (Fig. 13.4). Furthermore, an antegrade approach using a trochanteric entry point is needed in the skeletally immature patient. Good short-term results have been found from the age of 14-years when the entry-related defect of the apophyseal growth plate was bridged by the nail [7]. However, the exact lower age limit of applying a nail through the trochanteric physis is currently unknown. When the osteotomy is made proximal to the isthmus of the femoral diaphysis, the regenerate has a tendency to angulate slightly into varus and thereby compensate for the medialization of the knee joint, and a clinically important mechanical axis deviation might not occur in smaller lengthening.

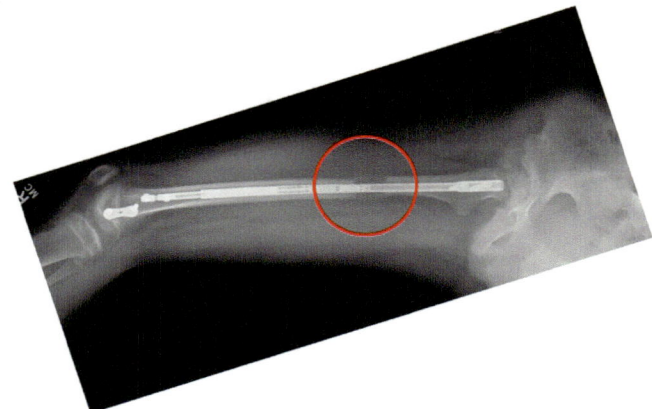

Fig. 13.4 In antegrade nailing, the level of the osteotomy can be chosen at the maximum of the femoral curvature in the lateral plane. This level can be located intraoperatively with fluoroscopy in the lateral view and allows for introduction of a straight lengthening nail into a curved bone. A possible minor extension at this level of the femur does not seem to introduce a clinical important sagittal plane deformity

The introduction of a straight nail into the curved femur is also assisted by an entry point in the anterior part of the femur. While the antegrade approach has the benefit of not violating the knee joint, it does penetrate the gluteal muscles. Consequently, preoperative and postoperative exercises focused on the hip abductors should be initiated.

In general, the retrograde approach is reserved for patients requiring lengthening with simultaneous deformity correction through the lengthening osteotomy (Fig. 13.22a–l). Another possible scenario for retrograde nail usage is in the patient with a large thigh. For the magnet powered nail, the retrograde nail position brings the magnet away from the thick proximal thigh and into the distal, thinner portion of the thigh. This more distal location allows the internal magnet to communicate with the magnets in the handheld device more easily.

Preoperative Radiographs

The following radiographs (Figs. 13.5, 13.6, 13.7, 13.8, 13.9, 13.10, and 13.11) are needed:

Fig. 13.5 Standing AP full length bilateral lower extremity with calibration. The clinical LLD is assessed to ensure that the patient has the correct lift under the short limb when taking the standing AP full length radiograph. Hereby both the correct LLD and limb axis are obtained

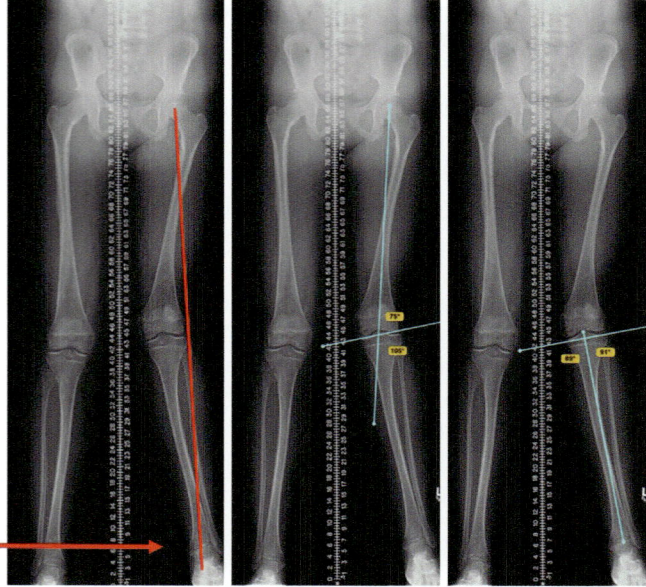

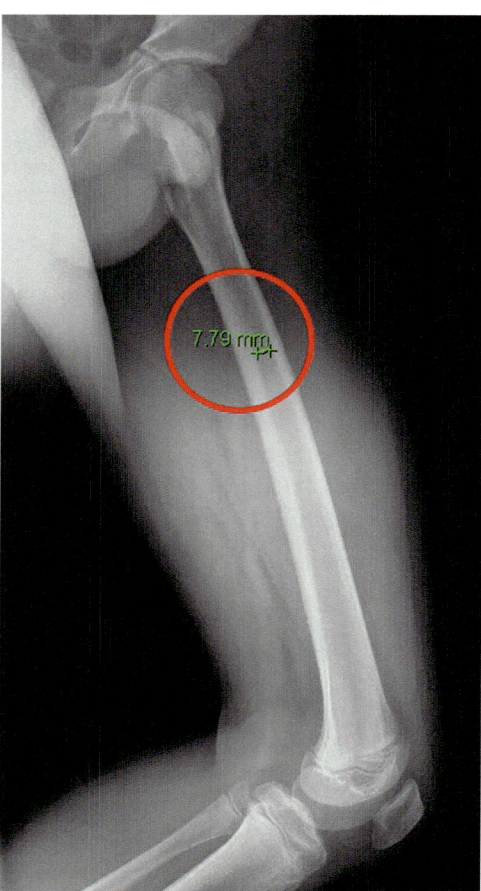

Fig. 13.6 Lateral femoral radiograph to ensure that a straight nail with chosen diameter can be inserted. Measurement indicates the diameter of the femoral canal at its narrowest point. (isthmus)

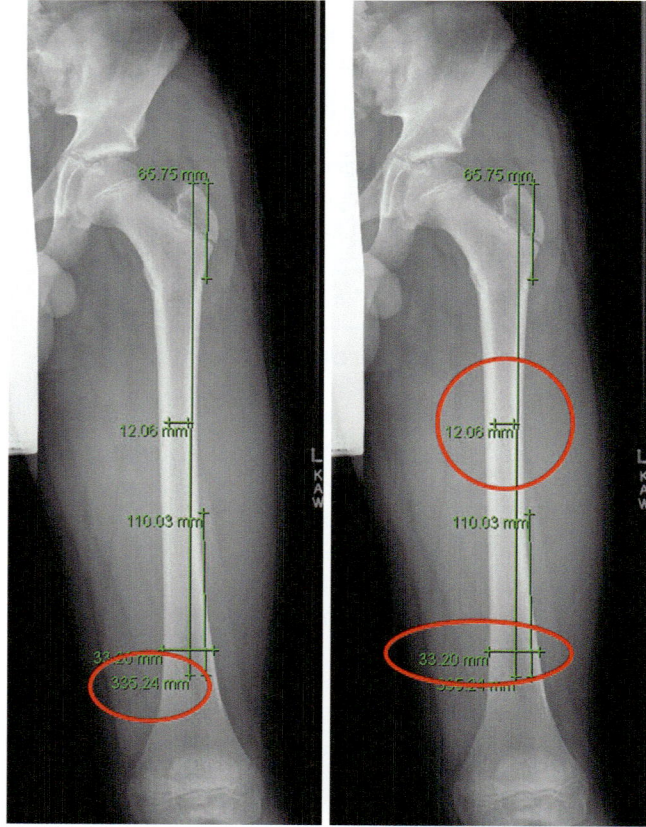

Fig. 13.7 The osteotomy level is chosen ensuring that the lengthening zone does not extend into the junctional part of the lengthening nail as this will destabilize the regenerate. (The distance = 8 cm + the desired lengthening amount)

13 Motorized Intramedullary Lengthening of the Femur: Antegrade and Retrograde

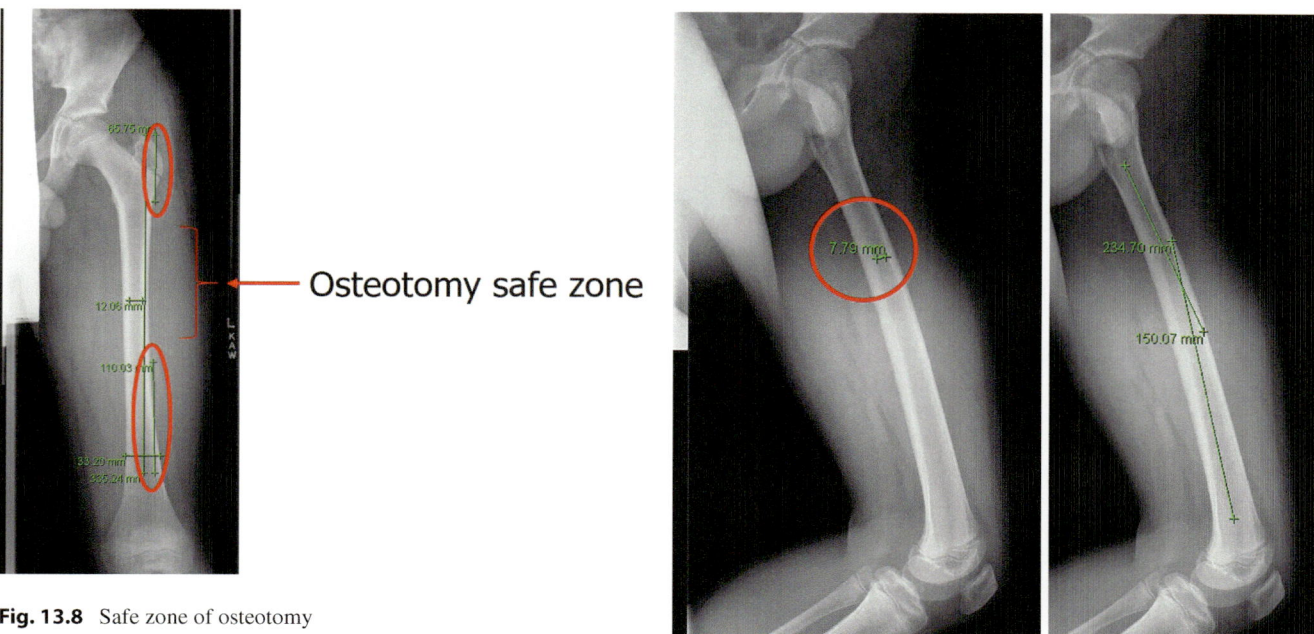

Fig. 13.8 Safe zone of osteotomy

Fig. 13.9 Osteotomy at maximum bending in lateral plane will ensure insertion of a straight nail into a curved femur

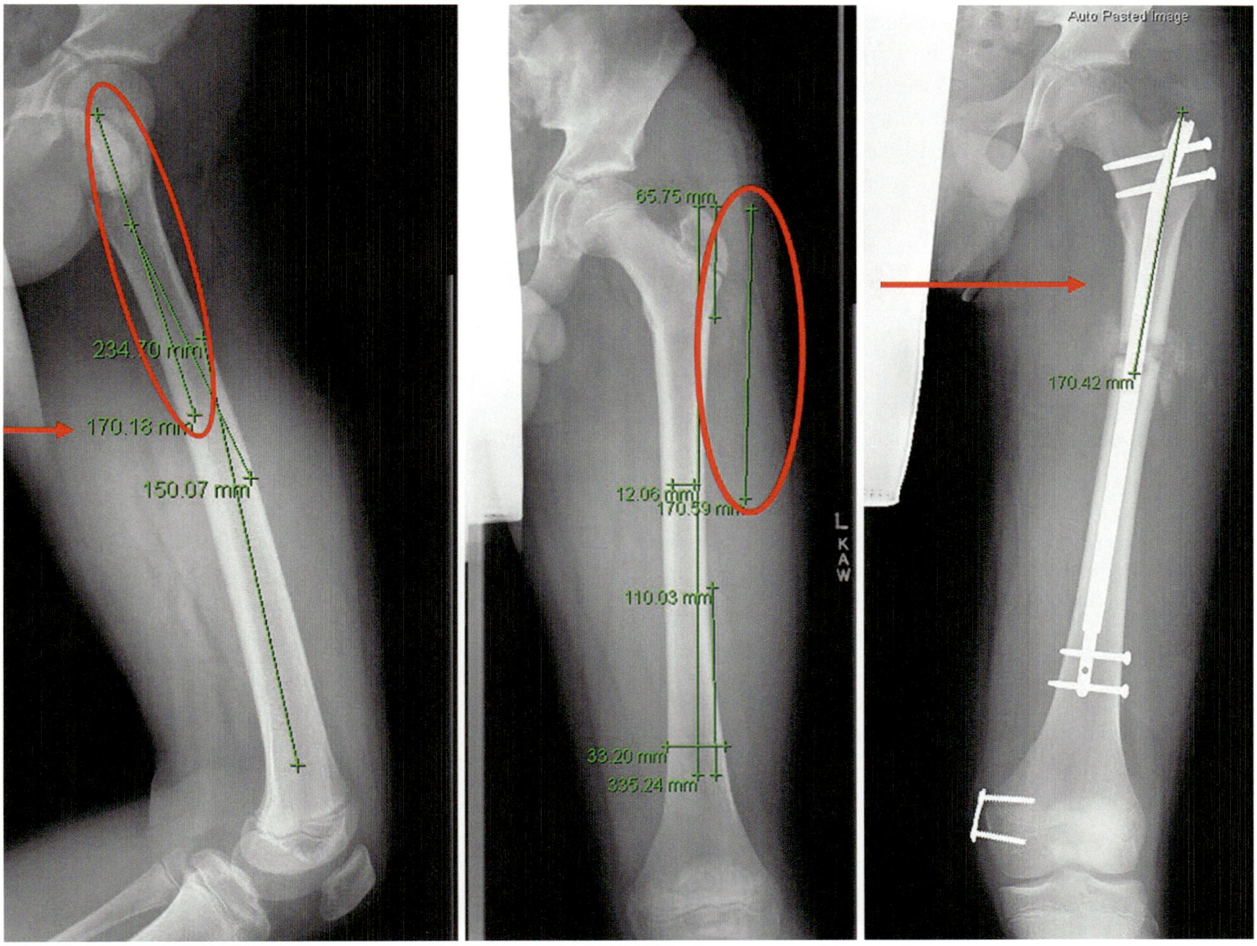

Fig. 13.10 Antegrade nail insertion and additional placement of guided growth plate to correct for distal valgus deformity

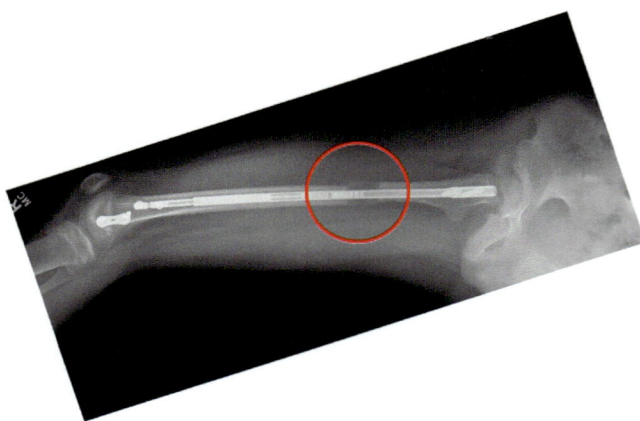

Fig. 13.11 The minimal extension at the osteotomy site does not produce a clinically relevant deformity

Preoperative Planning

A detailed preoperative plan is paramount to obtain the surgical goal. In most cases, the surgeon is aiming to achieve equal leg lengths with symmetric, neutral mechanical axes. Since the implant has no inherent capability of deformity correction other than distraction or compression, any angular or rotational deformities must be corrected acutely at the time of nail insertion. While distal deformity can potentially be corrected with a separate osteotomy (or guided growth in skeletally immature patients), antegrade femoral nails are ideally reserved for patients with leg length discrepancy and no additional deformity or a diaphyseal deformity. Inserting a straight nail allows acute correction of diaphyseal deformities nicely and can be combined with rotational corrections, if necessary.

Simple Antegrade Lengthening Without Deformity Correction

Intraoperative Pearls (Figs. 13.12, 13.13, 13.14, 13.15, 13.16, 13.17, 13.18, 13.19, and 13.20)

For antegrade nailing, the patient can be positioned either in a supine position or in the lateral decubitus position.

Reverse Planning Method

Baumgart has described the reverse planning method for preoperative planning using intramedullary lengthening nails [19]. Once the level of the osteotomy is determined, the desired final result after lengthening and deformity correction is simulated (Fig. 13.22a–l). The lengthening process is then virtually reversed along the axis of the planned nail position until the lengthening gap is closed. At this point, the needed translation or angulation at the osteotomy can be determined. The reverse planning method is particularly helpful when performing acute deformity correction and simultaneous intramedullary lengthening through the same osteotomy site. However, the preoperative planning can only be transferred to a successful clinical result if the planned nail position is replicated exactly intra-operatively. Since the lengthening will occur along the axis of the inserted nail any deviation from the planned position will result in either over- or under-correction. Using rigid rather than flexible reamers will help to keep the nail path true to its desired location.

It is also extremely important to guide the insertion of the nail along the proper path and to maintain the final position of correction with the use of blocking screws. Any space between the nail and the bone cortex in either the coronal or sagittal plane has the potential to allow migration of the nail in the canal. This migration will result in a loss of alignment over time. Blocking screws close this space and prevent loss of the desired correction. There is no universally agreed upon correct number of blocking screws to insert. Each case is evaluated on an individual basis and the number of screws necessary to secure the nail in the canal above and below the osteotomy site should be determined by the surgeon. (Fig. 13.22a–l).

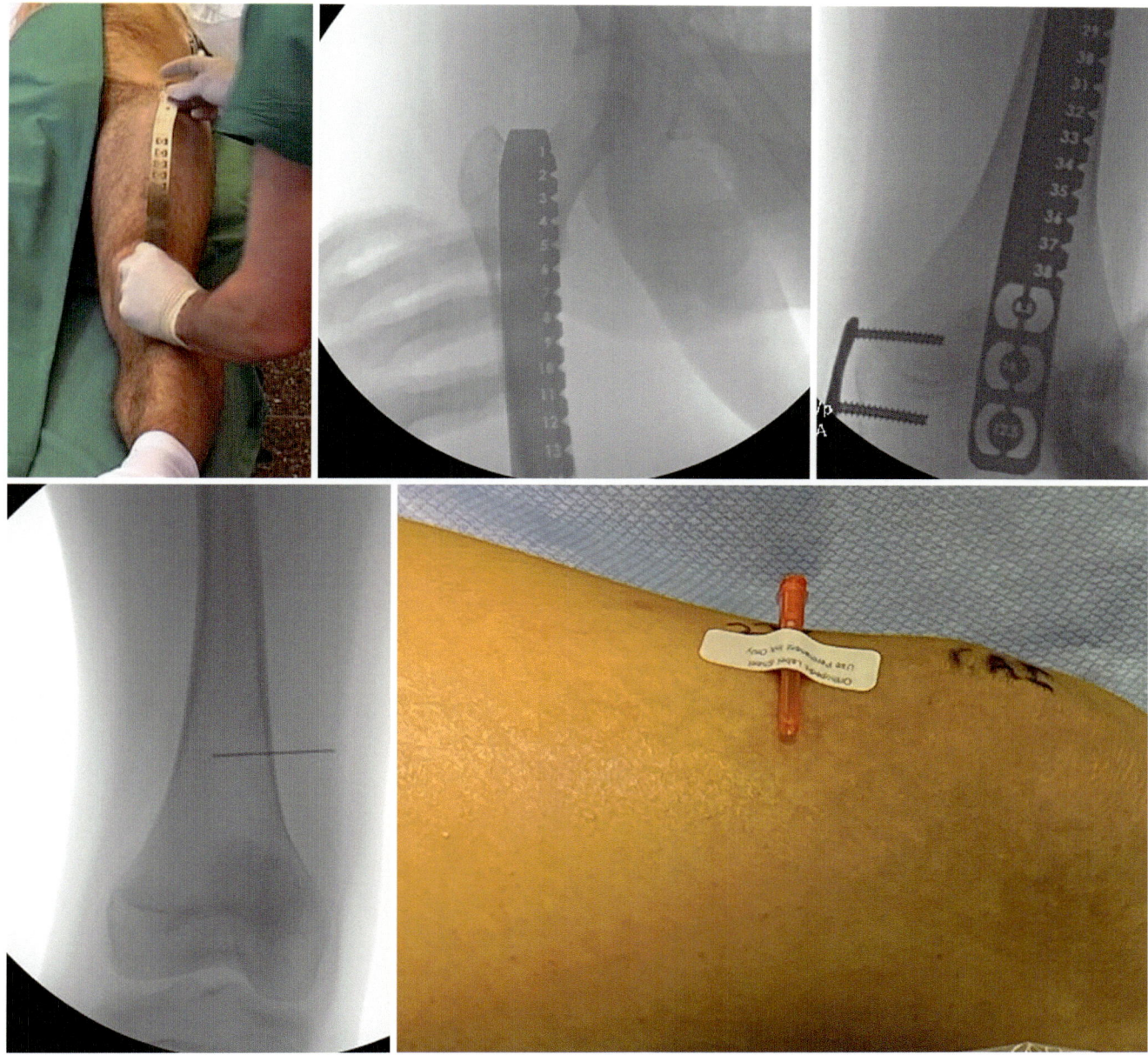

Fig. 13.12 The reaming depth, corresponding to a little longer than the length of the nail, is marked with a syringe needle taped to the skin

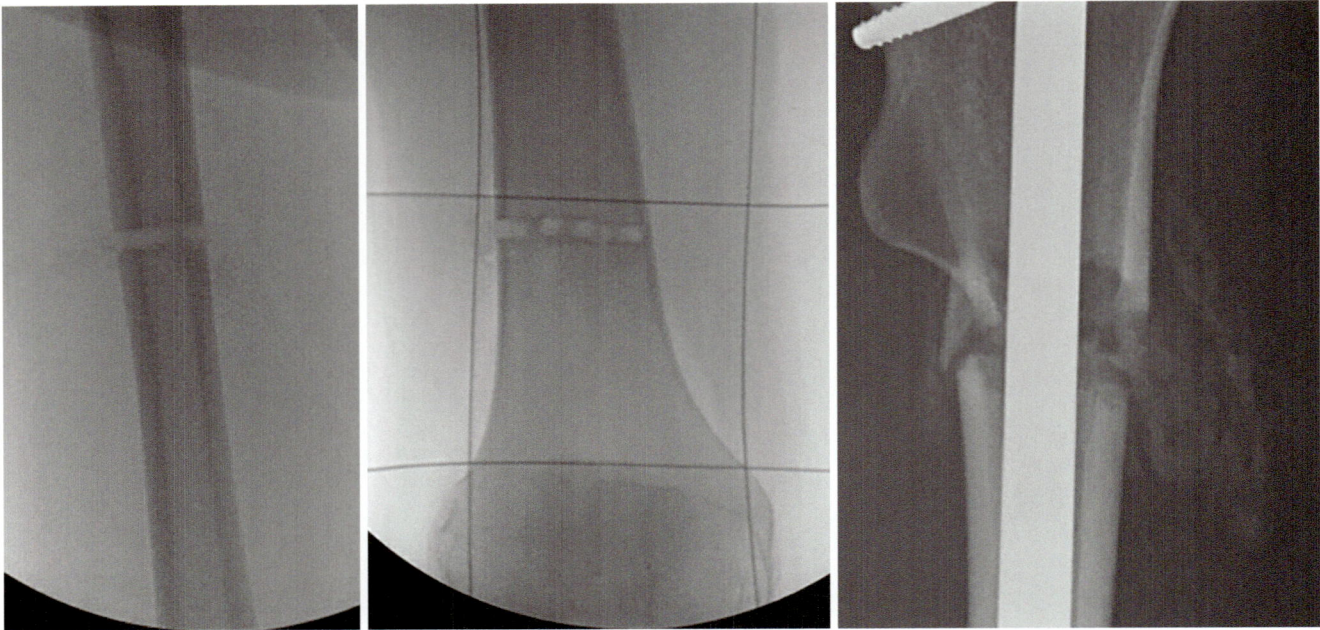

Fig. 13.13 At the planned osteotomy site, venting holes are made with a drill prior to reaming. The venting holes ensure that the intramedullary pressure during reaming is kept low to avoid fat embolism. In addition, the venting holes allow for autografting as the bone is deposited through the holes during reaming

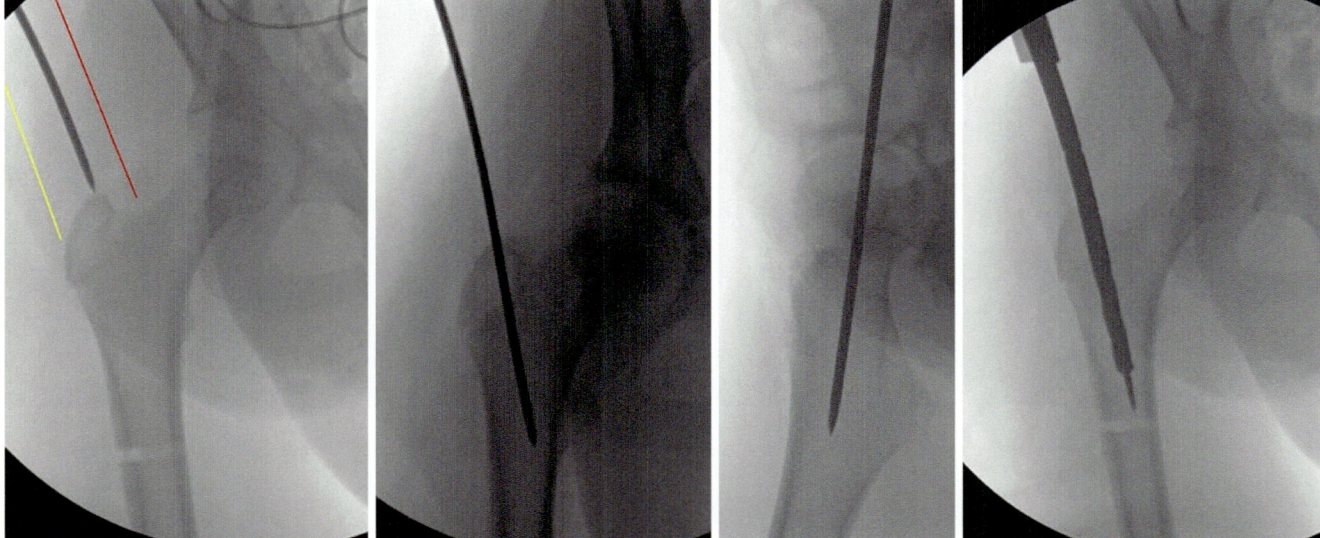

Fig. 13.14 The proper starting position of the guidewire will ensure that no secondary deformities are introduced during nail insertion and that the nail can be advanced. A too lateral entry point will result in a proximal varus deformity. A slightly anterior entry point in the sagittal plane ensures that the straight nail can be advanced into the center of the intramedullary canal

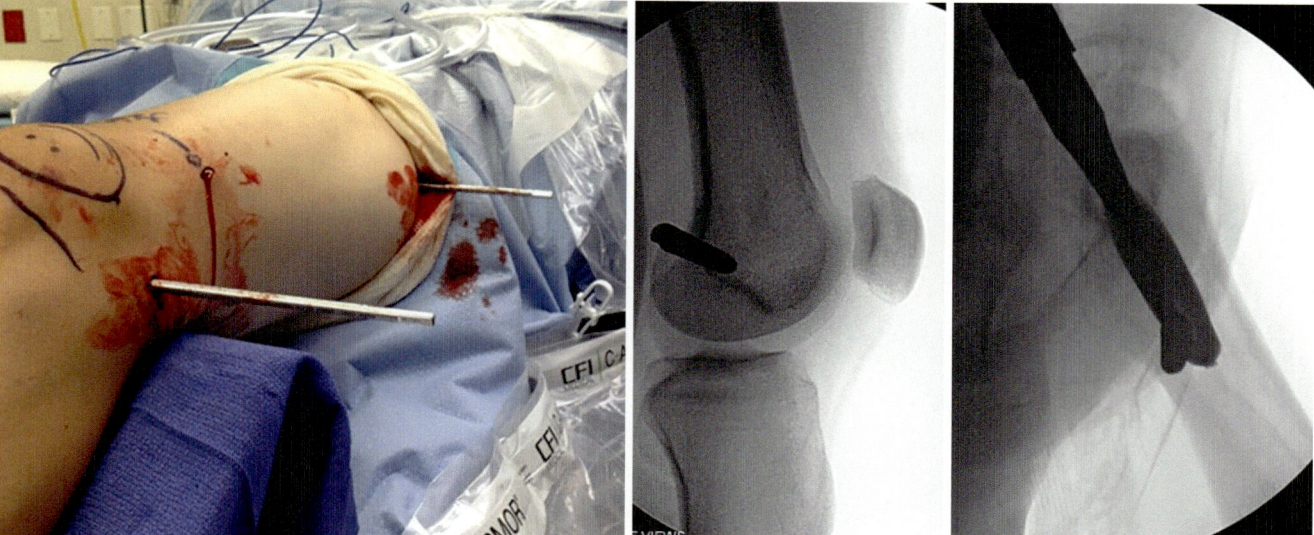

Fig. 13.15 Rotational markers are inserted proximal and distal for the planned osteotomy. These markers are used to ensure that a rotational deformity has not been introduced prior to locking screw insertion in the nail. The markers must be inserted posterior to the reamer in the proximal part. In the distal part, the marker can be inserted distal for the final reaming depth

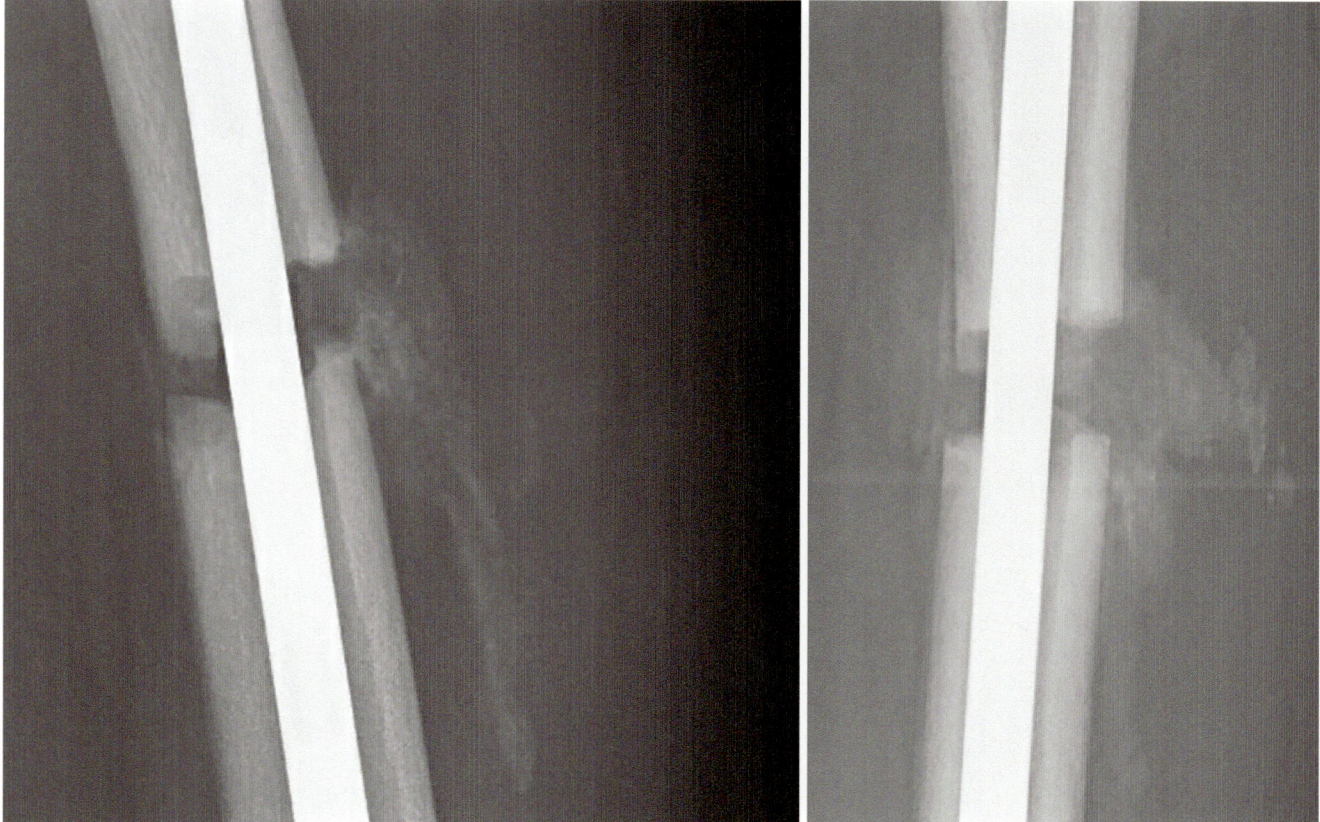

Fig. 13.16 Reaming is done slowly. When using flexible reamers, the femur is generally overreamed by 2 mm. Using straight (solid) reamers, the femur is overreamed by 1 mm. Note the abundance of autograft from the reamings that occurs at the osteotomy site

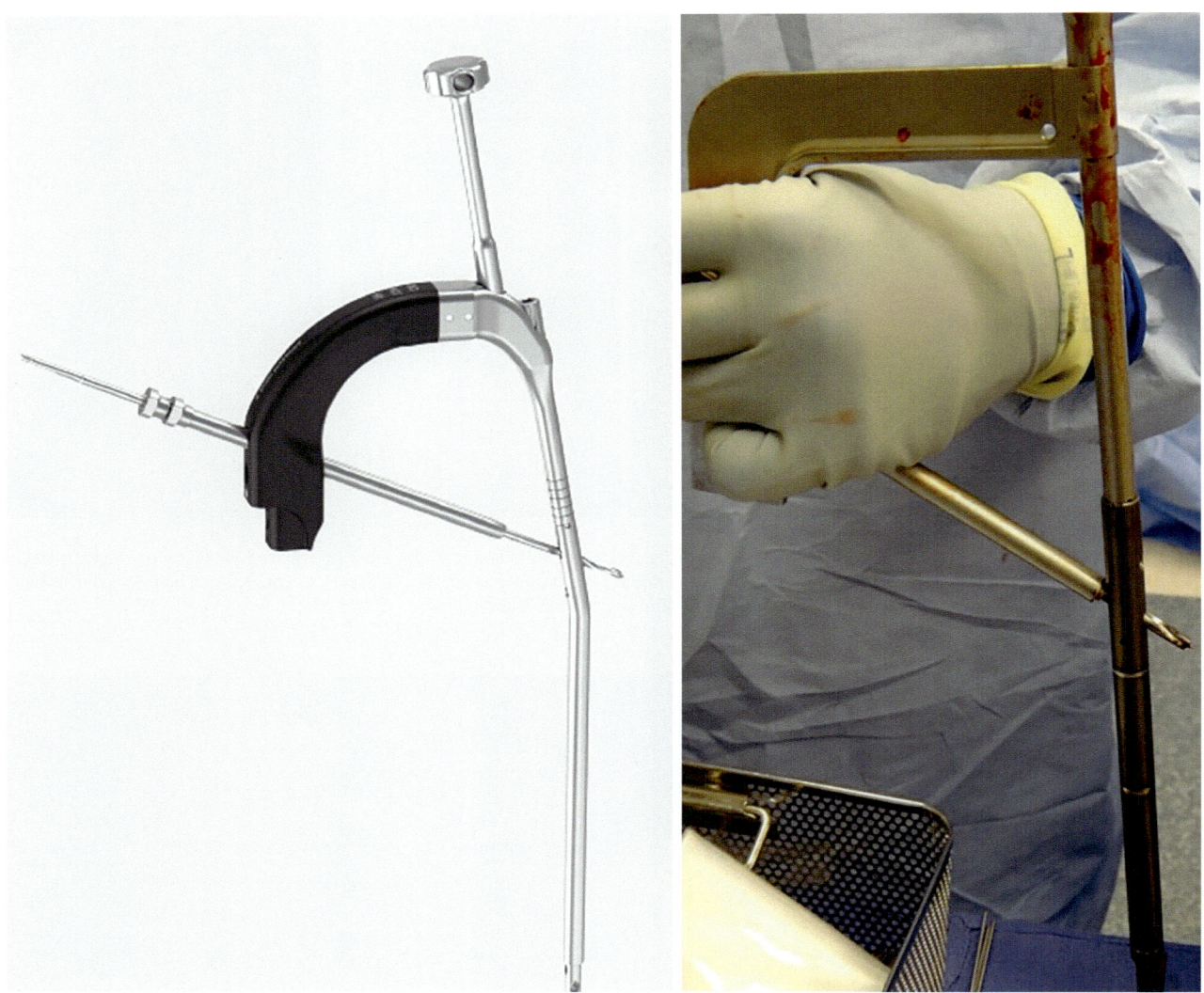

Fig. 13.17 The nail is assembled to the guide arm, and the correct guidance of the proximal locking screws are ensured

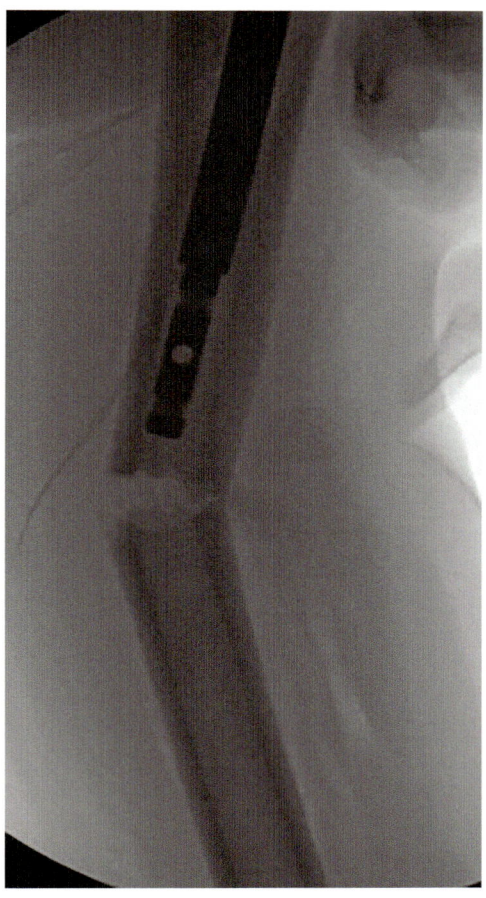

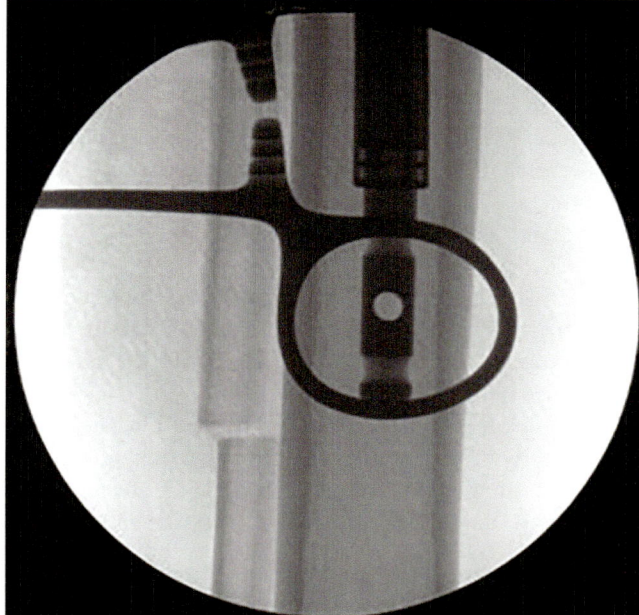

Fig. 13.19 Distal locking screws are inserted free hand after proximal screws have been inserted by use of guide-arm

Fig. 13.18 The solid nail is introduced after removal of the guide wire used for reaming. When the nail is at the level of the osteotomy, the osteotomy is completed with a chisel and the nail is further advanced. The nail should be advanced without hitting hard as this will damage the distraction mechanism. If problems are encountered during insertion further over-reaming should be performed

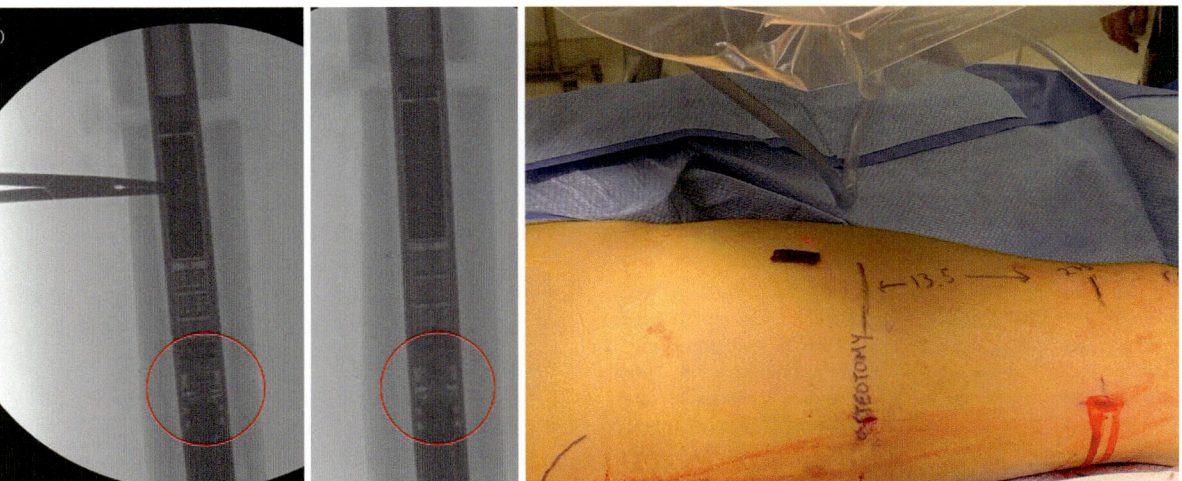

Fig. 13.20 The functionality of the nail is tested. The magnet location within the nail is marked on the skin. A C-arm picture is saved and 1 mm of acute intraoperative lengthening is performed without moving the C-arm or the leg. If the C-arm has a laser guide the position of the laser dot can be marked on the skin to ensure an exact image replica is obtained before and after the lengthening. The lengthening of the nail is demonstrated by comparing a new C-arm picture with the pre-lengthening picture. If in doubt, a second mm can be lengthened. The lengthening can be reversed if the bone gap becomes too large

Blocking Screws

Blocking screws or Poller screws can be used for:

1. Guidance of reaming according to preoperative planning
2. Prevention of angulation of the regenerate during lengthening
3. Increasing stability of the regenerate

Ad 1: When performing acute correction at the osteotomy site in the retrograde nail approach, blocking screws can be used to prevent the reamer from deviating from the preoperative planned nail canal (Fig. 13.21).

Straight reamers are used until the level of the osteotomy, and a cone with the same diameter as the reamed canal is introduced. Blocking screws can then be placed just distal to the osteotomy and in contact with the cone. The osteotomy is completed and reaming proximal to the osteotomy can be done through the cone. The blocking screw ensures that the direction of the distally reamed canal is kept during this proximal reaming. The blocking screws are kept in place as the nail is inserted to guide the nail into the reamed canal. Postoperatively, the blocking screws prevents the regenerate to angulate during lengthening.

Ad 2: Blocking screws can be placed to prevent angulation of the regenerate during lengthening. In general, blocking screws are placed on the concavity of the deformity (i.e., for a pre-operative varus deformity, the blocking screw is placed medial to the nail in the distal segment). The goal with blocking screws is to fill any space in the canal between the implant and the bone cortex. Empty space can possibly allow the bone to migrate and lose alignment over time. These blocking screws can be placed either prior to or after nail insertion. Placing the blocking screws after nail insertion ensures that the blocking screws can be placed in tight proximity to the nail. However, drilling and screw insertion very close to or in contact with the inserted nail carries the risk of nail damage. If the blocking screws are inserted prior to nail insertion, a reamer or a cone with same diameter or slightly larger diameter than the nail can be used to aim the blocking screw position after (Fig. 13.23a–r). Blocking screws can be placed on both sides of the osteotomy. When placing the osteotomy distal on the femur in the retrograde approach, the osteotomy will have a tendency to angulate into valgus, and blocking screws are placed on the medial side of the nail. With the retrograde approach and a distal osteotomy, it is also important to avoid that the distal segment angulates into flexion (procurvatum). A blocking screw is inserted distal to the osteotomy and posterior to the inserted nail (Fig. 13.22a–l). If the distal segment angulates into flexion during lengthening, it might change the access point for nail removal to a more anterior position than the original entry point. This flexion angulation might lead to extended cartilage damage at the time of nail removal.

Ad 3: In addition to preventing angulation of the osteotomy, blocking screws also add to the stability of the regenerate during lengthening. Hereby, the so-called "wind-sweeper" effect can be prevented, and the increased stability might be important to prevent delayed union of the regenerate.

The risk of corrosion might be increased when positioning different materials in tight contact. Thus, blocking screws with the same material as the inserted nail should ideally be used. Therefore, similar screws as the locking screws applied for the lengthening nail, can be applied. However, the nails are often removed within a short time period, and if a blocking screw of a different material is already in a good position after previous deformity correction, this different material blocking screw can be kept in place.

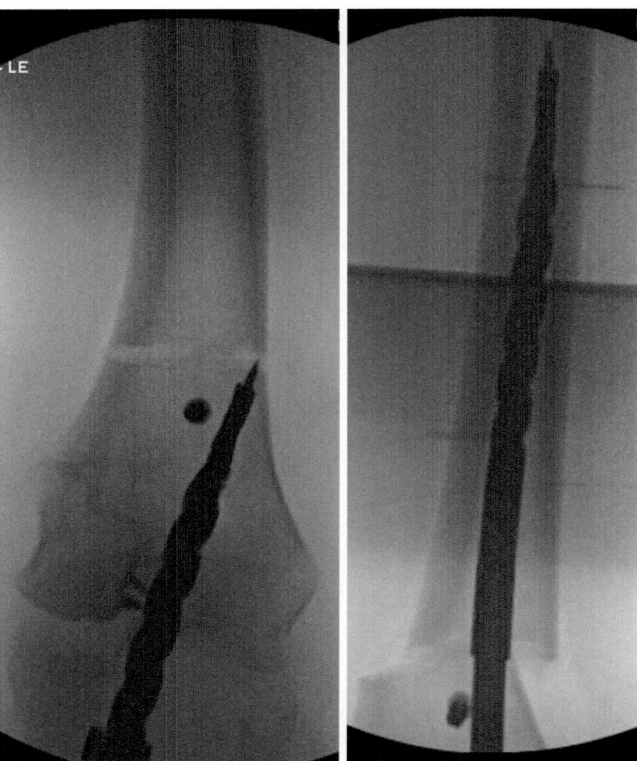

Fig. 13.21 Straight reamers are used until the level of the osteotomy, and a cone with the same diameter as the reamed canal is introduced. Blocking screws can then be placed just distal to the osteotomy and in contact with the cone. The osteotomy is completed and reaming proximal to the osteotomy can be done through the cone. The blocking screw ensures that the direction of the distally reamed canal is kept during this proximal reaming. The blocking screws are kept in place as the nail is inserted to guide the nail into the reamed canal. Postoperatively, the blocking screws prevents the regenerate to angulate during lengthening

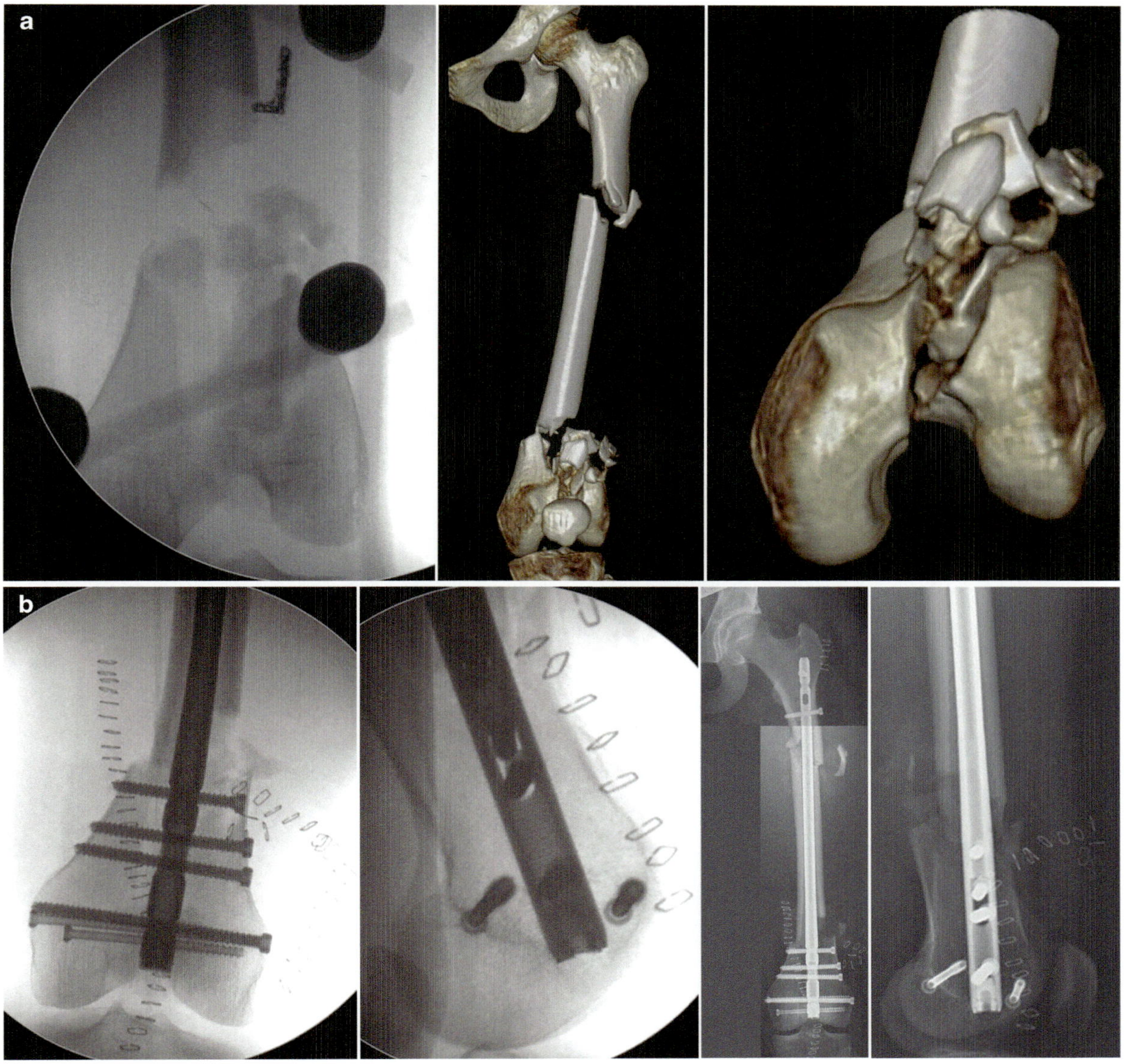

Fig. 13.22 (a) A 19-year-old female with a Gustilo IIIB segmental femoral fracture with distal bone loss. After initial debridement and temporary spanning external fixation, a two-stage procedure was planned. First goal was to obtain fracture healing without loss of joint motion. Second goal was to regain bone length and correct mechanical axis. (b) Ten days after initial debridement, the temporary external fixator was replaced. Open reduction and internal screw fixation were applied for the intra-articular fracture, and a retrograde trauma nail was inserted with intentional 50 mm shortening corresponding to the initial bone loss. The patient was allowed full weight-bearing after 6 weeks. (c) Status 6 months after trauma: The fractures are united. Full range of motion of knee and hip joint. 50 mm shortening with mild varus deformity both at proximal and distal fracture site. Medial mechanical axis deviation is accentuated by the shortening of the femur. No deformity in sagittal plane. No rotational deformity. (d) The lengthening and corrective osteotomy is planned at a 60 mm distance from the intercondylar notch. This allows for good purchase of the distal locking screws in a retrograde lengthening nail and allows for the needed bone correction in the frontal plane. (e) The reverse planning method introduced by Baumgart [19] was applied using the Bone Ninja™ App. The ideal mechanical axis of the lower limb is drawn. (f) The ideal position of the center of the femoral head is marked with a red dot, and the level of the distal osteotomy is marked with small blue dot. (g) The ideal position of the femur bone after acute correction and gradual lengthening along the anatomical axis. (h) The blue dotted line represents the overall lower limb mechanical axis after ideal correction and lengthening. (i) The "lengthening gap" is closed by sliding the proximal femur along axis of the nail to be inserted (red line in (h)). The blue dotted line represents the position of the nail to be inserted. (j) Postoperative radiograph after the initial trauma nail has been replaced with a 10.7 mm × 245 mm PRECICE straight retrograde lengthening nail. Red arrows mark the position of blocking screws inserted to: (1) Aid with the deformity correction, (2) Prevent deformity (distal varus and procurvatum) during lengthening, (3) Increase stability of the regenerate. The spring in the radiograph is from an external cooling device preventing excessive postoperative knee joint swelling. (k) Status after 80 days of bone lengthening. There is full range of motion of the hip and the knee joint. The overall lower limb mechanical axis is good. There is 10 mm shortening. The bone regenerate is judged to be sufficient; however, it is decided that only 5 mm of further lengthening will be applied. (l) Final follow-up 24 months after trauma and 6 months after removal of lengthening nail. The overall lower limb mechanical axis is good. There exists 5 mm of limb length discrepancy. There is full range of motion of the hip and the knee joint. The patient is capable of running without pain

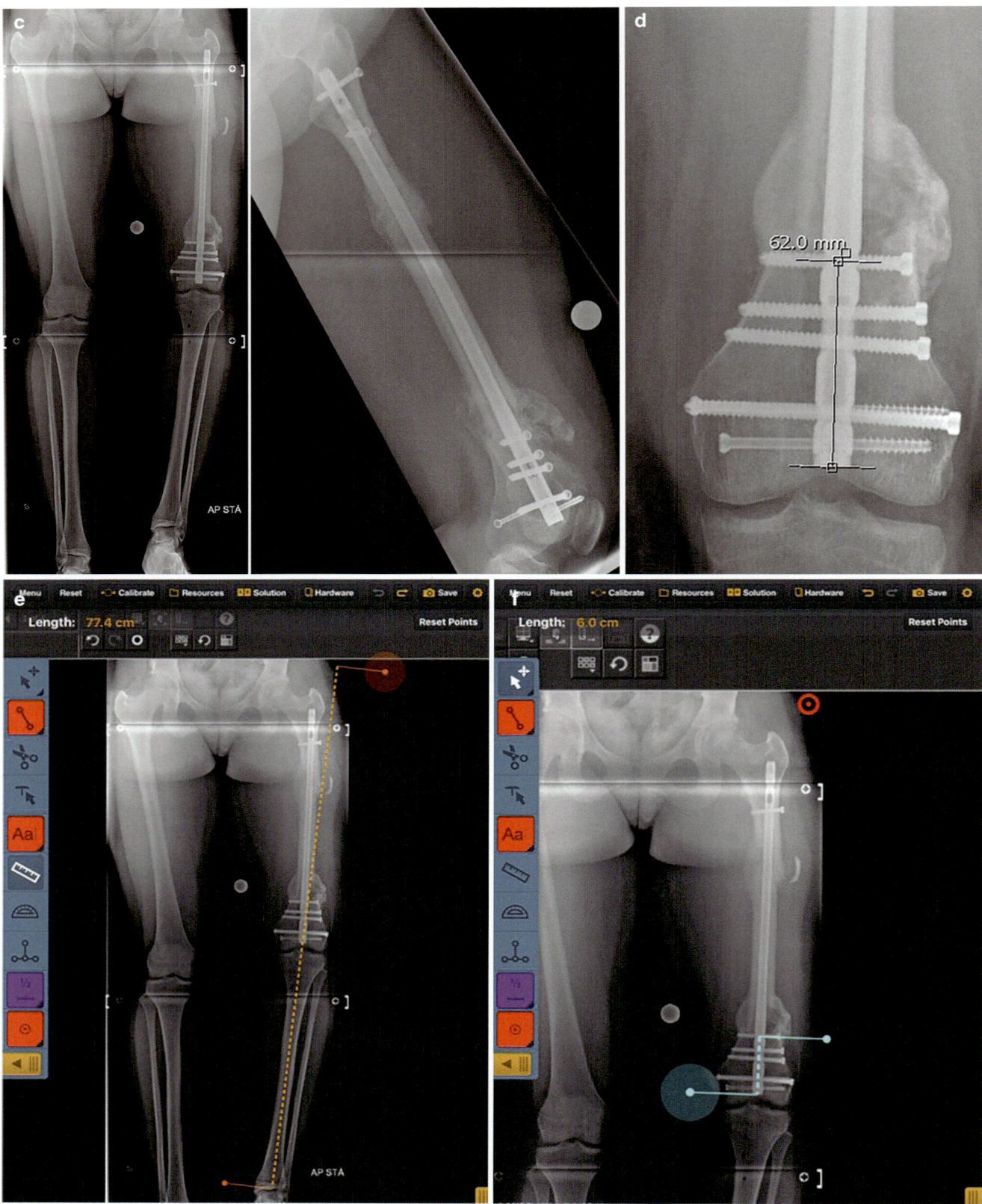

Fig. 13.22 (continued)

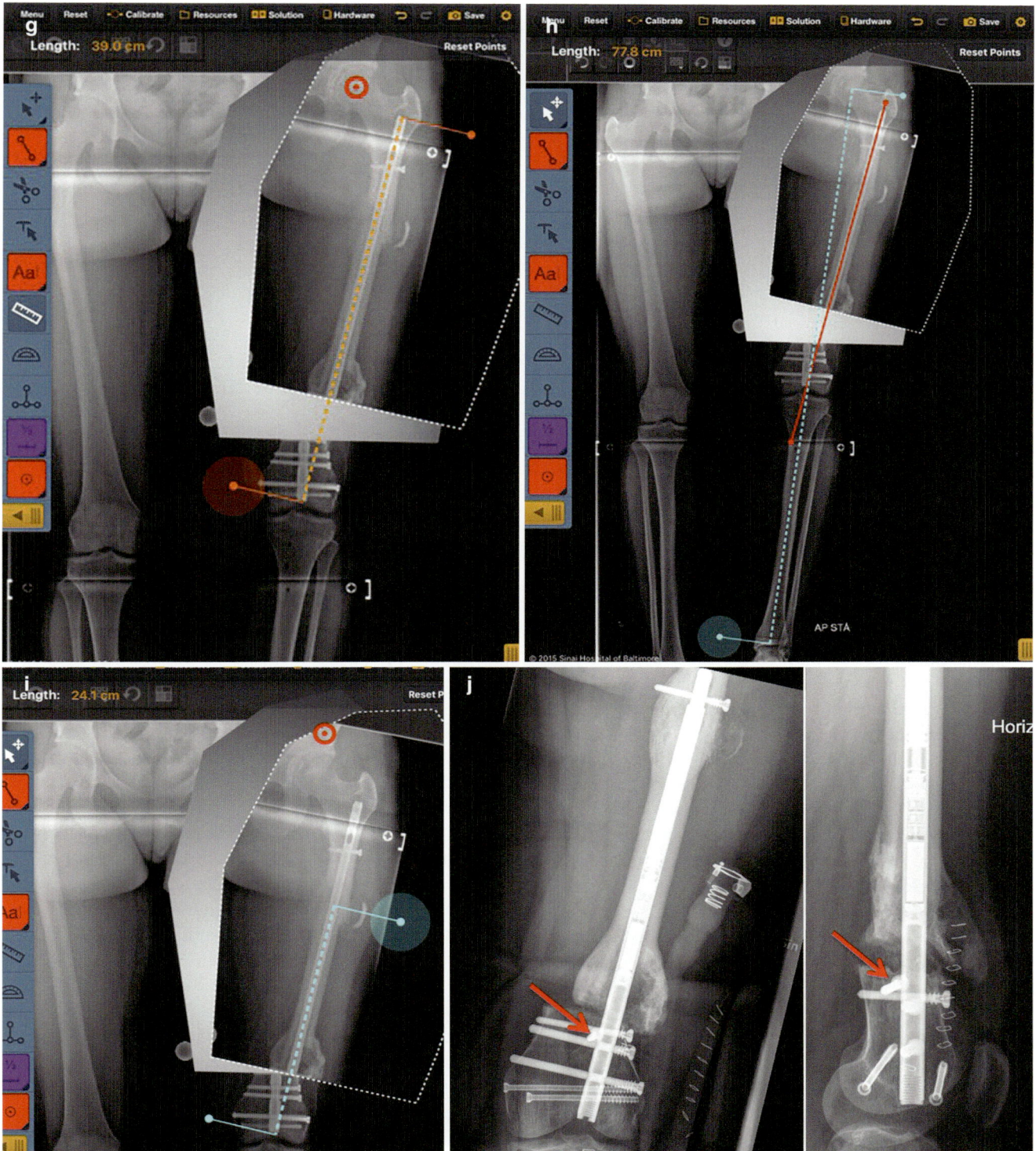

Fig. 13.22 (continued)

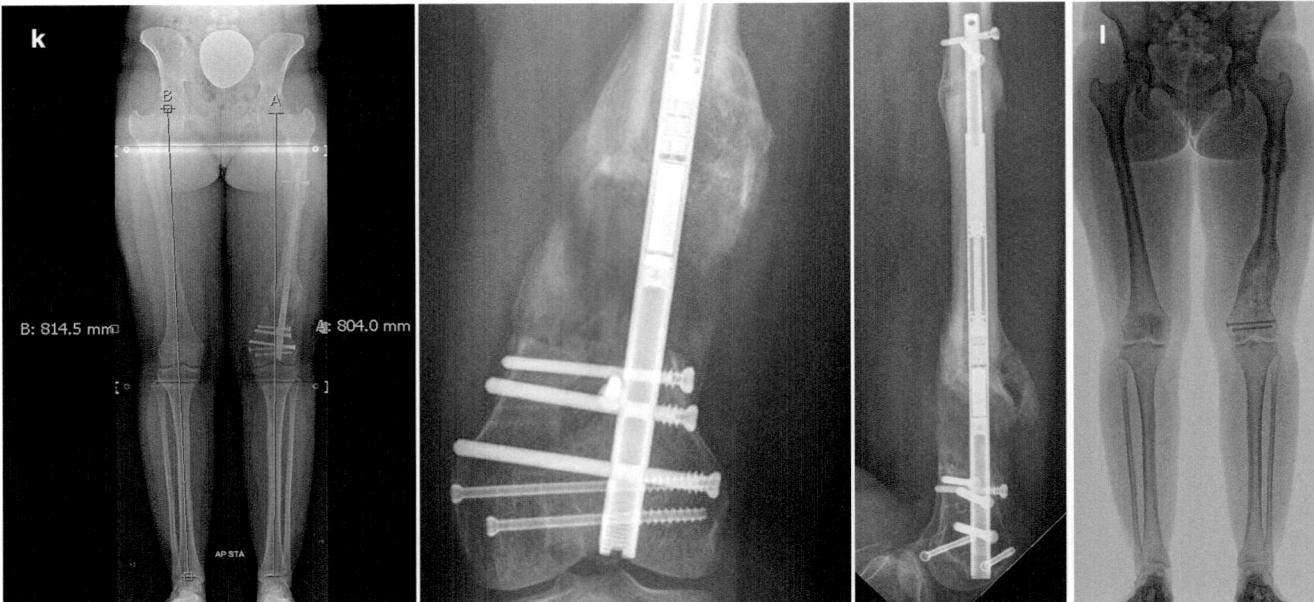

Fig. 13.22 (continued)

Deformity Correction

Simultaneous acute deformity correction and gradual lengthening can be performed through the same osteotomy. The sequence of performing the osteotomy and nail insertion can vary. The osteotomy can be corrected using blocking screws prior to reaming and insertion of the nail (Fig. 13.21) or the osteotomy can be corrected and held in place by temporary external fixation prior to nail insertion [20]. No comparison exists about which method that yields the most optimal results, and the choice of method is based on the preference of the surgeon. When avoiding temporary external fixation, it might be needed to reposition the blocking screws during final finetuning of the axis correction. Using temporary external fixation, the finetuning of the axis correction and positioning of the nail can be performed prior to insertion of blocking screws. Regarding bone healing, it has been found safe to perform acute correction and subsequent lengthening with angular deformities up to 15° and rotational deformities up to 30° [21]. However, the bone healing capacity after acute deformity will vary between patients and be dependent on the amount of bone contact between bone ends. After reaming, the endosteal blood supply is damaged leaving only the periosteal blood supply as the primary source of healing. Large acute angular or rotational corrections place further stress on the periosteal blood supply which can result in delayed healing. In larger corrections, the osteotomy site can be grafted not only from the reaming procedure into the ventilation holes but also from graft material harvested from the reamer.

Neurovascular structures at risk should be taken into consideration when performing large acute corrections. Particularly, performing a varus osteotomy at the very distal femur might place the peroneal nerve at risk. It might be safer to perform the osteotomy over staged procedures, often with a prophylactic peroneal nerve decompression, with subsequent lengthening at the final osteotomy.

Other possible reasons for choosing to go retrograde include: (1) a retrograde nail has previously been applied (Fig. 13.23a–r) or (2) if an antegrade approach might be technically demanding, i.e., in some patients with achondroplasia/hypochondroplasia or previous Perthes disease.

The retrograde approach often requires the insertion of blocking screws in order to avoid introducing clinically significant bone deformity during lengthening (Fig. 13.22a–l). Because the retrograde approach violates the knee joint, a correct entry point is critical. The nail should enter at the anterior border of Blumensaat's line to avoid damage to the cruciate ligaments and to allow penetration into the intramedullary femoral canal through the non-weightbearing portion of the articular surface. A tubular system should be used to protect the knee joint when reaming the bone (Fig. 13.23a–r). Special considerations exist when using the Fitbone™ nail in a retrograde approach as the wire from the nail must be tunneled from the femoral notch through the lateral femoral condyle to a subcutaneously placed receiver (Fig. 13.1). For both the Fitbone™ nail and the Precice™ nail it is recommended from the manufacturer that the nails are removed. This means that knee joint is violated twice doing the retrograde approach, both at insertion and later at removal, and

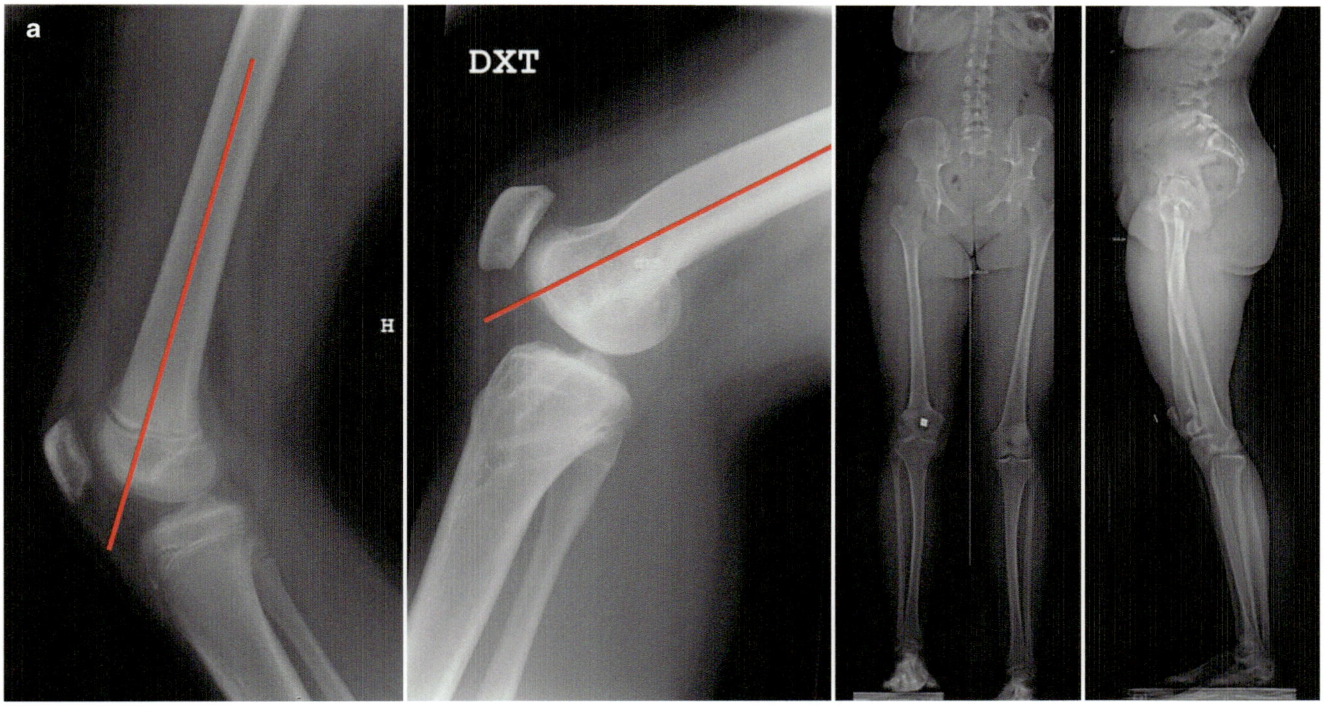

Fig. 13.23 (**a**) An 18-year-old female with shortening and distal procurvatum of right femur after growth plate injury in early childhood. 15° extension deficit of knee
a1: Sagittal femoral axis at the time of growth plate injury
a2: Sagittal femoral axis after partial growth arrest
a3: EOS anterior-posterior: LLD: 35 mm. No mechanical axis deviation in frontal plane
a4: EOS Sagittal plane. Lack of right knee extension
Two stage procedure planned. First stage: distal correction of procurvatum with retrograde nail. Second stage: retrograde lengthening nail through more proximal osteotomy
(**b**) Lateral fluoroscopy images at first stage surgery: Extension osteotomy with retrograde nail, entry point at Blumensaat's line and posterior blocking screw ensures correction. Red line is planned distal nail position. Osteotomy is performed just proximal to the suprapatellar articular surface to allow for maximal deformity correction with retrograde nail. (**c**) Healed osteotomy with restoration of full knee extension. No mechanical axis deviation in the frontal plane. Lengthening along the axis of a straight nail (red line) will ensure lengthening without introducing a deformity in the sagittal plane. (**d**) Intraoperative fluoroscopy at the second procedure. Level of secondary osteotomy marked by k-wire on AP view. K-wire on lateral view demonstrates ideal position of straight lengthening nail. (**e**) Nail removal using a similar technique as for removal of retrograde lengthening nail with protection sleeve and overreaming of the extraction point prior to nail removal. (**f**) Ventilation holes drilled at the planned osteotomy level prior to reaming. Ensures bone grafting from reaming through the holes and decreases risk of embolization from increased intramedullary pressure during reaming. (**g**) Intraoperative fluoroscopy in the sagittal plane showing straight reaming (using solid reamers) according to preoperative plan. (**h**) Two blocking screws are positioned proximal and distal for the osteotomy site posterior to prevent procurvatum. One blocking screw is positioned distal for the osteotomy at the medial side to prevent valgus deviation during lengthening. Blocking screws are inserted in close contact with 11 mm straight reamer prior to insertion of 10.7 mm lengthening nail. (**i**) Antirotation pins are placed proximal and distal for the osteotomy site prior to completing the osteotomy. (**j**) A retrograde PRECICE™ straight nail is inserted without translation or rotation of the osteotomy. (**k**) The position of magnet is marked intraoperatively. (**l**) The functionality is tested intraoperatively. (**m**) Intraoperative draping and position for insertion of retrograde femoral nail. (**n**) Transverse skin incision. Retrograde position of k-wire through patellar tendon. Longitudinal split of the patellar tendon. Insertion of protection sleeve. (**o**) Drilling ventilation holes at the planned osteotomy level prior to reaming. Insertion of anti-rotation pins prior to completing the osteotomy with chisel. (**p**) Ensuring correct rotation of the osteotomy after distal locking screws have been inserted and prior to insertion of proximal locking screws. The non-operated leg can be positioned on the c-arm to ensure sufficient lateral fluoroscopy of the proximal part of the operated leg. (**q**) Marking of magnet position of nail. Intraoperative test. (**r**) Postoperative lengthening by the patient. The external magnet is placed over the marked position of the nail magnet, and the external magnet is pressed firmly against the skin and soft-tissues to reduce the distance between the external and internal magnets

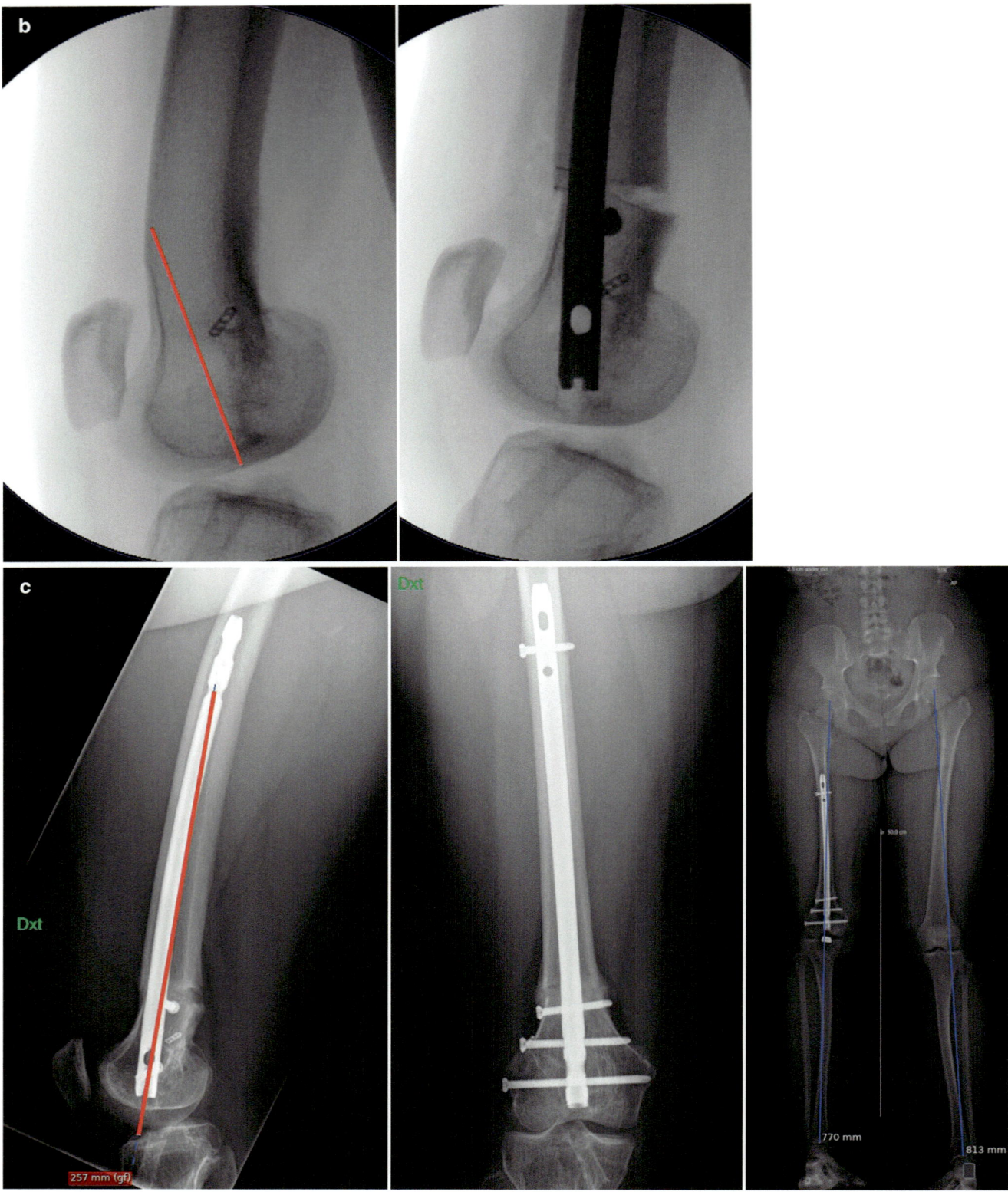

Fig. 13.23 (continued)

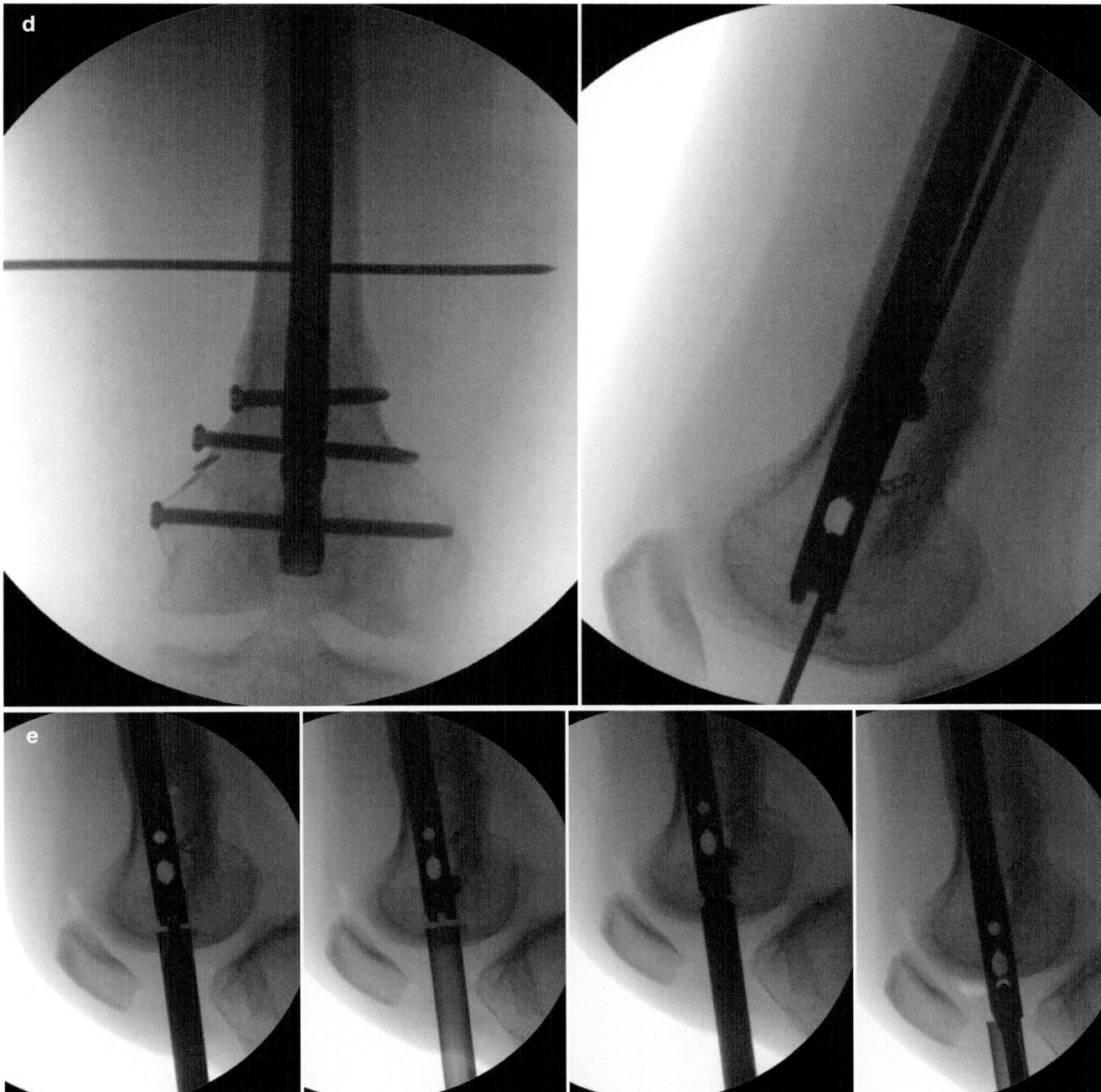

Fig. 13.23 (continued)

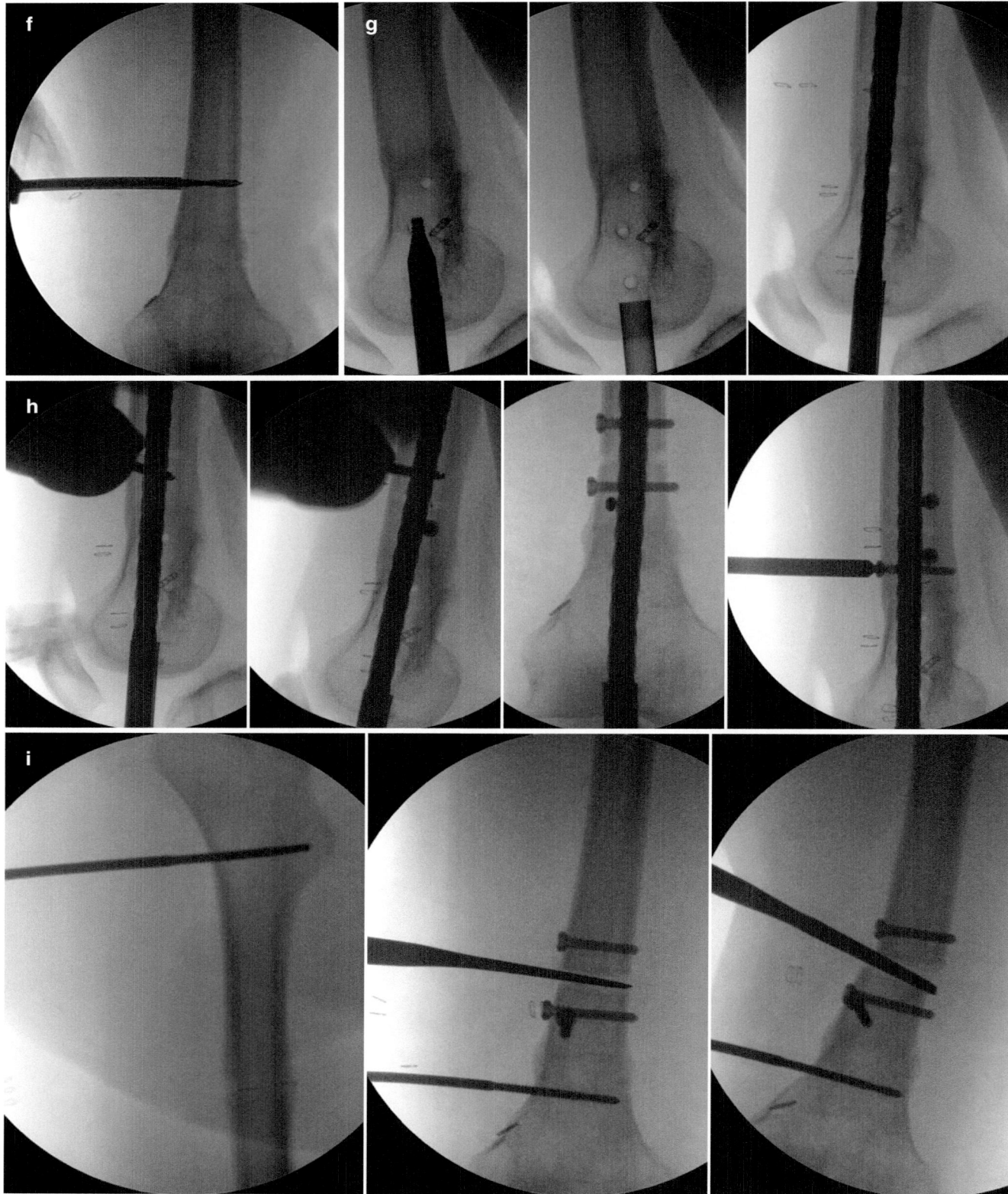

Fig. 13.23 (continued)

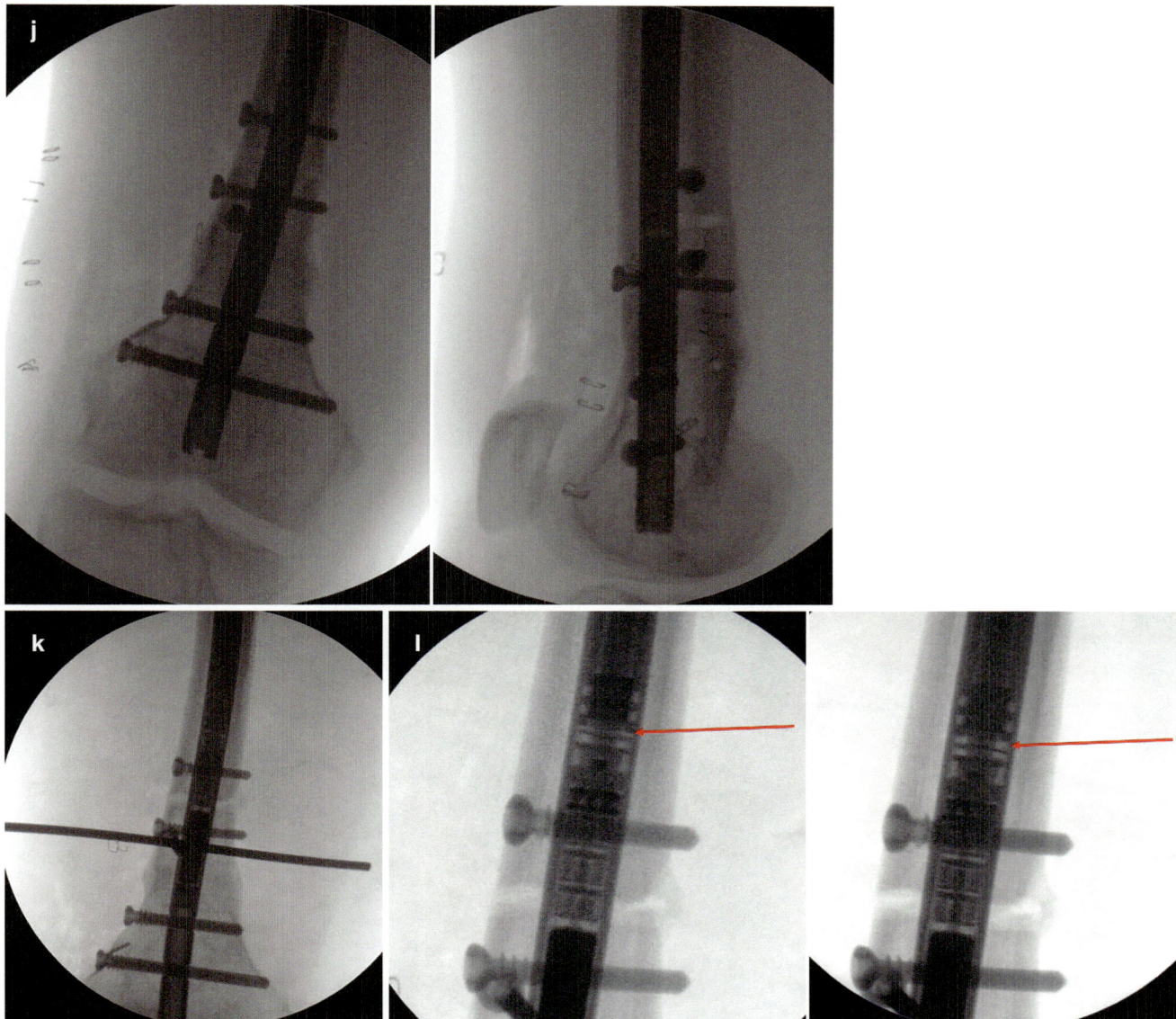

Fig. 13.23 (continued)

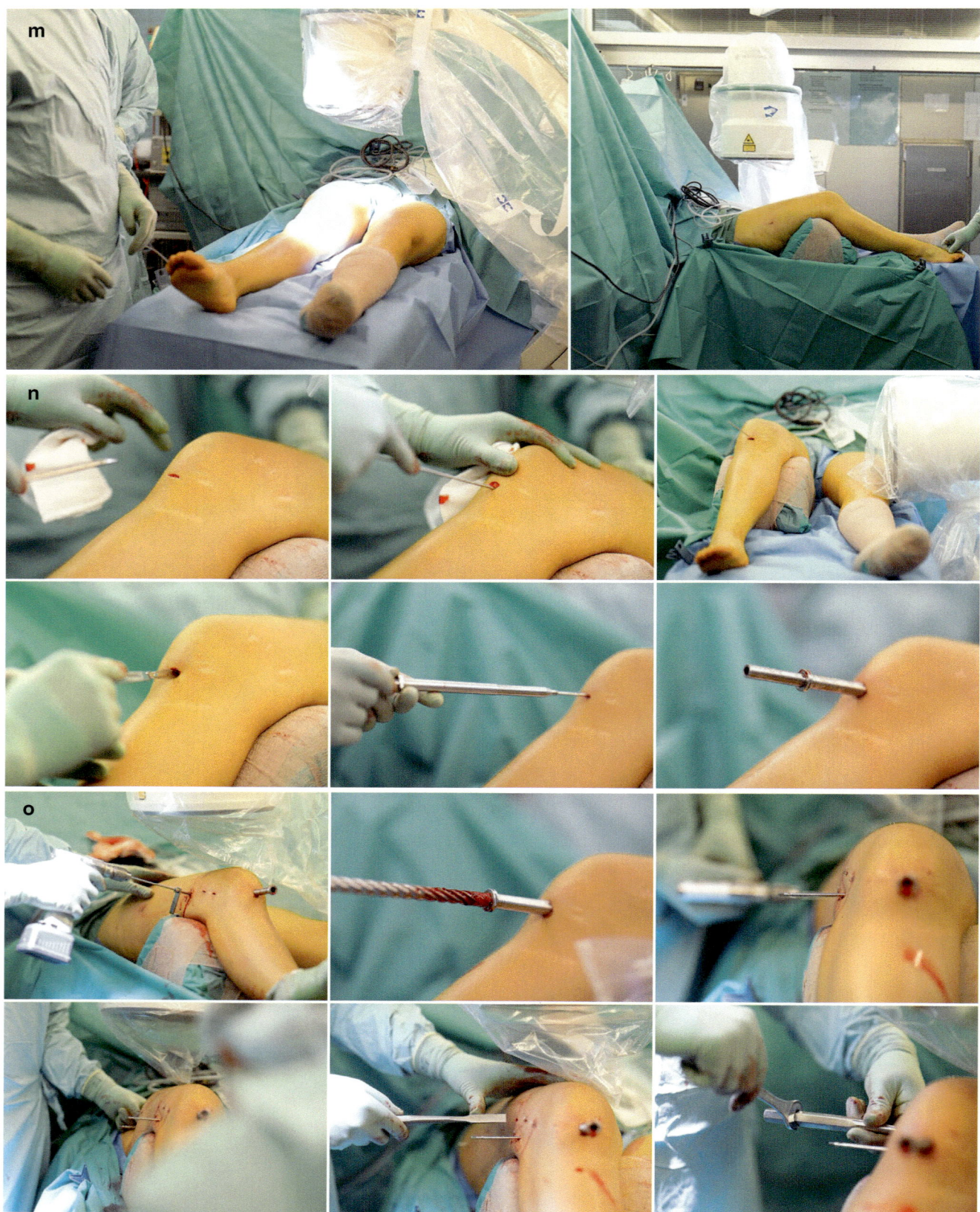

Fig. 13.23 (continued)

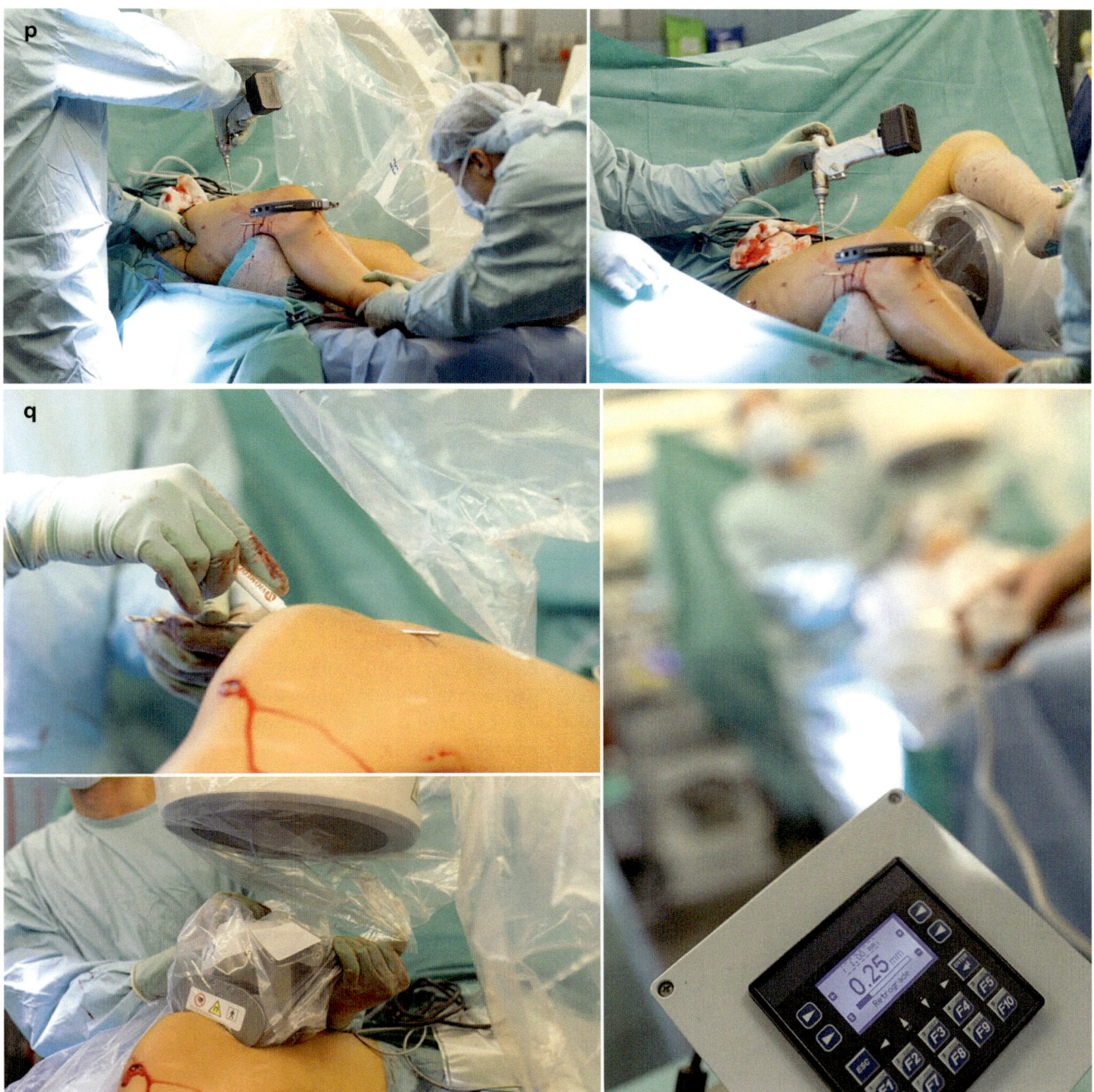

Fig. 13.23 (continued)

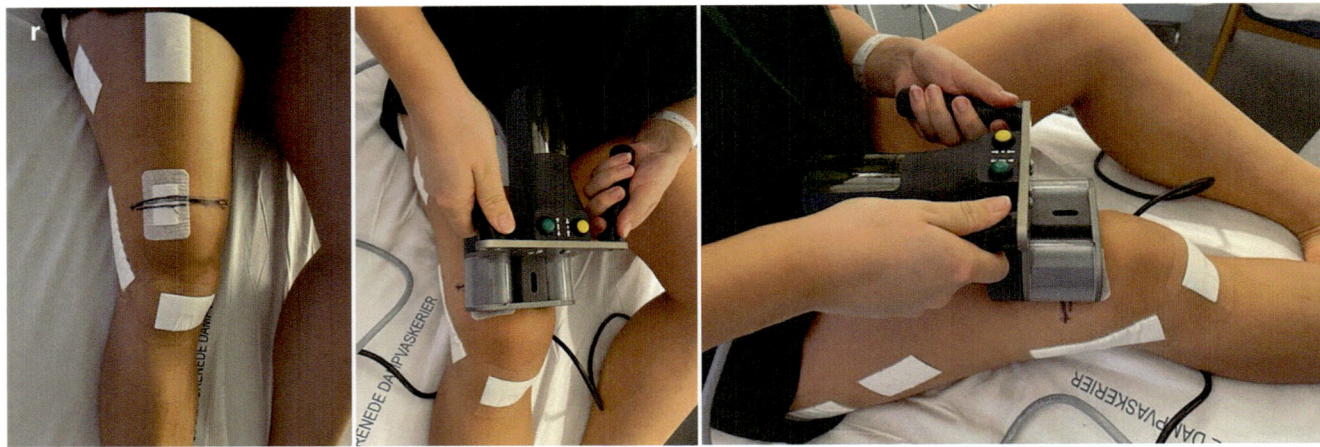

Fig. 13.23 (continued)

the retrograde approach might result in long term anterior knee pain. This knee pain is often mild and is typically present when the patient is kneeling.

Electric Versus Magnetic Nail: Pros and Cons

Differences between the electric Fitbone™ nail and the magnetic Precice™ nail are both due to differences in the powering of the lengthening mechanisms and due to other differences in nail designs (Table 13.2).

For the electric Fitbone™ nail, the subcutaneous receiver and the connecting cord into the nail poses certain limitations. A subcutaneous pouch must be made for the receiver, and in the retrograde approach, the wire must be tunneled through the lateral femoral condylar bone from the intraarticular nail to the subcutaneous receiver. When using a Fitbone™ nail, it is important to prevent swelling at the subcutaneous receiver site in order to allow the transducer to transmit energy sufficiently. Swelling is prevented by securing hemostasis in the subcutaneous pouch prior to insertion of the receiver and by applying ice and compression over the receiver site during the first postoperative days. In the case of excessive swelling, it might be difficult to locate the receiver and place the external transducer at the correct position on the femur. In these cases, the exact position of the receiver might be located by ultrasound.

For the magnetic Precice™ nail, the size of the magnet inside the nail limits the maximum distance that the external magnet can be placed from the nail and still appropriately drive the nail mechanism. At the end of nail insertion surgery, the position of the nail magnet is identified intraoperatively with fluoroscopy and this position is marked on the skin (Fig. 13.23a–r). When lengthening, the external magnet should be placed on the femur at this level and at the position with minimum soft-tissues between the magnet and the bone (Fig. 13.23a–r). The maximum allowable distances between the magnet and the nail are provided for the different nail diameters (Table 13.2). In case of uncertainty about the soft tissue volume, the distance between the bone and the outside can be assessed preoperatively by ultrasound or MRI. Ultrasound has the advantage that the ultrasound head can be compressed against the skin reducing the measured distance and thereby replicating the minimum distance that can be obtained when the external magnet is compressed against the skin.

At the time of this writing, the current nails do not provide feedback about the actual nail lengthening or the resistance force during lengthening. However, such feedback is expected to be introduced into the nail designs in the coming years. For the Precice™ nail, the current version of the external remote controller does indicate whether the nail magnet is connected and communicating properly with the magnets in the handheld device. Currently, intraoperative testing of nail functionality can be performed after insertion of the nail. The Fitbone™ nail is tested by placing a stethoscope externally on the femur over the nail site and a characteristic motor sound is heard when the nail is activated from the external applied transducer. The Precice™ nail is tested by performing a short intraoperative lengthening (i.e., 1 mm), and then the advancement of the nail is judged from fluoroscopy (Fig. 13.23a–r). This short intraoperative lengthening does not appear to affect the quality of the regenerate during later lengthening. However, if uncertain, the short lengthening can be partially reversed immediately intraoperatively.

For the magnetic Precice™ nail, the manufacturer does not recommend MRI examination of the patients; however, in case of acute need for MRI examination there does not appear to be a patient safety risk but there might be a risk of subsequent malfunction of the nail [22]. The risk of compli-

Table 13.2 Differences between the electric Fitbone™ nail and the magnetic Precice™ nail

Electric Fitbone™ nail	Magnetic Precice™ nail
Design <ul><li>Energy transferred transcutaneous from external transducer to subcutaneous receiver connected to the internal motor-unit through a chord</li><li>Stainless steel</li><li>Two locking screw options at the nail insertion site</li><li>One locking screw option at the tip of the nail going in the direction from lateral to medial</li><li>Femoral nail: Straight nail</li><li>Current nail diameters: 9 mm, 11 mm</li><li>The nail can be reversed by using a special designed transducer</li></ul> **Advantages** <ul><li>A stethoscope placed over the site of the lengthening nail enables real time feed-back at the time of lengthening. The sound of the motor-unit changes if the resistance at the lengthening site increases too much.</li></ul> **Disadvantages** <ul><li>Related to the receiver and the chord:<ul><li>Swelling around the receiver may inhibit the transfer of energy from the external receiver.</li><li>Infection of the receiver is a risk, and the infection may be spread along the cord to the knee joint in retrograde femoral lengthening.</li><li>Intraarticular placement of the cord in retrograde femoral lengthening may cause inflammation of the knee joint.</li><li>Tethering of the chord during lengthening may cause malfunction of the nail.</li><li>Difficulties may arise when removing the cord with the risk of intraarticular cord fragments into the knee joint in retrograde femoral lengthening.</li></ul></li></ul>	**Design** <ul><li>An externally placed magnet drives an internal magnetic stone in the nail</li><li>Titanium</li><li>Two locking screw options at the nail insertion site</li><li>Three locking screw options at the tip of the nail (distal portion with antegrade and proximal portion with retrograde) with 90 degrees angulation between screw options.</li><li>Femoral nails:<ul><li>Straight for antegrade piriformis or for retrograde insertion</li><li>Bend for retrograde insertion</li><li>Bend for antegrade trochanteric entry point</li><li>Current nail diameter: 8.5 mm, 10.7 mm, 12.5 mm</li></ul></li><li>The nail can be reversed by reversing the spinning direction of the external magnet.</li></ul> **Disadvantages** <ul><li>The magnet inside the nail will only rotate when the distance from the external magnet to the nail does not exceed certain limitations. Thus the volume of soft-tissues between external magnet and bone should be considered. Maximum recommended distances from magnet to nail are:<ul><li>For 8.5 mm diameter nail: 38 mm</li><li>For 10.7 mm diameter nail: 51 mm</li><li>For 12.5 mm diameter nail: 51 mm</li></ul></li></ul>

cations might be higher with the current Fitbone™ design due to the use of the subcutaneous receiver and the connecting cord between the receiver and the nail [23]. Particularly for the retrograde inserted Fitbone™ nail, an infection from the subcutaneous receiver might spread along the chord into the knee joint resulting in septic knee arthritis.

Post-operative Period

An efficient pain medication regimen is paramount to ensure sufficient exercises and range of motion of adjacent joints throughout the treatment. Regional anesthesia via continuous catheter can reduce the need for systemic opioids and may facilitate earlier hospital discharge [24]. Due to risk of catheters placed in the draped sterile area of implant insertion, the catheters are difficult to apply at the beginning of the surgical procedure. However, the catheters can be administered prior to awakening the patient. In some congenital cases, it can be difficult to administer and maintain the effect of continuous catheter infusions. In these cases, prolonged single-shot regional anesthesia blocks can be applied and re-administered if needed.

Paracetamol forms the base of analgetic treatment. It is supplemented with oral opioids when needed. The opioids can also be used for immediate pain relief or administered immediately prior to physiotherapy. No evidence exits whether non-steroid anti-inflammatory drugs compromise the bone formation with intramedullary lengthening nail. Swelling of the knee-joint and pain after retrograde nail insertion might be reduced by RICE (Rest, Ice, Compression, Elevation) including intermittent application of external cooling.

It is important to remember, that lengthening patients differ from other orthopaedic patients regarding the postoperative journey. The pain might be high and joint movement might be restricted immediately postoperatively and then proceed towards less pain and better joint movement. However, as the lengthening proceeds, the soft-tissues are tensioned, and the pain and restricted joint movement might rebound. Therefore, individualized follow-up of the patients is needed with special attention towards pain medication and joint movement. The majority of complications occur during the lengthening period, and a close follow-up of patients during this time period is mandatory. However, complications have been found to occur during all phases of treatment:

intraoperative, postoperative prior to lengthening, during lengthening, after lengthening and prior to nail removal, at nail removal, and after nail removal [23]. Therefore, a follow-up program should be made to assist the patient in all phases of treatment.

Deep venous thrombosis has been described after intramedullary lengthening, and anti-coagulant prophylaxis can be initiated based on the individual risk profile of the patient. At present, no evidence exists whether chemical thromboprophylaxis reduces the risk of venous thromboembolic complication, and a survey has shown a wide variability between treating surgeons both in terms of thromboprophylaxis risk assessment, choice of medications, and duration of treatment [19].

Postoperative Course

The three major objectives are:

1. Regenerate healthy bone
2. Maintain range of motion
3. Advance the weight bearing safely

Lengthening Protocols

The lengthening protocols are adapted from external lengthening as no clinical or experimental studies have determined the ideal protocols for intramedullary lengthening nails. Lengthening is initiated after a latency period ranging from 5 to 12 days on the femur depending on the clinical scenario. For example, in young and healthy patients with a simple osteotomy placing the bone ends in close contact, a shorter latency period (5–7 days) is recommended. On the other hand, in the older patient where simultaneous deformity correction has been performed, reducing the initial contact between bone ends, a longer latency period (8–12 days) is advised. Other factors such as comorbidities, previous surgery, and location of the osteotomy site (metaphyseal or diaphyseal) influence the latency period prior to initiating lengthening (Fig. 13.24).

The lengthening rate is adjusted based on the appearance of the regenerate bone on weekly or bi-weekly radiographs as well as the clinical examination. With the Fitbone™ nail,

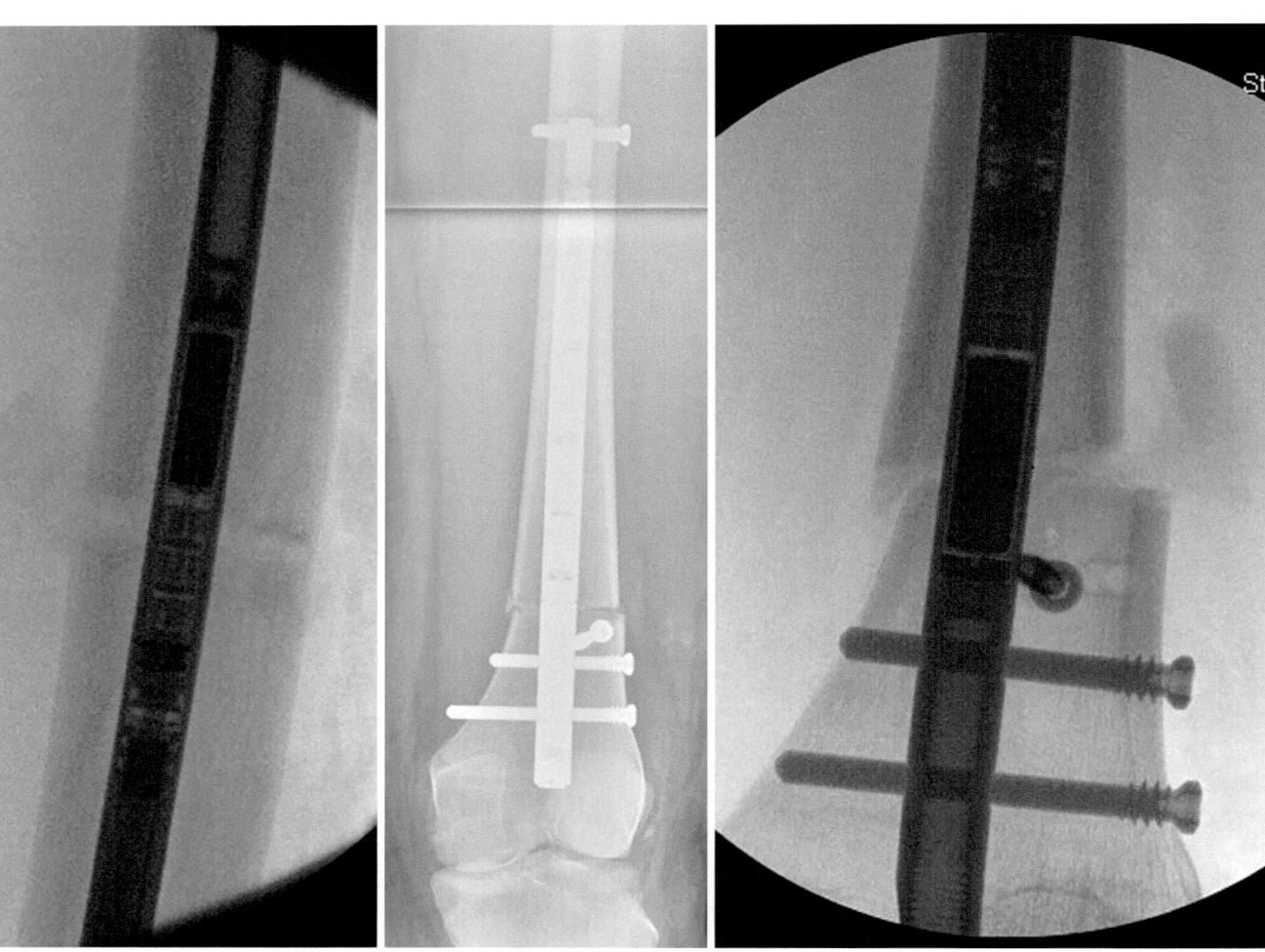

Fig. 13.24 Longer latency period is needed for diaphyseal than for metaphyseal osteotomy. Longer latency period with limited bone contact compared with good initial bone contact

the motor-unit sound detected by a stethoscope place externally on the femur over the lengthening nail can give information on how much resistance is present at the lengthening site.

The typical rates of lengthening described in the literature are 0.25 mm 4 times per day; 0.33 mm 3 times per day; 0.25 mm 3 times per day; 0.33 mm 2 times per day. The authors prefer to start the lengthening slowly at 0.20 mm 4 times a day. Once the patient demonstrates that healthy regenerate bone is forming, the surgeon can decide to speed up the rate and rhythm, if necessary. It is important that proper regenerate bone starts to form at the initiation of distraction. The goal is to avoid creating the dreaded radiographic "black hole" where there is a large distraction gap with no visible regenerate bone present. By monitoring the radiographs on a weekly basis, the surgeon can modulate the rate and rhythm faster or slower as dictated by the clinical results. It takes just a few seconds to re-program the external remote controller allowing the rate and rhythm to be continuously tailored to fit the patient's needs. It is critically important to be vigilant throughout the distraction phase. Train yourself and your team to assess the health of the regenerate bone on the radiograph each week. Do not lengthen blindly with a universal rate and rhythm the entire time. Adjust the rate and rhythm to avoid hypoplastic regenerate bone formation. Ideally, the time intervals between the lengthening should be equally distributed. However, in practice, a longer time interval is often present between the late evening lengthening and the early morning lengthening.

The goal is to have a lengthening rate that is sufficiently slow to allow formation of a healthy and homogeneous regenerate without risking premature consolidation. In addition to the radiographic appearance of the regenerate bone, the rate of lengthening might be affected by the range of motion in the adjacent joints. If the patient begins to lose hip or knee motion, then the lengthening rate my need to be slowed down or paused until the patient regains sufficient joint motion. In more severe cases of poor bone formation or compromised joint movement, the lengthening may need to be reversed. Shortening of the Precice™ nail can be done by reversing the direction of the external remote controller. The electric Fitbone™ nail can be reversed by using a specially designed transducer. If the bone regenerate or the joint movement does not benefit from reduced or reversed lengthening, it might be necessary to stop the lengthening prior to obtaining the desired bone length. With internal lengthening nails, the bone can be allowed to heal and the joint movement can resolve without a rush to remove the device, unlike an external fixator lengthening. The patient can then at a later point undergo a second lengthening (with the same nail or with a new nail) using a new osteotomy. This new osteotomy is preferable at a new site but can be through the previous bone regenerate if the reason for pausing was problems with joint movement. Other reasons for adjusting the lengthening protocol are other soft-tissue problems (such as uncontrollable pain or peripheral neurologic symptoms).

Postoperative Follow-Up

Radiographic and clinical follow-up are performed weekly or bi-weekly during the distraction phase and approximately every 4 weeks during the consolidation phase.

Clinical Examination

At each follow-up, the patient is asked about pain. In general, most patients are very comfortable during the entire lengthening process with internal lengthening nails. Non-narcotic pain medications are usually sufficient throughout the post-operative course. If the patient is having consistent, prolonged pain after surgery or develops pain when there wasn't previous pain, then a thorough investigation of possible sources should be performed. The pain quality and location are examined to capture the signs of peripheral neuropathy.

The most important feature to check at every visit is the joint range of motion as there are no easy rescues for these fixed joint contractures, subluxations or dislocations. Hip, knee, and ankle joint motions are examined and documented at each visit. In addition to assessing the quality of lengthening regenerate and hardware positioning, the clinician should train himself/herself to examine each radiograph, especially the lateral of the knee, for early evidence of joint subluxation (Fig. 13.25). If early changes are identified, then an aggressive approach to correcting the problem should be initiated.

Physical therapy is initiated at the hospital during the inpatient stay after surgery and it is important that the transfer to physical therapy outside the hospital happens without delay of treatment. Daily exercise programs are made, and if any signs of lost motion are observed, the physical therapy should be intensified and the lengthening rate should be adjusted. Smaller increments of lengthening are preferable to maintain range of motion.

It is up to the surgeon's discretion whether every femoral lengthening patient needs a brace. The authors recommend at a minimum that all congenital patients (or any other patients with unstable knee exam pre-operatively) use a knee brace during treatment. The patient should have a knee brace constructed before surgery to hold the knee in extension and to prevent knee contracture. The knee brace is worn at night and during the day when the patient is recumbent throughout the lengthening process.

Fig. 13.25 Lateral x-ray of the knee in normal position with center of the tibial plateau directly under the center of the femoral condyles. Lateral x-ray in retrograde nail lengthening showing postero-lateral subluxation of the knee joint. The lengthening must be stopped and the joint congruency and stability must be restored

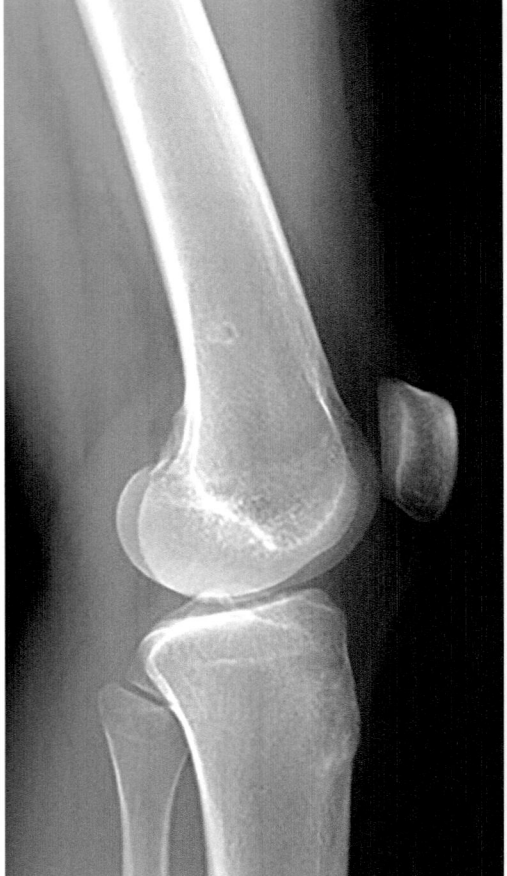
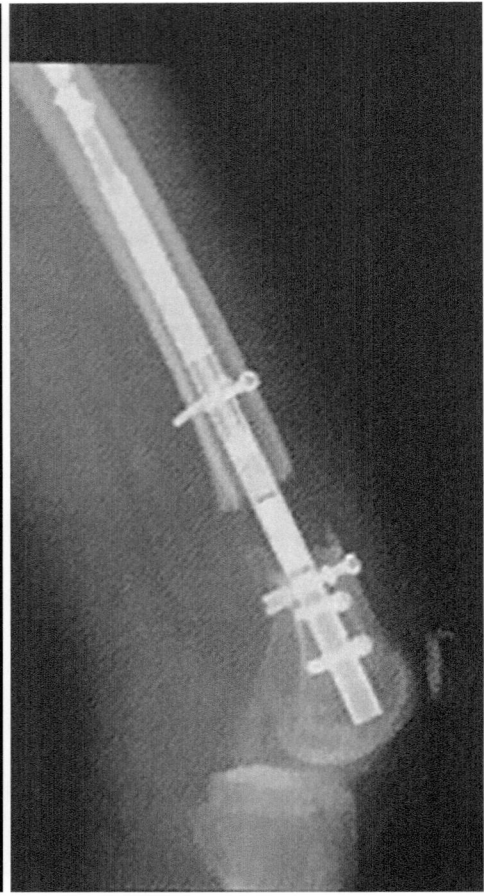

Contracture is prevented by both passive and active range of motion exercises as well as focus on avoiding hip and knee contracture during passive resting.

Radiographs

During the distraction and consolidation phase, radiographs in two planes (AP and lateral) of the osteotomy site are used to examine the quality of the bone regenerate, and to examine the lengthening progress (Fig. 13.26).

For a correct examination of both the bone quality and the opening of the osteotomy site, it is important that the radiographs are taken with the beam direction immediately over and orthogonal to the osteotomy site.

The regenerate formation is evaluated remembering that healing bone matures from outside in. The regenerated bone will ideally undergo the shapes from eggshell to hollow to fusiform.

The lengthening of the nail can be calculated from the advancement of the nail tip or from the internal nail mechanism (Fig. 13.27). These measurements should correlate with the amount of lengthening measured at the osteoplasty site.

The radiographs should also be examined for unplanned angulation of the lengthening segments, mechanical implant failure such as loosening (backing) or breakage of locking screws, nail bending or breakage or for tethering of the chord in the electric Fitbone nail.

In patients at high risk of joint subluxation, radiographs of the joints are taken separately and are examined for early signs of joint subluxation.

When Has Desired Limb Length Been Achieved?

During the distraction phase, a decision must be taken when the desired limb length has been achieved. This decision is not always easy to make. At the end of the distraction phase, it might be difficult for the patient to stand with the weight evenly distributed on both limbs and subtle contractures might be present. Thus, both the clinical examination and a long-standing weight-bearing radiograph might be misleading. Furthermore, at this early time of treatment, it is often difficult for the patient to judge whether the limb length feels correct. The authors base the decision on achieved limb length on the preoperatively decided lengthening goal. The

Two weeks

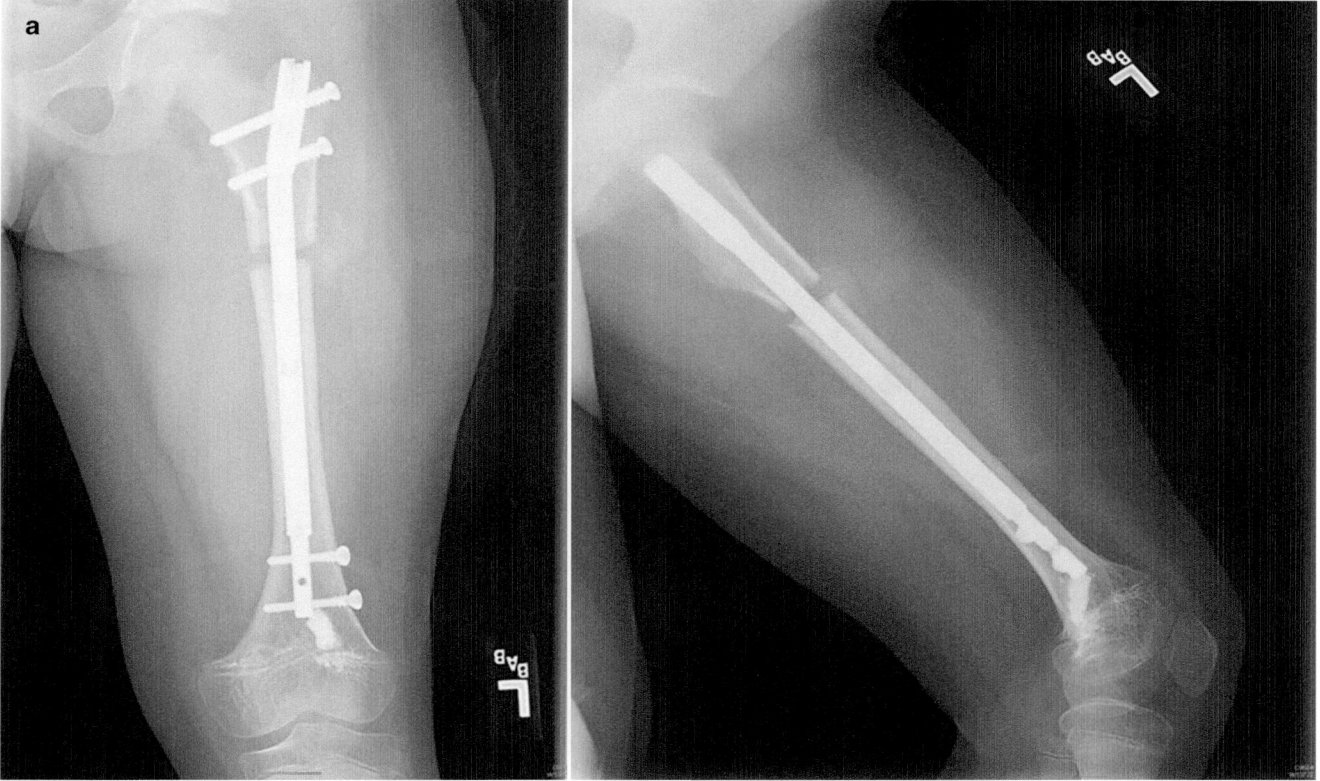

Three weeks

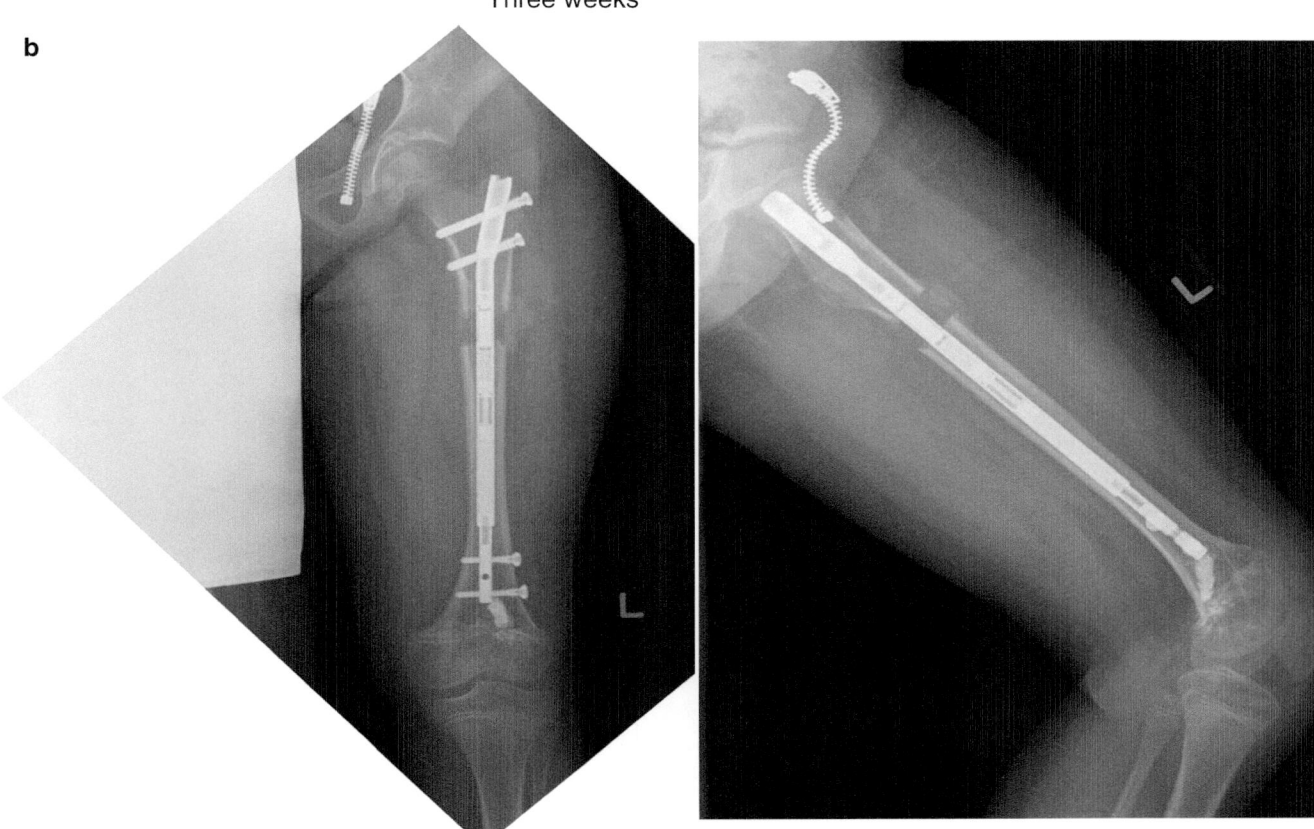

Fig. 13.26 The regenerate is usually not visible until the third week of distraction and absence of regenerate at this point requires slowing or pausing of distraction rate. The regenerate should be clearly visible by the fourth week

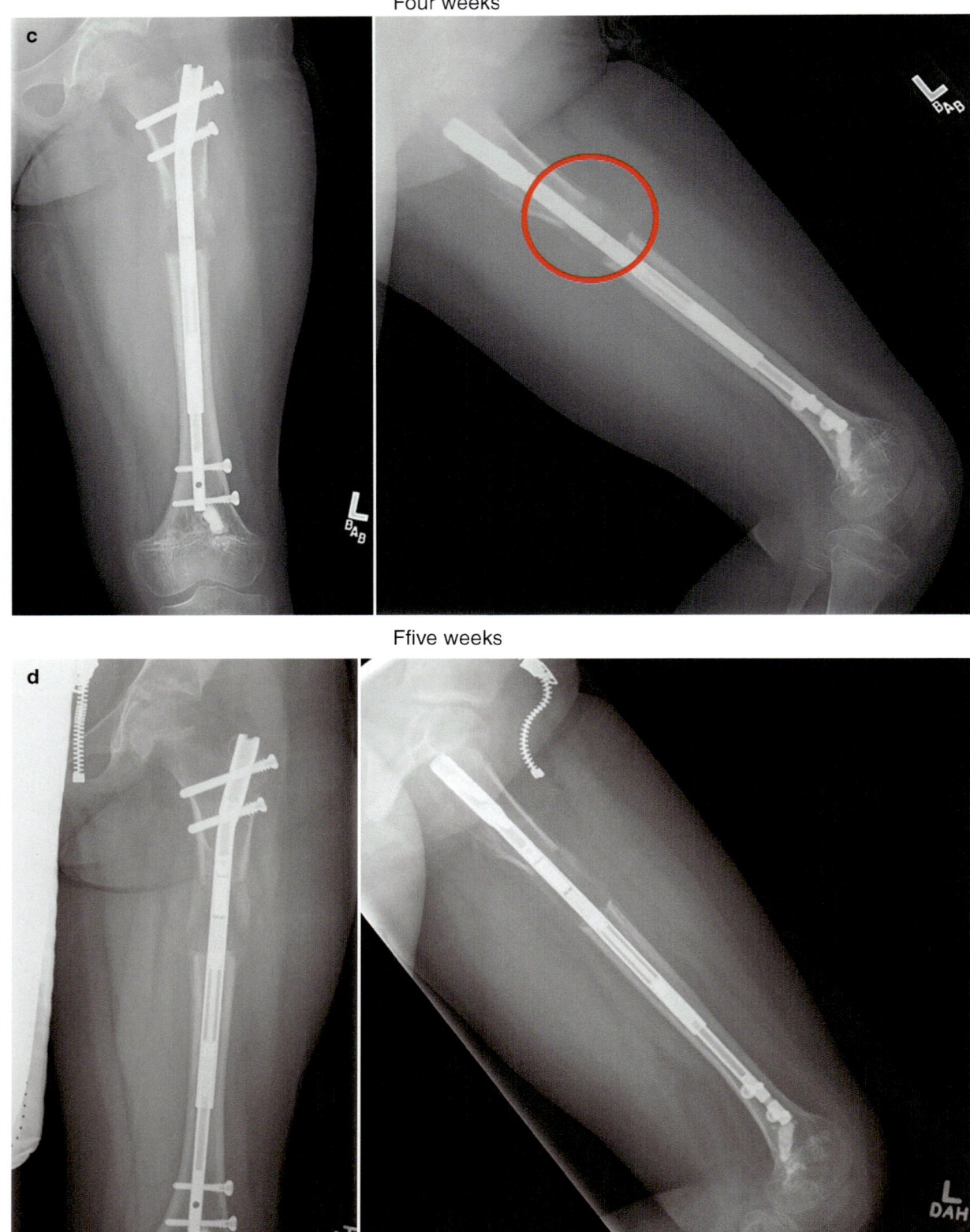

Fig. 13.26 (continued)

Six weeks

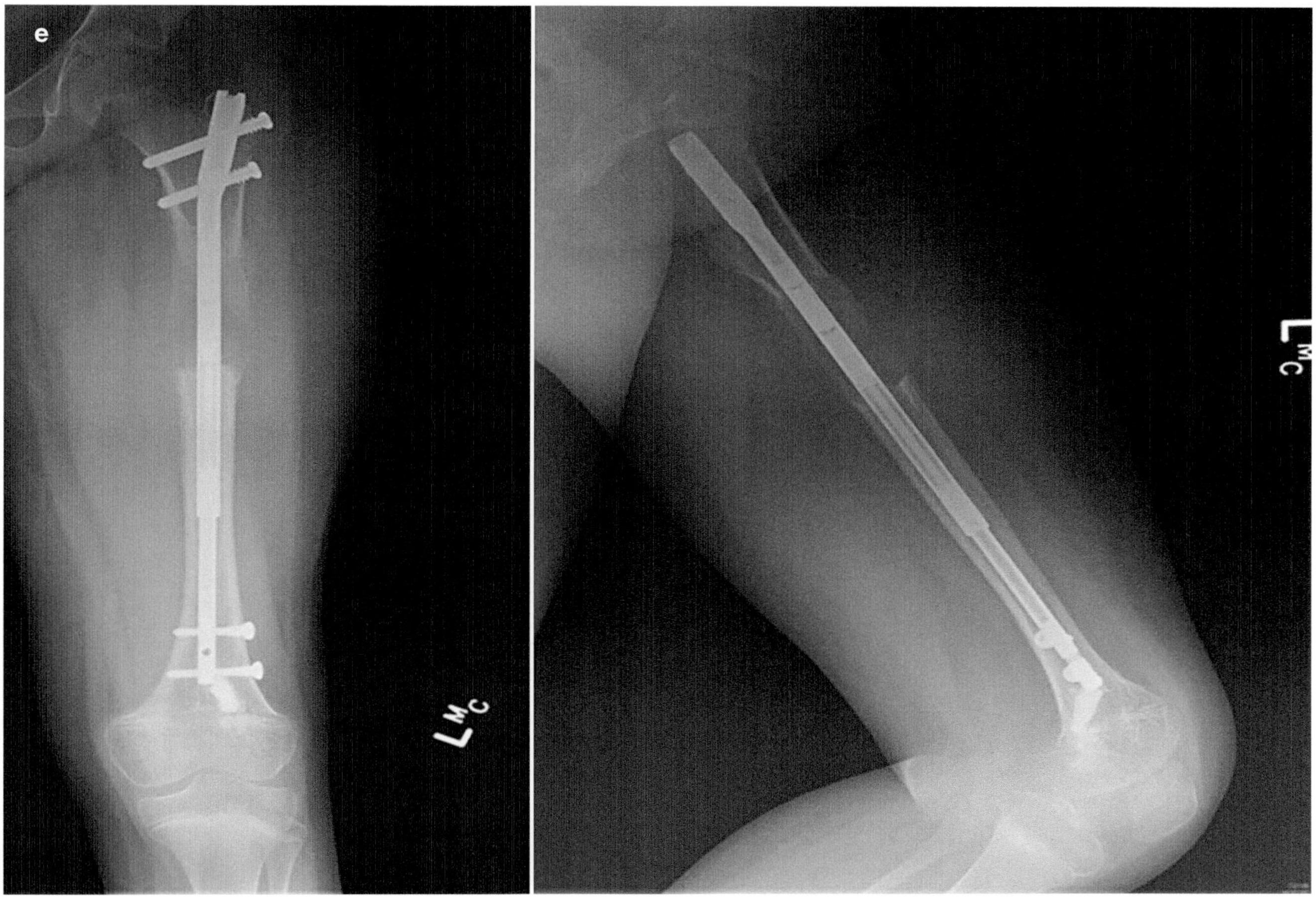

10 weeks

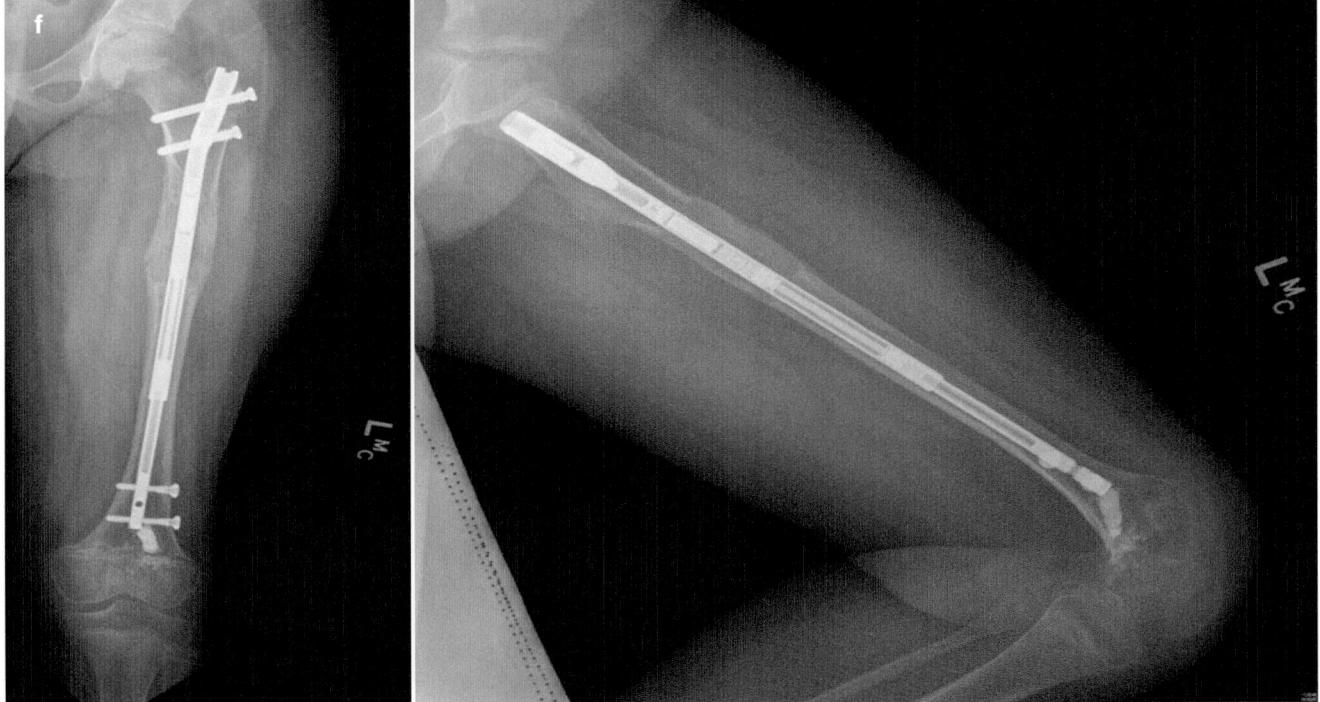

Fig. 13.26 (continued)

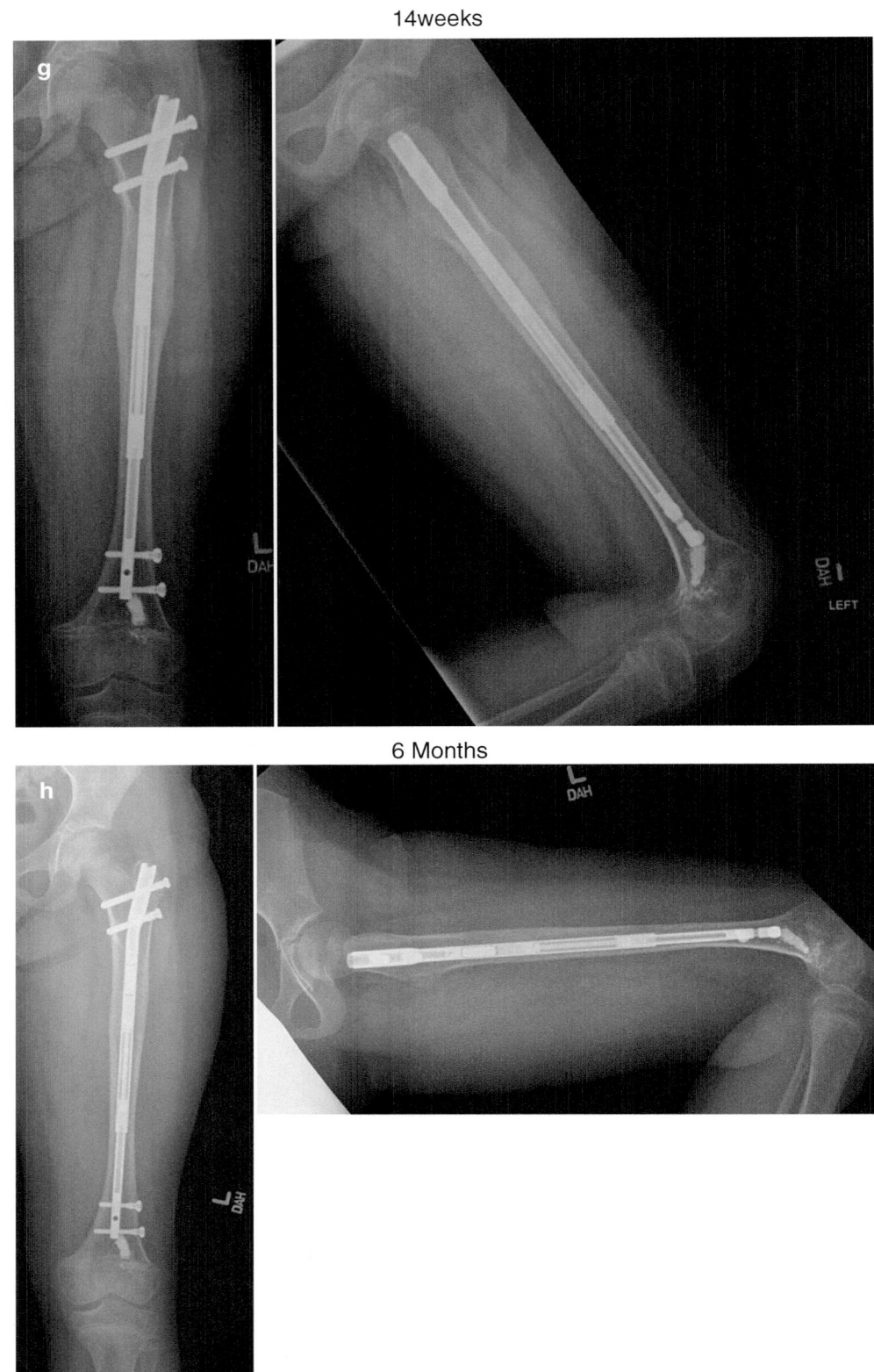

Fig. 13.26 (continued)

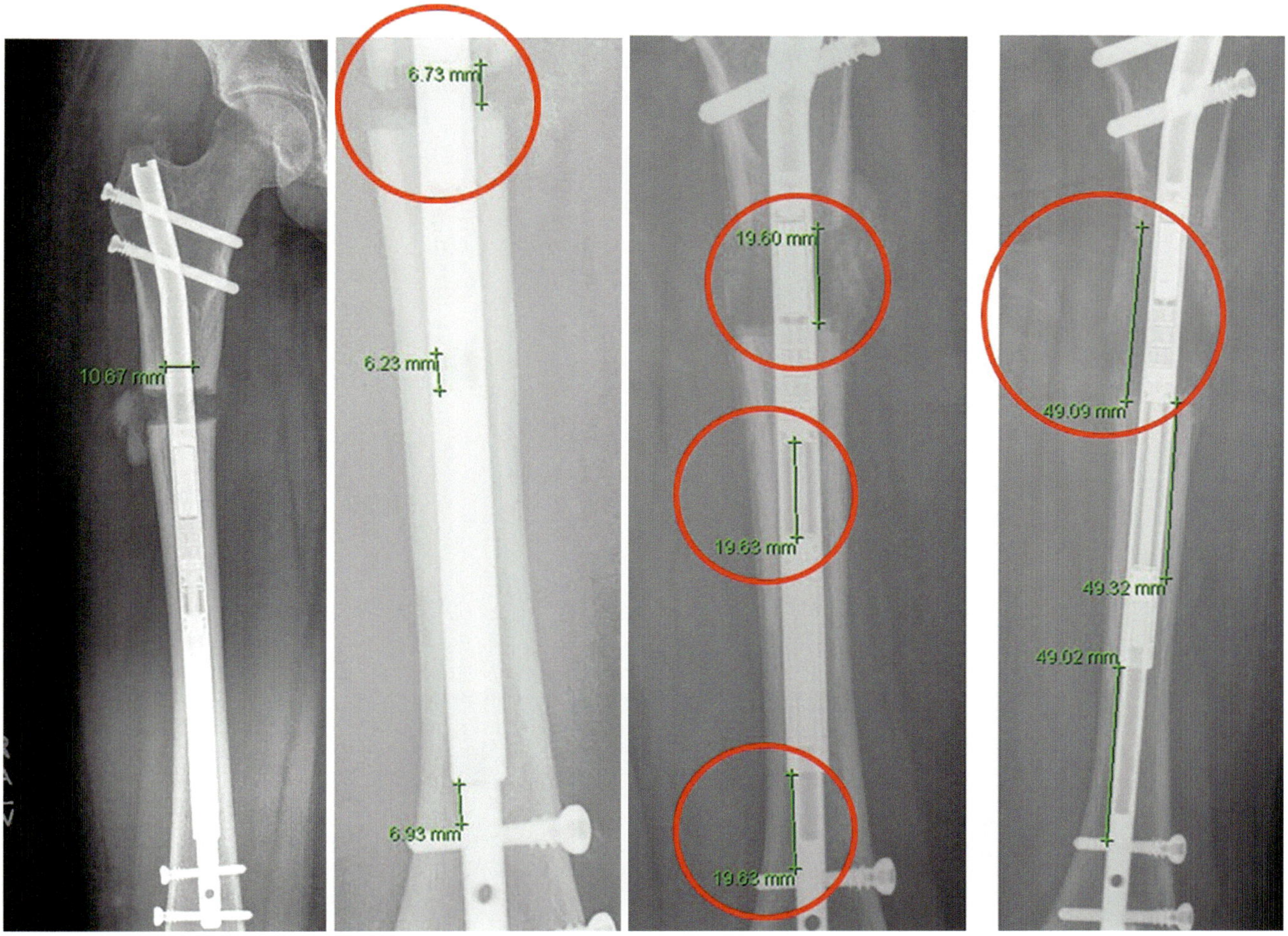

Fig. 13.27 The exact lengthening of the osteotomy site can be calculated by using the diameter of the inserted nail to calibrate for the magnification of the radiographs. This patient has a 10.7 mm diameter nail indicating there is no substantial magnification error that needs to be taken into account when making measurements on this radiograph

amount of achieved bone lengthening can be measured at the osteoplasty site from standard radiographs. Full-length radiographs of the femur might be needed to judge the amount of lengthening of the femoral mechanical axis if bone lengthening and deformity correction has been performed simultaneously. As it can be difficult to decide when the desired limb lengthening has been achieved, it is important to inform the patient prior to limb lengthening that a minor LLD can persist at the end of treatment.

Weight-Bearing Protocols

Immediate postoperative weight-bearing is individualized based on the stability and the strength of the inserted nail. Most nails allow for partial weight-bearing during the distraction phase where the weight allowed to be put onto the limb depends on the diameter of the nail. For the Fitbone™ nail (both diameter 9 mm and 11 mm), the recommended maximum weightbearing is 20 kg (44 lbs) during the distraction phase. For the Precice™ nail, the recommended maximum weightbearing during the distraction phase is 11 kg (24 lbs) for the 8.5 mm diameter nail; 22 kg (48 lbs) for the 10.7 mm diameter nail and 22 kg (48 lbs) for the 12.5 mm diameter nail. However, if the stability of the nail is compromised, the weight-bearing might be further reduced. When the distraction has ended, additional weight-bearing can be gradually increased as the consolidation of the regenerate bone increases (Fig. 13.28). The exact balance between restricted and full weight-bearing is currently unknown but the goal should be to advance weightbearing safely in order to stimulate bone formation. Using the pixel-value ratio, no adverse effects occurred when patients were allowed full weight-bearing when three out of the four cortices had a pixel-value ratio of at least 0.93 [25].

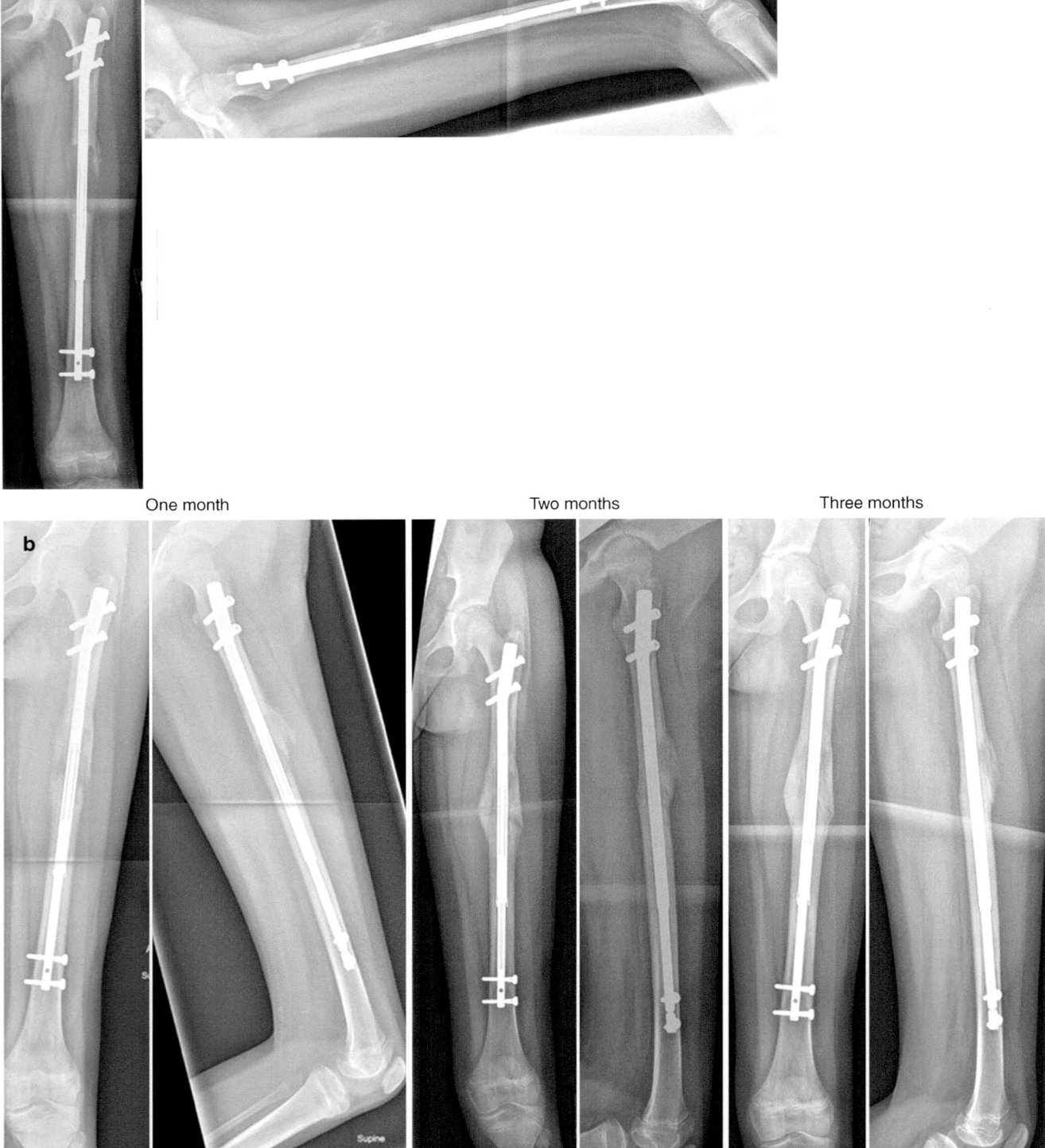

Fig. 13.28 Radiographs at end of distraction, and subsequent months during the consolidation phase

Physical Therapy

An individualized plan for physical therapy should be prescribed for patients undergoing bone lengthening with motorized intramedullary nails. The physical therapy is paramount in reducing complications. In addition, the restoration and maintenance of early limb function might contribute to improved bone healing and decreased pain. Patients should be given a daily home program of exercises to help prevent joint contracture. The frequency of outpatient physical therapy should be a minimum of 1–2 times per week during the lengthening phase to monitor the patient's status and reinforce the exercise and weight bearing protocol. The frequency of outpatient physical therapy can be increased if early signs of joint contracture occur and might be higher when performing lengthening in congenital shortening. If the range of motion falls below acceptable level cases, stop the lengthening and consider admitting the patient to the hospital for daily inpatient therapy until full range of motion returns. External bracing, both static and dynamic, can be supplemented in high-risk patients (such as congenital shortening).

Please, see separate Chap. 18 for detailed description of the applied physical therapy in limb reconstruction.

Nail Removal

Nail removal is recommended from the manufactures of both, the electric Fitbone™ nail and the magnetic Precice™ nail. For the electric Fitbone™ nail, the manufacturer recommends that the duration of implantation time in the patient should not exceed 2 years. For the Precice™ nail, the recommended maximum time of implantation is determined by the treating physician. For both the Fitbone™ and Precice™ nails, prolonged times of implantation have been reported, still with a low prevalence of radiological changes at the junctional interface [26].

The majority of nails are removed electively at the completion of treatment. This can be done as outpatient surgery. However, a more urgent nail removal is indicated for certain complications such as deep infection, fractures around the nail and breakage of nails. Complications have been reported to occur both intraoperatively during nail removal, and after nail removal [27]. Replacing the lengthening nail with a regular non-lengthening trauma nail can protect the bone regenerate after nail removal. This can be indicated when the risk of femoral fracture after nail removal is judged to be high such as in cases with fibrous dysplasia, previous radiation or poor regenerate.

A few tips at the time of nail insertion can ease the later recommended removal of the nail. Special attention is paid not to damage the screw head when inserting the locking screws. If any doubt about later difficulties in removing a locking screw due to damage of screw head or inner thread, the locking screw should be exchanged at the time of nail

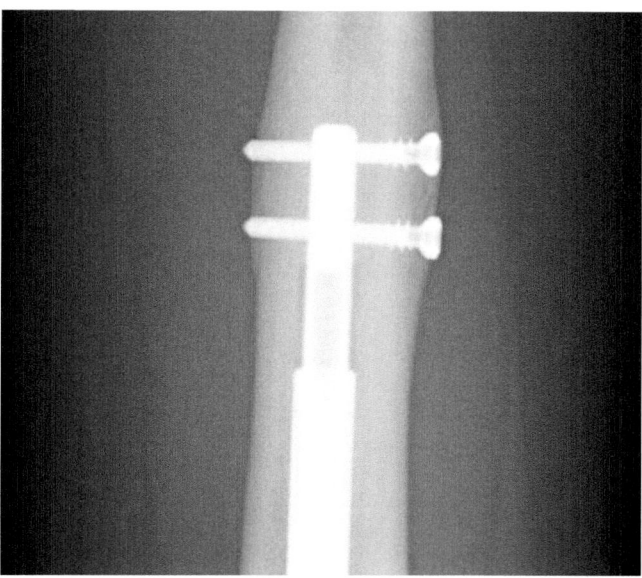

Fig. 13.29 Radiograph of implanted PRECICE™ nail immediately prior to nail removal. Bony overgrowth has occurred at the locking screw in the thin part of the nail. This may prevent the ability to perform a percutaneous screw removal in this patient

insertion. Leaving the screw head slightly proud at the time of insertion, but still with good capture of the threads into the bone, helps for later percutaneous palpation and capture during removal. Bony overgrowth over the screw heads might make a percutaneous removal of the screws difficult (Fig. 13.29) and make it necessary to use a more open approach with direct vision. A combination of osteotomes and curets can be used to carefully remove the overlying bone. Overly aggressive curettage of the screw head should be avoided as the interior threads may become damaged and prevent capture using the threaded retrieval device.

For the magnetic Precice™ nail, it is an option to insert an end-cap at time of implantation. However, the current authors do not apply an end-cap to the inserted nail. The later removal of the end cap seems unnecessarily difficult, and the protection of the integrity of the threads does not seem important as the conical nail retrieval devices are designed to aggressively cross thread into the end of the nail. During nail removal, it is an advantage that there is a direct access to the inner part of the nail for a guide wire placed with fluoroscopy (Fig. 13.30).

At antegrade nail removal, it is important to avoid being overly aggressive while hammering the nail as this could potentially cause a femoral neck fracture.

Complications

Fully implantable lengthening nails were introduced to reduce patient discomfort and complications in limb lengthening. However, complications still occur with bone lengthening nails, and the lengthening surgeon should be

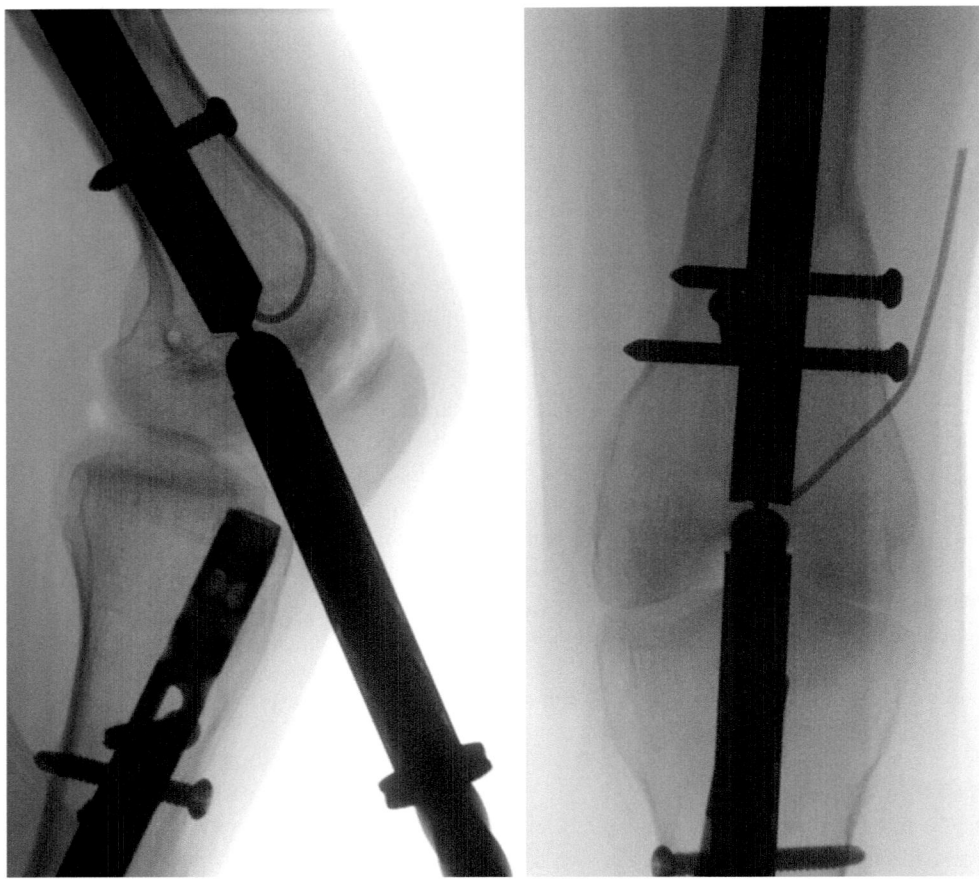

Fig. 13.30 A cannulated reamer is used to overream and remove any bony overgrowth at the site of insertion prior to nail removal

sufficiently trained in anticipating and dealing with these complications. The true incidence of complications with intramedullary lengthening nails on the femur is not known and will most likely differ between different patient groups. Thus, the risk of sustaining a severe complication will likely be smaller in a patient with stable joints and a relatively short lengthening without deformity correction compared with a patient with congenital femoral deficiency that has received multiple previous surgeries and has an unstable knee joint.

Data of complications extracted from published literature on femoral and tibial lengthening nails in 782 patients [23] showed that a complication occurred in 34% of lengthened segments. Regarding the severity of complications, 11% of the lengthened segments encountered a complication that could be resolved without further surgery. In 15% of the lengthened segments, further surgery was needed to resolve a complication, and the complication did not compromise the final outcome. In 5% of the lengthened segments, the final goal was not achieved. In 3% of the lengthened segments, the complication resulted in a new pathology or a permanent sequela, and these complications were mainly due to joint related complications (contracture, subluxation, dislocation).

The majority of complications with bone lengthening nails occur during the distraction phase, followed by the consolidation phase. However, complications can occur at any time including intraoperative, prior to nail removal, at nail removal (Fig. 13.31) and after nail removal. Regarding the origin of complications, the majority of reported complications in the literature either occurred due to failure of the inserted device or due to complications from the bone or the joints. Complications from the inserted lengthening nails have included malfunction of the distraction mechanism, breakage of the nail, and loss of fixation.

The most common complications with femoral bone lengthening nails include:

- Joint complications
  - Contracture of the knee or hip joint
  - Subluxation/luxation of the knee or hip joint
  - Anterior knee pain after retrograde nail insertion
- Bone complications
  - Delayed union/non-union
  - Premature consolidation
  - Secondary deformity
  - Fracture

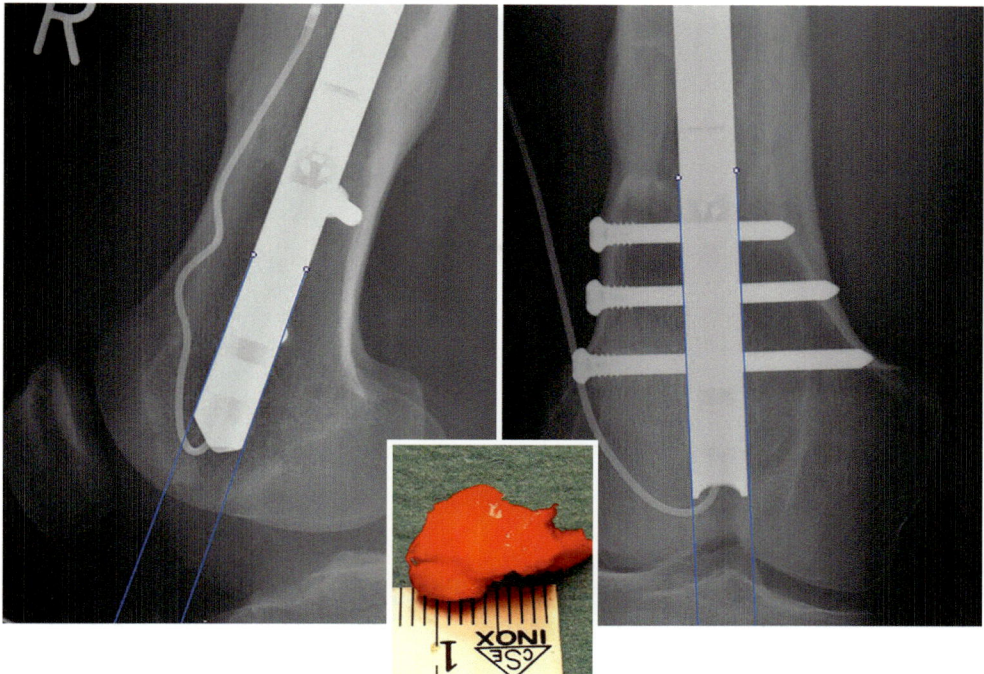

Fig. 13.31 If bone has overgrown or the entry point has changed slightly due to procurvatum during lengthening, there is a risk of producing a larger bone fragment into the knee joint

- Others
  - Malfunction of distraction mechanism
  - Loosening/breakage of screws and nails
  - Termination prior to lengthening goal achieved
  - Nerve palsy/paresthesia
  - Weakening/pain from gluteal muscle after antegrade nail insertion
  - Deep venous thrombosis/pulmonal embolism
  - Infection including osteomyelitis
  - Arterial vascular injury
  - Muscle hernia

Dealing with Complications

The best way to deal with a complication is to try to prevent them from occurring in the first place. Patients should be carefully screened for possible risk factors such as preoperative joint contracture or instability. Realistic goals for the bone lengthening should be agreed upon with the patient and caretakers. Furthermore, the post-operative program should be set-up to allow for timely monitoring of treatments to allow identification of issues before they become severe complications.

Dealing with premature consolidation: Carefully radiographic and clinical follow-up as described above is performed with short time intervals (weekly or bi-weekly during the distraction phase) to detect early signs of premature consolidation. If treated early, the premature consolidation might be avoided by increasing the lengthening rate for a brief period of time. However, if premature consolidation does occur, the patient will need to undergo a re-osteotomy. The re-osteotomy can be performed with the nail in situ. However, it is safer to temporarily remove the nail during the re-osteotomy, and then re-insert the nail using the same locking screw positions in the bone. In order to ensure healthy bone formation, the re-osteotomy should ideally be performed in close proximity to, but not at, the original osteotomy.

Dealing with delayed union/non-union: The bone regenerate is radiographically judged weekly or bi-weekly during the distraction phase to ensure that the bone formation is sufficient and homogeneous around the nail. With signs of poor bone formation, the lengthening rate can be either reduced, temporarily paused or even reversed. Delayed union or non-union might occur along the entire circumference of the nail; however, in the femur the lack of bone healing often occurs at the lateral and anterior cortices due to iatrogenic injury to the periosteum during the osteotomy. The need for additional interventions and the timing of such an intervention varies. If the stability of the nail is sufficient, the delayed bone healing site might heal without further intervention (Fig. 13.32).

If observation is chosen as the treatment for the delayed union site, the patient should be counselled about contacting the surgeon if increased pain occurs at the site. In addition, the patient should be followed by radiographs to look for compromised stability such as backing out, bending, or breaking of the interlocking screws. Stability might be increased by placing additional blocking screws in tight proximity to the nail, or by exchanging the lengthening nail to an intramedullary trauma nail with greater stability (larger

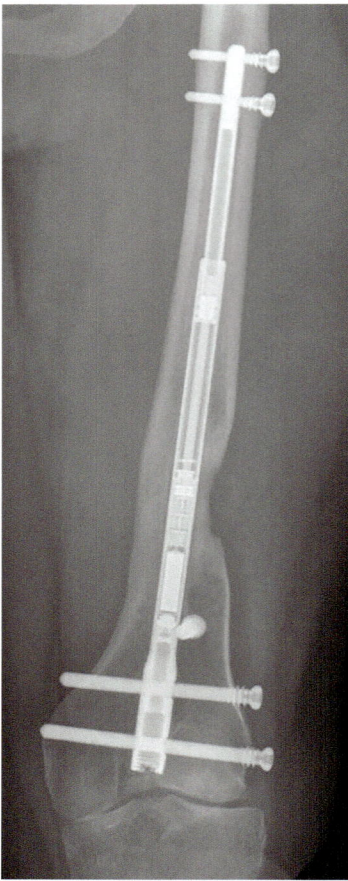

Fig. 13.32 Delayed bone healing with sufficient nail stability to proceed to bone healing without further intervention

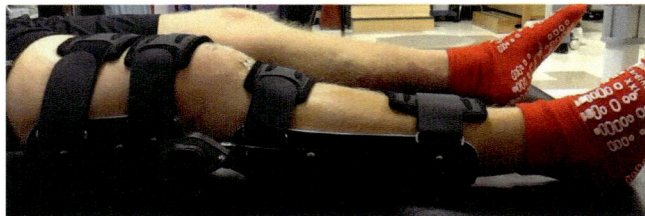

Fig. 13.33 Static or dynamic braces might be applied to maintain the knee joint in full extension in patients at high-risk of joint contracture. This is especially important in patients lacking cruciate knee ligaments to protect the knee from developing posterolateral subluxation

diameter of nail, longer nail, new and more locking screw positions). At the exchange procedure, the required reaming also adds to local autografting of the delayed healing site. Prior to reaming, the delayed healing site can be predrilled in a similar way as when making venting holes at the osteotomy site at primary nail insertion. The drilling removes fibrocartilaginous tissue at the delayed healing site, and the bone from later reaming procedure will be deposited at this site. The delayed healing site can also be grafted with autogenous bone graft or other stimulative agents, if necessary.

Dealing with joint complications: Physical therapy is paramount to avoid joint contractures. The rate of lengthening may need to be reduced to allow for sufficient joint mobility. A mild loss of joint mobility might be tolerated during the distraction phase if the clinician feels the contracture is mild enough to resolve later. However, the degree of contracture that can resolve after lengthening is difficult to predict.

When a joint contracture without joint subluxation occurs, the clinician should act quickly and aggressively to resolve it. The following steps are options for management of the contracture in gradually increasing intensity. Keep in mind that a combination of these recommendations may be necessary:

- Slowing or pausing of lengthening rate
- Increase frequency and intensity of physical therapy
- Apply a brace (Fig. 13.33)
- Admit to hospital for daily physical therapy and possible use of peripheral nerve catheters/blocks for pain management
- Stop distraction
- Reverse lengthening
- Consider soft-tissue release

If joints are dysplastic or have deformity pre-operatively, this adds to the risk of joint subluxation. In this situation, the surgeon should carefully plan how to control joint stability. If severe tibial deformities are present, it might be considered to correct these first. External frames are better tolerated on the tibia than on the femur, and the tibial frame might temporarily span the knee joint during deformity correction. Intraoperative release of the iliotibial band and the iliopsoas tendon during internal lengthening nail insertion should be considered if the patient demonstrates tightness on examination pre-operatively.

In case of joint subluxation that doesn't respond to non-operative management, it may be necessary to apply an external fixator to reduce the joint. If necessary, soft-tissue releases may be required as well. As a last resort, a shortening osteotomy can be performed to bring the joint into congruency.

Special Indications

Extramedullary Bone Lengthening with Motorized Lengthening Nail

Because internal lengthening nails are so much more comfortable for the patient than external fixators, it would be ideal if this option could be offered to every patient.

Fig. 13.34 Extramedullary lengthening with off-label use of the Precice nail allowing for internal lengthening in a young child with open growth plates and a narrow intramedullary canal

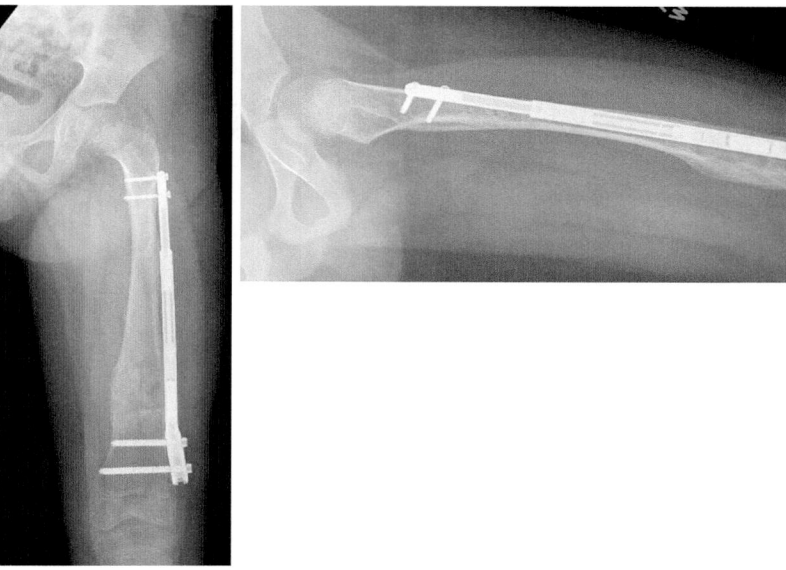

Unfortunately, for smaller or younger patients, the following limitations exist:

1. Due to the limited implant sizes, the length or intramedullary diameter of the femur may not allow safe implantation of the device in small patients.
2. Skeletally immature patients are at risk of avascular necrosis of the femoral head due to iatrogenic injury of the proximal femoral blood supply in antegrade nailing situations.
3. Retrograde femoral nailing requires the implant to be placed through an open physis in the skeletally immature patient.

Consequently, surgeons have begun to explore the concept of extramedullary bone lengthening (Fig. 13.34). In this case, the implant is placed under the soft tissue but outside the bone. Several different techniques for extramedullary lengthening have been described and the early results are encouraging. However, the surgeon must be aware that this is an off-label use of the device [28–30].

Bone Transport for Treatment of Segmental Femoral Defects

Segmental bone defects can be treated by fully implantable bone transport nails (Fig. 13.35).

Following patients to after nail removal, it has been shown that the frequency of complications is high with the FITBONE™ bone transport nail [31]. Further research is needed to optimize patient selection and nail design. The PRECICE™ bone transport nail has also been introduced to manage segmental defects of the femur [32]. Plate-assisted bone segment transport (PABST) using motorized lengthening nail in combination with an internal locking plate also enables treatment of segmental defects on the femur [33].

Stump Lengthening

Stump lengthening nails are available to increase the length of the femoral stump after high transfemoral amputation (Fig. 13.36). The increased stump length might enhance the functionality of a conventional suspended transfemoral prosthesis.

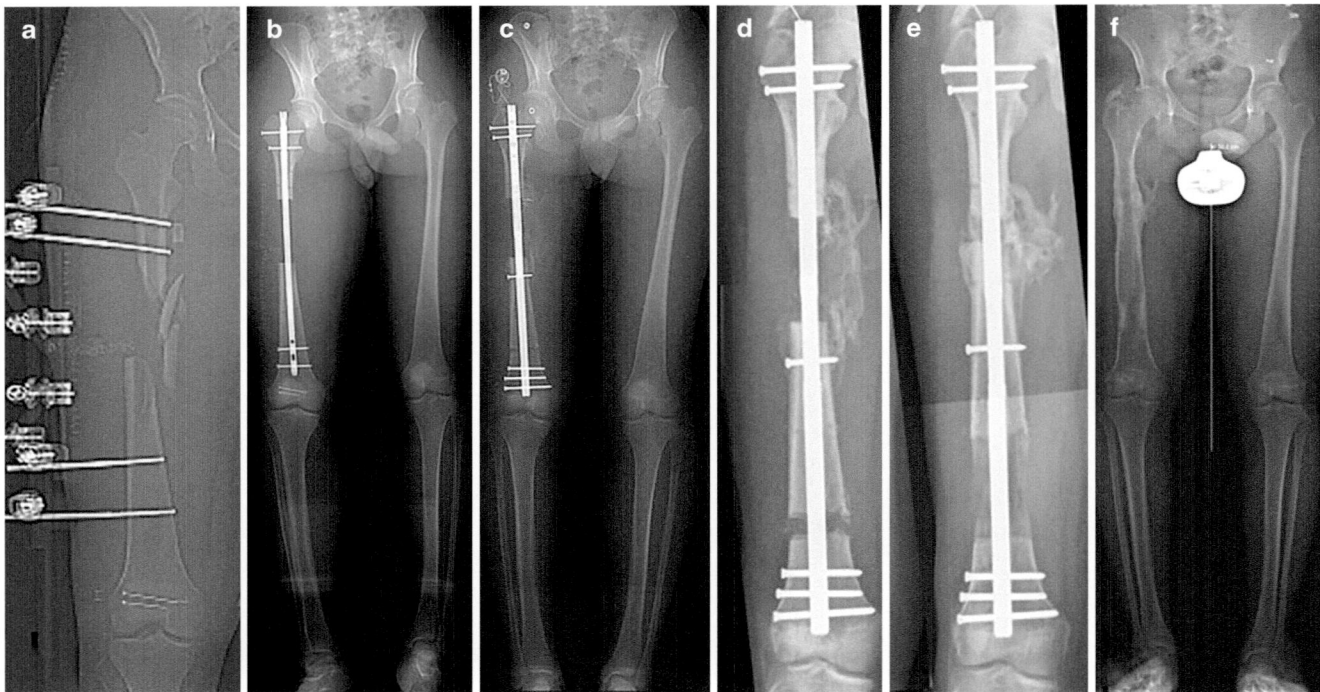

Fig. 13.35 A 22-year-old patient with open fracture of the right femoral shaft and segmental bone loss, primarily treated with external fixation. (**a**). After resection of non-vital bone, the femur with 10 cm bone defect was stabilized with a trauma nail within 14 days after trauma (**b**). The trauma nail is changed to Fitbone™ bone transport nail and distraction is started (**c**). Bone transport at 2 cm (**d**), and completed at 8 cm due to early callus formation at the docking site (**e**). Follow-up after nail removal (**f**), the remaining varus of proximal tibia is not changed [31]

Fig. 13.36 Stump lengthening in patient with traumatic transfemoral amputation. Limitation for lengthening is the soft-tissue padding at the tip of the stump

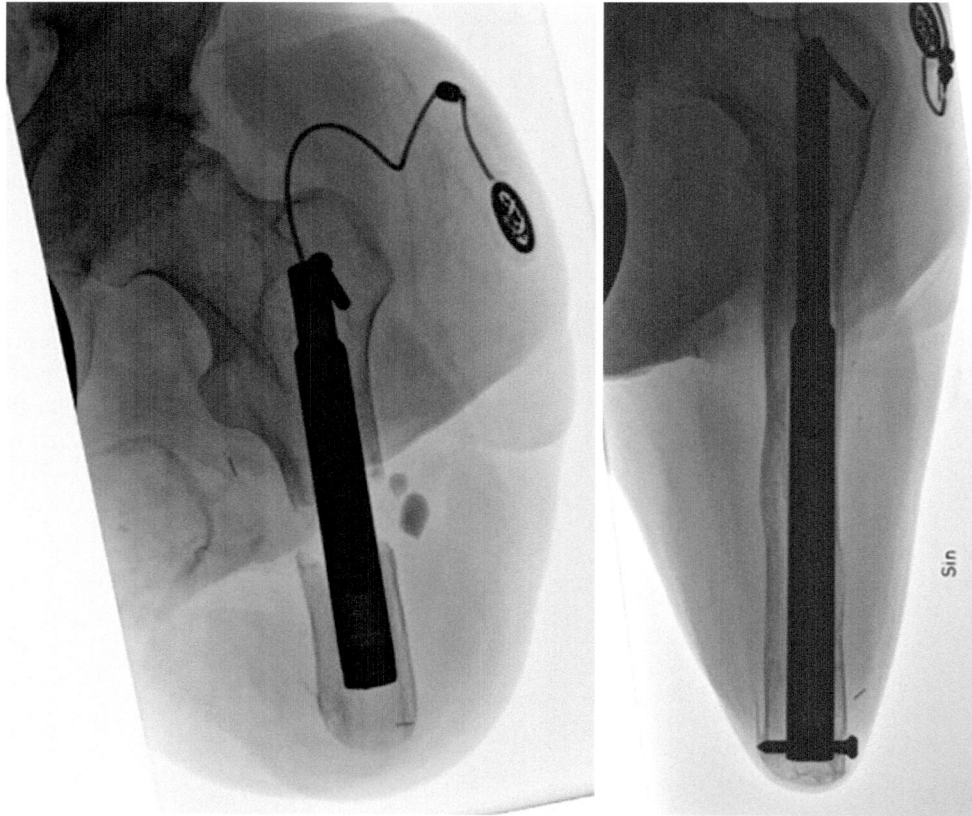

Future

Motorized intramedullary lengthening nails have revolutionized bone lengthening on the femur. However, it is still a highly individualized treatment where the surgeon must be well-trained in limb lengthening to foresee and deal with complications that are potentially very harmful. Further research is needed to gain information about benefits and complications for specific patient groups. The outcome measures should be relevant for the patient and at the same time reliable and sensitive. Patient and parent reported outcome measures are developed [34] and different classification systems are available for categorizing complications. The scientific community needs to agree upon common outcome measures in order to compare results between different patient groups and treatment algorithms. Multi-center clinical studies are needed to obtain sufficient numbers of patients for comparison. Experimental studies are needed to obtain basic knowledge about the optimal distraction osteogenesis with intramedullary lengthening nails. Post-marked surveillance of new implants is needed to monitor for unforeseen adverse events as exemplified with the PRECICE STRYDE™ nail resulting in adverse tissue reactions and pain due to unforeseen implant corrosion [35]. Further development and new nail designs might eliminate some of the drawbacks with current nail designs. Outcomes may improve if the strength of the nails can tolerate early full weight-bearing and if the nails do not need to be removed. Ideally, intramedullary nails should allow not just lengthening or compressing along the nail axis but also for a gradual deformity correction in any plane. Feedback mechanisms about the actual bone lengthening performed as well as the force needed to keep advancing the lengthening might optimize the patient journey towards a healthy bone regenerate without complications.

Commentary

Motorized Internal Femoral Lengthening Commentary

Mark T. Dahl
mdahl@gillettechildrens.com

Drs. Kold and Iobst describe the current foundational principles of motorized internal femoral lengthening. The authors discuss the basic requirements for success with this newer methodology, acknowledging a collective large worldwide clinical experience. They have written a cautionary chapter, emphasizing the need for the following preoperative assessments:

- Detailed preoperative history and physical examination relating to etiology and past history of interventions.
- Psychological evaluation noting any history of anxiety and or depression.
- Family dynamics to assess the fitness for the exacting follow-up requirements.
- Radiographic evaluation of lower extremities with a standing AP view with blocks leveling the pelvis.
- Associated joint deformities, contractures, instabilities including the spine (appendicular and axial skeleton).
- Soft tissue conditions that will affect distraction beyond the skeleton.
- Medical comorbidities that require treatment or may contraindicate the lengthening.
- Congenital etiologies carry considerable additional risk for joint injury.

Key Points in This Chapter
- The advantages and limitations of motorized internal femoral lengthening.
- Motorized internal lengthening nails have been safely employed in adults and children.
- This new technology, properly conducted, may diminish complications of limb lengthening.
- The surgeon must first understand the essential principles of limb lengthening.
- The surgeon must understand the principles and techniques of intramedullary nailing.
- Skeletal maturity, predicted discrepancy, and etiology inform treatment strategy.
- Complications common to any limb lengthening method, such as joint contracture, subluxation, and dislocation still exist.

Review of Ilizarov's Six Elements for Successful Distraction Osteogenesis

(a) Preservation of blood supply (endosteal and periosteal).
(b) Stable external fixation.
(c) A delay prior to initiating distraction ("Latency" phase).
(d) Slow fractionated distraction (~1 mm/day, varied as needed by continuous monitoring).
(e) A period of stable neutral fixation after lengthening.
(f) Physiologic use of the elongated limb.

These elements have been proven to be valid by Ilizarov, Aronson and others while using circular external fixation. However, modifications when using motorized internal lengthening are now required. This commentary describes rationale for these modifications, and introduces yet unpublished advancements of internal femoral lengthening.

Modifying Ilizarov's Six Elements of Distraction Osteogenesis for Motorized Internal Lengthening

1. The endosteal blood supply cannot be preserved while using an intramedullary nail because of the reaming process and the presence of the nail. However, a careful partial elevation of the periosteum with low-energy and low-heat drill corticotomy may best preserve the periosteal contribution to the corticotomy. This is particularly true in the tibia.
2. Strive to substitute "stable intramedullary fixation" for "stable external fixation" by secure nail fit in the following ways:
   (a) The nail chosen should have working length with isthmic contact of several centimeters.
   (b) The thick portion of the nail should extend at least 4 cm beyond the distal limit of the lengthening site at completion of lengthening.
   (c) The nail diameter should approximate the isthmic diameter measured on calibrated preoperative films.
   (d) Intraoperative chatter phenomenon signals an additional reaming of 1–2 mm is appropriate.
   (e) The commonly held reaming extent is said to be "2 mm greater than nail diameter with flexible reamers, and 1 mm greater with straight reamers". This "rule-of-thumb" is not laboratory or clinically proven, but it is logical that minimum reaming performed, provided prevention of femur fracture, osteotomy distraction, or nail damage at insertion may be best for regenerate formation. Varied bone density, cortical thickness, anterior bowing, nail starting point, and local anatomic variations are often too subtle for exacting recognition.
   (f) Professor Baumgart, the undisputed maven of motorized internal lengthening, applies sterile skin clips at the location of nail diameter transitions. Rigid reaming is then performed routinely to the planned nail diameter. Additional reaming is performed if a "dummy nail" does not pass with ease. This author reams ½ mm over for rigid reaming and 1 mm over for flexible reaming, with consistent ease of nail insertion. Thus, each case is not reamed to a predetermined point, but determined by the specific needs of the patient.
   (g) After corticotomy, with nail insertion performed by hand pressure and rotatory movement, one will recognize if the nail does not pass with ease, and thus require more reaming. We are always mindful that bone geometry and density differs among individuals and with varying etiologies.
   (h) A loose nail, with poor 'fit' allows the cut bone ends to 'waggle" during distraction, with the instability resulting in sheer and potential hypoplastic regenerate formation. Thoughtful use of blocking screws placed against the nail, generally on the concavity, will prevent most deformity during lengthening. Although not yet proven, blocking screws can be expected to improve regenerate. In capacious bone, such as wide metaphysis or metabolic bone disease, both sides of the lengthening site may benefit from blocking screws.
3. Latency period allows primary factors of fracture repair to accumulate at the corticotomy site before lengthening begins. Factors that negatively affect regenerate formation include: older age, poor soft tissue envelope, acute deformity correction, poor nutrition, medical comorbidities, prior surgery, prior lengthening, congenital or vascular etiologies, and diaphyseal corticotomy location. Thus, a longer latency period and a slower lengthening rate in such settings is advisable, but weekly radiographs and examination dictate re-adjusted rate as needed.

4. More fractionated distraction has been demonstrated to produce better regenerate, with highly fractionated (semi-automated) regenerate to be best. The readily adjustable rate and rhythm control possible with both the radiofrequency mechanism of the Fitbone and magnetic mechanism of the Precice, allows us to 'fractionate' whenever possible. We regularly instruct our patients to lengthen in smaller amounts, often at 1/8 mm per treatment, with the commonly stated rate of 1 mm per day reserved for the youngest and healthiest patient. We judge regenerate critically every visit, asking "is the bone regenerate hypotrophic, normotrophic, or hypertrophic?" The answer to this question combined with the patient's clinical status determines the next week's rate and rhythm.
5. Nail or screw breakage rates have not yet been thoroughly reported. The stable neutral period after lengthening completion is the time at which we expect advanced healing and progressive weight bearing by the patient. Conventional teaching beyond the initial limits of weight for the individual nail diameters state to restrict full weight bearing until 'three cortices' are evident. Kold and Iobst correctly point out that each motorized nail manufacturer identifies limits of weight bearing "until three cortices are evident on x-rays." Regenerate sites vary as they mature, and there is not yet a proven nor methodical way to advance weight bearing in the post-operative period on the basis of this vague guideline. In daily management of patients, we struggle to define what constitutes a cortex. Is corticalization a thicker portion of bone in the area of adjacent native cortex, or is it a rigid appearing margin on the outer new cortex? Bone volume, width, density, and/or pixel value ratio are all methods to improve these judgements, but none clearly guide this decision. Thus, we must further individualize, and incrementally advance weight bearing differently for each patient, considering their size, and individual ability to comply. We employ a bathroom scale in our clinics, teaching each patient how to recognize the extent of their weight bearing. Screw or nail breakage and migration is thus uncommon in this reviewer's experience, less than 1%, seeing six broken or bent nails from premature full weight bearing in over 1000 motorized intramedullary lengthenings.
6. The final tenant, physiological use of the limb is encouraged regarding range of motion, isometric exercises, static and dynamic stretching, yet the obligatory restriction of full weight bearing must be honored until the nail load can be adequately taken over by the maturing regenerate bone.

The Key Factors in Decision Making of Internal Femoral Lengthening
Etiology.
Magnitude of Discrepancy Now and at Maturity.
Unique anatomy of the femur, deformity, size, the effect of lengthening along the bone's axis.
Adjacent Joint Stability and Motion.
Neurovascular and Soft Tissue Status.
Condition of the entire limb and spine.
Medical Comorbidities.
Family and Social Dynamics.

Mentoring the Neophyte Lengthening Surgeon

A concept worthy of discussion is the role of mentoring for the neophyte limb lengthening surgeon. Both authors of this chapter and this reviewer have personally benefited from **limb lengthening mentors**. Every surgeon should create a preparatory pathway to success in limb lengthening and deformity correction. This must include education and mentorship prior to performing limb lengthening and complex deformity correction surgery by:

- Identifying an enduring interest in limb lengthening and complex deformity correction.
- Commitment to learning historical lessons of this uniquely difficult subspecialty.
- Visit experienced surgeons, and establish open relationships with such individuals.
- Attend fellowship training and education.
- Attend proprietary workshops.
- Define the limits of one's skill set, taking on cases of incremental complexity, building on less complex initial cases.
- Understand the expectations of the patient, matching them with your own realistic expectations.

New and Future Possibilities with Motorized Internal Limb Lengthening

Little is written about the limits of acute deformity correction with motorized internal lengthening nails. As safe limits of acutely performing angulation, translation, and rotation have not been established, and the risks of neurologic, vascular, skin, and soft tissue injury loom, we must use thoughtful anatomic considerations, and err on the side of caution. A comprehensive **Length and Deformity Correction Center** uses gradual correction via external fixation for the most extreme circumstances. This will commonly include valgus to varus knee correction greater than 10°–15°, acute foot, ankle, and leg corrections that risk wound injury or compartment syndrome. Bifocal lengthenings with motorized nails are possible, yet require additional treatment sites to be protected with internal fixation plates and intracortical screws avoiding nail impingement. Upper extremity lengthenings are less commonly necessary than lower extremity, and the bone size limits often restrict use of lengthening nails, but the surgeon must be ever vigilant to identify and expose neurovascular structures at the time of surgery, as the current nail inventory are not designed for these purposes.

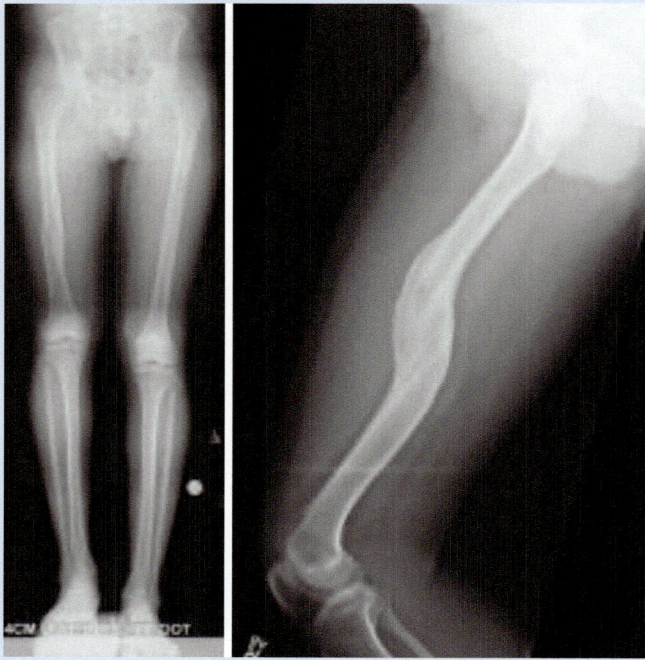

This 26-year-old male sustained a closed femur fracture at age 17, which healed with 4.5 cm of shortening, 8° varus, and 45 mm of lateral plane translation.

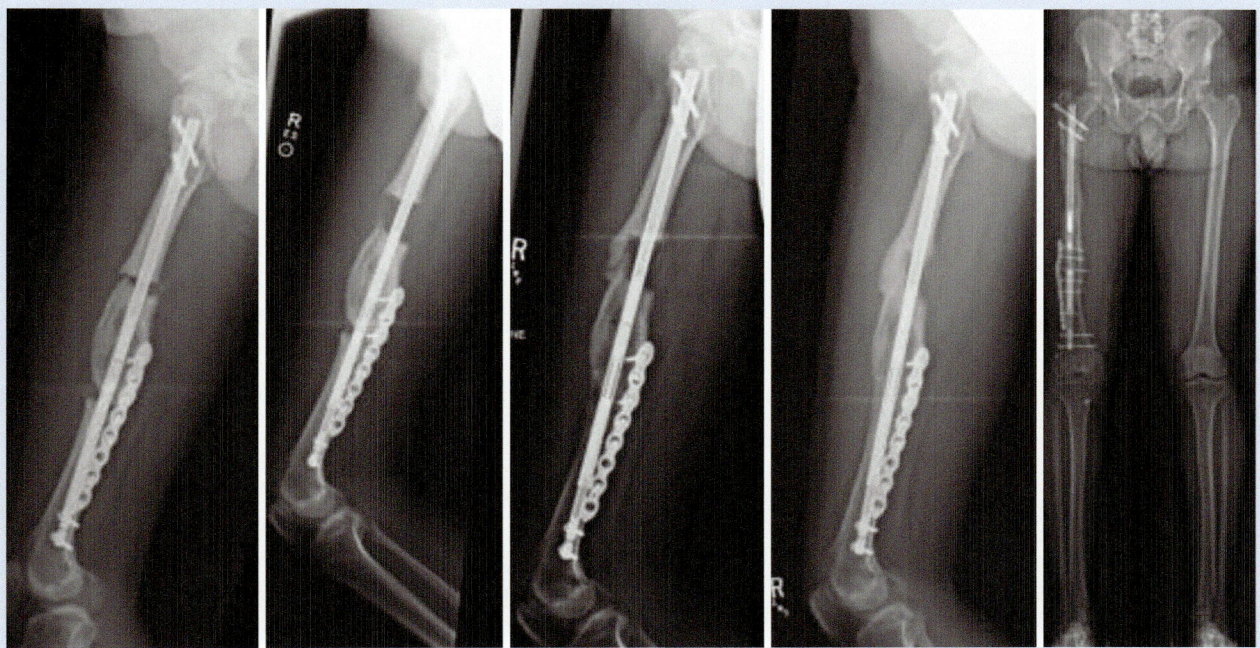

Bifocal oblique osteotomies were planned and performed, correcting each deformity at its apex and true plane, with the distal correction secured with a unicortical plating, and the proximal corticomy chosen as the lengthening site. Latency period was extended to 3 weeks, with atrophic bone formation noted at 20 mm of length. Lengthening rate was slowed to 0.5 mm per day in 4 doses of 1/8 mm each, with improvement in regenerate bone. Regenerate and cortilization is typically slowest on the side with greatest corticotomy separation (periosteal damage). Healing and full weight bearing at 5 months post-operatively.

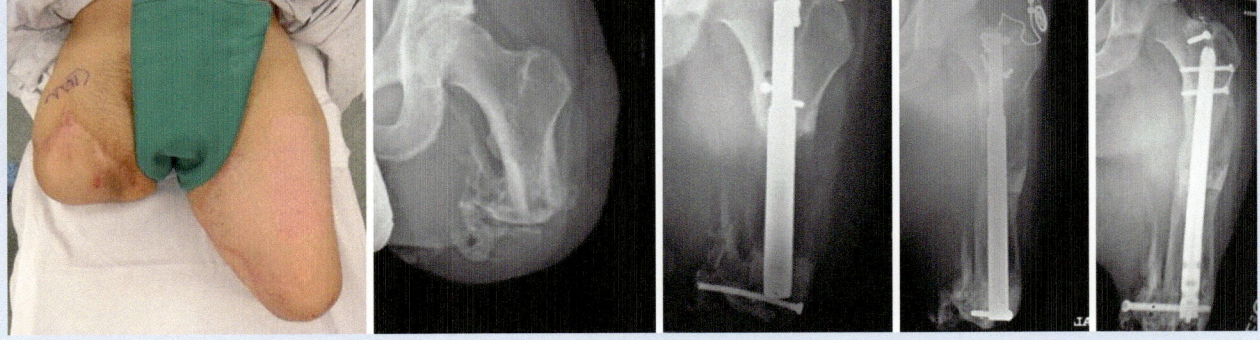

This 24-year-old special forces soldier stepped on an IED sustaining bilateral transfemoral amputations. The shorter limb could not be fit at transfemoral level, with two sequential 8 cm stump lengthenings performed. Note blocking screws used to provide stability and maximize regenerate formation. Trauma nail exchanged soon after second lengthening to expedite prosthetic fitting.

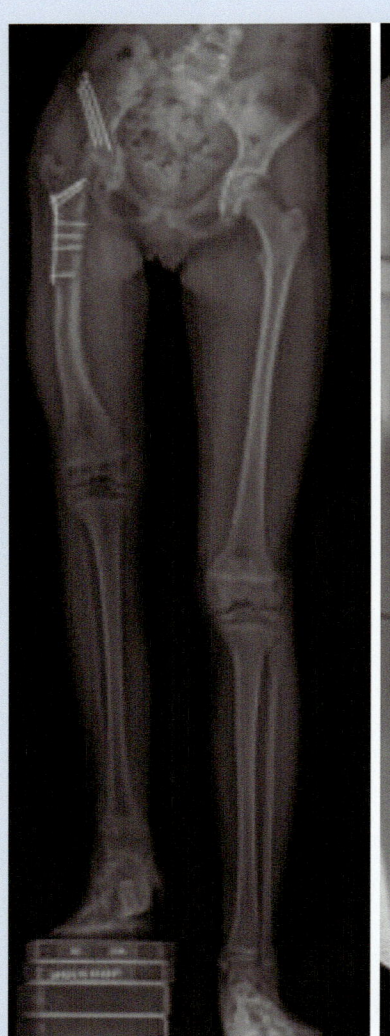
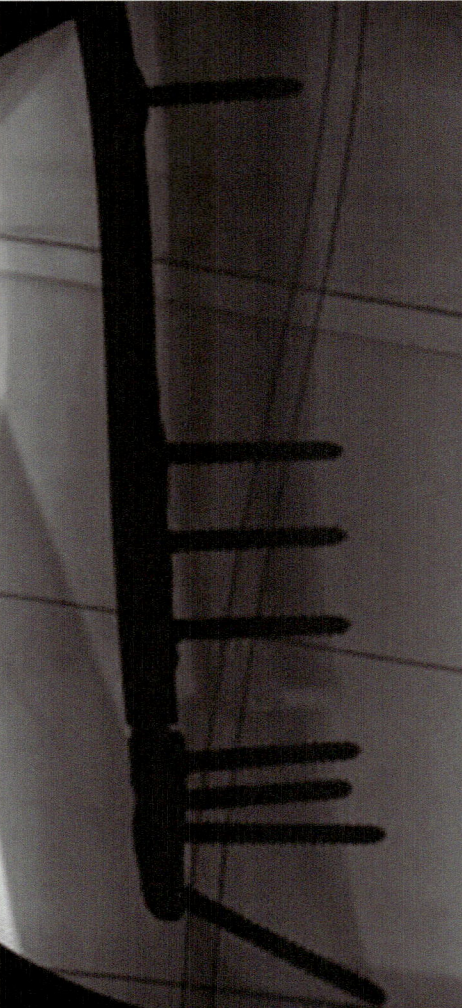
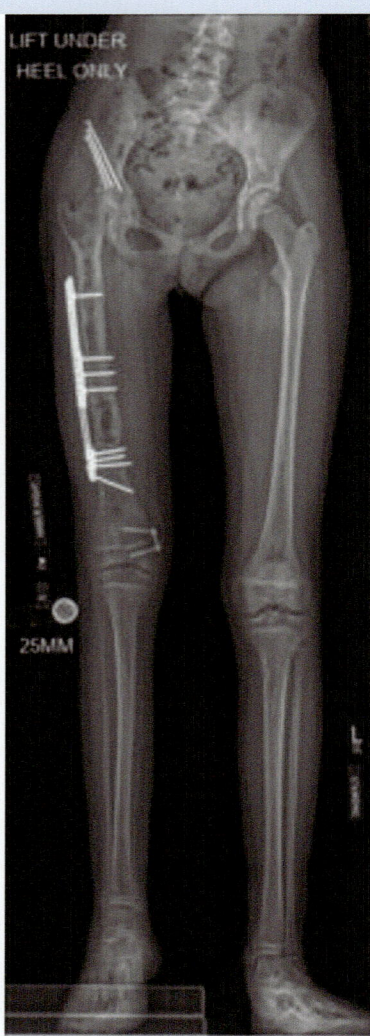

Future developments include extramedullary lengthening devices for younger children. This 8-year-old girl with congenital short femur had preparatory pelvic and proximal femoral osteotomies, followed by a "magnetic plate lengthener" to achieve acute correction of femoral varus and 4.5 cm of length.

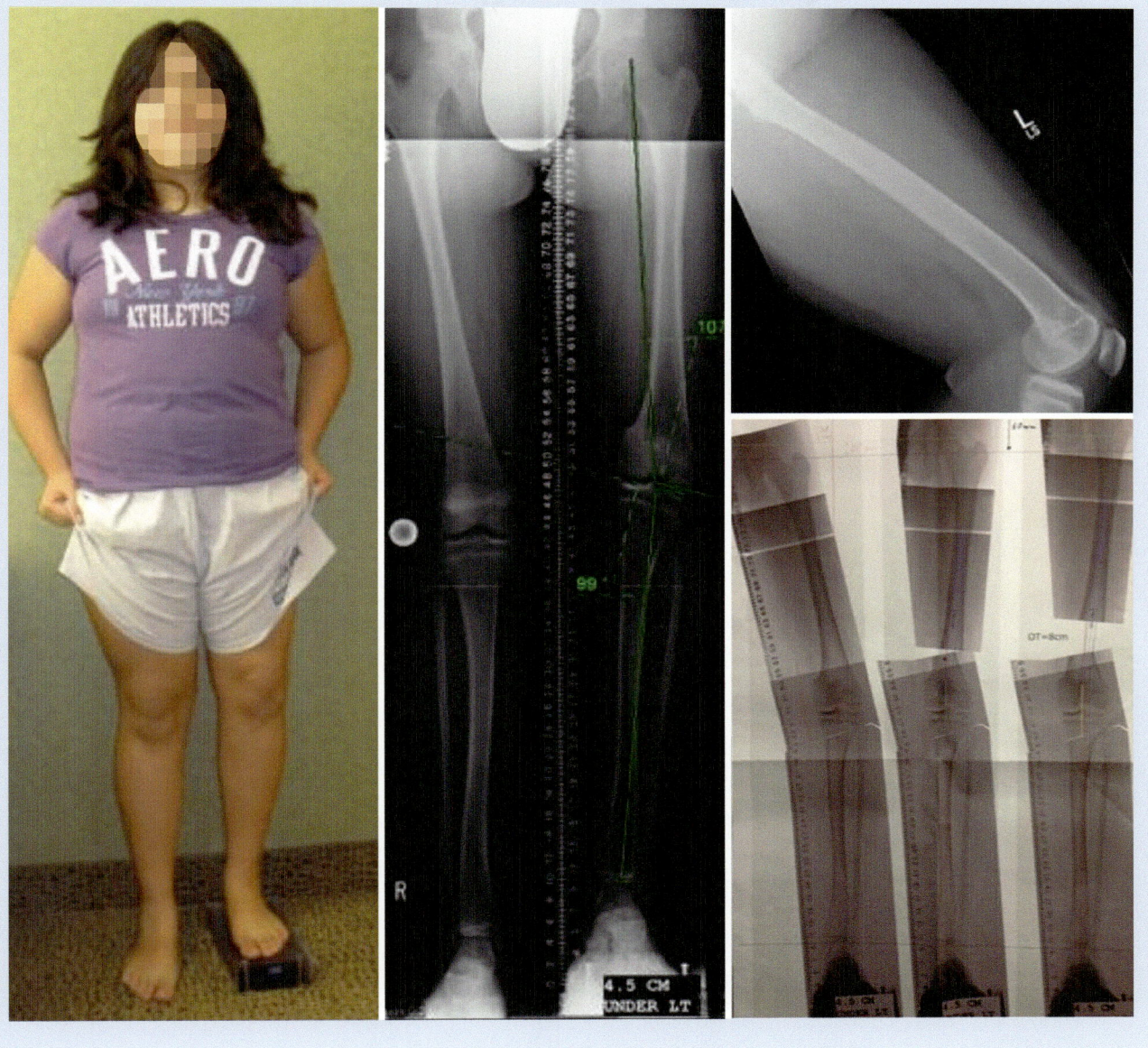

Trampoline injury caused distal femoral flexion, varus, and length deformity, and spontaneous valgus tibial compensatory growth. Single event surgery was planned that included varus tibial correction with plate fixation and retrograde femoral length and deformity correction. Planning with the reverse planning method as described by Baumgaart.

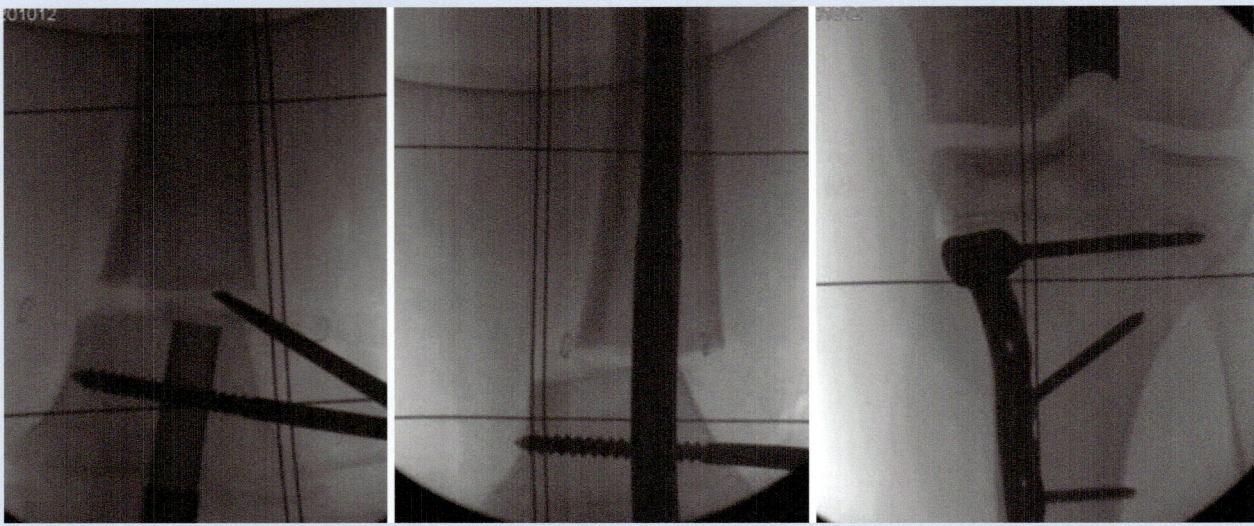

Despite indirect reduction of deformity, extreme corrections of angulation and translation result in periosteal damage and demand a prolonged latency of 3 weeks.

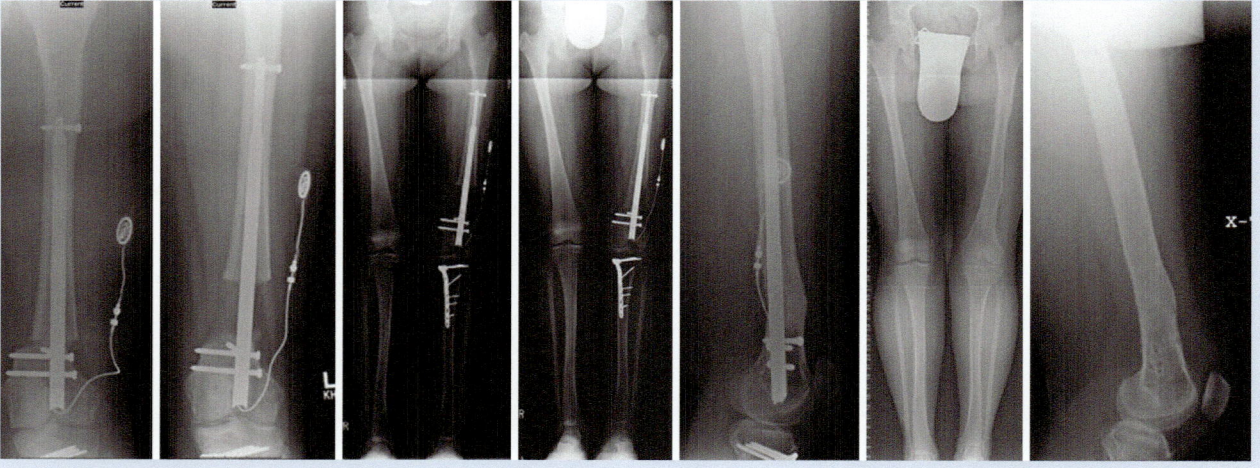

Lengthening rate must be slower and rhythm more highly divided and monitored and varied throughout treatment to achieve good healing without the need for supplemental grafting.

References

1. Birch JG. A brief history of limb lengthening. J Pediatr Orthop. 2017;37(6):S1–8.
2. Ilizarov GA. The tension-stress effect on the genesis and growth of tissues: part II. The influence of the rate and frequency of distraction. Clin Orthop Relat Res [Internet]. 1989;239:263–85. [cited 2021 Dec 8]. http://www.ncbi.nlm.nih.gov/pubmed/2912628
3. Horn J, Grimsrud Ø, Dagsgard AH, Huhnstock S, Steen H. Femoral lengthening with a motorized intramedullary nail. Acta Orthop [Internet]. 2015;86(2):248–56. http://www.tandfonline.com/doi/full/10.3109/17453674.2014.960647
4. Laubscher M, Mitchell C, Timms A, Goodier D, Calder P. Outcomes following femoral lengthening: an initial comparison of the precice intramedullary lengthening nail and the lrs external fixator monorail system. Bone Joint J. 2016;98-B(10):1382–8.
5. Küçükkaya M, Karakoyun Ö, Sökücü S, Soydan R. Femoral lengthening and deformity correction using the Fitbone motorized lengthening nail. J Orthop Sci. 2015;20(1):149–54.
6. Green SA. The evolution of remote-controlled intramedullary lengthening and compression nails. J Orthop Trauma. 2017;31(6):S2–6.
7. Frommer A, Roedl R, Gosheger G, Niemann M, Turkowski D, Toporowski G, et al. What are the potential benefits and risks of using magnetically driven antegrade intramedullary lengthening nails for femoral lengthening to treat leg length discrepancy? Clin Orthop Relat Res. 2022;480:790–803.
8. Hammouda AI, Jauregui JJ, Gesheff MG, Standard SC, Herzenberg JE. Trochanteric entry for femoral lengthening nails in children: is it safe? J Pediatr Orthop. 2017;37(4):258–64.
9. Knapik DM, Zirkle LG, Liu RW. Consequences following distal femoral growth plate violation in an ovine model with an intramedullary implant: a pilot study. J Pediatr Orthop. 2018;38(10):e640–5.
10. Abood AA, Rahbek O, Olesen ML, Christensen BB, Møller-Madsen B, Kold S. Does retrograde femoral nailing through a normal physis impair growth? An experimental porcine model. Strateg trauma limb Reconstr [Internet]. 2021;16(1):8–13. [cited 2022 Jan 24]. http://www.ncbi.nlm.nih.gov/pubmed/34326896
11. Paley D, Chong DY, Prince DE. Congenital femoral deficiency reconstruction and lengthening surgery. In: Pediatric lower limb deformities: principles and techniques of management. Springer US; 2016, pp. 361–425.
12. Calder PR, McKay JE, Timms AJ, Roskrow T, Fugazzotto S, Edel P, et al. Femoral lengthening using the Precice intramedullary limb-lengthening system: outcome comparison following antegrade and retrograde nails. Bone Joint J. 2019;101-B(9):1168–76.
13. Eltayeby HH, Alrabai HM, Jauregui JJ, Shabtai LY, Herzenberg JE. Post-retrieval functionality testing of PRECICE lengthening nails: the "sleeper" nail concept. J Clin Orthop Trauma [Internet]. 2021;14:151–5. https://doi.org/10.1016/j.jcot.2020.06.005.
14. Barakat AH, Sayani J, O'dowd-Booth C, Guryel E. Lengthening nails for distraction osteogenesis: a review of current practice and presentation of extended indications. Strateg Trauma Limb Reconstr. 2020;15(1):54–61.
15. Harkin E, Rozbruch SR, Liskutin T, Hopkinson W, Bernstein M. Total hip arthroplasty and femoral nail lengthening for hip dysplasia and limb-length discrepancy. Arthroplast Today [Internet]. 2018;4(3):279–86. https://doi.org/10.1016/j.artd.2018.03.001.
16. Wagner P, Burghardt RD, Green SA, Specht SC, Standard SC, Herzenberg JE. PRECICE magnetically-driven, telescopic, intramedullary lengthening nail: pre-clinical testing and first 30 patients. Sicot-J. 2017;3.
17. Richard HM, Birch JG, Nguyen DC, Roland S, Cherkashin AM SM. Pediatric limb lengthening and reconstruction: Risk factors impacting surgical outcomes. In: LLRS Annual Meeting July 26, 2014 Montreal, CA.; 2014.
18. Burghardt RD, Paley D, Specht SC, Herzenberg JE. The effect on mechanical axis deviation of femoral lengthening with an intramedullary telescopic nail. J Bone Joint Surg Br [Internet]. 2012;94(9):1241–5. http://www.ncbi.nlm.nih.gov/pubmed/22933497
19. Baumgart R. The reverse planning method for lengthening of the lower limb using a straight intramedullary nail with or without deformity correction. Oper Orthop Traumatol. 2009;21(2):221–33.
20. Iobst CA, Rozbruch SR, Nelson S, Fragomen A. Simultaneous acute femoral deformity correction and gradual limb lengthening using a retrograde femoral nail: technique and clinical results. J Am Acad Orthop Surg. 2018;26(7):241–50.
21. Karakoyun Ö, Küçükkaya M, Erol MF. Does lengthening after acute correction negatively affect bone healing during distraction osteogenesis? Acta Orthop Traumatol Turc. 2015;49(4):405–9.
22. Gomez C, Nelson S, Speirs J, Barnes S. Magnetic intramedullary lengthening nails and MRI compatibility. J Pediatr Orthop. 2018;38(10):e584–7.
23. Frost MW, Rahbek O, Traerup J, Ceccotti AA, Kold S. Systematic review of complications with externally controlled motorized intramedullary bone lengthening nails (FITBONE and PRECICE) in 983 segments. Acta Orthop. 2020;92(1):120–7.
24. Villalobos MA, Veneziano G, Iobst C, Miller R, Walch AG, Roth C, et al. Regional anesthesia for pain management after orthopedic procedures for treatment of lower extremity length discrepancy. J Pain Res. 2020;13:547–52.
25. Bafor A, Duncan ME, Iobst CA. Evaluating the utility of the pixel value ratio in the determination of time to full weight-bearing in patients undergoing intramedullary limb lengthening. Strateg Trauma Limb Reconstr. 2020;15(2):74–8.
26. Iobst CA, Frost MW, Rölfing JD, Rahbek O, Bafor A, Duncan M, et al. Radiographs of 366 removed limb-lengthening nails reveal differences in bone abnormalities between different nail types. Bone Joint J. 2021;103-B(11):1731–5.
27. Frost MW, Kold S, Rahbek O, Bafor A, Duncan M, Iobst CA. Complications in elective removal of 271 bone lengthening nails (FITBONE, PRECICE and STRYDE); 2021.
28. Iobst CA, Bafor A. Retrograde extramedullary lengthening of the femur using the PRECICE nail: technique and results. J Pediatr Orthop. 2021;41(6):356–61.
29. Dahl MT, Morrison SG, Laine JC, Novotny SA, Georgiadis AG. Extramedullary motorized lengthening of the femur in young children. J Pediatr Orthop. 2020;40(10):E978–83.
30. Shannon C, Paley D. Extramedullary internal limb lengthening. Tech Orthop. 2020;35(3):195–200.
31. Mikužis M, Rahbek O, Christensen K, Kold S. Complications common in motorized intramedullary bone transport for non-infected segmental defects: a retrospective review of 15 patients. Acta Orthop. 2021;92(4):485–92.
32. Kern T. Managing bone defects in the femur with a motorized intramedullary bone transport nail: case review with follow-up. J Orthop Trauma. 2021;35(10):S8–12.

33. Olesen UK, Nygaard T, Prince DE, Gardner MP, Singh UM, McNally MA, et al. Plate-assisted bone segment transport with motorized lengthening nails and locking plates: a technique to treat femoral and Tibial bone defects. JAAOS Glob Res Rev. 2019;3(8):e064.
34. Griffiths AL, Donnan LT, Iobst CA, Kelley SP, Bouchard M, Narayanan UG. The gait outcomes assessment list for children with lower limb difference (GOAL-LD): assessment of reliability and validity. J Pediatr Orthop. 2021;41(7):450–6.
35. Rölfing JD, Kold S, Nygaard T, Mikuzis M, Brix M, Faergemann C, et al. Pain, osteolysis, and periosteal reaction are associated with the STRYDE limb lengthening nail: a nationwide cross-sectional study. Acta Orthop. 2021;92(4):479–84.

Further Reading

Dahl MT. Motorized, telescopic, intramedullary lengthening nails for limb length and deformity correction. Tech Orthop. 2015;30(3):189–206.

Dahl MT, Georgiadis AG, Morrison SG. Motorized internal limb lengthening: an updated review. JPOSNA. 2020;2:67.

Georgiadis AG, Morrison SG, Dahl MT. Complications of limb lengthening using motorized nails. JAAOS. 2020;28:e803–9.

Green SA, Dahl MT. Intramedullary limb lengthening: principals and practice; 2018 https://www.springer.com/gp/book/9783319602967

Motorized Intramedullary Lengthening of the Tibia

14

Austin T. Fragomen

Introduction

The motorized internal lengthening nail (MILN) has revolutionized the ability to perform distraction osteogenesis without the use of circular external fixation. This group of implants uses an internal motor to precisely control lengthening through an electric antenna (Fitbone, Wittenstein/Orthofix, Igersheim, Germany) or through a magnetic coupling (Precice, NuVasive Specialized Orthopedics, San Diego, CA, USA). The Precice MILN is bidirectional and also provides the capability of compression through shortening. MILNs have transformed the world of limb lengthening and deformity correction in the femur where external fixation is poorly tolerated. Tibial lengthening and deformity surgery provides additional challenges when compared with the femur, and external fixation is still very useful in the lower leg. Use of the Precice MILN in patients with open growth plates is an off-label application of this device. This chapter will focus on indications, technical aspects, and outcomes of lengthening the tibia and fibula using the MILN.

Indications

Lengthening of the tibia bone can be accomplished with great success using a motorized internal lengthening implant. The indications for MILN lengthening are more restrictive than those for circular fixation tibial lengthening due to the limitations of the nail implant itself. Internal lengthening nails are fantastic at achieving length in long bones with little deformity. MILNs have more difficulty controlling the proximal tibial segment when the osteotomy is very proximal [1, 2]. Blocking screws are very helpful in steering the bone and preventing deformity [3]. Blocking screws are critical for acute deformity correction at the lengthening site at the time of osteotomy [4]. The indications for lengthening with an MILN can be expanded to acute deformity correction and lengthening because of the use of blocking screws. How much deformity can be corrected acutely without negatively impacting the bone's ability to form regenerate is unknown. As we know from limb lengthening with external fixators, congenital lengthening is more complicated than post traumatic lengthening as the distraction process places more stress on the nerves and tendons leading to symptomatic nerve entrapment and knee or ankle contractures. The amount of length that can be achieved varies based on anatomic considerations, the quality of regenerate (which forms less uniformly in the tibia compared to the femur), and the stroke length of the nail which is 8 cm for most magnetic lengthening products. Unlike frames, nails provide no ability to control the knee or ankle joint during the lengthening process. This makes congenital dysplastic conditions such as fibular hemimelia more difficult to treat with ILNs, and special considerations such as knee extension bracing and temporary ankle stabilization, for example, need to be made to prevent contractures or subluxations. Patients that are not expected to be excellent distraction osteogenesis candidates such as those with metabolic bone disease or advanced age can be treated with MILN but will likely develop poor regenerate. These patients may be better served with the lengthening and then nailing technique (LATN) [5] or may require exchange nailing after completion of the distraction phase to stimulate regenerate consolidation. Recent research has shown that the LATN technique produces superior bone regenerate and union rates over MILN in tibial lengthening [6]. *The ideal candidate for tibial lengthening is skeletally mature or close to maturity, has an intramedullary canal that can safely accept a nail, has the majority of the shortening originating from the tibia, and has little to no tibial deformity. In some cases, femur lengthening may be considered to treat a tibial shortening. If the tibia is unlikely to heal due to*

A. T. Fragomen (✉)
Limb Lengthening & Complex Reconstruction Service, Hospital for Special Surgery, New York, NY, USA
e-mail: FragomenA@hss.edu

trauma, infection, sclerosis, then the more reliable femur can reestablish normal limb length. This approach will result in knee height discrepancy which is well tolerated up to a few centimeters. For tibial shortening over 5 cm, a combined lengthening of both the femur and tibia will result in shortening the recovery time and improving the odds for successful regenerate formation at the two separate lengthening sites.

Contraindications for the MILN in the tibia have traditionally been a small intramedullary canal and open proximal tibial growth plates. The small canal issue has been circumvented in the femur using the MILN as an extramedullary lengthening device by placing it directly next to the diaphysis of the long bone underneath the soft tissue [7, 8]. *This method of extramedullary lengthening has been performed in the tibia as well to avoid growth plates and the narrow IM canal. [Shannon Paley TIO 2020 35(3):195–200]*

The ability to cross the physis of the proximal tibia and not generate a premature physeal closure has been the topic of much research interest and controversial discussions. The first strategy is to assume that the physeal insult is too minor to inhibit growth. A small series of adolescent tibias fractures with open growth plates treated with IM nailing did not result in physeal arrest or deformity despite passing directly through the physis [9]. Large animal studies have shown that the distal femur can tolerate damage of up to 7% of the physeal area without growth disturbance [10]. A clinical study looked at distal femur physeal violation during the treatment of fractures in children using a retrograde IM nail and found that there were no partial or complete growth arrests [11]. The patients were young (average age 10 years old), the physeal violation was 3%, and the follow up averaged 292 days (range 53–714). It is difficult to directly apply these distal femur results to the tibia where the entry point is far anterior and the area of the entry hole will violate a relatively larger portion of the tibial physis. The second strategy is to try to keep the hole created in the growth plate filled with the metal implant. Surgeons have claimed that if the metal nail occupies the hole created through the physis (usually achieved by using an end cap), then the growth plate will not create a bar and will continue to function normally. Maintaining the nail position across the physis may require additional surgery to insert a longer end cap as the nail migrates distally during growth to prevent closure of the epiphyseal entry hole. However, tibial lengthening with an MILN in patients with open physes is a risky endeavor and may be best postponed until physeal closure or left to circular external fixation where frame times are low and success rates are high. Many authors report waiting until their pediatric patients have closed their proximal tibial physis prior to using the tibial MILN [12, 13].

Technique

Pre Operative Planning

Use of the tibial MILN requires a good pre operative plan. Ideally, the surgeon will have a set of calibrated AP and Lateral X-rays of the tibia and have templates of the MILN available to plan the exact location that the nail will occupy. This is particularly important for finding the optimal start point for the nail and for deciding if a posterior blocking screw is needed and where to place it (Fig. 14.1). When the osteotomy is in the diaphysis, the blocking screw is usually not necessary. A proximal metaphyseal osteotomy will require a screw to prevent flexion both during nail insertion as well as during lengthening. A distal start point for the nail and no blocking screw will result in a flexion deformity even before the lengthening starts. A blocking screw may not prevent a flexion deformity particularly if the posterior cortex fractures during corticotomy or nail insertion [4]. Blocking screw placement is part of the pre operative planning process and can be the most important factor in executing an accurate deformity correction and in successfully preventing lengthening induced deformity [2]. The reverse-rule-of-thumbs method works well to determine reason where the screws should be placed [4, 14]. These radiographs will also serve to choose a corticotomy location. This decision must take into account various factors: an MILN will be better able to control both bone fragments through a diaphyseal osteotomy site, a metaphyseal osteotomy will heal more predictably than a diaphyseal osteotomy, sclerotic bone from a previous malunion will not produce an ideal regenerate, damaged skin over the osteotomy can increase the risk of a regenerate infection, a distal osteotomy may not leave enough of the large telescopic portion of the nail in the distal fragment during lengthening and consolidation.

A high quality, calibrated standing radiograph or EOS (EOS imaging, Paris, France) including the hip to ankle is

Fig. 14.1 (a) Shows the pre operative planning for MILN position in the right tibia. Using these templates, the nail length and width can be selected. The placement of a lateral blocking screw is determined. The screw is placed 1–2 cm proximal to the osteotomy site to prevent propagation of the corticotomy into the screw. The screw is also placed as distal as possible to have a maximal effect on controlling the nail and should be inserted directly next to the nail. The level of the osteotomy is also selected on this radiograph and measured from the joint line to allow for easier reproduction in the operating room. The solid metal ball to the left of the film is a 2.5 cm calibration ball. (b) shows the ideal start point for the MILN in the proximal tibia to avoid flexion. This entry point will need to be reproduced during the surgery. In this case the osteotomy site is distal enough that the nail will contact the posterior cortex without introducing flexion. There is no need for a blocking screw as the cortex acts in place of the screw. The calibration ball is again seen in this image anterior to the tibia

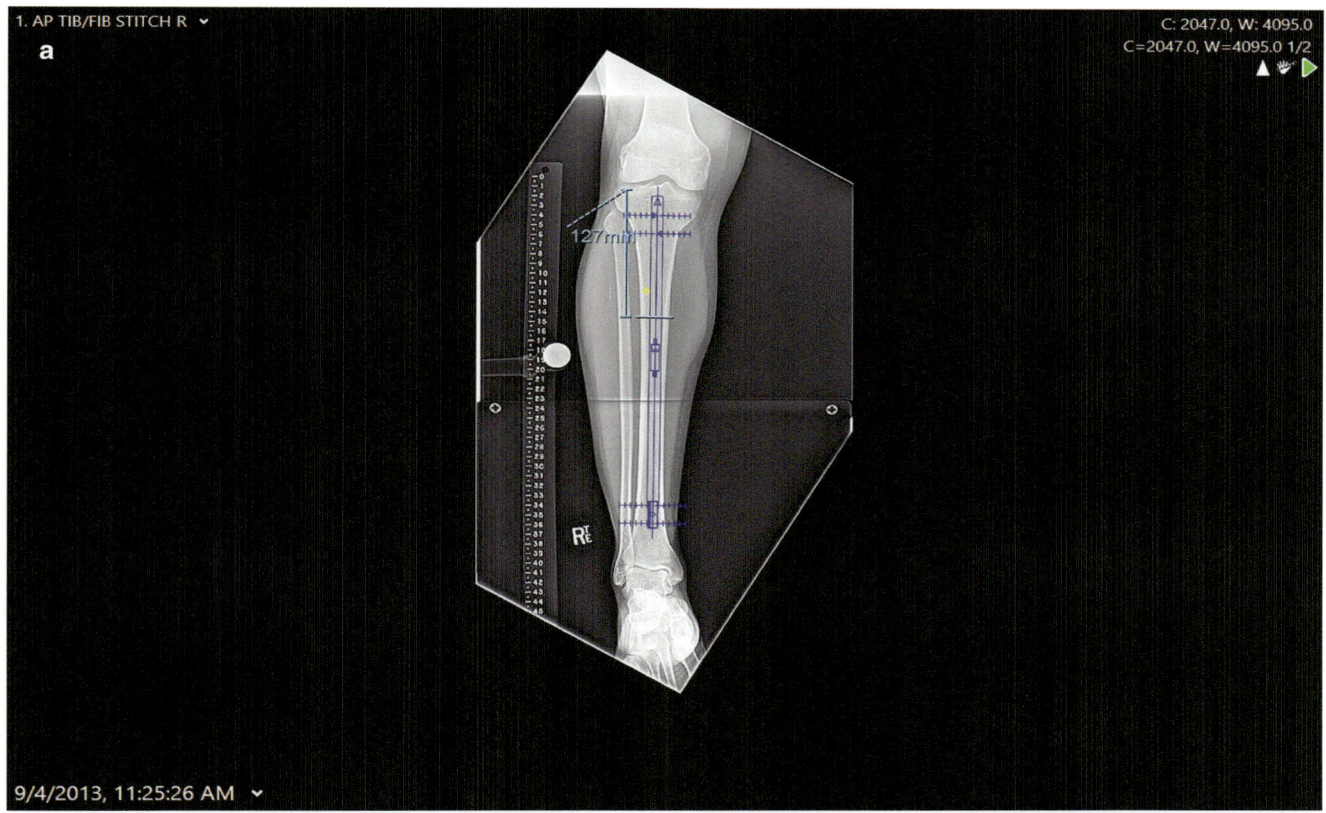
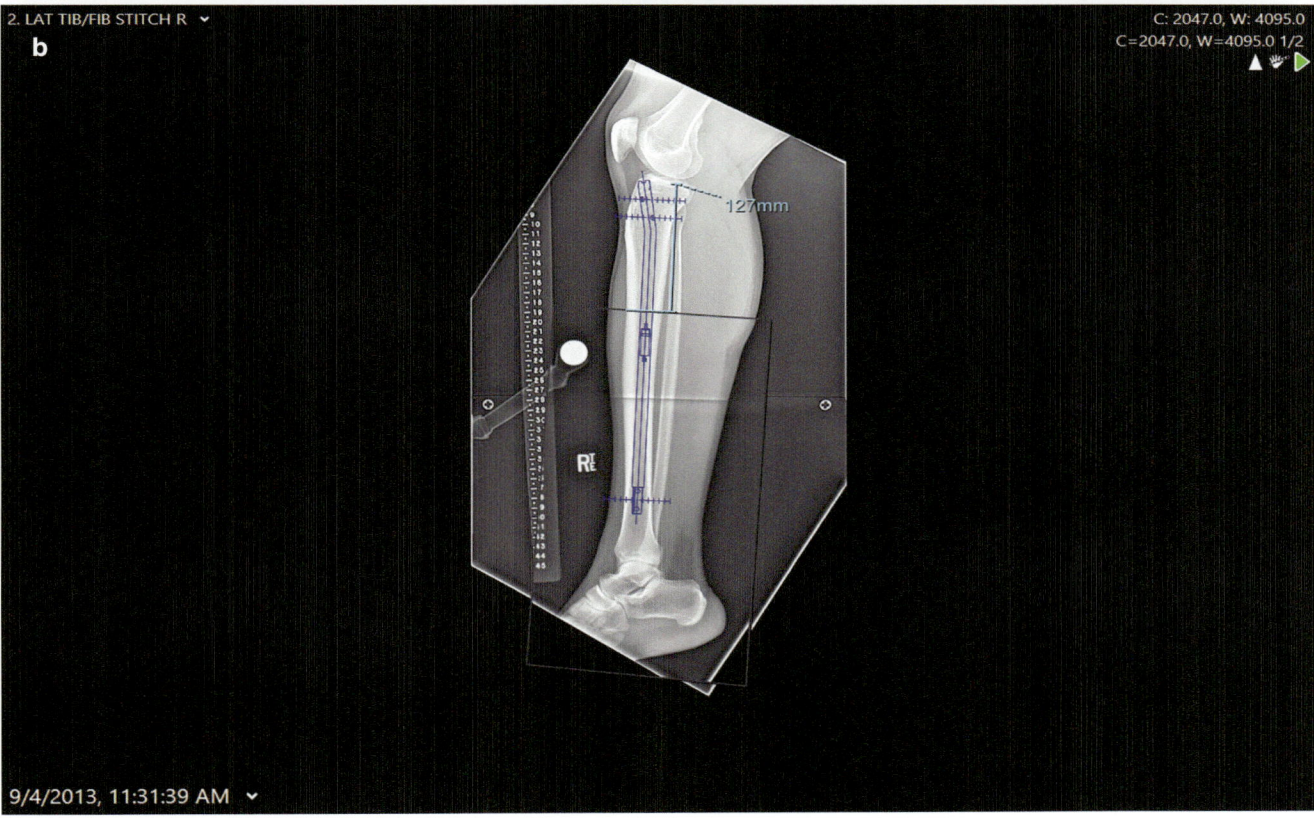

essential for measuring the leg length discrepancy and the desired amount of length. This X-ray will help determine the optimal start point for the nail to correct existing deformity. Slight lateralization of the planned start point will often serve well to mitigate lengthening induced valgus deformity. This AP radiograph, when overlaid with a template of the MILN, will provide the optimal location for a lateral blocking screw to help prevent valgus.

The length and diameter of the tibia MILN needs to be determined pre operatively. The nail should be long enough that a minimum of 5 cm of the thick barrel of the nail remains in the distal segment at the completion of lengthening. This is thought to be the minimal amount of thick portion of the telescopic nail needed to preserve the optimal biomechanical environment for regenerate healing. *If less than 5 cm of the thick portion of the nail remains in the distal fragment then the biomechanics of this over extended nail may lead to increased instability (with potential for implant fracture) and slower healing may occur* [15]. *A longer nail that provides >5 cm of thick barrel in the distal segment can be used as well and may better prevent lengthening induced deformity* (Fig. 14.2). The nail diameter should leave 5 mm of cortex on all sides of the diaphysis after reaming. Asymmetric reaming is common and very hard to control supporting the use of a nail that leaves greater than 5 mm of cortical thickness circumferentially.

Rotational deformity needs to be assessed on the prone physical exam. If necessary, any abnormality should be further investigated with a CT version study of bilateral knees and ankles where normal values can be compared and need for correction determined [16, 17].

Intra Operative Execution

The patient is laid supine on the radiolucent table and given adequate anesthesia. Tranexamic acid is used *in adults and in adolescents* to reduce intra op and post operative blood loss [18]. The limb is prepped and draped exposing the lower limb to mid thigh. The proposed osteotomy site is localized under fluoroscopy. Two small incisions are made: one is directly anterior on the tibial crest and the other is at the same axial level over the medial tibial crest. These incisions are 1 cm in length. The periosteum is elevated percutaneously where possible working through both approaches. A new drill bit is used to create multiple drill holes in one plane with the help of C-arm fluoroscopy. These holes will mark the osteotomy and provide venting of the canal during reaming (Fig. 14.3).

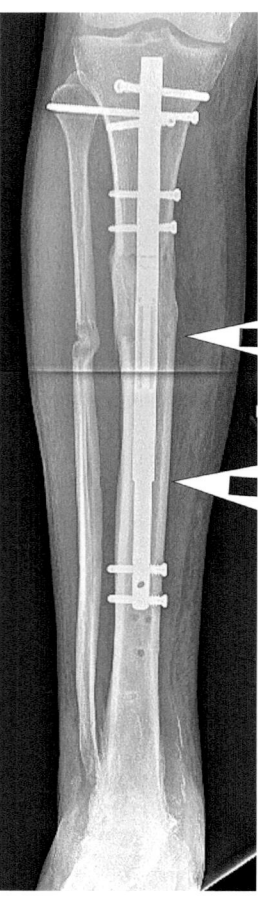

Fig. 14.2 The thick portion of the nail that remains in the distal fragment after lengthening is seen in between these two white arrows. This section should be at least 5 cm at the completion of tibial lengthening

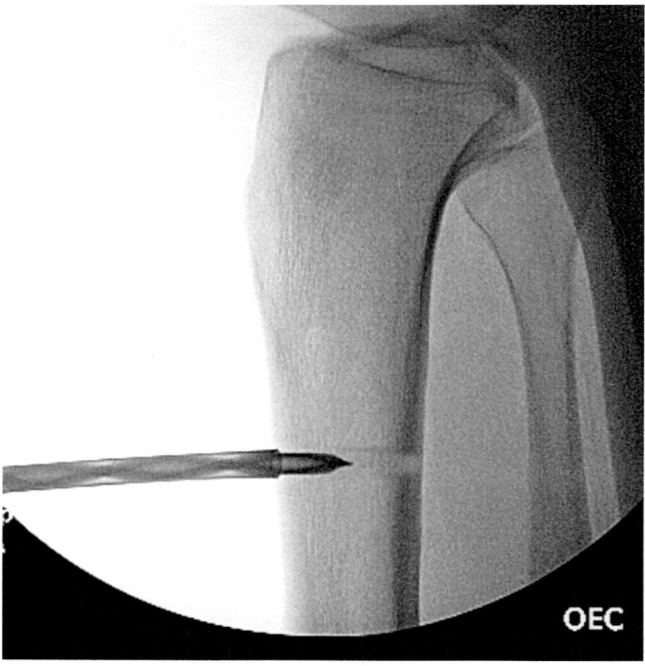

Fig. 14.3 A drill bit is used to prepare the osteotomy site for reaming and later for the osteotome. The drill is passed in multiple directions while staying in the same axial (transverse) plane. Many of the bone reamings will be deposited through these holes during canal preparation, which is believed to enhance the regenerate formation

The blocking screws are placed referencing from the corticotomy site which is visible on the image. The screw holes are pre drilled by mentally overlaying the pre operatively planned image over the real time fluoroscopic image. This technique is much like distal locking using perfect circles: it requires patience and precision. The rotational markers are now placed such that they are posterior to the planned path of the IM nail. This can be done using a cannulated technique if desired. The markers should be stiff enough to not be easily bent, which would cause a loss of all directional bearings. Typically, a 3.2 mm Steinmann pin or 5 mm Schantz pin are used (Fig. 14.4). The advantage of the Schantz pins is they can be grabbed and manipulated and can be locked in position with an external fixation bar for distal locking screw insertion.

The nail start point is now localized. There is no consensus for the best technique to insert a tibial IM nail, and this is surgeon preference. The suprapatellar (SP) insertion technique is outstanding in my experience as it allows for a semi extended knee position. This position provides an excellent fluoroscopic image of the proximal tibia during the entire nail insertion process and has improved my start point accuracy. A lateral release may be needed and is performed from inside-out. Alternatively, the lateral retinaculum can be "pie-crusted" in a similar fashion to create more space under the patella without committing to a full release. One of the commercially available SP nail insertion instrumentation systems should be used to place a protective sleeve and cannula through the joint for start point localization and reaming. A rigid guide wire is inserted according to the pre operative planning. An entry reamer is then used to create a metaphyseal pathway (Fig. 14.5).

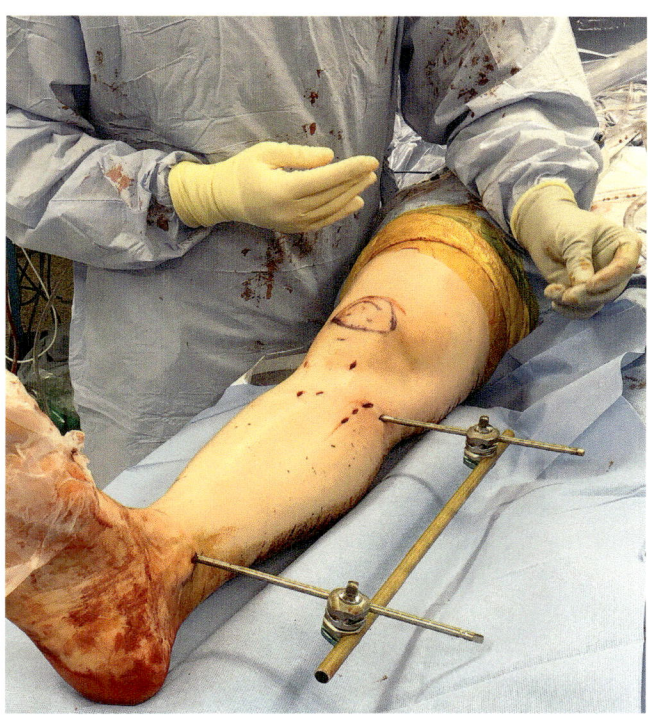

Fig. 14.4 This intraoperative photo shows an external fixator connecting two Schantz pins. The pins are marking the rotational orientation of the tibia. The pins can be grasped to control the bone segments after osteotomy and can be locked into position with the bar for distal locking screw insertion

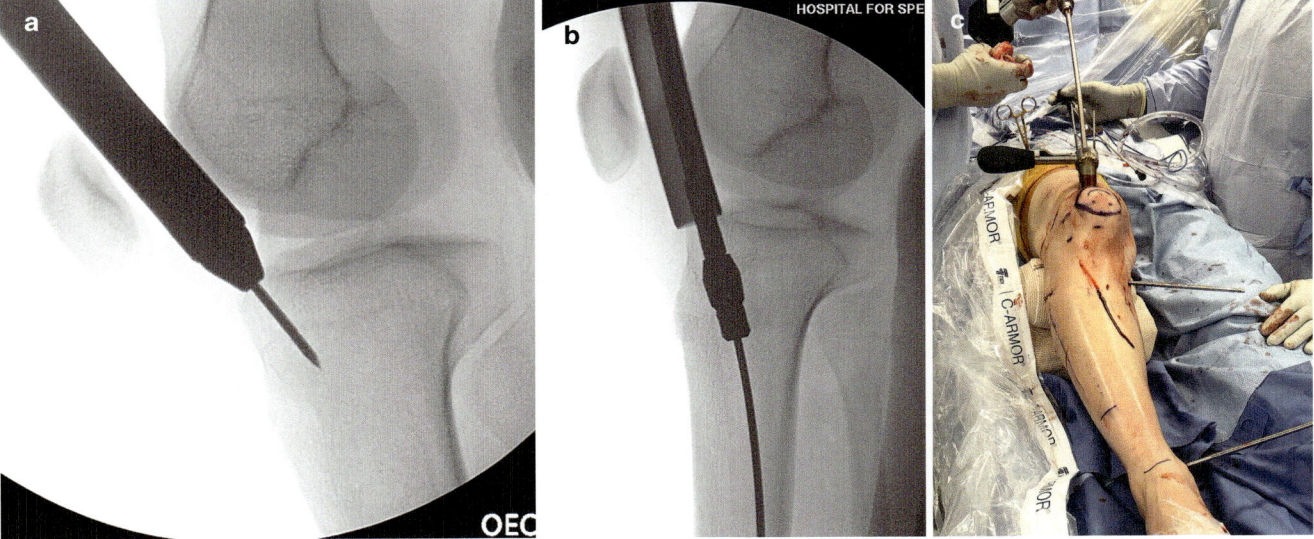

Fig. 14.5 (**a**) Shows the protective cannula placed through the patellofemoral joint and precisely aimed at the planned nail entry point. The guide wire is deployed through the cannula with outstanding control. (**b**) Shows the cannula protecting the joint and minimizing debris entry into the joint during flexible reaming. Figure 14.4c shows the set up for reaming through a suprapatellar canula

Reaming and Nail Insertion

Reaming of the IM canal can be done with either rigid or flexible reamers. Further, flexible reaming can be done before or after the corticotomy is completed. When correcting deformity through the proximal tibia, the corticotomy is often created and the deformity reduced prior to reaming. Alternatively, the reamers can be squeezed by the blocking screws prior to osteotomy and the deformity corrected upon nail insertion. The ball tipped guide wire is inserted to the distal epiphysis/physeal scar. Flexible reaming is performed until the canal has been reamed 2 mm over the diameter of the nail selected. The nail should be able to be inserted without a mallet. Nail insertion will often require further flexion of the knee when using a SP technique to take pressure off the trochlea. Insertion of the nail will finalize the coronal plane alignment and correct any deformity. Proximal locking is done with the targeting device. There are only two screws, so both must be inserted bicortically to prevent nail migration [2]. The targeting device is removed and coronal alignment is assessed with the tool of surgeon's choice: electrocautery cord, rigid stick, grid, or navigation. Any coronal plane malalignment should be either accepted or corrected at this time (Fig. 14.6). The rotational markers are then aligned and the distal locking can be performed using perfect circles. Rotation should be rechecked after each screw is inserted as imperfect screw placement will rotate the bone unintentionally. Leaving the fibula intact will help prevent any change in the rotational alignment. Once the nail is in place, the fibula can be cut using a percutaneous osteotomy under fluoroscopy. The fibula then needs to be stabilized with screws at either end. These fibular length stabilization screws (FLoSS) are inserted percutaneously and will prevent syndesmotic damage [15] (Fig. 14.7). A

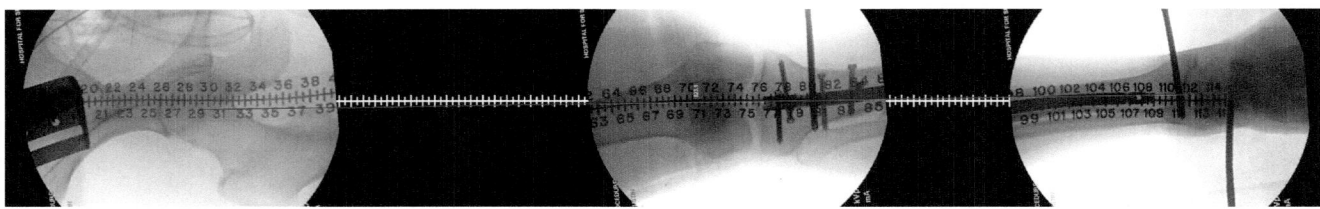

Fig. 14.6 While the total limb alignment can be measured by various methods, digital computer navigation can be employed to stitch fluoroscopic spot images together to recreate the mechanical axis and joint orientation angles. This image uses the RadLink (RadLink, Inc., El Segundo, California, USA) technology to confirm a neutral alignment at the end of an unrelated surgery

Fig. 14.7 The FLoSS screws are critical in ensuring proper lengthening of the fibula and in preventing fibular migration at the syndesmotic joints. (**a**) Shows a lateral image of the proximal fibula with the FLoSS screw (white arrow) centered in the fibular head and passing through the tibia posterior to the MILN and between the interlocking screws. This is the typical position for the proximal stabilization screw. (**b**) Shows the lateral image of the distal syndesmosis with the screw (white arrow) seen piercing both bones

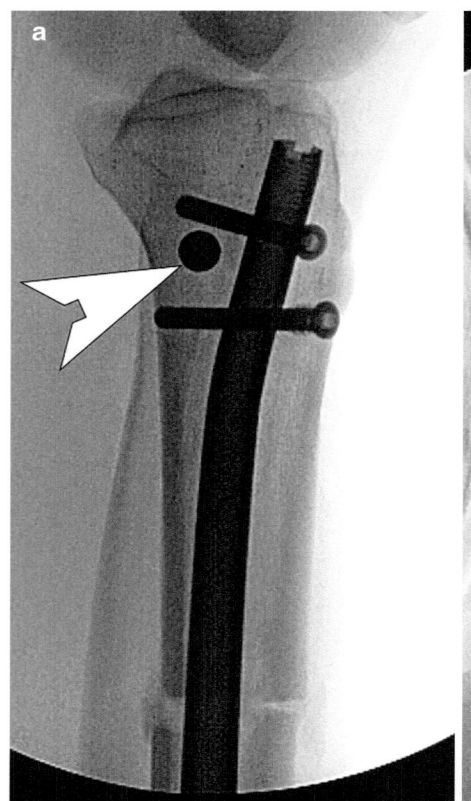
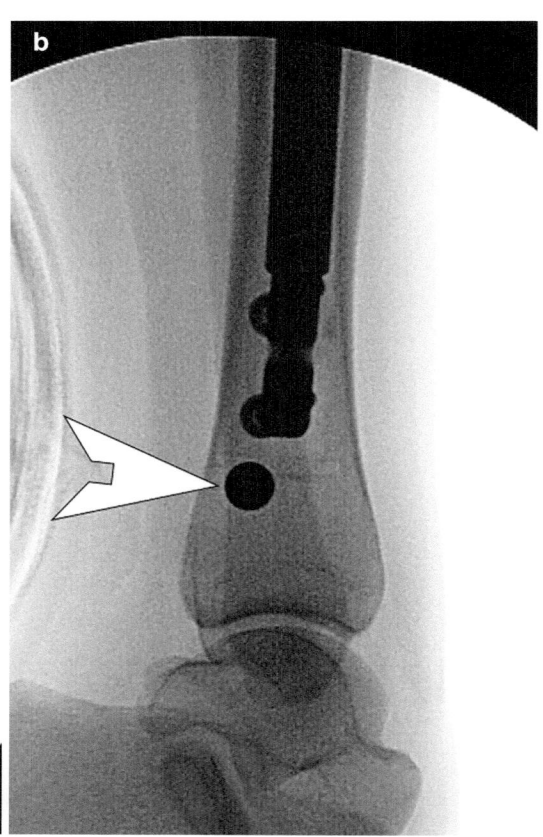

prophylactic anterior compartment fasciotomy is performed through a small anterior incision.

Magnet

The internal magnet is now localized using the fluoroscopy and a mark is made on the skin with a marking pen. The nail is then tested using an external magnet sterilely wrapped to lengthen the bone 0.5 mm. This test run will produce separation of the washer over the lead screw, which can be seen on the fluoroscopy to ensure the MILN is functional.

Post Op Recommendations

The amount of weight that the nails will support is dictated by the nail diameter and manufacturer recommendations. For tibial lengthening, a minimum latency of 7 days is typical for both children and adults. The lengthening in children can proceed at *0.15–0.20 mm* four times a day and adults lengthen at 0.15 mm four times a day. Follow up is every 1–2 weeks where X-rays are obtained and the regenerate is assessed (Fig. 14.8). Pain, nerve function, and joint mobility are evaluated. Rate of lengthening can be altered based on any of these metrics. Venous thrombus prophylaxis is recommended for patients over 16 years old. Once united, the implants should be removed typically 6–12 months post surgery. Non steroidal anti inflammatory drugs (NSAID) help reduce pain and the need for narcotics after osteotomy. Prolonged use may slow regenerate formation [19].

Outcomes

The results for tibial lengthening with the MILN are quite good with high surgeon and patient satisfaction reported [20–26]. One must keep in mind that the majority of MILN surgeries have been performed in the femur, so conclusions from the pooled data are truer for the femur and do not reflect the special circumstances of the tibia, namely, that the tibia heals more slowly than the femur and requires a longer latency and slower distraction rate [27]. Tibia lengthening surgery with an internal implant faces the well-known challenges unique to lower leg lengthening with external fixation including the need to protect the syndesmotic joints, the risk of peroneal nerve stretch injury, the risk of compartment syndrome, and the propensity for valgus and flexion deformity. Colleagues from the UK published a paper chronicling their experience with the MILN in the tibia calling attention to the tendency for the nail to veer into valgus both by moving laterally at the osteotomy site and by migrating medially at the entry point in the proximal tibia. Authors recommend a blocking screw be placed near the osteotomy on the lateral side of the nail and another on the medial side against the very proximal aspect of the nail [2, 28]. The MILN is also accompanied by mechanical complications unique to the nail [1]. Tibial regenerate healing has been cited as an obstacle to success [28]. The MILN was compared with classic external fixator lengthening and LATN methods revealing that the LATN provided the best circumstances for healing [6]. The superior healing of LATN was not surprising since the act of reaming through the regenerate at the completion of the lengthening phase is such a powerful stimulator of osteosynthesis [5]. *A slowly forming regenerate is best treated by early recognition and slowing the rate of distraction. Drilling the regenerate bone and injection with iliac crest bone marrow aspirate concentrate is the next level of regenerate stimulation. Open bone grafting with autograft and with bone morphogenic protein can also be used if needed. Exchange nailing will both accelerate bone formation and replace a weak implant with a biomechanically superior nail. Oscillation between distraction and compression (the accordion technique) may enhance bone formation but optional rate, rhythm, and excursion require further study.*

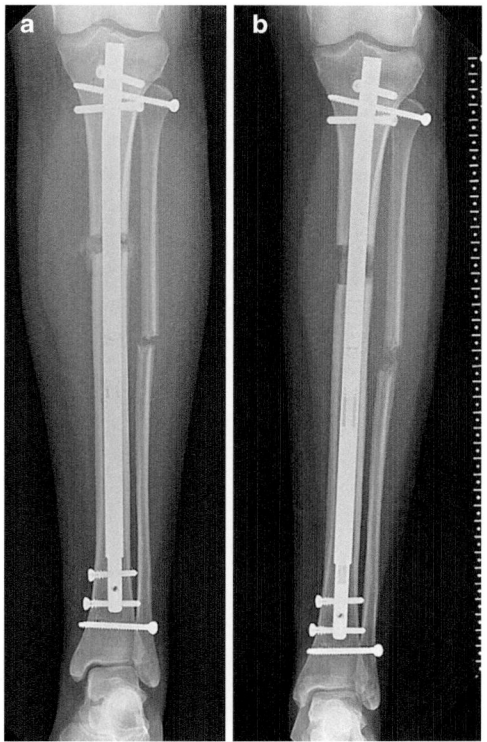

Fig. 14.8 A typical tibial lengthening set up is seen early after the index surgery (**a**) and then at the completion of the distraction phase (**b**). The diaphyseal cortex has prevented deformity during lengthening, and the FLoSS screws have protected the syndesmotic joints and ensured normal fibular lengthening. The patient will not be permitted full weight bearing until 2 of the 4 cortices are united

Pearls and Pitfalls

Take X-rays with a calibration ball to help with pre operative templating. Have your hospital obtain implant templates from the manufacturer for improved planning. After surgery, use the IM nail as the calibration tool since the nail diameter is known. This provides consistent measurements of length at each visit.

Translation of the pre op planning into the OR is a potential source of error in the execution of this technique. This is especially true when inserting blocking screws. A poorly placed screw will change the intended limb alignment significantly upon nail insertion. Perhaps computer navigation or blocking screw guides will make this step more reproducible in the future.

A slight lateral start point may leave the tibia in slight varus at the completion of nail insertion. This can be beneficial for longer lengthenings where strong valgus forces will work to straighten the limb to neutral. Beware when correcting varus tibia deformity with a MILN. Under-correct the deformity and add an additional lateral blocking screw after nail insertion to prevent over correction into valgus.

Use blocking screws to help direct the reamer and help prevent valgus and flexion during lengthening [2].

Acute correction of valgus tibial deformity may require a prophylactic peroneal nerve release. This is done at the discretion of the surgeon.

If the coronal plane is significantly malaligned after nail insertion this indicates that the blocking screws or the start point are off from the intended location. Correction of this would require nail removal, additional blocking screw placement, re-reaming, and nail re-insertion [3]. Spending extra time with proper planning and ensuring optimal nail start points and blocking screw location will avoid this frustrating experience.

MILN early malfunction is very rare [27] but easy to detect by simply testing the magnet in the operating room after nail insertion.

Lengthening rate varies among surgeons, but I suggest a slow rate for adults at 0.15 mm four times a day. This can be sped up at any time. A general rule is "the turtle always wins the race." The slowest possible lengthening will reduce complications, result in the most robust regenerate, and will have the quickest consolidation phase. Rapid consolidation in children requires faster distraction rates where joint contractures can be expected and therapy and bracing are very helpful.

Joint contracture is a common problem during tibial lengthening. As the gastrocnemius is stretched tightly, the knee flexes and the ankle is pulled into plantarflexion. In children, these contractures are worsened by the need to distract the bone quickly to avoid premature consolidation. The child tends to avoid stretching which is painful. The treatment is frequent stretching by parents and a physical therapist. Bracing can also help fight these contractures. Slowing the rate of bone lengthening is the best solution when possible. Soft tissue fractional lengthening of the gastrocnemius is a surgical solution when other methods are not successful. Temporary pinning of the calcaneus to the tibia is possible to prevent ankle contracture.

Conclusion

Tibial lengthening using MILN implants is an exciting and successful process for patients and surgeons. The Ilizarov method has been expanded to include this new internal technology, but distraction osteogenesis by any method is high maintenance and requires careful stewardship by the surgeon to ensure a safe experience and reliable outcome. Dedication to sophisticated pre operative planning prevents complications, and frequent follow up visits with a hypervigilant approach will allow for early identification and treatment of problems and obstacles.

Commentary

Motorized Intramedullary Lengthening of the Tibia

Peter Calder
Peter.calder@nhs.net

Introduction

Intramedullary lengthening offers major advantages over the traditional use of external fixators. An absence of wire and pin site complications, such as infection and soft-tissue tethering, produces an improved patient experience, increased tolerance of physiotherapy and joint rehabilitation, a reduction in mental health issues associated with external fixators and an improved quality of life.

The original lengthening nails involved ratchet systems. These were often associated with difficulties in lengthening due to pain associated with twisting of the osteotomy and lack of controlled lengthening. The motorized nails enable accurate sub-millimeter lengthening, and in the case of the magnetically driven nail, easy controlled retraction. With no rotation at the osteotomy site, the osteotomy does not need to be linear and so can be confidently performed using the De Bastiani or Ilizarov technique, accepting an irregular osteotomy line.

Indication

Open growth plates remain a relative contraindication for intramedullary lengthening. Some implants, such as lengthening rods in osteogenesis imperfecta, cross the growth plates but there is no published data on lengthening nails placed across the physis in a skeletally immature patient.

The principle of multiple short lengthening episodes should also be applied in intramedullary lengthening. This strategy is preferred to a single long lengthening episode, which is associated with increased complications including delayed and often inadequate bone healing, soft tissue issues such as joint stiffness and contracture, and a greater negative effect on mental well-being.

A limitation of intramedullary lengthening nails is the inability to bridge potentially unstable joints, seen in congenital limb deficiency, or prevent joint contractures such as ankle equinus due to tightness of the gastrocnemius. In these cases, the use of knee extension braces or ankle orthosis can be used during lengthening.

"Just because you can, doesn't mean you should"—the concept of extramedullary placement of the implant appears attractive, but published results involve small numbers. It may be advisable to wait for larger series of these techniques before adopting this as regular practice.

Technique

Careful pre-operative planning is essential to ensure an accurate entry point and position of the implant. Regenerate deformity has previously been recognized following lengthening using external fixators due to the eccentric placement of the subcutaneous tibia and pull of the muscles in the posterior and lateral compartments. Whereas, it may be assumed that a straight intramedullary nail would lengthen in a straight direction, valgus and procurvatum deformity unfortunately still occur in tibial lengthening. This has led to the insertion of blocking screws to maintain alignment during lengthening.

Using temporary k-wires to guide the intramedullary reamers and nail allows accurate placement to maintain the nail position or to aid deformity correction. If there is an error in placement and a new position is required, the residual hole is not as large as a screw hole which could make the new screw placement challenging.

The final placement of the blocking screws can be inserted by exchanging the k-wires, with the lengthening nail in situ, which ensures close apposition to the nail. Finally, be aware of the risk of the osteotomy propagating if the blocking wires/screw are placed too close to the osteotomy site. This is more likely to occur with placement of the posterior blocking screw, which can result in the screw becoming loose and failing to maintain the nail position.

Reaming and Nail Insertion

Debate remains over the need to vent the tibia during lengthening. My personal technique is to pre-drill the anteromedial cortex, but not pass the drill bit through the posterior cortex prior to reaming.

Further questions remain over the use of a prophylactic percutaneous fasciotomy, to reduce the risk of compartment syndrome favored by some surgeons. If this is performed, it is important to consent the patients for calf swelling as the muscle compartment expands. This may be an actual benefit in cases of congenital limb deficiency such as fibula hemimelia, or shortening associated with talipes equinovarus where the calf is clinically wasted.

During the insertion of the magnetically driven nail locking pegs, it is important to ensure that the threads are fully engaged with the cortex of the bone with the peg head fully down to the bone. It may be worth making the incision a little larger to visualize the peg head position. As the pegs only have threads under the head, failure to ensure full engagement can lead to loosening and the peg disengaging.

Post-Op Recommendations

With the risk of gastrocnemius tightness and risk of delayed bone regenerate healing, you can consider reducing the lengthening rate further to 0.33 mm twice per day. (i.e., 0.15 mm four times per day).

The use of a night splint can be used to maintain a plantigrade foot during the lengthening process.

There is a limitation in weight bearing, but patients should be encouraged to use a "shadow walk", which is a normal gait pattern with the majority of the weight taken through the crutches. This prevents knee flexion contractures, which occur if patients mobilize non-weight bearing and tend to lift the protected leg from the ground by flexing their hip and knee.

Once the length has been achieved, a gradual increase in weight through the leg could be considered. The first week 25% of body weight, the second 50%, third 75% and the fourth week 100%. An X-ray is taken at this time and if sufficient regenerate healing is noted then the patient can continue full weight bearing. If there is concern, then they return to partial weight bearing.

Outcomes
It is agreed that the tibia is not the same as the femur. The healing index is longer and intervention may be required, such as exchange nailing or bone grafting.

Pearls and Pitfalls
See above for tips, such as blocking screw insertion, brace treatment and lengthening rates.

References

1. Lee DH, Kim S, Lee JW, et al. A comparison of the device related complications of intramedullary lengthening nails using a new classification system. Biomed Res Int. 2017;2017:8032510. https://doi.org/10.1155/2017/8032510.
2. Wright SE, Goodier WD, Calder P. Regenerate deformity with the precice tibial nail. Strategies Trauma Limb Reconstr. 2020;15(2):98–105.
3. Furmetz J, Bosl S, Schilling J, et al. Blocking screws for alignment control in intramedullary lengthening. Injury. 2017;48:1597–602.
4. Dabash S, Zhang DT, Rozbruch SR, Fragomen AT. Blocking screw-assisted intramedullary nailing using the reverse-rule-of-thumbs for limb lengthening and deformity correction. Strategies Trauma Limb Reconstr. 2019;14(2):77–84. https://doi.org/10.5005/jp-journals-10080-1430.
5. Rozbruch SR, Kleinman D, Fragomen A, Ilizarov S. Limb lengthening and then insertion of an intramedullary nail. A case matched comparison. Clin Orthop. 2008;466(12):2923–32.
6. Fragomen AT, Falls TD, Suh J, Khabyeh-Hasbani N, Rozbruch SR. Tibial lengthening evolution: classic Ilizarov, lengthening and then nailing, motorized internal lengthening nail. J Limb Length Recon. 2020;6(1):13–9.
7. Dahl MT, Morrison SG, Laine JC, Novotny SA, Georgiadis AG. Extramedullary motorized lengthening of the femur in young children. J Pediatr Orthop. 2020;40(10):e978–83. https://doi.org/10.1097/BPO.0000000000001593.
8. Iobst CA, Bafor AJ. Retrograde extramedullary lengthening of the femur using the PRECICE nail: technique and results. Pediatr Orthop. 2021;41(6):356–61. https://doi.org/10.1097/BPO.0000000000001831.
9. Court-Brown CM, Byrnes T, McLaughlin G. Intramedullary nailing of tibial diaphyseal fractures in adolescents with open physes. Injury. 2003;34:781–5.
10. Knapik DM, Zirkle LG, Liu RW. Consequences following distal femoral growth plate violation in an ovine model with an intramedullary implant: a pilot study. J Pediatr Orthop. 2018;38:e640–5.
11. Benedick A, Bazar B, Zirkle L, Liu RW. Retrograde intramedullary nailing of pediatric femoral shaft fractures does not result in growth arrest at the distal femoral physis-a retrospective cases series. J Orthop Trauma. 2021;35(11):e405–10.
12. Radler C, Mindler GT, Stauffer A, Weiß C, Ganger RJ. Limb lengthening with precice intramedullary lengthening nails in children and adolescents. Pediatr Orthop. 2021;42:e192. https://doi.org/10.1097/BPO.0000000000002016. Online ahead of print.
13. Iliadis AD, Palloni V, Wright J, Goodier D, Calder P. Pediatric lower limb lengthening using the PRECICE nail: our experience with 50 cases. J Pediatr Orthop. 2021;41(1):e44–9. https://doi.org/10.1097/BPO.0000000000001672.
14. Muthusamy S, Rozbruch SR, Fragomen AT. The use of blocking screws with internal lengthening nail and reverse rule of thumbs for blocking screws in limb lengthening and deformity correction surgery. Strategies Trauma Limb Reconstruct. 2016;11(3):199–205.
15. Rozbruch SR. Tibial lengthening technique. Tech Orthop. 2020;35(3):176–82.
16. Gruskay JA, Fragomen AT, Rozbruch SR. Idiopathic rotational abnormalities of the lower extremities in children and adults. JBJS Rev. 2019;7(1):e3. https://doi.org/10.2106/JBJS.RVW.18.00016.
17. Vanhove F, Noppe N, Fragomen AT, Hoekstra H, Vanderschueren G, Metsemakers WJ. Standardization of torsional CT measurements of the lower limbs with threshold values for corrective osteotomy. Arch Orthop Trauma Surg. 2019;139(6):795–805.
18. Steinhaus ME, Buksbaum J, Eisenman A, Kohli M, Fragomen A, Rozbruch SR. Tranexamic acid reduces post operative blood loss in distal femoral osteotomy. J Knee Surg. 2020;33(5):440–4.
19. Fragomen A, Suh J, Matta K, McCoy TH Jr, Hart KL, Rozbruch SR. the variable effects of nsaids on osteotomy healing and opioid consumption. J Am Acad Orthop Surg Glob Res Rev. 2020;4(4):e20.00039. https://doi.org/10.5435/JAAOSGlobal-D-20-00039.
20. Green SA, Fragomen AT, Herzenberg JE, Iobst C, McCarthy JJ, Nelson SC, Paley D, Rozbruch SR, Standard SC. A magnetically controlled lengthening nail: a prospective study of 31 individuals (The Precice intramedullary nail study). J Limb Length Recon. 2018;4(2):67–75.

21. Horn J, Hvid I, Huhnstock S, et al. Limb lengthening and deformity correction with externally controlled motorized intramedullary nails: evaluation of 50 consecutive lengthenings. Acta Orthop. 2019;90(1):81–7.
22. Wagner P, Burghardt RD, Green SA, et al. Precice, magnetically-driven, telescopic, intramedullary lengthening nail: pre-clinical testing and first thirty patients. SICOT. 2017;3(19):1–7.
23. Accadbled F, Pailhé R, Cavaignac E, Sales de Gauzy J. Bone lengthening using the Fitbone(®) motorized intramedullary nail: the first experience in France. Orthop Traumatol Surg Res. 2016;102(2):217–22.
24. Kirane YM, Fragomen AT, Rozbruch SR. Precision of the Precice internal bone lengthening nail. Clin Orthop Relat Res. 2014;472(12):3869–78.
25. Krieg AH, Lenze U, Speth BM, Hasler CC. Intramedullary leg lengthening with a motorized nail. Acta Orthop. 2011;82(3):344–50.
26. Karakoyun O, Sokucu S, Erol MF, et al. Use of a magnetic bone nail for lengthening of the femur and tibia. J Orthop Surg. 2016;24(3):374–8.
27. Fragomen A. Motorized intramedullary lengthening nails: outcomes and complications. Tech Orthop. 2020;35(3):225–32. https://doi.org/10.1097/BTO.0000000000000458.
28. Frost MW, Rahbek O, Traerup J, Ceccotti AA, Kold S. Systematic review of complications with externally controlled motorized intramedullary bone lengthening nails (FITBONE and PRECICE) in 983 segments. Acta Orthop. 2021;92(1):120–7. https://doi.org/10.1080/17453674.2020.1835321. Epub 2020 Oct 27.

Part II

Related Concepts and Management Options

Biomechanically Based Clinical Decision Making in Pediatric Foot and Ankle Surgery

15

Jon R. Davids

Introduction

The understanding and classification of functional deviations and deficits at the ankle and foot are based upon an appreciation of normal function during the gait cycle [1–3]. The interaction between the ankle, foot, and the floor is a critical element of normal gait. Function of the ankle and foot is determined by a complex interaction of anatomy, physiology, and physics. Proper ankle and foot alignment is required for optimal function of the knee and hip during gait. Disruption of normal function of the ankle and foot may disrupt knee and hip function, compromising the energy efficiency of gait and in extreme cases precluding the ability to ambulate.

Clinical decision making for the management of ankle and foot deformities in children can be standardized by the use of a diagnostic matrix (Table 15.1) [4]. This paradigm is based upon the collection and integration of data from five sources: the clinical history, physical examination, plain radiographs, observational gait analysis, and in complex cases associated with certain disease processes (e.g., cerebral palsy, myelodysplasia, and hereditary sensorimotor neuropathies), quantitative gait analysis (which may include kinematic/kinetic analyses, dynamic electromyography (EMG), and dynamic pedobarography).

This chapter will begin with an overview of normal ankle and foot function during the gait cycle. This will provide a

Table 15.1 The diagnostic matrix for the assessment of the ankle and foot deformities

Source	Information
Clinical history	Pain
	Tripping
	In-/out-toeing
Physical examination	Gross foot shape weight-bearing/non weight-bearing
	Flexible/rigid
	Plantar callous pattern
Radiographic examination	Segmental alignment weight-bearing, AP and LAT views
Observational gait analysis	Foot contact with floor (3 rockers)
	Foot progression angle
	Foot clearance in swing phase
Quantitative gait analysis	Kinematics
	Kinetics
	Dynamic EMG
	Pedobarography

framework for the identification of common (or coupled), and uncommon (or uncoupled), segmental malalignments of the ankle and foot. This will be followed by an overview (principles and indications) of the most common interventions (i.e. guided growth, soft tissue surgery, and skeletal surgery) utilized to correct these segmental malalignments. Finally, a standardized approach for the preoperative, intraoperative, postoperative, and surveillance of ankle and foot alignment and function will be presented.

Ankle and Foot Function During Normal Gait

The understanding of ankle and foot function during normal gait is facilitated by considering the lower leg to consist of four segments: the tibial or shank segment, the hindfoot (talus and calcaneus), the midfoot (navicular, cuneiforms, and cuboid), and the forefoot (metatarsals and phalanges) [1–3, 5, 6] (Fig. 15.1a, b). It is also helpful to consider the

---

Supplementary Information The online version contains supplementary material available at https://doi.org/10.1007/978-3-031-55767-5_15.

J. R. Davids (✉)
Shriners Children's Northern California, Sacramento, CA, USA

Department of Orthopaedic Surgery, University of California Davis, Sacramento, CA, USA
e-mail: jdavids@shrinenet.org

foot to consist of two columns: the medial column (talus, navicular, cuneiforms, first and second toe metatarsal, and phalanges), and the lateral column (calcaneus, cuboid, third through fifth toe metatarsals, and phalanges) [7] (Fig. 15.2a–c). Standardized, consistent terminology is required to describe the alignment of the separate segments of the ankle and foot [8]. Movement of the plantar aspect of the segment in question during the gait cycle is described as *inversion or varus* (towards the midline) or as *eversion or valgus* (away from the midline). Movement of the distal aspect of the segment in question during the gait cycle is described as *adduction* (towards the midline) or *abduction* (away from the midline). *Supination* is a combination of inversion/varus and adduction. *Pronation* is a combination of eversion/valgus and abduction. Rotation of the segment about its longitudinal axis towards the midline is described as *internal rotation*. Rotation of the segment about its longitudinal axis away from the midline is described as *external rotation*.

The gait cycle is a period of time beginning with the initial contact of the reference foot with the ground, continuing through ipsilateral stance and swing phases until the subsequent ipsilateral initial contact. Stance phase occurs when the reference limb is in contact with the ground. Swing phase occurs when the reference limb is not in contact with the ground. The interaction of the ankle and foot with the ground during the stance phase of the gait cycle is described by the

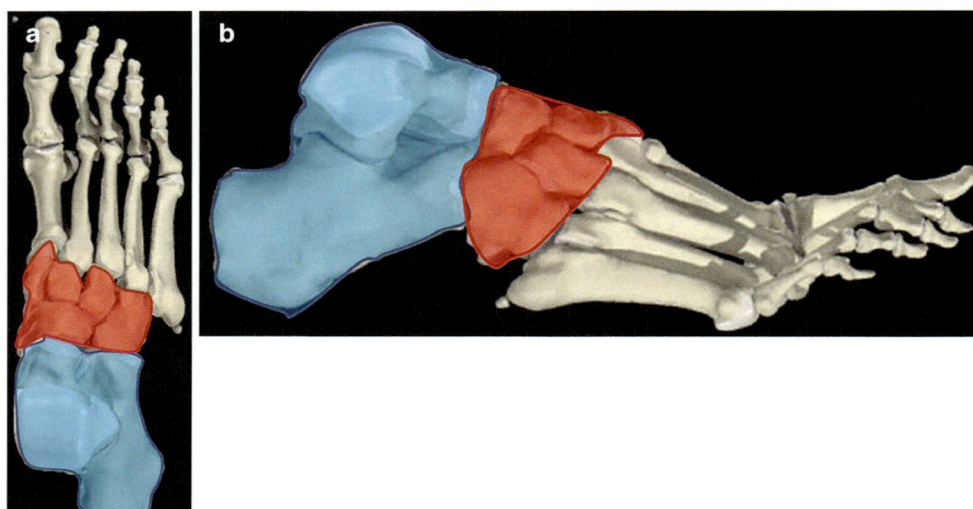

Fig. 15.1 Three segments of the foot. (**a**) Diagram of the anteroposterior view of the right foot. The hindfoot segment is *blue*, the midfoot segment is *red*, and the forefoot segment is *white*. (**b**) Diagram of the lateral view of the right foot. The hindfoot segment is *blue*, the midfoot segment is *red*, and the forefoot segment is *white*

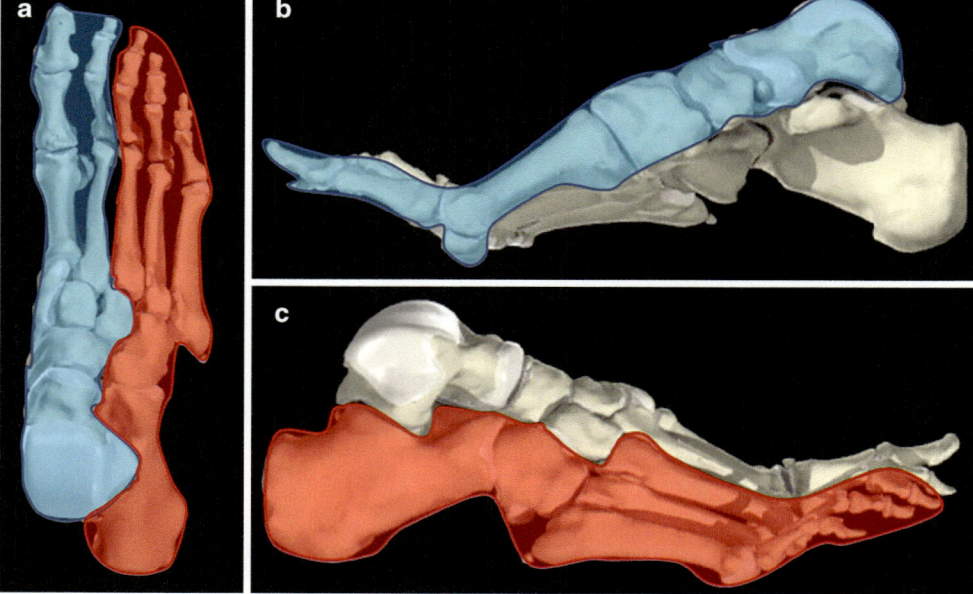

Fig. 15.2 Two columns of the foot. (**a**) Diagram of the anteroposterior view of the right foot. The medial column is *blue*, and the lateral column is *red*. (**b**) Diagram of the lateral view (medial side) of the right foot. The medial column is *blue*. (**c**) Diagram of the lateral view (lateral side) of the right foot. The lateral column is *red*

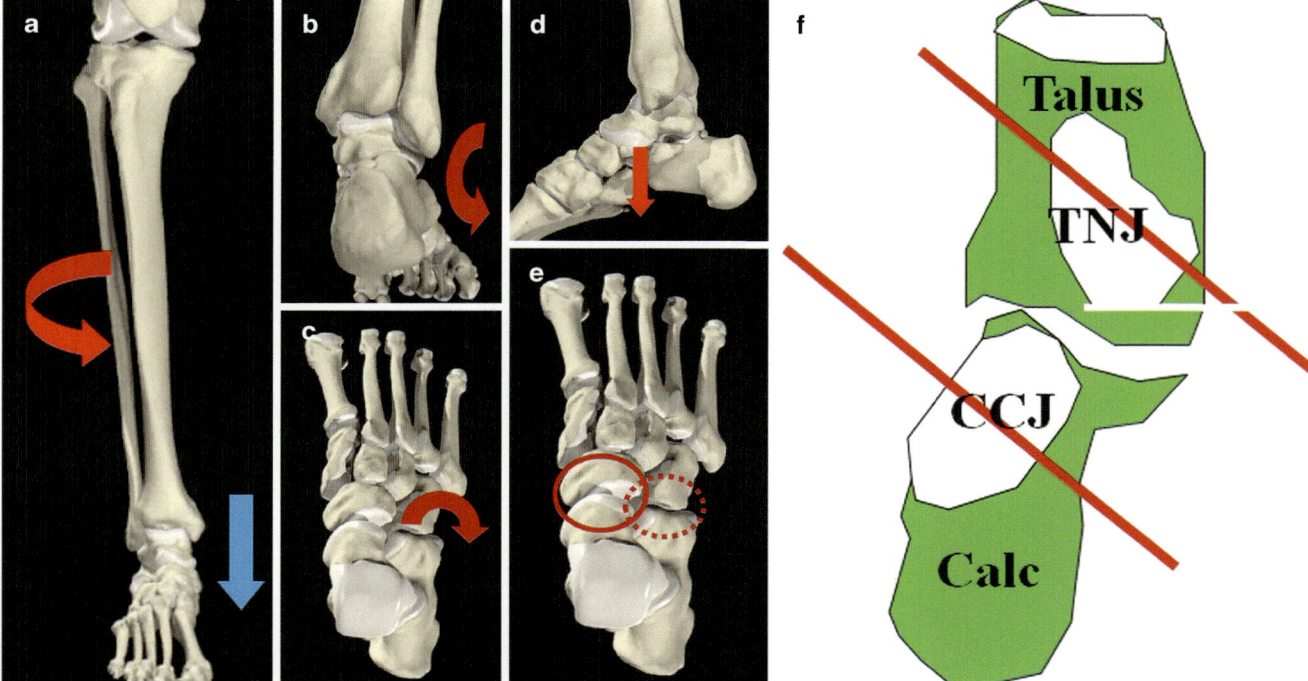

Fig. 15.3 Skeletal alignment of the lower extremity during the first rocker of stance phase. (**a**) The tibia is rotating internally (*red arrow*) and the ankle is plantarflexing (*blue arrow*). (**b**) Hindfoot alignment during the first rocker of stance phase consists of calcaneal eversion/valgus (*red arrow*). (**c**) Hindfoot alignment during the first rocker of stance phase consists of calcaneal abduction (*red arrow*). (**d**) Hindfoot pronation (eversion/valgus and abduction) forces the talus to plantarflex (*red arrow*) during the first rocker of stance phase. (**e**) This "unlocks" the primary joints of the midfoot (talo-navicular in *solid circle*, calcaneocuboid in *dashed circle*). (**f**) Coronal view of the articulation between the hindfoot and midfoot in the first rocker of stance phase. Lateral is to the left, medial is to the right. *TNJ* talo-navicular joint, *CCJ* calcaneocuboid joint, *Calc* calcaneus. The main axes of the TNJ and CCJ are parallel (*red lines*), which allows motion and "unlocks" the midfoot

concept of three rockers [2, 3]. In normal gait, the heel is the first part of the foot to contact the ground at initial contact. The ankle subsequently plantar flexes until the foot is flat on the floor. This motion is controlled by the eccentric activity of the ankle dorsiflexor muscle group. The *first, or heel rocker*, occurs from heel strike to foot flat during the loading response subphase of stance. As the body progresses forward, the tibia advances forward over the foot, which is achieved through ankle dorsiflexion. This motion is controlled by eccentric activity of the ankle plantar flexor muscle group. The *second, or ankle rocker*, occurs as the tibia advances over the foot during the midstance subphase of stance. The *third, or forefoot rocker*, begins immediately prior to the initial contact of the opposite foot, as the heel of the reference foot rises off the ground and dorsiflexion occurs through the metatarsophalangeal joints of the forefoot. The ankle begins to plantar flex as the limb is unloaded during the terminal stance subphase of stance. This motion is controlled by concentric activity of the ankle plantar flexor muscle group. This is an essential event during normal gait, as the largest moment generated by any single muscle group during the gait cycle is the internal plantar flexion moment generated by the ankle plantar flexor muscle group during third rocker in terminal stance [2, 3, 9].

In the stance phase of the normal gait cycle, the ankle and foot provide shock absorption during loading response (first or heel rocker), stability during midstance (second or ankle rocker), and a rigid lever during terminal stance (third or forefoot rocker) [2, 3]. During loading response, the tibial or shank segment rotates internally, and the ankle is plantarflexing (Fig. 15.3a). This results in eversion/valgus and abduction of the hindfoot, primarily through the subtalar joint (see Fig. 15.3b, c). Pronation of the hindfoot forces the talus to plantarflex, which "unlocks" the joints of the midfoot, which follows into pronation (see Fig. 15.3d, e, f) This coupled movement of the hindfoot and midfoot results in maximum flexibility of the foot, which allows the joints to contribute to shock absorption. During midstance, the tibial or shank segment is rotating externally, and the ankle is dorsiflexing (Fig. 15.4a). This results in inversion/varus and adduction of the hindfoot, primarily through the subtalar joint (see Fig. 15.4b, c). Supination of the hindfoot forces the talus to

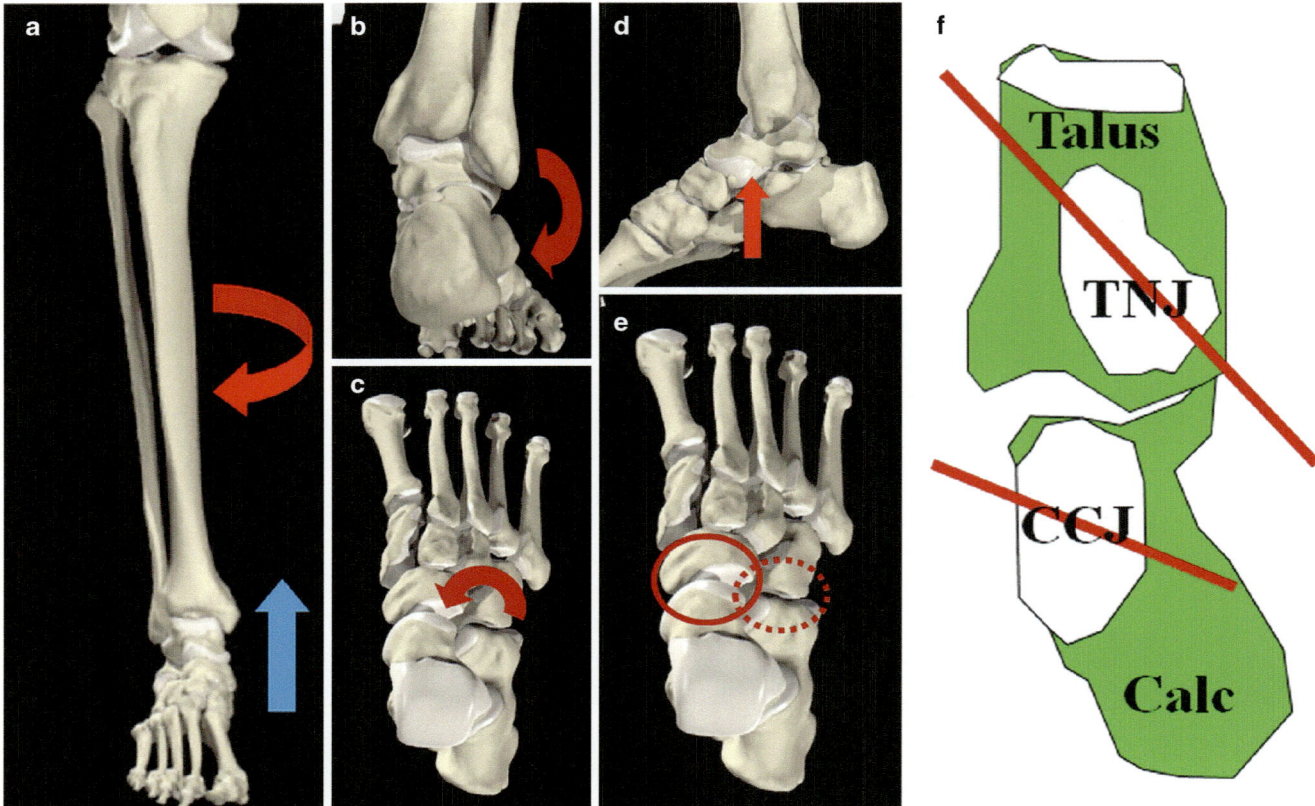

Fig. 15.4 Skeletal alignment of the lower extremity during the second rocker of stance phase. (**a**) The tibia is rotating externally (*red arrow*) and the ankle is dorsiflexing (*blue arrow*). (**b**) Hindfoot alignment during the second rocker of stance phase consists of calcaneal inversion/varus (*red arrow*). (**c**) Hindfoot alignment during the second rocker of stance phase consists of calcaneal adduction (*red arrow*). (**d**) Hindfoot supination (inversion/varus and adduction) forces the talus to dorsiflex (*red arrow*) during the second rocker of stance phase. (**e**) This "locks" the primary joints of the midfoot (talo-navicular in *solid circle*, calcaneo-cuboid in *dashed circle*). (**f**) Coronal view of the articulation between the hindfoot and midfoot in the second rocker of stance phase. Lateral is to the left, medial is to the right. *TNJ* talo-navicular joint, *CCJ* calcaneocuboid joint, *Calc* calcaneus. The main axes of the TNJ and CCJ are no longer parallel (*red lines*), which restricts motion and "locks" the midfoot

dorsiflex, which "locks" the joints of the midfoot, which follows into supination (see Fig. 15.4d, e, f) This coupled movement of the hindfoot and the midfoot results in restoration of the longitudinal arch of the foot and maximum rigidity of the foot, which enhances stability. During terminal stance, the tibial or shank segment continues to rotate externally, and the ankle continues to dorsiflex. As the body progresses forward, the center of pressure beneath the foot advances distally into the forefoot. Because the segments of the foot are aligned to promote maximum rigidity, the forefoot is stable as it is loaded. The rigidity of the foot segments provides an optimal lever arm to the ankle plantar flexor muscles during terminal stance. These typical, expected segmental alignment patterns of the ankle and foot during the stance phase of the gait cycle, as described above, are the consequence of coupled movements between the anatomical segments.

In the swing phase of the normal gait cycle, the foot and ankle contribute to clearance and pre-positioning for the subsequent stance phase [2, 3, 6]. During pre- and initial swing, the tibia or shank segment is rotating externally and the ankle is plantar flexing. The segments of the foot are "unlocked" as the limb is unloaded. During mid swing, the tibia or shank segment is rotating internally and the ankle is dorsiflexing. These coupled motions serve to functionally shorten the limb and promote clearance. During terminal swing, these coupled motions continue and the foot is maintained in a plantigrade alignment, perpendicular to the anatomical axis of the tibia or shank segment, through concentric activation of the ankle dorsiflexor muscles. This pre-positioning of the foot during terminal swing will result in a heel strike at the initial contact, which is the optimal alignment for the ankle and foot as the extremity enters the subsequent stance phase in loading response.

Box 15.1

- The lower leg consists of four segments: the tibial or shank segment, the hindfoot (talus and calcaneus), the midfoot (navicular, cuneiforms and cuboid), and the forefoot (metatarsals and phalanges).
- The interaction of the ankle and foot with the ground during the stance phase of the gait cycle is described by the concept of three rockers; first or heel rocker, second or ankle rocker, and third or forefoot rocker.
- In the stance phase of the normal gait cycle, the ankle and foot provide shock absorption during loading response (first or heel rocker), stability during midstance (second or ankle rocker), and a rigid lever during terminal stance (third or forefoot rocker).
- In the swing phase of the normal gait cycle, dorsiflexion of the foot and ankle contribute to clearance and pre-positioning for the subsequent stance phase.

Segmental Malalignment Patterns of the Ankle and Foot

Segmental malalignments of the ankle and foot may be categorized as coupled or uncoupled. *Coupled* segmental malalignments represent exaggerations of normal segmental alignments that occur during the gait cycle (as described above). The three most common coupled segmental malalignments are equinus, equinopronovalgus, and equinosupovarus. Equinus is characterized by excessive plantar flexion of the hindfoot relative to the ankle, with normal midfoot and forefoot alignment (Fig. 15.5a, b) Equinopronovalgus is characterized by equinus deformity of the hindfoot, coupled with pronation deformities of the midfoot and forefoot (Fig. 15.6a, b). The lateral column of the foot is functionally and/or structurally shorter than the medial column. Ankle valgus and hallux valgus deformities are frequently seen in association with equinopronovalgus foot segmental malalignment (see Fig. 15.6c, d) Equinosupovarus is characterized by equinus deformity of the hindfoot, coupled with supination deformity of the midfoot and variable malalignment of the forefoot (Fig. 15.7a, b) The lateral column is functionally and/or structurally longer than the medial column. Compensatory ankle valgus deformity may be seen in association with equinosupovarus foot segmental malalignment.

In all three coupled segmental malalignment patterns, heel strike at initial contact does not occur, disrupting the first or hindfoot rocker and shock absorption function in loading response. Equinus and equinosupovarus malalignment patterns disrupt the second or ankle rocker by blocking ankle dorsiflexion, compromising stability function in midstance. Equinopronovalgus malalignment maintains the mid- and forefoot segments in an "unlocked" alignment, compromising stability function in midstance, which may result in excessive loading of the plantar, medial portion of the midfoot. All three coupled segmental malalignments may compromise the ability of the ankle plantar flexor muscles to generate an adequate internal plantar flexion moment during third or forefoot rocker. The hindfoot malalignment associated with equinus and equinosupovarus malalignment patterns shortens the length of the plantar flexor muscles, compromising their ability to generate tension, as described by the length-tension curve for skeletal muscle [10, 11]. With equinopronovalgus, the moment generating capacity of the ankle plantarflexor muscles is further compromised by the malalignment of mid-and forefoot segments, which

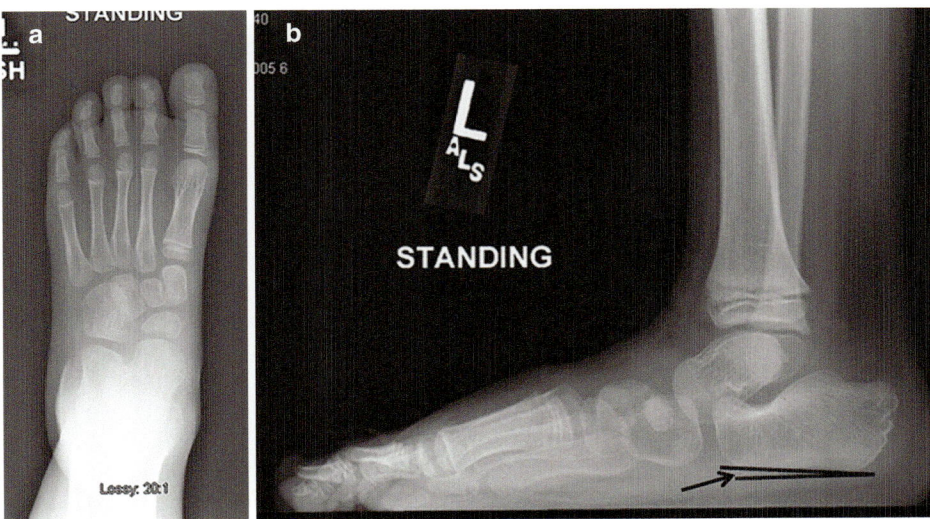

Fig. 15.5 Plain radiographs of the foot in a child with equinus deformity. (**a**) Anteroposterior view shows normal segmental alignment. (**b**) Lateral view shows hindfoot plantarflexion (diminished calcaneal pitch, indicated by *solid arrow* towards angle formed by *solid lines*, normal is approximately 20°), with otherwise normal foot segmental alignment

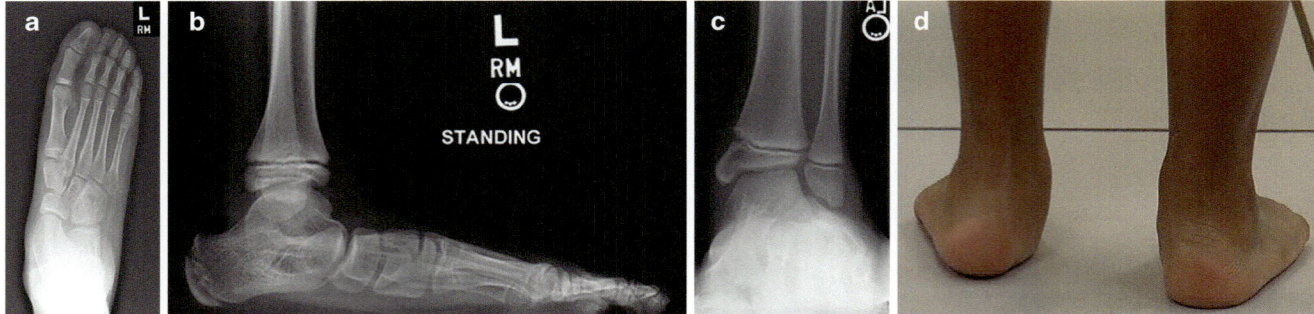

Fig. 15.6 Plain radiographs of the foot in a child with equinopronovalgus deformity. (**a**) Anteroposterior view shows hindfoot pronation, talonavicular uncoverage, forefoot abduction and hallux valgus. (**b**) Lateral view shows hindfoot plantarflextion, midfoot pronation (excessive naviculocuboid overlap), and forefoot pronation (excessive overlap of the metatarsals). (**c**) Anteroposterior view of the ankle shows ankle valgus deformity (increased tibiotalar angle, lateral wedging of the distal tibial epiphysis, and a high fibular station). (**d**) Clinical photograph of the left hindfoot in weight-bearing for this child. There is significant hindfoot valgus deformity, which the radiographs show to be a consequence of both tibiotalar (ankle) and talo-calcaneal (subtalar) valgus malalignments

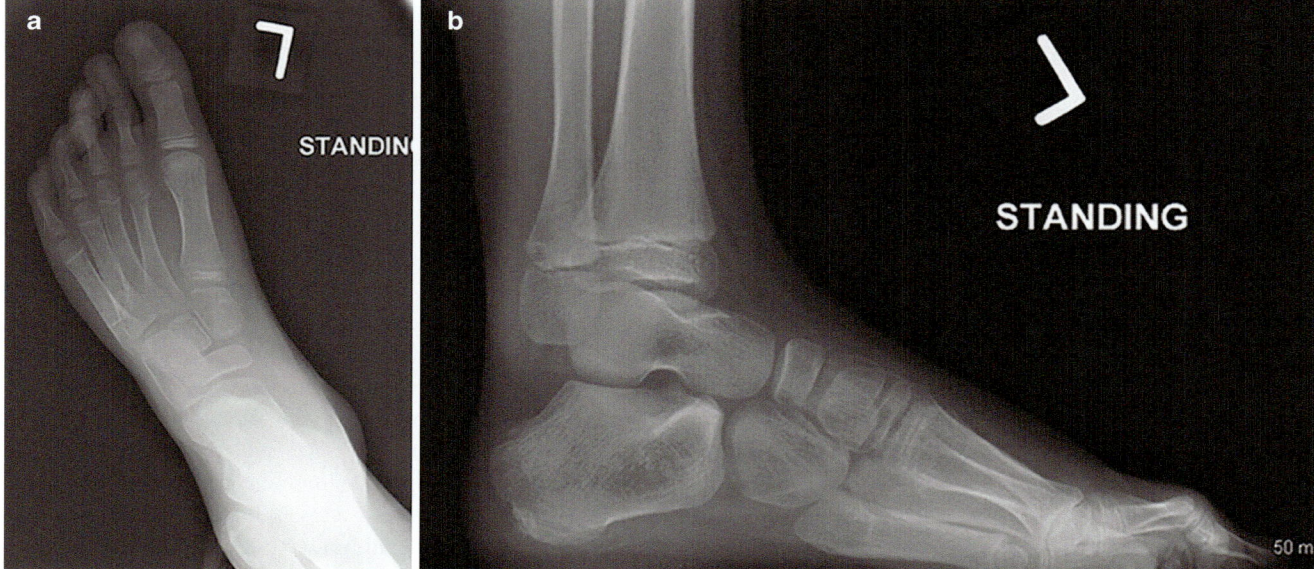

Fig. 15.7 Plain radiographs of the foot in a child with equionsupovarus deformity. (**a**) Anteroposterior view shows hindfoot supination (excessive overlap of the talus and calcaneus), and forefoot adduction (medial deviation of the great toe metatarsal relative to the talus). (**b**) Lateral view shows hindfoot varus (parallelism of the talus and calcaneus), midfoot supination (diminished naviculocuboid overlap), and forefoot supination (excessive stacking of the metatarsals)

effectively shortens the lever arm available to this muscle group during the third or forefoot rocker. All three segmental malalignment patterns of the ankle and foot may inhibit ankle dorsiflexion in swing phase, compromising clearance in midswing and proper positioning of the foot and ankle in terminal swing.

Uncoupled segmental malalignments are alignment patterns between the hind-, mid-, and forefoot that never occur during the gait cycle. Equinosupovalgus is an example of an uncoupled segmental malalignment pattern (Fig. 15.8a, b). Uncoupled segmental malalignments of the ankle and foot are relatively uncommon, and are frequently the consequence of deformity following previous surgery.

> **Box 15.2**
> - Segmental malalignments of the ankle and foot may be categorized as coupled or uncoupled. *Coupled* segmental malalignments represent exaggerations of normal segmental alignments that occur during the gait cycle. *Uncoupled* segmental malalignments are alignment patterns between the three segments of the foot that never occur during the gait cycle.
> - The three most common coupled segmental malalignments are equinus, equinopronovalgus, and equinosupovarus.

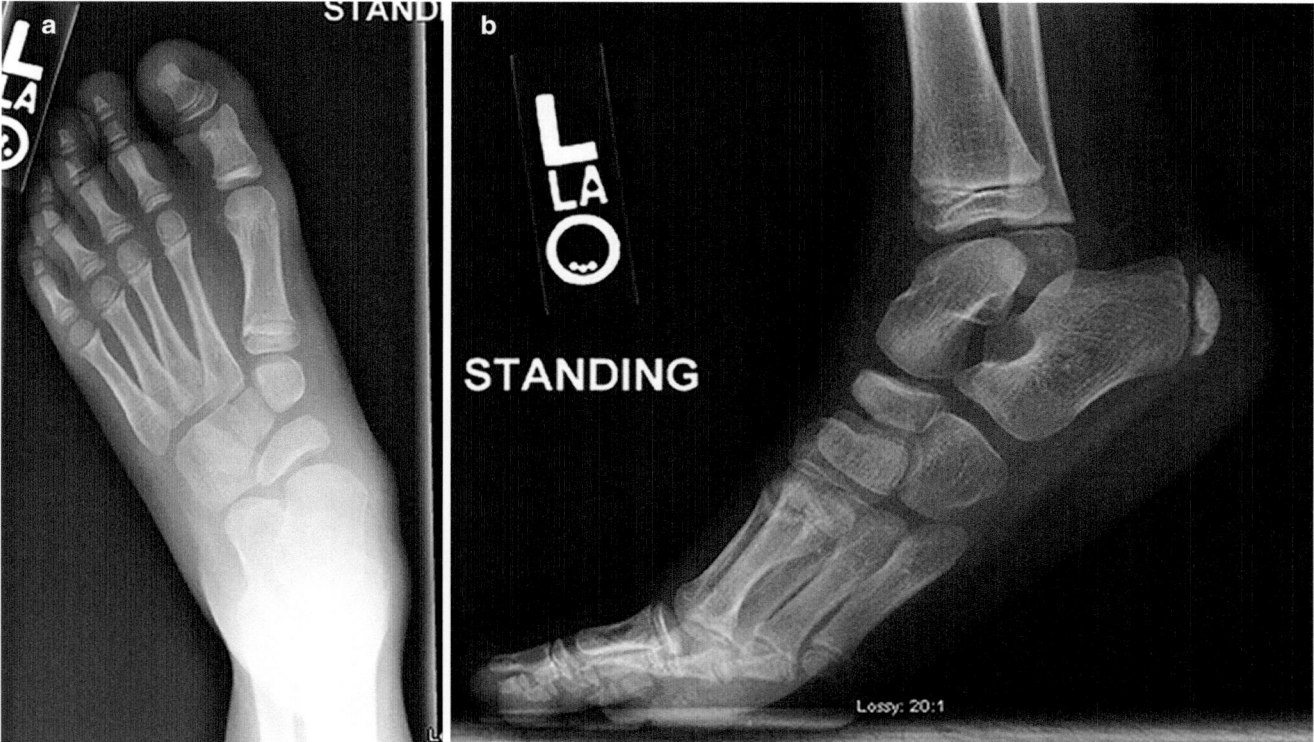

Fig. 15.8 Plain radiographs of the foot in a child with equinosupovalgus deformity, which is an example of an uncoupled malalignment. (**a**) Anteroposterior view shows hindfoot pronation, talonavicular uncoverage, forefoot abduction and hallux valgus interphalangeus. (**b**) Lateral view shows hindfoot varus (parallelism of the talus and calcaneus), midfoot supination (diminished naviculocuboid overlap), and forefoot supination (excessive stacking of the metatarsals). The normal coupling between the three segments of the foot is disrupted, as shown by the dissonance between anteroposterior and lateral radiographic views

Surgical Interventions

Interventions to correct foot deformities in children may be selected to improve function and/or cosmesis. Both of these goals may be achieved by surgeries designed to improve foot shape. It is presumed that improved foot shape following soft tissue and skeletal surgery can restore both the stability function of the foot during the second or ankle rocker in midstance and the skeletal lever arm function of the foot during the third or forefoot rocker in terminal stance [12–15]. However, it is important to recognize that increased foot stiffness associated with many skeletal surgical procedures (e.g., arthrodesis) utilized to improve foot shape may compromise shock absorption function of the foot during the first or ankle rocker in loading response [16]. Cosmetic improvements following foot surgery are related to improved visual assessment of static standing foot alignment (particularly restoration of the medial longitudinal arch and toe alignment) and improved foot progression angle during stance phase.

Soft tissue surgeries include release, lengthening, or shortening of muscles, tendons, ligaments, and joint capsules; or transfer of the muscle tendon unit. Release of soft tissue structures is generally reserved for fixed ankle and foot deformities associated with progressive disease processes in subjects who have significant impairment and whose goals are to improve static alignment in order to promote brace wear, shoe wear, or foot position in a wheelchair, and to facilitate transfer level motor activities. Lengthening of soft tissue structures is appropriate for fixed ankle and foot deformities associated with static or stable disease processes in subjects whose goals are to improve alignment to facilitate dynamic functional motor activities. It is important to recognize that in most cases there is preexisting weakness of the muscle tendon unit that is being lengthened, and that all lengthening surgical procedures result in additional weakening. When operating on muscles and tendons, selective surgical lengthening techniques that minimize the subsequent weakness of the muscle tendon unit are therefore favored [10, 11]. Surgical procedures that partially (also called "split") or completely transfer the muscle tendon unit are reserved for completely dynamic ankle and foot deformities associated with static or stable disease processes in subjects who have relatively lower levels of motor impairment

[17–19]. Partial and complete transfers are performed to address a dynamic muscle imbalance. Achieving perfect dynamic balance with all types of tendon transfer can be challenging. Over correction may occur with either partial or complete transfers, and under correction may be seen following partial transfers. Proper patient selection is essential.

Skeletal surgeries include guided growth, osteotomy, and arthrodesis. Guided growth can be utilized to correct ankle valgus deformity and metatarsus/phalangeal deformity associated with juvenile hallux valgus [20–22]. Typically two or more years of growth remaining is required to achieve correction by guided growth strategies. Osteotomy and arthrodesis techniques may correct deformity by addition (i.e., lengthening), subtraction (i.e., shortening), angulation, or rotation. Acute skeletal lengthening techniques are preferred as they utilize coupled segmental relations between the segments of the foot to achieve correction [12, 23, 24]. These procedures require a bone graft, and in most cases, internal fixation. The use of allograft is favored over autograft, though late allograft collapse during the re-ossification phase of graft incorporation has been reported [25]. Acute skeletal shortening procedures are used for the correction of the most rigid foot deformities, which are usually associated with congenital conditions (e.g., arthrogryposis) or peripheral neuropathies and myopathies (e.g., hereditary sensorimotor neuropathies and dystrophin deficient muscular dystrophies).

Clinical decision-making for surgery is guided by the classification of foot deformities into three levels (Table 15.2). Level I deformities are characterized by dynamic soft tissue imbalance. Skeletal anatomy is normal. Level II deformities are characterized by fixed or myostatic soft tissue imbalance. However, the underlying skeletal segmental malalignments are flexible and correctable on manipulation. Level III deformities are characterized by structural skeletal deformities that are usually associated with fixed or myostatic soft tissue imbalance. For foot deformities associated central nervous system conditions (e.g., cerebral palsy) it is not always possible to determine preoperatively if the deformity is level II or III. In such cases, sequential soft tissue lengthening is performed first, followed by intraoperative assessment of segmental foot alignment with stress radiographs under fluoroscopy (Fig. 15.9). If correction of alignment is determined to be insufficient, then sequential skeletal surgery, focused on the segment(s) that remain malaligned is performed.

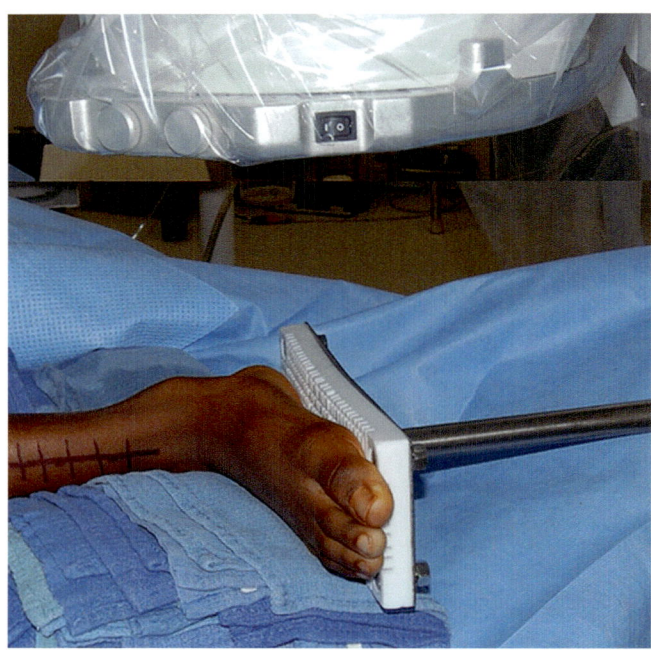

Fig. 15.9 Intraoperative clinical photograph of the use of a "foot pusher" to achieve simulated weight bearing lateral radiographs

Table 15.2 Levels of ankle and foot deformity and treatment options

| | Treatment options | | |
Levels of deformity	Pharmacologic/neurosurgery	Muscle tendon surgeries	Skeletal surgeries
I: Dynamic soft tissue imbalance, no skeletal deformities	Neuromuscular junction blockade	Partial or complete tendon transfers	Usually not necessary
	Selective dorsal rhizotomy		
	Intrathecal baclofen		
II: Fixed soft tissue imbalance, no fixed skeletal deformities	Not appropriate as isolated intervention	Sequential lengthening (Myotendinous Junction Recession, Tendon Lengthening)	Usually not necessary
III: Fixed soft tissue imbalance, with fixed skeletal deformities	Not appropriate as isolated intervention	Sequential lengthening	Osteotomy or arthrodesis
		Appropriate in conjunction with skeletal surgery	(Lengthening, shortening, angular, rotational)

Box 15.3
- *Soft tissue surgeries* include release, lengthening, or shortening of muscles, tendons, ligaments, and joint capsules; or transfer (partial or complete) of the muscle tendon unit.
- *Skeletal surgeries* include guided growth, osteotomy, and arthrodesis.
- *Clinical decision-making for surgery* is guided by the classification of foot deformities into three levels

Assessment Tools and Indications

Clinical decision making for the management of ankle and foot deformities in children integrates a range of data by the use of a diagnostic matrix (see Table 15.1) [4]. The integration of data from multiple sources results in a degree of redundancy that improves decision making and quality of outcomes. When the data is consistent across the fields, and the problem is common, the confidence in decision making should be high. When the data is apparently inconsistent across the fields, or the problem is unusual, then the confidence in decision making should be lowered. Surgical treatment paradigms for coupled segmental malalignments of the ankle and foot are more advanced and generally more effective than those for uncoupled segmental malalignments. The latter deformities are individually unique, and therefore require careful, case-by-case surgical planning and treatment.

Different types of ankle and foot deformities are best evaluated with different combinations of assessment tools at different points in the course of management (Table 15.3). Plain radiographic views at all points include standing anteroposterior and lateral views of the foot, and a standing anteroposterior view of the ankle. Additional views of the hindfoot (Cobey view) and subtalar joint (Harris heel view), while not part of the routine radiographic assessment paradigm, may be used to further assess for overall hindfoot alignment and the presence of a talocalcaneal coalition. In the case of the latter, computed tomography scan (CT) is required to confirm the diagnosis and for adequate planning prior to surgical management. True or simulated weight bearing is essential; foot segmental alignment may be dramatically different in loaded versus unloaded conditions, and non-weight bearing views are of little value. Qualitative and quantitative assessment of plain radiographs should be done is a systematic fashion, referring to normative data to objectively describe the ankle and foot segmental alignment (Table 15.4) [7, 26]. Accurate assessment of the causes of hindfoot alignment in the coronal plane (i.e., determining the relative contributions of deformity at the tibiotalar and talocalcaneal joints) requires analysis of the anteroposterior radiograph of the ankle in addition to the views of the foot [27] (see Fig. 15.6) For the *preoperative assessment* of the valgus and varus foot, kinematics is limited by the reliance on a single segment foot model that can not account for abnormal midfoot alignments [28, 29]. Dynamic electromyography (EMG) is only necessary for feet with dynamic varus deviations, to sort out the relative contributions of the gastrocsoleus complex, the tibialis posterior, and tibialis anterior muscles [30, 31]. Pedobarography is indicated for valgus and varus

Table 15.3 Assessment tools for the ankle/foot

Deformity	Assessment tools						
	History	Physical examination (ROM, OGA)	Standing/stress radiographs	Kinematics	Kinetics	EMG	Pedobarography
	Preoperative						
	Preoperative						
Equinus	X	X	X	X			
Valgus	X	X	X	Limited	X		X
Varus	X	X	X	Limited	X	X	X
	Intraoperative						
Equinus			X				
Valgus			X				
Varus			X				
	Postoperative						
Equinus	X	X	X				
Valgus	X	X	X		X		X
Varus	X	X	X		X		X
	Surveillance						
Equinus	X	X					
Valgus	X	X					
Varus	X	X					

ROM Range of motion, *OGA* Observational gait analysis, *EMG* Electromyography, *X* Appropriate tool to use

Table 15.4 Normal radiographic angle measurements [7, 26]

Ankle and foot segments and columns[a]	Normal mean ± 1 SD[a]	Increased value (>Mean + 1 SD)	Decreased value (<Mean − 1 SD)
Hindfoot			
Tibiotalar Angle (anteroposterior view, degrees)	1.1 ± 3.75	Eversion	Inversion
Calcaneal Pitch (lateral view, degrees)	17 ± 6.0	Calcaneus	Equinus
Tibiocalcaneal Angle (lateral view, degrees)	69 ± 8.4	Equinus	Calcaneus
Talocalcaneal Angle (lateral view, degrees)	49 ± 6.9	Eversion	Inversion
Midfoot			
Naviculocuboid Overlap (anteroposterior view, percentage)	47 ± 13.8	Pronation	Supination
Talonavicular Coverage Angle (anteroposterior view, degrees)	20 ± 9.8	Abduction	Adduction
Lateral Talo-First Metatarsal Angle (lateral view, degrees)	13 ± 7.5	Pronation	Supination
Forefoot			
Anteroposterior Talo-First Metatarsal Angle (anteroposterior view, degrees)	10 ± 7.0	Abduction	Adduction
Metatarsal Stacking Angle (lateral view, degrees)	8.2 ± 9	Supination	Pronation
Columns			
Medial-Lateral Column Ratio (lateral view)	0.9 ± 0.1	Abduction	Adduction

For direction on how to measure each angle or distance ratio on plain radiographs, see reference [7]
[a] See Fig. 15.2

malalignments [32]. The relation between static standing foot alignment (as indicated by plain radiographs) and dynamic foot loading (as indicated by pedobarography) is complex [33, 34]. The former is not always a good predictor of the latter, and when there is apparent discrepancy between the two modalities, priority should be given to the pedobarograph data as it is a closer measure of actual function [32, 34]. *Intraoperative assessment* relies primarily on stress radiographs, which requires the use of a "foot pusher" device to obtain simulated weight bearing views of the foot (see Fig. 15.9). *Postoperative assessment*, once recovery, healing, and rehabilitation following surgery have been completed, should be as quantitative as possible, mirroring the preoperative assessment to allow objective assessment of outcome in multiple domains. Finally, *surveillance* is guided by the history and physical examination, with additional assessment tools utilized only if a problem has been identified.

> **Box 15.4**
> - Clinical decision making for the management of ankle and foot deformities in children integrates a range of data by the use of a diagnostic matrix, which considers and integrates data from five domains.
> - Coupled segmental malalignments are easier to treat surgically than uncoupled segmental malalignments.
> - Different types of ankle and foot deformities are best evaluated with different combinations of assessment tools at different points in the course of management.

> **Commentary**
>
> **Biomechanically Based Clinical Decision Making in Pediatric Foot and Ankle Surgery: Commentary**
>
> Noman A. Siddiqui
> nsiddiqu@lifebridgehealth.org
>
> NAS is a paid consultant for Arthrex. The following organizations supported the institution of NAS: DePuy Synthes, Integra LifeSciences, NuVasive Specialized Orthopedics, Orthofix, OrthoPediatrics, Paragon 28, Pega Medical, Smith & Nephew, Stryker, Treace Medical Concepts, and WishBone Medical Inc.
>
> Foot and ankle biomechanics have been the cornerstone of knowledge, prior to surgical intervention, for musculoskeletal specialists. Understanding bipedal gait pattern is critical for deconstructing the deforming forces that can result in pathologic conditions. My own experiences in managing pediatric and adult patients, and the evolution of conditions from youth to adulthood, have shaped my approach to be concentrated on biomechanical forces. I have spent a great deal of time focusing on the work of Drs Inman, Sarrafian, and Hansen as I've developed my basis for approaching foot and ankle pathology. This chapter by Dr. Davids is an excellent addition to that body of work for the pediatric population.
>
> The opening portion of the chapter provides the reader a simple, yet effective, approach when evaluat-

ing a patient with foot and ankle pathology. The five categories (clinical history, physical exam, radiographic exam, observational gait exam, and quantitative gait analysis) give the practitioner a prescription to determine the source of pathology. Once the source(s) are identified, the appropriate intervention can be recommended.

An important concept in this chapter highlights the differences that sometimes are present during the various diagnostic components of the exam. It is not uncommon to have patients who present for pedal complaints that are clinically apparent but are not demonstrated on static radiographs. This mismatch can be misleading and pose a challenge for determining proper intervention. For such scenarios, the authors correctly advise the utility of a dynamic pedobarographic evaluation. I have found this to be the case in various pathologies such as juvenile pes planus, where a patient radiographically appears to have minor changes on plain films but demonstrates substantial pressure changes on a pedobarographic study.

These variances can be a challenge to manage, particularly as many juvenile patients will not always present with pain but have parents who are concerned about the long-term effect of the position. For these scenarios, I have been able to provide what I believe is the natural progression of a long-standing malalignment that traverses from youth to adulthood. In these situations, I often find myself discussing the benefits of a healthy lifestyle, proper weight management, supportive shoe gear/orthoses, and the potential for surgery.

I also have found that the same principle is applied in adults that may have been "treated" as juveniles for a particular condition. For example, adults with contrasting presentations such as a "high arch" or "fallen arches" will describe how they never had symptoms and were "treated" with observation. However, they developed different issues with their feet as they aged. Examples in patients with high-arch feet may include ankle sprains, fifth metatarsal fractures, and painful midfoot arthritis. Meanwhile, patients with low arches may complain of arch pain, difficulty with shoes, and hallux valgus.

The author provides an overview of the gait cycle and describes the action of the foot at the three different rocker positions during stance. This serves as the basis for determining if deformity is "coupled" or "uncoupled." The review of the gait cycle is an important refresher for specialists and serves as a basis to determine exaggeration of normal position during gait as coupled segmental malalignments. Therefore, exaggerated positions that do not occur in the normal course of gait are considered uncoupled and may be a result of prior intervention. Presenting biomechanics-related pathology as either "coupled" or "uncoupled" patterns makes it easier for the reader to approach problems with an algorithm for treatment. This concept is simple yet elegant, since patterns tend to emerge with certain disorders. Because normal gait is dependent on each structure of the foot performing a specific motion at each of the three rockers during stance, an overemphasis of movement in either pronation or supination will result in pathology of soft tissue, bone, or both. This chapter serves as a good overview of pedal mechanics and provides musculoskeletal specialists a stepwise approach during the pediatric evaluation. Furthermore, this approach may be similarly beneficial for management of adult foot and ankle disorders.

References

1. Davids JR. Normal function of the ankle and foot: biomechanics and quantitative analysis. In: Drennan J, McCarthy J, editors. Drennan's the child's foot and ankle. 2nd ed. Philadelphia, PA: Lippincott Williams and Wilkins; 2009. p. 54–63.
2. Inman VT, Ralston HJ, Todd F. Human walking. Baltimore, MD: Williams & Wilkins; 1981.
3. Perry J. Gait analysis: normal and pathological function. Thorofare, NJ: Slack Inc.; 1992.
4. Davids JR. Orthopaedic treatment of foot deformities. In: Gage J, Schwartz M, Koop S, Novacheck T, editors. The identification and treatment of gait problems in cerebral palsy. 2nd ed. London: MacKeith Press; 2009. p. 514–33.
5. Inman VT. The human foot. Manit Med Rev. 1966;46(8):513–5.
6. Inman VT. The influence of the foot-ankle complex on the proximal skeletal structures. Artif Limbs. 1969;13(1):59–65.
7. Davids JR, Gibson TW, Pugh LI. Quantitative segmental analysis of weight-bearing radiographs of the foot and ankle for children: normal alignment. J Pediatr Orthop. 2005;25(6):769–76.
8. Ponseti IV, El-Khoury GY, Ippolito E, Weinstein SL. A radiographic study of skeletal deformities in treated clubfeet. Clin Orthop. 1981;160:30–42.
9. Gage JR. The clinical use of kinetics for evaluation of pathologic gait in cerebral palsy. Instr Course Lect. 1995;44:507–15.
10. Delp SL, Statler K, Carroll NC. Preserving plantar flexion strength after surgical treatment for contracture of the triceps surae: a computer simulation study. J Orthop Res. 1995;13(1):96–104.
11. Firth GB, McMullan M, Chin T, Ma F, Selber P, Eizenberg N, et al. Lengthening of the gastrocnemius-soleus complex: an anatomical and biomechanical study in human cadavers. J Bone Joint Surg Am. 2013;95(16):1489–96.
12. Davids JR. The foot and ankle in cerebral palsy. Orthop Clin North Am. 2010;41(4):579–93.
13. Mosca VS. The child's foot: principles of management. J Pediatr Orthop. 1998;18(3):281–2.

14. Kadhim M, Holmes L Jr, Miller F. Long-term outcome of planovalgus foot surgical correction in children with cerebral palsy. J Foot Ankle Surg. 2013;52(6):697–703.
15. Shore BJ, Smith KR, Riazi A, Symons SB, Khot A, Graham K. Subtalar fusion for pes valgus in cerebral palsy: results of a modified technique in the setting of single event multilevel surgery. J Pediatr Orthop. 2013;33(4):431–8.
16. Astion DJ, Deland JT, Otis JC, Kenneally S. Motion of the hindfoot after simulated arthrodesis. J Bone Joint Surg Am. 1997;79(2):241–6.
17. Barnes MJ, Herring JA. Combined split anterior tibial-tendon transfer and intramuscular lengthening of the posterior tibial tendon. Results in patients who have a varus deformity of the foot due to spastic cerebral palsy. J Bone Joint Surg Am. 1991;73(5):734–8.
18. Hoffer MM, Barakat G, Koffman M. 10-year follow-up of split anterior tibial tendon transfer in cerebral palsied patients with spastic equinovarus deformity. J Pediatr Orthop. 1985;5(4):432–4.
19. Scott AC, Scarborough N. The use of dynamic EMG in predicting the outcome of split posterior tibial tendon transfers in spastic hemiplegia. J Pediatr Orthop. 2006;26(6):777–80.
20. Davids JR, McBrayer D, Blackhurst DW. Juvenile hallux valgus deformity: surgical management by lateral hemiepiphyseodesis of the great toe metatarsal. J Pediatr Orthop. 2007;27(7):826–30.
21. Davids JR, Valadie AL, Ferguson RL, Bray EW 3rd, Allen BL Jr. Surgical management of ankle valgus in children: use of a transphyseal medial malleolar screw. J Pediatr Orthop. 1997;17(1):3–8.
22. Stevens PM, Belle RM. Screw epiphysiodesis for ankle valgus. J Pediatr Orthop. 1997;17(1):9–12.
23. Mosca VS. Calcaneal lengthening for valgus deformity of the hindfoot. Results in children who had severe, symptomatic flatfoot and skewfoot. J Bone Joint Surg Am. 1995;77(4):500–12.
24. Yoo WJ, Chung CY, Choi IH, Cho TJ, Kim DH. Calcaneal lengthening for the planovalgus foot deformity in children with cerebral palsy. J Pediatr Orthop. 2005;25(6):781–5.
25. Danko AM, Allen B Jr, Pugh L, Stasikelis P. Early graft failure in lateral column lengthening. J Pediatr Orthop. 2004;24(6):716–20.
26. Westberry DE, Davids JR, Roush TF, Pugh LI. Qualitative versus quantitative radiographic analysis of foot deformities in children with hemiplegic cerebral palsy. J Pediatr Orthop. 2008;28(3):359–65.
27. Stevens PM. Effect of ankle valgus on radiographic appearance of the hindfoot. J Pediatr Orthop. 1988;8(2):184–6.
28. Davis RB, Jameson EG, Davids JR, Christopher LM, Rogozinski BM, Anderson JP. The design, development, and initial evaluation of a multisegment foot model for routine clinical gait analysis. In: Harris GF, Smith P, Marks R, editors. Foot and ankle motion analysis: clinical treatment and technology. Boca Raton, FL: CRC Press; 2007. p. 425–44.
29. Davis RBOS, Tyburski D, Gage JR. A gait analysis data collection and reduction technique. Hum Mov Sci. 1991;10:575–87.
30. Perry J, Hoffer MM. Preoperative and postoperative dynamic electromyography as an aid in planning tendon transfers in children with cerebral palsy. J Bone Joint Surg Am. 1977;59(4):531–7.
31. Sutherland DH. Varus foot in cerebral palsy: an overview. Instr Course Lect. 1993;42:539–43.
32. Jameson EG, Davids JR, Anderson JP, Davis RB 3rd, Blackhurst DW, Christopher LM. Dynamic pedobarography for children: use of the center of pressure progression. J Pediatr Orthop. 2008;28(2):254–8.
33. Cavanagh PR, Rodgers MM, Iiboshi A. Pressure distribution under symptom-free feet during barefoot standing. Foot Ankle. 1987;7(5):262–76.
34. Westberry DE, Davids JR, Anderson JP, Pugh LI, Davis RB, Hardin JW. The operative correction of symptomatic flat foot deformities in children: the relationship between static alignment and dynamic loading. Bone Joint J. 2013;95-B(5):706–13.

Congenital Foot Deformities

16

Mitzi L. Williams and Matthew B. Dobbs

This chapter will review some of the more common congenital foot and ankle deformities among children. Many of these deformities have a genetic influence while others may arise secondary to a failure in differentiation in utero. A complete pediatric history and physical exam is key in excluding any neurologic component. Some secondary diagnoses may not be identified at birth and may require monitoring as the child develops (Fig. 16.1).

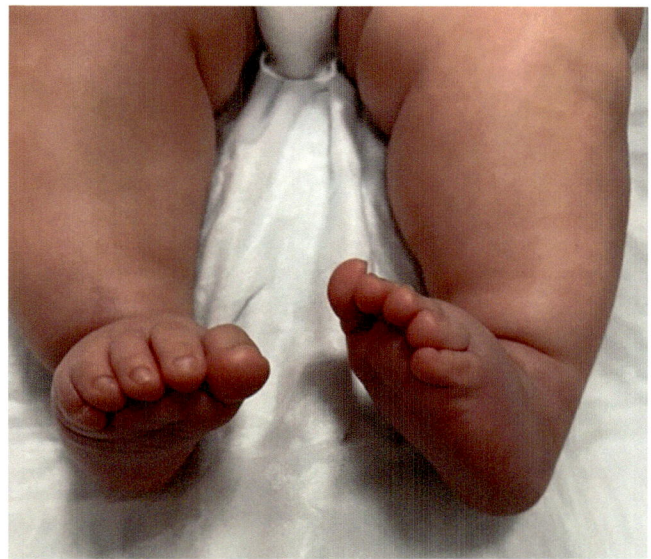

Fig. 16.1 Progressive foot deformity associated with Myelomeningocele

Introduction

Foot deformity in infants is one of the most common congenital musculoskeletal conditions. Diagnosis and treatment require sound knowledge of normal physiologic development, neurology, histopathology, and radiologic interpretation. While many pediatric conditions can be attributed to genetics and, in fact, assist with the diagnosis of various syndromes, others are a direct product of trauma or overuse. One must appreciate the delicate nature of these anatomic structures and the variation in which they present. With experience, and a firm understanding of normal pediatric lower extremity anatomy, one can delineate abnormal structural conditions in hopes of early treatment modalities. Early intervention for many diagnoses leads to improved functional outcomes.

Many congenital foot deformities will be noted in utero via ultrasound and furthermore reviewed with detailed ultrasounds and amniocentesis. One may find the foot deformity

M. L. Williams
Kaiser San Francisco Bay Area Foot and Ankle Residency Program, Department of Orthopedics and Podiatric Surgery, Kaiser Permanente, Oakland, CA, USA
e-mail: mitzi.l.williams@kp.org

M. B. Dobbs (✉)
Dobbs Clubfoot Center, Paley Institute,
West Palm Beach, FL, USA

Clinical Orthopaedics and Related Research, Park Ridge, IL, USA

United States Bone and Joint Initiative, Warrenville, IL, USA

Association of Bone and Joint Surgeons, Park Ridge, IL, USA

International Federation of Pediatric Orthopaedic Societies,
St. Louis, MO, USA
e-mail: mdobbs@paleyinstitute.org

to be a component of a syndrome identified via amniocentesis. However, both the formal diagnosis and the rigidity of many conditions such as talipes equinovarus (clubfoot) or congenital vertical talus (CVT) will only be verified once a clinical examination can be performed. An amniocentesis may be advised with high-risk pregnancies or if noninvasive testing reveals concerning results. If performed, the fluid from the sac surrounding the fetus is aspirated and sent for evaluation between the 15th–20th week of pregnancy.

Amniocentesis does not detect all birth defects, and this is important when counseling families. It can be used to detect Down syndrome, sickle cell, cystic fibrosis, muscular dystrophy, and Tay-Sachs, for example. With respect to foot deformities associated with various syndromes, an amniocentesis can be helpful in assessing for any connection to neural tube defects such as spina bifida and/ or chromosomal abnormalities. At the same time, one generally undergoes a detailed ultrasound that complements the amniocentesis in detecting any structural abnormalities such as heart defects or cleft palate.

Given the ossification pattern of the foot, X-rays in an infant may not be required unless difficulties with treatment exist, the diagnosis is unclear, or postoperative alignment is being reviewed, often with respect to the talus. X-rays, for example, are rarely indicated in the treatment of clubfoot unless there is difficulty with reduction in infancy. As for vertical talus, a stress plantarflexion lateral X-ray is utilized to either confirm or exclude the diagnosis from other conditions such as calcaneovalgus or oblique talus (Fig. 16.2).

Systemic and Local Bone Growth Factors

Bone growth can be influenced by systemic and local factors. Systemic factors include genetics, hormones, overall nutrition, and infection. Nutritional deficits may be linked to diet while may also be secondary to conditions associated with prematurity or systemic secondary diagnoses. Advances in neonatal care have significantly increased infant survival rates, especially among very low birth weight infants. These children should be followed closely as these bone growth deficiencies can be multifactorial. Likewise, any unusual growth disturbance can have an impact on limb length and/or lead to angular deformities.

Local factors influencing growth of a single epiphysis often include trauma, vascular insult, or osteomyelitis. Trauma can include obvious fractures or mechanical injuries while radiation may locally impact bone growth or lead to a growth hormone deficiency. Infections can also cause long-term harm with respect to bone growth. Caution should be taken with infection management including proper peripheral and central line care in infants. Line infections may lead to bone infections or possibly the premature closure of an isolated physis. Saphenous peripheral lines for example are near the distal tibia and can lead to future angular deformities if osseous infection ensues.

Normal Development

Parents quite often have worries with respect to their child's growth, development, and or gait. It remains important that throughout development, physicians recognize normal is a spectrum that changes. Physicians must educate parents that it is normal for the infant foot to be flat and supple. With age, the arch develops, and the osseous structures and intrinsic musculature matures. Therefore, it is normal for a young toddler or child to have flatfeet. This is different than a young child that has severely pronated feet or asymmetry.

It is important to exclude neurologic conditions associated with intoeing, cavus feet, and varus position. Equally, it is essential to understand how ligamentous laxity, connective tissue disorders, Down's syndrome, coalitions, and autism can often influence flatfeet. Identifying the underlying neurologic driving forces and recognizing the pathologic biomechanical influences are crucial to developing an appropriate management strategy (Figs. 16.3 and 16.4).

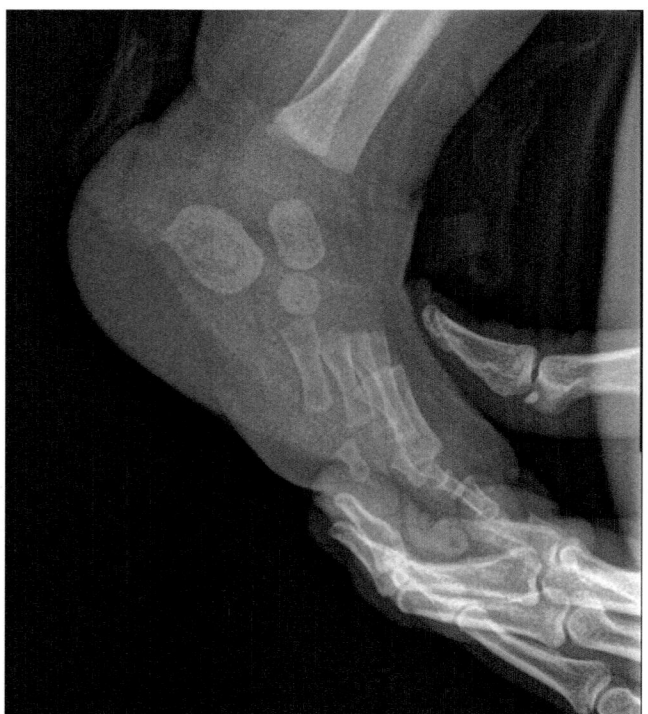

Fig. 16.2 Stress plantarflexion view excluding vertical talus

16 Congenital Foot Deformities

Foot Conditions and Developmental Limb Deformities

Curly Toe/Digital Flexion Contractures

Curly toe is a common congenital digital deformity which presents as a flexion deformity often involving the third, fourth, or fifth toes [1]. One or multiple toes may be affected. The affected toe is essentially plantarflexed, medially deviated and in varus rotation with the apex of the deformity involving the distal interphalangeal (DIP), or both DIP and proximal interphalangeal (PIP) joints. This condition can be hereditary, with a positive family history and autosomal dominant pattern of inheritance [2]. Still, despite the genetic influence for some, the etiology of the deformity is not completely understood. Children with excessive pronation or metatarsus adductus have presented more frequently with these flexion contractures [3], which may suggest that the flexor stabilization mechanism is an important driving force in this deformity (Fig. 16.5).

Curly toes are often noticed early in infancy and can be an early source of parental anxiety. At this stage, they are rarely symptomatic. Parental reassurance, education, and evaluation for any other neurologic manifestations are the main goals of that initial visit. Spontaneous self-correction of the deformity before the age of 6 occurs in up to 24% of the patients [4]. The remaining percentage of curly toes may per-

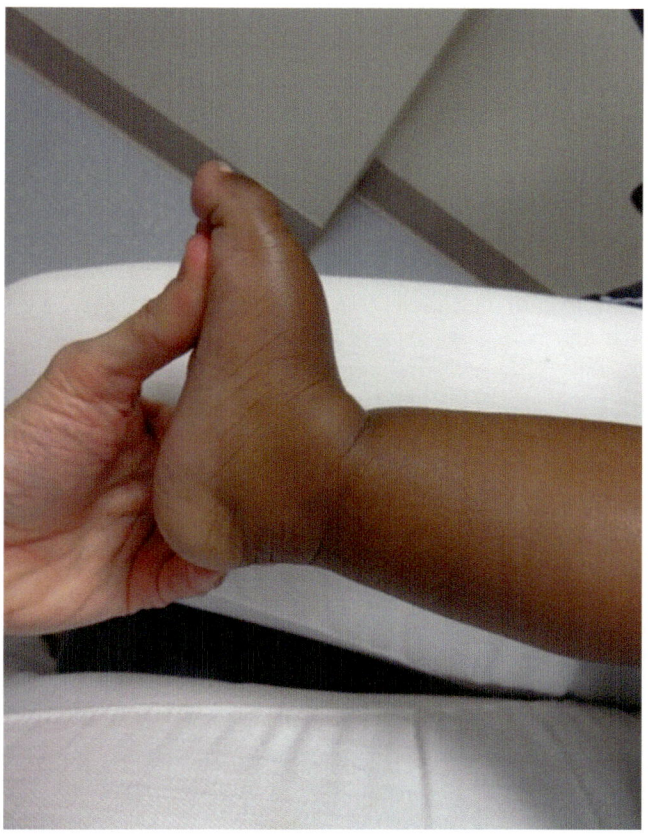

Fig. 16.3 Undeveloped arch at 2 years of age

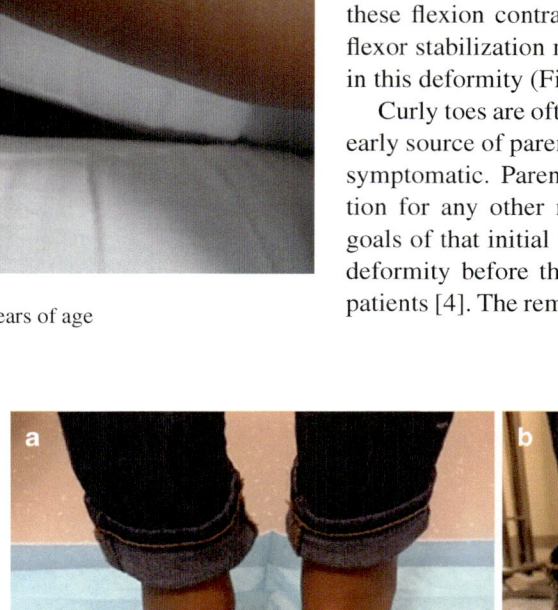
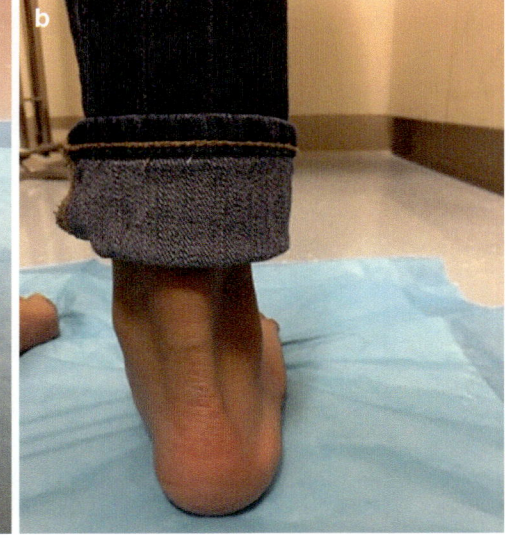

Fig. 16.4 (**a** and **b**) Pathologic flatfoot associated with middle facet coalition

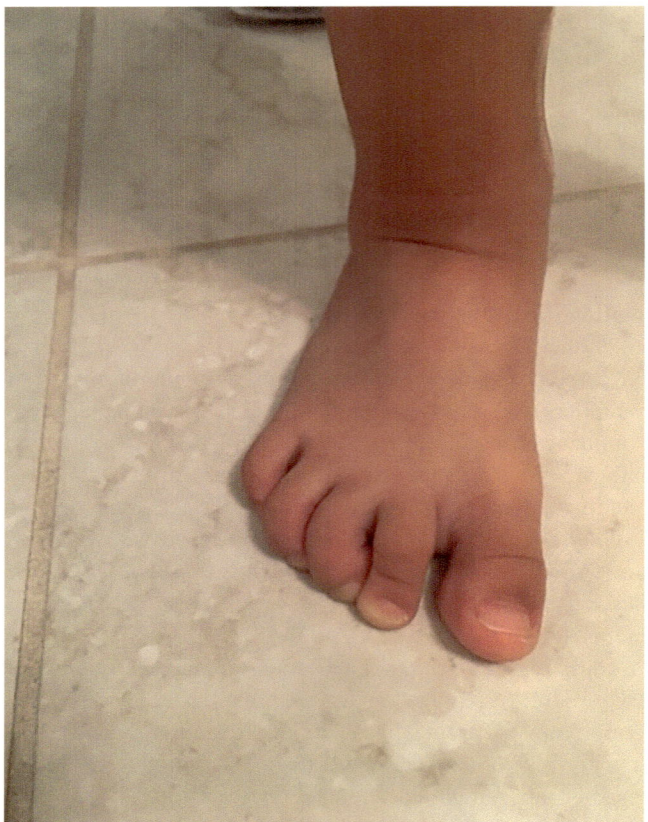

Fig. 16.5 Reducible curly toes in 3-year-old patient

sist to varying degrees. Therefore, delaying surgical intervention until the age of 6 is an option unless the presence of skin problems secondary to pressure, and/ or infections mandates the need for surgery prior to the age of 6. Likewise, children undergoing surgery under the age of 6 for other reasons may elect for surgical correction of the toe(s) to minimize future episodes of anesthesia. Finally, if the condition is becoming more semi-rigid and there is concern that one's window to perform a tendon release will be lost, then one may proceed sooner.

Treatment

Toe strapping is one of the available nonoperative treatment modalities, which can be attempted at any age [4]. Its effectiveness, however, is controversial. In a study by Turner, toe strapping was performed daily on 28 children over 5 months of age for an average of 13 months [5]. No statistically significant difference was noted in the improvement rates between the study group versus a control group, consisting of children, who received no treatment. In another study, Smith and colleagues performed daily toe strapping for 3 months on 68 children with underlapping and overlapping toes, all of whom were no older than 10 days [4]. The authors observed a 94% improvement rate, which led them to suggest that toe strapping may be more successful in younger children. It is important to recognize that children in time may improve without treatment. The authors do not advocate for routine strapping and/or taping of curly toes in infancy.

Surgical treatment ultimately is reserved for patients with persistent deformity and symptomatic deformities. Patients may present with blisters or calluses at the tip of the underlapping toe or the plantar aspect of the adjacent toe. Others may present with nail deformities or pain in shoes [6]. Waiting until the child is at least 6 years old to assess if a toe will self-correct is appropriate, provided the deformity is flexible. If the deformity is progressively becoming stiffer, from the ages of 2–6, one could proceed with surgery sooner to minimize the risk of an osseous procedure. If the deformity is flexible, tendon transfers and flexor tenotomies are performed. Arthroplasties, arthrodesis procedures, and phalangectomies are reserved for patients with semi-rigid or rigid contractures.

Girdlestone and Taylor have popularized flexor-to-extensor tendon transfer for treatment of clawtoes in 1951 [7]. The procedure allows recreating the dynamic pull of the intrinsic muscles and provides triplanar correction [8]. This procedure was shown to be effective for correction of central curly toes, 2, 3, and 4. The procedure is performed through a dorsolateral incision made over the extensor expansion. The long flexor is divided close to its insertion and transferred dorsolaterally, slightly distal to the extensor expansion, where it is attached under tension. Toe stiffness is a side effect following this procedure [1].

A flexor tenotomy is preferred to flexor-to-extensor tendon transfer to avoid postoperative toe stiffness. The procedure is performed through a small transverse stab incision on the plantar aspect of the toe [9]. The long and short flexor tendons are released. No sutures are needed with this type of small incision. Studies comparing flexor-to-extensor transfer and flexor tenotomy procedures suggest similar success rates with both procedures, with patient satisfaction being higher with flexor tenotomy [1, 10]. A flexor tenotomy is also preferred for treatment of the underlapping fifth toe, for which flexor-to-extensor tendon transfer is not indicated [6] (Fig. 16.6).

Polydactyly

Polydactyly is a congenital digital malformation characterized by formation of supernumerary digits. It can be classified as preaxial: extra hallux; postaxial (most common): extra fifth toe; and central (rarest): middle 3 toes involved [11]. While it is a common congenital deformity of the hand and foot, with incidence in the foot of approximately 1 per 1000 live births [12], the preaxial and central manifestations

Fig. 16.6 (**a**) Flexible curly toe. (**b**) Rigid curly toe

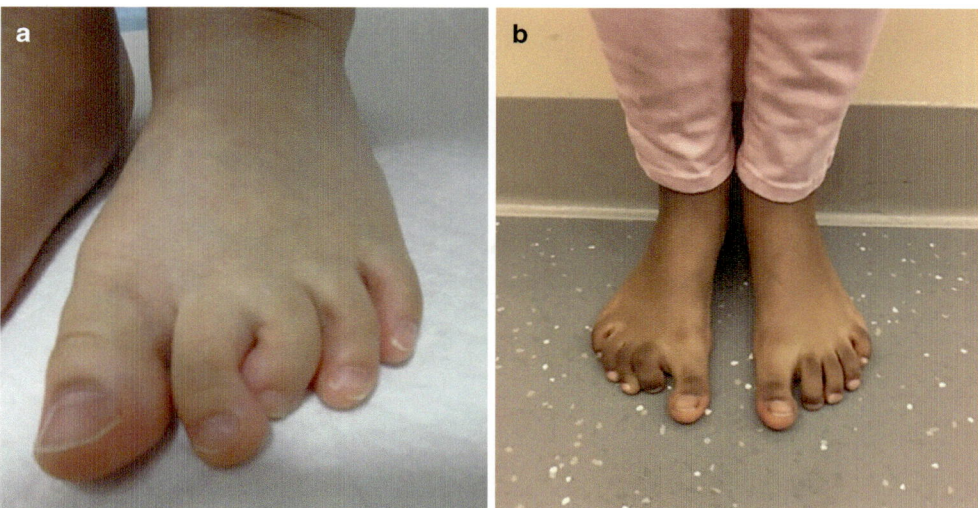

Fig. 16.7 (**a**) AP foot X-ray of 2-year-old male with polydactyly. Risks of angular deformity exist with growth. (**b**) AP foot X-ray of child's asymptomatic biological father demonstrating no history of surgical amputation

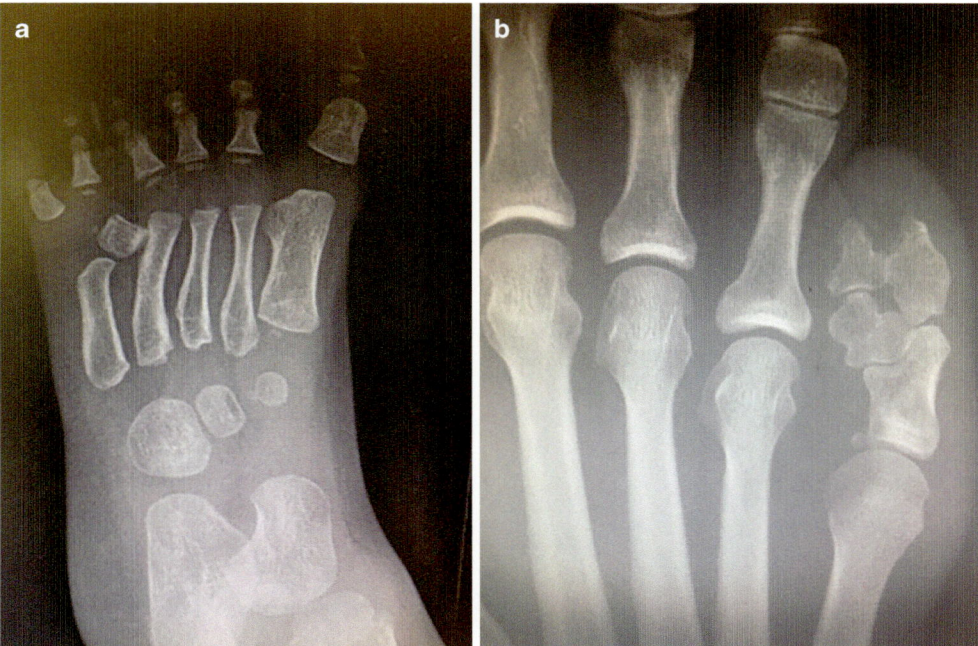

remain rare. Bilateral involvement is seen in 25% to 50% of patients [13]. No gender predilection is observed.

In addition to duplication of the phalanges, there may be a duplication of the metatarsals. X-rays are important in assessing the number of extranumerary bones while also assessing if the growth and position of such bones will cause problems to the remainder of the foot. These X-rays are often obtained just prior to surgery. Treatment must be individualized in accordance with the needs of the patient [14] (Fig. 16.7).

For example, the authors have met asymptomatic parents who did not undergo excision of simple extranumerary postaxial digits. Therefore, not every child must undergo surgical excision. Unfortunately, the duplication of metatarsals and rays do pose additional risk of angular growth deformities if not resected. Many find the extranumerary toe to eventually cause shoe irritation.

Polydactyly Surgical Pearls

- Most incisions can be elliptical in nature around the toe and carried out dorsally to remove any duplicated metatarsal.
- It is important to obtain hemostasis in the operating room since any void secondary to ray resections or toe amputations may lead to hematoma formation.
- Surgery is not advised in children less than 12 months of age unless the child is undergoing a concomitant proce-

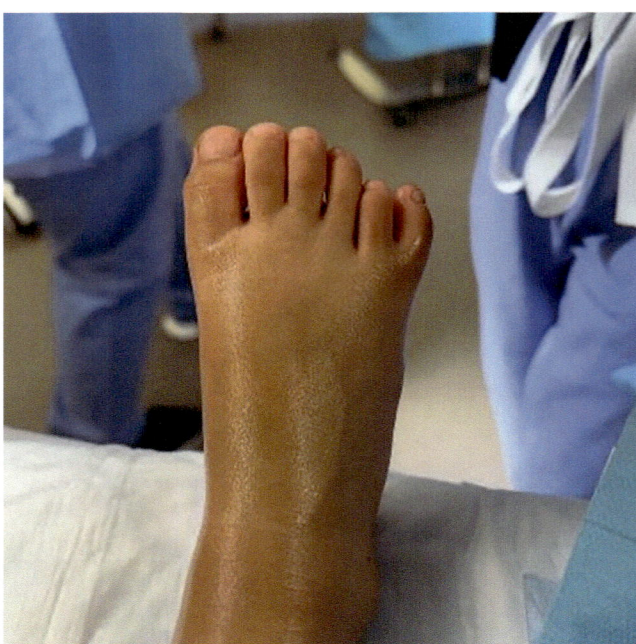

Fig. 16.8 Postaxial polydactyly

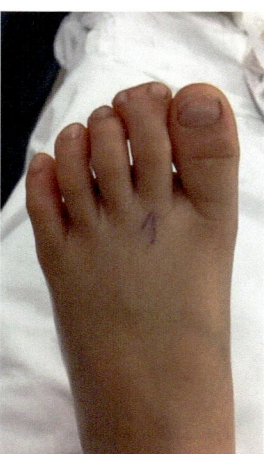

Fig. 16.9 Polydactyly

dure in need of anesthesia within this timeframe. If any of the soft cartilaginous structures are left behind and growth continues, it may require a subsequent surgery.
- Radiographic evaluation is key in determining which digit or portion of the ray should be removed. Often the goal is to preserve the most normal appearing toe. The most normal appearing toe is not always the most lateral or medial toe.
- One should be cautious using buried surgical suture knots in this location since there is a risk of developing suture abscesses (Figs. 16.8 and 16.9).

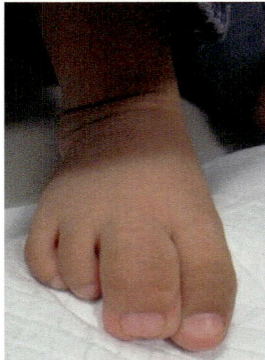

Fig. 16.10 Syndactyly in the absence of polydactyly

Syndactyly

Syndactyly of toes is a common inherited condition in which there is cutaneous webbing. The webbing may be complete or incomplete in nature. Quite often the second and third toes are conjoined. While this condition often causes parental anxiety and a consultation, the child often remains asymptomatic. For this reason, the authors do not advise desyndactylization unless pain and/or functional deficit exists secondary to the syndactyly of the digits (Fig. 16.10).

Syndactyly can be classified into two types. Type 1 (Zygosyndactyly) is a cutaneous webbing only. This condition is likely to not cause any shoe fitting problems or functional deficits. As for Type 2 (Polysyndactyly) is a more complex anatomical finding resulting from failure of differentiation of the apical ectodermal ridge during the first trimester [14]. The fourth and fifth toes are often conjoined with a postaxial duplicated fifth toe. The child often has a duplicated nail plate as well. This may cause some symptoms in children. With growth, some children do experience pain with shoes due to the increased width of the foot. The duplicated nail plate (synonychia) can also become inflamed causing pain or infections in young children. With symptomatic polysyndactyly the duplicated toe and/or ray is removed. It is important to educate parents that simple webbing of lesser digits is often not associated with functional deficits.

Macrodactyly

Macrodactyly is a rare congenital deformity of the hands and feet characterized by the enlargement of soft tissue and osseous elements of the digit [15]. The condition may occur as part of a syndrome, such as Klippel–Trenaunay–Weber, proteus, neurofibromatosis, or as an isolated phenomenon [16]. The etiology of the deformity is unknown, though some

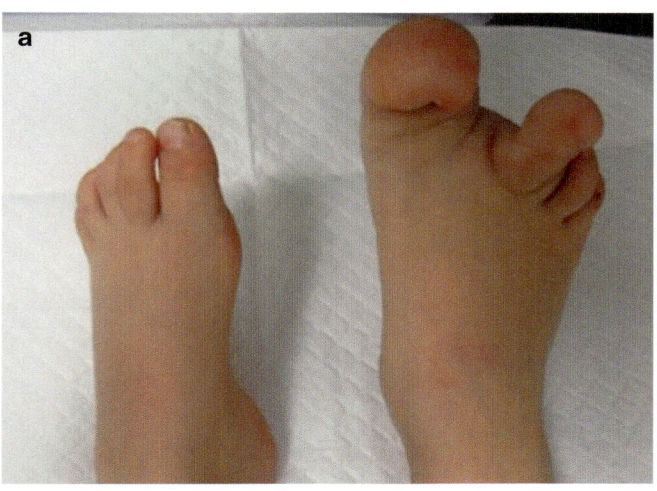 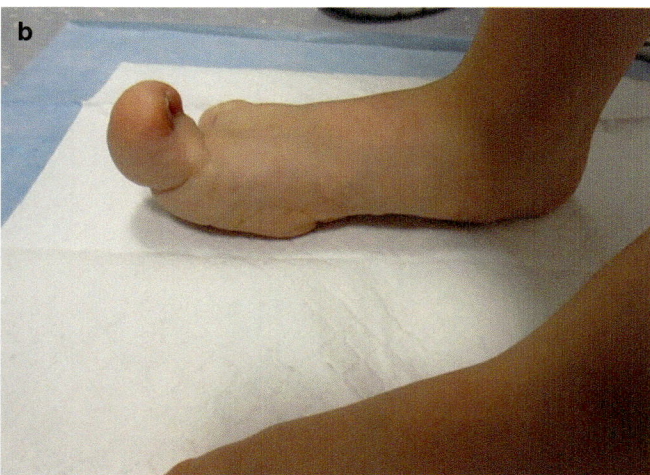

Fig. 16.11 (**a** and **b**) Macrodactyly

studies implicate hyperinduction of a neurotrophic mechanism responsible for normal pedal growth [17]. Slight male predilection has been noted [18]. Second and third digits are affected most often [18]. The enlargement of the bony phalanges and accumulation of the fibrofatty tissue defines the deformity (Fig. 16.11).

Two forms of the deformity exist. In the first, the toes are enlarged in proportion to a hypertrophied foot while the other presents with toes enlarged as compared to the rest of the foot. The amount of soft tissue involvement may be monitored via the metatarsal spread angle. The axes of the first and fifth metatarsals on an anteroposterior (AP) X-ray form this angle [19]. This angle may be compared to the contralateral foot. Shoe fitting problems can exist for both forms of macrodactyly and unfortunately obtaining a cosmetically acceptable foot is very challenging. Quite often this cannot be obtained, and functional partial foot amputations are most helpful.

Surgical options are utilized to promote improved function and to reduce pain. Reconstruction can be achieved by epiphysiodesis, amputation, resection of phalanges, or partial ray resections [20]. Debulking procedures may be used in conjunction with the above but it is often not helpful when performed alone. Parents must be educated that many of these procedures rely on the child's available growth for the unaffected toes and structures to obtain further length and size. While length may be affected with epiphysiodesis, the girth of the toe will likely remain enlarged.

Varus Fifth Toe

A varus fifth toe is present at birth and likely attributed to genetics. The fifth toe is noted to be overlapping the fourth toe in a dorsiflexed and adducted manner. The toenail itself is more laterally deviated and can remain a source of irritation in shoes. The authors find this deformity to be often bilateral in presentation and one in which treatment is surgical [21, 22] (Fig. 16.12).

For children under the age of 2, manipulation and gentle stretching may be utilized but has not proven to be successful at long-term deformity reduction. The authors have used casting to reduce this deformity in infants with good success. Plaster is used and must be molded to plantarflex the toe at the level of the metatarsophalangeal joint. Children over the age of 2 that have pain or shoe complaints associated with this deformity may progress toward surgery. Many children do require surgery given the challenges of shoe wear with this deformity and the time of initial presentation. The Butler procedure is most typically utilized. A racquet-shaped incision is fashioned to allow for circumferential release. The extensor tendon and entire dorsal metatarsophalangeal capsule is released. Vasospasm and vascular compromise can take place. Cooling techniques should be avoided postoperatively. Many children are placed into short leg casts if ambulatory to offload and maintain sterility.

Longitudinal Epiphyseal Bracket

A longitudinal epiphyseal bracket is a congenital condition in which the epiphysis is continuous from distal to proximal along often the medial aspect of the phalanx or first metatarsal. Historically, this condition was termed a delta phalanx for its U configuration and abnormal growth [23]. Growth of the abnormal epiphysis leads to a shortened, wide, and often triangular or trapezoidal bone. The etiology is not completely understood but thought to be a failure of proper fetal forma-

Fig. 16.12 (a and b) Varus fifth toe

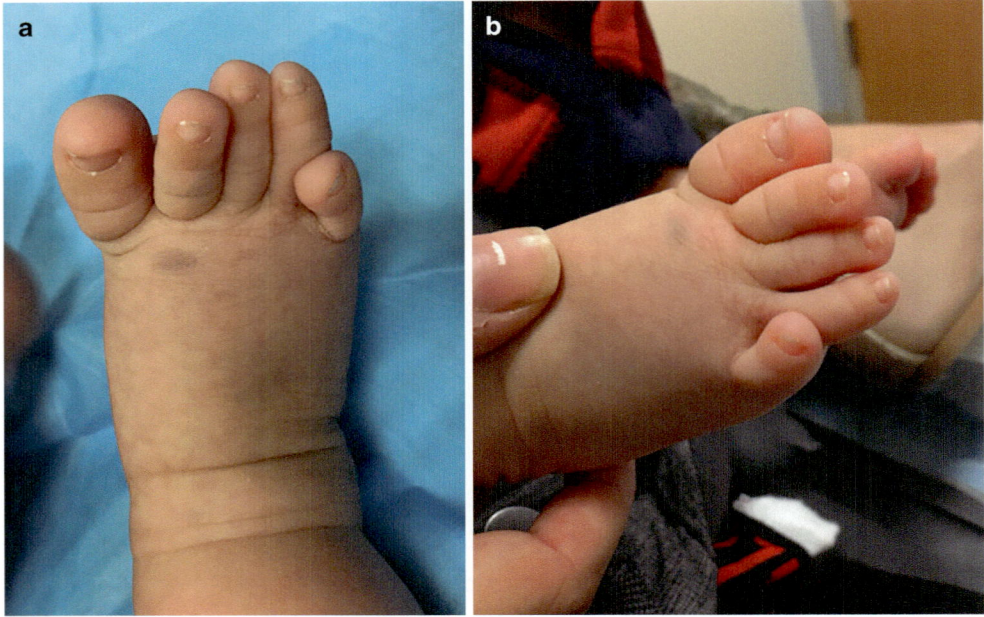

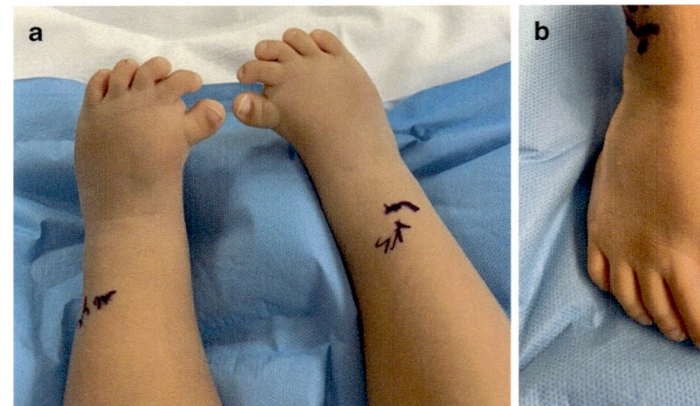
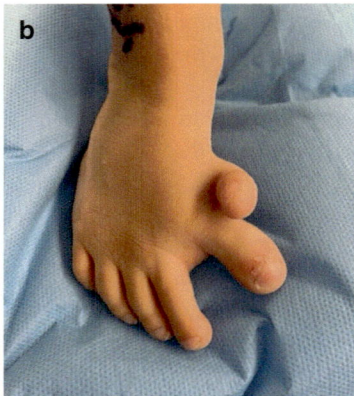
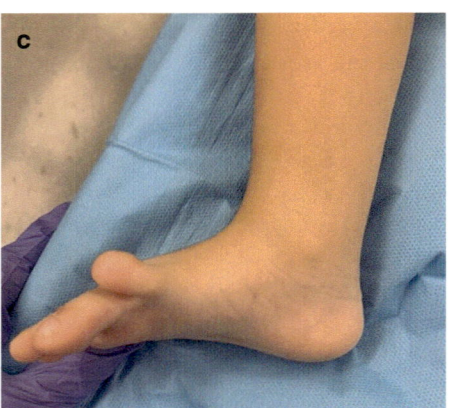

Fig. 16.13 (a–c) Longitudinal Epiphyseal Brackets

tion of the primary ossification centers from the apical ectodermal ridge [24, 25]. Many children present with coexisting deformities such as polydactyly, syndactyly, or coalitions. Others may present with Apert's syndrome. An MRI can help confirm the presence of a longitudinal epiphyseal bracket and its anatomic location (Fig. 16.13).

Longitudinal Epiphyseal Bracket Surgery Pearls

- Treatment is surgical often between 12–24 months of age.
- In infants the deformity may not be seen on X-rays, but it will be visible on MRI [26].
- Surgery: At a minimum, the abnormal longitudinal section of the epiphysis is resected. Smooth wires can be used to preserve the transverse extensions of the epiphysis proximally and distally during resection. One can interpose polymethylmethacrylate or fat. The authors believe it is important to achieve a complete resection of the longitudinal portion. An osteotomy with bone graft of the affected bone to assist with length and angular deformity can be utilized. Pinning of the first metatarsophalangeal joint and across the graft inserted into the first metatarsal is often performed with removal at 6 weeks.
- Mubarak et al. demonstrated improved longitudinal growth in the first metatarsal after surgery [26] (Fig. 16.14).

Longitudinal Epiphyseal Bracket Pitfalls

- Inappropriate graft positioning may lead to deformity often in the form of a plantarflexed or dorsiflexed metatarsal.
- Angular deformity of the metatarsal phalangeal joint can occur.
- Look for coexisting deformities such as polydactyly, syndactyly, and tarsal coalitions.

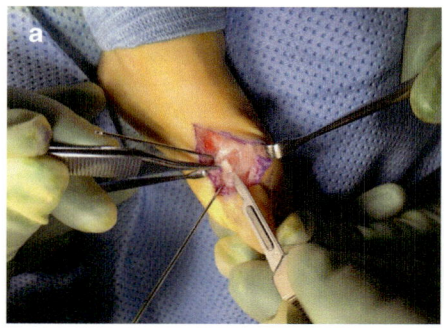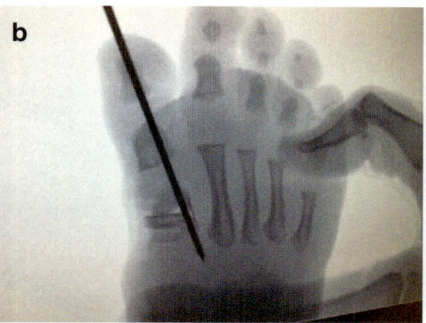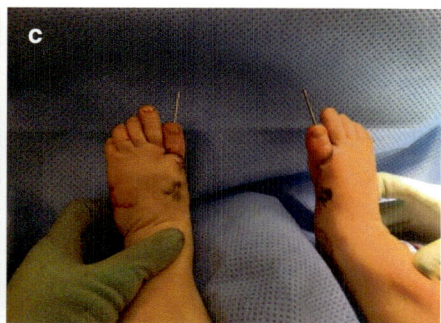

Fig. 16.14 (**a**) Surgical excision of longitudinal epiphyseal bracket. (**b**) AP radiograph demonstrating k wire fixation with graft placement post resection. (**c**) Clinical post operative photo

Subungual Exostosis

Subungual exostosis is a benign bone growth deep to the nail, which causes pain and toenail dystrophy. At times the nail becomes so traumatized by the bone growth that it falls off and the bone growth becomes visually apparent. Bone growth tends to involve the dorsomedial aspect of the distal phalanx with the hallux most typically affected [27].

Symptoms often include pain and toenail irritation leading to surgical excision. As this condition progresses, one may lose complete soft tissue or nail bed coverage of the exostosis, which makes surgical coverage of the distal phalanx difficult in nature. In many instances, the child must heal secondarily and granulate over the phalanx. Treatment is toenail removal with excision of the abnormal bone growth and repair of available nail bed. Recurrence risks are higher if the exostosis is not fully resected initially. The exostosis is essentially an osteochondroma and consists of trabecular bone capped by fibrocartilage.

Subungual Exostosis Pearls

- An Osteochondroma is capped with hyaline cartilage [28].
- Osteochondromas are the most common bone tumor of the foot [28].
- Saucerization: use of a high-speed burr to saucerize the cancellous bone following excision of the abnormal bone growth is advised.

Metatarsus Adductus

Any deformity that is associated with intoeing tends to cause concern and fear among parents. Many parents note a visual deformity of the foot at birth yet quite often flexible metatarsus adductus is overlooked. Upon inspection, metatarsus adductus produces medial deviation of metatarsals at the level of the tarsometatarsal joint. The infant's foot may appear to have a slightly higher arch with a valgus rearfoot and medially deviated metatarsals. Equinus is not present.

In a screening of 2401 neonates, Widhe and associates noted foot abnormalities in 4% of infants, with 1% having metatarsus adductus [29]. Around 0.7% of infants had calcaneovalgus. Wynne-Davies found an incidence of metatarsus adductus of 1 in 1000 births and reported that if 1 child were affected, the risk of deformity in a second child in the same family was 1 in 20 [29]. This alludes to a genetic component while etiology is not completely understood (Fig. 16.15).

It is important to distinguish metatarsus adductus from clubfoot. Equinus and varus of the heel do not exist with metatarsus adductus. Whereas Ponseti casting is employed for clubfoot regardless of the degree of stiffness, one must closely evaluate degree of flexibility of metatarsus adductus to determine treatment. If the deformity is flexible hence easily reducible one may closely monitor. This flexible type may reduce when the foot is stimulated into active eversion. Often these deformities will resolve gradually. Parents may be reassured and educated on how to gently stretch the foot.

There is debate over the semi-rigid metatarsus adductus foot deformity. Many physicians do not advocate for casting this group while others will cast to reduce the deformity. Braces utilized at night often follow casting. If the foot type is rigid and the deformity cannot be reduced, then casting is advised to assist with serial correction over time. Still this diagnosis always sparks debate over treatment with many questioning how much metatarsus adductus is pathologic as an adult.

In a 7-year follow-up of 130 untreated feet, Rushforth found that 10% had moderate deformity but were asymptomatic and that only 4% had residual deformity and stiffness

Fig. 16.15 (a and b) Flexible metatarsus adductus

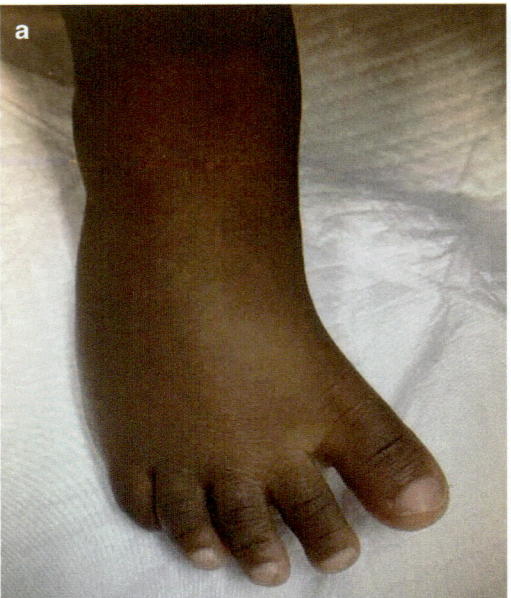
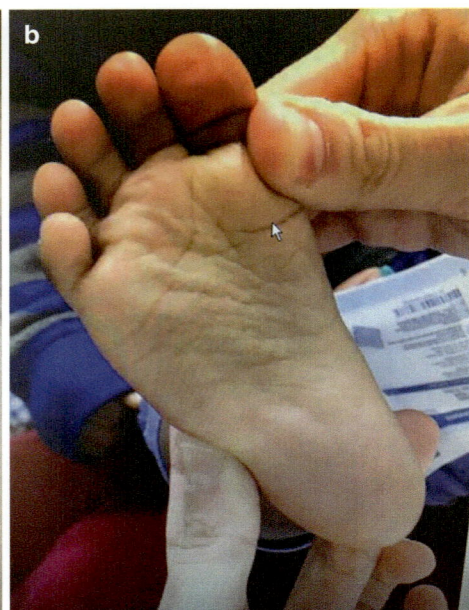

[30]. Long-term research would be beneficial in furthering our knowledge on this deformity and its effects into adulthood.

Proper manipulation of the deformity is key in creating a supple rectus foot. The correct manipulation is to hold the heel in neutral position while the forefoot is abducted. Counter pressure is applied to the calcaneocuboid joint, so the abduction occurs at the level of the tarsometatarsal complex. This is the same gentle stretch that parents may perform at home. The authors often encourage stretching with diaper changes, if advised. For the flexible and easily reducible deformity, one does not have to cast as this often improves with time. With semi-rigid and rigid metatarsus adductus, the authors recommend casting to gently manipulate the foot into a more corrected position. Care should be taken to not evert the forefoot when casting. Use of long leg casts with the knee flexed will minimize slippage. In older children between 6 months and 3 years of age, one may also utilize casting to minimize the deformity.

If the foot is resistant to casting and the deformity remains severe, then surgical intervention is an option. Often this rigid foot type has a significant medial crease and overactive abductor hallucis. Hence, surgical intervention includes release of the abductor hallucis, capsulotomy of the first tarsometatarsal joint, and serial cast correction [31]. The authors find these soft tissue procedures to be more typically executed between 2.5–4 years of age. Osseous procedures are often reserved for children near 8 years of age or older while this is not absolute. This often includes either midfoot osteotomies or metatarsal osteotomies with or without soft tissue release. Surgery is dependent on severity of angular deformity, stiffness of deformity, and functional deficit.

Metatarsus Adductus Pearls

- Long leg casting as described by Dr. Ponseti for metatarsus adductus.
- After casting, a shoe and bar brace is worn at nighttime until 2 years of age.
- Flexible deformity: monitor and instruct parents on stretching maneuvers.
- Semi-Rigid/ Rigid deformity: serial casting advised followed by shoe and bar brace for sleep until 2 years of age.
- Various casting materials may be utilized but plaster provides a better mold than fiberglass.
- Maneuver: hold the heel in neutral, apply counter pressure to the cuboid and abduct the forefoot.
- 2.5–4 y/o children who fail casting: consider abductor hallucis release, capsulotomy of the first tarsometatarsal joint and subsequent casting.
- Older children: may consider tarsometatarsal capsulotomies, metatarsal osteotomies, or opening wedge osteotomy of the medial cuneiform/closing osteotomy of cuboid.
- It is important to perform a hip exam and confirm that the hip is not dislocatable or dislocated. In the presence of metatarsus adductus and breech position, a hip ultrasound can be helpful in excluding infant hip pathology.

Metatarsus Adductus Pitfalls

- Eversion of the forefoot can cause unwanted deformity. Care should be taken to use the cuboid or CC joint as the fulcrum. If the talus is used, this also results in excessive hindfoot valgus.

- It is important to differentiate from congenital skewfoot.
- We do not fully understand the absolute degree of metatarsus adductus that is pathologic in adulthood.

Brachymetatarsia

Brachymetatarsia can be defined by the presence of an unusually shortened metatarsal. This is a congenital deformity, which does not always manifest in pain. Many patients present because the appearance of the short toe(s) is cosmetically unappealing. It is important that the clinician discerns which patients truly have pain or lesser metatarsalgia as compared to others with asymptomatic cosmetic complaints. While cosmesis may be a reason for surgery, the expectations of the patient should be addressed preoperatively. Risks of tissue necrosis, vasospasm, floating toe syndrome, and/or pain do exist.

Pathologic brachymetatarsia often presents as pain plantar to the adjacent metatarsal heads rather than the plantar aspect of the shortened metatarsal itself. The fourth metatarsal is often the shortened metatarsal with pain beneath the third and or fifth metatarsal heads. One may note a subluxation of the metatarsal phalangeal joint hence a floating toe. Of surgical note, the length of the shortened metatarsal needed to restore a more normal parabola must be assessed.

Conservative care includes rigid supportive shoes complimented by custom orthoses to offload the metatarsal heads. Beyond this, there is not a plethora of options outside of surgical intervention. Surgery is dependent on the length of the metatarsal needed to restore the metatarsal parabola. Compliance also plays a special role with these surgical candidates especially when external fixation is considered.

When 1–1.5 cm of length is needed, one may consider a one-stage procedure in which an osteotomy of the metatarsal is fashioned, and a graft is inserted. Structural allograft or autograft may be utilized. One should gradually distract the osteotomy prior to graft placement in the operating room with a deflated tourniquet. Stable internal fixation is utilized to secure the graft in place. The patient is non-weightbearing for 6 weeks. When more length is desired, callus distraction and use of external fixation are executed. Two half pins proximal to the osteotomy, 2 half metatarsal pins distal to the osteotomy, and 2 half pins in the proximal phalanx can assist with stabilization and purchase of the toe. This concept of bridging the adjacent joint helps control toe position and prevent compression of the metatarsophalangeal joint. The patient must be compliant and understand the directions with callus distraction to minimize a subsequent deformity.

The principles of callus distraction are key. Two pins are inserted on either side of the osteotomy. A pin guide and or the external fixator frame may be utilized. The osteotomy is performed in the proximal metaphysis of the shortened metatarsal. If the osteotomy is performed in the proximal metaphysis, distraction is typically started at approximately 7 days by use of a monorail. The rate and amount of distraction has been debated. Still the rate of 0.25 mm every 6 h for a total of 1 mm a day has shown to produce predictable bone remodeling. Some will start with a lower rate and alter such according to radiographic response. Histologic repair is ongoing and should not be stopped despite the radiographic lucency that often appears. One should continue with callus distraction until the desired length is achieved. The external fixator is left intact until osseous consolidation, which may be the time equivalent it took to obtain length. Hence, if it took 4 weeks to obtain length, the external fixator may be needed for a total length of 8 weeks. The authors find the external fixator frame is needed for a minimum of 4 weeks following desirable length.

Brachymetatarsia Surgery Pearls

- Callus distraction facilitates gradual lengthening of bone and provides sufficient time for the soft tissue to adapt.
- Place pins prior to osteotomy. Pins should be bicortical orthogonal to the plantar surface and parallel to one another. Use the external fixator as a guide for proper placement to avoid angulation. The latent period is generally 7 days prior to distraction.
- Turn 0.25 mm every 6 h/day to equal 1 mm/day.
- Smaller frequent turning intervals result in efficient osteogenesis.
- The osteotomy should be perpendicular to the metatarsal. Authors perform the osteotomy via drill holes followed by an osteotome. One must minimize osteonecrosis by irrigating to reduce heat from instrumentation.
- Pins attached to the external fixator, or a K-wire may be utilized in the digit itself to alter alignment.

Brachymetatarsia Pitfalls

- Overlengthening of the metatarsal results in dislocation of the metatarsal phalangeal joint.
- Necrosis, ulceration, vasospasm, ischemic changes, and loss of toe remain risks of surgery.
- Angular deformities may occur secondary to poor pin placement or osteotomy.
- Patients may be displeased with surgical outcome, as the phalanx may still appear short despite surgical lengthening of the metatarsal. It is important to address expectations of the patient prior to any surgical intervention.

Vertical Talus

Much like talipes equinovarus (clubfoot), congenital vertical talus (CVT) has undergone an incredible paradigm shift in treatment. Prior to the Dobbs Method, children who presented with CVT underwent large incisions and surgical releases in the absence of any serial casting. There was no attempt at serial casting or manipulation for this complex deformity. The deformity was thought to be irreducible without surgery. Children presented with various degrees of rigidity, angulation, and at times spasticity often in the setting of secondary neurologic conditions. In 2006, The Dobbs Method was published [32]. This less invasive approach focuses on a dorsolateral thrust upon the medial talar head and relocation of the talonavicular joint [32–35]. It remains key to scrutinize reduction in all planes. The foot is stretched serially into a maximal equinovarus position. Essentially, the final cast should mimic a clubfoot position. Following five weekly casts, children undergo a surgical tenotomy of the Achilles tendon and pinning of the talonavicular joint. Functional outcome scores and maintenance of alignment is noted to be good [35] (Fig. 16.16).

Etiology

In infancy, this rare deformity often resembles calcaneovalgus or a severe planovalgus foot type. Although the exact incidence of vertical talus is unknown, the estimated prevalence is 1 in 10,000 live births [36]. Due to the hindfoot valgus, equinus, and fixed dorsal dislocation of the navicular on the talus, many have referred to this deformity as a rocker-bottom flatfoot. Despite these findings, it is the rigidity of the deformity and true equinus that distinguishes itself from others such as positional calcaneovalgus or oblique talus. A true congenital vertical talus is generally not easily reduced nor passively corrected. The condition is defined by its inability to reduce, or in essence rigidity, along with equinus.

Recognition of this deformity is key as without treatment vertical talus can lead to significant disability with growth and persistence [34]. Without treatment, vertical talus can lead to pain and disability that hampers daily activities. The foot position can also place some children at greater risk for ulceration or a non-braceable foot. Traditional surgical management for vertical talus is extensive and fraught with both short-term and long-term complications. These complications include both under-correction and over-correction of the deformity, scarring, neurovascular injury, infection, wound dehiscence, and the need for multiple surgical procedures during growth. The scar tissue created with extensive soft tissue releases in a child's foot can lead to both stiffness and pain much like the consequences of a surgical clubfoot reconstruction. The Dobbs Method has proved successful in providing correction while avoiding the need for extensive soft tissue release procedures in many children.

In most cases, the etiology of vertical talus deformity remains unknown. Approximately one half of cases of vertical talus occur in conjunction with neurologic disorders [37] or genetic defects [38]. The remaining children present with further congenital anomalies are considered idiopathic or isolated cases [34]. The most common neurologic disorders associated with vertical talus are distal arthrogryposis and myelomeningocele [37]. The most common genetic defects include aneuploidy of chromosomes 13, 15, and 18 [39]. Genetic research has gained insight into pathogenesis with the discovery of mutations in the PITX1-TBX4-HOXC transcriptional pathways and their influence in familial clubfoot and vertical talus in a small number of families [40–42]. Subsequent studies continue to be performed [43]. Finally, of the 50% of cases of vertical talus that are isolated, almost 20% have a positive family history of vertical talus.

In most of the isolated cases, the condition is inherited in an autosomal dominant fashion [42]. This supports the notion that a significant number of isolated cases have a genetic etiology [40]. Still, while no one single gene defect has been held accountable of all cases of vertical talus, its

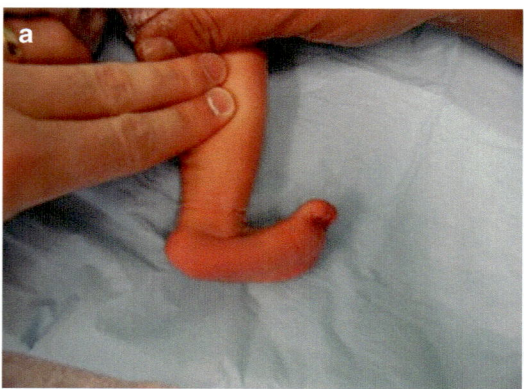 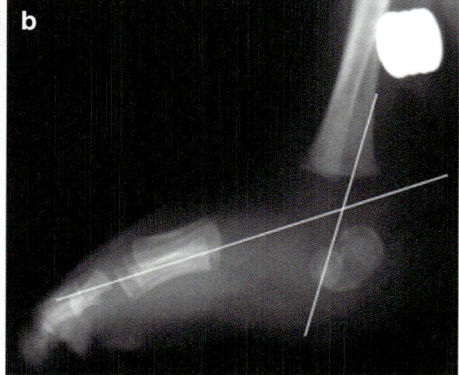

Fig. 16.16 (a) Vertical talus. (b) Vertical talus noted on stress plantarflexion radiograph

etiology is heterogeneous [44]. For example, in patients with myelomeningocele, a weak posterior tibialis muscle with strong ankle dorsiflexors could contribute to the deformity. Weakness of the foot intrinsics may play a role for other children with neurologic influence. Children with abnormal muscle biopsies such as arthrogryposis may be prone to vertical talus, given skeletal muscle abnormalities [38]. Congenital vascular insufficiency of the lower extremities has also been proposed as a potential cause of vertical talus based on magnetic resonance angiography findings that demonstrated congenital arterial deficiencies of the lower extremity in a group of patients with vertical talus [45]. Beyond its etiology, early detection is helpful in reduction of deformity and overall outcomes. Correction prior to the age of 12 months is thought to improve functional outcome scores [35].

Vertical Talus Clinical Features

Hindfoot equinus, hindfoot valgus, forefoot abduction, and forefoot dorsiflexion are present in all patients with vertical talus. The rigidity of the deformities is the key to differentiating vertical talus from the more common and less severe conditions, such as calcaneovalgus foot, posteromedial bowing of the tibia, and oblique talus (without an equinus contracture). If ankle dorsiflexion is not limited, then the deformity does not meet vertical talus criteria. Because of the frequency of neuromuscular and genetic abnormalities associated with vertical talus, it is important to perform a complete and careful physical examination of the entire patient.

Clinically, a congenital vertical talus foot has a convex plantar surface that results in a rocker-bottom appearance. The skin on the dorsum of the foot has a crease secondary to forefoot and midfoot dorsiflexion. The extreme dorsiflexion of the forefoot creates a gap dorsally where the navicular and talar head would articulate in a normal foot. If the gap reduces with plantar flexion of the forefoot, then the deformity has a degree of flexibility and may fall on the spectrum of oblique talus. This is important to assess because even if the talonavicular reduces in plantarflexion indicating an oblique talus, this does not mean that treatment is not needed. In this situation, the examiner must then assess for contracture of the Achilles tendon with the subtalar joint inverted. In our experience, oblique tali in the setting of a contracture of the Achilles tendon need treatment just like true vertical tali.

Vertical Talus Imaging

- *Stress plantarflexion X-ray (standard of care):* In vertical talus, the talus fails to align with the first metatarsal. The talus remains vertical when compared to the first metatarsal. In infancy, the navicular is not visible, therefore, the clinician should focus on the talus with respect to the first metatarsal. An oblique talus or calcaneovalgus will realign or essentially reduce.
- *Neutral lateral X-ray:* in vertical talus, the long axis of the talus is vertical when compared to the first metatarsal. The calcaneus is in equinus.
- *Stress dorsiflexion X-ray:* Persistent rigid hindfoot equinus is noted with vertical talus.

The Dobbs Method

Historically, large releases for this deformity were performed with persistent risks of stiffness, diminished function, and pain. The Dobbs Method is a less invasive approach that relies on serial manipulation and casting. Achieving correction without extensive surgery leads to more functional and flexible feet [38]. With the retracting fibrosis and abundance of collagen that forms, it is advantageous to avoid large releases at an early age and approach reduction from a less invasive standpoint. While most of the deformity correction is the result of manipulation and casting, the child does undergo at least an Achilles tenotomy and talonavicular joint pinning upon reduction.

Following Achilles tenotomy and talonavicular pinning, the foot is casted and monitored closely over the next 6 weeks following surgery. The wire is then removed and the child transitions to a boot and bar brace. The foot is held in a straight position. Boot and bar braces are utilized until the child is 2 years of age. The authors use the Easy Click bar, D Bar Enterprises, as there is no dorsiflexion bend in it unlike the other bars. It is important not to brace in dorsiflexion, as the feet are most tight dorsolateral. Since the introduction of the Dobbs Method in 2006 [32], many subsequent studies have demonstrated its efficacy in achieving initial correction in patients with isolated or nonisolated vertical talus [46–53].

Traditional management involved lengthening the contracted dorsolateral tendons, dorsolateral capsular contractures, and reducing both the talonavicular joint and subtalar joint. Lengthening both the Achilles and peroneals along with performing a posterolateral capsulotomy followed [54]. Many performed all procedures in a single-stage approach [55–60].

To perform this manipulation, the treating provider must have knowledge of the subtalar joint and experience in treating clubfoot with manipulation and casting. The ability to accurately locate the talar head is essential. All components of the deformity are corrected simultaneously except for the hindfoot equinus, which is corrected with release of the Achilles in the operating room.

The Dobbs Methods: Manipulation and Casting

- Manipulations are gentle and consist of stretching the foot into plantarflexion with one hand while counterpressure is applied as the thumb of the opposite hand gently pushes the talus dorsally and laterally (from the medial side of foot).
- Do not touch the calcaneus. The calcaneus needs to glide smoothly beneath the talus from its valgus position.
- After 1–2 min of manipulation, a long leg plaster cast is applied to hold the foot into this manipulated position. The cast is applied in two sections, with the short leg portion applied first. This allows for an appropriate mold of the foot.
- The foot should be held in position achieved by stretching while an assistant rolls the plaster.
- Mold carefully around the talar head, malleoli, and above the calcaneus posteriorly.
- Remove excess plaster dorsally to expose the toes.
- The cast is then extended above the knee with knee in 90° of flexion.
- Weekly casting is advised. An average of 5 casts is utilized to reduce the deformity. Hindfoot equinus still persists. In the final cast, the foot resembles a clubfoot. It is critical to achieve a maximal equinovarus position. This is analogous to achieving 70° of external rotation in a final clubfoot cast.
- When reduction of the talonavicular and calcaneocuboid joints is achieved, the child is scheduled for surgery. More may need to be performed in the operating room if the deformity cannot be fully corrected following 5 casts.

The Surgical Portion of The Dobbs Method

- Serial manipulation and casting are performed to improve the talonavicular and hindfoot alignment as described in the Dobbs Method for manipulation and casting.
- Surgery is performed in the operating room with full intention of performing a percutaneous Achilles tenotomy and talonavicular joint pinning.
- A complete Achilles tenotomy is performed. When performed first, this allows for the surgeon to fully stretch the joint capsules. This stretch is maintained for a few minutes prior to any pinning. Historically, when the Achilles tenotomy was performed in the office, possible future intention of talonavicular pinning subluxation was noted.
- When reduction of the medial column is achieved, a small dorsal medial incision is fashioned over the talonavicular joint. The surgeon confirms reduction of talonavicular joint. As the surgeon becomes more familiar with casting and manipulation, this incision may not be needed any further.
- If the joint is not completely reduced, a small capsulotomy is made in the anterior subtalar joint region to allow an elevator to be placed. This assists with talonavicular reduction. At times, some children with syndromes and or neurologic influence may require a vertical incision between the Extensor Hallucis Longus tendon and Extensor Digitorum Longus tendon to perform a sequential release: Dorsal lateral ankle and subtalar joint capsulotomy, calcaneocuboid capsulotomy, and tarsometatarsal capsulotomy. The extensors may be cut in children with functional deficit.
- A K-wire is placed from distal to proximal across the talonavicular joint. Central positioning of the 0.062 k wire in younger children and 2.0 pin in older children is utilized.
- The pin is distally inserted between the first and second metatarsal to capture the first metatarsal base, cuneiform, navicular, and talus. One's hand must be dropped down to capture these structures.
- The pin is often buried to minimize migration in young children.
- A long leg cast is applied with the ankle and foot in neutral position (foot is perpendicular to the lower leg).
- The cast is changed 2 weeks post-surgery to manipulate the ankle to 10° of dorsiflexion. This cast is left intact until 6 weeks following surgery.
- The K-wire is removed in the operating room at 6 weeks post-surgery. A final cast is applied for 1 week followed by boot and bar brace system 23-hours/day for 3 months. The child then wears the boot and bar system at night until 2 years of age. The boots are pointed straight ahead. Do not place a dorsiflexion bend in the bar.
- It is important to stretch the foot into plantarflexion and adduction.
- The authors use the Dobbs Easy Click bar. Some research has been performed with other bars [61].
- Not only should the talonavicular joint be reduced on the lateral radiograph but also on the anteroposterior view (Fig. 16.17).

Calcaneovalgus

Severe calcaneovalgus foot deformity is a deformity in which the foot is hyperdorsiflexed and often abutting the anterior aspect of the tibia. The forefoot is abducted with marked heel valgus. Plantarflexion is often restricted and limited to a neutral position. While parents may be very concerned about the appearance of this deformity, it often improves on its own. Most calcaneovalgus deformities will improve by 6–12 months of age without intervention. Caregivers can assist with gentle manipulations emphasizing plantarflexion

Fig. 16.17 (**a**) Lateral view status post the Dobbs Method. (**b**) AP view post the Dobbs method. (**c**) Lateral aspect of foot post pin removal. (**d**) AP view post pin removal

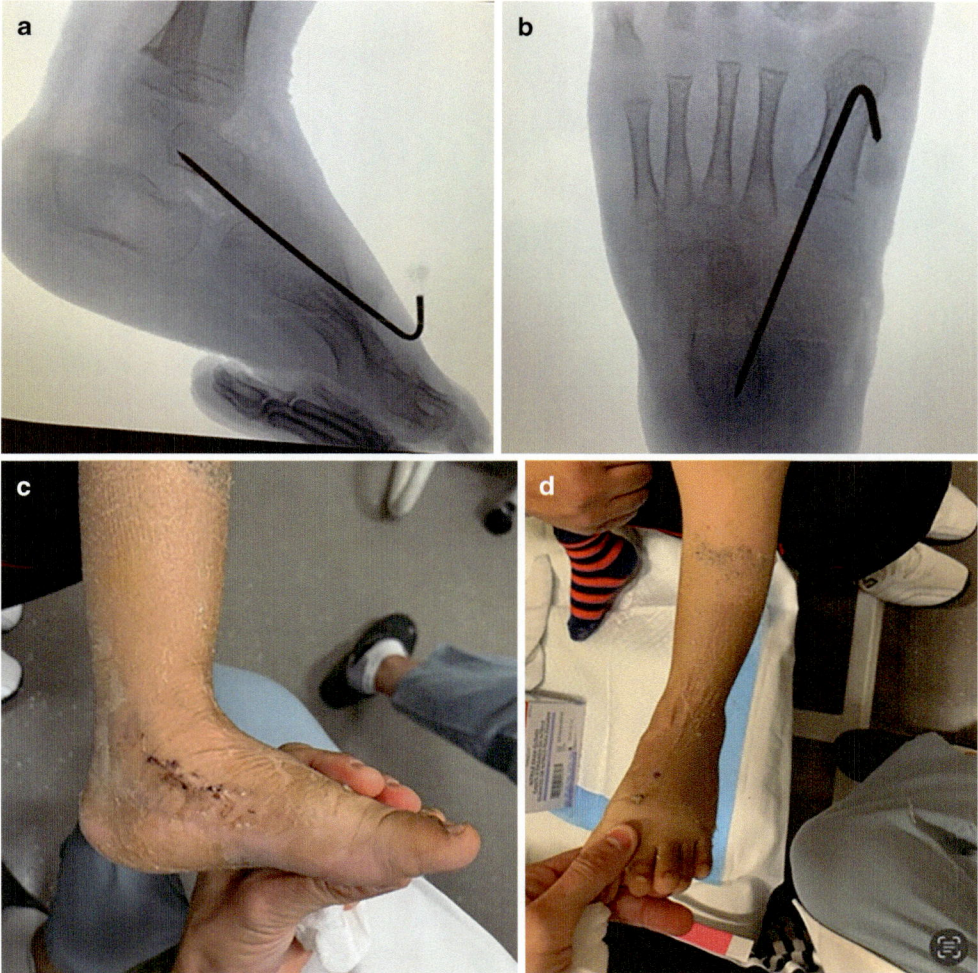

at the level of the ankle. Gentle inversion and adduction can also be helpful based on the deformity.

While calcaneovalgus most typically improves on its own, it is more important to exclude deformities associated with abnormal packing in utero such as hip dysplasia or posteromedial bowing of the tibia. It is important to recognize that the initial infant's hip exam may be normal while there is a greater association of hip dysplasia in children who have calcaneovalgus on one foot and metatarsus adductus on the contralateral foot. Advanced imaging in the form of ultrasound or X-rays, based on the child 's age, can be helpful in excluding a silent hip dysplasia.

One will note the calcaneus to be in equinus in vertical talus whereas the heel is easily palpable, void of equinus, and in a dorsiflexed position with calcaneovalgus. Stress plantarflexion radiographs are most helpful in distinguishing between the two deformities. In congenital vertical talus, the talus will not align with the first metatarsal while the deformity will reduce with calcaneovalgus (Fig. 16.18).

Generally, this deformity will improve in the first 6–12 months of life. Still given the small number of children that have persistent valgus deformities beyond this age group, casting can be utilized to assist with reduction of the deformity during the timeframe in which a child is not ambulatory. Bracing and manipulations for the more severe cases can follow serial casting. There is definite variation among clinicians with regards to casting, treatment modalities, and plan of care. For residual calcaneovalgus deformities that persist beyond 12 months, it is prudent to exclude any neurologic influence.

Oblique Talus

Oblique talus is less understood as compared to vertical talus. Oblique talus is noted by a talus that aligns well with the first metatarsal on a lateral radiograph. Some subsets of such will present with equinus. Equinus is diagnosed by inverting the subtalar joint while dorsiflexing at the level of the ankle joint. An inability to dorsiflex the ankle beyond perpendicular indicates equinus. The authors treat oblique talus with equinus via The Dobbs Method. These children

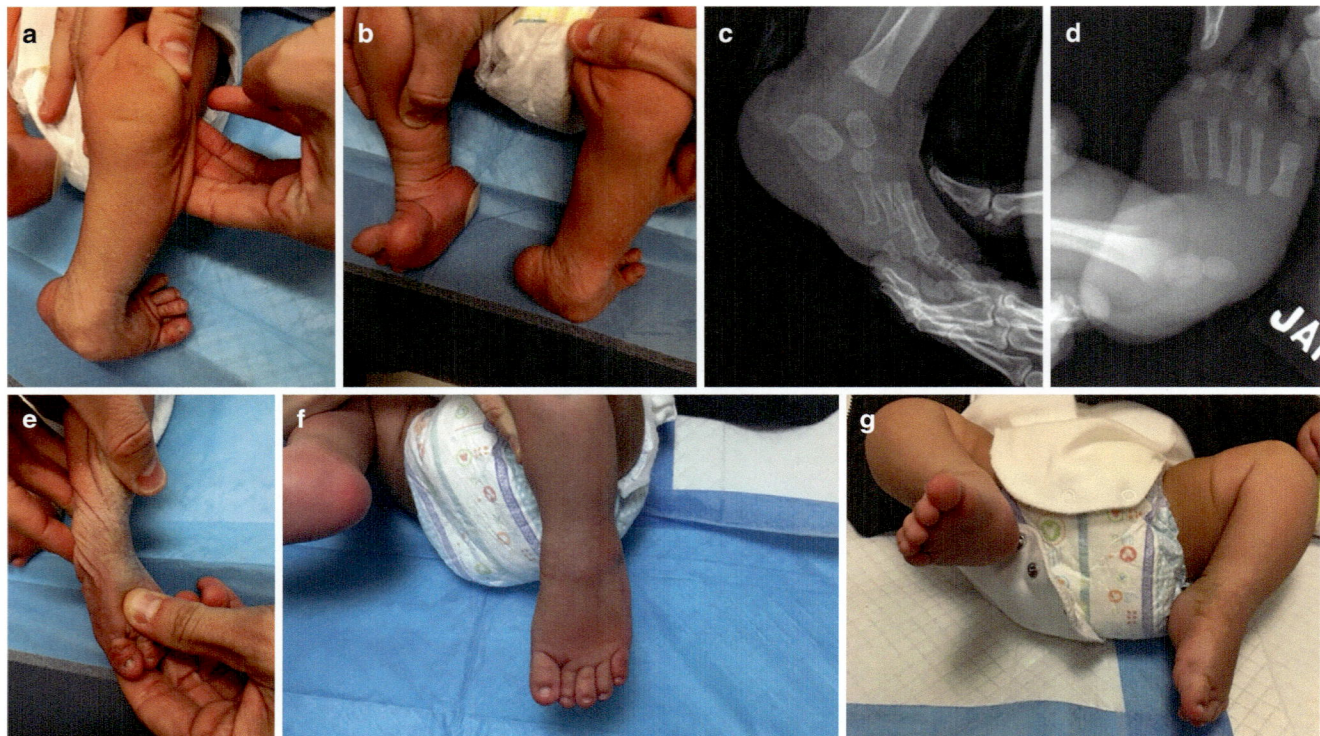

Fig. 16.18 (a) Calcaneovalgus in 1-week-old male. (b) Clubfoot right and calcaneovalgus left. (c) Stress plantarflexion radiograph demonstrating aligned talus and first metatarsal. (d) AP X-ray of calcaneovalgus. (e) Clinical manipulation of deformity. (f) After serial casting for calcaneovalgus. (g) post serial casting

often require two to three casts prior to surgical tenotomy of the Achilles and pinning of the talonavicular joint. Recognition of such deformity in infancy may reduce the risks for osseous procedures and symptomatic valgus feet with growth.

Tarsal Coalitions and Flatfoot Deformities

Despite the overall prevalence of tarsal coalitions being 1% to 2%, they appear frequently in high-volume pediatric foot and ankle clinics. Quite often this condition can be found in young patients presenting with pediatric pes valgus but they are not limited to this foot type alone. Likewise, many patients, prior to diagnosis, present with injuries, pain, stiffness, or flatfeet. Coalitions are unusual unions between foot bones that can restrict motion and cause adaptive arthritic changes to surrounding joints. The condition is due to a failure of segmentation of the primitive mesenchyme during development [62].

It is important to recognize that children may have more than one coalition present even in the same foot given the underlying developmental cause for this condition. Therefore, it is important to review all radiographic views and or advanced imaging studies. While coalitions can affect any joint, the most common tarsal coalitions of the foot include calcaneonavicular coalitions, middle facet talocalcaneal coalitions, and talonavicular coalitions in that order. Bilaterality has been reported in 50% of patients with talocalcaneal coalitions.

Physical Exam

Pediatric patients can present with various positional deformities in association with coalitions, yet the pronated flatfoot tends to be most common. Often when compared to an unaffected side, the foot will feel stiffer with limited subtalar joint motion. The patient often describes this stiffness as a "locked up" sensation when participating in pivoting activities. In the presence of a flatfoot, the deformity is often not reducible as compared to a pediatric pes planovalgus foot without a coalition. Pain often exists along the dorsal lateral aspect of the foot in the presence of calcaneonavicular coalition. A double medial malleolus sign or prominence inferior to the medial malleolus is typically present with talocalcaneal coalitions. The timing of symptoms tend to correspond with ossification of the tarsal bones [63].

Imaging and Diagnostic Studies

These images are utilized on patients with stiffness and/or pain of the foot when evaluating for tarsal coalitions. Bilateral X-rays are often helpful for comparison.

- Weightbearing anteroposterior bilateral foot X-rays.
- Weightbearing lateral bilateral foot X-rays.
- 45° internal oblique X-ray bilateral (detects calcaneonavicular coalitions).
- Harris and Beath bilateral X-rays (detects talocalcaneal coalitions).
- Hind foot alignment X-rays bilateral.

There are several radiographic signs often associated with coalitions; however, they are not specific to coalitions. Moraleda and Mubarak reviewed the prevalence of the C sign on lateral weightbearing X-rays and its association to talocalcaneal coalitions. In this study, a complete C sign was noted in 15% of talocalcaneal coalitions [64]. An interrupted C sign was present in 77% of talocalcaneal coalitions while also present in 45% of flexible pediatric flatfeet without a coalition [64]. Talar beaking may also be noted on the lateral radiograph with talocalcaneal coalitions while it is not exclusive to such deformity. As for calcaneonavicular coalitions, an anteater sign or elongated anterior process is often visualized on the lateral radiograph.

A CT scan is helpful in evaluating coalitions and joint involvement. Rozansky and colleagues described a radiologic classification of talocalcaneal coalitions [65]. This classification was based on the CT 3D reconstruction and remains very helpful in both the anatomic assessment of talocalcaneal coalitions and surgical planning. Long-term studies on prognosis are needed specifically following the middle facet coalition as compared to a more posteriorly deviated subtalar joint coalition.

While there is little controversy over the diagnosis of a tarsal coalition, the treatment modalities do vary especially with respect to talocalcaneal coalitions. The debate regarding the variation of surgical options lies in the decision to resect alone versus resection with realignment procedures, realignment alone, or the use of fusion and realignment procedures. There is also debate over the arthrodesis guidelines. In 1994, Wilde and colleagues reviewed their results from treating talocalcaneal coalitions and found unsatisfactory results in feet with a CT scan showing a relative coalition area greater than 50% [66]. In this study, patients had more than 16° of heel valgus, narrowing of the posterior talocalcaneal joint, and impingement of the lateral talar process on the calcaneus. Talar beaking was noted to be more of a traction spur and present in 33% of feet with a relative coalition size greater than 50% and in 70% of feet with smaller coalitions. They recommended arthrodesis as a result for patients in which the talocalcaneal coalition involved more than 50% of the joint [66].

Luhmann and Schoenecker reviewed results from 25 symptomatic talocalcaneal coalitions [67]. They recommended that all pediatric symptomatic talocalcaneal coalitions that failed nonoperative treatment and did not have an arthritic hindfoot be treated with resection as opposed to arthrodesis. They further reported satisfactory results in patients with greater than 50% joint involvement and greater than 21° of hindfoot valgus. The valgus of the heel was addressed post resection with an orthotic or surgical calcaneal osteotomy or lateral column lengthening procedure [67]. Arthrodesis was reserved for patients that failed the above and/or developed an arthritic hindfoot.

Mosca and colleagues reviewed 13 symptomatic talocalcaneal coalitions and concluded that a calcaneal lengthening osteotomy is a good alternative to triple arthrodesis for a painful foot with significant hind foot valgus and an unresectable solid talocalcaneal tarsal coalition [68]. Gantsoudes and colleagues found excision of the coalition to improve motion is the best solution to minimize impending pathology and alleviate pain. They also determined that correction of the preoperative valgus deformity could be necessary as a secondary procedure with good results in pain reduction [69].

As noted, there is variation to the surgical management of talocalcaneal coalitions. Literature supports multiple treatment pathways from a resection versus arthrodesis standpoint. Likewise, there is support from a staged resection standpoint followed by orthoses versus resection of coalition with realignment procedures. One should think of the coalition and valgus position as two separate deformities. In the younger population, restoring some motion can be helpful as the child develops. Evaluating the child for excessive hind foot valgus and or peri-talar subluxation should assist the surgeon in offering realignment procedures. In the presence of degenerative joint changes, arthrodesis should be considered (Fig. 16.19).

Authors Preferred Treatment

1. Resection of calcaneonavicular coalitions with or without fat graft interposition is performed.
2. Resection of talocalcaneal coalitions with fat graft interposition in skeletally immature patients with no severe valgus deformity is performed. This is complimented with orthoses if there is a mild valgus deformity.
3. Patients with a significant valgus deformity and/or peritalar subluxation undergo talocalcaneal coalition resection with fat graft interposition. In the absence of severe degenerative joint changes or severe valgus angulation,

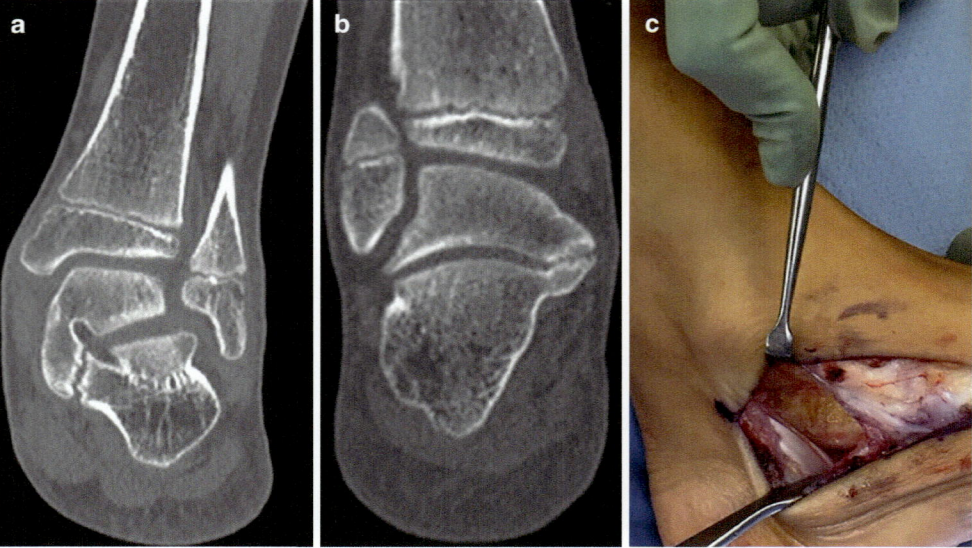

Fig. 16.19 (a) CT scan showing middle facet coalition with hindfoot valgus. (b) CT scan showing middle facet coalition fairly rectus. (c) Intraoperative talocalcaneal middle facet coalition

realignment procedures are often staged to promote motion and minimize recurrence of coalition. In 6–12 months, children are offered realignment procedures based on the deformity, if persistent symptoms. Often additional procedures performed include a gastrocnemius recession, calcaneal lengthening osteotomy, and possible medial cuneiform osteotomy. Some children do undergo both resection and realignment in one stage if the valgus is grossly pathologic. The authors pay close attention to peri-talar subluxation, hindfoot valgus, valgus ankle presence, and the role of equinus.

4. Arthrodesis procedures are offered to older patients with degenerative joint changes or patients who have failed resection with or without realignment procedures.
5. All coalition patients are educated on the risks of requiring an arthrodesis at some point in their lifetime. Likewise, coalitions occupying over 50% of the joint are educated that they are at increased risk for need for arthrodesis in their lifetime.

Surgical Technique

Talocalcaneal Coalition Resection:

1. Patient is positioned in the supine position.
2. Thigh tourniquet may be utilized.
3. The leg is prepped and draped with the ability to move the foot for intraoperative imaging. Buttocks region prepped for fat graft harvest.
4. A medial utility incision is fashioned from the medial malleolus along the medial subtalar joint transcending to the level of the talonavicular joint region. Care is taken to not fashion this incision too dorsal or plantar. This incision may be elongated posteriorly for Type 5 talocalcaneal coalitions.
5. The posterior tibial tendon is often retracted superior while the FDL is retracted inferior. The FHL and bundle will need to be retracted with Type 5 talocalcaneal coalitions.
6. Osteotomes are utilized to resect the coalition. This is continued until there is normal appearing cartilage. One may complement this resection by using a rongeur, curette, and/or burr.
7. Intraoperative motion is then assessed clinically and under fluoroscopy. Intraoperative CT scans can confirm adequate resection.
8. Fat graft is then placed into the site of coalition resection.
9. Tendon sheaths are repaired.
10. Tourniquet is deflated prior to closure if utilized.
11. Bulky Jones splint applied for 2 weeks, followed by weightbearing in a boot for 2–4 weeks prior to supportive shoes. Early range of motion is key once skin is healed.
12. The addition of realignment procedures requires 6 weeks of non-weightbearing with immobilization.

Calcaneonavicular Coalition Resection:

1. Oblique incision fashioned along the dorsal lateral aspect of the foot from the anterior process of the calcaneus to the navicular. Incision stops at the level of the extensors dorsally.
2. Extensor digitorum brevis is reflected.
3. Osteotomes are utilized to resect the entire coalition and most plantar bar.

4. Tourniquet is deflated prior to closure. Hemostasis is achieved prior to closure. This is important as some children will bleed following resection.
5. Fat graft may be inserted into the area of resection. The authors do not pack this void with any muscle belly. To minimize migration of the fat graft, the authors recommend not overpacking.
6. Layer closure.

Clubfoot

Congenital clubfoot (talipes equinovarus) is a complex multiplanar deformity involving cavus, adductus, varus, and equinus. Clubfoot is a heterogeneous disorder that despite what its name implies, is not an isolated foot problem. Instead, it is a developmental limb disorder and the amount of involvement of the soft tissue structures of the lower limb can be highly variable between patients. While a variety of deformities can present in infancy, clubfoot is truly defined by its hindfoot varus deformity in association with equinus. The condition affects 1 out of every 1000 live births with a male to female ratio of 2:1 [70]. It remains one of the most common birth defects. While many are isolated birth defects, approximately 20% are linked to neuromuscular and/or genetic conditions. Specifically, mutations in the PITX1-TBX4-HOXC transcriptional pathway have been noted to cause familial clubfoot and vertical talus in a small number of families [40]. In children, 50% present bilaterally. Hawaiians and Maoris have been reported to have the greatest prevalence at 7 per 1000 live births [70, 71] (Fig. 16.20).

Anatomically, this complex deformity involves the ankle, subtalar and midfoot joints. The anatomy of these joints is distorted and remains the focus during correction. Both osseous and soft tissue components contribute to the deformity. The talus and calcaneus are both positioned in equinus. The hindfoot is positioned in varus due to subtalar joint inversion as well as internal rotation and adduction. The talus is smaller than normal, and the body is laterally rotated within the mortise while the head and neck are medially and plantarly deviated. Adding to the hindfoot complexity, the calcaneus is internally rotated below the head and neck of the talus and in an equinus position. Along the transverse tarsal joint, the navicular is rotated medially around the talar head so much that it may contact the medial malleolus. The cuboid is translated medially in relation to the calcaneus. Instead of these joints being parallel to each other, they lie on top of one another. The midfoot and forefoot are adducted and plantarflexed on the hindfoot, creating a cavus. The forefoot is not as inverted as the hindfoot. Occasionally, internal tibial torsion or bowing of the tibia is present.

Fibrous hyperplasia of the posterior and medial structures has been described as myofibroblast-like cells and changes in muscle fibers, although this has been disputed [72–79]. Contractures of the posteromedial structures and leg atrophy have been described including contractures of the gastrocsoleus complex, tibialis posterior, flexor digitorum longus, flexor hallucis longus, ankle, subtalar and talonavicular joint capsules, and the deltoid ligament [80–83].

Pathogenesis

If untreated, the deformity becomes much more difficult to treat conservatively, and worsens over time. Patients may

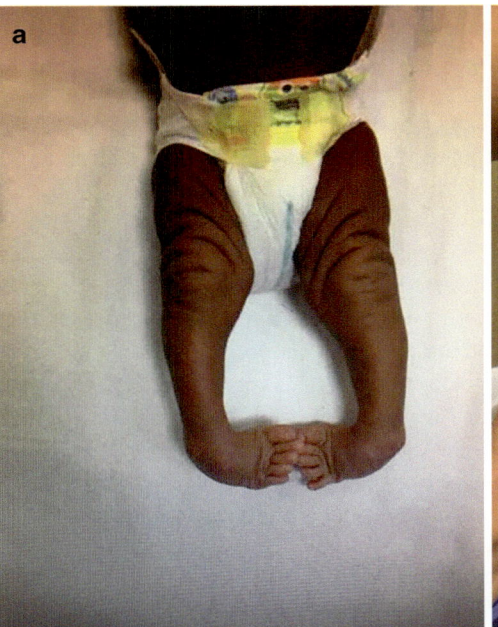
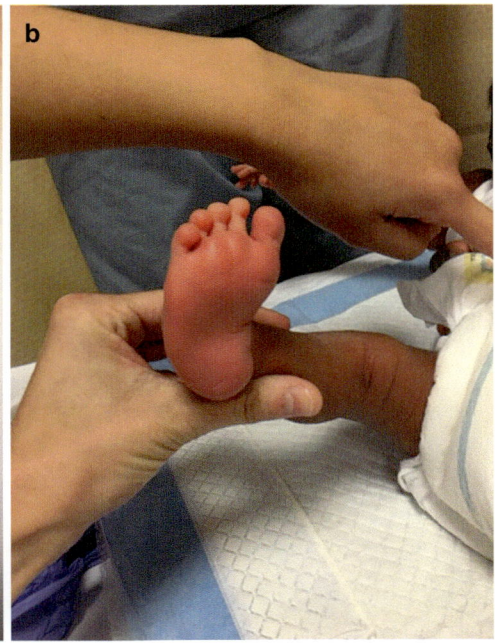

Fig. 16.20 (**a** and **b**) Infant with talipes equinovarus

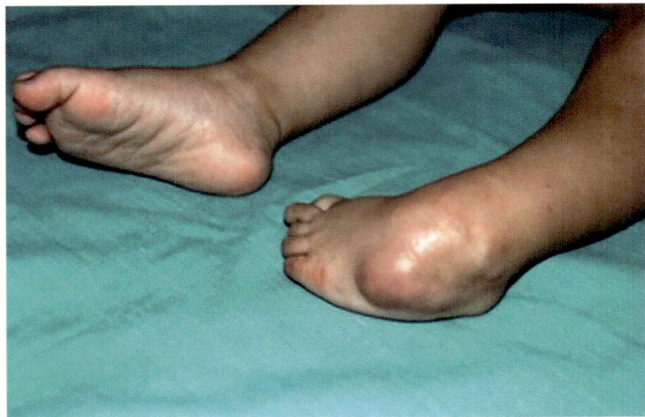

Fig. 16.21 Untreated clubfoot

have little to no pain during ambulation, but will eventually develop abnormal, thickened skin, and bursae on the dorsolateral foot. Children with neglected clubfeet are often unable to eventually wear shoes. Weakness of the lower extremity and a smaller calf size may decrease the ability to participate in sports and activity. Since the talus and calcaneus are notably plantarflexed, there is an equinus gait and compensation that occurs with knee hyperextension and hip external rotation. There is also an increase in knee and hip joint moments and decrease in ankle moments, likely due to a weak calf and plantar flexors. A weak posterior muscle group can lead to decreased push-off strength. Complete foot drop may also occur (Fig. 16.21).

Conservative treatment using the Ponseti technique has provided a functional, plantigrade foot in 85–95% of patients [80, 84–88]. It has been reported that even after treatment there is decreased ankle range of motion when compared to unaffected children, but overall, there is increased ankle range of motion and strength, as well as less pain, after casting [89]. This is accompanied by decreased peak pressures over the medial forefoot and hindfoot as well as increased pressure over the lateral midfoot. Residual intoeing is seen in up to 33% of children with moderate clubfoot using the Dimeglio scoring system [90]. Normal ankle sagittal plane motion may be obtained using casting or physical therapy in children with severe clubfoot, and almost two-thirds of patients have normal kinematic ankle motion if treated properly [90, 91].

Clubfoot may be associated with multiple other congenital disorders such as myelomeningocele, myelodysplasia, and arthrogryposis, most of which are neurologic [29]. While the true pathogenesis has not been elucidated, the origin is likely multifactorial. Many note that clubfoot has a partial genetic factor [40]. Since most cases are idiopathic and not associated with an additional congenital condition, it has been suggested that clubfoot is associated with a more complex trait, rather than a single gene. Current literature has examined the presence of mutations and deletions of transcription factor PITX [40, 92, 93]. The incidence among different races ranges from 0.39–7 per 1000 [94]. Chinese populations have been reported to have the lowest incidence. The male to female ratio is as high as 2.5:1 [91]. Twenty-four percent of cases have a positive family history and siblings have a 30-fold increased risk of congenital clubfoot. More recently, transcription factors have been tied to the etiology [40].

Additionally, factors such as abnormal muscle fiber ratio and nerve abnormalities, abnormal soft tissue, abnormal bone formation, and even vascular malformations have been described [95–98]. Cigarette smoking during pregnancy has an odds ratio of 1.34 for clubfoot [95].

Physical Exam

It is critical to perform a thorough physical exam on all clubfoot patients, which includes an examination of the hips, all four extremities, the neck, and spine to rule out other associated anomalies. Assessing for a sacral dimple is important to rule out spinal cord issues such as a tethered cord, sacral agenesis, or spina bifida. In terms of the feet, the treating physician must ensure an accurate diagnosis of clubfoot as well as rule out associated nerve or muscle problems indicative of atypical clubfoot. While all clubfeet share the same general characteristics, they are quite heterogeneous in etiology. Isolated clubfoot, those clubfeet that occur without other associated diagnoses, are the most common type, but this number is getting smaller. This is due to more careful physical examinations uncovering nerve and muscle abnormalities in many clubfoot children that were not diagnosed as infants in the past. To diagnose these nerve and muscle problems, a few simple exam techniques are required. Simply stimulating the bottom of the child's foot should elicit strong dorsiflexion and plantarflexion of the toes. If the infant cannot do this or does it weakly in any of the toes, this should raise the suspicion of underlying congenital nerve problem or muscle weakness. Similarly, stimulation of the plantar lateral aspect of the foot should elicit firing of the peroneus brevis. This exam tactic should be done at each cast change to get a clear picture of motor ability in the foot. This is important as those children with weak/absent dorsiflexion and/or eversion have a more difficult treatment course with higher relapse risk. This needs to be explained to parents and caregivers. The ability to perform a more careful physical examination will lead the treating physician and patient into the era of personalized medicine where risk of relapse will be able to be better predicted based on specific physical exam findings.

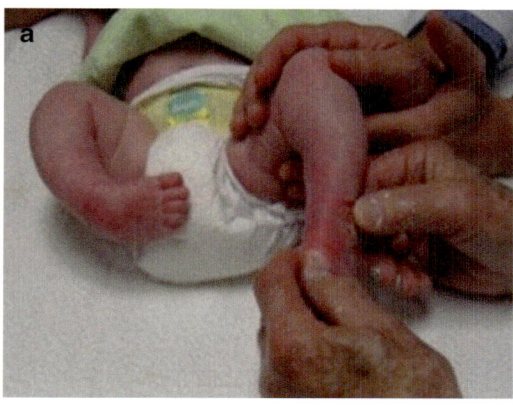 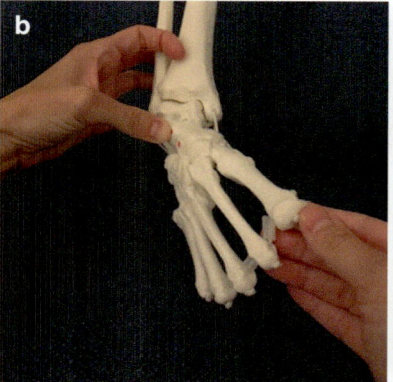 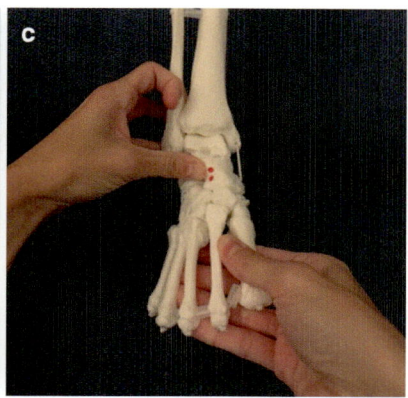

Fig. 16.22 (**a**) The Ponseti method. (**b**) The Magic Move. (**c**) The Ponseti method

Treatment

The Ponseti method has proven to be successful in the treatment of both isolated and non-isolated clubfoot. The method should be executed prior to any pediatric invasive procedures and likewise should be attempted with any pediatric recurrence [99]. Quite often, the method provides a stretch and can improve overall foot position minimizing procedures needed to obtain a plantigrade foot. Still, it is important to recognize that without proper bracing following, serial casting recurrence is likely [99, 100]. Despite the method's effectiveness, 40% of children will require some form of surgical intervention in their lifetime [99]. Proper use of the method can minimize the extent of procedures required or eliminate the need for surgery (Fig. 16.22).

The Ponseti Method

- A full musculoskeletal exam is performed prior to treatment.
- The Magic Move: A dorsiflexory force is applied beneath the first metatarsal head with counterpressure applied to the lateral talar head. This maneuver reduces the cavus and medial crease. This is performed, as the forefoot is not as inverted as compared to the hindfoot.
- Do not touch the calcaneus or cuboid.
- Upon resolution of the medial crease, the forefoot is abducted with counterpressure applied to the lateral talar head. Upon reduction of the adduction, inversion, and cavus, one can proceed with correction of the equinus. The goal is to hyperabduct the foot about 50°–70° with respect to the leg.
- A complete Achilles tenotomy is performed to reduce equinus if less than 10° of dorsiflexion is noted at the level of the ankle joint. A final cast is applied and left intact for 2–3 weeks.
- Abduction bar bracing is utilized until at least 4 years of age. The affected foot is externally rotated at 50°–70° to the lower leg and an unaffected foot is positioned to 30°–40° to the lower limb.

Casting Pearls

- A thin layer of webril or cast padding is utilized from the toes up to the groin.
- A well-molded cast is utilized and secured from the toes to just below the knee. Once completed, the cast is continued above the knee while maintaining 90°–110° of knee flexion to minimize cast slippage.
- Excess plaster or casting material is removed to expose the toes.
- Semi-rigid casting material may be utilized in place of plaster while proper manipulation is key.
- Often with recurrences, a well-molded plaster cast is fashioned below the knee and fiberglass is applied over the plaster and extends above the knee.
- It is essential to apply long leg casts, as below the knee casts will lead to slippage and or lack of correction.
- Soothing techniques: bottle feeds, sweet ease, pacifier, sound machines.
- Casts are changed weekly leading to Achilles tenotomy (Fig. 16.23).

Complex Clubfoot

Complex clubfeet are neurologically normal. Historically, this term was utilized interchangeably for the atypical subset. We now recognize that while the treatment is the same,

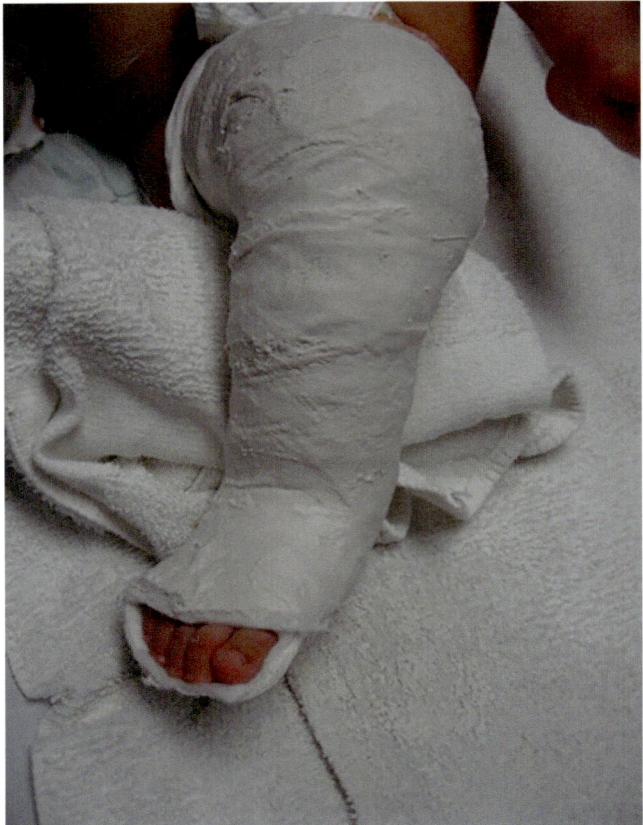

Fig. 16.23 Ponseti casting

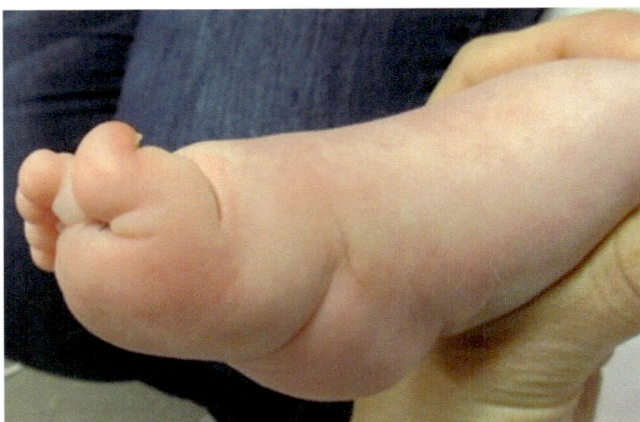

Fig. 16.24 Complex clubfoot

- Resistant to classic Ponseti Method.
- Often identified following cast slippage.
- This condition can also be the result of improper manipulation and casting.
- The 4-finger technique is utilized: Pushing upwards beneath the first and fifth metatarsals while applying a dorsiflexion force on the posterior superior aspect of the calcaneus.

the etiology is quite different. Complex clubfeet appear short and fat with a retracted first ray. Cast slippage is a common issue with these feet and if it continues to occur, a deep plantar crease is evident indicating entire midfoot cavus. Fortunately, Ponseti recognized this variation and developed a modified casting technique. The emphasis is on dorsiflexing the first and fifth ray to stretch the plantar crease. Serial casts result in achieving 30 to 40° of external rotation. At that time, a tenotomy is done and the foot casted in 50° of external rotation and 10° of dorsiflexion. Trying to externally rotate the foot further results in a midfoot breach laterally. Hyperflexion of the knee up to 110° is helpful to prevent cast slipping. Care should be taken to use posterior plaster slab for lower leg and dorsal slab for the knee to minimize the amount of plaster rolls. This technique leads to better molding. Foot abduction bracing is used after the casting, but care should be taken to set the feet at 50° of external rotation and not greater (Fig. 16.24).

Complex Clubfoot Pearls

- May present with deep plantar crease initially and extreme cavus. Hyperabduction may lead to tightening of the quadratus plantae and pulling of the flexors. This leads to worsening cavus.

Atypical Clubfoot

Atypical clubfoot, which is mistakenly used synonymously with complex clubfoot, is a different entity though the casting treatment is the same as it is for complex clubfoot. Atypical clubfeet share many of the same clinical features as complex clubfoot, but these are identifiable at birth and are associated with a neurologic condition. Patients with atypical clubfeet often have weak or absent active dorsiflexion of the toes and ankle as well as weak active eversion of the foot. This subset is associated with neurological and or motor deficits. Casting is done as for complex clubfoot, but these patients are at higher risk of relapse due to lack of motor strength.

Atypical Clubfoot Pearls

- Noted at birth.
- Weak or absent active dorsiflexion of the toes and ankle as well as weak active eversion of the foot.
- Associated with neurologic and/or motor deficits.
- Deep plantar crease initially and extreme cavus. Hyperabduction may lead to tightening of the quadratus plantae and pulling of the flexors. This leads to worsening cavus.
- Resistant to classic Ponseti Method.

Fig. 16.25 Bracing following Ponseti casting

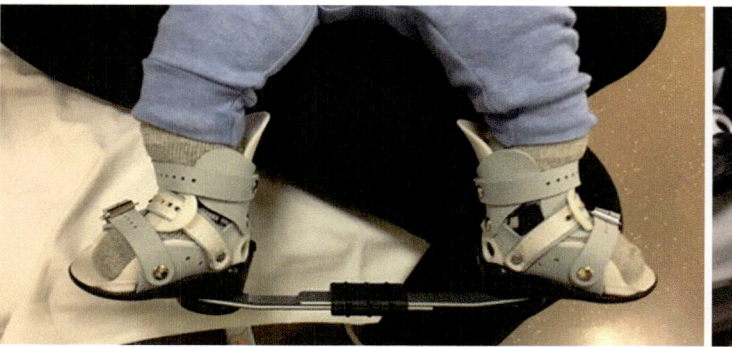

- The 4-finger technique is utilized: Pushing upwards beneath the first and fifth metatarsals while applying a dorsiflexory force on the posterior superior aspect of the calcaneus.
- Higher risks of relapse given motor strength deficit.

Bracing Period

In many ways the bracing period can be much more challenging for parents and families than the casting period. There is always a feeling of accomplishment and relief among parents with completion of casting. The adjustment period for braces can come as a surprise to the family. It is important to educate all caregivers on the importance of bracing and the high risks for recurrence of clubfoot without proper brace compliance. Immediately following the casting period, the child transitions to boots attached to an abduction bar. It is important to educate caregivers that while the braces do not cause pain, they are a change especially for an infant (Fig. 16.25).

Parents should attempt to soothe their child as compared to removing the braces while the child is crying. Demonstrating how the child can use their legs attached to the bar is often helpful as well. Boots should be snug while not too tight. Sores can develop if straps are too tight. If sores do arise, various products such as moleskin, molefoam, mepilex, lambs wool, athletic tape, etc. may be utilized to protect the skin. If ulcerations or tissue necrosis occurs, a bracing vacation may be needed with expectation of a return to casting. The feet and ankles are stretched daily, and ankle dorsiflexion is performed prior to brace application. It is important to remember that the braces do not correct any deformities. The braces simply maintain correction obtained from casting or surgery.

Surgical Management of Clubfoot

Up to 40% of patients with clubfoot treated successfully by the Ponseti method do experience a recurrence of deformity [40, 99]. Hence, it has become important not only to adhere to the strict details of the Ponseti method during the casting period but also to promote bracing compliance until 4–6 years of age. Some children, especially in the presence of neurologic influence require not only nighttime bracing but also daytime ankle foot orthoses in conjunction with nighttime abduction bar bracing. Still, despite successful execution of the method and bracing compliance, the deformity can still recur. The authors have studied symptomatic recurrence. Possible causes for recurrence include the intrinsic contractile nature of the soft tissues in clubfoot deformity, genetic and neuromuscular factors, casting techniques [101], different designs of braces [101], and variable brace wear time due to parental noncompliance [100].

While the syndromic foot or non-isolated clubfoot has an increased risk for symptomatic recurrence, along with an earlier age in which recurrence is noted, the isolated clubfoot can still reoccur. It is essential to follow this pediatric population after the age of 5 to minimize the severity of recurrence, if possible. In a study by van Praag et al., recurrence was seen in 19% [99] of 382 children who were eligible for the study and who were typically discharged after the age of 5 years from their clinic. This alludes to the importance of continued follow-up even after age 5 [99]. Treatment with casting for the recurrence was successful in many patients and may be a reasonable choice for recurrent idiopathic clubfeet [99].

Achilles Tenotomy

Most children with clubfoot will require an Achilles Tenotomy to reduce the equinus deformity. A topical anesthetic is utilized on the skin in the posterior ankle region. EMLA or Lidocaine plain are most commonly utilized anesthetics under occlusion. The authors do not inject any further local anesthesia prior to the procedure as this can obscure the margins of the Achilles tendon. With the foot held in dorsiflexion, a Beaver blade is introduced by the surgeon through the skin onto the medial edge of the tendoachilles about 1 cm proximal to its calcaneal insertion. The tendon is felt with the tip of the knife much like a probe. The knife is introduced in

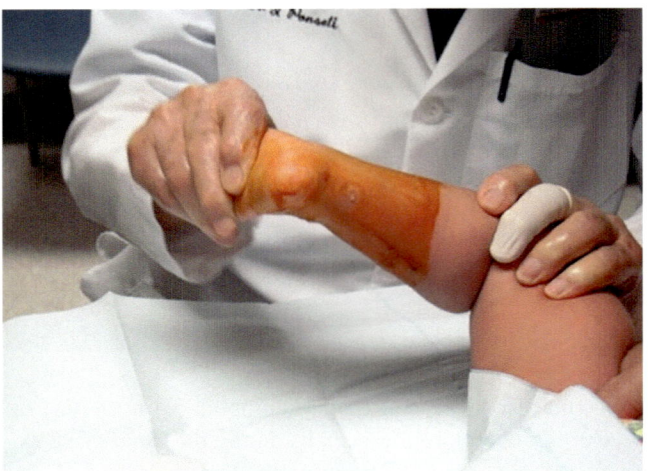

Fig. 16.26 Achilles tenotomy

front of the tendon and then rotated 45°. The angle of dorsiflexion of the ankle will suddenly increase about 10°–15° [102].

Advancing the blade too far laterally can place the peroneal artery or lesser saphenous vein at risk of being severed. After the tenotomy is performed and temporary dressing is applied, the child is monitored for good skin perfusion and digital refill over several minutes. The temporary dressing is removed, and gauze is applied. Local anesthesia may be utilized at this time. A well-molded long-leg plaster cast is then applied, maintaining the foot in maximum dorsiflexion and in about 70° of external rotation to the lower leg. The final cast is left intact for 2–3 weeks to allow for tendon healing (Fig. 16.26).

Using a more rounded beaver blade may reduce the risk of vascular injury. This makes palpation of the tendon edge easier. If the Achilles is easily palpable, the procedure may be performed in clinic without anesthesia. If serial Achilles tenotomies are performed for recurrence, the authors are more likely to perform a small open procedure in the operating room. Likewise, if patient's comorbidities or disposition make it unsafe to perform in clinic, the authors will perform the procedure in the operating room under general anesthesia. The majority of children under 12 months of age can undergo Achilles tenotomies in the office, provided the borders of the Achilles are easily palpable.

A thorough lower extremity vascular exam is recommended prior to performing a percutaneous Achilles tenotomy. This should include palpation of the dorsalis pedis and posterior tibial pulses. Doppler ultrasound may be considered in those patients with an absent dorsalis pedis or posterior tibial pulse [102]. If both are absent or diminished on Doppler, then consideration should be given to performing an arteriogram to assess whether the peroneal artery is the dominant supply to the foot [102]. If the peroneal artery is dominant, then consideration should be given to performing an open Achilles tenotomy.

Anterior Tibialis Tendon Transfer

Some children of walking age demonstrate supination during swing and stance phase of gait. While often not complaining of pain, one may see callus formation as a result of abnormal pressure and lateral column overload. This muscle imbalance is common among children with clubfoot given the overactivity of the supinating muscles and the underactivity of the everting muscles. While not every child born with clubfoot will require this procedure, it remains quite common.

Prior to the procedure, if the foot is not fully corrected, it is essential to proceed with serial Ponseti casting to obtain a well-corrected foot prior to tendon transfer. Casts at this time are still well-molded plaster casts with a fiberglass cast overlay up to the groin. The knee is flexed to minimize slippage and rotation. Many children are older than 3 years of age and continue to attempt ambulation in bilateral casts. It is important to educate caregivers on cast care to minimize blisters, skin breakdown, or infections that may delay this procedure.

Casting should be done prior to tendon transfer in all patients not fully corrected. On average of 3 casts are generally needed to fully achieve correction. The tendon transfer itself will only maintain correction—it cannot be used to achieve correction. The pre-operative casts are long leg bent 30° to allow full weight-bearing. After surgery, a long leg plaster cast is used with knee bent to 90 to prevent weight-bearing for 4 weeks. At that time, any external tendon button utilized is removed and a short leg weight-bearing cast is used for an additional 2 weeks. The external tendon button is often utilized in the younger patient with cartilaginous bone. Following cast removal, AFO bracing is helpful for 6 weeks along with nighttime stretching splint and physical therapy.

Anterior Tibialis Tendon Transfer Pearls

- Medial incision is fashioned over the first metatarsal cuneiform joint.
- The anterior tibial tendon is released from its insertion site.
- The tendon is reflected, and a whip stitch is performed to the anterior tibial tendon.
- The tendon is directed beneath retinacular tissue and transferred to the lateral cuneiform.
- A biotenodesis screw can be utilized, however, an external suture button is preferred in younger children given the immature ossific structures. Care is taken to not overtighten the button as maceration, ulceration, and skin

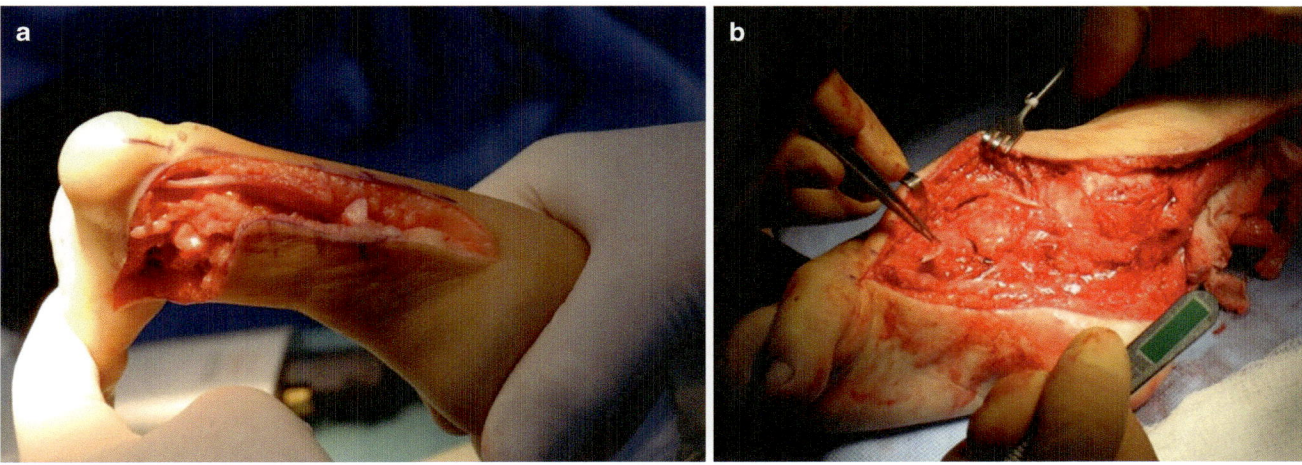

Fig. 16.27 (a) Posteriormedial release. (b) Retracting fibrosis

necrosis can occur. Overtightening of the tendon can also lead to limited plantarflexion.
- An Achilles lengthening procedure often is performed in conjunction with any persistent equinus.
- A long leg cast is applied with the knee flexed to 90°.
- It often takes 6 weeks for the tendon to incorporate into bone.

Posterior Medial Release

Historically, the posterior medial release was the treatment of choice prior to the Ponseti technique. Many young children underwent long incisions releasing tendons, joint capsules, and ligamentous structures of the posterior and medial compartments in an attempt to reduce the talonavicular and subtalar joints. After posterior medial releases, children had stiff feet with often-recurrent deformities that led to overall poorer functional outcome scores (Fig. 16.27).

A posterior medial release is performed upon failure of Ponseti casting or the presence of resistant recurrent deformity. The goal of releases is to use casting to reduce the deformity and then proceed with a small incision a la carte approach. One should strive to avoid large incisions and focus on the individual structures in need of release. The critical aspects of the deformity must be understood to distinguish which structures require release.

A complete posterior medial release requires extensive dissection of the posterior ankle and subtalar joints along with the medial, lateral, and plantar aspects of the foot. A medial incision is fashioned extending along the medial arch transcending posteriorly across the posterior aspect of the ankle to expose both the ankle and subtalar joints. This posterior arm of the incision may be a vertical or a transverse continuum from the medial incision. Care is taken to preserve neurovascular structures. A vessel loop is utilized to identify medial structures for retraction and protection. The medial plantar nerve is followed and protected while the abductor hallucis muscle is mobilized from the calcaneus and further released at the musculotendinous junction. The Achilles is lengthened or completely released based on the age of patient. The posterior tibial, flexor digitorum longus, and flexor hallucis longus tendons are lengthened proximal to the medial malleolus. Lengthening proximal to the porta pedis or proximal to the tarsal tunnel region may minimize adhesions. The talonavicular joint capsule, subtalar joint capsule, and calcaneocuboid capsules can then be released. Finally, the posterior ankle capsule is released to allow for the talus to rotate posteriorly into the ankle mortise when the ankle is dorsiflexed. This should be performed as an a la carte approach.

A plantar release is fashioned posterior to the neurovascular bundle. A plane is created between the subcutaneous tissue and plantar aponeurosis. Division of the aponeurosis allows for further correction of the cavus deformity. Following sequential soft tissue release, the talonavicular and subtalar joints are pinned to maintain alignment. One may utilize a 2 or 3 k-wire construct as needed for stability. A 0.062 smooth k wire is antegraded from the posterior talus into the talar head to transcend the reduced talonavicular joint. The base of the first metatarsal is slightly abducted and held. A subsequent K wire may be utilized across the subtalar joint. A third k wire may be utilized from the lateral column into the calcaneus. If a tourniquet is utilized, it is important to deflate prior to closure to assess for appropriate perfusion.

A splint or bivalved cast is applied to reduce motion while also minimize edema postoperatively. Immobilization is advised for a minimum of 4–6 weeks. Often the initial splint is left intact for 7–14 days based on the extent of the release followed by subsequent above the knee casting for the remaining period. Children with increased risks for skin necrosis such as loss of protective sensation are seen in shorter intervals. It remains important to monitor all children undergoing such releases given the risks of edema, tissue necrosis, vascular compromise, bleeding problems, and dehiscence.

A full posterior, medial, and lateral release can often be avoided if recurrence is casted early in life prior to osseous adaptive changes. Often, casting can be utilized to correct for the medial soft tissue contracture and if equinus and stiffness remain, a posterior release may be executed in resistant clubfeet.

Complications

Not only can complications arise from surgery but also from the casting process. Often, complications are linked to subsequent deformities resulting from poor casting technique. It is important not to evert the forefoot and, rather, to focus on supination of the forefoot initially. One should not solely abduct the foot until the medial crease has resolved. By pushing up under the first metatarsal head, one reduces the cavus and realigns the forefoot to the rearfoot. At times the four-finger technique may be utilized to further address the cavus. Please refer to the alternative maneuver for both atypical and complex clubfoot within this chapter.

One of the easiest means of minimizing complications is to never apply counterpressure to the calcaneocuboid joint. While Kite's maneuver promoted a noninvasive approach, it blocked the calcaneus from moving beneath the talus. Despite many recognizing the faultiness with Kite's maneuver, it is quite easy to block the calcaneus from moving beneath the talus if one's thumb is on the prominent anterior process. Blockage of the calcaneus will leave the heel inverted and in varus. This may also lead to a posteriorly deviated fibula or inability for the talus to move within the ankle joint. In general, forceful manipulation should be avoided because it can lead to an eventual flat top talus later in life or immediate distal tibial fractures. The flat top talus remains a challenging problem. The ability to restore normal morphology of the talus does not exist. Hence, the surgeon attempts to realign around a disfigured talus. Many attempt supramalleolar osteotomies, calcaneal osteotomies, or midfoot osteotomies with inconsistent results while striving toward a plantigrade foot.

It is important for the treating physician to recognize atypical and complex clubfoot types. Failure to identify these specific groups may lead to further edema, disfigurement, rigidity, and progressive challenging deformities. Hyperabduction with these groups will lead to the quadratus plantae pulling the flexors and worsening the cavus deformity.

Likewise, surgical complications can arise. Often this healthy, young population will heal; however, as with any surgery they are at risk of dehiscence, wound healing problems, infection, inability to close surgical sites, nerve problems, stiffness, pain, hardware problems, and recurrence. Parents and caregivers should be educated on these potential outcomes well prior to surgery. Infections, wounds, and unfortunate limb loss are all outcomes of clubfoot treatment that should be discussed with parents and caretakers. Children with coexisting syndromes carry increased risks with higher likelihood for poorer outcomes.

Skewfoot

Skewfoot is a complex congenital foot deformity. The foot presents with the hindfoot and midfoot in valgus while the forefoot is adducted. The talonavicular joint is often subluxed laterally. Metatarsus adductus is a component of skewfoot that can present with severe angulation. This condition can present as an isolated condition or may be associated with secondary diagnoses such as Marfan's syndrome or Freeman Sheldon syndrome. Skewfoot can also become an evolving deformity for patients treated via surgery for clubfoot.

In infancy, skewfoot can be improved upon via a specialized casting technique. This maneuver requires abduction at the level of the forefoot and counterpressure at the calcaneocuboid joint to improve the metatarsus adductus. This maneuver does not increase hindfoot valgus or midfoot valgus. If the calcaneocuboid counterpressure is not applied, one notes increase in talonavicular subluxation and hindfoot valgus. This maneuver may be viewed as not providing full correction of all aspects of the deformity while with growth it makes any subsequent procedure in childhood or adulthood easier to execute.

Skewfoot presenting in children closer to four or five years of age may benefit from surgical intervention including capsular release of the tarsometatarsal complex with pinning of the medial and lateral columns. With growth, the child would demonstrate a more flexible flatfoot. If any symptoms developed associated with pronation, the child would be evaluated for pediatric flatfoot reconstruction. The absence of metatarsus adductus makes this condition easier to correct in adolescence.

References

1. Pollard JP, Morrison PJ. Flexor tenotomy in the treatment of curly toes. Proc R Soc Med. 1975;68:480.
2. Wagreich C. Congenital deformities. In: Banks A, Downey, MS, Martin, DE, Miller, SJ, editor. Baltimore: Williams & Wilkins; 2001.

3. Downey MRL. Common pediatric digital deformities. In: De Valentine S, editor. Foot and ankle disorders in children. St. Louis: Mosby; 1992.
4. Smith WG, Seki J, Smith RW. Prospective study of a noninvasive treatment for two common congenital toe abnormalities (curly/varus/underlapping toes and overlapping toes). Paediatr Child Health. 2007;12(9):755–9.
5. Turner PL. Strapping of curly toes in children. Aust N Z J Surg. 1987;57(7):467–70.
6. Talusan PG, Milewski MD, Reach JS Jr. Fifth toe deformities: overlapping and underlapping toe. Foot Ankle Spec. 2013;6(2):145–9.
7. Taylor RG. The treatment of claw toes by multiple transfers of flexor into extensor tendons. J Bone Joint Surg. 1951;33-B(4):539–42.
8. Biyani A, Jones DA, Murray JM. Flexor to extensor tendon transfer for curly toes. 43 children reviewed after 8 (1-25) years. Acta Orthop Scand. 1992;63(4):451–4.
9. Ross ER, Menelaus MB. Open flexor tenotomy for hammer toes and curly toes in childhood. J Bone Joint Surg. 1984;66(5):770–1.
10. Hamer AJ, Stanley D, Smith TW. Surgery for curly toe deformity: a double-blind, randomised, prospective trial. J Bone Joint Surg. 1993;75(4):662–3.
11. Burger E, Baas M, Hovius S, Hoogeboom J, Nieuwenhoven C. Preaxial polydactyly of the foot. Acta Orthop. 2018;89(1):113–8.
12. Phelps DA, Grogan DP. Polydactyly of the foot. J Pediatr Orthop. 1985;5(4):446–51.
13. Fahim R, Thomas Z, DiDomenico LA. Pediatric forefoot pathology. Clin Podiatr Med Surg. 2013;30(4):479–90.
14. McCarty J, Drennan J. Drennan's the child's foot and ankle. 2nd ed. LWW; 2009.
15. Hop MJ, van der Biezen JJ. Ray reduction of the foot in the treatment of macrodactyly and review of the literature. J Foot Ankle Surg. 2011;50(4):434–8.
16. Barsky AJ. Macrodactyly. J Bone Joint Surg Am. 1967;49(7):1255–66.
17. Inglis K. Local gigantism (a manifestation of neurofibromatosis): its relation to general gigantism and to acromegaly; illustrating the influence of intrinsic factors in disease when development of the body is abnormal. Am J Pathol. 1950;26(6):1059–83.
18. Kalen V, Burwell DS, Omer GE. Macrodactyly of the hands and feet. J Pediatr Orthop. 1988;8(3):311–5.
19. Chang CH, Kumar SJ, Riddle EC, et al. Macrodactyly of the foot. J Bone Joint Surg Am. 2002;84:1189.
20. Grogan DP, Bernstein RM, Habal MB, et al. Congenital lipofibromatosis associated with macrodactyl of the foot. Foot Ankle. 1991;12:40.
21. Morris EW, Scullion JE, Mann TS. Varus fifth toe. J Bone Joint Surg Br. 1982;64:99.
22. Paton RW. V-Y for correction of varus fifth toe. J Pediatr Orthop. 1990;10:248.
23. Jones GB. Delta phalanx. J Bone Joint Surg Br. 1964;46(46):226.
24. Light TR, Ogden JA. The longitudinal epiphyseal bracket: implications for surgical correction. J Pediatr Orthop. 1981;1:299.
25. Stevens P. Toe deformities. In: Drennan J, editor. The child's foot and ankle. New York: Raven Press; 1992. p. 183.
26. Mubarak SJ, O'Brien TJ, Davids JR. Metatarsal epiphyseal bracket: treatment by central physiolysis. J Pediatr Orthop. 1993;13:5.
27. Landon GC, Johnson KA, Dahlin DC. Subungual exostoses. J Bone Joint Surg Am. 1979;61:256.
28. Franklin TP, Miguel MQ, Félix MR, Leydi MQ, Herbert PC. Subungual osteochondroma: review of the literature. MOJ Orthop Rheumatol. 2017;8(5):00327. https://doi.org/10.15406/mojor.2017.08.00327.
29. Wynne-Davies R. Family studies and the cause of congenital clubfoot, talipes equinovarus, talipes calcaneovalgus and metatarsus varus. J Bone Joint Surg Br. 1964;46:445.
30. Rushforth GF. The natural history of hooked forefoot. J Bone Joint Surg Br. 1978;60:530.
31. Thomson SA. Hallux varus and metatarsus varus: a five-year study (1954-1958). Clin Orthop Relat Res. 1960;16:109.
32. Dobbs MB, Purcell DB, Nunley R, Morcuende JA. Early results of a new method of treatment for idiopathic congenital vertical talus. J Bone Joint Surg Am. 2006;88(6):1192–200.
33. Alaee F, Boehm S, Dobbs MB. A new approach to treatment of congenital vertical talus. J Child Orthop. 2007;1(3):165–74.
34. Miller M, Dobbs MB. Congenital vertical talus: etiology and management. J Am Acad Orthop Surg. 2015;23:604–11.
35. Yang J, Dobbs M. Treatment of congenital vertical talus: Comparison of minimally invasive and extensive soft tissue release procedures at minimum five-year follow up. J Bone Joint Surg. 97(16):1354–65.
36. Jacobsen ST, Crawford AH. Congenital vertical talus. J Pediatr Orthop. 1983;3(3):306–10.
37. Sharrard WJ, Grosfield I. The management of deformity and paralysis of the foot in myelomenengocele. J Bone Joint Surg Br. 1968:50.
38. Merrill LJ, Gurnett CA, Connolly AM, Pestronik A, Dobbs MB. Skeletal muscle abnormalities and genetic factors releated to vertical talus. Clin Orthop Relat Res. 2011;469(4):1167–74.
39. Townes PL, Manning JA, Dehart GK Jr. Trisomy 18 (16-18) associated with congenital glaucoma and optic atrophy. J Pediatr. 1962;61:755.
40. Dobbs MB, Gurnett CA. The 2017 ABJS Nicolas Andry Award: advancing personalized medicine for clubfoot through translational research. Clin Orthop Relat Res. 2107(475):1716–25.
41. Alvarado D, McCall K, Hecht J, Dobbs M, Gurnett C. Deletion of 5' HOXC genes are associated with lower extremity malformations, including clubfoot and vertical talus. J Med Genet. 2016;53:250–5.
42. Dobbs M, Schoenecker P, Gordon J. Autosomal dominant transmission of isolated congenital vertical talus. Iowa Orthop J. 2002;22:25–7.
43. Tayebi N, Charng WL, Dickson P, Dobbs M, Gurnett C. Diagnostic yield of exome sequencing in congenital vertical talus. Eur J Med Genet. 2022;65:104,514.
44. Dobbs MB, Gurnett CA, Pierce B, et al. HOXD10 M319K mutation in a family with isolated congenital vertical talus. J Orthop Res. 2006;24(3):448–53.
45. Kruse L, Gurnett CA, Hootnick D, Dobbs MB. Magnetic resonance angiography in clubfoot and vertical talus: a feasibility study. Clin Orthop Res. 2009;467(5):1250–5.
46. Bhaskar A. Congenital vertical talus: treatment by the reverse ponseti technique. Indian J Orthop. 2008;42(3):347–50.
47. Aydin A, Atmaca H, Muezzinoglu US. Bilateral congenital vertical talus with severe lower extremity external rotational deformity: treated by reverse Ponseti technique. Foot (Edinb). 2012;22(3):252–4.
48. Khader A, Huntley JS. Congenital vertical talus in cri du chat syndrome: a case report. BMC Res Notes. 2013;6:270.
49. Eberhardt O, Fernandez FF, Wirth T. The talar axis-first metatarsal base angle in CVT treatment: a comparison of idiopathic and non-idiopathic cases treated with the Dobbs method. J Child Orthop. 2012;6(6):491–6.
50. Eberhardt O, Wirth T, Fernandez FF. Minimally invasive treatment of congenital foot defomrities in infants: new findings and midterm-results (German). Orthopade. 2013;42(12):1001–7.
51. Aslani H, Sadigi A, Tabrizi A, Bazavar M, Mousavi M. Primary outcomes of the congenital vertical talus correction using the

51. Dobbs method of serial casting and limited surgery. J Child Orthop. 2012;6(4):307–11.
52. Chalayon O, Adams A, Dobbs MB. Minimally invasive approach for the treatment of nonisolated congenital vertical talus. J Bone Joint Surg Am. 2012;94(11):e73.
53. Eberhardt O, Fernandez FF, Wirth T. Treatment of vertical talus with the Dobbs method (German). Z Orthop Unfall. 2011;149(2):219–24.
54. Walker AP, Ghali NN, Silk FF. Congenital vertical talus: the results of staged operative reduction. J Bone Joint Surg Br. 1985;67(1):117–21.
55. Seimon LP. Surgical correction of congenital vertical talus under the age of 2 years. J Pediatr Orthop. 1987;7(4):405–11.
56. Stricker SJ, Rosen E. Early one-stage reconstruction of congenital vertical talus. Foot Ankle Int. 1997;18(9):535–43.
57. Duncan RD, Fixsen JA. Congenital convex pes valgus. J Bone Joint Surg Br. 1999;81-B(2):250–4.
58. Kodros SA, Dias LS. Single stage surgical correction vertical talus. J Pediatr Orthop. 1999;19(1):42–8.
59. Oppenheim W, Smith C, Christie W. Congenital vertical talus. Foot Ankle. 1985;5(4):198–204.
60. Mazzocca AD, Thompson JD, Deluca PA, Romness MJ. Comparison of the posterior approach versus the dorsal approach in the treatment of congenital vertical talus. J Pediatr Orthop. 2001;21(2):212–7.
61. Garg S, Porter K. Improved bracing compliance in children with clubfeet using a dynamic orthosis. J Child Orthop. 2009;3(4):271–6. (endcvt).
62. Vincent KA. Tarsal coalition and painful flatfoot. J Am Acad Orthop Surg. 1998;6:274–81.
63. Olney BW. Tarsal coalition. In: McCarthy JJ, Drennan JC, editors. Drennan's the child's foot and ankle. New York: Wolters Kluwer/Lippincott Williams & Wilkins; 2010. p. 160–73.
64. Moraleda L, Gantsoudes GD, Mubarak SJ. C sign: talocalcaneal coalition of flatfoot deformity? J Pediatr Orthop. 2014;34:814–9.
65. Rozansky A, Varley E, Mubarak SJ, et al. A radiologic classification of talaocalcaenal coalitions based on 3D reconstruction. J Child Orthop. 2010;4:129–35.
66. Wilde PH, Torode IP, Dickens DR, et al. Resection for symptomatic talocalcaneal coalition. J Bone Joint Surg Br. 1994;76:797–801.
67. Luhmann SJ, Schoenecker PL. Symptomatic talocalcaneal coalition resection: indications and results. J Pediatr Orthop. 1998;18:748–54.
68. Mosca VS, Bevan WP. Talocalcaneal tarsal coalitions and the calcaneal lengthening osteotomy: the role of deformity correction. J Bone Joint Surg Am. 2012;94:1584–94.
69. Gantsoudes GD, Roocroft JH, Mubarak SJ. Treatment of talocalcaneal coalitions. J Pediatr Orthop. 2012;32:301–7.
70. Chung CS, Nemechek RW, Larsen IJ, Ching GH. Genetic and epidemiological studies of clubfoot in Hawaii. General and medical considerations. Hum Hered. 1969;19:321–42.
71. Beals RK. Club foot in the Maori: a genetic study of 50 kindres. N Z Med J. 1978;88:144–6.
72. Fried A. Recurrent congenital clubfoot: the role of the m. tibialis posterior in etiology and treatment. J Bone Joint Surg Am. 1959;41:243–52.
73. Hersch A. The role of surgery in the treatment of clubfeet. J Bone Joint Surg Am. 1967;49:1684–96.
74. Turco VJ. Surgical correction of the resistant club foot: one-stage posteromedial release with internal fixation. J Bone Joint Surg Am. 1971;53:477–97.
75. Fukuhara K, Schollmeier G, Uhthoff HK. The pathogenesis of clubfoot: a histomorphometric and immunohistochemical study of fetuses. J Bone Joint Surg Br. 1994;76:350–7.
76. Gray DH, Katz JM. A histochemical study of muscle in club foot. J Bone Joint Surg Br. 1989;63:417–23.
77. Ionasescu V, Maynard JA, Ponseti IV, Zellweger H. The role of collagen in the pathogenesis of idiopathic clubfoot. Helv Pediatr Acta. 1995;29:305–14.
78. Isaccs H, Handelsman JE, Badenhorst M, Pickering A. The muscles in clubfoot: a histological, histochemical, and electron microscopic study. J Bone Joint Surg Br. 1977;59:465–72.
79. Khan AM, Ryan MG, Gruber MM, et al. Connective tissue structures in clubfoot: a morphologic study. J Pediatr Orthop. 2001;21:708–12.
80. Ippolito E. Update on pathological anatomy of clubfoot. J Pediatr Orthop. 1995;4:17–24.
81. Howard CB, Benson MK. Clubfoot: its pathological anatomy. J Pediatr Orthop. 1993;13:654–9.
82. Irani RN, Sherman MS. The pathological anatomy of idiopathic clubfoot. Clin Orthop. 1972;84:14–20.
83. Ippolito E, De Maio F, Mancini F, et al. Leg muscle atrophy in idiopathic clubfoot congenital clubfoot: is it primitive or acquired? J Child Orthop. 2009;3:171–8.
84. Ponseti IV. Congenital clubfoot: fundamentals of treatment. Oxford University Press; 1996.
85. Laaveg SJ, Ponseti IV. Long-term results of treatment of congenital clubfoot. J Bone Joint Surg Am. 1980;62(1):23–31.
86. Abdelgawad AA, Lehman WB, van Bosse HJ, et al. Treatment of idiopathic clubfoot using the Ponseti method: minimum 2-year follow-up. J Pediatr Orthop B. 2007;16(2):98–105.
87. Bor N, Coplan JA, Herzenberg JE. Ponseti treatment for idiopathic clubfoot: minimum 5-year followup. Clin Orthop Relat Res. 2008;467(5):1263–70.
88. Banskota B, Yadav P, Rajbhandari T, et al. Outcomes of the Ponseti method for untreated clubfeet in Nepalese patients seen between the ages of one and five years and followed for at least 10 years. J Bone Joint Surg Am. 2018;100:2004–14.
89. Sinclair MF, Bosch K, Rosenbaum D, Bohm S. Pedobarographic analysis following Ponseti treatment for congenital clubfoot. Clin Orthop Relat Res. 2009;467:1223–30.
90. Gottschalk HP, Karol LA, Jeans KA. Gait analysis of children treated for moderate clubfoot with physical therapy versus the Ponseti cast technique. J Pediatr Orthop. 2010;30:235–9.
91. El-Hawary R, Karol LA, Jeans KA, Richards BS. Gait analysis of children treated for clubfoot with physical therapy or the Ponseti cast technique. J Bone Joint Surg Am. 2008;90:1508–16.
92. Alvarado DM, McCall K, Aferol H. Pitx1 haploinsufficiency causes clubfoot in humans and a clubfoot-like phenotype in mice. Hum Mol Genet. 2011;20:3943–52.
93. Alvarado DM, Buchan JG, Frick SL, et al. Copy number analysis of 413 isolated talipes equinovarus patients suggest role for transcriptional regulators of early limb development. Eur J Hum Genet. 2012;21:373–80.
94. Shimizu N, Hamada S, Mitta M, et al. Etiological considerations of congenital clubfoot deformity. In: Tachdjian MO, Simons G, editors. The clubfoot: the present and a view of the future. New York: Springer; 1993. p. 31–8.
95. Honein MA, Paulozzi LJ, Moore CA. Family history, maternal smoking, and clubfoot: an indication of a gene-environment interaction. Am J Epidemiol. 2000;152(7):658–65.
96. Dickinson KC, Meyer RE, Kotch J. Maternal smoking and the risk for clubfoot in infants. Birth Defects Res A Clin Mol Teratol. 2008;82(2):86–91.
97. Hootnick DR, Levinsohn EM, Crider RJ, et al. Congenital arterial malformations associated with clubfoot. A report of two cases. Clin Orthop Relat Res. 1982;167:160–3.
98. Levinsohn EM, Hootnick DR, Packard DS Jr. Consistent arterial abnormalitis associated with a variety of congenital malformations of the human lower limb. Investig Radiol. 1991;26(4):364–73.

99. van Praag VM, Lysenko M, Harvey B, Yankanah R, Wright JG. Casting is effective for recurrence following Ponseti treatment of clubfoot. J Bone Joint Surg Am. 2018;100:1001–8.
100. Dobbs MB, Rudzki JR, Purcell DB, Walton T, Porter K, Gurnett CA. Factors predictive of outcome after use of the Ponseti methods for the treatment of idiopathic clubfoot. J Bone Joint Surg. 2004;86-A(1):22.
101. Zhao D, Li H, Zhao L, Liu J, Wu Z, Jin F. Results of clubfoot management using the Ponseti method: do the details matter? A systematic review. Clin Orthop Relat Res. 2014;472(4):1329–36. Epub 2014 Jan 17.
102. Dobbs MB, Gordon JE, Walton T, Schoenecker PL. Bleeding complications following percutaneous tendoachilles tenotomy in the treatment of clubfoot deformity. J Pediatr Orthop. 2004;24(4)

Management of Pediatric Foot and Ankle Deformities: Gradual Correction

Bradley M. Lamm

Introduction

This chapter provides an overview and an update about the ever-evolving indications and applications of external fixation for the pediatric foot and ankle. During the last two decades, there have been many advances in technology and preoperative deformity planning. The principles of deformity correction have become an essential component for successful application of external fixation. Technology for external fixation has also improved such as computer-assisted external fixation, improved pin geometry and coatings, and fixator materials have expanded the indications and applications of external fixation.

External fixation can be utilized for gradual soft tissue correction or osseous correction. The effect of the rate and rhythm used in distraction osteogenesis (DO) has a significant effect on the expression of factors involved in the DO process [1–17]. Further, several experimental studies show improved bone regeneration with continuous versus intermittent distraction osteogenesis. Distraction begins at a specific rate and rhythm, typically 1.0 mm a day, divided into four increments. Although this is the classically cited rate, in clinical practice, the rate can vary (0.5 mm/day to 1 mm/day in the foot and ankle) based on multiple factors including patient age, health, medications, location, and type of osteotomy. Several experimental studies have shown improved bone regeneration using continuous versus intermittent distraction osteogenesis, with the former demonstrating up-regulation of several growth-stimulating genes. They found that there was decreased cellular staining of FGF, VEGF, and PDGF in the rapid distraction group starting on the first day of lengthening [14]. Many parameters have been implemented aiming to quantify the quality and speed of bone formation. The healing index (HI) is the most widely used parameter and is defined as the time needed for consolidation per cm of distracted osteotomy site. Consolidation time (CT) is defined as the time between the end of distraction and total consolidation or removal of hardware. The consolidation time is about twice as long as the distraction time in children, but may be three to four times longer in adults [12]. Thus, it usually amounts to 1 month/cm in children and 2–3 months/cm in adults [13].

The effect of bone lengthening on surrounding tissues especially on neurovascular structures must be taken into account. Neurovascular compromise is less of a concern then musculotendinous injury during the process of gradual bone lengthening. Nerves and vessels are able to adapt in length during the distraction process and recover from temporary degenerative changes within 2 months after the stopping of distraction [5, 6]. Neurovascular compromise is most often the result of surgical technique, such as pin placement, significant edema, and/or compartment syndrome. More commonly, bone distraction places increased tension on the muscles as the muscle length becomes relatively short compared to that of the bone, ultimately leading to muscle contractures. The muscles most frequently involved in contracture are those that cross two joints and are a result of an imbalance between the strength of the flexors and the extensors [15]. The mechanism of action of muscle groups can also be inhibited secondary to transfixation of the tendons or fascia via external hardware (i.e. pins, k-wires).

In addition to the previously mentioned neurovascular and musculoskeletal complications, one of the major drawbacks of distraction osteogenesis is the prolonged length of time needed to reach consolidation. This extended period of time in which the external fixator is left intact may increase the risk of complications, such as pin site infections, pain, discomfort, and psychological issues [6]. Numerous methods have been described in an attempt to accelerate the consolidation time, including the effect of mechanical loading induced by early weight-bearing. Other reported complications in DO include joint stiffness and subluxation, as well as axial deviation. During the lengthening process, there is a tendency for the bone segment being lengthened to gradually veer off its intended course due to muscle

B. M. Lamm (✉)
Foot and Ankle Surgery at St. Mary's Medical Center & Palm Beach Children's Hospital, West Palm Beach, FL, USA

Foot and Ankle Deformity Correction Center and Fellowship, Paley Orthopedic and Spine Institute, West Palm Beach, FL, USA
e-mail: blamm@paleyinstitute.org

imbalance or instability secondary to an inadequate external fixator construct [1, 5, 6]. Other complications encountered are related to the rate of consolidation at the distractions site. Premature consolidation occurs as a direct result of an excessive latency period in which significant callus healing is allowed to block the distraction of the osteotomy site. The most common foot bones to undergo premature consolidation are the midfoot and calcaneus as they are well-vascularized bones and require a 0.75 mm or 1 mm a day rate of distraction. The rate of distraction is less for metatarsal lengthening, usually around 0.5 mm a day. In contrast to premature consolidation, prolonged or delayed consolidation can occur secondary to technical factors including a traumatic corticotomy, thermal necrosis of bone during osteotomy, unstable external fixation, initial diastasis, or rapid distraction [5, 6]. Pin site infections, fracture after removal of the external fixator, and chronic regional pain syndrome have also been reported [15]. In addition, a disadvantage of external fixation is the surgical expertise that is required for construction and postoperative management. Complications such as pin site infections are common; however, most complications are minor and can be addressed non-operatively. Half pins or wires can cut through the skin during lengthening and create pin site drainage or infection in the short term and a scar line adjacent to the pin as a long-term consequence. Typically, when operative interventions are required, the distraction treatment can continue while the complications are being addressed [18].

Advantages of external fixation treatment are that surgeons have access to soft tissues for incision and wound care. External fixation allows fine-tuning of residual deformity correction during the postoperative period and allows for joint range of motion and early weight bearing. These advantages should decrease the risk of disuse osteoporosis and maintain the ability to perform joint range of motion. Theoretically, this joint motion allows joint fluid to bathe the cartilage with nutrients and allow for growth. However, despite the use of weight bearing on a walking ring, disuse osteopenia of the foot and ankle bones remains a problem even in children [19–22] (Figs. 17.1 and 17.2).

Gradual correction affords many benefits for the pediatric patient. The gradual nature of correction allows for a slow stretching of muscles and tendons while preserving joints and growth plates. The gradual correction is also beneficial to maintain limb length. Anatomical correction is the goal both from an osseous and soft tissue standpoint. When contractures occur, soft tissue distraction is performed gradually and in a joint sparing fashion using joint distraction techniques [19–22].

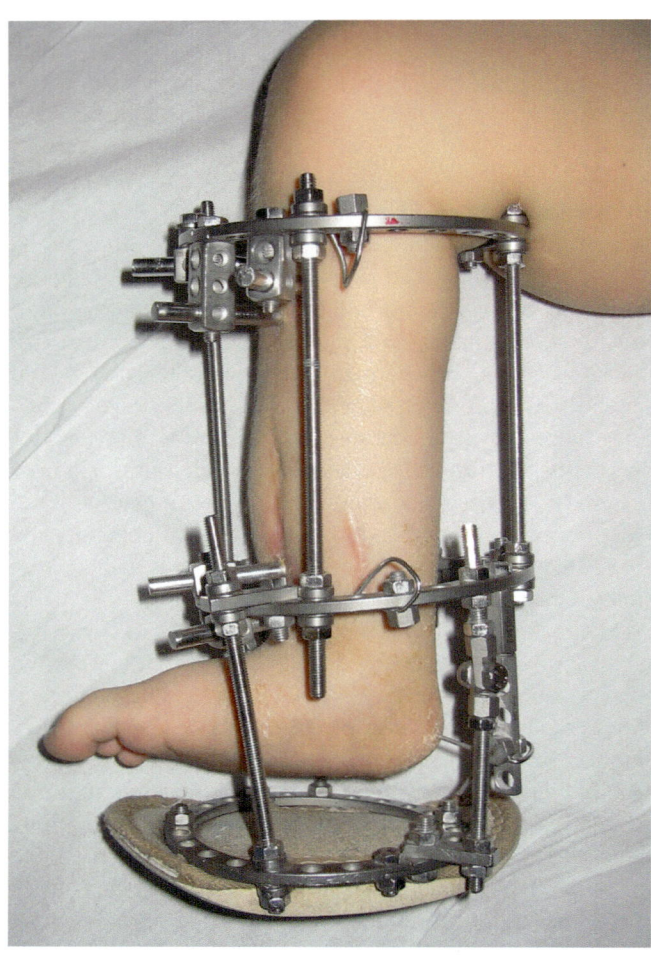

Fig. 17.1 Walking ring permits the patient to bear weight during the treatment

Fig. 17.2 (**a**, **b**) Disuse osteopenia can occur with extended treatment periods. (**a**) Preoperative lateral view radiograph of the foot and ankle shows normal bone density. (**b**) Generalized pedal osteopenia was observed in the lateral view radiograph after external fixation is removed. Thus, weight bearing is encouraged with external fixation

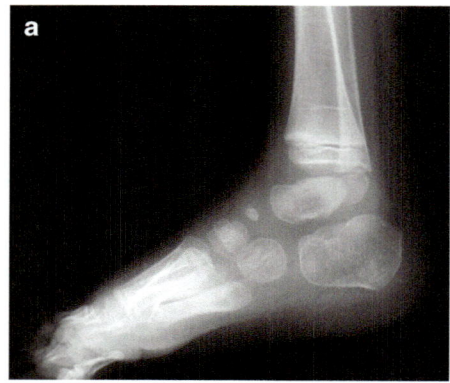
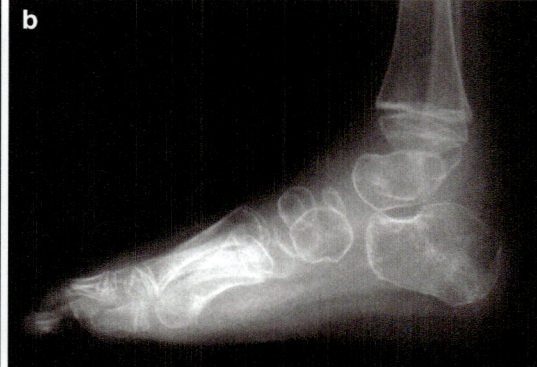

Update on Technology

In 1994, Dr. J. Charles Taylor and his brother, engineer Harold Taylor, developed the Taylor Spatial Frame (Smith &Nephew, Memphis, Tennessee). The Spatial Frame, which modified the Ilizarov apparatus, is a circular external fixator that uses a Stewart Platform and projectictive geometry by way of a computer program to allow for gradual, multiplanar deformity correction. Improved hardware and software have been developed specifically for the foot and ankle. Because of this computer-based programing, the Spatial Frame broadened the potential applications for complex deformity correction of the foot and ankle. More recently, other orthopedic companies have launched similar computer-generated software programs for their dynamic external fixation. Mobile applications are now available for patients and surgeons with automated adjustment reminders and tracking of the lengthening progress. In addition, automated smart robotic adjustable lengthening struts have also been introduced to minimize the chance of human error and improve the accuracy and reliability of bone generation [21].

Soft Tissue Contracture

Contractures of the soft tissue structures about the foot and ankle can result from a multitude of causes, including previous trauma, surgery, compartment syndromes, congenital abnormalities, burns, radiation, and a variety of neurologic conditions [23]. The contractures range from simple equinus of the ankle to complex multiplanar deformities with associated osseous malalignment and joint degeneration [24]. Osseous deformity can mimic soft tissue contracture [21]. For example, distal tibial procurvatum, forefoot equinus, and flattop talus can each present as an ankle equinus contracture. It is also important to recognize osseous deformities can coexist or contribute to soft tissue contractures.

Skeletal malalignment and soft tissue contractures can be treated simultaneously with external fixation, although the constructs can become very complex. The causes of soft tissue contractures can be further divided into extra-articular, intra-articular, or extra- and intra-articular. The extra-articular causes of ankle contractures might involve muscles.

Large acute corrections might require soft tissue expanders, extensive soft tissue release, shortening osteotomy, or microvascular free-tissue transfer to address soft tissue coverage. As an alternative, gradual correction allows for slow and better tolerated change of soft tissues and bone [21, 25]., especially in the presence of abnormal soft tissue such as scars burns and friable skin [21, 22, 26, 27]. External fixation allows for a gradual correction of abnormal soft tissues without extensive open exposures through them. The correction can be achieved purely through soft tissue distraction or can be combined with limited soft tissue releases. Avoiding tendon releases decreases the risk of overlengthening and excessively weakening the musculotendinous unit. Gradual correction of the foot and ankle is also less likely to compromise the nerves, muscles, and vascular supply. The risk can be further reduced by decompressing the posterior tibial neurovascular bundle and/or common peroneal neurovascular bundle, at the time of external fixation application. The author performs tarsal tunnel release prophylactically at the time of equinus contracture correction that is more than 5°, especially in the presence of associated varus or prior soft tissue compromise. Such releases can also be performed on an as-needed basis during the course of gradual external fixation correction. If any neurogenic compromise occurs during gradual correction, the rate of distraction can be slowed or temporarily stopped to allow for recovery. Nerve decompression should be considered when the nerve function does not improve or when any new motor deficit is noted. Typically, if a distraction holiday is undertaken either intermittently or for a short period of time, the regenerate bone can still successfully grow. Lengthy distraction holidays can result in premature consolidation of the regenerate. A soft tissue contracture should be overcorrected and held with a fixator for a minimum of 6 weeks to allow for soft tissue adaptation. The amount of overcorrection varies depending on the joint of correction. Typically, knee joint contractures require 10–15° of overcorrection whereas the ankle joint only needs 5–10° of overcorrection. However, the etiology of the deformity is an important factor to consider when deciding how much to overcorrect a soft tissue contracture. To prevent recurrence, the position should be maintained with a cast after removal of external fixation for approximately 4 weeks followed by continuous functional bracing thereafter. Any motor imbalance should be addressed by subsequent tendon transfer or tendon balancing to prevent soft tissue recurrence.

External fixators that are used to correct equinus contractures can be constructed using uniaxial hinge (constrained) or no hinge (unconstrained) designs. Dynamic external fixation correction using a hexapod is performed by means of a virtual hinge. The constrained fixator uses a single hinge on each side of the joint aligned on the center of the joint rotation being treated. For example, in the ankle, it is the transmalleolar axis or Inman's axis. The constrained fixator allows for range of motion of a joint during contracture correction. An ankle fixator should be constructed to allow for distraction of the ankle joint space during the deformity correction and lengthening. The fixation should be applied to the talus and calcaneus to prevent over or unwanted distraction of the subtalar joint. Unconstrained constructs are used for multi-axial multi-joint corrections such as clubfoot [21] (Fig. 17.3).

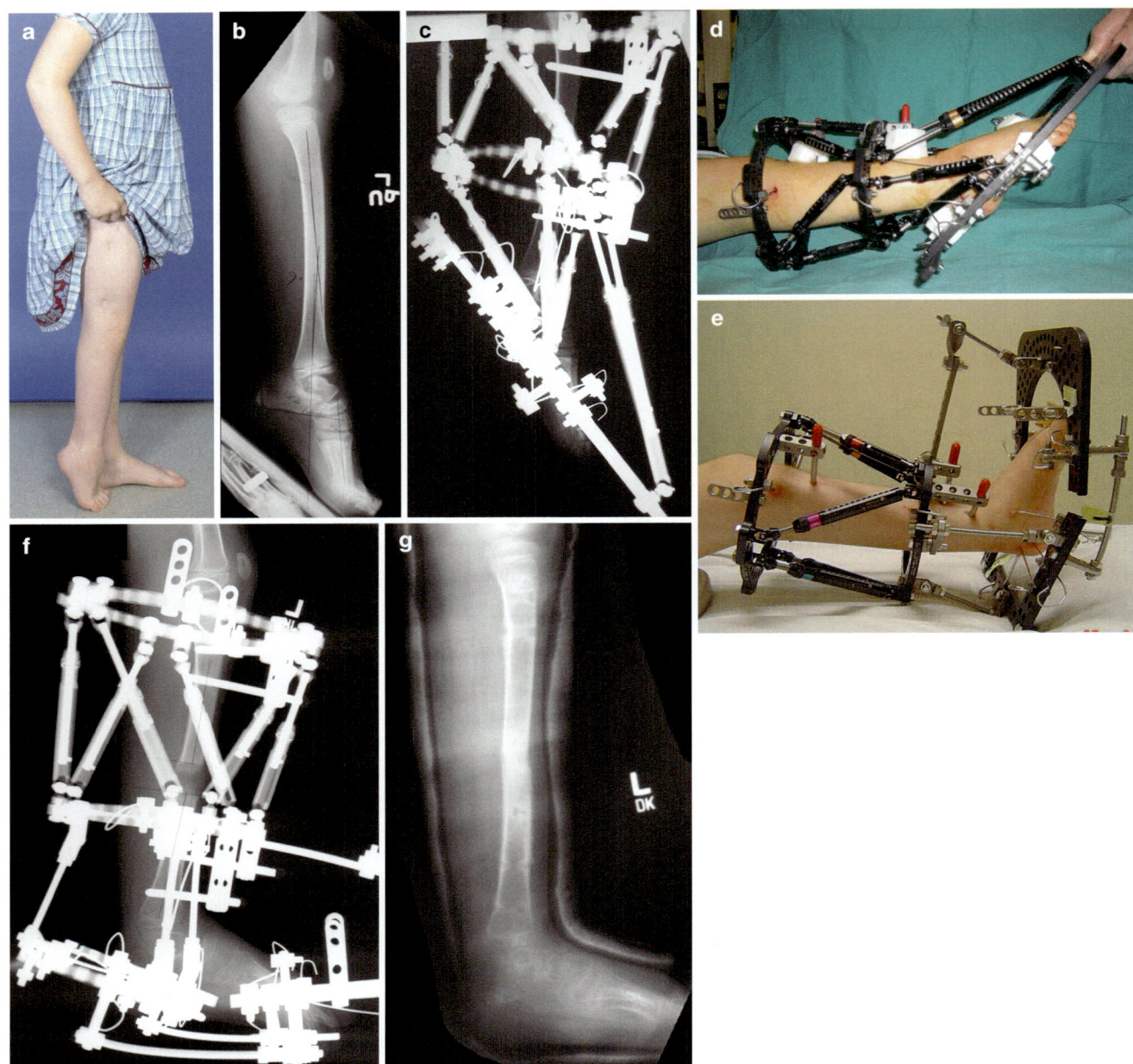

Fig. 17.3 (**a–g**) Patient with fibular hemimelia and a significant equinus and cavus foot deformity. (**a**) Preoperative clinical photograph. (**b**) Lateral view radiograph shows mid-tibial procurvatum deformity with severe equinus and cavus deformities. (**c**) Postoperative lateral view radiograph after the Taylor spatial frame was applied. (**d**) Postoperative lateral view clinical photograph of the Taylor spatial frame. Note that this fixator uses the virtual hinge (constrained) method. (**e**) After the equinus deformity is corrected, the foot ring is then cut (medial and lateral) to allow for correction of the cavus deformity. The gradual distraction is accomplished by adding pusher and puller Ilizarov rods. (**f**) Lateral view radiograph of the cavus deformity correction. (**g**) Postoperative lateral view radiograph shows a plantigrade foot in a short leg bivalved cast brace. The cast brace is worn for several months to maintain correction

Clubfoot

A primary indication is for children who have recurrent clubfoot deformities and have had previously undergone extensive open surgery. Gradual correction can also be used for older children who have residual clubfoot deformities. The treatment for these complex deformities in young children is performed with multiplanar external fixation in an unconstrained fashion [28–31]. Children less than 8 years could be treated by soft tissue and joint distraction, whereas children 8 years and older are typically treated with distraction osteotomies. Younger children are treated with soft tissue and joint distraction because they still possess some degree of biological plasticity, remodeling potential, of their bones and cartilage (Fig. 17.4).

The Ilizarov method of joint and soft tissue distraction is analogous to treating infants with serial casting. With casting, pressure is applied to the skin and the joints primarily experience compressive forces. In contrast, the Ilizarov method applies distraction forces across the joints. The tissues are stretched rather than surgically released, avoiding extensive intra-articular fibrosis and peri-capsular scarring. Treating a patient with tendon lengthening can alter the Blix curve of the musculotendinous unit and cause permanent weakness. This risk is largely avoided by using the distraction technique.

Ilizarov distraction is the preferred method to treat clubfoot with severe relapse after surgical treatment. These feet show extensive scar tissue formation, and to perform a repeat open surgery through the scar is a daunting task and can result in further complications. With Ilizarov techniques, the foot should be overcorrected by 5°–10° in the plane of correction because of the tendency for the deformity to reoccur. Once the deformity is corrected, the external fixation device should be held in the overcorrected position for 4–6 weeks. After removal, a long leg cast is applied to maintain the overcorrected position just as in the Ponseti technique. A custom-molded foot and ankle orthotic should be worn for the first six to 12 months. If dynamic recurrence occurs, then the appropriate tendon transfer should be considered. Rigid recurrences might require appropriate corrective osteotomies or arthrodesis.

Toe flexion contractures commonly occur during the gradual external fixation correction and often are caused by tightening of the intrinsic and extrinsic toe flexors. To prevent toe flexion contractures, the toe should be stretched with toe slings made from leather and elastic bands or with a plastic molded toe splint held to the fixator with Velcro straps. In addition, regularly performed physical therapy is required to prevent toe stiffness and contractures. For a pre-existing toe contracture, consider percutaneous flexor plantar tenotomy or flexor tendon lengthening. In older children, two wires can be used to gradually pull the toes upward and maintain a corrected digital position during correction (Fig. 17.5).

The gradual correction method is powerful and allows for anatomical realignment. However, in the pediatric patient, a risk of physiolysis or injury to the physis can occur with gradual correction. Therefore, it is important to protect the physis during the gradual correction process. In an immature skeleton, spontaneous fractures through the distal tibial physis can occur during distraction. Physiolysis can be avoided by inserting a transverse wire through the distal tibial epiphysis connected to the tibial external fixation device to stabilize the growth plate in position (Fig. 17.6).

The Ilizarov device and dynamic external fixation can also be used in conjunction with the principles described by Ponseti for correction of recurrent clubfoot deformity [32].

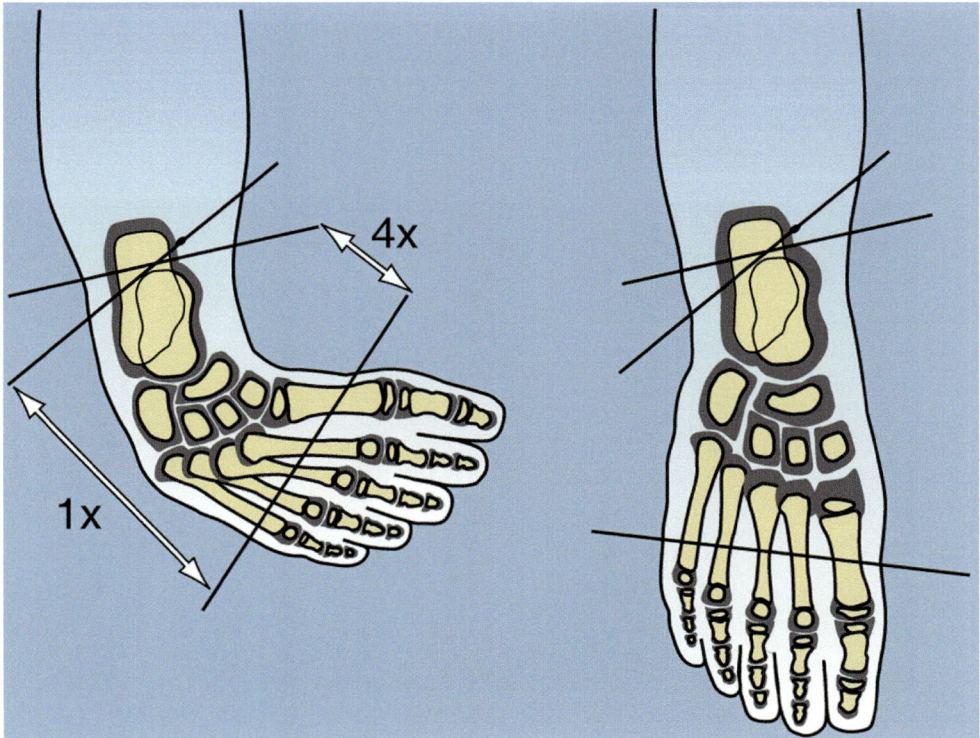

Fig. 17.4 Forefoot adduction correction with an Ilizarov fixator (4:1 adjustment ratio medial to lateral, respectively) in a child allows for anatomic formation of cartilage and bone

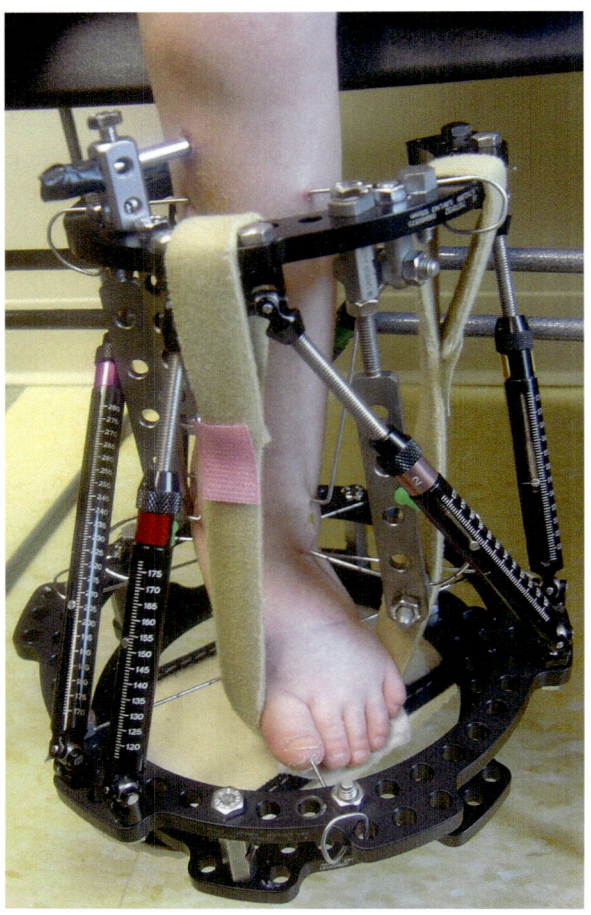

The forefoot position can be improved before surgery by a brief period of preoperative casting to allow for less complicated frame construction. In the Ponseti sequence, the foot is first externally rotated through the subtalar joint. The initial correction of the dynamic external fixation is programmed for external rotation and valgus correction. A lateral olive wire through the lateral aspect of the talar neck mimics the thumb of the Ponseti casting technique which is used for counterpressure. This wire is attached to the proximal tibia ring. After the foot is externally rotated approximately 40°, the talar neck olive wire is connected to the foot ring and then the ankle can be safely dorsiflexed. An additional computer-generated program is created to allow for ankle dorsiflexion with the external fixator and the position is maintained to hold the correction. This method is similar to the method used by Joshi, who developed an inexpensive, simple external fixator for clubfoot correction [33]. He similarly emphasizes correction of varus deformity with distraction followed by equinus correction. This unconstrained device permits the external rotation to occur through the calcaneal pedal block. This rationale can be explained as follows: unconstrained external rotation of the calcaneal pedal block allows for normal subtalar motion about its axis. Therefore, the calcaneal pedal block external rotation allows for the talus–foot realignment. After normal calcaneal–talus relationship is restored, the ankle can then be safely dorsiflexed. This combined subtalar and ankle joint motion is called kinematic coupling [32] (Fig. 17.7).

Fig. 17.5 Custom-molded forefoot plate with Velcro straps assists in the prevention of digital flexion contractures during deformity correction of the foot and ankle. Digital pinning can also be performed to correct or prevent toe flexion contractures

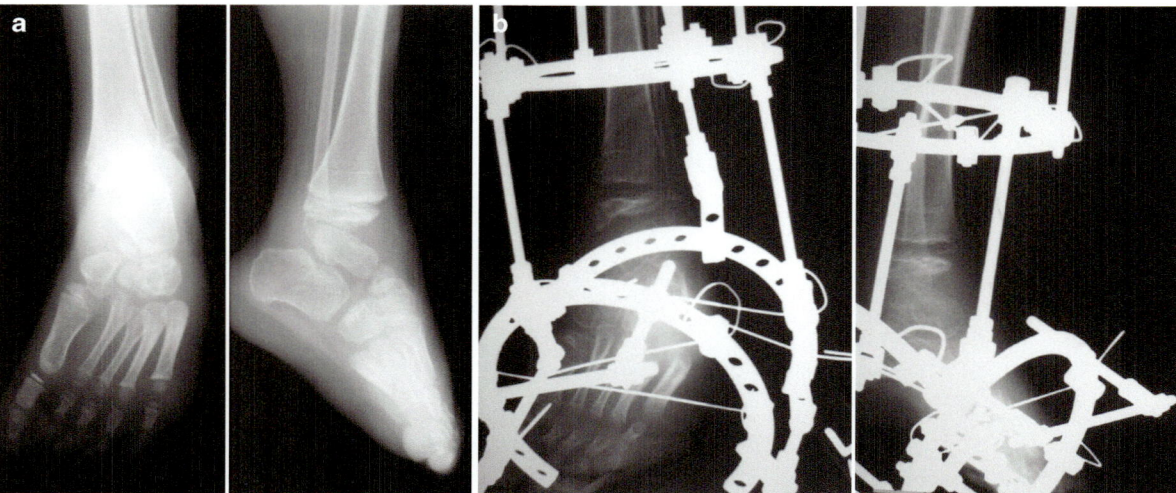

Fig. 17.6 (**a**, **b**) Physiolysis or distraction of the growth plate can occur when deformity correction is being performed about the foot and ankle. (**a**) Preoperative anteroposterior and lateral view radiographs of the left ankle. (**b**) Postoperative anteroposterior and lateral view radiographs of the left ankle. Note the radiographic distraction of the distal tibial physis

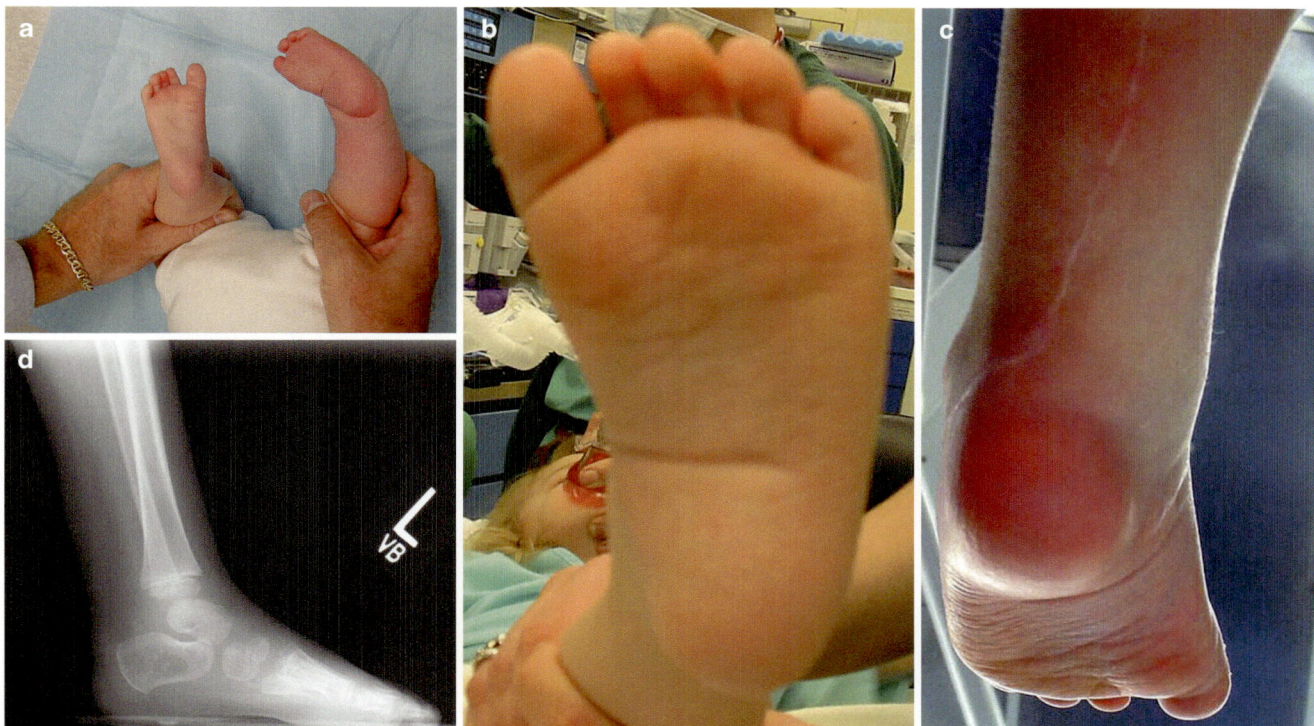

Fig. 17.7 (a–l) Relapsed clubfoot. (**a**) Clinical photograph of the left limb obtained when the infant initially presented. The photograph shows the equinus and varus deformity of the hindfoot and the adduction and supination deformity of the forefoot. (**b**) Plantar photograph showing the cavus and the adduction of the foot in this now 8-year-old residual clubfoot child. (**c**) Posterior photograph showing the residual varus clubfoot in this now 8-year-old child. (**d**) Lateral view radiograph shows the residual clubfoot in the 8-year-old child. (**e**) Anteroposterior view radiograph shows the residual clubfoot in the 8-year-old child. (**f**) Intraoperative fluoroscopy shows an olive wire inserted from lateral to medial through the talar neck. Also note the distal tibial epiphysial stirrup wire, which prevents physiolysis. (**g**) Postoperative photograph shows the talar neck wire attached to the tibial ring via plates. (**h**) Clinical photograph shows the completion of the first stage of treatment (foot external rotation). When the foot is externally rotated 40, the dorsiflexion of the ankle can begin. (**i**) Clinical photograph of the anteroposterior view of the foot. Note that the talar wire was detached from the tibial ring (plates removed) and reattached to the foot ring. (**j**) Lateral view radiograph of the foot. The ankle can now be safely dorsiflexed. (**k**) Lateral view clinical photograph of the foot with overcorrection of the ankle dorsiflexion, because rebound equinus is anticipated. (**l**) Final postoperative lateral view radiograph shows a plantigrade foot position

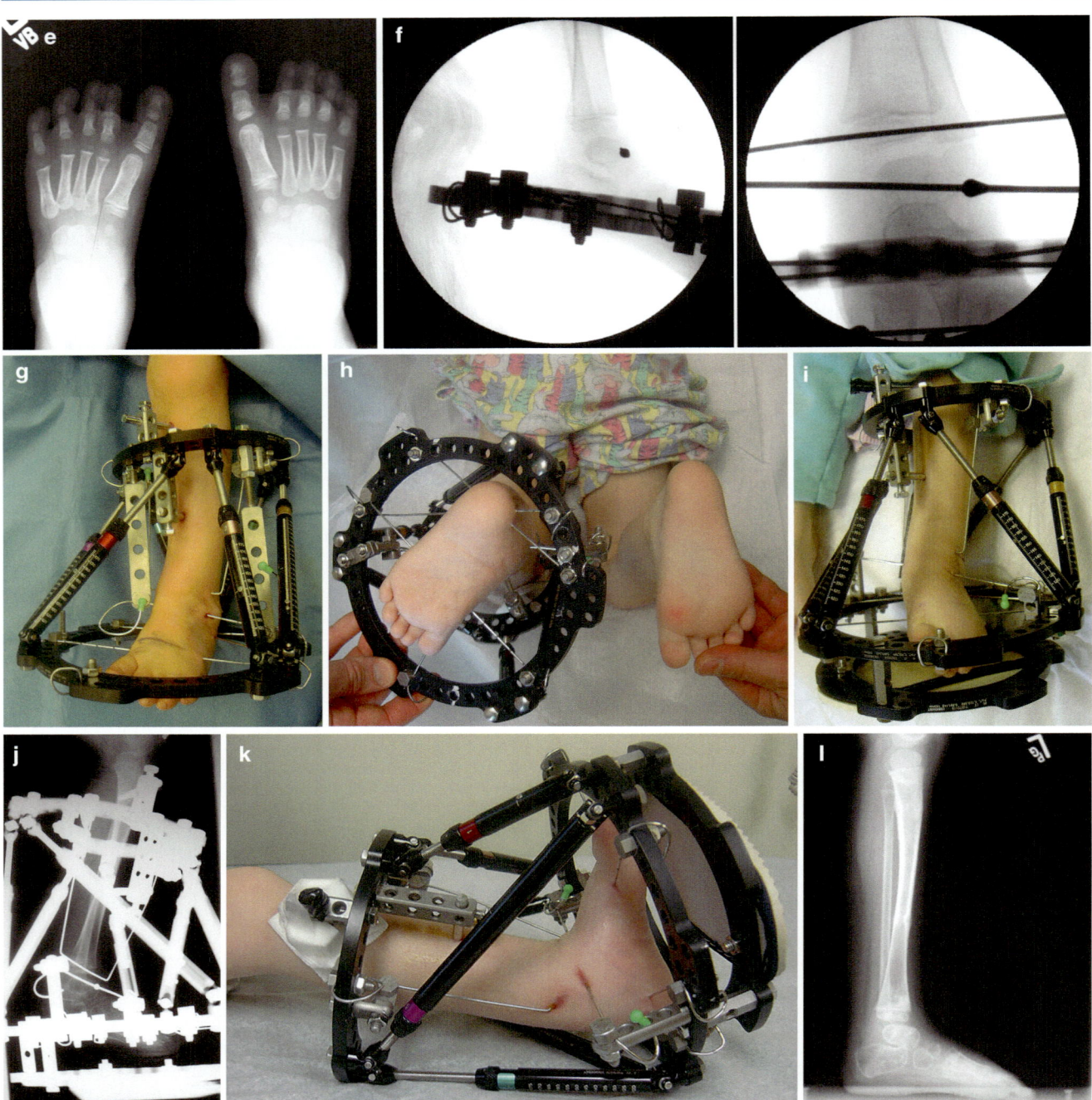

Fig. 17.7 (continued)

Equinuocavusvarus Deformity

In a case of equino-cavo-varus deformity, the treatment of gradual correction like the aforementioned clubfoot treatment is performed with an additional step. This additional step involves an external fixation modification at the end to correct the cavus deformity. The cavus deformity will exacerbate the equinus deformity. Thus, care must be taken to address these in a combined fashion. Equinus is corrected first, as the entire foot needs to be held in position for appropriate leverage to focus the forces on ankle dorsiflexion correction. Cavus can be then corrected after equinus is reduced. When a rigid midfoot is present, osteotomy is needed or the surgeon can except the cavus and just address the equinus. When a flexible midfoot is present, then gradual distraction of the forefoot to the hindfoot can be achieved. With the Ilizarov device, cutting (with a Gigli saw) the foot ring in half both medial and lateral to separate the forefoot and hindfoot can be done. Adding medial and lateral pusher threaded rods and anterior medial and lateral puller up threaded rods allow for cavus correction. The puller rods must pull 2 times faster than the pusher rods to ensure a dorsal foot hinge correction. Alternately, a computer-assisted dynamic external fixator can be used with the same external fixation frame modifications (separate forefoot ring and hindfoot ring fixation) [34].

Arthrogryposis

Many congenital syndromes cause severe foot deformities. For example, arthrogryposis can cause patients to experience severe clubfoot contractures that are associated with high surgical recurrence rates. These patients typically have very stiff joints. Treatment with external fixation using soft tissue and joint distraction in young children and distraction through osteotomies combined with joint arthrodesis in older children is a reasonable alternative for these severe stiff and often multiply operated feet.

Recurrences in arthrogryposis are common and might require arthrodesis or osteotomy. In such cases, the author generally performs extensive open and acute realignment correction of the hindfoot and ankle. The external fixation is then applied for simultaneous tibial lengthening and static fixation of the foot deformity correction. Alternatively, casting can also be performed in these acute correction cases [35, 36].

Osteotomy

The primary indication for correction through bone is a fixed bony deformity. In patients younger than 8 years, some remodeling can still be expected and attempts at joint distraction are reasonable. When bony deformity is present in patients older than 8 years, soft tissue releases and distractions have high rates of recurrence. Other indications for an osteotomy include neuromuscular imbalance. Occasionally, it is not possible to maintain correction obtained by distraction. In such cases, arthrodesis can be considered with osteotomy. Nonunion in the presence of previous fusions and severe stiffness of deformities are also indications for bony correction [30, 37]. Osteotomy provides osseous realignment with acute or gradual correction with use of external fixation or acute correction with internal fixation.

Supramalleolar osteotomies are indicated for deformities of metaphyseal or juxa-articular region deformities. Other indications include deformity at the level of a previous arthrodesis or deformity at the level of the talus or subtalar joint in the presence of an ankle ankylosis. Equinus, calcaneus, varus, and valgus deformities, tibial torsion and limb length discrepancies can be corrected through the metaphyseal or juxa-articular region. The level of an ankle osteotomy should be within 2.5 cm of the joint which is critical for providing realignment and reliable bone consolidation. In addition, the method with which the osteotomy is performed is important for bone formation. The author prefers either a percutaneous Gigli saw technique or a multiple drill hole osteotome osteotomy technique through the tibia and fibula [21]. The supramalleolar osteotomy with external fixation allows for gradual correction of length, angulation translation, and rotation. Although the procedure avoids performing surgery on the foot that has undergone multiple operation, it does not allow for correction of deformities between the hindfoot and forefoot. When the level of deformity is at a level different from that of the osteotomy, translation is required to prevent the creation of a secondary deformity [38].

The U osteotomy passes under the subtalar joint through the superior part of the calcaneus posteriorly and across the sinus tarsi and neck of the talar anteriorly. It is indicated when the deformity occurs in the talus, such as in a case of flat-topped talus. The foot can be repositioned into a plantigrade position while leaving the ankle mortise undisturbed. Although this osteotomy can be performed acutely, most deformities require gradual realignment with external fixation. The U osteotomy crosses the sinus tarsi and physically blocks the subtalar motion. The U osteotomy can correct foot height, Equinus, calcaneus, varus, and valgus deformities. It is unable to correct forms between the forefoot and hindfoot [19, 21, 39] (Fig. 17.8).

The V osteotomy is a double osteotomy, one osteotomy crosses the body of the calcaneus posterior to the subtalar joint and the other crosses the midfoot at the neck of the talus and calcaneus through the sinus tarsi, the cuboid-navicular row, and cuboid-cuneiform row. When the midfoot osteotomy is made across the neck of the talus and calcaneus, it converges with the posterior calcaneal osteotomy on the plantar aspect of the calcaneus. The procedure leaves a triangular wedge of calcaneus and subtalar joint connected by the posterior facet to the body of the talus. The triangular wedge must be fixed in place during distraction. This type of V osteotomy as indicated when deformities are present between the forefoot and hindfoot with an associated stiff subtalar joint. When preservation of subtalar joint motion is important, the anterior segment of the V should be made through the cuboid-navicular or cuboid-cuneiform rows. Hindfoot and forefoot osteotomies can correct all types of foot deformities including hindfoot and forefoot equinus, calcaneus, rockbottom, cavus, abductus, adductus, supination, pronation, and even bony deficiency of the hindfoot or forefoot. Again, this procedure is performed as a gradual correction with the use of external fixation. As an alternative, the same approach can be performed with using closing wedge correction of one or both osteotomies using internal or static external fixation.

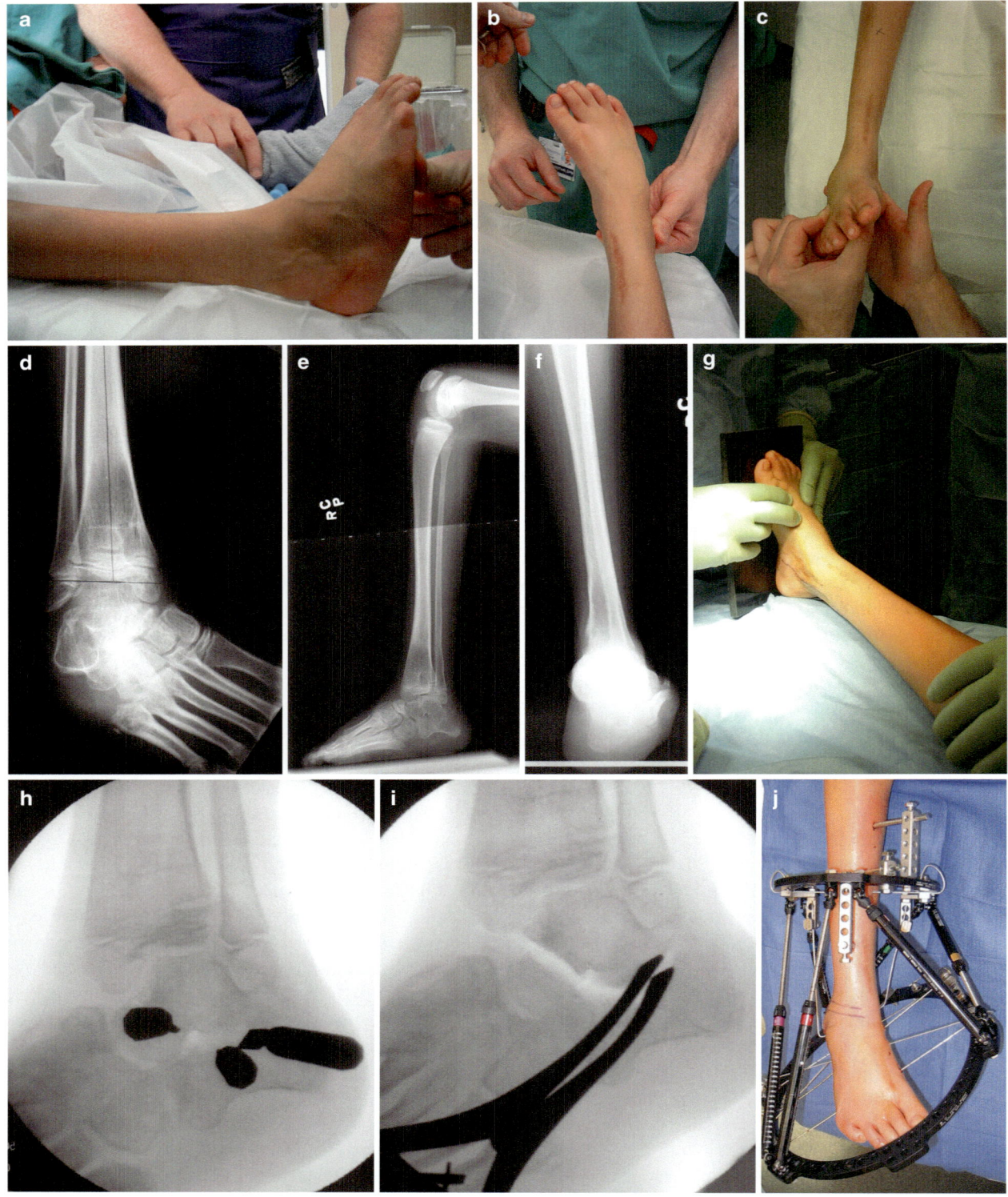

Fig. 17.8 (**a–p**) Residual clubfoot. (**a**) Clinical photograph shows a clubfoot that is stiff and has undergone previous operations. Note the equinus deformity. (**b**) Clinical photograph shows the forefoot abduction. (**c**) Clinical photograph shows the combined forefoot and hindfoot varus deformity. (**d**) Anteroposterior view radiograph shows normal ankle alignment. (**e**) Long standing, lateral view radiograph of the foot and ankle shows cavovarus deformity. (**f**) Long standing, calcaneal axial radiograph shows significant hindfoot varus. (**g**) A foot board is used intraoperatively to confirm the diagnosis of a combined forefoot and hindfoot varus deformity. (**h**) Fluoroscopy shows the multiple osteotome technique used to perform the U osteotomy, which is made beneath the sustentaculum tali and through the neck of the talus. (**i**) Under fluoroscopy, the osteotomy is visualized to ensure completion. (**j, k**) Postoperative clinical photographs show the limb after application of a Taylor spatial frame. (**l**) Postoperative anteroposterior view radiograph. (**m**) Postoperative lateral view radiograph. (**n**) Clinical photograph obtained after correction shows how the U osteotomy corrects the foot as a unit. Note the neutral heel position. (**o**) Clinical photograph shows the external rotation of the foot. (**p**) Clinical photograph shows a plantigrade position of the foot

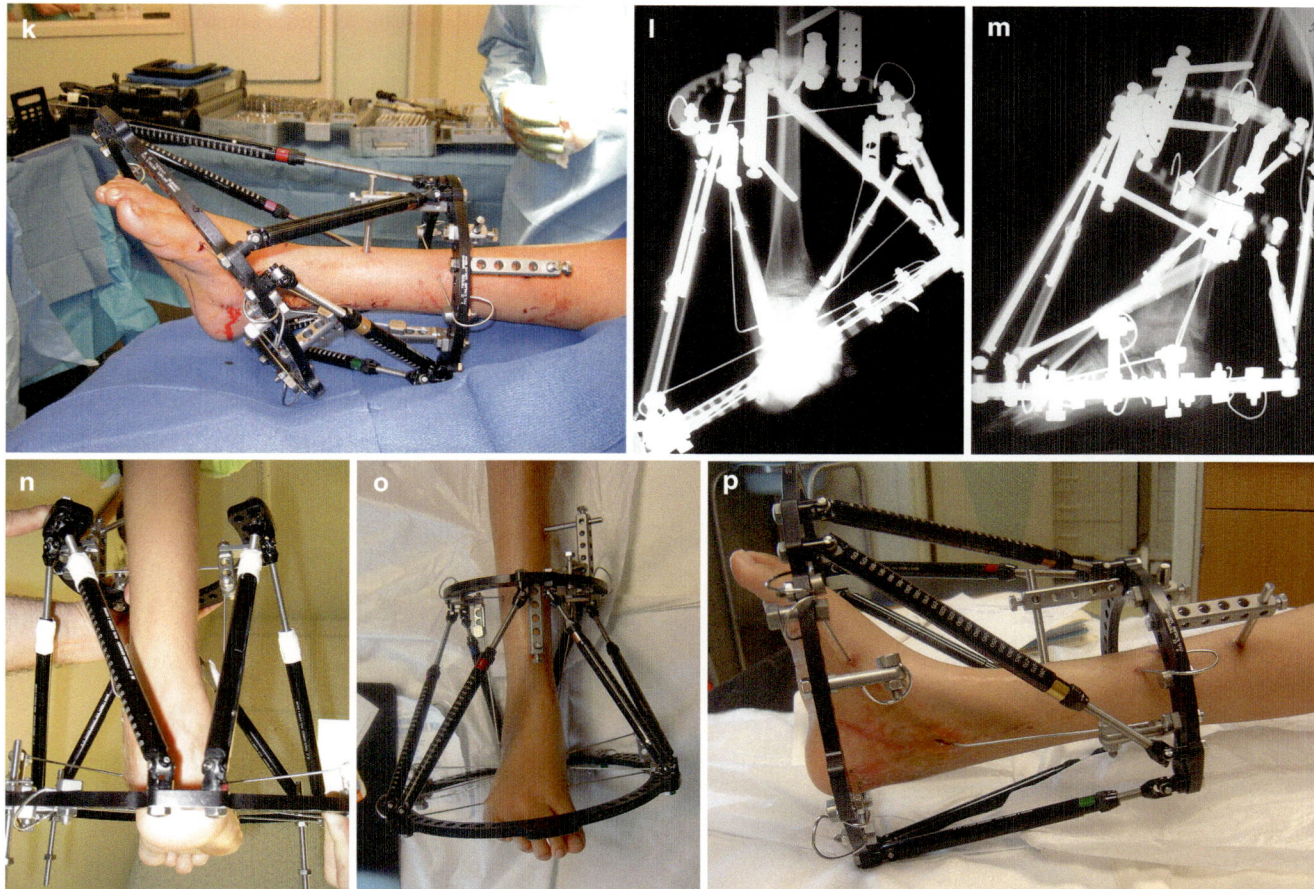

Fig. 17.8 (continued)

The posterior calcaneal osteotomy is essentially the posterior segment of the V osteotomy. It is used in cases of isolated deformities of the hind foot and can be combined with soft tissue correction of the forefoot. Posterior calcaneal osteotomys are performed acutely with pin or screw fixation and include the Dwyer (closing lateral wedge), medial, lateral, dorsal, and plantar displacement osteotomies. The dorsal opening wedge calcaneal osteotomy, however, is typically performed through gradual distraction, especially in complex realignment cases. Calcaneal bone deficiency due to congenital or post-traumatic causes can be treated by lengthening of the calcaneus through this osteotomy. Smooth wires or half pins can be inserted through the posterior calcaneus segment for fixation. Alternatively, olive wires can also be used. Smooth wires and half pins can cut through or pulled out of the calcaneus as the calcaneus becomes osteoporotic during the treatment. Therefore, careful postoperative monitoring is important. Ilizarov hinges should be placed at the apex of the angular correction and with dynamic external fixation, appropriate planning of a distal opening wedge osteotomy should be performed. In a short or stubby calcaneus, distraction of the calcaneal tuber in a posterior direction provides a great lever arm for the Achilles tendon and prevents the heel from slipping up out of the shoe [19, 21] (Fig. 17.9).

A midfoot osteotomy and talocalcaneal neck osteotomy are essentially to the anterior segment of the V osteotomy. It is used for correction of forefoot deformities in the presence of a stiff or ankylosed subtalar joint. When a mobile subtalar joint is present, a midfoot osteotomy across the cuboid-navicular bones or across the cuboid-cuneiform bones should be used. The author prefers to perform all three midfoot-type osteotomies using percutaneous Gigli saw technique. The Gigli saw should not be used to perform osteotomies across multiple metatarsals because of risk of neurovascular injury. A midfoot osteotomy can also be used to lengthen the forefoot. For a foot with normal mobile joints, a midfoot osteotomy is associated with creating a stiff midfoot; however, these midfoot joints normally have minimal mobility [19, 21, 37, 40].

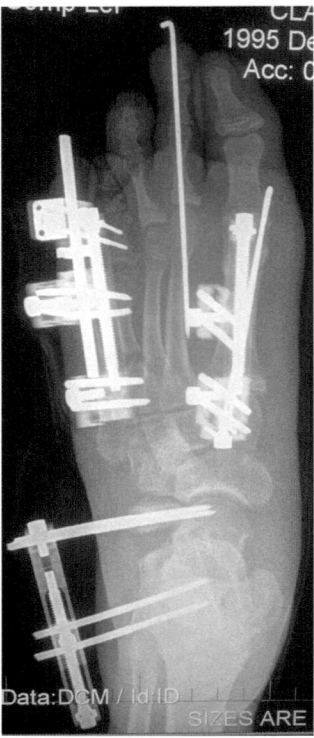

Fig. 17.9 Case of simultaneous gradual calcaneal neck lengthening and fourth metatarsal lengthening with external fixation. Note the gradual calcaneal/metatarsal lengthening can achieve larger corrections than the acute lengthening

Tibial Lengthening

Patients who have foot and ankle deformities often present with concomitant limb length discrepancies. Limb length discrepancy can be congenital, traumatic, secondary to previous surgery, arthrodesis, or malalignment. Limb lengthening is a challenging procedure that demands an experienced surgeon. Most tibial lengthenings are performed proximally through the metaphyseal diaphyseal junction below the tibial tuberosity with a multiple drill hole osteotome osteotomy or Gigli saw-type osteotomy. Fixation of the tibia and the fibula is important to avoid descent of the fibula or proximal migration of the distal fibula, therefore maintaining the ankle and knee joint congruency. When applying a fixator to the proximal tibia, care should be taken to avoid injury to the common peroneal nerve. Distal tibial lengthening is performed when a deformity is present at or proximal to the ankle joint. To prevent equinus deformity, the external fixator should be extended to the foot for distal tibial, double level, and longer lengthenings. Ankle equinus and knee contractures are common problems that can arise with limb lengthening. A 5 day per week combined land and aquatic physical therapy regimen is critical to avoid these joint contractures. In addition, dynamic knee extension and ankle dorsiflexion splints can be used. A prophylactic gastrocnemius recession can be performed in a case of high-risk patient or in the presence of a preoperative equinus contracture. Axial deviation such as a bony deformity can occur during lengthening. This deviation occurs secondary to the surrounding posterior and lateral muscle mass about the tibia. When the amount of tension is high enough, the bone deviates in the direction of the larger muscle mass and path of least resistance. In proximal tibial lengthening, procurvatum and valgus deformities together with lateral and posterior translation, respectively, can occur and will increase in severity with increasing amounts of tibial lengthening. Alignment should be assessed by using appropriate long leg weight-bearing radiographs during treatment to ensure proper alignment of the lengthen bone. In the case of an unstable ankle joint or ball and socket ankle joint, it is important to fix the foot with the lateral opposing olive wires to maintain foot position [21].

Acute Trauma

External fixation is important instrument for surgeons treating distal tibia, foot, and ankle trauma. These injuries are often associated with soft tissue compromise, especially in cases of open fracture or crush injury. External fixation can be used as a temporary splint to allow for reduction of soft tissue swelling before definitive internal fixation or as a neutralization device combined with internal fixation to maintain alignment and hold an osseous correction [41, 42]. High-energy injuries and injuries with compromised skin lend themselves well to correction by external fixation because the method limits further soft tissue disruption. External fixation provides stability to multiple bone segments, allowing access and healing to soft tissue wounds without compromising the bone healing. Modern external fixation devices allow for acute or gradual reduction of the fracture fragments. Another advantage of external fixation includes the prevention of soft tissue contractures during bone healing [42]. In most pediatric cases, fractures are typically treated with casts. However, in cases that involve complex distal tibial fractures, external fixation is an excellent instrument to treat children and adolescents. The dynamic external fixation or Ilizarov device allows for gradual correction or acute reduction in fractures that cannot be controlled with casting techniques alone. External fixation can be used in the treatment of complex midfoot, tarsal, and metatarsal dislocations and fractures, particularly in association with soft tissue severe injuries (Fig. 17.10).

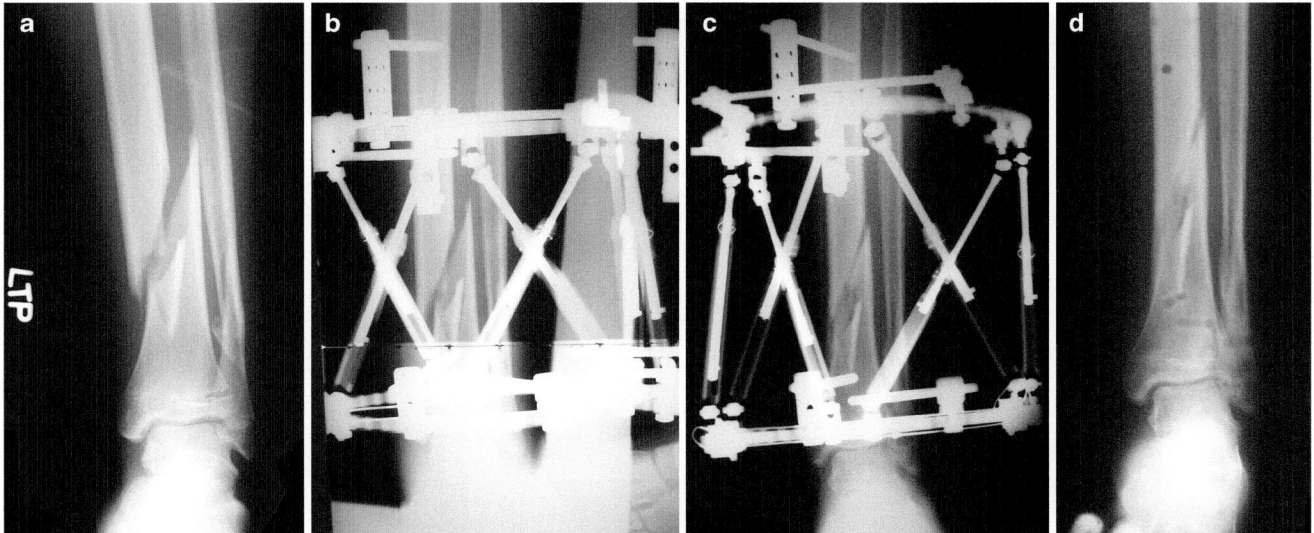

Fig. 17.10 (a–d) Case of a distal tibiofibular fracture. (**a**) Preoperative anteroposterior view radiograph shows a comminuted distal tibiofibular fracture. (**b**) Postoperative anteroposterior view radiograph shows the Taylor spatial frame and the distal tibial malalignment. (**c**) An anteroposterior view radiograph shows the anatomic alignment after gradual correction with the external fixator. (**d**) An anteroposterior view radiograph shows a healed, aligned distal tibia and fibula after removal of the external fixator

Metatarsal Lengthening

Brachymetatarsia is a complex deformity of a ray(s) of the foot that has both an osseous (metatarsal and the corresponding phalangeal bones) and soft tissue component. Congenital brachymetatarsia is metatarsal growth deficiency of length along with the corresponding phalangeal bones, whereas a traumatic metatarsal growth plate disturbance has normal length phalanges. Clinically the brachymetatarsia ray will have a shortened toe that sits more dorsal on the foot than the adjacent toes and the adjacent toes converge toward the short toe. Greater amounts of metatarsal shortening can cause deeper plantar skin creases. Brachymetapody is when there is more than one short metatarsal in a foot. The shortened metatarsal(s) induce an adverse appearance of the foot and abnormal foot function [43].

Various surgical techniques have been attempted for acute and gradual metatarsal lengthening [44–47]. The potential complications associated with lengthening metatarsals and the treatment of these complications have been published [43–49]. A commonly encountered complication of metatarsal lengthening is metatarsophalangeal joint (MTPJ) stiffness or dislocation/subluxation. To prevent this complication, bridging of the external fixation across the MTPJ during gradual callus distraction is utilized. This concept of bridging the joint has been utilized for decades in limb lengthening surgery in order to minimize stiffness and contracture of the joint postoperatively. The first publication to describe this technique for brachymetatrsia treatment was by Lamm in 2009 [50]. With greater amounts of lengthening, the joint is more susceptible to greater forces and thus increasing risk for joint subluxation, chondrolysis, and postoperative joint stiffness. The farther the osteotomy from the joint, the less forces, thus a proximal metaphyseal–diaphyseal junction ostetotomy is preferred. Stabilizing the digit to the metatarsal head via axial pinning creates negative side effects of cartilage injury to the joint and MTPJ stiffness regardless of the length of time the pin is maintained. The senior author's (BML) technique of spanning and protecting the MTPJ was devised to prevent postoperative subluxation, stiffness, and chrondrolysis of the joint. In addition, this bridging fixator provides acute digital deformity correction with simultaneous joint distraction to maintain mobility of the MTPJ for the long term [50–52].

Lengthening of the bone at the proper rate, rhythm, trajectory, and protecting the surrounding soft tissues can be a challenge to even the most experienced surgeons. As the amount of bone lengthening increases so does the associated potential risk for complications [53, 54]. Because there has been no consensus of methodology of lengthening for brachymetatarsia, the authors have developed a comprehensive anatomic classification system (Lamm Classification) which provides a surgical guide to treatment of each classification type [55].

Brachymetatarsia deformities range from purely short metatarsals to irregularities of specific regions of the bone, including the shaft, head, and joint. The Lamm Brachymetatarsia Classification is based on the normal foot radiographic measurements and angles [56]. Three broad classification categories have been defined: type A

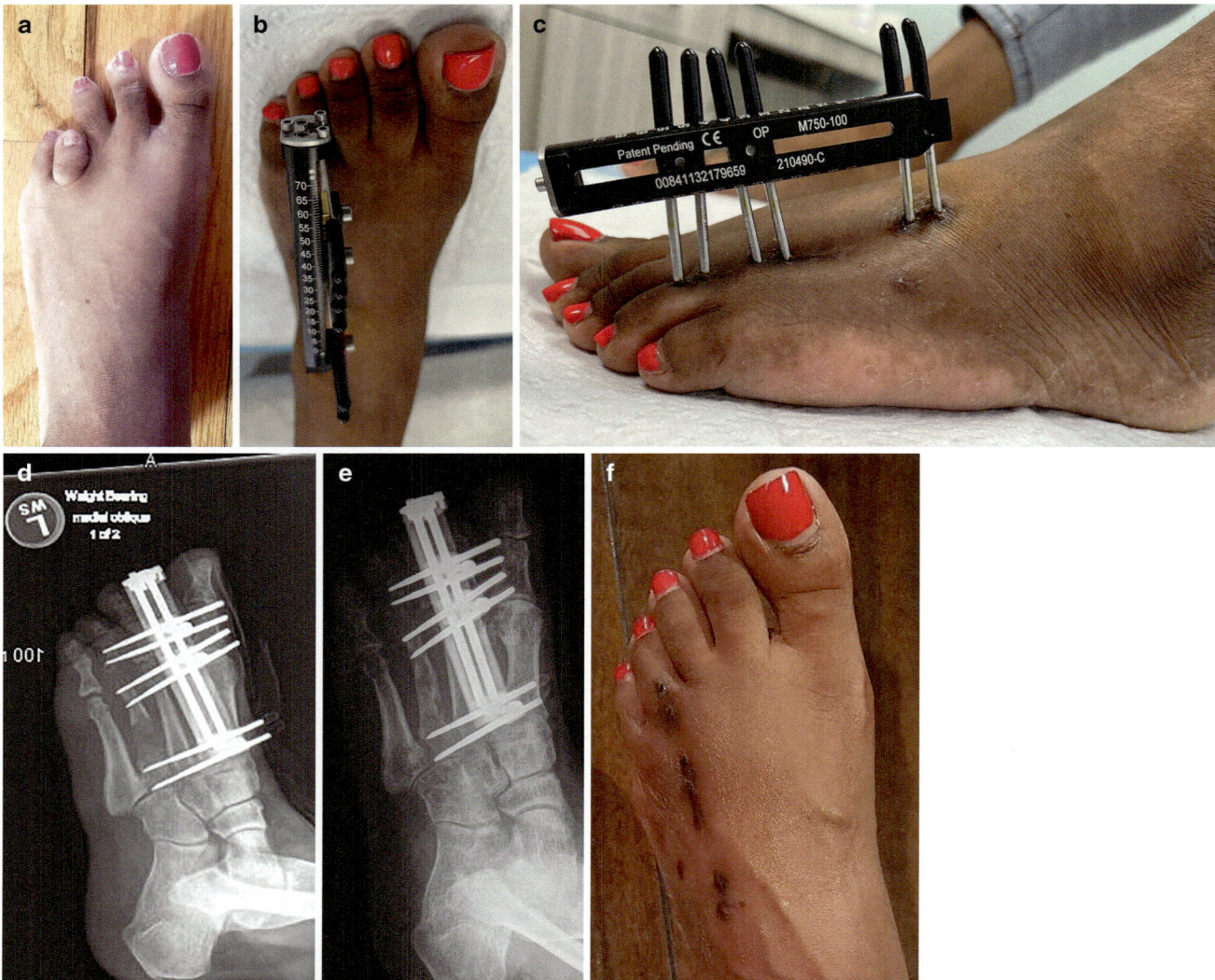

Fig. 17.11 (a–f) Congenital short fourth metatarsal lengthening. (a) Preoperative clinical photograph shows a fourth brachymetatarsia with an extension contracture of the fourth toe. (b) A clinical photograph after lengthening of the fourth metatarsal via gradual distraction osteogenesis with external fixation. Anteroposterior view radiograph shows a slight medial bowing of the fourth metatarsal. (c) Lateral clinical photograph shows that 6 half pins of which two are in the digit as to span the fixator across the metatarsophalangeal joint to prevent digital dislocation during lengthening. (d) Oblique radiographic view of the foot shows normotrophic bone regenerate formation of the fourth metatarsal with external fixation. (e) Oblique radiographic view of the foot shows healed normotrophic bone regenerate formation of the fourth metatarsal. (f) Postoperative clinical photograph shows a well aligned and lengthen fourth toe with minimal scar

(Axial distance deficiency) includes those metatarsals that are normal in all respects aside from their shortened length; type B (Bowing) involves angulation of the shaft of the affected metatarsal; and type C (Congruency), MTPJ congruency is associated with joint imbalances and metatarsal head and phalangeal base irregularity. The classification system provides one number (1–5) and 3 letters (A,B,C). The number indicates which metatarsal is short or hypoplastic. For example, a number 1 would indicate the first metatarsal, and 4 would indicate the fourth metatarsal. Therefore, for example, if a patient has is a short fourth metatarsal, bowing of the metatarsal shaft, and an incongruent MTPJ, this patient would be classified as a 4ABC [55] (Fig. 17.11).

Summary

Gradual correction of deformity has been well documented as a successful treatment of pediatric limb deformities. External fixation has many applications to the pediatric foot and ankle and lower limb. Additional applications of external fixation continue to be developed as technology and experience improve. External fixation should not be performed by a surgeon inexperienced in the technique. It is vital to gain knowledge from courses, lectures, seminars, and books about the topic. Surgeons who wish to use external fixation should visit and observe at a center where external fixation is frequently performed and obtain personal instruction from surgeons experienced in the field of external fixation and the principles of deformity correction.

Many surgeons prefer acute correction as the postoperative care is simplified and the operating time is decreased. The acute correction typically involves shortening of bone and soft tissues. This a novel concept that is extremely powerful for correction and can decrease operative and healing times. However, if joint preservation and soft tissue balancing is the goal, then gradual correction restores the normal anatomy. Restoring anatomy is paramount to allow for normal gait function. Ultimately, the surgeons experience and knowledge is the key for the success of the pediatric patient's outcome.

References

1. Aronson J, Harrison BH, Stewart CL, Harp JH Jr. The histology of distraction osteogenesis using different external fixators. Clin Orthop Relat Res. 1989;241:106–16.
2. Murray JH, Fitch RD. Distraction histiogenesis: principles and indications. J Am Acad Orthop Surg. 1996;4(6):317–27.
3. Jazrawi LM, Majeska RJ, Klein ML, et al. Bone and cartilage formation in an experimental model of distraction osteogenesis. J Orthop Trauma. 1998;12(2):111–6.
4. Frierson M, Ibrahim K, Boles M, et al. Distraction osteogenesis. A comparison of corticotomy techniques. Clin Orthop Rel Res. 1994;301:19–24.
5. Goldstein RY, Jordan CJ, McLaurin TM, et al. The evolution of the Ilizarov technique; part 2: the principles of distraction osteosynthesis. Bull Hosp Jt Dis. 2013;71(1):96–103.
6. Paley D. Problems, obstacles, and complications of limb lengthening by the Ilizarov technique. Clin Orthop Relat Res. 1990;250:81–104.
7. Aronson J, Harp JH. Mechanical forces as predictors of healing during tibial lengthening by distraction osteogenesis. Clin Orthop Relat Res. 1994;301:73–9.
8. Aronson J, Good B, Stewart C, et al. Preliminary studies of mineralization during distraction osteogenesis. Clin Orthop Relat Res. 1990;250:43–9.
9. Hasler C, Krieg A. Current concepts of leg lengthening. J Child Orthop. 2012;6:89–104.
10. Fischgrund J, Paley D, Suter C. Variables affecting time to bone healing during limb lengthening. Clin Orthop Relat Res. 1994;301:31–7.
11. Vauhkonen M, Peltonen J, Karaharju E, et al. Collagen synthesis and mineralization in the early phase of distraction bone healing. Bone Miner. 1990;10:171–81.
12. Herzenberg JE, Waanders NA. Calculating rate and duration of distraction for deformity correction with the Ilizarov technique. Orthop Clin North Am. 1991;22:601–11.
13. Ilizarov GA. The tension-stress effect on the genesis and growth of tissues. Part 1. The influence of stability of fixation and soft tissue preservation. Clin Orthop Rel Res. 1989;238:249–81.
14. Schiller JR, Moore DC, Ehrlich MG. Increased lengthening rate decreases expression of fibroblast growth factor 2, platelet-derived growth factor, vascular endothelial growth factor, and CD3 in a rat model of distraction osteogenesis. J Pediatr Orthop. 2007;27:961–8.
15. Velazquez RJ, Bell DF, Armstrong PF, et al. Complications of use of the Ilizarov technique in the correction of limb deformities in children. J Bone Joint Surg Am. 1993;75:1148–56.
16. Alzahrani MM, Anam EA, et al. The effect of altering the mechanical loading environment on the expression of bone regenerating molecules in cases of distraction osteogenesis. Front Endocrinol. 2014;5:1–11.
17. Handy RC, Rendon JS, Tabrizian M. Distraction osteogenesis and its challenges in bone regeneration. Bone regeneration. In Tech; 2012. p. 185–212.
18. Lamm BM, Standard SC, Galley IJ, Herzenberg JE, Paley D. External fixation for the foot and ankle in children. Clin Podiatr Med Surg. 2006;23:137–66.
19. Kirienko A, Villa A, Calhoun JH. Ilizarov technique for complex foot and ankle deformities. New York: Marcel Dekker; 2004.
20. Oganesyan OV, Istomina IS, Kuzmin VI. Treatment of equinocavovarus deformity in adults with the use of hinged distraction apparatus. J Bone Joint Surg Am. 1996;78(4):546–56.
21. Paley D. Ankle and foot considerations. In: Paley D, editor. Principles of deformity correction. 2nd ed. Berlin, Germany: Springer-Verlag; 2003. p. 571–645.
22. Paley D. Principles of foot deformity correction: Ilizarov technique. In: Gould S, editor. Operative foot surgery. Philadelphia: WB Saunders; 1994. p. 476–514.
23. Calhoun JH, Burke-Evans E, Herndon DN. Techniques for the management of burn contractures with the Ilizarov fixator. Clin Orthop. 1992;280:117–24.
24. Erdoğan B, Gorgu M, Girgin O, et al. Application of external fixators in major foot contrac-tures. J Foot Ankle Surg. 1996;35(3):218–21.
25. Lamm BM, Paley D, Herzenberg JE. Gastrocnemius soleus recession: a simpler, more limited approach. J Am Podiatr Med Assoc. 2005;95(1):18–25.
26. Paley D, Herzenberg JE. Applications of external fixation to foot and ankle reconstruction. In: Myerson MS, editor. Foot and ankle disorders, vol. 2. Philadelphia: WB Saunders; 2000. p. 1135–88.
27. Herzenberg JE, Paley D. Ilizarov applications in foot and ankle surgery. Adv Orthop Surg. 1992;16(3):162–74.
28. Franke J, Grill F, Hein G, et al. Correction of clubfoot relapse tusing Ilizarov's apparatus in children 8-15 years old. Arch Orthop Trauma Surg. 1990;110(1):33–7.
29. Grill F, Franke J. The Ilizarov distractor for the correction of relapsed or neglected clubfoot. J Bone Joint Surg Br. 1987;69(4):593–7.
30. Reinker KA, Carpenter CT. Ilizarov applications in the pediatric foot. J Pediair Orthop. 1997;17(6):796–802.
31. Wallander H, Hansson G, Tjenström B. Correction of persistent chubfoot deformities with the Ilizarov external fixator. Acta Orthop Scand. 1996;67(3):283–7.
32. Ponseti IV. Congenital clubfoot: fundamentals of treatment. New York: Oxford University Press; 1996.
33. Joshi BB. Correction of congenital talipes equino varus (CTEV) by controlled differential fractional distraction using Joshi's external stabilization system (JESS). 1st ed. Mumbai, India: JESS Research and Development Centre; 2001.

34. Paley D, Lamm BM. Correction of cavus foot using external fixation. Foot ankle Clin N Am. 2004;9:611–24.
35. Huang SC. Soft tissue contractures of the knee or ankle treated by the Ilizarov technique. Acta Orthop Scand. 1996;67(5):443–9.
36. Brunner R, Hefti F, Tgetgel JD. Arthrogryotic joint contracture at the knee and foot: correction with a circular frame. J Pediatr Orthop B. 1997;6(3):192–7.
37. Grant AD, Atar D, Lehman WB. Ilizarov technique in correction of foot deformities: a pre-liminary report. Foot Ankle. 1990;11(1):1–5.
38. Siddiqui NA, Herzeneberg JE, Lamm BM. Supramalleolar osteotomy for realignment of the ankle joint. Clin Podiatr Med Surg. 2012;29(4):465–82.
39. Gourdine-Shaw MC, Lamm BM, Paley D, Herzenberg JE. Distraction osteogenesis for complex foot deformities: U-osteotomy with external fixation. J Bone Joint Surg Am. 2012;94(15):1420–7.
40. Hentgnes M, Pugh E, Gesheff MG, Ernst JJ, Lamm BM. Realignment midfoot osteotomy: a preoperative planning method and intraoperative surgical technique. J Foot Ankle Surg. 2022;61(1):170–4.
41. Aktuglu K, Ozsoy MH, Yensel U. Treatment of displaced pylon fractures with circular external fixators of Ilizarov. Foot Ankle Int. 1998;19(4):208–16.
42. Kenzora JE, Edwards CC, Browner BD, et al. Acute management of major trauma involving the foot and ankle with Hoffman external fixation. Foot Ankle. 1981;1(6):348–61.
43. Lamm BM. Metatarsal lengthening. In: Rozbruch RS, Ilizarov S, editors. Limb lengthening and reconstruction surgery. New York: Informa Healthcare; 2007. p. 291–302.
44. Davidson RS. Metatarsal lengthening. Foot Ankle Clin. 2001;6(3):499–518.
45. Fox IM. Treatment of brachymetatarsia by the callus distraction method. J Foot Ankle Surg. 1998;37(5):391–5.
46. Lamm BM, Paley D, Herzenberg JE. Percutaneous distraction osteogenesis for treatment of Brachymetatarsia. In: Scuderi GR, editor. Minimally invasive surgery in orthopedics. AJ Tria Springer Science + Business Media; 2010. p. 435–42.
47. Lamm BM. Brachymetatarsia: distraction osteogenesis. In: Rozbruch RS, Hamdy RC, editors. Limb lengthening and reconstruction surgery case Atlas: trauma, foot and ankle. Springer International Publishing Switzerland; 2016.
48. Cordoba-Fernandez A, Vera-Gomez ML. Literature review on brachymetatarsia. Orthop Nurs. 2018;37(5):292–302.
49. Levine SE, Davidson RS, Dormans JP, et al. Distraction osteogenesis for congenitally short lesser metatarsals. Foot Ankle Int. 1995;16(4):196–200.
50. Lamm BM. Percutaneous distraction osteogenesis for treatment of brachymetatarsia. J Foot Ankle Surg. 2009;49(2):197–204.
51. Lamm BM, Moore KR, Knight JM, Pugh E, Baker JR, Gesheff MG. Intramedullary metatarsal fixation for treatment of delayed regenerate bone in lengthening of brachymetatarsia. J Foot Ankle Surg. 2018;57(5):987–94.
52. Lamm BM, Pugh ED, Knight JM. Pediatric brachymetatarsia. In: Butterworth ML, Marcoux JT, editors. The pediatric foot and ankle. Springer Nature Switzerland AG; 2020. p. 107–17.
53. Kim HS, Lee YS, Jung JH, Shim JS. Complications of distraction in brachymetatarsia: comparison between the first and fourth brachymetatarsia. J Foot Ankle Surg. 2019;25(2):113–8.
54. Lamm BM, Gourdine-Shaw MC. Problems, obstacles, and complications of metatarsal lengthening for the treatment of brachymetatarsia. Clin Pod Med Surg. 2010;27(4):561–82.
55. Lamm BM, Lamm TB. Brachymetatarsia: classification for surgical treatment. J Foot Ankle Surg. 2022;11
56. Lamm BM, Stasko PA, Gesheff MG, Bhave A. Normal foot and ankle radiographic angles, measurements, and reference points. J Foot Ankle Surg. 2016;55(5):991–8.

Further Reading

Bassett GS, Mazur KU, Sloan GM. Soft tissue expander failure in severe equinovarus foot deformity. J Pediatr Orthop. 1993;13(6):744–8.

Choudhury SN, Kitaoka HB, Peterson HA. Metatarsal lengthening: case report and review of literature. Foot Ankle Int. 1997;18(11):739–45.

Codivilla A. On the means of lengthening in the lower limbs, the muscles and tissues which are shortened through deformity. Am J Orthop Surg. 1905;2:353–63.

LaBianco GJ, Vito GR, Kalish SR. Use of the Ilizarov external fixator in the treatment of lower extremity deformities. J Am Podiatr Med Assoc. 1996;86(11):523–31.

Ohmori S. Correction of burn deformities using free flap transfer. J Trauma. 1982;22(2):104–11.

Paley D. Current techniques of limb lengthening. J Pediatr Orthop. 1988;8(1):73–92.

Paley D, Kovelman HF, Herzenberg JE. Ilizarov technology. In: Stauffer RN, editor. Advances in operative orthopaedics, vol. 1. St. Louis, MO: Mosby-Year Book; 1993. p. 243–87.

Paley D. Surgical reconstruction for fibular hemimelia. J Child Orthop. 2016;10(6):557–83.

Tachdjian MO. Clinical pediatric orthopedics: the art of diagnosis and principles of management. Stamford (CT): Appleton & Lange; 1997.

Pediatric Joint Contractures

Aaron J. Huser and David S. Feldman

Introduction

"Joint contractures" or limitation of joint movement of the lower extremities are present in a variety of congenital, developmental and acquired conditions including post-traumatic and infectious conditions. The treating physician must understand the etiology of the limitation of motion or "contracture" to adequately treat the underlying pathoanatomy: shortened muscles, contracted ligaments or capsule, pterygia or bony conditions such as deformity or arthritis. Understanding which factor or factors are involved will allow the physician to create an appropriate treatment plan. This chapter will discuss the general management of contractures at the hip, knee and ankle. The term "deformity" will be used to describe a joint without full range of motion whether the etiology is bony or soft-tissue. The term "contracture" will be used to mean the joint has limited motion due to shortened muscles, ligaments or other soft-tissues. This chapter will not discuss the management of contractures related to a spastic etiology as the authors believe spastic contractures and the imbalance of those muscles is a unique discussion and are reviewed in Chap. 23 in this book.

History/Examination

A thorough history should be performed with specific attention paid to birth, family and surgical/intervention history. The age and timing of onset is critical. Whether the limitation of motion is static, progressive or improving should be ascertained. Pain and the type pain as well as inciting factors need to be determined. The patient's ambulatory status is recorded as community, household, non-functional or as non-ambulators based on the work of Hoffer et al. [1].

The initial portion of the physical exam should focus on observation of the patient in general. Is the patient dysmorphic? Is the patient's speech impacted? If the answer is yes, then it is likely that the etiology is systemic and not isolated to a single joint. Does the patient's skin appear normal? Skin abnormality can suggest an underlying collagen disorder. Next, the patient's ambulation (if capable) is observed. Is there an obvious limp? An antalgic gait would suggest pain; Trendelenburg would suggest weakness, and short leg would suggest a limb length discrepancy or contracture. If they cannot walk, do they scoot on the floor to move around? The ability to scoot requires strong upper limbs.

Next, the range of motion for each of the major joints in the lower extremity is recorded. It is important to examine both lower limbs and not just the affected side.

The hip can be difficult to assess because of mobility through the lumbar spine and sacroiliac joints and because of the multiplanar motion that occurs through the joint. The patient should be placed in the supine position. The limb should be held in a neutral rotational position with the patella forward. If the patella is dislocated, this can be difficult and we recommend rotating the lower limb so that the flexion/extension axis is parallel to the floor. The anterior superior iliac spines (ASIS) should be palpated, and two fingers (usually thumb and index) should remain on the ASIS to monitor for motion while flexion of the hip is tested. Once your fingers sense motion at the ASIS, the patient's hip has reached maximal flexion. Extension is measured using the Thomas test. Both hips are flexed maximally with the knees to the chest or as far as the hip flexes while flattening the lumbar spine. One hip is allowed to extend maximally and this value is recorded and then repeated for the opposite side. Abduction and adduction are also tested in the supine position. Again, with two fingers on the ASIS, the hip is abducted until motion is sensed at the fingers on the ASIS and then hip adduction is similarly tested. It can be difficult

A. J. Huser (✉) · D. S. Feldman
Paley Orthopedic and Spine Institute, West Palm Beach, FL, USA
e-mail: ahuser@paleyinstitute.org; dfeldman@paleyinstitute.org

to separate abduction and external rotation. It is best to attempt to rotate the limb to a patella forward position with the hip in maximum extension when assessing adduction/abduction to limit the effect of multiplanar motion on your assessment. Finally, external and internal rotation are ideally assessed with the patient prone and the hip at full extension. While in the prone position, the knees are flexed 90° (if possible) and the thigh foot axis (a measure of tibial torsion/rotation) is determined as well as internal and external rotation of the hip. The hip is externally and internally rotated and measurements documented. When testing rotation, the greater trochanter is palpated and when it is horizontal/parallel to the ground, the extent of rotation at that point determines the anteversion/retroversion of the hip. If the patient is unable to lie prone because of a significant hip flexion contracture, this motion may be assessed with the patient supine and hip maximally extended. Hip rotation may also be assessed with the hip flexed, but this rotational profile does not mimic hip rotation during ambulation. Again, it is important to abduct/adduct the hip to neutral prior to assessment of axial plane contractures.

The patient is then placed in a lateral decubitus position and an Ober test is performed. The ipsilateral hip is extended and knee is flexed and the limb is let go and allowed to drop. A tight/contracted tensor fascia lata/Iliotibial band will maintain abduction of the lower limb. With the patient still on the side and the knee flexed, one can flex the hip and if there is simultaneous, obligate abduction, i.e. a positive reverse Ober test, suggesting a contracted Gluteus maximus [2].

Knee range of motion is tested with the hip flexed and extended to understand the contribution of biarticular muscles. Knee extension is assessed in the supine position with the hip extended and then with the hip flexed to 90° (popliteal angle). The short-head of the biceps femoris is the only hamstring muscle that does not cross the hip. Knee flexion is tested in the supine position with the hip flexed and in the prone position with the hip extended. The rectus femoris is the only quadriceps that crosses the hip joint.

Dorsiflexion of the ankle is tested with the knee extended and knee flexed (Silverskiold test). This allows one to differentiate between contracture of the gastrocnemius and the soleus muscle. Plantarflexion of the ankle can be examined with the knee in flexion or extension as ankle dorsiflexors do not cross the knee joint. In the assessment of toe walking or an equinus contracture, the physician first must differentiate between a habitual toe walker which is a child with no contracture of the Achilles tendon versus a true contracture. In unilateral toe walkers, differential diagnosis should include limb length discrepancy, hemiplegia and hip dislocation.

Any child with a contracture must be examined neurologically, specifically looking for weakness in strength testing and changes in deep tendon reflexes as seen in spastic conditions and muscular dystrophies.

Imaging

Following the physical examination, radiographs should be obtained to differentiate between a soft-tissue contracture and bony deformity. Suggested radiographs for the hip include a frontal view of the pelvis, false-profile views of the hips and frog lateral views of the proximal femurs. These images should be assessed for pincer/cam impingement, hip instability (subluxation/dislocation) and angular deformities of the proximal femurs.

For the knee, sagittal images of the lower limb in maximum flexion and maximum extension with the patella forward may provide more insight on the true measurements of the deformity. These images should include the entire length of the femur and tibia so that the posterior distal femoral angle (PDFA) and posterior proximal tibial angle (PPTA) can be measured. These angles are essential to determine how much of the clinical deformity is related to the bony deformity and how much is related to a soft-tissue contracture (see Fig. 18.1). Sagittal images of the ankle in maximum plantarflexion and dorsiflexion may also aid in determining the bony and soft-tissue components of a deformity as well as the extent of midfoot cavus which can mimic equinus. At least one lateral view should include as much of the tibia as possible in order to measure the anterior distal tibial angle (ADTA) [3].

Advanced imaging of the area concerning suspected soft-tissue contractures is not routine in the authors' practices. In the past, computed tomography (CT) has been used to assess rotational deformities of the femurs and separate those from soft-tissue contractures. However, the authors now advocate for lower radiation options such as magnetic resonance imaging (MRI) or EOS to quantify rotational deformities in bones [4]. If the patient cannot remain still for the MRI or unable to stand for the EOS, then CT imaging can still be used (see Fig. 18.2). MRI may be useful for assessing abnormal locations of the neurovascular structures when treating congenital deficiency etiologies or patients with multiple pterygium [5]. In patients with multiple congenital or developmental joint contractures or isolated congenital/developmental ankle contractures that are not associated with isolated clubfoot, we recommend a MRI of the lumbar spine to rule out tethered cord or other spinal cord abnormalities.

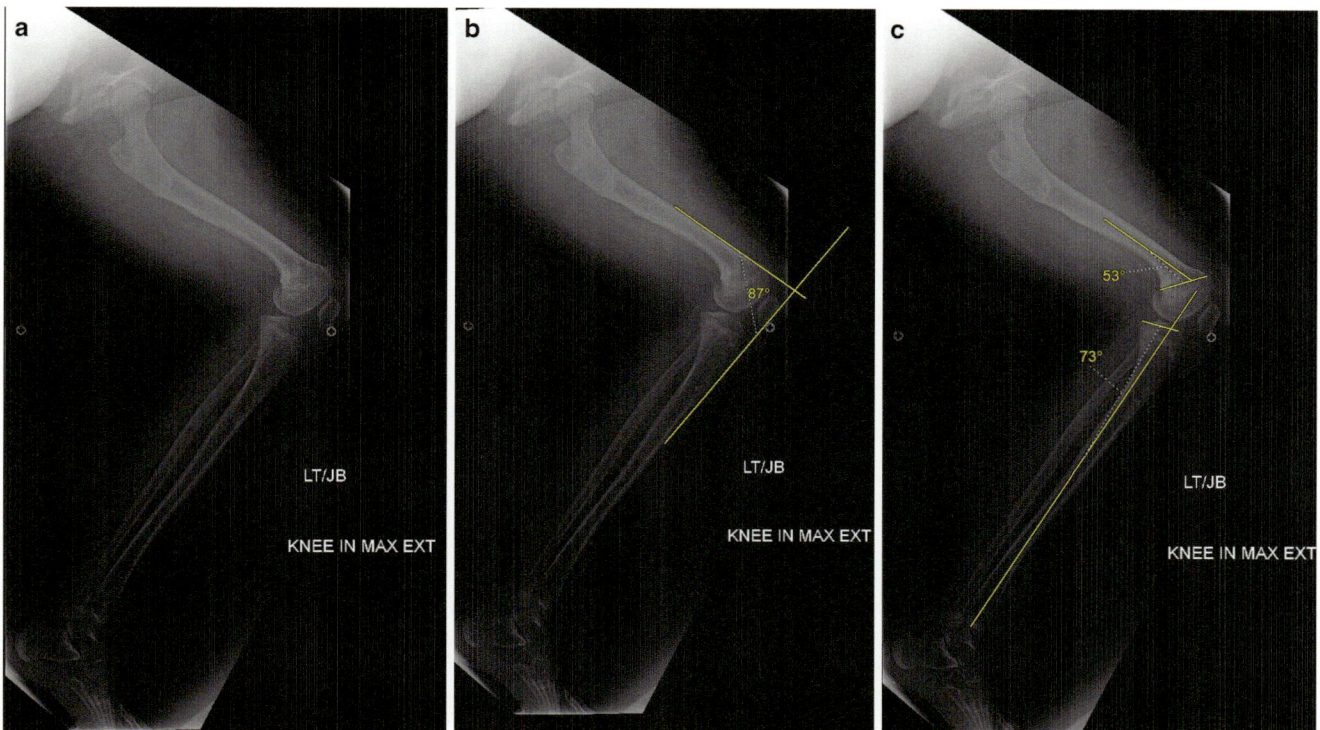

Fig. 18.1 A sagittal, maximally extended view of the left lower extremity of a patient who had neonatal sepsis as an infant (**a**). Measurement demonstrating the degree of flexion deformity (**b**), we take the supplement of 87° (180°–87°) which is 93° and would say that this patient has a 93° flexion deformity. Sagittal measurements of the PDFA (normal is 83°) and PPTA (normal is 81°) (**c**), this tells us that the distal femur contributes 30° to the flexion deformity and the proximal tibia contributes 8°. The actual soft tissue contracture of the knee in this patient is 55° (93° − 30° − 8° = 55°)

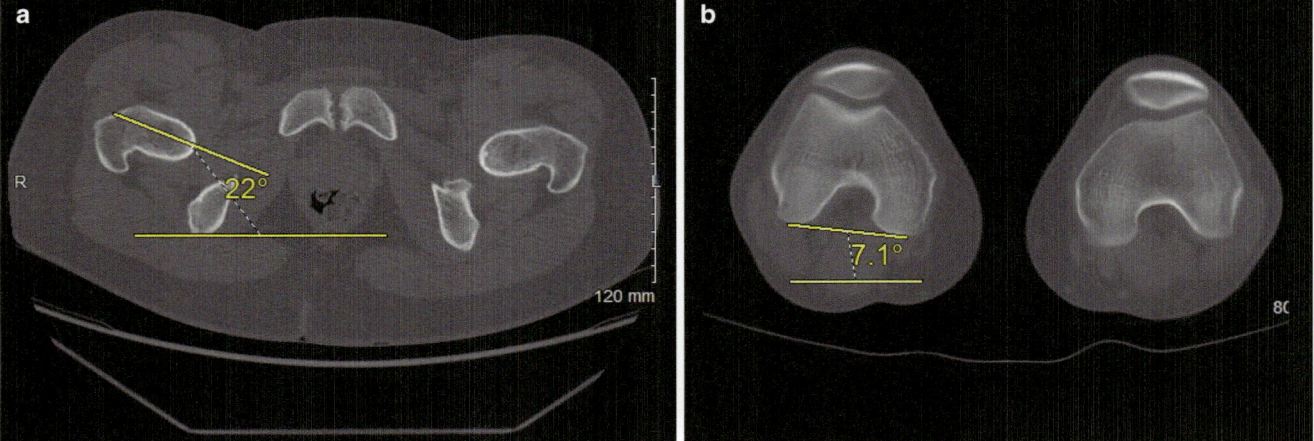

Fig. 18.2 Axial CT cuts of the pelvis (**a**) and the knees (**b**) to measure rotation. The patient did not move during the scan as that can affect the measurement. The measurement at the hip (**a**) is with a line down the neck and its angle to the horizontal. The measurement at the knee (**b**) is with a line tangential to the posterior condyles and the angle with the horizontal. The rotational deformity is determined by subtracting 22° from 7°. This gives a difference of −15° which would be a neutral version hip. Normal anteversion is 10–15°. If we calculate −15°−15° (normal anteversion) the difference is −30°. Thus, this patient has 30° of femoral retroversion

Principles of Treatment

1. The deformity discovered on physical examination must be separated into its soft-tissue contracture component and bony deformity component. For example, on examination of the knee, you discover the patient's range of motion is 35–140°. This patient has a 35° flexion deformity (lacks 35° of full extension). On imaging, this is confirmed with the patient's flexion/extension films. The PDFA is measured at 68° (normal 83°) and the PPTA is measured at 81° (normal 81°). This means that the distal femur is flexed 15°; if we subtract 15° from the original 35°, we have 20° remaining. The soft-tissue contracture, in this case, is responsible for 20° of the deformity. (see Fig. 18.1).
2. Bony deformity should be treated with bony surgery—osteotomies or guided growth. We perform osteotomies in skeletally mature patients and immature patients. Growth modulation procedures are performed in patients who are skeletally immature with at least 2 years of growth remaining and skeletal deformity measuring <25°.
3. Soft-tissue contractures are treated with soft-tissue interventions or osteotomy. Serial casting may be attempted. One must be careful not to cause a secondary contracture with casting in patients with fibrotic diseases like arthrogryposis. For instance, if one is casting a foot deformity with casting above the knee, the cast should be removed often for range of motion of the knee (preferably by a physical therapist). The surgical approach is a la carte. For shortened tendons, we recommend fractional lengthening, z-plasty or tenotomy. For contracted capsules, we recommend capsulotomy. For contracted ligaments, we recommend partial release to prevent joint instability.
4. The neurovascular bundle cannot be directly lengthened. If the bundle is preventing correction, consider bone shortening to relatively lengthen the bundle.

Non-operative Treatment

Patients with soft-tissue contractures as a result of a congenital or post-traumatic etiology may benefit from physical therapy and soft-tissue manipulation. We routinely see patients with congenital contractures; if the joints are reduced, participate from birth—3 years of age in serial casting and manipulations with physical therapy for their hips, knees and ankles. At age 2–3 years of age, if the contractures are functionally limiting and have not resolved in the hips and knees, we consider operative management.

Soft-tissue contractures of the ankles are treated differently. Often, soft-tissue contractures of the ankle are part of a larger foot deformity as seen in clubfoot or congenital vertical talus. In these cases, we encourage soft-tissue manipulation and casting as prescribed by Ponsetti and Dobbs [6, 7]. In isolated equinus contractures/toe-walkers, we recommend soft-tissue manipulation and casting. A recent study suggested that 80% of idiopathic toe-walking resolves by age 10 with non-operative modalities [8]. If these contractures do not resolve by age 8, patients are indicated for operative treatment.

Dorsiflexion contractures are often seen in children with calcaneovalgus deformity and myelomeningocele. In general, these contractures are less common. They can also occur from postoperative over-correction of equinus contractures. Casting may be attempted for non-iatrogenic dorsiflexion contractures.

Patients with contractures due to joint subluxation/dislocation or related to incongruous joints, such as seen in Larsen Syndrome and diastrophic dysplasia, should not be casted or stretched as the pressure on a dislocated joint may actually damage the cartilage or ligaments of the joints involved. These patients often require surgical reduction of their knees and hips.

Joint-Specific Operative Treatment

Hip

Surgical treatment and approach for the hip is based on the type of soft-tissue contracture and is focused on the inciting muscle(s) and/or ligaments/capsule.

For flexion, abduction and/or internal rotation contractures, we recommend an anterior approach utilizing the sartorious and tensor-fascia lata (TFL) interval. Once this interval is created, we identify the direct head of the rectus femoris and release it off the anterior inferior iliac spine (this is a complete tenotomy). Continuing to work in this interval, a hemostat is placed into the middle of the iliopsoas muscle belly with the tip pointing distal and then rotated to point posteriorly. The hemostat is pulled back to bring the iliopsoas tendon into the interval. Care is taken to not injure the femoral nerve which sits anterior and medial to the iliopsoas muscle belly while the tendon sits posterior and medial to the muscle belly. We routinely try to stimulate the tendon with a nerve stimulator to ensure we have isolated the tendon and not the nerve prior to release. If we are sure the structure we have is the tendon, a fractional lengthening is performed. Many hip flexion contractures also have an abduction contracture. Once we have released the direct head of the rectus and iliopsoas, we incise the iliac apophysis and elevate the periosteum off the outer and inner tables of the ilium. This facilitates release of the abduction contracture by relatively lengthening the gluteus medius, gluteus minimus and TFL from the outer table and harvest periosteum from the inner table. If the Iliopsoas was not yet lengthened, it can be released at the pelvic brim using the technique described above. If there is a residual hip flexion contracture >30°, the anterior capsule of the hip can be pie-crusted with horizontal incisions. Finally, the hip is brought to a neutral position (out of the abduction, flexion and internal rotation). The split iliac apophysis is assessed at the level of the outer table of the ilium. The prominent proximal portion of the iliac wing is resected so that the apophysis can be reapproximated with the hip in a neutral position and without tension.

For extension/external rotation contractures of the hip, we use a lateral approach. For the lateral approach, an incision is made in line with the femoral shaft and posterior third of the greater trochanter. The Iliotibial band is incised and the muscle belly of the vastus lateralis is retracted anteriorly exposing the femoral insertion of the gluteus maximus. The gluteus maximus tendon is tenotomized. The intermuscular septum is released as well as the posterior third of the iliotibial band. The femur is internally rotated to expose small external rotators. The piriformis tendon can be tenotomized with care not to disrupt the ascending branch of the medial femoral circumflex artery. If there is a residual extension contracture, the ischium can be visualized by retracting the gluteus maximus posteriorly and using a "rake" retractor to pull the greater trochanter/femur anteriorly. The quadratus femoris can be traced posteriorly to the ischium. Care should be taken as the sciatic nerve will be superficial to the quadratus femoris. The sciatic nerve should be visualized. The proximal origins of the hamstrings can be released.

Adduction contractures are treated using a medial approach. With the leg held in maximum abduction, a transverse incision is made over the adductor longus tendon. Hemostasis is achieved in the subcutaneous tissue and the fascia overlying the tendon is incised longitudinally. A right-angle clamp is used to isolate the adductor longus tendon remembering that the anterior branch of the obturator nerve sits deep to the adductor longus. A fractional lengthening is performed. If the contracture is still present, the adductor brevis, just deep to the anterior branch of the obturator nerve, may be released. The gracilis lies posterior to the adductors and may be released if the adduction contracture persists.

Knee

The treatment of knee flexion contractures is case and severity dependent.

Mild contractures of less than 25° may be treated with simple soft tissue releases such as hamstring, iliotibial band (ITB) and less frequently posterior capsulotomy. In a growing child, extension osteotomies should be avoided because recurrence of the deformity occurs rapidly. One may use guided growth with an anterior hemiepiphysiodesis in these more mild cases. In an adult, an extension distal femoral osteotomy is a reasonable option so long as the sacrifice of that many degrees of flexion will not adversely impact function.

In a patient with severe flexion deformity, a single-stage correction can be achieved [9]. The knee is approached via dual lateral and medial incisions (see Fig. 18.3). The purpose of the lateral incision is to perform decompression of the peroneal nerve, ITB lengthening, biceps femoris lengthening, lateral gastrocnemius head recession and posterior capsulotomy. Depending on the etiology, posterior pterygia may also have to be excised. The small medial incision allows lengthening/recession of the semitendinosus, semimembra-

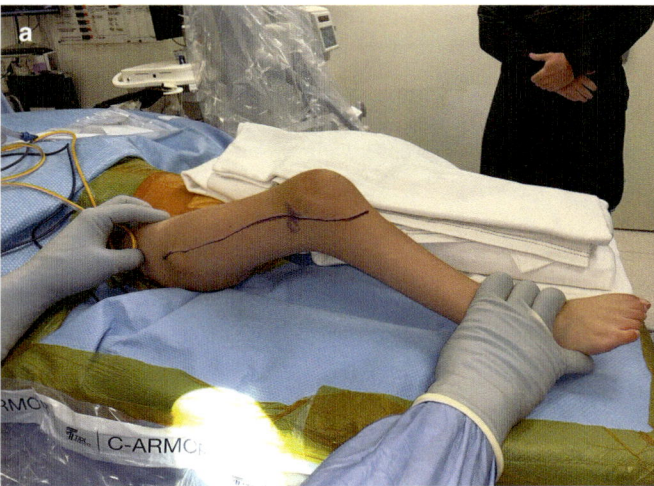
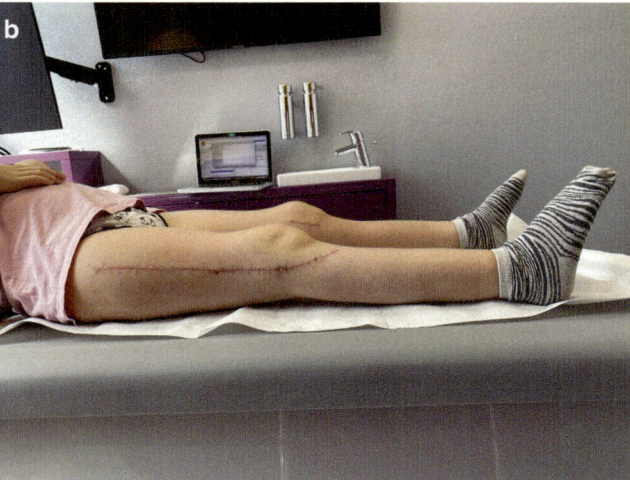

Fig. 18.3 Preoperative (**a**) and postoperative (**b**) clinical pictures of a patient who underwent acute flexion deformity correction. The incision prior to the surgery (**a**) and the postoperative scar can be seen (**b**).

Originally published in Feldman DS, Rand TJ, Huser AJ (2021) Novel Approach to Improving Knee Range of Motion in Arthrogryposis with a New Working Classification. Children 8:546

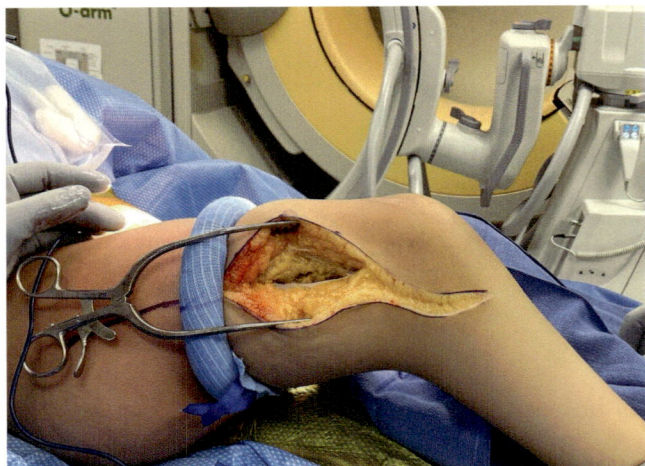

Fig. 18.4 The lateral incision is made and the first goal is to get to the femur. This is done prior to decompressing the peroneal nerve because the lack of muscle can be disorienting for the surgeon and this allows the surgeon to get their bearings. Originally published in Feldman DS, Rand TJ, Huser AJ (2021) Novel Approach to Improving Knee Range of Motion in Arthrogryposis with a New Working Classification. Children 8:546

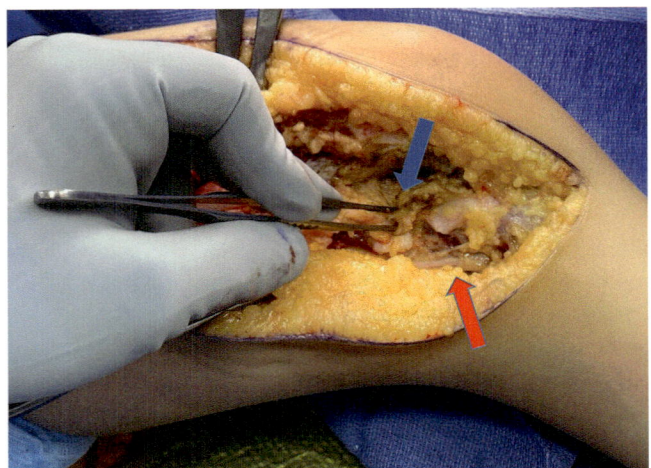

Fig. 18.5 After transection of the long head of the biceps femoris. The pickup is holding the proximal portion of the biceps femoris that has been transected (blue arrow). The red arrow is identifying the peroneal nerve

nosus, gracillis, medial head of the gastrocnemius and completion of the posterior capsulotomy.

The lateral incision is made first down to the ITB. The ITB is incised and the vastus lateralis is elevated anteriorly off the femoral shaft. Some patients with flexion contractures lack the vastus lateralis and care should be taken not to drift posteriorly (see Fig. 18.4). Once the femoral shaft is identified, the tendon of the biceps femoris is located posteriorly and attaching to the fibular head. The peroneal nerve runs posteromedial to the tendon of the biceps femoris. Using blunt dissection, the nerve is identified and decompressed as it curves around the neck of the proximal fibula and enters the lateral compartment. A transverse fasciotomy of the anterior and lateral compartments in the lower leg is performed to decompress the nerve. Any vertical septa are transected as they may cause compression of the nerve. Once the nerve is decompressed, the biceps femoris is lengthened (see Fig. 18.5). With the knee flexed, the lateral head of the gastrocnemius is recessed off the posterior capsule of the knee. An incision, proximal to the joint line/meniscus and posterior to the lateral collateral ligament, is made into the knee capsule and the posterior condyle of the femur identified. Using blunt dissection, a corridor is developed between the posterior capsule and proximal soft tissues. The meniscus may be adhered to the distal femur and will need to be detached for the femur. This will create a safe plane to perform the capsulotomy. Care should be taken to avoid the middle geniculate artery; however, if injured, it can be ligated or cauterized. Once the latera half of the posterior capsule has been transected, a freer elevator is placed into the lateral joint and out the medial joint tenting the skin to be

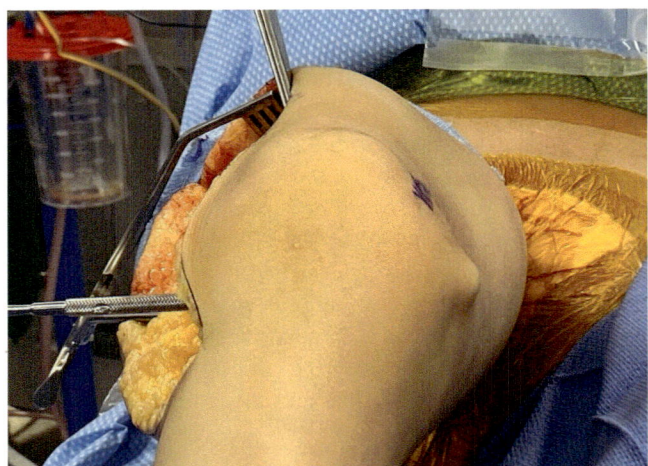

Fig. 18.6 The freer is passed from the lateral incision, through the back of the knee and tents the medial skin. The medial incision should be made where the skin is tented. Originally published in Feldman DS, Rand TJ, Huser AJ (2021) Novel Approach to Improving Knee Range of Motion in Arthrogryposis with a New Working Classification. Children 8:546

used as a landmark for the medial incision (see Fig. 18.6). Many times when attempting this maneuver, the freer will hit the intercondylar notch; to remedy this, the surgeon should move their hand anteriorly relative to the knee to slip around the posterior-medial femoral condyle.

Next, an incision is made over the tented skin medially. This incision typically measures five centimeters. A posterior flap is created with blunt dissection and the gracillis, semimembranosus and semitendinosus are identified and lengthened/recessed. The saphenous nerve is identified and protected. The freer, which was used to guide incision placement, can be

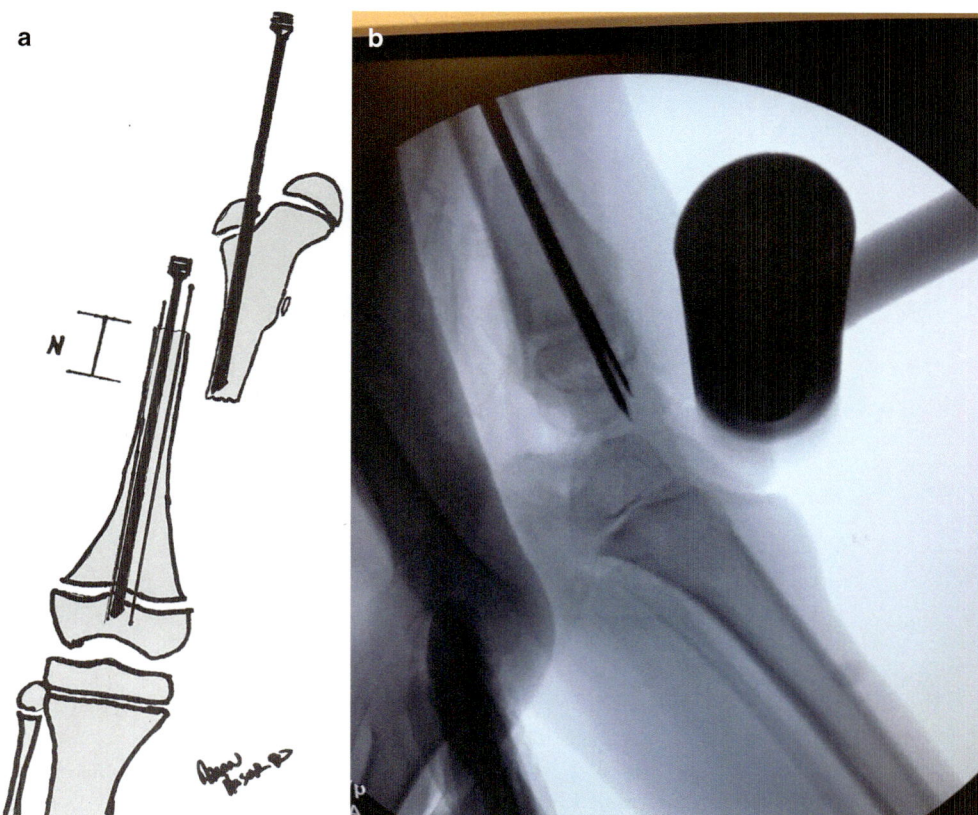

Fig. 18.7 Two intramedullary rods are used during the acute extension of the knee (**a**). One rod maintains control of the proximal fragment, while the other rod is used to aid extension of the knee. N denotes the overlap of the two fragments and the amount that will need to be shortened to take tension off the bundle. The fluoroscopic image (**b**) demonstrates the rod and wires across the physis to protect it during acute extension. Posterior translation is common. The wires and rod in the distal segment will be removed and the proximal rod (**a**) will be passed into the distal segment. Originally published in Feldman DS, Rand TJ, Huser AJ (2021) Novel Approach to Improving Knee Range of Motion in Arthrogryposis with a New Working Classification. Children 8:546

retracted laterally and an incision can be made where it once was. This will recess the medial head of the gastrocnemius and start the medial portion of the capsulotomy. Again, a corridor should be created between the capsule and posterior soft tissues to allow for safe transection of the capsule. Once the capsulotomy is complete, one should be able to easily pass a freer or small finger through the defect. One should not dissect both posteriorly and anteriorly on the distal femur as avascular necrosis of the distal femur may occur.

If residual contracture still exists, a proximal femoral shortening osteotomy can be performed by extending the lateral incision proximally. The osteotomy is performed proximally so as to allow a long lever arm for extension. After the bone is osteotomized, a rod and wires are placed intramedullary in the distal femoral fragment antegrade and across the distal femoral physis to protect the physis as the knee is brought into full extension (see Fig. 18.7). The rod and wires from the distal segment are removed. The amount of required shortening to achieve full extension is marked and resected.

The shortening osteoplasty is rotated for correction of anteversion/retroversion and can then be fixed with a combination intramedullary rod/plate construct. This construct is chosen to allow for immediate motion of the knee following surgery and without the need for immobilization (see Fig. 18.8).

Escobar Syndrome has proven difficult to treat with this method because the tibial nerve is the most posterior structure and no amount of reasonable shortening will allow this nerve to be freed for full extension. Slow correction with an external fixator can be performed across the knee but one must be prepared for an overall loss of arc of motion. As well the hip and or knee may subluxate/dislocate during this procedure. A combined approach of starting with external fixation and then performing the procedure above is also possible.

Routine use of external fixation is still in use at some centers for severe knee contractures; however, because of an overall loss of motion, we no longer use these methods in most patients [10, 11]. We have opted for constructs that allow for acute correction and immediate motion.

Extension contractures of the knee are less common than flexion types. The treatment is dependent upon the age of the patient, etiology and whether the knee joint is dislocated. Infants may benefit from a simple rectus tenotomy or VY plasty [12]. Older children and adolescents particularly with post-traumatic deformities may benefit from a la carte procedure which begins with arthrolysis of the joint with retinacular releases to a full Judet quadriceplasty. A VY plasty in these older patients has the risk of causing a permanent extensor lag.

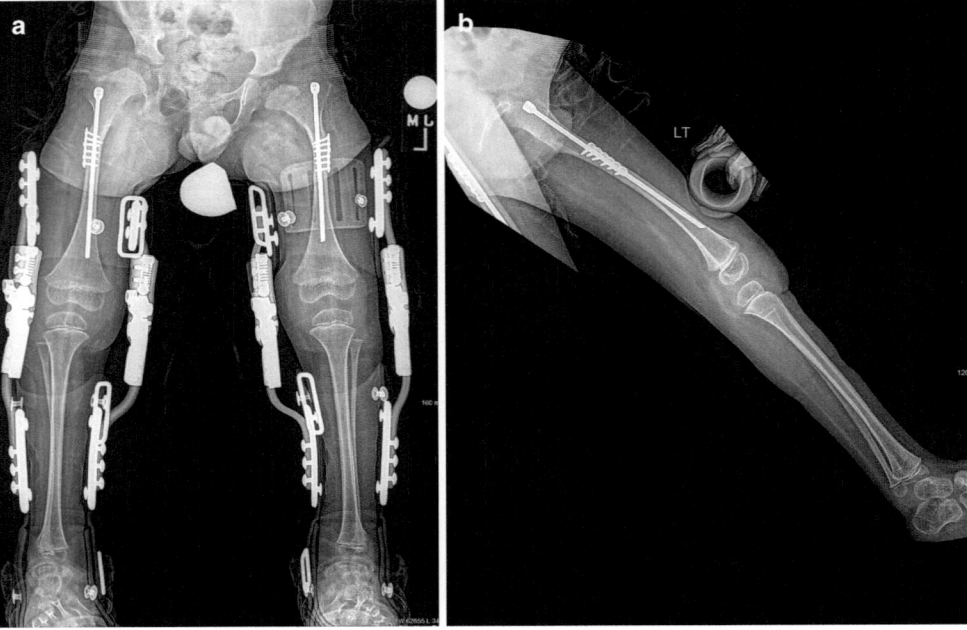

Fig. 18.8 AP (**a**) and lateral (**b**) radiographs at 1 year follow-up. Note the proximal migration of the femoral rod out of the distal femoral physis

The Judet quadriceplasty has been fraught with recurrence of the extension contracture over time even though full flexion is achieved in the operating room. Therefore, in patients with irreducible dislocated knees (such as Larsen Syndrome and diastrophic dysplasia) and arthrogryposis, we disconnect the patellar tendon from the tibia (elevation of the patellar tendon off the apophysis versus tibial tubercle osteotomy in skeletally mature patients) in order to gain access to the knee joint for a lysis of the adhesions. Additionally, if 90° of knee flexion is unable to be obtained with the release, a distal femoral shortening is performed to obtain at least 90° of flexion and reattach the patellar tendon. The shortening is secured with a retrograde, intramedullary rod and plate construct with the goal of immediate motion following surgery.

Ankle

Non-operative treatment failure for a pediatric equinus contracture requires surgical intervention. Before pursuing an intervention, we often recommend MRI of the lumbar spine to rule out intraspinal pathology such as a tethered cord and if found, may need to be addressed prior to surgical correction of the equinus deformity.

Initially, surgical correction of the pure equinus contracture is driven by the results of the Silfverskiold test. If positive, there is increased dorsiflexion of the ankle with the knee flexed when compared to the knee extended, we perform a gastrocnemius recession. If the Silfverskiold test is negative, then we perform a triple hemisection of the Achilles (Hoke type) and possible posterior tibial-talar capsulotomy. In these cases and if the equinus contracture is greater than 15° and the patient has neurogenic symptoms with forced dorsiflexion, we advocate for concomitant tarsal tunnel decompression to take tension off the neurovascular bundle.

In patients who have little passive and/or active motion of the ankle with a complex foot deformity and equinus contracture or in patients who have failed multiple non-operative and operative interventions, we have moved toward ankle arthrodesis, distal fibular excision and tarsal tunnel decompression (see Fig. 18.9). This can be done with a two or three incision technique. The two incision technique uses a posteromedial and lateral incision. The three incision technique uses a posteromedial incision, transverse anterior incision and posterolateral incision. Fixation is achieved in both techniques with percutaneous screws-driven retrograde from the calcaneus, into the talus and ending in the tibia. This technique obviates the need for an AFO and prevents recurrence. This technique can also be used in patients with dorsiflexion contractures without the need for tarsal tunnel decompression.

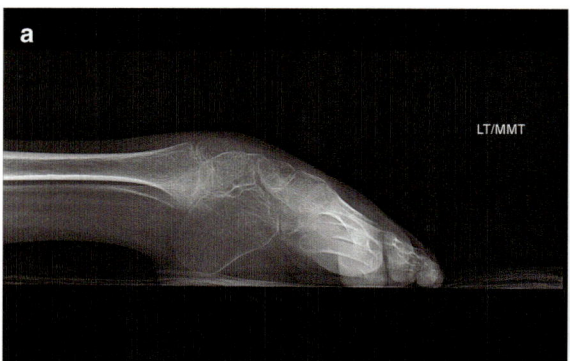 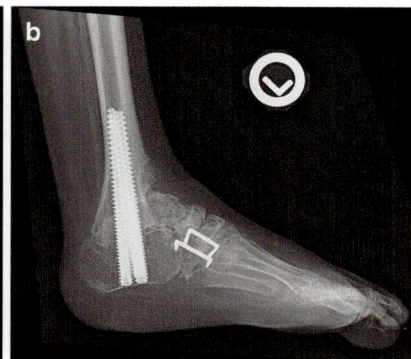

Fig. 18.9 Preoperative (**a**) and postoperative (**b**) lateral images after ankle fusion for recurrent contractures. Osteotomies and soft-tissue releases have also been performed on the foot

Conclusion

Treatment of lower extremity contractures is challenging. The goal of surgery is to improve position of the limb and maintain motion. After extensive release of offending muscles, ligaments and capsule, the neurovascular bundle is usually the only structure remaining as a limit to motion. Bone shortening is an effective solution to removing tension on the neurovascular bundle without causing irreparable harm.

Commentary

Richard Luzzi

The authors start the chapter "Joint Contractures" by defining and differentiating the terms "deformity" (a joint without full ROM due bony and/or soft tissue involvement) and "contracture" (when limited ROM whose origin is related exclusively to soft tissues).

History, physical examination and imaging methods are well discussed, and readers will find in detail how to identify subtle details that will greatly contribute to treatment. They focus this chapter on lower limb contractures, and exemplify with excellent images to differentiate the origin of deformity, with the respective bony versus soft tissue contribution.

When principles of treatment are explained, all presented topics of history, physical examination and imaging methods are put together, making treatment execution rational and reproducible.

In this obviously complex group of diagnosis with multiple etiologies—present in the daily practice of specialists in pediatric orthopedics—authors were able to deliver concise and relevant information. Among all objectives in this treatment, it is essential not only to gain a functional range of motion of the affected joint, but also to preserve the surrounding neurovascular structures.

I will focus primarily on knee contractures. These are very common and many good examples of strategies must be known by the surgeon, and sometimes decisions must be taken during surgery and strategies can change. When we analyze different kinds and different degrees of knee contractures, sometimes a simple soft tissue release and/or bone shortening may not be the ideal treatment. Some diseases associated with knee contractures—like scleroderma—or conditions like burns—including chemical burns—soft tissue release may not achieve the desired full extension. Surgeons must be comfortable to use circular frames and, in a more limited occasions, monolateral frames.

In severe knee contracture, due to spasticity in spinal cord injury, and with no possibilities to walk, a very simple monolateral frame can be installed using one half pin in lateral femur diaphysis and another in lateral tibia diaphysis. One motor unit is used to adjust the frame and increase the distance between clamps of a rail fixator. Half pins become hinges, and both working together will turn in a multicentrical hinge, extending the knee. Some complications may occur as half pin loosening and overdistraction on lateral side, with consequent varus. A stronger construct can be achieved by using at least two half pins in each segment and two shorter rails and a well-positioned hinge centered on the knee center of rotation—connecting both rails—with a posterior motor unit. The motor unit can be removed for physical therapy, and replaced in the same position to maintain the correction that is achieved. Special attention must be paid to the half pins insertion into the tibia to avoid inadvertent nerve damage.

Sometimes, in patients with good prognosis to walk, circular frames in my opinion must be used if all other attempts have failed to get the maximum extent. Frame installation starts with appropriately positioning the knee hinges. First, leave an unattached ring proximal to the knee. If the available frame has cannulated hinges, the proper place to insert a K wire from lateral to medial is the point where posterior femoral cortex crosses the Blumensaat line (or physis if still present). This hinge will be perfect to correct knee contractures up to 90°. Now, with K wire inserted, hinges can be mounted on it, ring attached to both hinges and this ring fixed orthogonal to the femur with half pins. Pay attention to not bend this wire during this process or secure the hinges by twisting the K wire. Connect distal parts of the hinges and on then a second ring. It will be easier if both rings have the same size. Positioning the second ring orthogonal to the tibia—so that now the device mimics the deformity. New elements can be added, like a half ring on proximal femur and an extra ring on distal tibia. If physis is open, another K wire must be inserted at the epiphysis to avoid physeal fracture during correction. If an equinus contracture coexist, this frame can be extended to correct this contracture also. One or two motor units can be connected to extend the knee and ankle. In the same way, motor units can be removed during physical therapy and replaced.

In contractures greater than 90°, the strategy must change, and a hexapod frame must be considered. The first steps are the same, and even using and hexapod, hinges can and must be fixed to the distal femur ring position. When some distraction, torsional, translation or any correction that is facilitated by hexapod ends, frame can be converted to a simple circular fixator by connecting hinges from distal femur ring to proximal tibia ring and motor unit. Struts are now removed. The big question is "Why turn a hexapod to a regular circular frame?" My answer is because physical therapy cannot be executed if struts are in place. Treatment is not about keeping the knee or ankle corrected, but allowing for the best function as possible. The sooner the joint can be mobilized, the better the prognosis and viability.

References

1. Hoffer MM, Feiwell E, Perry R, Perry J, Bonnett C. Functional ambulation in patients with myelomeningocele. J Bone Joint Surg Am. 1973;55(1):137–48.
2. Scully MWF, White KK, Song KM, Mosca VS. Injection-induced gluteus muscle contractures: diagnosis with the "reverse Ober test" and surgical management. J Pediatr Orthop. 2015;35(2):192–8.
3. Paley D, Herzenberg JE, Tetsworth K, McKie J, Bhave A. Deformity planning for frontal and sagittal plane corrective osteotomies. Orthop Clin North Am. 1994;25(3):425–65.
4. Folinais D, Thelen P, Delin C, Radier C, Catonne Y, Lazennec JY. Measuring femoral and rotational alignment: EOS system versus computed tomography. Orthop Traumatol Surg Res. 2013;99(5):509–16.
5. Huser AJ, Kwak YH, Rand TJ, Paley D, Feldman DS. Anatomic relationship of the femoral neurovascular bundle in patients with congenital femoral deficiency. J Pediatr Orthop. 2021;41(2):e111–5.
6. Church C, McGowan A, Henley J, Donohoe M, Niiler T, Shrader MW, et al. The 5-year outcome of the Ponseti method in children with idiopathic clubfoot and arthrogryposis. J Pediatr Orthop. 2020;40(7):e641–6.
7. Yang JS, Dobbs MB. Treatment of congenital vertical talus: comparison of minimally invasive and extensive soft-tissue release procedures at minimum five-year follow-up. J Bone Jt Surg. 2015;97(16):1354–65.
8. Engström P, Tedroff K. Idiopathic toe-walking: prevalence and natural history from birth to ten years of age. J Bone Jt Surg. 2018;100(8):640–7.
9. Feldman DS, Rand TJ, Huser AJ. Novel approach to improving knee range of motion in arthrogryposis with a new working classification. Children. 2021;8(7):546.
10. van Bosse HJP, Feldman DS, Anavian J, Sala DA. Treatment of knee flexion contractures in patients with arthrogryposis. J Pediatr Orthop. 2007;27(8):930–7.
11. Herzenberg JE, Davis JR, Paley D, Bhave A. Mechanical distraction for treatment of severe knee flexion contractures. Clin Orthop. 1994;301:80–8.
12. Roy DR, Crawford AH. Percutaneous quadriceps recession: a technique for management of congenital hyperextension deformities of the knee in the neonate. J Pediatr Orthop. 1989;9(6):717–9.

Physical Therapy During Limb Lengthening and Deformity Correction: Principles and Techniques

Anil Bhave, Erin Baker, and Mary Campbell

Introduction

Treating children who have lower limb deformities including leg length discrepancy can present challenges for the physical therapist. Whether the deformity is related to a congenital, developmental, or acquired etiology, these patients often present with biomechanical abnormalities and compensations in their movement strategies in order to be as independent as possible while performing daily functional activities. Besides assessing the child's psychosocial and support system, when planning treatment of their lower limb deformities, one must critically evaluate the mobility, strength, and stability across the weight-bearing joints to understand how mobility may be impacted during surgical correction. The goal of treatment for these children is primarily to improve their function and gait. In addition to physical abnormalities, these patients do suffer from body image issues [1]. Many patients report improved body image after limb lengthening [2].

In this chapter, we discuss the critical principles and techniques employed by the physical therapist while treating children undergoing limb lengthening and deformity correction with conventional techniques using external fixation as well as intramedullary (IM) lengthening nails. The technique of using an IM nail has become increasingly popular and poses unique challenges compared to limb lengthening performed with external fixation. We also discuss specific rehabilitation issues for patients with congenital shortening of the lower limb as well as certain other clinical conditions such as achondroplasia and Perthes disease.

Rehabilitation During Distraction Osteogenesis

Rehabilitation for limb lengthening and reconstruction surgery can be divided into four distinct phases: (1) inpatient phase (postoperative days 1–3), (2) lengthening or correction phase, (3) consolidation phase, and (4) post frame removal phase [3]. At author's institution, patients that are found to have pre-surgical muscle tightness or contractures are encouraged to start Physical Therapy prior to surgery, this also familiarizes patients with process and what to expect after surgery.

Inpatient Phase

Physical therapy begins on the first day following surgery. During this phase, the therapist teaches the patient and family correct positioning in bed as well as in the wheel chair, especially in cases of bilateral limb lengthening. Resting splints are made to apply gentle stretch and maintain correct positioning of the adjacent joints (Fig. 19.1). The patient and caretakers are instructed regarding active and active assisted range of motion exercises for a home program. The physical therapist is responsible for teaching the patient how to ambulate with assistive devices, to maintain weight-bearing precautions, and to maneuver stairs. Correct weight bearing can be easily taught by having the patient stand with the surgical leg on a scale and transferring weight gradually to the side until the correct weight is applied to the scale. This should be repeated multiple times to re-inforce the learning of the correct weight bearing. Equipment such as a walker, commode, wheelchair, and crutches are also ordered in preparation for

A. Bhave (✉)
Rubin Institute for Advanced Orthopedics, Sinai Hospital, Baltimore, MD, USA
e-mail: abhave@lifebridgehealth.org

E. Baker
OrthoNY, Albany, NY, USA
e-mail: ebaker@orthony.com

M. Campbell
Baltimore, MD, USA
e-mail: mary@truesortspt.com

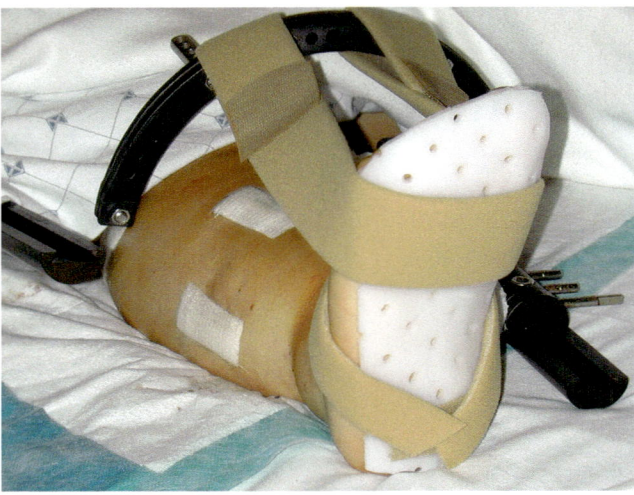

Fig. 19.1 Orthoplast custom foot splints are fabricated prior to discharge from the hospital. In case of monolateral fixators, a ring is attached to the fixator for easy application of the foot splint using Velcro straps. Patient and caretakers are educated to check the skin integrity periodically and to only tighten the strap to apply gentle pressure to maintain correct ankle positioning in the plantigrade position

discharge from the hospital. For patients undergoing limb lengthening, it is preferable to order wheelchairs with reclining back rests. This design avoids sciatic nerve stretch caused by having patients sit upright with their hips flexed 90° with the knee in full extension In addition, elevated leg rests are used to allow appropriate leg elevation. Removable armrests are also recommended for easy transfers to and from the wheelchair. It is recommended that the reclining back rest be at an angle of 45° when using the leg rest in full knee extension. Conversely, if the back rest is in an upright position, then patients are encouraged to keep the knees bent 70–90°.

Lengthening or Correction Phase

Based on variables such as the underlying diagnosis, the need for multi-segment lengthening, the amount of deformity, type of insurance coverage for post recovery therapy, and social considerations, there are three different rehabilitation pathways that most patients take after surgery: outpatient physical therapy with one to two sessions per day for 3 days per week, a day program with two sessions of therapy a day for 3–5 days a week, and inpatient rehabilitation with extensive physical therapy in a rehabilitation hospital [4]. Because of recent trends in insurance coverage, the third option of inpatient rehabilitation is not a viable option for most patients. This option is reserved for very special cases with significant mobility issues and still is only a short-term solution. The goals of physical therapy during the lengthening/correction phase are to maintain and maximize joint

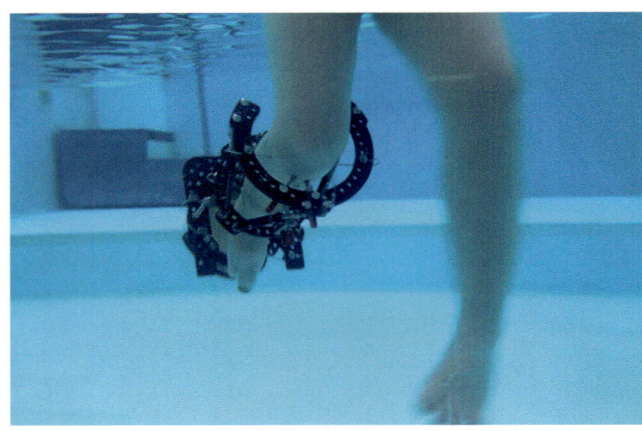

Fig. 19.2 Chlorinated, heated, hydrotherapy pool for promoting increased range of motion and muscle strength

range of motion and maintain muscle tone and flexibility. Early joint mobilization is imperative to prevent contractures. Barker et al. [5] found that greatest loss of motion across joints occurred between surgery and commencement of distraction indicating pain as the primary cause. As the lengthening proceeds, resultant contractures and loss of ROM is caused by inadequate accommodation by dense connective and myofascial tissue to change in length. Due to this fact, physical therapists have to use various techniques such as soft tissue techniques, therapeutic exercises, joint mobilization, and splinting. Astym therapy has shown promise in maximizing ROM during the lengthening phase. Aquatic therapy is also a good adjunct to land therapy for patients with multi-segment lengthening and those undergoing bilateral lower extremity lengthening when full weight bearing is not allowed (Fig. 19.2). Hydrotherapy promotes early recovery of active range of motion and neutralizes the weight of the fixator for ease of movement. Heated pool also helps with relaxation of muscles and dense connective tissue.

Consolidation Phase

In this phase, the goal of therapy is to maximize and achieve full range of motion and continue to improve strength. Weight bearing and exercises that promote axial loading of the bone are encouraged. If patients have lost substantial knee range of motion, such as the development of a flexion contracture after tibial or femoral lengthening, then aggressive splinting across the knee joint with customized bracing or casting is done (Fig. 19.3). It is best to treat these contractures before the removal of the external fixator since the treatment of the contracture after the removal of the fixator may lead to fractures due to excessive stress and unresolved soft tissue tension.

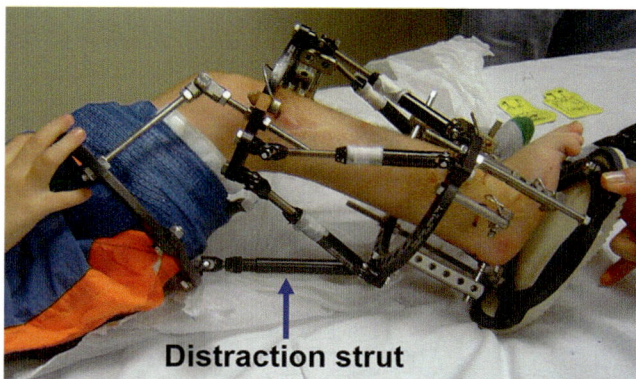

Fig. 19.3 Use of a Taylor Spatial Frame™ strut to apply an extension force in a patient who developed severe knee flexion contracture during tibial lengthening for fibular hemimelia. Thigh cuff using fiberglass casting is linked to the external fixator with hinges

> **Box 19.1 Complications During Limb Lengthening**
> - Muscle contractures
> - Muscle weakness
> - Joint stiffness
> - Nerve injury
> - Joint subluxation

Post Frame Removal

Gradual recovery of range of motion and functional strength through progressive exercises is the focus of physical therapy after removal of the fixator [4]. At this stage, there is a concern for fracture through the pin sites and at the newly formed bone of the lengthening regenerate [6]. It is recommended to be cautious in the first 4–6 weeks after fixator removal to allow for bone healing at these areas and therapy may be delayed for a month [7]. Casts and braces may be utilized during this phase for providing additional stability to the lengthened bone [4]. Once physical therapy is resumed, it is recommended that closed chain exercises be started before open chain exercises. Closed chain exercises are weight-bearing exercises, providing axial loading to further strengthen the lengthened bone segment. Open chain exercises are exercises where the distal limb segment moves around the proximal axis, this leads to increase torque and stress on the weaker newly lengthened bone segment. Careful stabilization of the bone segment as close to the joint line as possible is necessary to avoid bending stress on the bone during mobilization with physical therapy (Fig. 19.4). Manual mobilization with adequate stabilization of the lengthened bone is a safe and effective way to regain motion. Gait training and return to normative function are other additional goals during this phase. Recovery is slowest immediately following fixator removal and speeds up between 6 months to 1 year postoperatively. No further recovery is typically seen after 2 years following fixator removal [2]. During this period, a home exercise program and participation in activities play a big part in the final journey of return to full functionality.

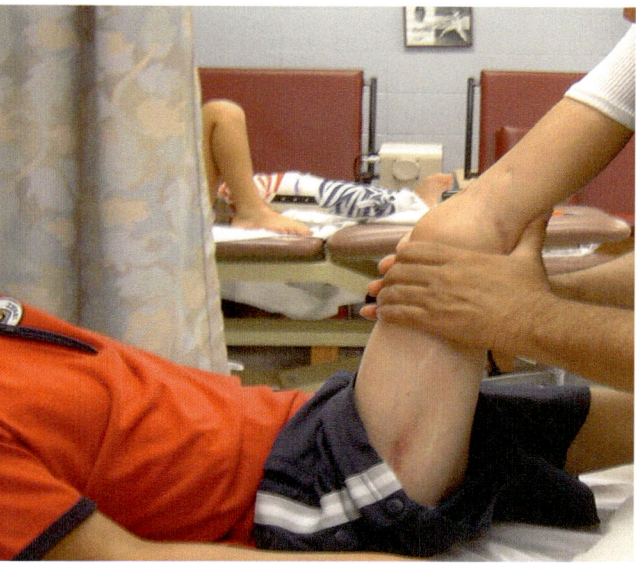

Fig. 19.4 Careful stabilization of the femur and tibia are critical during therapy after fixator removal. Patient receiving hamstring stretch with posteroanterior mobilization. Therapist's hands are placed as close to the joint line as possible

Role of Physical Therapy in Management of Complications

After the index surgery, patients may experience bone and/or soft tissue complications, which can compromise functional outcomes. Temporary soft tissue dysfunction occurs in almost all of the patients who undergo limb lengthening and deformity correction procedures. The severity of these complications and obstacles to lengthening are dependent upon the diagnosis, amount of lengthening or correction, soft tissue quality, level of osteotomy, technique and device used for surgical correction, and nerve complications [1]. In addition to physical causes of complications, there are social reasons such as poor pain tolerance, inadequate insurance coverage, or lack of family support that can lead to suboptimal results.

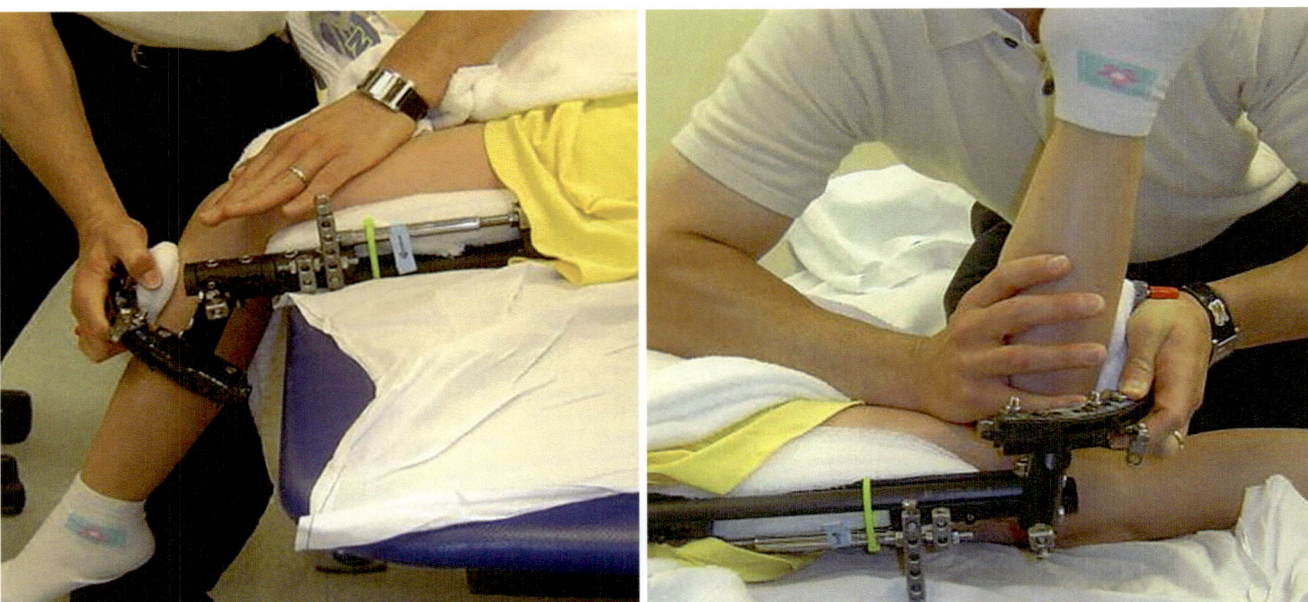

Fig. 19.5 Hand placement is critical for joint mobilization. Interior mobilization of the patella during knee flexion mobilization and correct posterior stabilization of the proximal tibia are important

Examples of soft tissue dysfunctions include contractures, muscle weakness, joint stiffness, nerve injury, joint subluxation, and dislocations. Bone complications include poor bone formation, angulation of the regenerate bone, and insufficiency fractures. Therapeutic intervention is crucial to avoid permanent dysfunctions. The physical therapist needs to have adequate handling techniques and the skill to apply appropriate forces and stabilization in order to focus treatment targeted at the appropriate tissues (Fig. 19.5). Therapists that are used to handling pediatric patients are best suited for this therapy, especially in a younger child. The magnitude of force application and tissue handling is an acquired skill and takes time and practice to develop. It is a fine balancing act since excessive forces can cause the bone to bend or fracture. The therapist must keep in mind that the stress–strain curve for tissues in the human body alters with age [8]. Pediatric patients deform their soft tissue with much less force than adults. Bone and soft tissue complications can occur during lengthening and consolidation phases, as well as after the removal of the external fixator.

Muscle Contractures

Contractures occur when elastic tissues and to a lesser extent contractile elements are unable to accommodate change in their length following limb lengthening and deformity correction. Myofascial tissues resist such elongation more than most other tissues and are therefore more prone to contractures. A relative shortening of biarticular muscles (crossing two joints) and the fascial component is often the cause of such contractures [1]. For example, the gastrocnemius develops passive tension much more rapidly in response to bony lengthening than does the soleus.

When muscles are kept in a shortened position, often due to postoperative pain early in the lengthening process, the muscle adaptively shortens by absorbing sarcomeres to maintain efficiency. Prolonged stretch through a muscle has been proven to add sarcomeres [8]. The therapist must devise a way to provide prolonged stretch of such muscles across adjacent joints without causing excessive pain. For such stretch to be effective, it must have four critical components: (1) adequate intensity, (2) long duration, (3) adequate frequency with multiple repetitions, and (4) an active stretch component [9].

Problematic muscles should be identified early in order to treat contractures effectively. In tibial lengthening, for example, problem muscles are the gastrocnemius and toe flexors. As a result, patients are prone to develop knee flexion, ankle plantar flexion, and toe flexion contractures. Likewise, during femoral lengthening, the quadriceps (especially the rectus femoris) and hamstring muscles are predisposed to develop contractures resulting in deficits of flexion and potential for fixed flexion deformity across the knee joint, respectively. In addition, especially hip adductors are prone to develop tightness followed by contracture in proximal or mid diaphyseal lengthening.

Soft tissue restriction can be further complicated by the presence of scars from previous surgery, as is often seen in patients with long-standing limb deformities. Scar tissue lacks the elasticity of the native tissue and scar fibers are often laid down in a much more disorganized, rigid pattern,

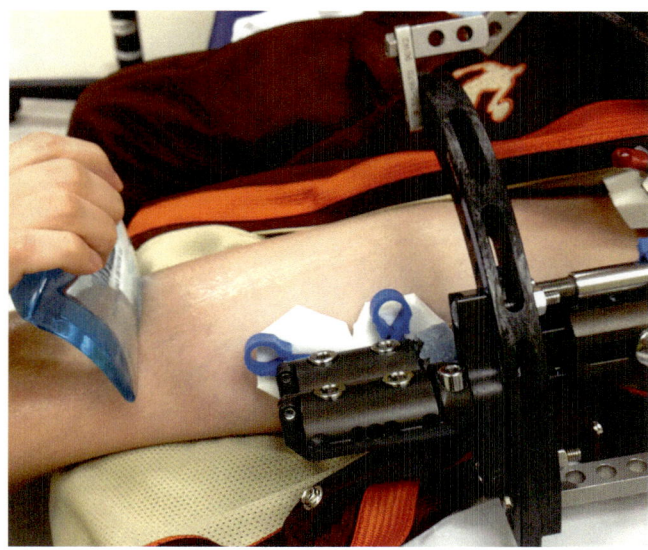

Fig. 19.6 ASTYM™ treatment for improving muscle flexibility and to promote remodeling of the fibrous tissue

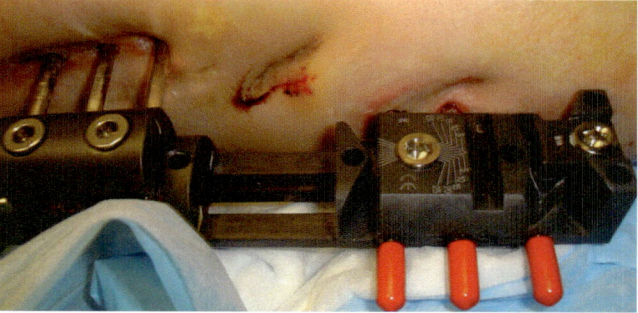

Fig. 19.7 Pin site around the hip joint can be painful due to movement of excess tissue during therapy. Massage around the pin site and use of tight wraps help reduce pain during therapy

especially when the tissue is immobilized due to pain or lack of motion. Utilizing soft tissue mobilization with implementation, such as ASTYM™ (Fig. 19.6) and Graston™, can break down scar tissue and establish a more organized, pliable scar [9].

Managing muscle contractures effectively is vital for a satisfactory clinical outcome following limb lengthening and deformity correction [1]. Passive stretching with end range holds and oscillating manipulations at end range is an effective way to manage soft tissue contractures. Per our protocol, moist heat is applied for 10–15 min prior to stretching to aid in collagen breakdown and improve the stretch of connective tissue [9]. Analgesic medications administered 30 min prior to therapy help patients tolerate the stretch better. Reciprocal inhibition, activating the antagonist muscle before stretching the agonist, also relaxes the muscle being stretched. Pin sites near the fascial and muscle planes are susceptible to inflammation. Thus, gentle soft tissue mobilization and massage help to manage tightness caused by adherent soft tissues around the pin. Another strategy to reduce pain around the pins during joint mobilization and stretching is to use tight pin wraps, especially at sites near the knee or hip joint (Fig. 19.7). The tight pin wraps reduce skin motion during therapy and significantly reduce pain (Fig. 19.8). Stretching of biarticular muscles ten times per session and uniarticular muscles five times a session with 20–30 s holds for each stretch is recommended. When stretching a biarticular muscle, stabilization at one joint is necessary during mobilization at the other joint to obtain maximum stretch. Ideally, a patient should have such treatments twice a day.

Positioning and splinting strategies should also be used to manage soft tissue contractures. Optimal positions vary by affected body part. For example, patients who have undergone tibial lengthening should be positioned in knee extension and ankle dorsiflexion (Fig. 19.9). Knee extension, along with hip abduction, is a desirable position for patients undergoing femoral lengthening. Commercially made static splints (Fig. 19.10) augment therapeutic passive stretching by counteracting the connective tissues' elastic response to passive stretching. Using a splint to place the muscle under tension helps prevent contractures by obtaining plastic response in the connective tissue. Dynamic splints produce optimal plastic elongation (permanent elongation) of the connective tissue through a low load prolonged duration stretch (Fig. 19.11). Dynamic splints offer constant force with gradual change in length, such a stretch also causes physiological remodeling of connective tissue through biochemical response. Dynamic splints work most effectively in treating knee and ankle contractures as they are a hinge joints. Be aware that splints work only in optimal positions.

Commercially made dynamic splints do not always provide the customization needed for an effective stretch. Therefore, the authors developed and utilize a custom knee device (CKD) for contracture management during or after external fixation (Fig. 19.12). This is a semi-rigid device made of a conformable polyester and fiberglass cast of the thigh and lower leg with hinges across the knee to allow for progressive stretching into the restricted range of motion. Elastic bands are utilized to provide the needed tension and the rigidity of the casting materials allows for minimal loss of the stretch energy to the desired tissues. Knee joint subluxation can also be managed utilizing the CKD with added straps at the knee joint to help approximate the joint and reduce the subluxation. The more the patient wears this device, the sooner the muscle truly lengthens and range of motion is restored. This concept can be utilized with tibial frames, as a thigh cast can be made with a half ring casted in and then attached to the tibial frame with a hinged joint. A telescoping strut can be added and the knee can be progressively straightened if a flexion contracture develops (Fig. 19.13). It is recommended to use these splints all night or at least 3–4 h/day.

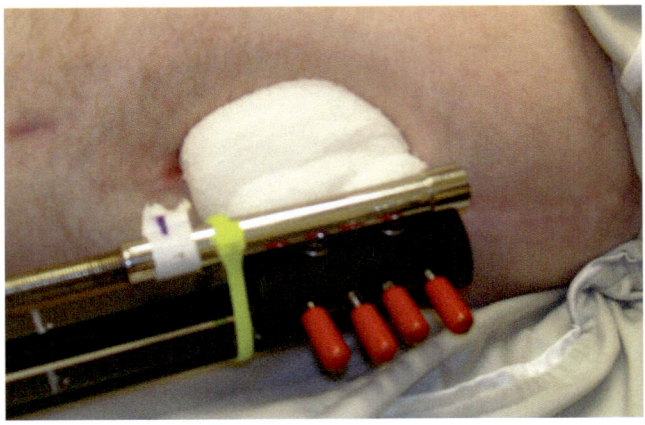

Fig. 19.8 A compression wrap around proximal femoral pins to avoid tissue motion during therapy. This technique reduces pain as well as risk of infection

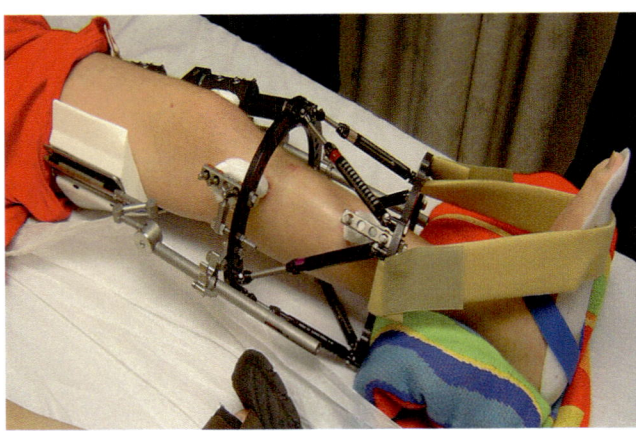

Fig. 19.11 Use of commercially available dynamic brace (Dynasplint™) attached to the proximal tibial ring to improve knee extension

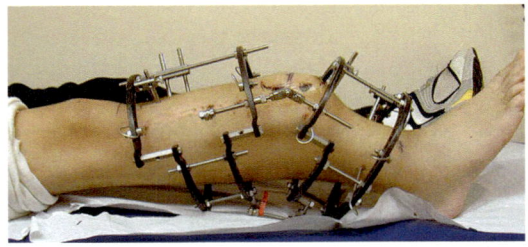

Fig. 19.9 Patient undergoing tibial lengthening and procurvatum deformity correction. Gastrocnemius and soleus contracture with lack of ankle dorsiflexion occurs commonly in these patients

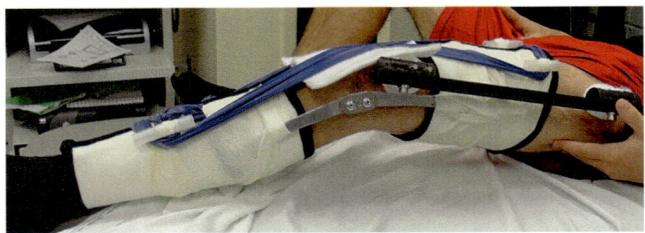

Fig. 19.12 Use of custom knee device (CKD) in a child with congenital femoral deficiency (CFD) undergoing femoral lengthening using monolateral fixator. Elastic bands offer continuous dynamic stretch in to extension. Patients are encouraged to use the device 8–14 h per 24-h period daily

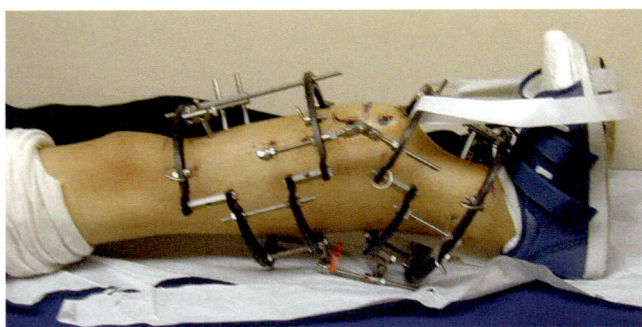

Fig. 19.10 Commercially available walking shoe modification with Velcro straps to keep ankle in neutral dorsiflexion position

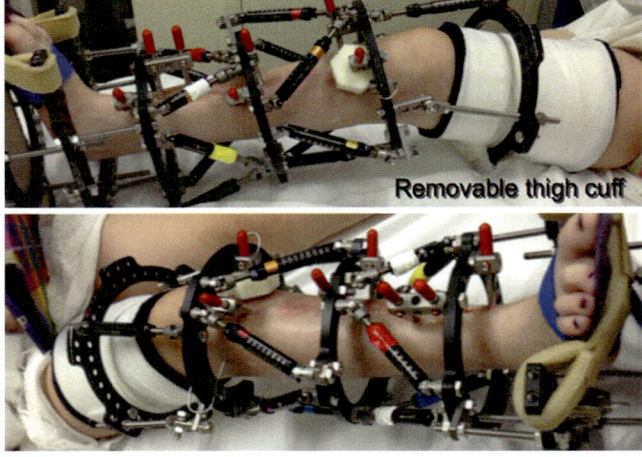

Fig. 19.13 Use of removable thigh cuff attached to tibial frame with hinges in a patient undergoing tibial lengthening. Spatial frame strut between ring incorporated in thigh cuff and proximal tibia ring allows for applying an extension stretch

Joint Stiffness

Muscle contractures, if not treated aggressively, lead to capsular and intra-articular adhesions. Contracture of biarticular muscles also introduces compressive force on the articular cartilage, which leads to a stiffness across adjacent joints [10]. Characteristics of a stiff joint include loss of motion and ease of movement within the joint's available excursion. Joint stiffness is best prevented with a large quantity of active and passive motion. Manual traction with joint mobilization is beneficial and recommended when feasible. However, such mobilization can only be performed on joints that are not included in the external fixation construct. If an internal lengthening patient develops stiffness, this is harder to handle than patients with external fixators since the ability to distract the knee joint by placing hinges across the joint is not available.

Muscle Weakness

Patients may experience muscle weakness due to disuse atrophy and neurogenic inhibition with associated pain. Electrical stimulation and hydrotherapy are two modalities that can be used to manage muscle weakness. Electrical stimulation is used as an adjunct to a strengthening program and to augment voluntary muscle contraction. The most common area for electrical stimulation is the quadriceps muscle (Fig. 19.14). In our experience, as long as there is no direct contact of electrodes to the half-pins, it has been safely tolerated by children undergoing conventional distraction osteogenesis treatment with external fixation.

At our center, typical electrical stimulation parameters are a biphasic pulse at a frequency of 35–70 Hz and pulse duration of 300–400 μs. In addition, an on-to-off ratio of 1:3 is recommended. Stimulation intensity should be adequate to cause strong contraction of the muscle. Patients tolerate newer electrical stimulation devices better using advanced frequency modulation software. Children tolerate higher intensity settings with these devices as compared to older devices. Family education for setup is recommended for incorporation of electrical stimulation into a home program.

Hydrotherapy helps avoid significant muscle weakness, especially in patients with bilateral external fixators or unilateral femur plus tibial fixators. Hydrotherapy also promotes increased active ROM (see Fig. 19.2). Buoyancy offsets fixator weight and facilitates muscle strengthening. Limb lengthening patients experience aquatic therapy in a heated, clinically chlorinated pool. Hydrotherapy allows for weight bearing early in the lengthening process, even if there are weight-bearing restrictions on land. With the water up to the nipple line, patients can utilize the buoyancy of the water to provide their bones with protection from gravity's compressive forces to walk for continued cardiovascular health and muscle memory. The heated water brings muscle relaxation and freedom of motion, which allows for exercise and standing mobility. The chlorine levels at our center are kept at level 5 since patients get in with open pin sites. Purulent drainage from a pin site is a contraindication for getting into the pool. Daily assessment of pin sites are done by the treating land therapist as well as the aquatics therapist.

During the recovery phase of limb lengthening, the use of a more recent technique known as Blood Flow Restriction Therapy (BFRT) (Fig. 19.15) has been found to be a very useful method for muscle fiber hypertrophy and recruitment of fast twitch muscle fiber. A BFRT utilized tourniquet is placed at the most proximal portion of the lower extremity. The tourniquet cuff is inflated to 80% occlusion for arterial flow and 100% venous occlusion is obtained. Patients then exercise at 20–40% of their max for up to 75 repetitions. BFRT allows for rapid muscle hypertrophy and strength gain without having to work at close to max levels which are difficult for patients to engage in the recovery phase. In the author's institution, we prefer to use a doppler controlled device for safety and this device allows for continuous monitoring and modulation of the cuff pressure through out the exercise.

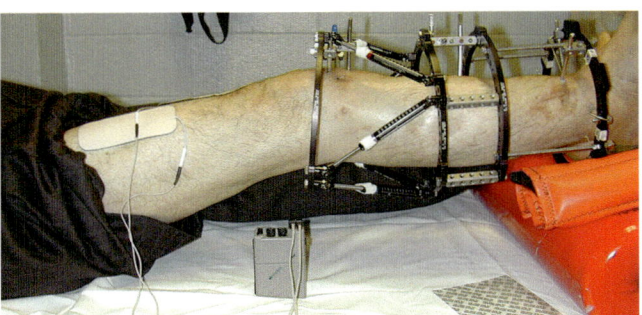

Fig. 19.14 Neuromuscular electrical stimulation of the quadriceps muscle using the heel propped position. This position allows for active stretch as well as augmented strengthening of the quadriceps

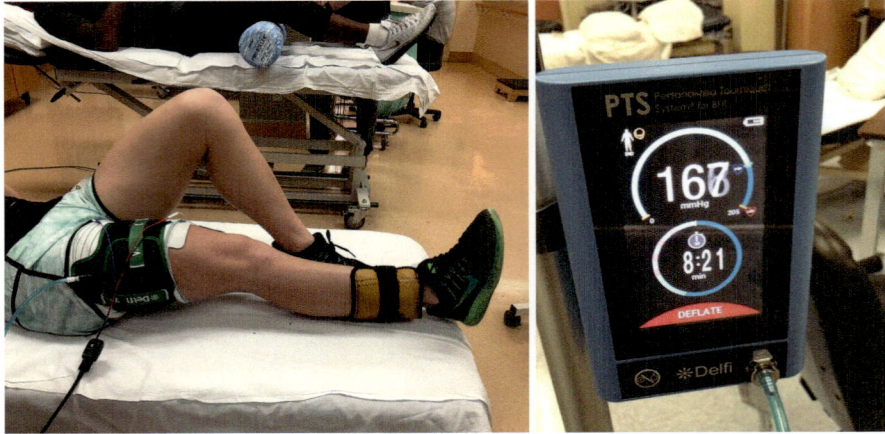

Fig. 19.15 Patient doing a Blood Flow Restriction therapy using a 3 pound weight at the ankle for straight leg raises. Torniquet is applied at the proximal thigh. Arterial occlusion at 80% of the max and 100% venous occlusion is performed using a doppler driven cuff. Patients exercise at a lower intensity, and high repetitions up to 75 reps per exercise in under 8 min. Patents typically perform three to four different exercises

Joint Subluxation

Joint subluxation is a dreaded complication of limb lengthening surgery. Subluxations are caused by lack of opposition of the joint surfaces, muscle and tendon contracture, and ligamentous laxity. If a subluxation is not recognized and treated early, it can result in permanent sequelae. This can lead to significant reduction in range of motion, pain, and early onset of arthritis due to articular cartilage erosion. Knee subluxation in patients who have undergone femur lengthening for congenital femoral deficiency usually involves posterolateral translation of the proximal tibia. Such patients may have cruciate deficient knee joints, hamstring contracture, quadriceps inhibition, tight iliotibial bands, and flexed knee posturing. The combined effect of these conditions leads to unopposed posterolateral pull on the proximal tibia and in some cases also lateral subluxation of the patella [1]. Knee joint subluxation can occur during femoral lengthening if the joint is not protected in the frame or during lengthening with an intramedullary lengthening device. It can also occur due to unresolved residual tension in the soft tissues post fixator removal. Due to the high frequency of subluxations in the congenital femoral lengthening, most surgeons prefer to extend the frame to the tibia with a hinge at the knee joint (Fig. 19.16) [1].

Treatment for knee subluxation starts with early detection. Usual signs include posterior slope of the tibia (commonly called the ski slope sign) (Fig. 19.17), anterior pain on knee extension, and overall sudden increase in stiffness and pain. Physical therapy treatment consists of vigorous knee extension with proper proximal tibia anterior tracking via slings and manual mobilization techniques. Soft tissue mobilization techniques and augmented tissue stimulation to the lower kinetic chain using ASTYM™ is particularly useful. If the patient has an external fixator with no extension to the

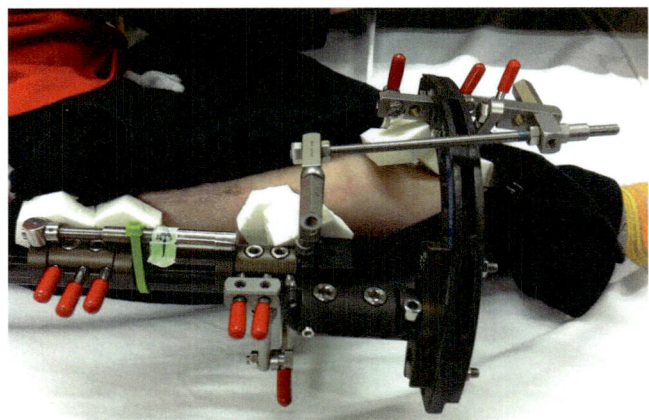

Fig. 19.16 Use of knee extension rod in a patient undergoing femoral lengthening for congenital femoral deficiency. Patients are recommended to use the extension rod all night long and 2 h on and 2 h off during day

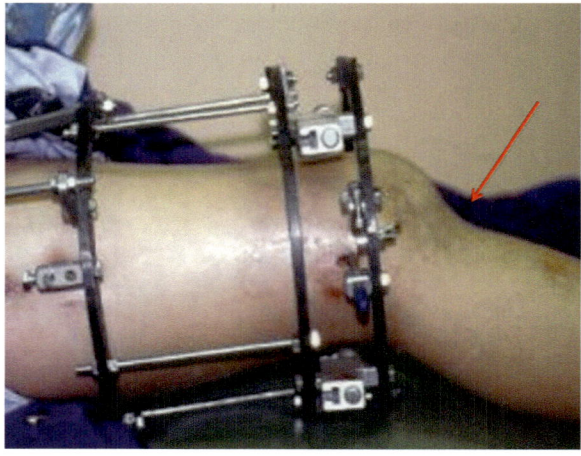

Fig. 19.17 Posterior subluxation of the knee in a patient undergoing femoral lengthening. The posterior subluxation of the tibia is demonstrated by the *arrow*. Due to prevalence of this complication, most surgeons use tibial frame linked to the femoral frame with hinges to prevent knee subluxation

tibia, then manual therapy with joint distraction can also be employed. At night, the patient may also use tibial traction and dynamic splints. In the author's experience, mild to moderate subluxations respond to conservative regimens, while more severe ones may need surgery that includes distal iliotibial band and biceps femoris releases.

Hip subluxation is a rare complication of femoral lengthening. It presents as posterolateral migration of the femoral head and usually occurs in patients with acetabular dysplasia in the face of an adductor contracture during proximal femur lengthening. Adductor stretching and an abduction pillow can help prevent hip subluxation in proximal femoral lengthening. When hip subluxation occurs, patients usually need additional surgery including adductor release, followed by tibial skin traction and intensive therapy.

Nerve Injury

During the lengthening process, as the bony segments slowly distract, the soft tissue often becomes taut and restricted. It was thought that bony distraction over-stretches the nerve, but Nogueira et al. [11] found this is not always the case as no correlation was noted between amount lengthened and the onset of nerve signs. Patients often present to therapy with numbness and tingling peripherally with burning pain along nerve distributions. The most commonly compromised nerve is the peroneal nerve, more prevalent in tibial lengthenings and corrections. Classic signs are numbness and burning pain on the dorsum of the foot, especially between the first and second toes. In more severe cases, the extensor hallucis longus (EHL) becomes weak or worse, the tibialis anterior muscle weakness leads to a foot drop. The sciatic nerve can also be over-stretched, especially in large femoral lengthenings or simultaneous femoral and tibial lengthenings. In foot corrections, as in clubfoot, the medial plantar nerve is at greatest risk for compromise, with burning and tingling on the plantar surface of the hallux. If nerve compromise is suspected, the authors utilize the pressure specified sensory device, or PSSD (Fig. 19.18). This device can reliably test the light touch sensation of various nerve distributions with 100% sensitivity and 87% specificity [11]. The device also has the capability to store data for later comparison. One drawback of such a device or any sensation testing is that the patient needs to be of an age or maturity to participate reliably in the test. Usually, this is reserved for patients aged 6 years and older. When sensory signs and symptoms of nerve compromise are present, the medical team will either slow down the lengthening or prescribe medications like Gabapentin (Neurontin™) or Lyrica™ to manage the pain associated with nerve problems. In some cases, especially those with motor weakness, urgent surgical release of the offending nerve is required. Considerations need to be made

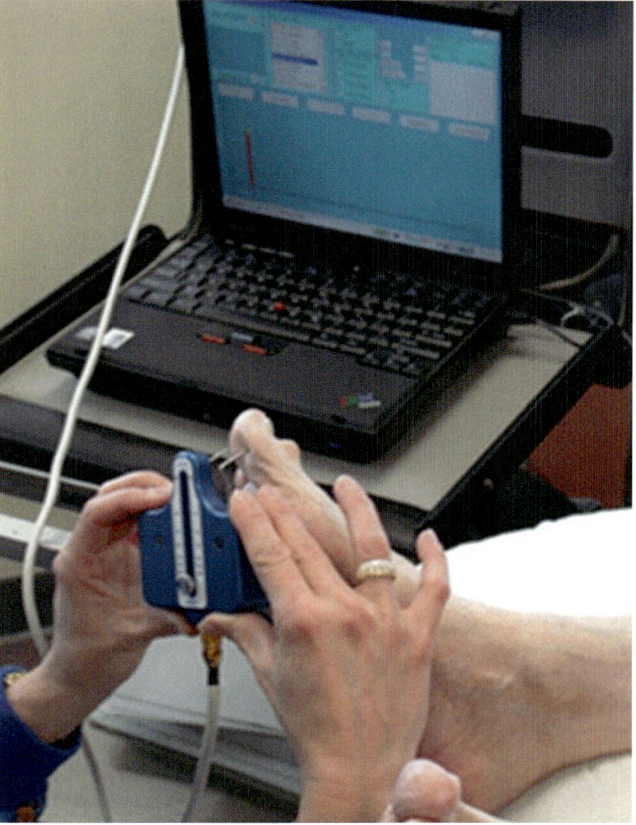

Fig. 19.18 Pressure specified sensory device (PSSD) (Sensory Management, Baltimore, MD). This device allows for invasive monitoring of sensory function during lengthening

when providing therapy to patients who have nerve compromise. Bi-articular stretches, such as straight leg raises, should be avoided in favor of mobilization at each individual joint of the lower leg. This allows for soft tissues to be lax on one end while the opposite end is treated.

Weight-Bearing Considerations

Functional mobility training will depend greatly on the level of weight bearing allowed. During the lengthening and consolidation phases, weight bearing may be permitted, dependent on the type of fixator or device used and the bone being lengthened [4]. A ring fixator (such as the Ilizarov and a hexapod-type fixator) generally provides the underlying bone with substantial support to allow for 50–100% weight bearing. In the classic Ilizarov frame where each segment has two rings and two wires are placed on each ring with specific tensile strength, all of the force that normally would go through the bone is transferred to the metal frame, protecting the osteotomy site and allowing for full weight bearing. The more recent versions of the circular frame utilize rings similar to that of the Ilizarov but favor half-pins instead of transosseous wires as fixation elements. These pins are generally better tolerated by the patients as they minimize the tethering of the soft tissue compartments. If the foot is incorporated into the frame, then a walking ring is added, fitted with a rubber tread to allow for safe ambulation (Fig. 19.19).

Monolateral rail fixators handle weight-bearing forces very differently. Typically, the majority of the forces on the bone are lateral for the femurs and medial for the tibia. Without any counter to distribute the forces evenly, weight bearing is restricted in such patients during lengthening to prevent loosening of the pins or worse, fracture at the pin site. Many monolateral fixators for femoral lengthening will have a hinge at the knee and an extension to the tibia, with a partial ring attached to pins in the tibia (see Fig. 19.16). This offers a great deal of additional stability at the osteotomy site, allowing for weight bearing as tolerated during the lengthening process.

Even in cases where monolateral rails are used without a counter as in stature lengthening, weight bearing with a walker is often allowed but for transfers only. The repetitive forces that occur with unrestricted weight bearing through these devices can weaken the bony interface. Restricted, controlled weight bearing for very short durations allows for stretching of the gastrocnemius muscles and the work induced is good for cardiovascular health.

These considerations around weight bearing will shape the plan of care in physical therapy. Ambulation during lengthening helps to maintain muscular and bony strength and may shorten the rehabilitation process after fixator removal [12].

Specific Musculoskeletal Disorders

Legg-Calve-Perthes Disease

Legg-Calve-Perthes disease (commonly referred to as Perthes disease) is usually seen in children aged 4–10 years and is more common in boys [13]. Perthes disease has been treated using the principle of "containment" by long periods of immobilization, historically using hip spica casting to hold the femoral head in a most congruous position within the acetabulum to allow the best reshaping of the femoral head. Hip spica casts often cause difficulty with maintaining mobility of the child as well as hygiene issues. Utilizing a hip distractor external fixator mitigates these issues as well as assures a congruous position of the hip (Fig. 19.20). They hold the hip in 15°–20° of abduction, 10° of flexion and 10° of external rotation. A partial ring over the pelvis provides stabilization to a hinged joint at the axis of the sagittal plane for hip motion and a distractor bar is attached to the monolateral rail. The femur is gently distracted over a period of 10–14 days and held in position for approximately 4 months to allow for re-ossification and reshaping of the femoral epiphyses. Utilizing this frame can lead to improved joint mobility and decreased pain [14].

The focus of rehabilitation immediately after surgery is on standing mobility training, family education, and establishing a home program for the patient. Since the legs are being held in abduction and weight bearing through the effected limb is limited, a wide rolling walker is often needed initially to aid in ambulation. Patients can progress to axil-

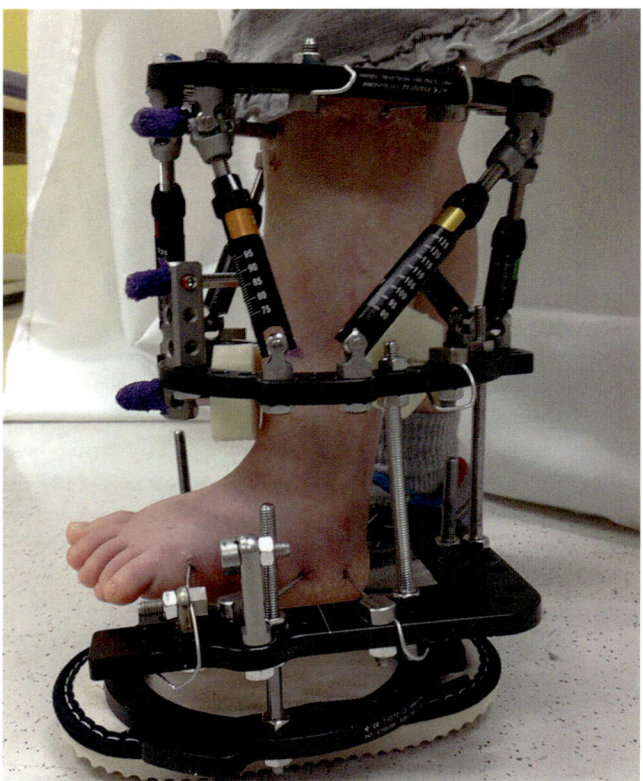

Fig. 19.19 Application of walking ring to the tibial frame allows for less painful-free weight bearing. The height of the walking ring can also be adjusted to accommodate the leg length difference

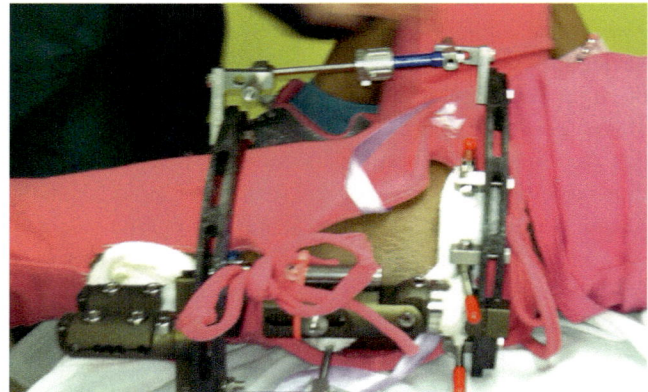

Fig. 19.20 Use of hip extension rod to maintain maximal hip extension in patient undergoing hip distraction for treatment of Perthes Diseases. Patients wear the rod all night

lary crutches eventually to allow for ambulation on stairs, but selection of crutches is a very individual choice, based on the patient's safety awareness and balance control. For long distances, these children still need a wheelchair, with consideration of the size of the patient and the extra width added by the frame laterally.

Only sagittal plane motion is allowed by the hip distractor. Therefore, only hip flexion and extension mobilization can be done while in the frame. The family needs to be educated in a home stretching program to maintain hip motion and prevent contractures from immobility and pain. A removable anterior telescoping bar is added to the frame to provide a progressive, sustained stretch across the hip into extension (see Fig. 19.20). After 4 months, the frame is removed and the role of physical therapy increases exponentially. For the first 6 weeks post removal, the patient is wearing a hip abduction brace nearly at all times, giving the patient a very wide stance in gait. Weight bearing is allowed at this point and gait training is needed to learn to ambulate without a device.

Without frontal and transverse planes of motion across the hip during external fixation, abduction/adduction and internal/external rotation motions are very limited after frame removal. Therapy focuses on regaining the hip motion, both passively through joint mobilization and actively through exercise and mobility training. Control of active hip motion is challenging in this population since the lumbar spine so readily provides foot placement in gait and movement in exercise—a compensatory strategy developed during the 4 months of non-use in the frame and potentially even longer, depending on how long the disease progressed prior to treatment. With an abduction contracture on the effected limb, the leg feels longer to the patient, and a compensatory trunk lean to the contralateral side is apparent. Furthermore, due to the young patient population, it becomes imperative that the family is involved in treatment, learning to cue the patient to aid in re-training and performing the exercise program at home. Normalization of gait can take several months. In our experience, integrating yoga and other treatment modalities that provide postural awareness help in the recovery of hip motion and strength, and ultimately allow a return to independent activity.

Congenital Femoral Deficiency

Lengthening the femur of a child with congenital femoral deficiency (CFD) can be one of the most difficult lengthenings to manage. Up to 95% of these children have deficient or absent cruciate ligaments in the knee and such instability can cause problems during lengthening [15]. In addition, many patients have lateral patellar instability due to a shallow lateral trochlea, external rotation of the femur, and a tight distal IT band. As the femur gets longer, the pull of the muscles increases, especially that of the hamstrings. With underdeveloped quadriceps and pain limiting motion, the pull of the hamstrings can cause a posterior subluxation of the tibia on the femur. Having a soft tissue reconstruction to address the cruciate deficiency prior to femoral lengthening in a patient with CFD associated with ligamentous laxity and patellar stabilization lowers the risk of postoperative subluxation [16]. If subluxation occurs, lengthening is slowed or stopped and knee extension mobilization needs to be done with posterior support to the proximal tibia.

The half pins used to anchor the fixator across the knee joint can be problematic with knee flexion mobilization. Therapists' hand placement is important for the safety of the patient. The knee cannot be mobilized into flexion from the distal tibia because that can cause loosening of the tibial pins. Anterior to posterior tibial mobilization must be done proximally, with a posterior counter force to prevent pin loosening and fracture of the bone (Fig. 19.21). The loss of leverage and inefficient grip can make this mobilization difficult for the therapist. Knee flexion is often where the greatest loss of motion occurs during CFD lengthening. If the flexion measures 40° or less, it is often recommended that

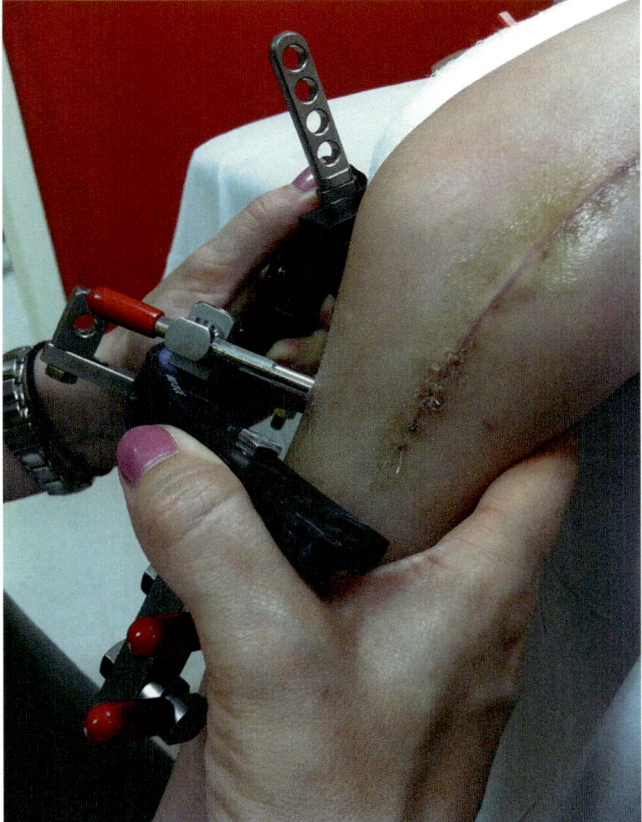

Fig. 19.21 Careful hand placement for knee flexion mobilization in a patient with femoral lengthening for CFD. The therapist's left hand is stabilizing the hinge and right hand applies flexion force as well as stabilizes posterior tibia

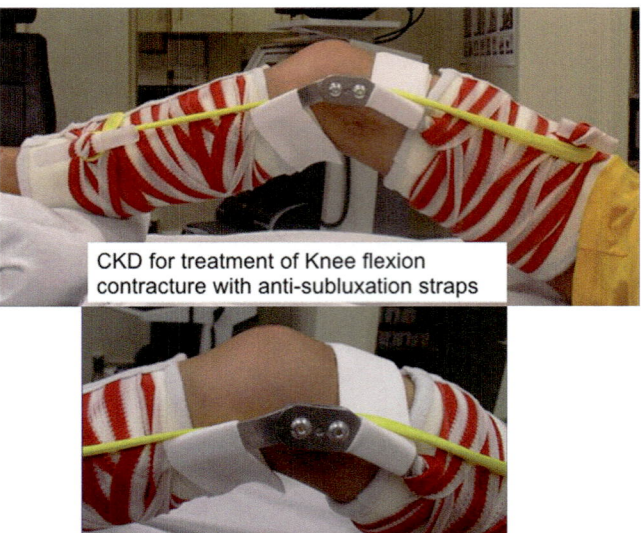

Fig. 19.22 Use of CKD bracing with special straps. The straps allow for an inferior mobilization of the distal femur and superior mobilization of the proximal tibia. The combination of CKD with an elastic band applying an extension stretch and elastic straps that are placed on the distal femur anteriorly and proximal tibial elastic straps posteriorly allow for simultaneous correction of knee flexion contracture and subluxation

lengthening be stopped, at least temporarily, until further joint mobility is gained [10].

After removal of the fixator, therapy can begin to focus on mobility training as well as regaining motion to the preoperative level. Often children with CFD have acetabular dysplasia and weakness around the hip, especially involving the abductors. Gait training and exercise that focuses on closed chain control of the hip and trunk are needed, but often difficult for the patient. Gaining normal strength of the abductors may not be a realistic goal—prior surgeries such as trochanteric entry intramedullary nails may have caused damage to the abductors and any residual underlying hip dysplasia may leave abductor weakness.

Treating a child or adolescent with an internal femoral lengthening device presents a similar set of potential problems, although the external fixation can provide stability to the knee and prevent subluxation. Often CKDs are made with the use of subluxation straps early in the process to encourage gentle knee extension and prevent posterior subluxation of the knee during such lengthening (Fig. 19.22).

Fibular Hemimelia

Fibular hemimelia is the most common lower extremity deficiency affecting males slightly more than females [17]. Tibial lengthening and deformity correction for the treatment of fibular hemimelia is commonly done with a circular fixator. Knee extension and ankle dorsiflexion are the motions most compromised. The foot can be in or out of the frame. In our experience, the patient is more apt to lose range of motion at the knee and ankle if the foot is not included in the frame.

The peroneal nerve is also at risk of being compressed or overstretched during tibial lengthening [1]. Neurogenic symptoms can worsen with knee extension. Patients with the foot included in the frame are at a higher risk of peroneal nerve palsy with tibial lengthening as they are unable to plantarflex the ankle to provide relief to the nerve at the fibular head. Surgeons will often prophylactically release the peroneal nerve in such cases.

Patients with fibular hemimelia often have altered mechanics of the ankle joint. The mobility of the ankle is generally limited in these patients with some compensation at the midfoot and forefoot due to some compensatory hyper flexibility at these distal joints. It is important for the physical therapist to consider these compensatory mechanisms as gait training advances following removal of the fixator. Rocker bottom shoes may help the patient achieve a more normal gait pattern despite lack of ankle mobility.

Achondroplasia

When approaching an achondroplasia patient undergoing limb deformity correction, it is important to take into consideration the unique morphologic features of this patient population. Skeletal characteristics in achondroplasia include but are not limited to increased lumbar lordosis with excessive anterior pelvic tilt, a more prominent sacrum, and a smaller spinal canal. These skeletal characteristics put the patient at an increase risk of symptomatic spinal stenosis during bilateral lower extremity lengthening. Besides neurologic deficits in the lower extremity, loss of bowel and bladder function can also occur due to tethering of the spinal cord and nerve roots. During treatment, the physical therapist should position the patient to compensate for these skeletal abnormalities while performing lower extremity mobilizations. This can be done by utilizing pillows and wedges to allow for hips to be in a flexed position and the spine to have decreased lordosis (Fig. 19.23). A prominent sacrum also puts patients at a higher risk of sacral wounds. It is important for patients to have time set during the day that they are lying prone to allow for decreased pressure on the sacrum to decrease risk of pressure wounds. Wheelchair cushions are also used to alleviate pressure on the sacrum in sitting.

Individuals with achondroplasia also present with unique soft tissue characteristics including ligamentous and joint laxity, and relatively redundant muscle tissue [18]. This relative laxity of the muscles decreases strength and leads to a waddle-type gait pattern. Often, there is a noticeable trunk

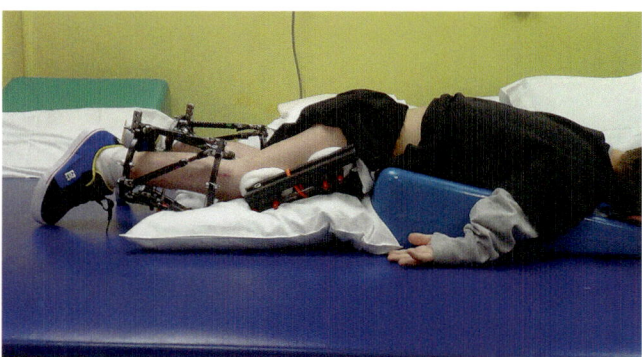

Fig. 19.23 Prone positioning in a patient with achondroplasia undergoing four-segment lengthening. Use of a wedge allows for reduction of the hyperlordosis in patients

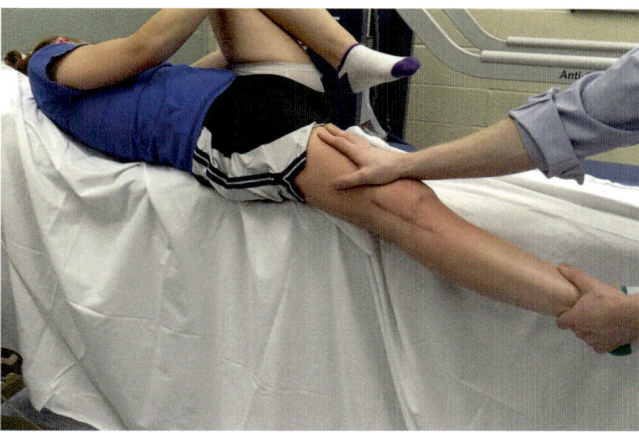

Fig. 19.24 Knee extension mobilization with hip in extension. This position allows for adequate knee extension stretch without compromising or stretching sciatic nerve

sway for compensation as well as a larger base of support during the gait cycle. These gait abnormalities provide the individual with increased stability without the use of core control and proper hip abductor mechanism function. Redundant muscle tissue along with ligamentous and joint laxity allows for increased flexibility early in the limb lengthening process, limiting the amount of motion lost in the early phase of lengthening.

While undergoing bilateral lower limb deformity correction/lengthening, patients are allowed weight bearing for transfers only. In addition to muscular and cardiovascular benefits mentioned earlier, transfer training gives the patient and family increased independence at home. Patients can use push up blocks to help provide upper extremity leverage during lateral and anterior/posterior transfers from wheelchair to bed. Assistance should be given to the lower extremities, lifting from the full tibia rings if available. Core stabilization exercises can help the patient control the spine for transfers, particularly important in head and neck control. Aquatics become an important physical therapy modality for strengthening and gait training while the patients are non-weight bearing.

Physical therapy is performed on a daily basis throughout lengthening, with the primary focus to limit loss of motion through the use of soft tissue and joint mobilization. If lengthening can be carried out simultaneously in all four segments (bilateral femur and tibia), these patients are at a high risk for joint contractures, despite their soft tissue laxity. Loss of motion often occurs in ankle dorsiflexion, hindfoot eversion, knee flexion/extension, hip flexion/extension, and hip abduction. Patients with monolateral rail lengthening of the femur may experience increased tension in the distal iliotibial band due to the tethering at the pin sites [18]. Mobilizations can be performed to the distal iliotibial band by performing a gentle varus mobilization of the knee. If circular fixators are being used for the tibia, then foot splints can be attached to the circular rings to help limit loss of dorsiflexion.

Four-segment lengthening also contributes to increased risk of nerve injury. The physical therapist must continue to monitor for early signs and symptoms of neuropraxia during the lengthening process. Knee extension stretching should be performed with the hip in less than 60° of flexion. In severe cases, the hip can be dropped over the side of the table into slight hip extension to avoid stressing the nerve pathway during knee extension mobilization (Fig. 19.24). Ankle dorsiflexion mobilization can be modified by being performed with the knee in slight flexion.

After lengthening is complete, patients remain in the external fixators until proper bone healing has occurred. During this consolidation phase, weight bearing is gradually increased and strengthening can be progressed. Loss of hip extension and ankle dorsiflexion during lengthening leads to an increase in lumbar lordosis while standing with a significantly flexed posture of the knees and hips. Standing stretches of the gastroc-soleus complex with use of tilt boards or wedges helps to improve erect posture and allow for the stretch-recoil necessary for proper push off during gait. Regaining hip extension is important to decrease the stress on the lumbar spine and spinal cord. Increasing hip extension also restores the stretch-recoil of the hip flexor mechanism to allow for appropriate propulsion of the lower extremity.

Immediately after the external fixators are removed, patients are non-weight bearing for approximately 4 weeks. During this non-weight-bearing phase, the patient's family performs gentle range of motion exercises. When sufficient bone healing has occurred and weight bearing is allowed, physical therapy resumes with an emphasis on gait training. Patients habitually have a wider base of support after fixator removal, both from compensatory gait prior to surgery and from having walked with external fixators. Treatment strategies should focus on normalizing the base of support, increasing stride length, and improving timing of hip musculature activation. Global lower extremity and core strengthening facilitates the patient's overall independence with their functional activities and gait.

Internal Lengthening Devices

There has been an increasing interest in performing "internal lengthening" of the lower extremity using intramedullary lengthening nails. Patients and families seem to prefer this method over using external fixators due to ease of after care and less pain.

In the past, use of intramedullary lengthening devices in femur or tibia was generally limited to patients who had reached skeletal maturity, had minimal or no angular deformity, and had adequate diameter of the intramedullary canal of the lengthened bone. In last 5 years, however, it has changed significantly due to three reasons

1. There are several smaller diameter nails available for the femur as well as for tibial lengthening,
2. The technique of combining acute correction of the deformity followed by gradual lengthening using a lengthening IM nail has been established, and
3. In patients as young as 4 or 5 years of age, the technique of using lengthening nail as an extramedullary device just sitting on the outer cortex with an additional small diameter rod in an IM fashion has been employed when the diameter of the bone is even smaller than the available nail diameter.

Weight bearing is usually 30–50 lb. during lengthening. It is also important to remember that it is not the magnitude of load but the frequency of loading that can have deleterious effects on the stability of the intramedullary lengthening implant. During the distraction phase, weight bearing is typically limited to activities of daily living only, whereas in the consolidation phase, weight bearing can be increased as maturation of the lengthening regenerate occurs.

Complications of internal lengthening are similar to that of the external fixator excluding pin site problems. The rate of complications or obstacles to lengthening using the ISKD™ device has been reported as high as 65% [19]. These rates are similar to rates reported in the limb lengthening performed with external fixator.

In addition, due to lack of external fixation stability, the risk of joint subluxation is increased with the lengthening nails. Knee flexion contracture with subluxation is a possible complication of internal femoral lengthening, especially in patients with a congenital etiology (Fig. 19.25). Prophylactic bracing and adequate physical therapy are critical to prevent joint subluxation and development of permanent contractures. The magnitude of the complications is also dependent upon the ability to control the rate of lengthening. If the internal lengthening device goes faster than 1–1.5 mm a day, the severity of complications is greater. The authors have successfully treated this problem of excessively rapid lengthening utilizing proper handling techniques as well as custom dynamic bracing (see

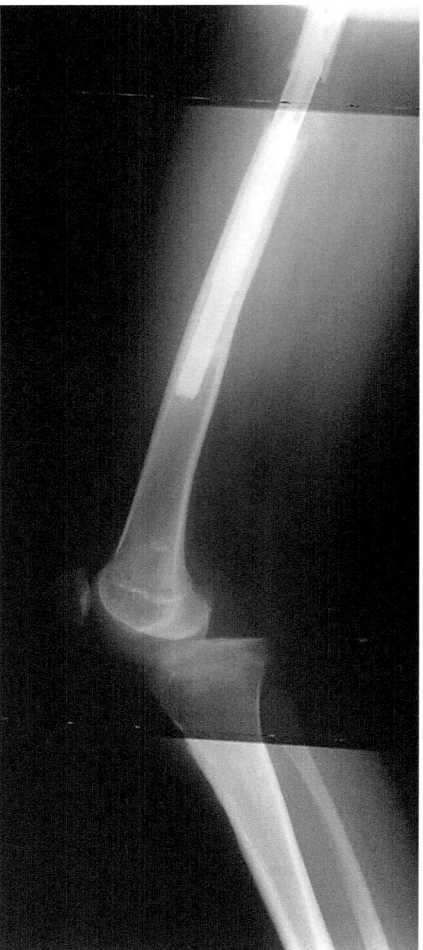

Fig. 19.25 Knee subluxation in a patient undergoing internal femoral lengthening for congenital femoral deficiency

Fig. 19.22). In a retrospective review of this approach in 20 patients (with 22 contractures, 9 subluxations), successful resolution of knee flexion contractures occurred in 19/20 patients (95% success) and 8/9 subluxations (88%) (Fig. 19.26) [20]. During femoral lengthening, there is significant knee joint compression due to contractures that develop in muscles around the knee. These compressive forces can cause arthritic changes that can be irreversible. In the case of an external fixator on the femur, a common strategy is to apply a tibial ring and put a hinge across the knee joint to keep the joint distracted. This type of hinging across the knee joint also can be used as splinting technique to keep the knee joint in full extension for extended periods of time. These advantages of external fixation are not possible with internal femoral lengthenings. The burden of maintaining good arthrokinematics of the knee joint depends on (1) Skill of therapist, (2) number of end-range manipulations throughout the PT session, (3) compliance with the home exercise program, and (4) the use of splints to apply gentle corrective force across the joint. Prophylactic early bracing to keep the knee joint in extension and an

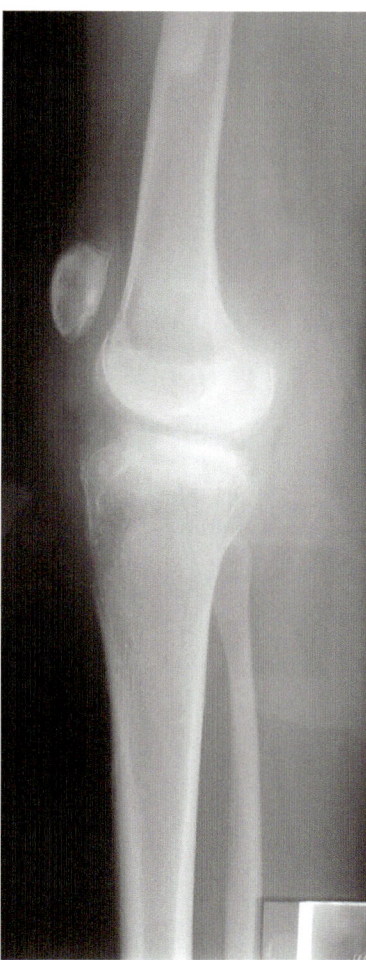

Fig. 19.26 Complete resolution and normal knee alignment of the patient in Fig. 19.25 after 6 weeks of customized therapy including joint and soft tissue mobilization, quadriceps electrical stimulation, and use of CKD with special straps for 16 h/day

increased dosage of therapy supplemented by a diligent home exercise program by caregivers are critical components of reducing joint stiffness and knee joint subluxation. At the author's institution, monitoring of the home exercise program compliance is done using an app-based augmented reality program called MirrorAR motion capture, www.mirrorar.io (US Patent No 11069144). This app-based program gives realtime feedback to patients about their range of motion as well as exercise compliance, and daily exercise and range of motion achieved is automatically downloaded to a portal that healthcare team can access. Lastly, it is critical that caregivers are vigorously involved in the management of the patient. In the current environment of reduced therapy coverage by insurance carriers, a diligently followed home program has become that much more critical. Counseling of the caregivers should be done pre-surgically. A lack of commitment to follow through on the home program usually results in a compromised functional result.

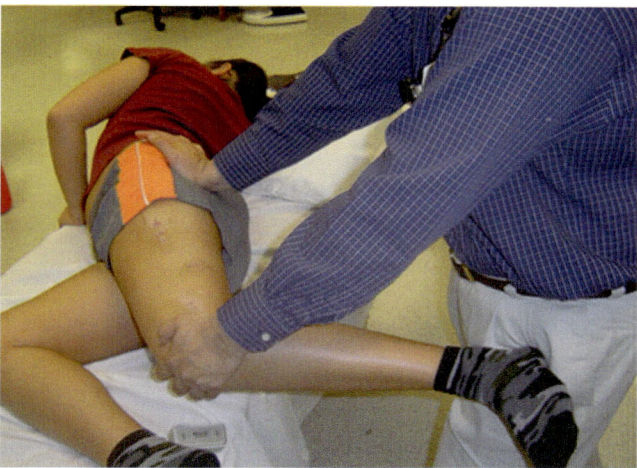

Fig. 19.27 Iliotibial band stretching in a modified Ober position

Knee flexion deficits are also a common obstacle to internal femoral lengthening. Restoration of motion is best achieved with daily therapy including patella and soft tissue mobilization. The authors prefer ASTYM™ to treat the entire kinetic chain for patients undergoing internal lengthening since there are no pins to interfere with the treatment. For femoral internal lengthening, special attention must be given to the tensor fascia lata and iliotibial band as well as the muscles that attach to the tensor fascia lata. Modified Ober positioning (Fig. 19.27) with gentle varus mobilization of the tibia as well as prone knee flexion with external rotation of the hip and simultaneous internal rotation of the tibia over femur are useful techniques to target these tissues. Patellar mobilization along with regaining knee joint mobility is paramount. Special emphasis should be given to inferior patella mobilization with knee flexion mobilization and superior patella mobilization with knee extension mobilization. Patellar taping techniques are also a useful adjunct to therapy (Fig. 19.28). The goal of patellar taping is to neutralize the lateral subluxation force due to tight lateral structures and encourage inferior movement of the patella. It is very rare that one needs a specialized orthosis to improve knee flexion. Most patients respond to a carefully planned therapy program. In case such devices are needed, it is recommended that one must wait until lengthening is finished before employing splints to apply a flexion stretch. If splints are applied during the lengthening phase, patients can experience significant retropatellar pain. It is best to also slow down lengthening so that muscle flexibility can keep up with the rate of lengthening and large losses of flexion range of motion do not occur.

In tibial lengthening with an internal device, common joint problems include knee flexion contracture and ankle equinus contracture. In cases in which the osteotomy is at the distal tibia, patients may also develop equino-varus contracture due to over pull of the tibialis posterior, in addition to the tightness of the gastrocnemius and soleus. Dynamic splints for prophylactic treatment are recommended. CKD bracing with ankle

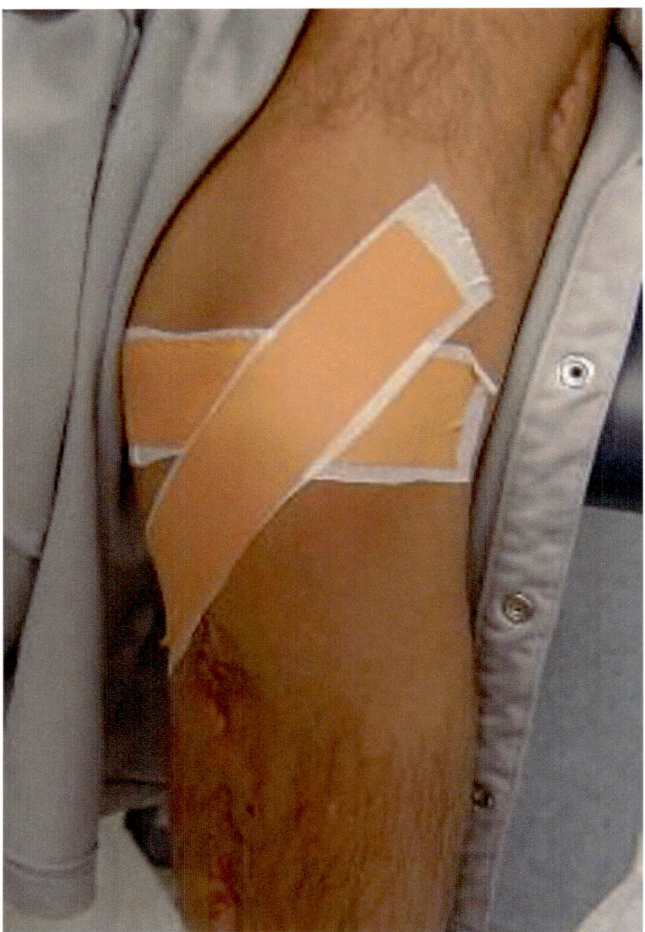

Fig. 19.28 Patients with femoral lengthening have a tendency for lateral subluxation of the patella and patella alta. Patellar taping is a useful adjunct to help mobilize the patella medially and inferiorly

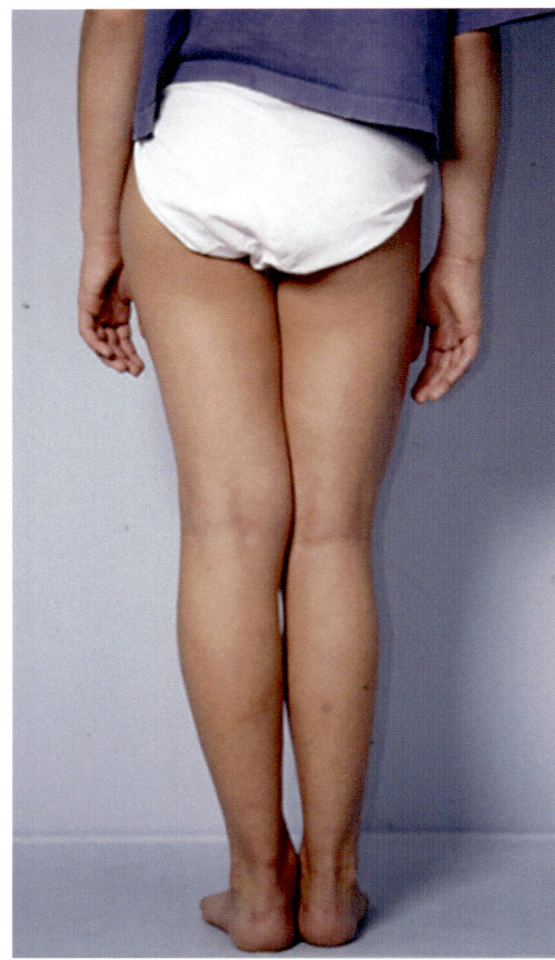

Fig. 19.29 Pelvic obliquity compensation for leg length difference. This results in hip abduction of the short limb and hip adduction of the longer limb

dorsiflexion is useful to manage this. Knee extension mobilization and simultaneous ankle dorsflexion mobilization in addition to subtalar and foot mobilization is instituted. Due to the foot being a small lever, the therapist has to use good foot stabilization technique to obtain an effective stretch. As with all patients undergoing limb lengthening, it is important to continue to work on strengthening the quadriceps and hip abductors since these muscles are often atrophied due to prior immobilization and limited weight bearing.

Gait Considerations

Children with leg length discrepancy (LLD) may also have skeletal deformities, muscle contractures, joint subluxations, and muscle weakness. In order to equalize their leg lengths, children with LLD intuitively use compensatory mechanisms such as (1) equinus posturing of the ankle on the short side, (2) pelvic tilt with lowering of the pelvis on the short side, and (3) knee flexion on the long side (Fig. 19.29). Short leg gait has the following characteristics: (1) stance time reduced on the short side, (2) stride length reduced on the short side, (3) cadence (steps/minute) increased, and (4) walking velocity marginally reduced. Limb equalization reduces these compensatory strategies and the gait becomes more symmetrical [21].

When working with a child with a congenital cause of limb length discrepancy, there are also angular deformities of the bones to consider when evaluating and treating gait abnormalities. At the hip, there may be coxa vara or coxa valga which can impact hip biomechanics and function of the hip abductors. Considering the length–tension relationship of muscles, the abductors rely on the normal femoral neck-shaft angle to be 120–135°. When this angle is changed, the muscles are unable to provide the trunk with a stable base of support at the pelvis, leading to a compensatory Trendelenberg gait pattern.

If there is a fixed flexion deformity of the femur and/or an anterior pelvic tilt, then the hip extension needed for proper propulsion at the end of swing is not available. The child will instead utilize their lumbar spine to allow their center of gravity to move over the stance limb. Even with compensation, the step length will be shorter on the affected side. An equinus contracture further compromises the child's propulsion.

During normal gait, knee range of motion provides shock absorption and stability in stance and toe clearance in swing. When one has a shortened limb, often the knee is quite stiff in gait, as there is limited need to flex it to clear the ipsilateral foot. Femoral deformities and small patellae can limit quadriceps muscles' ability to fully activate. Couple this with cruciate ligament deficiencies, and the affected child will generally lock his or her knee to prevent buckling and potential injury. Often the lack of range of motion at the knee does not affect these patients until their leg length has been equalized and they need to start functioning more normally.

Gastrocnemius tightness is certainly the most common problem at the ankle, leading to difficulty in toe clearance once the limb lengths are equalized and decreased propulsion in stance, since it is not able to stretch and recoil normally. Congenital problems of the lower leg may present with procurvatum or recurvatum of the distal tibia. If there is procurvatum of the distal tibia, then the patient will be in excessive dorsiflexion throughout the gait cycle and propulsion will be difficult. With a recurvatum of the tibia, the ankle is in a plantigrade position, thus preventing the knee from functioning normally in gait and preventing the body's weight from advancing over the foot. The knee will lock out early in gait and will decrease the stride length of the unaffected limb.

Rotational and angular deformities of the lower leg also present problems for all of the joints of the lower extremity. In these cases, the ground reaction forces will become unevenly distributed at each joint causing abnormal wear and tear and inefficient gait. Normal foot progression is difficult and the possibilities of running and sporting activities are greatly limited the more severe the deformity is.

Summary

Treating patients with limb length discrepancies before, during, and after limb lengthening can be incredibly challenging. It takes an understanding of the anatomy of the human body and how it interacts in mobility to effectively determine a proper plan of care for these patients. Customized therapy (Fig. 19.30) is the greatest tool to overcome the common pitfalls in lower limb lengthening and deformity correction to ensure the best clinical outcomes. Current therapy coverage for most patients is not adequate. One must consider limb lengthening surgery as a surgery that happens every day unlike any other MSK procedure that only happens once. Due to this difference, the physiologic needs of the lengthened tissue cannot be met by a standard routine of therapy three times a week to get the job done. The lengthened tissue needs more time to stretch per day (8–12 h/day). However, this can be achieved by formal therapy, a home program carefully carried out by caretakers, and the use of customized dynamic splinting.

Fig. 19.30 Successful outcome for children undergoing limb lengthening and deformity correction can only be obtained by a carefully designed protocol for the individual patient that involves daily therapy, static or dynamic splints, and strict adherence to a home exercise program with parent or caregiver participation

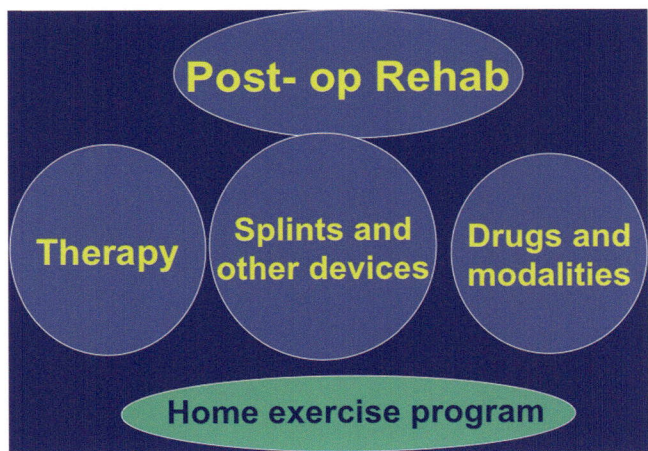

Commentary

Fran Guardo
fguardo@paleyinstitute.org

During the limb lengthening process and recovery, when range of motion is limited, it is always best practice to perform progressive motion throughout each session with each movement serving to prepare for the next. For instance, beginning the session with the patient performing a closed chain motion such as a seated stepper, gait training on a partial body weight supported treadmill, or standing positional stretches is helpful preparation for the following activity. Next, open chain active range of motion, or active assisted range of motion may be coupled with moist heat placed over target muscle groups which serves to further prepare soft tissue elongation and muscles for upcoming, and more intense movement. The next step is to progressively begin manual stretches with overpressure to the one joint muscles before incorporating the two joint muscles (i.e. the lower quadriceps stretched in a seated position before progressing to include the rectus femoris with the hip extended, or stretch of the soleus with the knee flexed before performing dorsiflexion with the knee fully extended). Soft tissue preparation either by use of the therapist's hands directly or a soft tissue tool, such as ASTYM, can be included as indicated throughout the session.

As the primary authors noted, joint mobilization is important, as appropriate, throughout the session. Once all of the preparatory active and passive motion has been addressed, followed by manual stretches with gradually intensifying overpressure have been performed on the shortest muscles, the patient is ready for multiple and progressive stretches toward end range on the relevant two joint muscles. When a session is conducted in this progressive manner, much less overpressure is needed to achieve soft tissue elongation and true end range of motion, thus decreasing the risk of increased pain and adverse events.

Management of anxiety by providing patient targeted activities and support throughout the session also serves to improve outcomes. Anxiety and fear increase pain and guarding which can become a vicious cycle. At our center, we use Child Life Specialists (CLS) to help train therapists and parents in order to meet the child at their developmental level, and to assist in one on one mental distraction when needed. We run a family-centered practice in which we encourage a caregiver to be present during the session to serve as a positive distraction and comfort to the child. There are instances, however, when this dynamic escalates pain behaviors instead and we encourage the caregiver to leave either briefly or for the session. Following all sessions, pediatric patients visit our treasure chest to pick out a prize. This leaves each child with a positive last moment before departing.

At our center, external fixator pin sites are no longer wrapped tightly as we have found that this can be associated with tissue necrosis around the pin due possibly to decreased blood flow. In order to decrease pin site pain, the therapist may either use hand placement or tape to approximate the skin toward the pin during stretch to avoid excessive tissue pulling. In some cases, the use of ASTYM scar stroke techniques has been very helpful in managing pain as reported by patients and can provide relief following the session up for to 24–48 h.

At our center, we began gradually permitting weight bearing as tolerated with an assistive device during the distraction phase for patients undergoing four segment limb lengthening with external fixation in 2013. We have not found it to be associated with increased pin loosening. Patients with unilateral external fixators are also allowed, in most cases to bear weight as tolerated and have not experienced increased pin loosening.

Below is a screening questionnaire that is given to patients with Achondroplasia prior to lengthening. If the patient answers "yes" to any of the questions, the patient will be screened by a spine specialist before lengthening is approved. If the patient is found to have spinal stenosis, spinal decompression surgery is indicated with adequate recovery prior to the patient undergoing the limb lengthening process.

Achondroplasia questionnaire:
1. Do you experience weakness in your legs and/or do you routinely have numbness or tingling in your legs when you walk or sit?
2. Do you have urinary or fecal incontinence—that is, are you unable to hold your urine or feces in?
3. Are you limited with how far you can walk? If so, how far can you walk before having to take a rest or sit down? How quickly after you take a rest does your weakness, numbness, or pain go away?
4. Do you find yourself squatting after walking a certain distance to alleviate the pain/weakness/numbness? Do you find yourself flexing forward, like leaning forward on a counter or grocery cart to alleviate pain or tiredness in your legs?

5. If you have a limit to how far you can walk, what seems to limit you? Meaning, do you become short of breath and that is why you have to stop or are your legs the limiting factor in how far you can walk? Do your legs become tired and/or weak and this is why you stop?
6. Do you snore, have you had a sleep study that showed central or obstructive sleep apnea?
   (Courtesy David Feldman MD)

Fracture Risk Management

As the primary authors have mentioned, fractures are a risk of limb lengthening and can even occur during PT sessions. In order to study the situation at our center, in collaboration with Nova Southeastern University (Dr. Alicia Fernandez-Fernandez), we conducted a retrospective chart review study in 2014 which consisted of review of patients who had experienced fractures during PT for limb lengthening/deformity correction (LL/DC) from June 2009 through October 2014 [22]. During this time period, of the more than 1000 of LL/DC patients treated, 11 subjects sustained fractures, ($N = 11$). Two controls were matched by gender, age, surgical procedure, type of fixation, and diagnosis ($N = 22$). Due to rarity of some diagnoses, similar matches were made. Exclusion criteria were fracture during surgery or trauma. Variables considered: Anthropometric and demographic characteristics, past medical history, prior level of function, repeat procedure, type of correction, fracture site and date, recent pin or hardware removal, weight-bearing history, characteristics of treating therapist, and patient compliance, among others. Data analysis: Stata® Multiple logistic regression model was used to compare Fracture (outcome), patient/provider attributes (predictors), with a $P < 0.05$. On average, fractures occurred 81 days after surgery (range 22–248 days). The following variables were significantly associated with fracture: Recent hardware removal within 3 months of fracture and, setting-specific years of experience for the treating therapist. No association with prior level of function, repeat procedure, weight-bearing history, patient compliance, and non-setting specific experience was found to be significant. There was insufficient data to conclude effect for distraction rate, or range of motion changes (reference below). Based on the outcomes of this study, changes were made in our practices. Increased specialized training time was provided for new therapists working with LL/DC patients. Protocols were modified to include the gradual, progressive techniques discussed earlier in my comments. All therapists must view the x-rays of the patient prior to treating the patient and become familiar with surgery including pin removal sites and stress risers.

It is my opinion that the collaborative effort of the multi-site authors of this chapter and its reviewing author are greatly needed in the progression of rehabilitation techniques in the LL/DC field.

References

1. Paley D. Problems, obstacles, and complications of limb lengthening by the Ilizarov technique. Clin Orthop Relat Res. 1990;250:81–104.
2. Moraal JM, Elzinga-Plomp A, Jongmans MJ, Roermund PM, Flikweert PE, Castelein RM, et al. Long-term psychosocial functioning after Ilizarov limb lengthening during childhood: 37 patients followed for 2–14 years. Acta Orthop. 2009;80(6):704–10.
3. Coglianese DB, Herzenberg JE, Goulet JA. Physical therapy management of patients undergoing limb lengthening by distraction osteogenesis. J Orthop Sports Phys Ther. 1993;17(3):124–32.
4. Simard S, Marchant M, Mencio G. The Ilizarov procedure: limb lengthening and its implications. Phys Ther. 1992;72(1):25–34.
5. Barker KL, Simpson AHRW, Lamb SE. Loss of knee range of motion in leg lengthening. J Orthop Sports Phys Ther. 2001;31(5):238–46.
6. O'Carrigan T, Nocente C, Paley D, Herzenberg JE. Fractures complicating limb lengthening. J Bone Joint Surg Br. 2005;87-B(Suppl III):312–3.
7. Launay F, Younsi R, Pithioux M, Chabrand P, Bollini G, Jouve JL. Fracture following lower limb lengthening in children: a series of 58 patients. Orthop Traumatol Surg Res. 2013;99:72–9.
8. Tabary JC, Tabary C, Tardieu C, Tardieu G, Goldspink G. Physiological and structural changes in cat's soleus muscles due to immobilization at different lengths by plaster casts. J Physiol. 1972;224(1):231–44.
9. Currier DP, Nelson RM. Dynamics of human biologic tissues. Philadelphia: FA Davis; 1992.
10. Herzenberg JE, Scheufele LL, Paley D, Bechtel R, Tepper S. Knee range of motion in isolated femoral lengthening. Clin Orthop Relat Res. 1994;301:49–54.
11. Nogueira MP, Paley D, Bhave A. Nerve lesions associated with limb lengthening. J Bone Joint Surg Am. 2003;85-A:1502–10.
12. Ilizarov G. Clinical application of the tension-stress effect for limb lengthening. Clin Orthop Relat Res. 1990;250:8–26.
13. Brech GC, Guarnieiro R. Evaluation of physiotherapy in the treatment of Legg-Calvé-Perthes disease. Clinics (São Paulo). 2006;61(6):521–8.
14. Laklouk MA, Hosny GA. Hinged distraction of the hip joint in the treatment of Perthes disease: evaluation at skeletal maturity. J Pediatr Orthop B. 2012;21(5):386–93.
15. Chomiak J, Podškubka A, Dungl P, Ošt'ádal M, Frydrychová M. Cruciate ligaments in proximal femoral focal deficiency: arthroscopic assessment. J Pediatr Orthop. 2012;32(1):21–8.
16. Paley D. Intra-articular osteotomies of the hip, knee, and ankle. Oper Tech Orthop. 2011;21(2):184–96.

17. Walker JL. Pediatric orthopaedics: fibular deficiency. Curr Orthop Pract. 2011;22(2):162–6.
18. Venkatesh KP, Modi HN, Devmurari K, Yoon JY, Anupama BR, Song HR. Femoral lengthening in achondroplasia. J Bone Joint Surg Br. 2009;91(12):1612–7.
19. Schiedel FM, Pip S, Wacker S, Pöpping J, Tretow H, Leidinger B, Rödl R. Intramedullary limb lengthening with the intramedullary skeletal kinetic distractor in the lower limb. J Bone Joint Surg Br. 2011;93(B):788–92.
20. Bhave A, Baker E, Specht S. Custom knee device (CKD) for the treatment of knee flexion contractures (KFC) after ISKD femoral lengthening. In: AAOS Annual Meeting Mar 2010, New Orleans, LA, Scientific Exhibit 60.
21. Bhave A, Paley D, Herzenberg JE. Improvement in gait parameters after lengthening for the treatment of limb-length discrepancy. J Bone Joint Surg Am. 1999;81-A(4):529–34.
22. Guardo F, Fernandez-Fernandez A, Paley D, Mylett C, McCarthy J, Cartwright K. Factors associated with fracture during physical therapy intervention in patients undergoing limb lengthening and/or deformity correction. In: International limb lengthening and reconstruction society (ILLRS) 2015 congress, Miami, FL. November 6, 2015. Oral presentation.

Amputation and Prosthetic Management: Amputation as a Reconstructive Option

John A. Herring

When a child presents with a major lower limb deformity, whether congenital or acquired, many treatment options must be considered. Modern limb lengthening techniques with external frames and intramedullary lengthening devices have greatly expanded the treatment. In many cases, these technological advances have enabled surgeons to effectively manage deformities which were untreatable in earlier times.

In a similar way, amputation and prosthetic strategies have also advanced dramatically in recent years. Over the last several decades, a remarkable increase in social acceptance of visible disabilities has come about. Many factors have contributed to this progress, including the Americans with Disabilities Act, inclusion of Paralympic sports in concert with the Winter and Summer Olympic Games, and an appreciation for the remarkable achievements of prominent athletes with limb deficiencies (Figs. 20.1 and 20.2). Children, who in the past sat quietly on the sidelines because of their "disabilities," are now competing as varsity athletes, cheerleaders, and team captains, using highly functional state-of-the-art prostheses.

Initial enthusiasm for limb lengthening reconstruction for congenital deformities was very high. As the difficulties and complications of such interventions came to light, especially those encountered with "heroic" lengthenings, a reconsideration of the role of amputation has been appropriate [1–7]. Let us consider the example of a child born with fibular hemimelia, or congenital absence of the fibula, and we will compare Syme amputation to correction with the Ilizarov method. A child with a fibular hemimelia with a well-formed, four ray foot and a 10% limb length discrepancy can expect an excellent result with one tibial lengthening and a contralateral epiphysiodesis and is not usually a candidate for amputation (Fig. 20.3). At the other end of the spectrum, a child with a very short tibia, marked anterolateral bowing, and a two ray foot can expect to achieve his or her full athletic potential with a single surgery and appropriate prosthetic management following amputation done at 11 months of age (Fig. 20.4a, b). An Ilizarov approach would require three or more periods of frame management, with considerable loss of childhood experiences, with an end result of compromised function and cosmesis. The decision for management of the child with a deformity in between these two extremes is more difficult. The decisions are complex and emotionally laden and require extensive knowledge of all aspects of proposed treatment, and consideration of family and social dynamics [8, 9].

J. A. Herring (✉)
Department of Orthopedic Surgery, Scottish Rite for Children, University of Texas Southwestern Medical School, Dallas, TX, USA
e-mail: tony.herring@tsrh.org

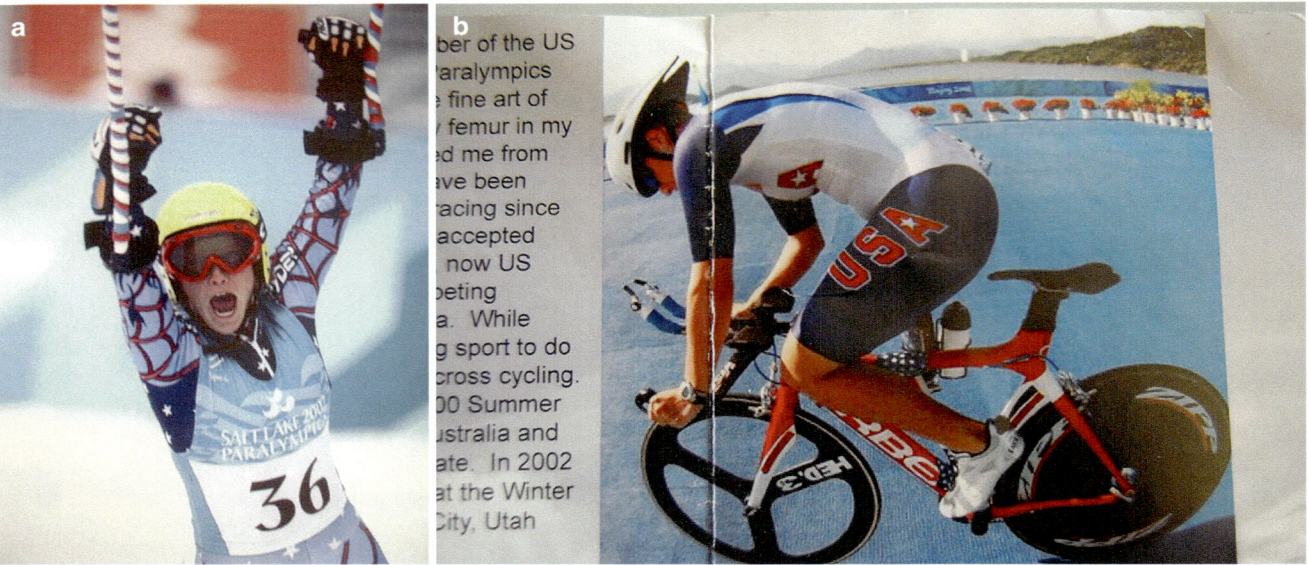

Fig. 20.1 (**a**) A young woman with proximal femoral deficiency. Her management was with Symes amputation and knee fusion. She is celebrating her first Paralympic gold medal in three-track skiing at Salt Lake City. (**b**) The same woman as she achieves another Paralympic medal, this time in track cycling. Overall, she has now medaled in four Paralympic games

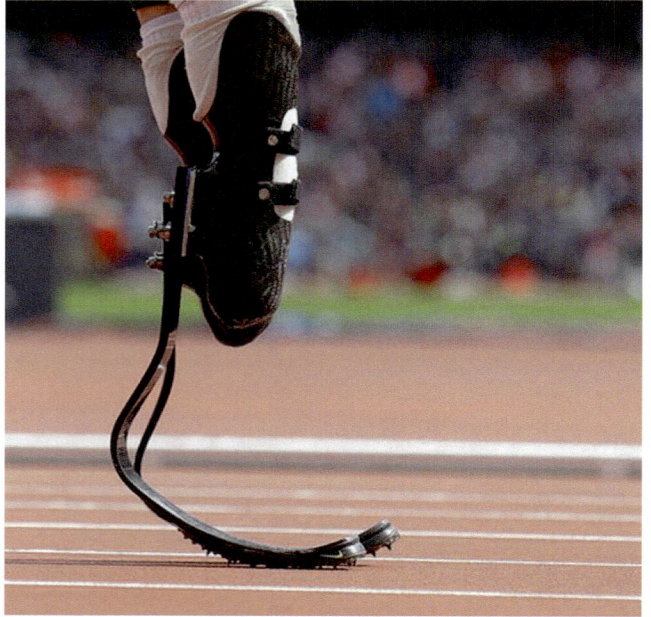

Fig. 20.2 Cheetah-type carbon blades. These enable highly competitive performance in a number of sports including track and field, basketball, and football

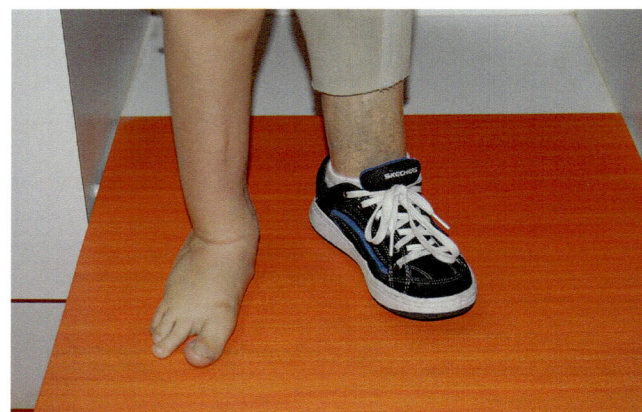

Fig. 20.3 A boy's foot with fibular hemimelia. This four-rayed foot was functional and had good mobility. Note the Symes prosthesis on the other side, which had a more severe fibular deficiency

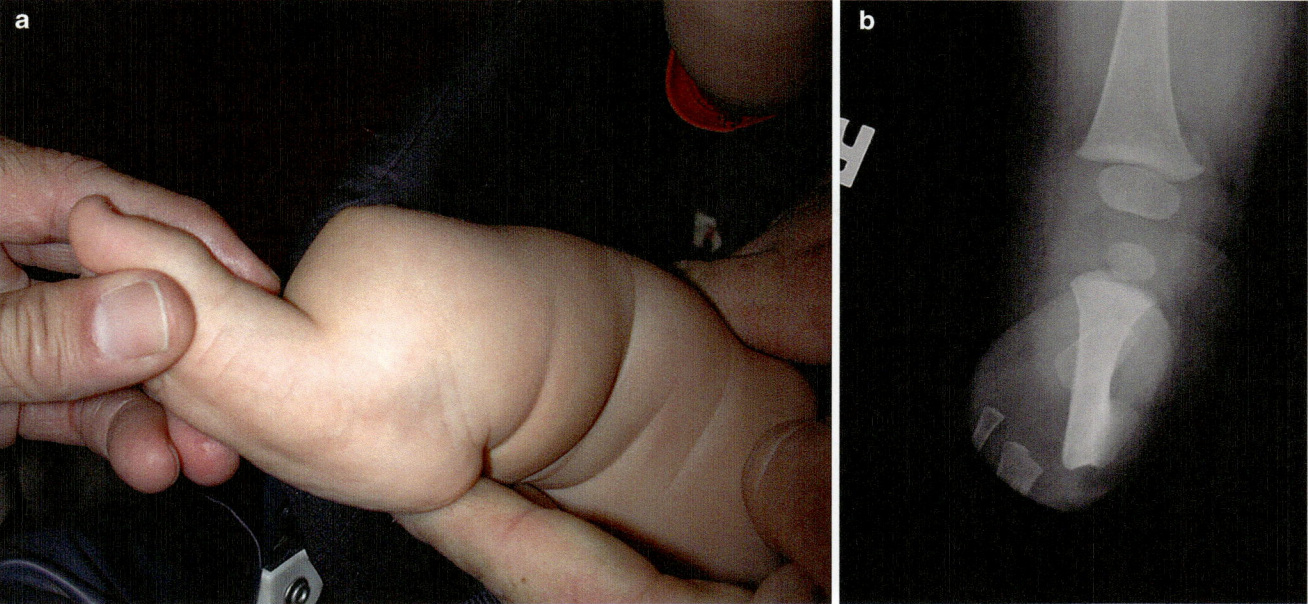

Fig. 20.4 (**a**) A more severe fibular hemimelia with marked shortening and angulation of the lower limb. The two-rayed foot was subsequently converted to a Symes amputation. (**b**) A radiograph of the same leg showing marked shortening and angulation of the tibia

Treatment Concepts

Congenital deficiencies involving the lower extremities present with varying degrees of severity, some of which are best treated with amputation. Amputation in this context is often one part of a complex strategy involving removal of some bony and soft tissue elements while reconstructing other anatomic components. When applied appropriately, amputation becomes a very positive step in achieving the best functional and cosmetic outcome for the child (Box 20.1). Conditions in which amputation is often useful include congenital femoral deficiency, fibular hemimelia, and tibial hemimelia. Amputation for congenital pseudarthrosis of the tibia may be appropriate after failure of other methods to obtain a stable union with a functional extremity, and occasionally amputation is chosen by the parents as the primary management for this condition.

Deformity and dysfunction following severe trauma may also be an indication for amputation, either primarily or following attempts at reconstruction. Primary amputation may be indicated in young children when major epiphyses are injured in such a way that future growth is severely limited.

Many methods of limb reconstruction are appropriately used to maintain lower extremity function after tumor excision. Allograft and internal prosthetic reconstruction have made a positive impact on the management of malignant and aggressive benign tumors in children. Amputation at times becomes a solution to intractable complications such as infection and implant failure after these initial efforts. Amputation remains the best primary treatment option when the size and location of the tumor exceeds the limits of reconstructive options [10–18]. In addition, amputation may be appropriate when the patient presents with wide-spread disease, and it can provide pain relief and the ability to ambulate over a shortened life span.

> **Box 20.1**
> Amputation as a positive event:
>
> - PFFD
> - Fibular hemimelia
> - Tibial hemimelia
> - Trauma
> - Others

Patient and Family Management

Management options for these abnormalities also vary greatly depending not only on the severity of the condition, but also on the available medical expertise and prosthetic support. Early on, the parents should be introduced to and educated about treatment methods which involve amputation as well as those which involve other methods of complex reconstruction. This education is markedly enhanced when such parents trying to make a decision for their child meet other parents, some of whose children are being managed by amputation and others by limb lengthening reconstruction. These encounters allow parents to ask other parents questions which they would not ask their doctors, and in fact, which the doctors are not really very good at answering.

Historically, amputation was a last resort, dreaded by the surgeon and feared by the patient and caretakers. As prosthetic devices have become more functional and cosmetic, and sports prostheses have allowed people with amputations to compete in sports at very high levels, the concept of amputation as a positive strategy has taken hold in society. Parents and children need to be informed about modern amputation techniques and prosthetic fitting which provide high function with a minimum number of surgical encounters and morbidity (Box 20.2). They will need the knowledge with which to compare amputation to limb lengthening reconstruction, typically requiring multiple procedures over time. They should be provided with honest information about complications and outcomes of all methods, frequency and duration of hospitalizations, and the availability and quality of prosthetic care.

> **Box 20.2**
> Education is essential:
>
> - By physician
> - By other parents (who have had a child with a similar diagnosis)
> - With psychologic support

The comparative financial costs of prosthetic management and complex reconstruction are difficult to assess. Several studies have shown conflicting conclusions and consideration of all relevant factors is difficult. A most important cost to consider is the lost childhood or adolescence which occurs with multiple episodes of frame application and hospitalizations to manage complications [19–21].

Decisions That Have to Be Made

The birth of a child with visible limb deformities or absences is a time of great and conflicting emotions for the parents and family. In many instances, the abnormalities have been noted before birth with ultrasound studies, while in others, there has been no anticipation of a problem. The parents want and need answers; why did this happen, might it happen again, were we at fault, how can things be fixed? The medical team must answer the questions with empathy and honesty. It is likely that there is no known etiology and, in most instances, subsequent pregnancies are not at risk, although there are known syndromes with Mendelian inheritance patterns.

Major anomalies happen in the first 2 months and are not due to some later event that may be concerning the parents.

The first responsibility for those of us who will provide care for the children is to help the family work through the sense of loss that they feel; that loss being the loss of the "perfectly normal" baby which they had expected. We should find ways in which we can help the parents bond with their child and work through the grieving process. Usually the initial shock is gradually replaced as the maternal and paternal instincts react to the baby's responses and activities. We need to honor this process and look for help when it goes awry.

In the early weeks of the child's life when we are consulted to assess and plan for the management of the limb issues, it is essential that we take a broad and comprehensive look at the child and family with an awareness of their social and cultural world. Teammates are essential and include family physicians, psychologists, therapists, social workers as well as experienced orthopedic surgeons.

The decision for type of definitive management boils down to what type of intervention for this child's anatomy will provide the best function and cosmesis with the least degree of lost childhood due to hospitalizations and interventions. The care team must find the right balance between the child's body parts, the physical and mental price of surgical correction, and the ultimate functional outcome of the proposed treatment. We surgeons rarely fully appreciate the difficulties that the patients experience as they recover from our interventions. Weeks in casts or frames seem inconsequential to us but are really challenging for a child and young family. We strive to be certain that the outcome for the patient is worth the hardships of the journey. We are also challenged knowing that the fruits our work have to last a lifetime.

Human Costs

The first question we should ask is what is the cost of each potential treatment method; how much interruption of school, sports, and family life will the treatment involve? How much pain, discomfort, and disruption of sports typically accompany the planned intervention(s)? How many surgeries are necessary and how will they be spaced through the years? These "costs" are not quantifiable and are easily overlooked in the planning process.

In addition, there are actual costs to calculate. What does a prosthesis cost the family? How much is the co-pay for a surgery? There are also costs which are more difficult to calculate, such as time off from work, transportation to the doctor, loss of school time, and decreased time and attention for siblings and spouses.

Result

The second question to ask is what does the result look like, and what is the range of outcomes from best to worst, and where does this patient's condition fall on the scale of difficulty? Clearly more severe deficits are more challenging to treat and are prone to an adverse outcome. It is not too difficult to correct a 6 cm deficit in femoral length, but much harder to make up 6 in.

Short/Long Term

The third question illustrates the conundrum of treating children; we must always consider how our interventions interact with growth. Will our work help or hinder the child's growth? How our management hold up over a lifetime of many decades. The challenge is to win on both accounts. Stated another way, the short-term sacrifices should be balanced by the long-term benefits.

Making the Decision

The Doctor's Role

You as the person responsible for the evaluation and treatment should first, based on your knowledge of the condition, knowledge of the literature, and understanding of the patient's circumstances, determine a plan outlining the best treatment options for the child. It is helpful to list them in the order of your preference. Noting that the ultimate decision is made by the parents and the patient, the next job is to educate the parents about the treatment methods. You should stress that the decision will always be theirs and the first step is for them to be fully informed about all the options and the advantages and disadvantages of each.

In our institution, we have a unique and effective strategy for working with new patients with limb differences. We have two multidisciplinary clinics which take place at the same time in adjacent clinics. The Ilizarov, or reconstruction clinic and the prosthetic clinic are staffed by surgeon experts in those disciplines. Other important staff in both include psychologists, physical and occupational therapists, social workers, and child life specialists. Each patient is the responsibility of a single surgeon. Hand surgeons are also available in adjacent areas.

In each of the clinics, the parents are told that our first purpose is to give them as much information and education about the available treatments as possible. They will hear this not just from us, but usually from a patient and family who will be peers for them. This family interaction is a great source of information about what having the condition and treatment is all about. This happens in both clinics and we usually tell the parents that they do not need to make a decision on this first visit. We encourage them to gather information from reliable sources before the next visit.

We will usually plan a second visit, often at 6 months, and at that time repeat most of the steps of education. After that we often find that the parents are favoring one path or the other. Sometimes especially with unusually complex disorders, both teams will suggest postponing major interventions pending further growth of the child and evolution of the deformity.

The great value of this approach is that the parents do not feel that they are being pressured into a treatment which they do not fully understand. Frequently we find that patients who initially state that they do not want an amputation ultimately decide that amputation is the best choice. In the peering process, the parent whose child has had an amputation will tell the new parents that the choice to "cut off my baby's foot" was the hardest decision he or she ever had to make. They will add that this was also the best decision they ever made. Frequently I hear professionals say that a parent from some particular social or religious category will never consider amputation. To the contrary, I have found that once parents fully understand the options and benefits of each treatment, they will often choose amputation in spite of their prior reluctance.

Specific Conditions

Congenital Femoral Deficiency

There is great variation of femoral anatomy among children with congenital femoral deficiency (CFD), and several classifications are useful. The Gillespie classification [19–21] is based on length of the femur at presentation (Fig. 20.5). In type A, the femur is at least 50% as long as the normal femur, and in type B, it is less than 50% of the normal length. In type C, there is almost no development of the proximal femur. The classification relates in general to treatment recommendations. The Hamanishi classification [22] illustrates the wide variety of anatomic presentations, but is not specifically tied to treatment (Fig. 20.6). The Paley classification [23] adds consideration of the mobility of the femoral head within the acetabulum, and is useful for some reconstruction methods (Fig. 20.7).

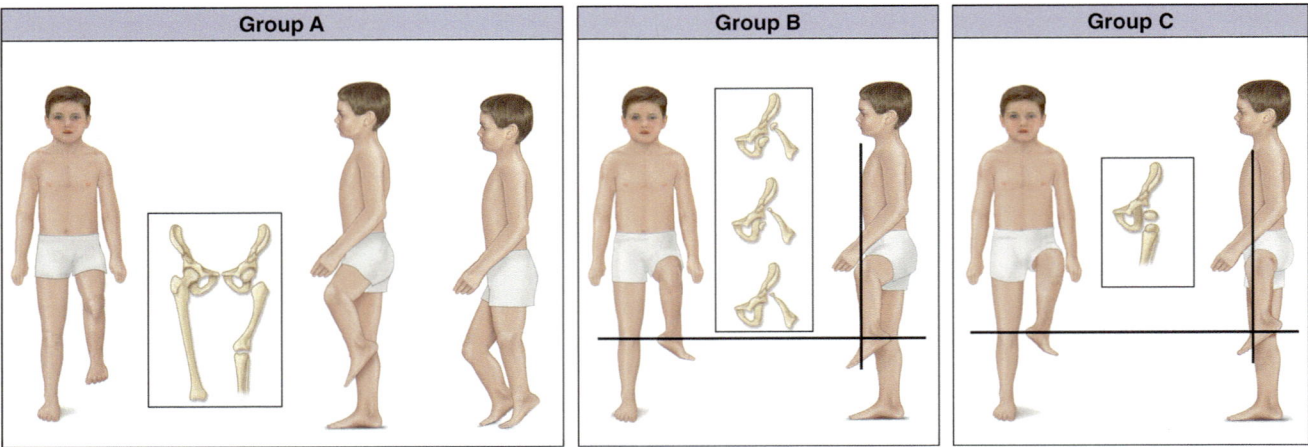

Fig. 20.5 The Gillespie classification of femoral deficiency. In type A, the femoral length is more than 50% of the normal side. In type B, the length of the femur is 50% or less than the other femur. In type C, there is almost no femoral length. This image was published in Tachdjian's Pediatric Orthopedics, Herring JA, Limb deficiencies, 965–974, Copyright Elsevier 2014

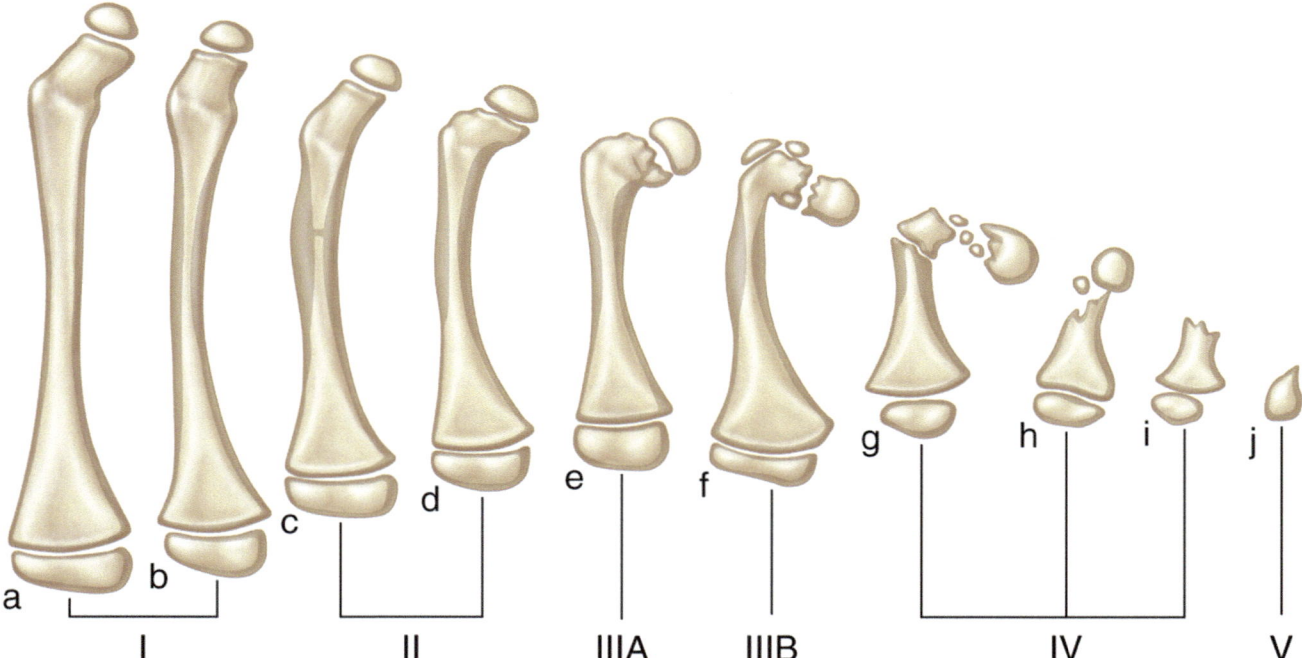

Fig. 20.6 The Hamanishi classification of femoral deficiency. This classification notes the multiple variations of the deformity. This image was published in Tachdjian's Pediatric Orthopedics, Herring JA, Limb deficiencies, 965–974, Copyright Elsevier 2014

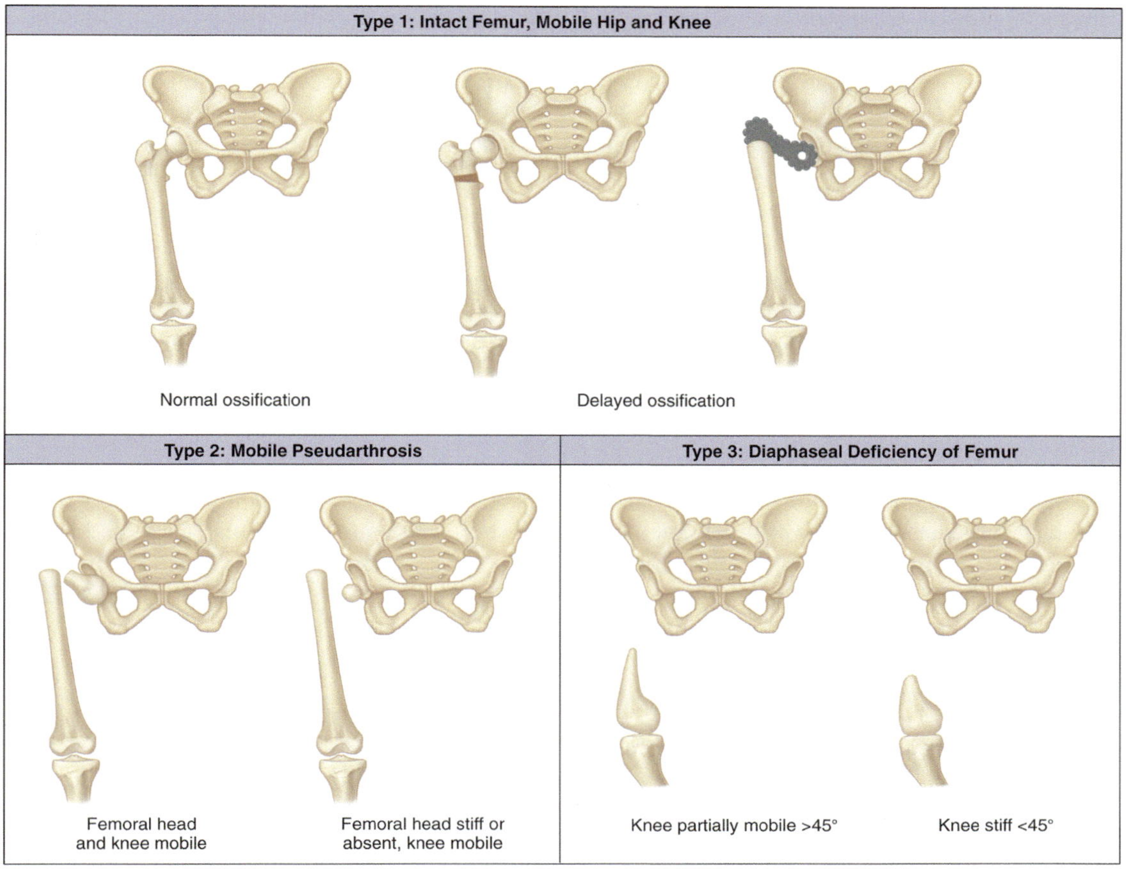

Fig. 20.7 The Paley classification of femoral deficiency. This classification takes note of hip and knee mobility. This image was published in Tachdjian's Pediatric Orthopedics, Herring JA, Limb deficiencies, 965–974, Copyright Elsevier 2014

Treatment in Gillespie Type A

These patients, with at least 50% of normal femoral length can usually be managed with lengthening and reconstructive methods. The outcome is best when the hip is stable and well formed, and when the upper femoral deformity or deficiency can be corrected. The greater the shortening of the femur, the greater is the number of corrective and lengthening procedures that will be required. The lengthening process in this condition is difficult and a number of authors report a high frequency of complications and failures because of shortening and contracture of all the tissues in the thigh [24–26].

Gillespie Types B and C

In these patients, the femur is less than 50% of the normal length, and lengthening and reconstruction will generally require three or more episodes of lengthening. Each of these will consume months of time, and complications often increase with successive lengthening. Likewise, the ultimate function likely decreases as the underlying anatomy is more deficient in cases with substantial femoral shortening. Thus, in this situation, some variation of amputation is usually

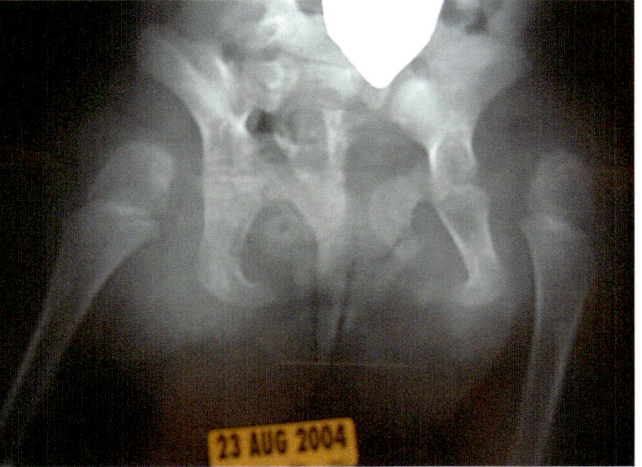

Fig. 20.8 A radiograph of severe bilateral femoral deficiency, Gillespie type C, in which there is no femoral formation and the tibias articulate with the pelvis. Treatment alternatives are minimal in these children. This image was published in Tachdjian's Pediatric Orthopedics, Herring JA, Limb deficiencies, 965–974, Copyright Elsevier 2014

appropriate (Box 20.3). Patients with bilateral femoral deficiency are almost never candidates for amputation, nor are those with major upper limb anomalies requiring the feet for manual activities (Fig. 20.8).

The treatment options in CFD can best be understood relative to the presenting anatomy. Factors to consider include (1) the anatomy of the hip and its musculature, (2) relative shortening of the femur, (3) the range of motion of the knee, and (4) the anatomy of the foot. The anatomy of the hip varies from relatively normal to severe deformity or sometimes absence of the femoral head and acetabulum. In young children, structures of the hip and knee may appear on radiographs to be absent when they are actually well-formed in cartilage. Often, MRI imaging will provide an excellent analysis of the relevant anatomy. With almost any treatment approach, the anatomy of the upper femur should be reconstructed to restore bony continuity of the femur and restore the femoral neck shaft angle whenever possible, and acetabular dysplasia should also be corrected (Fig. 20.9). When the femoral head has not developed, or there is no acetabular formation, hip reconstruction is generally not feasible.

Knee arthrodesis with or without Symes amputation has been used for many years when the femur is very short and the knee range of motion is poor. The child can be fitted with a prosthesis at walking age incorporating the foot in the prosthetic socket, or a Symes amputation can be done at walking age to facilitate prosthetic fitting. The arthrodesis of the knee is usually done at an older age, often age 3 or 4 years, when there is enough ossification of the distal femoral and proximal tibial epiphyses to achieve a fusion. The arthrodesis improves the gait by reducing the flexed position of the thigh segment and aligning the mechanical axis of the limb under the weight line of the body.

To have appropriate length of the thigh segment after arthrodesis, the entire distal femoral epiphysis is removed and the upper tibial epiphysis is fused to the distal femoral metaphysis (Fig. 20.10). The goal is for the end of the thigh segment to be about 10 cm shorter than the contralateral thigh to allow room for the prosthetic knee components. Because the distal femoral epiphysis is removed, the thigh will gradually relatively shorten as the contralateral distal femur continues to grow.

As an alternative, rotation of the distal limb to achieve a Van Nes effect may be done at the time of knee arthrodesis [27, 28]. However, when there is inadequate hip stability, the distal segment has a tendency to derotate with growth, and may have to be repeated.

When the proximal hip anatomy is not amenable to reconstruction, several procedures have been developed in an attempt to reduce the abductor limp which is usually quite noticeable. The most successful has been that developed by Ken Brown in which the femur is rotated 180° and fused to the pelvis in a vertical position [27, 28] (Fig. 20.11). In this position, flexion of the rotated knee becomes hip flexion. The fusion of the femur to the pelvis, with full rotation turns the foot backward with the toes facing posteriorly. The foot is placed in equinus into a prosthetic socket so that the ankle controls the prosthetic knee. When the ankle dorsiflexes the prosthetic knee flexes and when the foot plantar flexes, the knee extends. The anatomic ankle also provides proprioception of "knee" position which is an important advantage for the patient, for example when descending stairs.

Box 20.3
Options with amputation:

- Femoral length <50%
- Hip reconstruction
- Knee fusion
- Femoral-pelvic fusion
- Symes amputation
- Rotationplasty

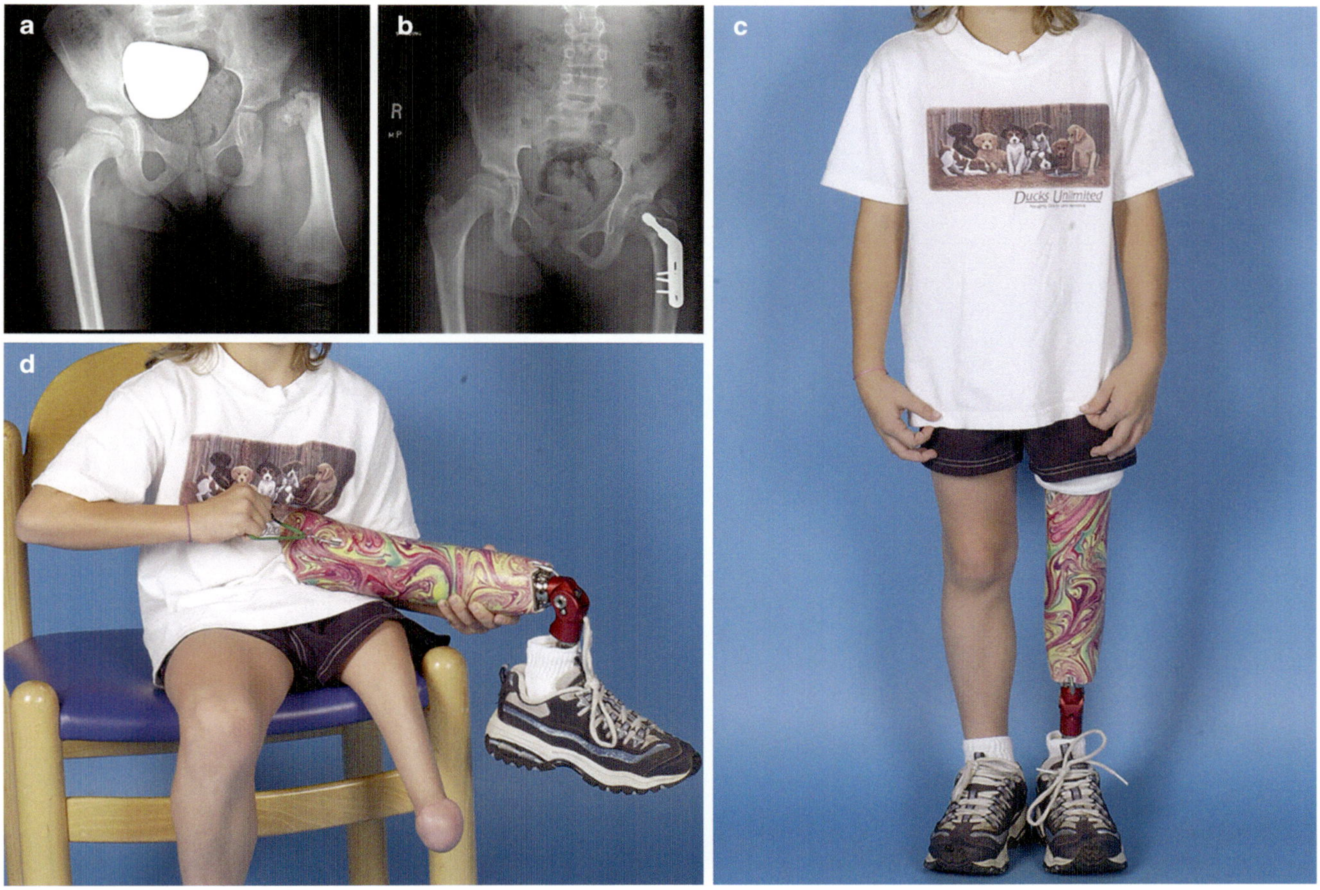

Fig. 20.9 (**a**) A Gillespie type B deficiency with less than 50% of femoral length. There is a short femoral neck with a marked varus deformity. (**b**) A radiograph of the pelvis after proximal femoral valgus osteotomy and acetabuloplasty. (**c**) The same patient with her prosthesis. Her anatomic knee is intact and flexes just at the top of the prosthesis. She is an active varsity cheerleader at a major university with no functional limitations. (**d**) Her shortened thigh segment is evident as she sits without her prosthesis

Fig. 20.10 (**a**) A radiograph of a type B femoral deficiency. Note the absence of femoral head or acetabular development. (**b**) The same patient after arthrodesis of the knee and Symes amputation

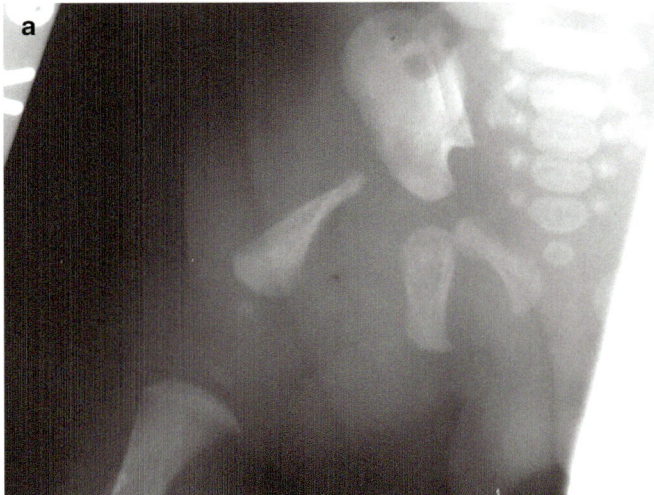
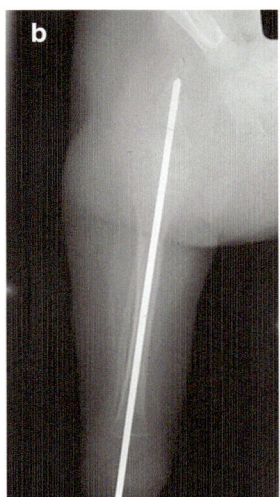

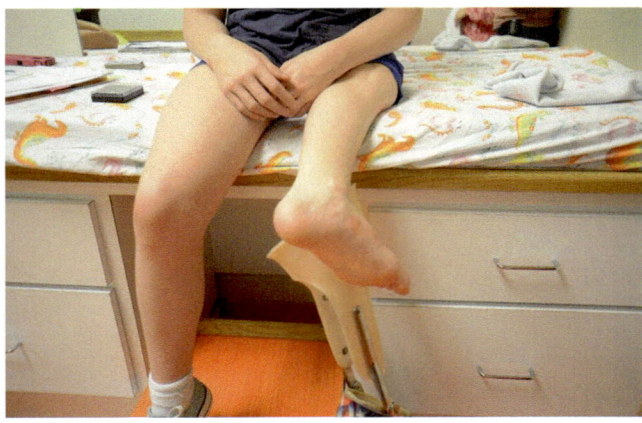

Fig. 20.11 A 10-year-old girl with a Van Nes-type rotationplasty after tumor resection. The foot is not in an ideal position and may require rotational realignment

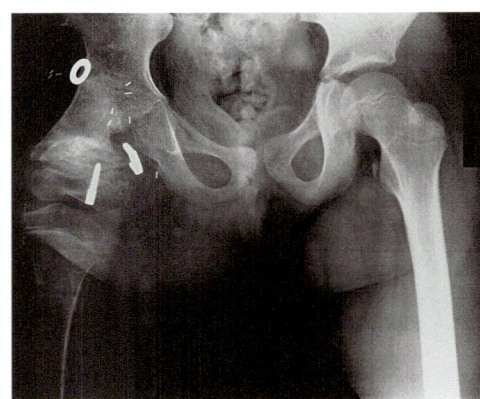

Fig. 20.12 A radiograph of a patient who had a Brown procedure. The proximal femur with a tumor was removed and the distal femur was rotated 180° and fused to the pelvis in an extended position. The staples are placed to stop the growth of the distal femoral epiphysis

Table 20.1 Proposed classification of congenital fibular deficiency based on clinical deformity and treatment based on classification[a]

Type	Characteristic	Treatment anticipated
Type 1 (foot preservable)		
1A	<6% inequality	No treatment or orthosis or epiphysiodesis
1B	6–10% inequality	Epiphysiodesis ± lengthening
1C	11–30% inequality	1 or 2 lengthenings ± epiphysiodesis or extension orthosis
1D	>30% inequality	>2 lengthenings or amputation or extension orthosis
Type 2 (foot nonpreservable)		
2A	Functional upper extremity	Early amputation
2B	Nonfunctional upper extremity	Consider salvage

[a] Shortening is calculated as a percentage relative to the contralateral limb. In bilateral cases, the longer limb is classified as Type 1A, and the shorter limb is classified as is done for unilateral cases

Congenital Fibular Deficiency

While several classifications of congenital fibular deficiency (or fibular hemimelia) are used, we prefer the Birch classification [29] which is based on the severity of the foot deformity and the limb length discrepancy (Table 20.1). In general, a patient whose foot can be made plantigrade and which has three or more rays, may be a candidate for lengthening. When the overall limb length inequality is 10% or less, lengthening is preferred. With discrepancies between 10 and 30%, either method may be appropriate. With discrepancies greater than 30%, often requiring more than two limb lengthening procedures, we usually recommend an amputation (Box 20.4) (see Figs. 20.4 and 20.12).

Our preferred amputation technique for fibular hemimelia is a variation of the Symes procedure in which the ankle is disarticulated without removing the medial malleolus [30]. The heel pad remains as an excellent weight-bearing structure, and the incision is anterior to the weight-bearing surface (Figs. 20.13 and 20.14). Some surgeons prefer the Boyd modification with fusion of the calcaneus to the distal tibial articular surface.

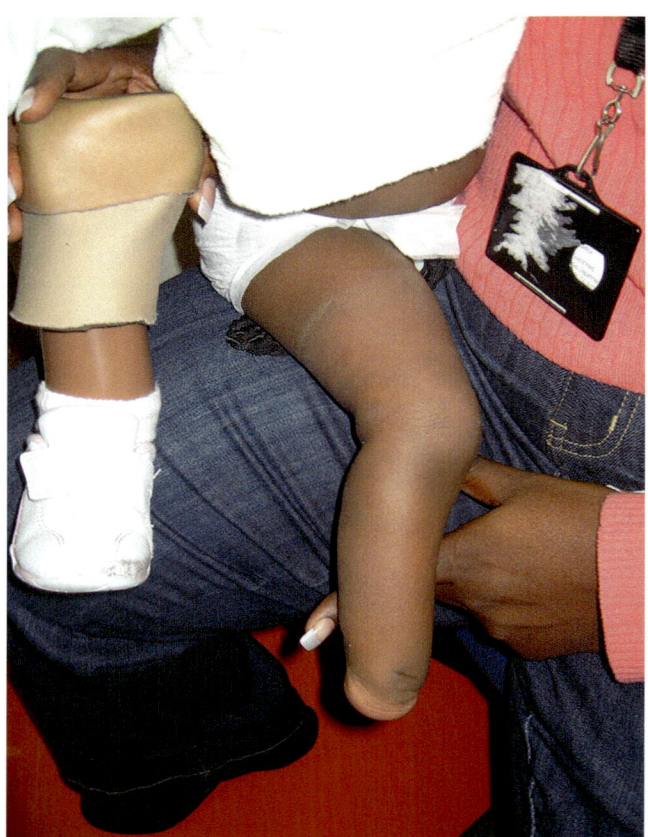

Fig. 20.13 A 2-year-old girl treated with Symes amputation for fibular hemimelia

The limb length discrepancy can easily be equalized by varying the length of the prosthetic limb. A moderately shorter limb is ideal so that there is room for prosthetic foot components. Most patients can ambulate well without the

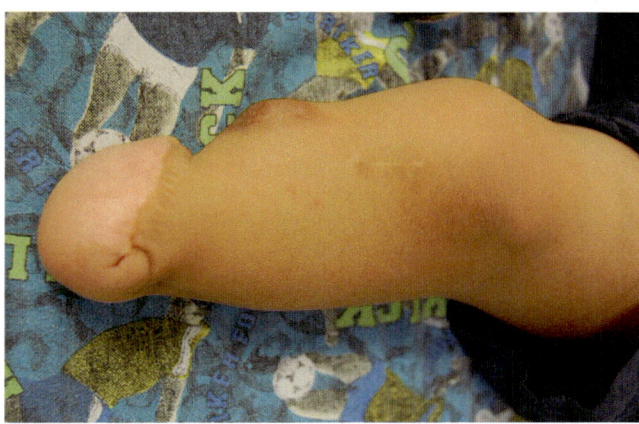

Fig. 20.14 Appearance of a Symes amputation for fibular hemimelia

prosthesis and compensate for more severe length discrepancy by walking with the other knee flexed.

> **Box 20.4**
> Amputation considered for:
>
> - Three-rayed foot or less
> - Limb length discrepancy >30%
> - Optional for LLD 10–30%
>   *Never with missing upper extremity function

We prefer to perform amputation when the child reaches the developmental stage of cruising, and is taking steps while holding on. The prosthesis can be fitted just as the child reaches walking age, and very little training is then necessary. Within a few hours the child comprehends, almost magically, what this addition to his or her anatomy is there for, and will simply begin to walk.

Congenital Tibial Deficiency

The Jones classification [31] is very useful in the management of congenital tibial deficiency (or tibial hemimelia) (Fig. 20.15) which presents with wide anatomic variability. In the type 1a, in which there is complete absence of the upper tibia, we consider amputation through the knee (knee disarticulation) to be the best management (Figs. 20.16 and 20.17) (Box 20.5). The absence of the extensor mechanics of the quadriceps and patella prevents functional reconstruction. Following amputation, the femoral length should be monitored as the child grows. A distal femoral epiphyseal arrest is often necessary during growth so that the femur is 6 or 8 cm shorter than the contralateral femur at skeletal maturity. This allows space for the prosthetic knee component so that the prosthetic and anatomic knees are at the same level.

The now-obsolete Brown procedure, in which the fibula was centered beneath a bulbar distal femur, was widely abandoned after studies showed almost universal long-term failure. Loder and Herring found that these created knees became stiff and non-functional over several years [32].

When the proximal tibia is present and the quadriceps actively extends the proximal tibial segment, as in the Jones type 1b and 2, a very functional reconstruction is available. In the young child, there may be a well-formed upper tibial segment which is not ossified and is therefore not seen on the radiograph, the type 1b. Careful physical examination and ultrasound or MRI evaluation will identify the tibial structure. When there is a functional proximal tibial segment, the ideal treatment is fusion of the fibula to the upper tibia. Because of the absence of the distal tibia and ankle, a Syme amputation is usually performed at the distal fibular level, while maintaining the heel pad. In the young child, the upper tibial portion may be mostly formed of cartilage. Fusion of the fibula to the tibial segment requires enough bone formation in the upper tibia to accomplish fixation and fusion. In this situation, we often will primarily amputate the foot to enable the child to ambulate in a prosthesis with support above the knee. As the tibial cartilaginous anlage ossifies, we perform a fusion of the fibula to the upper tibia with either pin or screw fixation. Once the fusion matures, the child will wear a Symes-type prosthesis and usually function at the same level as the child with fibular hemimelia (Fig. 20.18).

Jones type 3 anomalies are rare and the anatomy is variable. Some cases with radiographically absent upper tibias actually have cartilaginous upper segments and can be managed with synostosis procedure as in the type 2.

> **Box 20.5**
> Amputation appropriate for:
>
> - Jones 1a (knee disarticulation)
> - Jones 1b, 2 (Symes amputation, synostosis of tibia to fibula)
> - Jones 3, 4-variable indications

The Jones 4 type abnormality has a distal diastasis between the tibia and fibula. Some of these deformities are best managed with Syme amputation and others with reconstruction (Fig. 20.19). These abnormalities vary considerably, and treatment must be individualized for the given anatomy. Elements which may favor amputation include severe limb length discrepancy, lack of a distal tibial articular surface, and the relative size and stiffness of the foot. As with other conditions, the choice of treatment relative to the foot is between a complex and multistage reconstruction with an outcome which is hard to predict and a relatively simple amputation surgery which requires prosthetic wear for life.

Fig. 20.15 Jones classification of tibial deficiency. Redrawn with permission from Herring JA, Cummings, DR. The Limb Deficient Child. In: Morrissy RT, Weinstein SL, editors. Lovell and Winter's Pediatric Orthopedics, vol 2, ed 4. Philadelphia: Lippincott-Raven; 1996

Type	Radiologic Description	No. of limbs
1a	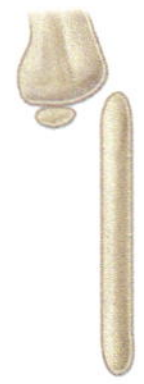 Tibia not seen / Hypoplastic lower femoral epiphysis	6
1b	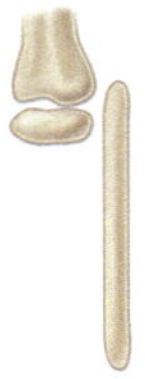 Tibia not seen / Normal lower femoral epiphysis	12
2	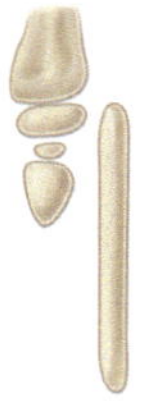 Distal tibia not seen	5
3	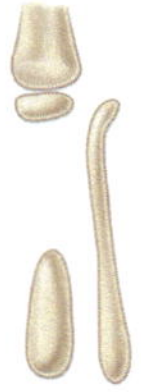 Proximal tibia not seen	2
4	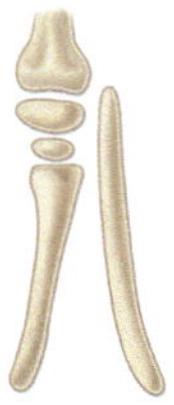 Diastasis	4

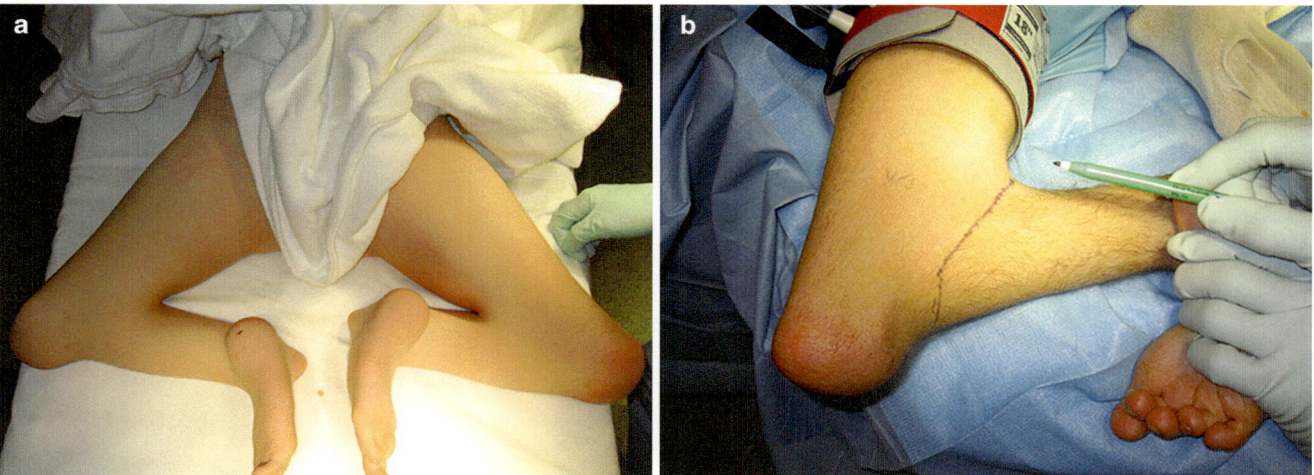

Fig. 20.16 (**a**) A 15-year-old boy with untreated complete tibial hemimelias, Jones type 1a. (**b**) Incision lines have been drawn for knee disarticulation surgery. The suture line does not impair the distal end bearing skin

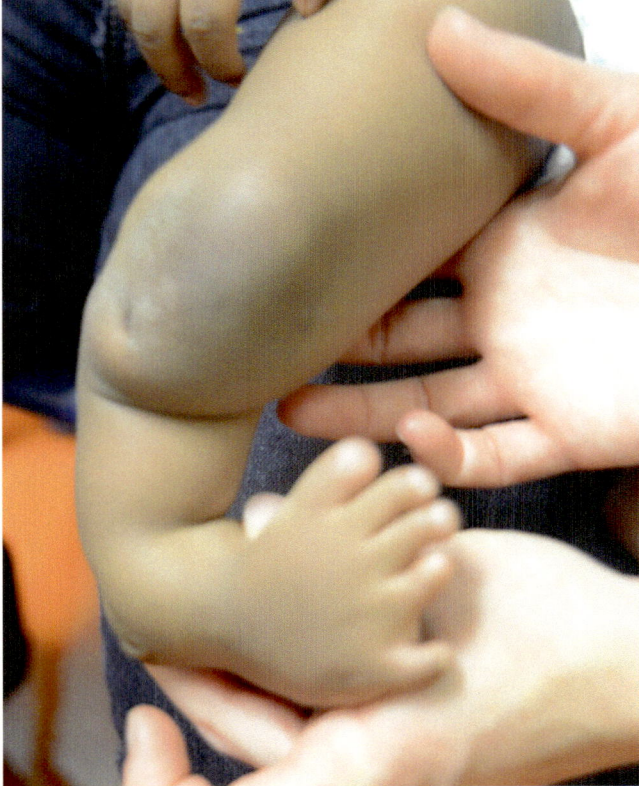

Fig. 20.17 A Jones type 2 tibial hemimelia. There is a proximal tibial segment which is powered by the quadriceps and hamstrings. The subsequent treatment was a fusion of the tibia to the fibula and a Symes amputation

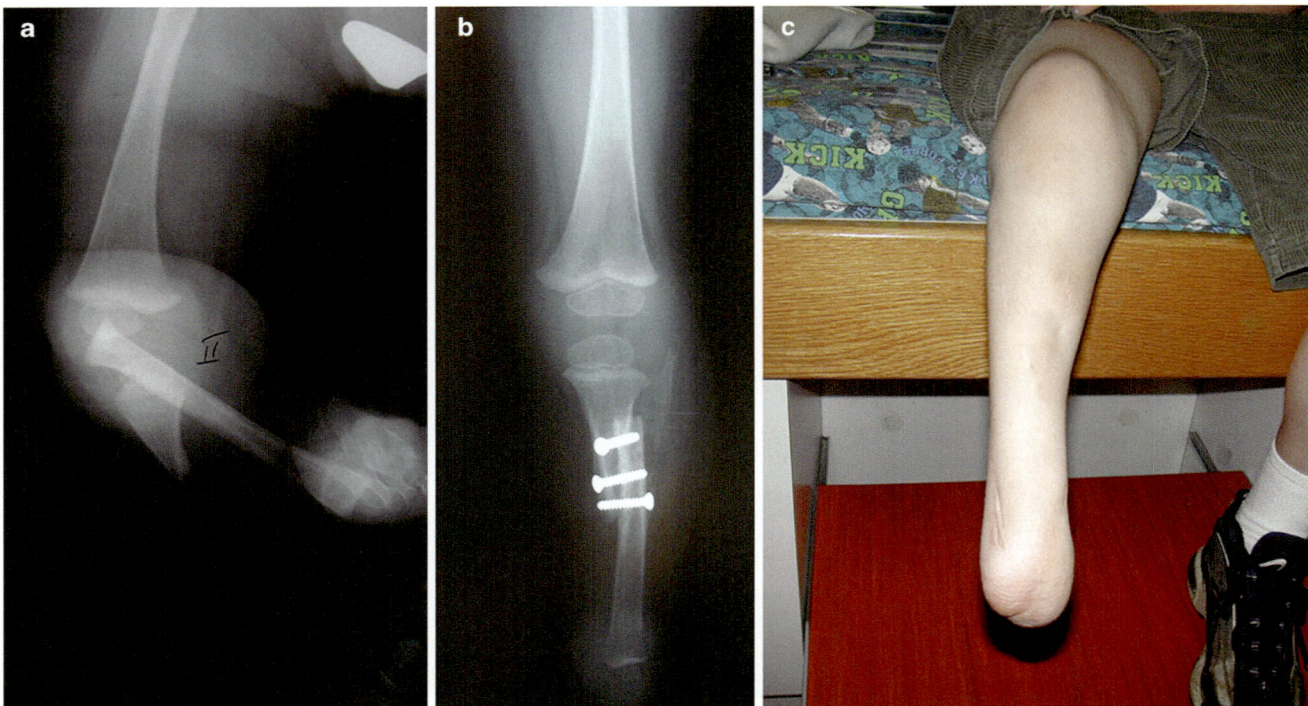

Fig. 20.18 (a) A Jones type 2 tibial hemimelia before treatment. (b) Radiograph of the limb after fusion of the fibula to the proximal tibial segment. (c) Appearance of the limb after fusion is complete. The patient had excellent athletic function

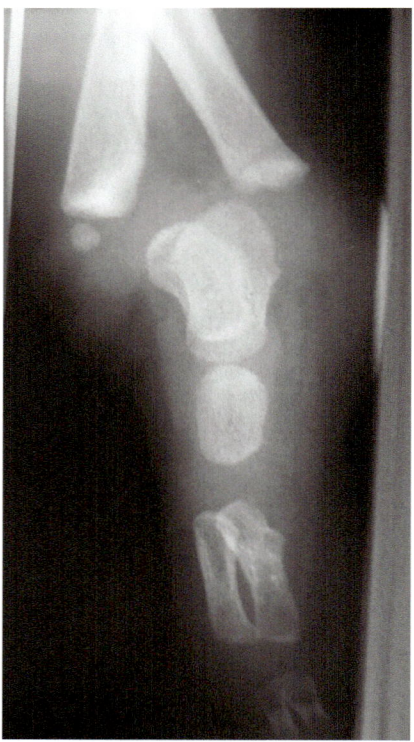

Fig. 20.19 A radiograph of a Jones type 4 tibial hemimelia with a distal diastasis between the tibia and fibula. In this instance, there was no distal tibial articular surface and a diminutive foot, and a Symes amputation was performed

Congenital Pseudarthrosis of the Tibia

In our experience, children with congenital pseudarthrosis of the tibia are candidates for amputation in two scenarios. The more common need for amputation arises following several surgical interventions with either failure to achieve union, or when refracture occurs and the parents do not wish to have more reconstructive surgery. In these cases, various types of surgery have been performed, and the likelihood of a subsequent procedure being successful is low (Fig. 20.20).

Over recent years, a small number of families have been referred to us who desire primary amputation for their young child. They have reasoned that the child with an amputation about the age of first walking will be able to function with prosthetic management and minimal future surgery, with no need for protection from vigorous life and sporting activities. We have performed such amputations after careful evaluation of the child and parents' understanding. In addition to meeting other children with similar amputations, our psychologists also evaluate and educate the family.

We perform the amputation in this disorder at the pseudarthrosis site. Some have recommended Syme amputation with the suggestion that the pseudarthrosis may heal [33]. In earlier years we had no such healing when we took this approach, and some patients had pain at the pseudarthrosis site requiring reoperation. In addition, current trends for sports prostheses require significant available space for blades and other components that cannot be used with a longer residual limb.

A modification we prefer for this amputation, which also we use for traumatic amputations, is to remove a short segment of cartilage-covered bone from the foot to block overgrowth of the tip of the residual limb. We will take a metatarsal head with a short segment of diaphysis and use this as an intramedullary osteochondral plug into the distal tibia. To block the fibular overgrowth, we usually use a phalanx from a toe for the same purpose. I should note that we have no firm evidence at this time of the efficacy of this maneuver.

Tumor Reconstruction

While a discussion of the available amputation options for patients requiring amputation for malignancy is beyond the scope of this chapter, certain procedures have proven to be very functional. For proximal femur resections, the procedure described by Ken Brown with rotation plasty gives excellent functional results [27, 28]. The distal femur is rotated 180° and fused to the pelvis in a vertical orientation. The anatomic knee, which is placed at the level of the pelvis, functions as a hip with hinge flexion and extension; the ankle and foot power the prosthetic knee. The resultant function is very good (Fig. 20.21) [34–37].

When a femoral lesion can be excised leaving the proximal femur and hip intact, fusion of the tibia to the proximal femur in a 180° rotated position also provides excellent function, again using the foot to power the prosthetic knee (Fig. 20.22).

With tumors distal to the knee, function of the knee joint should be preserved, if at all possible. In unusual circumstances the distal tibia can be "flipped" to be fused to a remaining proximal tibial segment (Fig. 20.23).

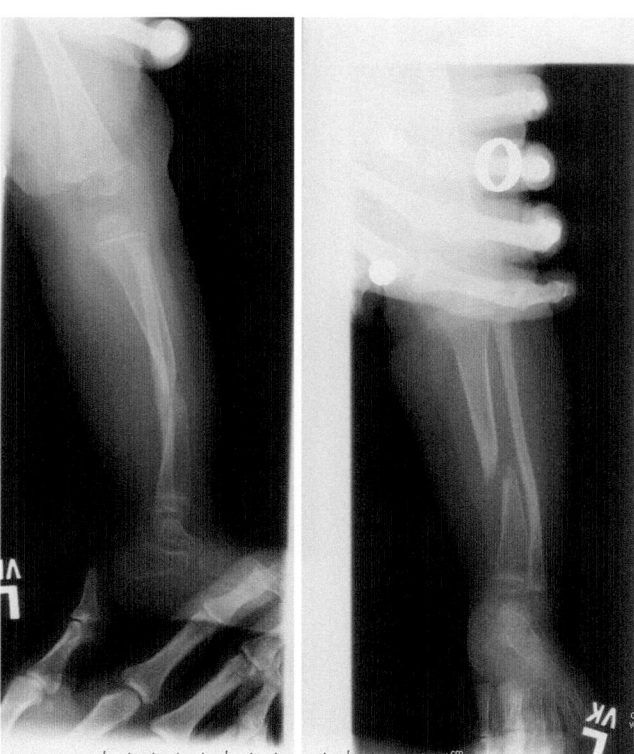

Fig. 20.20 A radiograph of a congenital tibial pseudarthrosis in a girl with neurofibromatosis. After a number of procedures, she developed a late recurrent pseudarthrosis and underwent trans-tibial amputation

Fig. 20.21 (a) A radiograph of a patient treated for a proximal femoral tumor. Her remaining femur was rotated 180° and fused to the pelvis. A revision will likely be necessary to shorten the femur and reduce the abducted position. (b) A photograph showing the rotated and very functional foot

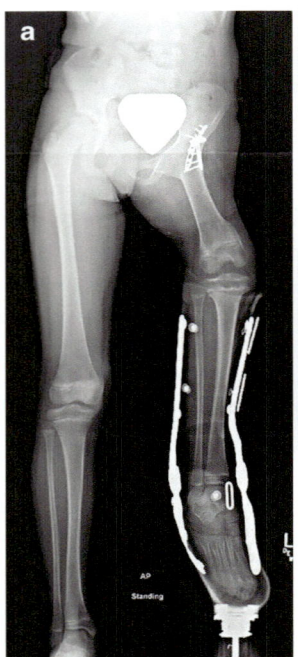
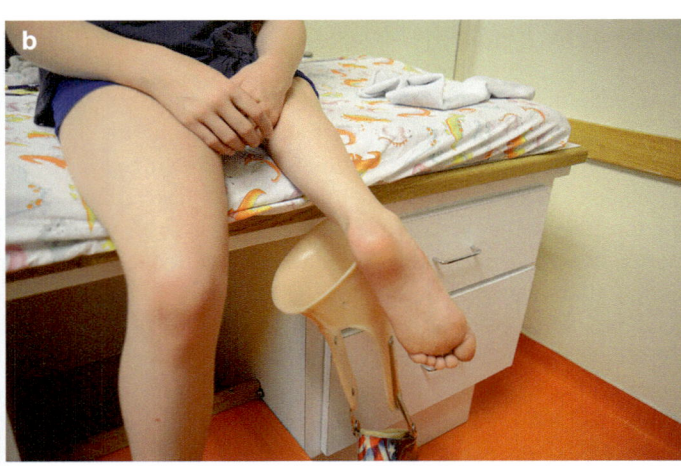

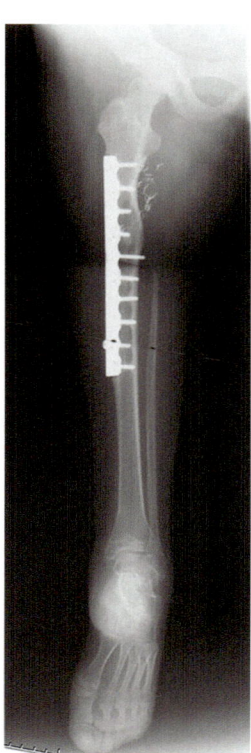

Fig. 20.22 A radiograph of a patient who had a distal femoral tumor excised and a fusion of the remaining proximal femur to the tibia, which was rotated 180°

Fig. 20.23 (**a**) A radiograph of a patient who presented with a painful valgus right knee deformity. The density in the proximal tibia was an osteosarcoma. (**b**) An AP radiograph showing a complex allograft reconstruction of the tibia. (**c**) A lateral radiograph showing a complex allograft reconstruction of the tibia. (**d**) A radiograph showing the allograft after removal of the fixation devices. Subsequent infection and non-union required consideration for amputation. (**e**) The proximal tibia was retained and the allograft removed. The distal tibial segment was reversed allowing fusion of the more healthy distal tibia to the proximal segment with pin fixation

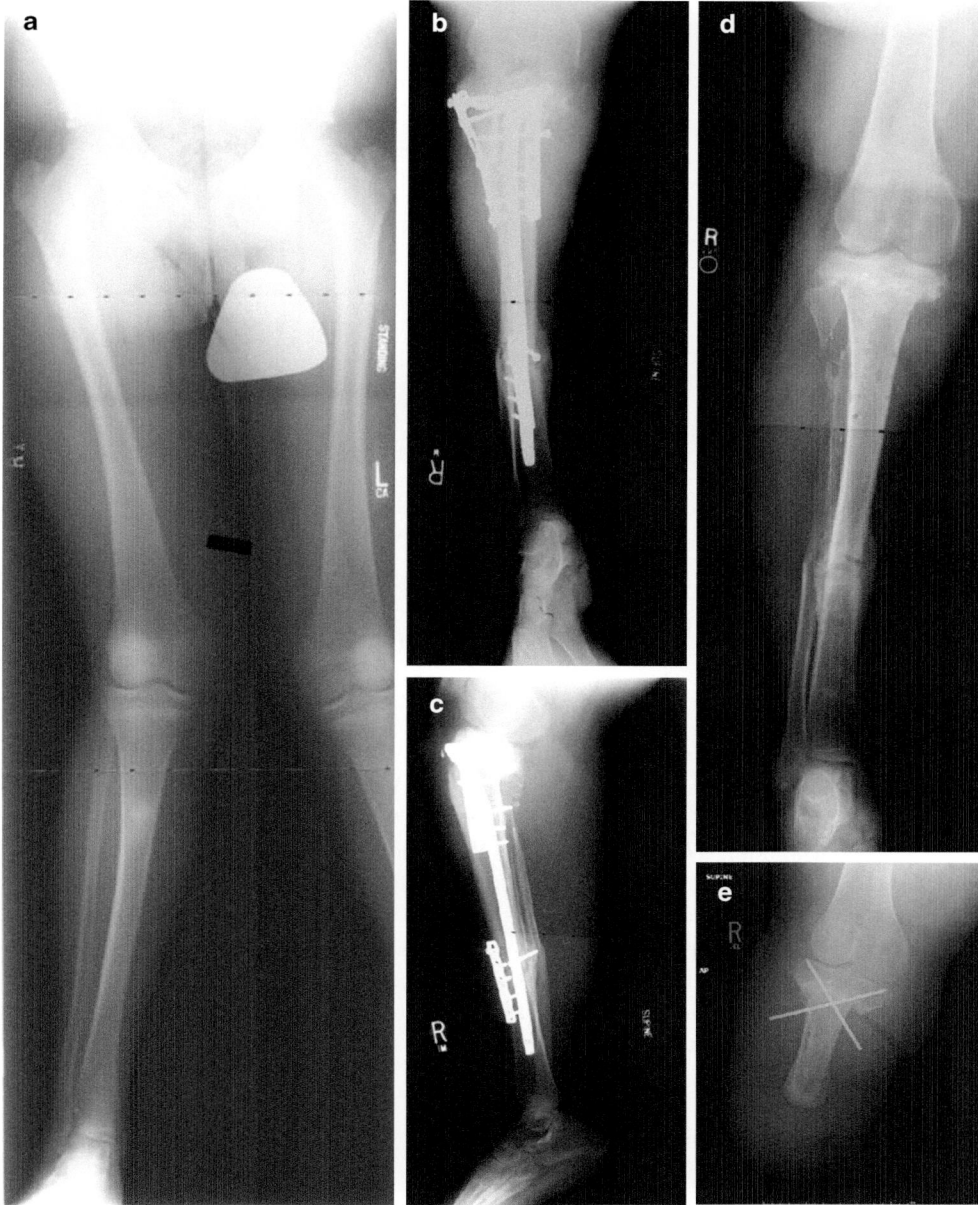

Volume Changes with Oncology

Patients undergoing chemotherapy or multiple other procedures may experience significant volume changes of their residual limb from either weight loss or, conversely, edema. These children may benefit from prostheses with sockets which can be expanded and contracted as necessary.

Amputation After Trauma

Whenever possible, the knee joint should be preserved at the time of amputation. Exposed, granulating areas on the upper tibia can be maintained with skin grafting. While some areas may break down, children have better healing properties than adults, and there is great functional benefit to maintaining the native knee joint (Fig. 20.24).

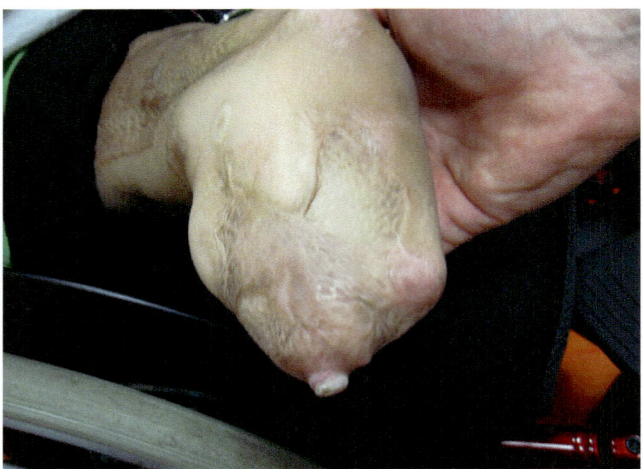

Fig. 20.24 A clinical photo of a knee and residual tibia following severe trauma. The patient had excellent function in spite of the compromised soft tissue coverage

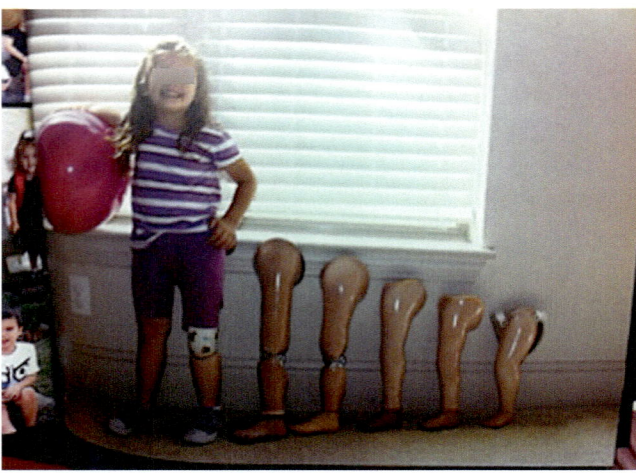

Fig. 20.25 A young girl standing beside all of her previous prostheses. In a growing child, a new prosthesis may be needed as often as every 12 months

Prosthetic Considerations

First Prosthesis

We prefer to perform indicated amputations at the time when the child is pulling up or beginning to take steps. We then fit the child with a prosthesis at the time when he or she would naturally begin walking. When the amputation is at the knee level or above, the initial prosthesis is constructed without a knee joint. We usually add the knee to the next prosthesis when the child is 18 months or older. With bilateral absences, we may wait longer to add an articulated knee to either one or both prostheses depending on the child's walking abilities and the length of the residual limb.

Prosthetic Replacement for Children

Children in their growing years will require new prostheses about every 12–18 months. Varying the thickness of socks and liners can sometimes prolong the useful life of a prosthesis. Children with end bearing residual limbs, such as knee disarticulations and Symes amputations, can often wear their prostheses well after they have grown a fair amount (Fig. 20.25). It is not uncommon for a child to prefer the "old" prosthesis to the "new" one, especially if changes in design have been made. Gradually, and often after some modifications, the child will prefer the new limb. When possible, the old limb can be modified to be used for swimming, water skiing, or other "rough" activities.

Length of the Residual Limb

A major advantage of the Syme or Boyd amputation is the ability of the patient to weight bear on the residual limb without a prosthesis. This provides the patient with options for activities without the prosthesis such as swimming, walking indoors, and mobility when the prosthesis is not available. The recent availability of prostheses with terminal devices such as the spring and blade devices have changed the desires of many patients. These powerful blades provide the ability to run, jump, and participate in sports up to and including the Olympic level, and require 10 or more cm of space below the end of the residual limb. Some patients with well-functioning Symes amputations have returned requesting more proximal amputation in order to use such terminal devices. Before doing such an operation we make sure that the patient understands the both the functional losses as well as the gains, especially relative to losing the ability to walk without the prosthesis.

Residual Limb Overgrowth

Overgrowth at the distal end of trans-tibial amputations as well as trans-femoral amputations and others produce annoying problems for prosthetic wear. Usually a slender spike of bone grows from the distal periosteum and becomes prominent or protrudes from the end of the limb. There is usually a bursa around this bony spicule, which is filled with fluid and bone and cartilage fragments. These are exquisitely painful and often prevent wear of the prosthesis (Figs. 20.26 and 20.27).

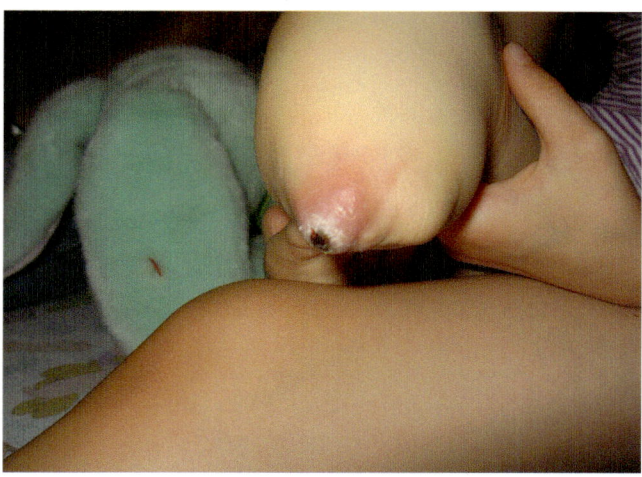

Fig. 20.26 A clinical photograph of a transtibial amputation with marked overgrowth of the fibula. It is remarkable that in spite of bone penetration of the skin, infection is very rare

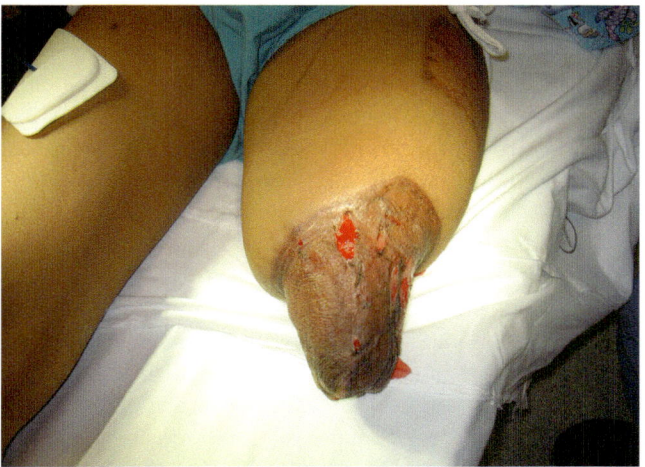

Fig. 20.27 A clinical photograph of a transfemoral amputation. In an effort to keep extra length, a segment of bone was covered with split skin graft. The extra femoral length was not needed and the wound healed after the poorly covered segment was removed

The first line of treatment is to resect the overgrowth and shorten the residual limb so that there is ample distal soft tissue coverage. Many efforts have been proposed to reduce the frequency of overgrowth. Placement of a bone and cartilage plug into the canal of the transected bone is sometimes effective. Iliac crest bone and cartilage graft has been used for this purpose, as well as biologic elements such as metatarsal heads which may be available at primary amputation. Excision of distal periosteum at the time of revision has also been advised. Blockage of the distal canal with cement, bone wax, polytetrafluoroethylene felt, and other substances has also been advised [38–46].

End Weight-Bearing

Amputation levels which allow end weight-bearing have a number of advantages, especially in growing children. We often see children who are functioning well in a prosthesis that they have outgrown. These are usually children with either knee disarticulation or Symes-level amputations. While they have grown up out of the prosthetic socket, the ability of the limb to tolerate full weight-bearing has allowed these children to function normally.

The Future of Prosthetics

Future developments will likely add much to our ability to help children with missing limbs. We can expect stronger and lighter materials for prosthetic manufacture. New prosthetic knee mechanisms which provide powered knee extension for stair climbing have just become available and will likely become useful. Running legs continue to be improved to the extent that super-normal performance may soon be achieved. While these powerful blades may make it difficult to determine fairness for sports competitions, the amputee athlete will enjoy greater success on the playing field. Hopefully we will see the development of prostheses which will have permeable components which allow passage of air and moisture to free the wearer from problems of odor and skin rash. Transmission of sensation from prostheses to the person is on the horizon for upper extremity devices and could be useful in lower limb prosthetics as well. Finally, better durability and water proofing would be much appreciated.

Osseointegration

In recent years, techniques have been developed for directly attaching prosthetic devices to long bones following amputation. This has primarily been done in the femur, tibia, and occasionally the humerus. The connection between the bone and the prosthesis is accomplished through bony ingrowth into a porous prosthetic stem which is inserted into the medullary canal of the long bone. With ongoing experience, a complex protocol has shown effectiveness and is termed OPRA, Osseointegrated Prostheses for the Rehabilitation of Amputees.

Current reports have noted improved patient satisfaction in a number of ways. The integrated prosthesis is self-suspended and rigidly attached to the limb, which relieves the patient of wearing suspension sleeves which are hot and uncomfortable. The integrated trans-femoral prosthesis allows the patient's thigh to rest flat on a surface in sitting. Patients also note a feeling of better sensory and positional input from the prosthesis-bone continuity.

The OPRA technique [47] developed in Sweden has been well-studied. Briefly, the technique has three main components, the fixture which anchors to the bone by osseointegration, the abutment which connects to the fixture, and a safety device which connects to the prosthesis. The treatment requires 2 surgeries separated by 6 months. In the first surgery, the intramedullary canal is reamed and the fixture is carefully positioned and installed. It remains in the bone for 6 months without any loading while the bony ingrowth occurs.

At the second surgery, all distal muscles are sectioned and sutured to the periosteum. A 5 mm portion of the bone is left protruding and is covered by a skin flap which has had the subcutaneous fat removed. This flap is attached to the end of the bone. The abutment is inserted through the skin into the fixture where it is secured with an abutment screw. From this point, the prosthesis is attached and the patient undergoes rehabilitation with gradually increased weight-bearing.

A significant and not fully solved problem is one of infection. The OPRA techniques involve careful management of the "stoma" where the prosthetic stem enters the skin. In spite of these techniques, infections have been frequent. Most infections have been superficial, but deep infections, some requiring implant removal, have been reported with the incidence varying from center to center.

Branemark and associates [47] reported a study of 51 patients with 55 trans-femoral prostheses. Patients' ages ranged from 20 years to 70 years. At 5-year follow-up, 92% retained their prosthetic fixation, but 55% had had revisions. Superficial infection occurred 70 times in 34 patients. Most resolved with oral antibiotics for 10 days, but 16 required longer treatment. Deep infections occurred in 14 instances with 9 being successfully treated with oral antibiotics. Mechanical failures also occurred with 43 instances in 15 patients in this study.

Reetz [48], whose group started using osseointegration in 2009, reported outcomes in 39 patients. Thirty patients (77%) had some kind of infection with 156 infection events. Eight events in four patients were considered severe infections. Soft-tissue refashioning was done 30 times in 14 patients, and there were two intramedullary stem fractures. Quality of life measures improved in most patients.

Ontario Health [49] reported a 13% incidence of osteomyelitis in a study of 69 patients treated in the OPRA method. They showed that the 10-year risk of osteomyelitis in all patients was 20%. They also noted that the 10-year risk that infection would lead to implant extraction was 9%.

Atallah [50] in a systematic review of 12 cohort studies noted that infection was reported in 29% of implants for transtibial amputees. Press-fit trans-femoral implants had a much lower rate of infection, 0–3%. Matthews [51], in a report of the UK trial for osseointegrated prostheses, noted that of 18 patients studied, 5 (28%) had been removed for infection. Superficial infection occurred in 11 (61%) who were successfully treated with antibiotics.

I have not found any studies of the use of osseointegration in children, and am not aware of a center where children have been so treated. The challenges in children include their vigorous activity levels, growth, and cooperation. Our goal with prosthetic management of children is that they should have no prescribed activity limitations. We want them to be free to play and compete at the highest levels, and let us repair the damage to the prosthetic. The fixation of the integrated prosthesis may or may not be able to meet the forces and challenges we want our children to achieve.

Integrated prostheses may be able to accommodate growth through modifications of the attached prosthesis. Revisions of the "stoma" will likely be needed. The biologic behavior of the of the bone attachment site, and the responses of the bone to stress over many years will require study.

In pediatric practice, it may be advisable to first consider osseointegration for skeletally mature patients who are not functioning well with standard prosthetics. Early efforts in younger children might be directed to those who are hard to fit due to very short residual bone structure. Those with fitting problems due to obese residual limbs may be more challenging for osseointegration from skin interface issues and superficial infections.

Commentary

Hugh G. Watts
hwatts@ucla.edu

The plea of medical personnel specializing in children's diseases is *"Don't treat a child as a small adult"*… they're not just smaller but have different needs and problems. Consequently, Herring aptly focusses this chapter on congenital lower limb deficiencies and gives excellent advice in their management as well as to amputations that can result in enhanced rehabilitation.

When dealing with congenital deficiencies of the limbs, there is a significant likelihood that there will be additional congenital deformities... of the spine and internal organs especially the heart. These aspects require careful evaluation *before* making plans about the lower extremities.

Not only are children's amputations commonly due to congenital anomalies, they are three times more likely to involve multiple limbs than amputations caused by trauma. Decisions about the lower extremities must include considering the possible difficulties to be encountered by the concomitant loss of function of an upper extremity. A child might be better off retaining a mobile, lower extremity which, by being shorter, can allow the foot to reach the mouth as a substitution for missing upper extremities.

The planning for an amputation requires a thorough understanding of the patterns of growth in children bones. A child born with a short femur that is 50% as long as the normal side will reach adulthood with the short side at 50% of the normal side. This has been called the Principle of Proportionality. Hoping that growth will eventually correct the difference is futile. X-rays in infancy (taken in the lateral position to obviate the illusion of added shortening due to associated hip and knee flexion deformities) can help to make the prediction.

Absence of growth from the physics, especially in the femur (where distal growth contributes 75% of the length) can turn an above knee amputation in a small child into a tiny residual limb that can only function as a hip disarticulation at adulthood. *Do everything possible to save the physis*... shorten the residual bone at mid-shaft to achieve skin coverage, or leave a stump open to granulate in or use split thickness grafts to gain coverage... things that can work in children.

Distal overgrowth after amputation in a child can prove to be a difficult and recurring problem. *Make every effort to prevent the problem* by performing disarticulations. Avoid cross-bone amputations, where possible. Save the left-overs such as metatarsals. If a disarticulation is not possible, save a viable bone-end from the distal tissue that would otherwise be discarded and attach it, together with its cartilaginous end covering. This can be especially useful in an elective amputation for a congenital problem or for tumors.

While the advice in Herring's chapter is excellent, he does view matters from a strong America-centric perspective. Many other cultures are more resistant to the use of amputations regardless of the improved function that can result. The importance and guidance of grandparent feelings can be more prevailing than in the USA. Additionally, the continuing worldwide problems caused by Explosive Remnants of War (i.e. land mines and unexploded bombs) may alter the statistics of the proportion of childhood amputees due to congenital causes versus acquired.

My only caveat concerning this chapter is the inclusion of an inordinately lengthy discussion concerning osteointegration. Osteointegration is a relatively new technique in adults and as Herring aptly points out, there have been no publications to date of its uses in children. The unnecessary emphasis about the subject suggesting that it adds a modern bent to current thinking about childhood amputees should be avoided.

References

1. Aston WJ, Calder PR, Baker D, Hartley J, Hill RA. Lengthening of the congenital short femur using the Ilizarov technique: a single-surgeon series. J Bone Joint Surg Br. 2009;91(7):962–7.
2. Catagni MA, Radwan M, Lovisetti L, Guerreschi F, Elmoghazy NA. Limb lengthening and deformity correction by the Ilizarov technique in type III fibular hemimelia: an alternative to amputation. Clin Orthop Relat Res. 2011;469(4):1175–80.
3. El-Sayed MM, Correll J, Pohlig K. Limb sparing reconstructive surgery and Ilizarov lengthening in fibular hemimelia of Achterman-Kalamchi type II patients. J Pediatr Orthop B. 2010;19(1):55–60.
4. Gordon JE, Manske MC, Lewis TR, O'Donnell JC, Schoenecker PL, Keeler KA. Femoral lengthening over a pediatric femoral nail: results and complications. J Pediatr Orthop. 2013;33(7):730–6.
5. Kim SJ, Agashe MV, Song SH, Song HR. Fibula-related complications during bilateral tibial lengthening: 60 patients followed for mean 5 years. Acta Orthop. 2012;83(3):271–5.
6. Oostenbroek HJ, Brand R, van Roermund PM, Castelein RM. Paediatric lower limb deformity correction using the Ilizarov technique: a statistical analysis of factors affecting the complication rate. J Pediatr Orthop B. 2014;23(1):26–31.
7. Papakostidis C, Bhandari M, Giannoudis PV. Distraction osteogenesis in the treatment of long bone defects of the lower limbs: effectiveness, complications and clinical results; a systematic review and meta-analysis. Bone Joint J. 2013;95-B(12):1673–80.
8. Aitken G. Proximal femoral focal deficiency: a congenital anomaly. In: Aitken G, editor. A symposium on proximal femoral focal deficiency: a congenital anomaly. Washington, DC: National Academy of Sciences; 1969. p. 1.
9. Aitken G. Osseous overgrowth in amputations in children. In: Swinyard C, editor. Limb development and deformity: problems of evaluaiton and rehabilitation. Springfield, IL: Charles C. Thomas; 1969.
10. Bekkering WP, Vliet Vlieland TP, Koopman HM, Schaap GR, Bart Schreuder HW, Beishuizen A, et al. Functional ability and physical activity in children and young adults after limb-salvage or ablative surgery for lower extremity bone tumors. J Surg Oncol. 2011;103(3):276–82.
11. Bhamra JS, Abdul-Jabar HB, McKenna D, Ng Man Sun S, Gillott E, Pollock R. Van Nes rotationplasty as a treatment method for Ewing's sarcoma in a 14-month-old. Int J Surg Case Rep. 2013;4(10):893–7.

12. Gupta SK, Alassaf N, Harrop AR, Kiefer GN. Principles of rotationplasty. J Am Acad Orthop Surg. 2012;20(10):657–67.
13. Harris JD, Trinh TQ, Scharschmidt TJ, Mayerson JL. Exceptional functional recovery and return to high-impact sports after Van Nes rotationplasty. Orthopedics. 2013;36(1):e126–31.
14. Mayerson JL. Living with rotationplasty—quality of life in rotationplasty patients from childhood to adulthood. J Surg Oncol. 2012;105(8):743–4.
15. Sawamura C, Hornicek FJ, Gebhardt MC. Complications and risk factors for failure of rotationplasty: review of 25 patients. Clin Orthop Relat Res. 2008;466(6):1302–8.
16. Sawamura C, Matsumoto S, Shimoji T, Ae K, Tanizawa T, Gokita T, et al. Indications for and surgical complications of rotationplasty. J Orthop Sci. 2012;17(6):775–81.
17. So NF, Andrews KL, Anderson K, Gozola MA, Shives TC, Rose PS, et al. Prosthetic fitting after rotationplasty of the knee. Am J Phys Med Rehabil. 2014;93(4):328–34.
18. Tiwari P, Agrawal N, Kocak E. The use of free microvascular techniques to improve the results of Van Nes rotationplasty. Ann Plast Surg. 2013;70(6):672–4.
19. Gillespie R. Principles of amputation surgery in children with longitudinal deficiencies of the femur. Clin Orthop Relat Res. 1990;256:29–38.
20. Gillespie R. Classification fo congenital abnormalities of the femur. In: Herring J, Birch J, editors. The child with a limb deficiency. Rosemont, IL: American Academky of Orthopaedic Surgeons; 1998. p. 63.
21. Gillespie R, Torode IP. Classification and management of congenital abnormalities of the femur. J Bone Joint Surg Br. 1983;65(5):557–68.
22. Hamanishi C. Congenital short femur. Clinical, genetic and epidemiological comparison of the naturally occurring condition with that caused by thalidomide. J Bone Joint Surg Br. 1980;62(3):307–20.
23. Paley D. Lengthening reconstruction surgery for congenital femoral deficiency. In: Herring J, Birch J, editors. The child with a limb deficiency. Rosemont, IL: American Academy of Orthopaedic Surgeons; 1998. p. 113.
24. Murray DW, Kambouroglou G, Kenwright J. One-stage lengthening for femoral shortening with associated deformity. J Bone Joint Surg Br. 1993;75(4):566–71.
25. Velazquez RJ, Bell DF, Armstrong PF, Babyn P, Tibshirani R. Complications of use of the Ilizarov technique in the correction of limb deformities in children. J Bone Joint Surg Am. 1993;75(8):1148–56.
26. Westin G, G G. Proximal femoral focal deficiency: a review of treatment experiences. In: Aitken G, editor. A symposium on proximal femoral focal deficiency: a congenital anomaly. Washington, DC: National Academy of Sciences; 1969. p. 100.
27. Brown K. Rotationplasty with hip stabilization in congenital femoral deficiency. In: Herring J, Birch J, editors. The child with a limb deficiency. Rosemont, IL: American Academy of Orthopaedic Surgeons; 1995. p. 103.
28. Brown KL. Resection, rotationplasty, and femoropelvic arthrodesis in severe congenital femoral deficiency. A report of the surgical technique and three cases. J Bone Joint Surg Am. 2001;83(1):78–85.
29. Birch JG, Lincoln TL, Mack PW, Birch CM. Congenital fibular deficiency: a review of thirty years' experience at one institution and a proposed classification system based on clinical deformity. J Bone Joint Surg Am. 2011;93(12):1144–51.
30. Herring J, e. Tachdjian's pediatric orthopaedics. Philadelphia, PA: Elsevier; 2014.
31. Jones D, Barnes J, Lloyd-Roberts GC. Congenital aplasia and dysplasia of the tibia with intact fibula. Classification and management. J Bone Joint Surg Br. 1978;60(1):31–9.
32. Loder R. Fibular transfer for congenital absence of the tibia (Brown procedure). In: Herring JA, Birch JG, editors. The child with a limb deficiency. Rosemont, IL: American Academy of Orthopaedic Surgeons; 1998. p. 233.
33. Guille JT, Kumar SJ, Shah A. Spontaneous union of a congenital pseudarthrosis of the tibia after Syme amputation. Clin Orthop Relat Res. 1998;351:180–5.
34. Cahan WG, Woodard HQ, et al. Sarcoma arising in irradiated bone; report of 11 cases. Cancer. 1948;1(1):3–29.
35. Hillmann A, Hoffmann C, Gosheger G, Krakau H, Winkelmann W. Malignant tumor of the distal part of the femur or the proximal part of the tibia: endoprosthetic replacement or rotationplasty. Functional outcome and quality-of-life measurements. J Bone Joint Surg Am. 1999;81(4):462–8.
36. Kotz R, Salzer M. Rotation-plasty for childhood osteosarcoma of the distal part of the femur. J Bone Joint Surg Am. 1982;64(7):959–69.
37. Merchan EC, Sanchez-Herrera S, Gonzalez JM. Secondary chondrosarcoma. Four cases and review of the literature. Acta Orthop Belg. 1993;59(1):76–80.
38. Abraham E. Operative treatment of bone overgrowth in children who have an aquired or congenital amputation. J Bone Joint Surg Am. 1996;78(8):1287–8.
39. Canavese F, Krajbich JI, LaFleur BJ. Orthopaedic sequelae of childhood meningococcemia: management considerations and outcome. J Bone Joint Surg Am. 2010;92(12):2196–203.
40. Davids JR, Meyer LC, Blackhurst DW. Operative treatment of bone overgrowth in children who have an acquired or congenital amputation. J Bone Joint Surg Am. 1995;77(10):1490–7.
41. Klimisch J, Carmichael KD, Muradov P, Evans EB. Prevalence of stump overgrowth in pediatric burn patient amputations. J Pediatr Orthop. 2011;31(2):216–9.
42. Michels F, De Smet L. Osseous overgrowth in congenital amputations of the upper limb: report of 3 cases treated with autologous stump plasty. Acta Orthop Belg. 2001;67(5):452–5.
43. O'Neal ML, Bahner R, Ganey TM, Ogden JA. Osseous overgrowth after amputation in adolescents and children. J Pediatr Orthop. 1996;16(1):78–84.
44. Tenholder M, Davids JR, Gruber HE, Blackhurst DW. Surgical management of juvenile amputation overgrowth with a synthetic cap. J Pediatr Orthop. 2004;24(2):218–26.
45. Weber M. Neurovascular calcaneo-cutaneus pedicle graft for stump capping in congenital pseudarthrosis of the tibia: preliminary report of a new technique. J Pediatr Orthop B. 2002;11(1):47–52.
46. Wheeler JS, Anderson BJ, De Chalain TM. Surgical interventions in children with meningococcal purpura fulminans— a review of 117 procedures in 21 children. J Pediatr Surg. 2003;38(4):597–603.
47. Branemark RP, Hagberg K, Kulbacka-Ortiz K, Berlin O, Rydevik B. Osseointegrated percutaneous prosthetic system for the treatment of patients with transfemoral amputation: a prospective five-year follow-up of patient-reported outcomes and complications. J Am Acad Orthop Surg. 2019;27(16):e743–e51.
48. Reetz D, Atallah R, Mohamed J, van de Meent H, Frolke JPM, Leijendekkers R. Safety and performance of bone-anchored prostheses in persons with a transfemoral amputation: a 5-year follow-up study. J Bone Joint Surg Am. 2020;102(15):1329–35.
49. Ontario H. Osseointegrated prosthetic implants for people with lower-limb amputation: a health technology assessment. Ont Health Technol Assess Ser. 2019;19(7):1–126.
50. Atallah R, Leijendekkers RA, Hoogeboom TJ, Frolke JP. Complications of bone-anchored prostheses for individuals with an extremity amputation: a systematic review. PLoS One. 2018;13(8):e0201821.
51. Matthews DJ, Arastu M, Uden M, Sullivan JP, Bolsakova K, Robinson K, et al. UK trial of the osseointegrated prosthesis for the rehabilitation for amputees: 1995-2018. Prosthetics Orthot Int. 2019;43(1):112–22.

Working in Resource-Challenged Environments

21

Scott C. Nelson and Philip K. McClure

Abbreviations

CBC	Complete blood count
EBV	Estimated blood volume
EtO	Ethylene oxide
FDA	Federal Drug Administration
HCT_f	Final hematocrit
HCT_i	Initial hematocrit
HINARI	Health InterNetwork Access to Research Initiative
MABL	Maximum allowable blood loss
RPM	Revolutions per minute
SIGN	Surgical Implant Generation Network
SUDs	Single-use devices
TSF	Taylor spatial frame
UN	United Nations
US	United States
WHO	World Health Organization

Introduction

Due to the considerable responsibility that we as pediatric limb deformity surgeons have to our patients and their families, we should never compromise our surgical principles based on the circumstances or location in which we perform operations. The techniques outlined throughout this book have applicability to every part of the world and thus will not be rewritten in this chapter. The limited resource environment presents some unique challenges which often create the need for improvisation and innovation, but this must not be allowed to compromise results. Indications and surgical techniques may vary based on the type and severity of limb deformities being treated, but surgical principles remain the same, independent of geographic location.

The global demand for limb deformity correction continues to expand. The potential reasons for increasing prevalence of congenital, post-traumatic, and post-infectious limb deformities in resource-limited locations include the following: lack of environmental regulation (teratogenic pollutants in the air, soil, and water), lack of education, urbanization, transportation-related injuries, natural disaster, lack of prenatal care, consanguineous relationships, and limited access to health care. As globalization, communication, and technology increase, so do our opportunities for treatment. Possibilities for education, development of international relationships, and ultimately enhanced patient care are greater than ever before. The world population is growing fastest in resource-limited environments where children account for a greater portion of the population than in developed countries. The population on this planet is now over eight billion people—more than double what it was in the 1970s and quadruple what it was in the 1930s. Income disparity between wealthy and poor also continues to increase (Table 21.1) [1, 2].

S. C. Nelson (✉)
Department of Orthopaedic Surgery, Loma Linda University School of Medicine, Loma Linda, CA, USA
e-mail: scnelson@llu.edu

P. K. McClure
International Center for Limb Lengthening, Rubin Institute for Advanced Orthopedics, Sinai Hospital of Baltimore, Baltimore, MD, USA

Table 21.1 Relative wealth ratio between nations in the upper and lower percentiles of economic prosperity showing a severely progressive disparity between the richest 20% and poorest 20% of countries in the world

Year	Wealth disparity
1820	3:1
1913	11:1
1950	35:1
2002	75:1

Worldwide healthcare expenditures continue to increase, as does disparity in spending. Per capita healthcare expenditures vary from a high of $10,623.85 in the United States to $18.51 in the Democratic Republic of the Congo. Within the Northern Hemisphere, Haiti has the lowest spending per capita at $64.25 [3]. In the United States and in other developed countries, the primary concern is toward the medical care of the aging population. Although the average age is also increasing in most low- and middle-income countries, the 0- to 14-year age group still accounts for a much greater proportion of the population than in high-income countries [4].

A primary objective of all physicians remains "first, do no harm." This phrase takes on additional meaning when practicing out of the surgeon's home environment. This ethos obviously includes the patients, but should also include the local infrastructure and environment. Few things can sabotage an otherwise successful mission more significantly than unintended collateral damage. A prime example involved UN forces in Haiti, which introduced cholera and untold suffering due to poor planning and execution [5–7].

As pediatric limb deformity surgeons, there is an increasing urgency to engage in service. International relationships and mutual understanding between healthcare providers around the world are necessary to build sustainable programs that will best be able to serve the needs of children with limb deformities. This chapter is written both for surgeons wishing to provide humanitarian service in foreign countries as well as practicing surgeons who are citizens of countries with limited resources.

Initial Steps: Selecting a Partnership

National and international collaboration between surgeons can be a rewarding experience, both for the host and visiting surgeons, and in the end, patient care is improved. Operating together with colleagues and other surgeons is a unique benefit of doing humanitarian work. Every opportunity to share knowledge and techniques with others should be sought, as it provides an opportunity for learning and expanding our ideas.

Good communication is essential to developing a working relationship between surgeons. This starts long before any planned time together and continues long afterward. In the era of electronic communication, it is now easy to do remote preoperative planning and provide consultation in the follow-up period. Personal preparation as well as preparation of material and supply needs can be optimized by detailed communication.

Commit to a Program

As limb deformity surgeons, we will be much more effective if we make a long-term commitment to a program in a resource-limited environment rather than making first-time visits to a wide variety of different locations. With repeat visits to a specific location, expectations are established, relationships exist, communication is simplified, and work can be done more effectively. Also, the value of long-term follow-up should be emphasized, both for the patient and for the surgeon. The quest for exploration and adventure is always intriguing and may be appropriate in certain situations. However, this should not be the motivating factor as such notions may dilute the quality and quantity of patient care.

Great Ways Volunteers Can Make a Positive Impact

1. Go primarily with a desire to learn and secondarily a willingness to teach. Inquire about local ways of doing things, learn about available equipment and supplies, and ask lots of questions. A humble attitude will build relationships and everyone will benefit.
2. Clearly communicate your team's capabilities and interests to the hosting surgeon and facility in the early phases of planning.
3. Understand that your brief trip is likely only one of a continuous flow of volunteers for the host. The nurses and staff may not be enthusiastic about operating late every night and getting as many cases done as possible. Situations vary, and this may not be a mistake in all situations. However, relationships should be ultimately prioritized over pure production. As much as it pains the volunteer surgeon to leave behind a child with a deformity that could be corrected, it is sometimes best deferred to a more favorable time for the team and local staff.
4. Use materials and supplies sparingly. Opening multiple packs of sutures, extra gloves, and other materials that may not be essential to the operation is wasteful and may be offensive to the local staff. Many of these items that we take for granted in our own countries are in short supply and are used very sparingly. Even if they are materials brought by yourself, it is best to respect the use of supplies with the local standard of discrimination since these items can be saved and used for future cases.
5. Donating equipment and supplies is greatly appreciated in resource-depleted hospitals. Financial donations are often helpful but should be discussed specifically. Patient volume is often increased as are overhead costs for the

hospital; as a result, volunteers coming to do charity work can be a financial burden on the hosting institution. It is wonderful if the hosting institution can afford to provide transportation, food, and lodging, but in many situations they simply do not have the resources to do this and the mature volunteer should realize that it is often necessary to help with these expenses.

Host Responsibilities

1. Be responsive to pre- and post-trip communications. Even in the era of modern communication, our lives are busy and sometimes important emails and phone messages unfortunately go unanswered.
2. Have patients prepared and available for surgery. Hosts should understand that a visiting surgical team has likely sacrificed thousands of dollars of lost income to come and do charity work. It can be very frustrating if controllable factors have not been appropriately managed to make the most of the trip. Preoperative evaluation for anemia and other endemic diseases is often needed; the visiting team may be unaware of these considerations.
3. Know the capabilities of the visiting group and avoid planning operations that are not appropriate for the skills of the volunteers. Adequate pre-trip communication and/or long-term relationships are invaluable.
4. Make sure that equipment is organized and in as best working condition possible. This is a key factor for assuring the highest quality surgery possible. If equipment and materials exist, then it is important to know where they are at the moment they are needed. If essential stock is lacking, this can be communicated ahead of time to the visiting teams who often have access to the needed items.

Understand Potential Repercussions of Good Work

Human needs sometimes may call for you to help in a situation where you are needed but not wanted. Our acts of charity can be of great benefit but also can have secondary repercussions. For example, how does a local pharmacist feel when foreigners bring a box of free medications to distribute and now his income is undermined? How do the surgeons across town feel when an organization offers free surgery to patients potentially capable of paying? How does a hosting hospital recuperate costs from taking care of an increased quantity of nonpaying patients? Although licensing regulations for physicians and import taxes on gifts in kind are often annoying and have been subject to corrupt government processes, it should be understood that the basis behind this is to protect the economic infrastructure of the medical community. There are no easy solutions to these challenges as the needs of the people are often dire and the barriers can seem insurmountable. An important concept to keep in mind when navigating these issues is to go with the idea that you are helping more than just individual patients. Go with the idea that you are going to help a doctor, an institution, a medical community, and a country in addition to the individual patient. Remember: we are all committed to "first, do no harm."

Keep Your Motives Pure

There are many reasons to do charity work. Travel, adventure, learning, publicity, and a feeling of well-being are some reasons that may motivate surgeons to volunteer, but should be secondary to the sincere desire to provide a needed service in the most effective way. Is it OK to have ulterior motives as long as we are doing good work and people are getting helped? This is similar to having a conflict of interest with a particular implant company or letting personal economics affect your surgical decision-making. Yes, patients can still be helped in a good way, but this can lead to poor judgment and places the priority on benefitting yourself more than the patient. Beware of these secondary gains, and know their presence can reduce your impact.

Credentialing and Liability

Credentialing and medico-legal concerns vary widely around the globe. Often, the credentialing process is rather simple or does not exist at all, but other times it can be quite burdensome. Although it can be liberating to practice in environments where bureaucracy and liability issues do not take precedence over patient care, this freedom should not be used carelessly. Proper communication and doing what is right for the patient are guiding principles. A surgeon should not work beyond his expertise and/or perform procedures that he is not licensed to do in his home country. As a guest surgeon, respecting the credentialing rules of a host institution and country is important. Many resource-limited countries have licensing provisions for surgeons coming for short periods of time to do charity work. The general motive of the licensing entity in these countries is to protect the economic viability of local surgeons and make sure that there is a minimum standard of quality among foreign healthcare workers.

Medico-legal issues are usually less concerning outside of North America. Nonetheless, a few precautions are warranted. The issues vary greatly depending on the cultural norms, types of patients being treated, and organizational affiliations. Most legitimate organizations can provide some information on the subject and have provisions in place to protect volunteer surgeons. Many times, in these environments it is the hospital or international organization rather than the individual surgeon that carries the burden of malpractice. However, one unique and potentially serious issue is the situation of a US surgeon operating on a US citizen in another country. There have been reports of such cases being litigated in the US court system.

Aside from the subject of formal litigation, disgruntled patients often access social media. This provides an easy and cost-free way to damage the reputations of doctors and institutions. Whether the allegations are perceived or real, these types of patients can do significant damage. In any part of the world, maintaining good communication with patients can help to sustain a strong reputation and prevent misunderstandings and negative consequences.

Operative Challenges: Improvise, Don't Compromise

Indications

In general, operative indications should follow the same basic principles in any part of the world. This involves evaluating whether or not the benefits outweigh the risks. As circumstances vary, so does the relative relationship between benefit and risk. Some of the most difficult questions center around how to balance quality in a scenario where resources are limited. In general, each patient needs to be looked at as an individual and efforts should be made to obtain the necessary equipment and expertise to do the highest quality operation possible. The principles "do it right or don't do it at all" and "something is better than nothing" should both be taken into consideration and adapted for the situation. It is the authors' strong preference to respect the philosophy of not doing an operation unless it can be done well.

Economics have to be considered but should not be the most important factor. Ironically, in resource-challenged environments the re-use of costly hexapod fixators can provide opportunity for treatment that might otherwise be cost prohibitive in countries like the United States where re-use may not be an option. When third-party payors are not scrutinizing the cost of components, additional fixator parts can be added without regard to cost. External fixators are a renewable resource in many resource-challenged environments and lighten the burdens of implant cost and supply chain issues. Operating room time is also significantly less expensive in these environments which makes it easy to take patients back to the operating room to adjust fixators, manipulate joints, or perform other needed procedures.

The indications for limb salvage versus amputation make for complex decisions even in our home country where we understand the economics and many of the cultural issues. The relative importance of functional outcome, cultural views, and cost of reconstructive procedures versus cost of lifetime prosthetic maintenance take a paradigm shift and differ greatly from country to country depending on the availability of prosthetic services. Often, the expectation of performance is different in less developed environments. In economically privileged countries, the debate centers on what option is best for high performance in sports and long-distance running. In resource-limited environments, difficulty with prosthetic access and care may be a major obstacle, and the preservation of a limb is often preferable even if high demand activities will be adversely affected. The surgeon must consider the distinct possibility that a prosthetic will never be obtained, or that the first may be the last and only. A stiff plantigrade limb is useful, whereas multiple attempts to salvage a painful, unstable, or severely deformed limb usually are not justified. Patients must be included in this decision-making process, as well as a translator if necessary.

In a situation where fluoroscopy is not available, certain procedures are impossible to perform. Indications may change based on whether or not fluoroscopy may be available in the near future or at another accessible location. Compensation for a lack of fluoroscopy can be achieved by making larger incisions and/or performing more traditional operations, such as open instead of closed epiphysiodeses. Performing open approaches to the hip allows visualization of the femoral head and neck for cases that could otherwise be done in a more minimally invasive fashion if fluoroscopy were available.

Perioperative and Anesthetic Considerations

Maintaining a wide safety margin in areas where an extensive infrastructure does not exist can be difficult. This calls for a careful preoperative evaluation, additional intraoperative precautions, and careful postoperative vigilance.

Preoperative evaluation should be done by both the surgeon and anesthesia staff. Anemia can be common in areas where nutritional deficiencies and parasitic diseases are endemic. Even when preoperative laboratory evaluations are not routinely indicated in first-world settings, it may be prudent to do additional work-up in other settings. Sometimes, local bureaucracy requires seemingly unnecessary testing despite limited resources which must be respected by volunteer staff. There are several point of care devices which can be extremely helpful in these situations. The HemoCue device (HemoCue AB, Ängelholm, Sweden) (Fig. 21.1a) is a relatively inexpensive piece of equipment and is an efficient and cost-effective way to evaluate preoperative hemoglobin levels. The i-STAT (Abbott Laboratories, Abbott Park, IL) (Fig. 21.1b) can perform a variety of tests including CBC, chemistry panels, and blood gases.

Even if it does not involve a piece of paper, informed consent should always be obtained. It is important to communicate the plan of the procedure and possible risks and complications to patients, family members, and local staff. This is especially important for ablative procedures, complex surgery that involves considerable risk, and for procedures that involve gradual corrections and limb lengthening which require additional patient and family commitment.

Intra-operative blood loss needs to be minimized and carefully assessed. The following formula can be used to calculate the maximum allowable blood loss (MABL):

$$MABL = EBV \times (HCT_i - HCT_f / HCT_f)$$

$$EBV - \text{Estimated blood volume} \left[\text{average blood volume} (mL/kg) \times \text{weight} (kg) \right]$$

Average blood volume
- Neonates 85 mL/kg
- Infants 80 mL/kg
- Adult men 75 mL/kg
- Adult women 65 mL/kg

HCT_i – Initial hematocrit

HCT_f – Final hematocrit (lowest acceptable at end of operation)

A healthy patient with a normal starting hematocrit can usually tolerate an acute loss of one-third of their blood volume. If you consider that a total EBV is approximately 70 mL/kg (slightly more in infants and less in adult females), then a short way to estimate MABL is to divide 70 mL/kg by 3, which is just over 20 mL/kg. **Most patients who are healthy and have normal starting hemoglobin will tolerate 20 mL/kg blood loss without needing transfusion.** In many situations, blood may not be available and when it is, it may take days to obtain. Thus, a wide margin of safety regarding surgical blood loss is warranted and one must always be prepared for the worst possible scenario.

By using these calculations, objective and well-informed decisions can be made regarding performing multiple procedures in one operation versus staging procedures to decrease blood loss. This is especially applicable to children with significant deformities in bilateral lower extremities such as osteogenesis imperfecta, skeletal dysplasias, and rickets. Using the Esmarch bandage as a sterile tourniquet is a safe and effective method of controlling blood loss. Care must be taken to apply it as a wide band, tight enough to avoid a venous tourniquet but not overly tight to cause bruising or injury. Any time an Esmarch is used, an audible alarm is set to avoid inadvertently leaving it in place beyond 2 h and risking irreversible injury.

Pharmaceutical minimization of blood loss can be sought using tranexamic acid, which has been heavily studied in total joint arthroplasty. Recently, oral administration has been shown to be comparable to intravenous administration in spine surgery [8]. Extrapolation of these data to the care of patients undergoing deformity correction seems reasonable. Intravenous administration has been shown to reduce blood loss in high tibial osteotomies and reduce transfusion rates in pelvic osteotomy [9, 10]. Oral tranexamic acid is both affordable and easily transported, making it an ideal medication for use in resource-limited environments.

The WHO has created a Surgical Safety Checklist (Fig. 21.2) in the interest of reducing surgical deaths and operative morbidity. This is not meant to be a regulatory document, but rather a guide to reinforce accepted principles of surgical safety and to promote teamwork and communication. The principles outlined here are basic elements for performing safe operations and should be implemented in every surgical venue.

Post-operative management varies widely in different parts of the world. In North America, pain is said to be the

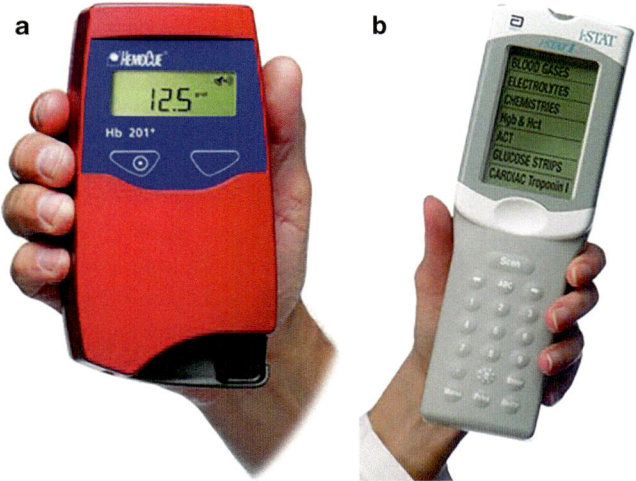

Fig. 21.1 (a) HemoCue. [With permissions from HemoCue America] (b) I-STAT. [With permissions from Abbott Point of Care]

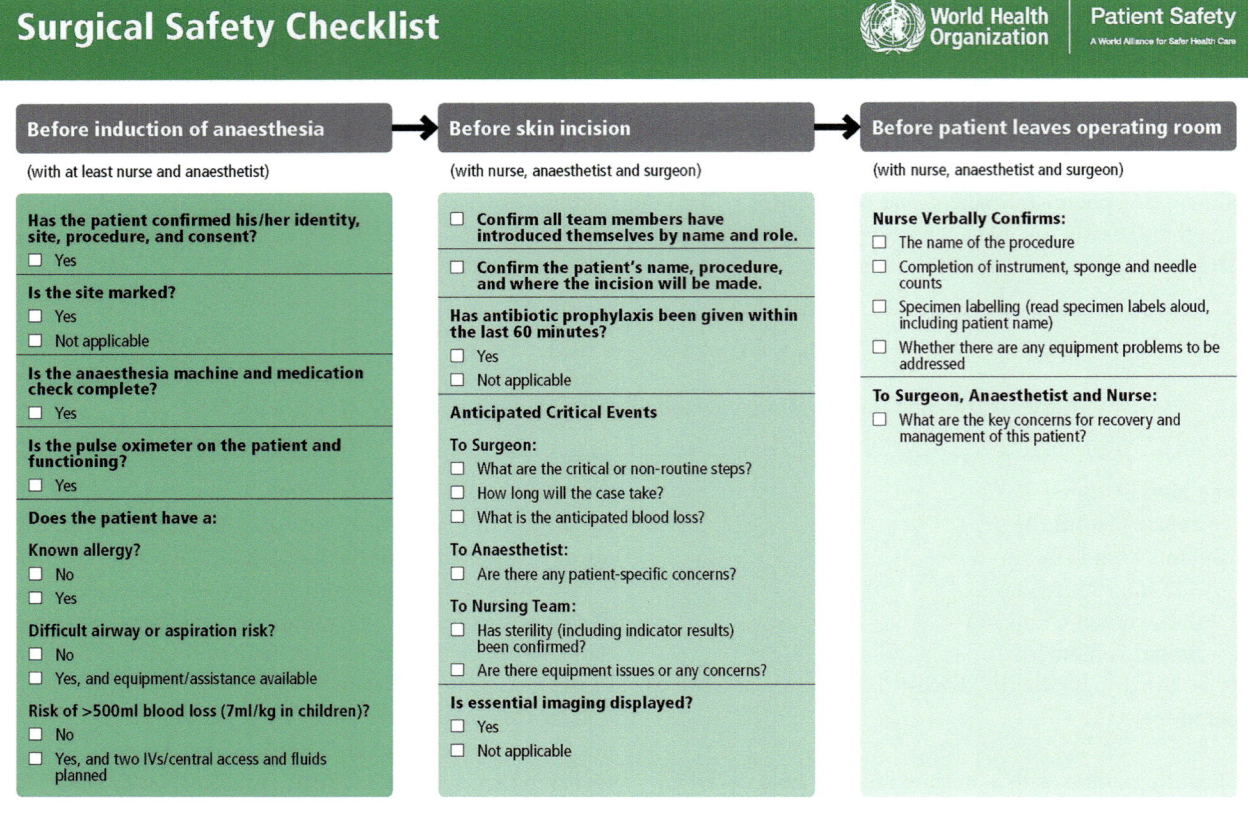

Fig. 21.2 WHO Surgical Safety Checklist. Available at http://www.who.int/patientsafety/safesurgery/en. Copyright World Health Organization, 2008, all rights reserved

fifth vital sign and there is a belief that less is always better than more. When specifically considering patient safety, this is actually not the case, especially in locations where patient monitoring may not be adequate, nurses may not be well-trained in resuscitation, or the code cart is missing or not well stocked. Until an entire infrastructure can be created to remedy these issues, some level of discomfort may be necessary to prioritize patient safety. Fortunately, in these environments patients expect that major surgery will involve some pain and they are much more tolerant of it. As surgeons working in this environment, we also need to be trained and updated on resuscitation credentials as we cannot always depend on those around us to do the task.

Sterility

Surgeons are not typically involved in the process of sterilization but do hold the ultimate responsibility for patient outcomes; thus, it is helpful to have a knowledge of the basics and know the options available in resource-challenged settings. For something to be considered sterile with autoclave processing, it must reach 121 °C/250 °F with a pressure of 15 psi/100 kPa for 15 min. Longer times (up to 2 h) or higher temperatures are needed to completely eradicate certain types of biofilms [11]. Thorough mechanical washing of instruments to reduce bio burden prior is important for effective sterilization. Indicators are available for heat and gas sterilization methods and should be used routinely. They are an easy and compact addition to the list of essential surgical materials that can be taken on a trip. This can be especially important in situations where aging autoclaves and maintenance schedules may not be strictly followed [12]. If a reliable autoclave is not available, some portable stovetop units can be acquired and their cost is not prohibitive (Fig. 21.3). These units come in various sizes and can hold a variety of surgical instruments; larger sizes can accommodate larger instruments and implants but are not able to contain full-size instrument trays. Dry heat sterilization is another valid method and is no more complicated than baking in an oven. It requires higher temperatures and longer exposure times because heat transfer is 12 times slower with hot air than steam at 121 °C. Heat transfer is also affected by the wrapping and packaging of instruments.

Cidex (Johnson & Johnson, New Brunswick, NJ) is a disinfectant that comes in three different variations: Cidex

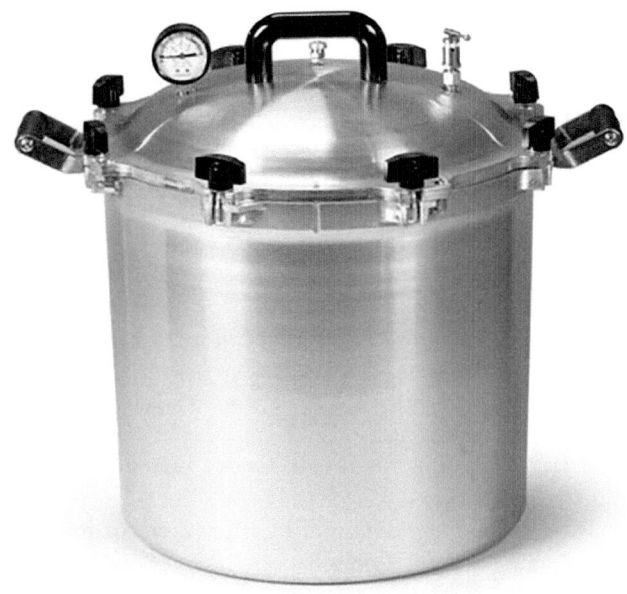

Fig. 21.3 All-American stovetop sterilizer autoclave. [With permissions from Wisconsin Aluminum Foundry]

14-Day (glutaraldehyde), Cidex Plus 28-Day (glutaraldehyde), and Cidex OPA (ortho-phthalaldehyde). These provide a fast and effective method of sterilization for a wide variety of instruments, external fixator parts, et cetera. It can be useful for heat-sensitive materials that are not destroyed by submersion. Cidex is bactericidal, fungicidal, tuberculocidal, and sporicidal when used appropriately. Although it can be quite effective, it is very sensitive to dilution, storage methods, expiration dates, and duration of use [13]. Similar to opening a carton of milk, it has an expiration date and a limited period of use once opened and poured into a sterilization tray. Due to this variability, it must not be used indiscriminately and we do not use it for implant sterilization. There are indicator strips available which can be helpful to prove efficacy of sterilization.

Ethylene oxide (EtO), known by the trade name Anprolene (Andersen Sterilizers, Haw River, NC), is especially useful for sterilizing heat-sensitive materials. EtO is considered a gold standard for high-level sterilization of implants. It is a highly toxic and explosive gas which was used for making bombs in World War II. It can provide safe and effective sterilization of heat-sensitive materials such as gowns, drapes, gloves, Esmarch bandages, Ioban drapes (3M, Saint Paul, MN), cautery pencils, suction tubing, bulb syringes, suture packs (nylon, Monocryl [Ethicon, Raritan, NJ], Vicryl [Ethicon]), and electronic devices (drill, camera, et cetera). Practically, any item (apart from food, drugs, and liquids) can be sterilized with EtO. There are some commercially available processing units that provide ventilation pumps, purge pumps, aeration, and monitors that track cycle progress. Special plastic sterilization bags and EtO ampules are marketed to be used with these units. For emergencies and stark conditions, these plastic sterilization bags and ampules can be used safely without the processing units if appropriate precautions are taken.

Operating Room Set Up

Optimizing every controllable factor includes arranging the operating room furnishings before an operation for it to proceed as smoothly as possible. Many operating rooms are small. In order to comfortably operate and prevent people from contaminating the field, it is important to remove all nonessential pieces of equipment from the room and arrange the remaining furnishings in an ideal position to work effectively. Difficult operations in difficult circumstances become unnecessarily more difficult when modifiable factors are not idealized. Avoid this by preparing the proper instruments, organizing them on an adequately sized table, positioning a C-arm (if available) and other equipment appropriately, assuring adequate lighting or a headlamp is in available and the patient is well positioned and draped. Additional efforts on the part of the surgeon are often necessary when working in unfamiliar settings where a team may not be familiar with these details.

Operating room heating, ventilation, and air conditioning (HVAC) systems have an important role in minimizing airborne bacterial colony-forming units [14]. These systems are complex, and the requirements in modern settings are difficult to replicate in limited resource settings. However, some parameters can be controlled by simple means. Operating room temperature is ideally 68–75 °F (20–24 °C) with relative humidity 20–60%. Stringent standards in North America require 20 room air exchanges per hour with at least four air exchanges of outdoor air. In addition, ventilation is calibrated to create positive pressure which helps prevent airborne particulate from entering the room. Sophisticated systems are not practical in limited resource settings, but some simple measures can be taken to emulate the principles. This may include the use of portable HEPA (high-efficiency particulate air) filters which can theoretically remove 99.97% of dust, pollen, mold, and bacteria down to 0.3 μm. If properly positioned, they can potentially create some positive pressure and bring in some outside air.

In environments where cleaning standards may be lacking, it is preferable to do infected cases at the end of the day in a separate room designated for infections. For infected cases, negative pressure rooms are ideal and can be created by placing an exhaust fan that vents to the outside. This concept is used for isolation rooms in modern hospitals and effectively isolates the room from adjacent indoor areas.

It is essential that equipment is well organized, cleaned, and maintained. It is unfortunate when available instruments, materials, or implants are either overlooked or not prepared for use when needed. Often, the burden of making sure the proper equipment is prepared for surgery falls on the surgeon. It is also helpful to have one or more back-up plans should the operation take a different direction than anticipated. This sometimes requires spending extensive amounts of time in the storage room organizing equipment and preparing for cases.

Performing Operations in Resource-Challenged Environments

The ability to provide post-operative care and manage potential complications must be considered when planning operations. Limb lengthening surgery, gradual corrections, and management of computer-programmed hexapod fixators are examples of cases that may present challenges for the local infrastructure if the surgeon is not physically available. Highly invasive operations with potential medical complications that the local infrastructure is not prepared to deal with could be disastrous. In the scenario of short-term trips, it is usually best to perform the larger cases earlier in the week.

Internal vs. External Fixation in Resource-Challenged Environments

Acute correction of deformities provides a "one and done" operation which is often preferable over the more diligent follow-up needed for gradual corrections. Ways to safely use internal fixation with acute corrections should always be explored. However, in resource-challenged settings there are some distinct advantages of using external fixation with either acute or gradual corrections.

Benefits of internal fixation
- Less post-operative maintenance necessary
- No pin site infections and less risk of late osteomyelitis
- Less soft tissue irritation allowing easier range of motion
- May result in earlier return to function
- Better for treatment for femoral deformities due to less soft tissue concerns
- Often does not need to be removed

Benefits of external fixation
- Can be applied with minimal incisions and blood loss
- When equipment can be re-used:
  - Inventory is more easily maintained
  - Expenses are minimized
- Enables gradual corrections, lengthening or bone transport in appropriate situations
- Facilitates intentional displacement of osteotomies that are performed away from the apex of deformity
- Post-operative alignment can be more easily adjusted

Another option is to consider the use of Steinmann pins or K-wires for fixation. This is a very economical approach to osteotomy fixation. In extreme situations, bicycle or motorcycle spokes have been sharpened with a small bench grinder, sterilized, and used for fixation. In addition to the biological benefits for making osteotomies in metaphyseal bone, the larger surface area provides more stability and also facilitates stable pin/wire fixation methods. These can be buried under the skin if there is a high risk of infection, but this obligates another procedure for removal. If left in a percutaneous position, a large portion of wire (2 cm or more for most situations) should be left outside the skin and generously bent in order to prevent migration and an otherwise unnecessary return trip to the operating room.

Re-use of Implants and External Fixation Components

The re-use of implants (including plates, screws, intramedullary rods, and bone fixation half pins) is not something that can be universally recommended due to variability in implant strength, size, material, and variability in the magnitude of stress as well as number of cycles to which these are subjected. Catastrophic failure can occur when cyclic stresses that exceed the endurance limit of a metal are applied to an implant over a given amount of time. The endurance limit is an amplitude of stress below which it appears that even with an indefinitely large number of loading cycles failure will not occur. The endurance limit is usually about half of the ultimate tensile strength of an implant, unless it is notched, which can significantly decrease the endurance limit. Some metals such as aluminum do not have an endurance limit, and even small amounts of cyclic stress will eventually cause failure. Titanium and the ferrous alloys like stainless steel are materials that *do* have an endurance limit, meaning that small amplitude (below endurance limit) loading cycles theoretically will not cause failure. Practically speaking, it is not possible to know the magnitude of stress and number of cycles to which an implant has been subjected nor is it possible to visually decipher this with the naked eye. Ultimately, the risks and benefits of re-using an implant must be left up to the judgment of the surgeon. If an implant is re-used, it is advisable to carefully examine it, and consider using more robust constructs to decrease the amount of stress on an implant thus increasing the number of cycles to failure.

Using common sense and appropriate reprocessing methods, most implants can be re-used without complication.

The implications of re-using external fixators in resource-limited environments are different from North America due to perceptions and medico-legal issues. The real question is as follows: What is safe and effective for the patient? In parts of Europe (where resources are not severely limited) and in developing countries, fixators are re-used on a regular basis. In the United States, many external fixators are labeled "single-use only." Due to an interest in cost containment and social responsibility, many institutions in North America have sought ways to reprocess single-use devices (SUDs). The Federal Drug Administration (FDA) has thus classified SUDs into three categories: noncritical risk (level 1), semi-critical risk (level 2), and critical risk (level 3) [15]. The re-use of fixator clamps and bars that do not penetrate the skin is considered level 1 SUDs by the FDA. There are approved reprocessing protocols for these devices. They include cleaning with various solutions to remove all biologic material, dismantling the device, inspection of components for defects or fatigue cracks (usually with magnification or microscope), and re-sterilization.

Biomechanical effects of cyclic loading and patient outcomes with the re-use of fixators have been studied. Matsuura et al. report the effects of various magnitude and quantity of load cycles on the EBI Dynafix external fixator [16]. They loaded one group with 100–450 N of compressive force for three million load cycles to simulate three uses of the device. They found that 17% of initial stiffness was lost and that some fatigue cracks began to develop at three million cycles. Another group was subjected to higher loads, and it was found that fatigue of the device occurred much sooner. Their advice is that external fixators should only be re-used a limited number of times and should be carefully inspected. Fixators with more articulating parts are more prone to failure than simple rods and rings. Also, fixators that are applied to large patients, highly active patients, and fixators that have been left in place for prolonged periods of time have a higher risk of failure vs. those applied for damage control orthopedics and have only been left in place for a few days or weeks. Several clinical studies have been published showing no loosening of components, no loss of fixation, no increase in pin site infections, and no mechanical failures when re-using fixators [17, 18]. Even if there is a failure of an external fixation device, it can usually be resolved with noninvasive and frequently non-operative means.

In spite of these results, commentaries have been published against the re-use of external fixation devices which are not scientifically based, do not apply to limited resource environments and add fuel to medico-legal fears [19]. **The re-use of external fixators can be safely done if the appropriate inspection and reprocessing methods are implemented.**

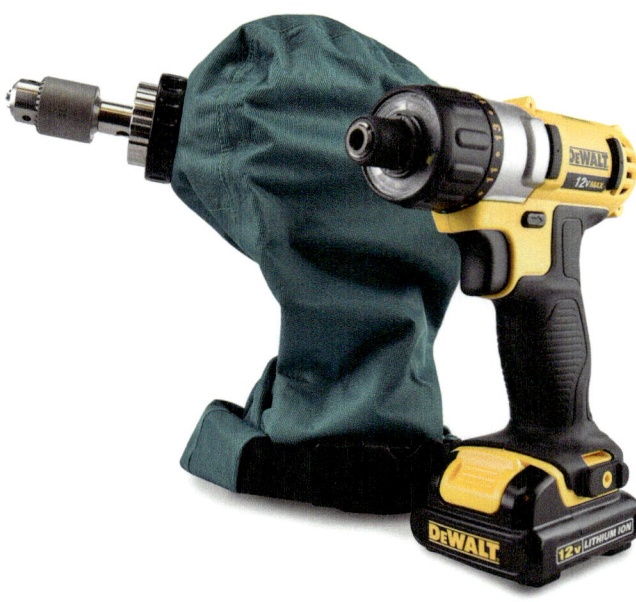

Fig. 21.4 12v cordless variable speed drill with cover and surgical chuck

Cordless Power

Many orthopedic operations require a power drill. In limited resource environments, the prohibitive costs of the systems that are on the market have led to the development of safe and effective alternatives. The Dewalt 12v variable speed cordless drill (Leola, PA) pictured in Fig. 21.4 runs at up to 1050 RPM (revolutions per minute). The torque and velocity are similar to surgical grade orthopedic power systems. Drills that function at RPMs above 1500 in general are not appropriate for orthopedics as they create excessive heat and can cause osteonecrosis. The stainless steel surgical chuck can withstand the demands of harsh solutions and repeated cycles of steam sterilization. It is integrated into an impervious cover that also can be autoclaved. Arbutus Medical (Vancouver, Canada) also offers a variety of similar products including oscillating saws and reamers. Theoretically, any drill or hardware store power tool could be made sterile using EtO and thus not require special covers and surgical grade chucks; however, fluids and biomaterials can easily enter vent holes and damage the internal components of the drill. In addition, hardware store quality drill chucks used in this fashion do not stand up to the rigors required for appropriate cleaning and reprocessing.

Post-operative Care

Documentation standards are often relaxed in places that do not have a lot of medico-legal concerns. Nonetheless, writing clear orders, an operative note with all significant aspects of the operation including implants used, and some clear post-operative instructions is essential. We have found it helpful to use a pre-made form for a detailed post-operative plan that includes dates of follow-up, physical therapy instructions, casting, dressing, and suture removal instructions as well as any specific needs such as antibiotics (Fig. 21.5). If you are not likely to be present at the time of follow-up, it is even more important to leave detailed instructions and contact information that can be easily understood by local staff. Most importantly, the patient must be able to easily access someone who is knowledgeable of the operation and capable of managing any possible complications. Thankfully, the ease and accessibility of international communication allows us to follow-up remotely in ways that were not previously possible.

Protocole Opératoire/Operative Note

Nom/Last Name	Prénom/First Name	Date/Date:
Numéro de Dossier/Medical Record #:	Date de Naissance/Date of Birth:	Age/Age:
Diagnostique/Diagnosis:		
Trouvailles opératoires/Operative Findings:		
Chirugien/Asistant(e)/Surgeon/Assistant(s):		
Anestésie/Anesthesia:		
Protocole/Title of Operation		
Description/Description:		
	Perte de sang/EBL: _____	
Etat post opératoire/Post Operative Condition:	Spécimen/Specimen(s)	

Signature: _____

Plan Post opératoire: Voir au verso de cette page/See other side for post operative plan

Fig. 21.5 Bilingual operative note with post-operative plan

POST OP PLAN

☐ SORTIE MÊME JOUR QUE LA CHIRURGIE/DISCHARGE SAME DAY OF SURGERY

☐ SUIVI PAR LE MÉDECIN/FOLLOW UP APPOINTMENT_____ (Date)

☐ ACTIVITÉS/ACTIVITIES   ☐ pas de restriction   ☐ pas d'appuis   ☐ appuis partiel
                          (no restrictions)   (non-weight-bearing)   (partial weight-bearing)

_____

☐ CHANGEMENT DE GAZES/DRESSING CHANGES _____

Instructions speciales/Special Instructions _____

_____

☐ PLÂTRE/CAST   1er plâtre/1st cast _____ (nombre de semaines/duration in weeks)

                  2eme plâtre/2nd cast _____ (nombre de semaines/duration in weeks)

                  3eme plâtre/3rd cast _____ (nombre de semaines/duration in weeks)

TOTAL DE SEMAINES DE PLÂTRE/TOTAL WEEKS IN CAST_____

☐ RETIRER SUTURES/REMOVE SUTURES _____ (# semaines après la chirurgie/# of weeks after surgery)

☐ RETIRER K-WIRE (BROCHE)/ REMOVE K-WIRE)_____ (# semaines après la chirurgie/# of weeks after surgery)

☐ INSTRUCTIONS SPÉCIALES OU NOTES/SPECIAL INSTRUCTIONS OR OTHER NOTES :

Fig. 21.5 (continued)

Other Aspects of Orthopedics in the "Wild"

There may be a certain attraction to performing difficult operations in the most austere of conditions. Perhaps, it is appropriate in certain situations, but, in general, emphasis should be placed on adhering to some minimum requirements for safely performing operations. These include running water and reliable electricity and lighting, as well as an intact operating room which provides a well-protected barrier to the outside elements. As previously discussed, safe sterilization, safe anesthesia, adherence to basic principles of sterile technique, and stable orthopedic fixation are essential. These are factors that the surgeon should have control over. Surgical risk and the difficulty of performing operations are increased when doing surgery in the "wild." Some of these factors are modifiable, and others are not. Factors such as biology, patient compliance, and limitations in available resources and personnel are largely uncontrollable. The surgeon must optimize all modifiable factors and take extra precautions to assure patient safety and stable fixation in spite of other uncontrollable risk factors. This may mean added points of fixation—extra bone pins on a fixator or more robust plating patterns than would otherwise be necessary.

Communication is often difficult, requiring extra effort to interact effectively with local staff and patients. Patience is of paramount importance, and interpreters are necessary. Pictures and drawings can be invaluable to convey concepts across linguistic barriers, just as they have merits when relating to patients who may share your language but possess zero medical knowledge. For deformity correction, anticipated results may be illustrated with the aid of paper cutouts or software such as the iPad (Apple, Cupertino, CA) application Bone Ninja (International Center for Limb Lengthening, Rubin Institute for Advanced Orthopedics, Sinai Hospital of Baltimore, Baltimore, MD) (Fig. 21.6). Sincere efforts to learn the local language are often greatly appreciated and may help to generate strong relationships and trust.

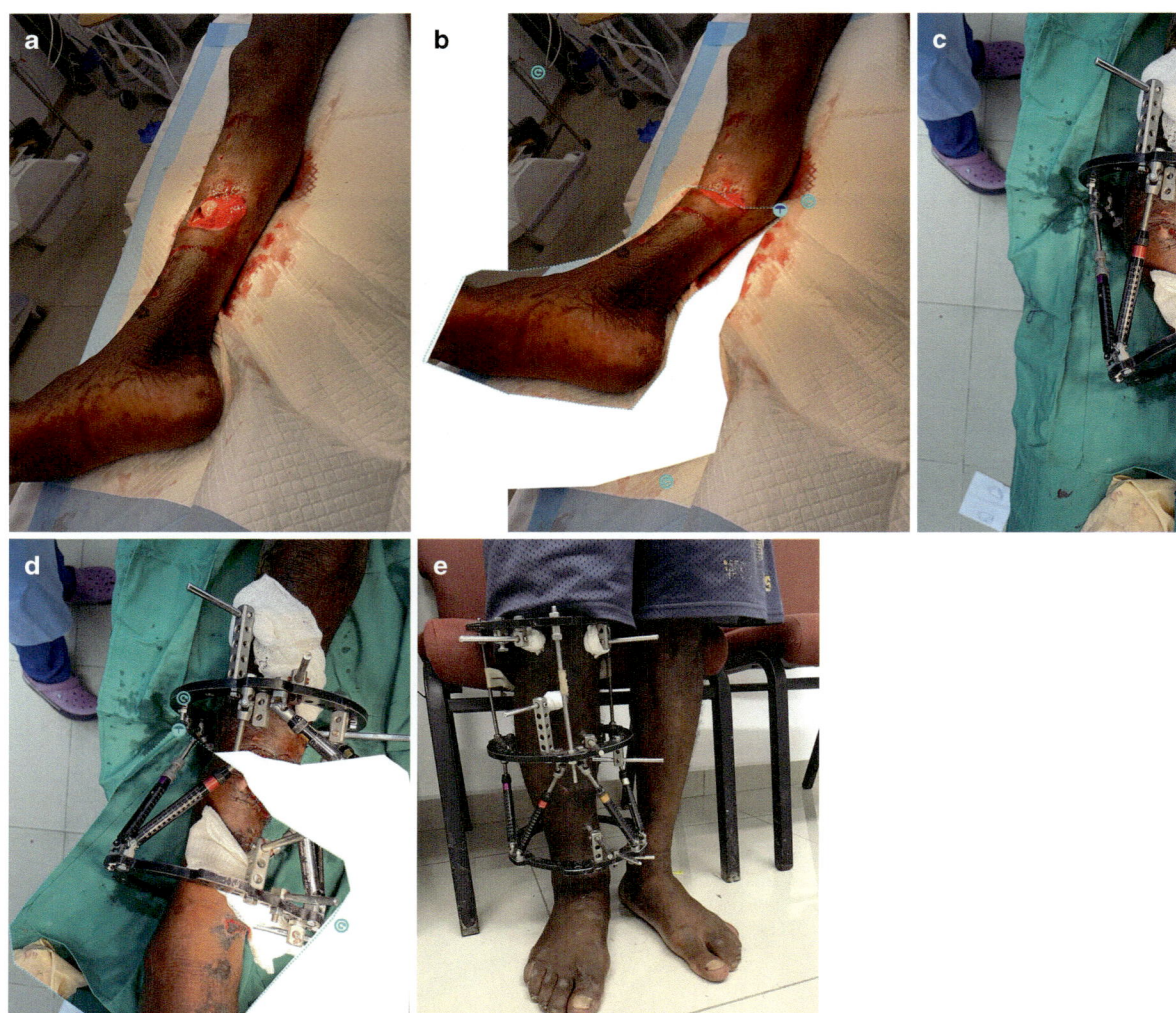

Fig. 21.6 (**a**) An open tibia fracture with soft tissue loss in a 55-year-old man. The patient was strongly against amputation, and a complex discussion regarding various reconstructive techniques was required. (**b**) Bone Ninja was used to aide in discussion with the patient through a translator to demonstrate how the wound could be closed by temporarily deforming the leg, and then restrengthened after wound healing. (**c** and **d**) Another discussion was had after placement to show him how the leg would straighten back out with the external fixator. (**e**) Restoration of alignment through correction of induced deformity 3 weeks after wound closure. Transition was made at that time to a bone transport construct to restore lost length in the setting of slow bone healing in the defect

Specific Techniques

Clubfoot

Clubfeet seen in resource-limited environments are not usually like the ones typically seen by surgeons in North America (Fig. 21.7). In many locations, the success of Ponseti casting is making the operative treatment of clubfoot a lost art. In more austere environments, severe clubfeet are often present in older children, some of whom have had prior surgery. For this reason, a review of the surgical options for clubfoot is briefly described here.

The Ponseti treatment for clubfoot has revolutionized the treatment of clubfoot around the world. The results of this treatment have been shown to be superior to previous methods of casting and/or surgery [20–22]. The most rapid corrections with Ponseti casting are seen in newborns; however, the technique continues to be effective in older children as well. When performing casting, it is important to follow all the details of the Ponseti technique to get the very best

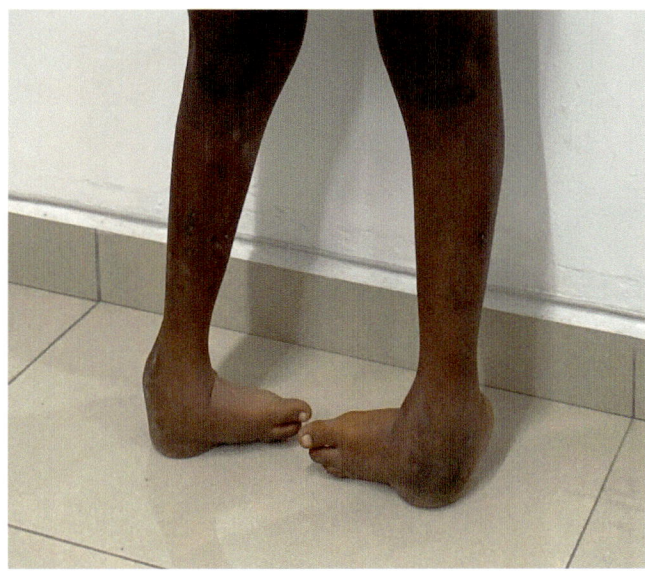

Fig. 21.7 A 16-year-old girl with severe neglected clubfeet in Haiti

results. These include supinating the forefoot to lock the metatarsal cuneiform joints in order to concentrate forces at the subluxed talonavicular joint, placing long leg casts in order to provide sufficient abduction of the forefoot, and performing percutaneous Achilles tenotomy in nearly all cases.

Neglected and recurrent clubfeet are a common cause of disability in developing countries. The stigma of this deformity often prevents those who have it from going to school, integrating into society, and having a job. In older children and adolescents, the correction of the deformity has been shown to be worthwhile for social reasons even when function and mobility may not be significantly improved [23].

The excellent results of effectively implementing the Ponseti method add complexity to surgical decision-making when patients in limited resource environments are unable to return for weekly casting, or when short-term humanitarian surgical trips do not permit the luxury of providing treatment over time. Ultimately, the best outcome for the child is what should be sought. No child has ever died because they had a clubfoot, and a poor surgical result is worse than a deformity not previously operated. Thus, immediate operative treatment may not be in the best interest of all patients. Every possible effort should be made to cast clubfeet even if an operation will ultimately be necessary. In situations where casting is logistically difficult, an accelerated program has been described where casting is done every 5 days and has been shown to give similar results to the typical 7-day protocol [24]. One-day protocols have been proposed, with reported good outcomes as well [25–27]. In the authors' opinion, this should be approached cautiously as there may be an increased risk of swelling and adverse casting events.

In cases where operations are required, casting can be a helpful preoperative adjunct to surgery. Sometimes, even just a few days of casting can improve operative results, decrease wound complications, and facilitate the ease of an operation. A hybrid approach can be taken where a minimal release (including posterior tibialis tenotomy, plantar fasciotomy, and Achilles lengthening) is combined with pre- and postoperative casting for cases where extensive casting is difficult or not practical. There is much debate about the maximum age limit for effective casting. In reality, there is no specific age at which casting becomes ineffective, although the time and materials required to correct the clubfoot deformity significantly increase with age and stiffness of the foot. This is due to progressive ossification of the foot bones. As the child ages, there will be less cartilage and less remodeling potential.

Prior to the popularization of the Ponseti method, posteromedial release was traditionally considered a standard treatment for clubfoot. In severe, recurrent, or neglected clubfoot, it is still a viable option. For children with significant adductus, posteromedial release can be combined with a lateral column shortening osteotomy (either a Lichtblau anterior calcaneal resection, calcaneal cuboid wedge resection, or calcaneal shortening osteotomy). Talus decancellation with or without posterior release is an effective way to correct residual equinus, especially in the younger population with a flat top talus. Known as the Verebelyi-Ogston procedure, it involves removing a rectangular window of cortex on the lateral talus, then curetting out the interior to collapse the dome and allow increased dorsiflexion and valgus [28]. We have used it regularly with the modification demonstrated in Fig. 21.8a–d which involves a triangular window with an additional cut starting from the superior corner of the triangle that traverses the dorsum of the talus to allow for a more complete collapse of the dome. In older children with severe deformities, triple arthrodesis is often necessary. This can be done in children as young as 8 years old, especially in bilateral cases where discrepancy in foot size is not a concern. For cases with severe cavus, a dorsal closing wedge midfoot osteotomy followed by possible posterior release can be performed. These and other options for residual deformities are outlined in Table 21.2.

The temptation to correct recurrences and residual deformity, particularly in the 5- to 12-year-old age group, needs to be weighed against expected results, risk, and recuperation time. In most cases, it is best to avoid repeated surgery to fine-tune less than perfect feet in this age group. A definitive operation like triple arthrodesis at an age closer to skeletal maturity may be less prone to recurrence. A detailed description of the options and techniques for neglected clubfeet is available in the literature [23].

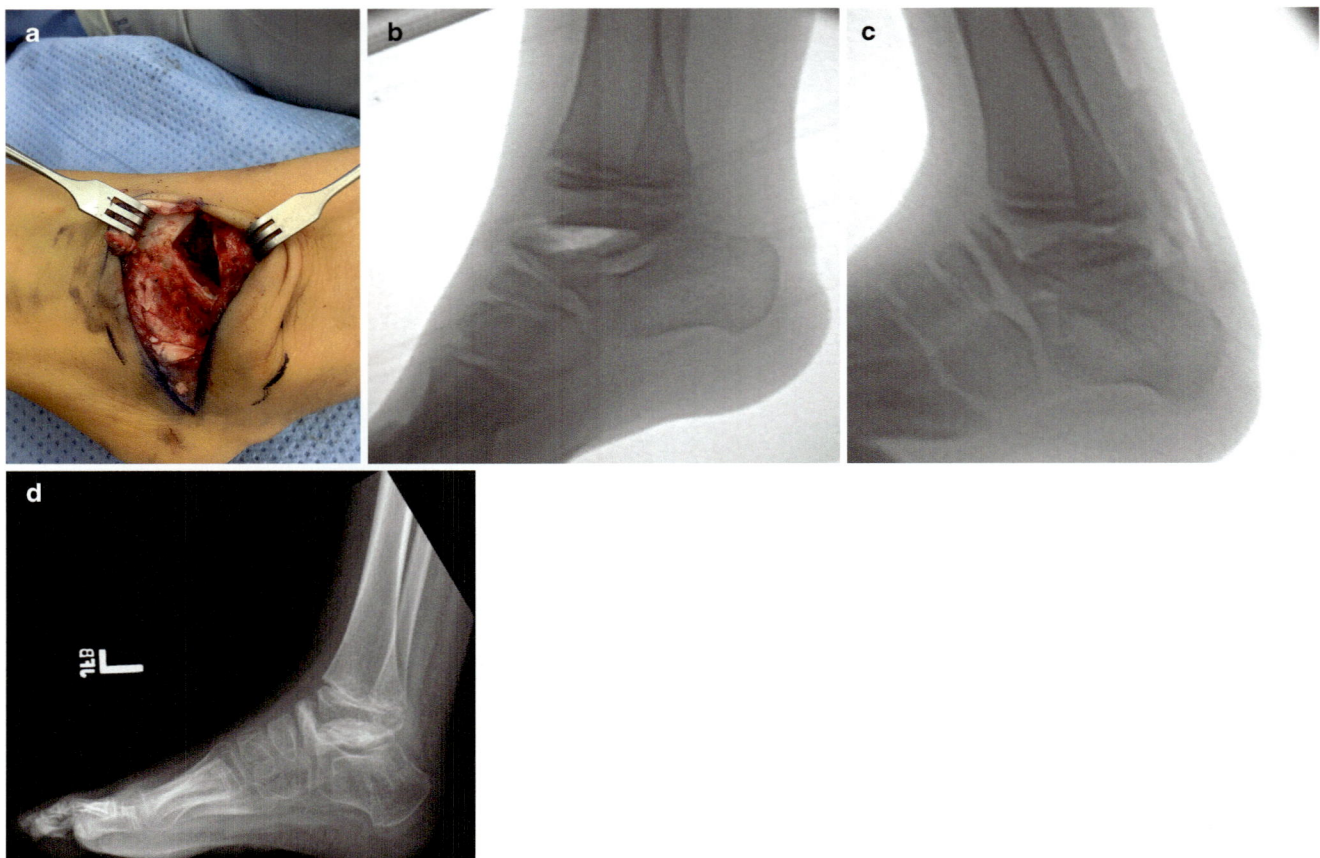

Fig. 21.8 Modified Verebelyi-Ogston talar decancellation. A triangular cortical window is removed through an Ollier incision. (**a**, **b**) At the superior corner, the dorsal cortex of the talar neck is cut in a lateral to medial direction to allow the roof to more easily and completely collapse to correct equinus. This is usually combined with a heel cord tenotomy. By removing the lateral window and leaving the cortex intact on the medial side, the varus deformity is also corrected (**c**) Three month post operative image (**d**)

Table 21.2 Surgical options for neglected and recurrent clubfoot

Posteromedial release	Soft tissue release for cavus, adductus, varus, and equinus	• Cincinnati • 2 incision • Turco
Additional procedures	Treatment of residual adductus	• Calcaneal closing wedge • Lichtblau calcaneal resection • Calcaneocuboid wedge resection/arthrodesis
	Treatment of residual equinus	• Excision head of talus • Naviculectomy • Distal tibia osteotomy
	Treatment of residual heel varus	• Calcaneal osteotomy (lateral slide)
	Treatment of residual supination	• Tibialis anterior transfer • Medial cuneiform osteotomy • Trans cuneiform osteotomy
	Wound closure difficulty	• Leave wound open • Immobilize under-corrected then serial casting post-operatively • Dorsal foot rotational flap • Distal tibia shortening osteotomy
Salvage procedures (for severe and recurrent clubfoot)	Older child with stiff/severe deformity	• Triple arthrodesis—Lambrinudi modification • Posterior release with midfoot dorsal closing wedge
	Arthrogryposis and myelomeningocele	• Talectomy
External fixation	Ilizarov or Taylor spatial frame for recurrent/residual deformities and severe clubfoot	• Soft tissue distraction • Distraction osteogenesis (osteoplasty)

With permissions from: Penny NJ. The neglected clubfoot. *Tech Orthop* 2005; 20(2):153–166

Previously operated and neglected clubfoot can also be managed with the use of external fixation. Two basic methods of foot deformity correction using Ilizarov techniques are as follows: (1) soft tissue stretching (correcting through joints) and (2) bony correction (osteotomies) with or without distraction osteogenesis. Due to the improved ability to correct rotational deformity with hexapod fixators over traditional Ilizarov fixation, we have applied these to clubfeet in a fashion that simulates Ponseti casting (correction through soft tissue) (Fig. 21.9). Other fixator configurations with or without osteotomies are also effective (Fig. 21.10). Any of these methods require experience and an infrastructure that can support close follow-up and post-operative management. One of the biggest risks with external fixation is the risk of recurrent deformity. This can be largely avoided by stretching soft tissues slowly (<1 mm/day), overcorrecting, and once the correction is complete the fixator should stay in place approximately twice as long as the correction phase. This is followed by another few weeks of casting. The long treatment time, psychological effects, and commitment to follow up need to also be considered when entertaining the use of gradual distraction with external fixation.

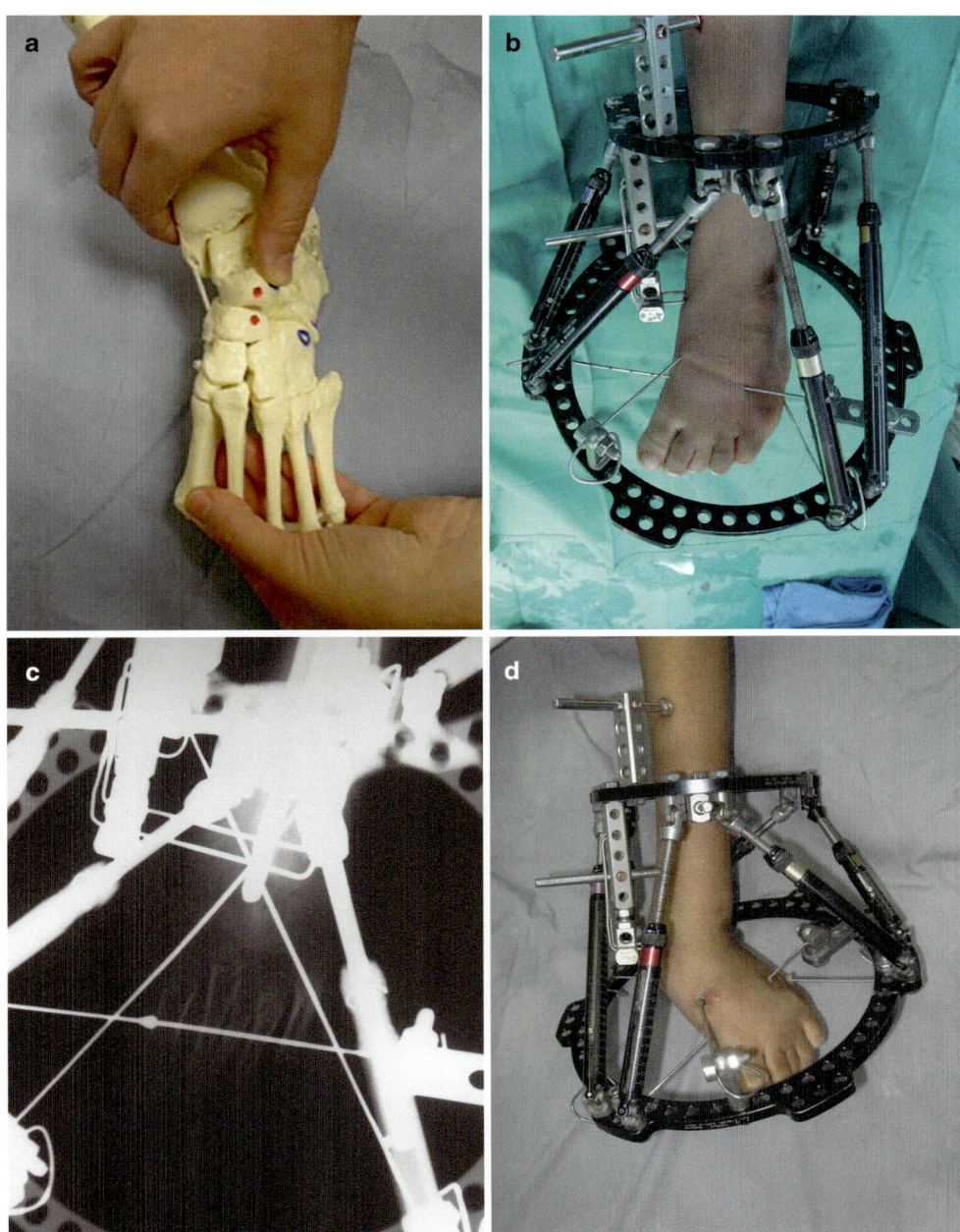

Fig. 21.9 A TSF can be used to simulate Ponseti correction. (**a**) One wire is placed through the neck of the talus and initially connected to the proximal segment of the fixator. In this example, (**b, c**) the wire was placed from lateral to medial, and then, a 180° bend was placed in the remaining wire laterally. A small incision is then made, and the wire is tapped through the neck of the talus with a mallet and connected to a post-stabilized by a half pin in the tibia and connected to the proximal ring. Distal segment foot wires are placed in the forefoot to abduct. If the midfoot deformity is not severe, the foot wires may capture some hindfoot as long as the talus is avoided. Once the foot is abducted to the desired position and varus deformity is corrected (**d**) then the talar neck wire is disconnected from the proximal segment and connected to the distal ring. This does not involve manipulation of the foot and can be done in clinic. A program is then created to correct equinus. We have not noticed additional benefit of heel cord tenotomy when doing external fixator corrections

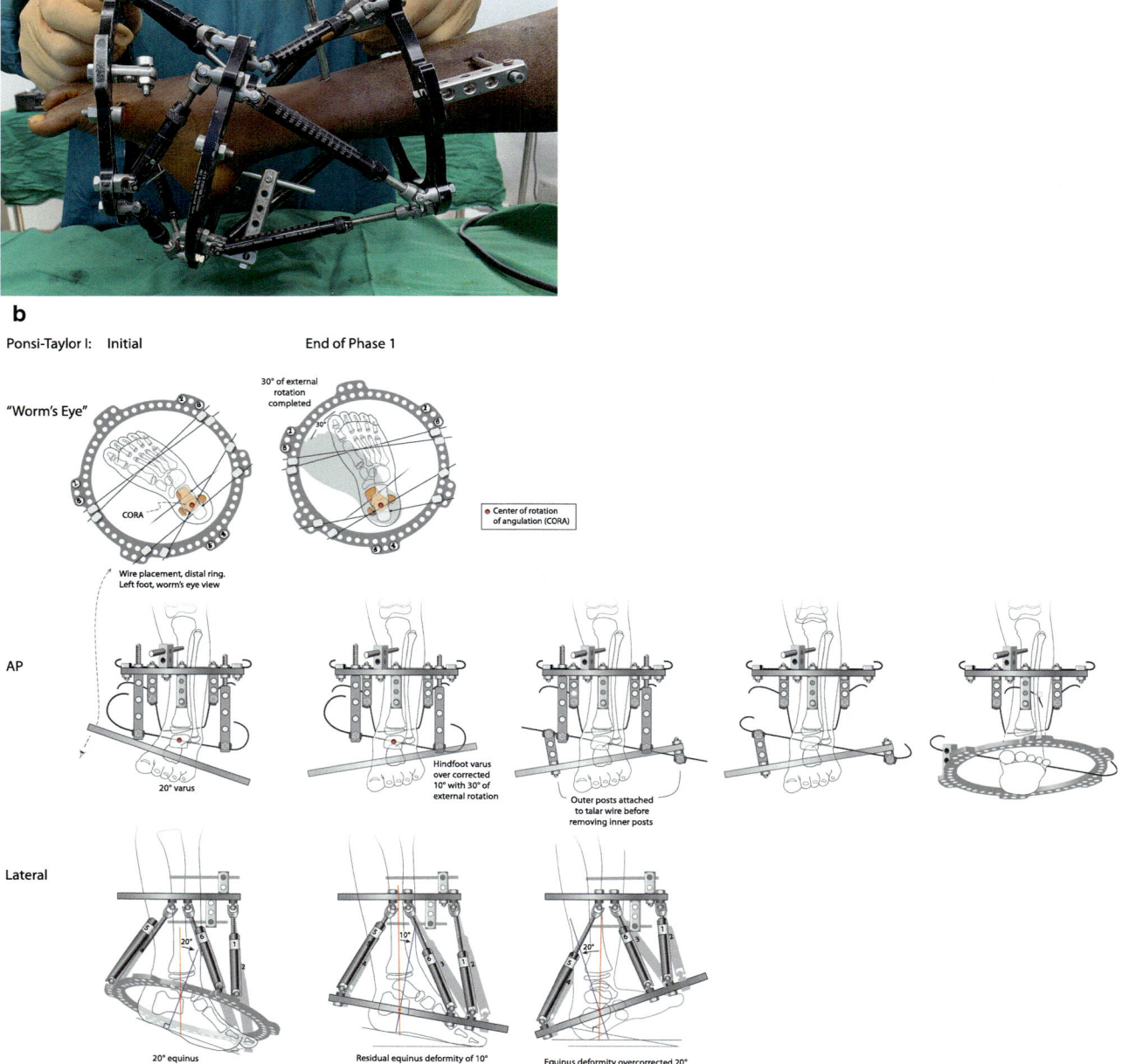

Fig. 21.10 This rigid clubfoot correction of the 16-year-old girl in Fig. 21.9 was treated with a Lambrinudi triple arthrodesis. Even with the described removal of large bone wedges, it can be difficult to obtain a complete correction. In this situation rather than forcibly correcting the foot and risking soft tissue breakdown, it is preferable to gradually correct residual deformity. This can be done with a cast or external fixation. In this case, a TSF miter frame (**a**) can simultaneously correct both hindfoot and midfoot deformity. Image (**b**) demonstrates the correction technique termed "Ponsetaylor" in which the Ponseti manipulation sequence is executed using an external fixator for gradual treatment of severe recalcitrant clubfoot deformity. Reproduced with permission from Sinai Hospital of Baltimore, Inc.

SIGN Nail

SIGN (Surgical Implant Generation Network) is a nonprofit organization that makes an intramedullary locking nail which can be implanted without fluoroscopy. It is made specifically for use in limited resource environments and is available for surgeons and institutions at minimal cost. This has revolutionized long bone fracture care around the world with more than 350,000 cases performed. SIGN has established programs in more than 50 countries where they have provided training to surgeons and equipped them with instrumentation. Accountability, quality control and maintenance of a sustainable inventory are realized through the use of a database that requires uploading of pre- and post-operative images as well as input of case data and implant use. There is a learning curve to using the system, which has some unique features enabling distal interlocking without X-ray guidance (Fig. 21.11). This system is useful for correcting limb deformities often with the aid of intra-operative external fixation (fixator-assisted nailing) or for performing lengthening over nail surgery. Fluoroscopy is required to perform accurate and minimally invasive fixator-assisted nailing. When using the SIGN nail for this, additional blocking screws should be used to stabilize the deformity as the interlocking options are not as versatile as most modern nail systems. In addition, the slotted locking screw holes in the SIGN nail do not provide tight control of angulation between the nail and the locking screws. There is a pediatric version of the SIGN nail available; however, the standard nail is suitable for a trochanteric entry and may be used in older children. The pediatric nail is more useful for fractures and has a unique distal interference fit without a distal interlocking option. The standard adult nail comes in sizes as small as 8 × 200 mm, making it versatile for deformity corrections in relatively small patients.

Spica Cast

Many pelvic and femoral osteotomy surgeries involve the use of a post-operative spica cast. It is mentioned here to highlight the fact that a specialized spica table is not necessary nor may it be available in many resource-challenged environments. Spica casts can be applied on a simple arm board (Fig. 21.12) [29]. A plank of wood or other material ideally about ½" thick and about 4" wide can be slid under the pad on the operating table and be used for both an arm board and spica table. To do this, the board is placed at 90° to the table under a thin mattress and sticks out to the side like a diving board. One person stabilizes the proximal end of the board onto the table as well as the torso of the child who is placed over the side of the bed on the opposite end of the board. Bilateral and unilateral spica casts can be placed on any size child with the appropriate size arm board.

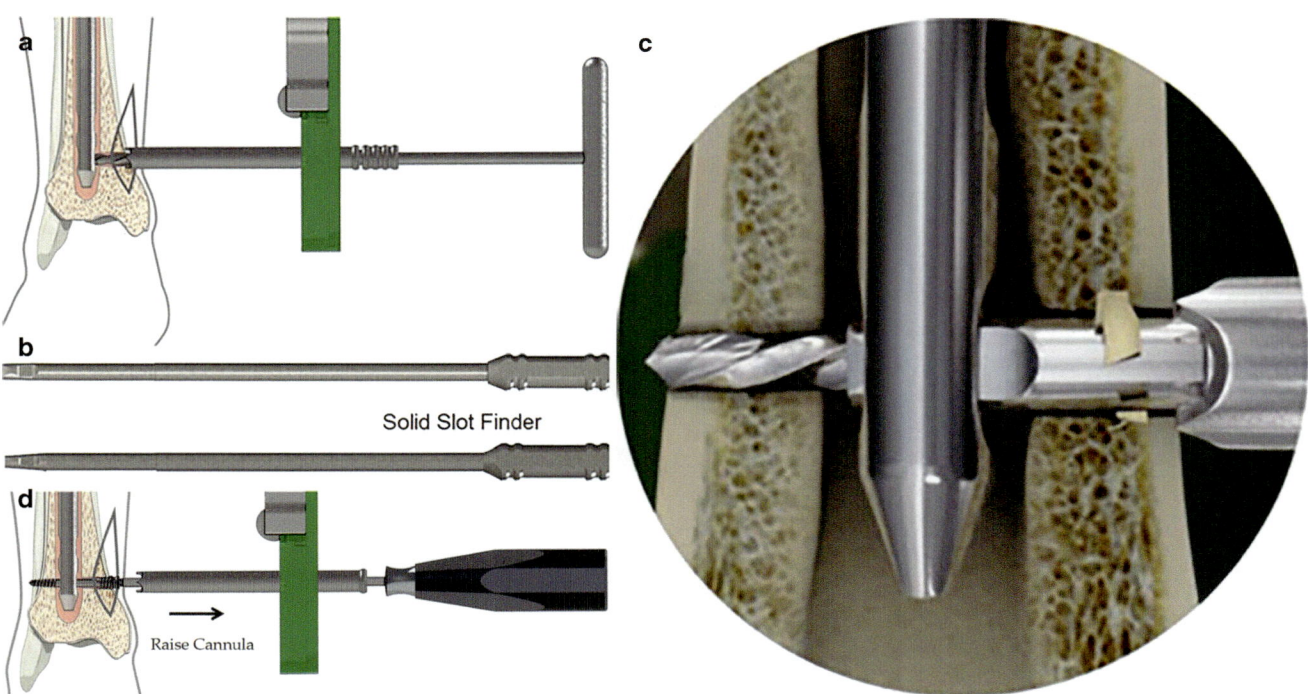

Fig. 21.11 The SIGN nail interlock technique allows for proximal and distal locking without the use of fluoro. (**a**) A near cortex hole is made with the large drill bit. (**b**) The slot finder is used to confirm the slotted hole in the nail. (**c**) Once this is done, the cannulated slot finder can be used to direct the small drill bit. (**d**) The screw with threads on the tip as well as the head is placed through the nail with secure fixation

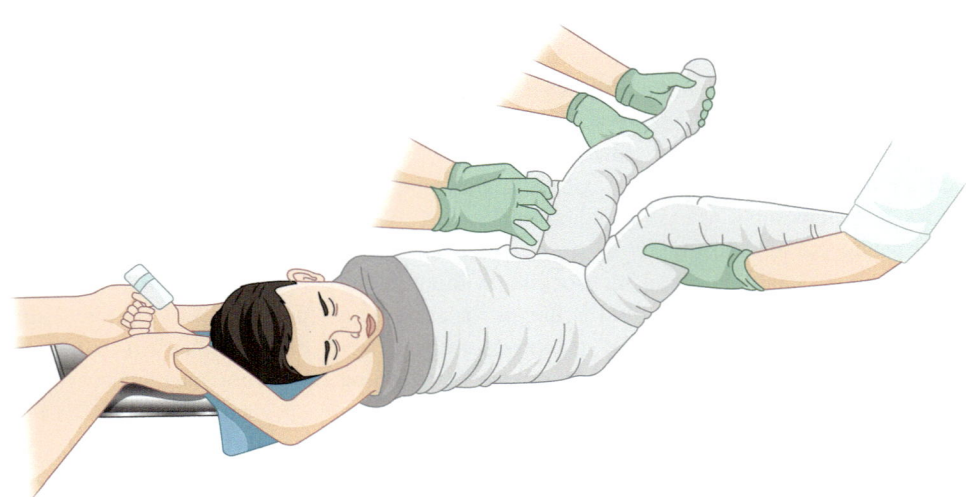

Fig. 21.12 Hip spica application. After appropriate anesthesia, the patient's torso is placed supine on the end of the arm board. Three assistants are used to stabilize and position the patient's arms/head region and each of the lower extremities. Standard casting materials, including a temporary towel to pad the patient's back, are used to complete the hip spica cast. [With permissions from Pasque C, Harbach G. Hip spica application using an operating table arm board. *J Pediatr Orthop* 2000; 20(6)]

Educational Resources

Having a collection of orthopedic textbooks available on a laptop or tablet is very helpful when performing orthopedics in resource-challenged environments. Demands are made often to perform difficult operations that one may not commonly perform. Conscientious surgeons will find it necessary to frequently consult the literature on the wide variety of challenging cases that they face. A review of operative details and often a consult from a colleague can greatly facilitate the quality and effectiveness of an operation. Fortunately, most textbooks are now available in electronic formats which can allow one to maintain an entire orthopedic library on a small electronic device. The Global Help website (www.global-help.org) has a wide variety of textbooks and monographs available for free. They have an excellent monograph on the Ponseti treatment of clubfoot which has been translated into more than 20 languages and serves as an educational tool both for surgeons and parents. Other patient-specific educational materials are available on this site as well. An excellent resource is their "Pediatric Orthopedic Library" DVD disk which contains the *Atlas of Pediatric Orthopaedics Surgery* (3rd Edition) [Morrissy & Weinstein]; *Bibliography of Orthopaedic Problems in Developing Countries* [Spiegel]; *Lovell & Winter's Pediatric Orthopaedics* (5th Edition) [Morrissy & Weinstein]; *Neuromuscular Disorders; Practice of Pediatric Orthopaedics* [Staheli]; *Sequelae of Septic Arthritis of the Hip* [Spiegel, Penny, & Shrestha]; *Standards in Pediatric Orthopaedics* [Hensinger]; *The Easter Seal Guide to Children's Orthopaedics* [The Easter Seal Society]; and *What Parents Should Know About Flatfeet* [Staheli, Staheli, & Mosca]. The cost is $1.00 USD.

HINARI (Health Inter Network Access to Research Initiative) is a WHO program which provides free or very low-cost online access to up to 35,000 information sources/journals in biomedical and related social sciences to local, nonprofit institutions in developing countries. This functions as an institutional subscription to journals referenced by PubMed and others. An application process is required, and in the most resource-challenged countries, subscriptions are completely free of charge, whereas in other developing countries, a small fee is assessed. More information and application materials can be obtained at www.who.int/hinari/en.

Summary

Working with limited resources and/or in unfamiliar locations can be one of the most challenging but also most rewarding experiences in life. Many of these operations are life-changing for patients. Basic principles should never be compromised; every effort should be made to obtain outcomes equal to those where ample resources exist. This often requires more robust fixation, extra precautions to avoid complications, and clear communication. As orthopedic surgeons with education and resources, we should consider it our obligation to help those who are in need regardless of their ability to compensate us. This can be in our own country or another. By going beyond mundane and repetitive routines, new perspectives are gained, new relationships are built, and lives are changed for the better.

Commentary

David A. Spiegel
spiegeld@chop.edu

This outstanding chapter addresses the many challenges in providing orthopedic surgical services in settings with limited resources, specifically the scenario in which a limb deformity surgeon from a high-income environment becomes involved in a surgical mission trip or teaching/training activities in a resource-limited setting. The chapter is replete with useful insights, philosophic pearls, and practical tips illustrating the extensive experience of the lead author who has dedicated a significant portion of his career to providing orthopedic surgical care to populations with limited resources. Deficiencies in access to health services are due to a number of barriers including physically being able to get to a facility (geospatial), availability of services, ability to afford services, and whether the services are culturally acceptable. Such barriers often result in delays in presentation, and orthopedic pathologies such as limb deformities commonly present at a late stage and require more complex treatment strategies. Challenges in treatment are compounded by limitations in all aspects of service delivery including imaging, equipment, and supplies, sterile operating room environment, anesthesia and perioperative care, and the ability to provide follow-up care. Orthopedic surgeons practicing in resource-rich environments are often unfamiliar with the challenges of working in settings with limited resources, and the wealth of information covered will be of value to any health provider who finds themselves in similar circumstances.

The authors emphasize the importance of developing sustainable relationships between individuals and/or institutions, a "win-win" situation for providers and patients. This cannot be overemphasized. As a visiting surgeon, we should consider ourselves a guest, and qualities which will enhance our ability to contribute in a positive way include humility, having an open mind and a desire to learn, flexibility, and a willingness to share knowledge and skills. It is not enough just to show up, getting the most out of such an experience requires adequate preparation and above all, a knowledge of the local context. It is imperative that we have adequate preparation for the experience, namely an understanding of the local context including pathology, resources available, cultural issues, health system, and expectations for our involvement. The most appropriate treatment will depend upon the pathology, the availability of equipment and supplies, access to orthoses, assistive devices and rehabilitation services, reliability of follow-up care, experience of the surgeon, and local cultural variables. While the principles remain the same and our goal is to achieve the same outcome as we would in a setting with unlimited resources, there is commonly a "need for improvisation and innovation."

The most appropriate orthopedic surgical services are therefore based on the local context. The authors emphasize the commitment to "first, do no harm," and surgeons must carefully calculate the risk to benefit ratio for each individual patient and never assume that "something is better than nothing." Stay within your skill set and err on the side of minimizing risk, and attempt to address modifiable elements within the system to enhance safety and improve outcomes. Lack of an image intensifiers mandates changes in surgical technique, often requiring at least a modified open approach. Care must be taken to anticipate blood loss and be able to calculate what volume of blood loss can be tolerated, and if safe blood products are unavailable, the surgery may need to be staged. The surgeon needs to not only have a plan A, but also plans B and C. Donations of equipment and supplies may be welcome, but the donor should ensure that the equipment can be maintained and supplies can ideally be replenished.

A number of other issues are easily taken for granted when participating in service-oriented activities such as credentialing and liability, risks associated with anesthesia and coexisting medical conditions, anticipating and addressing potential need for transfusion, balancing post-operative analgesia with safety, the basics of sterilization, and setting up the operating room. Informed consent is often a challenge and is facilitated by local colleagues and family members. It is also important to promote a culture of safety, and one way is to introduce a surgical safety checklist. Narcotics and sedatives must be carefully titrated, balancing the goal of adequate analgesia with potential complications related to oversedation, especially when adequate monitoring cannot be assured. The availability of multimodal pain therapy including local or regional blocks would be ideal. A rudimentary understanding of techniques for sterilization is helpful, and alternatives to an autoclave include portable stovetop units, dry heat sterilization, and/or the use of disinfectants. Portable HEPA filters can be considered in the absence of HVAC systems to reduce airborne bacterial colony formation. Infected cases can be performed after clean cases or in an operating room designated for such cases.

While a "one and done" intervention is most desirable from the perspective of the patient and the health system, open surgical interventions have an increased risk of infection when sterility is questionable, and the pros and cons of an acute versus gradual correction, and what type of fixation, must be weighed in each limb deformity case. Necessity dictates that many implants be re-used to service more patients and save resources/reduce costs, and each surgeon must balance implant needs with the knowledge that fatigue failure will occur after a certain number of loading cycles. He or she must consider the material properties of the implant, number of times the implant has been used, future loading expected, and whether the implant is notched on visual inspection, when making decisions for reimplantation. Other variables of importance for external fixators include the size of the patient and their anticipated demands/activity level, how long the implant must be left in place, and how many articulating parts are present. It is also essential to ensure adequate communication and documentation, especially when local providers will be tasked with post-operative management, coordinating physical therapy, providing for orthoses or assistive devices, etc. Newer technologies, including online platforms, should enhance the ability to communicate, assuming there is access to the Internet, and should facilitate the delivery of longitudinal care even for patients treated by visiting surgeons or surgical teams. Surgical mission trips focusing on service delivery can represent a double-edged sword: Many individual patients may derive benefit from the services but remember that there is the potential for damage to the local healthcare ecosystem.

I applaud the efforts of the authors and feel this chapter should become essential reading for any orthopedic surgeon who plans to participate in their field in a resource-challenged environment!

References

1. Sachs J. The end of poverty: economic possibilities for our time. New York: Penguin Press; 2005.
2. The Jimmy Carter Presidential Library and Museum. Nobel Peace Prize Lecture. https://www.jimmycarterlibrary.gov/about_us/nobel_peace_prize_lecture.
3. The World Bank. Current health expenditure per capita (current US$). https://data.worldbank.org/indicator/SH.XPD.CHEX.PC.CD?most_recent_value_desc=false.
4. Ritchie H, Rose, M. Age structure. Our World in Data 2019. https://ourworldindata.org/age-structure.
5. Fraulin G, Lee S, Bartels SA. "They came with cholera when they were tired of killing us with bullets": community perceptions of the 2010 origin of Haiti's cholera epidemic. Glob Public Health. 2021:1–15.
6. The Lancet Global Health. The UN in Haiti: an adulterated vision of accountability. Lancet Glob Health. 2016;4:e872.
7. Enserink M. Despite sensitivities, scientists seek to solve Haiti's cholera riddle. Science. 2011;331:388–9.
8. Yu CC, Fidai M, Washington T, Bartol S, Graziano G. Oral is as effective as intravenous tranexamic acid at reducing blood loss in thoracolumbar spinal fusions: a prospective randomized trial. Spine. 2022;47:91–8.
9. Ma J, Lu H, Chen X, Wang D, Wang Q. The efficacy and safety of tranexamic acid in high tibial osteotomy: a systematic review and meta-analysis. J Orthop Surg. 2021;16:373.
10. Levack AE, McLawhorn AS, Dodwell E, DelPizzo K, Nguyen J, Sink E. Intravenous tranexamic acid reduces blood loss and transfusion requirements after periacetabular osteotomy. Bone Joint J. 2020;102-B:1151–7.
11. Almatroudi A, Tahir S, Hu H, Chowdhury D, Gosbell IB, Jensen SO, Whiteley GS, Deva AK, Glasbey T, Vickery K. Staphylococcus aureus dry-surface biofilms are more resistant to heat treatment than traditional hydrated biofilms. J Hosp Infect. 2018;98:161–7.
12. O'Hara NN, Patel KR, Caldwell A, Shone S, Bryce EA. Sterile reprocessing of surgical instruments in low- and middle-income countries: a multicenter pilot study. Am J Infect Control. 2015;43:1197–200.
13. Hune SR, DiGeorge Foushee A-M, Ervin MC, Anderson SJ, Ervin MD, Mallory AM. An analysis of the effectiveness of high-level disinfection for surgical instruments used by Department of Defense austere surgical teams. Mil Med. 2021;186:122–8.
14. Weiser MC, Moucha CS. Operating-room airflow technology and infection prevention. J Bone Jt Surg. 2018;100:795–804.
15. Food and Drug Administration. Medical devices; reprocessed single-use devices; termination of exemptions from premarket notification; requirement for submission of validation data. 2005. https://www.federalregister.gov/documents/2005/09/29/05-19510/medical-devices-reprocessed-single-use-devices-termination-of-exemptions-from-premarket-notification.
16. Matsuura M, Lounici S, Inoue N, Walulik S, Chao EYS. Assessment of external fixator reusability using load- and cycle-dependent tests. Clin Orthop Relat Res. 2003;406:275–81.
17. Dirschl DR, Smith IJ. Reuse of external skeletal fixator components: effects on costs and complications. J Trauma. 1998;44:855–8.
18. Sung JK, Levin R, Siegel J, Einhorn TA, Creevy WR, Tornetta P 3rd. Reuse of external fixation components: a randomized trial. J Orthop Trauma. 2008;22:126–30.

19. Beck DJ, Seligson D. External fixator parts should not be reused. J Orthop Trauma. 2006;20:39–42.
20. Halanski MA, Davison JE, Huang J-C, Walker CG, Walsh SJ, Crawford HA. Ponseti method compared with surgical treatment of clubfoot: a prospective comparison. J Bone Joint Surg Am. 2010;92:270–8.
21. Richards BS, Faulks S, Rathjen KE, Karol LA, Johnston CE, Jones SA. A comparison of two nonoperative methods of idiopathic clubfoot correction: the Ponseti method and the French functional (physiotherapy) method. J Bone Joint Surg Am. 2008;90:2313–21.
22. Ippolito E, Farsetti P, Caterini R, Tudisco C. Long-term comparative results in patients with congenital clubfoot treated with two different protocols. J Bone Joint Surg Am. 2003;85:1286–94.
23. Penny JN. The neglected clubfoot. Tech Orthop. 2005;20:153–66.
24. Morcuende JA, Abbasi D, Dolan LA, Ponseti IV. Results of an accelerated Ponseti protocol for clubfoot. J Pediatr Orthop. 2005;25:623–6.
25. Ahmad AA, Aker L. Accelerated Ponseti method: first experiences in a more convenient technique for patients with severe idiopathic club feet. Foot Ankle Surg. 2020;26:254–7.
26. Ahmad AA, Ghanem AF, Hamaida JM, Maree MS, Aker LJ, Abu Kamesh MI, Berawi SN, Abu Hamdeh MS. Magnetic resonance imaging of severe idiopathic club foot treated with one-week accelerated Ponseti (OWAP) technique. Foot Ankle Surg. 2021;S1268-7731(21):00091–6.
27. Elbatrawy YA. One-week accelerated Ponseti method in the management of idiopathic clubfeet. J Limb Lengthen Reconstr. 2020;6:131–6.
28. Gross RH. The role of the Verebelyi-Ogston procedure in the management of the arthrogrypotic foot. Clin Orthop. 1985:99–103.
29. Pasque CB, Harbach GP. Hip spica application using an operating table armboard. J Pediatr Orthop. 2000;20:757–8.

Part III
Underlying Conditions

Metabolic Disorders

Ali Bas, Mehmet Kocaoglu, Levent Eralp, and F. Erkal Bilen

General

Deficiency in the shape, strength, and structure of bone tissue due to altered bone mineral homeostasis is called *metabolic bone disease* [1]. The major factors affecting this homeostasis can be thought of as the three 3s: the intracellular and extracellular levels of *three* ions (calcium, phosphorus, and magnesium), which are controlled by *three* hormones (parathyroid hormone, calcitonin, and 1, 25-dihydroxyvitamin D) and act upon *three* tissues (bone, gut, and kidney) [1, 2]. Common clinical manifestations of metabolic bone disease in children include electrolyte disturbances, fractures, bone deformity, abnormal gait, and short stature.

Commonly encountered forms of metabolic bone disease in children are the various types of rickets and renal osteodystrophy. Other less common but important pediatric metabolic conditions include osteoporosis, malabsorption syndromes, and inherited diseases such as hypophosphatasia, X-linked hypophosphatemia, and various forms of vitamin D-dependent rickets [1, 3] (Box 22.1).

> **Box 22.1**
> - Metabolic problems related to vitamin D must be addressed prior, during, and after the surgical treatment.
> - There are various forms of metabolic bone diseases. Thus, collaboration with the pediatric/internal medicine department is essential.

Pathophysiology

Although there are several types of *rickets*, the basic pathogenesis is a relative decline in calcium or phosphorus (or both) of a large enough amount so that it interferes with physeal growth and mineralization of the bone matrix in the growing child [1, 3, 4]. Mineralization defects are classified into two major groups according to the predominant mineral deficiency: calcipenic rickets and phosphopenic rickets. Calcipenic rickets occurs most commonly due to vitamin D deficiency [5]. Other rare causes are defects in the metabolic pathway of vitamin D (as in liver pathology, 25-α-hydroxylase deficiency, and chronic kidney disease) and end-organ resistance to 1,25-dihydroxy vitamin D ($1,25(OH)_2D$). In phosphopenic rickets, the defect usually results from increased renal excretion of phosphate. Phosphate wasting can be a part of generalized renal tubular dysfunction (as in Fanconi syndrome) or secondary to increased fibroblast growth factor 23 (FGF-23) metabolic pathway [6].

In renal osteodystrophy, glomerular damage leads to phosphate retention, and tubular damage causes decreased production of the active form of vitamin D (i.e., $1,25(OH)_2D$) due to the absence of 1-α-hydroxylase activity. These two factors severely impede intestinal calcium absorption and reduce serum-ionized calcium. The subsequent hypocalcemia generates secondary hyperparathyroidism, which remains ineffective in increasing intestinal absorption of calcium. Consequently, the body's only means of increasing

A. Bas (✉)
Department of Orthopedics and Traumatology, Koç University Hospital, Istanbul, Turkey
e-mail: albas@kuh.ku.edu.tr

M. Kocaoglu
Istanbul Faculty of Medicine, Unimed Center, Istanbul, Turkey

L. Eralp
Istanbul Faculty of Medicine, Istanbul University, Istanbul, Turkey

F. E. Bilen
Macka EMAR Medical Center, Istanbul, Turkey

serum calcium levels is bone resorption. Metabolic acidemia may further deteriorate this condition (Figs. 22.1 and 22.2) [1, 3, 4].

In patients with *osteoporosis*, the bone is structurally normal but is reduced in overall amount. In children, osteoporosis may be idiopathic as in juvenile osteoporosis or may be due to disuse or chronic corticosteroid administration. The mechanism is uncertain, but numerous theories include increased bone resorption versus decreased bone formation, possibly due to deficient $1,25(OH)_2D$ or calcitonin or due to a significant interruption in the transduction of mechanical forces that stimulate new bone formation [1, 3].

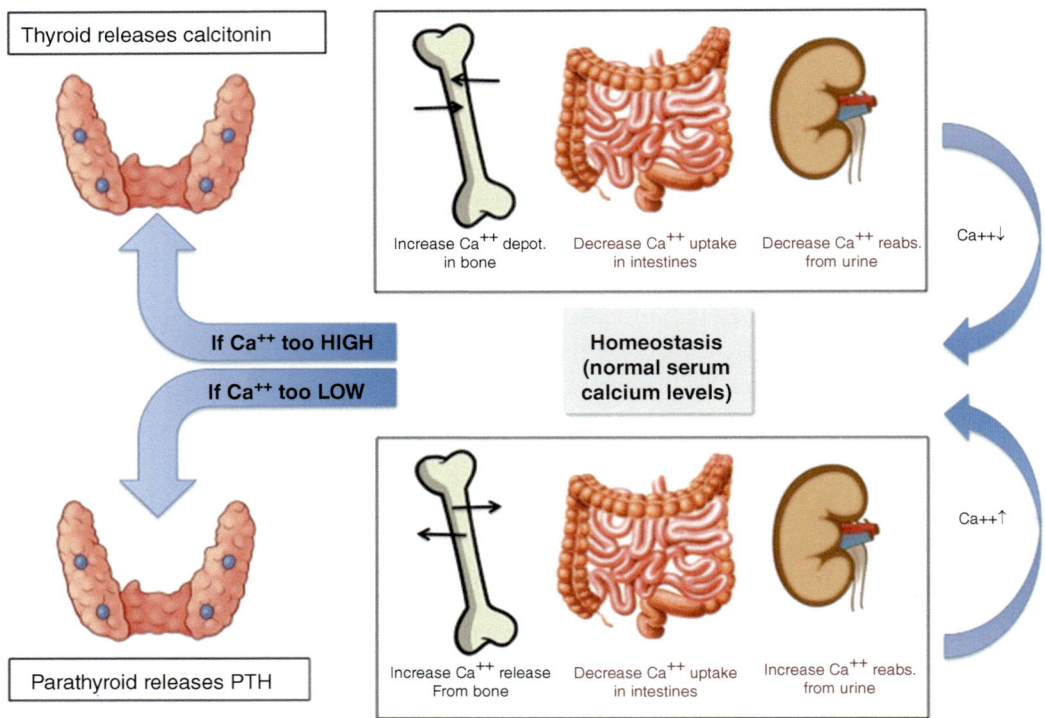

Fig. 22.1 Metabolic control of calcium levels

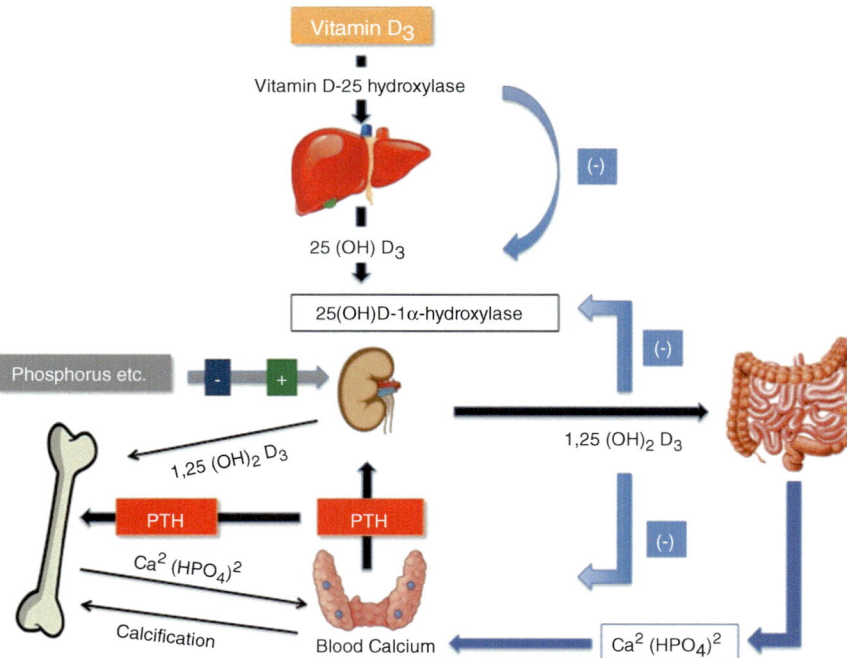

Fig. 22.2 Vitamin D metabolism

Hypophosphatasia results from a genetic error in the alkaline phosphatase (ALP) synthesis, the enzyme necessary for the maturation of the primary spongiosa in the physis. This condition leads to normal production of osteoid tissue but inadequate mineralization, with resultant skeletal deformities that resemble rickets [1, 3, 4].

Rickets

General

Rickets, a common, worldwide disease, affects the overall health and growth of children and adolescents and usually occurs secondary to deficiencies of calcium or phosphate, two major constituents of the crystalline component of bone and essential for mineralization and bone growth. The organic component of the extracellular bone matrix, produced by osteoblasts, must be mineralized by calcium salts for bone maturation. Deficient mineralization in the zone of provisional calcification disrupts the conversion of the growth plate into primary bone spongiosa. Simultaneously, the progression of chondrocyte proliferation causes hypertrophic zone enlargement and columnar disorganization of physis. This process results in the accumulation of unmineralized osteoid adjacent to the growth plate and gradually leads to softness in the bone [6–8].

Skeletal symptoms including deformities, bone pain, and slight prominence around the knee and ankle are generally similar in most types of rickets. The type and location of deformity depend on the deforming forces acting on the lower extremities at the time of the bone structure weakness and the child's age. Forearm deformities and posterior bowing of the distal tibia are common in infants. Exaggeration of physiological genu varum or bow leg is a characteristic finding in the toddler. Genu valgum and coxa vara can be seen in older children [9, 10]. As rickets continues, tubular bone growth insufficiency leads to short stature [10].

Diagnosis is based on serum biochemical studies in patients with characteristic clinical features and radiographic findings. The initial evaluation should include the measurements of serum parathyroid hormone (PTH), inorganic phosphorus, calcium, ALP, 25-hydroxy vitamin D (25(OH)D), $1,25(OH)_2D$, and urinary calcium, phosphate, and creatinine [9] (Table 22.1). If the serum PTH is elevated and phosphorus is normal or low, then a provisional diagnosis of calcipenic rickets can be made. Calcium levels may be low, especially in the advanced stage of the disease, or normal due to a compensatory increase in PTH in calcipenic rickets [9]. 25(OH)D serves differential diagnosis of calcipenic rickets, caused by vitamin D deficiency from other calcipenic rickets forms [5]. Chronic renal failure is also one of the causes of calcipenic rickets via altering the vitamin D metabolism and will be discussed under a separate topic below. PTH and inorganic phosphorus help to distinguish calcipenic rickets from phosphopenic rickets. If the serum PTH is normal or elevated and the phosphorus is low, then phosphopenic rickets should be considered. Elevated serum ALP level confirms the diagnosis of rickets in patients with radiologic and clinical features. It indicates the disease activity and excludes all the differential diagnoses of abnormal metaphysis and bone deformities such as Blount disease and metaphyseal dysplasia [9, 11]. ALP levels in phosphopenic rickets tend to be moderately high when compared to much higher levels in calcipenic rickets [9]. Other biochemical parameters can vary in terms of rickets type and severity of the disease.

Treatment is based on the management of the primary underlying etiology.

Table 22.1 Laboratory findings of rickets

	Type	Calcium	Phosphorus	ALP	PTH	25(OH)D	1,25(OH)2D
Calcipenic rickets	Nutritional rickets (Vitamin D-deficient rickets)	↓/N	↓/N	↑/↑↑	↑	↓[a]	↑/N [a]
	Vitamin D-dependent rickets type I (VDDR type I)	↓	↓/N	↑↑	↑	↑	↓↓
	Vitamin D-dependent rickets type II (VDDR type II)	↓	↓/N	↑↑	↑	N/↑↑	↑↑↑
Phosphopenic rickets	Hereditary hypophosphatemic rickets (VDRR)	N	↓↓	↑	N	N	N/↓

VDDR type I consists of 1-α-hydroxylase deficiency (type IA) and the 25-α-hydroxylase deficiency (type IB)
VDDR type II, hereditary resistance to vitamin D
VDRR (vitamin D-resistant rickets), X-linked hypophosphatemia, and other hypophosphatemic disorders mediated by FGF23
[a] In Vitamin D-deficient rickets, Vitamin D level is best indicated by serum 25(OH)D (calcidiol). In contrast, the level of the 1,25(OH)2D is not helpful since it may be usually normal or elevated

Nutritional Rickets

Treatment

Vitamin D administration (cholecalciferol) represents the mainstay of nutritional rickets treatment, and calcium supplementation is essential to avoid "hungry-bone syndrome" [5, 6]. Calcification occurs with treatment, and radiographic appearance normalizes gradually. Radiographs typically display improved mineralization within 2–4 weeks of initiating medical treatment [10]. There is no specific orthopedic treatment for nutritional rickets besides follow-up to ensure acceptable lower limb alignment since the residual deformities are rarely seen with the appropriate medical treatment.

Hereditary Hypophosphatemic Rickets

The term vitamin D-resistant rickets (VDRR) was initially used to describe a syndrome of hypophosphatemia and rickets that resembled vitamin D deficiency but did not respond to vitamin D replacement. This disorder is known as hereditary hypophosphatemic rickets because the main pathophysiological problem is phosphate wasting rather than true vitamin D resistance. Various forms of hereditary hypophosphatemic rickets include X-linked, autosomal-dominant, and autosomal-recessive diseases and hypophosphatemic rickets with hypercalciuria. The X-linked form is the most common. An acquired disorder, tumor-induced osteomalacia, has similar clinical manifestations to hereditary syndromes. In addition to hypophosphatemia, normal serum levels of calcium and normal or modestly elevated levels of PTH are also seen in this disorder. In addition, elevated serum fibroblast growth factor 23 (FGF23) is detected in most of these patients, causing phosphate wasting.

X-Linked Hereditary Hypophosphatemic Rickets (XLH)

XLH is the most common form of heritable rickets [12] and the most common cause of inherited phosphate wasting, with an incidence of 3.9 per 100,000 live births and a prevalence ranging from 1.7 per 100,000 in children [13]. Renal phosphate wasting disorder is caused by mutations in the **PH**osphate-regulating gene with homologies to **E**ndopeptidases on the **X** chromosome (PHEX) gene, inherited x-linked dominant fashion [14, 15]. Its expression is highest in osteoblasts and osteocytes [13]. PHEX mutations encode a protein, an unknown physiologic function, and lead to increased serum FGF23 [12, 13]. At the kidney, FGF23 results in renal phosphate wasting via downregulation of sodium-phosphate cotransporters in the proximal tubules, decreasing 1,25(OH)$_2$D via impaired 1-α-hydroxylation, and consequently impaired skeletal mineralization and rickets [12, 14, 16, 17].

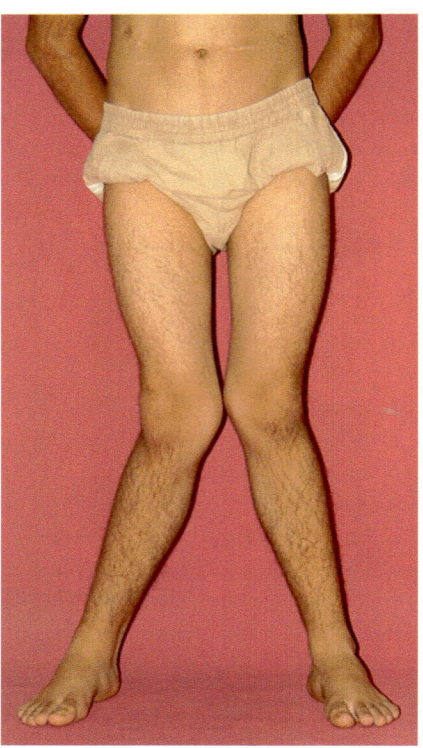

Fig. 22.3 Photograph of a patient with severe genu valgum deformity

The deformities are much more severe when compared to nutritional rickets and typically become evident between the ages of 1 and 2 years, slightly older than nutritional rickets. Clinical features include progressive lower limb deformities (varus/valgus) (Figs. 22.3 and 22.4), torsion deformities (in-toeing/ex-toeing), delayed walking, or waddling gait, which could not be evident in early childhood until the second year of life [13, 18]. Dental abscesses are common in patients >3 years of age, and in adulthood, typical clinical findings include short stature, osteomalacia, bone pain, pseudofractures, stiffness, enthesopathy, and poor dental condition [13]. Short stature is also a feature of hypophosphatemic rickets, with their standing height often being two standard deviations below the mean for their peers [19], and a disproportionate height ratio can occur due to impaired limb growth with rela-

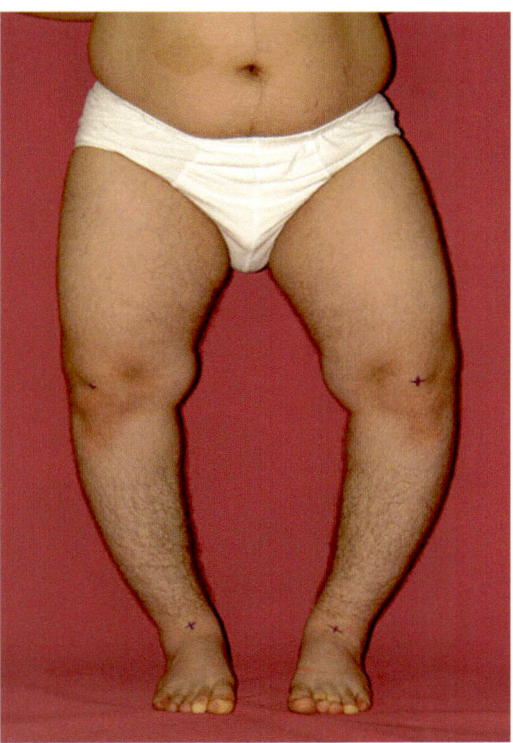

Fig. 22.4 Photograph of a patient with severe genu varum deformity

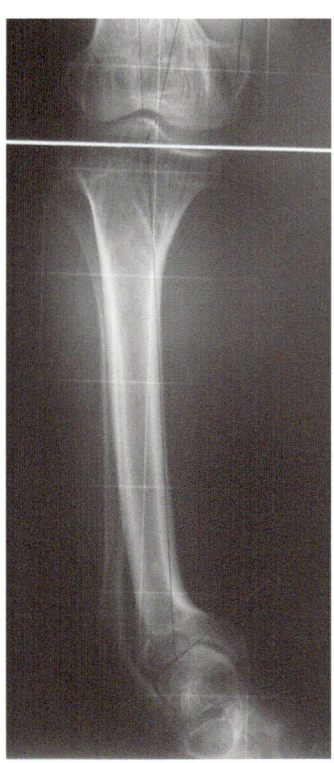

Fig. 22.5 X-ray showing distal tibial varus deformity

tively preserved trunk growth [13]. In addition, valgus deformities of the legs or a windswept (valgus deformity of one leg and varus deformity of the other) deformity can be seen [12, 20, 21].

The characteristic radiologic findings of long bones are similar to nutritional rickets. However, it differs from them by often thickening of cortical bone and lack of bone resorption. Deformities occur at sites of rapid growth and typically involve the lower limb shaft of the long bones [13]. The physes are widened. Genu varum and coxa vara with anterolateral femoral bowing may occur. Furthermore, a varus deformity of the distal tibia often leads to varus malalignment of the ankle joint (Fig. 22.5). The upper extremities are involved, to a lesser degree, as well [4].

The laboratory finding of XLH is summarized in Table 22.1.

Treatment

A patient-centered multidisciplinary care model, consisting of medical, surgical, and non-pharmacological treatments, should be initiated in childhood and maintained into adulthood. The goals of treatment are optimizing the quality of life, decreasing bone deformities and pain, improving linear growth, mobility, and physical activity, and minimizing school absenteeism [14] (Fig. 22.6).

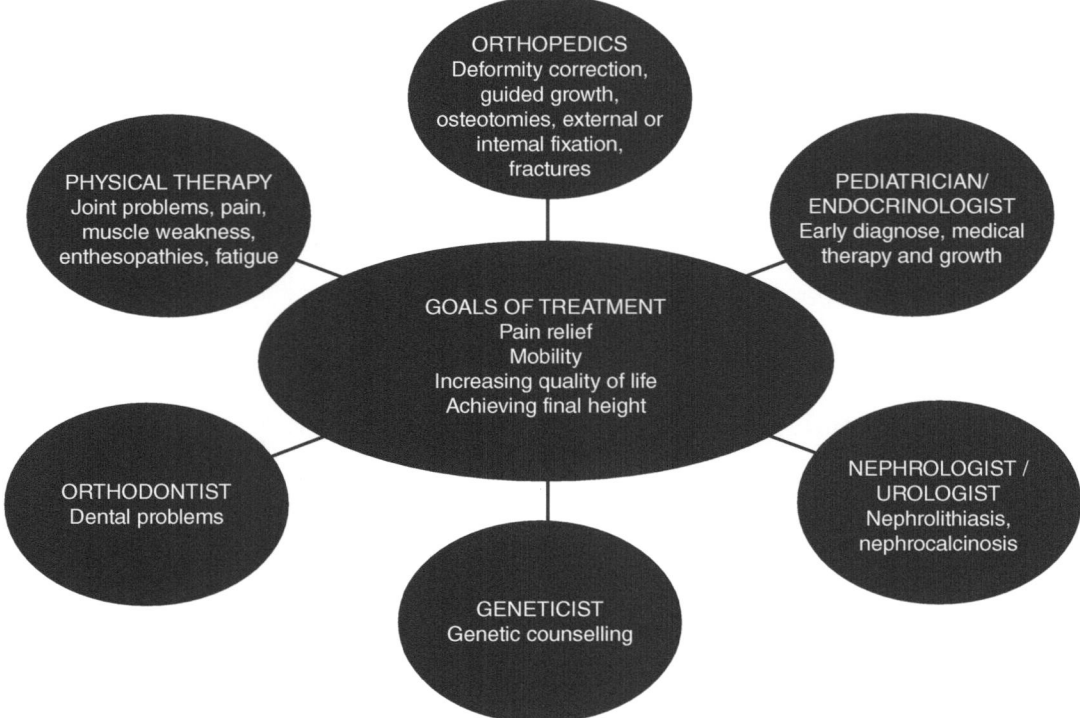

Fig. 22.6 Multidisciplinary care and treatment goals of XLH

Medical Treatment

Optimized medical therapy is the cornerstone of the treatment and may provide the reducing necessity of surgical interventions, alleviating deformities, and improving attained height [4, 12, 22]. In addition, early diagnosis and treatment are associated with better outcomes. That is why it should be started as soon as it is diagnosed [14, 18, 23].

No consensus exists on conventional therapy doses (phosphate and calcitriol) and depends on age and disease severity. The therapy suggestion in children is a 20–30 ng/kg dose of calcitriol (1,25-dihydroxycholecalciferol) and 20–60 mg/kg elemental phosphorus with split multiple doses to provide steady serum levels to optimal bone mineralization and to reduce the gastrointestinal side effects of phosphate [13, 18, 24]. Medical treatment in children has been recommended before elective surgery for at least 12 months [14].

The United States Food and Drug Administration (FDA) and the European Medicines Agency (EMA) approved Burosumab in 2018. This human monoclonal FGF23 antibody seems effective for the XLH treatment in 1-year-old children and older [13, 24, 25], especially for untreated children with moderate or severe rickets. Its efficiency has been demonstrated in randomized clinical trials compared with conventional therapy. Treatment with Burosumab revealed improvement in biochemical parameters (i.e., decreasing serum ALP levels and renal phosphate wasting) and clinical outcomes, including decreasing pain, increasing mobility and linear growth velocity, and decreasing lower extremity deformities radiologically without potential complications of conventional therapy such as nephrocalcinosis and hyperparathyroidism [13, 14]. Therefore, Burosumab should be considered an alternative therapy in children previously treated with conventional therapy but who did not respond. It should not be administered to patients with severe renal impairment and in combination with conventional therapy [14].

Final heights are reduced by up to 60% of XLH patients. The recombinant human growth hormone (rhGH) has improved predicted height for treating short stature with the improvement of final height, z-score, bone density, and phosphate retention [14, 26, 27]. Nevertheless, available studies do not support the routine administration of rhGH therapy for short stature. If it is considered, optimal control of rickets, PTH, and ALP levels should be achieved before the administration [13].

One of the recent studies is about sclerostin protein, which is produced primarily in osteocytes, suppresses bone formation, and is elevated in XLH patients. Sclerostin antibodies increase serum phosphate levels, bone mass, and strength, and suppress significantly circulating FGF23 levels in Hyp mice [28]. However, the genetic ablation of osteopontin improves bone mineralization in Hyp mice. This protein is independent of phosphate-regulating factors and a substrate for PHEX enzymatic activity. It typically accumulates in the extracellular matrix of bone and teeth despite medical treatment, inhibiting bone mineralization [29].

Non-pharmacological Treatment and Rehabilitation

Targeted rehabilitation is highly recommended due to the limited range of motion in the lower limbs and spine and gait abnormalities [13, 14, 18]. In addition, the individuals are encouraged to be involved in sports activities with low risk of trauma, such as Pilates, dancing, and swimming, to improve and preserve muscle strength, range of motion of joints, postural control, and core stability and to reduce XLH-related disabilities [13, 14]. The use of casts, insoles, and orthotic management of deformities in these patients have been unsuccessful [13].

Specific gait abnormalities are common in patients with XLH, such as internal tibial rotation and external hip rotation, resulting in impaired gait scores. Therefore, instrumented gait analysis in conjunction with the assessment of deformity parameters of the lower limb, including radiographic angles and mechanical axis, is helpful in adequately evaluating the effectiveness of conservative and surgical treatment [30].

Orthopedic Treatment

Orthopedic interventions performed in early childhood have been associated with high recurrence rates and complications [13]. With current improvements in medical care, most limb deformities improve in patients, while some others persist or progress to a more severe deformity [13]. The orthopedic management should be coordinated by an orthopedic surgeon along with an expert in metabolic bone diseases and trained in deformity analysis, correction, and different surgical procedures [13, 14, 31]. Surgical procedures should be considered for persistent and progressive deformities despite optimized medical treatment and the presence of symptoms such as pain and gait abnormality with functional impairment [4, 13, 14, 32]. The surgical treatment goals are to obtain equal-length extremities, to correct alignment, to preserve, or to improve joints' range of motion. If possible, it should be achieved with minimal time away from school or educational activities, a minimum number of surgeries, and no complication and functional loss [13]. Despite the improvement of surgical procedures and more sophisticated implants, the overall complications and reoperation rate

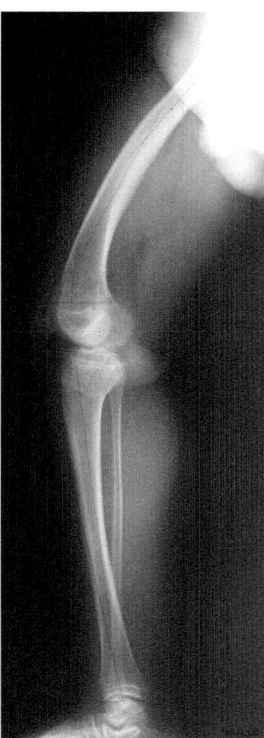

Fig. 22.7 X-ray of a patient with an anterior bowing of the femur

remain high. Surgical interventions can be done before or after skeletal maturity. The surgery's timing depends on the child's overall condition and the size of the bone; an individualized surgical treatment plan for severe deformities can be performed as early as the second year of life [33].

The most common deformity seen in this patient group is a gradual anterolateral bowing of the femur accompanied by tibia vara (Figs. 22.7 and 22.8). Multilevel osteotomies are often necessary in order to reach a physiologic lower extremity alignment [4, 16, 32, 34]. The mechanical axis can be slightly overcorrected during surgery. The suggested fixation modality varies among reports. While external fixation allows fine-tuning of the alignment postoperatively [35] (Fig. 22.9), surgical procedures consisting of intramedullary fixation (solid or flexible), plate fixation, and a combined technique consisting of an Ilizarov external fixator have also been reported [16, 34, 36–38] (Fig. 22.10; Table 22.2). Combined osteosynthesis with Ilizarov and flexible intramedullary nail reduces the complication rate related to external fixation and external fixator time. Flexible intramedullary nails protect the diaphyseal segment of the bone from recurrent deformities. However, new deformities in the proximal tibia and distal femur metaphysis may occur during growing up [16]. Regardless of the type of implants utilized, careful surgical preoperative planning for these multiplanar deformities is obligatory to reestablish the alignment of the lower extremity successfully.

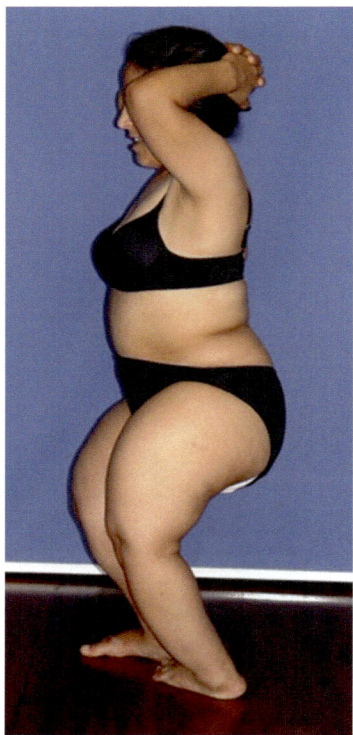

Fig. 22.8 Photograph of a patient with severe anterior bowing of the femur

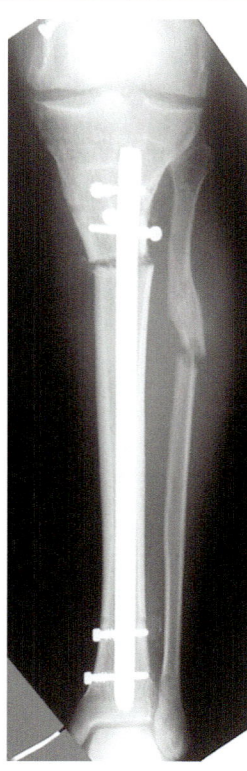

Fig. 22.10 Intramedullary fixation of a tibial deformity correction

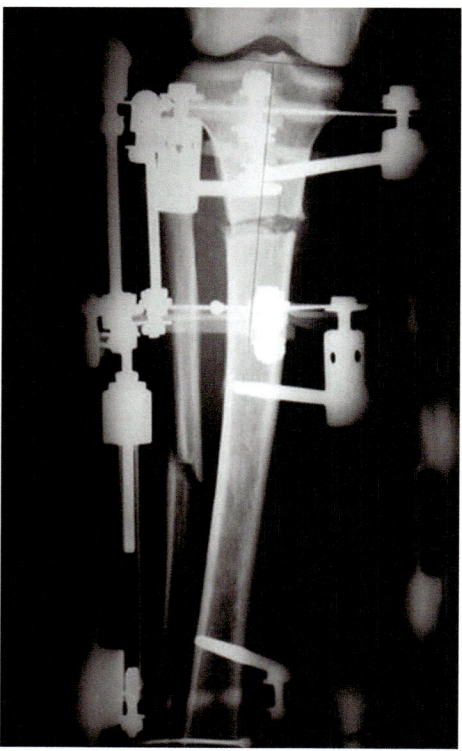

Fig. 22.9 X-ray of external fixation for the tibial deformity

The recurrent deformity is a common sequela of osteotomies in patients [4, 34, 36] (Fig. 22.11). As expected, younger patients have a higher risk of recurrence. The guided growth technique may correct the mild deformities in young children [12]. The guided growth technique by hemiepiphysiodesis is a successful and minimally invasive method for coronal plane deformities. It may be an alternative to invasive methods (such as intramedullary nailing, circular external fixators, or combined techniques) requiring osteotomy [13, 14, 39]. It depends on the growth potential of the patient and is advised to be carried out at least 2–3 years before skeletal maturity. Also, it aims to correct the deformity from the physeal level before the diaphyseal deformity occurs [13]. Torsional deformities cannot be treated with this method, but the method can be repeated safely despite failure [31]. This technique is recommended in early childhood since invasive surgeries using complex osteotomies before puberty have a higher risk for deformity recurrence [13]. More invasive methods such as osteotomies should be recommended, after multidisciplinary assessment and medical optimization in patients with severe deformities or for residual deformities after skeletal maturity [40].

Lower limb long bones are deformed and mechanically less resistant. Therefore, intramedullary devices with a telescopic mechanism seem to be the most suitable implants for children. The deformity correction and intramedullary stabili-

Table 22.2 Review of literature

Authors	Journal (year)	Title	Number of patients	Results
Rubinovitch et al.	Clin Orthop Relat Res (1988)	Principles and results of corrective lower limb osteotomies for patients with vitamin D-resistant hypophosphatemic rickets	10 (44 osteotomies)	Osteotomies were combined with shortening and compression plating. Recurrence of the deformity occurred in 27% of the cases. While osteotomies were safe and provided dramatic improvement to limb deformity, postoperative control of vitamin D metabolism was the one constant factor for the maintenance of correction
Stanitski	Clin Orthop Relat Res (1994)	Treatment of deformity secondary to metabolic bone disease with the Ilizarov technique	8 (18 segments)	Complications were limited to several pin-tract infections and mild translational deformity in two patients. The healing index averaged approximately twice that seen in pediatric femoral lengthening and was 25% greater than for patients undergoing tibial lengthening. The lack of implants requiring removal, modularity, and reasonable treatment time make this technique an attractive alternative to conventional osteotomy for the management of limb-length deformity associated with metabolic bone disease
Kanel et al.	J Pediatr Orthop (1995)	Unilateral external fixation for corrective osteotomies in patients with hypophosphatemic rickets	9 (29 segments)	Corrective osteotomies were performed on 29 bones in nine children with hypophosphatemic rickets. The use of the Orthofix external fixator enabled precise correction of the deformities without interruption of medical management
Eralp et al.	J Bone Joint Br (2004)	A correction of windswept deformity by fixator-assisted nailing	2 (7 segments)	Seven segments in two patients with vitamin D-related metabolic bone disease were treated by fixator-assisted nailing technique. All deformities were accurately corrected, and there was no consolidation problem at the osteotomy sites. The total treatment time was found to be less than with other techniques
Song et al.	Acta Orthopedica (2006)	Deformity correction by external fixation and or intramedullary nailing in hypophosphatemic rickets	20 (55 segments)	55 segmental deformities (20 femora, 35 tibiae) from 20 patients were examined retrospectively. Distraction osteogenesis was used in 28 segments and acute deformity correction in 27 segments. External fixation was applied in 24 segments, intramedullary nailing in 6 segments, and external fixation and intramedullary nailing in 25 segments. Recurrent deformity or refracture occurred in 10 of 21 segments with distraction osteogenesis by external fixation only, 4 of 6 with acute correction by intramedullary nailing, and 1 of 25 with distraction osteogenesis or acute correction by external fixation and intramedullary nailing. External fixation and intramedullary nailing can be recommended to prevent complications during or after deformity correction in hypophosphatemic rickets
Fucentese et al.	J Child Orthop (2008)	Metabolic and orthopedic management of X-linked vitamin D-resistant hypophosphatemic rickets	12	Eight patients were operated. Single bilateral surgical correction was performed in six patients; one patient each had three and five corrections. Bone lengthening was performed in three patients. At the last follow-up, the height of seven operated patients was within normal range. In addition, the leg axis was normalized in six patients with mild genu varum in two patients. Bone healing was excellent: Surgical complications were rare. In case of bone deformity, surgery can safely be performed, independent of age or bone maturation
Petje et al.	Clin Orthop Relat Res (2008)	Deformity correction in children with hereditary hypophosphatemic rickets	10 (53 segments)	37 corrective operations were performed on ten children. Depending on the patient's age, external fixation was used in 53 segments: Kirschner wires in 18 segments, DynaFix in 3 segments, the Taylor spatial frame device in 13 segments, and the Ilizarov device in 19 segments. Internal fixation with intramedullary nailing was performed in 12 segments. Deviation of the mechanical axis and knee orientation lines was increased at the follow-ups conducted during 5–12 months. Additional follow-ups revealed a recurrence rate of 90% after the first corrective procedure and 60% after a second procedure

(continued)

Table 22.2 (continued)

Authors	Journal (year)	Title	Number of patients	Results
Popkov	International Orthopaedics (2010)	Results of deformity correction in children with X-linked hereditary hypophosphatemic rickets by external fixation or combined technique	47	The results were compared in children with XLH, who underwent simultaneous deformity correction in the femur and tibia and were treated with either the Ilizarov device alone or combined technique (Ilizarov fixator with hydroxyapatite-coated flexible intramedullary nailing) followed-up for 5–9 years. There was no difference between groups statistically in terms of correction accuracy. Recurrent deformities were observed in the Ilizarov group. However, new deformities at the metaphyseal zone of the distal femur and proximal tibia occurred in the combined group without recurrent deformity in parts of bone reinforced by elastic nails while the child continues to grow. Both fixator time and complication rate were decreased in the combined group
Kocaoglu et al.	J Bone Joint Surg Br (2011)	Combined technique for the correction of lower limb deformities resulting from metabolic bone disease	17 (43 segments)	43 segments in 17 patients with metabolic bone disease underwent surgical treatment by the fixator-assisted nailing technique. The deformity correction was achieved with a low complication rate. The use of intramedullary nail prevented the recurrence of deformity and refracture

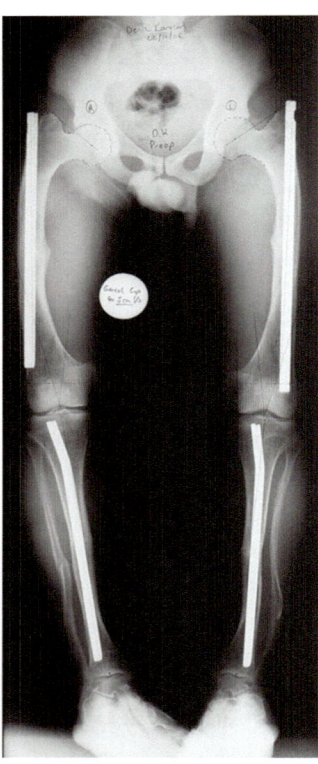

Fig. 22.11 Note the recurrence of the deformities in a patient despite the intramedullary nails

zation provide pain relief, fracture risk reduction, functional improvement, and minimization of traumatic events [33]. However, patients treated with deformity correction and bone lengthening have higher complication risks such as recurrent deformity and refracture when compared to others who had deformity correction alone. Therefore, even in children, intramedullary nailing combined with an external fixator or nailing after the external fixator treatment is recommended [12]. Intramedullary nailing provides long-term support allows the patients to walk on stable lower extremities [33] and has become the mainstay of treatment, especially in adults.

Short stature is also noted among children with hypophosphatemic rickets. The common indication for long bone lengthening is a shortening of the entire or segment of the limb in one or both legs [32]. The procedure can be performed by monolateral or circular external fixators, by lengthening over an intramedullary nail (LON) (Fig. 22.12) [34] or using intramedullary lengthening implants. The application of flexible intramedullary nails in limb lengthening for children is also an alternative with multiple advantages [41]. This technique also respects the bone biology that is essential during limb lengthening. In addition, intramedullary lengthening nails allow acute deformity correction and then lengthening. However, the technical limitations of these devices are the severe bowing of the femur and tibia often seen in XLH patients [31].

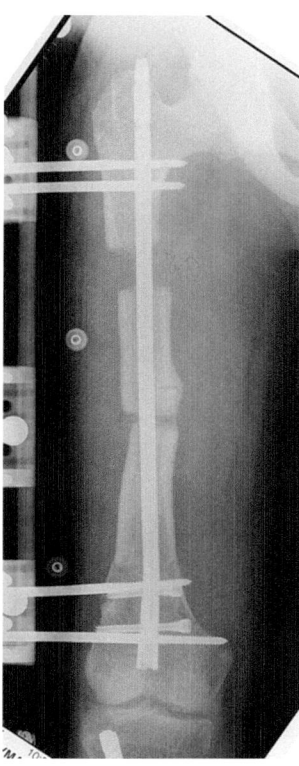

Fig. 22.12 Following deformity correction (fixator-assisted nailing) lengthening over the nail was performed at the femur

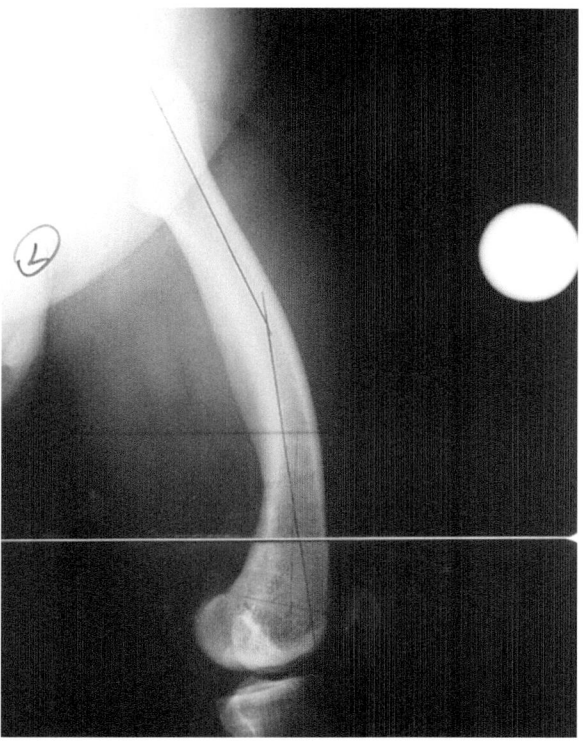

Fig. 22.13 Long sagittal bowing deformity at the femur: Note there are multiple centers of rotation in these types of deformities

Author's Preferred Method, Tips, and Tricks

The pathological change caused by hypophosphatemic rickets occurs very close to the growth plate, often leading to juxta-articular multiplanar deformities and severe malalignment. Preoperative assessment usually reveals multiple centers of rotation of angulation (CORA) (Fig. 22.13); thus, several osteotomies may be required to fully correct the multiapical deformities. Many methods of treatment have been described. The most common involve acute or gradual correction, using either circular or monolateral external fixators, which can secure accurate correction of the deformity and address the limb-length discrepancy. However, these methods are uncomfortable for the patient, especially when both legs are involved. There are further disadvantages, such as the need for daily adjustments, weekly follow-ups, a high rate of pin-track infection, and a long duration of external fixation.

We use the fixator-assisted nailing technique described by Paley and Herzenberg [42], with osteotomies created at the center(s) of the deformity(ies), followed by correction using a monolateral fixator and stabilization with locked intramedullary nailing (Figs. 22.14, 22.15, and 22.16). Removal of the external fixator at the end of the operation reduces post-

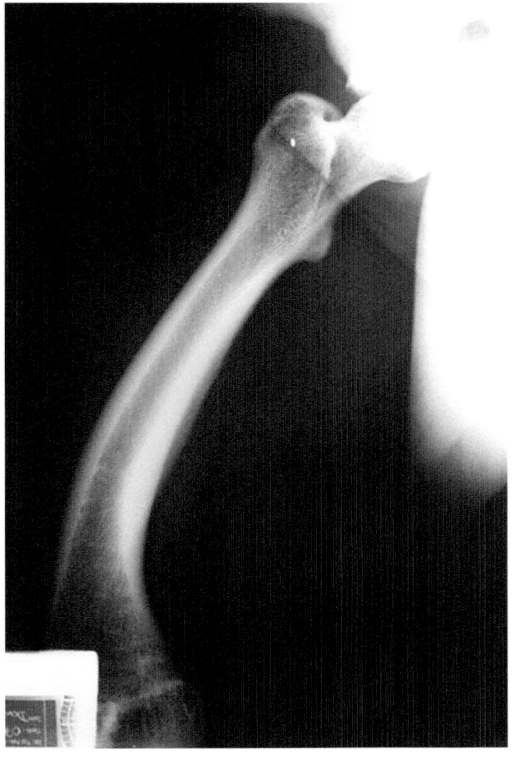

Fig. 22.14 X-ray showing a varus bowing deformity at the femur

operative discomfort and avoids pin-track infections, except where patients require additional postoperative lengthening over the nails. However, this technique does not allow residual correction or adjustment postoperatively. Thus, careful analysis of the deformity and preoperative planning are crucial. We recommend using this technique for a patient, who has essentially reached skeletal maturity. Flexible intramedullary nails (elastic nails) can be used in the pediatric age group [41].

Osteotomies in the long bones can be executed through limited incisions percutaneously either by the Gigli saw technique (Fig. 22.17) or by the multiple drill hole technique (Fig. 22.18). This technique combines the accuracy, minimal invasiveness, and safety of external fixation with the patient convenience of internal fixation. The use of an intramedullary nail prevents the recurrence of the deformity of the stabilized bone segment, which is especially important in patients with metabolic bone diseases who are prone to recurrence of the deformity as the metabolic problem continues. In addition, the surgeon must be familiar with both

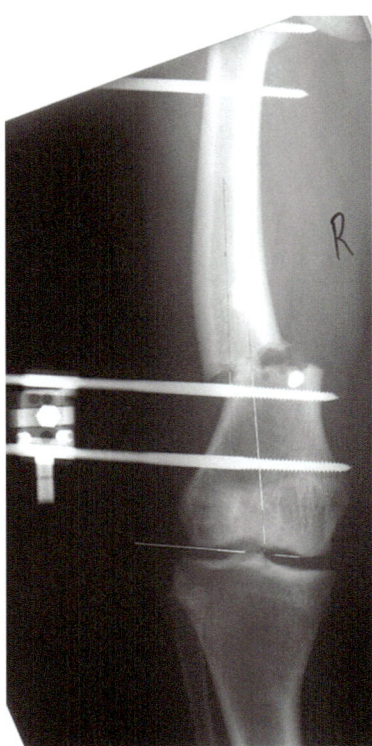

Fig. 22.15 Deformity has been acutely corrected with the use of a unilateral external fixator

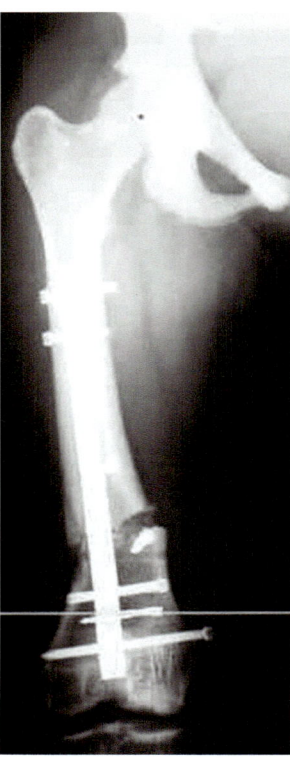

Fig. 22.16 Once the satisfactory correction was achieved, intramedullary static fixation was performed (FAN procedure)

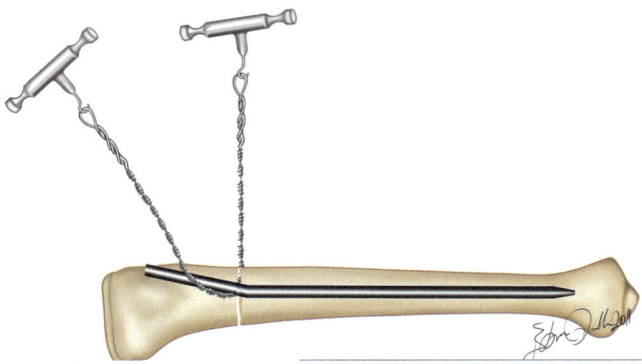

Fig. 22.17 Gigli saw osteotomy technique

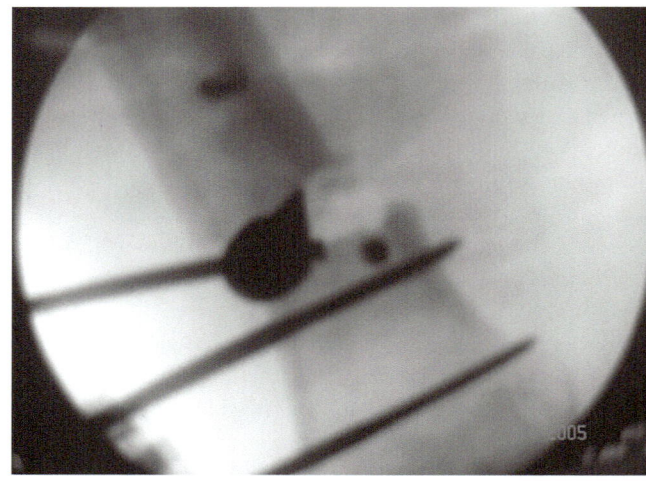

Fig. 22.18 Drill hole technique which is completed by an osteotome

external fixation and intramedullary nailing techniques, as well as combined techniques, which can be technically demanding.

Surgical Technique

The patient is placed supine on a radiolucent table and the lower limb is checked for imaging on the radiography table from the hip joint to the ankle joint on both frontal and side views (Fig. 22.19). In patients with genu valgum, resulting both from the femur and/or the tibia, mini-open release of the peroneal nerve is performed prior to correction of the deformity to avoid neurapraxia due to traction. Two 6-mm conical Schanz screws are placed into the proximal and distal segments above and below the planned osteotomy to maintain the stability, perpendicular to the anatomical axis, taking care to leave enough space for inserting an intramedullary nail without making contact with the screws (Figs. 22.20, 22.21, and 22.22). The level of osteotomy is chosen based on preoperative planning and performed percutaneously using the multiple drill hole technique for the femur or a Gigli saw for the tibia. Following the osteotomies, the deformity is corrected using a monolateral external fixator (Fig. 22.23). The correction is confirmed by obtaining frontal and side view long radiographs. If the desired correction is not achieved, it is adjusted and then confirmed by obtaining further X-rays. Once the surgeon is satisfied with the correction, the intramedullary nailing is performed through a 2 cm transverse incision over the ligamentum patellae (Fig. 22.24). The standard ligament split approach is used to open the tibial or femoral canals under fluoroscopic control. Over a guide wire, the medullary canal is over-reamed 1 mm larger than the diameter of the nail to be used (Fig. 22.25). Interference-blocking screws are placed before or after nail insertion to reduce the larger diameter of the medullary canal at the metaphyseal level to prevent the motion of the nail (Fig. 22.26). The nail is inserted and locked both proximally and distally if no lengthening is planned. The positions of the nail and the Schanz screws and the deformity correction are once again confirmed under fluoroscopic control, and then, the fixator is removed (Figs. 22.27 and 22.28) (Box 22.2).

Fig. 22.19 Long X-rays for deformity analysis provided by a radiolucent table

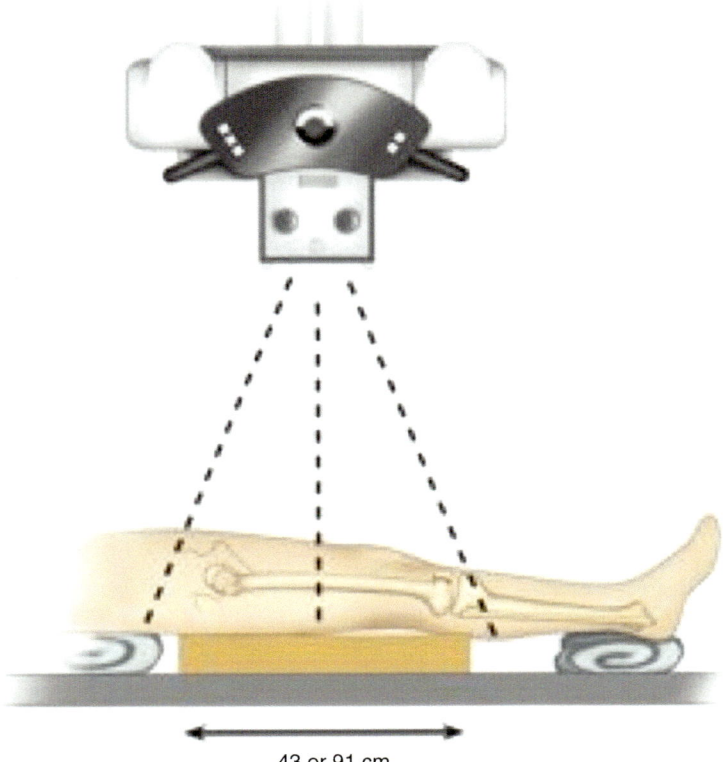

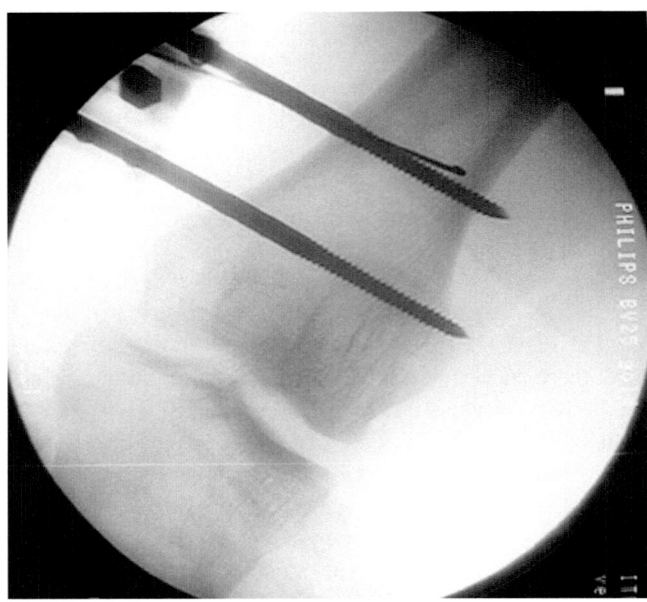

Fig. 22.20 Two parallel Schanz screws distally at the femur

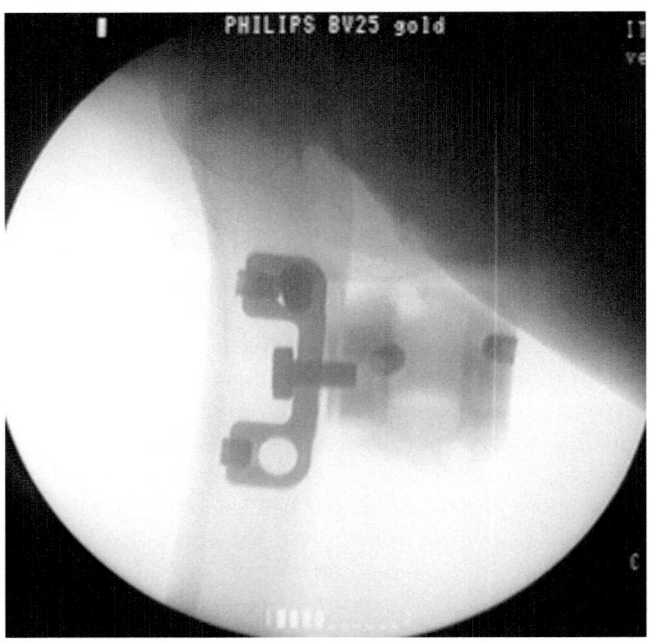

Fig. 22.22 Schanz screws must leave enough space for intramedullary nailing

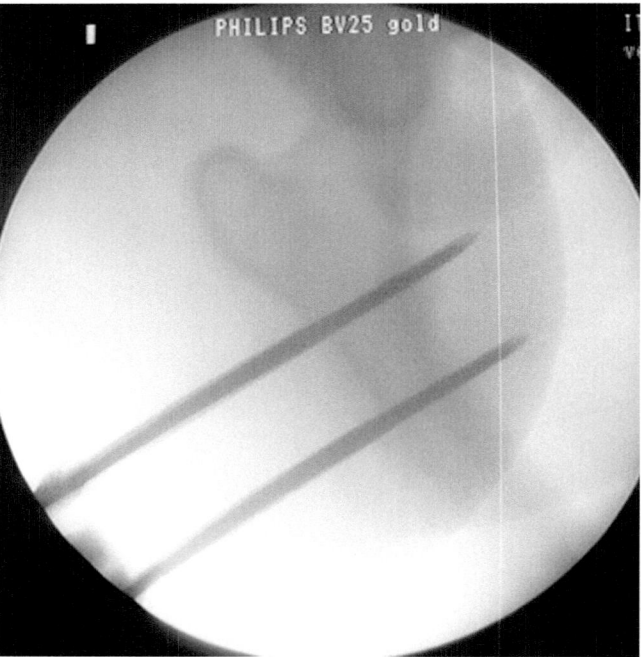

Fig. 22.21 Two parallel Schanz screws proximally at the femur

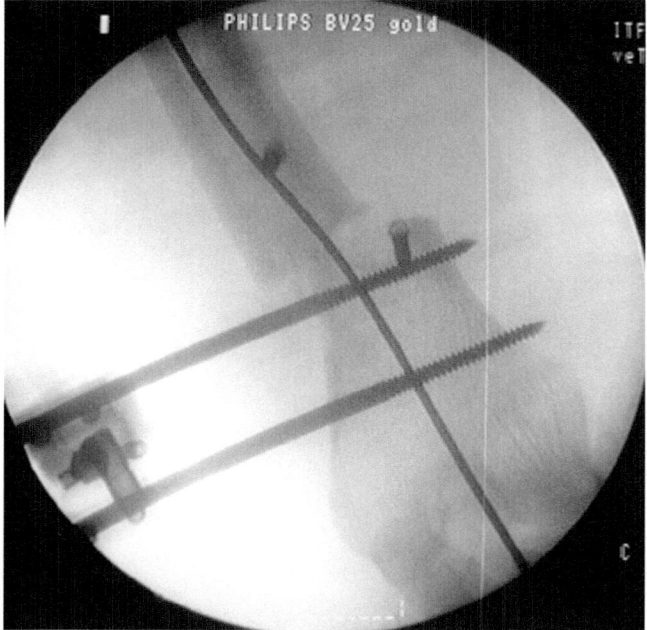

Fig. 22.23 Following osteotomy, the correction is performed and maintained by a monolateral external fixator

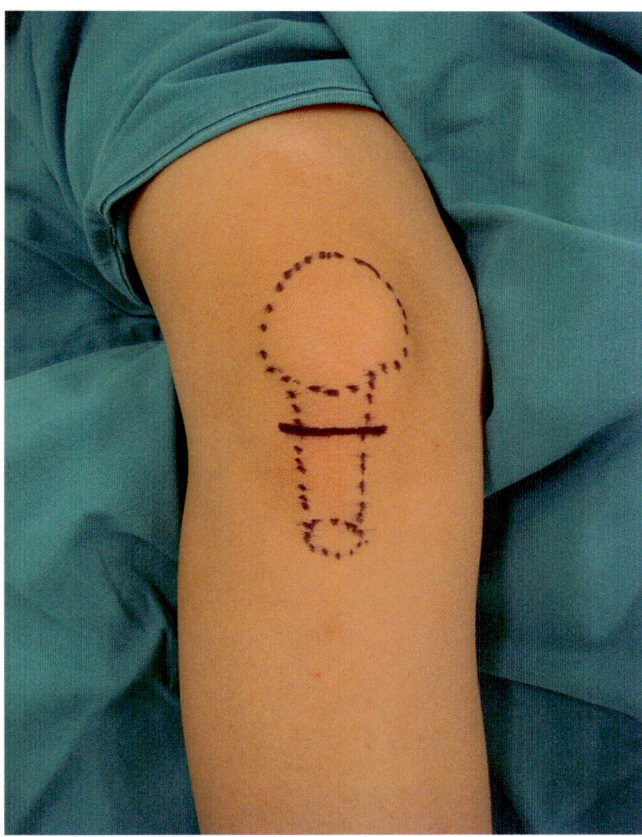

Fig. 22.24 Transverse skin incision over the ligamentum patella

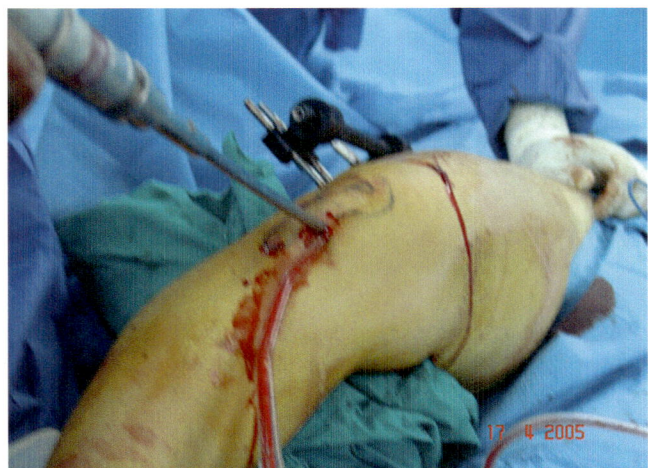

Fig. 22.25 The over-reaming of the intramedullary canal by 1 mm larger than the nail diameter

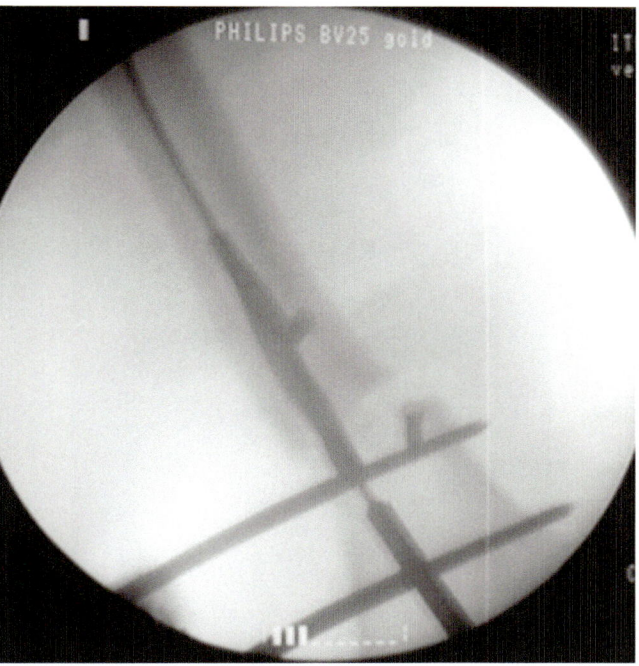

Fig. 22.26 Using the interference screws to help maintain the correction

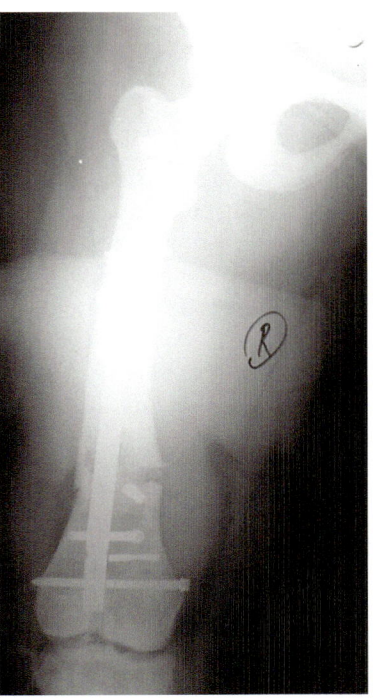

Fig. 22.27 AP view following intramedullary static fixation

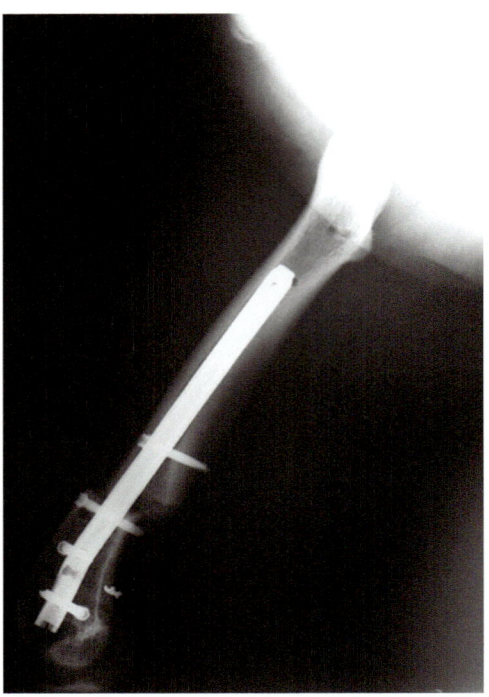

Fig. 22.28 Lateral view following intramedullary static fixation

Box 22.2
- The deformities are multiapical (long bowing) and tend to recur.
- Intramedullary nailing should be always performed, if possible, to prevent recurrence.
- Preoperative planning is of paramount importance and should contain paper-tracing to simulate the surgical procedure. It will increase the precision of the procedure while shortening the surgical time.
- Fixator-assisted nailing is very effective for accurate deformity correction and prevention of recurrences.

Follow-Up

Isometric exercises are begun postoperatively, and partial weight-bearing is allowed with crutches as tolerated. Full weight-bearing is allowed only after achieving the consolidation of three of four cortices on AP and lateral radiography (approximately 3 months).

The postoperative management should be done in close collaboration with the attending nephrologist or endocrinologist since calcium levels tend to increase suddenly with postoperative immobilization. It is recommended to reduce the medical dose to half for a week to avoid hypercalcemia and vitamin D toxicity and then increase to a full dose with patient mobilization [12].

Renal Osteodystrophy

General

As the use of renal transplantation for treating renal failure in children has increased, the prevalence of renal osteodystrophy has also climbed. Manifestations of renal osteodystrophy are present in 66–79% of children with renal failure [43]. Renal osteodystrophy is noticeably different from either nutritional or hypophosphatemic rickets. It is often driven by the presence of secondary hyperparathyroidism, which leads to the activation of osteoclasts and resorption of bone [2, 4]. Features of both rickets and hyperparathyroidism are present in children with renal osteodystrophy.

Children affected by renal osteodystrophy are often short-statured and have fragile bones. These patients often have bone pain, and fractures occur easily. The most common orthopedic manifestations are skeletal deformities, usually genu valgum, periarticular enlargement of long bones, slipped capital femoral epiphysis (SCFE), muscle weakness, and Trendelenburg gait, especially if SCFE is present [4]. In severe and persistent renal failure, aggressive lytic areas in long bones may develop (*brown tumor*). Since many patients with renal failure, especially those who undergo renal transplantation, are treated with steroids, osteonecrosis can also develop.

Treatment

Medical Treatment

The treatment of causal renal disease is of crucial importance. Dialysis and renal transplantation prolong the survival of these patients. Medical therapy is initiated with 1,25 dihydroxy form of vitamin D. The use of calcitriol significantly decreases serum PTH levels and delays secondary bone changes [44]. The treatment of acidosis with sodium bicarbonate also improves metabolic bone disease.

Decreased skeletal growth and short stature are significant problems, probably due to disturbances in the growth hormone-insulin-like growth factor axis. rhGH restores growth in these children.

Orthopedic Treatment

Patients with renal osteodystrophy are generally referred to the orthopedic surgeon for the treatment of three pathologies: angular deformity of lower extremity long bones, SCFE, and avascular necrosis [4]. Any surgical intervention in this patient population should be carefully considered, as the perioperative risks are amplified due to associated anemia, hypertension, bleeding tendencies, and electrolyte imbalances. The risk of infection is additionally increased in patients with a renal transplant who are on immunosuppressive therapy.

Angular Deformity

Angular deformities of the lower extremity occur in renal osteodystrophy because the long bones are soft, undermineralized, and prone to bend with weight-bearing. Genu valgum is the most common deformity, but genu varum or a windswept deformity may also occur [4, 21]. If renal osteodystrophy occurs before 4 years of age, varus deformity may develop because the normal alignment of the leg is in slight varus, which then is accentuated when the bone becomes weak. Similarly, older children are prone to the development of genu valgum because of the physiologic valgus alignment of the lower extremities. Valgus at the ankle may also accompany the genu valgum [45].

Some milder deformities will be corrected with medical treatment of renal osteodystrophy [4, 45]. However, these deformities do not respond well to bracing. If the patient becomes symptomatic and has had optimum medical treatment without resolution of the deformity, surgical management with guided growth or corrective osteotomy should be attempted [4, 45, 46]. Usually, the greatest deformity is in the distal femoral metaphysis, but sometimes, a supplementary proximal tibial osteotomy is also needed. Internal or external fixation may be used. While external fixators have been successfully applied by taking care of achieving stable constructs and utilizing hydroxyapatite-coated Schanz pins, bone healing may be delayed [47]. Deformity recurrence is common in patients with continuing metabolic pathology, so medical treatment should be adjusted before and continued after corrective osteotomy. Elevation of serum alkaline phosphatase concentration above 500 U/L is a worthy marker of ongoing metabolic bone disease [4, 45]. Milder deformities may respond to hemiepiphysiodesis [46].

Slipped Capital Femoral Epiphysis

The clinical picture of a child with SCFE secondary to renal osteodystrophy differs from the usual cases of SCFE. Often, these patients are younger, and obesity is not a part of the clinical picture. Bilaterality is also very common. Radiologic pathology in the physis is more pronounced, accompanied by physeal widening and generalized osteopenia [48].

Standard management of SCFE aims to prevent further deformity and promote early closure of the proximal femoral physeal growth plate. However, cessation of proximal femoral growth may not be desirable in a young child with renal osteodystrophy. Moreover, physeal healing is compromised due to the underlying metabolic pathological condition. Fortunately, the pain and physeal widening resolve with appropriate medical treatment. However, if the slip is displaced or symptoms continue despite medical treatment, fixation should be performed with a screw that provides stability by crossing the physis before the physeal closure.

Avascular Necrosis

The prolonged use of corticosteroids is the likely cause. Avascular necrosis frequently occurs bilateral, affecting the hip. Treatment is usually symptomatic [4].

Hypophosphatasia

General

Hypophosphatasia is a rare genetic defect of alkaline phosphatase production, resulting in pathologic mineralization of bone. There is a wide variation in the severity of the disease, and the prognosis depends on the age of onset; perinatal, infantile, childhood, and adult hypophosphatasia can occur [4, 49]. The genetic defect for this disorder is determined to be in the tissue-nonspecific alkaline phosphatase gene (*TNSALP*), and many different mutations have been described [50].

Treatment

Before the availability of Asfotase alpha, bone-targeted enzyme replacement therapy developed by recombinant DNA technology in Chinese hamster ovary cell line, medical treatment of hypophosphatasia was limited. FDA and EMA approved in 2015 for treatment of pediatric-onset forms, administered subcutaneously three times a week. Studies in a limited number of patients showed improvement in patient survival, radiological skeletal changes, growth, mobility, and bone mineral densitometry; however, there is no consensus for the treatment criteria worldwide [10].

Fractures and deformities need orthopedic management. Fracture healing is commonly delayed. Multiple osteotomies with intramedullary fixation are often required to correct the bowing and provide structural support to the long bones [4]. Thus, when possible, it is advised to utilize an intramedullary nail in all corrected bone segments.

Medical control of the underlying disease is of paramount importance as deformities tend to recur in various metabolic bone diseases. Therefore, consultation with the endocrinologist should be done preoperatively and continued after the surgical intervention.

Idiopathic Genu Valgum

High rates of obesity associated with idiopathic genu valgum among children have been seen. The severity of the deformity is directly related to skeletal maturation and body mass index, which plays an etiological role in obesity in the development and progression of the deformity. Treatment with the guided growth technique before skeletal maturity can correct the deformity and reduce the osteoarthritis risk in adulthood [51].

Example Cases

Case 1: Figures 22.29, 22.30, 22.31, 22.32, 22.33, 22.34, and 22.35 show the treatment sequences of a patient (hypophosphatemic rickets) with a profound bilateral femoral varus deformities.

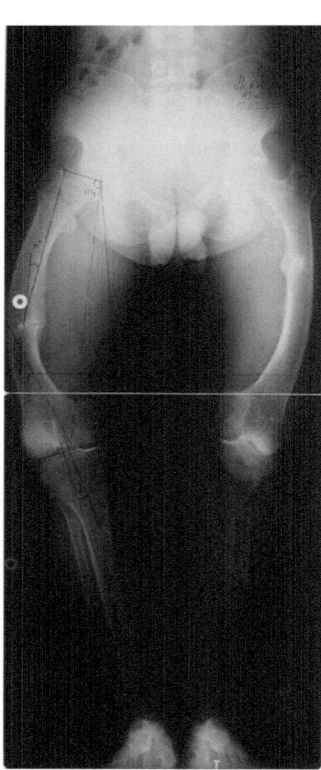

Fig. 22.29 A patient's orthoroentgenogram showing severe varus deformities

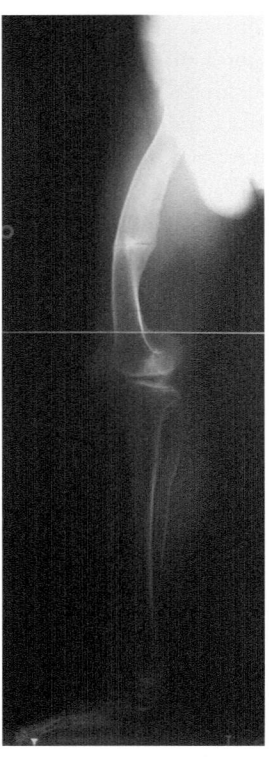

Fig. 22.30 Right lateral orthoroentgenogram shows anterior femoral bowing deformity. Note there is a pending stress fracture at the femoral diaphyseal level

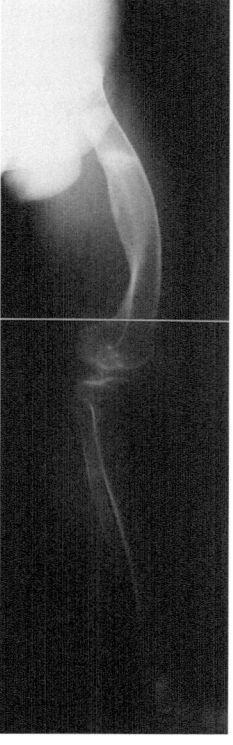

Fig. 22.31 Left lateral orthoroentgenogram shows anterior femoral bowing deformity

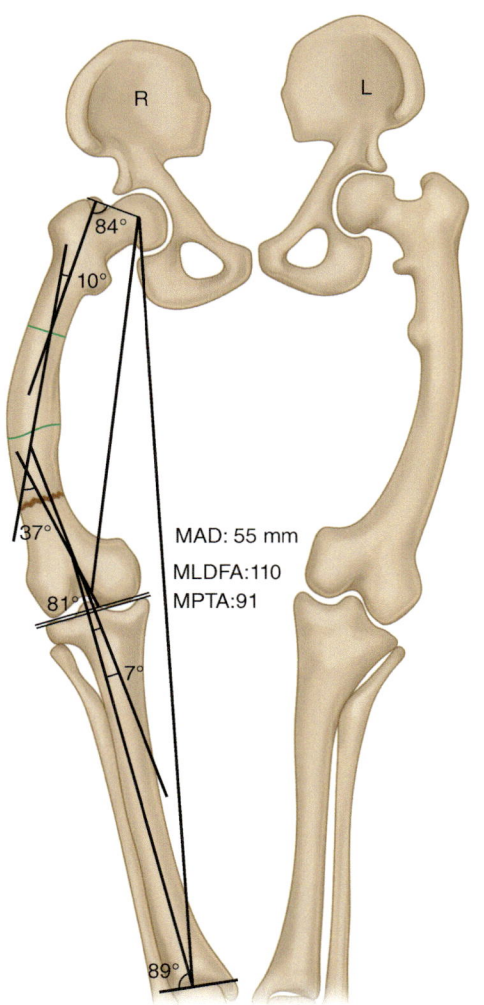

Fig. 22.32 Paper-tracing for deformity analysis

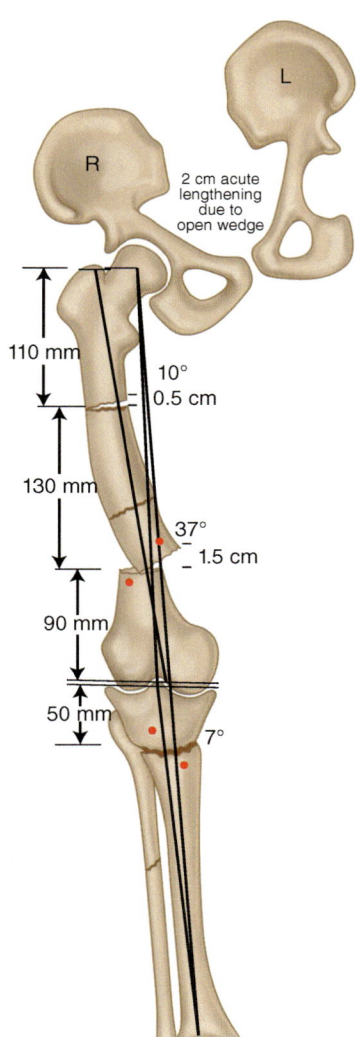

Fig. 22.33 Paper-tracing for surgical simulation

Case 2: Figures 22.36, 22.37, 22.38, 22.39, 22.40, 22.41, 22.42, 22.43, and 22.44 show the treatment sequences of a patient (hypophosphatemic rickets) with a profound genu valgum deformity.

Case 3: Figures 22.45, 22.46, 22.47, 22.48, 22.49, 22.50, 22.51, 22.52, and 22.53 show the treatment sequences of a patient (hypophosphatemic rickets) with a profound genu varum deformity.

Case 4: Figures 22.54, 22.55, 22.56, and 22.57 show the treatment sequences of a patient (XLH rickets) by guided growth technique.

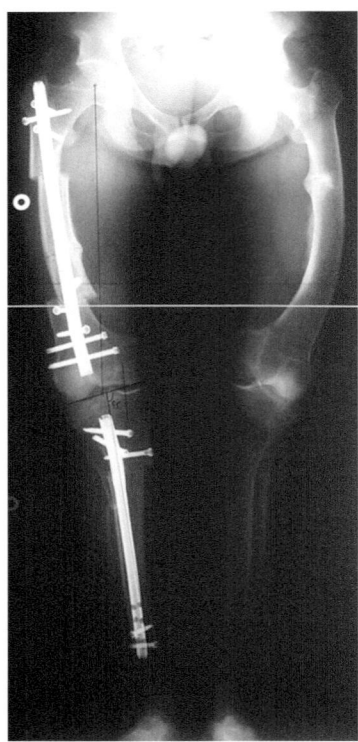

Fig. 22.34 Orthoroentgenogram following FAN procedure at the femur and tibia on the right

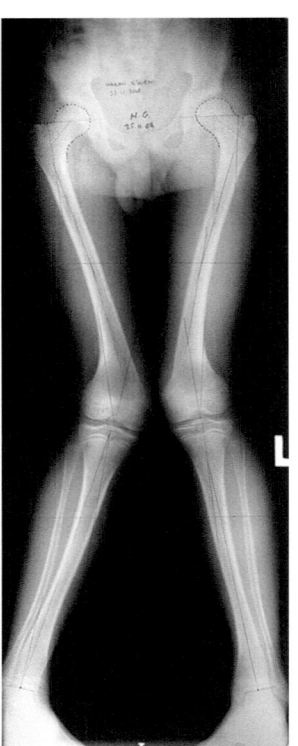

Fig. 22.36 Orthoroentgenogram of a patient with severe genu valgum deformity

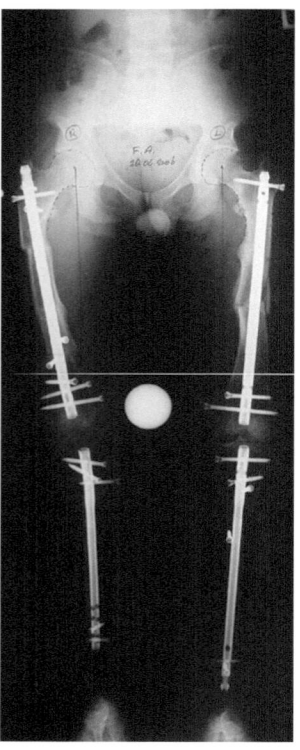

Fig. 22.35 Orthoroentgenogram following final FAN procedure at the femur and tibia on the left

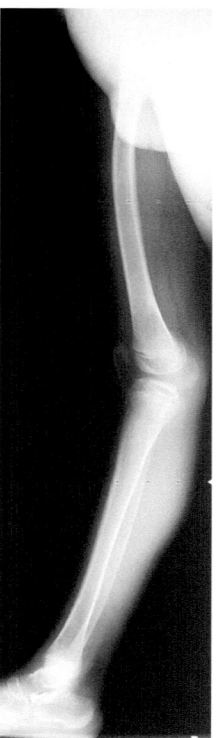

Fig. 22.37 Right lateral orthoroentgenogram of the same patient

22 Metabolic Disorders

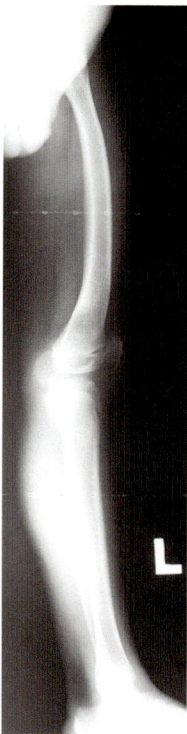

Fig. 22.38 Left lateral orthoroentgenogram of the same patient

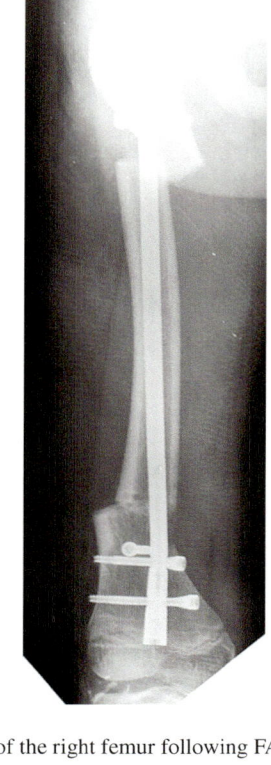

Fig. 22.40 X-ray of the right femur following FAN procedure

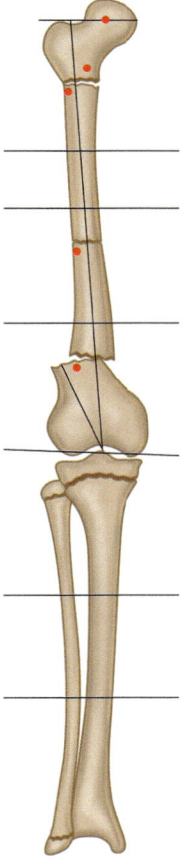

Fig. 22.39 Paper-tracing for surgical planning

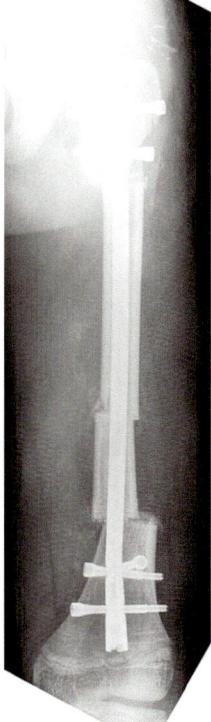

Fig. 22.41 X-ray of the left femur following FAN procedure

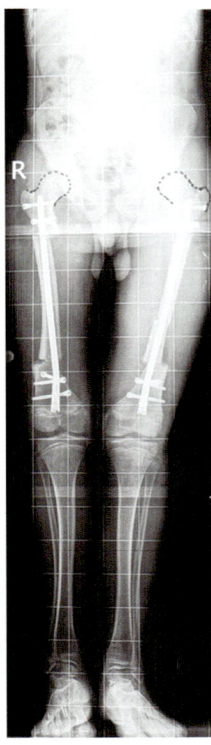

Fig. 22.42 Orthoroentgenogram at the end of the treatment

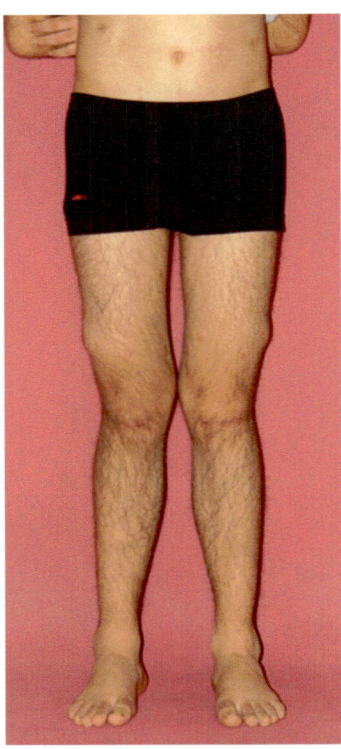

Fig. 22.44 Clinical view of the same patient after the treatment

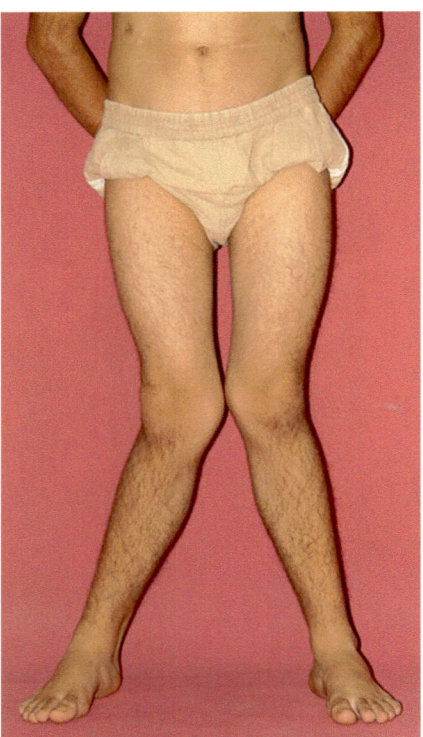

Fig. 22.43 Clinical view of the same patient prior to surgery

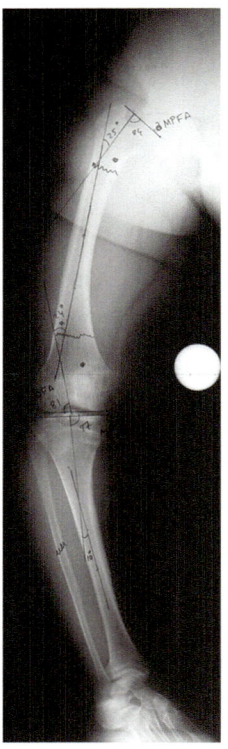

Fig. 22.45 Right frontal orthoroentgenogram showing severe genu varum

22 Metabolic Disorders

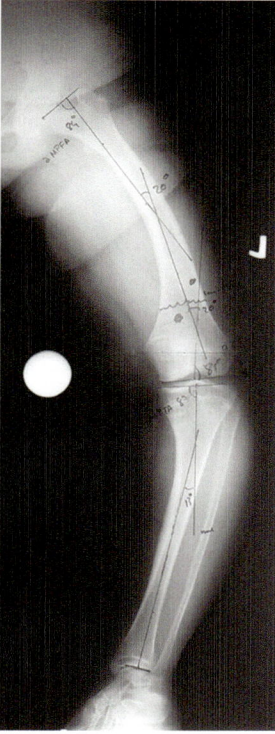

Fig. 22.46 Left frontal orthoroentgenogram of the same patient showing severe genu varum

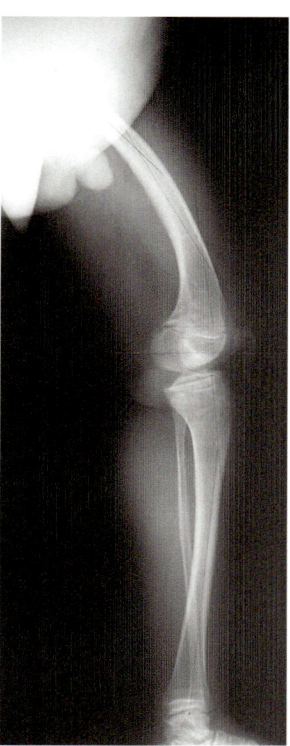

Fig. 22.48 Left lateral orthoroentgenogram showing anterior bowing (same patient)

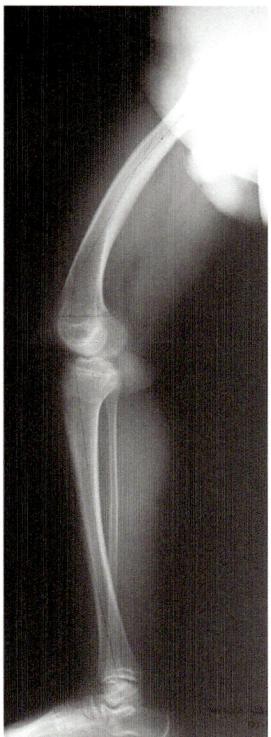

Fig. 22.47 Right lateral orthoroentgenogram showing anterior bowing (same patient)

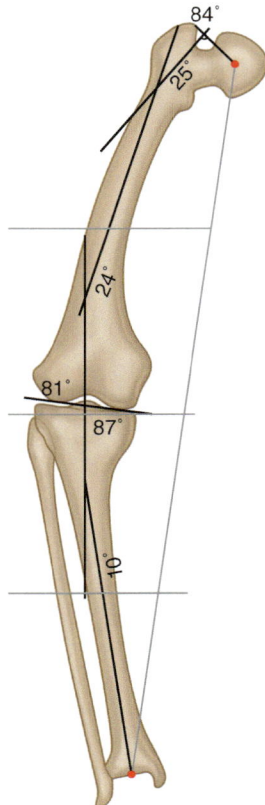

Fig. 22.49 Paper-tracing for deformity analysis on the right

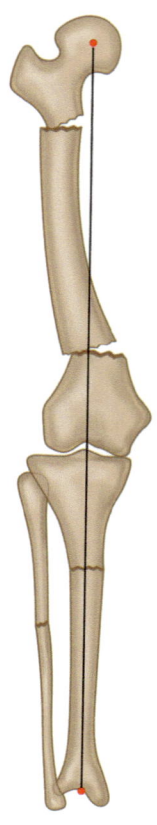

Fig. 22.50 Paper-tracing for surgical simulation

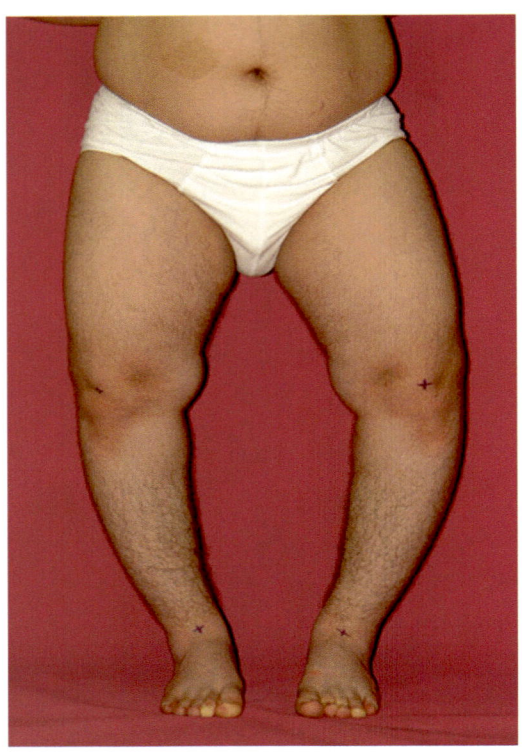

Fig. 22.52 Clinical view of the same patient prior to surgery

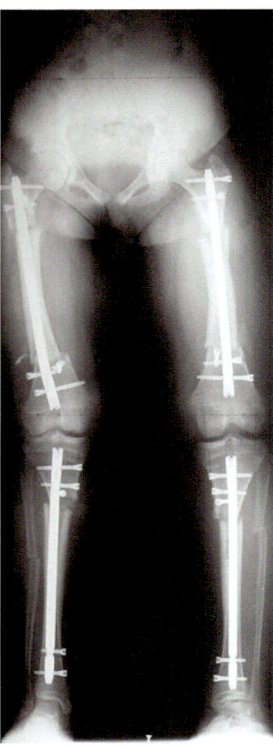

Fig. 22.51 Orthoroentgenogram at the end of the treatment

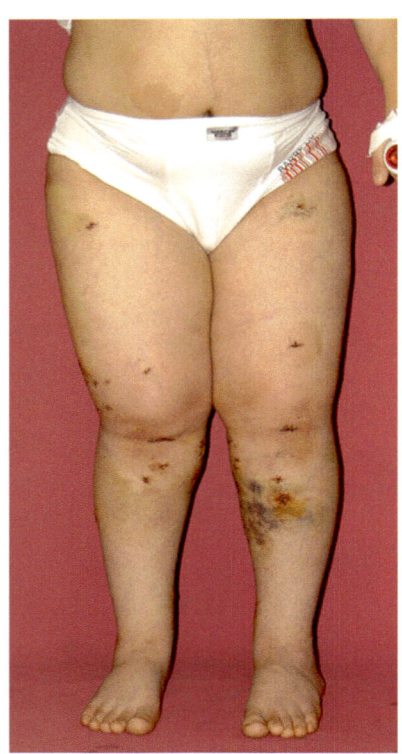

Fig. 22.53 Clinical view of the same patient after the treatment

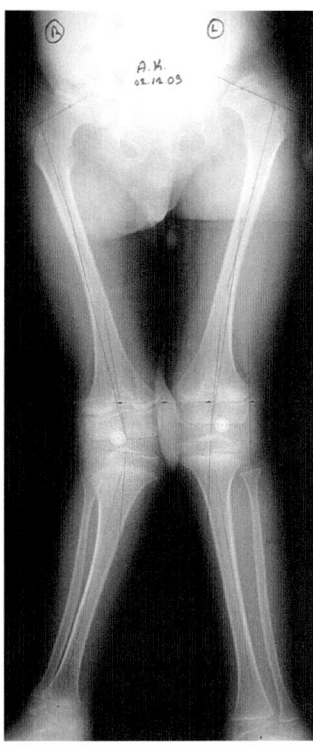

Fig. 22.54 Orthoroentgenogram of a patient with XLH rickets prior to treatment

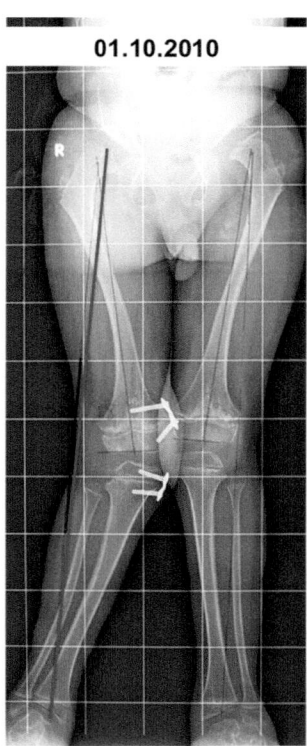

Fig. 22.56 Orthoroentgenogram of the same patient 3 months later

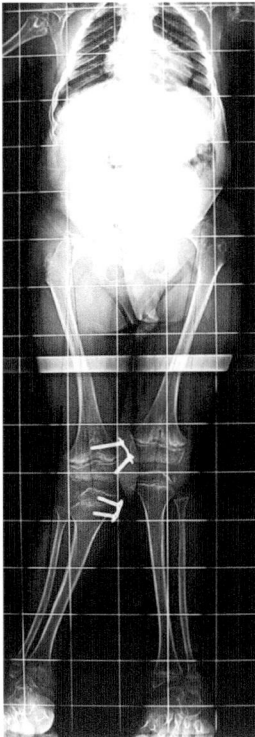

Fig. 22.55 Orthoroentgenogram of the same patient after application of hemiepiphysiodesis

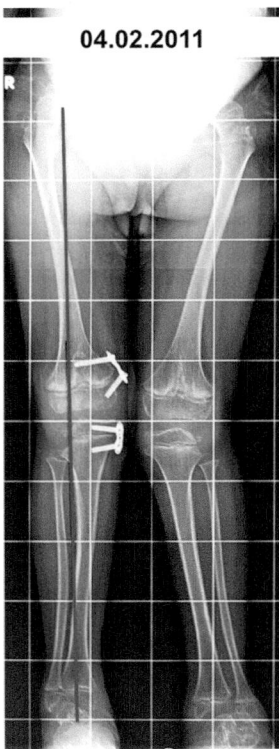

Fig. 22.57 Orthoroentgenogram of the same patient 7 months later. Please note the correction of the mechanical axis

Commentary

Jill C. Flanagan
Jill.Flanagan@choa.org

The authors do an excellent job describing metabolic bone disorders, including potential deformities, and strategies for medical and surgical treatment. It is imperative for the orthopedic surgeon treating these conditions to understand this information, as it will improve the likelihood of success. For metabolic bone disease, the surgeon should work closely with the endocrinologist and/or nephrologist to ensure that the patient is as medically optimized as possible preoperatively. Healthier bones will allow the surgery to be easier, as the bone will be easier to work with, and there will be an improved chance of healing and consequently less chance of hardware failure.

Surgical Indications: For deformities secondary to rickets in younger children that are progressive despite optimal medical treatment, surgery may be indicated. With the introduction of Burosumab for XLH rickets, this author agrees that this medication has been very effective at treating rickets both at the chemical level and at the macroscopic level when looking at the bones on radiographs. Physeal width improves, and deformities are less severe when given in the younger age group. Similarly, Asfotase alfa has been revolutionary in the treatment of hypophosphatasia. In general, for mild deformities where the coronal plane dominates, especially in younger age groups (under 10), this author utilizes guided growth treatment given the appeal of less invasiveness. Osteotomies are indicated for failure of guided growth in patients where deformities are causing pain and/or functional limitation. The use of telescopic nails in younger children is ideal for rickets and hypophosphatasia as it can help maintain deformities and prevent significant recurrences in the future. Note that there is no rotational control with most telescopic nails, so additional mini-plate fixation may be needed to control rotation. In older patients, nailing is preferred over plating for two important reasons. A load-sharing device such as an intramedullary nail will decrease the incidence of osteolysis of the bone. Secondly, there can be a higher risk of secondary fracture at the end of a plate. The nail should span the entire length of the long bone, in order to maintain the correction and protect the bone from secondary fracture and possibly recurrent deformity.

Surgical Planning: If a more traditional intramedullary nail will be used, it is imperative to measure the anticipated length and diameter of the nail preoperatively. As these patients are short in stature, the nail may need to be custom-ordered for length. Most telescopic nails are cut in the surgical field and should not be a problem. If bilateral limbs have deformity, this author prefers operating on one side at a time and staging the operations. That way, one limb can still be free for weight-bearing. Standard deformity analysis, as discussed in the chapter, works well as the surgeon needs to anticipate the location and number of osteotomies planned. The application of a temporary spanning external fixator (aka "fixator-assisted nailing") proximal and distal to the osteotomies can be an invaluable tool to help obtain and maintain acute correction of these complex deformities.

Surgical Positioning: This author prefers to use a radiolucent table. Ensure that the patient is positioned with the operated side close to the edge of the table to help facilitate the start point for an antegrade femur surgery. A sheet can be placed around the groin and then tied to a post on the side of the table to allow for countertraction which may be needed during surgery. Tranexamic acid, cell saver, and other modalities may be utilized to decrease blood loss. While a tourniquet can be used for the tibia, ensure that the tourniquet is down for reaming to decrease the risk of thermal injury.

Postoperative: If your institution has a pool, aqua therapy may be a very nice alternative to traditional physical therapy. Patients with rickets may have prolonged healing time following an osteotomy, so this is a great modality to allow an early range of motion and simulate walking without true weight-bearing. A zero-gravity treadmill may be another such option. Splinting time should be minimized for osteotomies to decrease the incidence of disuse osteopenia.

References

1. Staheli LT, Song KM. Rickets and metabolic disorders. In: Staheli LT, editor. Pediatric orthopedic secrets. 3rd ed. Philadelphia, PA: Elsevier; 2007. p. 551–9.
2. Mankin HJ. Rickets, osteomalacia, and renal osteodystrophy. An update. Orthop Clin North Am. 1990;21(1):81–96.
3. Zaleske DJ, Doppelt SH, Mankin HJ. Metabolic and endocrine abnormalities of the immature skeleton. In: Morrissey RT, editor. Lovell and winter's pediatric orthopaedics. 3rd ed. Philadelphia, PA: JB Lippincott; 1990. p. 203–61.
4. Herring JA. Metabolic and endocrine bone diseases. In: Herring JA, editor. Tachdjian's pediatric orthopaedics. 4th ed. Philadelphia, PA: Elsevier; 2008. p. 1917–82.
5. Gentile C, Chiarelli F. Rickets in children: an update. Biomedicines. 2021;9(7):738. https://doi.org/10.3390/biomedicines9070738.

6. Chanchlani R, Nemer P, Sinha R, Nemer L, Krishnappa V, Sochett E, et al. An overview of rickets in children. Kidney Int Rep. 2020;5(7):980–90. https://doi.org/10.1016/j.ekir.2020.03.025.
7. Rauch F. The rachitic bone. Endocr Dev. 2003;6:69–79. https://doi.org/10.1159/000072770.
8. Sabbagh Y, Carpenter TO, Demay MB. Hypophosphatemia leads to rickets by impairing caspase-mediated apoptosis of hypertrophic chondrocytes. Proc Natl Acad Sci USA. 2005;102(27):9637–42. https://doi.org/10.1073/pnas.0502249102.
9. Lambert AS, Linglart A. Hypocalcaemic and hypophosphatemic rickets. Best Pract Res Clin Endocrinol Metab. 2018;32(4):455–76. https://doi.org/10.1016/j.beem.2018.05.009.
10. Kim HKW, Seikaly MG. Metabolic and endocrine disorders of bone. In: Herring JA, editor. Tachdjian's pediatric orthopaedics: from the Texas Scottish Rite Hospital for Children. 6th ed. Philadelphia: Elsevier; 2021. p. 1928–75.
11. Baroncelli GI, Bertelloni S, Ceccarelli C, Amato V, Saggese G. Bone turnover in children with vitamin D deficiency rickets before and during treatment. Acta Paediatr. 2000;89(5):513–8. https://doi.org/10.1080/080352500750027763.
12. Sharkey MS, Grunseich K, Carpenter TO. Contemporary medical and surgical management of X-linked hypophosphatemic rickets. J Am Acad Orthop Surg. 2015;23(7):433–42. https://doi.org/10.5435/JAAOS-D-14-00082.
13. Haffner D, Emma F, Eastwood DM, Duplan MB, Bacchetta J, Schnabel D, et al. Clinical practice recommendations for the diagnosis and management of X-linked hypophosphataemia. Nat Rev Nephrol. 2019;15(7):435–55. https://doi.org/10.1038/s41581-019-0152-5.
14. Laurent MR, De Schepper J, Trouet D, Godefroid N, Boros E, Heinrichs C, et al. Consensus recommendations for the diagnosis and management of X-linked hypophosphatemia in Belgium. Front Endocrinol (Lausanne). 2021;12:1–20. https://doi.org/10.3389/fendo.2021.641543.
15. Holm IA, Huang X, Kunkel LM. Mutational analysis of the PEX gene in patients with X-linked hypophosphatemic rickets. Am J Hum Genet. 1997;60(4):790–7.
16. Popkov A, Aranovich A, Popkov D. Results of deformity correction in children with X-linked hereditary hypophosphatemic rickets by external fixation or combined technique. Int Orthop. 2015;39(12):2423–31. https://doi.org/10.1007/s00264-015-2814-7.
17. Razzaque MS, Lanske B. The emerging role of the fibroblast growth factor-23-klotho axis in renal regulation of phosphate homeostasis. J Endocrinol. 2007;194(1):1–10. https://doi.org/10.1677/JOE-07-0095.
18. Linglart A, Biosse-Duplan M, Briot K, Chaussain C, Esterle L, Guillaume-Czitrom S, et al. Therapeutic management of hypophosphatemic rickets from infancy to adulthood. Endocr Connect. 2014;3(1):R13–30. https://doi.org/10.1530/EC-13-0103.
19. Steendijk R, Hauspie RC. The pattern of growth and growth retardation of patients with hypophosphataemic vitamin D-resistant rickets: a longitudinal study. Eur J Pediatr. 1992;151(6):422–7. https://doi.org/10.1007/BF01959355.
20. Al Kaissi A, Farr S, Ganger R, Klaushofer K, Grill F. Windswept lower limb deformities in patients with hypophosphataemic rickets. Swiss Med Wkly. 2013;143:w13904. https://doi.org/10.4414/smw.2013.13904.
21. Eralp L, Kocaoglu M, Cakmak M, Ozden VE. A correction of windswept deformity by fixator assisted nailing. A report of two cases. J Bone Joint Surg Br. 2004;86(7):1065–8. https://doi.org/10.1302/0301-620x.86b7.14923.
22. Makitie O, Doria A, Kooh SW, Cole WG, Daneman A, Sochett E. Early treatment improves growth and biochemical and radiographic outcome in X-linked hypophosphatemic rickets. J Clin Endocrinol Metab. 2003;88(8):3591–7. https://doi.org/10.1210/jc.2003-030036.
23. Quinlan C, Guegan K, Offiah A, Neill RO, Hiorns MP, Ellard S, et al. Growth in PHEX-associated X-linked hypophosphatemic rickets: the importance of early treatment. Pediatr Nephrol. 2012;27(4):581–8. https://doi.org/10.1007/s00467-011-2046-z.
24. Carpenter TO, Imel EA, Holm IA, Jan de Beur SM, Insogna KL. A clinician's guide to X-linked hypophosphatemia. J Bone Miner Res. 2011;26(7):1381–8. https://doi.org/10.1002/jbmr.340.
25. Lamb YN. Burosumab: first global approval. Drugs. 2018;78(6):707–14. https://doi.org/10.1007/s40265-018-0905-7.
26. Baroncelli GI, Bertelloni S, Ceccarelli C, Saggese G. Effect of growth hormone treatment on final height, phosphate metabolism, and bone mineral density in children with X-linked hypophosphatemic rickets. J Pediatr. 2001;138(2):236–43. https://doi.org/10.1067/mpd.2001.108955.
27. Saggese G, Baroncelli GI, Bertelloni S, Perri G. Long-term growth hormone treatment in children with renal hypophosphatemic rickets: effects on growth, mineral metabolism, and bone density. J Pediatr. 1995;127(3):395–402. https://doi.org/10.1016/s0022-3476(95)70070-6.
28. Carpenter KA, Davison R, Shakthivel S, Anderson KD, Ko FC, Ross RD. Sclerostin antibody improves phosphate metabolism hormones, bone formation rates, and bone mass in adult Hyp mice. Bone. 2021;154:116201. https://doi.org/10.1016/j.bone.2021.116201.
29. Hoac B, Ostergaard M, Wittig NK, Boukpessi T, Buss DJ, Chaussain C, et al. Genetic ablation of Osteopontin in Osteomalacic Hyp mice partially rescues the deficient mineralization without correcting hypophosphatemia. J Bone Miner Res. 2020;35(10):2032–48. https://doi.org/10.1002/jbmr.4101.
30. Mindler GT, Kranzl A, Stauffer A, Haeusler G, Ganger R, Raimann A. Disease-specific gait deviations in pediatric patients with X-linked hypophosphatemia. Gait Posture. 2020;81:78–84. https://doi.org/10.1016/j.gaitpost.2020.07.007.
31. Raimann A, Mindler GT, Kocijan R, Bekes K, Zwerina J, Haeusler G, et al. Multidisciplinary patient care in X-linked hypophosphatemic rickets: one challenge, many perspectives. Wien Med Wochenschr. 2020;170(5–6):116–23. https://doi.org/10.1007/s10354-019-00732-2.
32. Fucentese SF, Neuhaus TJ, Ramseier LE, Ulrich EG. Metabolic and orthopedic management of X-linked vitamin D-resistant hypophosphatemic rickets. J Child Orthop. 2008;2(4):285–91. https://doi.org/10.1007/s11832-008-0118-9.
33. Wirth T. The orthopaedic management of long bone deformities in genetically and acquired generalized bone weakening conditions. J Child Orthop. 2019;13(1):12–21. https://doi.org/10.1302/1863-2548.13.180184.
34. Kocaoglu M, Bilen FE, Sen C, Eralp L, Balci HI. Combined technique for the correction of lower-limb deformities resulting from metabolic bone disease. J Bone Joint Surg Br. 2011;93(1):52–6. https://doi.org/10.1302/0301-620X.93B1.24788.
35. Kanel JS, Price CT. Unilateral external fixation for corrective osteotomies in patients with hypophosphatemic rickets. J Pediatr Orthop. 1995;15(2):232–5.
36. Rubinovitch M, Said SE, Glorieux FH, Cruess RL, Rogala E. Principles and results of corrective lower limb osteotomies for patients with vitamin D-resistant hypophosphatemic rickets. Clin Orthop Relat Res. 1988;237:264–70.
37. Petje G, Meizer R, Radler C, Aigner N, Grill F. Deformity correction in children with hereditary hypophosphatemic rickets. Clin Orthop Relat Res. 2008;466(12):3078–85. https://doi.org/10.1007/s11999-008-0547-2.
38. Song HR, Soma Raju VV, Kumar S, Lee SH, Suh SW, Kim JR, et al. Deformity correction by external fixation and/or intramedullary nailing in hypophosphatemic rickets. Acta Orthop. 2006;77(2):307–14. https://doi.org/10.1080/17453670610046073.

39. Horn A, Wright J, Bockenhauer D, Van't Hoff W, Eastwood DM. The orthopaedic management of lower limb deformity in hypophosphataemic rickets. J Child Orthop. 2017;11(4):298–305. https://doi.org/10.1302/1863-2548.11.170003.
40. Gizard A, Rothenbuhler A, Pejin Z, Finidori G, Glorion C, de Billy B, et al. Outcomes of orthopedic surgery in a cohort of 49 patients with X-linked hypophosphatemic rickets (XLHR). Endocr Connect. 2017;6(8):566–73. https://doi.org/10.1530/EC-17-0154.
41. Popkov D, Popkov A, Haumont T, Journeau P, Lascombes P. Flexible intramedullary nail use in limb lengthening. J Pediatr Orthop. 2010;30(8):910–8. https://doi.org/10.1097/BPO.0b013e3181f0eaf9.
42. Paley D, Herzenberg JE, Bor N. Fixator-assisted nailing of femoral and Tibial deformities. Tech Orthop. 1997;12(4):260–75.
43. Fassier F, St-Pierre M, Robitaille P. Renal osteodystrophy in children: correlation between aetiology of the renal disease and the frequency of bone and articular lesions. Int Orthop. 1993;17(4):269–71. https://doi.org/10.1007/BF00194194.
44. Morii H, Ishimura E, Inoue T, Tabata T, Morita A, Nishii Y, et al. History of vitamin D treatment of renal osteodystrophy. Am J Nephrol. 1997;17(3–4):382–6. https://doi.org/10.1159/000169125.
45. Davids JR, Fisher R, Lum G, Von Glinski S. Angular deformity of the lower extremity in children with renal osteodystrophy. J Pediatr Orthop. 1992;12(3):291–9. https://doi.org/10.1097/01241398-199205000-00004.
46. Yilmaz G, Oto M, Thabet AM, Rogers KJ, Anticevic D, Thacker MM, et al. Correction of lower extremity angular deformities in skeletal dysplasia with hemiepiphysiodesis: a preliminary report. J Pediatr Orthop. 2014;34(3):336–45. https://doi.org/10.1097/BPO.0000000000000089.
47. Stanitski DF. Treatment of deformity secondary to metabolic bone disease with the Ilizarov technique. Clin Orthop Relat Res. 1994;301:38–41.
48. Barrett IR, Papadimitriou DG. Skeletal disorders in children with renal failure. J Pediatr Orthop. 1996;16(2):264–72. https://doi.org/10.1097/00004694-199603000-00026.
49. Bardin T. Renal osteodystrophy, disorders of vitamin D metabolism, and hypophosphatasia. Curr Opin Rheumatol. 1992;4(3):389–93. https://doi.org/10.1097/00002281-199206000-00018.
50. Cai G, Michigami T, Yamamoto T, Yasui N, Satomura K, Yamagata M, et al. Analysis of localization of mutated tissue-nonspecific alkaline phosphatase proteins associated with neonatal hypophosphatasia using green fluorescent protein chimeras. J Clin Endocrinol Metab. 1998;83(11):3936–42. https://doi.org/10.1210/jcem.83.11.5267.
51. Walker JL, Hosseinzadeh P, White H, Murr K, Milbrandt TA, Talwalkar VJ, et al. Idiopathic genu Valgum and its association with obesity in children and adolescents. J Pediatr Orthop. 2019;39(7):347–52. https://doi.org/10.1097/BPO.0000000000000971.

Osteogenesis Imperfecta

Reggie C. Hamdy, Yousef Marwan, Frank Rauch, Kathleen Montpetit, and François R. Fassier

Introduction

Osteogenesis imperfecta (OI), commonly known as "brittle bone disease," is a group of hereditary disorders characterized by increased bone fragility, leading to multiple fractures and bone deformities [1]. It is most often caused by mutations in one of the two collagen type I encoding genes that lead to a wide spectrum of skeletal and nonskeletal manifestations. Over the last 15 years, due to advances in molecular testing, many more genes involved in causing an OI phenotype have been identified [2].

Population-based studies on OI have found an incidence of around 1:10,000 [1]. Life expectancy and prognosis depend on the severity of the condition that varies from absence of symptoms to lethality in the newborn period [3].

Diagnosis

The diagnosis of OI can typically be made based on clinical and radiological appearance. The diagnosis should then be confirmed and refined by molecular genetic testing, which usually detects a disease-causing abnormality in one of the OI-associated genes [4]. As genetic testing is becoming more widely used, it has emerged that a significant proportion of children with recurrent low-trauma fractures have pathogenic variants in an OI-associated gene, even if the clinical appearance is not typical for OI [5]. It may therefore be useful to perform genetic testing in children with recurrent low-trauma fractures regardless of the clinical phenotype.

Differential Diagnosis

In babies, the most significant condition that may sometimes present some difficulty in diagnosis is non-accidental injury [6]. In older children, several other genetic disorders such as juvenile osteoporosis and hypophosphatasia may lead to frequent fractures and therefore can give rise to an OI-like appearance [7].

Classification

As the severity and the genetic causes of OI vary widely, several classifications of the disorder have been developed. The 2019 Nosology and Classification of Genetic Skeletal Disorders distinguishes five clinically recognizable OI types which are summarized in Table 23.1 [8]. Among the various OI types, OI type I is by far the most prevalent, representing about 70% of cases in a population-based study [9].

Apart from this phenotype-based classification, an alternative approach uses the results of genetic testing to classify OI into additional types. In this approach, a new OI type is attributed to each new gene that is linked to an OI phenotype, in the order that the association between the genes and OI is discovered [2]. At the time of writing, the Online Mendelian Inheritance of Man database lists 21 different OI types based on genetic test results (http://www.ncbi.nlm.nih.gov/omim/).

R. C. Hamdy (✉) · Y. Marwan · F. Rauch · K. Montpetit
F. R. Fassier
Shriners Hospital for Children – Canada and McGill University Health Centre, Montreal, QC, Canada
e-mail: rhamdy@shriners.mcgill.ca; frauch@shriners.mcgill.ca; kmontpetit@shrinenet.org; ffassier@shrinenet.org

Table 23.1 Types of OI based on the 2019 nosology and classification of genetic skeletal disorders

Type	Main features
I	The mildest phenotype that is usually associated with straight limbs and a body height within or slightly below the reference range
II	The most severe form of the disease, usually leading to death shortly after birth due to respiratory failure
III	The most severe form of OI in individuals surviving the neonatal period. It is associated with severe short stature, limb deformities, and scoliosis
IV	Intermediate in disease severity, between OI types I and III. With adequate care, most individuals with OI type IV are ambulatory, but usually have short stature and develop scoliosis
V	Associated with distinctive characteristics, such as hyperplastic callus formation and ossification of the interosseous membrane of the forearms

Pathogenesis

The mutations affecting collagen type I production have consequences on various levels [2]. On the cellular level, mutations in collagen type I encoding genes often lead to stress in the endoplasmic reticulum, thereby disturbing the function of collagen type I-producing cells, such as osteoblasts. These cells produce abnormal extracellular bone matrix which leads to abnormal mineralization, making the bone brittle. At the same time, growth factors that are normally stored in the extracellular matrix, such as transforming growth factor beta (TGF-β), are more easily released by the abnormal extracellular matrix, which further disturbs bone cell function. Defective osteoblasts produce fewer and thinner trabecula, as well as thin bone cortices. Decreased periosteal bone formation gives rise to a decreased diameter of the diaphysis of long bones and ribs.

Clinical and Radiological Features

The clinical and radiological manifestations of OI depend on the type and severity of the condition [1, 2]. The mildest forms of the disease can present with almost no detectable changes in the bone density, while the more severe types can cause severe shortening, deformities, and thinning of the bone with very little cortical bone formation.

As OI is mostly a disease of collagen formation, any tissue containing collagen type I may be affected, with various amounts of severity [1, 2]. This results in skeletal and non-skeletal manifestations.

The nonskeletal manifestations include:

- Blue sclera and other ocular problems
- Hearing defects
- Dentinogenesis imperfecta
- Hyperlaxity of ligaments, skin, and joints
- Hearing impairment
- Cardiac and pulmonary involvement

The musculoskeletal manifestations include:

- Fractures with poor bone remodeling
- Deformities of long bones (Fig. 23.1)
- Coxa vara (Fig. 23.1)
- Protrusio acetabuli (Fig. 23.1)
- Spine deformities and compression fractures (Fig. 23.2)
- Basilar invagination
- Short stature
- Muscle weakness
- Ligamentous laxity
- Congenital radial head dislocation
- Soft-tissue contractures

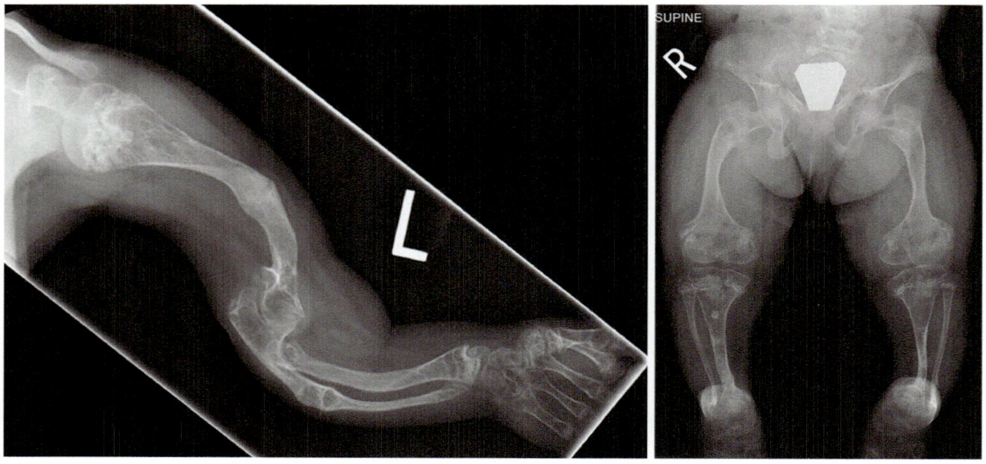

Fig. 23.1 Deformities of the upper and lower extremities in OI. In the upper extremity, severe bowing of the long bones is present. In the lower extremities, in addition to bowing, there is acetabular protrusion, coxa vara, and popcorn appearance of the epiphysis

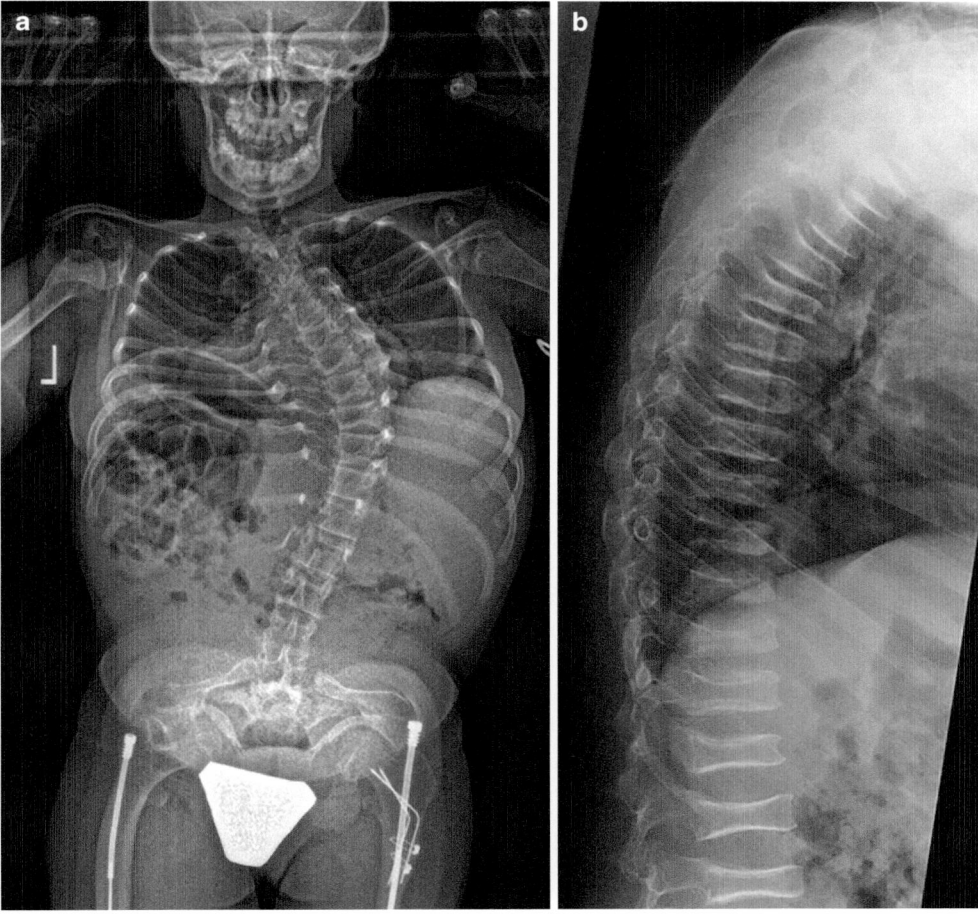

Fig. 23.2 (**a**) Scoliosis in a patient with OI. (**b**) Multiple compression fractures of the spine in a patient with OI

Management of OI

The overall goal of treatment is to improve mobility and function, hence improving the quality of life of these children. This goal is best obtained by a multidisciplinary clinic, capable of offering the various services needed by these patients and their families. Medical treatment aims at making the bones stronger, surgical treatment aims at making bones straighter, and rehabilitation aims at improving mobility and muscle strength. In addition, other teams should be available to provide further care for OI patients, such as nutritional, dental, and social services.

Medical Treatment

As the disease-causing genetic defect cannot be repaired at present, the medical treatment of OI aims at symptomatic improvements. At a very basic level, medical treatment involves avoiding deficiencies in vitamin D and calcium intake that might aggravate the bone abnormalities caused by the genetic defect. More specific treatment approaches aim at increasing bone mineral density using drugs from the class of bisphosphonates, which has been the most widely used medical treatment for OI since the 1990s [10]. Both orally and intravenously administered bisphosphonates are available, but studies suggest that the oral approach is less effective in children with OI [11, 12], and therefore, intravenous bisphosphonates are the usual treatment modality [1]. Intravenous bisphosphonate treatment increases bone mineral density through its effect on both trabecular and cortical bone, leading to more trabecula and thicker cortices [13]. Long-term treatment with intravenous bisphosphonates in growing children can lead to the reshaping of vertebrae that are affected by compression fractures [14].

In contrast to their good effect on the shape of growing vertebrae, bisphosphonates do not seem to prevent the development of scoliosis. Two large studies found that intravenous bisphosphonate treatment slowed down the progression rate of scoliosis in the most severely affected patients, but the prevalence of scoliosis at maturity was not influenced by bisphosphonate treatment history [15, 16].

Most observational studies report that the bisphosphonate treatment decreases the fracture rates of long bones by 30% to 60% [12, 14, 17, 18]. Even though this means that many long-bone fractures still occur, it has been observed that intravenous bisphosphonate treatment can improve mobility, especially when started early in life [19].

Regarding potential adverse events of bisphosphonate treatment, the delayed healing of osteotomy sites seems to be more common in patients receiving intravenous bisphosphonate therapy [20]. Avoiding bisphosphonate treatment in the 4 months following surgery seems to decrease the percentage of osteotomy sites that heal with delay or not at all [21]. Another potential adverse event linked to bisphosphonate therapy is osteonecrosis of the jaw. However, systematic reviews have not identified any confirmed occurrence of this problem in OI [22].

Rehabilitation

The physical therapist (PT) and occupational therapist (OT) are important members of the multidisciplinary team as they are dedicated to enhancing mobility, function, and independence [23–25]. Their involvement begins with diagnosis and continues on an intense basis from the newborn period through to age 3 years.

Therapy in this period focuses on teaching appropriate handling, holding, and positioning, thus promoting minimization of fracture risk, good alignment, and prevention of deformities. This early intervention and monitoring can be seen as preparation for eventual surgery.

Therapists continue to follow children with all types of OI closely through childhood and adolescence with the key episodes/time points being presurgery and postsurgery, postfracture, and at school entry. Outside these episodes, the PT and OT follow the child with OI at regular intervals (customized to the type of OI and individual needs) throughout growth to monitor development, establish goals, and support the youth's ability for lifelong activity and fitness. As such, they play a key role in assessing the child's readiness for lower limb rodding. With the surgeon, a thorough evaluation of fracture history, deformities, and functional needs is necessary to determine the appropriateness and timing for lower limb surgery. Specifically, therapists will assess the child's:

- Ability to sit independently and pull to standing
- Cognitive and language development and the ability to participate in the postoperative rehabilitation program
- Deformity and function of upper extremities and their role in ambulation

Therapies with children who are having surgery can be divided into three stages: (1) presurgery, (2) immediate postsurgery, and (3) ongoing rehabilitation and bracing.

Presurgery

Therapists will advise caregivers on how to safely manage transfers and vehicle transportation during the immobilization period. It is highly recommended to measure baseline function, joint's range of motion, and muscle strength preoperatively with standardized validated outcome measures.

Immediate Postsurgery

The intense rehabilitation following lower limb rodding begins once the surgeon ascertains that the osteotomies/fractures are well healed, and the mobilization can be initiated. Initiating early mobilization as soon as possible is widely acknowledged. The rehabilitation program should focus on muscle strengthening and active-assisted range of motion followed by active-only range of motion, gradual weight-bearing, and balance training. Hydrotherapy is an excellent venue for strengthening muscles and facilitating range of motion, but it should always be done in conjunction with land-based therapy as weight-bearing through bone is critical for healing.

Orthotics/Bracing

Bracing remains a controversial topic and the evidence for or against various bracing options is poor. Expert opinion does agree that the use of orthotics is based on individual needs and in all cases should be kept to a minimum, so the active use of muscles is optimized. That being said, the use of knee-ankle-foot orthosis (KAFO) post-rodding in young children ambulating for the first time allows the child to bear weight and step while still gaining quadriceps strength. Knee joints can be unlocked, and eventually, the thigh portion is removed as the child progresses. Ankle-foot orthosis (AFO) allows dorsiflexion and/or plantarflexion while maintaining the alignment during healing post-tibial rodding. Supramalleolar orthotics provide support for a weak ankle or hypermobile foot. When bracing, a fracture proximal to the brace should be expected in some cases.

Surgical Treatment

In a child with no bony anomalies and normal bony geometry, the majority of fractures heal within the standard time of 4–6 weeks and, depending on the age of the child and the fracture type, most fractures in the pediatric age do not need surgical intervention, and the conservative treatment is usually satisfactory. Even in the presence of mild deformities and angulation, remodeling of the fracture usually occurs and corrects the bony alignment. However, that is not the case in children with OI, where the structure and geometry of bone are abnormal due to defective collagen or other bony protein mutations [2]. Without straightening the bone (following a fracture or deformity) and maintaining that correction with some form of internal fixation, not only will remodeling not occur, but the inherent bony weakness, together with the unequally distributed muscular forces, will eventually lead to delayed union or nonunion of the fractures and increase in the degree of deformities (Fig. 23.3). Hence, the golden and standard rule in these children with systemic bony osteopenia is to correct any bony deformity and maintain that correction during the growing years. In many cases, this can only be attained with internal implants. Today, it has been well established that the best implants in such a context are intramedullary rods as they protect the whole length of the bone and are not stress risers like plates (Fig. 23.4). The overall aim of rodding in children with OI is for the rod to act as an internal tutor during the bone-growing years and to prevent or at least to decrease the incidence of fractures and deformities (see Box 23.1).

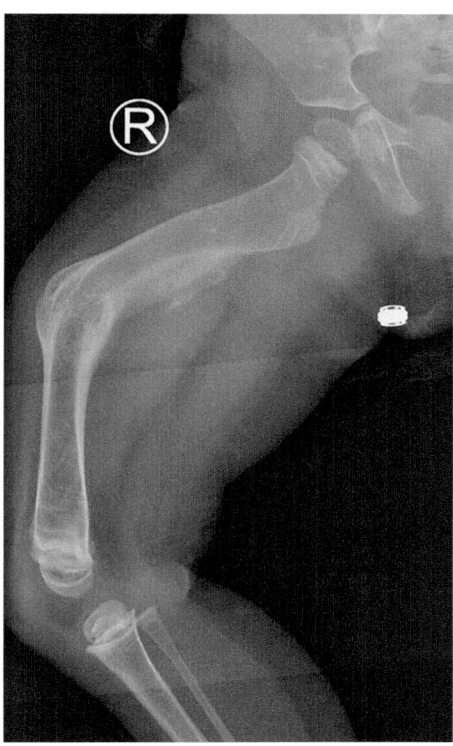

Fig. 23.3 A healed right femur fracture with poor remodeling in a 17-month-old child with OI. This fracture was immobilized in a hip spica cast without correction of the alignment

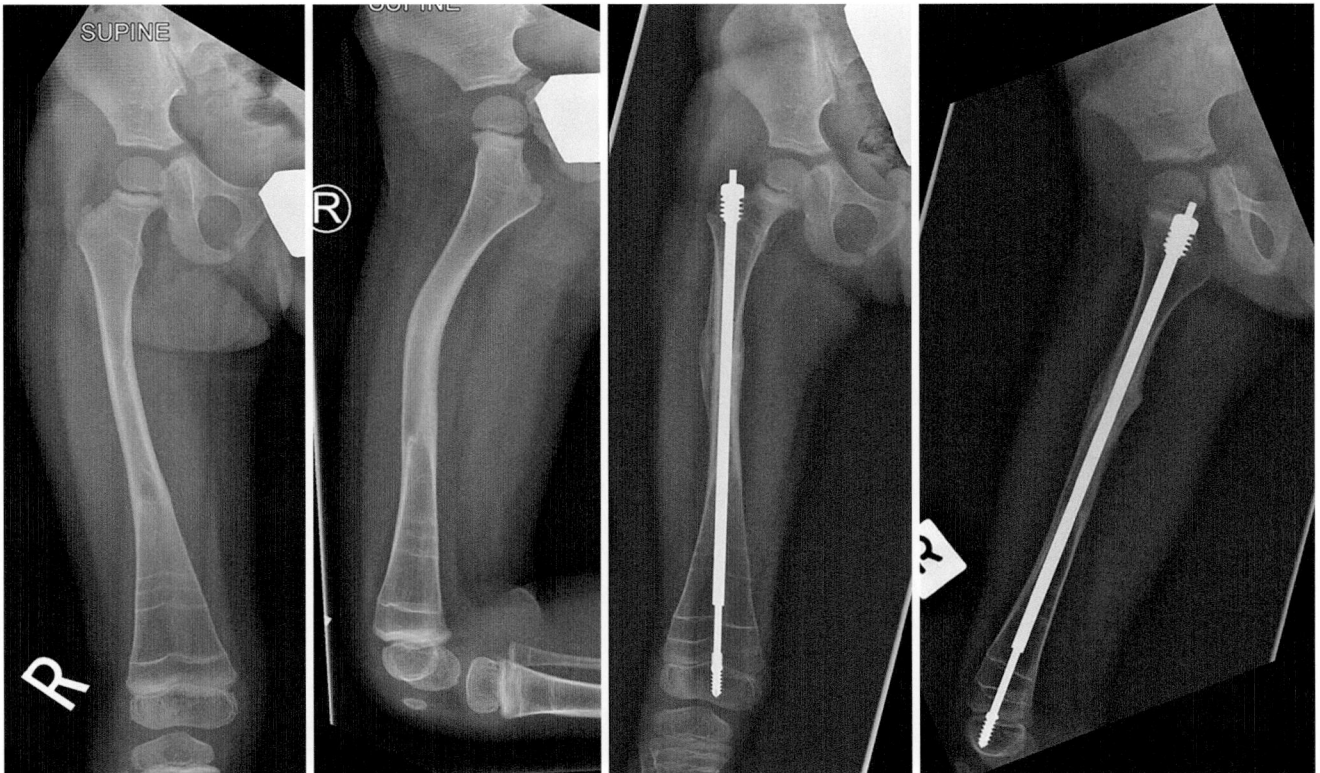

Fig. 23.4 Example of femoral deformity correction with osteotomy and telescopic rodding in a patient with OI

> **Box 23.1 Indications for Lower Extremity Intramedullary Rodding in Children with OI**
>
> 1. Lower limb (or bone segment) angular deformity of more than 30°
> 2. Long-bone severely displaced fractures
> 3. Multiple bone fractures
> 4. Repeated fractures in the same bone segment
> 5. Persistent pain in the lower limbs unresponsive to medical treatment

Perioperative Considerations

Soft-Tissue Problems

Soft tissues play an important role in the development of bone curvatures in OI. During growth, the soft tissue resists the elongation of the bone. The tether effect leads to a pattern of deformities defined by the most important muscle groups.

In the femur, the posteromedial hamstrings are the most resistant muscles, and therefore, the femur bows anterolaterally. In the tibia, most muscles are posterior and lateral, hence the anteromedial bow of the tibia (Fig. 23.5). This "rule" can be modified according to the antenatal position of the fetus; for instance, a child with OI born in a breech position may be born with a recurvatum deformity of the femur due to the extended knee with a flexed hip.

These soft-tissue problems can, and will, cause difficulties at the time of surgical correction of the deformities. Generally speaking, beyond 30° of angulation, it is advisable to shorten the bone (closing wedge resection) in order to be able to straighten it without too much tension in the muscles and to avoid neurovascular compromise.

General and Anesthesia-Related Considerations

Bisphosphonate therapy should be planned perioperatively. Fracture healing does not seem to be affected by the administration of bisphosphonates, while osteotomy healing (slow remodeling process) is often delayed [20, 21]. Therefore, the following should be considered with the multidisciplinary team:

- The medication can be given 48 h before surgery (no bisphosphonates in the bloodstream 48 h after infusion).
- No infusion for 4 months postoperatively or until clear evidence of bone healing is seen on X-rays.

The patient/family must be aware of the risk of complications that can be seen with any type of surgery, but also specific complications related to the OI:

- Malignant hyperthermia [26, 27].
- Difficult intubations (big head, big tongue).
- Ventilation problems (deformed thorax).
- Fracture: The risk is always present during the transfer of patients, while finding an IV access, positioning on the OR table, and during the surgical manipulations.
- Neurologic complications (basilar invagination and hydrocephalus in some cases).
- Hemorrhage: Excessive bleeding is common in some patients with OI.

Preoperative Planning

The structure of the bone in children with OI is affected; the deformed bone gets thinner in the frontal plane and wider in its sagittal plane (Fig. 23.6). As a consequence, the medullary canal is deceptively narrow, and the evaluation of the size of an implant is challenging. The cross section of the bones (femur and tibia) is more "rib-shaped," and the triangular aspect of the normal bone has disappeared. Measuring the size of the implant on a single view only may, therefore, lead to an overoptimistic size for a rod and intraoperative problems.

One fundamental aspect of OI bone surgery is that the child needs more bone than metal; reaming to enlarge the medullary canal should be limited as it removes bone, and a large implant takes most of the biomechanical stress leading to bone resorption around the rod. This could be a very challenging situation. Prevention is the best way to deal with this problem.

In addition to the medullary canal diameter, the length of the bone segment should be measured and studied. This helps prepare rods that appropriately match the length of the bone. In OI, the bone might be very short, limiting the use of specific implants.

As long-bone deformities in patients with OI are often multisegmental, multiapical, and multiplanar, the bony deformity must be carefully analyzed, and a detailed step-by-step plan for intervention has to be established preoperatively (Fig. 23.7). The bone deformity is a 3D problem; the 2D pre-op imaging gives a limited understanding of the complexity of the deformity (Fig. 23.8). In our institution, we have recently been using 3D-printed models of the deformed bone to help in the analysis of complex bony deformities to ease the surgical planning for osteotomies and the amount of bony resection required (Fig. 23.9). Intraoperatively, prior to making an incision, it is useful to analyze the deformity with fluoroscopy. This allows us to precisely define the apex (or apices) of the deformity (or deformities) and choose wisely where to perform the osteotomy (or osteotomies) (Fig. 23.10).

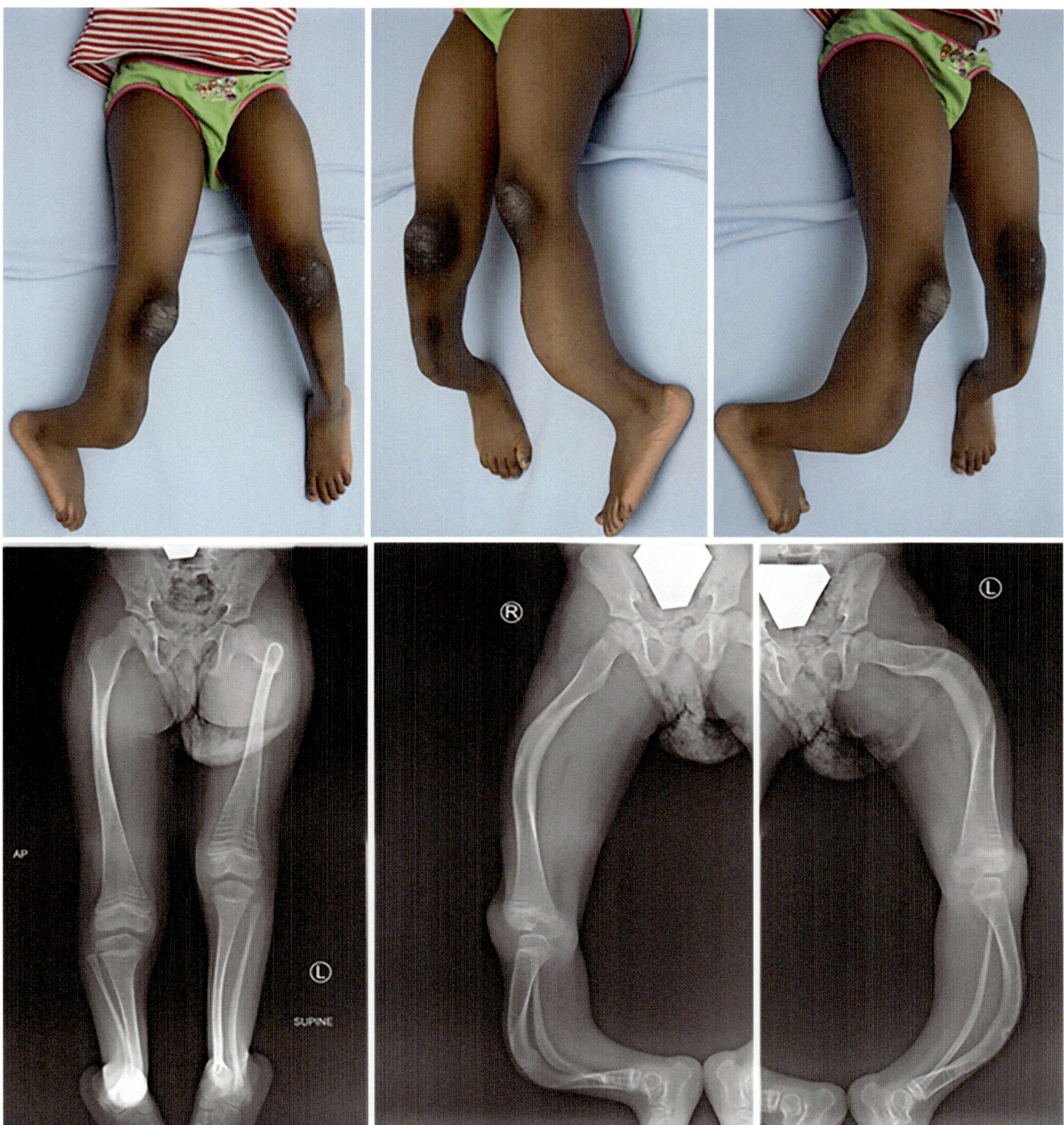

Fig. 23.5 Clinical and radiological images showing lower limb deformities in OI. In the femur, there is anterolateral bowing, while in the tibia, there is anteromedial bowing

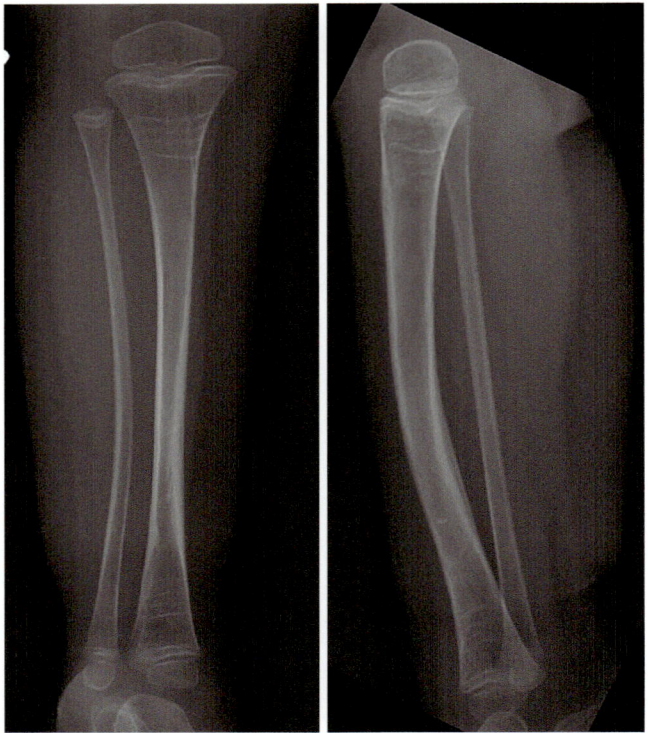

Fig. 23.6 X-ray images of a tibia in a patient with OI showing a larger diameter medullary canal in the lateral view compared to the anteroposterior view

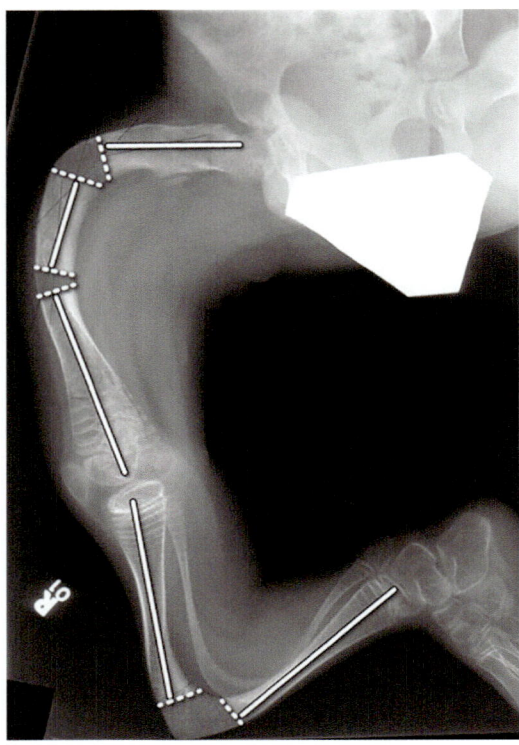

Fig. 23.7 X-ray image of the lower extremity of a patient with OI. Preoperative understanding of the deformities and planning for multiple osteotomies of the femur and tibia

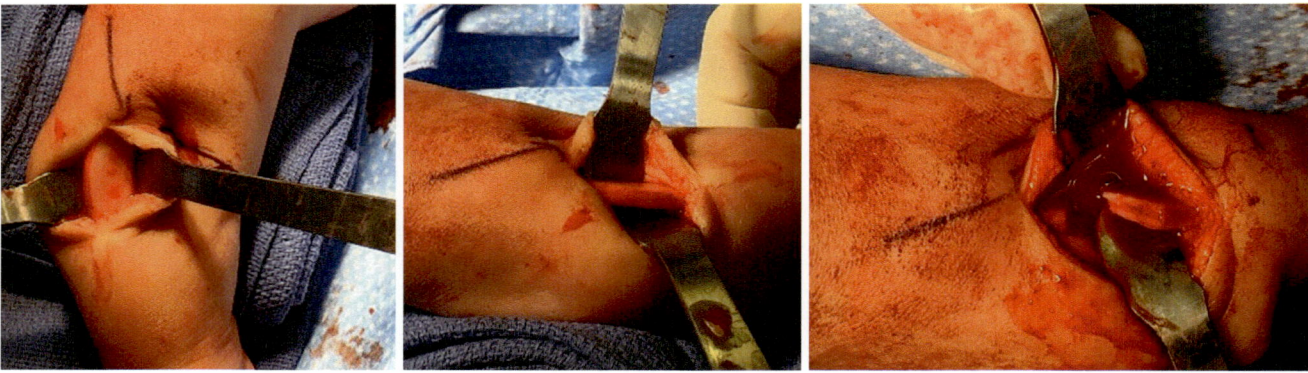

Fig. 23.8 Intraoperative clinical images of a tibia of a patient with OI showing that the tibia is very flat in one plane, very thin in another plan, and very narrow (almost nonexistent) in the transverse plane

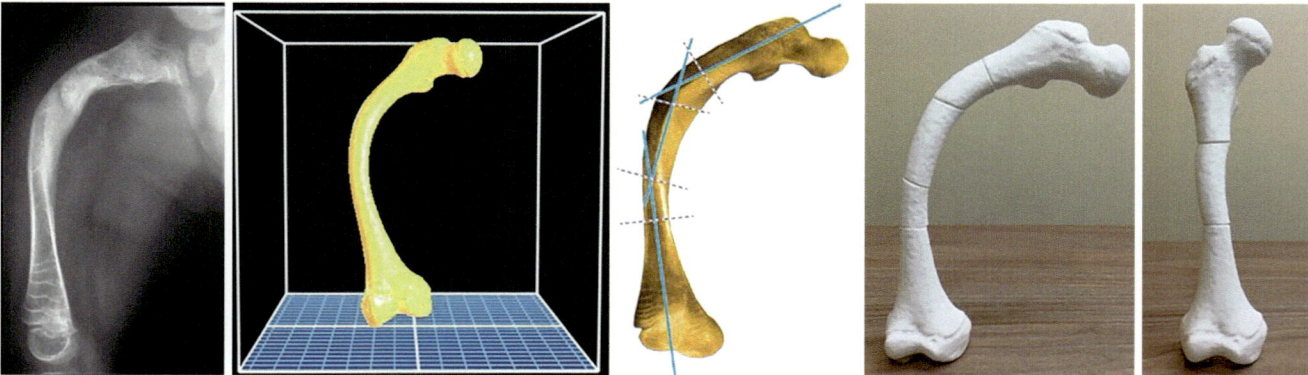

Fig. 23.9 3D printing for preoperative planning of deformity correction surgery in OI

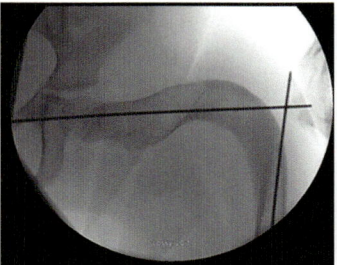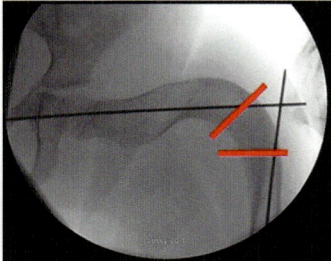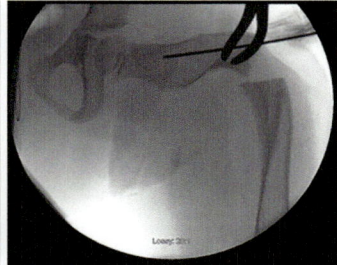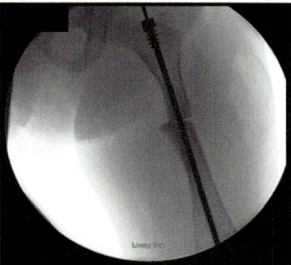

Fig. 23.10 Intraoperative planning of the corrective osteotomies for an OI femur using fluoroscopy before starting the surgery

Surgery

Why?

A deformed bone (particularly when weak due to OI) loses its biomechanical properties and is likely to break at the apex of the deformity. Usually, the deformity gets worse after a fracture, leading to a vicious circle of fracture/deformity/fracture.

When?

Rodding before walking age is technically more difficult, and postoperative rehabilitation can be challenging. Since the introduction of bisphosphonates, stronger bones can be obtained in a few months, and therefore, the need to operate on children before walking age is rare.

There is no consensus regarding the best time for the first rodding surgery. The generally accepted timing for rodding of lower extremities is when the child with bowed bones or repeated fractures pulls to stand (about 18–24 months of age). However, in cases of very young children with multiple repeated fractures, rodding may be indicated. The disadvantage of rodding at an early age is that the child may require revision rodding earlier, and more often revision surgery [28]. However, the advantages of earlier rodding and earlier protection of the bone may outweigh the disadvantages [28].

How?

"Guided growth" with hemiepiphysiodesis using nonlocking plates or staples is quite popular for managing angular deformities of the lower extremities in children. This technique is very effective when the angulation originates close to the growth plate, and the growth plate has a normal growth potential. It is unlikely to work on a diaphyseal angulation like OI and with a limited function of the growth plate. Therefore, the indications of hemiepiphysiodesis in OI are relatively rare.

The use of IM rods was initially proposed by Sofield and Millar in 1959 [29]. The rod acts as a tutor in the bone, preventing progressive deformity during growth. It reduces the fracture rate, and if a fracture happens, it eases the treatment, preventing the displacement of the bone fragments.

The application of plates alone is generally not indicated in patients with OI, since the plate creates a rigid segment and the bone is likely to break above or below the implant [30]. Furthermore, under the plate, the bone is not submitted to any stress and resorbs (Fig. 23.11). Nevertheless, the use of plates in conjunction with intramedullary nails is becoming popular, as the addition of a small plate at the fracture or osteotomy site provides additional rotatory stability that may be present in most cases when a telescoping rod is used alone. This concept is further discussed in this chapter later.

Types of Rods

Regular rods (e.g., K-wires, Rush rods, and elastic nails) have the advantage of being readily available and relatively inexpensive and come in varying diameters from 1 mm up (K-wires). The telescopic rods introduced by Dubow-Bailey [31] have been modified by Sharrard [32] Karbowski [33] and Cho [34]. A new concept of the telescopic rod, known as the Fassier-Duval (FD) rod, without the need for arthrotomies has been later introduced, with improved results [35]. These implants are more expensive and need to be ordered (and currently not available in all countries), and the smallest diameter is 3.2 mm, which is sometimes too large for small children. The major advantage of telescopic (or growing rods) is that the implant gets longer as the child grows, reducing the need for reoperation (which is needed every second or third year with non-telescopic rods because the bone deforms under the tip of the nail during growth) [36, 37]. If a telescopic rod is not available, it is also possible to use "sliding rods"; two regular rods (Rush or elastic nails) are inserted, one from the proximal epiphysis-distally and the other rod from the distal epiphysis-proximally. As each of the two rods is inserted from a distinct epiphysis, these implants move away from each other during growth. Unfortunately, they do

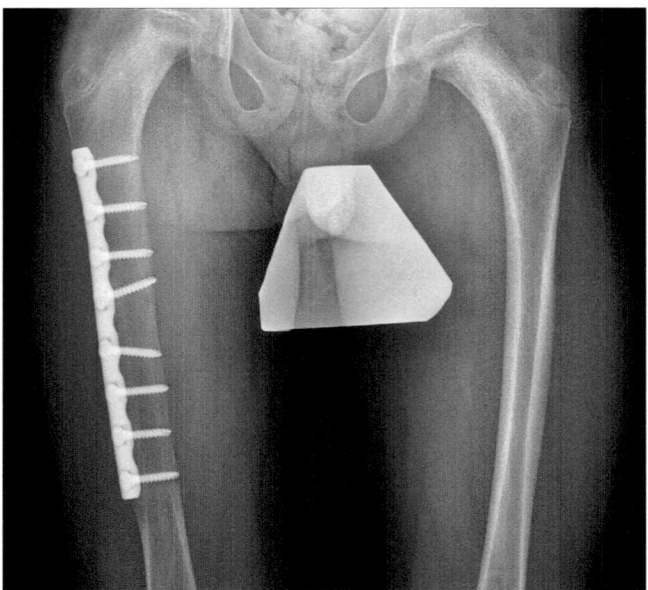

Fig. 23.11 OI femur showing periprosthetic resorption of the bone mainly at the medial cortex

not provide the same stability as telescopic nails, and it is common to see the bone deform during growth (Fig. 23.12). Additionally, the Slim nail is a non-telescopic rod with one side head and threads that can be used for small-diameter bone with added stability at the epiphysis. In the chapter, the FD rodding technique will be described later as this is the preferred method of fixation for the authors.

Patient Positioning

Most children with OI are smaller than average, and the soft-tissue tightness can lead to intraoperative difficulties. A good way to stay out of trouble is to have the patient semi-supine, with a radiolucent cushion (such as a saline bag) under the ipsilateral buttock and another support under the ipsilateral shoulder (Fig. 23.13). The patient is brought to the edge of the radiolucent table. This maneuver has two major advantages. First, at the beginning of the surgery, the leg can hang off the edge of the table, allowing good control of the proximal femur deformity and ruling out a "pseudo coxa vara" (see next section on Coxa Vara). The second advantage is to be able by flexing, adducting, and internally rotating the hip to get a lateral view of the femur without changing the C-arm position. Beware during positioning that the contralateral arm is not left parallel to the trunk, as the hand will be in the C-arm field during the surgery. Verify as well that towel clips, suction tubes, cautery cables, or plates do not prevent a good imaging of the knee during surgery. Another major advantage of this position is at the time of the introduction of the femoral nail through the greater trochanter, it is much easier to manipulate the long tools as they can be "outside" the OR table and often lean lower than the level of the table (which would be impossible if the patient was in the middle of the OR table).

Osteotomy

Osteotomy can be performed open or percutaneously. Whenever possible, osteotomy should be done percutaneously as it results in less scars and decreased soft-tissue trauma (including less blood loss and less postoperative pain), but this can be technically more demanding.

The use of an oscillating saw for performing the osteotomy in patients with OI is not recommended; it burns the bone ends, and as these patients receive bisphosphonates (which reduces the number of osteoclasts), the remodeling is slow. It takes time to remove the dead bone, and this may lead to delayed union or nonunion. It is best to perform a low-energy osteotomy by preparing the bone with multiple drill holes and then completing the osteotomy with sharp osteotomes (Fig. 23.14). Moreover, when manipulating the bone for realignment, it is important to have the patient fully relaxed with proper anesthesia to avoid fractures.

Technique for Femoral FD Rodding (See Box 23.2)

The FD telescopic rod is inserted from the GT, and the introduction of the male driver is done first. A K-wire (same diameter as the male nail) is pushed up in the buttock from the osteotomy, and the male driver is pushed down on the K-wire as a guide (the K-wire can be placed from the tip of the GT instead from the osteotomy site if the alignment of the femur allows). When the driver is at the level of the osteotomy, the K-wire is removed and replaced with the nail. After the reduction of the osteotomy, the male nail is pushed down in the shaft until it reaches the growth plate and screwed into the epiphysis. The position of the distal tip of the rod in the epiphysis is critical as this affects rod survival [38]; the nail should be in the middle third of the epiphysis both on AP and lateral views. It is relatively simple to be centered on AP, but in lateral, any mild bow of the femur will drive the nail to be too anterior. In such a case, the nail is withdrawn a few centimeters, a percutaneous metaphyseal osteotomy is done, and the nail is pushed into the center of the epiphysis (Fig. 23.15). The male driver is removed while maintaining pressure on the nail to avoid dislodging it. The female nail is measured, from the ossified proximal femoral metaphysis to 1 cm above the distal femoral growth plate. The threads of the female nail are left above the ossified metaphysis of the proximal femur (the measurement of the

Fig. 23.12 Sliding rods. (**a**) Early after fixation. (**b**) After 4 years, progressive varus deformity aggravated by a proximal femoral fracture

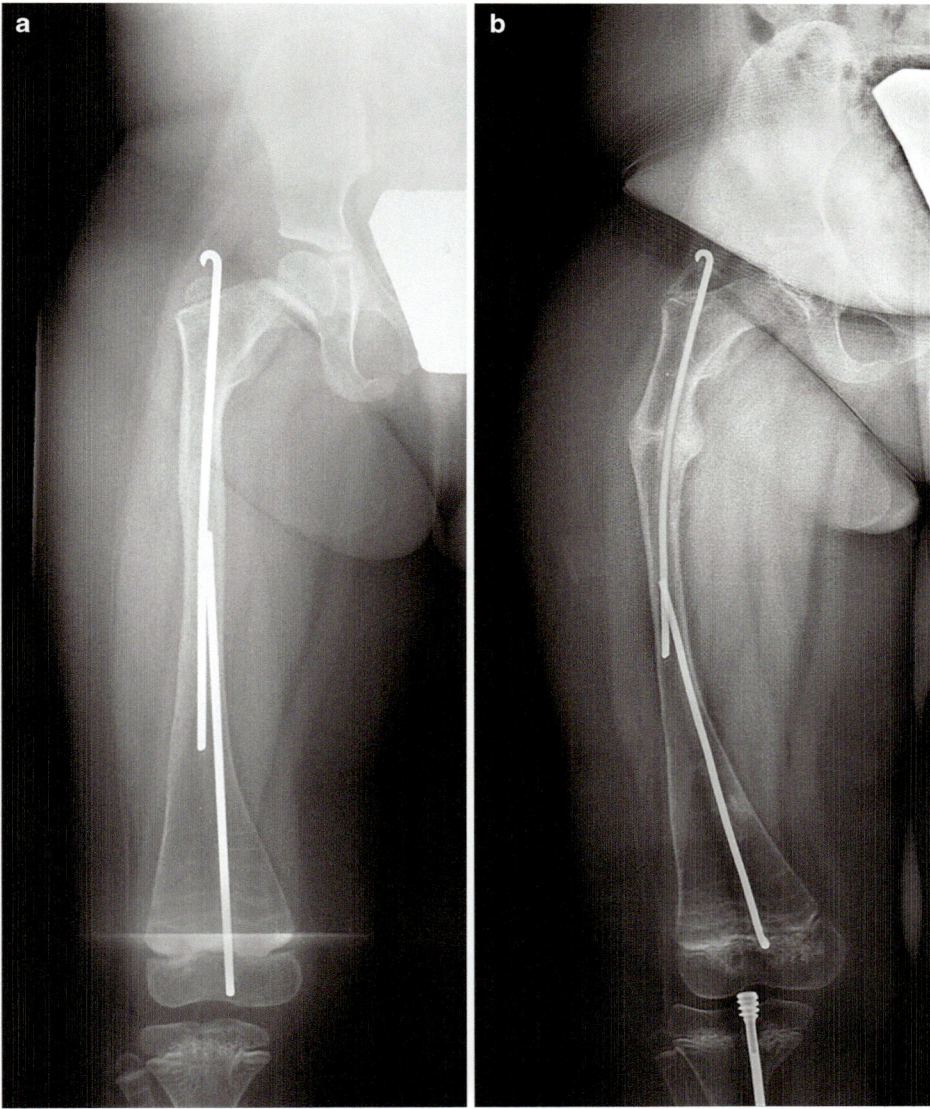

nail length does not take the threads of the female nail into consideration.) (Fig. 23.15). When the female nail has been cut (Midas Rex®) and the lumen of the nail cleaned to allow a smooth telescoping, the female nail is pushed down over the male nail. At the moment the proximal end of the nail disappears inside the wound, a careful X-ray measurement is done to verify that the distance between the distal end of the female nail and the "aisles" of the male nail ("A" in Fig. 23.16) is greater than the distance between the proximal threads of the female nail and the proximal metaphysis ("B" in Fig. 23.16). If "B" is greater than "A," while screwing the female nail in the non-ossified GT, one will push the male nail into the knee joint. The male nail is cut above the female, and the smoothness of the section is checked with a little probe to ensure that the male nail slides smoothly and distally during growth.

Box 23.2 Summary of Femoral Fassier-Duval Rod Technique
1. Male rod introduced with a male driver.
2. Male rod positioned in the middle third of the distal epiphysis on both AP and LAT intraoperative fluoroscopic views.
3. Remove the male driver, keeping pressure on the nail.
4. Measurement of the female rod, which is cut intraoperatively (Midas Rex®).
5. Female rod introduced: Verify that the rod is not too long, as when screwing it in the GT you may push the male distally, into the knee joint.
6. The female rod threads are left proximal to the ossified metaphysis.
7. Cut the male rod above the female, and check the smoothness of the rod (as it has to slide down into the hollow female nail).

Fig. 23.13 Positioning of the patient on the OR table. The operated side is raised, as is the ipsilateral shoulder. (**a**) This position allows to do lateral shoot-through of the knee without changing the C-arm position. (**b**) One must be sure that objects such as the patient's upper extremity, suction tube, and cautery cable will not interfere with adequate intraoperative fluoroscopic visualization of the operative field

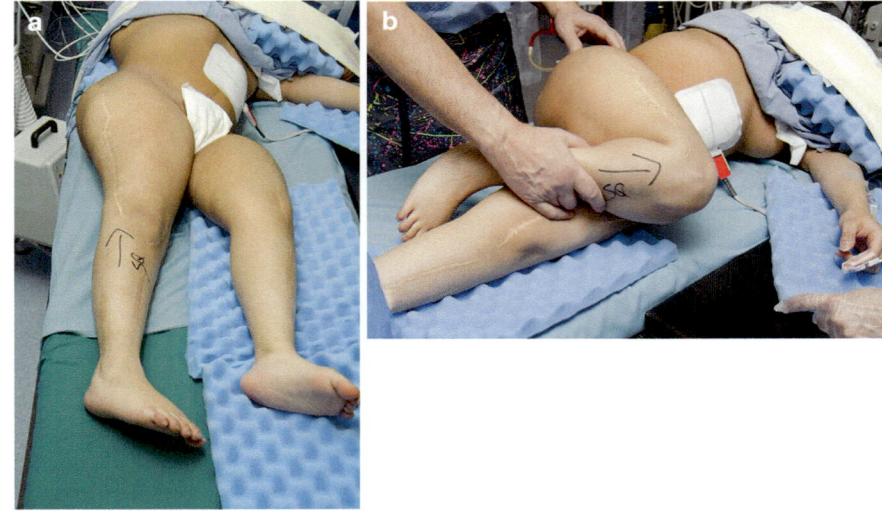

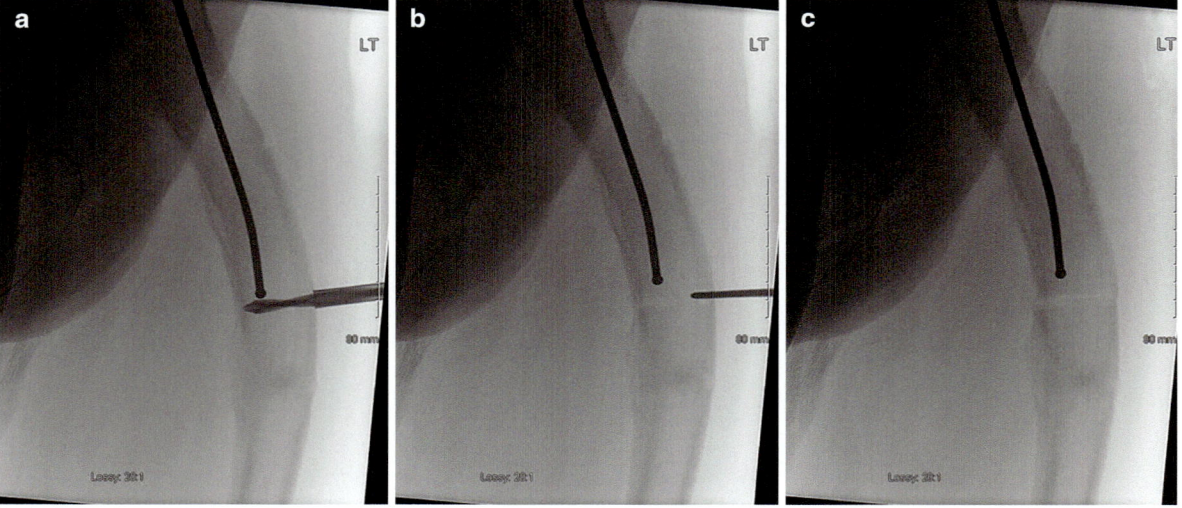

Fig. 23.14 Percutaneous osteotomy of the femur in a patient with OI. (**a**) Multiple drill holes are created at the apex of the deformity; (**b**) osteotomes are used to complete the osteotomy; and (**c**) osteotomy is completed

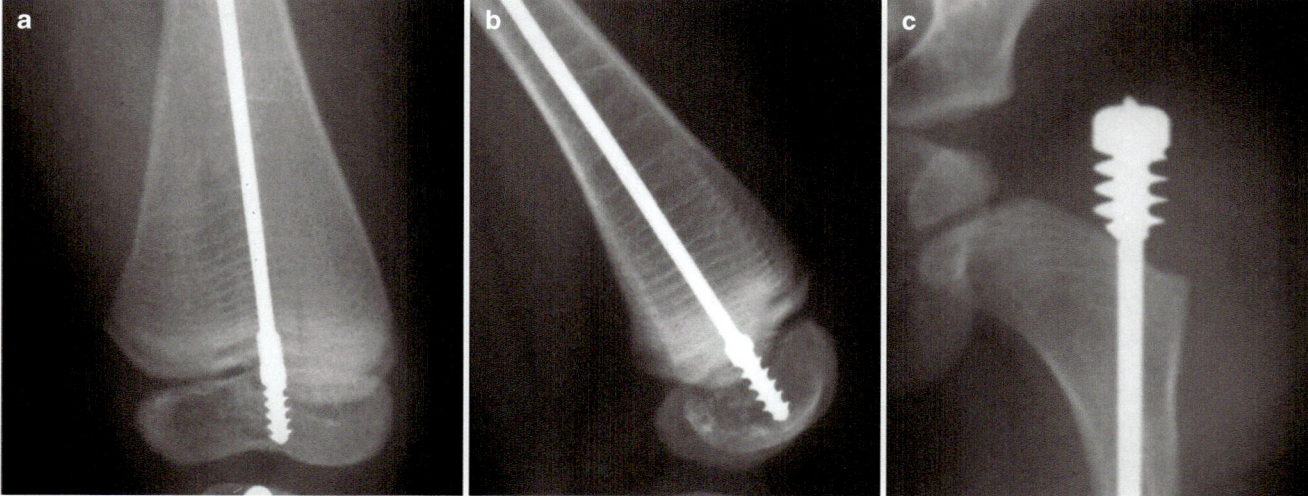

Fig. 23.15 "Ideal" positioning of the FD rod in the femur at the distal (**a**, **b**) and proximal ends (**c**)

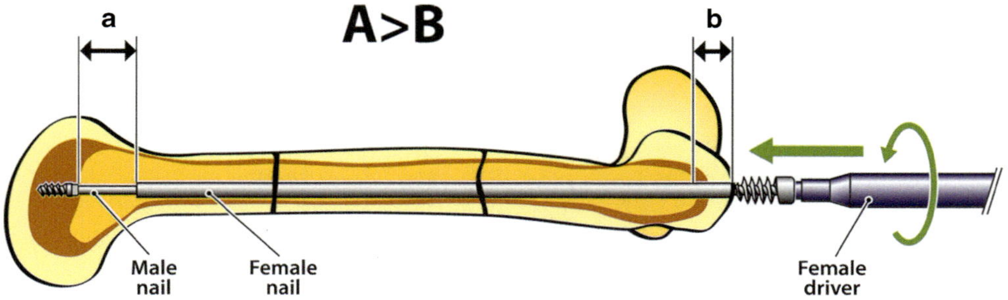

Fig. 23.16 FD rodding. Before screwing the female nail in the non-ossified greater trochanter, verify (via C-arm) that the distance between the distal end of the female nail and the aisles of the male nail A is greater than the distance between the proximal threads of the female nail to the ossified metaphysis B. If B > A, the male nail will be pushed distally

Technique for Tibial FD Rodding (See Box 23.3)

The principles for tibial rodding are the same regardless of the rod used. The nail is introduced through a medial parapatellar tendon incision. The entry point of the nail is behind the patellar tendon, on the edge of the proximal tibial epiphysis (which is extra-articular). A pre-bent K-wire is useful to find the medullary canal. If the tibia is deformed into valgus, it is better to use a lateral parapatellar tendon approach. The direction of the rod will be more in varus, allowing a better correction of the deformity. Figure 23.17 shows the "ideal" position of the FD rod in the tibia, proximally and distally.

> **Box 23.3 Summary of Tibial Fassier-Duval Rod Technique**
> 1. Use a bent K-wire to find the medullary canal.
> 2. Ream over the K-wire (beware of posterior tibial cortex breach if the entry point is too anterior).
> 3. The male driver is pushed down, and the male nail is positioned in the middle third of the distal tibial epiphysis.
> 4. The male driver is removed, keeping the male nail in place.
> 5. Cut the male nail.
> 6. Measure the female nail.
> 7. Slide the female nail over the male.
> 8. Check that the knee extension is not limited by the male nail.

Technique for Coxa Vara Correction

This deformity is present in about 60% of type III OI patients and may progressively develop after IM rodding of the femur [39]. True coxa vara must be differentiated, on X-rays, from "pseudo"-coxa vara due to the projection of an anteriorly bowed proximal femur [39]. To do so, the patient is positioned on the edge of the table (semi-lateral as for femoral rodding) (Fig. 23.18), and before surgery, a true AP view of the hip is obtained by letting the leg hang out of the table. In addition, the "adduction test" will give a precise idea of how much correction can be obtained. The surgical technique for coxa vara correction is illustrated in Fig. 23.19 [40]. The advantages of such a technique are that it is adaptable to varying bone sizes and that the implants (K-wires and cerclage wires) are available in most operating rooms. Depending on the stability of the fixation in the bone, in most cases, there is no need for postoperative spica cast (which both the patient and parents appreciate). For bilateral cases, an "A" frame can be used, particularly in young patients (Fig. 23.20). No weight-bearing for 6 weeks followed by a week of intensive physiotherapy starting in the pool allows the patient to recuperate quickly. The results of this technique [40] show that an average of 30° of correction of the neck-shaft angle can be obtained (Fig. 23.21).

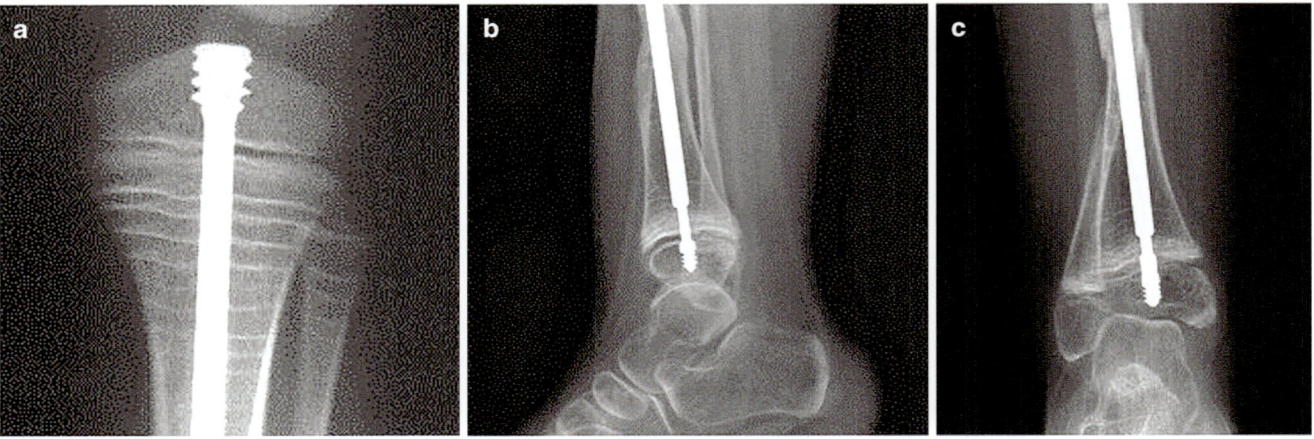

Fig. 23.17 "Ideal" positioning of the FD rod in the tibia at the proximal (**a**) and distal ends (**b**, **c**)

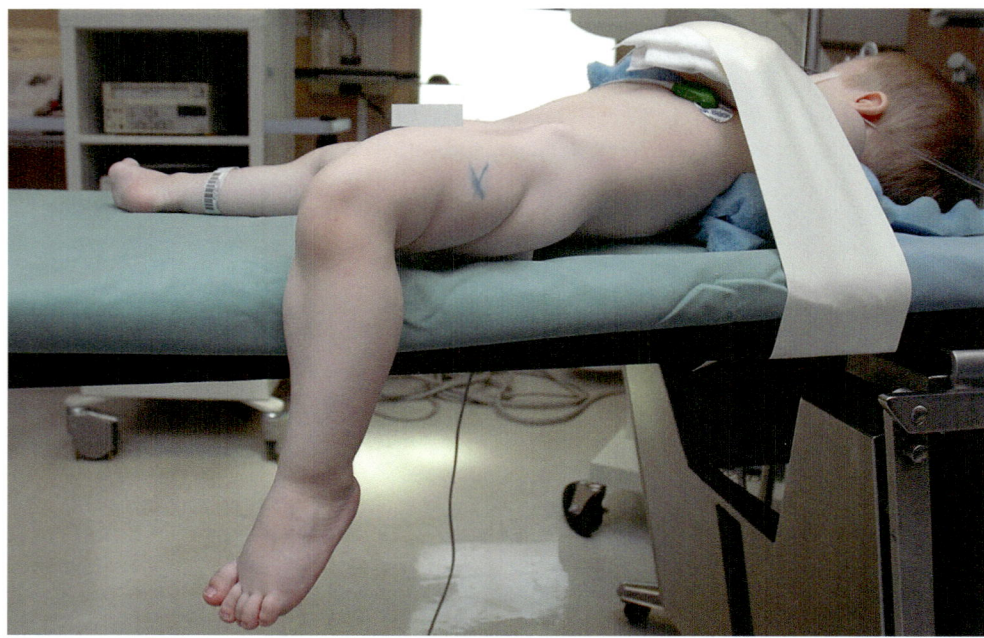

Fig. 23.18 Before correcting a coxa vara, a true AP view of the hip is obtained with the ipsilateral hip extended off the edge of the table. The anterior bow of the femur is eliminated, and a true assessment of the neck-shaft angle is appreciated

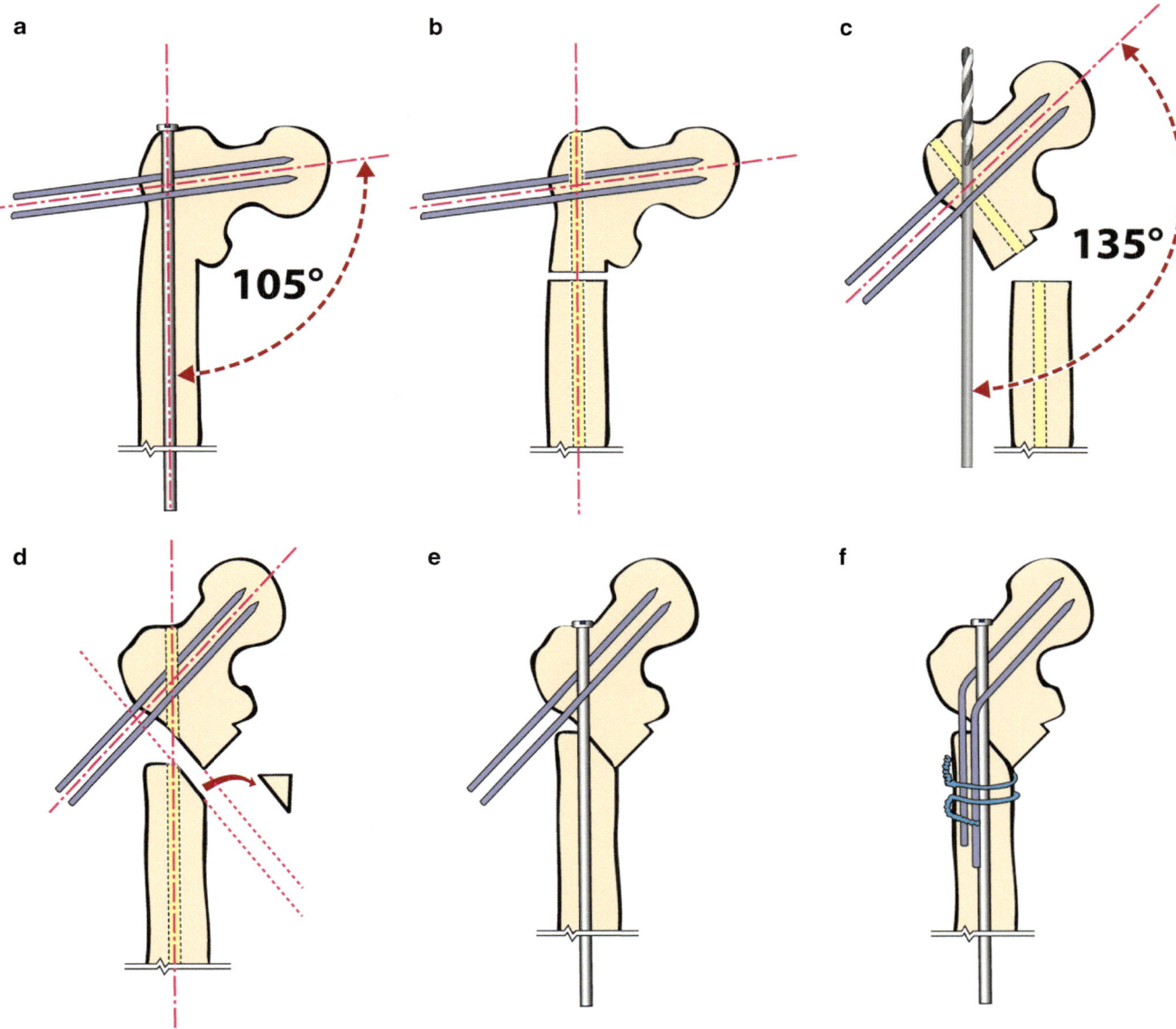

Fig. 23.19 The sequential steps of the coxa vara correction: The two K-wires can be used as a joystick (**a, b**) and the reaming of the proximal fragment is done through the *lateral* cortex (**c**). The angle between the drill bit and the K-wires determines the final neck-shaft angle. The removal of a medial wedge of bone from the distal bone fragment (**d**) allows better stability of the fixation with rodding and cerclage wire (**e, f**)

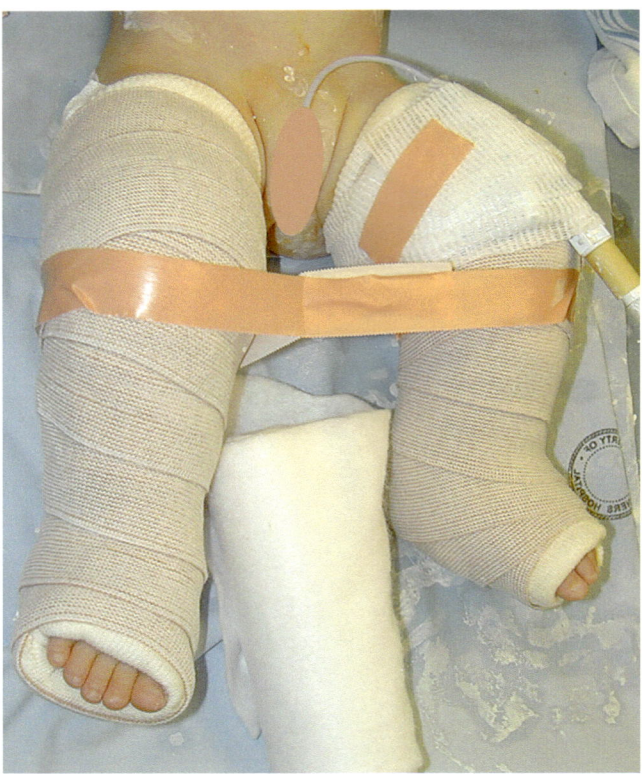

Fig. 23.20 Postoperative immobilization after bilateral femoral and tibial rodding. The tape between the legs avoids spontaneous external rotation of the hips

Fig. 23.21 (a) Preoperative and postoperative (b) radiographs of the femur of a patient with coxa vara associated with type IV OI

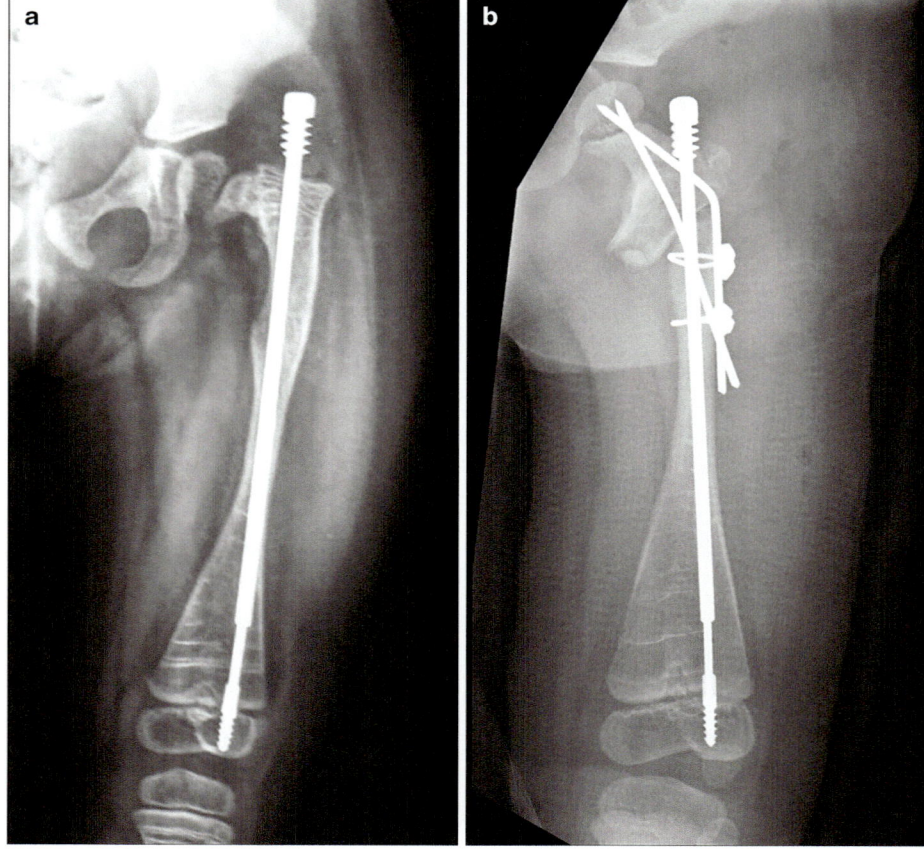

Results and Complications

The combination of medical treatment, surgical realignment rodding, and postoperative rehabilitation has proven to improve ambulation, gross motor function, self-care, and mobility at short- and long-term follow-up [19, 25, 36, 41]. The outcomes of sliding rods or telescopic rods are superior to a single rod with regard to the longevity of the rod [42, 43]. However, complications are frequent, and the reoperation rate is high as, despite bisphosphonates, the bone remains brittle though harder [44, 45]. The children feel better, and their level of activity raises, and with it, the risk of fracture increases. During growth, the rod can migrate through the cortex (Fig. 23.22), requiring revision surgery. In other cases, particularly with telescopic rods (if the female rod threads are screwed in the ossified metaphysis), the greater trochanter grows proximally and the tip of the FD rod becomes completely sunk into the bone. The indications for the reoperation in such a case are not clear [46] as the patient may be completely asymptomatic. Retrieving the rod in the bone without an osteotomy is challenging despite rescue tools, and a common solution is to wait until a significant complication (such as a fracture) occurs to change the rod. No telescoping may occur after a fracture or spontaneously (progressive bowing of the bone and the rod). In such cases, the rod behaves as a regular rod. The indication for revision should then be the same as for solid rods (angulation, fracture, and migration of the implant beyond the confines of the bone). Moreover, periprosthetic fractures can happen around such implants. This complication can be very challenging to manage in some locations (Fig. 23.23).

Delayed union/nonunion rate was as high as 20% in OI before the era of bisphosphonates [47]; but with these medications, the risk is much higher [20] and the treatment of such a complication remains challenging. In many patients, the pseudo-arthrosis is mildly symptomatic (recurrent pain after minimal trauma), while in others the pain is debilitating. To improve the biomechanical environment for the bone to heal, unicortical plates have been recently used at the osteotomy or fracture site, especially in cases of severe deformity, fracture nonunion, and revision surgery (Fig. 23.24) [48, 49].

Another challenge for the surgeon is the long and thin bone often seen in adolescents with severe OI. In such cases, a single Rush rod can be used, but a locking nail is a safer implant with no need for post-op immobilization. Unfortunately, most locking nails are 8.5 mm in diameter and greater, which may be too large for patients with OI. The

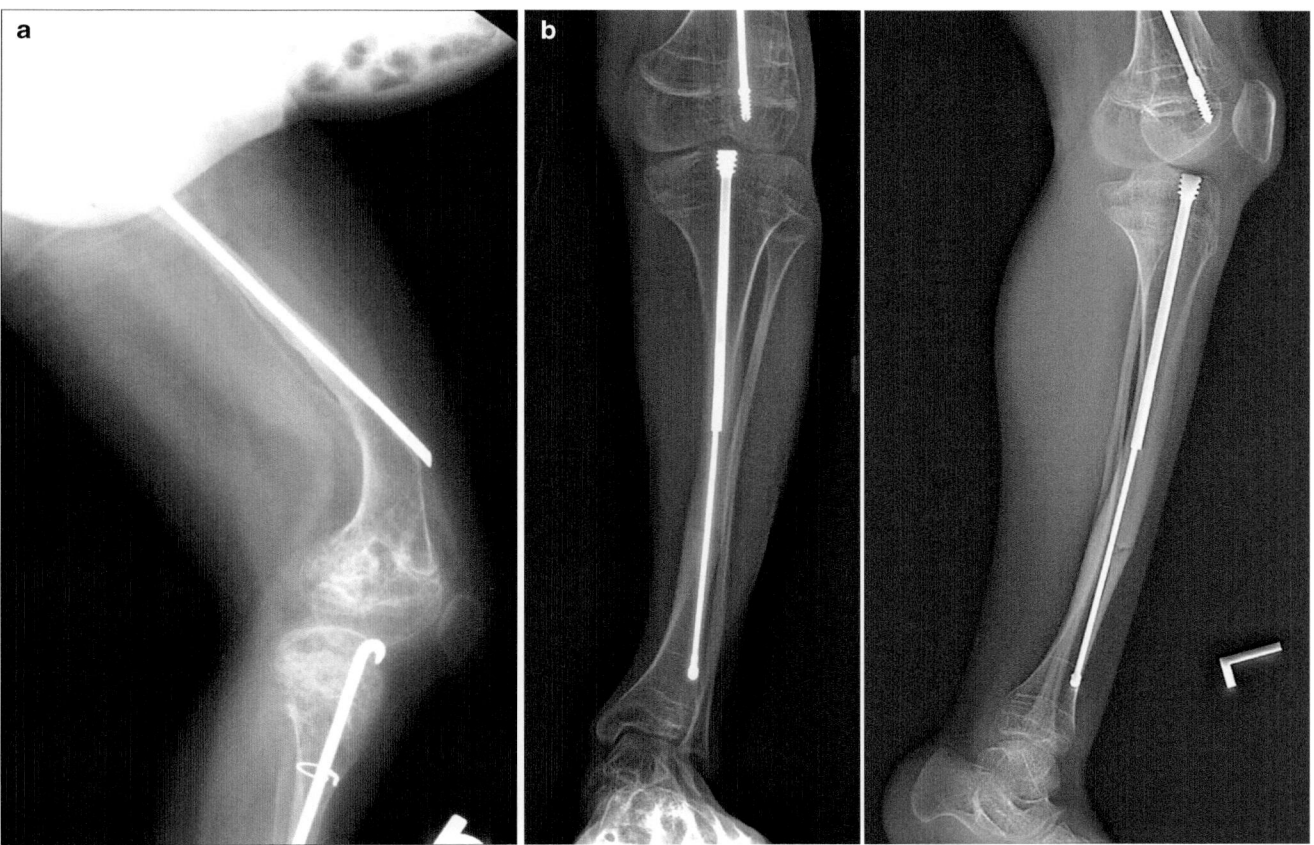

Fig. 23.22 Examples of rod migration in non-telescopic (**a**) and telescopic (**b**) rods in OI patients with bone growth

Fig. 23.23 (a) Proximal femur periprosthetic fracture next to FD rod in an OI patient. (b) This was managed with revision FD rodding and proximal femur fixation using the coxa vara correction technique

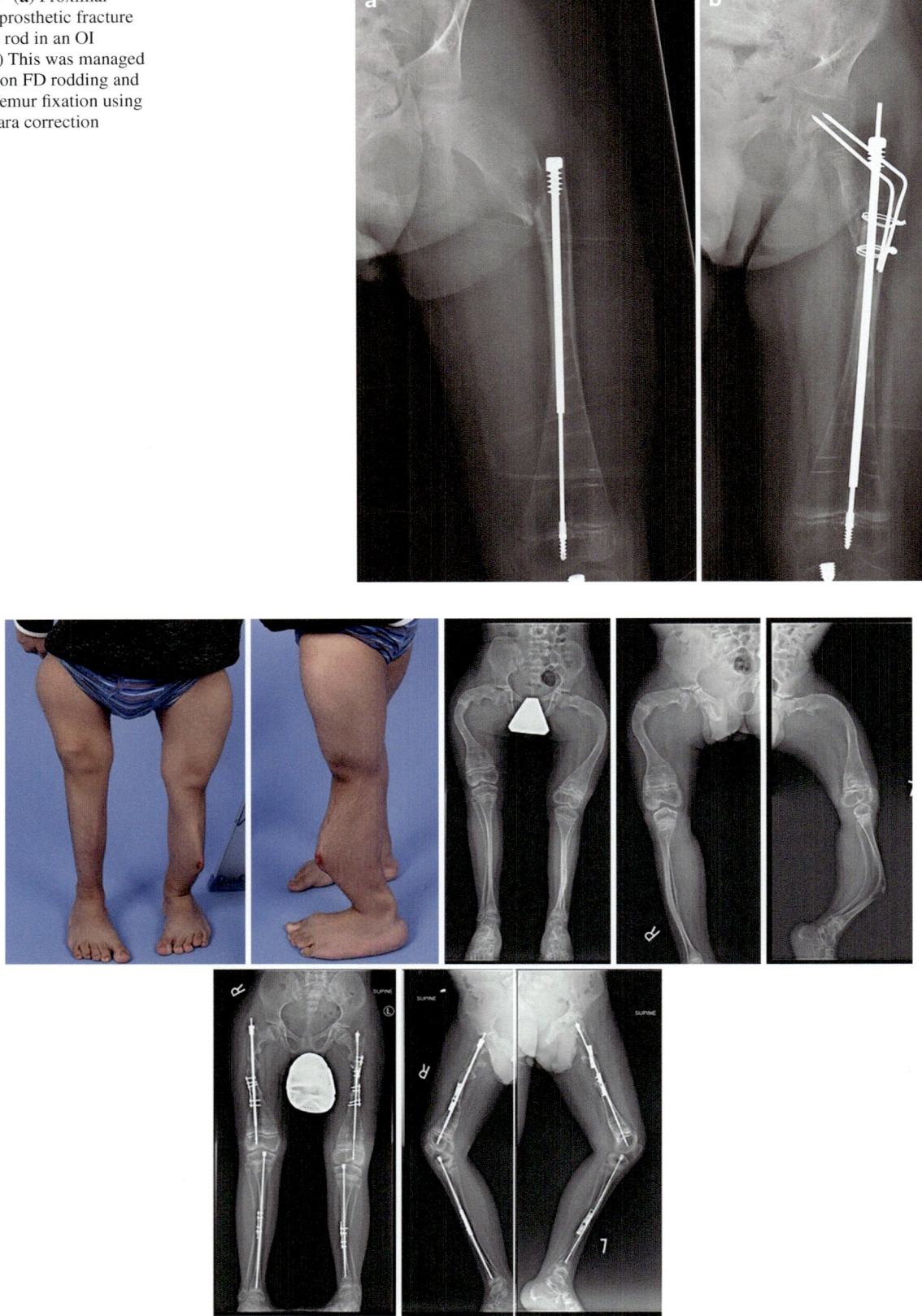

Fig. 23.24 Example of a patient with OI with severe lower extremity deformities that were managed with osteotomies, rodding, and supplemental plate fixation around the osteotomy sites to improve the stability of the bones

gap nail developed by Drs. Galban and Para [50] seems promising in such cases (with diameters between 4.8 and 8 mm) (Fig. 23.25). In addition, the Simple Locking Intra Medullary (SLIM) nail (threads for epiphyseal fixation at one end; diameter as small as 2.0 mm) is a good option that can be used for small canals in skeletally mature and immature patients with OI (Fig. 23.26).

Surgical correction of the lower limb deformities in OI has become more frequent since these patients benefit from medical treatment, including the use of bisphosphonates. In the future, the development of new medications will likely further improve the bone quality in such patients, while awaiting other advances such as gene therapy for this condition. The challenge for the orthopedic surgeon is to continue to develop improved surgical techniques and better implants until metallic implants are no longer necessary for patients with OI.

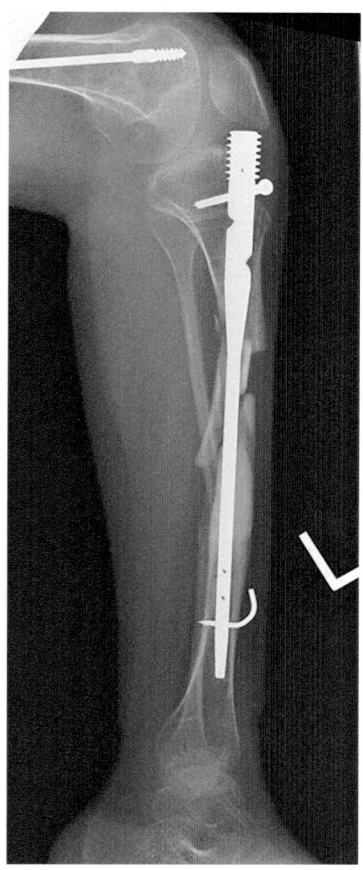

Fig. 23.25 Example of gap nail used for a complex revision surgery of FD rod migration with fracture and bowing of the tibia

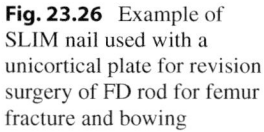

Fig. 23.26 Example of SLIM nail used with a unicortical plate for revision surgery of FD rod for femur fracture and bowing

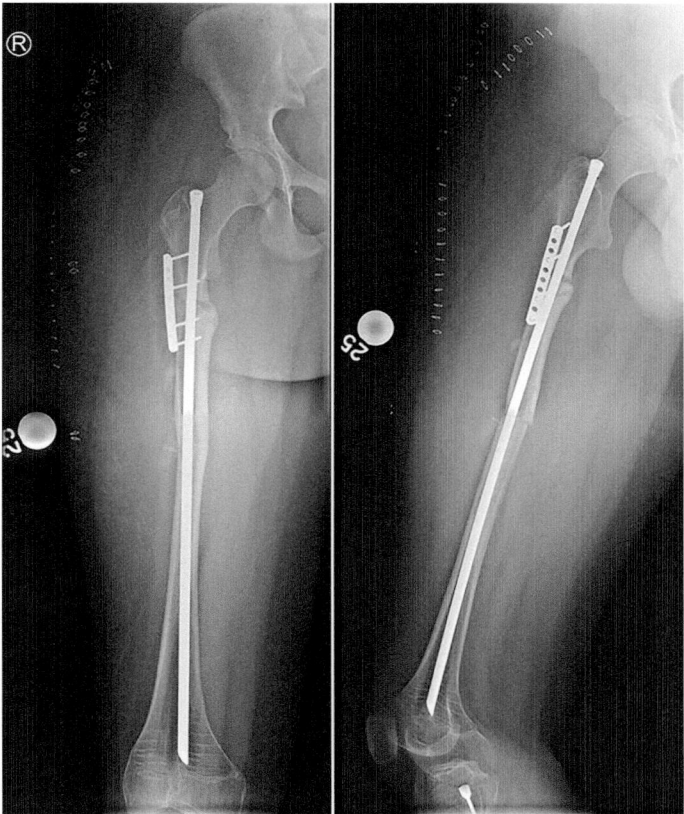

Commentary

Jeanne M. Franzone
Jeanne.Franzone@nemours.org

Professors Hamdy et al. deliver a comprehensive review of both modern osteogenesis imperfecta (OI) care and many developments put forth by their team and center over the years. The Montreal Center has been a giant in the field of OI care and research, and there are many pearls within the chapter that deserve special attention.

OI is a complex condition with many skeletal and nonskeletal manifestations. Comprehensive multidisciplinary care is critical for success and to optimize surgical outcomes. One may consider orthopaedic surgery reconstructive procedures but one small piece of the overall care of an OI patient; the underlying medical care and planning for and attention to the rehabilitation process is critical for an optimized outcome. An additional challenge within OI care and research is the heterogeneity of the condition and a broad range of clinical severity.

As is also well noted in the chapter, despite our current multidisciplinary care, there is, at this time, no cure for OI. The medical treatments are aimed at symptomatic improvements. The surgical procedures are fraught with challenges due to the poor bone quality. It is imperative to discuss with families that several surgical interventions will be necessary during growth and often beyond. Furthermore, one may take that a step further, and as OI surgeons, with each procedure, we are planning for the next one, planning for the revision. The attention to technical detail with each procedure has ramifications on future revisions; i.e., a carefully planned starting point for a threaded rod as that starting point will be used for a lifetime, attention to tension across the osteotomy sites, and soft-tissue tension as both affect healing and future deforming forces and rod size selection.

Regarding rod size selection, a few points within the chapter are to be emphasized. Attempting to measure a planned rod diameter based on preoperative radiographs is fraught with error as OI bones have a saber shape and the canal may be deceptively smaller than it appears on a two-dimensional projection. The decision regarding rod size is best made intraoperatively with an appreciation for the true canal size either based upon direct visualization (with an open osteotomy) or reamer fit (with a percutaneous osteotomy or closed osteoclasis). Our best rule of thumb is currently as stated by Professor Fassier: *"One fundamental aspect of OI bone surgery is that the child needs more bone than metal."* At this juncture, we do not have a more scientific statement, and this pearl guides practice. If rods are too small, they have a propensity to bend and break. If a rod is too large, a worse problem ensues—excessive reaming removes cortical bone and with the large-diameter implant stress shielding ensues, rendering future revision procedures quite challenging. Rod diameter selection is therefore akin to a "Goldilocks" phenomenon, not too big, not too small, but just right per Professor Fassier's statement.

Although 3D printed models from preoperative CT scans may be helpful for particularly challenging or unique cases, I would caution against the routine use of them due to the radiation considerations.

As the authors indicate, guided growth techniques, such as an instrumented hemiepiphysiodesis, have a limited role in the correction of deformities arising from a significant diaphyseal bow. For more mildly affected patients with genu varus or valgus, however, arising from a deformity closer to the physis, instrumented hemiepiphysiodesis has been reported and successful in the setting of OI.

As noted, a saw is not recommended for osteotomies in the setting of OI. When performing percutaneous osteotomies (preferable when possible due to maintenance of surrounding soft tissues and healing biology), it is important to understand the personality of the bone. If the percutaneous osteotomy falls at a sclerotic area of bone, attention to sufficient drill holes and use of an osteotome is important to avoid the bone breaking during manipulation at a different level than planned where the bone may be less sclerotic.

Regarding the indications for upper extremity realignment and rodding, particular attention is to be paid to upper extremity functional abilities. In following and publishing functional measures on a routine basis, the Montreal OI team has contributed to our understanding of the impact of addressing the upper extremities in the OI population. Particularly considering the dependence on upper extremity use for wheelchair ambulators for both self-care and recreational activities, it is imperative to consider upper extremity intervention as a part of wholistic OI care.

Supplemental plate and screw constructs have proven a useful way to introduce rotational control at an osteotomy or nonunion site as needed. A locking plate is preferable as the fixation does not rely on compression of the underlying bone. A locking plate additionally permits the use of unicortical screws and would recommend a locking plate with variable angle technology to facilitate bicortical fixation when possible around an intramedullary rod. It is recommended to keep the supplemental plates small in size and as emphasized to avoid a stand-alone plate and screw construct in the setting of OI. The removal of the supplemental plate and screws following healing is currently controversial, and further research and follow-up on the topic are necessary and underway.

The small-diameter bones such as the tibias in young patients undergoing an initial rodding procedure and the long and thin bones seen in many adolescent OI patients do pose a challenge regarding implant options. The small-diameter fixed length threaded nail option (SLIM) has been a useful addition for both of these situations and for skeletally mature patients not requiring the telescopic feature. A critical point, however, that resonates throughout the chapter is that surgery for OI patients should be performed based on patient indications and principles, not at a particular age or wedded to a specific implant.

It is an exciting time in OI care given recent and upcoming medical advances and the surgical techniques described by Professor Hamdy et al. and the large OI centers are working together to push forward surgical care with an emphasis on patient-reported outcome measures.

References

1. Tauer JT, Robinson ME, Rauch F. Osteogenesis imperfecta: new perspectives from clinical and translational research. JBMR Plus. 2019;3:e10174.
2. Forlino A, Marini JC. Osteogenesis imperfecta. Lancet. 2016;387:1657–71.
3. Folkestad L, Hald JD, Canudas-Romo V, Gram J, Hermann AP, Langdahl B, Abrahamsen B, Brixen K. Mortality and causes of death in patients with osteogenesis imperfecta: a register-based nationwide cohort study. J Bone Miner Res. 2016;31:2159–66.
4. Bardai G, Moffatt P, Glorieux FH, Rauch F. DNA sequence analysis in 598 individuals with a clinical diagnosis of osteogenesis imperfecta: diagnostic yield and mutation spectrum. Osteoporos Int. 2016;27:3607–13.
5. Robinson ME, Rauch F. Mendelian bone fragility disorders. Bone. 2019;126:11–7.
6. Shur NE, Summerlin ML, McIntosh BJ, Shalaby-Rana E, Hinds TS. Genetic causes of fractures and subdural hematomas: fact versus fiction. Pediatr Radiol. 2021;51:1029–43.
7. Bronicki LM, Stevenson RE, Spranger JW. Beyond osteogenesis imperfecta: causes of fractures during infancy and childhood. Am J Med Genet C Semin Med Genet. 2015;169:314–27.
8. Mortier GR, Cohn DH, Cormier-Daire V, Hall C, Krakow D, Mundlos S, Nishimura G, Robertson S, Sangiorgi L, Savarirayan R, Sillence D, Superti-Furga A, Unger S, Warman ML. Nosology and classification of genetic skeletal disorders: 2019 revision. Am J Med Genet A. 2019;179:2393–419.
9. Lindahl K, Astrom E, Rubin CJ, Grigelioniene G, Malmgren B, Ljunggren O, Kindmark A. Genetic epidemiology, prevalence, and genotype-phenotype correlations in the Swedish population with osteogenesis imperfecta. Eur J Hum Genet. 2015;23:1042–50.
10. Glorieux FH, Bishop NJ, Plotkin H, Chabot G, Lanoue G, Travers R. Cyclic administration of pamidronate in children with severe osteogenesis imperfecta. N Engl J Med. 1998;339:947–52.
11. Ward LM, Rauch F, Whyte MP, D'Astous J, Gates PE, Grogan D, Lester EL, McCall RE, Pressly TA, Sanders JO, Smith PA, Steiner RD, Sullivan E, Tyerman G, Smith-Wright DL, Verbruggen N, Heyden N, Lombardi A, Glorieux FH. Alendronate for the treatment of pediatric osteogenesis imperfecta: a randomized placebo-controlled study. J Clin Endocrinol Metab. 2011;96:355–64.
12. Bishop N, Adami S, Ahmed SF, Anton J, Arundel P, Burren CP, Devogelaer JP, Hangartner T, Hosszu E, Lane JM, Lorenc R, Makitie O, Munns CF, Paredes A, Pavlov H, Plotkin H, Raggio CL, Reyes ML, Schoenau E, Semler O, Sillence DO, Steiner RD. Risedronate in children with osteogenesis imperfecta: a randomised, double-blind, placebo-controlled trial. Lancet. 2013;382:1424–32.
13. Rauch F, Travers R, Plotkin H, Glorieux FH. The effects of intravenous pamidronate on the bone tissue of children and adolescents with osteogenesis imperfecta. J Clin Invest. 2002;110:1293–9.
14. Palomo T, Fassier F, Ouellet J, Sato A, Montpetit K, Glorieux FH, Rauch F. Intravenous bisphosphonate therapy of young children with osteogenesis imperfecta: skeletal findings during follow up throughout the growing years. J Bone Miner Res. 2015;30:2150–7.
15. Sato A, Ouellet J, Muneta T, Glorieux FH, Rauch F. Scoliosis in osteogenesis imperfecta caused by COL1A1/COL1A2 mutations—genotype-phenotype correlations and effect of bisphosphonate treatment. Bone. 2016;86:53–7.
16. Anissipour AK, Hammerberg KW, Caudill A, Kostiuk T, Tarima S, Zhao HS, Krzak JJ, Smith PA. Behavior of scoliosis during growth in children with osteogenesis imperfecta. J Bone Joint Surg Am. 2014;96:237–43.
17. Sakkers R, Kok D, Engelbert R, van Dongen A, Jansen M, Pruijs H, Verbout A, Schweitzer D, Uiterwaal C. Skeletal effects and functional outcome with olpadronate in children with osteogenesis imperfecta: a 2-year randomised placebo-controlled study. Lancet. 2004;363:1427–31.
18. Lindahl K, Kindmark A, Rubin CJ, Malmgren B, Grigelioniene G, Soderhall S, Ljunggren O, Astrom E. Decreased fracture rate, pharmacogenetics and BMD response in 79 Swedish children with osteogenesis imperfecta types I, III and IV treated with Pamidronate. Bone. 2016;87:11–8.
19. Montpetit K, Palomo T, Glorieux FH, Fassier F, Rauch F. Multidisciplinary treatment of severe osteogenesis imperfecta: functional outcomes at skeletal maturity. Arch Phys Med Rehabil. 2015;96:1834–9.
20. Munns CF, Rauch F, Zeitlin L, Fassier F, Glorieux FH. Delayed osteotomy but not fracture healing in pediatric osteogenesis imperfecta patients receiving pamidronate. J Bone Miner Res. 2004;19:1779–86.
21. Anam EA, Rauch F, Glorieux FH, Fassier F, Hamdy R. Osteotomy healing in children with osteogenesis imperfecta receiving bisphosphonate treatment. J Bone Miner Res. 2015;30:1362–8.
22. Hernandez M, Phulpin B, Mansuy L, Droz D. Use of new targeted cancer therapies in children: effects on dental development and risk of jaw osteonecrosis: a review. J Oral Pathol Med. 2017;46:321–6.
23. Mueller B, Engelbert R, Baratta-Ziska F, Bartels B, Blanc N, Brizola E, Fraschini P, Hill C, Marr C, Mills L, Montpetit K, Pacey V, Molina MR, Schuuring M, Verhille C, de Vries O, Yeung EHK, Semler O. Consensus statement on physical rehabilitation in children and adolescents with osteogenesis imperfecta. Orphanet J Rare Dis. 2018;13(1):158.
24. Sakkers RJ, Montpetit K, Tsimicalis A, Wirth T, Verhoef M, Hamdy R, Ouellet JA, Castelein RM, Damas C, Janus GJ, Nijhuis WH,

24. Panzeri L, Paveri S, Mekking D, Thorstad K, Kruse RW. A roadmap to surgery in osteogenesis imperfecta: results of an international collaboration of patient organizations and interdisciplinary care teams. Acta Orthop. 2021;92(5):608–14.
25. Marr C, Seasman A, Bishop N. Managing the patient with osteogenesis imperfecta: a multidisciplinary approach. J Multidiscip Healthc. 2017;10:145–55.
26. Posborg P, Astrup G, Bendixen D, Lund AM, Ording H. Osteogenesis imperfecta and malignant hyperthermia. Is there a relationship? Anaesthesia. 1996;51:863–5.
27. Bojanic K, Kivela JE, Gurrier C, Deutsch E, Flick R, Sprung J, et al. Perioperative course and intraoperative temperatures in patients with osteogenesis imperfecta. Eur J Anaesthesiol. 2011;28(5):370–5.
28. Rodriguez Celin M, Kruger KM, Caudill A, et al. A multicenter study of intramedullary rodding in osteogenesis imperfecta. JB JS Open Access. 2020;5(3):e20.00031.
29. Sofield HA, Millar EA. Fragmentation, realignment, and intramedullary rod fixation of deformities of the long bones in children: a ten-year appraisal. J Bone Joint Surg Am. 1959;41:1371–91.
30. Enright WJ, Noonan KJ. Bone plating in patients with type III osteogenesis imperfecta: results and complications. Iowa Orthop J. 2006;26:37–40.
31. Bailey RW, Dubow HI. Studies of longitudinal bone growth resulting in an extensible nail. Surg Forum. 1963;14:455–8.
32. Stokely I, Bell MJ, Sharrard WJ. The role of expanding intramedullary rods in osteogenesis imperfecta. J Bone Joint Surg Br. 1989;71(3):422–7.
33. Karbowski A, Schwitalle M, Brenner R, Lehman H, Pontz B, Worsdorfer O. Experience with Bailey-Dubow rodding in children with osteogenesis imperfecta. Eur J Pediatr Surg. 2000;10(2):119–24.
34. Cho TJ, Choi IH, Chung CY, Yoo WJ, Lee KS, Lee DY. Interlocking telescopic rod for patients with osteogenesis imperfecta. J Bone Joint Surg Am. 2007;89(5):1028–35.
35. Fassier F, Glorieux FH. Osteogenesis imperfecta. Surg Tech Orthop Traumatol. 2003;SS-0S0 D-30:8.
36. Ruck J, Dahan-Oliel N, Montpetit K, Rauch F, Fassier F. Fassier-Duval femoral rodding in children with osteogenesis imperfecta receiving bisphosphonates: functional outcomes at one year. J Child Orthop. 2011;5(3):217–24.
37. Rosemberg DL, Goiano EO, Akkari M, Santili C. Effects of a telescopic intramedullary rod for treating patients with osteogenesis imperfecta of the femur. J Child Orthop. 2018;12(1):97–103.
38. Holmes K, Gralla J, Brazell C, et al. Fassier-Duval rod failure: is it related to positioning in the distal epiphysis? J Pediatr Orthop. 2020;40(8):448–52.
39. Aarabi M, Rauch F, Hamdy RC, Fassier F. High prevalence of coxa vara in patients with severe osteogenesis imperfecta. J Pediatr Orthop. 2006;26(1):24–8.
40. Fassier F, Sardar Z, Aarabi M, Odent T, Haque T, Hamdy R. Results and complications of a surgical technique for correction of coxa vara in children with osteopenic bones. J Pediatr Orthop. 2008;28(8):799–805.
41. Nicolaou N, Bowe JD, Wilkinson JM, Fernandes JA, Bell MJ. Use of the Sheffield telescopic intramedullary rod system for the management of osteogenesis imperfecta: clinical outcomes at an average follow-up of nineteen years. J Bone Joint Surg Am. 2011;93(21):1994–2000.
42. Benjamin J, Gleeson R, Chandra KB. The choice of intramedullary devices for the femur and the tibia in osteogenesis imperfecta. J Pediatr Orthop B. 2005;14:311–9.
43. Azzam KA, Rush ET, Burke BR, Nabower AM, Esposito PW. Midterm results of femoral and Tibial osteotomies and Fassier-Duval nailing in children with osteogenesis imperfecta. J Pediatr Orthop. 2018;38(6):331–6.
44. Cox I, Al Mouazzen L, Bleibleh S, et al. Combined two-centre experience of single-entry telescopic rods identifies characteristic modes of failure. Bone Joint J. 2020;102-B(8):1048–55.
45. Musielak BJ, Woźniak Ł, Sułko J, Oberc A, Jóźwiak M. Problems, complications, and factors predisposing to failure of Fassier-Duval rodding in children with osteogenesis imperfecta: a double-center study. J Pediatr Orthop. 2021;41(4):e347–52.
46. Frick SL, Sponseller PD, Leet A. Pediatric limb reconstruction in osteogenesis imperfecta. In: Shapiro JR, editor. Osteogenesis imperfecta—a translational approach to brittle bone disease. New York: Elsevier; 2014. p. 443–51.
47. Gamble JG, Rinsky LA, Strudwick J, Bleck EE. Non-union of fractures in children who have osteogenesis imperfecta. J Bone Joint Surg Am. 1988;70:439–43.
48. Cho TJ, Lee K, Oh CW, Park MS, Yoo WJ, Choi IH. Locking plate placement with unicortical screw fixation adjunctive to intramedullary rodding in long bones of patients with osteogenesis imperfecta. J Bone Joint Surg Am. 2015;97(9):733–7.
49. Franzone JM, Kruse RW. Intramedullary nailing with supplemental plate and screw fixation of long bones of patients with osteogenesis imperfecta: operative technique and preliminary results. J Pediatr Orthop B. 2018;27(4):344–9.
50. Galban M. Intramedular rodding in adult with osteogenesis imperfecta developing of a new device. In: Anticevic D, editor. 11th international conference on osteogenesis imperfecta final program & abstract book. Dubrovnik: Croatian Pediatric Orthopaedic Society of Croatian Medical Association; 2011. p. 81.

Lower Limb Deformity in Neuromuscular Disorders: Pathophysiology, Assessment, Goals, and Principles of Management

Unni G. Narayanan

This chapter will highlight common neuromuscular conditions that arise from primary pathology in different parts of the neural-muscular axis (brain, spine, peripheral nerve to the muscle). Cerebral palsy, a static encephalopathy (upper motor neuron disorder), is associated with progressive secondary musculoskeletal deformities during growth. Spina bifida (mixed lower motor neuron and upper motor neuron features) is a congenital deficiency of the neural tube that presents with musculoskeletal deformities both at birth and acquired later during growth. Charcot-Marie-Tooth (CMT), an inherited peripheral neuropathy, falls under a group of hereditary sensory motor neuropathies (HSMN) and is associated with specific lower extremity deformities of the foot and dysplasia of the hip. The muscular dystrophies, of which Duchenne's muscular Dystrophy (DMD) is the most severe and common, is a group of genetic disorders of skeletal muscle associated with progressive weakness.

Cerebral Palsy

Cerebral Palsy (CP) encompasses a large group of disorders of movement and posture that arise from a disturbance to the developing fetal or infant brain. The primary pathology is permanent but not progressive and can be accompanied by deficits of sensation, perception, cognition, and communication; by seizure disorders; and secondarily acquired musculoskeletal deformity [1, 2].

CP accounts for the most common cause of chronic childhood disability, with a prevalence of 2–3 per thousand, and is associated with a wide range of etiologies [3]. Prematurity is one common risk factor due to the fragility of the cerebral vasculature and immaturity of the autonomic nervous system that controls cerebral perfusion. Some additional risk factors include congenital brain malformations, intrauterine infections, placental malformations, prenatal brain hemorrhages or strokes, perinatal causes of hypoxic-ischemic encephalopathy and hyperbilirubinemia, postnatal strokes, infections or traumatic and other kinds of brain injuries. A number of genetic disorders (Rett syndrome, Fragile X syndrome, Familial or hereditary spastic paraparesis) and metabolic disorders (mucopolysaccharidoses, phenylketonuria, etc.) can mimic features of CP.

Classification of CP

CP is best classified by the five-level Gross Motor Function Classification System (GMFCS), which is reliable, valid, stable, and highly prognostic [4–6] (Fig. 24.1). Children functioning at GMFCS level I walk independently without a walking aid and can perform most activities of typically developing children, with some difficulties with speed, balance, and coordination. At level II, children are independently ambulant without a walking aid, but require support in more challenging situations such as on uneven surfaces or while climbing stairs. At GMFCS level III, children rely on walking aids such as crutches or walkers for at least some of their functional mobility. Some may use wheelchairs for longer distances. Children in GMFCS levels IV and V rely on a wheelchair for their functional mobility. Children at level IV can usually sit without support and do some functional weight-bearing for transfers. Walking, if possible, is limited to short distances with a supportive walker, for exercise purposes. Children classified as level V are unable to sit without support, and weight-bearing is limited to supported weight-bearing in a stander for exercise rather than functional

U. G. Narayanan (✉)
Department of Surgery and Rehabilitation Sciences Institute, University of Toronto, Toronto, ON, Canada

Division of Orthopaedic Surgery and Child Health Evaluative Sciences Program, The Hospital for Sick Children, Toronto, ON, Canada
e-mail: unni.narayanan@sickkids.ca

Fig. 24.1 GMFCS levels. (Reproduced with permission copyright © Kerr Graham, Bill Reid, and Adrienne Harvey, The Royal Children's Hospital, Melbourne)

GMFCS E & R Descriptors and Illustrations for Children between their 6th and 12th birthday

GMFCS Level I

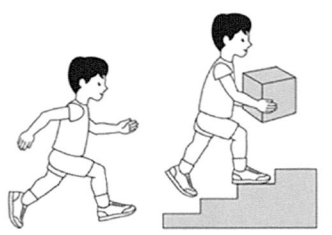

Children walk at home, school, outdoors and in the community. They can climb stairs without the use of a railing. Children perform gross motor skills such as running and jumping, but speed, balance and coordination are limited

GMFCS Level II

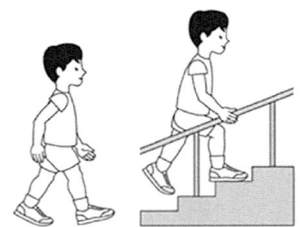

Children walk in most settings and climb stairs holding onto a railing. They may experience difficulty walking long distance and balancing on uneven terrain, inclines, in crowded areas or confined spaces. Children may walk with physical assistance, a hand-held mobility device or use wheeled mobility over long distances. Children have only minimal ability to perform gross motor skills such as running and jumping.

GMFCS Level III

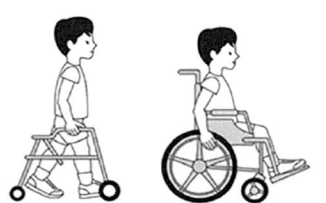

Childen walk using a hand-held mobility device in most indoor settings. They may climb stairs holding onto a railing with supervision or assistance. Children use wheeled mobility when traveling long distances and may self-propel for shorter distances.

GMFCS Level IV

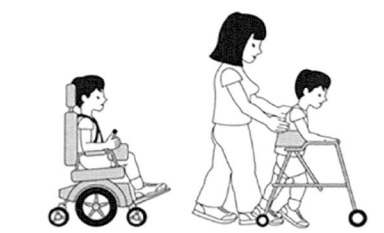

Children use methods of mobility that require physical assistance or powered mobility in most settings. They may walk for short distances at home with physical assistance or use powered mobility or a body support walker when positioned. At school, outdoors and in the community children are transported in a manual wheelchair or use powered mobility.

GMFCS Level V

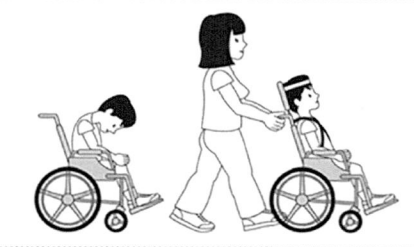

Children are transported in a manual wheelchair in all settings. Children are limited in their ability to maintain antigravity head and trunk postures and control leg and arm movements.

GMFCS descriptors copyright © Palisano et al. (1997) Dev Med Child Neurol 39:214-23
CanChild: www.canchild.ca

Illustrations copyright © Kerr Graham, Bill Reid and Adrienne Harvey, The Royal Children's Hospital, Melbourne purposes. These children depend on a caregiver for much of their activities of daily living.

CP is also classified by the type of abnormal tone or movement disorder. The location and extent of brain involvement account for the type and severity of the abnormal tone and movement disorder as well as the topographical distribution of involvement of the trunk and limbs. Lesions involving the pyramidal tract are associated with spasticity or velocity-dependent hypertonia; whereas lesions of the basal ganglia are associated with dyskinesias including dystonia or choreoathetosis. Dystonia is characterized by jerky involuntary movements of the limbs or trunk and neck. Choreoathetosis is characterized by involuntary writhing movements. Cerebellar involvement is associated with ataxia and hypotonia. Some children have features of more than one type or "mixed" tone abnormalities. The commonly used topographical classification: hemiplegic, diplegic (lower extremities involved more than upper extremities), and quadriplegic or total body involved, has some clinical and prognostic utility, but these terms are not very reliable. Instead, the regional involvement may be categorized as being "Unilateral" or "Bilateral," which can be symmetric or asymmetric with one side more involved than the other.

Pathophysiology of Musculoskeletal Deformity in Cerebral Palsy

Musculoskeletal deformities in CP are acquired secondarily. Characteristically, upper motor neuron disorders are associated with hypertonia, hyperreflexia, and co-contraction of agonist-antagonist muscles. Other features can include loss of selective motor control, poor centrally mediated balance and coordination, and muscle weakness [7]. These children often have a delay in the development of the motor milestones.

Hypertonia is associated with "dynamic" muscle contractures. Muscles are taut due to the increased muscle tone, but they are of sufficient length. Muscles grow in response to the stimulus of stretch. In a child with CP, developmental delay prevents the child from engaging in the typical physical activities that would provide the source of stretch. The hypertonia further impedes the extent of any stretch. Consequently, muscle growth is impaired relative to bone growth. This results in the development of "static" contractures where the muscles are both tight and too short [8]. The acquisition of motor milestones, from rolling over into the prone position, sitting upright, crawling, pulling up to stand, cruising, and walking, typically occur during the first 12–15 months of a child's life. The growing skeleton undergoes significant changes during this time, in response to the natural stresses applied to the skeleton. The delay in motor milestones, or in some cases failure to achieve them at all, deprives the skeleton of these important corrective forces, resulting in the retention of infantile morphology of the skeleton (e.g., increased femoral anteversion and coxa valga in the proximal femur). Furthermore, the abnormal muscular forces acting on the growing skeleton contribute additionally to the development of bony deformities and joint instability over time. Joint instability in these patients is often a consequence of both the bony deformity and the unbalanced forces of the agonist-antagonist muscles that traverse a joint. The skeletal deformities result in lever arm dysfunction [9]. In the lower extremity, the interaction of joint contractures, muscle weakness, bony deformities, and joint instability at multiple levels is associated with inefficient (higher energy consuming) pathologic and compensatory gait patterns in ambulant children. This leads to limitation in physical function or symptoms such as pain and fatigue. In nonambulatory children, contractures and deformities of the lower limbs contribute to discomfort, difficulties with care, positioning and mobility, and poorer quality of life. Although the primary lesion in the brain is not progressive, the secondary musculoskeletal consequences become worse with growth [10–13] (Fig. 24.2).

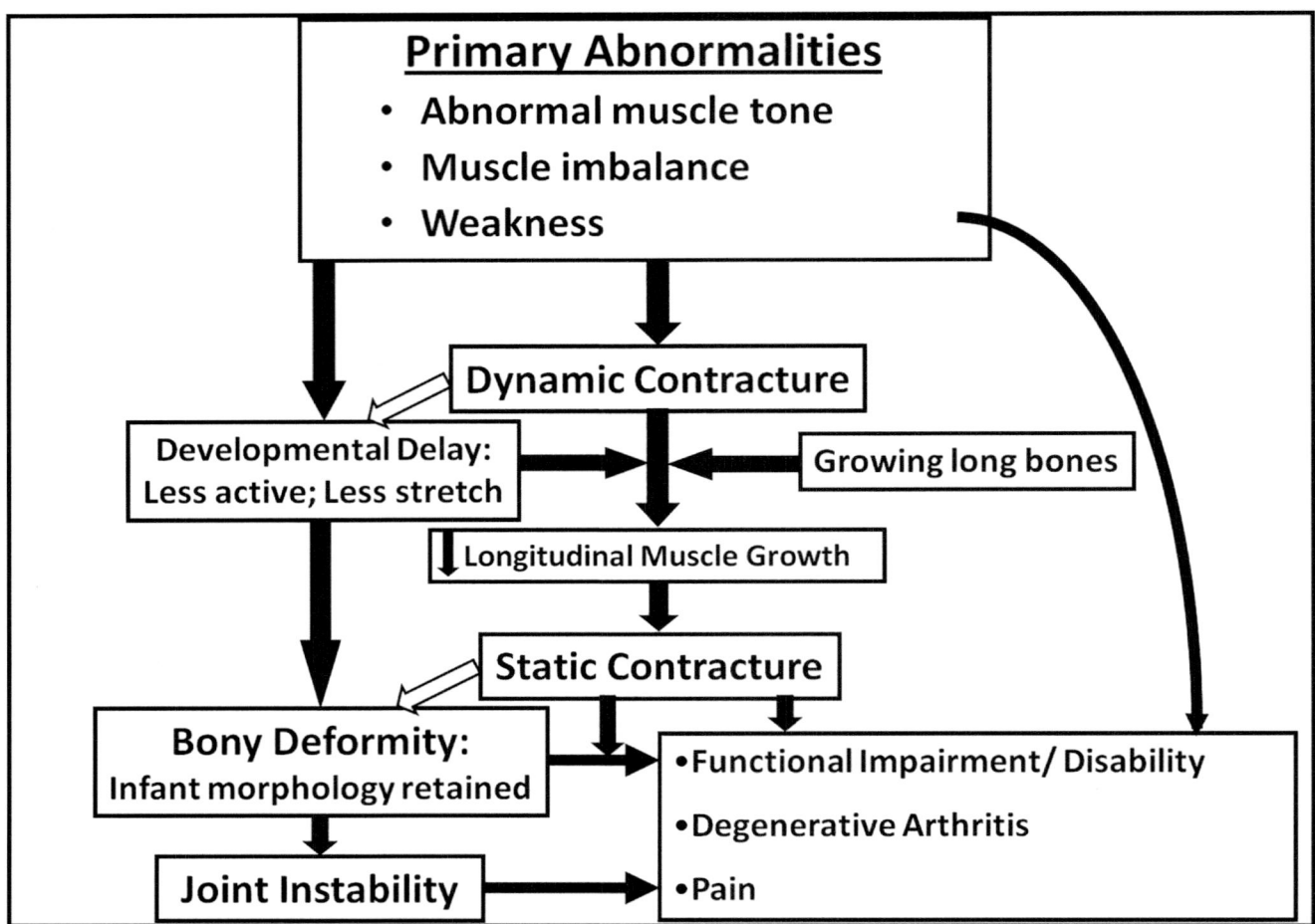

Fig. 24.2 Pathway to secondary musculoskeletal pathology in cerebral palsy. (Adapted from Noordin, S & Narayanan, U. Chapter 64. Neuromuscular Disorders in Mercer's Textbook of Orthopaedics and Trauma, 10th Edition, CRC Press 2012)

Specific Deformities of the Lower Extremity

Pelvis and Hip

Across the hip joint, adductors and flexors are typically more involved, overpowering their antagonist counterparts, the hip abductors, and hip extensors. This muscle imbalance results in adduction and flexion contractures of the hip. The hip flexion contracture arising from the iliopsoas can be accompanied by anterior pelvic tilt with associated lumbar lordosis. Anterior pelvic tilt might also be secondary to weak hip extensors or weak anterior abdominal muscles or a combination of these [14, 15]. In contrast, contracted hamstrings can pull down on the ischium resulting in a relative posterior tilt of the pelvis. In the transverse plane, the hip commonly lies internally rotated. This is more likely due to increased femoral anteversion rather than an internal rotation contracture [16]. In bilaterally involved children, the muscle contractures and bony deformities may not be symmetric. The more severely involved side might be more adducted and internally rotated. If this is accompanied by relative abduction and/or external rotation of the contralateral side, the deformity is described as "windswept" toward the abducted/externally rotated side (Fig. 24.3).

In CP, the morphology of the proximal femur is characterized by an increase in the neck–shaft angle in the coronal plane (coxa valga) and excessive femoral anteversion in the transverse plane (Fig. 24.4a). Femoral anteversion is the angle in the transverse plane, by which the neck of the femur is directed (forward) from the transcondylar or coronal plane [17] (Fig. 24.4b). The terms femoral anteversion and femoral (medial) torsion are used interchangeably, the latter term suggesting that the orientation of the proximal femur relative to the coronal plane is a consequence of torsion occurring along the shaft of the femur rather than in the neck [18–20]. In the new born, both femoral anteversion and neck–shaft angle are increased. This might be related to the fetal position. As the growing infant begins to roll over and crawl and pull up to stand and walk, the progressive extension of the hip is believed to push back the femoral neck axis to the normal values of anteversion seen in older children and adults by the age of 1 or 2 years. The developmental delay associated with CP removes the benefits of these corrective forces resulting in the retention of the infantile morphology of the proximal femur [21]. This is borne out by the finding that the mean neck–shaft angle increases with the severity of CP by GMFCS level from 135.9° (range: 130° to 145°) at GMFCS level I to 163.0° (range: 151–178°) at level V [22]. Femoral anteversion also increases with GMFCS level but seems to plateau at level III to level V, where it averages 40.0° (range: 25–67.5°). Whether the abnormal proximal femoral geometry is further affected by the abnormal forces associated with adduction/flexion contractures is less clear. The reduced femoral head coverage associated with increased femoral anteversion is compensated for by increased internal rotation of the femur and the increased anterior tilt of the pelvis [16].

At birth, the hip joint is typically normal in children with CP. Hip instability is usually acquired due to the interaction between the adduction and flexion contractures with the increased neck–shaft angle and anteversion, contributing to the posterolateral displacement of the femoral head. The magnitude of the hip displacement (subluxation) is quantified using the Reimer's migration percentage (MP) [23] (Fig. 24.5). The "hip at risk" is defined as the hip that is likely to progress to hip dislocation if left untreated. The proportion of children with CP who will develop progressive hip displacement is strongly associated with increasing GMFCS level in population-based studies [24–26]. Using 30% MP as the definition of hip at risk, the incidence is virtually 0% for GMFCS level I but increases to 90% for level V [26]. When a threshold of 40% is used to define a hip at risk, the incidence is 65% for GMFSC level V [25]. Approximately one-third of hips with a MP between 33 and 40% will improve spontaneously or will not deteriorate [25]. Progressive subluxation is very likely if the MP is greater than 40% in a child still growing (Fig. 24.6a–c). A higher head–shaft angle (HFA) has also been shown to increase the risk of progressive hip displacement [27]. This has led to the development of predictive models that use the age, GMFCS level, current MP, and HFA to predict the probability of progression of MP to at least 40% [28]. The displaced femoral head pushes up against the superolateral surface of the acetabulum leading to increasing acetabular dysplasia, measured by the acetabular index (AI) when the triradiate cartilage is open, or by the acetabular angle of Sharp, when the triradiate cartilage is closed [29]. In association with hip flexion contracture, the acetabular deficiency tends to be more posterior [21]. Initially

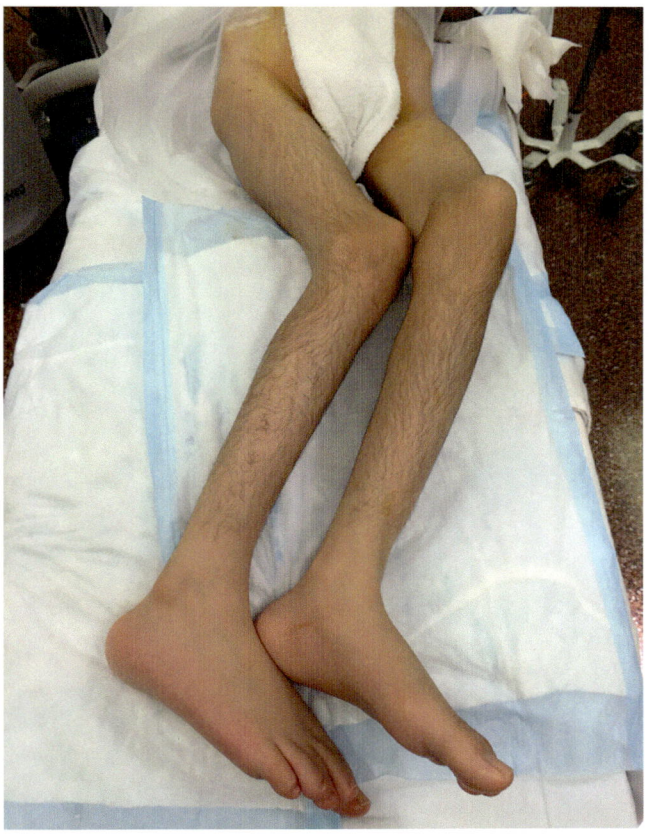

Fig. 24.3 Windswept hips

Fig. 24.4 (a) Coxa valga. (b) Femoral anteversion. (Adapted from Narayanan, Unni G Chapter 26 in Volume 2, Part 4: Pediatrics in Operative Techniques in Orthopaedic Surgery. Ed. Weisel. S.W. Wolters Kluwer, Lippincott Williams & Wilkins, 2011. Philadelphia)

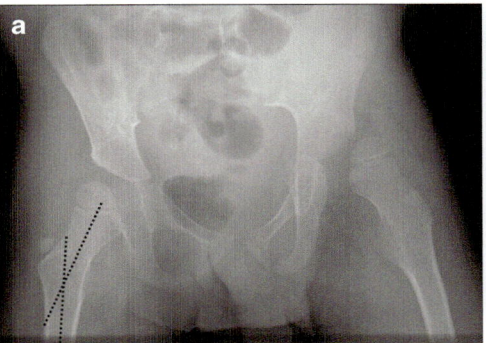
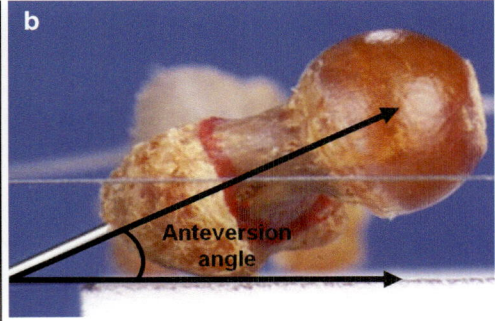

Fig. 24.5 AP radiograph of the pelvis with radiographic parameters quantifying hip displacement and acetabular dysplasia

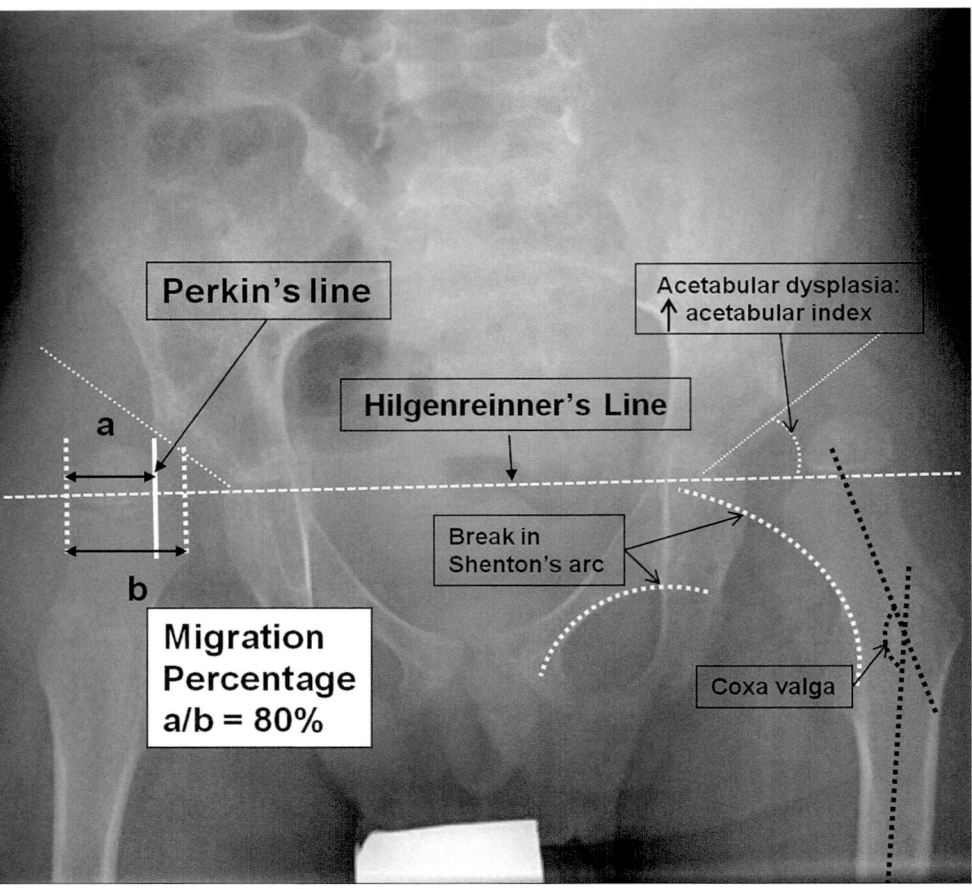

Fig. 24.6 (**a–c**) Hip at risk progressing to increased subluxation and acetabular dysplasia. (**d–e**) Dislocated femoral head leading to loss of sphericity and advanced degenerative changes

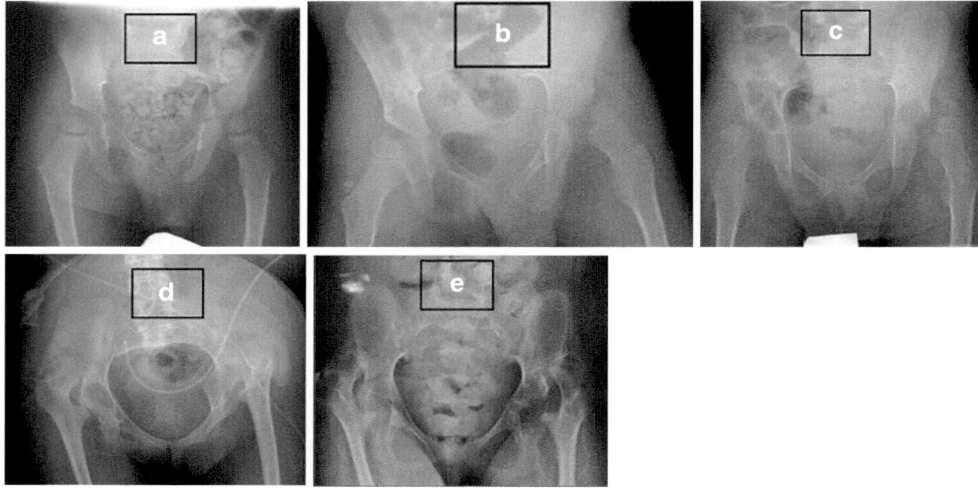

the subluxated femoral head might reduce in the abducted position, but eventually the dislocation becomes irreducible. The uncovered femoral head is subject to the abnormal forces of the overlying capsule and abductors draped over the superolateral surface of the femoral head (Fig. 24.6d). This leads to loss of sphericity and progressive flattening of this surface leading to increasing femoral head deformity. Ultimately, there is erosion of the articular cartilage and degenerative changes consistent with osteoarthritis (Fig. 24.6e).

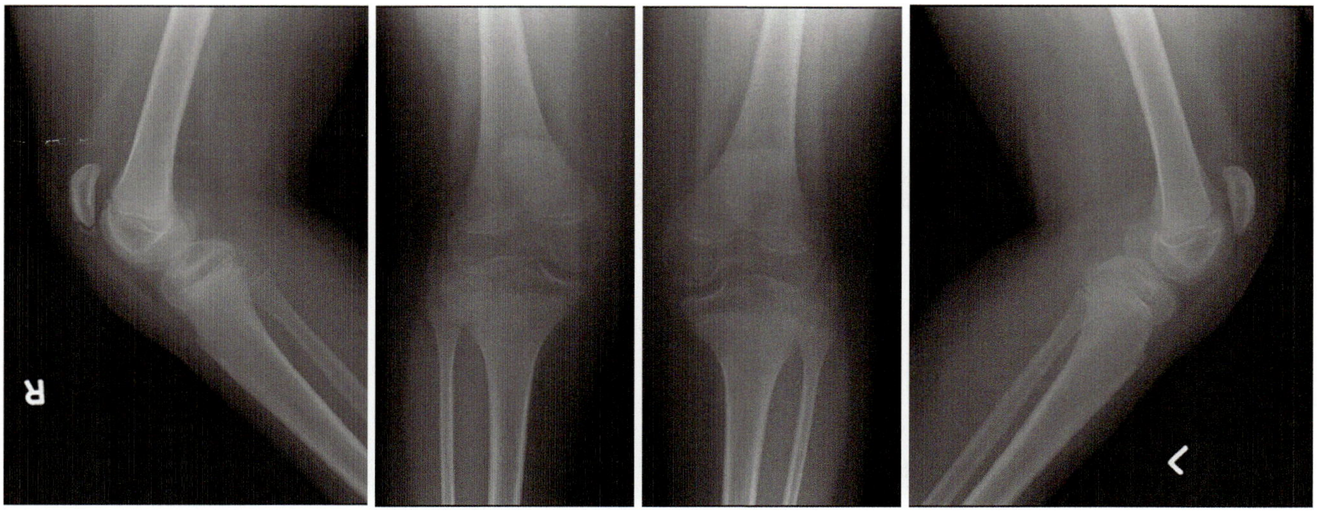

Fig. 24.7 Bilateral patella alta due to longstanding crouch with avulsion fractures of the inferior pole of patella

Knee and Lower Leg Segment

At the knee, the most common deformity is a flexion deformity. The knee flexion deformity has a wide range of etiologies. It can arise from contracture of the medial and/or lateral hamstrings. Since the medial hamstrings (semitendinosus and semimembranosus) and part of the lateral hamstrings (long head of biceps femoris) take origin on the ischium which is above the hip joint, a "functional" contracture of the hamstrings is possible even in the presence of normal or even excessive length of the hamstrings when there is an associated anterior pelvic tilt that raises the origin of these muscles [14, 15, 30]. Knee flexion deformity might also be due to a weak gastrocsoleus complex leading to the forward translation of the tibial shank over the foot, leading to the ground reaction force passing posterior to the knee resulting in an (external) knee flexion moment that has to be counteracted with a corresponding (internal) extension moment using the quadriceps. These are the features of a crouch gait pattern. If the knee extensors are weak, the knee goes into progressively increased flexion. A gastrocnemius contracture can also lead to flexion deformity of the knee to take the tension off the gastrocnemius, especially if the foot is being held plantigrade in a brace. Often a combination of these factors may be present. Excessive knee flexion present during weight-bearing or walking may not initially be associated with a fixed flexion contracture. Over time, passive extension is likely to become restricted with increasing fixed knee flexion contracture due to insufficient length of the hamstrings and/or a posterior capsular contracture. Weight-bearing in the crouch position increases the joint reaction force on the patellofemoral joint which can cause anterior knee pain, patella alta, and avulsion fractures of the inferior pole of the patella (Fig. 24.7).

> **Multiple Etiologies of Knee Flexion Deformity**
> True contracture of the hamstring/s.
> "Functional" contracture of hamstring/s: Increased anterior pelvic tilt due to any cause, raises the origin (ischial tuberosity) of the medial hamstrings and long head of biceps, which in turn contributes to flexion at the distal insertion. Excessive anterior pelvic tilt can be due to:
>
> Hip flexion contracture
> Weak hip extensors
> Weak anterior abdominal muscles
> Compensatory strategy for excessive anteversion
>
> Weak plantar flexion—knee extension couple leads to forward lean of the tibia shank over the foot, leading to the ground reaction force passing posterior to the knee, causing an increased external flexion moment. Reasons for this include:
>
> Weak gastrocsoleus complex, often iatrogenic due to over-lengthened tendo-Achilles, in a child with spastic diplegia.
> Hindfoot valgus with midfoot break and forefoot abduction
> Excessive external tibial torsion
>
> Gastrocnemius contracture (dynamic or static): knee bends to allow foot to be plantigrade by taking the stretch off the contracted gastrocnemius
> Posterior capsular contracture
> Combinations of above

True coronal plane deformity at the knee is uncommon. However, the internal rotation of the hip due to increased femoral anteversion is characterized by a corresponding medial rotation of the knee (patella), which creates an apparent (pseudo) valgus appearance of the (flexed) knee. This appearance is exacerbated if the femoral anteversion is accompanied by external tibial torsion below the knee. The tibial segment can be associated with normal torsion, increased external or increased internal tibial torsion. At birth, the torsion of the tibia is relatively internal, with the bimalleolar axis typically being neutral in the transverse plane. The tibia undergoes external rotation maximally during the first 4 years, and about 1° per year until skeletal maturity when it reaches average of 28° external [31]. In some children with CP, the infantile internal torsion may persist due to the failure of the natural lateral rotation to occur. In others, significantly increased external tibial torsion can occur often in association with valgus hindfoot, flattening of the midfoot, and forefoot abduction. This is associated with a poor lever arm for push off in gait and is often accompanied by crouch position at the knee due to the weak plantarflexion-knee extension couple (Fig. 24.8).

Ankle and Foot

Equinus of the ankle is the most common deformity of the lower extremity in CP. Equinus arises from an imbalance between the hypertonic and/or contracted plantar flexors (gastrocsoleus complex) that overpower the weak dorsiflexors (tibialis anterior). What begins as a dynamic contracture due to spasticity is likely to become fixed when the gastrocnemius-soleus complex fails to keep up with the tibial growth. In bilateral CP, the gastrocnemius is usually more involved than the soleus. Consequently, the ankle might have sufficient dorsiflexion when the knee is flexed but demonstrates an equinus contracture when the knee is extended due to the proximal stretch of the gastrocnemius muscle at its origin above the knee (Fig. 24.9). In unilateral CP (hemiplegia), the soleus is usually just as involved as the gastrocnemius, so that the equinus contracture does not alter much

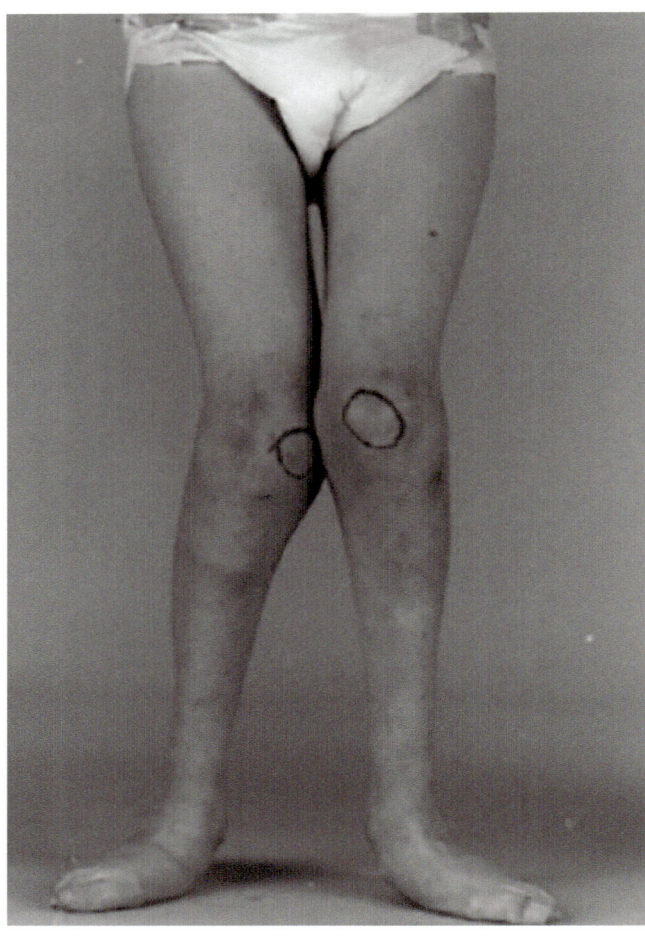

Fig. 24.8 Torsional malignment: pseudo-valgus due to increased femoral internal torsion and increased external tibial torsion

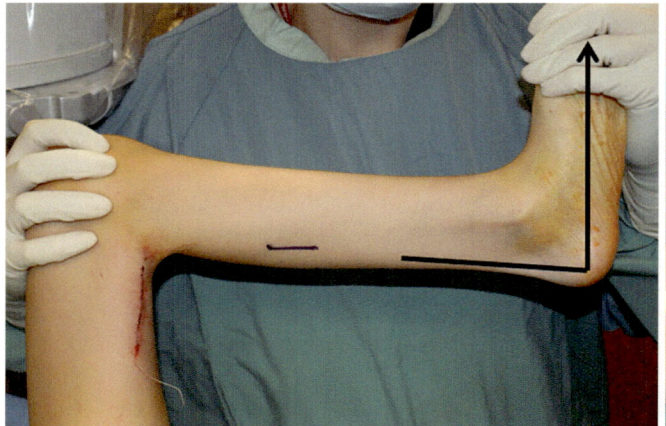
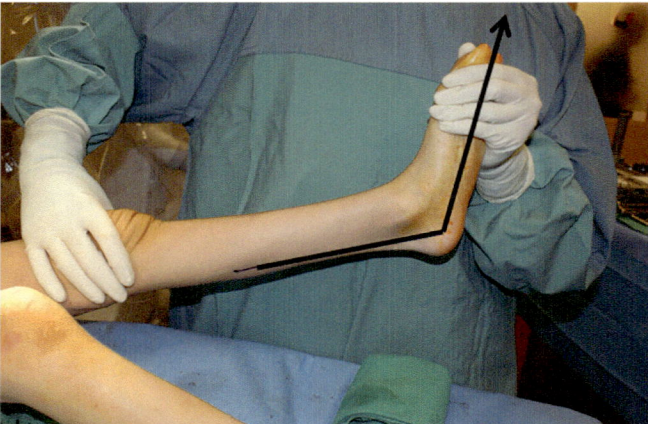

Fig. 24.9 Equinus contracture involving the gastrocnemius more than the soleus (Silverskiold test)

with changes in knee position. This distinction is important to assess, as it will influence at which level the gastrocnemius-soleus complex should be targeted: gastrocnemius alone, both the gastrocnemius and the soleus separately, or jointly through the Achilles tendon.

In the coronal plane, the hind foot might be in physiologic valgus position, or in excessive valgus or varus. These coronal plane deformities typically arise in combination (coupled) with ankle equinus. Equinovalgus deformities are more common in bilateral CP (diplegics). With the hindfoot in valgus, the talus and calcaneus are typically plantarflexed. There is a collapse of the subtalar joint (mid-foot break) with the prominence of the head of the plantarflexed talus, the midfoot is everted taking the forefoot with it into an abducted position (Fig. 24.10a, b). There is a flattening of the longitudinal arch and a pronated appearance, although the foot might in fact supinated relative to the hind foot to compensate for the valgus. Passive correction of the hindfoot out of the valgus position unmasks the supinated position of the foot. The abducted forefoot is often accompanied by a hallux valgus deformity that is believed to be acquired over time due to the foot rolling off the medial border during push-off. To test the true dorsiflexion of the ankle, the hindfoot valgus must be passively corrected to lock the subtalar joint prior to dorsiflexing the ankle. Failing to do so allows dorsiflexion to occur about the unlocked subtalar joint and provide a spurious estimate of dorsiflexion. The equinovalgus foot with forefoot abduction provides a very ineffective lever arm to generate any power during push-off (Fig. 24.11a, b). The tibial shank falls forward over the foot due to dorsiflexion through the subtalar joint, and shifts the ground reaction force behind the knee resulting in a flexed knee or crouched position.

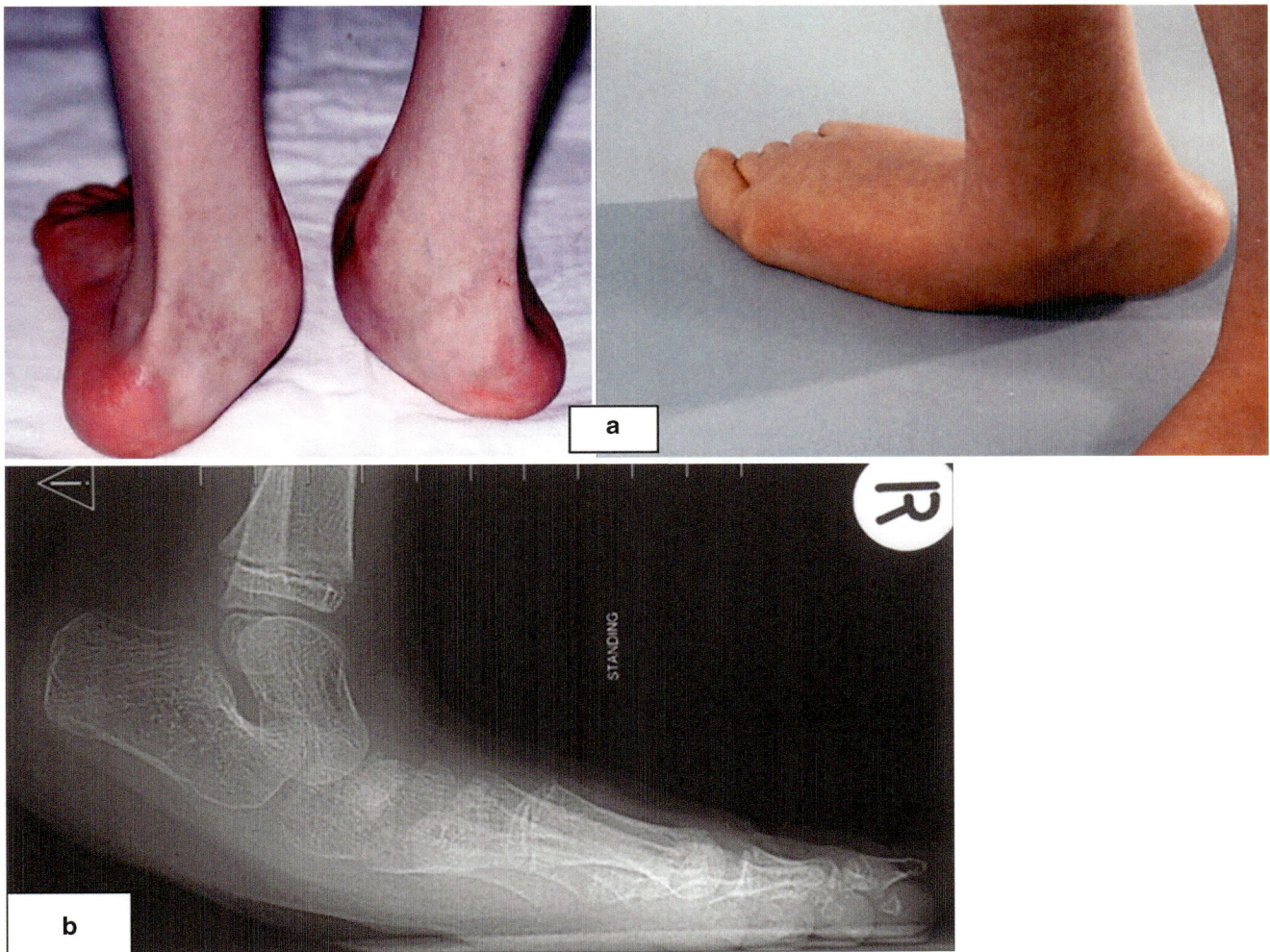

Fig. 24.10 (a) Equinoplanovalgus deformity with hindfoot valgus, midfoot break, forefoot abductus, hallux valgus. (b) Weight-bearing lateral radiograph of equinoplanovalgus deformity

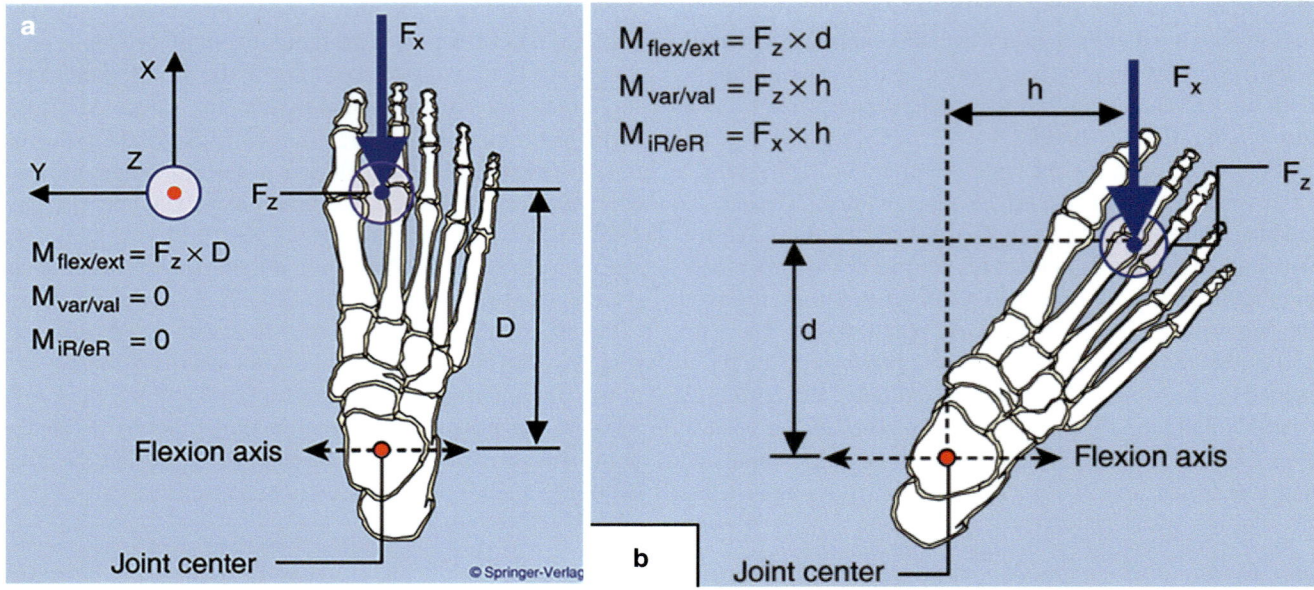

Fig. 24.11 (a) Lever arm of the normal foot. (Reproduced with permission from Paley 2003. Springer-Verlag Berlin Heidelberg 2003). (b) Lever arm deficiency of the equinoplanovalgus and abducted foot. (Reproduced with permission from Paley 2003. Springer-Verlag Berlin Heidelberg 2003)

Equinovarus deformities are more common in unilateral CP (hemiplegics). The hindfoot varus might be a consequence of an overactive tibialis posterior and/or tibialis anterior muscle in combination with weak peroneals. The deformity might be flexible or rigid. The hindfoot varus might be accompanied by midfoot cavus due to the tight plantar fascia or intrinsic muscles of the foot, and forefoot adductus. Weak tibialis anterior along with overactive peroneus longus might lead to increased plantar flexion of the first ray. This might result in a compensatory hindfoot varus to maintain a weight-bearing tripod. This can be tested using the simulated Coleman block test. In the prone position, the lateral border of the foot is pushed down on to simulate standing on the Coleman block [32]. The hindfoot varus corrects to normal valgus and the increased plantar flexion of the first metatarsal ray becomes apparent relative to the remaining rays, confirming that the hindfoot varus is secondary to the plantarflexed first ray. The hindfoot varus leads to increased weight-bearing along the lateral border of the foot leading to callus formation and even stress fractures causing discomfort and difficulties with brace and shoe wear (Fig. 24.12).

Fig. 24.12 Equinocavovarus deformity in a hemiplegic child. Note the plantarflexed first ray and the stress fracture of the fifth metatarsal due to excessive loading of the lateral border

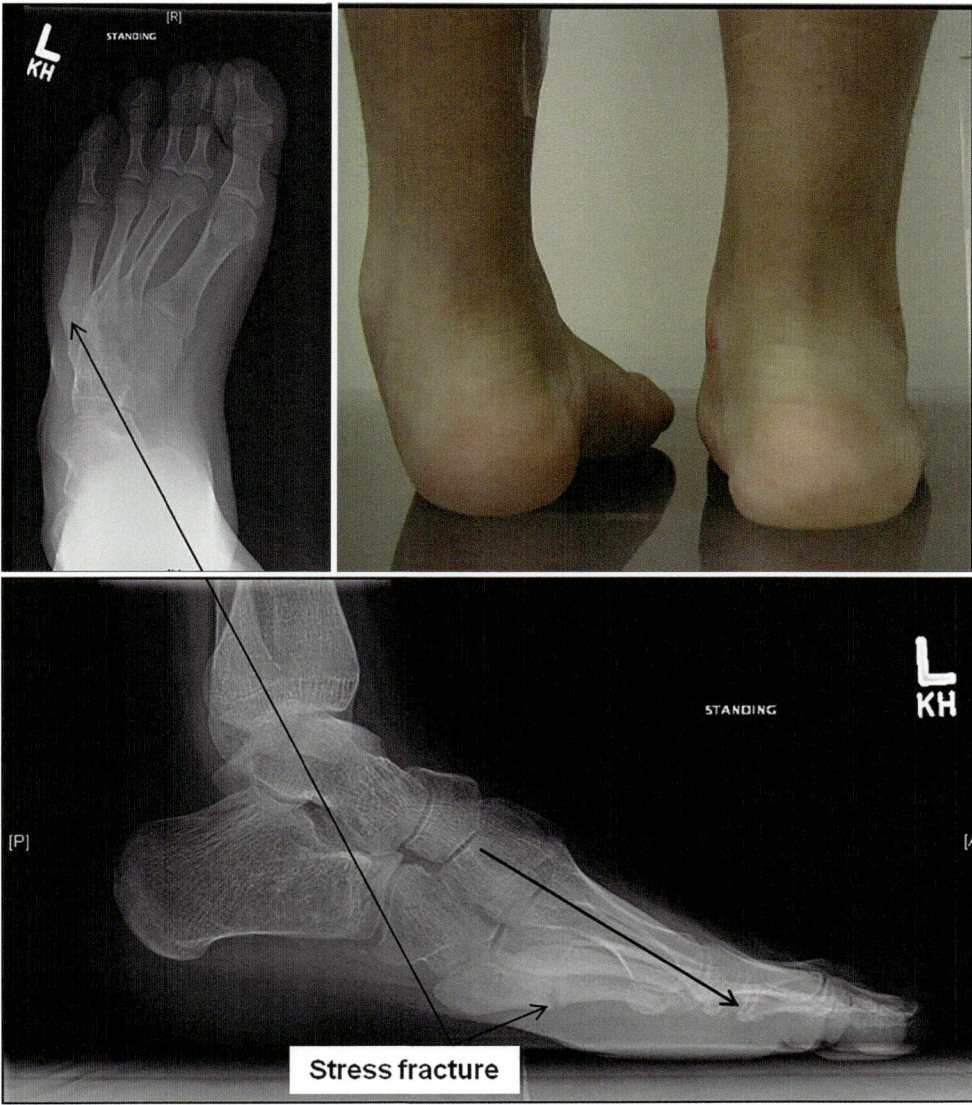

Lower Limb Assessment in the Ambulant Child (GMFCS Levels I–III)

The assessment of an ambulant child with CP who presents with gait-related problems should begin with an inquiry about how the child gets around at home, school, and in the community, which establishes the GMFCS level and allows the elicitation of specific gait-related problems of concern. The physical examination of the ambulant child begins with a visual assessment of the gait to identify abnormal gait patterns and specific problems. This dynamic assessment is followed by an on-table systematic examination of the muscle tone and muscle length, range of motion, and skeletal alignment at each segment to explain the gait abnormalities identified during walking. These should in turn be linked to specific gait-related problems reported by the child or their parents.

Assessment of the Ambulatory Child
Generate gait-related problem list from child and parent/s
    Observational assessment of the gait: dynamic exam
        With and without orthotics
        With and without walking aids if possible
    Examination on the table: static exam
        Muscle tone
        Muscle length: Passive range of motion
            Fast stretch (R1_
            Slow stretch (R2)
        Muscle strength
        Selective control
        Bony alignment
    Radiographic imaging
    Video and 3-D gait analysis

Observation of Gait: Observe the child's walk from the front/back and from the side to best estimate the gait abnormalities in all three planes. The child should walk both in their usual orthotics and footwear as well as barefoot if possible. The assessment is both qualitative and quantitative. A useful framework to evaluate the global quality of the gait is to assess the five prerequisites or attributes of gait [33, 34]: (1) Stability in stance; (2) (Foot) clearance in swing; (3) Correct prepositioning of foot for the next step; (4) Adequate step length; and (5) Energy efficiency (minimizing the excursion of the body's center of mass during walking). This is followed by a systematic assessment for specific abnormalities at each level: foot and ankle, the knees, hips and pelvis, the trunk and upper extremities, with due consideration of the coronal, sagittal, and transverse planes to explain the abnormalities noted with any of the five priorities of gait. This quantitative assessment can be greatly enhanced by capturing the gait with video (ideally split screen to see the frontal and sagittal planes simultaneously and in slow motion) [35].

> **Five Prerequisites of Gait**
> Stability of the weight bearing side during stance
> Clearance of the foot in swing phase
> Appropriate prepositioning of the swing phase foot for the next step
> Adequate step length
> Energy conservation

Three-dimensional gait analysis in a motion laboratory provides a more sophisticated assessment of gait patterns and deviations. Gait parameters include the step lengths (for each side), the gait velocity, and cadence. Kinematics describe the dynamic position of each limb segment in each of the three planes over the course of the gait cycle. Kinetics during stance reveal the moments, generated externally by the position of the ground reaction force relative to each joint, accompanied by the corresponding internal moments of the muscles to counteract the external moment; and powers about the joints. Dynamic electromyography documents the activation-specific muscles during the gait cycle. Pedobarographs capture the weight-bearing distribution pattern of the stance phase foot. 3-D gait analysis provides insight beyond what is derivable from observational analysis alone, and can help distinguish primary abnormalities (which might benefit from treatment) from secondary abnormalities that are compensatory responses that require no treatment [36, 37]. Gait analysis has identified recognizable gait patterns which can be classified and used for making treatment decisions [38–40]. 3-D gait analysis has been shown to influence or alter treatment decisions for at least some patients [41–43]. Finally, the effectiveness of these interventions can be assessed objectively using gait analysis as a measure of gait outcomes [44].

Abnormal Gait Patterns in Cerebral Palsy

In bilateral CP, there are broadly recognizable patterns [38] (Fig. 24.13).

True equinus is characterized by the absence of a heel strike and a toe-toe pattern because the ankle remains plantarflexed throughout stance phase. If the equinus is not severe, initial contact may be with the forefoot and the heel might even come in contact with the ground in mid stance. The knee can be flexed during stance phase to accommodate the equinus, or it may come to full extension or even hyperextend to allow the plantarflexed foot to remain flat on the ground for more stability (Fig. 24.14a) True equinus can be associated with poor stability due to the narrow base of support; poor clearance if the knee does not flex enough to facilitate clearance of the plantar flexed foot, leading to foot drag and tripping. Step length is typically shortened because the plantarflexed foot leads to an early forefoot strike. This might also be a consequence of poor stability on the stance phase limb forcing the contralateral swing phase limb to contact the ground sooner.

Jump gait pattern is characterized by equinus at the ankle accompanied a flexed knee and flexed hip, resembling someone preparing to jump. All five priorities of gait are affected in this pattern. Step length is further compromised as the swing phase knee might not be able to extend if increased hamstring activity prevents the knee from reaching full extension in terminal swing.

In *Apparent equinus* pattern, the child's heels do not come in contact with the ground even though the ankle is not in equinus (Fig. 24.14b). This typically happens when there is a flexion deformity of the knee and the ankle has only sufficient range to come to neutral dorsiflexion. If the feet were flat on the floor in the presence of an uncorrectable flexed knee, the child's center of gravity would fall well behind the base of support. To stop from falling backward the body is forced to shift the center of gravity forward by flexing the hip and increasing forward trunk lean or tipping forward on tip toe. This pattern may affect all five priorities of gait.

Crouch gait is characterized by flexed knee during stance phase accompanied by dorsiflexion of the ankle or foot segment relative to the tibial shank. This dorsiflexion can occur through the ankle (true calcaneus) when there is excessive range of dorsiflexion of the ankle, which could be iatrogenic from overlengthening and weakening of the gastrocsoleus complex from tendo-Achilles lengthening (Fig. 24.15a). Alternatively, the dorsiflexion may occur through the subta-

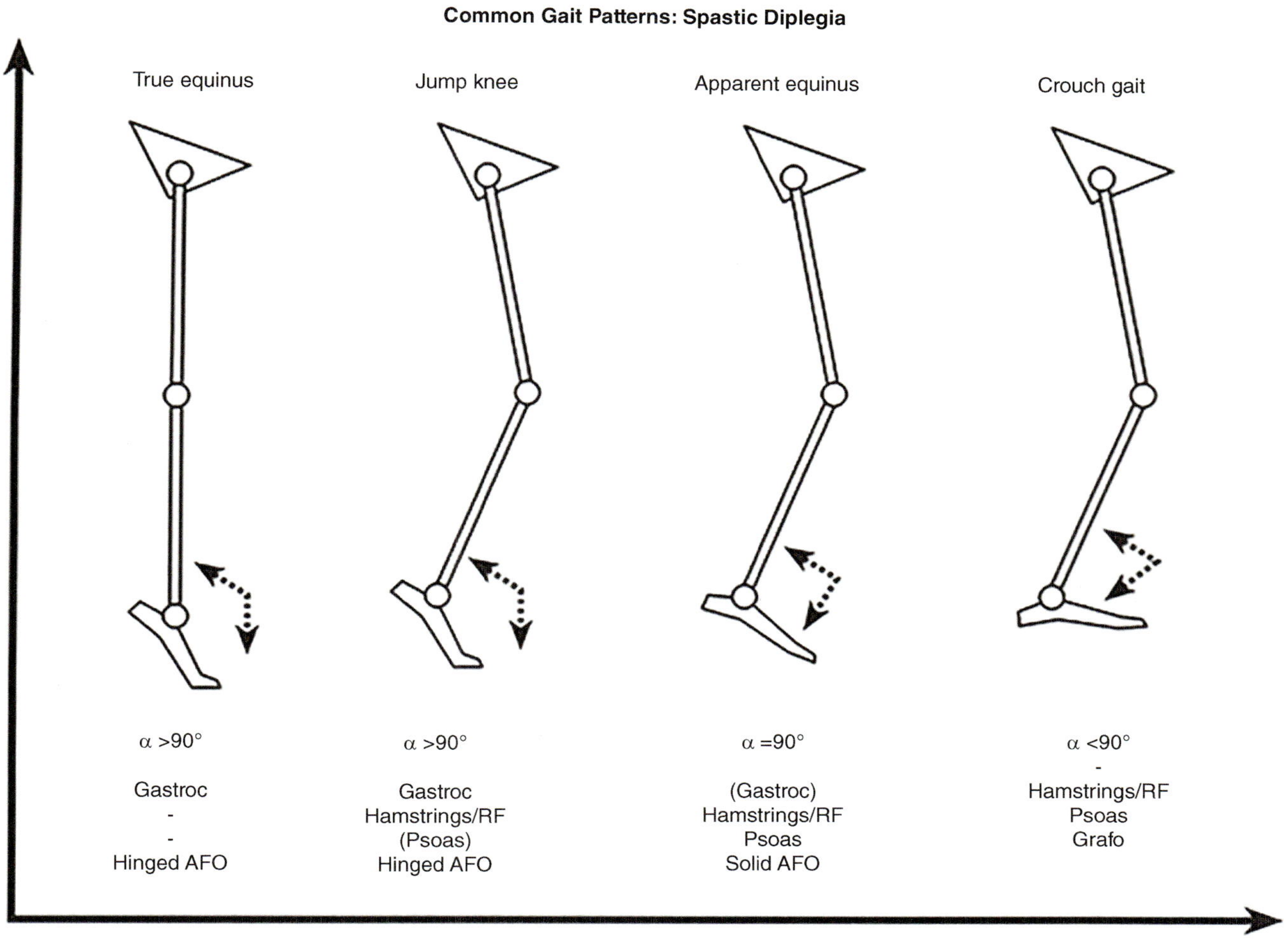

Common Gait Patterns: Spastic Diplegia

True equinus	Jump knee	Apparent equinus	Crouch gait
α >90°	α >90°	α =90°	α <90°
Gastroc	Gastroc	(Gastroc)	-
-	Hamstrings/RF	Hamstrings/RF	Hamstrings/RF
-	(Psoas)	Psoas	Psoas
Hinged AFO	Hinged AFO	Solid AFO	Grafo

Fig. 24.13 Common gait patterns in bilateral (diplegic) cerebral palsy. (Reproduced with permission from Rodda, J. and H.K. Graham, *Classification of gait patterns in spastic hemiplegia and spastic diplegia: a basis for a management algorithm*. Euro J Neurol, 2001. 8(Suppl 5): p. 98–108)

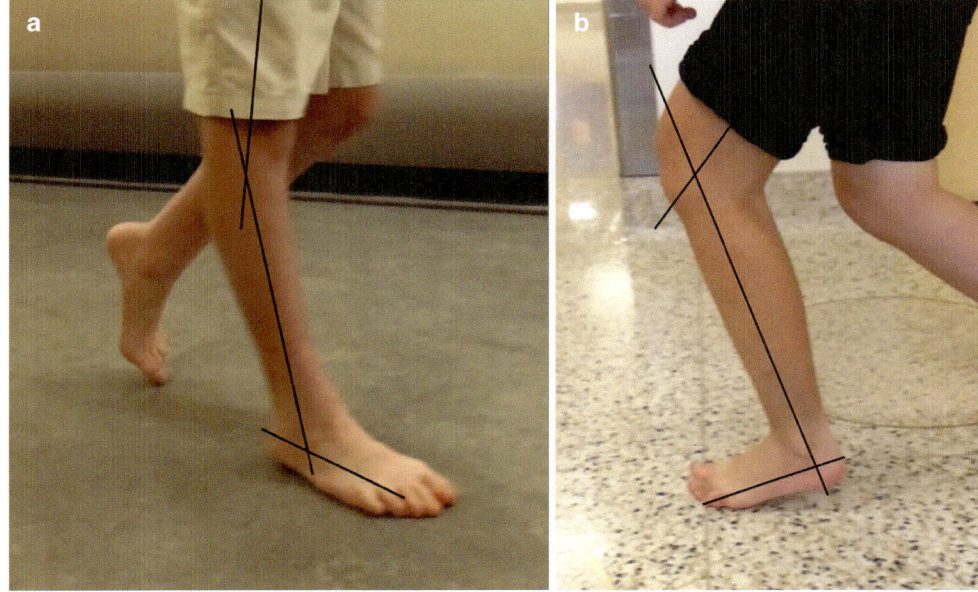

Fig. 24.14 (a) Knee hyperextended to accommodate equinus contracture with flatfoot contact despite plantarflexed position of ankle. (b) Forefoot contact (apparent equinus) to accommodate fixed flexion deformity of the knee

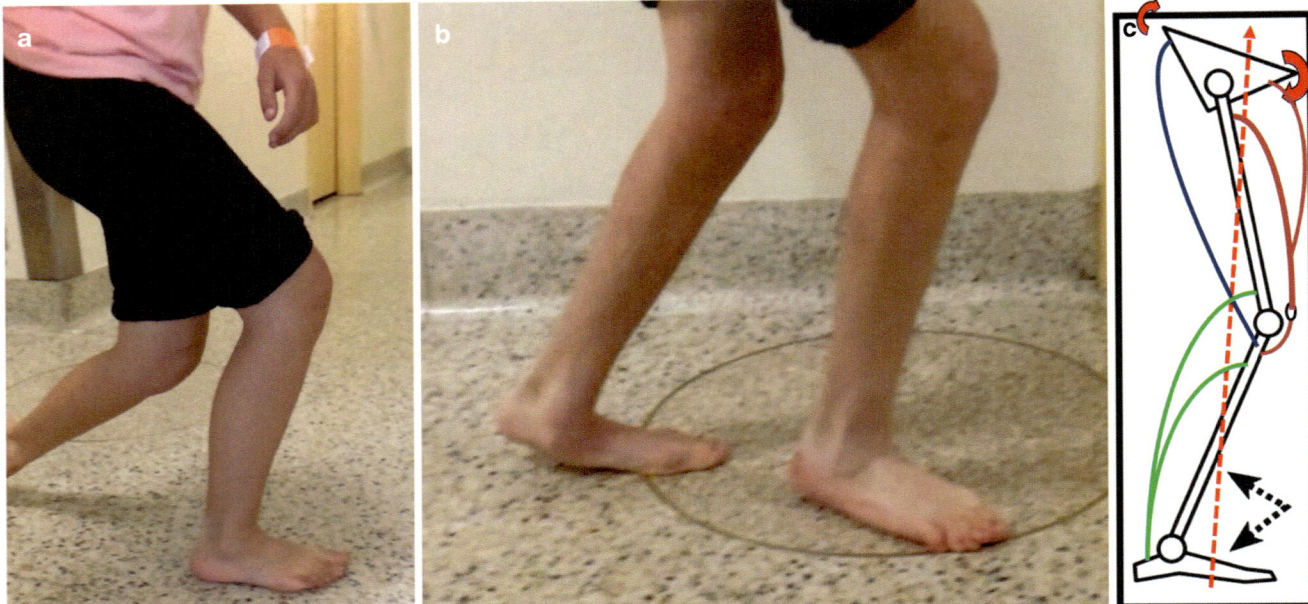

Fig. 24.15 (a) Crouch gait pattern: flexed knee with forward translation of the tibia over the dorsiflexed ankle. (b) Crouch gait pattern in the presence of equinovalgus foot. (c) When in crouch, the ground reaction force passes in front of the ankle, behind the knee and in front of the hip, resulting in ankle plantarflexion, knee extension, and hip extension (internal) moments to counteract the abnormal external moments generated by the ground reaction force

lar joint, in the presence of equinus of the hind foot along with increased hindfoot valgus (Fig. 24.15b). The subtalar joint collapses creating a midfoot break and a rocker bottom deformity, and the forefoot is often abducted. In either situation, the tibial shank is flexed forward over the foot segment throughout stance. This shifts the ground reaction force well behind the knee creating an external flexion moment that has to be countered by a corresponding internal extension moment generated by the quadriceps. In order to keep the center of gravity over the base of the support, the hips must flex (Fig. 24.15c). This crouch pattern is also a consequence of the natural history in children with more severe bilateral CP (GMFCS III or greater). All five priorities of gait are affected, and the energy consumption associated with this pattern is substantial. Weight-bearing in the crouch position increases the joint reaction force on the patellofemoral joint which can cause anterior knee pain, patella alta, and avulsion fractures of the inferior pole of the patella [45].

Stiff knee gait is characterized by limited knee excursion into flexion, often due to the spasticity or contracture of the rectus femoris, which prevents the knee from adequately flexing at the beginning of swing phase, which is important to facilitate clearance of the plantarflexed foot immediately after toe-off. Consequently, the foot might drag, slowing gait, causing tripping, and increased shoe wear. Stiff knee pattern might accompany the other gait patterns.

Any of the gait patterns can be associated with transverse plane abnormalities that can arise from one or more of the following levels: the forefoot (adductus or abductus), hindfoot (varus or valgus), tibial torsion (internal or external), femoral anteversion (or torsion), hip rotation (internal or external), or pelvic rotation (protraction or retraction). The foot position can be quantified by the foot progression angle (FPA), normally an average of 5° external [46]. The knee progression angle (KPA) should also be assessed as this will help determine the source of rotational abnormality. A normal FPA does not rule out torsional malalignment. In children with bilateral CP, it is not unusual to have increased internal rotation of the hips due to increased femoral anteversion characterized by internal KPA (patella points medially) and apparent "scissoring" (Fig. 24.16). FPA may be internal, normal or even external if accompanied by increased external tibial torsion, hindfoot valgus, and abducted foot. Internal rotation of the hip in the face of external rotation of the tibial segment creates a pseudo-valgus appearance at the knee (miserable malalignment).

In unilateral CP (hemiplegia), four types of gait pattern have been described [38, 39] (Fig. 24.17).

Type 1 pattern is characterized by equinus in swing phase only. This is a drop foot pattern due to weakness of the tibialis anterior which is unable to adequately dorsiflex the ankle against gravity during swing phase. Initial contact might be with the forefoot but the heel comes in contact with the ground early in stance with adequate dorsiflexion in mid stance. *Type 2* pattern is characterized by equinus both in swing and stance phase with a toe-toe or toe-heel pattern in stance phase. This is due to a contracture of the gastrocsoleus complex which might be dynamic due to spasticity or fixed due to static contracture. In *Type 3* pattern, the knee is involved as well, showing abnormal flexion (jump) or stiff knee pattern. Finally, in *Type 4,* there is additional proximal involvement at the hip, including varying combinations of hip adduction, flexion and internal rotation, and pelvic obliquity. This pattern can be particularly troublesome as it is often accompanied by progressive hip displacement and dysplasia.

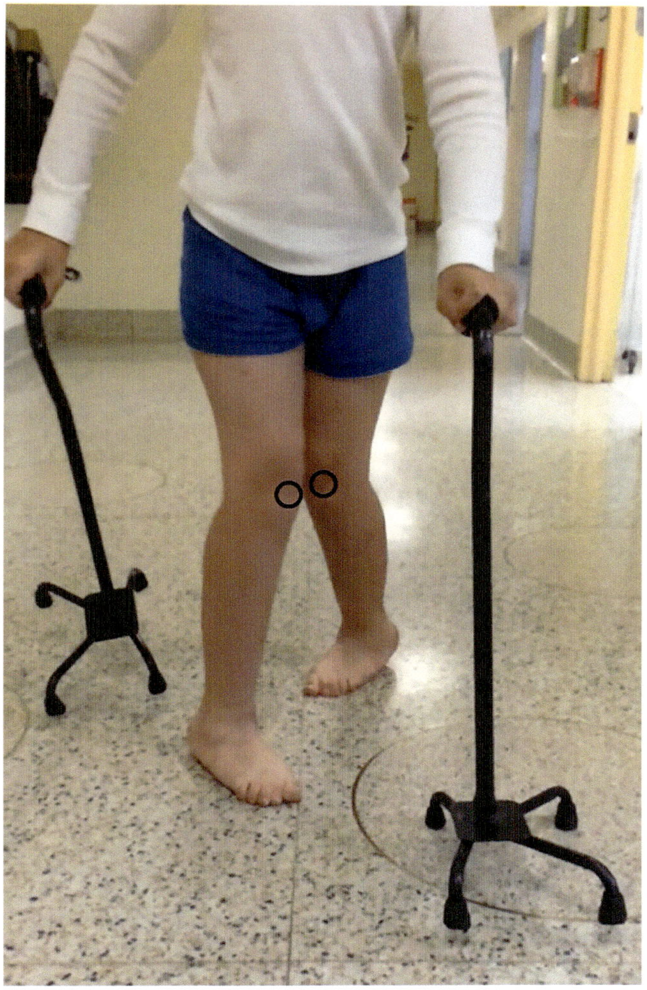

The distinctions between these different gait patterns in CP may not always be clear with many permutations and combinations involving one or both lower extremities.

On-Table Physical Examination

The static examination (on the table) includes assessment of muscle tone and length, bony alignment, muscle strength, and selective control.

Assessment of Muscle Tone and Length

Spasticity is velocity-dependent hypertonia. Muscle tone is therefore assessed for each muscle group by testing the passive range of motion with a fast stretch that elicits a catch (R1), as well as the maximal passive range obtained by a slow, sustained stretch (R2) [47, 48]. In the presence of spasticity, the R1 catch is noted early and a large gap between the

Fig. 24.16 Internal rotation gait pattern

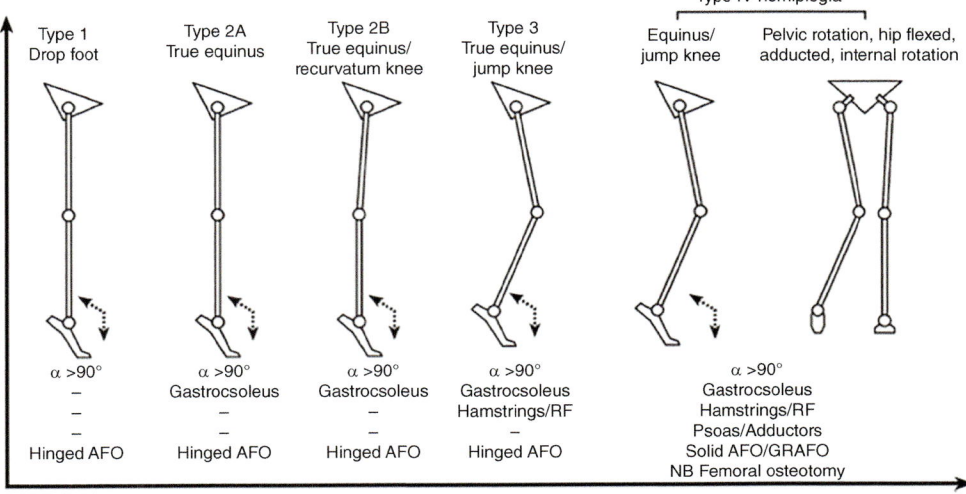

Fig. 24.17 Common gait patterns in unilateral (hemiplegic) cerebral palsy. (Reproduced with permission from Rodda, J. and H.K. Graham, *Classification of gait patterns in spastic hemiplegia and spastic diplegia: a basis for a management algorithm.* Euro J Neurol, 2001. **8** (Suppl 5): p. 98–108)

R1 and R2 represents the dynamic component of the contracture, which is more amenable to spasticity management. R2 represents the functional muscle length. When the range of motion is reduced, and R2 is close to R1, that is indicative of a static contracture or reduced length of the muscle tendon unit (in addition to tightness). In CP, biarticular muscles are more involved than muscles that cross only one joint. It is therefore important to separately test the tone and length of both groups of muscles (e.g., gastrocnemius and the soleus) to target interventions more precisely.

The following specific joints (muscle groups) of the lower extremity are tested in the supine position. Hip flexors are tested by extending the hip (Thomas test) while the opposite hip is held sufficiently flexed to neutralize the anterior pelvic tilt and, but not over correct, the lumbar lordosis. Hip abduction is tested first with the knees flexed to test the length of the adductor muscles. Abduction is then tested with the hips and knees held in extension to assess the additional contribution of the gracilis which is a hip adductor and a knee flexor. The Galeazzi sign assesses the relative lengths of the thigh segment. A shorter thigh segment in combination with an adduction contracture might be indicative of hip subluxation on that side. Knee extension is quantified to rule out a knee flexion contracture. This could be due to one or more of the following: shortened hamstrings, shifted hamstrings due to increased anterior pelvic tilt, shortened proximal gastrocnemius or a posterior contracture of the knee joint capsule. The popliteal angle tests the functional length of the hamstrings. This is first done unilaterally (one leg at a time) with the hip on the tested side held in 90° of flexion, while the contralateral hip is held in full extension. The bilateral popliteal angle or the hamstring shift test requires testing the popliteal angle with the contralateral hip and knee flexed to neutralize the pelvic tilt similar to the Thomas test [30]. This is a measure of the "true" hamstring contracture (Fig. 24.18). A large reduction in the popliteal angle (increased available hamstring length) suggests that the anterior pelvic tilt might be responsible for the relative elevation of the origin of the medial hamstrings and the long head of the biceps femoris, and that hamstring length is sufficient. Ankle dorsiflexion is tested both with the knee flexed and the knee extended (Silverskiold test) to distinguish contractures arising from the gastrocnemius alone from those where the soleus is involved as well. At the time of testing ankle dorsiflexion, any hindfoot valgus must be corrected to neutral by supinating the foot to ensure that the subtalar joint is "locked" to ensure that dorsiflexion is occurring through the ankle joint rather than spuriously through the subtalar joint (Fig. 24.9). Hindfoot is tested for its flexibility to correct any valgus or varus. If a cavovarus foot deformity is present, simulate a Coleman block test, as described earlier, to identify whether the hind foot varus is fixed or not and if not confirm that it is secondary to the plantarflexed deformity of the first metatarsal ray or a primary problem [32]. In a cavovarus foot, the hindfoot might be in equinus, neutral or even in relative calcaneus with the forefoot plantarflexed relative to the hindfoot.

In the prone position, knee flexion is tested rapidly and then slowly for the Duncan Ely (DE) sign. A positive sign would be associated with a significant elevation of the buttock off the table, due to an increase in hip flexion and anterior pelvic treat created when the spastic or short rectus femoris is being stretched and pulls down on its origin at the anterior inferior iliac spine. The rectus femoris contracture might be responsible for the stiff knee pattern observed during walking.

Assessment of Bone Alignment

Assessment of the bony alignment includes the examination of the torsional profile of the lower limb in the prone position

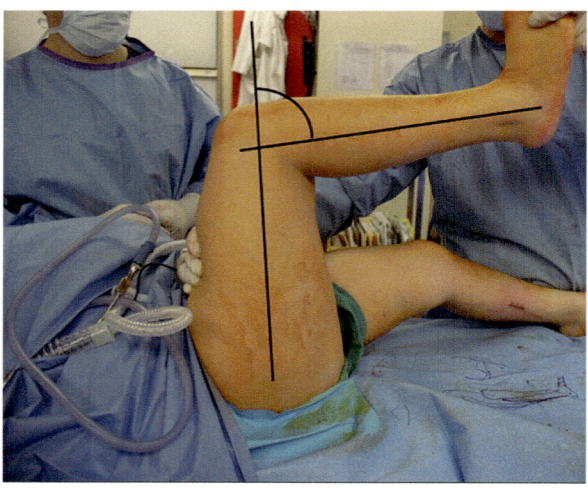
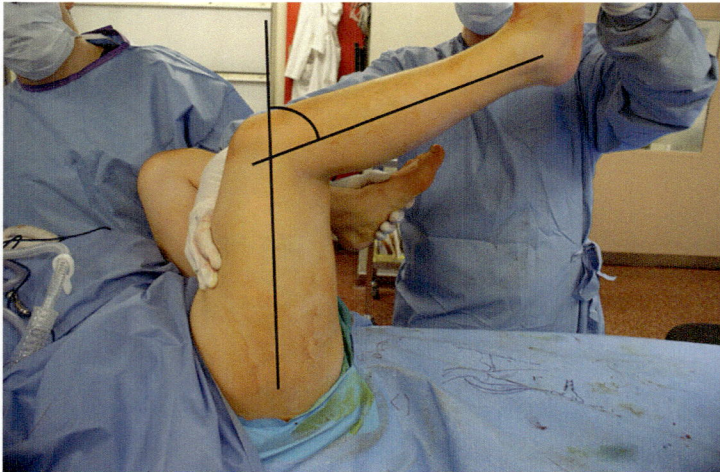

Fig. 24.18 Unilateral and bilateral popliteal angles: the hamstring shift test

Fig. 24.19 Femoral anteversion with trochanteric palpation test: (**a**) prone and neutral (baseline) (**b**) prone and maximal internal rotation until the prominence of the greater trochanter is palpated most laterally

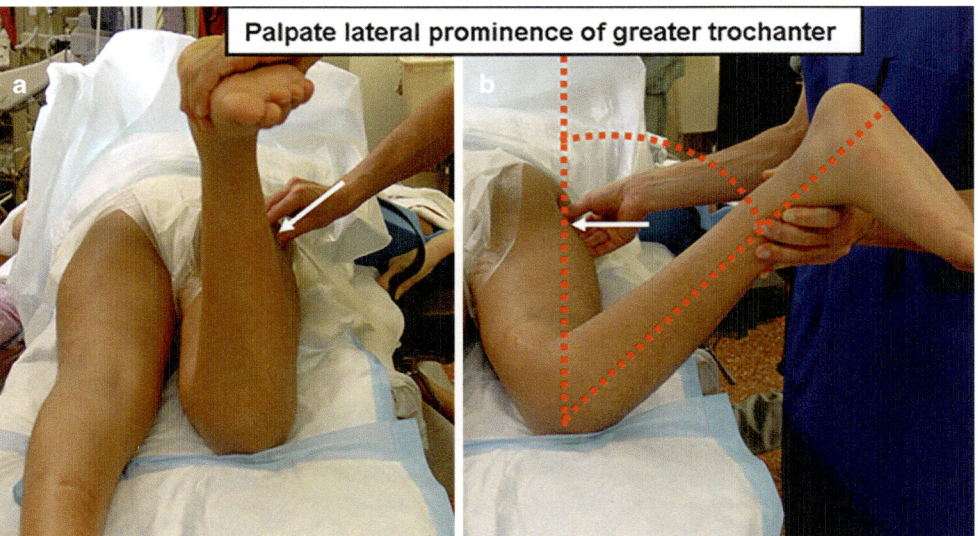

to evaluate for excessive femoral anteversion and tibial torsion. The magnitude of femoral anteversion can be estimated using the trochanteric palpation test. In the prone position, the knee is flexed to 90° and the lower leg held upright perpendicular to the examination table. In this baseline position, the patella is pointing directly "anterior" into the table. The maximum prominence of the greater trochanter is palpated in the proximal lateral thigh, and should be situated more posteriorly. The lower leg (tibia) serves as a goniometer. The lower leg is rotated outward which corresponds to internal rotation of the hip, until the prominence of the greater trochanter is palpated most laterally, which corresponds to when the femoral neck (axis) is horizontalized and parallel to the floor. The number of degrees of outward rotation of the tibia relative to the vertical position at baseline represents the femoral anteversion on that side [49, 50] (Fig. 24.19).

Tibial torsional alignment is based on thigh foot angle (TFA) and the transmalleolar (bimalleolar) axis (TMA). With the ankle held in neutral dorsiflexion, the TFA is the angle between the long axis of the foot (heel bisector to second toe) and the thigh axis, which is usually between 10 and 20° external [46]. If the lateral border of the foot is straight, one can infer that there is no deformity arising from the forefoot and that an abnormal TFA is arising from the torsional alignment of the tibia and fibula. This is best quantified by the TMA which is the angle between the trans(bi)malleolar axis and the transverse knee axis, which is usually between 10 and 30° external. TMA less than or greater than this range represents internal and external tibial torsion respectively [51] (Fig. 24.20).

Assessment of Muscle Strength and Selective Control

In children with CP, there is increasing evidence that muscles are weak, and that motor function is directly associated with muscle strength [52]. It is therefore important, whenever possible, to assess muscle strength for prognostication and clinical decision-making [53]. Muscle strength is tested for each of the lower limb muscle groups using manual muscle testing (MMT) [54]. These tests are somewhat subjective and reliant on the examiner's experience, and are only possible in older children who are capable of cooperating with the manual testing. In the gait laboratory and in research settings, isometric muscle strength testing using dynamometers or isokinetic evaluations have some value.

Selective motor control is impaired in children with CP and contributes to ambulatory function and patterns [55, 56]. The ability to isolate movements can be graded into three levels of control. 0: No ability; 1: Partial ability; and 2:

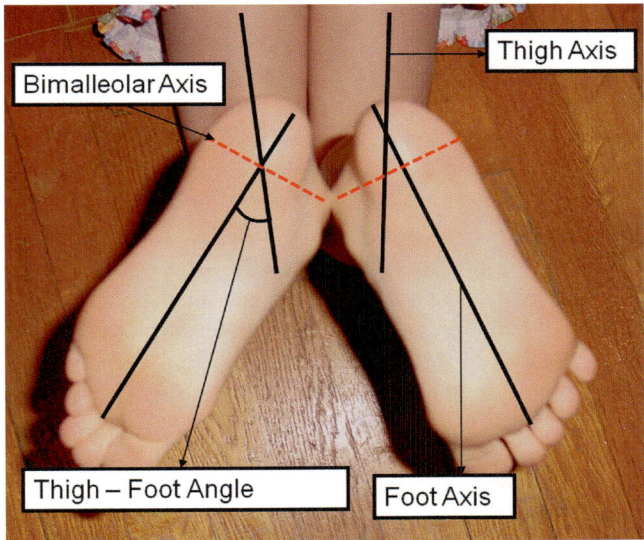

Fig. 24.20 Assessment of tibial torsional profile: the TFA and TMA

Normal ability to isolate movements [57]. These are tested and reported along with the strength for each muscle group tested.

Lower Limb Assessment in the Nonambulant Child (GMFCS Levels IV–V)

The musculoskeletal assessment of the nonambulant child with CP should begin with an inquiry about signs of discomfort, challenges with caregiving, positioning, transfers, and mobility. It is important to contextualize these with some knowledge about the overall health of the child, since nonambulatory children often experience multiple comorbidities including seizure disorders, cognitive impairments, communication difficulties, visual and hearing impairments, swallowing difficulties, drooling, risk of aspiration and pneumonias, gastroesophageal reflux, malnutrition necessitating tube feeding, constipation, and incontinence. The physical examination should include an assessment of the child seated in the wheelchair or seating system, and assessment lying on the table. In the chair, specific attention is paid to the presence, flexibility, and impact of any spinal deformity in the coronal (scoliosis) and sagittal (kyphosis/lordosis) planes; and pelvic inclination on sitting balance, ischial weight-bearing, skin integrity, and hygiene. Particular areas that are vulnerable to skin breakdown are over prominences including those due to kyphoscoliosis, sacrococcygeal area, the ischial weight-bearing area, and the prominences of the greater trochanter or dislocated femoral heads in the lateral proximal thigh. Additionally, in the presence of a large and rigid scoliosis, there can be skin break down on the side of the concavity where the inferior aspect of the rib cage might rest against the iliac crest and skin crease in the flank might be hard to reach or maintain hygiene due to stiffness of the deformity.

The lower extremity examination of the nonambulant child is done in the supine position. The examination of the hip joint, knee joint, and foot and ankle is identical to that described for ambulant children. Usually, there is little value in turning the child prone to assess the torsional profile, as these can be reasonably assessed supine. Whenever possible, and particularly in children functioning at GMFCS level IV, an effort should be made to examine the child in a supported weight-bearing position, as the ability to bear weight for transfers might be an important functional ability to preserve.

Goals of Treatment in Cerebral Palsy by GMFCS Level

For ambulatory children (GMFCS Levels I–III), the primary goals of treatment are to optimize gait efficiency in order to preserve or improve independence and physical function that will permit increased participation in their daily lives. Functional problems of gait impact walking distance, speed, balance and stability, endurance and are often accompanied by fatigue and pain. Improving the appearance of gait and minimizing the reliance on walking aids and orthotics are also identified as important priorities by children with CP and their parents [58].

> **Goals of Treatment: Ambulatory CP (GMFCS Levels I–III)**
> Optimize gait efficiency (correct biomechanics) in order to optimize energy conservation
>   Preserve or improve physical function
>   Walk longer distance
>   Walk faster
>   Decrease fatigue
>   Better stability: reduced tripping and fewer falls
>   Keep up with friends
>   Pain relief or pain prevention and increased endurance
>   Preserve or increase activities and participation
>   More physically active
>   More independence
>   More participation in sports/recreational activity
> Improve appearance of gait
>   Reduced reliance on walking aids
>   Reduced use of orthotics
>   Feet flat on the ground
>   Feet pointing forward
>   Reduced dragging of feet
>   Stand and walk taller (knees less bent)
>   More symmetry

Goals of treatment for nonambulatory children (GMFCS IV and V) are different from those for ambulatory children. These more severely involved children are at high risk of developing joint contractures, progressive hip displacement and spinal deformity that interfere with comfort and caregiving, positioning, transfers, mobility, and seating. The musculoskeletal involvement occurs in the context of other associated comorbidities. The goals of treatment are to prevent or relieve pain, facilitate caregiving, improve health, and optimize the quality of life [59].

> **Goals of Treatment: Nonambulatory CP (GMFCS Levels IV–V)**
> Relieve or prevent pain and discomfort
>   Facilitate ease of care
>   Dressing; toileting; bathing/hygiene
>   Positioning: seating and lying down
>   Transfers and mobility
> Preserve or improve health
> Improve quality of life

Management of Lower Extremity Problems: Principles of Treatment and Techniques

In general, the principles of treatment include (1) prevention or slowing the development of progressive joint contractures, bony deformities, and joint instability in the younger child; and (2) correction of these clinically significant bony deformities and joint instability when these have already occurred. These objectives are best achieved using a multidisciplinary approach.

Early intervention focuses on dealing with dynamic contractures in order to delay the need for more extensive surgical procedures (Fig. 24.21). Multiple strategies are used including physical therapy to strengthen and stretch muscles, orthotics (braces) to maintain stretch or stabilize joints, and serial casting in an attempt to simulate the stretch that would normally arise from typical physical activity. Stretch is facilitated by local or systemic tone management by pharmacologic (botulinum toxin-A, phenol injections) or neurosurgical methods (selective dorsal rhizotomy, intrathecal baclofen). Effective tone management improves range of motion, tolerance of brace wear, and might prevent or delay the onset of static contractures and bony deformities [60–65]. Severe spasticity involving bilateral lower extremities in children with good balance and muscle strength might benefit from more extensive spasticity control from selective dorsal rhizotomy (SDR), which has been shown in randomized trials to produce significant reduction in muscle tone, but only modest benefits on physical function [66–69]. SDR does not necessarily reduce the need for subsequent orthopedic surgery [70–73]. In a systematic review, the functional effects and benefits of SDR in the long term remain uncertain, despite appearing promising in small series of selected patients [73–75]. Baclofen is a GABA agonist that can reduce hypertonia. The relatively large oral doses required for any meaningful effect, can be associated with undesirable side effects. When administered intrathecally, very small doses (micrograms) are required to reduce severe generalized hypertonia due to spasticity or dystonia. Intrathecal baclofen administered continuously by an implantable pump is usually reserved for more severely involved children (GMFCS level V), as it can be associated with significant complications [76–78].

Established deformities are most efficiently addressed with Single-Event Multilevel orthopedic Surgery (SEMLS) using a combination of fractional muscle or intramuscular or tendon lengthening, tendon transfers and corrective osteotomies, and joint stabilization procedures to address bony deformities and joint instability that contributes to lever arm dysfunction [79–81]. Surgery is delayed until the gait patterns have matured and any functional gains from the natural history have plateaued [82]. The optimal timing is sometime between 7 and 11 years of age, to reduce the likelihood of recurrence of deformity with further growth, necessitating repeat surgery (Fig. 24.21). In the short term, SEMLS is associated with significant improvements in gait quality, with more modest corresponding functional improvements [83–86]. In general, the children with more abnormal gait patterns stand the most to gain, but about 25% show little measurable benefit. It is unclear whether these patients would have deteriorated further without the intervention [87]. There is limited information in the literature about the long-term effects of multilevel orthopedic surgery at skeletal maturity or adulthood [83, 88–91].

Table 24.1 summarizes the most common surgical procedures for cerebral palsy and their indications.

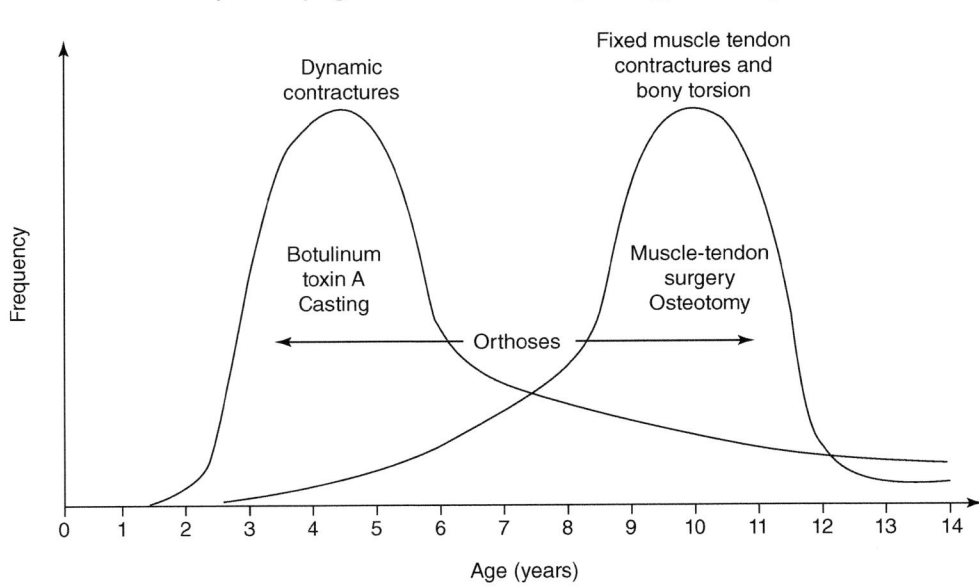

Fig. 24.21 Management strategies and timing principles. (Reproduced with permission from Bache CE SP, Graham HK. The management of spastic diplegia. Current Orthopaedics. 2003;17:88–104)

Table 24.1 Common soft tissue and bony procedures performed during multilevel surgery for cerebral palsy

	Indications for surgery	Procedure
Hip flexion contracture: psoas	**Ambulatory child** • Reduced hip extension in terminal stance • Excessive anterior pelvic tilt + lordosis • Hip flexion contracture >20° • Hip subluxation • Kinematic: excessive anterior pelvic tilt with double bump pattern in diplegia; single bump pattern in hemiplegia • Kinetics: delay in transition from hip-extensor (internal) moment to hip flexor (internal) moment (beyond the typical 25% of gait cycle) **Nonambulatory child** • As part of the management of hip displacement	**Ambulatory child** Selective intramuscular lengthening of the psoas tendon over the brim of the pelvis (spare the iliacus) Note: Proximal femoral derotational osteotomy done above the lesser trochanter can functionally lengthen the psoas **Nonambulatory child** Ilio-psoas tenotomy or release off the lesser trochanter
Hip adduction contracture: adductors* Note: during normal gait, the arc of hip motion in the coronal plane is from 10° of abduction to 10° of adduction. About 15° of abduction is sufficient for normal gait	**Ambulatory child** • Decreased abduction in swing phase (scissoring) • Adduction contracture: <15° **Nonambulatory child** • Adduction contracture interfering with care: dressing, toileting, perineal hygiene • As part of the management of hip displacement	**Ambulatory child** Percutaneous or open release of adductor longus alone is usually sufficient **Nonambulatory child** Open release of adductor longus, adductor brevis, gracilis + iliopsoas tenotomy
Hip internal rotation: anteversion	**Ambulatory child** • Excessive internal rotation of the hip due to increased femoral anteversion • Increased "scissoring" with knees rubbing • Internal foot progression angle causing tripping **Nonambulatory child** • As part of the management of hip displacement	**Ambulatory child** Proximal femoral (intertrochanteric) derotational osteotomy with internal fixation; Alternative: distal femoral derotational osteotomy **Nonambulatory child** Combined proximal femoral derotation + varus osteotomy with stable internal fixation
Proximal femur: coxa valga and hip subluxation	• Increased neck–shaft angle • Migration percentage >40% • Break in Shenton's arc • Increased anteversion	Proximal femoral (intertrochanteric) varus and external derotational osteotomy (VDRO)
Pelvis: acetabular dysplasia	• Acetabular index >30° • Subluxated hip • Older than 5 years	Periacetabular pelvic osteotomy (e.g., Dega) to restore posterolateral coverage

Knee flexion: hamstrings	**Ambulatory child**
	• Decreased knee extension in terminal swing
	• Increased popliteal angle, provided that
	  – Bilateral popliteal angle >50°
	• Kinematics:
	  – Posterior pelvic tilt
	  – Decreased knee extension in terminal swing
	Nonambulatory child
	• Knee flexion contractures due to hamstring contracture interfering with care, dressing, seating, and positioning. Goal is to decrease contracture (and popliteal angle) and not to straighten the knee entirely
		Ambulatory child
		Medial hamstring lengthening: intramuscular tenotomies of the gracilis, semitendinosus; aponeurotic lengthening (striping) of semimembranosus.
		Lateral hamstring lengthening: fascial striping of the biceps femoris aponeurosis. This is avoided unless there is posterior pelvic tilt present to prevent excessive weakness of hip extensors.
		Nonambulatory child
		Percutaneous or open hamstring lengthening: medial and lateral

Knee flexion contracture	• Knee flexion contractures >20° despite hamstring lengthening, or • Hamstring length is sufficient (normal) • Older children (closer to skeletal maturity): >12 years • Significant crouch pattern in gait (GMFCS II–III) or during standing for transfers (GMFCS IV)	Distal femoral extension osteotomy. This must be accompanied by patella tendon shortening or patellar tendon distal advancement to restore tension of the elongated knee extensors following the extension osteotomy
Stiff knee: rectus femoris	• Stiff knee pattern: limited flexion at initial swing • Foot drag resulting in poor clearance • Positive Duncan Ely sign • Kinematic: Peak knee flexion in initial swing is decreased in amplitude and delayed • EMG: RF active throughout gait cycle • Avoid in more severe GMFCS III and IV	Rectus femoris tendon is separated from the underlying vasti and the detached tendon is tenodesed to the semitendinosus, gracilis or sartorius

Table 24.1 (continued)

	Indications for surgery	Procedure
Tibial torsion: external	• External torsion: bimalleolar axis >30° external – Out-toeing: external foot progression angle > 30° – Foot drag – With planovalgus/abducted foot – Relatively normal foot progression angle in the presence of increased femoral anteversion that is being corrected by external derotation of the femur	Distal tibial internal derotational osteotomy to correct bimalleolar axis to 10° external (Concomitant fibular osteotomy may not be needed for derotation of <30°)
Tibial torsion: internal	• Internal torsion: bimalleolar axis >10° internal – In-toeing: internal foot progression angle > 10° internal – Tripping	Distal tibial external derotational osteotomy to correct bimalleolar axis to 10° external (Concomitant fibular osteotomy may not be needed for derotation of <30°)
Equinus: gastrocnemius-soleus	**Ambulatory child** • Equinus in stance phase: poor stability • Equinus in swing: poor clearance • Tripping and falling • Poor tolerance of AFO • Increased shoe wear **Nonambulatory child** • Contracture interfering with bracing or footwear necessary for weight-bearing for transfers (GMFCS IV) • Contracture interfering with bracing or footwear, or resting of feet on the foot-plate of wheelchair (GMFCS V) Note: These apply to any foot deformity in nonambulatory children	Gastrocnemius contracture alone (Silverskiold): isolated lengthening of the gastrocnemius (Strayer technique) Gastrocnemius > soleus contracture (Silverskiold test): Strayer + Soleus fascial lengthening by striping the aponeurosis leaving muscle intact; or gastrocsoleus aponeurotic lengthening (e.g., Baker, Vulpius)
Equinus: tendo-Achilles	• Fixed equinus contracture involving both gastrocnemius and soleus, seen commonly in hemiplegia	Tendo-Achilles lengthening is the most aggressive method of lengthening the gastrocsoleus complex. This can be done by 2 or 3 hemitenotomy sliding lengthening techniques or open Z-lengthening
Equino (plano)valgus	• Increased hindfoot valgus with collapse of subtalar joint (rocker bottom) and abducted forefoot. – Poor push off (tendency to crouch) – Pain with weight-bearing – Blistering or callosity over medial prominence of talar head – Loss of flexibility: unbraceable	Lateral column lengthening through the calcaneus; along with plantar flexion osteotomy of first ray. May needs lengthening of peroneus brevis; lengthening of gastrocsoleus as needed to address the unmasked equinus after correction of hindfoot valgus. Triple C osteotomy: medial slide osteotomy of calcaneus; opening wedge osteotomy of cuboid: closing wedge osteotomy of medial cuneiform
Equino (cavo) varus	• To prevent or correct weight-bearing on lateral border of the foot which leads to – Poor stability in stance – Pain and callosity – Difficulty with brace and shoe wear – Stress fracture of the fourth or fifth metatarsal – Poor clearance in swing • Flexible hind foot varus is amenable to tendon transfers • Fixed contractures of tibialis posterior requires lengthening • Hindfoot varus driven by presence of plantarflexion of the first ray (confirmed by the Coleman block test)	Split tibialis anterior tendon transfer to the cuboid if hindfoot varus is flexible and occurs primarily in swing phase Split tibialis posterior tendon transfer to the peroneus brevis when the hindfoot varus is flexible but occurs in stance phase as well Requires lengthening of tibialis posterior: intramuscular tenotomy. Tibialis posterior tendon lengthening may be combined with the split tibialis anterior tendon transfer Plantar fascia release along with extension osteotomy of the base of 1st metatarsal or medial cuneiform; consider transfer of the peroneus longus to the peroneus brevis. These may be combined with tibialis posterior tendon lengthening. All of these may require gastrocsoleus or tendo-Achilles lengthening as needed to address the equinus contracture

Orthopedic Procedures at the Hip

Iliopsoas Lengthening: The indication for psoas lengthening in ambulatory children is controversial [15, 92]. In the presence of a hip flexion contracture accompanied by increased anterior pelvic tilt, reduced hip extension in terminal stance can be addressed with selective intramuscular lengthening of the psoas (sparing the iliacus) over the brim of the pelvis [93]. In nonambulatory children with hip displacement, iliopsoas tenotomy is performed at the level of insertion into the lesser trochanter.

Adductor Releases: In ambulatory children, adductor lengthening is only necessary if the adduction contracture is severe. During normal gait, the coronal plane arc of motion of the hip is limited from 10° of abduction to 10° of adduction. Abduction of 15° is compatible with normal gait [94]. In the ambulatory child with CP, adductor surgery is usually restricted to percutaneous or open release of the adductor longus alone. A proximal release of the gracilis may be added if the range of hip abduction is further reduced with the knee in maximal extension. More extensive adductor releases to include the adductor brevis are seldom indicated in ambulant children unless there is a more severe adduction contracture associated with increased hip displacement [94]. In a nonambulant child, adductor releases help to relieve adduction contractures that can interfere with care, dressing, perineal hygiene, and are routinely lengthened when the contracture is associated with increased hip displacement either in isolation or along with proximal femoral osteotomies to center the hip. The adductor longus, the adductor brevis, and gracilis are typically released from their origins through a medial transverse groin incision just distal to the groin crease, centered over the adductor longus tendon. The same approach allows access to the iliopsoas tendon insertion at the lesser trochanter. Adductor releases alone are insufficient to stabilize hip subluxation and for GMFSC level IV and V level children, with recurrent or progressive hip displacement occurring in more than 75% of patients, requiring additional operations including bony reconstructive surgery [95].

Femoral Derotation and Varus Derotational Osteotomy: When there is a clinically significant internal rotation gait due to increased anteversion, the excessive anteversion can be corrected by derotational osteotomy proximally (intertrochanteric) or distally [96–99]. The proximal osteotomy allows for the addition of varusization when there is coxa valga and any subluxation [100] (Fig. 24.22a). When the osteotomy is proximal to the insertion of the iliopsoas on the lesser trochanter, some functional lengthening of the psoas may occur with external rotation of the lesser trochanter. The proximal osteotomy can be done supine or prone, the latter having the advantage of providing reliable (bilateral) intraoperative assessment of the torsional profile. Internal fixation with a blade plate or locking plate provides sufficient stability to avoid postoperative casting (Fig. 24.22b,c). Proximal femoral derotational osteotomies can also be performed in the subtrochanteric diaphysis using a minimally invasive technique and internally fixed using elastic intramedullary nailing [101].

Windswept deformities are not uncommon in more severely involved nonambulatory children. These hips require an approach that addresses the asymmetric deformity. The adducted and internally rotated side requires releases of the adductors, flexors, and hamstrings along with an external derotational osteotomy of the femur. On the abducted and externally rotated side, the abductors, iliotibial band, and lateral hamstrings may have to be released, and derotational osteotomies of the femur are based on whether and by how much the femur is anteverted. The "abducted" side may just be less adducted and require similar but less extensive procedures than on the more adducted side.

Periacetabular Pelvic Osteotomy: In the presence of hip subluxation, acetabular dysplasia develops secondary to the mechanical pressure of the subluxating femoral head. The acetabular deficiency is usually posterolateral. Following

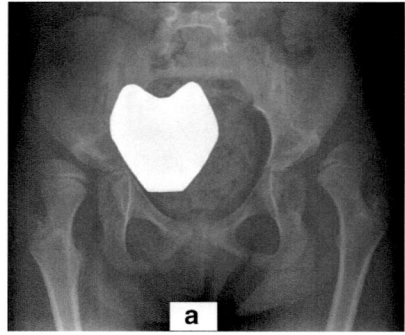
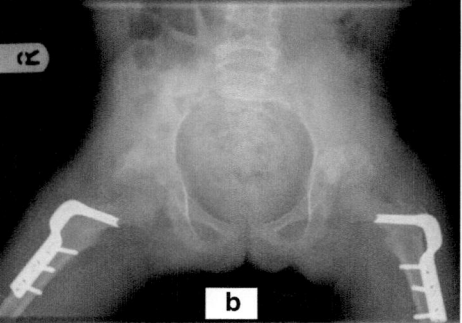
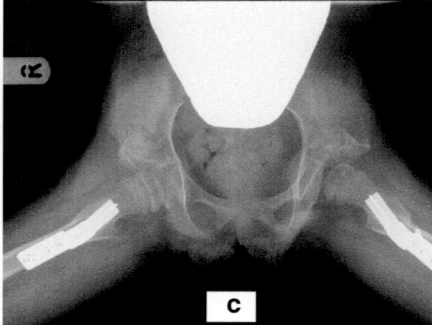

Fig. 24.22 (a) Eight-year-old girl with bilateral hip subluxation, coxa valga, and acetabular dysplasia. (b) AP radiographs after bilateral proximal femoral varus derotational osteotomy with blade plate fixation; and periacetabular pelvic osteotomy (Dega). (c) Frog-leg lateral radiograph after bilateral proximal femoral varus derotational osteotomy with blade plate fixation; and periacetabular pelvic osteotomy (Dega)

Fig. 24.23 (a) Deformation of the dislocated femoral head with loss of sphericity and flattening of superolateral surface. (b) Femoral head resection, subtrochanteric valgus osteotomy of the proximal femur

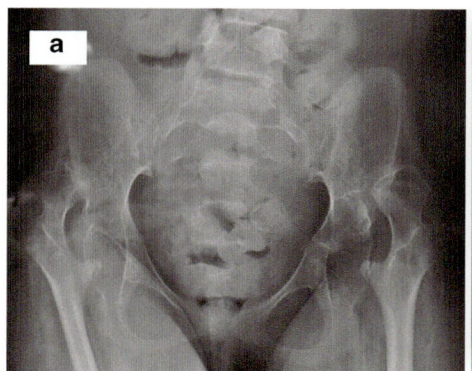
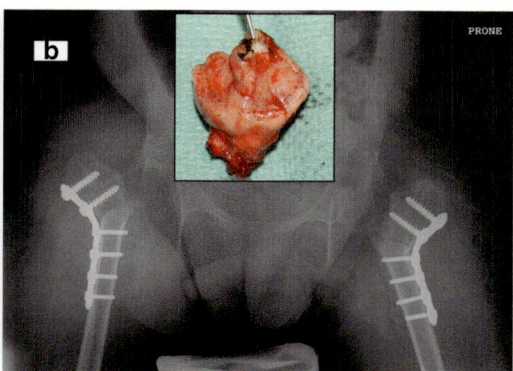

proximal femoral varus derotational osteotomy to redirect the femoral head into the center of the acetabulum, posterolateral coverage is improved with a Dega type periacetabular osteotomy or one of its adaptations, which comprises a lateral opening wedge osteotomy through the outer table, hinging on or just proximal to the triradiate cartilage [102, 103]. Autologous bone graft is derived from the proximal femoral varus osteotomy and/or the anterior iliac crest. Tricortical allograft can also be used if sufficient amount of structural autograft is not available (Fig. 24.21b,c). Internal fixation is typically not required.

Femoral Head Resection and Related Procedures: Salvage procedures are indicated for long standing hip dislocations that are painful but not reconstructible because of the advanced changes associated with the long-standing dislocation including loss of sphericity of the femoral head and severe acetabular dysplasia. The femoral head typically deforms along its exposed superolateral surface due to the pressure from the overlying abductors (Fig. 24.23a). In general, salvage procedures are not as effective as reconstructive procedures at achieving the goals of pain relief. Proximal femoral head resection at the base of the neck, along with a subtrochanteric valgus osteotomy of the femur, tenodesis of the ligamentum teres to the lesser trochanter, and capsular closure, in addition to the adductor and psoas lengthening is an effective strategy to provide sufficient abduction for perineal hygiene, pain relief from the previous dislocation but not without a significant period of recovery [104] (Fig. 24.23b). Heterotopic ossification or proximal migration is uncommon with this procedure but occurs more frequently with other salvage procedures that involve more extensive proximal femoral resections.

Orthopedic Procedures at the Knee and Lower Leg Segment (Tibia)

Hamstring Lengthening: In ambulant children, hamstring lengthening is indicated when there is a true contracture (reduced length) of the hamstrings contributing to a flexed knee gait or shorter step length due to decrease knee extension in terminal swing or initial contact [105]. In ambulant children, only the medial hamstrings are usually lengthened [94, 105, 106]. Using a posteromedial approach (patient supine) or posterior midline approach (patient prone), intramuscular tenotomies of the gracilis and semitendinosus and fractional lengthening of semimembranosus aponeurosis can be performed. Lateral hamstrings (biceps femoris) lengthening is avoided in ambulatory children due to the increased risk of knee hyperextension and weak hip extension [107]. Transfer of the tenotomized semitendinosus to the adductor tubercle might preserve hip extension and prevent increased anterior pelvic tilt, but the indications and effectiveness of this procedure remain uncertain [94, 105]. In nonambulant children, hamstring lengthening can be performed percutaneously. Hamstring lengthening is often performed in conjunction with hip reconstructive surgery, to reduce the tension on the relocated hips and to address knee flexion contractures that might be interfering with positioning, seating, dressing or caregiving.

Distal Femoral Extension Osteotomy: In the presence of fixed knee flexion contractures (15–45°), a distal femoral extension osteotomy might be the only way to achieve full "extension" of the knee acutely [108, 109]. This has been shown to be an effective procedure to address crouch gait [110]. An anteriorly based closing wedge (shortening) osteotomy is performed through a lateral incision using a subvastus approach to the distal femur stabilized with a fixed angle blade plate or locking plate for internal fixation [111] (Fig. 24.24a–e). The sciatic/peroneal nerves are at risk of stretch injury with acute corrections (extension) of knee flexion contractures intraoperatively or in the immediate postoperative period, which can result in dysesthesias in the lower extremity [112]. To reduce this risk, the apex of the closing wedge should be at the level of the nerve (well behind the posterior cortex), such that the wedge resected is trapezoidal in shape. Shortening of the femur by resecting a segment of distal femur has also been described to be effective for crouch gait [113, 114]. Intraoperative neuromonitoring has been reported to be useful to mitigate this risk [115].

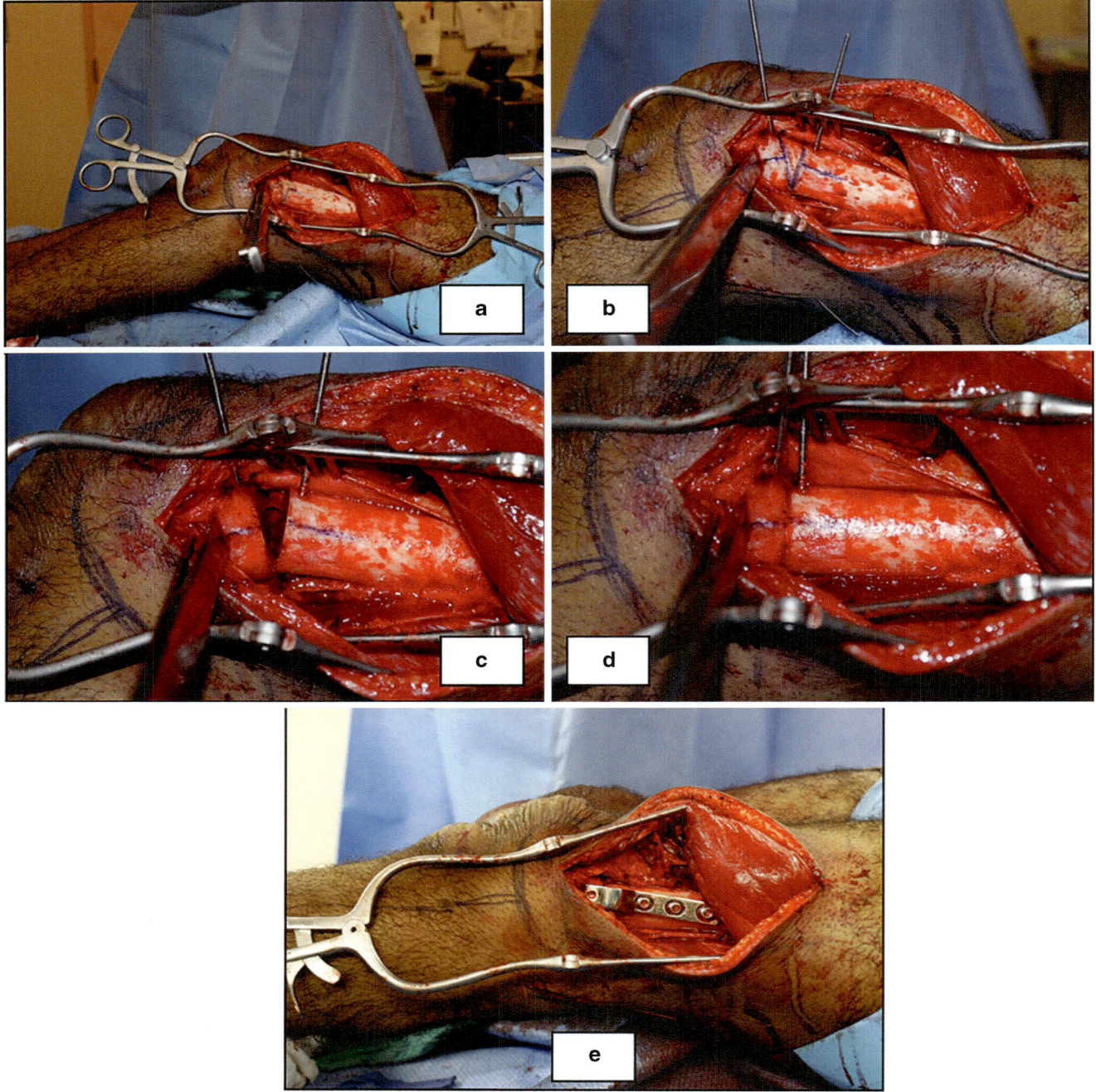

Fig. 24.24 (a–e) Distal femoral extension osteotomy with blade plate fixation

Postoperative immobilization in some flexion is recommended for a few days following surgery especially if an indwelling epidural catheter is in place, before the knee is brought to full extension after the epidural has been removed. Up to 30° of external rotation can be included with the extension osteotomy to address increased anteversion if present [108].

Patellar Tendon Shortening (PTS) or Advancement (PTA): This procedure is usually done in combination with the distal femoral extension osteotomy to re-tension the relatively lengthened quadriceps following the osteotomy. It might also be indicated for patella alta without a knee flexion contracture. PTS is by an infrapatellar shortening procedure of the patella tendon [116, 117]. Alternately, patellar tendon advancement may be performed by a distal transfer of the tibial tubercle in the skeletally mature child or the anterior portion of the tibial tubercle apophysis, in a skeletally immature child [111].

Fig. 24.25 Distal tibial derotational osteotomy

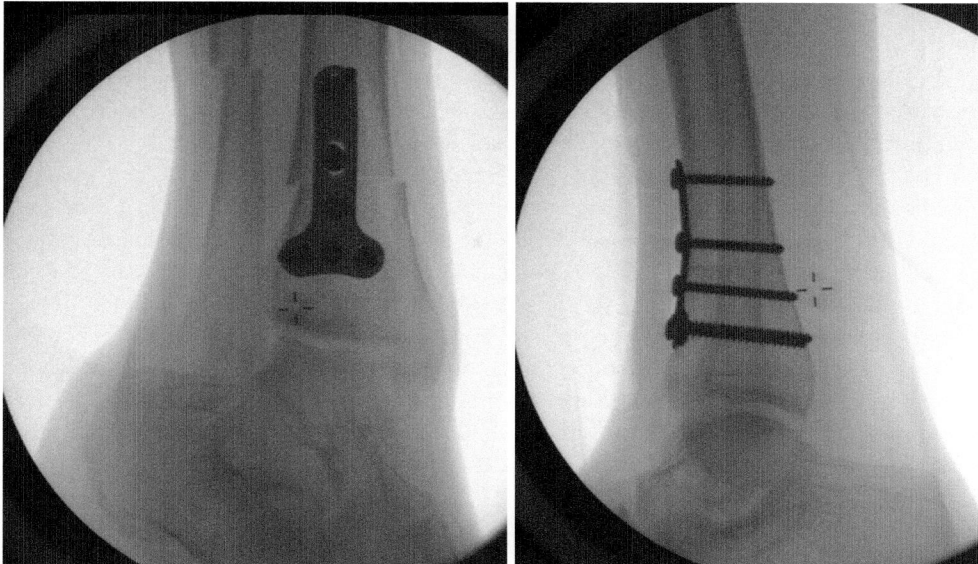

Anterior Hemiepiphysiodesis of Distal Femoral Physis: Guided growth with the use of anterior staples or extraperiosteal tension band plates might gradually correct fixed flexion deformities in children who have sufficient growth remaining. The long-term effectiveness of these procedures remains uncertain [82]. These implants have also been associated with irritation to the knee making some of these poorly tolerated. Anteriorly placed transphyseal screws from proximal to distal have been promoted as an alternate method to achieve anterior hemiepiphysiodesis [118].

Rectus Femoris Transfer or Releases: Co-spasticity of the rectus femoris and the hamstrings is associated with a stiff knee gait pattern, characterized by decreased knee flexion in early swing phase resulting in poor foot clearance or foot drag [119]. The Duncan Ely sign is positive on the physical examination [120]. Gait kinematics show decreased amplitude and delay of the peak knee flexion in swing. Dynamic EMG shows abnormal activation of the rectus femoris throughout swing. Rectus femoris transfer is indicated to improve knee flexion in early swing in order to improve foot clearance [120, 121]. The rectus femoris tendon is separated from the underlying vasti; the detached tendon is transferred medially over the surface of the vastus medialis and tenodesed to the semitendinosus, gracilis or sartorius. Early postoperative range of motion (immediate CPM) is important to prevent adhesions. Postoperative rehabilitation including muscle strengthening is crucial for the success of this procedure. This procedure has been shown to be more effective in higher functioning ambulatory children who are motivated and capable of participating in a rehabilitation program [119, 122, 123]. A distal rectus femoris release instead of a transfer has been promoted as an alternative, and the comparative effectiveness of these two approaches is not well established [124].

Distal Tibial (Supramalleolar) Derotational Osteotomies: Excessive external or internal torsion of the tibia can result in abnormal foot progression angle, associated with foot drag and a poorer lever arm of the foot for push off. Torsional deformities are corrected through distal tibial derotational osteotomies and stabilized with internal fixation (ideally plates/screws) [125] (Fig. 24.25). A concomitant osteotomy of the fibula is usually only necessary when the tibial derotation exceeds 30° [126]. No fixation is required for the fibula osteotomy.

Orthopedic Procedures at the Ankle and Foot

Gastrocnemius and Soleus Lengthening: Lengthening of the gastrocsoleus is indicated for equinus gait in ambulatory children with CP [127]. The soleus typically contributes less to equinus than the gastrocnemius in children with bilateral CP, whereas in hemiplegics the soleus is usually just as involved in the contracture. Based on the relative contributions of both muscles, options include selective lengthening of the gastrocnemius alone [128], with complete sparing of the underlying soleus; addition of the aponeurotic striping of the underlying soleus; combined gastrocsoleus lengthenings; and tendo-Achilles lengthening [129]. Tendo-Achilles lengthening in bilateral CP has been implicated in development of iatrogenic crouch, and should be avoided unless the contracture is severe and involves both gastrocnemius and the soleus [130–133]. Surgery in children under 8 years is associated with increased risk of recurrence and overcorrection. The gastrocnemius lengthening is performed at the junction of the proximal and mid-calf, at the level of the inferior border of the muscle bellies of the medial and lateral heads of the gastrocnemius, where the aponeurosis of the gastrocnemius is separable from the underlying soleus [128]. In older children with long-standing equinus, there may be additional, though milder contracture of the soleus. In these children, it is possible to obtain additional dorsiflexion by dividing the aponeurosis of the soleus immediately deep to the divided gastrocnemius, while preserving the underlying muscle fibers of the soleus [82]. In hemiplegics, both gastrocnemius and soleus are usually equally tight and therefore a tendo-Achilles lengthening can be performed by a percutaneous or mini-open sliding technique (Hoke or White) or open z-lengthening [134]. Recurrence of equinus is the most common complication of a tendo-Achilles lengthening in a hemiplegic, and is usually more likely when done in children less than 8 years old.

Tibialis Posterior Tendon Lengthening or Split Tibialis Posterior Tendon Transfer (SPOTT): Equinovarus deformities are more common in unilateral CP or hemiplegia. Fixed contractures need lengthening of the tibialis posterior tendon. An intramuscular tenotomy of the tibialis posterior at the distal calf is effective and distal z-lengthenings are seldom required. When the contracture is dynamic and the hind foot is passively correctable to normal, a split tibialis posterior tendon transfer to the peroneus brevis ensures maintenance of the varus correction [135]. Transfers are more likely to be effective and last longer when done in younger children.

Split Tibialis Anterior Tendon Transfer (SPLATT)

If the hindfoot varus deformity occurs primarily in swing phase of gait and positions the foot to land on its lateral border, a split tibialis anterior tendon transfer to the cuboid can be very effective [136]. In the situation of a fixed equinovarus contracture, a tibialis posterior tendon lengthening can be combined with a SPLATT and tendo-Achilles lengthening [137]. The goal is to achieve a braceable, plantigrade foot in stance so that weight-bearing is distributed on the plantar surface rather than along the lateral border, and to prevent difficulties with foot clearance in swing phase.

Foot Osteotomies: Foot osteotomies are indicated for fixed deformities, evaluated clinically and radiographically [138]. Equino planovalgus deformities are more common in bilateral CP. A lateral-based opening wedge calcaneal osteotomy just proximal to the anterior process will lengthen the lateral column, correcting the hindfoot valgus and forefoot abductus and restoring the medial arch. Bone graft (iliac crest or allograft) is used to fill the gap at the osteotomy site.

Peroneal brevis tendon lengthening is usually necessary. Gastrocsoleus recessions might be needed to address any unmasked equinus when the valgus is corrected [139]. To minimize the chance of a recurrent deformity, medical procedures are often added, such as capsulodesis of the talonavicular joint, and advancement of the tibialis posterior tendon. Plantar flexion osteotomy of the first ray to restore the normal tripod of the weight-bearing plantigrade foot might be necessary if following the correction of the hind foot valgus, mid/forefoot supination becomes apparent. An alternative to the lateral column lengthening strategy is the "triple C" method which includes (1) a closing wedge varus producing osteotomy of the calcaneus along with some medial slide all done from the lateral approach; (2) an opening wedge osteotomy of the cuboid using a wedge of autologous bone graft obtained from (3) a plantar-based closing wedge osteotomy of the medial cuneiform [140]. More severe or rigid varus or valgus deformities of the hindfoot are best managed by calcaneal osteotomies using closing wedge or sliding osteotomies. Once the hindfoot deformity is corrected, a subtalar (extraarticular) arthrodesis can be performed to correct and hold the deformity permanently [141]. A talonavicular arthrodesis may accomplish the same objective.

In the presence of a plantarflexed first ray, plantar fascia release and extension osteotomy of the medial cuneiform or base of the first metatarsal will address a midfoot cavus and secondarily eliminate the compensatory hindfoot varus. The peroneus longus tendon is tenodesed to the peroneus brevis to prevent further plantarflexion of the first metatarsal. Hallux valgus deformities are only addressed if painful or are interfering with shoe or brace wear. Correction of the deformity should be accompanied by an arthrodesis of the first metatarsophalangeal joint.

Summary

The musculoskeletal consequences of CP in the lower extremity are significant both in ambulant and nonambulant children. The goals for these two groups are quite different (See highlight boxes). These goals are best achieved using a multidisciplinary approach, of which orthopedic surgery plays an important role. Orthopedic surgery deals with the peripheral consequences of CP while the primary pathology in the brain remains unaddressed. There is an imperative for stronger evidence for the effectiveness of many of these interventions based on outcomes that are meaningful to this population [59, 142–146]. The longevity of these outcomes up to and beyond skeletal maturity into adulthood needs to be established [88]. Improved understanding of the biology of brain development, neuroplasticity and repair, and epidemiological research might provide the means to prevent or mitigate many of the etiological causes of CP. Until that time, orthopedic surgery will continue to play an important role in the management of the deformities associated with CP.

Myelomeningocele (Spina Bifida)

Deficient closure of the neural tube in the first month of embryonic life leads to a spectrum of neural tube defects, which affects about 0.5–1.0/1000 pregnancies in the United States [147]. The overall incidence has declined with oral folic acid supplementation and termination of pregnancy that is facilitated by maternal prenatal screening with ultrasound and elevated levels of α-fetoprotein and β-human chorionic gonadotrophin levels. The neurologic deficit has both motor and sensory components and the specific musculoskeletal deformities of the lower extremity depend on the level of the lesion and the resulting imbalance between the effects of neurologic deficit present at the level (mixed upper and lower motor neuron) and below the level (lower motor neuron) of the lesion and the relatively unopposed action of the uninvolved neurologic levels above the lesion (Table 24.2). Unlike in cerebral palsy, where the deformities are absent at birth, many of the musculoskeletal deformities associated with spina bifida might be present at birth, and not unlike CP, become worse with growth.

Hip Dysplasia

Hip dysplasia is most common with higher level lesions (thoracic and high lumbar) and is often present at birth and generally more resistant to reduction than idiopathic developmental hip dysplasia. The management of hip dysplasia in this population is controversial. Reconstructive approaches to relocate and stabilize the hips are unnecessary for the nonambulant children as pain is generally not a feature of hip dislocation in spina bifida. In ambulant children, gait function may be more affected by the presence of contractures than the instability of dislocated hip. Furthermore, complications associated with surgery (decrease in strength and increased fracture risk), may outweigh the benefits of reduction [148].

Knee Flexion Deformity and Tibial Torsion

Functional walking is reliant on the presence of some quadriceps action (present in lower lumbar lesions and more distal neurologic levels). In the presence of knee flexion deformity, the excessive external flexion moment at the knee cannot be adequately counteracted by an extension moment generated by the weak knee extensors. The use of knee-ankle-foot orthoses (KAFO) might facilitate some walking in these children. Fixed flexion deformities are amenable to radical posterior capsular releases which might provide some functional benefits in ambulatory children with low lumbar

Table 24.2 Musculoskeletal deformities by level of lesion in myelomemingocele (Adapted with permission from Narayanan, U.G. & Caird, M.S.: Neuromuscular disorders in children. Chapter 67 in Orthopaedic Knowledge Update (OKU) 11. Ed. Canada, L.K. AAOS. 2014. Rosemont, IL)

Level	Motor examination	Orthopedic manifestations	Functional manifestations
Thoracic	• Flaccid lower extremities	• Scoliosis (neuromuscular, congenital) • Kyphosis • Possible clubfeet, hip dislocations	• Household ambulation with HKAFO bracing when small • Wheelchair when bigger
Upper lumbar	• Hip flexion/adduction partially intact • Knee flexion/extension, ankle power, hip extension/abduct-tion absent	• Hip dislocation from unbalanced muscles common • Clubfoot deformities	• Ambulation with HKAFO bracing when small • Often wheelchair when bigger
Lower lumbar	• Knee extension intact (L4—quadriceps) • Ankle dorsiflexion possible (L5—tibialis anterior)	• Clubfeet • Calcaneus (L5) • Hip dislocation or subluxation sometimes	• Ambulation with KAFO bracing
Sacral	• Hip flexion/adduction, knee flexion/extension, ankle power present • Hip extension/abduction partially intact • Gastroc and foot weakness	• Cavovarus foot deformity • Hip dislocation much less common • Ulcers may lead to osteomyelitis	• Very good ambulation with AFO bracing

or sacral lesions who are in crouch [148, 149]. There may also be a role for addressing knee flexion contractures in nonambulatory patients with higher level lesions, to facilitate standing. Marked external tibial torsion may contribute to gait-related difficulties in ambulatory children who can benefit from tibial derotational osteotomies.

Ankle and Foot Deformities

A variety of specific foot deformities are associated with neurologic level of the neural tube defect [150, 151]. Some deformities are present at birth (e.g., equinovarus or clubfeet) while others are acquired over time. Common deformities include equinovarus (clubfoot) most often seen in patients with the higher spinal level lesions; cavovarus is often seen with L-4 lesions; calcaneus and calcaneovalgus with L-5 lesions. Pure equinus might arise from isolated reflex segments of the cord causing spasticity. A late onset cavus deformity that is progressive with growth might be associated with tethered cord. Goals of management in children with myelomeningocele are to maintain a stable, plantigrade foot for weight-bearing while minimizing the risk of ulceration of insensate areas of the weight-bearing areas of the foot. Neurogenic equinovarus deformities are stiffer than idiopathic clubfeet, but can still be successfully managed with serial casting using the Ponseti method in some cases, with careful attention paid to the health of the skin during casting [152]. A well balanced but floppy foot does not need surgery but can be successfully managed with a brace as can a passively correctable deformity. Surgery is indicated for persistent or recurrent deformity in children who can walk. In general, proximal deformities should be corrected before distal ones and soft tissue releases are done before corrective osteotomies. Equinus is often correctable with a tendo-Achilles tenotomy. Severe equinovarus deformities often require extensive posteromedial releases, which might be facilitated by excision of the talus. There is little role for tendon transfers in this population. Recurrent deformities might benefit from talectomy or triple arthrodesis. Cavovarus deformities can be managed by plantar fascia releases, calcaneal osteotomy, and osteotomy of the bases of the metatarsals. Ankle valgus can be managed by supramalleolar osteotomy or distal medial tibial hemiepiphysiodesis with a transphyseal screw or guided growth extraperiosteal plate [150, 151].

Poliomyelitis

Poliomyelitis is an acute enteroviral infection affecting the anterior horn cells of the spinal cord and the brain stem motor nuclei. The musculoskeletal deformities associated with polio provided the mainstay of clinical practice of pediatric orthopedic surgeons in the last century. With the advent of widespread vaccination since the 1950s, polio was on the brink of eradication. Wild poliovirus cases have decreased from an estimated 350,000 cases in 1988 in more than 125 endemic countries, to six reported cases in 2021 [153]. There are few remaining endemic areas in South Asia, Nigeria, and Afghanistan, where the penetration of vaccination has been suboptimal. Failure to eradicate polio from these last remaining strongholds could result in a global resurgence of the disease [153].

This pure motor condition manifests in three stages. The *acute stage* is characterized by initial gastrointestinal symptoms and fever, followed by meningeal symptoms and an asymmetric paralysis within 48 h, which affects the lower extremity more commonly than the upper extremity, particularly the glutei, hip flexors, quadriceps, tibialis anterior and medial hamstrings. During the acute phase, management involves bed rest, positioning, and range of motion to avoid contractures. During the *convalescent stage,* muscle strength improves, much of it in the first month, but this can last up to 2 years. During this time, treatment includes range of motion, splinting and bracing (orthoses) to prevent fixed contractures, and strengthening of the affected muscle groups. However, overactivity of muscles in the convalescent phase has the potential to inhibit recovery of function. The *chronic stage* begins 2 years from the onset of the disease, and no further muscle recovery is expected. The paralysis is associated with flaccid joints or active joints with muscle imbalance. Flaccid joints will develop contractures only if left immobile in abnormal positions for long periods of time. These joints are best treated with stretching exercises and orthoses to maintain the joint in neutral position. Active joints, on the other hand, are prone to develop fixed contractures over time and secondary bony deformities. These are treated by dynamic braces to counteract the unopposed muscle actions. Surgical treatment includes muscle-balancing procedures, such as tendon lengthening and transfers, [154] and corrective osteotomies to address fixed deformities and to stabilize joints (Table 24.3). These are ideally done when the child is older, so that optimal growth potential has been achieved [154–156].

Table 24.3 Common deformities of the lower extremity associated with poliomyelitis and their surgical management

Deformity	Surgical management
Quadriceps femoris paralysis	Biceps femoris and semitendinosus transfer to the patella
Flexion contracture of the knee	Soft tissue release or distal femoral extension osteotomy
Genu recurvatum	Tibial osteotomy Soft tissue triple tenodesis
Flail knee	Orthosis with drop-lock knee and arthrodesis
Equinus	Achilles tenotomy
Cavus	Plantar fascia release; calcaneal osteotomy and base of metatarsal osteotomies
Ankle valgus	Medial distal tibial hemiepiphysiodesis Supramalleolar osteotomy
Hindfoot (subtalar) valgus	Calcaneal osteotomy (medial slide); extraarticular arthrodesis of the subtalar joint (Grice); triple arthrodesis
Convex pes valgus (rocker bottom foot)	Open reduction with transfer of tibialis anterior and peroneus brevis and lengthening of the tendo-Achilles

---

Principles of Tendon Transfer

The joint of interest must be free of fixed deformity, with an acceptable range of passive motion.

Any deformity will require correction prior to transfer.

Muscle strength of tendon to be transferred must be at least grade 4, as the transfer is associated with a decrease in strength by one grade.

The line of excursion and strength of transferred muscle should be similar to the one being replaced. Linear line of action is preferable.

Synergistic muscle (in-phase transfer) is preferred over an antagonistic muscle (out of phase transfer).

Paratenon of the transferred tendon should be preserved.

Neurovascular supply to the transferred muscle should be preserved.

Preferable to run in one muscle compartment with a smooth gliding channel.

Transfer is applied under adequate tension.

Firm fixation to bone is preferable to tendon.

Hereditary Motor Sensory Neuropathy (HSMN)

These are a group of hereditary neuropathies with sensory and motor involvement of the peripheral nerves. These can usually be diagnosed by one or more of the following investigations: blood tests for genetic testing, nerve conduction studies, and nerve biopsies. The most common such neuropathy is HSMN type 1 or Charcot-Marie-Tooth disease type 1. CMT type 1A is autosomal dominant and associated with demyelination of the peripheral nerves due to a duplication of peripheral myelin protein (PMP22) that resides on chromosome 17. The typical clinical presentation is usually not evident until the second decade characterized by progressive atrophy, muscle weakness, loss of balance and contractures involving the intrinsic muscles of the foot which are the first nerves to become involved. Sensory loss occurs first in the distal legs followed by the distal upper extremity. Sensory and motor findings gradually worsen. Nerve conduction velocities are slowed in children even before the clinical onset of disease. Motor amplitudes decrease gradually. Nerve biopsy typically demonstrates age-related loss of myelinated axons and disability correlates with axonal loss [157]. There are numerous additional subtypes of CMT 1 caused by different mutations resulting in demyelination of the peripheral nerves. In contrast, HSMN Type 2 or Charcot-Marie-Tooth type 2 (CMT2) is an axonal (nondemyelinating) peripheral neuropathy which is characterized by distal muscle weakness and atrophy, mild sensory loss, clinically similar to CMT1 but less severe, and nerve conduction velocities are typically normal. Peripheral nerves are not enlarged or hypertrophic. There are many subtypes of CMT2 (15 genetic mutations) which are clinically indistinguishable and differentiated only by genetic testing [158].

Foot Deformities (Fig. 24.26)

The earliest and most common deformities involve the intrinsic muscles of the foot leading to clawed toes. This is followed by weakness of the peroneus brevis and tibialis anterior, while the peroneus longus and tibialis posterior are spared. This pattern of weakness results in cavus and hindfoot varus, associated with weight-bearing on the lateral border of the foot resulting in callosities and difficulties with shoe wear. A high stepping gait facilitates clearance of a drop foot. Examination reveals mild sensory disturbances and absent reflexes [159].

Treatment is initially symptomatic and supportive, and custom orthotics or AFOs can play a useful role in the management of flexible deformities. Surgery is indicated when orthotics fail to manage symptoms. For cavus deformities that are not fixed, an open plantar fascia release is done, but usually in combination with an extension osteotomy of the first metatarsal (or medial cuneiform) to address the plantarflexed deformity of the first ray. The peroneus longus may be transferred to the peroneus brevis. Flexibility of the hindfoot varus is preoperatively assessed using the Coleman block test. This test usually reveals that the plantarflexion of the first ray is the driving force of the hind foot varus, and rules out the need for a calcaneal osteotomy if the hind foot

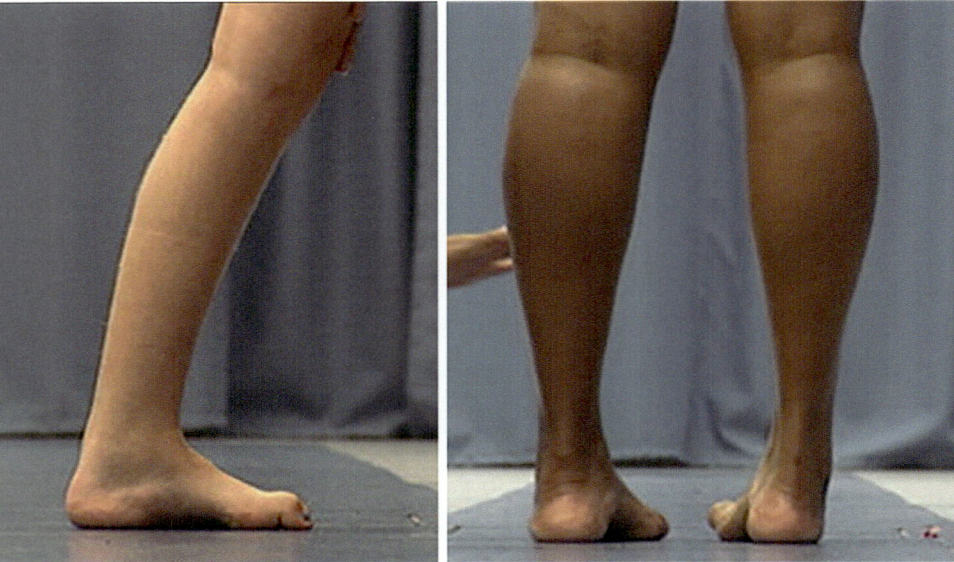

Fig. 24.26 Cavovarus foot deformity in Charcot-Marie-Tooth disease

varus corrects into valgus. A rigid cavus associated with forefoot equinus might require extension osteotomies of additional metatarsals. More severe cavus might require a mid-foot or tarsal osteotomy. Rigid hindfoot varus may need a calcaneal osteotomy (lateral based closing wedge or lateral slide). Claw toe deformities can be addressed with transfers of the extensor hallucis longus to the neck of the first metatarsal and the common extensor tendon to the lateral cuneiform along with flexor tenotomies or transfer of the toe flexors to the extensor hood. Triple arthrodesis is ideally avoided because of longer term risk of arthritis in the ankle but may be necessary for severe fixed deformities [160].

Hip Deformities

The onset of hip dysplasia occurs relatively late in HSMN, most commonly seen in patients affected with CMT1, presenting first in adolescence [161, 162]. Since the development of dysplasia is insidious and asymptomatic, annual radiographs are recommended to monitor the hips once a diagnosis of CMT1 has been established. Radiographs usually reveal a dysplastic acetabulum characterized by smaller lateral and anterior center-edge angles; decreased femoral head coverage; and increased acetabular anteversion; and abnormal proximal femur characterized by increased coxa valga [163] (Fig. 24.27). Pelvic osteotomies to correct the acetabular dysplasia and proximal femoral osteotomies are indicated when hips become symptomatic or the acetabular dysplasia becomes progressive. Stable internal fixation is recommended to avoid prolonged immobilization which can cause profound weakness. Postoperative nerve palsy are reported more common in HMSN [161].

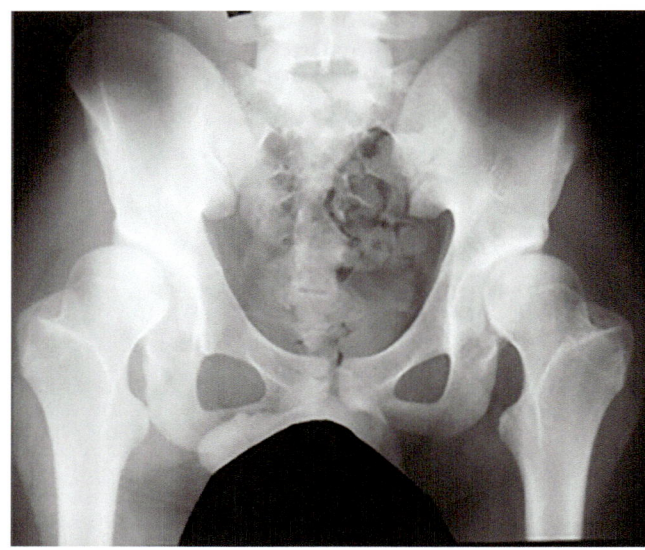

Fig. 24.27 Older onset hip dysplasia in Charcot-Marie-Tooth disease

Muscular Dystrophies

These are a group of more than 30 genetic diseases characterized by progressive skeletal muscle weakness. Duchenne's muscular dystrophy (DMD), the most common form, affects approximately 1 in 5000 to 1 in 6000 male births worldwide [164, 165]. DMD is an X-linked recessive condition due to mutations of the DMD gene on the short arm (p) of the X chromosome (Xp21.2) that regulates the production of dystrophin, a protein involved in the stabilization and integrity of the cell membrane of skeletal and cardiac muscle cells [166]. The cell membrane becomes permeable to creatine kinase (CK) which is elevated in the blood, and muscle fibers degenerate and are replaced with fibrofatty tissue. In DMD, there is a complete lack of dystrophin. Decreased or truncated dystrophin is a feature of Becker muscular dystrophy which is less severe dystrophinopathy. CK levels are elevated but are not as high as in DMD. Diagnosis is confirmed by molecular genetic tests or muscle biopsy.

DMD presents sometime between 2 and 6 years of age in boys. Initial presentation is characterized by history of some delay in the onset of walking, with abnormal stiff knee gait, or toe-walking, lumbar lordosis, and difficulty in going up stairs. Physical examination often reveals pseudohypertrophy of the calf, and a positive Gower sign, due to the greater weakness of the proximal muscles (pelvic girdle and hip extensors) than the distal lower extremity muscles [164, 166]. Toe-walking, Trendelenburg gait, and lumbar lordosis are essentially compensatory strategies to minimize the moments about the weight-bearing joints and maintain balance while standing and walking. Over time, fixed lower extremity contractures including equinus or equinovarus deformities of the foot can develop. The natural history is one of rapid decline with most boys unable to walk by 12 years of age, progressive scoliosis, and cardiorespiratory decline until death in the early twenties.

The use of corticosteroids, prednisone or deflazacort (approved by the FDA in 2017), has been shown to stabilize the cell membrane and slow the rate of deterioration of muscle strength, prolongation of independent ambulation, decrease the risk of scoliosis in childhood, and preserve pulmonary function by several years [167, 168]. More recently, the FDA has approved a new class of drugs called antisense oligonucleotides, to treat those patients with DMD who have confirmed mutations of the dystrophin gene that are amenable to skipping specific exons, specifically exon 51 (eteplirsen), exon 53 (golodirsen, viltolarsen), and exon 45 (casimersen) skipping, respectively. These drugs help improve muscle symptoms, and although approved by the FDA await definitive clinical trials to confirm their effectiveness in DMD, using condition-specific patient-reported outcome measures that can evaluate outcomes that are important and aligned with the goals of this population [169]. Lower extremity joint contractures are managed with bracing or surgically with tendon lengthening, the indications must serve to preserve function, assist seating or improve comfort with foot wear. Instrumented posterior spinal fusion that was necessary to treat scoliosis early is less frequently required with these new treatments reducing the risk of scoliosis in childhood.

Conclusion

This chapter provides an overview of the lower limb musculoskeletal consequences of the various neuromuscular disorders. Although the etiology, pathophysiology, and natural history vary widely across these conditions, there are some common principles of management that apply to most of these conditions. Orthopedic surgery plays an important role in management of these conditions, most effectively in the context of a multidisciplinary approach along with physical therapists, developmental pediatricians, physiatrists, neurologists, orthotists, and other specialists. Although our interventions have been shown to make significant differences, much work remains to be done to define the effectiveness and longevity of the outcomes, in terms that are relevant and meaningful to these populations. These conditions are chronic, permanent, and currently have no cures. Future advances will stem from basic research to understand the embryology and biology of the neural axis and the musculoskeletal system, and the pathophysiology of these heterogenous disorders; and epidemiologic research that will unravel the risk factors will eventually provide the strategies to mitigate or reverse the effects of these conditions, or prevent them from occurring in the first place.

Commentary

David B. Frumberg
david.frumberg@yale.edu

This chapter eloquently provides a framework for how one should approach the evaluation and treatment of limb deformities caused by neuromuscular disorders. The musculoskeletal differences caused by these conditions are secondary problems to the underlying pathology of the central nervous system. Thus, treatment aimed at counteracting deforming forces, or rerouting them, is the mainstay of treatment. There is notable responsibility on the orthopedic surgeon to get it right, as barriers tend to prevent patients with neuro-orthopedic conditions from finding orthopedic care once they graduate the pediatric world.

Neuromuscular deformity analysis is unique and challenging because it requires consideration of both osseous and muscular structures. These two parts of the lower limb can work independently or in synergy to cause dysfunction. A good example of this is deformity of the hip in spastic conditions. The immature bony architecture works in concert with unbalanced muscle forces to impair the hip's development. The resultant triplanar hip deformity may be best treated by addressing both musculotendinous and osseous structures. Contemporary management prefers a proactive approach rather than a reactive approach to hip dysplasia, because salvage options for the dislocated hip have far worse outcomes than a native joint preservation strategy as discussed in the chapter.

It is paramount to understand the biomechanics of the muscle-tendon unit. Classically, tight muscles have been treated with some form of lengthening of the muscle-tendon unit. However, such lengthening can result in weakness. Overlengthening of these muscle-tendon units can have a profoundly negative effect on gait efficiency and generate secondary gait dysfunction. One example is the overlengthening caused by hamstrings lengthening for knee flexion contracture. This treatment may result in a straighter knee in the short-term, but as the hamstrings originate at the pelvis, there may be a long-term development of anterior pelvic tilt that can be detrimental later in life. Hypertonic muscles are typically still weak muscles. Pubertal growth spurts may uncover this underlying weakness, particularly in children that rely on their spasticity to ambulate and stay erect.

The chapter articulates the importance of proper muscle tone management for hypertonic disorders. Strategies including local or systemic antispasmodic medication, and neurosurgical intervention can all be of benefit. It is important to optimize muscle tone management prior to surgery, and this is best addressed via a multidisciplinary approach.

Neuromuscular conditions that cause dystonia as the primary motor pattern need special consideration. Dystonia, which is an involuntary movement disorder, can sometimes be difficult to appreciate on physical examination. However, treatment of deformity caused by or complicated by dystonia has less predictable outcomes, particularly with soft tissue procedures alone. As it is not a spastic pattern, chemodenervation has less utility. Osseous procedures have been shown to be more efficacious.

The chapter contains a fantastic list of the multiple aspects of assessment of an ambulatory child. This list recommends starting with a gait-related problem list, as the family's perceived issues may be different from what is objectively noted by the clinician. Treatment recommendations should include the synthesis of all data: gait exam, tabletop static and dynamic exams, and objective tests such as imaging and instrumented gait analysis. When multiple lower limb segments have deformities that necessitate correction, the standard of care is for single-event multilevel surgery (SEMLS) so that there is one major surgical event with a single rehabilitation effort and less interruptions to the child's psychosocial development. This has the added benefit of correcting all deformities contributing to gait inefficiency at the same time. Table 24.1 lists many of the commonly included procedures that can be employed in such a surgical event.

Deformity correction surgery for nonambulatory (GMFCS IV–V) children is just as meaningful as those done for gait improvements in GMFCS I–III children. The goals of surgery listed in the chapter are worthy of pursuit. As nonambulatory adolescents shift their focus toward independent ambulation in early adulthood, deformity correction that enhances their ability to stand or pivot-transfer can enhance their capacity to perform instrumental activities of daily living (IADLs).

For low muscle tone or hypotonic conditions including certain muscle disorders and neuropathies, treatment of limb deformity is nicely delineated in the chapter. Supportive bracing and treatment should enable the acquisition of independence and mobility as much as possible throughout childhood. Tables 24.2 and 24.3 are concise compilations of some of these interventions.

Neuromuscular lower limb deformity should be analyzed in three planes like any other limb deformity. This chapter gave examples of uniplanar deformities (e.g., ankle equinus, knee flexion contracture, torsional malalignment, coxa valga) and their treatment, but also highlighted more complex multiplanar deformities (e.g., cavovarus foot). The successful identification and correction of osseous and soft tissue deformities can have a profound and lasting impact on the quality of life and mobility of children with these disorders.

References

1. Bax M, Goldstein M, Rosenbaum P, Leviton A, Paneth N, Dan B, et al. Proposed definition and classification of cerebral palsy, April 2005. Dev Med Child Neurol. 2005;47(8):571–6.
2. Rosenbaum P, Paneth N, Leviton A, Goldstein M, Bax M, Damiano D, et al. A report: the definition and classification of cerebral palsy April 2006. Dev Med Child Neurol Suppl. 2007;109:8–14.
3. Stanley FAE, Blair E. Cerebral palsies: epidemiology and causal pathways. London: Mac Keith; 2000.
4. Palisano R, Rosenbaum P, Walter S, Russell D, Wood E, Galuppi B. Development and reliability of a system to classify gross motor function in children with cerebral palsy. Dev Med Child Neurol. 1997;39(4):214–23.
5. Wood E, Rosenbaum P. The gross motor function classification system for cerebral palsy: a study of reliability and stability over time. Dev Med Child Neurol. 2000;42(5):292–6.

6. Palisano RJ, Rosenbaum P, Bartlett D, Livingston MH. Content validity of the expanded and revised gross motor function classification system. Dev Med Child Neurol. 2008;50(10):744–50.
7. Gage JR. The neurological control system for normal gait. In: Gage JR, editor. Gait analysis in cerebral palsy. London: MacKeith Press; 1991. p. 37–60.
8. Ziv I, Blackburn N, Rang M, Koreska J. Muscle growth in normal and spastic mice. Dev Med Child Neurol. 1984;26(1):94–9.
9. Gage JR, Schwartz M. Pathologic gait and lever arm dysfunction. In: Gage JR, editor. The treatment of gait problems in cerebral palsy. London: Mac Keith: Distributed by Cambridge University Press; 2004. p. 180–204.
10. Bell KJ, Ounpuu S, DeLuca PA, Romness MJ. Natural progression of gait in children with cerebral palsy. J Pediatr Orthop. 2002;22(5):677–82.
11. Johnson DC, Damiano DL, Abel MF. The evolution of gait in childhood and adolescent cerebral palsy. J Pediatr Orthop. 1997;17(3):392–6.
12. Murphy KP, Molnar GE, Lankasky K. Medical and functional status of adults with cerebral palsy. Dev Med Child Neurol. 1995;37(12):1075–84.
13. Bottos M, Feliciangeli A, Sciuto L, Gericke C, Vianello A. Functional status of adults with cerebral palsy and implications for treatment of children. Dev Med Child Neurol. 2001;43(8):516–28.
14. Delp SL, Arnold AS, Speers RA, Moore CA. Hamstrings and psoas lengths during normal and crouch gait: implications for muscle-tendon surgery. J Orthop Res. 1996;14(1):144–51.
15. DeLuca PA, Ounpuu S, Davis RB, Walsh JH. Effect of hamstring and psoas lengthening on pelvic tilt in patients with spastic diplegic cerebral palsy. J Pediatr Orthop. 1998;18(6):712–8.
16. Arnold AS, Komattu AV, Delp SL. Internal rotation gait: a compensatory mechanism to restore abduction capacity decreased by bone deformity. Dev Med Child Neurol. 1997;39(1):40–4.
17. Rogers SP. A method for determining the angle of torsion of the neck of the femur. J Bone Joint Surg Am. 1931;13(4):821–4.
18. Dunlap K, Shands AR Jr, Hollister LC Jr, Gaul JS Jr, Streit HA. A new method for determination of torsion of the femur. J Bone Joint Surg Am. 1953;35-A(2):289–311.
19. Rogers SP. Observations on torsion of the femur. J Bone Joint Surg Am. 1934;16(2):284–9.
20. Ryder CT, Crane L. Measuring femoral anteversion; the problem and a method. J Bone Joint Surg Am. 1953;35-A(2):321–8.
21. Beals RK. Developmental changes in the femur and acetabulum in spastic paraplegia and diplegia. Dev Med Child Neurol. 1969;11(3):303–13.
22. Robin J, Graham HK, Selber P, Dobson F, Smith K, Baker R. Proximal femoral geometry in cerebral palsy: a population-based cross-sectional study. J Bone Joint Surg Br. 2008;90(10):1372–9.
23. Miller F, Bagg MR. Age and migration percentage as risk factors for progression in spastic hip disease. Dev Med Child Neurol. 1995;37:449–55.
24. Connelly A, Flett P, Graham HK, Oates J. Hip surveillance in Tasmanian children with cerebral palsy. J Paediatr Child Health. 2009;45(7–8):437–43.
25. Hagglund G, Andersson S, Duppe H, Lauge-Pedersen H, Nordmark E, Westbom L. Prevention of dislocation of the hip in children with cerebral palsy. The first ten years of a population-based prevention programme. J Bone Joint Surg Br. 2005;87(1):95–101.
26. Soo B, Howard JJ, Boyd RN, Reid SM, Lanigan A, Wolfe R, et al. Hip displacement in cerebral palsy. J Bone Joint Surg Am. 2006;88:121–9.
27. Hermanson M, Hägglund G, Riad J, Wagner P. Head-shaft angle is a risk factor for hip displacement in children with cerebral palsy. Acta Orthop. 2015;86(2):229–32.
28. Hermanson M, Hägglund G, Riad J, Rodby-Bousquet E, Wagner P. Prediction of hip displacement in children with cerebral palsy: development of the CPUP hip score. Bone Joint J. 2015;97-B(10):1441–4.
29. Sharp IK. Acetabular Dysplasia. The acetabular angle. J Bone Joint Surg Br. 1961;43-B(2):268–72.
30. Hoffinger SA, Rab GT, Abou-Ghaida H. Hamstrings in cerebral palsy crouch gait. J Pediatr Orthop. 1993;13(6):722–6.
31. Kristiansen LP, Gunderson RB, Steen H, Reikerås O. The normal development of tibial torsion. Skeletal Radiol. 2001;30(9):519–22.
32. Price BD, Price CT. A simple demonstration of hindfoot flexibility in the cavovarus foot. J Pediatr Orthop. 1997;17(1):18–9.
33. Gage JR. Gait analysis in cerebral palsy. London: MacKeith Press; 1991.
34. Gage JR. The role of gait analysis in the treatment of cerebral palsy. J Pediatr Orthop. 1994;14(6):701–2.
35. Kulkarni VA, Kephart D, Olleac R, Davids J. Enhancing observational gait analysis–techniques and tips for analyzing gait without a gait lab. Curr Concept Rev. 2(3).
36. Davids JR, Ounpuu S, DeLuca PA, Davis RB 3rd. Optimization of walking ability of children with cerebral palsy. Instr Course Lect. 2004;53:511–22.
37. Narayanan UG. The role of gait analysis in the orthopaedic management of ambulatory cerebral palsy. Curr Opin Pediatr. 2007;19(1):38–43.
38. Rodda JM, Graham HK, Carson L, et al. Sagittal gait patterns in spastic diplegia. J Bone Joint Surg Br. 2004;86:251–8.
39. Winters TF Jr, Gage JR, Hicks R. Gait patterns in spastic hemiplegia in children and young adults. J Bone Joint Surg Am. 1987;69(3):437–41.
40. Rethlefsen SA, Blumstein G, Kay RM, et al. Prevalence of specific gait abnormalities in children with cerebral palsy revisited: influence of age, prior surgery, and gross motor function classification system level. Dev Med Child Neurol. 2017;59:79–88.
41. DeLuca PA, Davis RB 3rd, Ounpuu S, Rose S, Sirkin R. Alterations in surgical decision making in patients with cerebral palsy based on three-dimensional gait analysis. J Pediatr Orthop. 1997;17(5):608–14.
42. Kay RM, Dennis S, Rethlefsen S, Reynolds RA, Skaggs DL, Tolo VT. The effect of preoperative gait analysis on orthopaedic decision making. Clin Orthop Relat Res. 2000;372:217–22.
43. Cook RE, Schneider I, Hazlewood ME, Hillman SJ, Robb JE. Gait analysis alters decision-making in cerebral palsy. J Pediatr Orthop. 2003;23(3):292–5.
44. Chang FM, Seidl AJ, Muthusamy K, Meininger AK, Carollo JJ. Effectiveness of instrumented gait analysis in children with cerebral palsy—comparison of outcomes. J Pediatr Orthop. 2006;26(5):612–6.
45. O'Sullivan R, Horgan F, O'Brien T, et al. The natural history of crouch gait in bilateral cerebral palsy: a systematic review. Res Dev Disabil. 2018;80:84–92.
46. Staheli LT, Corbett M, Wyss C, King H. Lower-extremity rotational problems in children. Normal values to guide management. J Bone Joint Surg Am. 1985;67(1):39–47.
47. Haugh AB, Pandyan AD, Johnson GR. A systematic review of the Tardieu Scale for the measurement of spasticity. Disabil Rehabil. 2006;28(15):899–907.
48. Sanger TD, Delgado MR, Gaebler-Spira D, Hallett M, Mink JW. Classification and definition of disorders causing hypertonia in childhood. Pediatrics. 2003;111(1):e89–97.
49. Davids JR, Benfanti P, Blackhurst DW, Allen BL. Assessment of femoral anteversion in children with cerebral palsy: accuracy of the trochanteric prominence angle test. J Pediatr Orthop. 2002;22:173–8.

50. Ruwe PA, Gage JR, Ozonoff MB, DeLuca PA. Clinical determination of femoral anteversion. A comparison with established techniques. J Bone Joint Surg Am. 1992;74:820–30.
51. Novacheck TF, Trost JP, Sohrweide S. Examination of the child with cerebral palsy. Orthop Clin North Am. 2010;41(4):469–88.
52. Damiano DL, Vaughan CL, Abel MF. Muscle response to heavy resistance exercise in children with spastic cerebral palsy. Dev Med Child Neurol. 1995;37(8):731–9.
53. Damiano DL, Dodd K, Taylor NF. Should we be testing and training muscle strength in cerebral palsy? Dev Med Child Neurol. 2002;44(1):68–72.
54. Kendall HO, Kendall FP, Wadsworth GE, editors. Muscle testing and function. 2nd ed. London: Williams and Wilkins; 1971.
55. Fowler EG, Staudt LA, Greenberg MB. Lower-extremity selective voluntary motor control in patients with spastic cerebral palsy: increased distal motor impairment. Dev Med Child Neurol. 2010;52(3):264–9.
56. Fowler EG, Staudt LA, Greenberg MB, Oppenheim WL. Selective control assessment of the lower extremity (SCALE): development, validation, and interrater reliability of a clinical tool for patients with cerebral palsy. Dev Med Child Neurol. 2009;51(8):607–14.
57. Trost JP. Clinical assessment. In: Gage JR, Schwartz M, Koop SE, Novacheck TF, editors. The identification and treatment of gait problems in cerebral palsy. 2nd ed. London: Mac Keith Press; 2009. p. 179–203.
58. Rang M. Cerebral palsy. In: Lovell WW, Winter RB, editors. Lovell and winter's pediatric orthopaedics. Philadelphia: Lippincott; 1990. p. 465–506.
59. Narayanan UG, Fehlings D, Weir S, Knights S, Kiran S, Campbell K. Initial development and validation of the caregiver priorities and child health index of life with disabilities (CPCHILD). Dev Med Child Neurol. 2006;48(10):804–12.
60. Ade-Hall RA, Moore AP. Botulinum toxin type a in the treatment of lower limb spasticity in cerebral palsy. Cochrane Database Syst Rev. 2000(2):CD001408.
61. Bjornson K, Hays R, Graubert C, Price R, Won F, McLaughlin JF. Botulinum toxin for spasticity in children with cerebral palsy: a comprehensive evaluation. Pediatrics. 2007;120(1):49–58.
62. Dumas HM, O'Neil ME, Fragala MA. Expert consensus on physical therapist intervention after botulinum toxin a injection for children with cerebral palsy. Pediatr Phys Ther. 2001;13(3):122–32.
63. Lannin N, Scheinberg A, Clark K. AACPDM systematic review of the effectiveness of therapy for children with cerebral palsy after botulinum toxin a injections. Dev Med Child Neurol. 2006;48(6):533–9.
64. Molenaers G, Desloovere K, De Cat J, Jonkers I, De Borre L, Pauwels P, et al. Single event multilevel botulinum toxin type a treatment and surgery: similarities and differences. Eur J Neurol. 2001;8(Suppl 5):88–97.
65. Scholtes VA, Dallmeijer AJ, Knol DL, Speth LA, Maathuis CG, Jongerius PH. The combined effect of lower-limb multilevel botulinum toxin type a and comprehensive rehabilitation on mobility in children with cerebral palsy: a randomized clinical trial. Arch Phys Med Rehabil. 2006;87(12):1551–8.
66. McLaughlin J, Bjornson K, Temkin N, Steinbok P, Wright V, Reiner A, et al. Selective dorsal rhizotomy: meta-analysis of three randomized controlled trials. Dev Med Child Neurol. 2002;44(1):17–25.
67. McLaughlin JF, Bjornson KF, Astley SJ, Graubert C, Hays RM, Roberts TS, et al. Selective dorsal rhizotomy: efficacy and safety in an investigator-masked randomized clinical trial. Dev Med Child Neurol. 1998;40(4):220–32.
68. Steinbok P, Reiner AM, Beauchamp R, Armstrong RW, Cochrane DD, Kestle J. A randomized clinical trial to compare selective posterior rhizotomy plus physiotherapy with physiotherapy alone in children with spastic diplegic cerebral palsy. Dev Med Child Neurol. 1997;39(3):178–84.
69. Wright FV, Sheil EM, Drake JM, Wedge JH, Naumann S. Evaluation of selective dorsal rhizotomy for the reduction of spasticity in cerebral palsy: a randomized controlled trial. Dev Med Child Neurol. 1998;40(4):239–47.
70. Hagglund G, Andersson S, Duppe H, Lauge-Pedersen H, Nordmark E, Westbom L. Prevention of severe contractures might replace multilevel surgery in cerebral palsy: results of a population-based health care programme and new techniques to reduce spasticity. J Pediatr Orthop B. 2005;14(4):269–73.
71. Steinbok P. Outcomes after selective dorsal rhizotomy for spastic cerebral palsy. Childs Nerv Syst. 2001;17(1–2):1–18.
72. Thomas SS, Buckon CE, Piatt JH, Aiona MD, Sussman MD. A 2-year follow-up of outcomes following orthopedic surgery or selective dorsal rhizotomy in children with spastic diplegia. J Pediatr Orthop B. 2004;13(6):358–66.
73. Grunt S, Becher JG, Vermeulen RJ. Long-term outcome and adverse effects of selective dorsal rhizotomy in children with cerebral palsy: a systematic review. Dev Med Child Neurol. 2011;53(6):490–8.
74. Langerak NG, Lamberts RP, Fieggen AG, Peter JC, van der Merwe L, Peacock WJ, et al. A prospective gait analysis study in patients with diplegic cerebral palsy 20 years after selective dorsal rhizotomy. J Neurosurg Pediatr. 2008;1(3):180–6.
75. Langerak NG, Tam N, Vaughan CL, Fieggen AG, Schwartz MH. Gait status 17-26 years after selective dorsal rhizotomy. Gait Posture. 2012;35(2):244–9.
76. Albright AL. Intrathecal baclofen in cerebral palsy movement disorders. J Child Neurol. 1996;11(Suppl 1):S29–35.
77. Butler C, Campbell S. Evidence of the effects of intrathecal baclofen for spastic and dystonic cerebral palsy. AACPDM treatment outcomes committee review. Panel DevMedChild Neurol. 2000;42(9):634–45.
78. Campbell W, Ferrel A, McLaughlin J, Grant G, Loeser J, Graubert C, et al. Long-term safety and efficacy of continuous intrathecal baclofen. DevMedChild Neurol. 2002;44(10):660–5.
79. Nene AV, Evans GA, Patrick JH. Simultaneous multiple operations for spastic diplegia. Outcome and functional assessment of walking in 18 patients. J Bone Joint Surg Br. 1993;75(3):488–94.
80. Norlin R, Tkaczuk H. One session surgery on the lower limb in children with cerebral palsy. A five year follow-up. Int Orthop. 1992;16(3):291–3.
81. McGinley JL, Dobson F, Ganeshalingam R, Shore BJ, Rutz E, Graham HK. Single-event multilevel surgery for children with cerebral palsy: a systematic review. Dev Med Child Neurol. 2012;54(2):117–28.
82. Bache CESP, Graham HK. The management of spastic diplegia. Curr Orthop. 2003;17:88–104.
83. Gough M, Eve LC, Robinson RO, Shortland AP. Short-term outcome of multilevel surgical intervention in spastic diplegic cerebral palsy compared with the natural history. Dev Med Child Neurol. 2004;46(2):91–7.
84. Narayanan UG. Management of children with ambulatory cerebral palsy: an evidence-based review. J Pediatr Orthop. 2012;32(Suppl 2):S172–81.
85. Thomason P, Baker R, Dodd K, Taylor N, Selber P, Wolfe R, et al. Single-event multilevel surgery in children with spastic diplegia: a pilot randomized controlled trial. J Bone Joint Surg Am. 2011;93(5):451–60.
86. Wren TA, Otsuka NY, Bowen RE, et al. Outcomes of lower extremity orthopedic surgery in ambulatory children with cerebral palsy with and without gait analysis: results of a randomized controlled trial. Gait Posture. 2013;38(2):236–41.
87. Rutz E, Donath S, Tirosh O, Graham HK, Baker R. Explaining the variability improvements in gait quality as a result of sin-

gle event multi-level surgery in cerebral palsy. Gait Posture. 2015;38(3):455–60.
88. Saraph V, Zwick EB, Auner C, Schneider F, Steinwender G, Linhart W. Gait improvement surgery in diplegic children: how long do the improvements last? J Pediatr Orthop. 2005;25(3):263–7.
89. Thomason P, Selber P, Graham HK. Single event multilevel surgery in children with bilateral spastic cerebral palsy: a 5 year prospective cohort study. Gait Posture. 2013;37(1):23–8.
90. Firth GB, Passmore E, Sangeux M, Thomason P, Rodda J, Donath S, et al. Multilevel surgery for equinus gait in children with spastic diplegic cerebral palsy: medium-term follow-up with gait analysis. J Bone Joint Surg Am. 2013;95(10):931–8.
91. Dreher T, Thomason P, Svehlik M, et al. Long-term development of gait after multilevel surgery in children with cerebral palsy: a multicentre cohort study. Dev Med Child Neurol. 2018;60:88–93.
92. Novacheck TF, Trost JP, Schwartz MH. Intramuscular psoas lengthening improves dynamic hip function in children with cerebral palsy. J Pediatr Orthop. 2002;22(2):158–64.
93. Sutherland DH, Zilberfarb JL, Kaufman KR, Wyatt MP, Chambers HG. Psoas release at the pelvic brim in ambulatory patients with cerebral palsy: operative technique and functional outcome. J Pediatr Orthop. 1997;17(5):563–70.
94. Novacheck TF. Orthopaedic treatment of muscle contractures. In: Gage JR, Schwartz MH, Koop SE, Novacheck TF, editors. The identification and treatment of gait problems in cerebral palsy. London: Mac Keith Press; 2009.
95. Shore BJ, Yu X, Desai S, Selber P, Wolfe R, Graham HK. Adductor surgery to prevent hip displacement in children with cerebral palsy: the predictive role of the gross motor function classification system. J Bone Joint Surg Am. 2012;94(4):326–34.
96. Kay RM, Rethlefsen SA, Hale JM, Skaggs DL, Tolo VT. Comparison of proximal and distal rotational femoral osteotomy in children with cerebral palsy. J Pediatr Orthop. 2003;23(2):150–4.
97. Pirpiris M, Trivett A, Baker R, Rodda J, Nattrass GR, Graham HK. Femoral derotation osteotomy in spastic diplegia. Proximal or distal? J Bone Joint Surg Br. 2003;85(2):265–72.
98. Ounpuu S, DeLuca P, Davis R, Romness M. Long-term effects of femoral derotation osteotomies: an evaluation using three-dimensional gait analysis. J Pediatr Orthop. 2002;22(2):139–45.
99. McCarthy J, Shrader MW, Graham HK, et al. Establishing surgical indications for hamstring lengthening and femoral derotational osteotomy in ambulatory children with cerebral palsy. J Child Orthop. 2020;14:50–7.
100. Bobroff ED, Chambers H, Sartoris DJ, Wyatt MP, Sutherland DH. Femoral anteversion and neck-shaft angle in children with cerebral palsy. Clin Orthop. 1999;364:194–204.
101. Thompson N, Stebbins J, Seniorou M, Wainwright AM, Newham DJ, Theologis TN. The use of minimally invasive techniques in multi-level surgery for children with cerebral palsy. J Bone Joint Surg Br. 2010;92-B(10):1325–480.
102. Karlen JW, Skaggs DL, Ramachandran M, Kay RM. The Dega osteotomy: a versatile osteotomy in the treatment of developmental and neuromuscular hip pathology. J Pediatr Orthop. 2009;29(7):676–82.
103. McNerney NP, Mubarak SJ, Wenger DR. One-stage correction of the dysplastic hip in cerebral palsy with the San Diego acetabuloplasty: results and complications in 104 hips. J Pediatr Orthop. 2000;20(1):93–103.
104. McHale KA, Bagg M, Nason SS. Treatment of the chronically dislocated hip in adolescents with cerebral palsy with femoral head resection and subtrochanteric valgus osteotomy. J Pediatr Orthop. 1990;10(4):504–9.
105. Kay RM, McCarthy J, Narayanan U, et al. Finding consensus for hamstring surgery in ambulatory children with cerebral palsy using the Delphi method. J Child Orthop. 2022;16:55–64.
106. Thometz J, Simon S, Rosenthal R. The effect on gait of lengthening of the medial hamstrings in cerebral palsy. J Bone Joint Surg Am. 1989;71(3):345–53.
107. Kay RM, Rethlefsen SA, Skaggs D, Leet A. Outcome of medial versus combined medial and lateral hamstring lengthening surgery in cerebral palsy. J Pediatr Orthop. 2002;22(2):169–72.
108. Rutz E, Novacheck T, Dreher DJ, et al. Distal femoral extension osteotomy and patellar tendon advancement or shortening in ambulatory children with cerebral palsy: a modified Delphi consensus study and literature review. J Childrens Orthop. 2022;16:442.
109. Rodda JM, Graham HK, Nattrass GR, Galea MP, Baker R, Wolfe R. Correction of severe crouch gait in patients with spastic diplegia with use of multilevel orthopaedic surgery. J Bone Joint Surg Am. 2006;88(12):2653–64.
110. Boyer ER, Stout JL, Laine JC, et al. Long-term outcomes of distal femoral extension osteotomy and patellar tendon advancement in individuals with cerebral palsy. J Bone Joint Surg Am. 2018;100:31–41.
111. Novacheck TF, Stout JL, Gage JR, Schwartz MH. Distal femoral extension osteotomy and patellar tendon advancement to treat persistent crouch gait in cerebral palsy. Surgical technique. J Bone Joint Surg Am. 2009;91(Suppl 2):271–86.
112. Inan M, Sarikaya IA, Yildirim E, et al. Neurological complications after supracondylar femoral osteotomy in cerebral palsy. J Pediatr Orthop. 2015;35:290–5.
113. Joseph B, Reddy K, Varghese RA, et al. Management of severe crouch gait in children and adolescents with cerebral palsy. J Pediatr Orthop. 2010;30:832–9.
114. Klotz MCM, Hirsch K, Heitzmann D, et al. Distal femoral extension and shortening osteotomy as a part of multilevel surgery in children with cerebral palsy. World J Pediatr. 2017;13:353–9.
115. Erdal OA, Gorgun B, Sarikaya IA, et al. Intraoperative neuromonitoring during distal femoral extension osteotomy in children with cerebral palsy. J Pediatr Orthop B. 2022;31:194–201.
116. Sossai R, Vavken P, Brunner R, et al. Patellar tendon shortening for flexed knee gait in spastic diplegia. Gait Posture. 2015;41:658–65.
117. Klotz MCM, Krautwurst BK, Hirsch K, et al. Does additional patella tendon shortening influence the effects of multilevel surgery to correct flexed knee gait in cerebral palsy: a randomized controlled trial. Gait Posture. 2018;60:217–24.
118. Shore BJ, McCarthy J, Shrader MW, et al. Anterior distal femoral hemiepiphysiodesis in children with cerebral palsy: establishing surgical indications and techniques using the modified Delphi method and literature review. J Child Orthop. 2022;16:65–74.
119. Chambers H, Lauer A, Kaufman K, Cardelia JM, Sutherland D. Prediction of outcome after rectus femoris surgery in cerebral palsy: the role of cocontraction of the rectus femoris and vastus lateralis. J Pediatr Orthop. 1998;18(6):703–11.
120. Kay RM, Rethlefsen SA, Kelly JP, Wren TA. Predictive value of the Duncan-Ely test in distal rectus femoris transfer. J Pediatr Orthop. 2004;24(1):59–62.
121. Gage JR, Perry J, Hicks RR, Koop S, Werntz JR. Rectus femoris transfer to improve knee function of children with cerebral palsy. Dev Med Child Neurol. 1987;29(2):159–66.
122. Rethlefsen S, Tolo VT, Reynolds RA, Kay R. Outcome of hamstring lengthening and distal rectus femoris transfer surgery. J Pediatr Orthop B. 1999;8(2):75–9.
123. Saw A, Smith PA, Sirirungruangsarn Y, Chen S, Hassani S, Harris G, et al. Rectus femoris transfer for children with cerebral palsy: long-term outcome. J Pediatr Orthop. 2003;23(5):672–8.
124. Ounpuu S, Muik E, Davis RB 3rd, Gage JR, DeLuca PA. Rectus femoris surgery in children with cerebral palsy. Part II: a comparison between the effect of transfer and release of the distal rectus femoris on knee motion. J Pediatr Orthop. 1993;13(3):331–5.
125. Dodgin DA, De Swart RJ, Stefko RM, Wenger DR, Ko JY. Distal tibial/fibular derotation osteotomy for correction of tibial torsion:

126. Ryan DD, Rethlefsen SA, Skaggs DL, Kay RM. Results of tibial rotational osteotomy without concomitant fibular osteotomy in children with cerebral palsy. J Pediatr Orthop. 2005;25(1):84–8.
127. Strayer LM. Recession of the gastrocnemius. An operation to relieve spastic contracture of the calf muscles. J Bone Joint Surg. 1950;32-A:671–6.
128. Rutz E, McCarthy J, Shore BJ, et al. Indications for gastrocsoleus lengthening in ambulatory children with cerebral palsy: a Delphi consensus study. J Child Orthop. 2020;14:405–14.
129. Tinney A, Khot A, Eizenberg N, Wolfe R, Graham HK. Gastrocsoleus recession techniques: an anatomical and biomechanical study in human cadavers. Bone Joint J. 2014;96-B:778–82.
130. Dietz FR, Albright JC, Dolan L. Medium-term follow-up of Achilles tendon lengthening in the treatment of ankle equinus in cerebral palsy. Iowa Orthop J. 2006;26:27–32.
131. Rose SA, DeLuca PA, Davis RB 3rd, Ounpuu S, Gage JR. Kinematic and kinetic evaluation of the ankle after lengthening of the gastrocnemius fascia in children with cerebral palsy. J Pediatr Orthop. 1993;13(6):727–32.
132. Steinwender G, Saraph V, Zwick EB, Uitz C, Linhart W. Fixed and dynamic equinus in cerebral palsy: evaluation of ankle function after multilevel surgery. J Pediatr Orthop. 2001;21(1):102–7.
133. Borton DC, Walker K, Pirpiris M, Nattrass GR, Graham HK. Isolated calf lengthening in cerebral palsy. Outcome analysis of risk factors. J Bone Joint Surg Br. 2001;83(3):364–70.
134. Graham HK, Fixsen JA. Lengthening of the calcaneal tendon in spastic hemiplegia by the white slide technique. A long-term review. J Bone Joint Surg Br. 1988;70:472–5.
135. Green NE, Griffin PP, Shiavi R. Split posterior tibial-tendon transfer in spastic cerebral palsy. J Bone Joint Surg Am. 1983;65(6):748–54.
136. Hoffer MM, Barakat G, Koffman M. 10-year follow-up of split anterior tibial tendon transfer in cerebral palsied patients with spastic equinovarus deformity. J Pediatr Orthop. 1985;5(4):432–4.
137. Barnes MJ, Herring JA. Combined split anterior tibial-tendon transfer and intramuscular lengthening of the posterior tibial tendon. Results in patients who have a varus deformity of the foot due to spastic cerebral palsy. J Bone Joint Surg Am. 1991;73(5):734–8.
138. Davids JR, Shilt J, Kay R, et al. Assessment of foot alignment and function for ambulatory children with cerebral palsy: results of a modified Delphi technique consensus study. J Child Orthop. 2022;16:111–20.
139. Mosca VS. Calcaneal lengthening for valgus deformity of the hindfoot. Results in children who had severe, symptomatic flatfoot and skewfoot. J Bone Joint Surg Am. 1995;77(4):500–12.
140. Rathjen KE, Mubarak SJ. Calcaneal-cuboid-cuneiform osteotomy for the correction of valgus foot deformities in children. J Pediatr Orthop. 1998;18(6):775–82.
141. Dennyson WG, Fulford GE. Subtalar arthrodesis by cancellous grafts and metallic internal fixation. J Bone Joint Surg. 1976;58-B:507.
142. Goldberg MJ. Measuring outcomes in cerebral palsy. J Pediatr Orthop. 1991;11(5):682–5.
143. Narayanan U, Moline R, Encisa C, Yeung G, Weir S. Validation of the GOAL questionnaire: an outcome measure for ambulatory children with cerebral palsy. Dev Med Child Neurol. 2015;57:29–9.
144. Thomason P, Tan A, Donnan A, Rodda J, Graham HK, Narayanan U. The gait outcomes assessment list (GOAL): validation of a new assessment of gait function for children with cerebral palsy. Dev Med Child Neurol. 2018;60:618–23.
145. Paul SM, Siegel KL, Malley J, Jaeger RJ. Evaluating interventions to improve gait in cerebral palsy: a meta-analysis of spatiotemporal measures. Dev Med Child Neurol. 2007;49(7):542–9.
146. Butler C, Chambers H, Goldstein M, Harris S, Leach J, Campbell S, et al. Evaluating research in developmental disabilities: a conceptual framework for reviewing treatment outcomes. 1999. http://www.aacpdm.org/index?service=page/treatmentOutcomesReport.
147. Shaer CM, Chescheir N, Schulkin J. Myelomeningocele: a review of the epidemiology, genetics, risk factors for conception, prenatal diagnosis, and prognosis for affected individuals. Obstet Gynecol Surv. 2007;62(7):471–9.
148. Thomson JD, Segal LS. Orthopedic management of spina bifida. Dev Disabil Res Rev. 2010;16(1):96–103.
149. Moen TC, Dias L, Swaroop VT, Gryfakis N, Kelp-Lenane C. Radical posterior capsulectomy improves sagittal knee motion in crouch gait. Clin Orthop Relat Res. 2011;469(5):1286–90.
150. Davies MB, Smith TWD. Neuromuscular foot deformities in childhood. Curr Orthop. 2002;16:96–103.
151. Drennan JC. Foot deformities in myelomeningocoele. AAOS Instr Course Lect. 1991;40:287–91.
152. Janicki JA, Narayanan UG, Harvey B, Roy A, Ramseier LE, Wright JG. Treatment of neuromuscular and syndrome-associated (nonidiopathic) clubfeet using the Ponseti method. J Pediatr Orthop. 2009;29(4):393–7.
153. World Health Organization (WHO). 2022. https://www.who.int/news-room/fact-sheets/detail/poliomyelitis.
154. Mortens J, Pilcher MF. Tendon transplantation in the prevention of foot deformities after poliomyelitis in children. J Bone Joint Surg Br. 1956;38-B(3):633–9.
155. Sharrard WJ. The distribution of the permanent paralysis in the lower limb in poliomyelitis; a clinical and pathological study. J Bone Joint Surg Br. 1955;37-B(4):540–58.
156. Watts HG. Orthopedic techniques in the management of the residua of paralytic poliomyelitis. Tech Orthop. 2005;20(2):179–89.
157. Krajewski KM, Lewis RA, Fuerst DR, Turansky C, Hinderer SR, Garbern J, et al. Neurological dysfunction and axonal degeneration in Charcot-Marie-tooth disease type 1A. Brain. 2000;123(Pt 7):1516–27.
158. Shy ME, Lupski JR, Chance PF, Klein CJ, Dyck PJ. Hereditary motor and sensory neuropathies: an overview of clinical, genetic, electrophysiologic, and pathologic features. In: Dyck PJ, Thomas PK, editors. Peripheral neuropathy. 4th ed. Philadelphia: Saunders; 2005. p. 1623–58.
159. Yagerman SE, Cross MB, Green DW, Scher DM. Pediatric orthopedic conditions in Charcot-Marie-Tooth disease: a literature review. Curr Opin Pediatr. 2012;24(1):50–6.
160. Wukich DK, Bowen JR. A long-term study of triple arthrodesis for correction of pes cavovarus in Charcot-Marie-tooth disease. J Pediatr Orthop. 1989;9(4):433–7.
161. Kumar SJ, Marks HG, Bowen JR, MacEwen GD. Hip dysplasia associated with Charcot-Marie-tooth disease in the older child and adolescent. J Pediatr Orthop. 1985;5(5):511–4.
162. Walker JL, Nelson KR, Heavilon JA, Stevens DB, Lubicky JP, Ogden JA, et al. Hip abnormalities in children with Charcot-Marie-tooth disease. J Pediatr Orthop. 1994;14(1):54–9.
163. Novais EN, Bixby SD, Rennick J, Carry PM, Kim YJ, Millis MB. Hip dysplasia is more severe in Charcot-Marie-tooth disease than in developmental dysplasia of the hip. Clin Orthop Relat Res. 2014;472(2):665–73.
164. Duan D, Goemans N, Takeda S, et al. Duchenne muscular dystrophy. Nat Rev Dis Primers. 2021;7:13. https://doi.org/10.1038/s41572-021-00248-3.

165. Mah JK, et al. A systematic review and meta-analysis on the epidemiology of Duchenne and Becker muscular dystrophy. Neuromuscul Disord. 2014;24:482–91.
166. Mercuri E, Bonnemann CG, Muntoni F. Muscular dystrophies. Lancet. 2019;394:2025–38.
167. Alman BA, Raza SN, Biggar WD. Steroid treatment and the development of scoliosis in males with Duchenne muscular dystrophy. J Bone Joint Surg Am. 2004;86-A(3):519–24.
168. King WM, Ruttencutter R, Nagaraja HN, Matkovic V, Landoll J, Hoyle C, et al. Orthopedic outcomes of long-term daily corticosteroid treatment in Duchenne muscular dystrophy. Neurology. 2007;68(19):1607–13.
169. Propp R, McAdam L, Davis A, Salbach N, Weir S, Encisa C, Narayanan UG. Development and content validation of the muscular dystrophy child health index of life with disabilities questionnaire for children with Duchenne muscular dystrophy. Dev Med Child Neurol. 2019;61(1):75–81.

Arthrogryposis

Reggie C. Hamdy, Yousef Marwan, Khaled Abu Dalu, and Noémi Dahan-Oliel

Arthrogryposis is a group of disorders characterized by non-progressive, multiple joint contractures and muscle weakness, present at birth [1]. The word "arthrogryposis" is derived from the Greek language (arthro = joint and gryp = curved), referring to the multiple congenital contractures inherent to this category of disorders [2]. Most individuals with arthrogryposis have normal or above normal intelligence and normal sensation. Arthrogryposis can be seen in isolation or in association with other congenital abnormalities as part of a syndrome with or without visceral and/or central nervous system involvement [3]. There are over 300 different syndromes associated with congenital contractures [4], the most common being amyoplasia affecting all four limbs [5]. Contractures typically affect two or more areas of the body and limit children's mobility, self-care, and daily activities.

Prevalence

The overall prevalence of arthrogryposis has been estimated at 1 in every 3000 live births [6]. Recently, the prevalence of arthrogryposis was reported to range from 1 in 2000 in Leicester, UK [7], to 1 in 5100 in Alberta, Canada [8].

Etiology

The main cause of arthrogryposis is diminished fetal movements, resulting from either fetal or maternal abnormalities. The decreased fetal movements ultimately lead to the development of multiple joint contractures, as connective tissue around the joint limits joint mobility, leading to contractures [2, 7]. During pregnancy, a limb will not achieve optimal growth when in utero movement is restricted for several months [2]. There are numerous causes of diminished fetal movements, including neuropathic, muscle or connective tissue abnormalities, space limitations of the fetus, intrauterine vascular compromise, and maternal diseases [2, 7]. Prenatal diagnosis may be possible by using repeated ultrasound studies to evaluate fetal movements and characteristic fetal positions.

Classification

Two main classification systems for arthrogryposis exist. The first classification system by Dr. Judith G. Hall was first published in 1997 and classifies arthrogryposis into three main groups, according to the presence or absence of associated visceral and central nervous systems [3] (Table 25.1). A more recent classification system by Dr. Bamshad and colleagues [5] divides arthrogryposis into three main entities, including amyoplasia, distal arthrogryposis, and syndromic (Fig. 25.1). The main difference among those two classification systems is the inclusion of different types of distal

Table 25.1 Hall classification of arthrogryposis

Group	Type of involvement
Group 1	Mainly limb involvement (four limbs, lower limbs, or upper limbs)
Group 2	Limbs are affected with involvement of other parts of the body
Group 3	Limbs are affected with central nervous system involvement

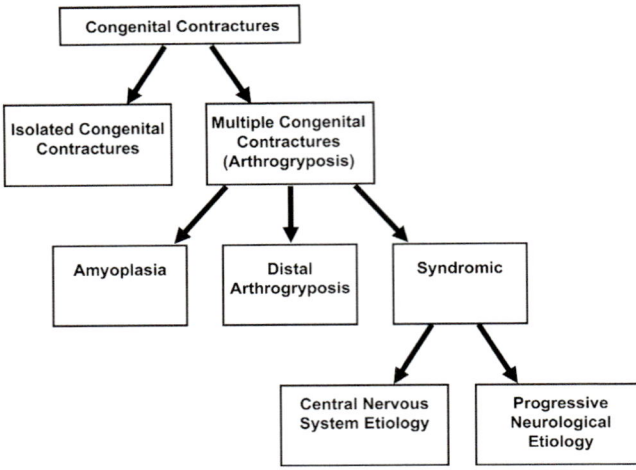

Fig. 25.1 Types of congenital contractures [4]. (Reproduced with permission from Bamshad M, Van Heest AE, Pleasure D. Arthrogryposis: a review and update. J Bone Joint Surg Am. 2009 Jul;91 Suppl 4:40–6)

arthrogryposes together, as in the newer classification, or as separate entities depending on involvement of body areas, as in the Hall classification. In this chapter, the different disorders encompassed by the umbrella term arthrogryposis are presented using Hall's classification [3].

Group 1: Disorders Affecting Mainly the Four Limbs

The most common disorder of this group is amyoplasia (a = no, myo = muscle, plasia = growth) meaning no muscle growth. It is the most common form of arthrogryposis, and represents one third of all cases. Most affected individuals have all four limbs involved. It has not been observed to recur in siblings [2].

Distal arthrogryposes (DA), as the name indicates, involve the distal joints, and do not involve a primary neurological and/or muscle disease. Distal arthrogryposes share a pattern of hand and foot involvement, limited involvement of proximal joints, and variable expressivity [5]. These disorders are inherited as autosomal dominant traits. Currently, distal arthrogryposes are subdivided into ten types, depending on the number and nature of additional features [5]. Of these, type 5 can be further divided into several subtypes based on additional phenotypic features [9, 10]. Type I (DA1) is characterized by a typical positioning of the hands with medially overlapping fingers, clenched fists, ulnar deviation of the fingers and camptodactyly, and clubfoot. The degree of joint deformity is highly variable. The other types of distal arthrogryposes involve other body parts (e.g., eyes, mouth), and hence are presented as part of group 2 arthrogryposes.

There are other types of arthrogryposis involving mainly the limbs and which are included in group 1, such as contractural arachnodactyly and symphalangism [2].

Both amyoplasia and distal arthrogryposis type I have been found to respond well to physical therapy [11, 12] and these disorders are usually seen by orthopedic surgeons.

Group 2: Disorders Affecting the Limbs with Involvement of Other Parts of the Body

Distal arthrogryposes (DA) other than type 1 are included in this group as in addition to contractures of the hands and feet, they involve other body parts. Type 2 can be further separated into two subtypes, Freeman–Sheldon syndrome (FSS or DA2A) and Sheldon–Hall syndrome (SHS or DA2B) [5]. The defining characteristic in FSS is that oropharyngeal abnormalities, scoliosis, and a very small oral orifice, puckered lips, and dimple in the chin, hence the name "whistling-face syndrome" (Fig. 25.2). SHS has similar congenital contractures present in DA1, with the addition of more prominent nasolabial folds, palpebral fissures, and a small mouth [5]. DA3 and DA4 are very rare. DA5 is unique in that ocular abnormalities are present in addition to muscle contractures. Other types of DA are very rare and have distinguishing features, such as very short stature and cleft palate

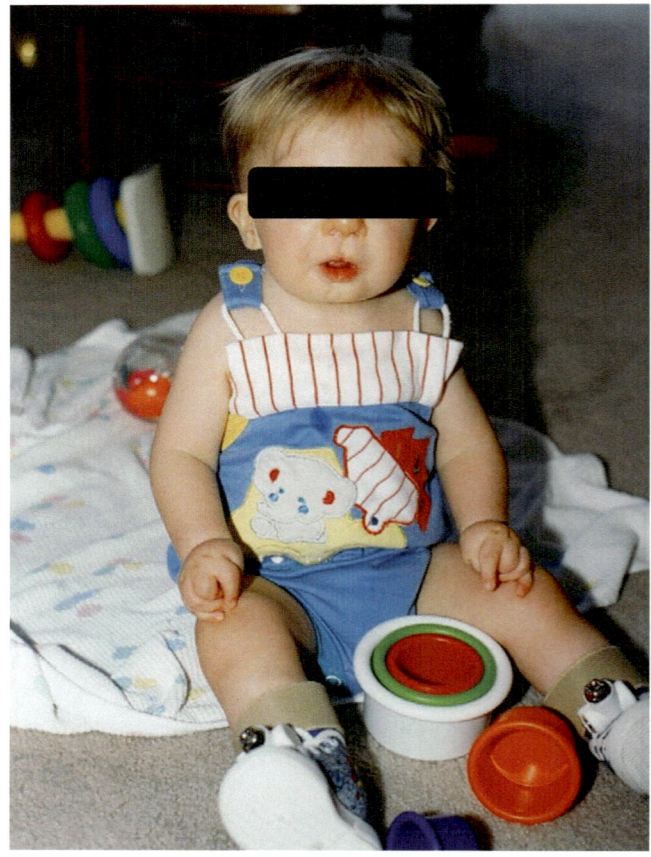

Fig. 25.2 Photograph of a toddler with Freeman–Sheldon syndrome showing typical facies. (Reproduced with permission from Bamshad M, Van Heest AE, Pleasure D. Arthrogryposis: a review and update. J Bone Joint Surg Am. 2009 Jul;91 Suppl 4:40–6)

Fig. 25.3 (a, b) Eleven-year-old boy with popliteal pterygium syndrome

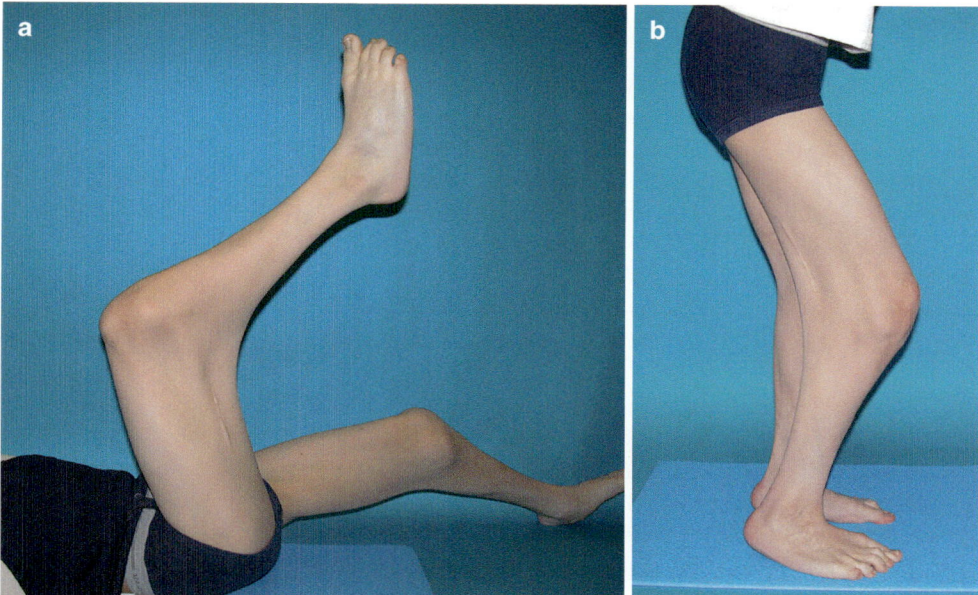

in DA6, and inability to fully open the mouth and pseudo-camptodactyly in DA7 [5].

In addition to DA, there are many different syndromes involving muscle contractures and other body areas [3], such as multiple pterygium syndromes, diastrophic dysplasia, and Larsen syndrome. Multiple pterygium syndromes involve a web or triangular membrane that forms across a joint [3]. Different pterygium syndromes have different forms of inheritance and features. Popliteal pterygium syndrome is the most common of the multiple pterygium syndromes, but is very rare and affects 1 in 300,000 live births. It is inherited as autosomal dominant with a wide pattern of expression. Key features include genitourinary, craniofacial, and extremity malformations in association with popliteal webs that vary greatly in severity. The fixed knee and ankle deformities render ambulation difficult (Fig. 25.3). Diastrophic dysplasia involves contractures of the shoulders, elbows, interphalangeal joints, and hips [2, 3]. This type of dwarfism has an autosomal recessive inheritance. Other features include cystic masses involving the external ear and cleft palate [2]. Mortality rate is increased during infancy, but life expectancy is normal past infancy. Larsen syndrome involves a distinctive facial appearance with flattening of the face, prominent forehead, depressed nasal bridge, widely spaced eyes, and ligamentous hyperlaxity, as well as flexed hips and hyperextended knees [2]. Often, there are multiple joint dislocations (hips, knees, shoulder, and elbows), hand deformities with long cylindrical fingers, feet deformities in the form of equinovarus or equinovalgus, and a high incidence of spine anomalies, specifically cervical kyphosis caused by marked hypoplasia of one or two vertebral bodies. Congenital cardiac and respiratory anomalies may also be present. The management of the orthopedic problems is usually surgical.

Group 3: Disorders Affecting the Limbs with Involvement of the Central Nervous System

Numerous syndromes with involvement of the central nervous system can have associated congenital contractures [3]. These may be caused by developmental abnormalities of the forebrain in utero, chromosomal deletions or rearrangements, or genetic mutations. These disorders are the most common cause of severe arthrogryposis [5]. Nerve conduction studies and EMG may be indicated in the case of neuromuscular disorders associated with arthrogryposis [5].

Genetic Aspects of Arthrogryposis

Multiple congenital contractures are present in a number of genetic syndromes. Many specific types of arthrogryposis have been mapped to loci in human chromosomes [2, 3]. The disorder may be caused by a single gene, in which case the disorder can be autosomal dominant, autosomal recessive, or X-linked. Rarely, disorders have a much higher risk of recurrence, such as mitochondrial inheritance. The presence of chromosomal abnormalities is prominent in cases of multiple congenital contractures with intellectual disability. Recent studies have identified several genetic mutations responsible for different forms of arthrogryposis [13–16]. Some types of arthrogryposis are sporadic, such as amyoplasia, in which genetics does not play a role in its inheritance. Prenatal testing and genetic counseling are indicated for parents with a higher risk of having another affected child.

Intellectual Skills

Intelligence is normal in many forms of arthrogryposis, including amyoplasia, distal arthrogryposis type I, diastrophic dysplasia, and Larsen syndrome. Patients with certain forms of arthrogryposis associated with chromosomal abnormalities or with CNS involvement may have decreased cognitive function [2].

Workup of a Child with Arthrogryposis

Any infant or child seen with multiple contractures should have a thorough clinical evaluation including a comprehensive family history, physical examination, and if necessary, further workup. In the physical examination, it should be determined first if arthrogryposis involves only the limbs or if it involves also other parts of the body, specifically the central nervous system. Second, it is important to determine which part of the limbs is involved, and to what extent. The range of motion of each joint should be carefully recorded. Radiographs of the spine, hips, and feet should be obtained. Bone mineral density appears to be lower in children with arthrogryposis compared to age-matched peers [17], and should be investigated.

It is essential to determine if this condition is genetic or nongenetic, not only for management purposes but also for counseling the parents on the risk of future pregnancies. Genetic investigations should include both blood cells and skin fibroblasts as, in some cases, mosaicism may exist (when chromosomal studies on blood cells are normal but an abnormality is detected in the skin fibroblasts). The most common form of arthrogryposis, amyoplasia, is not a hereditary condition and no specific genetic diagnosis can be made in this condition.

The focus of this chapter is on lower limb deformities as it pertains to amyoplasia, as it is the most common form of arthrogryposis.

Clinical Picture

A child with amyoplasia presents with a typical clinical picture. In the upper limbs, the shoulders are internally rotated and adducted; the elbows are extended, the forearms are pronated, the wrist and fingers are flexed (Fig. 25.4). This pattern of upper extremity involvement is often described as a policeman's hand or a waiter's tip hand (Fig. 25.5). In the lower limbs, the foot is most commonly affected (about 90% of cases), followed by knee deformities (about 70% of cases) and then hip deformities in about 40% of patients. Flexion, abduction, and external rotation contractures of the hips are typically observed (Fig. 25.6) (Box 25.1). Often, there is loss of skin creases across the joints and dimpling at the sites of

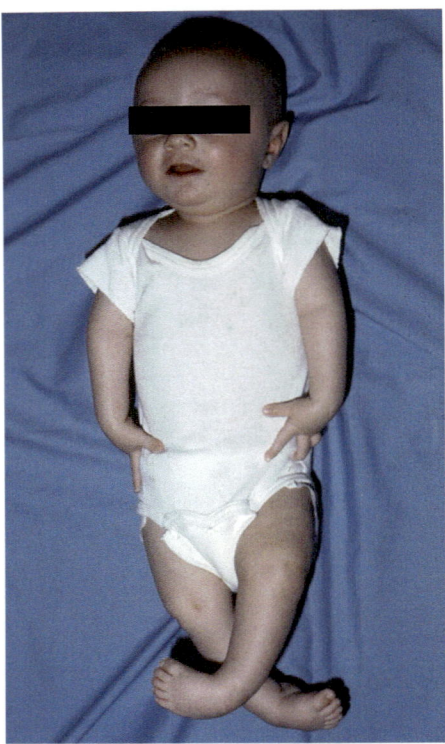

Fig. 25.4 Photograph of a 5-month-old baby with arthrogryposis showing bilateral clubfeet, extension contractures of the knees, and upper limb involvement with extended elbows and flexed wrists

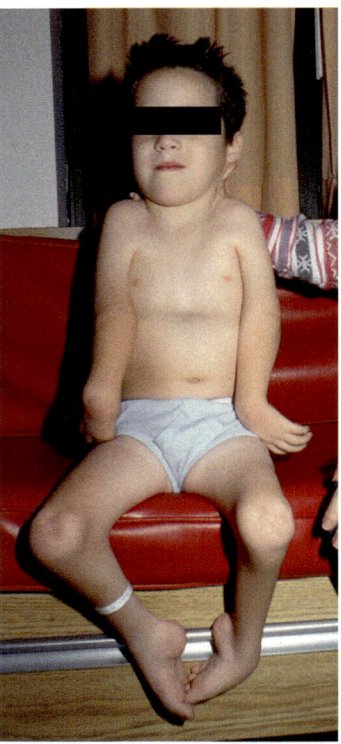

Fig. 25.5 Photograph of a 5-year-old child with arthrogryposis showing typical upper and lower limb deformities, including policeman tip position with flexed wrist and extended elbows in the upper limb, clubfeet and knee flexion contractures in the lower limb

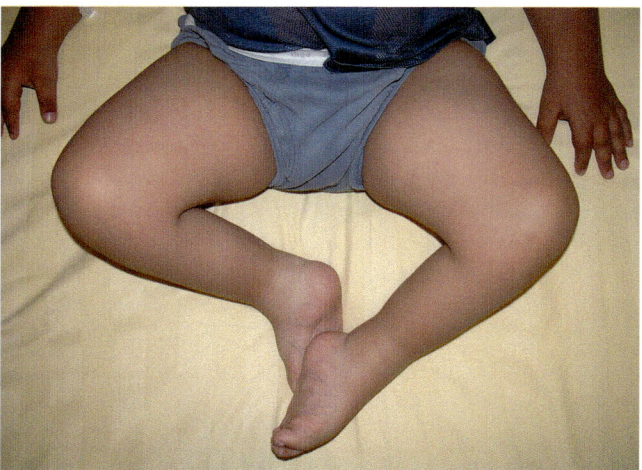

Fig. 25.6 Photograph of a 2-year-old child showing typical flexion abduction and external rotation contractures of the hips

the joints. The muscles are severely atrophied. Children with amyoplasia have normal IQ and normal sensation [18].

> **Box 25.1 Diagnostic Approach for the Lower Limbs in a Child with Amyoplasia**
> - The deformities are present at birth.
> - All four limbs are usually affected.
> - Sensation is normal.
> - Muscular atrophy and weakness is present.
> - Normal intelligence.
> - The feet are most commonly affected.
> - Knee flexion contractures are more common than extension contractures.
> - Hip flexion, external rotation, and abduction contractures of the hip, hip subluxation, or dislocation may be present.

Prognosis

The functional long-term prognosis is usually very good for most patients with amyoplasia, unlike other neuromuscular conditions. The contractures are usually most severe at birth and then gradually improve with life. The overall good prognosis should be clearly explained to the parents. Long-term ambulatory status and functional outcome at skeletal maturity are not necessarily correlated with the severity of arthrogryposis at birth, warranting early intensive treatment and rehabilitation in these children [19, 20].

General Management

Early intervention, in the form of aggressive physiotherapy including stretching, joint mobilization, and range of motion exercises, as soon as possible after birth, can facilitate optimal long-term functional outcome [5, 18–20]. Surgical interventions may also be indicated during the first year of life, as outlined below. Regular and frequent follow-up (every few weeks) is recommended during the first year of life to monitor progression and plan surgical interventions. This is followed by regular visits, typically every 6 months. Children with arthrogryposis should be followed in a multidisciplinary clinic. The overall goal in the management of these children is to improve function and ambulation while fostering optimal development. It is often recommended that the foot deformities be treated first, followed by the knee and finally the hip deformities [18].

Lower Limb

Involvement of the lower limb is common in arthrogryposis [12], and presents a challenging problem to the pediatric orthopedist [21]. Lack of joint motion may be due to inadequate muscle development, lack of normal and mobile skin and tissue, and contractures with fibrous connective tissue. These issues must be considered when devising the treatment plan, and include the affected joints (e.g., foot, knee, and hip) (Box 25.2). Range of motion of the knee and hip may be improved with treatment, thereby facilitating ambulation [22].

Foot

Clubfoot deformity or talipes equinovarus is the most common foot deformity in arthrogryposis and is present in over 90% of infants with amyoplasia [23]. Talipes equinovarus is much more common and is more rigid than the standard idiopathic clubfoot. It may be associated with knee contractures and hip contractures, subluxation, or dislocation (Fig. 25.7).

The goal in the management of feet deformities is to obtain a pain-free, plantigrade foot. Treatment should start immediately after birth with the Ponseti technique. Previous studies have reported that clubfeet in children with arthrogryposis are usually stiff and resistant to standard treatment and may require talectomy as a first-line treatment [24, 25]. However, more recently, it has been shown that tenotomy of the tendo Achilles before the start of the Ponseti technique may facilitate the manipulations and may yield good results with the Ponseti technique [26]. We recommend this approach as the initial treatment. In cases of failure of the Ponseti technique, a formal posteromedial release is recommended [27] even though the recurrence rate is high (Fig. 25.8). In cases where a posteromedial release is not sufficient to obtain a plantigrade foot, then a talectomy is advisable [24, 25]. The Verebelyi-Ogston procedure, which involves curettage of the subchondral cancelleous bone of the talus and cuboid followed by manipulation to collapse the bones and correct the foot deformity, is an alternative surgical option to talectomy in severe cases [28]. In cases of recurrent deformities, repeat soft tissue releases could be dangerous as the anatomy is completely distorted and neurovascular damage may ensue. Consideration should be given to correction through multiple osteotomies. The use of gradual correction with external fixators is another viable option (Fig. 25.9). A standard Ilizarov circular fixator could be used [29] or a Taylor Spatial Frame with the foot program [30]. In patients near or at skeletal maturity presenting with residual or recurrent foot deformities, triple arthrodesis may be the best option [31].

Conservative treatment in the form of the Ponseti technique, as described above, should be considered first. In case of recurrence or substantial residual deformity, a radical posteromedial release may be necessary around the age of 1 year followed by prolonged splinting to prevent or minimize recurrence of deformities [26, 30]. It should be clearly explained to the family that, while such surgical treatment will eventually correct the deformity, the foot remains stiff, with a high likelihood of needing subsequent surgeries as the recurrence rate is very high [24, 32]. If there is recurrence of the equinus deformity only in the skeletally immature patient, anterior distal tibial hemiepiphysiodesis could be a reasonable option to correct the anterior distal tibial angle and obtain a platigrade foot (Fig. 25.10) [32, 33].

Congenital vertical talus is reported to occur in approximately 2–12% of patients with arthrogryposis, most com-

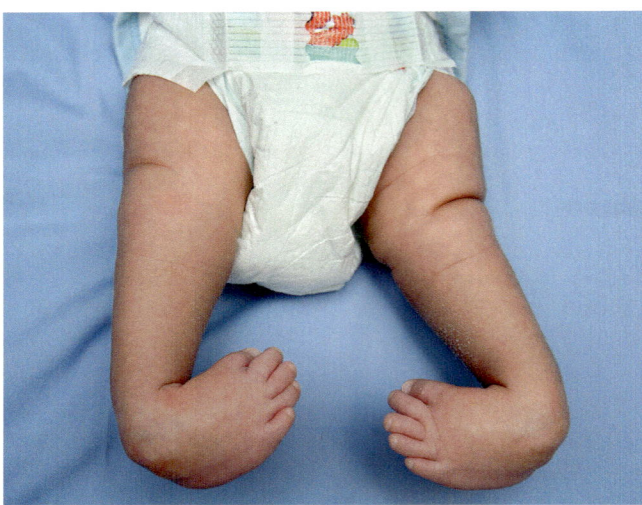

Fig. 25.7 Photograph of a 3-week-old infant with arthrogryposis showing right knee extension contracture, left knee subluxation, and bilateral clubfeet

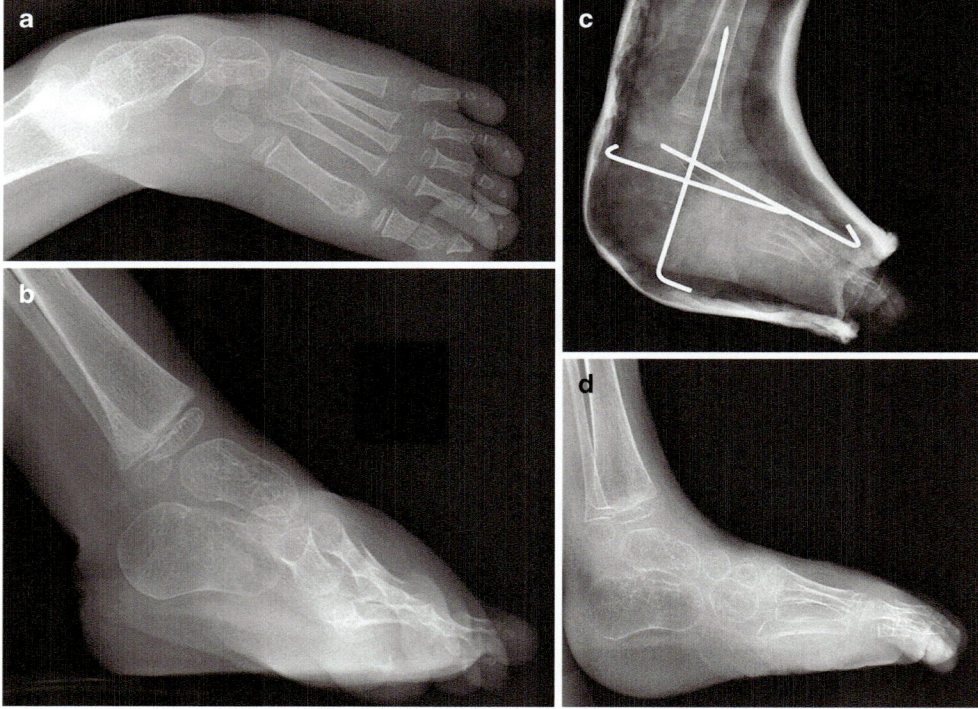

Fig. 25.8 (**a**, **b**) Radiographs of a 4-year-old child with arthrogryposis showing left clubfoot. (**c**) Postoperative radiograph following radical posteromedial release of the left foot after a failed Ponseti technique. (**d**) Three-month postoperative radiograph showing adequate correction

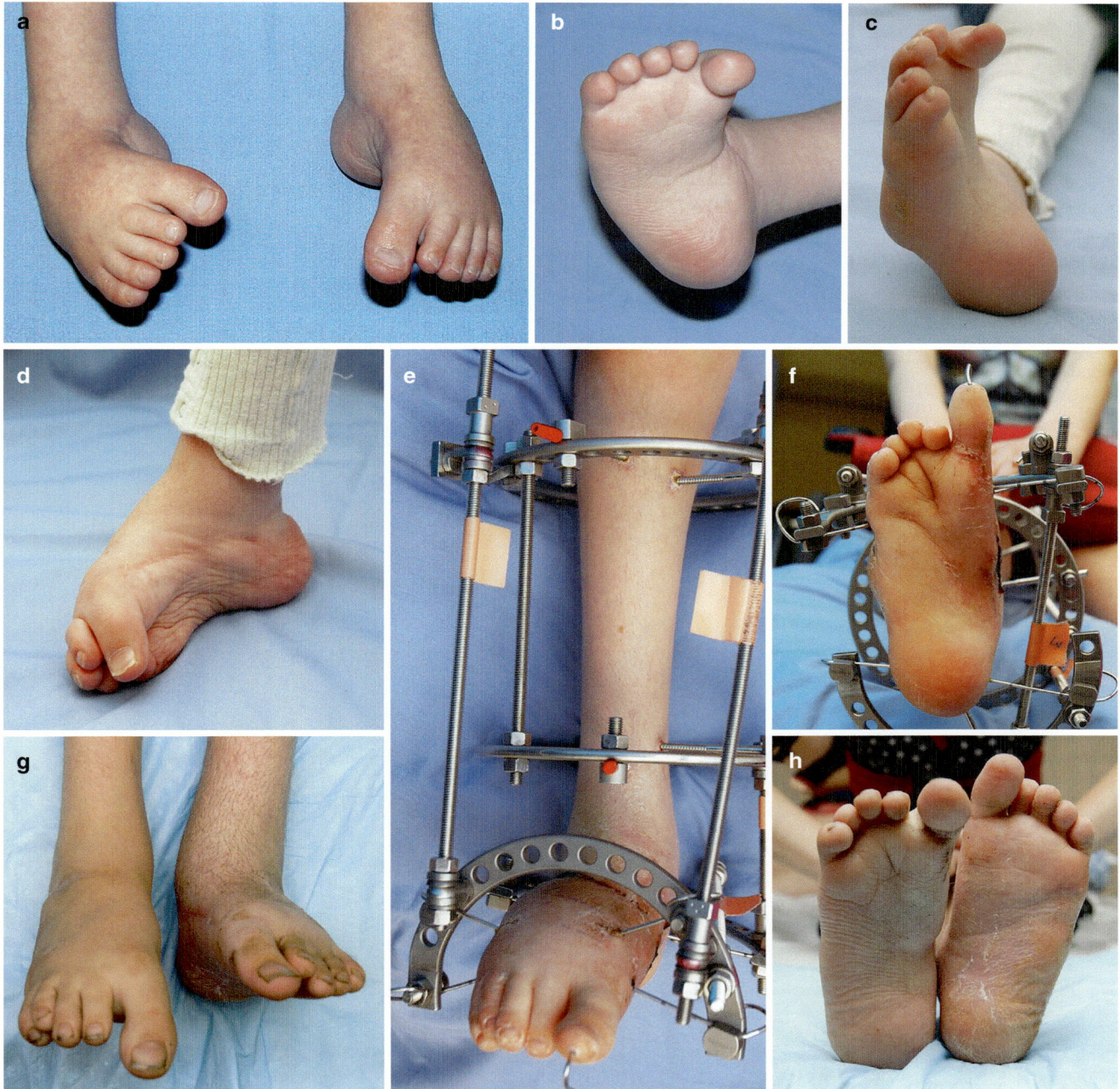

Fig. 25.9 Photographs (**a**, **b**) showing severe deformities of the right foot in a 3-year-old girl. The right foot is severely supinated at age 9 (**c**, **d**). Treatment of deformity with Ilizarov external frame (**e**, **f**). (**g**, **h**) Satisfactory alignment of the right foot post-Ilizarov removal at age 11

monly in distal arthrogryposis [34]. Because many of these patients have the potential to ambulate, the congenital vertical talus should be treated early, before walking age. Immediately after birth, the modified Ponseti technique should be initiated as described by Alaee, Boehm, and Dobbs [35]. This may be successful in the correction of the deformity. However, if the congenital vertical talus is rigid, then more aggressive treatment in the form of a one-stage release is usually recommended. A tibialis anterior transfer to the talar neck with or without Grice subtalar fusion is also recommended [36]. In very stiff feet and recurrent deformities, surgical options include excision of the navicular, talectomy, multiple osteotomies, and gradual correction with an external fixator (Fig. 25.11). If the patient is near skeletal maturity and has severe deformities, then a triple arthrodesis may be considered [36].

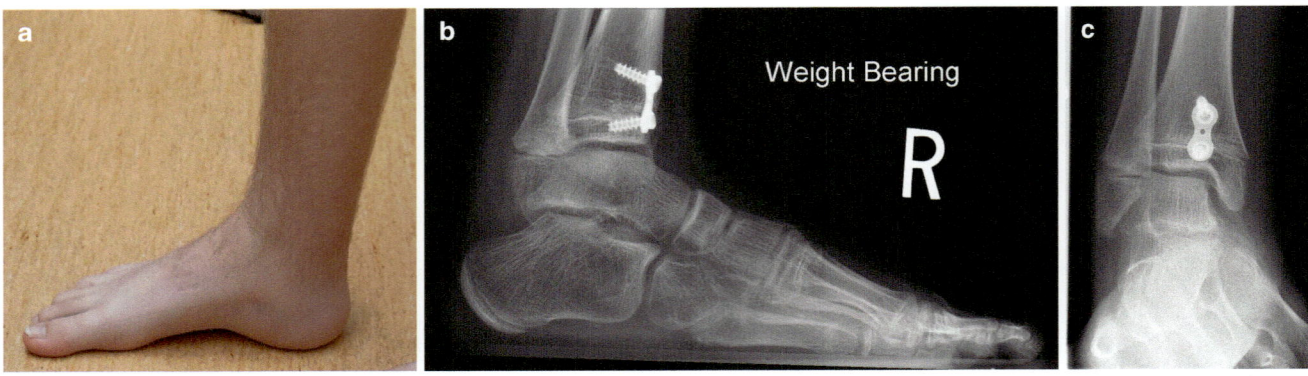

Fig. 25.10 Clinical (**a**) and radiological (**b** and **c**) images showing plantigrade foot position following equinus treatment with anterior distal tibial hemiepiphysiodesis

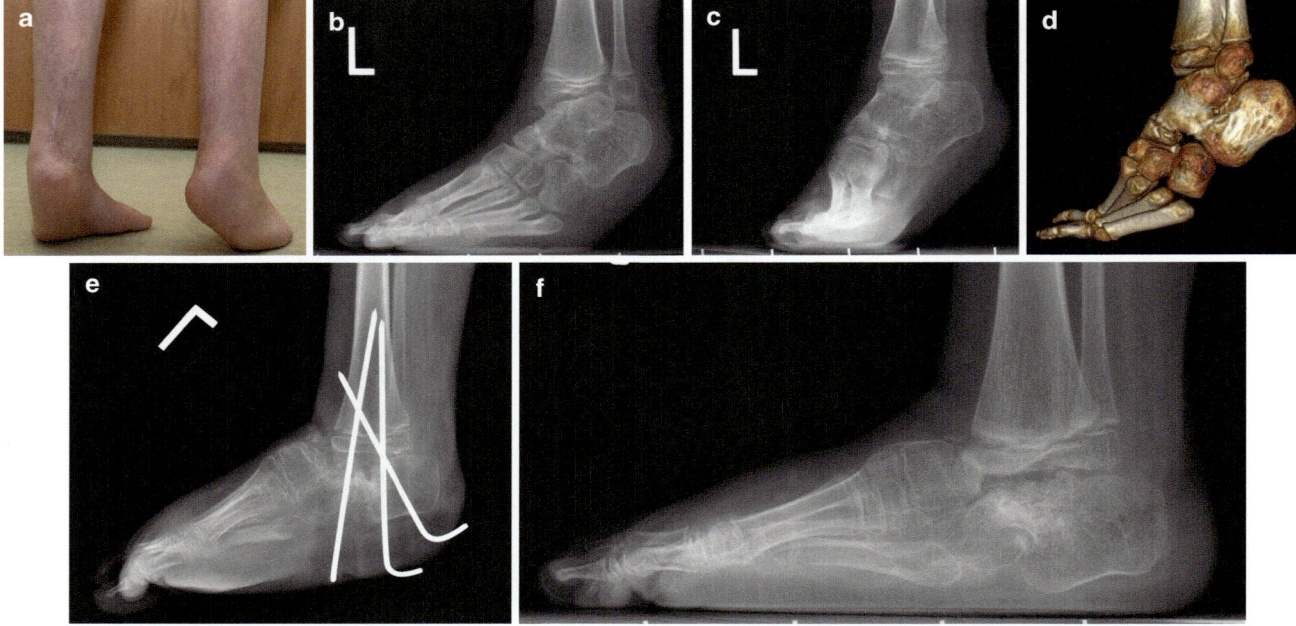

Fig. 25.11 A 6-year-old girl with arthrogryposis and feet contractures which failed previous surgical interventions and underwent talectomy to gain plantigrade feet position. (**a**) Clinical photograph of the feet deformity; (**b** and **c**) Lateral and transmalleolar radiographs of the left ankle/foot obtained preoperatively; (**d**) 3D-CT scan of the left ankle/foot showing detailed bony anatomy of the deformity; (**e**) Radiograph obtained 6 weeks following talectomy; (**f**) Weightbearing radiograph obtained 6 months following talectomy showing plantigrade position of the foot

Knee

The knee is the second most commonly affected lower extremity joint in amyoplasia (38–90% of patients) [37]. Knee contractures can be the most disabling deformity as they prevent motion and anatomical limb alignment [38]. Among knee deformities, flexion contractures are the most common in arthrogryposis [39, 40] and are also more disabling than extension contractures [39]. The goal in the management of flexion deformities is to facilitate ambulation, sitting, and standing (Table 25.2). Knee

Table 25.2 Indications of management for knee contractures

Knee contracture severity	Degrees	Management
Mild	0–20	• Physiotherapy • Stretching • Serial casting
Moderate	20–40	• Anterior distal femoral hemiepiphysiodesis • Soft tissue release
Severe	40–60	• Femoral extension osteotomy
Very severe	60+	• Gradual distraction

deformities may be more difficult to treat than other deformities and, more importantly, present some of the most challenging problems causing gait disturbances and may render ambulation very difficult [37, 38]. Contrary to extension deformities that may not interfere with walking, flexion contractures of more than 20–30° usually interfere with ambulation and should be treated. In fact, the presence of knee flexion contractures is the single most important indicator of the potential for ambulation. We and others have shown that correction of knee flexion deformities has a direct positive impact on the ambulation potential of these children [20, 40]. In our own series of patients where knee flexion contractures were treated with supracondylar osteotomies (Fig. 25.12) or with gradual correction using an Ilizarov circular frame, we reported that ambulation gains were maintained in most patients despite some loss in correction with time in many patients [20]. However, quadriceps strength should also be taken into account in the management of knee deformities as quadriceps weakness (noted in about 60% of patients) [41] may preclude any gains in ambulation despite correction of knee flexion deformity [37].

The fact that there are several options for the treatment of knee flexion deformities emphasizes the challenge that these deformities present [38]. Treatment of knee deformities should start at birth with intensive stretching exercises and bracing. If the flexion deformity exceeds 30° and is not responsive to physiotherapy, serial casting or braces with hinges may be used in order to gradually stretch the contracture. If these conservative measures fail to decrease the contracture to 20° or less, more aggressive techniques should be used such as soft tissue releases, femoral supracondylar osteotomy with or without shortening, anterior hemiepiphysiodesis of the distal femur, and gradual correction of the deformity using external fixators. However, some of these techniques have a high rate of recurrence in the skeletally immature patient and the natural history of knee flexion deformity is typically one of progression [42].

Soft tissue releases of the hamstrings alone are usually not enough to correct the flexion deformity, and the release should include the posterior capsule of the knee joint. The surgical dissection is not easy as much of the muscle is replaced by fibrous tissues and it may be difficult to identify the neurovascular structures. The posterior capsule has to be released in most cases as it is very thick and is believed to be one of the main factors in recurrence of the deformity [37]. Anterior hemiepiphysiodesis of the distal femur is another excellent option that has been recently described [42]. This technique is minimally invasive and should be used as a first-line treatment of flexion deformities in the skeletally immature patient with mild to moderate deformities—less than 45° [37, 43]. Care should be taken in the placement of the tension-band plates so as not to interfere with the patellofemoral joint (Fig. 25.13). Supracondylar extension osteotomy with distal femoral shortening is another excellent option in the treatment of knee flexion deformities as it avoids extension soft tissue dissection around the knee. The main problem with this technique is that it does not increase the range of motion of the knee—it only changes the arc of motion. Therefore, an increase in extension of the knee leads—at the same time—to a decrease in flexion, and this may interfere with the sitting position and getting in and out of a car [37]. Hence, careful planning of the treatment intervention is necessary, as well as a discussion with the patient and family preoperatively regarding the expectations of the surgery. Because of the rapid remodeling that occurs follow-

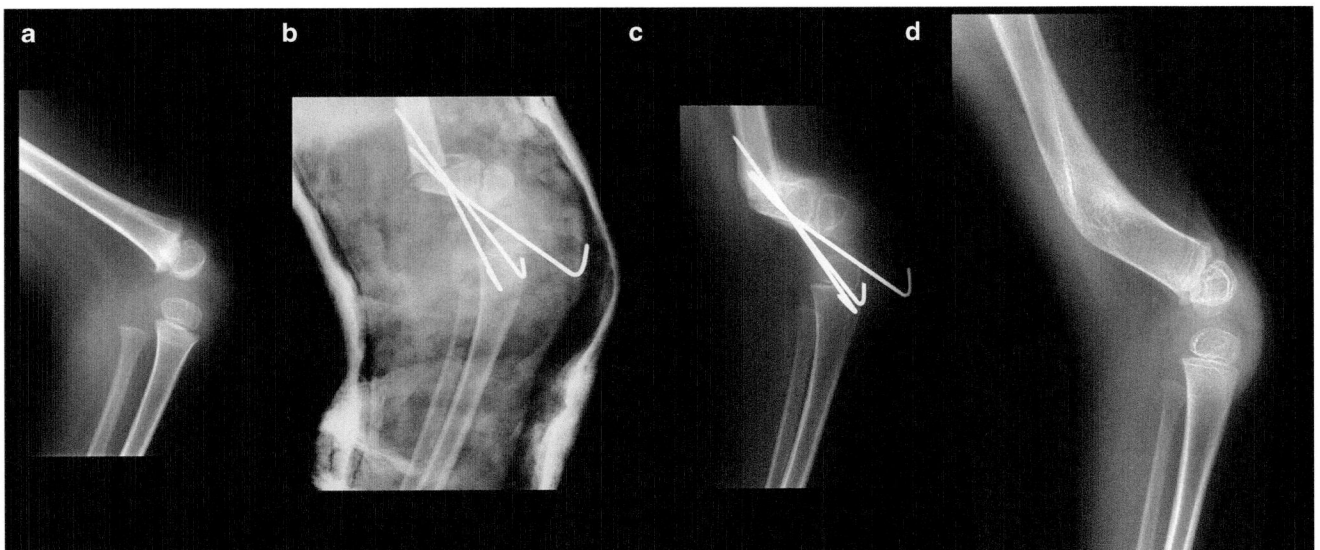

Fig. 25.12 (a) Preoperative radiograph showing a severe knee flexion deformity in a 5-year-old child with arthrogryposis. (b) Postoperative radiograph after supracondylar osteotomy was performed. (c) Radiograph obtained 2 months postoperatively. (d) Radiograph obtained 1 year postoperatively showing remodeling

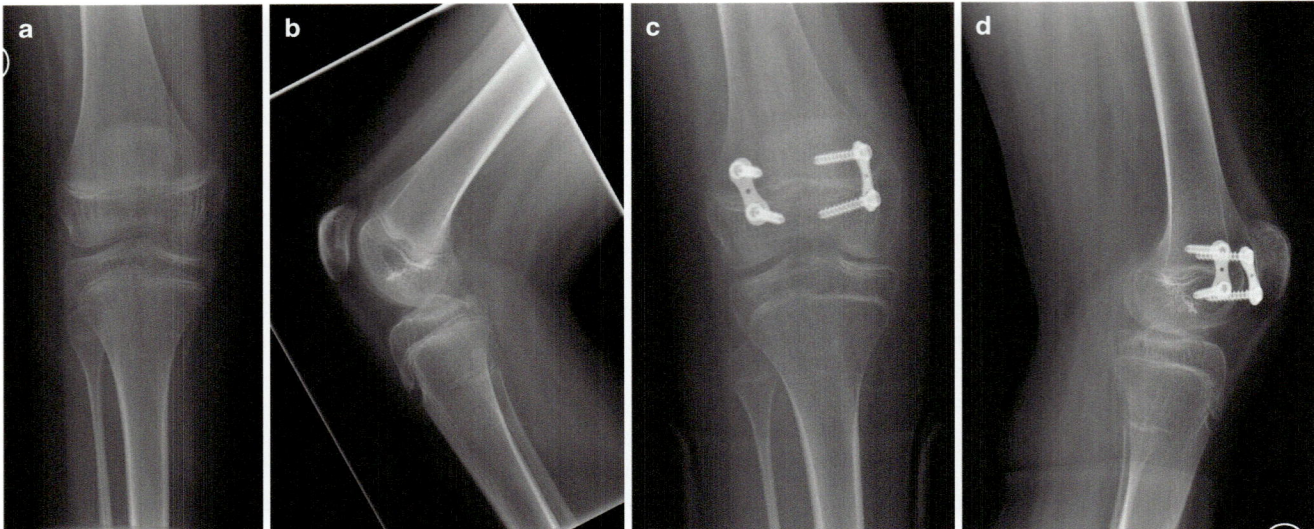

Fig. 25.13 Preoperative (**a** and **b**) and postoperative (**c** and **d**) radiographs of the right knee demonstrating correction of knee flexion contracture by anterior distal femoral hemiepiphysiodesis

ing these extension osteotomies (about 1° a month) [44], this technique has a high recurrent rate of flexion deformities and it is therefore preferable to reserve that technique for patients closer to skeletal maturity [38].

In severe knee flexion deformities of more than 60°, it may be safer to use gradual correction with external fixators [40] (Fig. 25.14). This has the advantage of protecting the neurovascular structures from sudden stretching, unless a concomitant shortening is performed with the supracondylar osteotomy. Posterior soft tissue release could be performed before the application of the external fixator [40]. Furthermore, gradual distraction may lead to an increase in the arc of motion of the knee. Attention to details of placement of the hinges when standard Ilizarov circular fixator is used is important in order to prevent subluxation of the knee or compression of the articular cartilage [37]. Gradual distraction may be associated with several complications, including fractures, exacerbation of the osteoporosis already present in these patients, knee subluxation, pin tract infection, pain, and recurrence of the deformity [40]. In older children who have underwent previous surgeries to correct knee flexion contractures, it is important to properly assess the radiological images to determine the center of the deformity as this may be coming from the bone, and therefore, requiring realignment osteotomy (Fig. 25.15).

Box 25.2 Management of the Lower Limb Deformities in Amyoplasia
- Early aggressive physiotherapy
- Feet
  - Early tenotomy of the tendo Achilles plus the Ponseti technique
  - If the Ponseti technique fails, consider posteromedial release
  - In recurrent equinus deformity, consider anterior distal tibia hemiepiphysiodesis
  - In severe and recurrent cases, talectomy or multiple osteotomies with acute or gradual distraction are indicated
- Knee flexion deformities
  - Stretching
  - Bracing
  - Casting following posterior soft tissue releases
  - Anterior hemiepiphysiodesis of the distal femur
  - Distal femoral extension osteotomies
  - Gradual soft tissue distraction
- Knee extension contractures
  - Stretching
  - Casting
  - Quadricepsplasty
- Hip flexion contractures
  - Physiotherapy
  - Soft tissue releases
  - Subtrochanteric extension osteotomy
- Hip instability
  - Reduce unilateral hip dislocation
  - In bilateral hip dislocation, surgical treatment depends on mobility of the hip
- The potential for ambulation is not related to the severity of deformities at birth; warranting early intervention for optimal long-term function

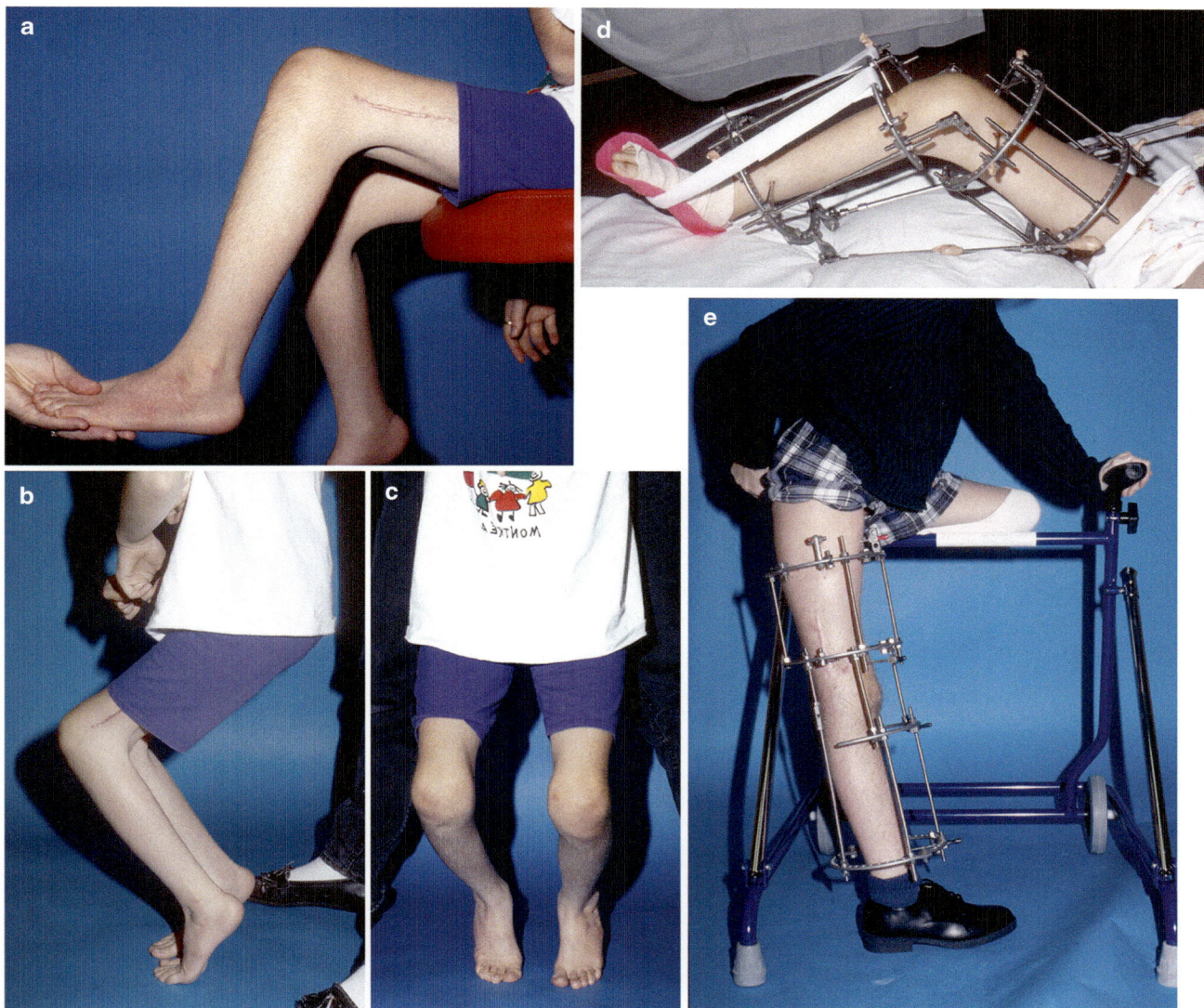

Fig. 25.14 (a) Photograph shows a severe knee flexion deformity in a 10-year-old patient with arthrogryposis (scar shows previous soft tissue releases). (b, c) Photographs show that the patient had difficulty standing with this degree of knee flexion contracture. (d) Photograph shows gradual correction with a circular external fixator. (e) Photograph shows full correction has been obtained

An alternative surgical option to improve the range of motion of the knee for cases of flexion contractures has been recently described [45]. The procedure involves peroneal nerve decompression, posterior knee release and proximal femoral shortening, in addition to early postoperative physiotherapy to maximize the gain in range of motion [45]. This surgical intervention achieved the desired outcomes even in cases with severe knee flexion contracture of more than 60°. This single stage acute correction can increase the range of motion by a mean of 34°, obtain full extension and improve ambulatory status of the patients at 2 years postoperatively [45].

Knee extension contractures are less common [37] and may vary from full extension of the knee with no flexion, knee recurvatum, and anterior knee subluxation to frank knee dislocation [37]. Long-standing deformities may lead to abnormal loading on the articular cartilage with subsequent damage and deformities of the epiphysis. Treatment of these contractures and/or dislocations should also start immediately after birth and include passive stretching, casting, and bracing. If knee extension contracture is associated with a clubfoot deformity, then corrective casting could be performed on both the foot and knee simultaneously [37]. If surgical correction of the foot is required, then sufficient amount of knee flexion is necessary in order to maintain the position of the foot, and hence knee surgery could be performed at the same time as the foot surgery [37]. In cases of failure of conservative treatment for knee extension contractures, a quadricepsplasty is indicated when less than 35° flexion is present despite nonoperative measures [46]. Most authors suggest that surgery should be performed early,

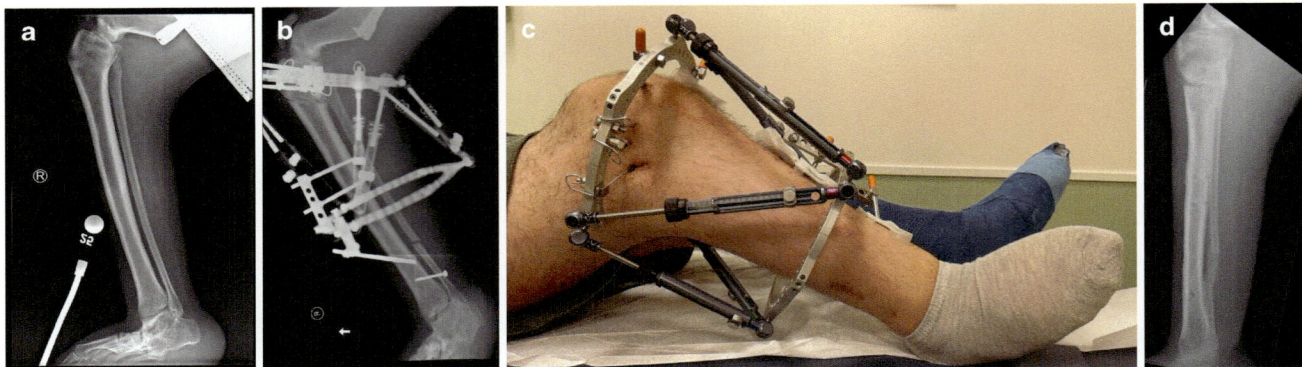

Fig. 25.15 Proximal tibia procurvatum deformity in an 18-year-old boy with arthrogryposis corrected with proximal tibia osteotomy and gradual correction with hexapod circular external fixator frame. (**a**) Preoperative radiograph; (**b**) Radiograph during treatment; (**c**) Clinical photograph of the leg during treatment; (**d**) Radiograph showing the final correction following removal of the frame

between 3 and 6 months of age [46]. Numerous techniques of quadricepsplasty have been described, including percutaneous, mini-incision, and open techniques [37]. Care should be taken not to over lengthen the quadriceps tendon [37]. Knee dislocations usually require surgery and should be reduced before 6 months of age [37].

Hip

Hip involvement is common in patients with amyoplasia and has been reported to range from 50 to 90% [19, 47]. Contractures may occur as isolated flexion or external rotation contractures, or as a combination of flexion, external rotation, and abduction contractures. Stretching exercises should start immediately after birth. It is difficult to apply orthoses for hip flexion contractures. An increased lumbar lordosis may compensate for a hip flexion deformity. However, if there is persistent hip flexion contracture of more than 30° despite physiotherapy, surgical treatment is usually required as such contractures may interfere with walking [48]. Soft tissue release should be considered, although it is very difficult to obtain complete correction of the contracture with soft tissue release only. Alternatively, subtrochanteric extension femoral osteotomy may be considered, but the recurrence rate is high [49]. For these reasons, it is preferable to wait until skeletal maturity before performing a subtrochanteric extension osteotomy. External rotation contractures may be beneficial as they widen the base of stance and in most of the cases do not need special treatment [18].

Hip dislocations occur in about 10–30% of patients with amyoplasia [50] and are almost always teratologic. Almost all authors agree that a unilateral hip dislocation needs to be treated in order to prevent pelvic obliquity, scoliosis, and unequal sitting pressure. On the other hand, the management of bilateral hip dislocation in children with amyoplasia is controversial. Some authors believe that attempts at surgical reduction of bilateral dislocations have a high rate of complications, including increased stiffness, avascular necrosis, and the possibility of redislocation and hence recommend no treatment. On the other hand, we and others favor reduction of bilateral dislocation as this may help function and ambulation [27, 47].

Closed reduction or the use of Pavlik harness is often unsuccessful [51, 52] and open reduction is usually necessary (Fig. 25.16). We prefer to use a Smith-Peterson approach, although a medial approach is advocated by others [23]. A complete capsulotomy near the acetabular brim is necessary, together with a pelvic osteotomy, usually an acetabuloplasty. A high rate of avascular necrosis, up to 70% in some series, has been reported [51]. Postoperatively, a hip spica should be kept for 8–12 weeks, followed by part-time bracing for another 12 weeks [18]. Bilateral stiff hip dislocations with limited abduction may interfere with toileting, and in such cases bilateral valgus osteotomies are recommended. (Fig. 25.17).

In patients with severe, multiplanar, arthrogrypotic hip contractures that restrict sitting or ambulation, proximal femur reorientation osteotomy that aims to align the lower extremity with the body without changing the femoral-acetabular relationship has been found to have good outcomes [53, 54]. This procedure can also be done for children with dislocated hips where relocation surgery is not feasible due to old age or severe stiffness, as well as for children with severely limited hip total flexion-extension arc that is not appropriately positioned for sitting and not improved with soft tissue releases. This osteotomy is done at the intertrochanteric level, correcting the hip contracture by altering the range of motion but not the total arc of motion, and is stabilized with a 90° angles blade plate. Patients with severe arthrogryposis may present with multiple severe lower extremity deformities that require several surgeries. In such cases, meticulous planning must be done as performing mul-

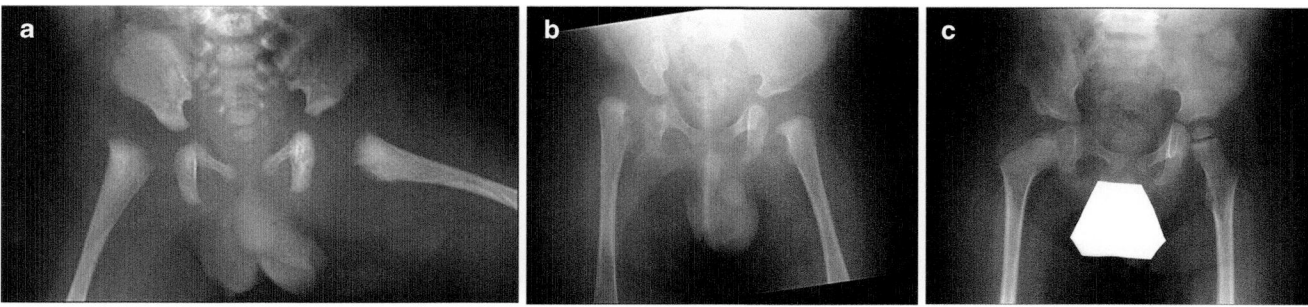

Fig. 25.16 (a) Radiograph shows a unilateral hip dislocation in a neonate with arthrogryposis. The contralateral hip shows limited abduction. (b) Radiograph shows failed closed reduction of the right hip and the limited abduction of the contralateral hip has been successfully treated with physiotherapy. (c) Postoperative radiograph obtained after open reduction showing avascular necrosis of the right hip

Fig. 25.17 (a) Radiograph of a young girl with arthrogryposis showing a bilateral abduction contracture of the hips. (b) Radiograph showing bilateral valgus osteotomies with increased abduction

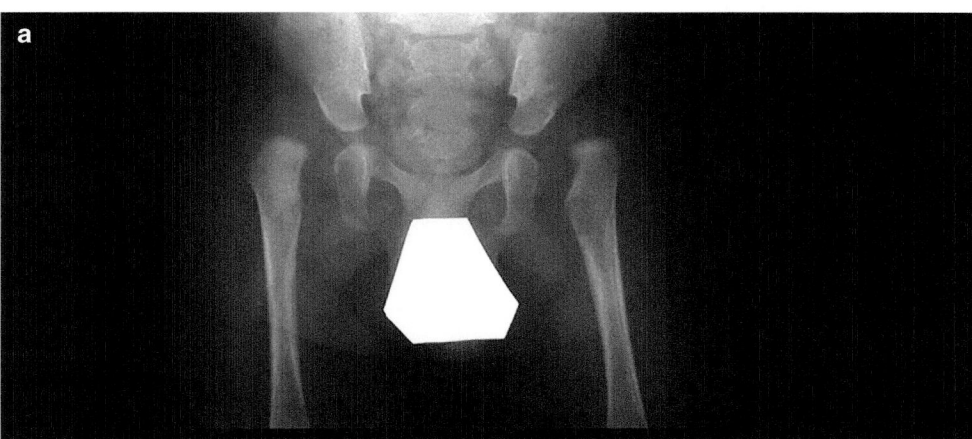
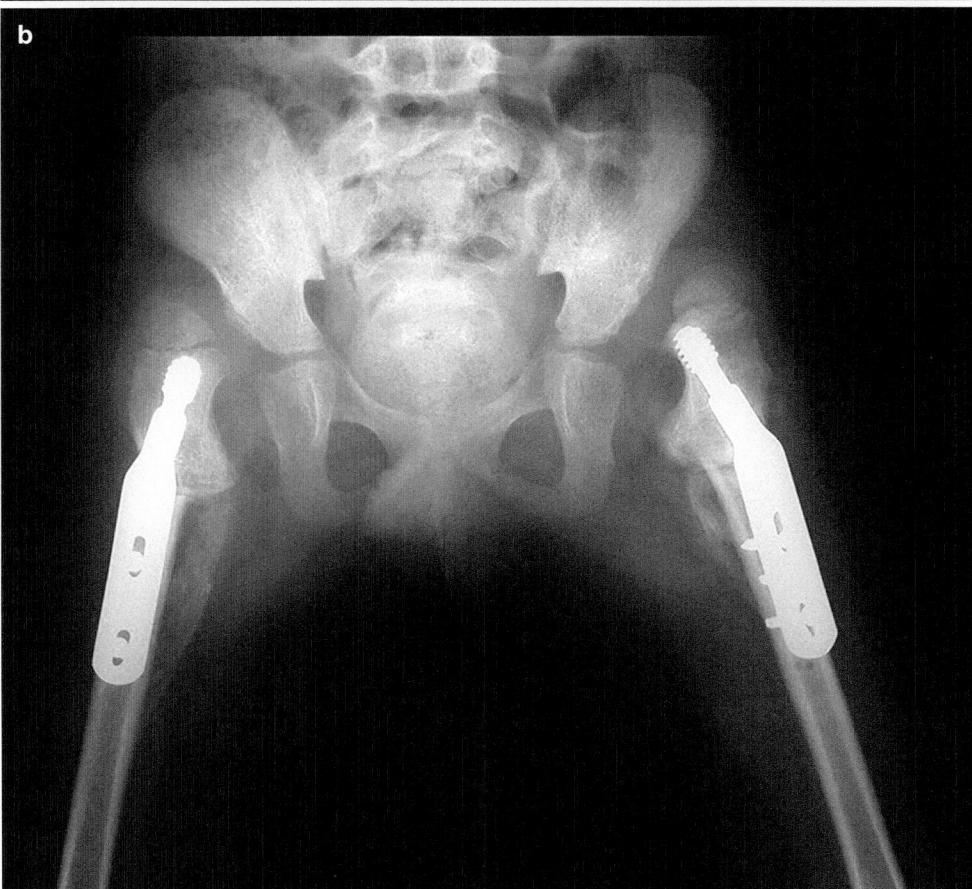

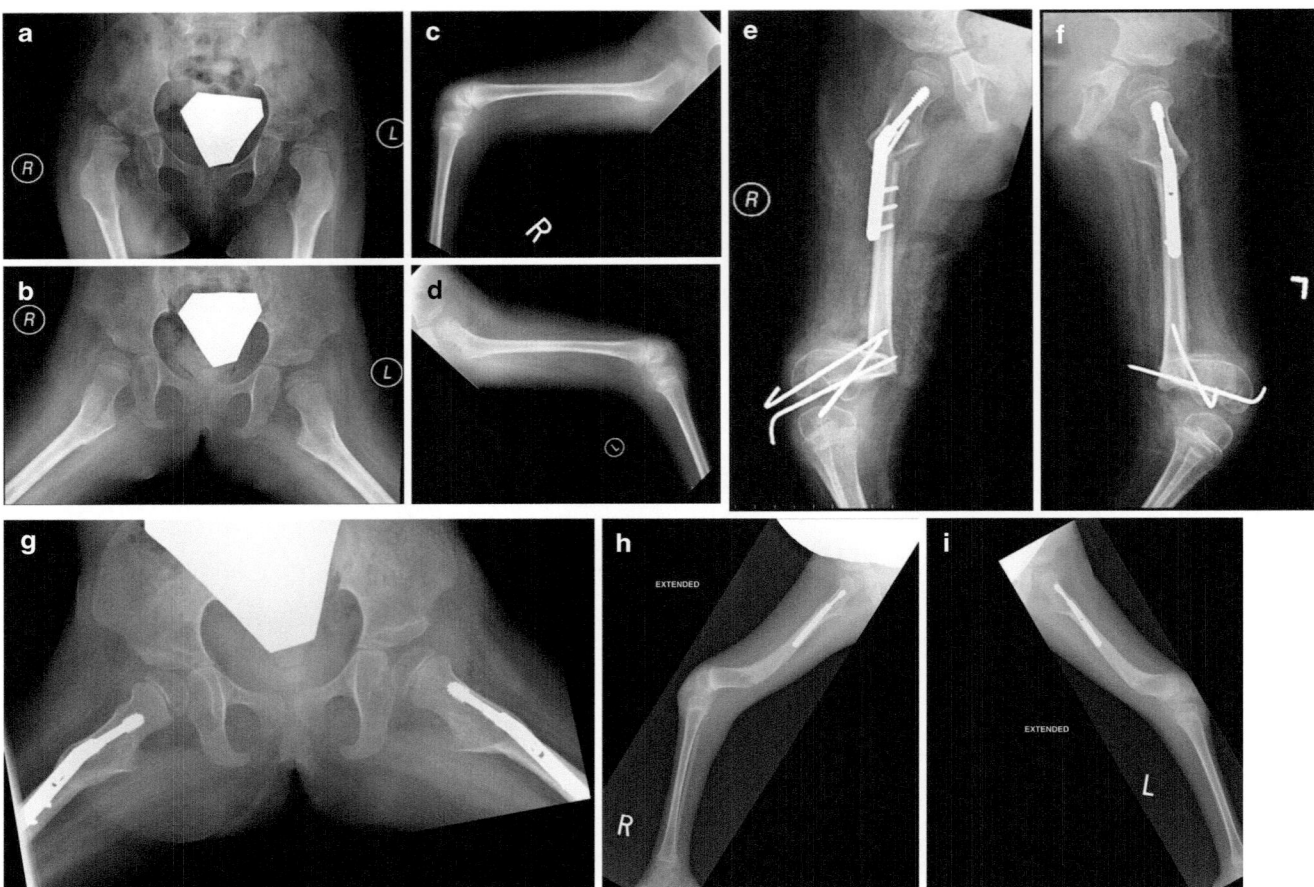

Fig. 25.18 Radiographs of a 5-year-old girl with arthrogryposis with bilateral hips and knees flexion contractures which were corrected simultaneously with proximal and distal femur osteotomies. (**a–d**) Preoperative radiographic views of the hips and knees; (**e** and **f**) Early postoperative radiographs; (**g–i**) Radiographs obtained 1 year postoperatively

tiple surgeries in different sittings will prolong the rehabilitation period and delay the functional gain. Therefore, simultaneous correction of multiple joints contractures should be considered. For example, hip and knee contractures can be corrected simultaneously with proximal and distal femur osteotomies [55] (Fig. 25.18).

Upper Limb

The classical upper limb deformities in arthrogryposis include adduction and internal rotation of the shoulder, extension of the elbow, flexion and ulnar deviation of the wrist, and stiff fingers with thumb-in-palm deformity. The goal in the management of upper limb deformities is to maximize functional independence by positioning the limbs for optimum use. For a long time, it was believed that the best position of the upper limbs should be one limb in full extension and one in flexion. However, absence of a strong unilateral grasp renders the use of bimanual function necessary, and therefore a bimanual use pattern of the upper limbs is recommended. Preservation of available elbow and wrist motion is essential [56]. Early surgical treatment is warranted if bony changes of normal elbow joints occur early on, and if development and independence in daily activities may be promoted through correction of the upper limbs [57]. Ideally, the upper limbs should be positioned at tabletop level in order to facilitate self-care, self-feeding, and the use of computers.

Scoliosis

The reported incidence of scoliosis in arthrogryposis is 20–30% [58]. About one third of children with amyoplasia have scoliosis. There is no single curve that is typical in these patients; congenital, paralytic, and idiopathic-like curves have been reported, and spinal deformity varies from minimal to severe [58]. Scoliosis is typically not present at birth but is usually detected during the first few years of life. Early onset, a paralytic curve pattern, and pelvic obliquity are poor prognostic patterns for curve progression. Bracing is usually ineffective in controlling the curve and most children with severe scoliosis will require surgical treatment. Combined anterior and posterior fusion seems to give the best curve correction with the least loss of correction after surgery. Children with arthrogryposis should have a physical examination of the spine early on with regular follow-ups, including upright radiographs to avoid an undetected severe deformity that is difficult to treat.

Orthopedic Management of Specific Conditions

Popliteal Pterygium Syndrome

Conservative treatment in the form of physiotherapy, traction, and casting is usually unsuccessful. Careful preoperative planning with MRI examination is essential in order to delineate the exact anatomical position of the sciatic nerve. When the popliteal webbing is mild, multiple skin Z plasties, excision of the posterior fibrotic band, hamstring lengthening, posterior capsulotomy, and tendo Achilles lengthening are recommended. When the flexion deformity is severe, femoral shortening and extension osteotomy with soft tissue release may be one option [59]. Another option that seems to give good results in severe deformities is gradual correction using a circular fixator, excision of the dense fibrotic band and multiple Z plasties of the skin.

Larsen Syndrome

Conservative treatment is typically unsuccessful in stabilizing the knees and surgery, including lengthening the quadriceps is recommended. The treatment of bilateral hip dislocations is controversial. Equinovarus deformities are treated with posteromedial release. Conservative methods are recommended for the correction of hip dislocations, knee deformities, and clubfeet, and operative correction should be performed once the child's general health is stable [60]. Because of the potential morbidity and mortality associated with cervical kyphosis, early posterior spinal fusion is indicated for patients with mild and flexible cervical kyphosis. Children with Larsen syndrome should be screened with radiographs at their first visit for early detection of cervical kyphosis to enable timely surgical management with posterior fusion [61].

Timing for the Management of Lower Limb Deformities

Many patients will have involvement of the feet, knees, and hip joints. The treatment should be individualized. However, early aggressive treatment, starting with the feet, then progressing proximally to the knees and then the hips is recommended. Intensive physiotherapy throughout the treatment process is strongly emphasized. We do not recommend simultaneous correction of multiple joint deformities at the same time because of the lengthy surgical intervention involved with such a procedure and the different rehabilitation programs for each joint.

Ambulation in Children with Amyoplasia

Most of the lower limb deformities are worst at birth and several studies have shown that many children with amyoplasia are able to ambulate, despite having had numerous surgeries [19, 48]. As previously mentioned, correction of severe knee flexion deformities facilitates ambulation. Muscle strength, specifically that of the quadriceps, may affect ambulation to a greater extent that the severity of the deformities [48] and hence the importance of muscle strengthening exercises. The importance of adequate bracing and its role in helping children ambulate cannot be overemphasized (Fig. 25.19). Other factors that may affect ambulation include upper limb function and the child's and caretakers' motivation. Although amyoplasia is not a progressive disorder, there is a tendency for recurrence of the deformities after correction.

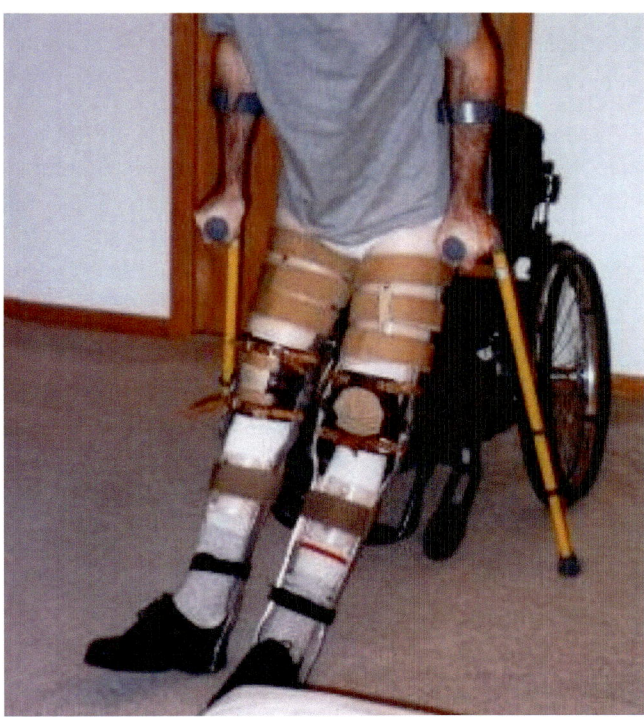

Fig. 25.19 Bracing and the use of canes to facilitate functional ambulation as well as transfers from a wheelchair

Rehabilitation

Multiple joint contractures usually affect the child's capacity of performing daily activities, such as feeding, dressing, grooming, toileting, mobility, and transfers. Decreased function in daily activities had a linear relationship with ambulatory level in 30 children aged 5–18 years of age with amyoplasia or nonsyndromic arthrogryposis, but normal scores in happiness and pain/comfort were reported [17]. Participation in sports and physical activity was found to be reduced in children with arthrogryposis compared to peers [17, 62, 63], demonstrating the need for rehabilitation in these children. The main objective of rehabilitation professionals is to maximize the child's potential and autonomy at home, at school and in the community. Stretching and bracing starting early in infancy is critical to optimize range of motion. Physical therapists focus on improving gross motor skills and mobility. Assistive devices (e.g., cane, walker, and wheelchair) are recommended depending on the severity of contractures and involvement of joints in order to promote independent mobility. Technical aids and other customized adaptations such as adapted utensils, raised working surface and adapted toys, and access to computers are provided to compensate for decreased function and facilitate autonomy in activities of daily living (e.g., feeding, writing, play, computer use). Occupational therapists focus on fine motor skills and activities of daily living. Splints or braces may be indicated to improve or maintain range of motion and joint alignment, to prevent contractures, and to maximize function in everyday activities such as eating, writing, or walking. Speech therapy, nutrition, and other rehabilitation areas may be warranted depending on the child's underlying needs. An individualized treatment plan delivered throughout the lifespan of the affected child with arthrogryposis via a multidisciplinary team is essential to promote each child's full potential during infancy, pre-school, school-age, and adolescence (Table 25.3). Adequate transitioning to adult health care services and preparation for independent living is recommended when the child is nearing discharge from the pediatric hospital center.

Table 25.3 Goals in rehabilitation during the lifespan

Lifespan years	Rehabilitation goals	Frequency of therapy
Infancy	• Increase range of motion and maintain gains • Positioning • Educate and reassure parents and family about handling and caring for their child	Weekly
Pre-school and school-age	• Maintaining range of motion • Strength training • Promoting independence in functional activities • Assistive devices to assist mobility • Technical aids and customized adaptations to maximize function in self-care, handwriting, computer, and leisure activities	Weekly or monthly for follow-up
Adolescence	• Therapy following surgery to improve range of motion and strength • Maximize independence in school and community • Transitioning to adult health care • Preparation for independent living	Intensive therapy postsurgery Consultation and monitoring as needed (e.g., driving)

Summary

Arthrogryposis is a general term that encompasses a multitude of different disorders with the commonality of multiple congenital contractures. The lower limbs are often affected, requiring surgical interventions and intense and long-term rehabilitation. Clubfoot deformity or talipes equinovarus is the most common foot deformity in arthrogryposis. The knee is the second joint most commonly affected. Knee contractures can be the most disabling deformity as they prevent motion and anatomical limb alignment. Treatment must be individualized and all the affected joints of the upper and lower limbs and spine should be comprehensively evaluated. Multidisciplinary treatment of the child with arthrogryposis with a focus on early and continued clinical evaluation is warranted for a positive prognosis and to optimize the affected child's integration in society and improve his or her quality of life.

Commentary

Harold J. P. van Bosse
Harold.vanBosse@Health.SLU.edu

The chapter by Hamdy et al. on arthrogryposis for the textbook Pediatric Lower Limb Deformities is a concise and thoughtful review on the current concepts. And it reminds us how arthrogryposis is big tent label for the more than 400 conditions that lead to a baby born with multiple contractures. As such, the term arthrogryposis cannot really be used as a diagnosis, since it is not specific for any of the individual conditions or diagnoses responsible for the formative fetal akinesia. Often, the most common form of arthrogryposis, Amyoplasia, is confused as the "true" form of the condition. The prevalence of Amyoplasia is estimated to be a third of all cases, but probably constitutes the majority of patients with arthrogryposis that a pediatric orthopaedist will see. It is important that all patients whose phenotype matches the agreed definition of arthrogryposis (a baby born with joint contractures of two or more body parts) are recognized as having arthrogryposis. Considering that the incidence of arthrogryposis (1:3000 births) is rarer than cerebral palsy (1–4:1000) but on par with myelomeningocele (2–5:5000), and more common than osteogenesis imperfecta (1:20,000), arthrogryposis seems to be relatively underrepresented in the orthopaedic literature, and in only the recent decades has it experienced a gradual increase in attention. Very often, practitioners would generalize what they knew of other conditions to develop a treatment plan for a child with arthrogryposis. Yet, the overlap of some arthrogrypotic deformities with deformities of other conditions has spurred awareness, such as when the Ponseti technique was found to be effective for arthrogrypotic clubfeet. This chapter helps to present, if not a uniform viewpoint, at least the most agreed upon treatment techniques and algorithms. For this commentary, I will include my own experiences to help broaden the subject.

The work-up to determine the specific diagnosis underlying a child's arthrogryposis is important from the standpoint of (1) providing the parents with information of possible heredity, should they be planning a larger family, (2) helping to determine a child's prognosis, which may change the treatment algorithm, and (3) help the patients themselves for planning their own family in time. Amyoplasia is the most common type of arthrogryposis, felt to be both a non-genetic condition and a diagnosis of exclusion. Most practitioners feel that a child with a classic Amyoplasia phenotype does not need an expensive and potentially uncomfortable work-up, unless findings arise that put the diagnosis into question. For other forms of arthrogryposis, the work-up has become much more specific and accessible, particularly with genetic testing. Although arthrogryposis panels can be helpful, they are limited by the number of conditions they include; whole genome sequencing has a higher rate of sensitivity for making a diagnosis. Luckily, current practice has largely abandoned routine acquisition of muscle biopsies, due to low diagnostic yields. Protocols to make pre-natal diagnoses more routine are needed, so that parents and practitioners can be prepared for the child, and curtail potential for misinformation. This likely will require coordinated efforts with obstetrics' groups to determine best practices for pre-natal ultrasound screenings, surveilling for fetal akinesia.

There are several treatment algorithms favored by those with expertise in arthrogryposis, which reflects both the importance of treating patients as individuals by creating a program that fits their specific presentation and needs, and the different philosophies and experiences of treating practitioners. The algorithms discussed in the chapter are well thought out and beneficial. My own algorithm is largely similar with a few differences. In general, my practice is to consider the constellation of contractures and deformities, rather than the specific kind of arthrogryposis the child may have. The exception is when other characteristics of their conditions will affect outcomes. For example, children with Wieacker–Wolff syndrome (ZC4H2 gene abnormality) often have congenital hip dislocation, but their prognosis for ambulation is guarded, therefore I will monitor their strength and coordination for an extended period before determining if they are suitable for a hip relocation. In general, my treatment plan is to address the foot deformities early on. After 1 or 2 years of age, I address the hip contractures and/or congenital dislocations. The knee flexion contractures are initially treated with knee-ankle-foot orthoses (KAFO), delaying surgery until they are anatomically large enough for surgery, usually about 4 years of age.

Treatment of foot deformities should start in infancy, but timing is not as crucial as we once thought. Many of us have experience correcting arthrogrypotic foot deformities with serial casting on children adopted at an older age from abroad who had no previous treatment. Providing the parents with even a few months to become acquainted with their newborn prior to starting treatment can be emotionally very beneficial. Relapses, particularly of clubfeet, are very common, regardless of the method of treatment (casting, surgery) and parents should be informed that multiple series of casting may be needed over the early childhood. Gradually, the interval between castings becomes longer, until the feet finally maintain their shape. The incidence of talectomies and posterior-medial clubfoot releases is luckily becoming less, as practitioners become more comfortable with obtaining clubfoot correction by casting. Unfortunately, relapses continue to occur after surgical treatment, and although a post-surgical relapse can be treated with casting, often the initial practitioner will continue with more invasive and ablative surgeries instead. An important characteristic of arthrogrypotic clubfeet is their association with moderate to severe external tibial torsion. This may cloud judgement of correction adequacy, for example when the foot seems well corrected relative to the leg yet the ankle mortise is facing laterally. Derotational osteotomies of the tibia are not unusual to maintain appropriate foot positioning.

My experience is that hip contractures inhibit ambulation worse than foot deformities or knee contractures in children with arthrogryposis, because the typical flexion-abduction contracture precludes positioning the feet under the body. By correcting hip contractures early, weight bearing can be begun. The treatment of the hip in arthrogryposis continues to evolve, particularly related to congenital dislocations. Previously the recommendation was not to surgically correct bilateral hip dislocations, due to concerns of stiffness and pain. These concerns were not substantiated in the literature, and were more a legacy of expert opinions. Our own unpublished data indicates that dislocated hips have a decreased range of motion pre-treatment, and on average only 4° of flexion-extension arc is lost on long-term followup. The most difficult hips to treat are those that lack hip flexion prior to treatment. The overpowering hip extensor musculature confounds attempts to stretch the hips into flexion, and gradually causes an anterior subluxation of the femoral head, complicating sitting.

Flexion contractures are the more common knee deformity. Prior to correcting the knees, the child's legs can be stabilized with KAFOs so they can learn to stand and walk. Heel wedges on the shoes worn over the braces can be extremely important in helping the patient balance over their flexed knees. In correcting the severe knee flexion contractures, we have found that gradual knee correction/distraction with an external fixator can adequately address pterygia without the need for Z-plasties. KAFOs and intensive physical therapy are required to maintain post-surgical correction and knee range of motion for both knee flexion and extension contracture treatment. Casting of knee extension contractures can be very rewarding, but great care needs to be exercised in understanding the anatomy before applying stretching casts, particularly if the casts are also addressing clubfoot deformities. The hips often have external rotational contractures, so that the medial femoral epicondyle is directly forward. The prominence of the epicondyle can be confused with the patella, so that attempts to flex the knee create a deforming valgus moment across the knee instead. In severe knee hyperextension conditions, especially those associated with Larsen syndrome, it may be necessary to place transarticular cross-pins to prevent the knee from subluxating during post-surgical casting.

Scoliosis presents a number of issues specific to children with arthrogryposis. A presentation nearly unique to arthrogryposis are babies born with a spinal curve. This is not a congenital scoliosis in the typical sense, as there are no vertebral malformations underlying the curve. Instead, it is a direct result of severe fetal akinesia, where the spine contracture mirrors the unchanging position of the fetus in the uterus. We coined the term "prenatal scoliosis" to help differentiate the curves from congenital scoliosis. Often these curves remain stable into mid childhood before progressing and needing surgical treatment. We have found serial spinal casting to be effective in slowing curve progression, allowing children further growth prior to undergoing surgical procedures; unfortunately, spinal casting in arthrogrypotic scoliosis rarely improves a curve. Expandable implants have made a meaningful change in treatment protocols of young children with arthrogryposis and scoliosis, although issues with stiffness and premature spontaneous spinal fusion can be problematic, particularly in children with Escobar syndrome. Children with Escobar syndrome have nearly a 100% incidence of scoliosis, of which there is a malignant variety, where the curve progresses to greater than 50° before 4 years of age, requiring early surgical intervention and occasionally an early spinal fusion.

References

1. Dahan-Oliel N, Cachecho S, Barnes D, et al. International multidisciplinary collaboration toward an annotated definition of arthrogryposis multiplex congenita. Am J Med Genet C Semin Med Genet. 2019;181(3):288–99.
2. Hall JG. Overview of arthrogryposis. In: Staheli LT, Hall JG, Jaffe KM, Paholke DO, editors. Arthrogryposis: a text atlas. Cambridge, UK: Cambridge University Press; 1998. p. 1–24.
3. Hall JG. Arthrogryposis multiplex congenita: etiology, genetics, classification, diagnostic approach, and general aspects. J Pediatr Orthop B. 1997;6(3):159–66.
4. Hall JG. Arthrogryposes (multiple congenital contractures). In: Rimoin DL, Connor JM, Pyeritz RE, Korf BR, editors. Emery and Rimoin's principles and practice of medical genetics, vol. 3. 5th ed. Philadelphia: Churchill Livingstone-Elsevier; 2007. p. 3785–856.
5. Bamshad M, Van Heest AE, Pleasure D. Arthrogryposis: a review and update. J Bone Joint Surg Am. 2009;91(Suppl 4):40–6.

6. Fahy MJ, Hall JG. A retrospective study of pregnancy complications among 828 cases of arthrogryposis. Genet Couns. 1990;1(1):3–11.
7. Navti OB, Kinning E, Vasudevan P, Barrow M, Porter H, Howarth E, et al. Review of perinatal management of arthrogryposis at a large UK teaching hospital serving a multiethnic population. Prenat Diagn. 2010;30(1):49–56.
8. Lowry RB, Sibbald B, Bedard T, Hall JG. Prevalence of multiple congenital contractures including arthrogryposis multiplex congenita in Alberta, Canada, and a strategy for classification and coding. Birth Defects Res A Clin Mol Teratol. 2010;88(12):1057–61.
9. Beals RK, Weleber RG. Distal arthrogryposis 5: a dominant syndrome of peripheral contractures and ophthalmoplegia. Am J Med Genet A. 2004;131(1):67–70.
10. Coste B, Houge G, Murray MF, Stitziel N, Bandell M, Giovanni MA, et al. Gain-of-function mutations in the mechanically activated ion channel PIEZO2 cause a subtype of distal arthrogryposis. Proc Natl Acad Sci USA. 2013;110(12):4667–72.
11. Hall JG, Reed SD, Greene G. The distal arthrogryposes: delineation of new entities—review and nosologic discussion. Am J Med Genet. 1982;11(2):185–239.
12. Sells JM, Jaffe KM, Hall JG. Amyoplasia, the most common type of arthrogryposis: the potential for good outcome. Pediatrics. 1996;97(2):225–31.
13. Alvarado DM, Buchan JG, Gurnett CA, Dobbs MB. Exome sequencing identifies an MYH3 mutation in a family with distal arthrogryposis type 1. J Bone Joint Surg Am. 2011;93(11):1045–50.
14. Attali R, Warwar N, Israel A, Gurt I, McNally E, Puckelwartz M, et al. Mutation of SYNE-1, encoding an essential component of the nuclear lamina, is responsible for autosomal recessive arthrogryposis. Hum Mol Genet. 2009;18(18):3462–9.
15. Hofmann K, Becker J, Heller R, Boute O, Andrieux J, Hoyer J, et al. 7 Mb de novo deletion within 8q21 in a patient with distal arthrogryposis type 2B (DA2B). Eur J Med Genet. 2011;54(5):e495–500.
16. Shaheen R, Al-Owain M, Khan A, Zaki M, Hossni H, Al-Tassan R, et al. Identification of three novel ECEL1 mutations in three families with distal arthrogryposis type 5D. Clin Genet. 2013;85:568–72.
17. Spencer HT, Bowen RE, Caputo K, Green TA, Lawrence JF. Bone mineral density and functional measures in patients with arthrogryposis. J Pediatr Orthop. 2010;30(5):514–8.
18. Bernstein RM. Arthrogryposis and amyoplasia. J Am Acad Orthop Surg. 2002;10(6):417–24.
19. Fassier A, Wicart P, Dubousset J, Seringe R. Arthrogryposis multiplex congenita. Long-term follow-up from birth until skeletal maturity. J Child Orthop. 2009;3(5):383–90.
20. Yang SS, Dahan-Oliel N, Montpetit K, Hamdy RC. Ambulation gains after knee surgery in children with arthrogryposis. J Pediatr Orthop. 2010;30(8):863–9.
21. Hamdy RC, van Bosse H, Altiok H, et al. Treatment and outcomes of arthrogryposis in the lower extremity. Am J Med Genet C Semin Med Genet. 2019;181(3):372–84.
22. Eriksson M, Gutierrez-Farewik EM, Broström E, Bartonek A. Gait in children with arthrogryposis multiplex congenita. J Child Orthop. 2010;4(1):21–31.
23. Staheli LT, Chew DE, Elliott JS, Mosca VS. Management of hip dislocations in children with arthrogryposis. J Pediatr Orthop. 1987;7(6):681–5.
24. Cassis N, Capdevila R. Talectomy for clubfoot in arthrogryposis. J Pediatr Orthop. 2000;20(5):652–5.
25. Drummond DS, Cruess RL. The management of the foot and ankle in arthrogryposis multiplex congenita. J Bone Joint Surg Br. 1978;60(1):96–9.
26. van Bosse HJ, Marangoz S, Lehman WB, Sala DA. Correction of arthrogrypotic clubfoot with a modified Ponseti technique. Clin Orthop Relat Res. 2009;467(5):1283–93.
27. Zimbler S, Craig CL. The arthrogrypotic foot plan of management and results of treatment. Foot Ankle. 1983;3(4):211–9.
28. Gross RH. The role of the Verebelyi-Ogston procedure in the management of the arthrogrypotic foot. Clin Orthop Relat Res. 1985;194:99–103.
29. Brunner R, Hefti F, Tgetgel JD. Arthrogrypotic joint contracture at the knee and the foot: correction with a circular frame. J Pediatr Orthop B. 1997;6(3):192–7.
30. Eidelman M, Katzman A. Treatment of arthrogrypotic foot deformities with the Taylor spatial frame. J Pediatr Orthop. 2011;31(4):429–34.
31. Chang CH, Huang SC. Surgical treatment of clubfoot deformity in arthrogryposis multiplex congenita. J Formos Med Assoc. 1997;96(1):30–5.
32. Iskandar HN, Bishay SN, Sharaf-El-Deen HA, El-Sayed MM. Tarsal decancellation in the residual resistant arthrogrypotic clubfoot. Ann R Coll Surg Engl. 2011;93(2):139–45.
33. Ebert N, Ballhause TM, Babin K, et al. Correction of recurrent Equinus deformity in surgically treated clubfeet by anterior distal Tibial Hemiepiphysiodesis. J Pediatr Orthop. 2020;40(9):520–5.
34. Aroojis AJ, King MM, Donohoe M, Riddle EC, Kumar SJ. Congenital vertical talus in arthrogryposis and other contractural syndromes. Clin Orthop Relat Res. 2005;434:26–32.
35. Alaee F, Boehm S, Dobbs MB. A new approach to the treatment of congenital vertical talus. J Child Orthop. 2007;1(3):165–74.
36. Hamdy RH. Chapter 4.3: Congenital vertical talus. In: Cramer KE, Scherl SA, Tornetta III P, Einhorn TA, editors. Pediatrics (orthopaedic surgery essentials series). Philadelphia: Lippincott Williams & Wilkins; 2003. p. 24–31.
37. Lampasi M, Antonioli D, Donzelli O. Management of knee deformities in children with arthrogryposis. Musculoskelet Surg. 2012;96(3):161–9.
38. Ho CA, Karol LA. The utility of knee releases in arthrogryposis. J Pediatr Orthop. 2008;28(3):307–13.
39. Murray C, Fixsen J. Management of knee deformity in classical arthrogryposis multiplex congenita (amyoplasia congenita). J Pediatr Orthop B. 1997;6:186–91.
40. van Bosse HJP, Feldman DS, Anavian J, Sala DA. Treatment of knee flexion contractures in patients with arthrogryposis. J Pediatr Orthop. 2007;27:930–7.
41. Södergård J, Ryöppy S. The knee in arthrogryposis multiplex congenita. J Pediatr Orthop. 1990;10(2):177–82.
42. Al-Aubaidi Z, Lundgaard B, Pedersen NW. Anterior distal femoral hemiepiphysiodesis in the treatment of fixed knee flexion contracture in neuromuscular patients. J Child Orthop. 2012;6(4):313–8.
43. Palocaren T, Thabet AM, Rogers K, Holmes L Jr, Donohoe M, King MM, et al. Anterior distal femoral stapling for correcting knee flexion contracture in children with arthrogryposis—preliminary results. J Pediatr Orthop. 2010;30(2):169–73.
44. DelBello DA, Watts HG. Distal femoral extension osteotomy for knee flexion contracture in patients with arthrogryposis. J Pediatr Orthop. 1996;16(1):122–6.
45. Feldman DS, Rand TJ, Huser AJ. Novel approach to improving knee range of motion in arthrogryposis with a new working classification. Children (Basel). 2021;8(7):546.
46. Fucs PM, Svartman C, de Assumpção RM, Lima Verde SR. Quadricepsplasty in arthrogryposis (amyoplasia): long-term follow-up. J Pediatr Orthop B. 2005;14(3):219–24.
47. St Clair HS, Zimbler S. A plan of management and treatment results in the arthrogrypotic hip. Clin Orthop Relat Res. 1985;194:74–80.
48. Stilli S, Antonioli D, Lampasi M, Donzelli O. Management of hip contractures and dislocations in arthrogryposis. Musculoskelet Surg. 2012;96(1):17–21.
49. Huurman WW, Jacobsen ST. The hip in arthrogryposis multiplex congenita. Clin Orthop Relat Res. 1985;194:81–6.
50. Sarwark JF, MacEwen GD, Scott CI Jr. Amyoplasia (a common form of arthrogryposis). J Bone Joint Surg Am. 1990;72(3):465–9.

51. Canavese F, Sussman MD. Orthopaedic manifestations of congenital myotonic dystrophy during childhood and adolescence. J Pediatr Orthop. 2009;29(2):208–13.
52. Wada A, Yamaguchi T, Nakamura T, Yanagida H, Takamura K, Oketani Y, et al. Surgical treatment of hip dislocation in amyoplasia-type arthrogryposis. J Pediatr Orthop B. 2012;21(5):381–5.
53. van Bosse HJ, Saldana RE. Reorientational proximal femoral osteotomies for Arthrogrypotic hip contractures. J Bone Joint Surg Am. 2017;99(1):55–64.
54. van Bosse HJP. Reorientational proximal femoral osteotomies for correction of hip contractures in children with arthrogryposis. JBJS Essent Surg Tech. 2017;7(2):e11.
55. Hamdy R, Dahan-Oliel N. Case 81: simultaneous correction of hip and knee flexion contractures in a 5 year old with arthrogryposis. In: Rozbruch SR, Hamdy RC, Iobst C, editors. Limb lengthening and reconstruction surgery case atlas. Pediatric deformity. Cham: Springer; 2015. https://doi.org/10.1007/978-3-319-18023-6.
56. Ezaki M. Treatment of the upper limb in the child with arthrogryposis. Hand Clin. 2000;16(4):703–11.
57. Axt MW, Niethard FU, Döderlein L, Weber M. Principles of treatment of the upper extremity in arthrogryposis multiplex congenita type I. J Pediatr Orthop B. 1997;6(3):179–85.
58. La Grone M. Spine. In: Staheli LT, Hall JG, Jaffe KM, Paholke DO, editors. Arthrogryposis: a text atlas. Cambridge, UK: Cambridge University Press; 1998. p. 51–3.
59. Oppenheim WL, Larson KR, McNabb MB, Smith CF, Setoguchi Y. Popliteal pterygium syndrome: an orthopaedic perspective. J Pediatr Orthop. 1990;10(1):58–64.
60. Staheli LT. Lower extremity management. In: Staheli LT, Hall JG, Jaffe KM, Paholke DO, editors. Arthrogryposis: a text atlas. Cambridge, UK: Cambridge University Press; 1998. p. 55–73.
61. Sakaura H, Matsuoka T, Iwasaki M, Yonenobu K, Yoshikawa H. Surgical treatment of cervical kyphosis in Larsen syndrome: report of 3 cases and review of the literature. Spine (Phila Pa 1976). 2007;32(1):E39–44.
62. Amor CJ, Spaeth MC, Chafey DH, Gogola GR. Use of the pediatric outcomes data collection instrument to evaluate functional outcomes in arthrogryposis. J Pediatr Orthop. 2011;31(3):293–6.
63. Dillon ER, Bjornson KF, Jaffe KM, Hall JG, Song K. Ambulatory activity in youth with arthrogryposis: a cohort study. J Pediatr Orthop. 2009;29(2):214–7.

Limb Lengthening and Deformity Correction in Patients with Skeletal Dysplasias

Mihir M. Thacker, Colleen Ditro, W. G. Stuart Mackenzie, and William G. Mackenzie

Introduction

Skeletal dysplasias include a wide and varied array of disorders, all characterized by an abnormality in the formation of bone and cartilage. There are many (>400 types) skeletal dysplasias and most are caused by specific mutations in genes involved in skeletal development [1] (Table 26.1). These disorders are often associated with short stature (proportionate or disproportionate), angular deformities of long bones, joint surface irregularity, and ligamentous laxity/instability [2–5]. Patients with skeletal dysplasias may have spinal deformities and/or instability which can be a cause of morbidity. In addition to skeletal manifestations, these individuals may also have substantial systemic involvement, which often is the cause of premature mortality [2, 5] (Table 26.2). Extremity involvement can be quite disabling and affect quality of life. Treatment of these children must involve a multidisciplinary team familiar with both skeletal and extra-skeletal concerns. There is a paucity of literature regarding the natural history of many of these disorders but there has been a recent surge in interest in many of these disorders, particularly mucopolysaccharidoses [6–9]. With improved understanding of the mechanisms involved in the genesis of these disorders, better medical treatments are being formulated [10, 11]. As a result of improved longevity, management of the skeletal issues is even more critical in maintaining mobility and quality of life.

Skeletal abnormalities in patients with skeletal dysplasias can be a source of considerable morbidity and often need surgical correction [5, 12]. These may result from:

(a) Shortening of specific limb segments (rhizomelic, mesomelic, and acromelic) characteristic of many disproportionate skeletal dysplasias associated with short stature.
(b) Unequal growth rates of paired long bones in the forearm and leg (for example, relatively long fibula in achondroplasia associated with genu varum; and relatively short fibula in chondro-ectodermal dysplasia associated with genu valgum).
(c) Angular deformity due to asymmetric physeal involvement.
(d) Joint contractures, deformities, and instability: Joint contractures result from angular deformation centered at the joints rather than in the adjacent physeal and metaphyseal regions of the developing bones. These are almost always in flexion and are particularly characteristic of diastrophic dysplasia. Joint instability can result from a combination of generalized ligamentous laxity and structural epiphyseal abnormality.

M. M. Thacker (✉) · C. Ditro · W. G. S. Mackenzie
W. G. Mackenzie
Department of Orthopedic Surgery, Nemours Children's Hospital, Delaware, Wilmington, DE, USA
e-mail: mthacker@nemours.org; colleen.ditro@nemours.org; Stuart.mackenzie@nemours.org; William.G.Mackenzie@nemours.org

Table 26.1 Genetics of skeletal dysplasias

Dysplasia	Gene defect	Mode of inheritance
Diastrophic dysplasia	DTDST gene (5q32-q33.1)	AD
Multiple epiphyseal dysplasia (MED) Type I Type II	COMP (Chr19) COL9A2	AD, less commonly AR
Pseudoachondroplasia	COMP (chromosome 19q13)	AD
Ellis van Creveld syndrome	EVC gene (chromosome 4p16)	AR
Achondroplasia	FGFR3	– 80% sporadic mutation – 20% AD
Hypochondroplasia	FGFR3/IGF-1	– Spontaneous mutation, less commonly AD
Spondyloepiphyseal dysplasia (SED)	Type II collagen	– Congenita: AD – Tarda: x-linked recessive
Kniest syndrome	Type II collagen	AD
Metaphyseal chondrodysplasias – Schmid type – Jansen type – McKusick	– Collagen type X A1 chain deletion – PTHRP (chromosome 3p22-p21.1) – RMPR (chromosome 9)	– AD – AD – AR
Cleidocranial Dysostosis	RUNX2/CFBA1gene (chromosome 6)	AD
Morquio syndrome (type IV Mucopolysaccharidosis)	GALNS/GLB1 gene defect	AR

Table 26.2 Selected systemic abnormalities in patients with skeletal dysplasias

System involved	Pathologic condition	Skeletal dysplasia
Head	Hydrocephalus	Achondroplasia
Eye	– Cataracts – Retinal detachment	– Morquio syndrome – SED congenital, Kneist
Ear	– Recurrent otitis media – Hearing loss	– Achondroplasia, Kneist – Kneist
Cardiac	– Congenital heart defects – Acquired (cardiomyopathy, valvular disease)	– Ellis van Creveld Dysplasia – Morquio syndrome
Respiratory	– Laryngotracheomalacia – Central +/– obstructive sleep apnea – Restrictive lung disease	– Camptomelic dysplasia, diastrophic dysplasia – Achondroplasia – Metatropic dysplasia, Thanatophoric dysplasia, Ellis van Creveld dysplasia
Immunologic	– T-cell impairment, neutropenia, anemia	McKusick metaphyseal chondrodysplasia

Lower Extremity Deformity in Skeletal Dysplasia

Individuals with skeletal dysplasias are not only shorter in stature than the average population, but each dysplasia has its own set of unique skeletal abnormalities. In addition, the natural history of these dysplasias is highly variable and influences decision making. Characteristic deformities at various bones and joints are seen in skeletal dysplasias (Table 26.3).

The challenges of deformity correction in skeletal dysplasia patients include:

- Multifocal, and often multiplanar deformities (sagittal, coronal, rotational, and translational)
- The abnormalities in ossification can impair visualization of the chondro-osseous structures and joint lines on plain radiographs, adding another level of difficulty to planning the deformity correction. This may necessitate additional imaging studies such as MRIs (often needing sedation or anesthesia, which is not without its difficulties) and CT scans as well as liberal use of intraoperative arthrograms.
- Deformity at one site (so also its correction) may influence the development and/or progression of deformities at adjacent sites (for example, coxa vara correction in SED can make the genu valgum at the knee worse due to the lateral shift of mechanical axis). Other challenges include deciding which deformities need to be managed surgically and which can be accommodated by adjacent correction.

Skeletal dysplasias can affect bone and cartilage quality. Therefore, it is imperative to understand the pathophysiology and natural history of these conditions. These differences can affect the types of correction and fixation used. The size and quality of bone often may influence implant selection and necessitate creativity in the operating room to accomplish the desired surgical goals.

Table 26.3 Characteristic deformities of various skeletal dysplasias

Deformity	Skeletal dysplasia
Acetabular dysplasia	Diastrophic dysplasia MED Morquio syndrome
Coxa vara	Cleidocranial dysplasia MED Pseudoachondroplasia SED congenita Schmid metaphyseal chondrodysplasia
Coxa Valga	Morquio syndrome
Hip degenerative disease	Pseudoachondroplasia MED SED
Genu varum	Achondroplasia McKusick metaphyseal chondrodysplasia (mild) Pseudoachondroplasia Schmid metaphyseal chondrodysplasia
Genu valgum	Diastrophic dysplasia Ellis-van Creveld syndrome MED Morquio syndrome Pseudoachondroplasia SED congenita
Internal tibial torsion	Achondroplasia Schmid metaphyseal chondrodysplasia
External tibial torsion	
Ankle varus	Achondroplasia McKusick metaphyseal chondrodysplasia (mild) Schmid metaphyseal chondrodysplasia
Talipes equinovarus	SED (supple) Diastrophic dysplasia (rigid)

MED multiple epiphyseal dysplasia; *SED* spondylo-epiphyseal dysplasia

Surgical Considerations

Pre-operative Evaluation

Evaluation of a child with skeletal dysplasia is best performed by a multidisciplinary team (including Orthopedic surgery, Genetics, physical, and occupational therapists and other necessary specialists such as Otorhinolaryngology, Neurosurgery, Ophthalmology, and Dentistry) familiar with these conditions [5, 13]. A thorough history, including questions regarding pain, endurance, gait abnormalities, activities of daily living and recreation, provides clues to functional limitations. A detailed systemic evaluation is also indicated and may identify major, sometimes life-threatening, issues (Table 26.2). The extremities should be examined for range of motion, ligamentous laxity, joint contractures, or malalignment (in all planes). Examination of the spine for sagittal and coronal plane deformities and a thorough neurological examination are needed because of the frequent incidence of spinal deformities, instability, and neurological compromise in certain dysplasias such as Morquio syndrome, Spondylo-epiphyseal dysplasia (SED), etc. Cervical spine instability is common in the mucopolysaccharidoses, SED, diastrophic dysplasia, pseudoachondroplasia, and chondrodysplasia punctata. Flexion-extension radiographs (and if needed, flexion-extension MRI (Magnetic Resonance Imaging) [15] to evaluate spinal cord compression) are useful in evaluating these patients at risk for instability, especially if they have symptoms of neck pain and long track signs. Plain radiographs may be difficult to interpret in this population given the delayed ossification, odontoid hypoplasia, limited neck motion and abnormal anatomy seen in many of these patients. Additionally, the bony landmarks used for measurement may be obscured by overlapping shadows cast by the mandible, occiput, and foramen magnum. Any patient with back or radicular pain, neurogenic claudication, incontinence, or objective neurologic findings (hypertonia, brisk reflexes, clonus, motor weakness) should be evaluated with an MRI [14]. The child's gait is assessed by observing the child walk, run, and play [16]. Gait analysis can be helpful in these patients. Discussion with the family is critical to establish the goals of treatment as well as to manage expectations appropriately.

Imaging

A skeletal survey is often performed at the initial visit to identify the skeletal features that aid in diagnosis. At our institution, a skeletal survey for skeletal dysplasia typically includes antero-posterior (AP) and lateral radiographs of the cervical thoracic and lumbar spine, AP view of the upper extremities and lower extremities as well as the pelvis and feet. We add further radiographs as clinically indicated. AP and lateral full-length radiographs of the lower extremities (preferably weight bearing views) are mandatory prior to surgical intervention. These allow for an evaluation of the overall alignment and location of deformities. It is also imperative to obtain dedicated weight-bearing radiographs of the specific joints to allow for appropriate deformity analysis. Full-length radiographs alone will not always allow for an accurate quantitative determination of the magnitude of deformity. For example, the magnitude of ankle deformity can be misjudged based on full-length radiographs centered at the knee because of the parallax of the x-ray beam. Additional three-dimensional studies such as computed tomography and/or magnetic resonance imaging may be performed for detailed evaluation of bone and cartilage anatomy, measurement of torsional abnormalities, assessment of joint condition, etc. However, these are static studies and may not always reflect the alignment of the limb in conditions of dynamic loading (gait). We often perform a 3-dimensional gait analysis in these patients as an adjunct to x-rays to aid in pre-operative decision making. Such dynamic evaluation helps to quantify the forces across the various joints and helps us compare pre- and post-operative functions.

Anesthesia

Preparation of the patient for the surgical procedure is at least as important as the surgical procedure itself. Given the fact that many of these patients have small and "difficult" airways, pre-operative anesthesia consultations and discussion of the various issues specific to that patient are very useful. There may be minor surgical procedures but there is no "minor anesthesia" for these patients. Anesthesia should be performed by an anesthesiologist familiar with various medical comorbidities associated with this patient population. Our institution has described a "difficult" airway management in these patients as one which requires two anesthesia providers when ventilating with a facemask. One provider applies the face mask while maintaining anterior mandibular displacement and cervical stabilization while the other ventilates with positive pressure [17]. Care must be taken to protect the neck in patients with cervical instability by using in-line cervical traction [18]. In addition, specialized tools such as video laryngoscope and fiberoptic intubation should be readily available in these situations. Given the fact that each anesthetic session poses a certain risk to the patient, we prefer to combine as many procedures as feasible under the same anesthetic.

Regional anesthesia is often used for pain control and to reduce the amount of narcotics needed during and after surgery. Caudal epidural analgesia is preferred over lumbar epidurals in patients with known vertebral anomalies, prior fusions, and thoracolumbar kyphosis that can co-exist with these conditions. Typically, caudal epidural may be administered to those patients of 10 years of age and younger who undergo lower extremity osteotomies. Careful dosing of the blocks and regular neurovascular checks are essential to avoid missing the diagnosis of early compartment syndrome. We have moved away from using epidural infusions in our patients since we often use neuromonitoring for these cases. We do use peripheral nerve blocks, and this can be done at the end of the procedure. An alternate strategy is to place a dry catheter at the beginning of the procedure and then dose it at the end.

Positioning and Neuromonitoring

Positioning these patients is also critical as patients with severe kyphosis are at risk for developing paraparesis/paraplegia with prolonged supine position. The pathogenesis of this phenomenon is poorly understood at this time [19]. Neuromonitoring should be considered in long procedures in the high-risk patients (exaggerated thoracic kyphosis, spinal stenosis at any level on MRI). We usually perform neuromonitoring for cases that involve supine positioning for more than 45 min. This may be in orthopedic or non-orthopedic procedures.

The neuromonitoring typically involves monitoring for spinal cord function. Our usual protocol utilizes motor evoked potentials (MEPs) as the primary monitoring modality. The muscle groups used are: First Dorsal Interosseous, (control group and also monitors cervical down to T2 level), Iliopsoas muscle group, (monitors down to L1 spinal cord level, therefore below the typical area of kyphosis apex and spinal cord watershed), Tibialis anterior, Abductor hallucis (these are robust responses used in all spinal cord monitoring). They allow for the recognition of the typical pattern we look for in spinal cord insults whereby the Abductor hallucis response is spared (sacral sparing) but loss or significant attenuation of Tibialis anterior and also the Iliopsoas would be present. They also monitor the sciatic distribution from a peripheral nerve perspective. Somatosensory Evoked potentials are recorded from the ulnar nerves (control and also monitors arm position) and the posterior tibial nerve from the medial malleolus in the lower extremity (monitors dorsal column function up through the spinal cord and over the thoracic kyphosis and also the tibial division of the sciatic distribution).

Implant Size and Design

Surgical implant size and design need to be considered in pre-operative planning. Some of these patients are extremely small (primordial dwarfism) and appropriately sized implants are critical to the successful execution of the preoperative plan. The popular commercially available pre-contoured implants will rarely accommodate the morphology of bones in patients with skeletal dysplasias. Given the poor bone quality in some of the patients, locking plate and screw constructs may be useful when performing acute corrections. These are especially useful when the osteotomy is away from the apex of the deformity and translation needs to be built into the construct (Fig. 26.6). Even while planning deformity correction with external fixators, this should be kept in mind. For example, the appropriate fit of a Taylor Spatial Frame (Smith & Nephew; Memphis, Tennessee, USA) may necessitate use of extra-extra short struts (which may need to be ordered pre-operatively). Frequently, given the multifocal nature of the deformities, more than one osteotomy, and therefore, fixation options may be needed in the same bone. Having an appropriate inventory of instruments and implants saves the surgeon from frustration and improves patient outcome.

Methods of Deformity Correction

The principles of deformity correction in the dysplasia population are no different from those without dysplasias. However, the multifocal and multiplanar nature of the deformities, issues with size and quality of the bone, ligamentous laxity and growth potential make deformity correction extremely challenging in these patients. Many of these patients have significant delays in ossification, making the planning and correction of deformities even more challenging. It has been demonstrated that the choice of osteotomy often changes based on the results of intraoperative arthrography, particularly in patients under 8 years of age [20]. We use arthrography liberally during surgery to mitigate some of these issues. This helps us not only to visualize the cartilaginous anatomy, but also helps evaluate the dynamic stability of the joint with stress views in the operating room (see Fig. 26.5).

Deformity correction in these patients can be accomplished via acute or gradual methods.

Acute Correction

Acute methods of deformity correction include use of osteotomies with immediate correction and fixation via various methods. In general, these techniques follow the same principles as those patients without skeletal dysplasias. Care should be taken to be familiar with the various deformities associated with particular conditions (Table 26.3). For example, genu varum is present in the majority of achondroplastic children by 5 years of age and 90% of achondroplastic adults [21]. The genu varum can be secondary to distal femoral varus, lateral joint line opening, proximal and distal tibial varus and is almost always associated with internal tibial torsion. Progressive varus, symptomatic gait abnormalities, lateral thrust are our typical indications of genu varum correction. One or all of these deformities may be present, so careful pre-op planning must be done prior to surgical correction. The deformity in young children usually is due to proximal tibial varus, lateral joint line opening, and internal tibial torsion. These children can be successfully treated with a proximal tibial osteotomy with fibular shortening osteotomy (we prefer removal of a segment of the fibula) via acute correction. Care must be taken to displace the proximal tibia to maintain a neutral mechanical axis and correct the typical internal tibial torsion. With this method, acceptable correction can be attained [22]. Recurrence is common in very young children and if there is under correction. It has been suggested that the preferred treatment for skeletally mature individuals with achondroplasia and distal tibial varus is an acute opening distal tibial osteotomy combined with a shortening distal fibula. Displacement usually is required to correct the mechanical axis [22]. The authors have typically used a shortening, derotation osteotomy to manage this deformity. With acute deformity correction, one can re-establish normal mechanical alignment, but not perform additional limb lengthening. In addition, acute corrections, particularly of the proximal tibia, have been associated with complications including peroneal nerve palsy, vascular injury, and compartment syndrome [23].

Gradual Correction with Guided Growth

Gradual deformity correction is a powerful tool for angular realignment and/or lengthening in the skeletal dysplasia population. This can be done by way of guided growth techniques or external fixation. We have demonstrated that growth modulation using a tension band plate and screw system, or staples is an effective way to provide deformity correction in a variety of skeletal dysplasias [24]. It is a relatively simple surgery that has a low risk of damage to the physis or mechanical failure. We have also found that despite an abnormal epiphysis and metaphysis, the screw purchase has been reliable. An exception is pseudoachondroplasia where it can be difficult to achieve epiphyseal fixation given the frequent delay in ossification. This technique can also be used in very young patients [24]. Guided growth via hemiepiphyseal stapling in patients with MED has also been studied. In these children, stapling has been effective for angular deformity correction. However, the response of the physis after staple removal is unpredictable, necessitating avoidance of excessive overcorrection and close monitoring until skeletal maturity [25]. We have also demonstrated that the risk factors for rebounding after correction of genu valgum in the skeletal dysplasia population includes primary procedure at an early age and a high growth velocity. Overcorrection does not reliably protect against rebound deformity [26]. There are some skeletal dysplasias that are associated with extremely slow growth or have significant joint laxity, which can affect correction. Slow growth, all cartilaginous epiphysis, and a large magnitude of skeletal deformity is a combination that will likely lead to failure of correction when using guided growth treatment in such patients. The ease of the procedure, along with postoperative recovery and the fact that it can be repeated for recurrent/rebound deformities, makes guided growth an attractive option for deformity correction in children with skeletal dysplasias.

Gradual Correction with External Fixation

Gradual deformity correction can also be accomplished using external fixators [27, 28]. This approach has two main advantages. Primarily, the multifocal and multiplanar deformities that are associated with skeletal dysplasias can be addressed at one surgery. Some of the gradual correction devices also allow for simultaneous multiplanar correction, addressing coronal, sagittal, and axial deformities without the need for complex osteotomies that are prone to error. Secondly, this method also allows for concurrent limb lengthening in this patient population with varying degrees of short stature. Patients must be counseled about their care and management pre-operatively if this is going to be undertaken as limb lengthening can be associated with several complications [29, 30]. However, with appropriate instruction and care, external fixators are extremely useful for correction of most complex deformities. We prefer to use computer aided deformity correction with hexapod external fixators for more complex deformities. These allow for placement of a virtual hinge at the apex of the deformity to allow appropriate angulation and translation with the osteotomy through a more convenient part of the bone. They also have the advantage of being able to fine tune the correction after the initial correction has been completed.

Controversies in Lengthening for Stature

Limb lengthening (without the correction of angular deformities) in short-statured individuals has been a subject of debate [29–34]. The achondroplastic population has been the most studied to date. The motivation to lengthen limbs in the skeletal dysplasia population has been to improve functional disabilities associated with difficulty in locomotion [35]. Other concerns, particularly in the idiopathic short-statured patient, have been related to aesthetic, social, and psychological concerns.

Medical and surgical treatments to address short stature in achondroplasia have been studied. Growth hormone (GH) administration has led to variable results [36]. In trials, early gains in height after commencement of GH treatment have been seen to varying degrees. However, the effects have not been as promising with continued administration. There are also concerns of aggravating the disproportionate nature of limb segment shortening. Surgical techniques for stature lengthening in achondroplasia have addressed femora, tibiae, and humeri via distraction osteogenesis. This method has reliably been able to provide an increase in height, but with potential risk for complications [32].

The average gain in height through multiple episodes of surgical limb lengthening in patients with achondroplasia has been reported to be 18–23 cm resulting in an average total patient height of 140 cm [29, 35, 37]. Though traditionally these procedures have been staged, a recent study recommended all four bones (bilateral femurs and tibias) simultaneous moderate lengthening which could be repeated later. Another study did report lengthening up to 30 cm in patients with achondroplasia using four bone lengthening as well as staged humeral lengthening [38]. This, however, does not completely ameliorate the disproportionate trunk height [39]. There are several drawbacks to limb lengthening purely for increased stature, including prolonged treatment time and high complication rate (reported up to 100%). Song et al. reported decreased growth in the proximal tibial physis after extensive lengthening of the tibia in patients with achondroplasia. It is unclear as to whether this improves the patient's quality of life [33]. Kim, et al., showed that there was an improvement in self-esteem (using the Rosenberg self-esteem questionnaire), but there was no difference in physical or functional scores (using the SF-36 and AAOS lower extremity scores) when comparing patients with achondroplasia, who underwent lengthening versus those who did not undergo surgical treatment [29]. There may be a role for stature lengthening in the carefully selected patient who is well-aware of the long and arduous nature of the process and the potential for significant complications. However, the patient must be counseled that the gain in height may not correlate to an improvement in quality of life [30].

Post-operative Considerations

There are several aspects of the post-operative course specific to short-statured patients that should be taken into consideration. This is particularly true when utilizing external fixation for deformity correction. These children typically require more support because of their limited upper extremity reach. It is important to work with physical and occupational therapists to provide appropriate assistive devices and strategies for activities of daily living.

The psychosocial aspect of deformity correction should not be overlooked in patients with skeletal dysplasias. These children may have preexisting self-image concerns because of their underlying conditions. With external fixators in place, these self-conscious feelings can be amplified. It may be useful to involve mental health professionals in the pre-operative evaluation and post-operative care of these patients.

The skeletal dysplasia population often travels to referral centers for these complicated deformity corrections. We prefer to keep these patients local during the timeframe of distraction and/or correction. This allows us to follow them in the clinic on a weekly or biweekly basis and to appropriately address any complications that may arise. This oftentimes entails working with local or national charities, such as the Ronald McDonald House, for lodging and other necessities. In addition, the caregivers of these children need ample time to plan for the required post-operative stay if they are not locally based.

Planning for the Future

When planning these corrections, care must be taken to consider the long-term effects that they may have. Many individuals with skeletal dysplasias, such as Multiple Epiphyseal Dysplasia (MED), Spondylo-epiphyseal Dysplasia (SED), pseudoachondroplasia, diastrophic dysplasia, and Morquio syndrome (MPS IVA) are predisposed to premature osteoarthritis. These patients often need total joint arthroplasty (TJA) at a relatively young age. This must be considered when performing osteotomies that may make TJA more difficult. We recommend routinely removing hardware (blade plates/screw side plates) from the proximal femur in patients who may need a subsequent hip arthroplasty. This may be combined with any of their other surgical procedures to minimize anesthetic risk. The surgeon needs to consider various obstacles when performing TJA in these patients. For instance, in total knee arthroplasty, customized implants and constrained designs are often needed because of patient size and a lack of ligamentous constraints associated with the underlying pathologies [40, 41]. When considering total hip arthroplasty, the surgeon needs to evaluate the need potential acetabular augmentation secondary to bony deficiency, extensive soft tissue releases because of contractures, tortuous and narrow proximal femoral intramedullary canal and need for custom implants due to small stature [42, 43]. When proper preoperative planning is executed, good results can be achieved with total joint arthroplasty in patients with skeletal dysplasia, though complication rates can be high [40, 42].

Specific Skeletal Dysplasias and Their Associated Deformities

Achondroplasia

Achondroplasia is the most frequently encountered form of skeletal dysplasia with an incidence of approximately one in 10,000 live births [44]. This results from a mutation in the FGFR3 gene. This overactivity of FGFR3 results in abnormalities in endochondral ossification, whereas intramembranous ossification is not affected. This therefore results in involvement of the base of the skull (resulting in foramen magnum stenosis) and the extremities. There are predictable patterns of deformity in this population. In the upper extremity, elbow flexion contractures are common and caused by distal humeral recurvatum. Associated severe rhizomelia can result in marked limitation in reach and humeral lengthening can improve function in these individuals [45]. In the lower extremity, hip flexion contracture and knee deformities occur. The most addressed deformity is genu varum, which is often associated with internal tibial torsion and occasionally genu recurvatum. A common misconception is that uncorrected genu varum in children with achondroplasia results in knee osteoarthritis later in life. In fact, osteoarthritis is rare, and the knee joint is usually not a source of functional limitation in these patients. Spine problems such as central stenosis of the lumbar segments often result in limited function. The etiology of genu varum is unclear. Several mechanisms have been proposed, including ligamentous laxity, obesity, asymmetric growth of the proximal tibial physis, and asymmetric growth of the fibula relative to the tibia [46–48]. As mentioned earlier, varus deformity can exist in the distal femur, the knee joint, and proximal and distal tibia. Indications for surgical correction of genu varum and internal tibial torsion in these children include knee pain, progressive deformity, lateral thrust during gait, and rarely, cosmesis. Genu valgum, though uncommon, may be seen in some patients. However, the valgus deformity is rarely severe enough to warrant surgical correction.

Several techniques for correction of genu varum in achondroplastic patients have been described previously. Fibular epiphysiodesis or shortening may be useful in young patients (5–8 years old) with mild deformity [22, 49]. In the young child (less than 10 years of age) with achondroplasia, we have used growth modulation with good success (Fig. 26.1a–c). However, long-term data on this technique is lacking. Acute correction in young children with an oblique proximal tibial osteotomy (Fig. 26.2a–k), simultaneously correcting the tibial varus and internal rotation, has achieved reliable results with a low recurrence rate if the joint line and mechanical axis are brought to a neutral position [50, 51].

In older children and adolescents, we prefer gradual correction of the proximal tibia with a hexapod fixator for severe deformities. Concurrent varus deformity in the distal femur and distal tibia are corrected as needed. The authors tend to use acute correction of these associated deformities. This approach allows for simultaneous correction of multiple sites of deformity, as well as multiple planes of deformity [27, 52]. Gradual tensioning of loose lateral collateral knee ligament has been described but the authors do not use this technique.

When considering isolated distal tibial varus correction, we do very careful pre-operative planning to determine that there is no clinically significant proximal tibial deformity. Concurrent untreated proximal tibial varus, even if mild, will result in poor patient satisfaction.

Bifocal tibial osteotomies (Fig. 26.3a–d) can be utilized to correct both the proximal and distal tibial varus deformities and internal rotation and simultaneously gain length with an acceptable complication risk (mostly equinus contractures with more than 15% lengthening through the distal tibial osteotomy) [53].

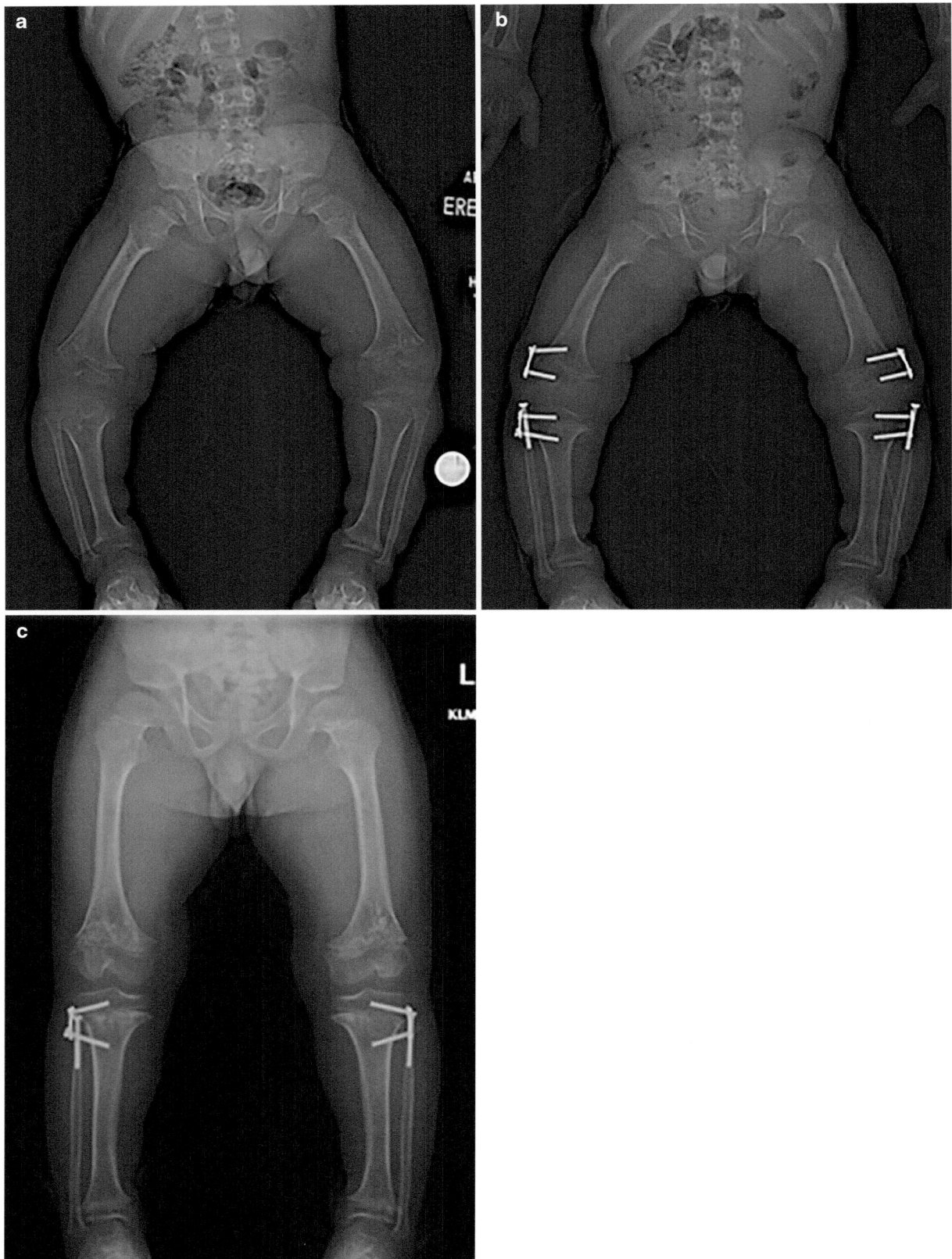

Fig. 26.1 Achondroplasia-growth modulation. (**a–c**) Lower extremity radiographs (pre-operative, immediate post-operative, and at follow up) demonstrating use of growth modulation in the proximal tibia and fibula to correct the varus deformity in a child with achondroplasia

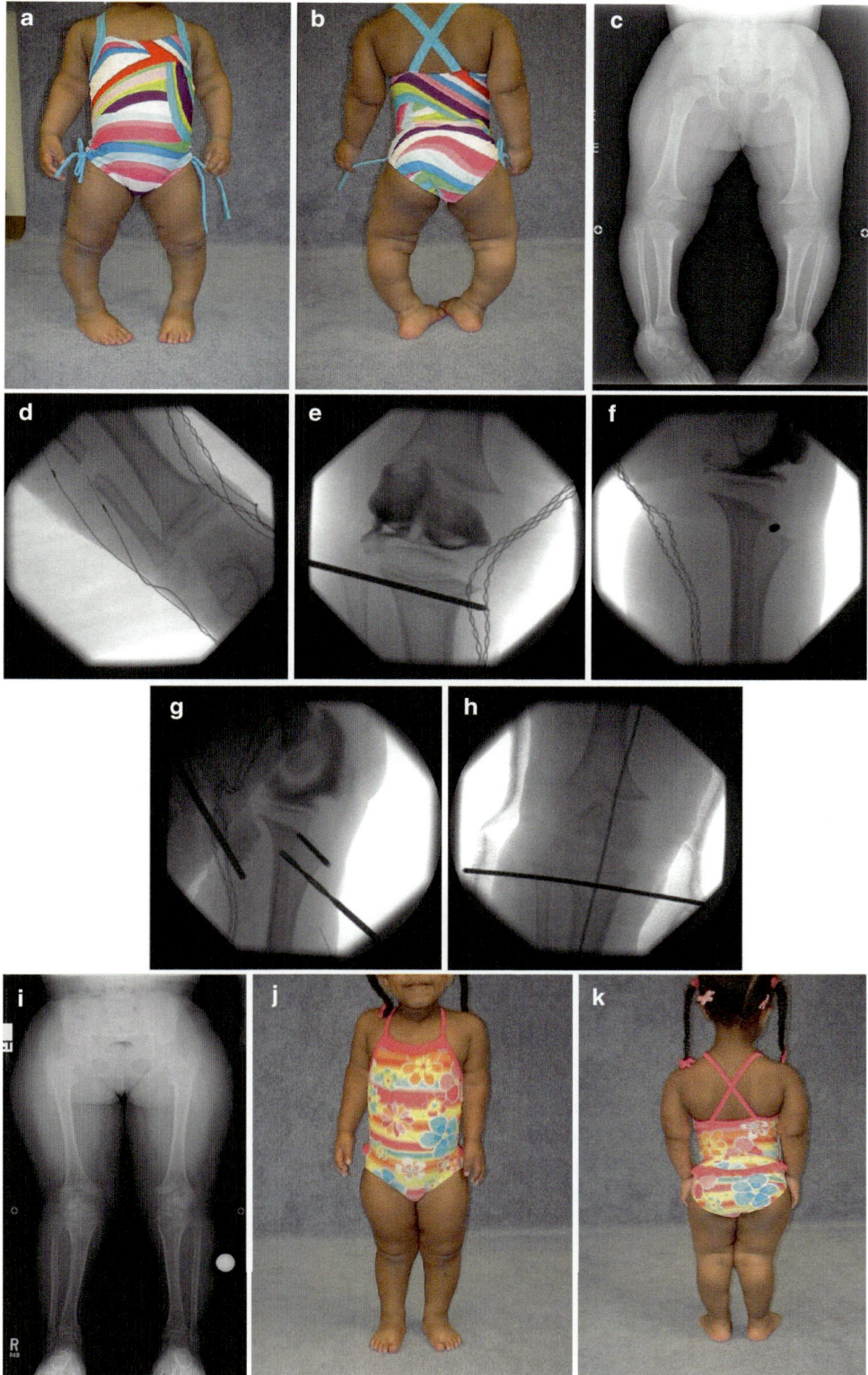

Fig. 26.2 Achondroplasia-acute correction. (**a**, **b**) Clinical photographs of a patient with achondroplasia with bilateral genu varum and internal tibial torsion. (**c**) Anteroposterior (AP) radiograph of bilateral lower extremities, showing characteristic bone changes with genu varum, long fibula. (**d**) Acute correction of proximal tibial varus and internal rotation. The first step is fibular shortening. (**e**, **f**) The next step is an arthrogram to delineate the joint surface and placement of a K wire parallel to the joint surface. (**g**) Oblique plane osteotomy of the proximal tibia. (**h**) Intraoperative fluoroscopy, confirming adequate correction using the Bovie cord technique. (**i**) Postoperative radiographs after healing and cast removal demonstrate excellent alignment. (**j**, **k**) Clinical photographs of the patient in Fig. 26.1a, b after correction of genu varum deformity

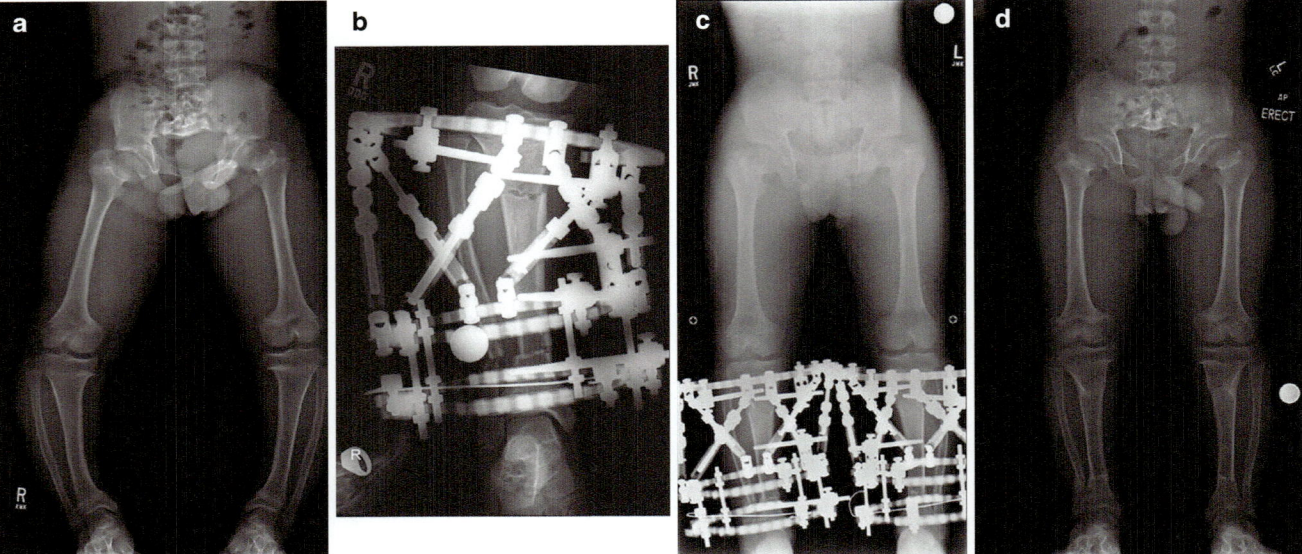

Fig. 26.3 Achondroplasia-gradual correction in a 13-year-old boy. (**a**) AP radiograph of bilateral lower extremities demonstrating varus in the proximal and distal tibia bilaterally. (**b**) Application of bilateral circular fixators with bilevel tibial osteotomies for gradual correction of the proximal tibial deformity and acute correction of the distal tibial deformity. (**c, d**) Radiographs of bilateral lower extremities after correction of the deformities and after removal of the frames demonstrating correction of the mechanical axis

Spondyloepiphyseal Dysplasia Congenita (SEDC)

Spondyloepiphyseal dysplasia congenita (SEDC) results in a short trunk type of disproportionate dwarfism (Fig. 26.4a, b). As the name suggests, both the axial and appendicular skeleton are involved. The genetic cause for this condition involves an abnormality in Type II collagen [54]. Lower-extremity problems include coxa vara, femoral retroversion, hip flexion contracture, genu valgum, and foot deformities, such as equinovarus and planovalgus. As the genetic defect is in Type II collagen, articular cartilage is affected. This results in premature osteoarthritis that manifests in the second-third decade of life [55].

Severe coxa vara, with neck-shaft angles less than 90°, is often present in patients with SEDC. This deformity can be difficult to judge radiographically because of delayed ossification of the capital femoral epiphysis [56]. We have described the use of the Hilgenreiner-Trochanteric angle for assessment of coxa vara in these children [47]. The epiphyseal deformity of the hip can result in femoral head flattening, hinge abduction, and lateral subluxation [56]. Indications for correction of coxa vara include hip pain and reduced function, Trendelenberg gait, a neck-shaft angle of less than 100°, progressive varus, Hilgenreiner-epiphyseal (H-E) angle greater than 60°, Hilgenreiner-trochanteric (H-T) angle of less than 0° [57–59]. Correction is performed through a proximal femoral valgus osteotomy. Femoral retroversion and hip flexion contracture (which are almost always present) can be addressed concurrently through this valgus-extension-derotation osteotomy. Fixation can be achieved with a blade plate or locking plate system (Fig. 26.5a–g). Ideally, the fixation is placed across the trochanteric apophysis to achieve closure to minimize the risk of recurrent varus. If there is a triangular medial metaphyseal

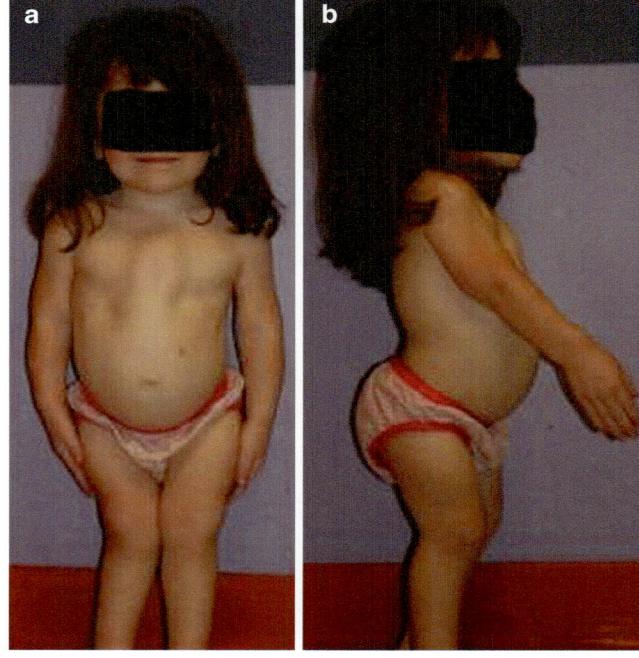

Fig. 26.4 (**a, b**) Clinical photographs of a girl with Spondyloepiphyseal dysplasia congenita (SEDC) showing characteristic clinical findings of kyphoscoliosis, lumbar hyperlordosis, pectus carintum, genu valgum

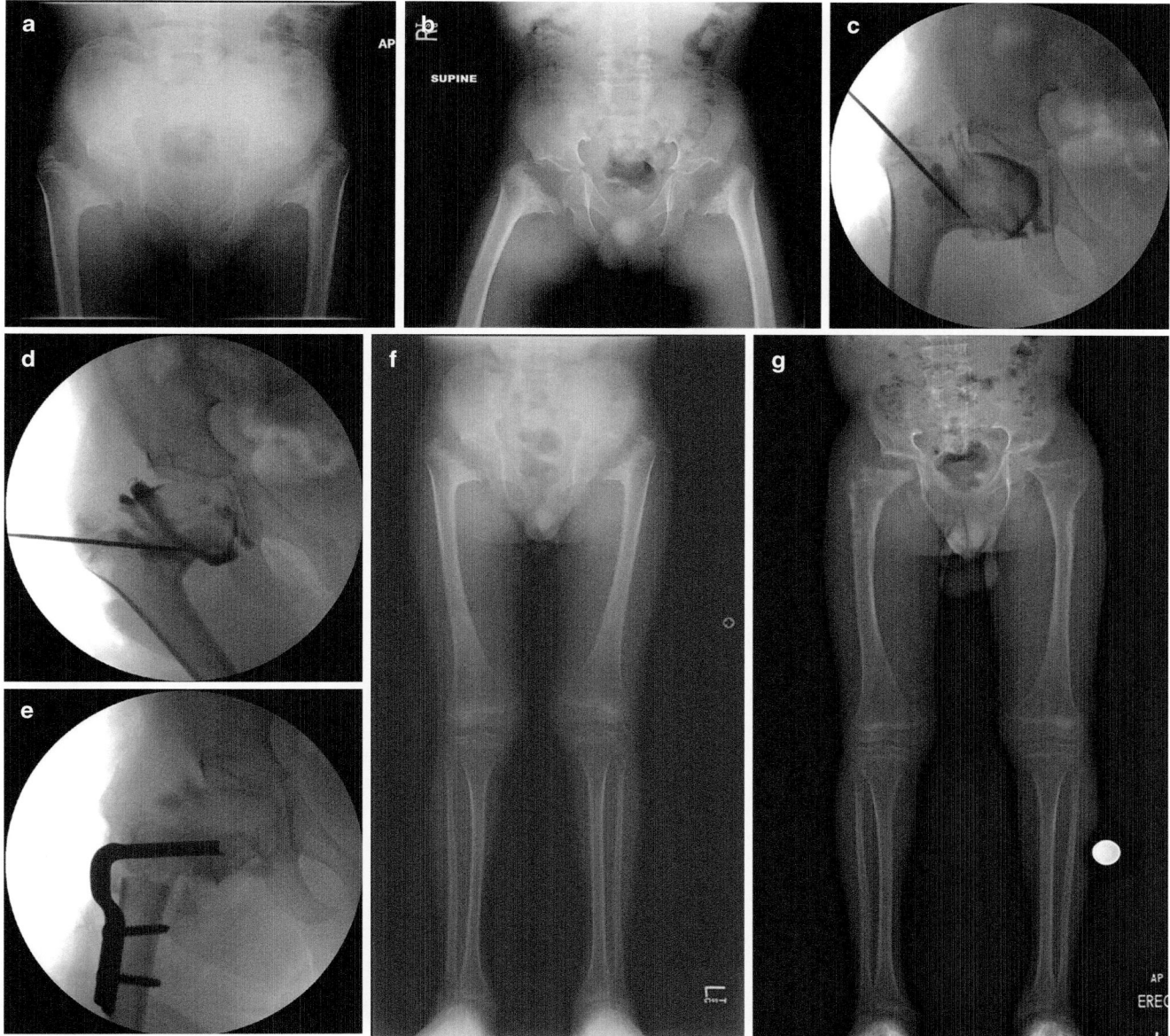

Fig. 26.5 (**a, b**) Preoperative AP and frog leg lateral radiographs in a patient with SEDC demonstrating coxa vara and delayed ossification of the femoral heads bilaterally. (**c**) Intraoperative fluoroscopy images showing use of the arthrogram to demonstrate the cartilaginous portion of the femoral head. The guidewire is placed through the trochanteric apophysis at the desired angle (90°—the degree of desired correction, if using a 90° blade plate). (**d**) The use of the adduction view to simulate the correction and assess the coverage of the femoral head. (**e**) Use of blade plate to achieve correction of the varus as well as the flexion and rotation deformities. It is important to leave the blade somewhat proud in order to achieve adequate lateral translation needed to centralize the mechanical axis. (**f, g**) AP radiographs of bilateral lower extremities before and after correction

proximal femoral fragment, we try to achieve fixation of the fragment. Radiographic measurements associated with low recurrence of coxa vara after proximal femoral valgus osteotomy are H-E angle less than 38° and H-T angle greater than 13° [57] and epiphyseal ossification. Open reduction of the hip may be necessary at the same surgical procedure, but this is rare. Correction of the hip deformity should precede correction of knee deformity, as surgical correction of coxa vara may add valgus force to the knee. Also, it is important for patients and their parents to be aware that correction of this proximal femoral deformity may result in an aggravated appearance of genu valgum [60]. Care should be taken to lateralize the shaft adequately while performing the valgus proximal femoral osteotomy. Lining up the shaft under the medial aspect of the greater trochanter is desirable to facilitate subsequent hip arthroplasty which is often needed in these patients. We therefore also recommend hardware removal routinely, after osteotomy healing in these patients.

Genu valgum is another common deformity seen in SEDC. The valgus can be attributed to the distal femur, proximal tibia, or both segments. The magnitude of genu valgum is often related to the severity of coxa vara. This deformity can often be corrected by distal medial femoral and/or proximal medial tibial hemiepiphysiodesis. If inadequate growth is remaining to achieve correction through growth modulation, then realignment osteotomy at the appropriate level can be performed (Fig. 26.6a–d). This can also address any knee flexion and/or tibial torsion at the same time.

Symptomatic valgus deformities of the ankle and hindfoot can be treated with supramalleolar tibial and fibular osteotomies and hindfoot procedures as needed. The symptomatic, flexible foot deformities in patients with SEDC are typically managed with orthotics. Stiff equinovarus feet are managed by techniques similar to idiopathic clubfeet.

Multiple Epiphyseal Dysplasia (MED)

Multiple epiphyseal dysplasia is a skeletal dysplasia with wide variations in clinical presentation and skeletal manifestations [61, 62]. It is caused by mutations in multiple genes including those for cartilage oligomeric protein COMP, type IX collagen, and matrilin-3 and results in symmetric changes of the epiphyses of long bones [61]. Spine involvement is absent in these patients. They have mild short stature and often present with lower extremity joint pain, angular deformities, gait deformities, or stiffness [63, 64]. The epiphyses in these patients are often small and fragmented. Avascular necrosis like changes may complicate fragmentation of the femoral head in up to 50% patients with MED [65, 66]. Individuals with MED are predisposed to premature osteoarthritis, particularly severely affecting the hips [67]. Hip deformity usually mimics that seen in Legg-Calve-Perthes disease. Treatment of these deformities is like that for Perthes disease [56].

Joint pain and stiffness are quite common in these children. Anti-inflammatory medications, exercise in warm water, stretching, and physical therapy can help to improve these symptoms.

Genu valgum is the most frequent knee deformity [68]. Prior to skeletal maturity, this can be addressed effectively with guided growth techniques (Fig. 26.7a–e). In patients after or nearing skeletal maturity, osteotomy at the site of deformity (distal femur and/or proximal tibia) should be undertaken. Ankle valgus can be managed with guided growth if enough growth is remaining [24].

Diastrophic Dysplasia

Diastrophic dysplasia is an autosomal recessive condition caused by a mutation in DTDST gene which encodes for a sulfate transporter protein [69, 70]. There is a wide variation in the phenotype of this condition. Common lower extremity

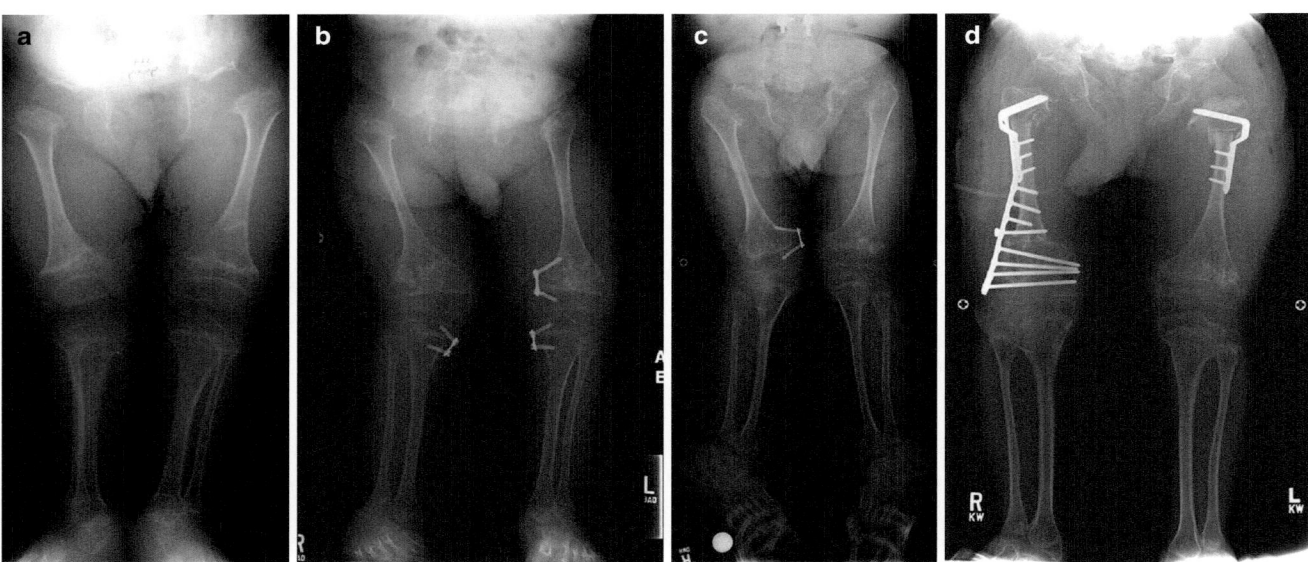

Fig. 26.6 (a–c) Radiographs of bilateral lower extremities demonstrating bilateral genu valgum in a patient with SEDC. And its correction using growth modulation. There is incomplete correction on the right side. (d) Correction of the distal femoral valgus using acute correction. The use of a locking plate allows for adequate translation needed to maintain appropriate correction of the mechanical axis. Note the limited bone available for fixation with the proximal femoral blade plate in situ

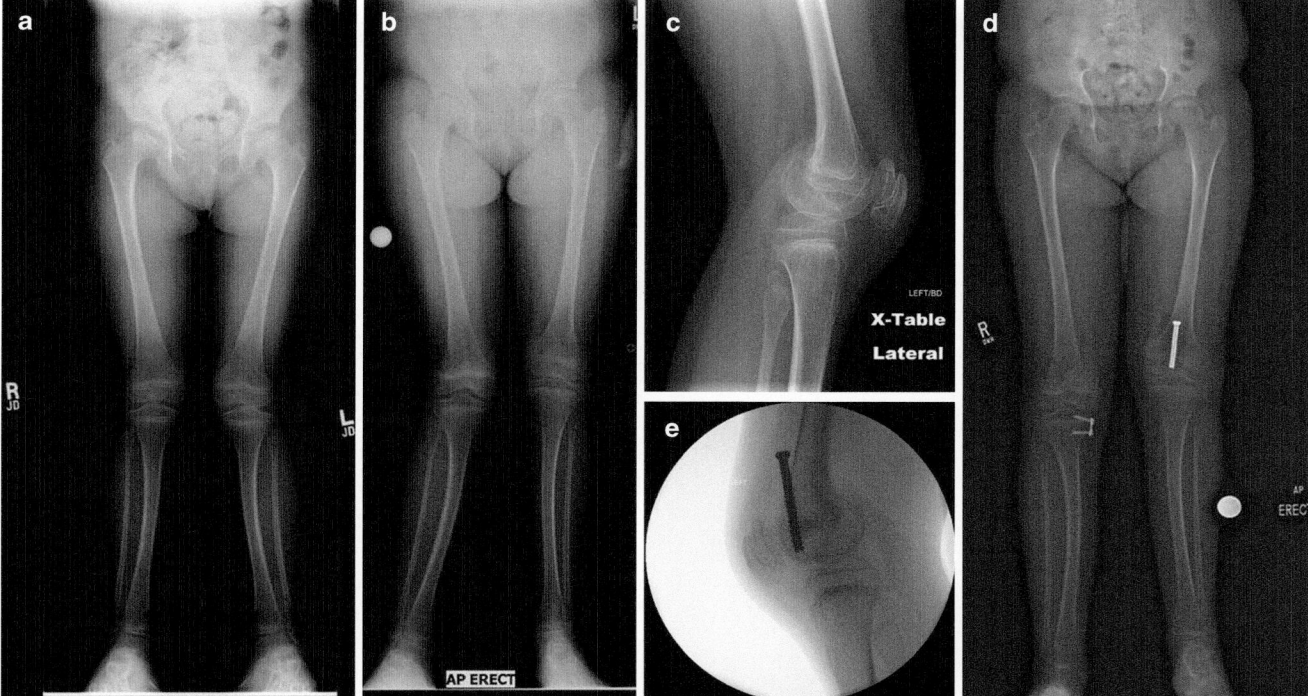

Fig. 26.7 (**a**, **b**) Progressive genu valgum, over 6 years, in a patient with multiple epiphyseal dysplasia. (**c**) Double layered patella in a patient with multiple epiphyseal dysplasia. (This is typically seen in patients with homozygous mutations of the diastrophic dysplasia sulfate transporter gene, one of the less common autosomal recessive variants of multiple epiphyseal dysplasia). This may be a source of knee pain if there is instability in between the two fragments. (**d**) Anterior distal femoral epiphysiodesis for correction of distal femoral procurvatum deformity. (**e**) Genu valgum corrected after proximal medial tibial hemiepiphysiodesis

bony deformities include hip dysplasia with or without hip dislocation, genu valgum, and rigid foot deformities (Fig. 26.8a, b). Soft tissue problems include hip and knee flexion contractures, as well as lateral patellar dislocation [5, 71].

Hips in these patients are notoriously difficult to reduce and reconstruct. They are also difficult to assess radiographically because of a marked delay in ossification of the proximal femur. The severity, deformity, and degree of hip flexion contracture increase with age [72]. The deformities present can include severe acetabular dysplasia, a shortened femoral neck, a wide, irregular femoral head, and (relative) trochanteric overgrowth. These deformities often lead to painful and restricted motion along with hinge abduction. Premature arthritis requiring total joint replacement in young adulthood-middle age can be expected.

Open reduction of these hips is technically difficult because of the severe acetabular dysplasia and short femoral neck. Function with hip dislocation is usually satisfactory in the short term but osteoarthritis and joint replacement are inevitable. Surgical hip dislocation and femoral head reduction has been successful in the short term for painful irregular movement in the authors' experience.

Knee problems in children with diastrophic dysplasia are universal. Genu valgum is present, oftentimes with a laterally dislocated patella (25% of patients) [5] (Fig. 26.9a, b). Progressive knee flexion contracture is often a clue as to the presence of abnormal patellar mechanics. The authors prefer to reduce the patella at an early age to allow for remodeling and to alleviate valgus force at the knee. Patellar realignment procedures that we utilize include an extensive lateral release with lengthening of the ilio-tibial band and biceps femoris with medial plication and a vastus medialis obliquus (VMO) advancement (Fig. 26.10a–f). Medialization of the insertion of the patellar tendon insertion is often required. Anatomical variations include a shallow, irregular intercondylar grove and the medial femoral condyle can be covered with synovium.

Rigid foot deformities are typically seen in diastrophic dysplasia [73]. Deformities described in these children vary from tarsal valgus and metatarsus adductovarus in 43%, equinovarus and adductus in 29%, equinus in 8%, metatarsus adductovarus in 13% and normal in 7%. These feet are not like idiopathic clubfeet. The main difference is that the navicular is displaced laterally [73]. Serial manipulation and casting using the Ponseti technique can be effective in infancy,

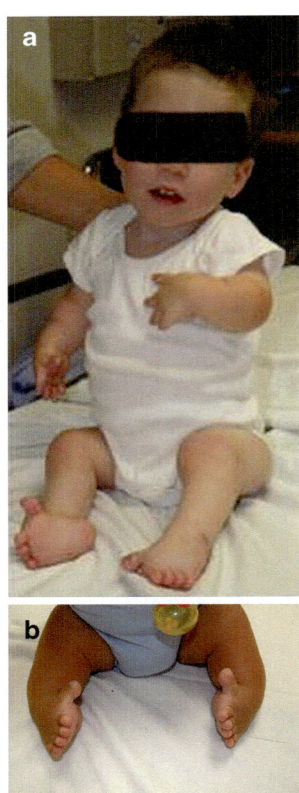

Fig. 26.8 (**a**) Hitch hiker thumb deformity in diastrophic dysplasia. (**b**) Rigid clubfeet with hallux varus in a patient with diastrophic dysplasia

but these feet often need surgical correction which must be customized to the deformity [74]. Recurrent equinus is the most common long-term complication. The feet are often scarred, and further soft tissue release doomed to failure. The authors have been managing equinus with supramalleolar extension tibial and fibular osteotomies (Fig. 26.11a–c). Recurrence in the growing child is common.

Morquio Syndrome

Mucopolysaccharidosis Type 4, also known as Morquio Syndrome, is an autosomal recessive condition attributable to an abnormality of the N-acetylgalactosamine-6-sulfatase (GALNS) gene or the B-galactosidase (GLB1) gene [75–77]. Deficiency of these enzymes leads to accumulation of keratin sulfate and chondroitin sulfate in lysosomes. Onset of clinical symptoms (Fig. 26.12a, b) is between 1 and 3 years of age, with severe early growth limitation and genu valgum being the most apparent features. A waddling gait and flat feet are seen around 3 years of age.

The hips have incomplete ossification of the proximal femoral epiphyses and acetabular dysplasia. This leads to progressive hip subluxation and femoral head deformation (coxa valga, coxa magna, and coxa brevis) [78, 79]. The result of their untreated hip pathology is oftentimes premature osteoarthritis in early adulthood [80].

Fig. 26.9 (**a**, **b**) Flexed knees secondary to dislocated patellae in a child with diastrophic dysplasia

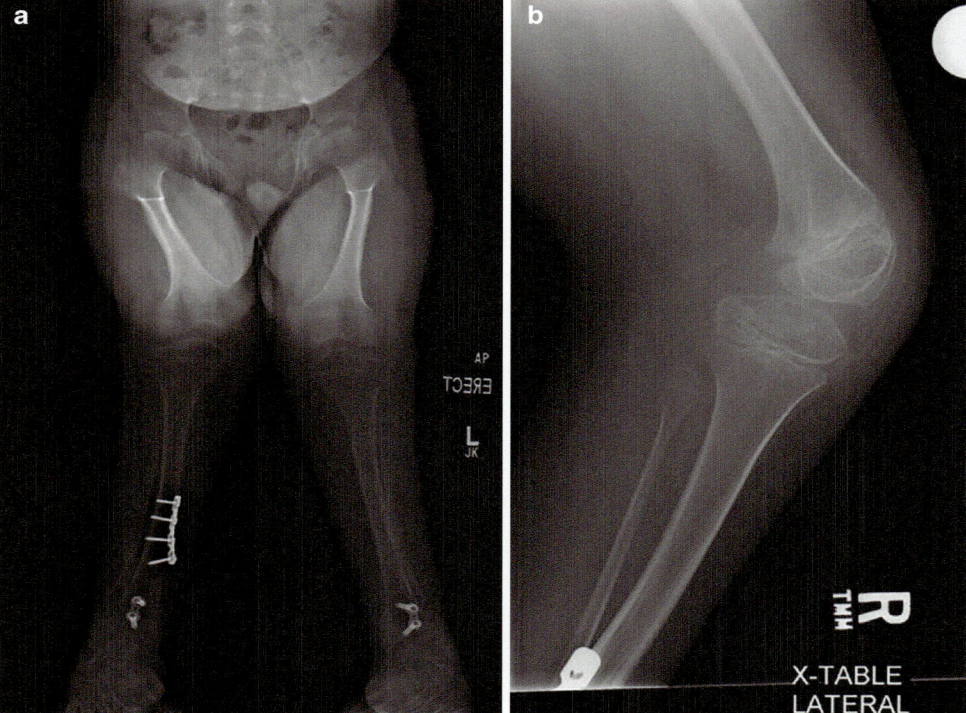

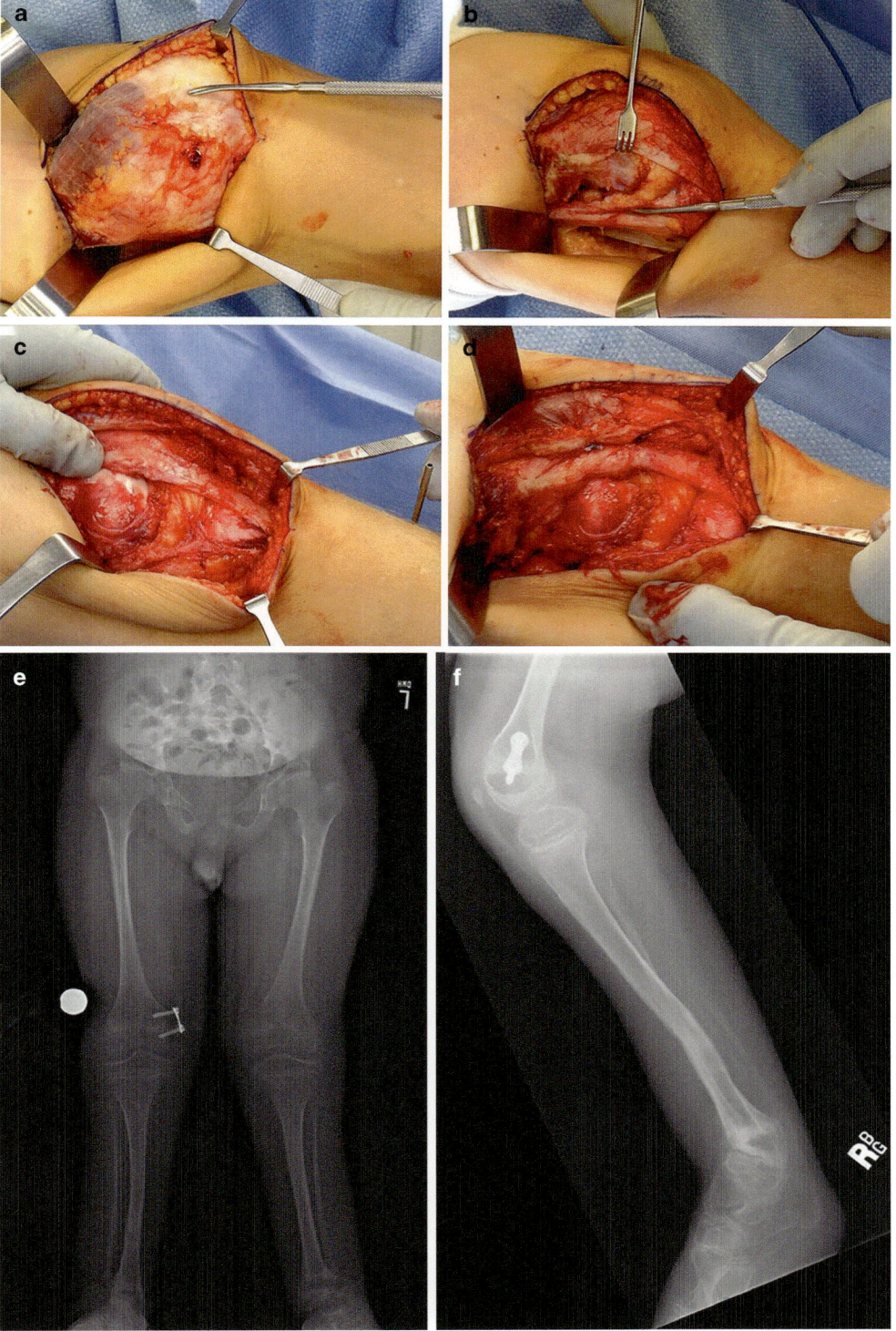

Fig. 26.10 Operative correction of patellar dislocation in a patient with diastrophic dysplasia. (**a**) Patella is dislocated laterally with the vastus medialis draped over the anterior surface of the knee. (**b**) Lateral release: Freer elevator pointing to the thickened, tight iliotibial (IT) band. (**c**) Patella relocated after extensive lateral release. (**d**) Patella stabilized with vastus medialis obliquus advancement. (**e**, **f**) Postoperative AP and lateral radiographs demonstrating correction of genu valgum with growth modulation and the patella is appropriately located on both views

To assess the complex deformities of the hip joint that may warrant operative reconstruction, preoperative computed tomography scanning [6] and intraoperative arthrography are especially useful. Isolated proximal femoral varus osteotomies or redirectional acetabular osteotomies have not prevented progressive dysplasia and subluxation. The acetabular bony roof is short with a large limbus. The limbus does not ossify normally, likely secondary to the accumulation of proteoglycans. Realignment procedures include a proximal femoral osteotomy with an acetabular procedure to improve coverage [7, 79, 81]. The authors use a large shelf harvested from the inner wall of the ilium (Fig. 26.13a–d).

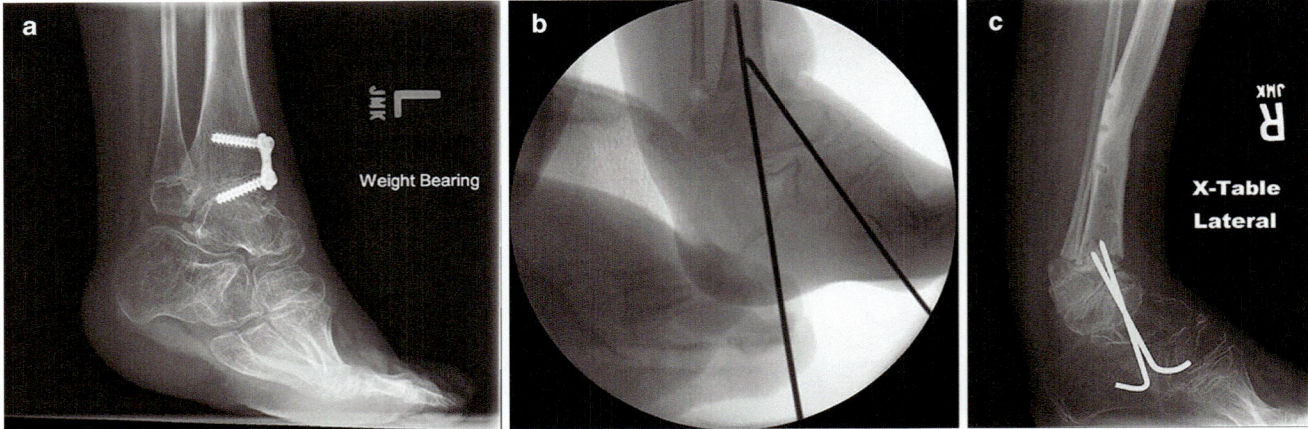

Fig. 26.11 Equinovarus foot deformity in a patient with diastrophic dysplasia. (**a**) Lateral radiograph of the ankle demonstrates the rigid deformity and an attempt to use growth modulation done at an outside facility, which did not work. (**b**) Supramalleolar osteotomies of the tibia and fibula for shortening and acute correction of the deformity. Note the posterior translation of the distal fragment. (**c**) Lateral radiograph of the ankle demonstrating healing in plantigrade position. These have a high recurrence rate

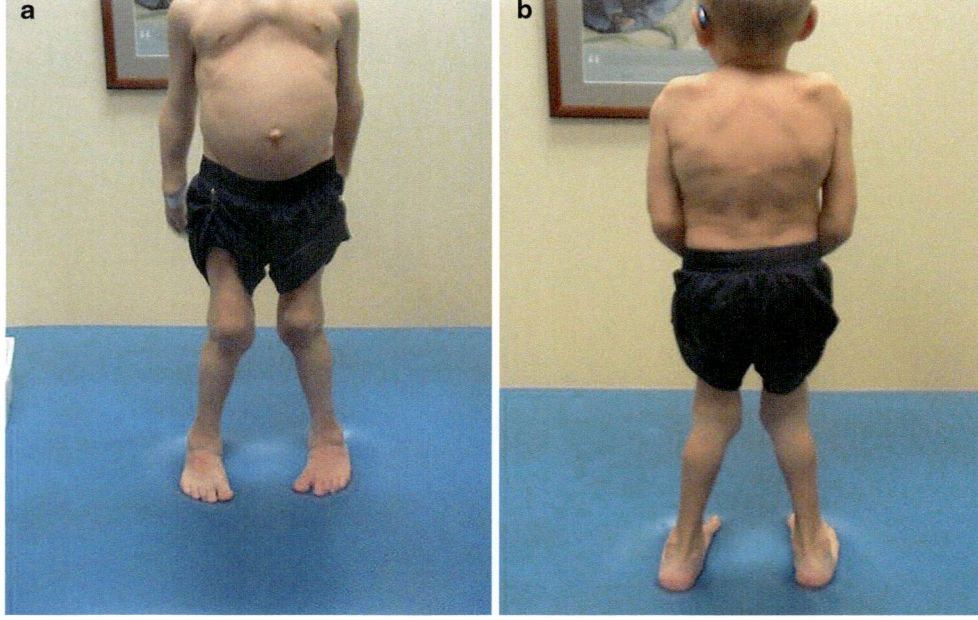

Fig. 26.12 (**a**, **b**) Clinical photographs of a boy with Morquio syndrome showing characteristic pectus carinatum, thoracolumbar kyphosis, genu valgum, and planovalgus feet

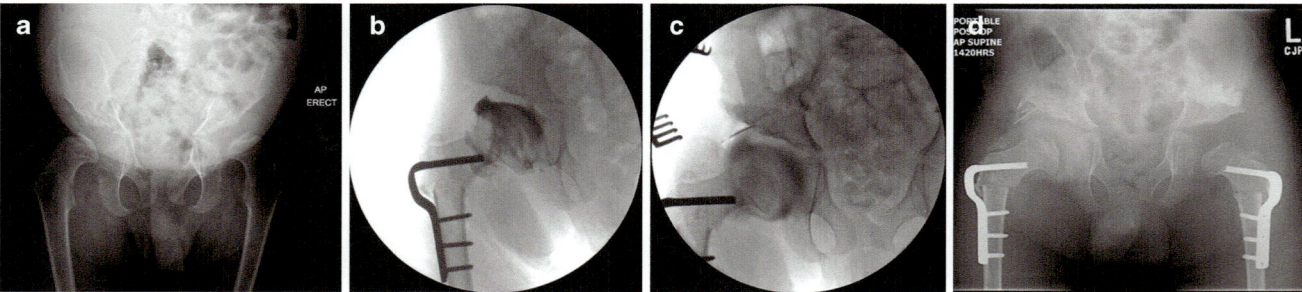

Fig. 26.13 (**a**) AP pelvis radiograph in a child with Morquio syndrome, showing bilateral coxa valga, small femoral epiphysis, acetabular dysplasia, and lateral subluxation. (**b**) Arthrogram after proximal femoral varus osteotomy highlights the unossified portions of the acetabular cartilage, which makes a volume altering osteotomy such as a Pemberton/Dega type osteotomy less appealing. (**c**) Improved coverage using a shelf (harvested from the inner table of the ilium) acetabuloplasty. (**d**) Postoperative AP pelvis radiograph showing better femoral head coverage, after proximal femoral osteotomy and shelf acetabuloplasty

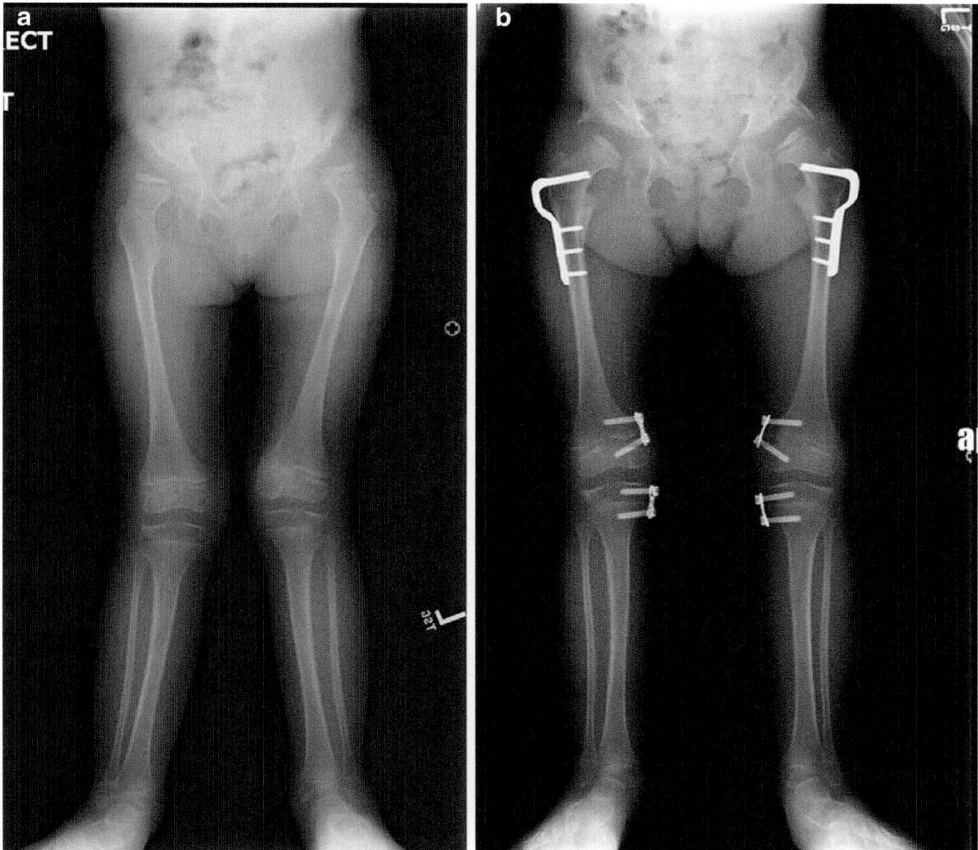

Fig. 26.14 (a, b) Genu valgum correction in a child with Morquio syndrome using growth modulation

This strategy has helped keep the femoral heads covered at intermediate to long follow up. The femoral heads do deform over time and there is proximal migration within the reconstructed acetabulum, but this strategy has helped minimize dislocation of the femoral heads.

Bilateral genu valgum is a prominent feature of Morquio syndrome. This is a result of progressive deformation due to incomplete ossification of the distal femoral and proximal tibial epiphyses, in combination with generalized ligamentous laxity [7]. Intraoperative knee arthrography is extremely helpful in planning corrective surgery about the knee. A distal femoral and/or proximal tibial realignment osteotomy has been advocated [3, 79]. The authors have found success using guided-growth techniques in the young child (less than 13 years of age) (Fig. 26.14a, b) [24]. We typically combine hip reconstruction (proximal femoral varus and derotation osteotomy, shelf acetabuloplasty) with guided growth at the distal femur and proximal tibia (using tension band plates) and ankle valgus correction (with a medial malleolar screw epiphysiodesis) under the same anesthetic. This is done using a two-surgeon team at our institution, which helps minimize surgical time. We also routinely perform neuromonitoring during these procedures.

The pes planovalgus feet seen universally in those children with Morquio syndrome can usually be managed very well using functional foot orthoses. If conservative treatment with these orthoses fails, lateral column lengthening or subtalar fusion in combination with medial column reconstruction is an option [7]. However, the long-term results of these procedures are not known.

Metaphyseal Chondrodysplasia

These are a group of dysplasias resulting from failure of uniform ossification of the cartilage columns, with persistence of cartilage islands, underdevelopment of the cartilage, resulting in deformities of the affected bones. The epiphyses are preserved and the metaphyses are the most severely affected. The differential diagnoses include rickets and hypophosphatasia. These are usually associated with genu varum, ankle varus, and coxa vara of variable severity. There are three major types of metaphyseal chondrodysplasia.

Schmid type is the most common type of metaphyseal chondrodysplasia. It is an autosomal dominant condition which results from a heterozygous mutation of the COL10A1 gene on chromosome 6q21-q22.3. This causes a defect in the α1 chain of type X collagen (which is essential for calcification of the hypertrophic zone of chondrocytes) [82].

Fig. 26.15 (a–c) Characteristic severe widening of the physes and bowing of the long bones of the lower extremities in a patient with Jansen metaphyseal chondrodysplasia

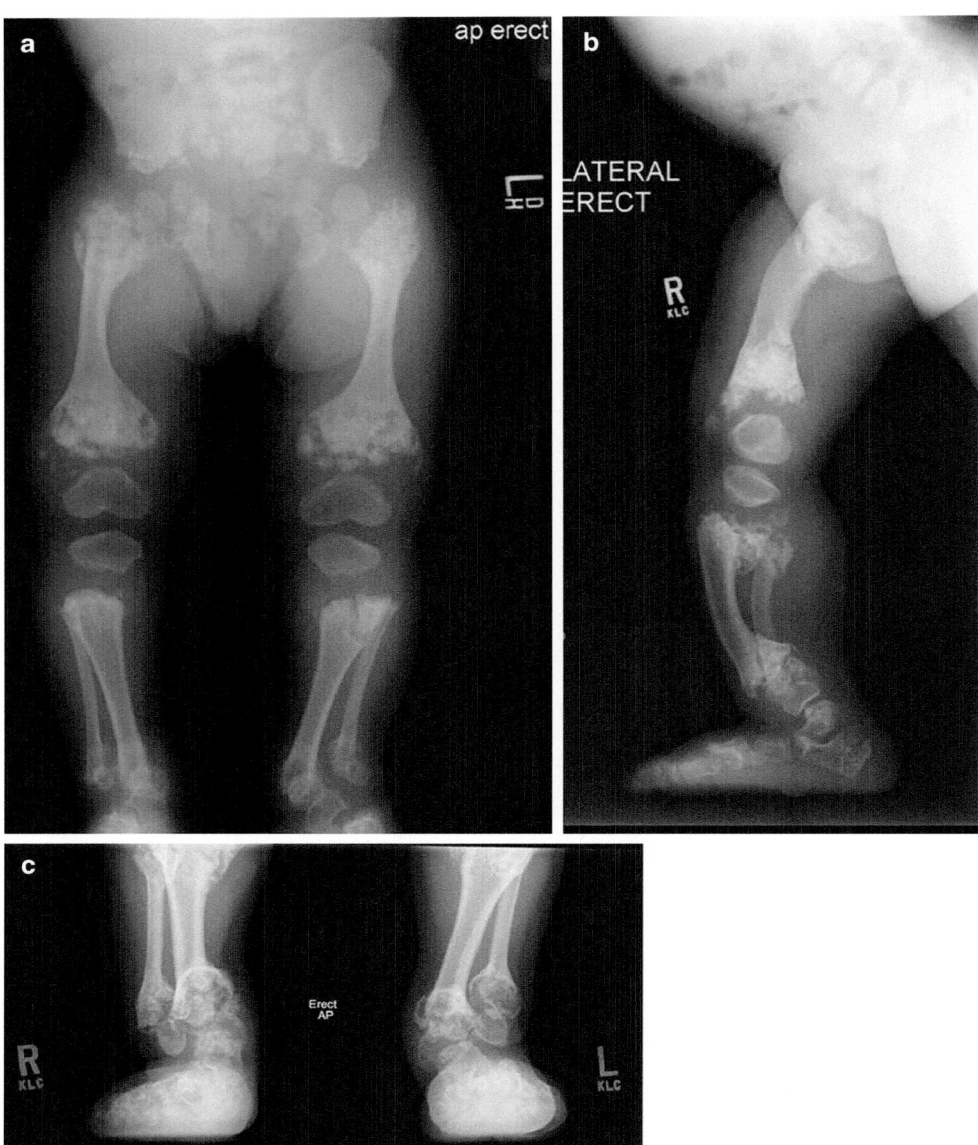

McKusick type of chondrodysplasia (also known as *cartilage hair hypoplasia*) is an autosomal recessive disorder due to a defect in the RMRP gene on chromosome 9p13.3. This results in milder genu varum and coxa vara and is also associated with decreased immunity, varying degree of anemia and characteristic cone shaped epiphyses in the phalanges [83, 84].

Jansen type (Fig. 26.15a–c) is a rare but severe, autosomal dominant, form of chondrodysplasia resulting from a mutation (at 3p21.31) resulting in ligand independent activation of parathyroid hormone related protein receptor I (PTHRP1). This results in hypercalcemia and hypophosphatemia [85, 86].

Treatment of deformities in these patients varies by type and severity. Patients with Schmid type dysplasia may show some spontaneous improvement in the first decade, but persistent or severe deformities may need correction using guided growth or osteotomies. Patients with McKusick type usually have mild deformities and rarely need treatment. Patients with Jansen type dysplasia often have severe deformities and need earlier and more aggressive treatment and are also at the highest risk of recurrence.

Ellis van Creveld Syndrome (EvC) or Chondroectodermal Dysplasia

Ellis van Creveld (EvC) syndrome is a rare autosomal recessive skeletal dysplasia that is characterized by short ribs and disproportionate short stature, ectodermal dysplasia (includ-

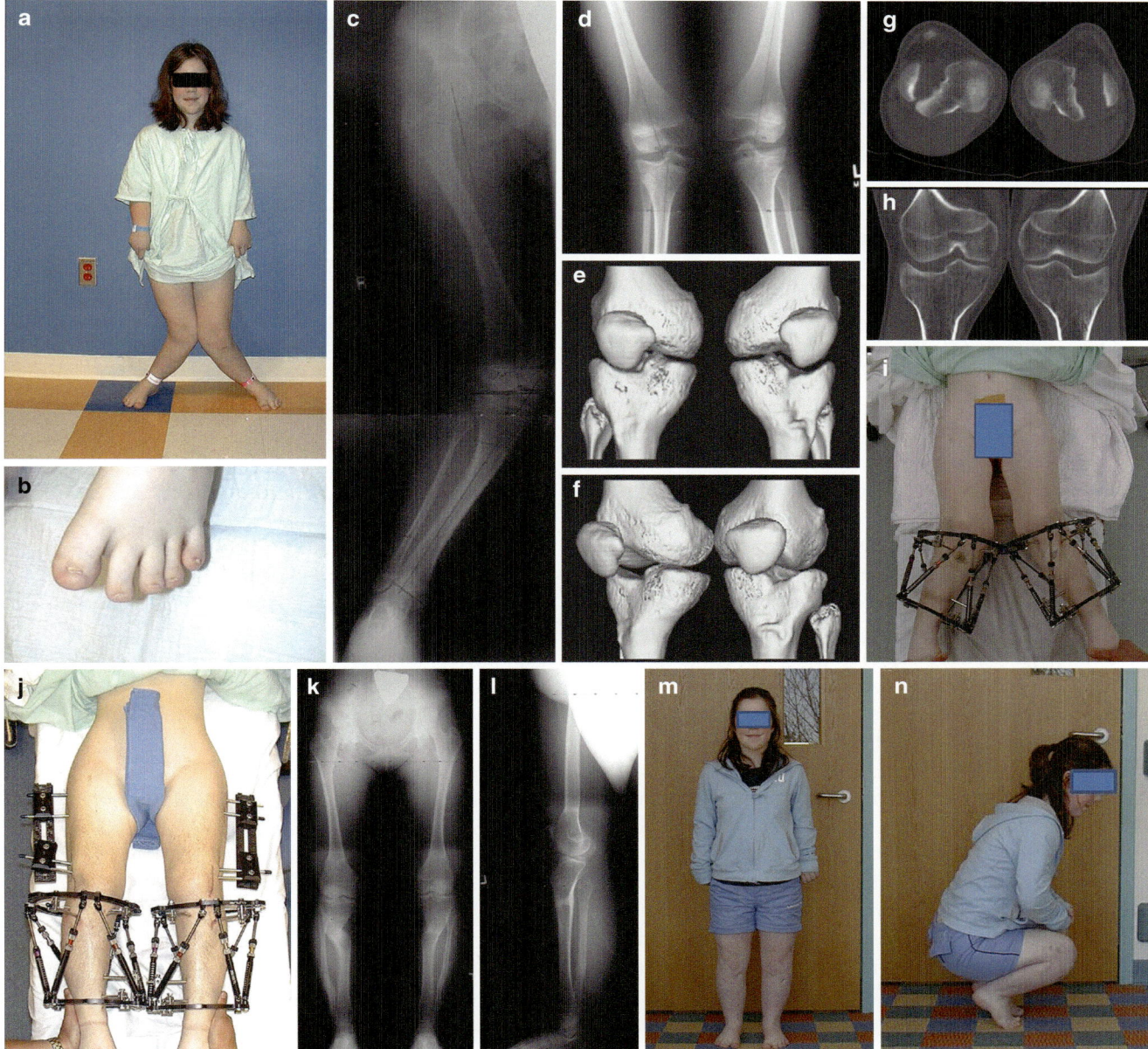

Fig. 26.16 (a) Clinical photograph of a girl with Ellis van Creveld syndrome (EvC) showing characteristic severe genu valgum. (b) Clinical photograph demonstrates dystrophic nails. EvC is also known as Chondroectodermal dysplasia. (c) AP radiograph of the right lower extremity demonstrating multifocal valgus in the lower extremity (distal and proximal femur, proximal tibia). (d) AP radiographs of the knee demonstrate genu valgum with characteristic depression of the lateral tibial plateau. (e–h) Computed tomography (CT) scan of the knee, axial, coronal views as well as 3D reconstructions demonstrate the central depression of the lateral tibial plateau. This makes plateau elevation unappealing. (i, j) Clinical photographs of the same patient with bilateral hexapod frames for computer aided deformity correction of the genu valgum as well as external tibial torsion, before and after correction. The distal femoral valgus deformity has been corrected with an external fixator. (k, l) Postoperative radiographs showing correction of the deformities in the frontal and sagittal planes. (m, n) Clinical photographs after correction demonstrating correction of the deformities and improved function

ing characteristic nail and tooth changes), post-axial polydactyly, and congenital cardiac defects (most commonly atrial septal defects) (Fig. 26.16a–n). This results from a homozygous mutation of the EvC gene located on chromosome 4p16. Orthopedic issues include post-axial polydactyly, genu valgum, patellar instability, as well as a characteristic depression of the lateral tibial plateau. The genu valgum in these patients comes from both the distal femur as well as the proximal tibia and frequently needs correction on both sides of the knee. The accompanying external tibial torsion, which can be fairly severe, makes the use of guided growth less appealing. Correction of angular deformities (often gradual), with or without lateral tibial plateau elevation, soft tissue releases, including peroneal nerve decompression, are important components of correcting and maintaining appropriate patellar tracking [87].

Summary

Limb deformities are a common source of morbidity and pain in patients with skeletal dysplasia. These patients need a comprehensive evaluation of both their skeletal as well as their systemic abnormalities by a multidisciplinary team of providers who are familiar with these issues. Correction of limb deformities is frequently needed in these patients and despite adequate correction, recurrences are common. Growth modulation has become a valuable tool in our armamentarium, given its ease and potential to repeat it, if needed. The cervical spine should be carefully evaluated preoperatively, especially in patients at risk for cervical instability (most dysplasias except achondroplasia). Anesthesia can be quite a challenge in these patients and appropriate equipment and expertise are paramount to safely putting these patients to sleep for their orthopedic procedures and waking them back up. Combining procedures to minimize episodes of anesthesia should be strongly considered to minimize anesthesia risk. Prolonged procedures, especially in patients with severe kyphosis, may place the cord at risk for stretching and neuromonitoring must be considered during these procedures (even if they do not involve the spine). Limb deformities should be carefully evaluated as most are multifocal and multiplanar. Appropriate equipment and size appropriate fixation devices must be available during deformity correction surgery for these patients. Deformity correction in these patients can offer relief of symptoms and improvement in their mobility. Early arthritis may be seen in some dysplasias (COMP abnormalities, etc.) and methods of deformity correction should not compromise the subsequent arthroplasty once the joint is irreversibly damaged.

Enzyme replacement therapy (ERT) has become standard in treatment of some dysplasias (particularly the mucopolysaccharidoses) [10, 88, 89]. ERT, unfortunately, does not seem to alter the musculoskeletal, ophthalmologic, and neurologic manifestations of the disease. Improvement in the understanding of the molecular mechanisms and pathways involved in the genesis of dysplasias may enable us to intervene at a molecular level early on and potentially prevent/blunt some of the musculoskeletal manifestations of the disease, and hopefully this will translate into less morbidity and better quality of life for our patients.

Commentary

Klane K. White
Klane.white@childrenscolorado.org

The collective knowledge about the etiology, pathophysiology, and clinical care for patients with skeletal dysplasia has expanded tremendously in the past 20 years. With over 400 phenotypes described, with at last count 96% having an identified genetic etiology, orthopedic surgeons should make themselves aware of the increasing nuances of care among this highly heterogeneous group. These patients present not only complex orthopedic challenges but are often quite medical complex as well. The orthopedic surgeon would be wise to enlist the insights and opinions of their medical subspecialist colleagues prior to embarking on a potentially fateful care episode.

Proper evaluation of airway by pulmonology and sleep medicine, cardiology, otolaryngology, genetics, physiatry, and anesthesia before surgical intervention is mandatory. Perioperative management not typically employed for average stature children, such as advanced airway equipment, spinal cord monitoring, and postoperative intensive care should all be considered for each case. At the very least, consider one level of postoperative care higher than that usually employed (i.e., for day surgery, consider admission; for surgical floor patients, consider an intensive care bed).

Regarding deformity correction, there is now greater acceptance of guided growth techniques. For children over age eight, it is worthwhile to study the individual growth charts to ensure that the child has growth potential based on the past and current growth trajectory. Hand bone age films can be helpful, but in many cases, are not reliable for predicting the amount of growth remaining. Furthermore, most children with skeletal dysplasia do not have the benefit of a prepubertal growth spurt to aid in the deformity correction achieved by guided growth, and to the contrary, often have a deceleration of growth as they approach puberty.

For children with little remaining growth, or those who are too small for tension banding plates, osteotomy still remains the treatment of choice. Acute correction or gradual corrective measure are well described in this chapter, and should be individualized based on the surgeon's best judgement. While the skeletal elements are typically smaller than those of average stature children, bone quality and healing are not generally a problem for patients with skeletal dysplasia, despite the common misconception that this is the case.

Finally, it is incumbent on the orthopedic surgeon to be aware of advancements in medical and therapeutic technologies for these patients. Several growth augmentation medications are in development or have been approved for achondroplasia. This development will have obvious consequences on the use of guided growth. Enzyme replacement therapy for the MPS, or in the case of Hurler Syndrome (MPS type IH) hematopoietic stem cell transplantation, have changed the medical care, function, quality of life, and even the life expectancy for these disorders. There are many other therapies in the pipeline for an array of skeletal dysplasia that may have a significant impact on how these children are cared for. Continued scholarly vigilance is paramount in the care of these medically complex children.

References

1. Baitner AC, Maurer SG, Gruen MB, Di Cesare PE. The genetic basis of the osteochondrodysplasias. J Pediatr Orthop. 2000;20(5):594–605.
2. Bassett GS. Lower-extremity abnormalities in dwarfing conditions. Instr Course Lect. 1990;39:389–97.
3. Kopits SE. Orthopedic complications of dwarfism. Clin Orthop Relat Res. 1976;114:153–79.
4. Nelson MA. Orthopaedic aspects of the chondrodystrophies. The dwarf and his orthopaedic problems. Ann R Coll Surg Engl. 1970;47(4):185–210.
5. Shapiro F. Review of specific skeletal dysplasias. Pediatric orthopaedic deformities. Academic Press; 2001. p. 733–870.
6. Borowski A, Thacker MM, Mackenzie WG, Littleton AG, Grissom L. The use of computed tomography to assess acetabular morphology in Morquio-Brailsford syndrome. J Pediatr Orthop. 2007;27(8):893–7.
7. Dhawale AA, Thacker MM, Belthur MV, Rogers K, Bober MB, Mackenzie WG. The lower extremity in Morquio syndrome. J Pediatr Orthop. 2012;32(5):534–40.
8. Dhawale AA, Church C, Henley J, Holmes L Jr, Thacker MM, Mackenzie WG, et al. Gait pattern and lower extremity alignment in children with Morquio syndrome. J Pediatr Orthop B. 2013;22(1):59–62.
9. White KK. Orthopaedic aspects of mucopolysaccharidoses. Rheumatology (Oxford). 2011;50(Suppl 5):v26–33.
10. Nan H, Park C, Maeng S. Mucopolysaccharidoses I and II: brief review of therapeutic options and supportive/palliative therapies. Biomed Res Int. 2020;2020:2408402. https://doi.org/10.1155/2020/2408402.
11. Peracha H, Sawamoto K, Averill L, Kecskemethy H, Theroux M, Thacker M, Nagao K, Pizarro C, Mackenzie W, Kobayashi H, Yamaguchi S, Suzuki Y, Orii K, Orii T, Fukao T, Tomatsu S. Molecular genetics and metabolism, special edition: diagnosis, diagnosis and prognosis of Mucopolysaccharidosis IVA. Mol Genet Metab. 2018;125(1–2):18–37.
12. Hunter AG. Perceptions of the outcome of orthopedic surgery in patients with chondrodysplasias. Clin Genet. 1999;56(6):434–40.
13. Al KA, Ganger R, Roetzer KM, Schwarzbraun T, Klaushofer K, Grill F. Re-alignment-procedures for skeletal dysplasia in three patients with genetically diverse syndromes. Orthop Surg. 2013;5(1):33–9.
14. Fernandes JA, Devalia KL, Moras P, Pagdin J, Jones S, Mcmullan J. Screening for spinal stenosis in achondroplastic patients undergoing limb lengthening. J Pediatr Orthop B. 2014;23(2):181–6.
15. Mackenzie WG, Dhawale AA, Demczko MM, Ditro C, Rogers KJ, Bober MB, Campbell JW, Grissom LE. Flexion-extension cervical spine MRI in children with skeletal dysplasia: is it safe and effective? J Pediatr Orthop. 2013;33(1):91–8.
16. Inan M, Thacker M, Church C, Miller F, Mackenzie WG, Conklin D. Dynamic lower extremity alignment in children with achondroplasia. J Pediatr Orthop. 2006;26(4):526–9.
17. Theroux MC, Nerker T, Ditro C, Mackenzie WG. Anesthetic care and perioperative complications of children with Morquio syndrome. Paediatr Anaesth. 2012;22(9):901–7.
18. Shetty GM, Song HR, Unnikrishnan R, Suh SW, Lee SH, Hur CY. Upper cervical spine instability in pseudoachondroplasia. J Pediatr Orthop. 2007;27(7):782–7.
19. Pruszczynski B, Mackenzie WG, Rogers K, White KK. Spinal cord injury after extremity surgery in children with thoracic kyphosis. Clin Orthop Relat Res. 2015;473(10):3315–20.
20. Fraser SC, Neubauer PR, Ain MC. The role of arthrography in selecting an osteotomy for the correction of genu varum in pediatric patients with achondroplasia. J Pediatr Orthop B. 2011;20(1):14–6.
21. Hunter AG, Bankier A, Rogers JG, Sillence D, Scott CI Jr. Medical complications of achondroplasia: a multicentre patient review. J Med Genet. 1998;35(9):705–12.
22. Beals RK, Stanley G. Surgical correction of bowlegs in achondroplasia. J Pediatr Orthop B. 2005;14(4):245–9.
23. Pinkowski JL, Weiner DS. Complications in proximal tibial osteotomies in children with presentation of technique. J Pediatr Orthop. 1995;15(3):307–12.
24. Yilmaz G, Oto M, Thabet AM, Rogers KJ, Anticevic D, Thacker MM, et al. Correction of lower extremity angular deformities in skeletal dysplasia with hemiepiphysiodesis: a preliminary report. J Pediatr Orthop. 2014;34(3):336–45.
25. Cho TJ, Choi IH, Chung CY, Yoo WJ, Park MS, Lee DY. Hemiepiphyseal stapling for angular deformity correction around the knee joint in children with multiple epiphyseal dysplasia. J Pediatr Orthop. 2009;29(1):52–6.
26. Ulusaloglu AC, Asma A, Rogers KJ, Thacker MM, Mackenzie WGS, Mackenzie WG. Risk factors for rebound after correction of genu Valgum in skeletal dysplasia patients treated by tension band plates. J Pediatr Orthop. 2022;42(4):190–4.
27. Bell DF, Boyer MI, Armstrong PF. The use of the Ilizarov technique in the correction of limb deformities associated with skeletal dysplasia. J Pediatr Orthop. 1992;12(3):283–90.
28. Kim SJ, Cielo B, Song SH, Song HR, Song SY. Gradual bilateral genu varum correction in skeletal dysplasia using the Ilizarov method. J Orthop Sci. 2011;16(4):405–12.
29. Kim SJ, Balce GC, Agashe MV, Song SH, Song HR. Is bilateral lower limb lengthening appropriate for achondroplasia?: midterm

29. analysis of the complications and quality of life. Clin Orthop Relat Res. 2012;470(2):616–21.
30. Song SH, Kim SE, Agashe MV, Lee H, Refai MA, Park YE, et al. Growth disturbance after lengthening of the lower limb and quantitative assessment of physeal closure in skeletally immature patients with achondroplasia. J Bone Joint Surg Br. 2012;94(4):556–63.
31. Ganel A, Horoszowski H. Limb lengthening in children with achondroplasia. Differences based on gender. Clin Orthop Relat Res. 1996;332:179–83.
32. Novikov KI, Subramanyam KN, Muradisinov SO, Novikova OS, Kolesnikova ES. Cosmetic lower limb lengthening by Ilizarov apparatus: what are the risks? Clin Orthop Relat Res. 2014;472(11):3549–56.
33. Song SH, Agashe MV, Huh YJ, Hwang SY, Song HR. Physeal growth arrest after tibial lengthening in achondroplasia: 23 children followed to skeletal maturity. Acta Orthop. 2012;83(3):282–7.
34. Venkatesh KP, Modi HN, Devmurari K, Yoon JY, Anupama BR, Song HR. Femoral lengthening in achondroplasia: magnitude of lengthening in relation to patterns of callus, stiffness of adjacent joints and fracture. J Bone Joint Surg Br. 2009;91(12):1612–7.
35. Aldegheri R, Dall'Oca C. Limb lengthening in short stature patients. J Pediatr Orthop B. 2001;10(3):238–47.
36. Kanaka-Gantenbein C. Present status of the use of growth hormone in short children with bone diseases (diseases of the skeleton). J Pediatr Endocrinol Metab. 2001;14(1):17–26.
37. Peretti G, Memeo A, Paronzini A, Marzorati S. Staged lengthening in the prevention of dwarfism in achondroplastic children: a preliminary report. J Pediatr Orthop B. 1995;4(1):58–64.
38. Shabtai L, Jauregui JJ, Herzenberg JE, Gesheff MG, Standard SC, McClure PK. Simultaneous bilateral femoral and tibial lengthening in achondroplasia. Children (Basel). 2021;8(9):749.
39. Paley D. Extensive limb lengthening for achondroplasia and hypochondroplasia. Children (Basel). 2021;8(7):540.
40. Kim RH, Scuderi GR, Dennis DA, Nakano SW. Technical challenges of total knee arthroplasty in skeletal dysplasia. Clin Orthop Relat Res. 2011;469(1):69–75.
41. Sewell MD, Hanna SA, Al-Khateeb H, Miles J, Pollock RC, Carrington RW, et al. Custom rotating-hinge primary total knee arthroplasty in patients with skeletal dysplasia. J Bone Joint Surg Br. 2012;94(3):339–43.
42. Ain MC, Andres BM, Somel DS, Fishkin Z, Frassica FJ. Total hip arthroplasty in skeletal dysplasias: patient selection, preoperative planning, and operative techniques. J Arthroplast. 2004;19(1):1–7.
43. Guenther D, Kendoff D, Omar M, Cui LR, Gehrke T, Haasper C. Total hip arthroplasty in patients with skeletal dysplasia. J Arthroplast. 2015;30(9):1574–6.
44. Foldynova-Trantirkova S, Wilcox WR, Krejci P. Sixteen years and counting: the current understanding of fibroblast growth factor receptor 3 (FGFR3) signaling in skeletal dysplasias. Hum Mutat. 2012;33(1):29–41.
45. Balci HI, Kocaoglu M, Sen C, Eralp L, Batibay SG, Bilsel K. Bilateral humeral lengthening in achondroplasia with unilateral external fixators: is it safe and does it improve daily life? Bone Joint J. 2015;97-B(11):1577–81.
46. Ain MC, Shirley ED, Pirouzmanesh A, Skolasky RL, Leet AI. Genu varum in achondroplasia. J Pediatr Orthop. 2006;26(3):375–9.
47. Bailey JA. Orthopaedic aspects of achondroplasia. J Bone Joint Surg Am. 1970;52(7):1285–301.
48. Stanley G, McLoughlin S, Beals RK. Observations on the cause of bowlegs in achondroplasia. J Pediatr Orthop. 2002;22(1):112–6.
49. Ponseti IV. Bone formation in achondroplasia. Basic Life Sci. 1988;48:109–22.
50. Kruse RW, Bowen JR, Heithoff S. Oblique tibial osteotomy in the correction of tibial deformity in children. J Pediatr Orthop. 1989;9(4):476–82.
51. Laurencin CT, Ferriter PJ, Millis MB. Oblique proximal tibial osteotomy for the correction of tibia vara in the young. Clin Orthop Relat Res. 1996;327:218–24.
52. Myers GJ, Bache CE, Bradish CF. Use of distraction osteogenesis techniques in skeletal dysplasias. J Pediatr Orthop. 2003;23(1):41–5.
53. Vaidya SV, Song HR, Lee SH, Suh SW, Keny SM, Telang SS. Bifocal tibial corrective osteotomy with lengthening in achondroplasia: an analysis of results and complications. J Pediatr Orthop. 2006;26(6):788–93.
54. Murray LW, Rimoin DL. Abnormal type II collagen in the spondyloepiphyseal dysplasias. Pathol Immunopathol Res. 1988;7(1–2):99–103.
55. Balint G, Szebenyi B. Hereditary disorders mimicking and/or causing premature osteoarthritis. Baillieres Best Pract Res Clin Rheumatol. 2000;14(2):219–50.
56. Crossan JF, Wynne-Davies R, Fulford GE. Bilateral failure of the capital femoral epiphysis: bilateral Perthes disease, multiple epiphyseal dysplasia, pseudoachondroplasia, and spondyloepiphyseal dysplasia congenita and tarda. J Pediatr Orthop. 1983;3(3):297–301.
57. Oh CW, Thacker MM, Mackenzie WG, Riddle EC. Coxa vara: a novel measurement technique in skeletal dysplasias. Clin Orthop Relat Res. 2006;447:125–31.
58. Carroll K, Coleman S, Stevens PM. Coxa vara: surgical outcomes of valgus osteotomies. J Pediatr Orthop. 1997;17(2):220–4.
59. Kim HT, Chambers HG, Mubarak SJ, Wenger DR. Congenital coxa vara: computed tomographic analysis of femoral retroversion and the triangular metaphyseal fragment. J Pediatr Orthop. 2000;20(5):551–6.
60. Shim JS, Kim HT, Mubarak SJ, Wenger DR. Genu valgum in children with coxa vara resulting from hip disease. J Pediatr Orthop. 1997;17(2):225–9.
61. Briggs MD, Hoffman SM, King LM, Olsen AS, Mohrenweiser H, Leroy JG, et al. Pseudoachondroplasia and multiple epiphyseal dysplasia due to mutations in the cartilage oligomeric matrix protein gene. Nat Genet. 1995;10(3):330–6.
62. Briggs MD, Chapman KL. Pseudoachondroplasia and multiple epiphyseal dysplasia: mutation review, molecular interactions, and genotype to phenotype correlations. Hum Mutat. 2002;19(5):465–78.
63. Makitie O, Mortier GR, Czarny-Ratajczak M, Wright MJ, Suri M, Rogala P, et al. Clinical and radiographic findings in multiple epiphyseal dysplasia caused by MATN3 mutations: description of 12 patients. Am J Med Genet A. 2004;125A(3):278–84.
64. Sebik A, Sebik F, Kutluay E, Kuyurtar F, Ademoglu Y. The orthopaedic aspects of multiple epiphyseal dysplasia. Int Orthop. 1998;22(6):417–21.
65. Mackenzie WG, Bassett GS, Mandell GA, Scott CI Jr. Avascular necrosis of the hip in multiple epiphyseal dysplasia. J Pediatr Orthop. 1989;9(6):666–71.
66. Mandell GA, Mackenzie WG, Scott CI Jr, Harcke HT, Wills JS, Bassett GS. Identification of avascular necrosis in the dysplastic proximal femoral epiphysis. Skeletal Radiol. 1989;18(4):273–81.
67. Treble NJ, Jensen FO, Bankier A, Rogers JG, Cole WG. Development of the hip in multiple epiphyseal dysplasia. Natural history and susceptibility to premature osteoarthritis. J Bone Joint Surg Br. 1990;72(6):1061–4.
68. Miura H, Noguchi Y, Mitsuyasu H, Nagamine R, Urabe K, Matsuda S, et al. Clinical features of multiple epiphyseal dysplasia expressed in the knee. Clin Orthop Relat Res. 2000;380:184–90.
69. Hastbacka J, de la Chapelle A, Mahtani MM, Clines G, Reeve-Daly MP, Daly M, et al. The diastrophic dysplasia gene encodes a novel sulfate transporter: positional cloning by fine-structure linkage disequilibrium mapping. Cell. 1994;78(6):1073–87.
70. Superti-Furga A, Hastbacka J, Rossi A, van der Harten JJ, Wilcox WR, Cohn DH, et al. A family of chondrodysplasias caused by

mutations in the diastrophic dysplasia sulfate transporter gene and associated with impaired sulfation of proteoglycans. Ann N Y Acad Sci. 1996;785:195–201.
71. Weiner DS, Jonah D, Kopits S. The 3-dimensional configuration of the typical hip and knee in diastrophic dysplasia. J Pediatr Orthop. 2010;30(4):403–10.
72. Vaara P, Peltonen J, Poussa M, Merikanto J, Nurminen M, Kaitila I, et al. Development of the hip in diastrophic dysplasia. J Bone Joint Surg Br. 1998;80(2):315–20.
73. Weiner DS, Jonah D, Kopits S. The 3-dimensional configuration of the typical foot and ankle in diastrophic dysplasia. J Pediatr Orthop. 2008;28(1):60–7.
74. Ryoppy S, Poussa M, Merikanto J, Marttinen E, Kaitila I. Foot deformities in diastrophic dysplasia. An analysis of 102 patients. J Bone Joint Surg Br. 1992;74(3):441–4.
75. Morris CP, Guo XH, Apostolou S, Hopwood JJ, Scott HS. Morquio a syndrome: cloning, sequence, and structure of the human N-acetylgalactosamine 6-sulfatase (GALNS) gene. Genomics. 1994;22(3):652–4.
76. Oshima A, Yoshida K, Shimmoto M, Fukuhara Y, Sakuraba H, Suzuki Y. Human beta-galactosidase gene mutations in morquio B disease. Am J Hum Genet. 1991;49(5):1091–3.
77. Tomatsu S, Montano AM, Nishioka T, Gutierrez MA, Pena OM, Tranda Firescu GG, et al. Mutation and polymorphism spectrum of the GALNS gene in mucopolysaccharidosis IVA (Morquio a). Hum Mutat. 2005;26(6):500–12.
78. Kanazawa T, Yasunaga Y, Ikuta Y, Harada A, Kusaka O, Sukegawa K. Femoral head dysplasia in Morquio disease type A: bilateral varus osteotomy of the femur. Acta Orthop Scand. 2001;72(1):18–21.
79. Mikles M, Stanton RP. A review of Morquio syndrome. Am J Orthop (Belle Mead NJ). 1997;26(8):533–40.
80. Heisel J, Hesselschwerdt HJ. [Endoprosthetic joint replacement in Morquio-Brailsford syndrome]. Z Orthop Ihre Grenzgeb 1996;134(2):189–94.
81. Tomatsu S, Montano AM, Oikawa H, Smith M, Barrera L, Chinen Y, et al. Mucopolysaccharidosis type IVA (Morquio A disease): clinical review and current treatment. Curr Pharm Biotechnol. 2011;12(6):931–45.
82. Wallis GA, Rash B, Sykes B, Bonaventure J, Maroteaux P, Zabel B, et al. Mutations within the gene encoding the alpha 1 (X) chain of type X collagen (COL10A1) cause metaphyseal chondrodysplasia type Schmid but not several other forms of metaphyseal chondrodysplasia. J Med Genet. 1996;33(6):450–7.
83. Mckusick VA, Eldridge R, Hostetler JA, Ruangwit U, Egeland JA. Dwarfism in the Amish. II. Cartilage-hair hypoplasia. Bull Johns Hopkins Hosp. 1965;116:285–326.
84. Bonafe L, Schmitt K, Eich G, Giedion A, Superti-Furga A. RMRP gene sequence analysis confirms a cartilage-hair hypoplasia variant with only skeletal manifestations and reveals a high density of single-nucleotide polymorphisms. Clin Genet. 2002;61(2):146–51.
85. Cohen MM Jr. Some chondrodysplasias with short limbs: molecular perspectives. Am J Med Genet. 2002;112(3):304–13.
86. Schipani E, Kruse K, Juppner H. A constitutively active mutant PTH-PTHrP receptor in Jansen-type metaphyseal chondrodysplasia. Science. 1995;268(5207):98–100.
87. Weiner DS, Tank JC, Jonah D, Morscher MA, Krahe A, Kopits S, et al. An operative approach to address severe genu valgum deformity in the Ellis-van Creveld syndrome. J Child Orthop. 2014;8(1):61–9.
88. Marzin P, Cormier-Daire V. New perspectives on the treatment of skeletal dysplasia. Ther Adv Endocrinol Metab. 2020;11:2042018820904016.
89. Sawamoto K, Álvarez González JV, Piechnik M, Otero FJ, Couce ML, Suzuki Y, Tomatsu S. Mucopolysaccharidosis IVA: diagnosis, treatment, and management. Int J Mol Sci. 2020;21(4):1517.

Lower Extremity Benign Bone Lesions and Related Conditions

27

Lori Karol and Daniel E. Prince

Introduction

Pediatric benign bone lesions comprise a group of diseases where the presence of abnormal tissue within or on the surface of the growing bone may create skeletal deformities of the lower limb, including pain, functional limitations, deformity, and limb length discrepancy. In conditions such as fibrous dysplasia and osteofibrous dysplasia, changes in the mechanical strength of bone lead to pain, angular deformity or pathologic fracture. In the growing child, angular deformity may also result from abnormal physeal growth as seen in multiple hereditary exostoses. Limb length discrepancy may result from disturbances in physeal function as seen in such conditions as enchondromatosis. This chapter will discuss the most common pathologic bony lesions seen in children that are associated with lower limb deformity.

Nonossifying Fibroma

A nonossifying fibroma is the most common benign bone lesion found in children. It is a solitary lytic lesion which is characterized by replacement of the normal bone with bland fibrous tissue. The lesions are usually asymptomatic and are diagnosed either coincidentally on a radiograph obtained following an injury or at the time of pathologic fracture [1, 2]. They are usually diagnosed in the first two decades of life [3].

Nonossifying fibromas appear as cortically-based, lytic lesions that are eccentric in the metaphyseal regions of growing bones (Fig. 27.1a). They typically appear lobulated with distinct sclerotic margins, but without periosteal reaction. They are contained within the bone and do not typically expand the width of the bone but may thin the cortex from within via endosteal scalloping. The lesion is lytic, lacking calcification, and are most often solitary. They occur most frequently in the long bones, with the most common sites being the medial aspect of the distal femur, the medial proximal tibia, and lateral distal tibia.

Biopsy is often not necessary given the characteristic radiographic appearance without malignant features. Histopathologic evaluation of nonossifying fibromas shows sheets of bland fibroblasts with small nuclei without pleomorphism.

Treatment of nonossifying fibromas is nonsurgical in the vast majority of patients, as structural integrity is rarely compromised. A NOF greater than 50% of the width of the bone and greater than 3 cm in length has been identified to increase the risk of pathologic fracture, though smaller lesions have been noted to lead to stress fractures too, albeit rare [4, 5]. Pathologic fractures heal with immobilization and may lead to resolution of the lesion. Surgical indications include progressive pain with weight bearing, a large nonossifying fibroma located in a weight-bearing bone, or a displaced pathologic fracture. Surgical treatment typically involves intra-operative biopsy or frozen section for diagnostic confirmation, curettage of the lesion without adjuvant treatment, and bone grafting, though internal fixation is typically required with surgical intervention. The natural history of nonossifying fibromas is that they ossify during adulthood, occasionally resulting in an ossified fibromatous lesion similar to an enostosis or bone island. Treatment typically eradi-

---

Lori Karol was deceased at the time of publication.

L. Karol (Deceased)
Department of Orthopedic Surgery, Texas Scottish Rite Hospital, Dallas, TX, USA
e-mail: lori.karol@tsrh.org

D. E. Prince (✉)
Division of Orthopaedic Oncology, Department of Surgery, Memorial Sloan Kettering Cancer Center, New York, NY, USA
e-mail: princed@mskcc.org

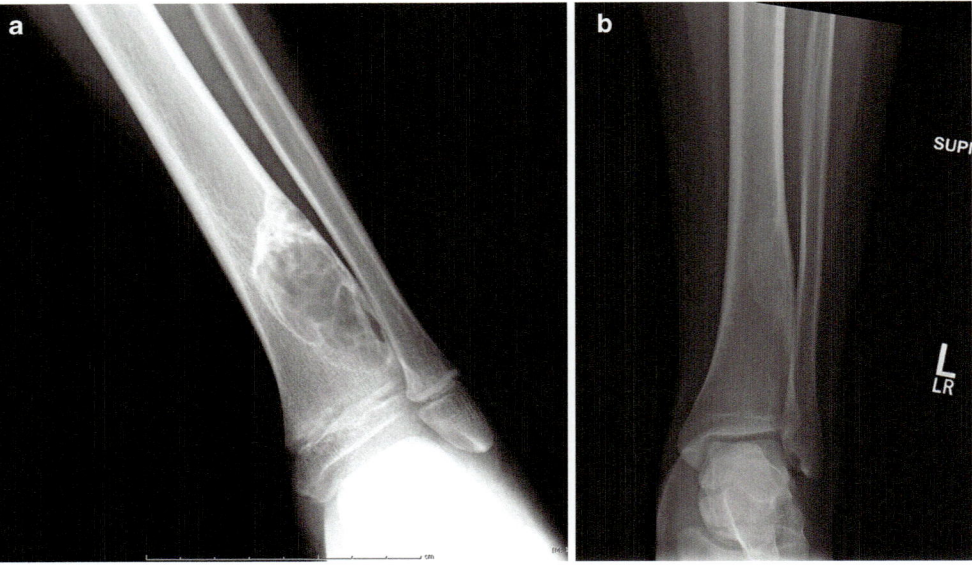

Fig. 27.1 (a) Radiograph of the ankle of a 7-year-old boy with ankle pain. Note the eccentric lobulated contained lesion which thins the surrounding cortex. Biopsy at the time of surgery confirmed the diagnosis of a nonossifying fibroma. (b) Radiograph 8 years following curettage and bone graft shows resolution of the lesion. The boy is asymptomatic and participates in contact athletics

cates the lesion and allows for return to full athletic participation [6, 7] (see Fig. 27.1b).

Box 27.1 Nonossifying Fibroma

Age at presentation: first or second decade.
  Location: Eccentric metaphyis.
  Number: solitary.
  Presenting symptoms: usually none, occasional fracture.
  Rx: none unless large.
  Malignant degeneration: none.

Fibrous Dysplasia, McCune Albright Syndrome

Fibrous dysplasia is a phenotypically varied, non-inherited condition defined by the replacement of normal trabecular bone by fibrous tissue and immature disorganized osteoid as well as eradication of normal hematopoetic bone marrow [8]. Significant progress has been made in understanding the underlying genetics and pathophysiology of this condition, although this knowledge has not yet translated into optimal treatment strategies [9]. McCune Albright Syndrome is the rare combination of FD, café-au-lait pigmentation, and endocrinological abnormalities, which are a result of widespread distribution of the constitutively stimulated Galphas mutation described in further detail. Mazabraud Syndrome is the association of fibrous dysplasia with muscular myxomas and is even more rare.

Fibrous dysplasia and related conditions are the result of a sporadic, post-zygotic somatic mutations in the GNAS locus on chromosome 20, which encodes for five transcripts, including the GAlpha-stimulating protein, part of the transmembrane heterotrimeric G protein which functions to tranduce signals from ligand-bound G protein-coupled receptors on the cell surface to intracellular effectors [10, 11]. All the known pathogenic mutations in FD/MAS result in the production of a constitutively active Galpha-signaling protein that upregulates cyclic AMP production by adenylyl cyclase and activating protein kinase A [12]. More than 95% of Galphas mutations occur at the R201 position of exon 8, while 5% occur at the Q227 position of exon 9 [10, 13, 14], though mutations in either codon inhibit the G protein conversion to its inactive state, leading to protracted downstream signaling including:

- Decreased osteoblastic differentiation
- Increased cellular proliferation
- Increased marrow fibrosis
- Increased woven bone formation
- Impaired mineralization
- Hormone over-production

The phenotypic outcome of these varied downstream biochemical processes results in replacement of bone with immature, fibroblast-like, osteoprogenitor cells that hyperproliferate; produce excessive bone matrix as woven bone; and show increased osteoclastogenesis mediated by increased IL-6 production—all resulting in abnormal accelerated bone resorption and formation. The distribution of lesions is quite variable, as dysplastic lesions may be present in one or many bones, traditionally named monostotic and polyostotic fibrous dysplasia, respectively. The distribution of FD/MAS is likely due to the timing of the post-zygotic GNAS mutation and the subsequent distribution of these abnormal osteoprogenitor cells throughout the skeleton. The most likely scenario given current evidence would postulate the mutational change occurring between the morula and blastocyst stage of embryogenesis, which is consistent with FD lesions appearing in bones from different embryonal origins: the femur and craniofacial bones are the most common sites for FD though they originate from the mesoderm and neural crest ectoderm, respectively [15, 16].

Correlating to phenotypic severity, FD is diagnosed at any age though the majority of lesions are present by age 15 and clinical bone lesions usually present by 5 years of age [17]. Presenting symptoms of fibrous dysplasia include limp, pathologic fracture, or bone pain [18]. The peak incidence of fractures occurs between 6 and 10 years of age [19], though rarely patients present with angular deformity.

The true prevalence of FD and MAS are difficult to estimate given the number of asymptomatic patients with clinically insignificant FD lesions and the number of patients identified with FD who do not undergo extensive testing for endocrinological abnormalities confirming the diagnosis of MAS. There is no identifiable prevalence of FD/MAS in different populations nor geographic areas, which suggests a random mutational event, rather than environmental or genetic factors that might predispose individuals [9].

MAS-associated precocious puberty affects 85% of girls, presenting as painless vaginal bleeding, but only 15% of boys, manifesting as testicular abnormalities and macroorchidism. Patients with MAS also have characteristic café-au-lait pigmentation on their skin, present from birth or infancy, with irregular borders described as "coast of Maine" (Fig. 27.2). Other endocrinopathies associated with McCune Albright syndrome include hyperthyroidism, growth hormone excess, and Cushing's disease [20, 21]. Children with MAS require referral at the time of diagnosis to pediatric endocrinologists for medical management [22, 23].

The radiographic appearance of fibrous dysplasia is of one or more ill-defined lesions in the metaphysis or diaphysis, as epiphyseal involvement is atypical. The borders of the lesions are a gradual transition radiographically and microscopically from areas with high concentration of abnormal cells and fibrous tissue to normal mineralization and macrostructure, and thus lack a sclerotic rim frequently seen in other benign bone cysts. Within the lesion, the bony trabeculae are replaced by fibrous tissue, creating a blurred and indistinct pattern on radiographs, coined "ground glass" appearance. The lesions can be expansile and may thin the cortices of the native bone though they do not create a periosteal reaction (Fig. 27.3). Large lesions in weight-bearing bones may result in bowing of the bone, with coxa vara of

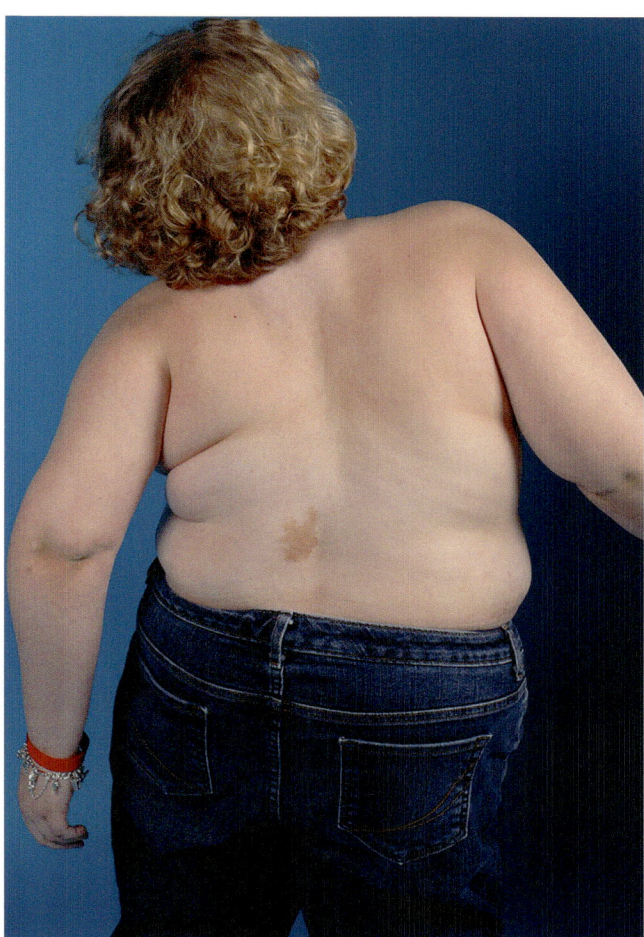

Fig. 27.2 Clinical photograph of a girl with McCune Albright syndrome. Note the skin macule which is hyperpigmented and has irregular borders. The child has spinal involvement and scoliosis

the femur and anterior bowing of the tibia being most dramatic examples of the remodeling deformities.

The craniofacial bones are most commonly affected in patients with polyostotic FD, affecting up to 87% and typically manifesting by 3 years of age, though one series found 36% of patients with craniofacial bone involvement were asymptomatic [17, 24, 25]. However, given the high concentration of vital structures, serious complications can arise: optical nerve entrapment, dental crowding and other problems, sensorineural and conductive hearing loss (22%), Chiari I malformation (7.6%), cranium deformity and assymetry, sinus congestion, nasal constriction, and malocclusion. Computed tomography is the most effective way to visualize FD in the craniofacial bones and axial skeleton. Patients with skull involvement should be evaluated by craniofacial specialists, neurosurgery, and endocrinology as bony enlargement and overgrowth can lead to cosmetic disfigurement and optic foraminal sclerosis may progress to blindness.

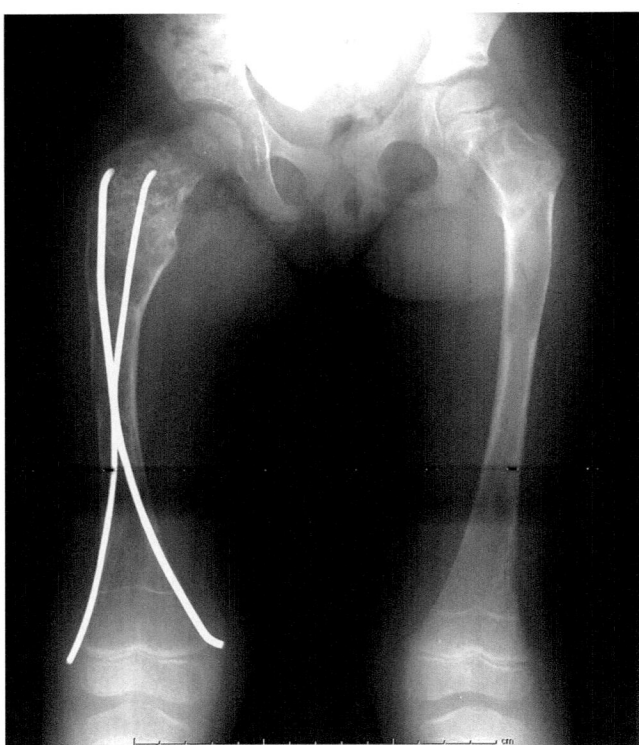

Fig. 27.3 Anteroposterior radiograph of a 3-year-old female with polyostotic fibrous dysplasia. Poorly defined lytic areas are present throughout both femora and the right hemipelvis. The right femoral neck is expanded, and an early shepherd's crook deformity is present. Intramedullary fixation is present due to previous pathologic fracture

The axial skeleton, including the spine and pelvis, is commonly involved in polyostotic FD, affecting up to 63% of patients and causing scoliosis in 52%, the severity of which is associated with total overall disease burden [26–28]. Rib involvement is common and can cause pain [26, 27]. Scoliosis correction and fusion with instrumentation can be extremely challenging due to the bony fragility, limited fixation options, and bleeding due to the hypervascular FD lesions. However, successful results of posterior spinal fusion have been published [27]. The efficacy of scoliosis bracing in fibrous dysplasia has not been proven, and the concurrent presence of rib lesions precludes its use in most patients.

The differential diagnosis in patients with monostotic fibrous dysplasia includes simple and aneurysmal bone cysts, eosinophilic granuloma, and when the tibia is involved, osteofibrous dysplasia. Radiographically, FD lesions can usually be differentiated from bone cysts as the edges of the lesion are less distinct, there is absence of the "fallen leaf" sign (seen with pathologic fractures when a portion of the cyst wall falls into the intramedullary defect), and an opaque matrix in FD lesions. Some authors recommend a technetium bone scan to identify the presence of polyostotic disease not readily recognized radiographically as all affected sites can be identified on bone scan by 6 years of age, though 2D radiographic imaging has been shown to be satisfactory [18].

The diagnosis of polyostotic FD is usually made both clinically and radiographically, therefore biopsy is only required when there is a concern for malignant transformation or to rule out other conditions with multiple lesions, such as metastatic cancer. The fibrous dysplasia lesion is filled with tissue rather than fluid, differentiating it from bone cysts, though there may be cystic areas. On gross examination, tissue from fibrous dysplasia lesions appears firm and gray with a gritty texture to palpation. Microscopic examination shows stellate, retracted osteogenic cells rimming the bone trabeculae surface depositing abnormally oriented perpendicular Sharpey's collagen bundles, abundant fibrous stroma, large lacunae filled with multiple developing osteocytes, and vast swaths of immature osteoid with disproportionate mature trabeculae. Comparatively, in craniofacial FD, the lesions are predominantly thick, interconnected, non-lamellar trabeculae and less fibrous stroma, similar in appearance to Paget's Disease.

The natural history of fibrous dysplasia in the skeletally immature patient is that of slow progression of osseous lesions and subsequent deformity. Characteristic deformities include coxa vara due to the "shepherd's crook" deformity of the femur, "windswept" angular deformity at the knee, and procurvatum of the tibiae. As the mechanical strength of the bone is diminished due to progressive replacement of mature, organized lamellar bone with fibrous tissue and erratic, woven bone, the weight-bearing bones gradually deform. Pain may present at the sites of increased stress or transitional zones secondary to microfractures. Limb length discrepancy and malalignment may develop. In polyostotic disease, gait becomes more difficult, with the median age at which patients require assistive devices to walk being 7 years [17].

The orthopedic management of FD/MAS is aimed towards preventing and correcting osseous deformity, prevention and stabilization of pathologic fractures, and palliation of pain. Bony lesions do not require operative intervention unless associated with pathologic fracture, deformity, or unremitting pain that does not respond to conservative measures including physical therapy, activity modification, anti-inflammatory medication, acupuncture, or anti-resorptive bone medications.

Curettage and bone grafting of fibrous dysplasia leads to recurrence of the lesions, and the bone graft (allograft or autograft) is eventually replaced again by the fibrous tissue characteristic of fibrous dysplasia. Cortical bone grafts have been used, with hopes of less resorption and greater improvement of mechanical strength of the bone [29]. Unfortunately, these grafts also resorb, although in a more delayed fashion compared to morselized bone graft. Curettage and bone grafting is typically recommended only for small lesions [30].

Pathological fractures occur most frequently in the first decade of life between the ages of 6 and 10 years with the femur most likely to sustain a fracture [19]. Fractures occurring through dysplastic bone may be treated nonoperatively in the upper extremity if alignment can be maintained with a low tolerance of angulation or displacement, given limited remodeling potential, but lower extremities fractures usually benefit from surgical treatment. Load-sharing intramedullary implants allow earlier weight bearing, which is important due to the underlying bone fragility, and are recommended over plate fixation [31–34]. Any residual deformity should be fully corrected, as FD bones have decreased remodeling potential and residual angulation will predispose to future fractures. Nonunion is infrequent in fibrous dysplasia. Normal fracture callous initially develops, but is ultimately replaced with fibrous tissue. Titanium IMN are recommended over stainless steel given their modulus of elasticity is closer to native bone, and evidence that stainless steel implants have a higher incidence of failure [30].

The shepherd's crook deformity of the proximal femur is particularly challenging to treat [29, 35]. Progressive coxa vara leads to a waddling gait, hip pain, and eventually pathologic stress fractures when the neck-shaft angle is less than 120°. Proximal femoral valgus osteotomy can correct the deformity, but fixation in the dysplastic bone is extremely challenging. Plate fixation frequently leads to either pathologic fracture at the end of the plate where stress transition occurs or loss of fixation due to screw pullout from weakened bone. Hip screw with side plate fixation may migrate out of the femoral neck as the dysplastic bone remodels and the deformity recurs. Our preference is an intramedullary nail, with the goal of achieving reasonable proximal femoral fixation to allow the osteotomy to heal, yet providing load-sharing along the entire length of the bone (Figs. 27.4 and 27.5).

Osteotomies for deformity correction require meticulous preoperative planning. The deformities are typically multiplanar, and more than one osteotomy may be required for passage of intramedullary devices, given the inherent fragility of the bone. The use of temporary intraoperative external fixation to attain and maintain alignment during stabilization is recommended. There is frequently no patent intramedullary canal in the dysplastic bone; often the intramedullary canal may require drilling for proper nail placement to avoid inadvertent cortical penetration or propagation of a pathologic fracture. Additionally, a large amount of blood loss should be anticipated from these hypervascular lesions.

Unfortunately, normal growth leads to recurrent deformity as does persistence of active FD lesions and revision surgery should be expected even past skeletal maturity in

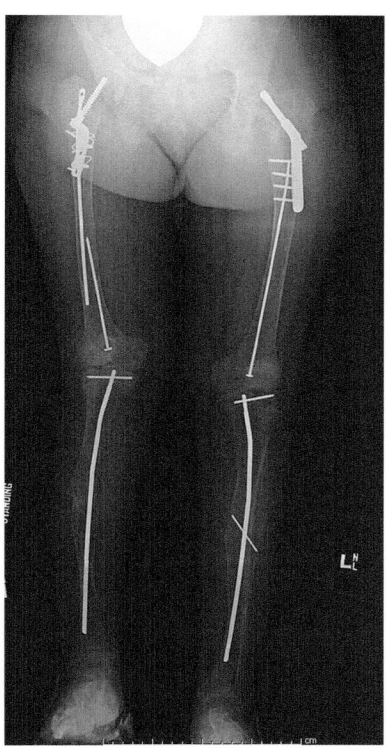

Fig. 27.4 Anteroposterior radiograph of the lower extremities of an 11-year-old girl with McCune Albright syndrome. She has undergone intramedullary fixation of the femora and tibiae as treatment of repetitive pathologic fractures. Note the proximal femoral fixation for treatment of coxa vara and shepherd's crook deformities. There is also a leg length discrepancy

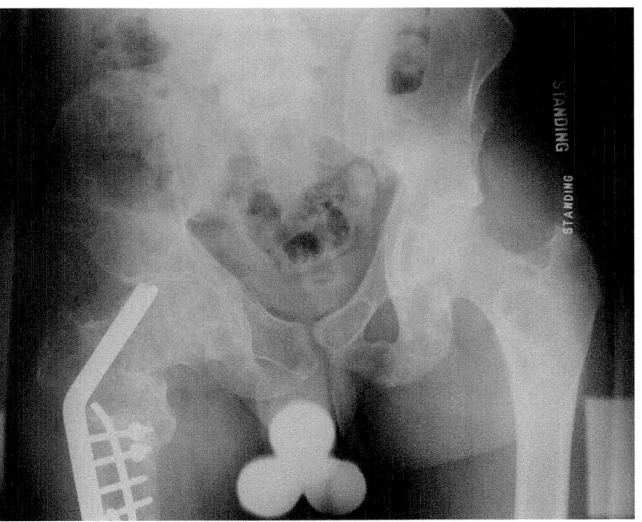

Fig. 27.5 Pelvis radiograph of a 21-year-old male who has undergone multiple surgeries for treatment of right femoral fractures and coxa vara. Note the expansion of the femoral neck, the lytic appearance of the femoral neck and head, and the superior migration of the implant in the femoral neck. There is shortening of the length of the limb on the right

Fig. 27.6 (a) AP radiograph of the lower extremities of a 9-year-old girl with polyostotic fibrous dysplasia. She has undergone a right proximal femoral allograft replacement due to marked bony enlargement suspicious for malignancy, a left proximal femoral osteotomy, and right tibial osteotomy with intramedullary fixation. (b) Two years later, the tibia has undergone great expansion and angular deformity has worsened with recurrent bone pain with weight bearing

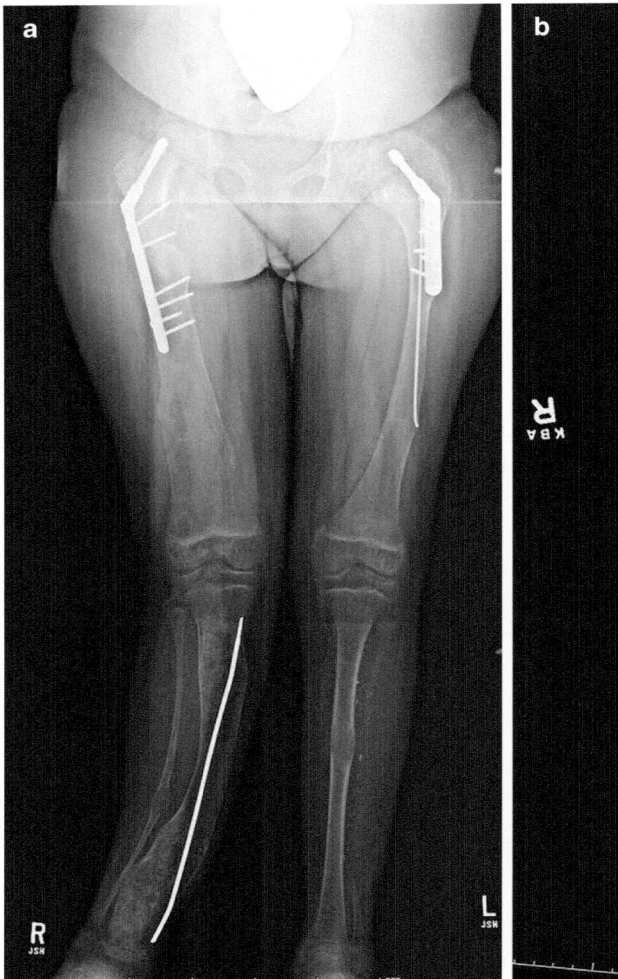
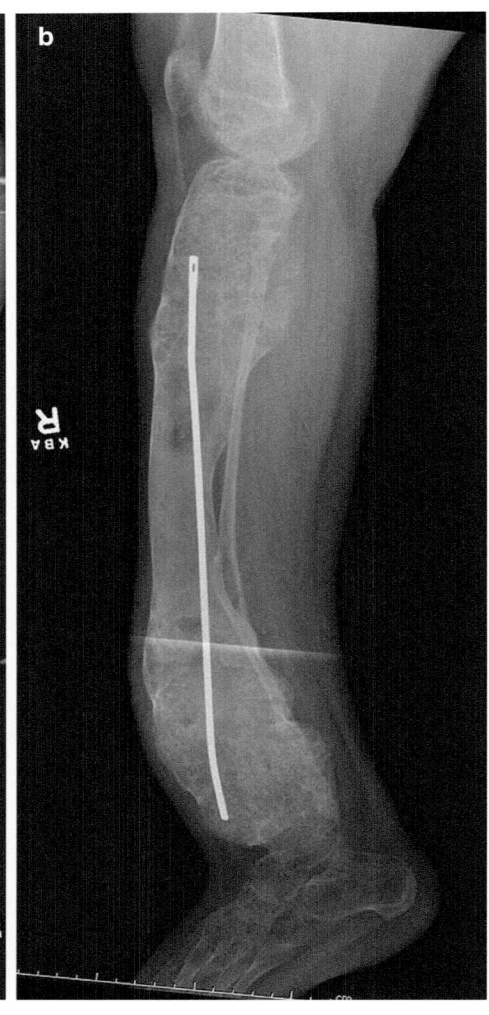

severely affected adults. Progression of the fibrous dysplasia can lead to enlargement of the bone, recurrent angulation, and increasing bone pain due to bone fragility (Fig. 27.6a, b).

Limb length discrepancy is seen most frequently in children with severe polyostotic disease. Lengthening is usually fraught with complications due to the poor mechanical properties of the dysplastic bone. Contralateral epiphysiodesis may be offered, though it compounds the patient's underlying short stature inherent to FD.

Pain in patients is typically multifactorial, though a pragmatic approach can divide pain into two elements: a structural component due to bone malalignment, joint deformity, impending fracture or stress related pain; and a physiologic component due to increased bone metabolism inherent in the constitutively activated lesional tissue. Medical treatment of FD pain should begin with correction of phosphate, calcium, and Vitamin D levels. Second line medical treatment, after other conservative measures have failed, can include bisphosphonates though they have shown mixed results [36–39]. A randomized, double blind, placebo-controlled trial of high dose oral alendronate at 40 mg daily found an increase in bone mineral density and a decrease in bone resorption marker NTX-telopeptide, but no significant effect on pain nor functional parameters and therefore should not be considered routinely [30, 40]. However, intravenous bisphosphonate use has been found to decrease pain and normalize bone metabolism markers, though studies have not shown to alter the progression of the disease [41]. New clinical studies using Denosumab, a receptor activator of nuclear factor kappa-B ligand (RANKL) inhibitor, have shown promise in influencing the progression of bone disease in FD specifically and shows promise though more experience is required before routine use can be recommended [42–45].

The development of cystic lesions most closely resembling aneurysmal bone cysts may occur within the dysplastic bone. Rapid enlargement of the lesions coupled with increasing pain is usually present. Malignant degeneration has been documented in rare patients with fibrous dysplasia [46, 47]. Malignant degeneration is most common in adulthood and has been associated with previous irradiation, which is now contraindicated in patients with fibrous dysplasia. Painful enlargement of the dysplastic bone may also be present. In

> **Box 27.2 Fibrous Dysplasia**
>
> Age at presentation: First or Second decade.
> Location: Long bones most frequent, metaphyis or diaphysis.
> Number: solitary or polyostotic.
> Presenting symptoms: limp, pathologic fracture, bone pain.
> Rx: intramedullary fixation of fractures, deformity correction, bisphosphonates for pain.
> Malignant degeneration: rare in adulthood.

Osteofibrous Dysplasia

Osteofibrous dysplasia, also known as Campanacci's disease, is a peculiar bone dysplasia which is typified by both sclerotic and lytic lesions most commonly present in the tibia in children and adolescents [48, 49]. It is usually not genetically transmitted. Osteofibrous dysplasia is bimodal in presentation. It can present in early infancy with apparent anterior bowing in the tibia [50, 51]. In such cases, it must be distinguished from anterolateral bow of the tibia as associated with congenital pseudarthrosis of the tibia and neurofibromatosis. The fibula in patients with infantile osteofibrous dysplasia is usually uninvolved, and pathologic fracture is rare. The condition is nearly always unilateral and does not involve the rest of the skeleton. Osteofibrous dysplasia is not typically genetically transmitted, but a rare form has been published in which several family members were affected [52, 53].

Osteofibrous dysplasia-like adamantinoma is a rare, confounding bone lesion that presents in late childhood or adolescence, typically involving the tibia with radiographic characteristics nearly identical to OFD and its relationship to OFD and adamantinoma has yet to be full elucidated [54]. Currently, the existing literature supports OFD-like AD as a benign condition without evidence of metastatic disease in numerous studies.

Radiographs of osteofibrous dysplasia show bubbly lytic lesions scattered throughout the anterior diaphysis of the tibia [55]. There is usually anterior bowing, and the limb may be somewhat shorter than the contralateral leg. The cortex may appear thickened in areas (Fig. 27.7).

The differential diagnosis of osteofibrous dysplasia includes monostotic fibrous dysplasia, congenital pseudarthrosis of the tibia, osteofibrous dysplasia-like adamantinoma, and adamantinoma.

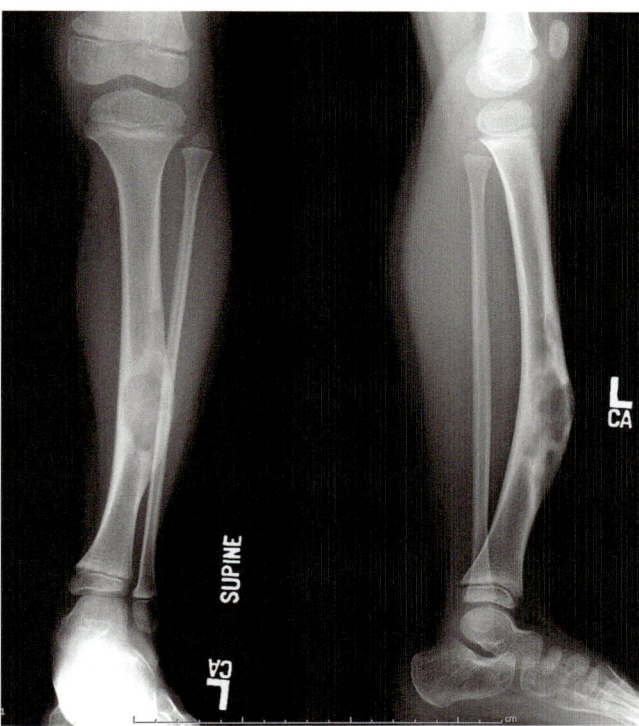

Fig. 27.7 AP and lateral radiograph of a 7-year-old female with progressive anterior bowing of the tibia. The lateral view shows loculated lytic lesions in the anterior cortex of the tibia typical for osteofibrous dysplasia

Pathological examination of tissue from osteofibrous dysplasia shows fibrous tissue with areas of immature osteoid, as is seen in fibrous dysplasia. The histological distinction from fibrous dysplasia is that the osteoid is rimmed in osteoblasts in osteofibrous dysplasia, which is its characteristic histologic finding. Cells stain positively for cytokeratin, which is also present in adamantinoma, supporting a relationship between the two lesions [55–59].

Treatment of osteofibrous dysplasia is controversial. Spontaneous resolution of osteofibrous dysplasia in children has been described, so treatment in these infants should be observation in the absence of pathologic fracture, pain, or progressive deformity [60]. If fracture does occur, intramedullary fixation such as is performed in congenital pseudarthrosis of the tibia, combined with autograft at the fracture site, usually is successful in obtaining and maintaining union [61].

Older children with osteofibrous dysplasia have undergone various forms of treatment. Observation of radiographically stable lesions may be chosen when the patient is asymptomatic. Marginal resection with curettage has been shown to lead to recurrence and is not recommended. Those surgeons who have concern that osteofibrous dysplasia may evolve into malignant adamantinoma have performed aggressive resection of the affected tibial area, with reconstruction as needed. Bone segment transport with proximal corticotomy and external fixation and treatment with free vascularized fibular graft have met with success in very rare instances [62, 63].

> **Box 27.3 Osteofibrous Dysplasia**
> Age at presentation: infantile or first or second decade.
> Location: anterior tibial diaphysis.
> Number: solitary.
> Presenting symptoms: bowing, enlargement, pain.
> Rx: controversial, possible en bloc excision.
> Malignant degeneration: associated with adamantinoma.

Enchondromatosis

Enchondromatous tumors encompass a wide array of chondroid lesions, including enchondromas, Ollier's Disease, and Maffucci's Syndrome. Enchondromas are solitary, benign hyaline cartilaginous lesions typically present within the metaphysis. Solitary enchondromas are common and rarely symptomatic, whereas Ollier's Disease is rare but its lesions are more often symptomatic. Maffucci's syndrome includes multiple enchondromas with soft tissue hemangiomatosis and carries a much bleaker oncologic prognosis. Enchondromatosis is not genetically transmitted but may be the result of a somatic mosaic mutation in isocitrate dehydrogenase 1 or 2 [64]. The incidence of Ollier's disease is estimated at 1 per 100,000.

Presenting complaints in multiple enchondromatosis are usually bone pain due to mechanical insufficiency, pathologic fracture through the lesions, angular deformity at the knee or fingers, or limb length discrepancy [65]. The condition typically presents in the first or second decade of life.

The radiographic appearance of multiple enchondromatosis is quite distinct (Fig. 27.8). Streaky lytic lesions are seen in the metaphysis of the bones. At the knee, the elongated areas of enchondroma give a "fan-like" appearance to the metaphysis. There are areas of fine calcification within the lesions due to ossification of the periphery of cartilaginous tissue. The lesions seem to stop at the physis. It is common that multiple enchondromas are seen, and that they tend to present unilaterally. The cortex of the bone is intact in the absence of pathologic fracture. Angular deformity at the knee and limb length discrepancy can be appreciated (Fig. 27.9) [66].

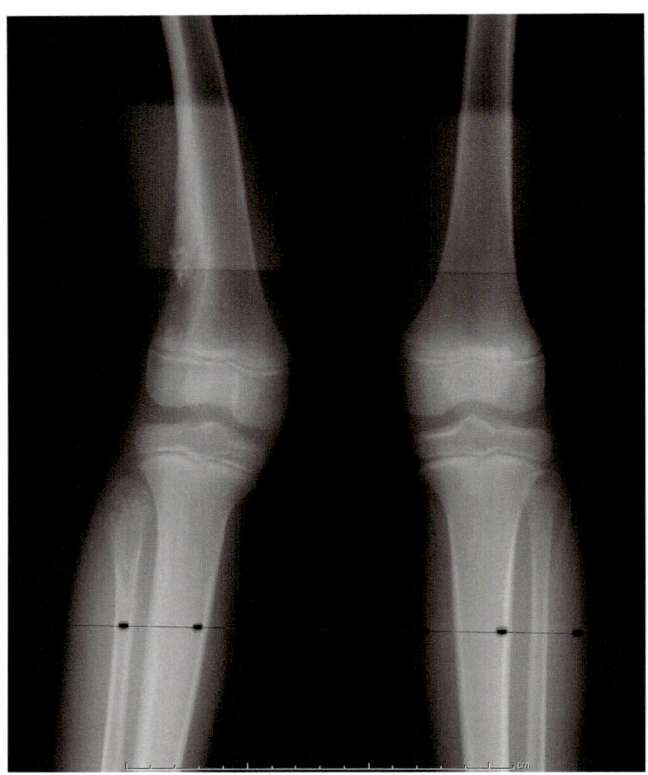

Fig. 27.8 Radiographic appearance of enchondromatosis of the distal femur and proximal tibia in a 7-year-old male. Note the eccentric location of the metaphyseal femoral lesion, and the presence of intralesional calcification which is typical of cartilage tumors. The right proximal fibula is also involved

Biopsy reveals a pearly white to bluish-white specimen. Microscopic examination shows bland cartilaginous tissue, with nests of plump chondrocytes. The nuclei are uniform, and mitotic figures may be seen in children but should be few in number. Calcification within the lesion can be appreciated on palpation, which renders the specimen slightly gritty.

Treatment of children with solitary enchondromas is merited if there is angular deformity, while small asymptomatic lesions in the lower extremities may be observed. Multiple enchondromatosis presents for orthopedic treatment more frequently. Curettage and bone grafting of the enchondromas is in large part ineffective due to the extensive nature of the disease, but may be of some benefit in the hand. Children with Ollier's disease have significant angular deformities, with a predisposition towards distal femoral varus [66]. The angular deformity is usually accompanied by varying amounts of limb shortening which may measure up to 25 cm at maturity (Fig. 27.10) [65]. In the lower extremity, angular correction with or without lengthening may be undertaken. Standard fixation with internal devices such as plates and

Fig. 27.9 (**a**) Asymmetric genu valgum and limb length discrepancy in a young boy with Ollier's disease. (**b**) A close-up of the left knee shows the streaky lytic lesions characteristic of enchondromatosis

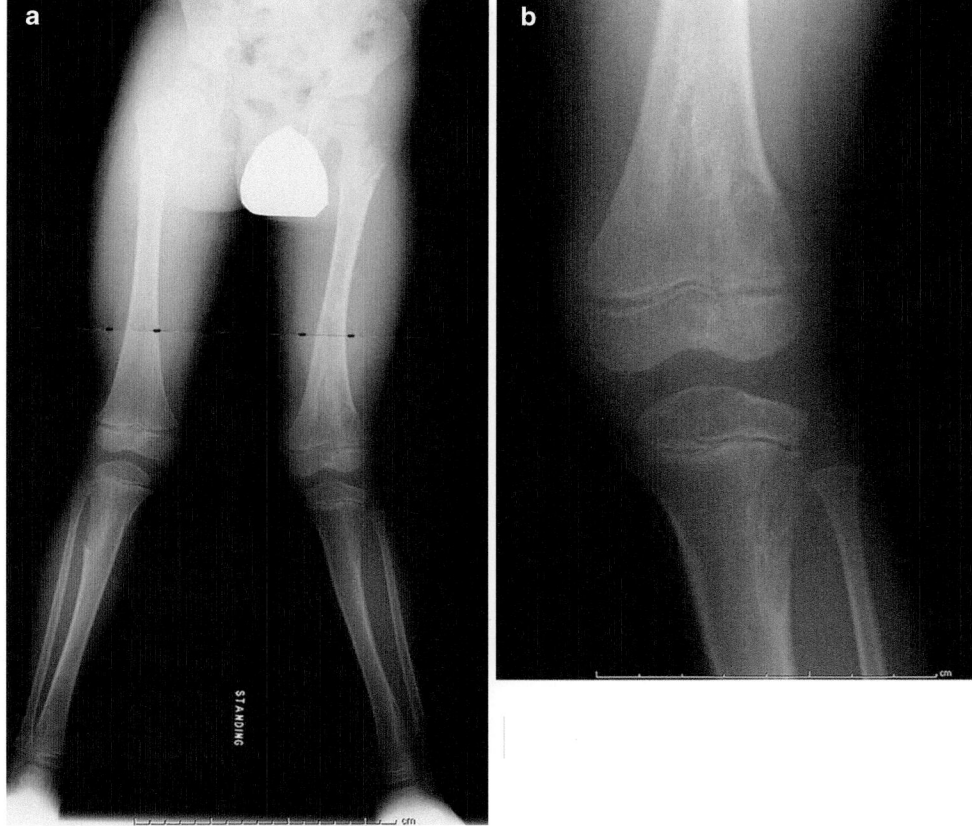

screws may be compromised by poor bony integrity due to the large cartilaginous lesions. Gradual deformity correction using external fixation devices with fine wire bony fixation has been successful [67–71]. When pins or wires are inserted intralesionally, fixation can usually be maintained; however it should be expected that the regenerate will contain enchondromatosis tissue (Fig. 27.11a, b) [70]. Lengthening with intramedullary devices has also been reported [72].

Malignant transformation has been described in enchondromatosis in up to 20–30% of patients by the age of 40. Patients with significant expansion of a lesion or with increasing pain should be suspected. Chondrosarcoma is the most frequent malignant tumor seen in up to 25–30% of adult patients with enchondromatosis [73, 74]. Histologic overlap between benign enchondromas seen in Ollier's disease and low-grade chondrosarcoma makes the diagnosis of malignant degeneration challenging. Remote non-bony malignancies are associated with Maffucci's syndrome, which carries a nearly 100% incidence of the development of a malignant tumor [75]. These children must be carefully monitored throughout their lifetime for the appearance of cancerous lesions.

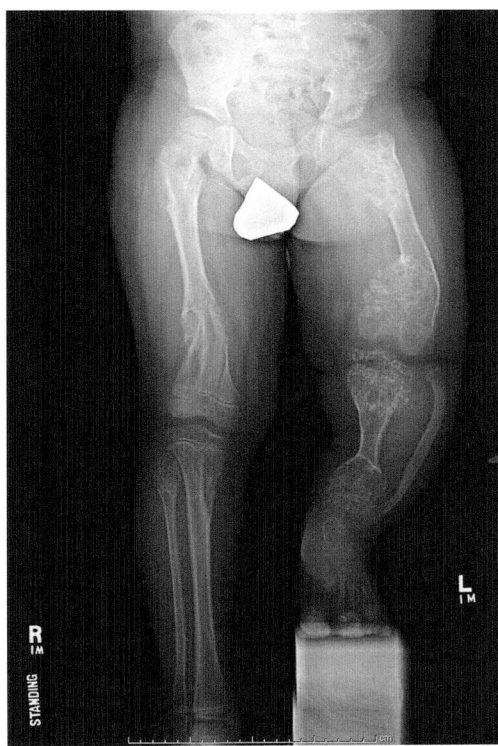

Fig. 27.10 Severe limb length discrepancy measuring greater than 15 cm and varus deformity of the left distal femur in 7-year-old male with Ollier's disease. Note the presence of enchondromas in bilateral femora and tibias as well as the pelvis. The extent of involvement is asymmetric

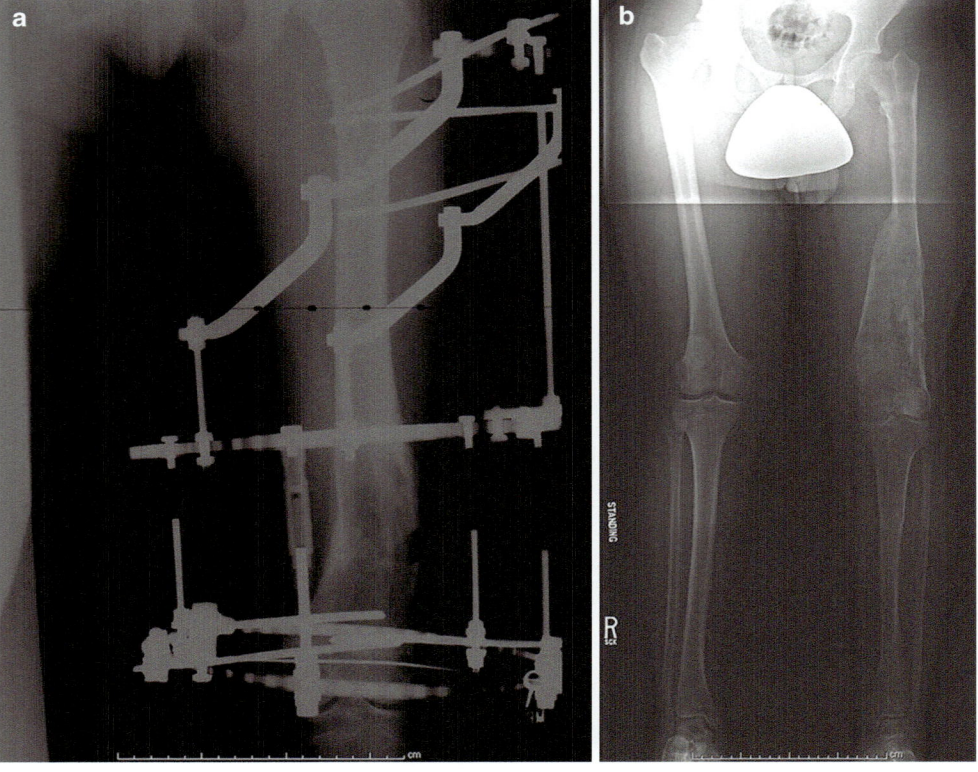

Fig. 27.11 (**a**) Varus osteotomy of the distal femur in patient with Ollier's disease. External fixation with half-pins and fine wires was successful in stabilizing the osteotomy. (**b**) Standing radiograph 1.5 years following removal of the external fixator shows satisfactory alignment but a persistent limb length discrepancy

---

Box 27.4 Enchondroma

Age at presentation: first or second decade.
  Location: metaphyis, predisposition to asymmetry.
  Number: solitary or multiple (Ollier's disease).
  Presenting symptoms: bone pain, pathologic fracture, angular deformity, limb length discrepancy.
  Rx: osteotomy for deformity correction, lengthening, in hand may curettage and bone graft.
  Malignant degeneration: chondrosarcoma in 25–30% of Ollier's disease.

Solitary Osteochondromas and Multiple Hereditary Exostoses

An osteochondroma is a common benign bone growth which protrudes from the surface of the native bone and is capped with cartilage. Osteochondromas occur in the metaphyseal area and have been hypothesized to be the result of sequestration of a fragment of physis which causes the outgrowth. The bone of an osteochondroma is normal bone and is in continuity with the host bone. Osteochondromas may occur in any bone, including the pelvis, spine, and fingers, but are most common in the distal femur, proximal tibia, and proximal humerus [76].

Multiple hereditary osteochondromatosis or exostoses (MHE) are an inherited condition typified by the presence of multiple osteochondromas scattered throughout the skeleton. It is genetically transmitted as an autosomal dominant trait with a very high (96%) penetrance but variable phenotypic expression. The number and location of osteochondromas can vary among family members. The tumor suppressor genes EXT1, EXT2, and EXT3 for MHE have been localized on chromosomes 8, 11, and 19 [77–79]. Patients with MHE have a loss of function of these genes, thereby allowing growth of the osteochondromas. Patients with EXT1 mutations generally have more severe phenotypical expression and shorter stature than those with EXT2 mutations [80–84]. It is believed that patients with solitary osteochondromas have somatic, but not generalized, mutations in the EXT gene. The incidence of multiple osteochondromas is 1 per 50,000. Ninety percent of patients with MHE have a positive family history and demonstrable mutations in the EXT 1 or 2 genes [85].

Patients with a single osteochondroma often present in the first or second decade for evaluation of a painless periarticular mass. Patients with MHE usually present in early childhood with multiple small masses. The median age of presentation in MHE is 3 years [86]. The presence of a positive family history generally creates a heightened awareness of the condition in parents and therefore an earlier presentation. Patients may complain of pain if there has been trauma in the area of the osteochondroma, or if the mass is sufficiently large to create symptoms due to impingement of overlying muscle or tendons. In many cases, the patient is asymptomatic, but the lesion has been identified coincidentally on a radiograph obtained for another reason. Patients with MHE tend to be of mildly short stature with one study finding 58% of patients shorter than the 25th percentile [83]. Additionally, the extremities will appear shorter than the trunk does, with the amount of shortening being linked to the size of osteochondromas present in the limb segment [87]. Angular deformity, such as genu valgum and ankle valgus, may be present.

Radiographs show a bony protrusion in the periarticular area originating from the metaphyseal region (Fig. 27.12). Osteochondromas are not epiphyseal. The cortex of the osteochondroma is in continuity with the native bone, and the trabeculae within the osteochondroma are similarly in continuity with the metaphysis. Osteochondromas may be pedunculated, with a distinct bony stalk, or sessile, where the lesion is broad-based. When pedunculated, osteochondromas typically grow away from the joint.

Osteochondromas vary extensively in number, location, and size. Large osteochondromas in two-bone segments, such as the lower leg and forearm, can cause deformity and limited range of motion. At the ankle, this typically manifests with ankle valgus, while in the forearm this is noticeable with diminished supination or pronation. Osteochondromas in the distal femur, proximal tibia, and/or proximal fibula are seen in 94% of children with MHE. Proximal humerus masses are present in 50% of cases, the scapula and ribs in 40%, the distal radius and ulna in 30%, the proximal femur in 30%, the phalanges in 30%, the distal fibula in 25%, and the distal tibia in 20% of MHE patients [86].

The radiographic appearance of an osteochondroma is sufficiently distinct that biopsy is not needed. When osteochondromas are excised for relief of symptoms, pathologic evaluation of the mass should be obtained. The bone of an osteochondroma is histologically normal bone. The junction of the bone and the cartilage cap shows endochondral ossification. It is important to evaluate the cartilaginous cap of the lesion. In a benign osteochondroma, the cartilage cap is thin (<2 cm) and the chondrocytes histologically bland, without mitotic figures or nuclear pleomorphism. In some instances, the cartilaginous portion of the osteochondroma can undergo malignant transformation into secondary chondrosarcomas. The incidence of malignant transformation is less than 1% and is more likely in mature patients and those located in axial skeleton, especially pelvic lesions. An increase in pain and a rapid increase in size should merit workup including contrast-enhanced MRI and/or CT scan to evaluate the cartilaginous cap of the osteochondroma, followed by biopsy. The cartilage cap in an osteochondroma that has become malignant is thickened, and the nuclei of the chondroid cells are pleomorphic with multiple chondroid cells within each lacunae. It is the combination of the histological appearance of the cartilage cap combined with its thickness that leads to the diagnosis of chondrosarcoma [88].

Treatment of a solitary osteochondroma is excision if the lesion is causing pain or mechanical symptoms due to its size. Recurrence is unlikely with complete excision. Patients with MHE should be offered excision of symptomatic lesions, and observation if the masses are asymptomatic. Due to the number of osteochondromas that many of these children have, excision of all the lesions is impractical and unnecessary; however recent validated outcome questionnaires have highlighted the complaints of musculoskeletal pain in children with MHE [89–91]. Masses that are creating secondary deformities, such as large distal tibial lesions that are producing fibular deformity (see Fig. 27.12), may benefit from excision. Advanced imaging of larger lesions prior to surgery may be helpful in identifying the location of neurovascular structures that may be displaced by the osteochondromas. In particular, the peroneal nerve is frequently

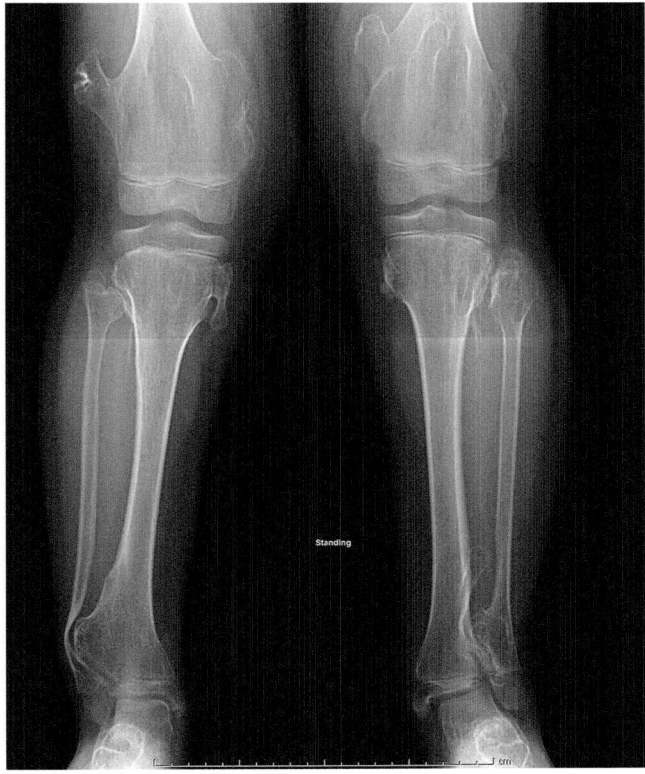

Fig. 27.12 Radiograph of a 10-year-old boy with multiple hereditary exostoses. Note the numerous sessile lesions, such as that seen at the distal tibia, and the pedunculated lesions as seen at the distal femur and proximal tibia. Ankle valgus is present at the left ankle, and an intraosseous osteochondroma from the right tibia deforms and thins the fibula

thinned or displaced by proximal fibular lesions, and should be identified and protected if the proximal fibular osteochondroma is to be excised. Even so, postoperative peroneal nerve palsy frequently results from excision of fibular lesions [92, 93], and preoperative counselling of the patient and family about the possibility of a foot drop necessitating use of an ankle-foot orthosis should be performed. Additionally, venous thromboembolism following excision of lesions behind the knee has been seen in rare cases [94].

Angular deformity of the lower extremities may be present in patients with MHE. Growth modulation via hemiepiphysiodesis in skeletally immature patients may be quite useful, especially about the knee. When preoperative planning growth modulation, consideration for inaccuracies in bone age should be made [95]. Most often, the knee assumes a valgus position due to proximal tibial involvement [87]. Patellar instability may be associated with genu valgum in some children [96]. Medial proximal tibial and distal femoral growth modulation can be useful (Fig. 27.13a, b). Skeletally mature patients may rarely require osteotomy. In such cases, the peroneal nerve is prone to postoperative palsy, so fibular osteotomy should be approached with great caution.

Ankle valgus is also frequently present in patients with MHE due to distal tibial and fibular lesions and abnormal physeal growth [97]. Radiographs show relative shortening of the distal fibula and distal tibial valgus tilt with narrowing of the epiphysis laterally, contributing to the valgus deformity. Gradual deformity correction via hemiepiphyseodesis of the medial distal tibia physis with insertion of a two or four hole-plate, staple, tension band plate, or fully threaded medial malleolar screw in skeletally immature patients has been shown to be effective [98, 99], but the authors find that correction of the ankle is frequently very slow and often incomplete. However, the ankle deformity is rarely sufficiently symptomatic to merit osteotomy. Other children with MHE may complain of ankle deformity due to a large distal tibial osteochondroma which exerts pressure on the distal fibula, leading to erosions, bowing of the fibula, and in some instances, arthrodesis of the distal tibia and fibula. Excision of the osteochondroma can relieve symptoms, and the fibula will typically remodel following excision of the tibial mass.

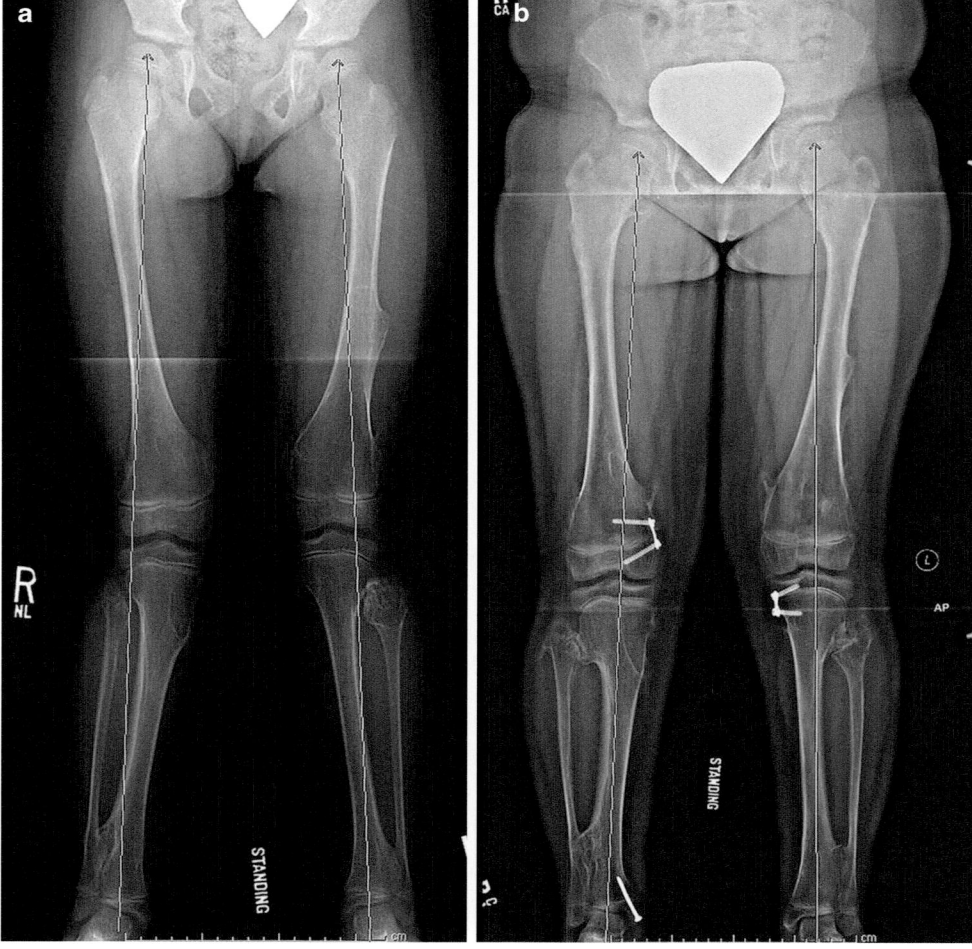

Fig. 27.13 (a) Valgus deformity in an 8-year-old male with multiple hereditary exostoses. (b) Radiograph 4 years following growth modulation shows correction of the valgus deformity. Note the medial malleolar screw placed for the treatment of ankle valgus

A long-term study of adults with ankle valgus secondary to osteochondromas linked persistent excessive ankle valgus with limitations in recreational activities and with the development of arthritis [100].

Progressive hip dysplasia due to the presence of proximal femoral osteochondromas has been seen in a minority of patients with MHE [101, 102]. Surgical reconstruction via excision of the osteochondromas combined with proximal femoral osteotomy as needed for containment can be useful when uncoverage of the acetabulum is accompanied by severe femoral neck valgus.

There have been published studies which have raised awareness of the presence of spinal osteochondromas in patients with MHE [103, 104]. The incidence of clinically important spinal osteochondromas remains quite rare, but it is imperative that the lower extremity surgeon be aware of their occurrence. The patient who presents with numbness or tingling in the lower extremity, or with difficulty with ambulation, should have a careful neurologic assessment. It is enticing to explain the symptoms by the presence of osteochondromas either in the popliteal fossa or at the proximal fibula, but consideration for a spinal etiology of the symptoms should be given. Spinal osteochondromas are readily seen via either CT or MRI scanning. Excision of a space-occupying lesion in the spinal canal should be offered.

As mentioned above, malignant transformation of an osteochondroma may occur in up to 1–2% of patients [88, 105–107]. Warning signs include a crescendo of pain, pain at rest, and unusually rapid growth of a lesion, particularly in a skeletally mature patient. Lesions in the pelvis and shoulder girdle are most prone to malignant degeneration. Preoperative imaging of the cartilaginous cap with MRI can support the suspicion of malignancy if the cap is greater than 2 cm in maximal thickness. Referral to an orthopedic oncological surgeon is merited in such cases. Treatment is typically wide surgical resection.

Finally, there are several case reports of popliteal artery pseudoaneurysms in association with large osteochondromas in the posterior knee area. In such cases, vascular repair is needed in conjunction with excision of the mass [108, 109].

> **Box 27.5 Osteochondroma**
> Age at presentation: First or second decade.
>   Location: metaphyseal.
>   Number: solitary or multiple.
>   Presenting symptoms: painless mass, mechanical symptoms.
>   Rx: excision of symptomatic lesions.
>   Malignant degeneration: chondrosarcoma in ≤1%.
> Under treatment: correction of angular deformity.

Dysplasia Epiphysealis Hemimelica (Trevor's Disease)

Dysplasia epiphysealis hemimelica is a condition where intra-articular osteocartilaginous lesions develop, originating from the epiphysis in skeletally immature children. Lesions are solitary in one-third of patients and multiple in two-thirds. Lesions in those patients with multiple epiphyseal involvement tend to be unilateral and to involve only one side (i.e., either the medial or lateral) of the epiphyses (Fig. 27.14). The disease is not genetically inherited but is more common in boys than girls [110, 111].

Patients present either in the first or second decade of life with a limited range of motion of involved joints which lead to gait disturbances. The most common sites are the distal femur, distal tibia, talus, and navicular. Lower extremity involvement is more common than upper extremity involvement. When the condition affects the distal tibia or talus, the presentation is usually of fixed equinus, while at the knee, a flexion position is adopted. Range of motion may be somewhat painful owing to the presence of the intra-articular mass. When present in the hip, the lesions are typically from the acetabulum and can lead to subluxation, if sufficiently large.

Radiographs may initially be normal, as the cartilaginous masses in the very young child are difficult to detect. As the child grows older, the lesions resemble those of osteochondromas, but the masses originate from the epiphysis and point towards the joint rather than away. Small lesions may be difficult to fully appreciate on plain radiographs, but MRI shows the cartilaginous extent of the lesion [112].

Histologically, lesions are made up of normal bone and varying amounts of overlying cartilage. The cells in both the bone and cartilage are benign in appearance and mitotic figures are not seen.

The intra-articular lesions grow in the skeletally immature patient. Treatment consists of excision of symptomatic lesions [113]. Unfortunately, due to the intra-articular nature of the masses, complete excision is difficult. While MRI may show delineation between the lesion and the native epiphysis, there is most often no visible distinction intraoperatively between the mass and the native articular cartilage, which is problematic for the surgeon in deciding on the margins of the excision. Recurrence is common. Residual joint incongruity leads to early degenerative arthritis. Excision of hip lesions is particularly challenging but may be successful via surgical hip dislocation [114–117] (Fig. 27.15). Limb length discrepancy owing to premature physeal closure may be present and require treatment.

Malignant transformation in dysplasia epiphysealis hemimelica has not been described.

Fig. 27.14 Dysplasia hemimelica epiphysealis (Trevor's disease) affecting the distal fibula and lateral midfoot. Note the enlargement of the distal fibular epiphysis and intra-articular exostoses

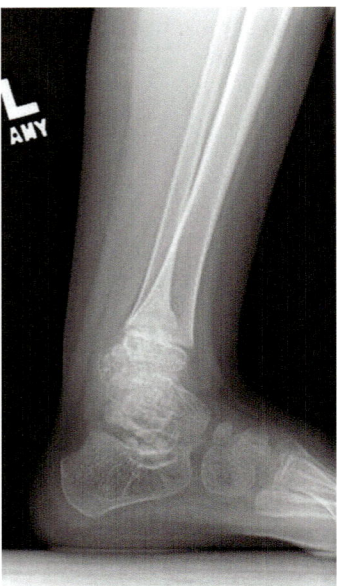
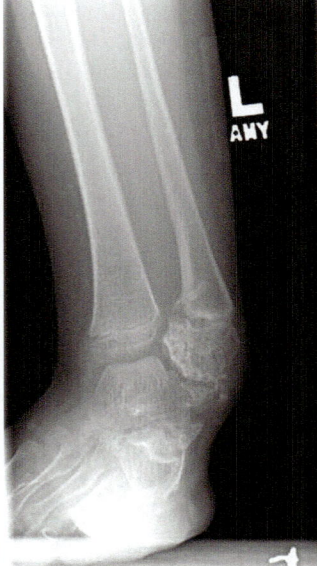
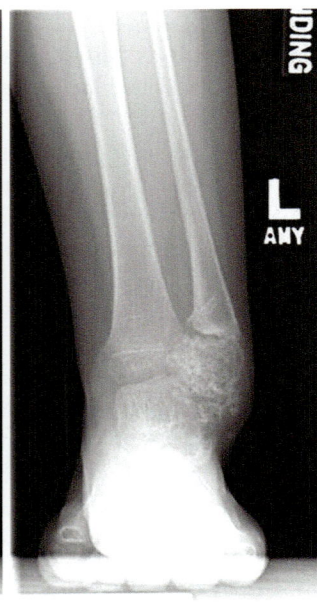

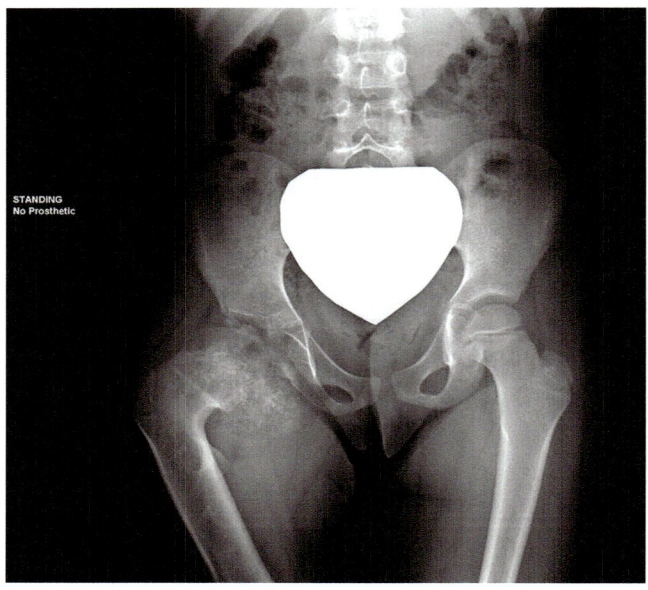

Fig. 27.15 Trevor's disease of the right hip of a 5-year-old male. Note the exostoses emanating from the femoral head and acetabulum leading to lateralization of the hip

Commentary

Alexandre Arkader
arkadera@chop.edu

Nonossifying Fibroma

This lesion is best seen as a developmental defect of the bone rather than a neoplastic process, hence the synonym *fibrous cortical defect*. Pathologic fractures are the most common indication for intervention and these can be in the form of either chronic stress fractures or acute injuries. Location seems to play a role in the likelihood of pathologic fractures associated to NOFs. The distal tibia, especially in syndesmosis based lesions, has the highest rate of fracture compared to any other location and, therefore, may warrant treatment more often [118].

Fibrous Dysplasia, McCune Albright Syndrome

Progressive deformity in the setting of fibrous dysplasia (FD) can be a challenging problem. The best "grafting" material is internal fixation, as the potential for replacement of graft material in FD is quite high. Load sharing devices are always preferred, but in very small children with pathologic fracture or progressive deformity, a combination of a flexible elastic nail and plating may be needed due to size constraints.

Understanding the natural history is important for long-term planning, as isolated lesions tend to stabilize with skeletal maturity. Polyostotic disease, however, will continue to progress beyond that point.

Often, the femoral head is the only adequate bone in a Shepherd's crook deformity of the proximal femur, and, therefore, epiphyseal fixation is recommended. Physeal sparing devices, such as telescoping screws or smooth tip implants may be preferred for very young children. Expect to be required to revise the fixation for these children as they continue to grow and the deformity recurs around the nail.

Cystic degeneration of FD can be quite challenging to manage. Treatment of painful cystic lesions, recurrent fractures or progressive deformity will require bone grafting since fibrous dysplastic bone is preferred over the fluid found with cystic degeneration [119].

Osteofibrous Dysplasia

This lesion has the potential to cause significant anterior bowing of the tibia (resembling a tibia sabre deformity) and recurrent pathologic fractures. Prevention or delay of progressive deformity is often successful with the use of a clamshell brace starting at a young age.

Curettage of the lesion and grafting, especially in skeletally immature patients, is associated with almost 100% recurrence rate, similar to fibrous dysplasia. It is recommended that definitive treatment be delayed until close to maturity.

Correction of the tibial alignment, with the associated changes in the biomechanical forces, may lead to improvement of the bone quality and decrease the chances of worsening deformity and potential fracture.

Enchondromatosis

Recurrent pathologic fracture and progressive deformity are the two main issues associated with Ollier's disease or enchondromatosis. Similar to fibrous dysplasia, load sharing devices are preferred. These lesions, however, tend to be intra-medullary and nailing can be challenging.

The use of guided growth devices can be successful in gradual correction of the angular deformities, unless the lesion directly involves the physis, in which case, de-tethering of the physis can be considered, but the results are mixed. Limb lengthening through an enchondroma tends to be successful with adequate bone regenerate formation.

Solitary Osteochondromas and Multiple Hereditary Exostoses

While isolated osteochondromas may cause pain and mechanical symptoms requiring excision, MHE is associated with a much broader myriad of symptoms, and yearly surveillance is recommended for growing children.

In the upper extremities, the development of forearm lesions, especially in the distal ulna, can cause progressive deformity and decrease forearm rotation. Over time, this may lead to radial head subluxation and dislocation, causing pain and functional impairment.

Knee and ankle valgus are the most common deformities associated to MHE, but coxa valga can be an important contributor to an abnormal mechanical axis, and, therefore, surveillance is important. While guided growth is usually successful, these children have a high rate of recurrence and repeat hemiepiphysiodesis may be needed.

Routine spinal advanced imaging is not usually recommended, as patients with intra-canal lesions who require intervention, will present with an abnormal physical exam. Therefore, a detailed history and thorough exam will help select patients who require advanced imaging [120, 121].

Dysplasia Epiphysealis Hemimelica (Trevor's Disease)

Joint congruency can be severely affected by Trevor's disease but other issues such as angular deformity and mechanical symptoms can occur. Guided growth can be helpful in some instances. Excision of the lesion can be challenging, and for the growing child, it is usually limited to lesions causing extra-articular mechanical impingement. Joint degeneration, limited motion, and limb length discrepancy are some of the long-term outcomes seen with Trevor's Disease.

References

1. DeMattos CBR, Binitie O, Dormans JP. Pathological fractures in children. Bone Joint Res. 2012;1:272–80.
2. Dormans JP, Pill SG. Fractures through bone cysts: unicameral bone cysts, aneurysmal bone cysts, fibrous cortical defects, and nonossifying fibromas. Instr Course Lect. 2002;51:457–67.
3. Betsy M, Kupersmith LM, Springfield DS. Metaphyseal fibrous defects. J Am Acad Orthop Surg. 2004;12:89–95.
4. Arata MA, Peterson HA, Dahlin DC. Pathological fractures through non-ossifying fibromas. Review of the Mayo Clinic experience. J Bone Joint Surg Am. 1981;63:980–8.

5. Shimal A, Davies AM, James SL, Grimer RJ. Fatigue-type stress fractures of the lower limb associated with fibrous cortical defects/non-ossifying fibromas in the skeletally immature. Clin Radiol. 2010;65:382–6.
6. Moretti VM, Slotcavage RL, Crawford EA, Lackman RD, Ogilvie EM. Curettage and graft alleviates athletic-limiting pain in benign lytic bone lesions. Clin Orthop Relat Res. 2011;469:283–8.
7. Easley ME, Kneisl JS. Pathologic fractures through nonossifying fibromas: is prophylactic treatment warranted? J Pediatr Orthop. 1997;17:808–13.
8. Parekh SG, Donthineni-Rao R, Ricchetti E, Lackman RD. Fibrous dysplasia. J Am Acad Orthop Surg. 2004;12:305–13.
9. Hartley I, Zhadina M, Collins MT, Boyce AM. Fibrous dysplasia of Bone and McCune-Albright syndrome: a bench to bedside review. Calcif Tissue Int. 2019;104(5):517–29. https://doi.org/10.1007/s00223-019-00550-z. Epub 2019 Apr 29.
10. Lumbroso S, Paris F, Sultan C, European Collaborative Study. Activating Gsalpha mutations: analysis of 113 patients with signs of McCune-Albright syndrome—a European collaborative study. J Clin Endocrinol Metab. 2004;89:2107–13. https://doi.org/10.1210/jc.2003-031225.
11. Tabareau-Delalande F, Collin C, Gomez-Brouchet A, Decouvelaere AV, Bouvier C, Larousserie F, et al. Diagnostic value of investigating GNAS mutations in fibroosseous lesions: a retrospective study of 91 cases of fibrous dysplasia and 40 other fibro-osseous lesions. Mod Pathol. 2013;26:911–21.
12. Hilger D, Masureel M, Kobilka BK. Structure and dynamics of GPCR signaling complexes. Nat Struct Mol Biol. 2018;25(1):4–12. https://doi.org/10.1038/s41594-017-0011-7. Epub 2018 Jan 8.
13. Idowu BD, Al-Adnani M, O'Donnell P, Yu L, Odell E, Diss T, Gale RE, Flanagan AM. A sensitive mutation-specific screening technique for GNAS1 mutations in cases of fibrous dysplasia: the first report of a codon 227 mutation in bone. Histopathology. 2007;50(6):691–704. https://doi.org/10.1111/j.1365-2559.2007.02676.x.
14. Bianco P, Riminucci M, Majolagbe A, Kuznetsov SA, Collins MT, Mankani MH, Corsi A, Bone HG, Wientroub S, Spiegel AM, Fisher LW, Robey PG. Mutations of the GNAS1 gene, stromal cell dysfunction, and osteomalacic changes in non-McCune-Albright fibrous dysplasia of bone. J Bone Miner Res. 2000;15(1):120–8. https://doi.org/10.1359/jbmr.2000.15.1.120.
15. Riminucci M, Liu B, Corsi A, Shenker A, Spiegel AM, Robey PG, Bianco P. The histopathology of fibrous dysplasia of bone in patients with activating mutations of the Gs alpha gene: site-specific patterns and recurrent histological hallmarks. J Pathol. 1999;187(2):249–58. https://doi.org/10.1002/(SICI)1096-9896(199901)187:2<249::AID-PATH222>3.0.CO;2-J.
16. Riminucci M, Fisher LW, Shenker A, Spiegel AM, Bianco P, Gehron Robey P. Fibrous dysplasia of bone in the McCune-Albright syndrome: abnormalities in bone formation. Am J Pathol. 1997;151(6):1587–600.
17. Hart ES, Kelly MH, Brillante B, Chen CC, Ziran N, Lee JS, Feuillan P, Leet AI, Kushner H, Robey PG, Collins MT. Onset, progression, and plateau of skeletal lesions in fibrous dysplasia and the relationship to functional outcome. J Bone Miner Res. 2007;22(9):1468–74. https://doi.org/10.1359/jbmr.070511.
18. Stanton RP, Ippolito E, Springfield D, Lindaman L, Wientroub S, Leet A. The surgical management of fibrous dysplasia of bone. Orphanet J Rare Dis. 2012;7:S1.
19. Leet AI, Chebli C, Kushner H, Chen CC, Kelly MH, Brillante BA, Robey PG, Bianco P, Wientroub S, Collins MT. Fracture incidence in polyostotic fibrous dysplasia and the McCune-Albright syndrome. J Bone Miner Res. 2004;19(4):571–7. https://doi.org/10.1359/JBMR.0301262. Epub 2003 Dec 22.
20. McCune DJ. Osteitis fibrosa cystica: the case of a nine year old girl who also exhibits precocious puberty, multiple pigmentation of the skin and hyperthyroidism. Am J Dis Child. 1936;52:743–4.
21. Albright F, Butler AM, Hampton AO, Smith PH. Syndrome characterized by osteitis fibrosa disseminate, areas of pigmentation and endocrine dysfunction, with precocious puberty in females, report of five cases. N Engl J Med. 1937;216:727–46.
22. Collins MT, Singer FR, Eugster E. McCune-Albright syndrome and the extraskeletal manifestations of fibrous dysplasia. Orphanet J Rare Dis. 2012;7:S4.
23. Zacharin M. Paediatric management of endocrine complications in McCune-Albright syndrome. J Pediatr Endocrinol Metab. 2005;18:33–41.
24. Lee JS, FitzGibbon E, Butman JA, Dufresne CR, Kushner H, Wientroub S, Robey PG, Collins MT. Normal vision despite narrowing of the optic canal in fibrous dysplasia. N Engl J Med. 2002;347(21):1670–6. https://doi.org/10.1056/NEJMoa020742.
25. Becelli R, Perugini M, Cerulli G, Carboni A, Renzi G. Surgical treatment of fibrous dysplasia of the cranio-maxillo-facial area. Review of the literature and personal experience form 1984 to 1999. Minerva Stomatol. 2002;51(7–8):293–300.
26. Leet AI, Magur E, Lee JS, Wientroub S, Robey PG, Collins MT. Fibrous dysplasia in the spine: prevalence of lesions and association with scoliosis. J Bone Joint Surg Am. 2004;86(3):531–7.
27. Mancini F, Corsi A, De Maio F, Riminucci M, Ippolito E. Scoliosis and spine involvement in fibrous dysplasia of bone. Eur Spine J. 2009;18(2):196–202. https://doi.org/10.1007/s00586-008-0860-1. Epub 2009 Jan 8.
28. Berglund JA, Tella SH, Tuthill KF, Kim L, Guthrie LC, Paul SM, Stanton R, Collins MT, Boyce AM. Scoliosis in fibrous dysplasia/McCune-Albright syndrome: factors associated with curve progression and effects of bisphosphonates. J Bone Miner Res. 2018;33(9):1641–8. https://doi.org/10.1002/jbmr.3446. Epub 2018 May 22.
29. Enneking WF, Gearen PF. Fibrous dysplasia of the femoral neck. Treatment by cortical bone-grafting. J Bone Joint Surg Am. 1986;68:1415–22.
30. Javaid MK, Boyce A, Appelman-Dijkstra N, Ong J, Defabianis P, Offiah A, Arundel P, Shaw N, Pos VD, Underhil A, Portero D, Heral L, Heegaard AM, Masi L, Monsell F, Stanton R, Dijkstra PDS, Brandi ML, Chapurlat R, Hamdy NAT, Collins MT. Best practice management guidelines for fibrous dysplasia/McCune-Albright syndrome: a consensus statement from the FD/MAS international consortium. Orphanet J Rare Dis. 2019;14(1):139. https://doi.org/10.1186/s13023-019-1102-9. Erratum in: Orphanet J Rare Dis. 2019 Nov 21;14(1):267.
31. Ippolito E, Bray EW, Corsi A, DeMaio F, Exner UG, Robey PG, et al. Natural history and treatment of fibrous dysplasia of bone: a multicenter clinicopathologic study promoted by the European Pediatric Orthopaedic Society. J Pediatr Orthop B. 2003;12:155–77.
32. Ippolito E, Caterini R, Farsetti P, Potenza V. Surgical treatment of fibrous dysplasia of bone in McCune-Albright syndrome. J Pediatr Endocrinol Metab. 2002;15:S939–44.
33. O'Sullivan M, Zacharin M. Intramedullary rodding and bisphosphonate treatment of polyostotic fibrous dysplasia associated with the McCune-Albright syndrome. J Ped Orthop. 2002;22:255–60.
34. Stanton RP, Ippolito E, Springfield D, Lindaman L, Wientroub S, Leet A. The surgical management of fibrous dysplasia of bone. Orphanet J Rare Dis. 2012;7 Suppl 1(Suppl 1):S1. https://doi.org/10.1186/1750-1172-7-S1-S1. Epub 2012 May 24.
35. Guille JT, Kumar SJ, MacEwen GD. Fibrous dysplasia of the proximal part of the femur. Long-term results of curettage and bone-grafting and mechanical realignment. J Bone Joint Surg Am. 1998;80:648–58.

36. Charpurlat RD, Hugueny P, Delmas PD, Meunier PJ. Treatment of fibrous dysplasia of bone with intravenous pamidronate: long-term effectiveness and evaluation of predictors of response to treatment. Bone. 2004;35:235–42.
37. Kelly MH, Brillante B, Collins MT. Pain in fibrous dysplasia of bone: age-related changes and the anatomical distribution of skeletal lesions. Osteoporos Int. 2008;19:57–63.
38. Plotkin H, Rauch F, Zeitlin L, Munns C, Travers R, Glorieux FH. Effect of pamidronate treatment in children with polyostotic fibrous dysplasia of bone. J Clin Endocrinol Metab. 2003;88:4569–75.
39. Parisi MS, Oliveri B, Mautalen CA. Effect of intravenous pamidronate on bone markers and local bone mineral density in fibrous dysplasia. Bone. 2003;33:582–8.
40. Boyce AM, Kelly MH, Brillante BA, Kushner H, Wientroub S, Riminucci M, Bianco P, Robey PG, Collins MT. A randomized, double blind, placebo-controlled trial of alendronate treatment for fibrous dysplasia of bone. J Clin Endocrinol Metab. 2014;99(11):4133–40. https://doi.org/10.1210/jc.2014-1371. Epub 2014 Jul 17.
41. Majoor BC, Appelman-Dijkstra NM, Fiocco M, van de Sande MA, Dijkstra PS, Hamdy NA. Outcome of long-term bisphosphonate therapy in McCune-Albright syndrome and Polyostotic fibrous dysplasia. J Bone Miner Res. 2017;32(2):264–76. https://doi.org/10.1002/jbmr.2999. Epub 2016 Nov 8.
42. Boyce AM, Chong WH, Yao J, Gafni RI, Kelly MH, Chamberlain CE, Bassim C, et al. Denosumab treatment for fibrous dysplasia. J Bone Miner Res. 2012;27:1462–70.
43. de Castro LF, Burke AB, Wang HD, Tsai J, Florenzano P, Pan KS, Bhattacharyya N, Boyce AM, Gafni RI, Molinolo AA, Robey PG, Collins MT. Activation of RANK/RANKL/OPG pathway is involved in the pathophysiology of fibrous dysplasia and associated with disease burden. J Bone Miner Res. 2019;34(2):290–4. https://doi.org/10.1002/jbmr.3602. Epub 2018 Nov 29.
44. Meier ME, Clerkx SN, Winter EM, Pereira AM, van de Ven AC, van de Sande MAJ, Appelman-Dijkstra NM. Safety of therapy with and withdrawal from denosumab in fibrous dysplasia and McCune-Albright syndrome: an observational study. J Bone Miner Res. 2021;36(9):1729–38. https://doi.org/10.1002/jbmr.4380. Epub 2021 Jun 10.
45. Majoor BCJ, Papapoulos SE, Dijkstra PDS, Fiocco M, Hamdy NAT, Appelman-Dijkstra NM. Denosumab in patients with fibrous dysplasia previously treated with bisphosphonates. J Clin Endocrinol Metab. 2019;104(12):6069–78. https://doi.org/10.1210/jc.2018-02543.
46. Yabut SM, Kenan S, Sissons HA, Lewis MM. Malignant transformation of fibrous dysplasia. A case report and review of the literature. Clin Orthop Relat Res. 1988;228:281–9.
47. Ruggieri P, Sim FH, Bond JR, Unni KK. Malignancies in fibrous dysplasia. Cancer. 1994;73:1411–24.
48. Campanacci M, Laus M. Osteofibrous dysplasia of the tibia and fibula. J Bone Joint Surg Am. 1981;63:367–75.
49. Van Delm I, Fabry G. Osteofibrous dysplasia of the tibia: case report and review of the literature. J Pediatr Orthop. 1999;8:50–3.
50. Cetinkaya M, Ozkan H, Koksal N, Sarisozen B, Yazici Z. Neonatal osteofibrous dysplasia associated with pathological tibia fracture: a case report and review of the literature. J Pediatr Orthop B. 2012;21:183–6.
51. Komiya S, Inoue A. Aggressive bone tumorous lesion in infancy: osteofibrous dysplasia of the tibia and fibula. J Pediatr Orthop. 1993;13:577–81.
52. Karol LA, Brown DS, Wise CA, Waldron M. Familial osteofibrous dysplasia. A case series. J Bone Joint Surg Am. 2005;87:2297–307.
53. Hunter AG, Jarvis J. Osteofibrous dysplasia: two affected male sibs and an unrelated girl with bilateral involvement. Am J Med Genet. 2002;112:79–85.
54. Schwarzkopf E, Tavarez Y, Healey JH, Hameed M, Prince DE. Adamantinomatous tumors: long-term follow-up study of 20 patients treated at a single institution. J Surg Oncol. 2020;122(2):273–82. https://doi.org/10.1002/jso.25950. Epub 2020 Apr 25.
55. Kahn LB. Adamantinoma, osteofibrous dysplasia and differentiated adamantinoma. Skel Radiol. 2003;32:245–58.
56. Springfield DS, Rosenberg AE, Mankin HJ, Mindell ER. Relationship between osteofibrous dysplasia and adamantinoma. Clin Orthop Relat Res. 1994;309:234–44.
57. Gleason BC, Liegl-Atzwanger B, Kozakewich HP, Connolly S, Gebhardt MC, Fletcher JA, et al. Osteofibrous dysplasia and adamantinoma in children and adolescents: a clinicopathologic reappraisal. Am J Surg Pathol. 2008;32:363–76.
58. Most MJ, Sim FH, Inwards CY. Osteofibrous dysplasia and adamantinoma. J Am Acad Orthop Surg. 2010;18:358–66.
59. Ramanoudjame M, Buinebretiere JM, Mascard E, Seringe R, Dimeglio A, Wicart P. Is there a link between osteofibrous dysplasia and adamantinoma? Orthop Traumatol Surg Res. 2011;97:877–80.
60. Ozaki T, Hamada M, Sugihara S, Kunisada T, Mitani S, Inoue H. Treatment outcome of osteofibrous dysplasia. J Pediatr Orthop. 1998;7:199–202.
61. Andrisano A, Soncini G, Calderoni PP, Stilli S. Critical review of infantile fibrous dysplasia: surgical treatment. J Pediatr Orthop. 1991;11:478–81.
62. Kosuge DD, Pugh H, Ramachandran M, Barry M, Timms A. Marginal excision and Ilizarov hemicallotasis for osteofibrous dysplasia of the tibia: a case report. J Pediatr Orthop B. 2011;20:89–93.
63. Karita M, Tsuchiya H, Sakurakichi K, Tomita K. Osteofibrous dysplasia treated with distraction osteogenesis: a report of two cases. J Orthop Sci. 2004;9:516–20.
64. Amary MF, Damato S, Halai D, Eskandarpour M, Berisha F, Bonar F, McCarthy S, et al. Ollier disease and Maffucci syndrome are caused by somatic mosaic mutations of IDH1 and IDH2. Nat Genet. 2011;43:1262–5.
65. Shapiro F, Ollier's disease. An assessment of angular deformity, shortening, and pathological fracture in twenty-one patients. J Bone Joint Surg Am. 1982;64:95–103.
66. Chew DK, Menelaus MB, Richardson MD. Ollier's disease: varus angulation at the lower femur and its management. J Pediatr Orthop. 1998;18:202–8.
67. Jesus-Garcia R, Bongiovanni JC, Korukian M, Boatto H, Seixas MT, Laredo J. Use of the Ilizarov external fixator in the treatment of patients with Ollier's disease. Clin Orthop Relat Res. 2001;382:82–6.
68. Popkov D, Journeau P, Popkov A, Haumont T, Lascombes P. Ollier's disease limb lengthening: should intramedullary nailing be combined with circular external fixation? Orthop Traumatol Surg Res. 2010;96:348–53.
69. Tsuchiya H, Morsy AF, Matsubara H, Watanabe K, Abdel-Wanis ME, Tomita K. Treatment of benign bone tumours using external fixation. J Bone Joint Surg Br. 2007;89:1077–83.
70. Watanabe K, Tsuchiya H, Sakurakichi K, Yamashiro T, Matsubara H, Tomita K. Treatment of lower limb deformities and limb-length discrepancies with the external fixator in Ollier's disease. J Orthop Sci. 2007;12:471–5.
71. D'Angelo G, Petas N, Donzelli O. Lengthening of the lower limbs in Ollier's disease: problems related to surgery. Chir Organi Mov. 1996;81:279–85.

72. Baumgart R, Burklein D, Hinterwimmer S, Thaller P, Mutschler W. The management of leg-length discrepancy in Ollier's disease with a fully implantable lengthening nail. J Bone Joint Surg Br. 2005;87:1000–4.
73. Sun TC, Swee RG, Shives TC, Unni KK. Chondrosarcoma in Maffucci's syndrome. J Bone Joint Surg Am. 1985;67:1214–9.
74. Liu J, Hudkins PG, Swee RG, Unni KK. Bone sarcomas associated with Ollier's disease. Cancer. 1987;59:1376–85.
75. Schwartz HS, Zimmerman NB, Simon MA, Wroble RR, Millar EA, Bonfiglio M. The malignant potential of enchondromatosis. J Bone Joint Surg Am. 1987;69:269–74.
76. Stieber JR, Dormans JP. Manifestations of hereditary multiple exostoses. J Am Acad Orthop Surg. 2005;13:110–20.
77. Cook A, Raskind W, Blanton SH, Pauli RM, Gregg RG, Francomano CA, et al. Genetic heterogeneity in families with hereditary multiple exostoses. Am J Hum Genet. 1993;53:71–9.
78. Wuyts W, Van Hul W, DeBoulle K, Hendrickx J, Bakker E, Vanhoenacker F, et al. Mutations in the EXT1 and EXT2 genes in hereditary multiple exostoses. Am J Hum Genet. 1998;62:346–54.
79. Wu YQ, Heutink P, deVries BB, Sandkuijl LA, van den Ouweland AM, Niermeijer MF, et al. Assignment of a second locus for multiple exostoses to the pericentromeric region of chromosome 11. Hum Mol Genet. 1994;3:167–71.
80. Alvarez CM, DeVera MA, Heslip TR, Casey B. Evaluation of the anatomic burden of patients with hereditary multiple exostoses. Clin Orthop Relat Res. 2007;462:73–9.
81. Porter DE, Lonie L, Fraser M, Dobson-Stone C, Porter JR, Monaco AP, et al. Severity of disease and risk of malignant change in hereditary multiple exostoses: a genotype-phenotype study. J Bone Joint Surg Br. 2004;86:1041–6.
82. Pedrini E, Jennes I, Tremosini M, Milanesi A, Mordenti M, Parra A, et al. Genotype-phenotype correlation study in 529 patients with multiple hereditary exostoses: identification of "protective" and "risk" factors. J Bone Joint Surg Am. 2011;93:2294–302.
83. Clement ND, Duckworth AD, Baker AD, et al. Skeletal growth patterns in hereditary multiple exostoses: a natural history. J Pediatr Orthop B. 2012;21:150–4.
84. Carroll KL, Yandow SM, Ward K, Carey JC. Clinical correlation to genetic variations of hereditary multiple exostosis. J Pediatr Orthop. 1999;19:785–91.
85. Bovee JV. Multiple osteochondromas. Orphanet J Rare Dis. 2008;3:3.
86. Schmale GA, Conrad EU, Raskind WH. The natural history of hereditary multiple exostoses. J Bone Joint Surg Am. 1994;76:986–92.
87. Shapiro F, Simon S, Glimcher MJ. Hereditary multiple exostoses. Anthropometric, roentgenographic, and clinical aspects. J Bone Joint Surg Am. 1979;61:815–24.
88. De Andrea CE, Kroon HM, Wolterbeek R, Romeo S, Rosenberg AI, De Young BR, et al. Interobserver reliability in the histopathological diagnosis of cartilaginous tumors in patients with multiple osteochondromas. Mod Pathol. 2012;25:1275–83.
89. Darilek S, Wicklund C, Novy D, Scott A, Gambello M, Hecht J. Hereditary multiple exostosis and pain. J Pediatr Orthop. 2005;25:369–76.
90. Chhina H, Davis JC, Alvarez CM. Health-related quality of life in people with hereditary multiple exostoses. J Pediatr Orthop. 2012;32:210–4.
91. Goud AL, deLange J, Scholtes VA, Bulstra SK, Ham SJ. Pain, physical and social functioning, and quality of life in individuals with multiple hereditary exostoses in The Netherlands: a national cohort study. J Bone Joint Surg Am. 2012;94:1013–20.
92. Abdel MP, Papagelopoulos PJ, Morrey ME, Wenger DE, Rose PS, Sim FH. Surgical management of 121 benign proximal fibula tumors. Clin Orthop Relat Res. 2010;468:3056–62.
93. Wirganowicz PZ, Watts HG. Surgical risk for elective excision of benign exostoses. J Pediatr Orthop. 1997;17:455–9.
94. Sabharwal S, Zhao C, Passanante M. Venous thromboembolism in children: details of 46 cases based on a follow-up survey of POSNA members. J Pediatr Orthop. 2013;33:768–74.
95. Loder RT, Sundberg S, Gabriel K, Mehbod A, Meyer C. Determination of bone age in children with cartilaginous dysplasia (multiple hereditary osteochondromatosis and Ollier's enchondromatosis). J Pediatr Orthop. 2004;24:102–8.
96. Nawata K, Teshima R, Minamizaki T, Yamamoto K. Knee deformities in multiple hereditary exostoses. A longitudinal radiographic study. Clin Orthop Relat Res. 1995;313:194–9.
97. Snearly WN, Peterson HA. Management of ankle deformities in multiple hereditary osteochondromata. J Pediatr Orthop. 1989;9:427–32.
98. Rupprecht M, Spiro AS, Rueger JM, Stucker R. Temporary screw epiphyseodesis of the distal tibia: a therapeutic option for ankle valgus in patients with hereditary multiple exostosis. J Pediatr Orthop. 2011;31:89–94.
99. Tompkins M, Eberson C, Ehrlich M. Hemiepiphyseal stapling for ankle valgus in multiple hereditary exostoses. Am J Orthop. 2012;41:E23–6.
100. Noonan KJ, Feinberg JR, Levenda A, Snead J, Wurtz LD. Natural history of multiple hereditary osteochondromatosis of the lower extremity and ankle. J Pediat Orthop. 2002;22:120–4.
101. Porter DE, Benson MK, Hosney GA. The hip in hereditary multiple exostoses. J Bone Joint Surg Br. 2001;83:988–95.
102. Felix NA, Mazur JM, Loveless EA. Acetabular dysplasia associated with hereditary multiple exostoses. A case report. J Bone Joint Surg Br. 2000;82:555–7.
103. Johnston CE, Sklar F. Multiple hereditary exostoses with spinal cord compression. Orthopedics. 1988;11:1213–6.
104. Roach JW, Klatt JW, Faulkner ND. Involvement of the spine in patients with multiple hereditary exostoses. J Bone Joint Surg Am. 2009;91:1942–8.
105. Lin PP, Moussallem CD, Deavers MT. Secondary chondrosarcoma. J Am Acad Orthop Surg. 2010;38:608–15.
106. Ahmed AR, Tan TS, Unni KK, Collins MS, Wenger DE, Sim FH. Secondary chondrosarcoma in osteochondroma: report of 107 patients. Clin Orthop Relat Res. 2003;411:193–206.
107. Nystrom LM, DeYoung BR, Morcuende JA. Secondary chondrosarcoma of the pelvis arising from a solitary exostosis in an 11-year-old patient: a case report with 5-year follow-up. Iowa Orthop J. 2013;33:213–6.
108. Rangdal SS, Behera P, Bachhal V, Raj N, Sudesh P. Pseudoaneurysm of the popliteal artery in a child with multiple hereditary exostosis: a rare case report and literature review. J Pediatr Orthop B. 2013;22:353–6.
109. Pellenc Q, Capdevila C, Julia P, Fabiani JN. Ruptured popliteal artery pseudoaneurysm complicating a femoral osteochondroma in a young patient. J Vasc Surg. 2012;55:1164–5.
110. Rosero VM, Kiss S, Terebessy T, Kollo K, Szoke G. Dysplasia epiphysealis hemimelica (Trevor's disease): 7 of our own cases and a review of the literature. Acta Orthop. 2007;78:856–61.
111. Keret D, Spatz DK, Caro PA, Mason DE. Dysplasia epiphysealis hemimelica: diagnosis and treatment. J Pediatr Orthop. 1992;12:365–72.
112. Tyler PA, Rajeswaran G, Saifuddin A. Imaging of dysplasia epiphysealis hemimelica (Trevor's disease). Clin Radiol. 2013;68:415–21.
113. Bahk WJ, Lee HY, Kang YK, Park JM, Chun KA, Chung YG. Dysplasia epiphysealis hemimelica: radiographic and magnetic resonance imaging features and clinical outcome of complete and incomplete resection. Skeletal Radiol. 2010;39:85–90.

114. Haddad F, Chemali R, Maalouf G. Dysplasia epiphysealis hemimelica with involvement of the hip and spine in a young girl. J Bone Joint Surg Br. 2008;90:952–6.
115. Tschauner C, Roth-Schiffl E, Mayer U. Early loss of hip containment in a child with dysplasia epiphysealis hemimelica. Clin Orthop Relat Res. 2004;427:213–9.
116. Link LC, Buckup K, Kalchschmidt K. Dysplasia epiphysealis hemimelica (Trevor's disease) of the acetabulum. Arch Orthop Trauma Surg. 2005;125:193–6.
117. Skaggs DL, Moon CN, Kay RM, Peterson HA. Dysplasia epiphysealis hemimelica of the acetabulum. A report of two cases. J Bone Joint Surg Am. 2000;82:409–14.
118. Baghdadi S, Nguyen JC, Arkader A. Nonossifying fibroma of the distal tibia: predictors of fracture and management algorithm. J Pediatr Ortho. 2021;41(8):e671–9.
119. Baghdadi S, Arkader A. Fibrous dysplasia: recent developments and modern management alternatives. J Pediatr Orthop Soc N Am. 2020;2(2):84. https://www.jposna.org/ojs/index.php/jposna/article/view/84.
120. Meza BC, Obana KK, Talathi NS, Shah AS, Lightdale-Miric N, Arkader A. Predicting radial head instability in multiple hereditary exostoses (MHE): a multicenter analysis of risk factors. J Pediatr Orthop. 2020;40(7):e656–61.
121. Jackson TJ, Shah AS, Arkader A. Is routine spine MRI necessary in skeletally immature patients with MHE? Identifying patients at risk for spinal osteochondromas. J Pediatr Orthop. 2019;39(2):e147–52.

Management of Juxtaphyseal Malignant Bone Tumors Around the Knee Joint: New Concepts in Limb-Sparing Surgery

Hidenori Matsubara and Hiroyuki Tsuchiya

Introduction

There are various kinds of malignant bone tumors in pediatrics. Osteosarcoma is the most common primary malignant bone tumor in children. Prior to the 1970s, amputation or joint disarticulations were the standard treatment and the only choice of treatment. However, now over 90% of osteosarcoma resections are limb-sparing surgeries due to advancements in chemotherapy, medical imaging, and implant technology [1–3]. Options for limb salvage reconstruction after wide resection include osteoarticular allografts, allograft prosthetic composites, recycled autograft, and modular or custom-made endoprostheses. However, the limb function often remains limited and deteriorates over time. Complications such as infections, nonunion of grafts, and bone resorption could eventually lead to amputation. Therefore, the aim of biological reconstruction is to achieve better limbs and almost normal limb function, and to reduce complications.

We first performed transepiphyseal osteotomy and resected a malignant bone tumor followed by reconstruction using the distraction osteogenesis technique (DO method) [4–6] and massive frozen tumor-bearing bone treated with liquid nitrogen (LN method) [7, 8]. In this chapter, we introduce our two original biological reconstruction procedures for malignant tumors.

Supplementary Information The online version contains supplementary material available at https://doi.org/10.1007/978-3-031-55767-5_28.

H. Matsubara · H. Tsuchiya (✉)
Department of Orthopedic Surgery, Kanazawa University Hospital, Kanazawa, Ishikawa, Japan
e-mail: ortho331@staff.kanazawa-u.ac.jp; tsuchi@med.kanazawa-u.ac.jp

Indication

To facilitate decision making for reconstruction in cases of juxta-articular malignant bone tumor around the knee joint, we developed a new system for classifying tumor excision (Table 28.1, Fig. 28.1) [9]. Cases indicated for the DO method should have tumors of Types I to IV according to our classification system, of no more than a 15 cm defect after the tumor resection (resulting in a treatment time of less than one year), and with a good response to chemotherapy. Theoretically, the DO method can be applied even in cases with Types V and VI tumors combined with arthrodesis. Currently, however, it has been replaced with the LN method. The LN method can be indicated in all cases. For chemotherapy responders, this enables preservation of the maximum amount of healthy tissue, such as soft tissue, growth plates, and joint surfaces, to provide excellent limb function [3].

Table 28.1 Decision making for reconstruction based on location and extent of tumor

Type I: Tumor at diaphyseal location or metaphyseal location over 2 cm from the epiphyseal plate
Type II: Tumor at metaphyseal location extending to less than half of the epiphyseal growth plate
Type III: Tumor at metaphyseal location extending to the whole growth plate
Type IV: Metaphyseal tumor extending through the growth plate into part of the epiphysis at least 10 mm from the articular surface
Type V: Tumor extending into less than half of the epiphysis less than 1 cm away from the articular surface
Type VI: Tumor extending into more than half of the epiphysis less than 1 cm away from the articular surface

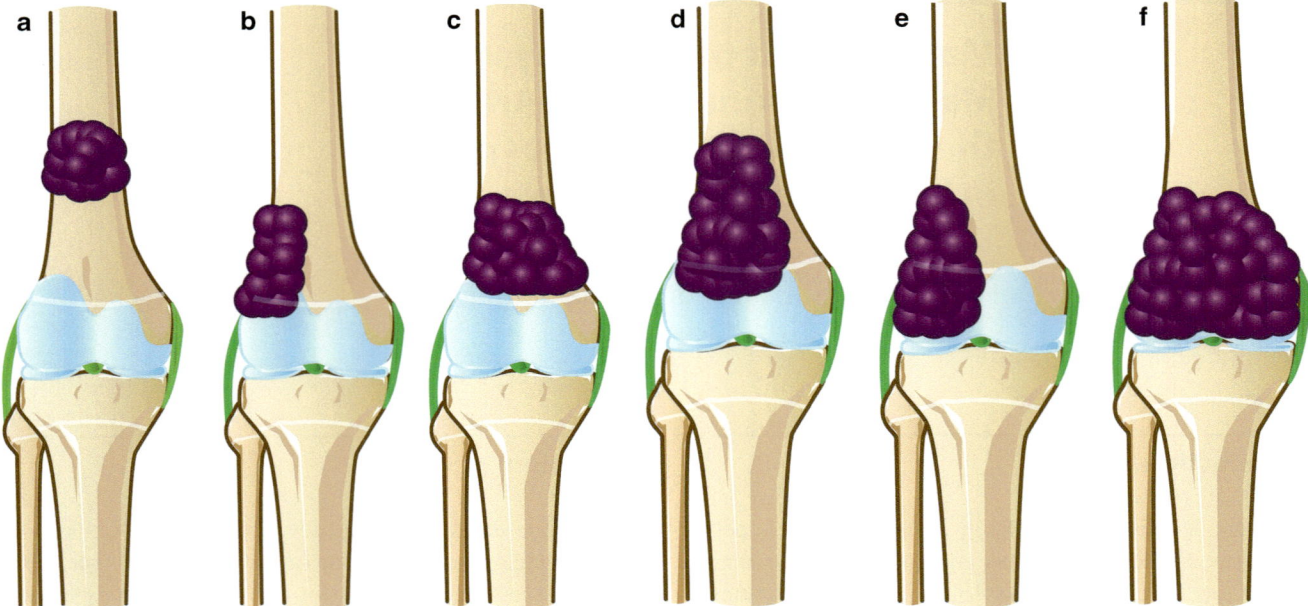

Fig. 28.1 Classification of tumor excision. (**a**) Type I. (**b**) Type II. (**c**) Type III. (**d**) Type IV. (**e**) Type V. (**f**) Type VI

Surgical Techniques

Type I: DO Method (Fig. 28.2)

In Type I, the tumor is diaphyseally or metaphyseally located over 2 cm away from the epiphyseal plate. The operative technique of the DO method consists of en bloc tumor excision with preservation of the epiphyseal plate and articular surface. An external fixator is applied and osteotomy is performed for postoperative bone transport. After docking bone transport, we usually perform bone graft at the docking site. Shortening-distraction is indicated if acute shortening is possible during the operation. Optional intramedullary nailing, if feasible, or plate conversion, is also used to shorten the external fixation time [5, 6].

Type I: LN Method (Fig. 28.3)

One-site osteotomy and pedicle freezing method are applied in the Type I LN method. After transdiaphyseal osteotomy, soft tissue is removed, and the tumor is curetted after thorough isolation to prevent fracture during freezing. Bony lesions connected to the limb are then rotated and frozen in liquid nitrogen for 20 min, thawed at room temperature for 15 min, and then thawed in distilled water for 10 min. Reconstructions are performed by osteosynthesis using double plates [8].

Type II: DO Method (Fig. 28.4)

In Type II, the tumor is located metaphyseally and extends to less than half of the epiphyseal growth plate. There is also a possibility of joint deformity due to unequal growth after reconstruction. The operative technique of the DO method consists of hemicortical en bloc tumor excision. An external fixator is applied, and proximal hemicortical osteotomy is performed for postoperative bone transport. Epiphysiodesis of the other side of the growth plate is one option to avoid future angular deformities for young patients. After docking bone transport, we usually perform a bone graft at the docking site. At that time, plate conversion is optionally used to shorten the external fixation time. If a deformity occurs in the future, correction with or without lengthening is performed.

Type II: LN Method (Fig. 28.5)

Hemicortical resection and a free-freezing method are applied for Type II resections. After transepiphyseal and hemicortical resection, soft tissue is removed, and the tumor is curetted after thorough isolation. The tumor-bearing bone is frozen in liquid nitrogen and thawed as usual. Reconstruction is performed by osteosynthesis using a single-locking plate [7].

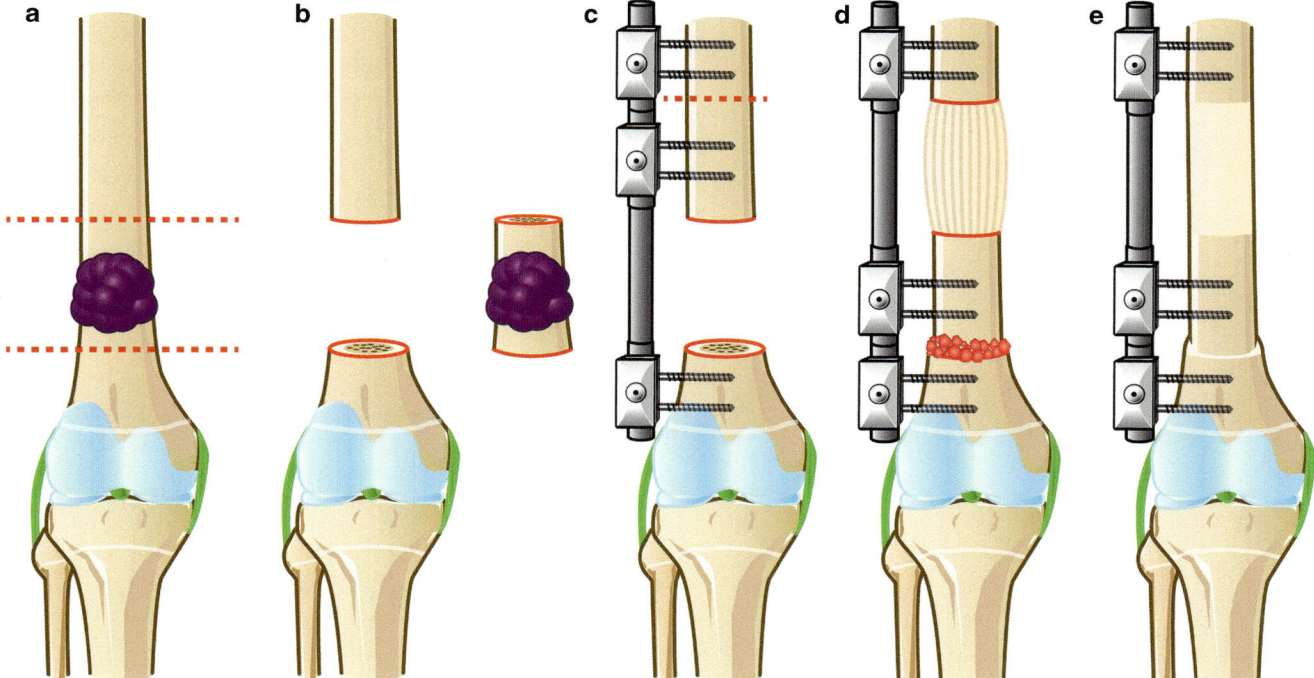

Fig. 28.2 Type I: DO method. (**a**) Resection line. (**b**) Tumor resection. (**c**) Application of external fixator and osteotomy for lengthening. (**d**) Bone grafting at docking site. (**e**) After bone consolidation

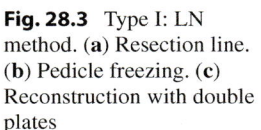

Fig. 28.3 Type I: LN method. (**a**) Resection line. (**b**) Pedicle freezing. (**c**) Reconstruction with double plates

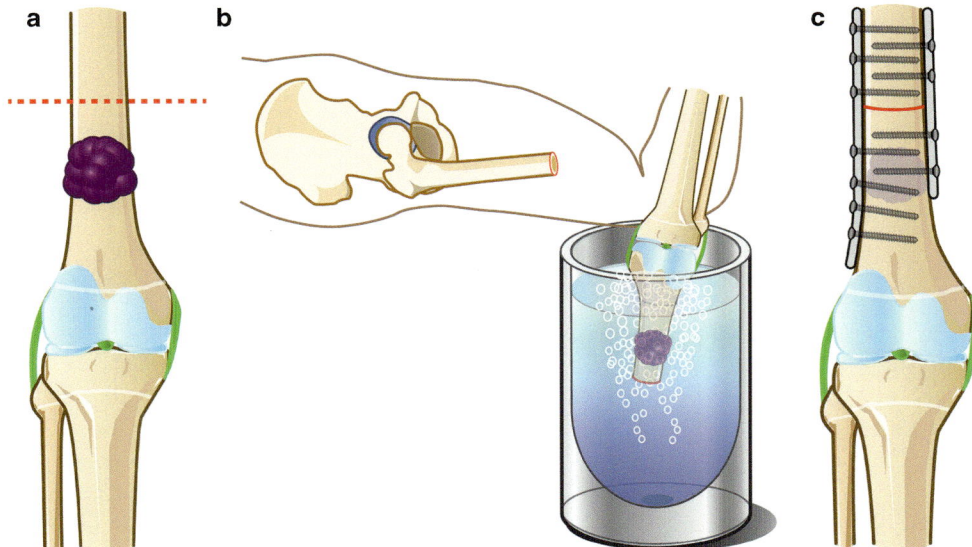

Type III: DO Method (Fig. 28.6)

In Type III, the tumor is metaphyseally located and extends to the whole growth plate. Limb length discrepancies are anticipated in immature patients, which may be managed surgically if necessary. The operative technique of the DO method consists of transepiphyseal and intercalary en bloc tumor excision with the growth plate. Surgical technique is basically the same as in the Type I DO method.

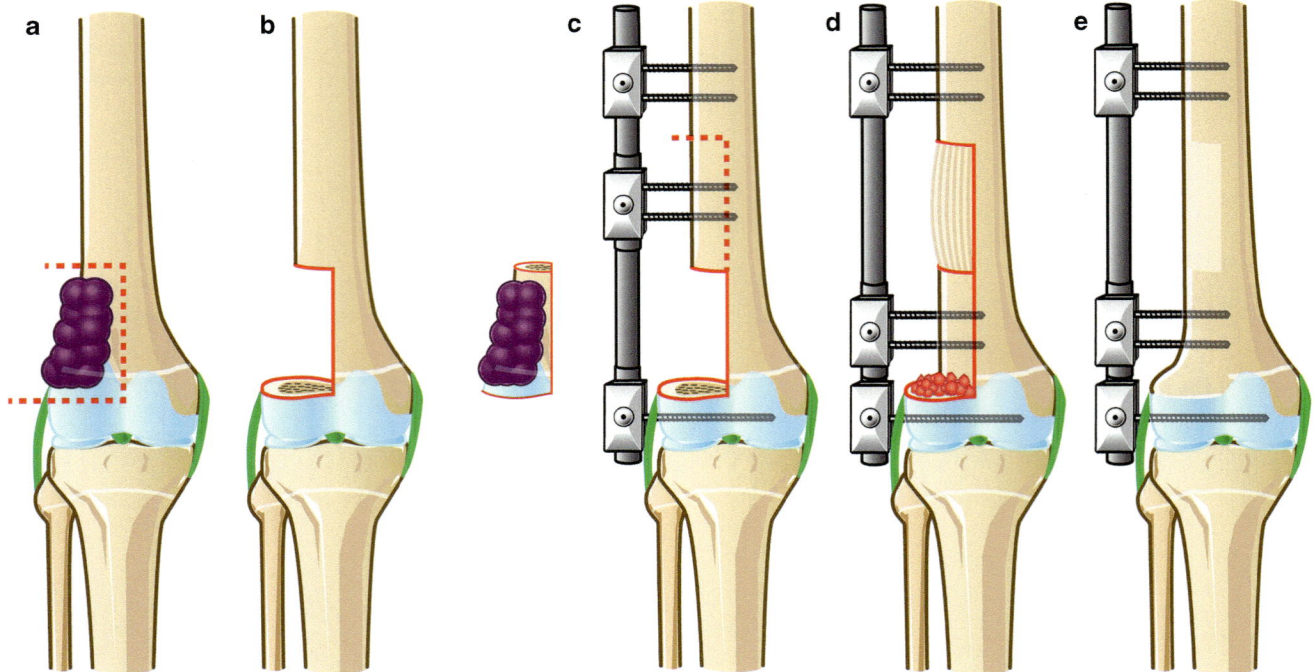

Fig. 28.4 Type II: DO method. (**a**) Resection line. (**b**) Tumor resection. (**c**) Application of external fixator and osteotomy for lengthening. (**d**) Bone grafting at docking site. (**e**) After bone consolidation

Fig. 28.5 Type II: LN method. (**a**) Resection line. (**b**) Freezing tumor-bearing bone. (**c**) Reconstruction with single plate

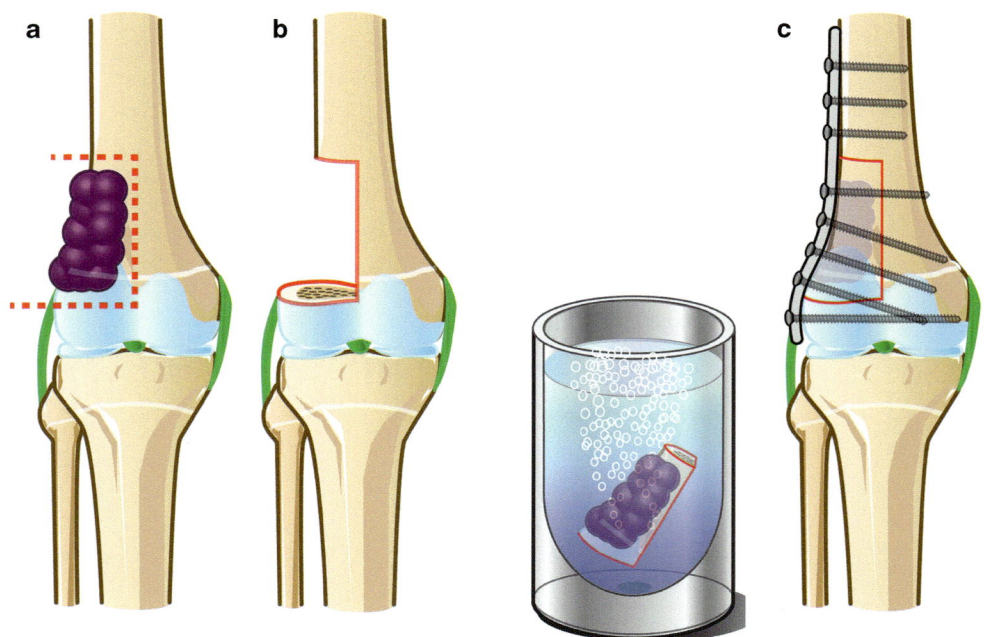

Type III: LN Method (Fig. 28.7)

Intercalary resection and the free-freezing method are applied for Type III resection. After transepiphyseal and intercalary resection, free freezing is performed in the same way as in the Type II LN method. Reconstruction is performed by osteosynthesis using double plates.

Type IV: DO Method (Fig. 28.8)

In Type IV, the tumor is metaphyseally located and extends to the whole growth plate into part of the epiphysis at least 10 mm away from the joint line. Limb length discrepancies are anticipated in immature patients, which may be managed surgically if necessary. The operative technique of the DO

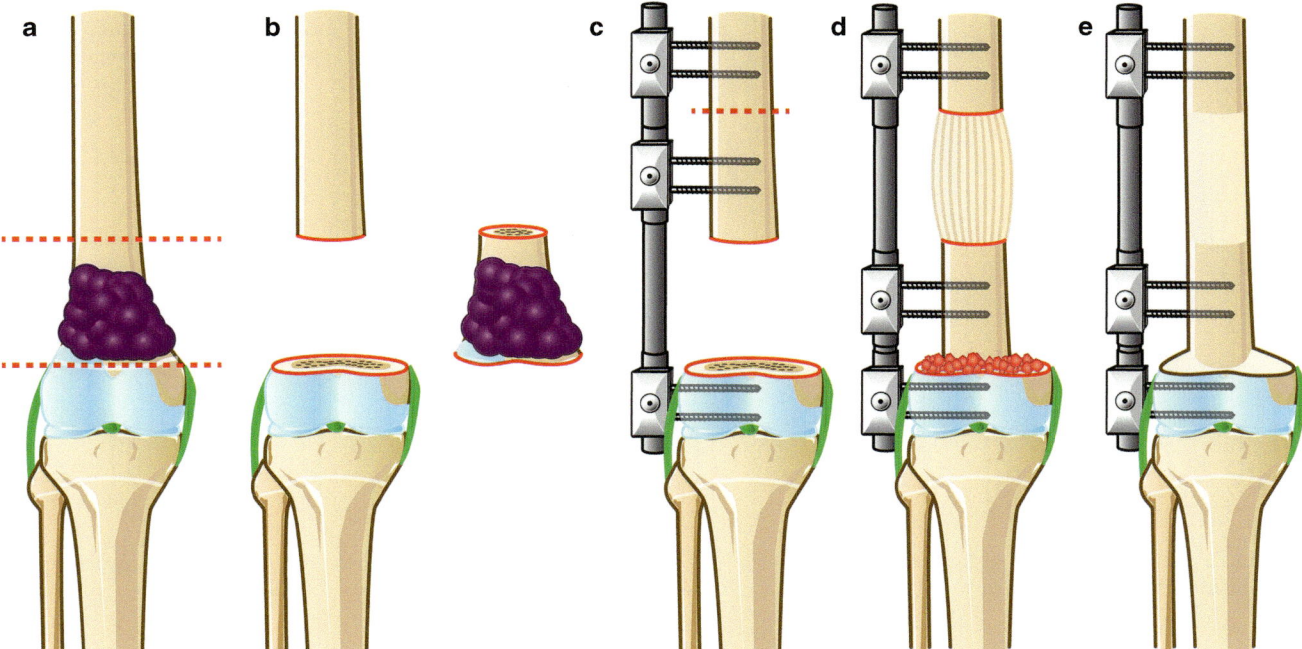

Fig. 28.6 Type III: DO method. (**a**) Resection line. (**b**) Tumor resection. (**c**) Application of external fixator and osteotomy for lengthening. (**d**) Bone grafting at docking site. (**e**) After bone consolidation

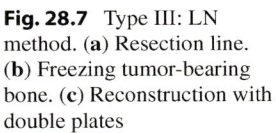

Fig. 28.7 Type III: LN method. (**a**) Resection line. (**b**) Freezing tumor-bearing bone. (**c**) Reconstruction with double plates

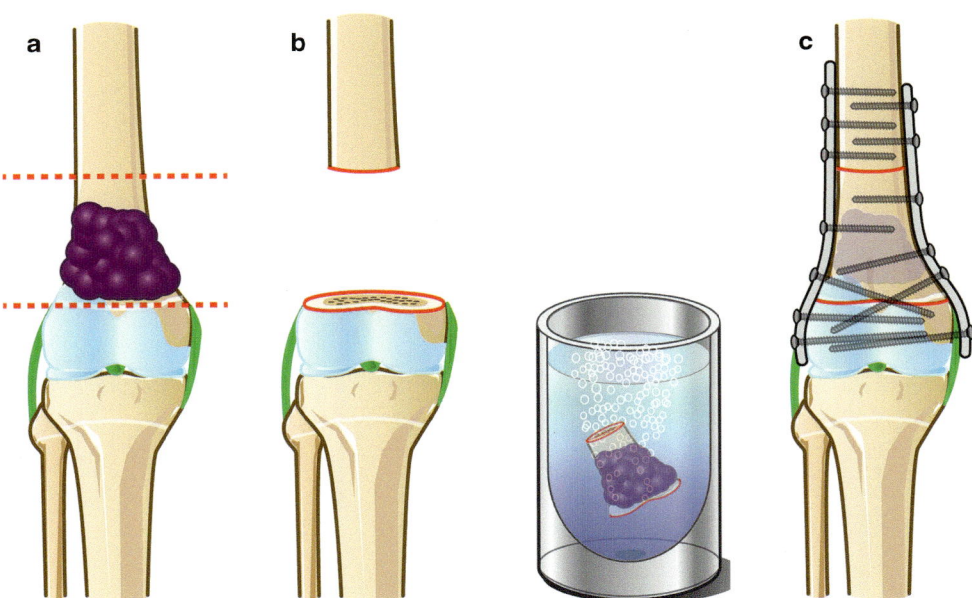

method consists of transepiphyseal and intercalary en bloc tumor excision with the growth plate, and with preservation of the articular surface. The periarticular structure should be stabilized immediately to prevent joint contracture. If only a thin epiphysis or articular surface is preserved, a free bone cylinder should be taken from the diaphysis and fixed to the remaining epiphysis with a bone graft and a spike washer and screw, in order to stabilize and reconstruct the periarticular structure. The newly created diaphyseal defect is restored by bone transport. If feasible, optional plate conversion is also used.

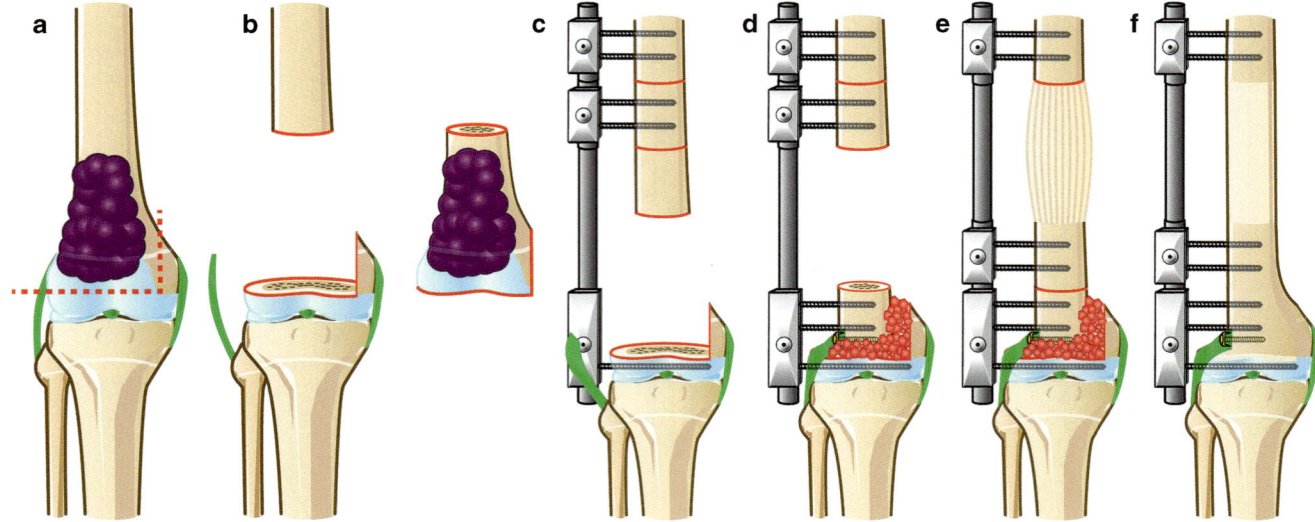

Fig. 28.8 Type IV: DO method. (**a**) Resection line. (**b**) Tumor resection. (**c**) Application of external fixator and osteotomy for lengthening. (**d**) Reconstruction of periarticular structure with diaphyseal bone cylinder. (**e**) After docking. (**f**) After bone consolidation

Fig. 28.9 Type IV: LN method. (**a**) Resection line. (**b**) Freezing tumor-bearing bone. (**c**) Reconstruction with double plates and spike wisher

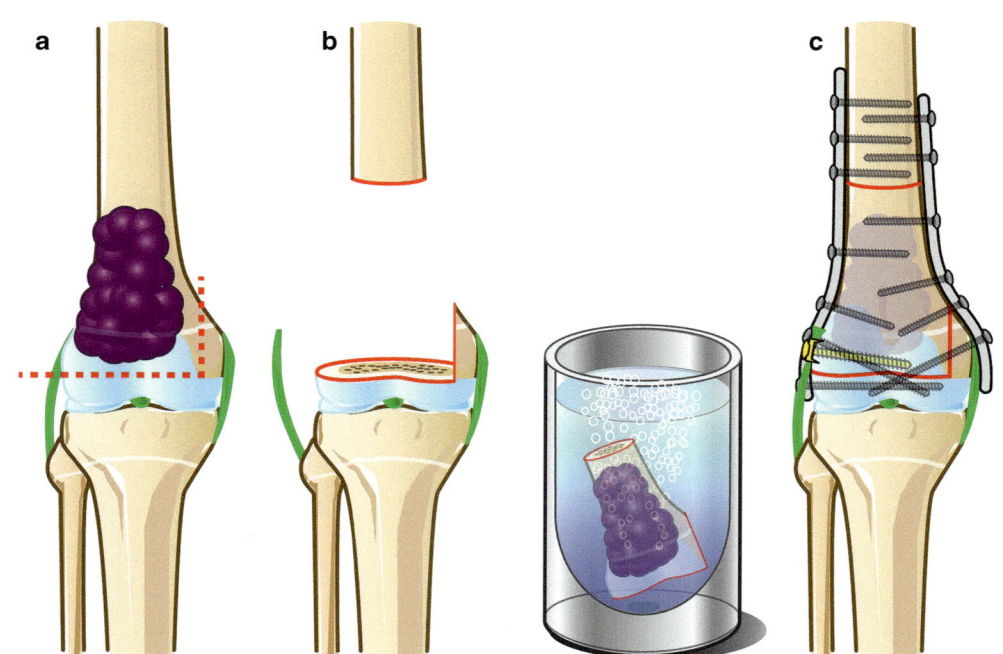

Type IV: LN Method (Fig. 28.9)

Intercalary resection and free-freezing method are applied for Type IV resection. After transepiphyseal and intercalary resection, the tumor-bearing bone is frozen and thawed in the same way as above. Reconstruction is performed with double plates. When the ligament is detached from the tumor-bearing bone, it is reconstructed with a spike washer and screw.

Type V: LN Method (Fig. 28.10)

In Type V, the tumor extends into less than half of the epiphysis. There is a possibility of joint deformity due to unequal growth after reconstruction. The operative technique of the LN method consists of hemicortical resection with the osteoarticular surface, and the free-freezing method is applied for Type V. After resection of the hemicondyle, soft tissue is removed, and the tumor is curetted after thorough isolation.

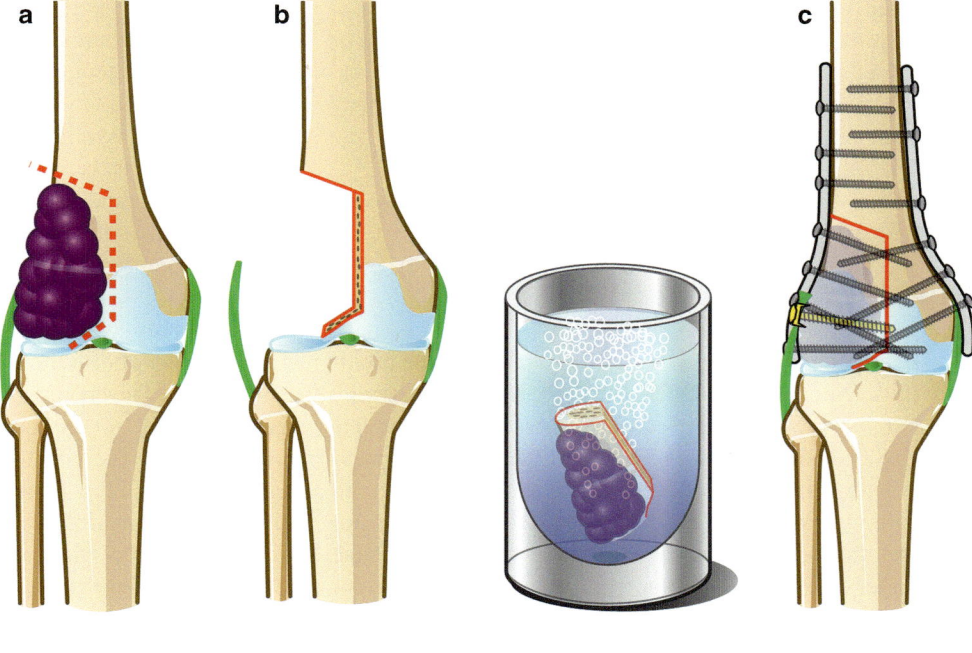

Fig. 28.10 Type V: LN method. (**a**) Resection line. (**b**) Freezing tumor-bearing bone. (**c**) Reconstruction with double plates and spike wisher

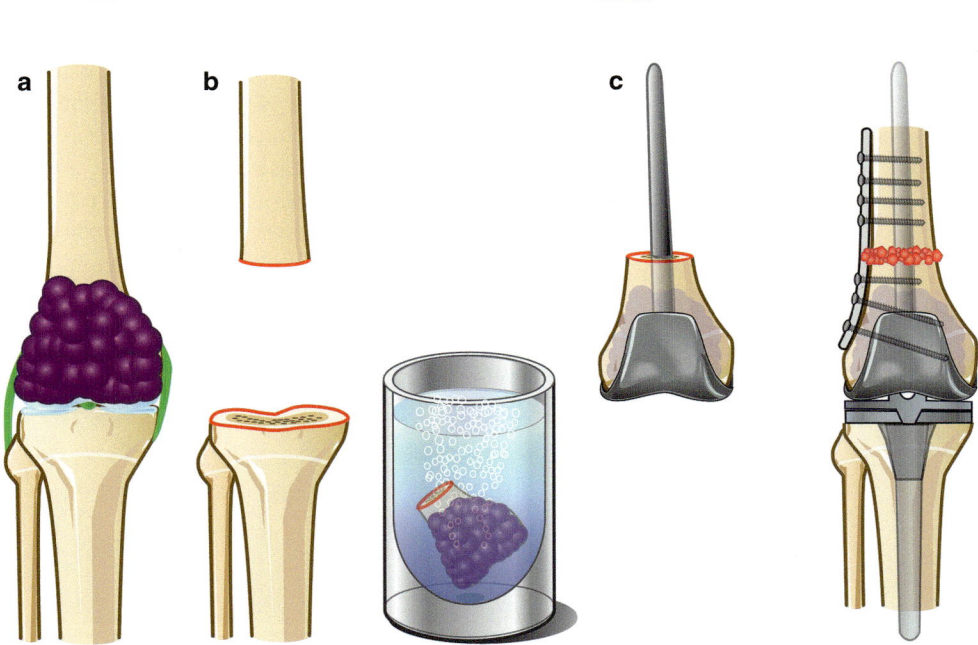

Fig. 28.11 Type VI: LN method. (**a**) Resection line. (**b**) Freezing tumor-bearing bone. (**c**) Reconstruction with surface arthroplasty with or without a locking plate and bone graft

The tumor-bearing bone is frozen in liquid nitrogen and thawed in the same way as above. Reconstructions are performed by osteosynthesis using single or double plates, a spike washer, and screws. Frozen osteoarticular grafts tend to undergo osteoarthritis changes; therefore, an optional composite autograft indicated for Type VI is also applied to avoid future operations. Otherwise, UKA or TKA is carried out for degenerative arthrosis.

Type VI: LN Method (Fig. 28.11)

In Type VI, the tumor extends into more than half of the epiphysis. There is no possibility of preservation of the whole joint. There is also a possibility of joint deformity and limb length discrepancy after reconstruction. The operative technique of the LN method consists of en bloc resection with the osteoarticular surface, and the free-freezing method is applied for Type VI. Reconstruction is performed by a combination of frozen grafts and surface arthroplasty with or without a locking plate and bone graft. Strictly speaking, these are partially biological reconstructions; however, they can preserve bone stock.

Case Examples

Case 1 (Type I: DO Method) (Fig. 28.12)

A 17-year-old boy presented with osteosarcoma of the proximal tibia. Neoadjuvant caffeine-potentiated chemotherapy was administered, and the clinical effect was a complete response with significant ossification of the soft-tissue mass of the lateral tibia. We planned intercalary resection and reconstruction with the DO method (bone transport). After the operation, gradual lengthening was started and bone transporter docking was completed. As of the seven-year follow-up, the patient is free of disease, and can run without any pain.

Case 2 (Type IV: LN Method) (Fig. 28.13) (Video 28.1)

A 19-year-old female presented with osteosarcoma of the distal femur. Neoadjuvant chemotherapy was administered, and the clinical effect was a partial response with significant ossification and necrosis of the soft-tissue mass of the femur. We planned transepiphyseal and intercalary resection and reconstruction with the LN method. Reconstruction was performed by osteosynthesis using three locking plates. The resection margins were tumor free, and pathological evaluation indicated grade III/IV on the Rosen and Huvos evaluating system. As of the 82-month follow-up, the patient is free of disease. She has no extension lag. The range of motion of the knee was 0–60°.

In summary, we introduced limb-salvage surgery for reconstruction after tumor resection using distraction osteogenesis and a frozen autograft method utilizing liquid nitrogen, according to the tumor site, size, and response to chemotherapy. The advantages of the DO method include regeneration of living bone with sufficient strength and durability, biological affinity, resistance against infection, and lifelong restored function. The disadvantages include delayed union at the docking site and pin- or wire-tract infection, as well as the fact that the procedure is time consuming (Table 28.2). The advantages of the LN method are simplicity, osteoinduction, osteoconduction, a short treatment time, a perfect fit, sufficient biomechanical strength, and easy attachment of tendons and ligaments. The disadvantage is basically dead bone at the time of reconstruction. Moreover, revitalization takes a long time, and degeneration of the preserved cartilage matrix occurs over time (Table 28.3). Possible complications with the DO method include pin-site

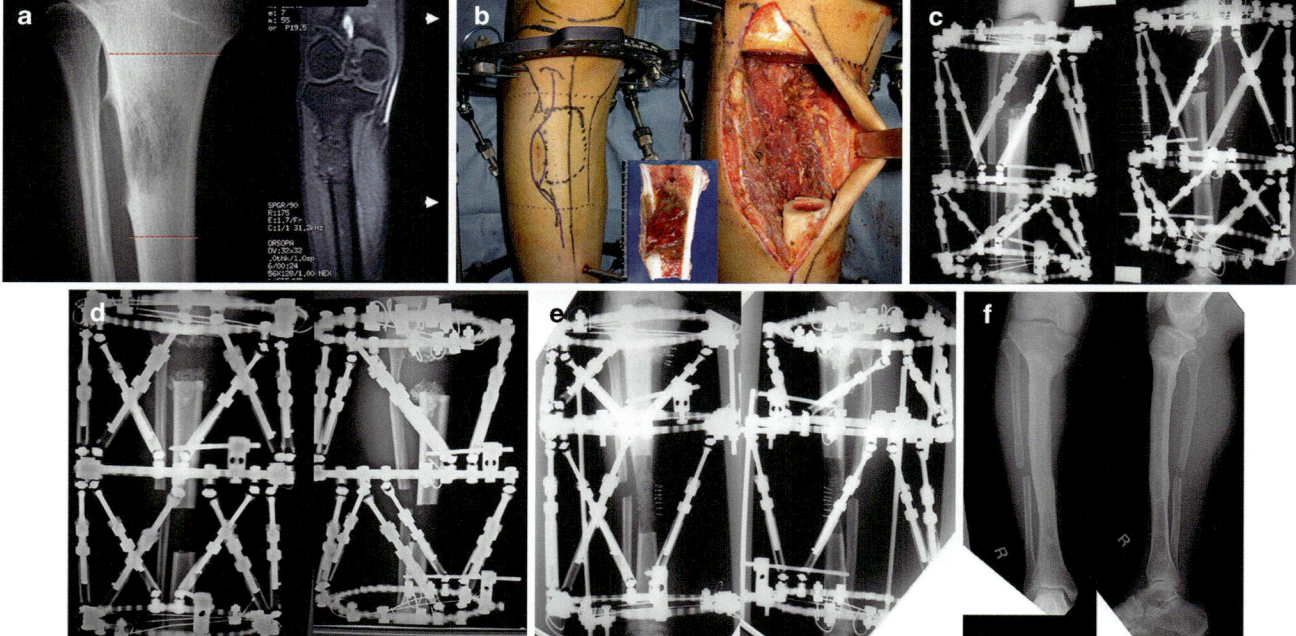

Fig. 28.12 Case (Type I: DO method). A 17-year-old boy with an osteosarcoma of the proximal tibia. (**a**) Preoperative X-ray and MRI scan. Osteotomy line (*broken lines*). (**b**) After tumor resection with intercalary osteotomies. (**c**) X-ray after the operation. (**d**) X-ray during bone transport. (**e**) X-ray at the complication of docking of bone transporter. (**f**) X-ray at 26 months after the operation

infection managed with antibiotics or removal of pins, docking-site nonunion or delayed union, and delayed consolidation of regenerated tissue treated with bone graft. Complications with the LN method are late infection and nonunion of frozen bone, which are managed with bone graft combined with rigid fixation. There are two important points in obtaining better functional results when either method is selected: firstly, the surgeon should try to preserve the epiphysis if possible; and secondly, it should be attempted to perform biological reconstruction as much as possible.

In future, there may be greater use of biological reconstruction methods to obtain better and earlier functional results, because a natural limb is the best option. To achieve this, we have to aim to facilitate bone regeneration and revitalization much faster, and to adopt biological soft-tissue reconstruction, through advances in tissue engineering, such as with regard to osteogenic and angiogenic growth factors, or with stem cell implantation.

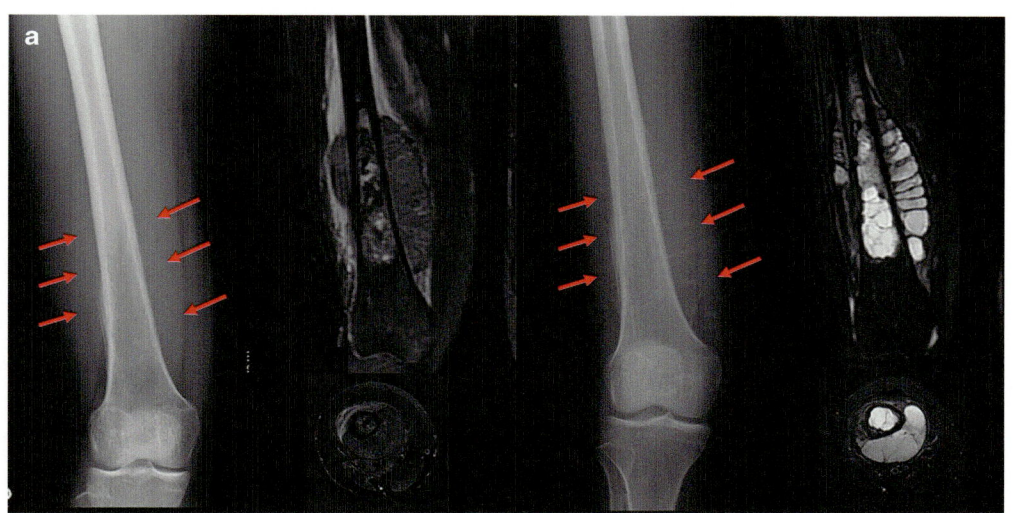

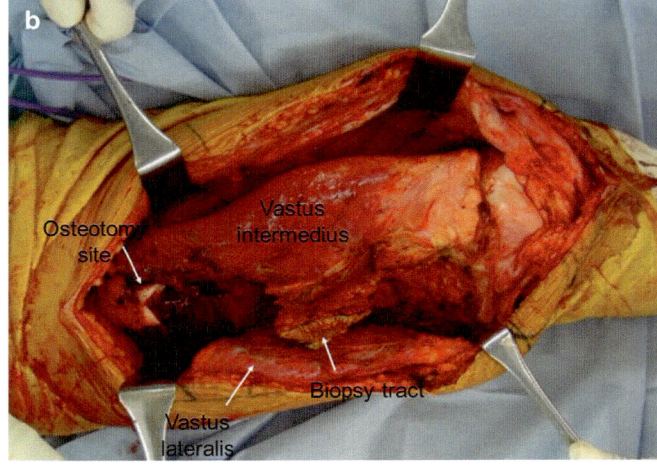

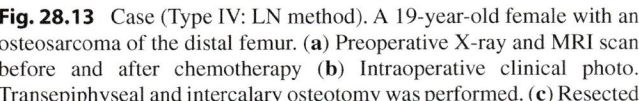

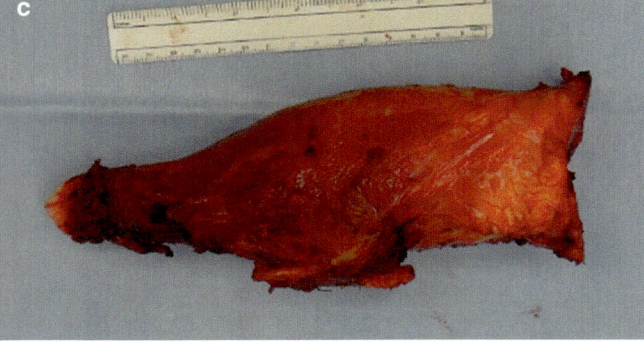

Fig. 28.13 Case (Type IV: LN method). A 19-year-old female with an osteosarcoma of the distal femur. (**a**) Preoperative X-ray and MRI scan before and after chemotherapy (**b**) Intraoperative clinical photo. Transepiphyseal and intercalary osteotomy was performed. (**c**) Resected tumor. (**d**) Freezing in liquid nitrogen. (**e**) After freezing. (**f**) Osteosynthesis with plates and screws. (**g**) Radiograph 82 months after reconstruction. Host-graft junctions achieved complete union

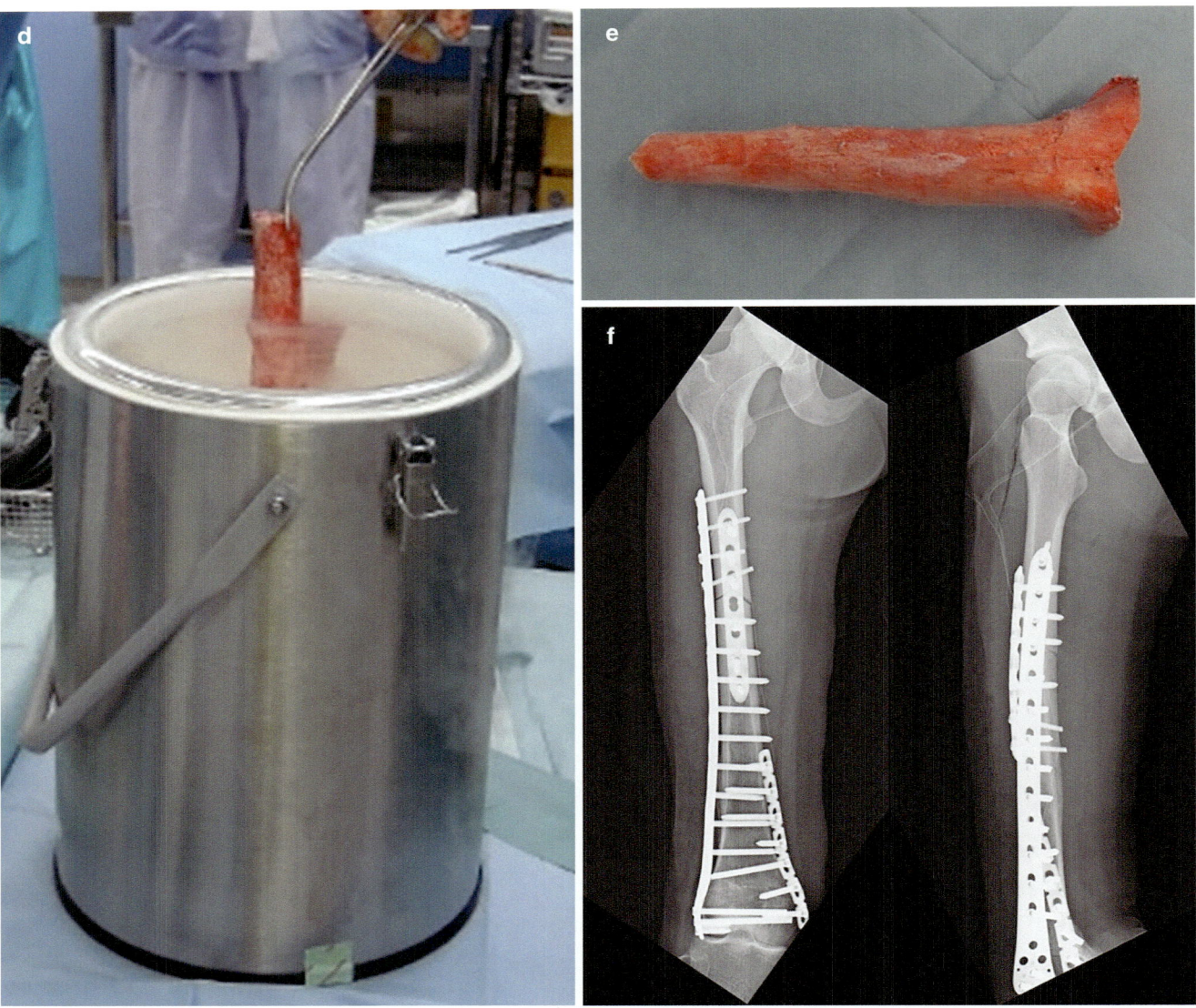

Fig. 28.13 (continued)

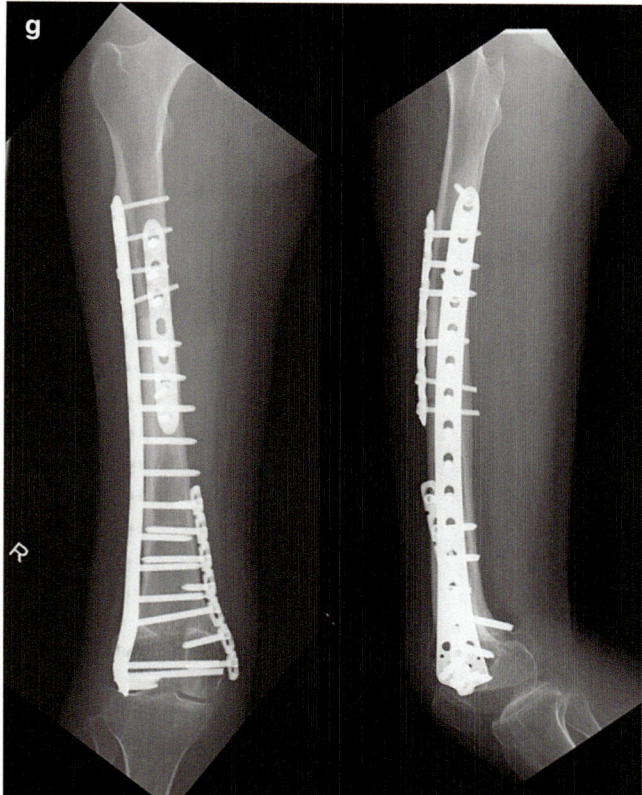

Fig. 28.13 (continued)

Table 28.2 Advantages and disadvantages of the DO method

Advantage	Disadvantage
Living bone regeneration	Lengthy external fixation
Sufficient strength	Patient's burden
Biological affinity	Delayed consolidation
Resistance against infection	Delayed consolidation
Lifelong restored function	Delayed union of docking site

Table 28.3 Advantages and disadvantages of the LN method

Advantage	Disadvantage
Simple procedure	Dead bone reconstruction
Reattachment of soft tissue (tendon and ligament)	Long time to be revitalized
Osteoinduction and osteoconduction	Cartilage degeneration over time
Perfect fit	Delayed union at host-graft junction
Sufficient biomechanical strength	Bone absorption
No contagion	
No harmful denatured protein	

Commentary

Tom Scharschmidt
thomas.scharschmidt@osumc.edu

Limb-salvage surgery for malignant bone tumors around the knee can be accomplished in >90% of cases and is the standard of care if oncologically clear margins can be obtained. These resections often require removal of large portions of bone and surrounding musculature. As such, reconstruction can be challenging but is fundamentally important to maximize the long-term function for these patients.

Traditionally, reconstruction options after limb-salvage include mega-prosthesis, allograft, or biologic autograft. Overall ten-year implant survival of these options is usually reported around 60% at best. Clearly, more durable robust options are needed as oncologic outcomes continue to improve. The authors of this chapter present their two original techniques for consideration as limb salvage options: transepiphyseal osteotomy followed by reconstruction using the distraction osteogenesis technique (DO method) and massive frozen tumor-bearing bone treated with liquid nitrogen (LN method). In addition, a new classification system is presented based on resection level.

The goal of the proposed classification system is to assist in surgical decision making based on the location and extent of the tumor in relation to the growth plate. Involvement of the epiphyseal plate adds an additional degree of challenge to the reconstruction as future growth of the limb needs to be taken in to consideration. The distal femoral growth plate will typically contribute up to 1 cm of growth per year to the patients' overall height, so the younger the child is the more significant this becomes. Consideration for a biologic reconstructive option in this population is attractive from the potential to minimize potential for future growth discrepancies.

Distraction osteogenesis (DO) is gaining popularity in multiple fields of orthopaedic surgery. There has been some hesitancy in oncologic indications due to inherent wound healing challenges in this population. Use of chemotherapy (often indicated in malignant bone tumors) contributes to delayed wound healing. Pin-site infection in the immunocompromised patient is also an area of concern. Despite these concerns, growing literature has demonstrated not only the technical aspects, but also the safety of this procedure in the oncologic setting. The authors nicely illustrate their indications and technique of distraction osteogenesis, adding to the body of support of this method of reconstruction.

The authors next describe their technique for liquid nitrogen freezing combined with either single or double osteotomies. This method of oncologic cryoablation has been published with good results both in terms of local tumor control and reconstruction. Complications including non-union and infection due to the devitalized bone should be anticipated, are similar in prevalence to untoward events following other complex limb-salvage options.

Biologic reconstruction options for juxta-articular malignant tumors around the knee are emerging techniques which can be added to the armamentarium of surgeons when developing treatment plans for these challenging tumors. The benefits of biologic reconstruction include a durable reconstruction and potentially less risk of infection and need for revision surgery. These are advanced surgical techniques and both are associated with potential complications. As such, these complex surgeries should be performed at centers specialized in these procedures.

References

1. Tomita K, Tsuchiya H. Intermediate results and functional evaluation of limb-salvage surgery for osteosarcoma: an intergroup study in Japan. J Surg Oncol. 1989;41(2):71–6.
2. Tsuchiya H, Tomita K. Prognosis of osteosarcoma treated by limb-salvage surgery: the ten-year intergroup study in Japan. Jpn J Clin Oncol. 1992;22(5):347–53.
3. Tsuchiya H, Tomita K, Mori Y, Asada N, Yamamoto N. Marginal excision for osteosarcoma with caffeine assisted chemotherapy. Clin Orthop Relat Res. 1999;358:27–35.
4. Tsuchiya H, Tomita K, Shinokawa Y, Minematsu K, Katsuo S, Taki J. The Ilizarov method in the management of giant-cell tumours of the proximal tibia. J Bone Joint Surg Br. 1996;78(2):264–9.
5. Tsuchiya H, Tomita K, Minematsu K, Mori Y, Asada N, Kitano S, Limb salvage using distraction osteogenesis. A classification of the technique. J Bone Joint Surg Br. 1997;79(3):403–11.
6. Tsuchiya H, Abdel-Wanis M, Kitano S, Sakurakichi K, Yamashiro T, Tomita K. The natural limb is best: joint preservation and reconstruction by distraction osteogenesis for high-grade juxta-articular osteosarcomas. Anticancer Res. 2002;22(4):2373–6.
7. Tsuchiya H, Wan SL, Sakayama K, Yamamoto N, Nishida H, Tomita K. Reconstruction using an autograft containing tumour treated by liquid nitrogen. J Bone Joint Surg Br. 2005;87:218–25.
8. Tsuchiya H, Nishida H, Srisawat P, Shirai T, Hayashi K, Takeuchi A, et al. Pedicle frozen autograft reconstruction in malignant bone tumors. J Orthop Sci. 2010;15(3):340–9.
9. Tsuchiya H, Abdel-Wanis ME, Tomita K. Biological reconstruction after excision of juxta-articular osteosarcoma around the knee: a new classification system. Anticancer Res. 2006;26(1B):447–53.

Part IV
Congenital and Developmental Disorders

Congenital Femoral Deficiency Reconstruction and Lengthening Surgery

Dror Paley and Claire E. Shannon

Introduction

Epidemiology

The often-cited incidence of congenital femoral deficiency (CFD) is 1 in 52,029 based on a review of the Edinburgh Register of the Newborn by Rogala et al. published in 1974 [1]. In retrospect, this may not be accurate, as the incidence is based on the only case identified during the 4.5-year collection period from 1964 to 1968, notably, after thalidomide use was discontinued. This survey is also representative of a relatively homogenous population, of which no information is given regarding race, age, environmental exposure, medication usage, or socioeconomic status of the population. More modern population studies cite the current incidence as 1:50,000 to 1:200,000 [2].

Embryology

Fetal growth and the development of the lower extremities are controlled by a complex cascade of growth factors that are expressed in a particular sequence and at various concentrations during development in order to produce a normal limb. In the process of limb patterning, mesenchymal cells in the limb bud integrate positional information from the three axes (proximal-distal, medial-lateral, and ventral-dorsal) [3–5].

Limb bud development occurs 4–8 weeks after fertilization, and the majority of congenital anomalies occur during this important period of time. The limb begins with the lateral migration of two layers of mesoderm and outgrowth into the overlying ectoderm. Cells from the underlying somitic mesoderm ultimately form the muscle tissue of the limb, while cells from the lateral plate mesoderm form cartilage and bones. Distinct but coordinated molecular pathways primarily control each axis. In the process of limb patterning, mesenchymal cells in the limb bud integrate positional information from the three axes, indicating a complex interplay of the responsible factors [5–7].

Development of the proximal-distal axis is at least partially controlled by fibroblast growth factors (FGF) secreted by the apical ectodermal ridge (AER) [6]. The AER is a thickened layer of the ectoderm that forms over the distal edge of the limb bud. FGF secreted by the AER stimulates proximal-distal growth of the limb via differentiation of the underlying mesoderm. As part of a complex positive feedback loop, the signal to produce FGF is supplied by the underlying mesoderm. The AER signaling center is responsible for the differentiation of the underlying mesoderm and the development of the limb in the proximal-to-distal direction. Removal of the AER results in the arrest of limb outgrowth. Furthermore, ectopic implantation of the AER results in the formation of an extra limb. The AER also contributes to interdigital necrosis, allowing separation of the initially webbed hand [8]. Defects in the AER lead to anomalies such as limb truncation, transverse deficiencies, and syndactyly [9]. The genetics of the apical ectodermal ridge have been further elucidated as a complex interplay of related genes. Five paralogous gene families, named Hox 9 through Hox 13, from Hox A and Hox D gene groups, come together co-linearly (HoxA-9 to HoxA-13 and HoxD-9 to HoxD-13) and play important roles in the mesoderm.

The development in the anteroposterior axis is patterned by the secretion of sonic hedgehog (SHH) from the zone of polarizing activity (ZPA), a collection of cells along the posterior aspect of the limb bud. Transplantation of the ZPA from the posterior aspect to the anterior aspect of the limb bud causes the creation of a mirrored duplication of the ulnar aspect of the hand. In addition to its primary role in the development of the anterior-posterior axis, the ZPA also contributes to the maintenance of proximal-to-distal limb development and participates in the feedback loop of the AER [6]. Mutations in Indian hedgehog, SHH, and PITX1 in humans

D. Paley (✉) · C. E. Shannon
Paley Orthopedic and Spine Institute, West Palm Beach, FL, USA
e-mail: dpaley@paleyinstitute.org; cshannon@paleyinstitute.org

have been implicated in lower extremity polydactyly, while mice studies have shown an interaction between the expression of each factor [3, 10].

The development in the dorsal-ventral axis is regulated by the Wingless-type (Wnt) signaling pathway within the dorsal ectoderm [4]. The Wnt pathway induces the underlying mesoderm to develop dorsal characteristics and is blocked in the ventral ectoderm, allowing the development of ventral characteristics. In mice, inactivation of the Wnt signaling pathway results in the development of biventral limbs. The Wnt pathway also contributes to the regulation of SHH, reflecting the complex interaction and coordination among the three-dimensional pathways responsible for limb development [6, 8].

It is unlikely that CFD is caused solely by a defect in the overall function of the AER, as the distal portion of an extremity affected by CFD is often normal. It is more likely that the defect is in the underlying mesodermal layer, within the complex interplay of developmental proteins at a point more downstream in the differentiation of the limb.

Pathophysiology and Genetics

A single underlying genetic cause for CFD has not been elucidated. In treating more than 1000 patients with unilateral CFD, the senior author (DP) has had only one patient who had a parent with unilateral CFD. In contrast, in a smaller group of multi-limb congenital deficiencies, including cases of bilateral CFD, it was more common to find a history of a first- or second-degree relative with a congenital limb anomaly. Several authors have postulated a genetic cause given the presence of the condition at birth, the association with other abnormalities that have known genetic conditions, occasional bilateral involvement, and reports of familial cases. These are all supporting evidence for an underlying inheritable genetic defect with incomplete penetration or an autosomal recessive pattern of inheritance [11–13]. It should be noted that phenotype has been used to diagnose and classify patients with CFD, despite varied clinical and radiographic presentations. As genetic and molecular understanding of the disease progresses, it is likely that grouping all patients into a single diagnosis of CFD will not be sufficient. Some of the reported abnormalities associated with CFD are fibular hemimelia, femoral-fibular-ulnar complex, patella aplasia/hypoplasia, absence of the fourth or fifth ray, unusual facies, Pierre-Robin sequence, and syndactyly of the toes. Considering the other congenital conditions that present in select individuals with CFD, the underlying pathophysiology and, therefore, genetic causes are likely to be distinct in this group of patients. In other words, one must be careful to assume that all patients *diagnosed* by today's criteria with "CFD" will have the same underlying causality.

An inheritable genetic defect or susceptibility to other risk factors or exposures at a particular stage in the lower extremity development of the fetus would commonly present with bilateral involvement; however, bilateral involvement is rare and associated with other known genetic defects, such as Pierre-Robin sequence. The Pierre-Robin sequence is primarily an anatomical defect of mandibular outgrowth that impacts on oropharyngeal volume and patency of the palate. No single genetic abnormality has been identified in Pierre-Robin, though recent evidence shows that Sox9 may be a crucial step in the pathway [14]. Similarly, it is likely that a variety of inheritable genetic defects are responsible for a common resultant phenotype with similar but varied congenital abnormalities. Conversely, a recent report of a child with Pierre-Robin and bilateral CFD found that the array's comparative genomic hybridization analysis showed no abnormalities at 1543 loci while whole-exon analysis identified no mutations suspected to be causative for the patient's condition [15].

A subset of bone morphogenetic proteins (BMPs), known as growth/differentiation factors (GDFs), affect several skeletal processes, including endochondral ossification, synovial joint formation, and tendon and ligament repair. Studies in mice have suggested that GDF-5 deficiency affects the composition and material properties of cortical bone tissue in the femur, but the detailed mechanisms by which this occurs remain to be determined [6]. Boden et al demonstrated severely disordered development of the proximal femoral physis in a 21-week fetus with CFD [16]. The cartilaginous anlage appeared normal; however, the histopathology demonstrated failure of the physis to migrate proximal, as well as a lack of normal cellular organization. This inability of the physis to gain proper organization inhibits the endochondral ossification of the cartilaginous femoral neck, resulting in the inability to convert the cartilage to bone. The degree of disorganization probably correlates with the delay in ossification of the femoral neck that we observe in Paley type 1b cases. The secondary ossification center of the femoral head normally appears between 4 and 6 months after birth [17]. In other pediatric orthopedic conditions with delayed ossification, such as hip dysplasia, ossification of the femoral head is delayed. With restoration of hip stability and loading, ossification catches up. It is a reasonable assumption then that restoration of normal anatomy and biomechanics in type 1b CFD would lead to ossification of the femoral neck and subtrochanteric region.

Other investigators have supported a teratogenic cause for CFD as the phenotype is similar to the effects of thalidomide exposure in utero [18]. These effects imply that at a particular stage in fetal growth an exposure in utero occurs causing a downstream effect on the remaining growth of the affected lower extremity. The exact stage in development at which the abnormality occurs could determine the severity of involvement. While a teratogenic exposure is possible as the underlying cause, the explanation would have to involve a teratogen with transient effect only at the time of exposure given the embryological pathway of the limb. Thus, fetuses exposed to the teratogenic agent at only the time of proximal femur formation might have only mild CFD, while those fetuses with more severe involvement might have undergone more persistent exposure to the teratogenic agent.

Endogenous retinoids, including vitamin A and retinoid acid (the active form of vitamin A), have long been implicated in limb development and abnormalities [7–9]. Embryological studies of quail, rats, and mice demonstrate a role for retinoic acid in the organization of the dorsoventral axis [9, 19]. These results suggest that a combination of maternal vitamin A supplementation and excess vitamin A in the neonatal period could potentially be unfavorable for cartilage development. It can be speculated that neonatal vitamin A supplementation may be beneficial for bone only if the mother's vitamin A status is low.

In summary, the embryologic and genetic data point toward a somatic mutation disorder of cells within the developing limb bud as opposed to a germ cell mutation (hereditary, familial) disorder for unilateral CFD. In contrast, multi-limb cases may be related to a germ cell mutation.

Deformity and Pathoanatomy

Osseous Deformities

CFD was initially grouped with cases of congenital coxa vara, as this is the most obvious deformity in the majority of cases [20]. Cases were often separated into congenital short femur, in mild presentations, and proximal femoral focal deficiency (PFFD), for more severe cases. Recognition that these were a spectrum of pathology of the same congenital deficiency leads to a consensus name change to CFD [21]. Although the femoral deformity and deficiency are the most obvious, non-femoral structures are also involved. These include the acetabulum, musculature, vessels, ligaments of the knee, tibia, fibula, and foot. In utero ultrasounds have shown both a shortened femur and a shallow acetabulum [22]. As with other pediatric proximal femur pathologies, dysplasia of the acetabulum whether initially present or not is progressive [23].

Delayed ossification has long been noted in patients with CFD. Sanperra and Sparks discussed this finding and its effect on classifying patients with CFD using the more traditional methods. As the patients got older, many of them had ossification of the previously cartilaginous femoral neck [24]. The disordered development of the physis results in the delayed ossification of the femoral neck [16], which can occur in varying degrees of severity. The variation in cellular structure and therefore time to ossification likely contribute to the varying degrees of deformity seen in CFD type 1.

Paley et al. reported on a series of 106 SUPERhip procedures performed on patients with delayed ossification of the proximal femur (Paley type 1b2 and 1b3). BMP2 (Infuse, Medtronic, Memphis, TN) was used to induce ossification of the cartilaginous femoral neck in 38/106 femurs. This reduced the rate of persistent delay in ossification from 41% in the non-BMP2 group to 13% in the BMP2 group [25] (p2).

The deformities of the femur vary from coxa valga in very mild cases to a very severe greater than 90° multiplanar complex angular deformity wrongly described as coxa vara in more involved cases (Fig. 29.1a–d). There is a varus, flexion, and retroversion deformity of the upper femur. The distal femur demonstrates a valgus deformity, often referred to as a hypoplastic lateral femoral condyle since the distance from the physis to the knee joint line is smaller laterally than medially. In other words, there is a greater valgus convergence between the joint line and the distal femoral physis. The deformity of the proximal femur will be discussed in greater detail in a later section.

The bony morphology of the pelvis is also affected in children with CFD. Musielak et al. demonstrated that the affected side has a smaller acetabulum with decreased anteversion and inclination compared to the unaffected side of the body, as well as a less upright ilium and more laterally curved ischium, imparting a rotated appearance to the pelvis [26]. The more severe the type of CFD, the greater the differences in shape between the sides of the body [26].

The ratio of growth in length of the short limb compared to the long limb remains relatively unchanged throughout growth [27–29]. This enables the final discrepancy in leg length to be predicted from the initial radiographs [30] This pattern of increasing leg length discrepancy (LLD) is referred to as Shapiro type 1 [31]. On this basis, the Paley multiplier method is able to accurately calculate the predicted LLD at skeletal maturity [32, 33].

Ligamentous Structures

Anterior-posterior instability of the knee is common in CFD, but the severity is variable. Modern era studies utilizing MRI and arthroscopy have evaluated the ligamentous structures at the knee in patients with various degrees of CFD [34–36]. The results support the conclusion that like the hip, the distal femur and proximal tibia require interaction of both bony and soft tissues to develop normally.

Manner et al. [34] performed a radiographic study of 34 knees associated with CFD with radiographs and MRI. The anterior cruciate ligament (ACL) was affected in all knees studied, with 15% hypoplastic and 85% absent. The PCL was hypoplastic in 21% and absent in 24%. The most common type (14 knees, 41%) was aplasia of the ACL and a normal PCL. The cruciate ligament dysplasia was differenti-

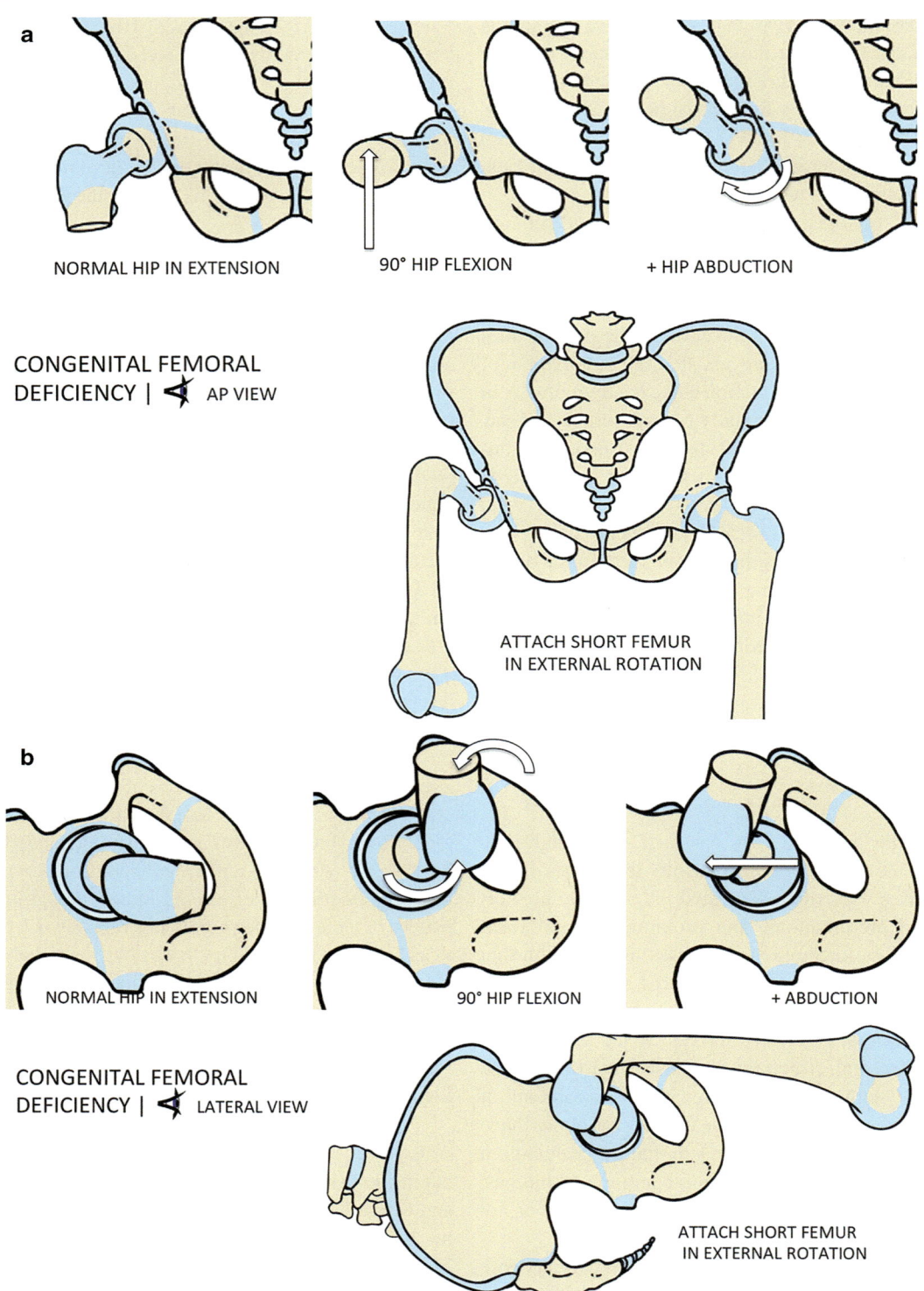

Fig. 29.1 Anteroposterior (**a**), lateral (**b**), and inferior (**c**) views of pelvis and hip joints. These illustrations serve to simulate and recreate the proximal femoral deformity seen with severe CFD on the right hip. The model is based on a normal proximal femur with a 130° neck-shaft angle. First, flex the proximal femur 90° relative to the pelvis. Next, abduct the flexed proximal femur 45° relative to the pelvis. Now, reconnect the distal femur to the proximal femur. The distal femur should be placed in 45° of external rotation relative to the pelvis. The resulting deformity is the CFD femur deformity typically seen in most type 1b and some type 1a cases. Note that the femoral neck appears to be retroverted due to the 90° hip flexion of a 130° neck-shaft angle femur. Just the flexion makes it appear to have 50° of retroversion. Since the distal femur is fixed to the proximal femur in external rotation, this retroversion is increased even more. Also, note that the varus deformity is caused by the abduction of the proximal femur with the hip flexed. The hip flexion places the greater trochanter facing posteriorly. The proximity of the greater trochanter to the ilium and to the sacrum in this position explains why the gluteus medius and minimus and piriformis muscles are short. (**d**) The deformity is seen from AP, lateral, and 45° oblique views (Copyright: The Paley Foundation. Reproduced with permission. All rights reserved.)

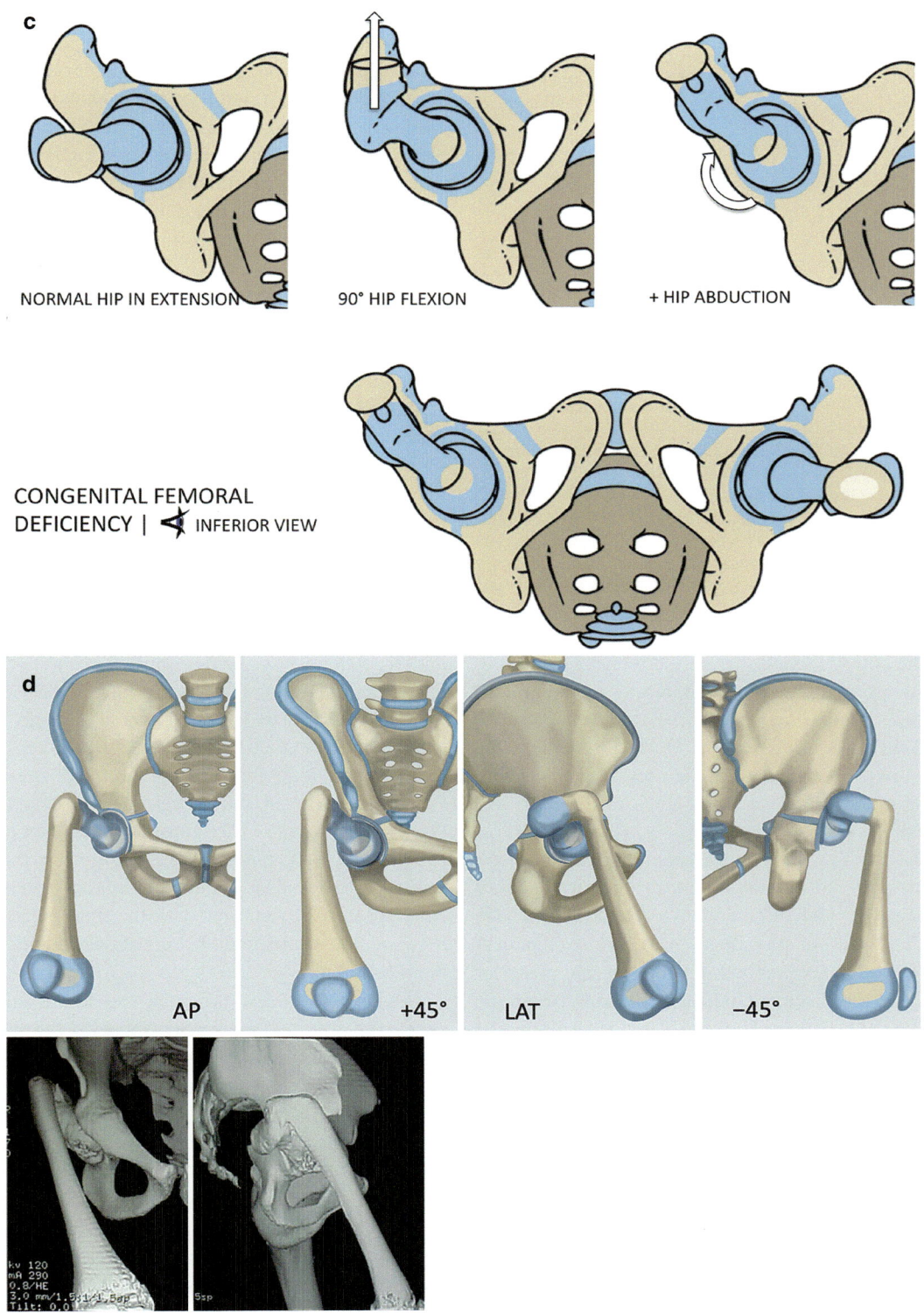

Fig. 29.1 (continued)

ated into three groups (Fig. 29.2). Type I had a hypoplastic or absent ACL and a normal PCL. The intercondylar notch width and height were decreased compared to the normal side, and the lateral tibial spine was hypoplastic. Type II knees had aplasia of the ACL and hypoplasia of the PCL. They had even narrower and shorter intercondylar notches, and both tibial spines were hypoplastic. Type III knees had aplasia of both cruciate ligaments. The intercondylar notch was absent and covered with hyaline cartilage, and both tibial spines were aplastic. The distal femoral joint surface is concave, matching the convex tibial plateau like a ball and socket. Three of these cases had discoid meniscus.

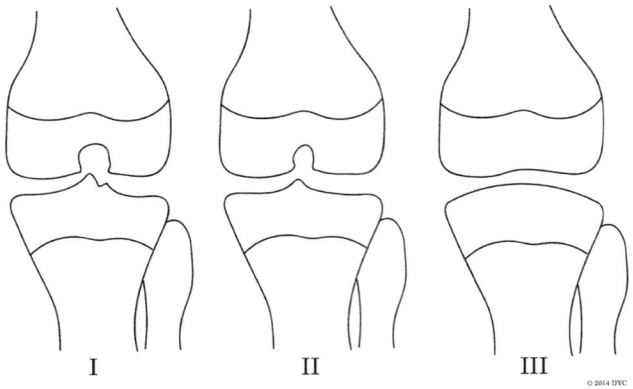

Fig. 29.2 Knee classification of intercondylar notch: (i) Type I: The intercondylar notch width and height are decreased compared to the normal side. The lateral tibial spine is hypoplastic. This corresponds to a hypoplastic or absent ACL and a normal PCL. (ii) Type II: Narrower and shorter intercondylar notch with hypoplasia of both tibial spines. This corresponds to aplasia of the ACL and hypoplasia of the PCL. (iii) Type III: The intercondylar notch is absent and covered with hyaline cartilage, and both tibial spines are aplastic. The distal femoral joint surface is concave, matching the convex tibial plateau. This corresponds to aplasia of both cruciate ligaments (Copyright: The Paley Foundation. Reproduced with permission. All rights reserved.)

Overall, the authors found that on the tunnel-view radiographs, narrowing or absence of the femoral notch and flattening of tibial eminences corresponded to a hypoplasia or deficiency of the cruciate ligaments. Thus, the shape of the distal femur and proximal tibia can be used to predict, with relative accuracy, the presence or absence of the ACL and PCL ligaments.

These radiographic studies have been validated with the use of arthroscopy to directly confirm the presence or absence of the ACL and PCL. Johansson and Aparisi [35] published a case series of six patients with cruciate ligament dysplasia. Three patients had both an anterior and posterior drawer sign, and arthroscopy confirmed aplasia of both the ACL and PCL. Three patients had an isolated anterior drawer and had ACL aplasia on arthroscopic examination. All knees were found to have hypoplastic tibial spines on radiographs.

Chomiak [36] looked at a larger series of 21 patients with clinical and arthroscopic examinations. All patients were found to have an anterior drawer sign, and nine patients (43%) had a posterior drawer sign. Four patients (19%) had medial instability, including one patient who also had lateral instability. The instrumented and clinic drawer tests were not found to be reliable enough, leading the authors to recommend imaging of the cruciate ligaments prior to lengthening to avoid knee dislocation. The majority of patients (38%) were found to be completely deficient in both the ACL and PCL. The ACL was completely deficient in 16 (71%) and hypoplastic in 3 (14%) patients. The PCL was completely deficient in 10 (48%) and hypoplastic in 3 (14%) patients. Only one patient had an intact ACL and PCL.

In the majority of patients, both menisci were intact, with only three (14%) being hypoplastic and unrelated to the cruciate ligaments. Changes in the intercondylar notch and tibial eminences were noted in some patients, but it was not specifically studied, as the authors felt that they were not as appreciable in patients under 6 years of age. They did note that the femoral intercondylar notch developed in some patients who had aplasia of both cruciate ligaments.

Muscle Pathoanatomy

Despite the wide spectrum of CFD, the underlying muscular anatomical differences appear relatively consistent. Pirani et al. used MRI to quantitatively assess musculature in patients with Aitken types A through D. The muscles were all present but altered in their size, structure, and location [37]. The majority of muscles were found to be smaller: gluteus maximus, gluteus medius, gluteus minimus, quadriceps, adductor magnus, adductor longus, adductor brevis, pectineus, semimembranosus, semitendinosus, and biceps femoris. The exception is the sartorius muscle that was found to be hypertrophied, which was attributed as the underlying cause of the deformities of the proximal femur, given the orientation of the sartorius [37, 38]. The obturator externus was found to be elongated and the muscle belly extended almost entirely to its insertion. The short external rotators had a larger cross-sectional diameter and were found to insert on the posteromedial greater trochanter. Overall, the course of the muscles was more perpendicular and proximal than normal, inserting onto the proximally migrated femur. The gluteus medius and gluteus minimus were found to be shorter than the unaffected side and lie between the ilium and the proximal femur, which abuts them from below.

We have also found this to be true in our surgical experience: The musculature is present with the muscle bellies extending nearly to their insertion with very short or absent tendons, and the course of the muscles is proximal. Panting and Williams had previously noted similar findings, including the hypertrophied sartorius muscle, the relatively normal gluteal muscles, and a hypoplastic quadriceps muscle [38]. Biko et al. also used MRI in seven patients to primarily evaluate the osseous structures and reported a qualitative decrease in the size of the musculature in general. At the level of the triradiate cartilage, the cross-sectional size of the gluteus muscles was significantly smaller in comparison to the uninvolved contralateral limb [39].

Pirani et al. postulated that the muscles became the primary stabilizers of the deformed hip joint, since the osseous structures did not impart inherent stability [37]. This is inconsistent with the authors' experience. Even in the complete absence of the femoral head and neck, the very thick fibrous femoral neck anlage gives ample static stability preventing proximal femoral migration. It is more likely that the muscular attachments at the upper femur act in conjunction with the fibrous anlage to transfer weight across the hip joint, acting like the rotator cuff of the shoulder to counter the proximal migration of the upper femur.

Vascular Pathoanatomy

The normal embryological development of the arteries of the lower extremity parallels the formation of limb buds, occurring between the 4th and 8th weeks of gestation. The limb begins with a single axial dorsal artery that continues as the ischiadic artery and onto the popliteal artery. The external iliac artery arises at 5 weeks of gestation and bifurcates into the inferior epigastric artery and the femoral artery, which then bifurcates at 6 weeks of gestation into lateral and medial branches. The medial branch becomes the deep femoral artery (profunda femoris) and gives rise to the medial and lateral circumflex arteries and connects to the ischiadic artery, while the lateral branch develops into the superficial femoral artery. By 7.5 weeks, the superficial femoral artery caliber is larger than the ischiadic artery and becomes the major blood supply to the popliteal artery and leg. After full development, the dorsal axial artery remains as the inferior gluteal artery while the ischiadic artery remains as the arteria comitans nervi ischiadici, running as the vasa vasorum of the sciatic nerve [40].

The vascular anatomy is often abnormal in an extremity affected by CFD. Chomiak et al. reported the results of 21 patients with various degrees of CFD studied with computed tomography (CT) angiograms to identify vascular abnormalities [41]. They reported that more severe cases of CFD had a smaller diameter and a shorter length of the superficial femoral artery; however, the severity of osseous abnormalities did not directly correlate with the topographical vascular anatomy abnormalities. All patients, at the least, had differences compared to the contralateral unaffected extremity: mainly with smaller vessel caliber, decreased number of vessels to the thigh, and more proximal bifurcation of the external iliac into superficial and deep femoral arteries. Despite this, 19 of the 21 patients had the blood supply to the femur and pseudoarthrosis from branches of the deep femoral artery, which originated from the external iliac artery. Notably, Chomiak found 2 of the 21 patients with a persistent ischiadic artery as the dominant vascular supply to the leg and a diminutive superficial femoral artery that supplied solely the medial thigh [41]. This is an extremely unusual finding in otherwise normal humans, but is seen in other mammals [42]. Fuller et al noted the presence of a dominant ischiadic artery and absent superficial femoral artery in 1/19 (5.3%) of severe CFD (mostly Paley type 3) cases undergoing rotationplasty [43]. It is critical to identify these vascular anomalies preoperatively, especially when reconstruction using rotationplasty is considered. An MR angiogram (MRA) is indicated, especially prior to rotationplasty.

> **Box 29.1 CFD Pathology**
> - The incidence of CFD is approximately 1 in 50,000–200,000.
> - Limb bud formation is affected by a complex interplay of signaling, including AER, ZPA, and Wnt.
> - CFD is likely caused by a somatic mutation during the development of the limb bud, but some cases may be caused by an inherited germ cell mutation.
> - CFD often presents with proximal coxa vara, flexion and retroversion, and distal femoral valgus.
> - Cruciate ligament deficiency is common and can often be identified on radiographs.
> - Generally, most muscles around the pelvis are present and hypoplastic, though the sartorius may be hypertrophied.
> - An ischiadic artery may be present and more dominant than the femoral artery in very severe cases of CFD.

Evaluating the Child with CFD

History

Most children born with unilateral CFD have no family history of this or other congenital anomalies. Nevertheless, inquiry should be made into family history, exposure to drugs, medications, radiation, or infectious diseases during the first trimester. Many cases of CFD are now identified with prenatal ultrasound early in the pregnancy by measuring the lengths of the two femurs. In such cases, the predicted leg length discrepancy at birth and maturity can be calculated using the multiplier method [44].

Physical Exam

There is an obvious leg length discrepancy. Associated fibular hemimelia (FH) may be present. The hips, knees, and ankles should be examined for range of motion and flexion contractures. Neonates and young infants normally have such contractures for the first 3–6 months. At the hip, patients may have external rotation and fixed flexion deformity (FFD), as well as limited abduction due to the proximal femoral deformity. At the knee, patients may have flexion contractures, hypoplastic patella with possible lateral subluxation or dislocation of the patella, and AP or rotary instability of the knee.

Muscle length tests should be recorded to identify preexisting potential contractures that could affect lengthening. These tests include the Ely test for rectus femoris length (Fig. 29.3a), popliteal angle measurement for hamstring tightness (Fig. 29.3b), and Ober sign for fascia lata-iliotibial band contracture (Fig. 29.3c).

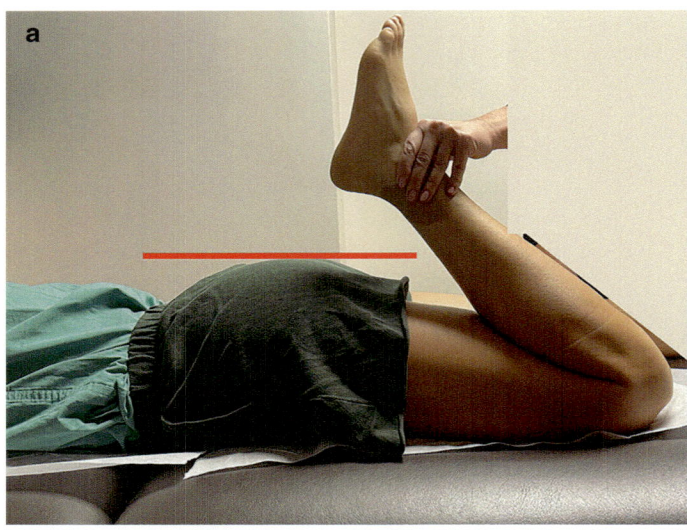
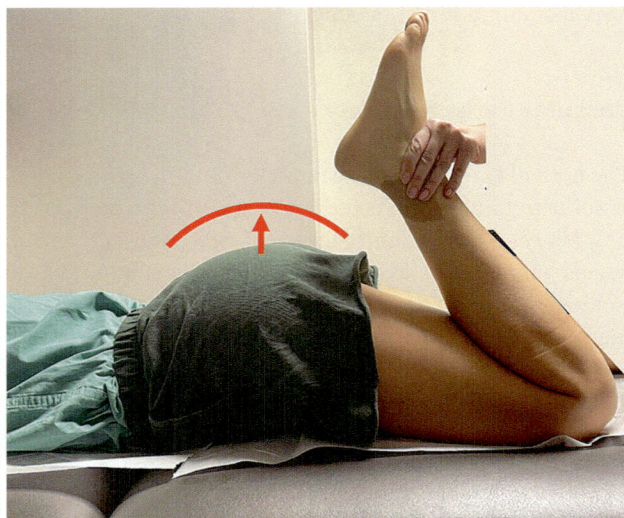
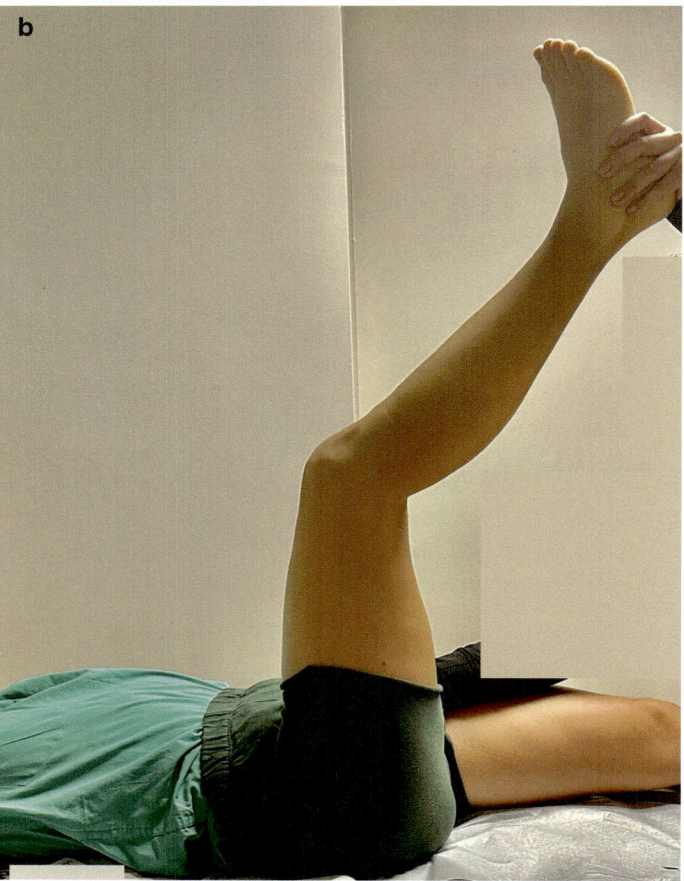

Fig. 29.3 Muscle length testing: (**a**) The Ely test checks for rectus femoris tightness, demonstrating pelvic flexion with prone knee bend if positive. Note the change in the pelvic position on the right, compared to the neutral pelvis on the left. (**b**) The popliteal angle is the angle between the vertical and the line of the tibia with the hip at 90° flexion and the knee maximally extended; (**c**) the Ober test checks for fascia lata tightness; a positive sign is the thigh going into an abduction position when the hip is hyperextended and the knee flexed to 90° (Copyright: The Paley Foundation. Reproduced with permission. All rights reserved.)

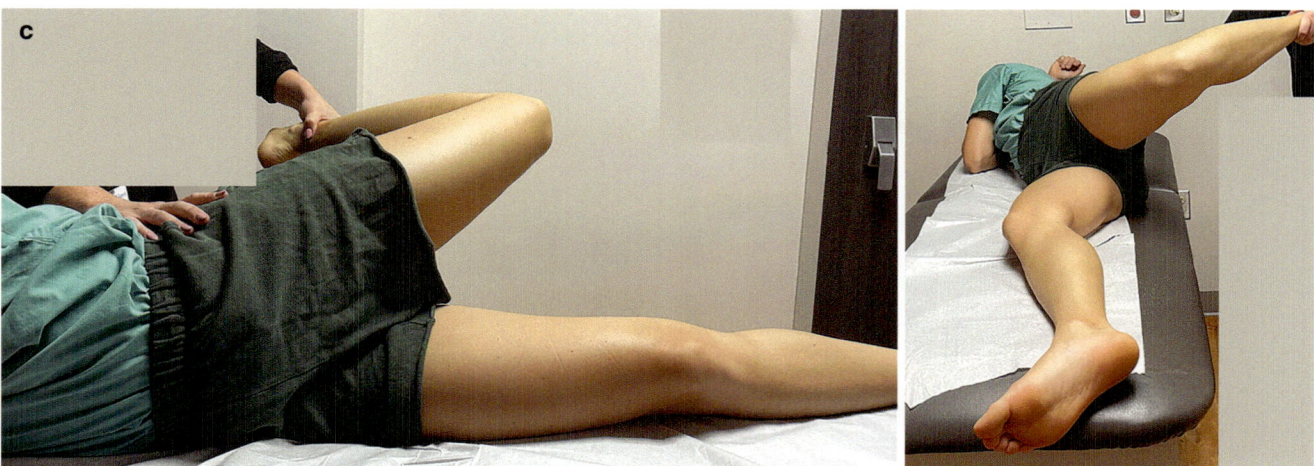

Fig. 29.3 (continued)

Box 29.2 Physical Examination Findings in Patients with CFD
- Hip: External rotation (ER) deformity or increased ER versus internal rotation (IR); fixed flexion deformity (FFD) of hip; and limitation of abduction.
- Knee: Fixed flexion deformity (FFD) of knee; no limitation of knee flexion; hypoplastic patella; lateral tracking, subluxation, or dislocation of patella; anteroposterior instability of knee; rotary instability of knee; anterior dislocation of tibia on femur with knee extension followed by reduction of knee with attempted flexion; hypermobile meniscal clunks; and temporary locking of the knee during flexion.
- Ankle: Limitations of ankle dorsiflexion; obligatory eversion and hindfoot valgus with dorsiflexion; hypermobility of ankle with increased eversion; and hypoplastic lateral malleolus at the level of the medial malleolus.

Imaging

Radiographic Examination

Radiographs should include a full-length anteroposterior (AP) standing legs with the patellae pointing forward (Fig. 29.4a, b). In children who are unable to stand, a pull-down X-ray may be performed (Fig. 29.4c). This allows measurement of the length of the femurs and tibia, though it does not include foot height. Long lateral leg radiographs in maximum extension allow for the evaluation of knee flexion contractures and more accurate length measurement (Fig. 29.4d). A supine AP pelvis allows more accurate measurement of hip coverage (can measure center-edge angle (CEA) of both hips, acetabular index, femoral head extrusion index, etc.). The AP pelvis radiograph is also useful to assess the ossification and deformity of the entire proximal femur (Fig. 29.4e). It is important that the pelvis be level for more accurate measurement.

Magnetic Resonance Imaging

Magnetic resonance imaging (MRI) is useful to assess the integrity of the proximal femur. It can help determine whether the femoral head is joined to the shaft of the femur via a cartilaginous femoral neck. In case of an absent femoral neck, the MRI can help determine if the cartilage of the femoral head is fused to the acetabular cartilage. This is best seen in the axial cuts since the fusion is usually between the ischium and the femoral head, distal to the triradiate cartilage (Fig. 29.5a). When severe proximal femoral deformity is present the sagittal cuts demonstrate the maximum deformity plane best (Fig. 29.5b). For more optimal imaging, the cuts of the proximal femur should be reformatted in an oblique plane to see the entire proximal femur as a single image. MRI can also help outline the intra-articular pathology of the knee, identifying deficiency of the cruciate ligaments and outlining the shape of the joint surfaces in the frontal and sagittal plane.

Computerized Tomography (CT)

CT is only useful at an older age (age 6 and older) when the acetabulum and proximal femur are more ossified. Three-dimensional (3D) CT reconstruction is useful to compare the normal acetabulum with the dysplastic side. In older children, 3D CT can nicely show the three-dimensional deformity of the proximal femur. 3D CT is also very useful for assessment of the orientation of the acetabulum which is usually hypoplastic and retroverted [26] (Fig. 29.6).

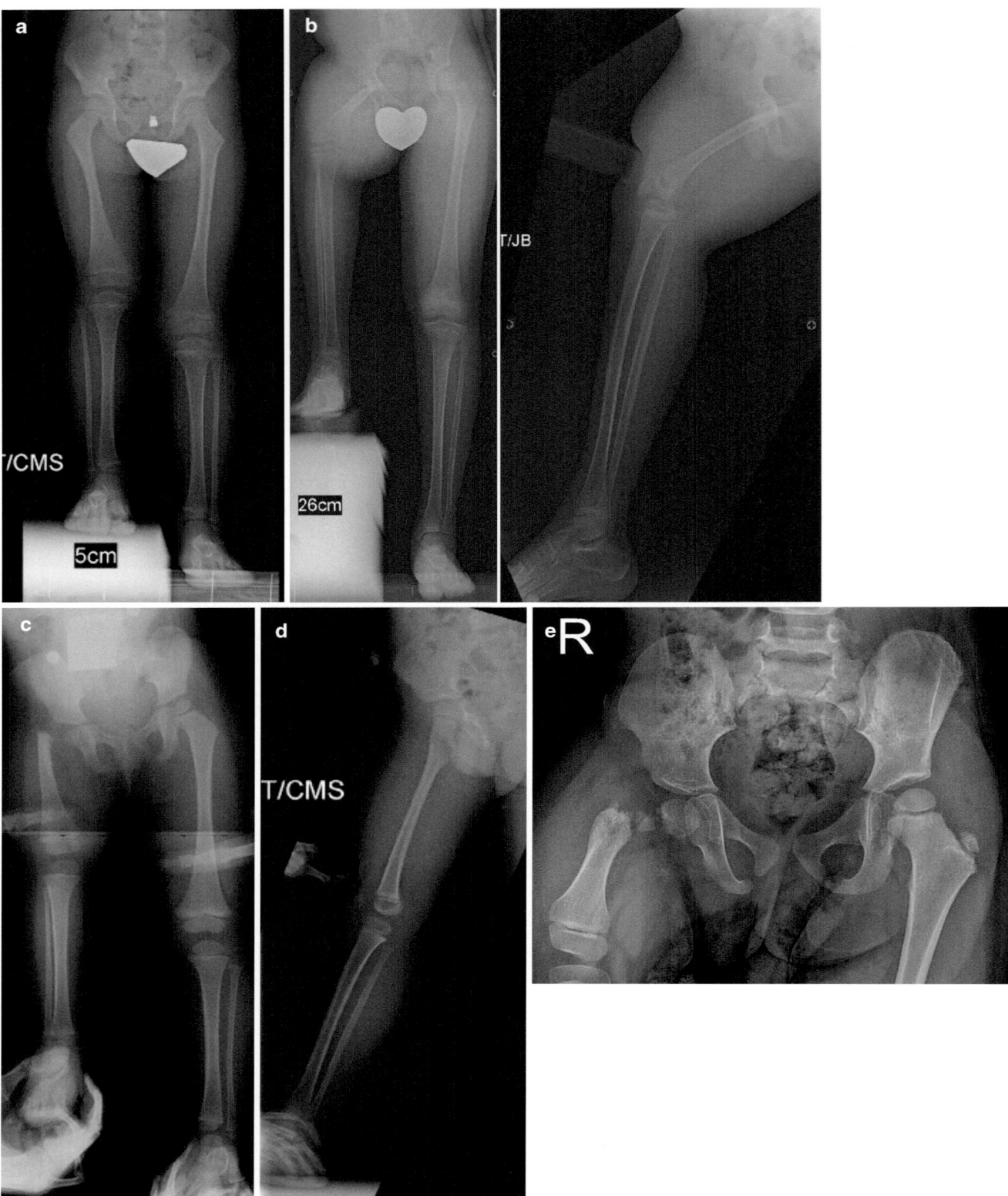

Fig. 29.4 (a) Erect leg AP radiograph (EL) of a child with Type 1a CFD. The patellae are pointed forward and a lift of known amount is placed under the short leg to level the pelvis. (b) EL radiograph in a child with type 3a CFD standing on lift, with knee maximally extended (left) and long lateral showing knee flexion deformity with knee maximally extended (right). (c) AP pull-down X-ray of a child with type 1b CFD. The foot height is not accounted for when measuring leg length difference. (d) Long lateral X-ray of patient in (a) with the knee in maximal extension, evidenced by the hand pushing back on the femur. (e) AP pelvis radiograph of a child with type 1b CFD taken supine to allow the pelvis to lie level (Copyright: The Paley Foundation. Reproduced with permission. All rights reserved.)

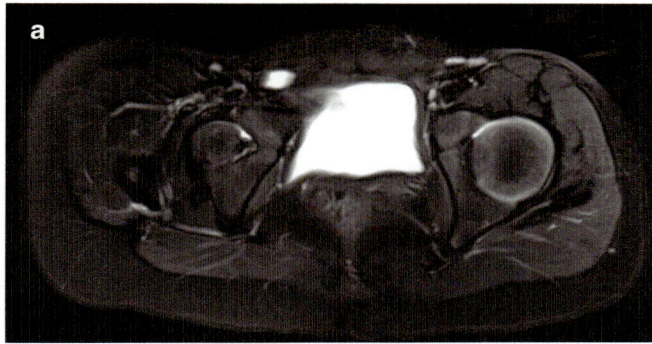
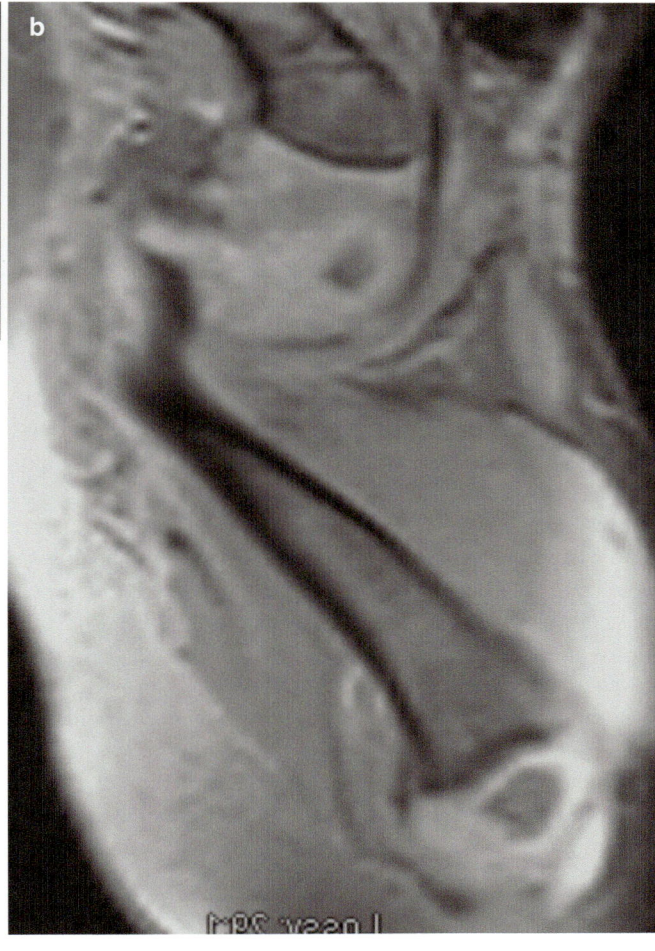

Fig. 29.5 (**a**) Axial MRI of a child with type 2b CFD showing a posterior fusion of the femoral head to the ischium. (**b**) Sagittal MRI of a patient with type 1b2 CFD demonstrating the cartilaginous femoral neck and deformity of the proximal femur (Copyright: The Paley Foundation. Reproduced with permission. All rights reserved.)

Fig. 29.6 3D CT of a 13-year-old boy with CFD type 1b1 (Copyright: The Paley Foundation. Reproduced with permission. All rights reserved.)

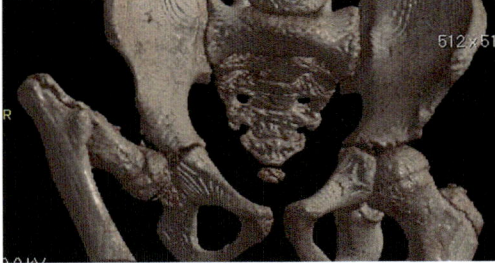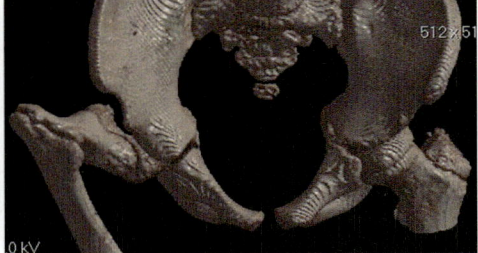

Box 29.3 Evaluating the Child with CFD
- CFD can be bilateral; check the contralateral side as well.
- The hip, knee, and ankle should all undergo thorough physical examinations.
- Fibular hemimelia is commonly associated with CFD.
- Radiographic imaging should include a full-length AP legs (standing or pull-down), long leg laterals in maximum extension, and a supine AP pelvis.
- MRI is useful to evaluate whether there is a cartilaginous vs a fibrous connection (true pseudarthrosis) between the femoral head and the intertrochanteric region. It is also useful to determine if there is a fusion of the femoral head to the acetabulum in cases with a true pseudarthrosis of the femoral neck.
- CT is useful in children over the age of 6 to assess the version of the acetabulum

Classification Systems

The purposes of a classification are to (1) divide cases according to a logical sequence of pathoanatomy with increasing deficiency; (2) to allow for comparison between studies (apples to apples); (3) guide treatment; and (4) guide prognosis. Multiple classification systems for CFD have been described over the years in attempts to categorize the pathology and direct surgical treatment (Aitken 1959 [45], Fixsen and Lloyd-Roberts 1974 [46], Hamanishi 1980 [18], Pappas 1983 [47], Gillespie and Torode 1983 [48], Kalamchi 1985 [49], and Paley 1998 [50].) The Aitken and Pappas were the two most commonly used classification systems until recently, when Sanpera and Sparks showed that patients classified with the Aitken, Fixsen and Lloyd-Roberts and Hamanishi systems will change types according to ossification of the proximal femur over time [24]. Newer classification systems incorporate modern imaging modalities, specifically MRI, which allows detailed evaluation of osseous, cartilaginous, and soft-tissue structures, including the non-ossified femoral head, non-ossified acetabulum, labrum, presence of a pseudoarthrosis, and musculature present [39]. The ability to perform MRI under anesthesia for infants allows for interpretation of these images with better reliability at younger ages. As a result, MRI dramatically improves the ability to correctly categorize patients over conventional radiographs alone [51]. Unfortunately, all of these classifications failed to achieve all of the tenets of a useful classification scheme.

The Paley classification (1998) [50] (Fig. 29.7) is based on increasing proximal femoral deficiency, from the least dysplastic and deficient to the most dysplastic and deficient: types 1–3, respectively. Type 4 was added to address a congenitally short femur with a distal deficiency. Type 1 has an intact femur with a hip and knee joint, where the femoral head, neck, and shaft are all connected by means of bone or cartilage. Type 2 has a true pseudarthrosis between the femoral head and the femoral shaft, but the greater trochanter apophysis is present. Radiographically, type 1b can appear the same as type 2 due to the non-ossification of the femoral neck. An MRI is needed to differentiate between these two types. Type 3 has a severe deficiency of the proximal femur with the absence of the greater trochanteric apophysis, and the femoral head may or may not be present. Type 4 has a distal femoral condylar deficiency. The Paley classification has replaced all of the previous classification systems in most major textbooks due to its adherence to the four principles outlined above. The types are logically divided in ascending order by increased pathology, the types are easily recognized which makes comparisons to other studies more consistent, and the treatments and outcomes are completely predicated on the diagnosis of type [52–56].

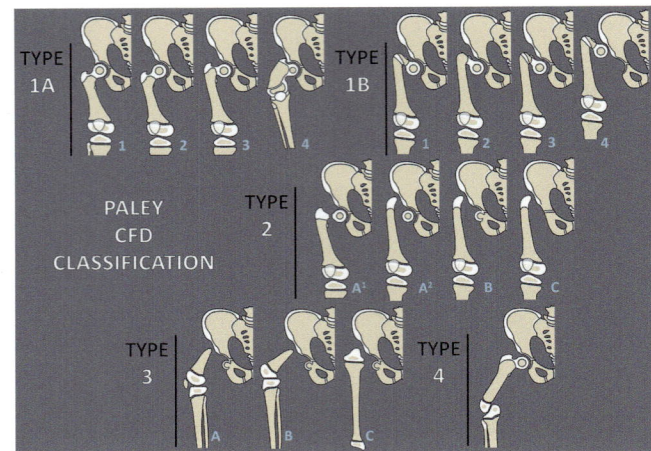

Fig. 29.7 Paley classification of congenital femoral deficiency. There are four types of CFD: Type 1 has an intact femur with normal ossification (1A) or delayed ossification (1B); type 2 has a mobile pseudoarthrosis of the proximal femur; type 3 has a diaphyseal deficiency; and type 4 has a distal deficiency (Copyright: The Paley Foundation. Reproduced with permission. All rights reserved.). Paley types 1, 2, and 3 have several subtypes: $1A_1$—normal-shaped short femur with mild genu valgum; $1A_2$—normal-shaped short femur with mild genu valgum and retroversion; $1A_3$—coxa vara, retroversion, and mild genu valgum; $1A_4$—delta femur; $1B_1$—delayed ossification of the subtrochanteric region; $1B_2$—delayed ossification of the femoral neck; $1B_3$—combined subtrochanteric and neck type; $1B_4$—delayed ossification with dislocation of hip joint; 2A—mobile femoral head within the acetabulum; 2B—partially fused femoral head within the acetabulum; 2C—completely fused femoral head; 3A—mobile knee joint with >45° arc of motion; 3B—stiff knee with <45° arc of motion; and 3C—absent femur or fused knee joint. (Copyright: The Paley Foundation. Reproduced with permission. All rights reserved.)

Treatment Options

Outlining a "Life Plan" for the Family

At the initial consultation, a surgical reconstructive strategy or "life plan" projected to skeletal maturity should be outlined for the child and the family. It is often helpful to write this down for the family to refer to in the ensuing years. The strategy is based on the type of CFD, the projected LLD at maturity, and the reconstructive potential of the hip and knee. In cases with combined CFD and FH, the strategy for FH must be combined with that of the CFD [50, 57, 58]. At the first consultation, based on X-rays, the type of CFD is classified. An MRI may be needed to confirm whether a type 1b vs type 2 is present. Once the type is determined, the next consideration is LLD, both current and at maturity. The calculation is done using the multiplier method, which allows reasonably accurate prediction from a single measurement. Knowing the LLD at maturity allows determination of the number of lengthening surgeries required. Each lengthening gains between 5 cm and 8 cm. Finally, the timing of each lengthening is determined so that there are 3- to 4-year intervals between lengthening. The parents leave the first consultation knowing whether they need a preparatory surgery, such as a pelvic osteotomy, SUPERhip, and SUPERknee , and at what age the preparatory surgery will be performed. They are informed that the first lengthening will be one year after the preparatory surgery and then every 3–4 years throughout the childhood. They are informed whether the lengthenings will be with internal or external devices and at what ages. Armed with a scope of treatment that spans their child's growing years through skeletal maturity, they have realistic expectations and can better prepare for the future.

Nonoperative Management

Shoe lifts, orthoses, and prostheses are used for the nonoperative management of LLD. All children should receive a shoe or prosthesis with a lift when they begin to cruise. A simple shoe lift of an amount equal to 1 cm less than the LLD is used in most cases in which LLD is less than 10 cm.

It is helpful to supplement the lift with an articulated ankle–foot orthosis (AFO) for ankle support from the long lever arm of the shoe lift. If the lift is more than 10 cm, a prosthetic foot with a pilon connected to an articulated AFO is preferred both to reduce weight and improve cosmesis. Avoid using a quadrilateral socket. This is unnecessary even when hip and knee FFD exists. Most patients can be fitted with an articulated AFO prosthesis (also known as foot-on-foot prosthesis) (Fig. 29.8). The clinician should avoid splinting the foot in the equinus because it might lead to an equinus contracture. In children younger than 4 years, a limb length radiograph should be obtained every 6 months to assess LLD and prescribe a new lift. After age 4 years, annual assessment and prescription are adequate.

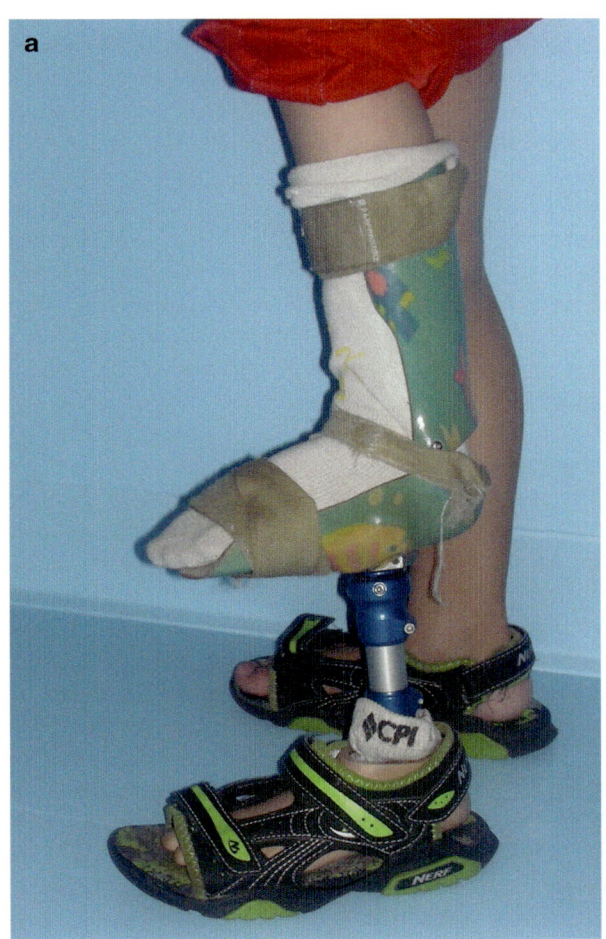
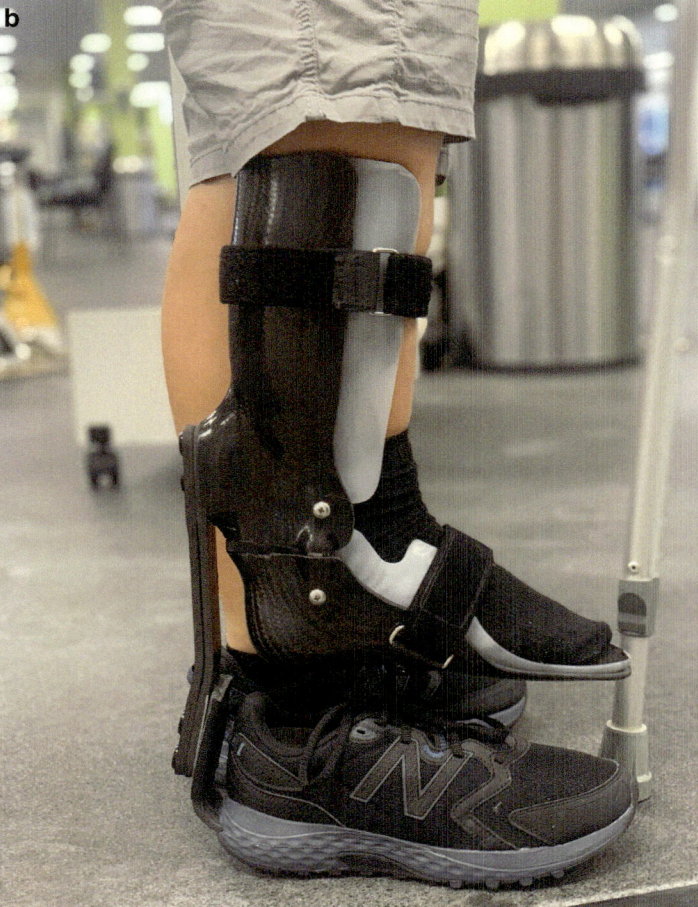

Fig. 29.8 (a) Articulated AFO (foot-on-foot) prosthesis with a tibial pilon construct. (b) A lower profile carbon fiber shoe mounted foot-on-foot prosthesis, also with articulated AFO. The ankle motion in both styles aids with walking (Copyright: The Paley Foundation. Reproduced with permission. All rights reserved.)

Treatment Options for CFD

Surgical treatment for CFD can be divided into two groups: (1) lengthening reconstruction surgery (LRS) and (2) prosthetic reconstruction surgery (PRS). The former are methods to equalize limb length discrepancy combined with surgery to correct associated bone and joint deformities and deficiencies. The latter are procedures to modify the limb so that one can better use a prosthetic limb. The prosthetic limb equalizes the leg length difference.

Lengthening Reconstruction Surgery

The treatment algorithm for lengthening reconstruction involves two main components. The first is preparatory surgery to stabilize the joints (hip, knee, and ankle) for lengthening. Each patient requires an individual assessment to determine the specific procedures required. The specific procedures recommended, such as SUPERhip 1 versus SUPERhip 2, are predicated on the specific type of CFD. The details of the surgical procedures will be discussed below.

The second component is limb length equalization. This can be accomplished with the lengthening of the short leg or shortening of the long leg via epiphysiodesis and, in some cases, with a combination of both. There are multiple methods to lengthen the femur in CFD, including via an external fixator, an intramedullary lengthening nail, or an extramedullary lengthening nail or plate. The indications and specific techniques for these methods will be further elucidated in the following sections of the chapter.

> **Box 29.4 Classification and Treatment**
> - Multiple classification schemes exist but are of primarily historical purposes
> - The Paley classification is separated into types and subtypes based on increasing degrees of deficiency that also determine surgical treatment options for reconstruction.
> - In the properly selected patient, limb lengthening often has good outcomes, but can have significant complications. However, these untoward events can be mitigated by prophylactic joint stabilization.
> - Rotationplasty has been used historically on severely shortened femurs with good results and continues to offer a highly functional outcome in patients with severe femoral deficiency.

Preparatory Surgery

Treatment for Paley Type 1 CFD

Preparatory Surgery of the Hip

Prior to undergoing lengthening, the hip and knee joints must be assessed for instability or deformity that requires treatment before initiating limb lengthening. At the hip, if the acetabulum has an acetabular index with a comparable slope to the normal contralateral side, a center-edge angle (CEA) $\geq 20°$, and a neck-shaft angle (NSA) $\geq 120°$, no separate hip surgery is required before the first lengthening [59]. If the acetabulum shows signs of dysplasia, then a pelvic osteotomy should be performed prior to lengthening. Increased slope of the sourcil (acetabular roof) or acetabular index compared to the other side is a subtle but sensitive sign of acetabular dysplasia. Coxa vara should be corrected prior to lengthening if the NSA is less than 120° [60]. Similarly, external rotation deformity of the hip is a factor to consider for correction at the same time as the acetabular dysplasia. If a unicortical iliac osteotomy is chosen, then there is usually a gain of about 1 cm in leg length. Associated hip deformities of retroversion, flexion contracture, and abduction contracture should be simultaneously addressed. The flexion contracture of the hip is treated by recession of the psoas tendon and release of the rectus femoris tendon. Bony flexion and retroversion deformities are treated with a proximal femoral extension and rotation osteotomy. The abduction contracture is treated by lengthening or resection of the fascia lata and, if necessary, an abductor muscle slide at the iliac crest. When all of these deformities are present together, the reconstructive procedure is called the SUPERhip procedure [54, 57, 58].

Other factors should also be examined prior to lengthening. The proximal femur should be normally ossified for the patient's age. Often, severe cases of CFD have delayed ossification of the femoral neck or subtrochanteric region, and off-label use of bone morphogenic protein (BMP2) may be added to the femoral neck to promote ossification [25]. The fascia lata is a thin but very tough limiting membrane that resists lengthening and applies pressure across the knee joint and the distal femoral growth plate. Thus, it should always be removed or released before lengthening. It can also be used to reconstruct absent knee cruciate ligaments if SUPERhip is done concurrently with a SUPERknee procedure. The SUPERknee surgery (detailed in the section below), much like the SUPERhip, combines multiple procedures to address knee instability. The ACL ligament is reconstructed in an extra-articular (Macintosh procedure) or intra-articular fashion using the ITB. Rotational instability can be treated by performing the reverse Macintosh procedure since it wraps the iliotibial band medially instead of laterally around the knee joint [55, 57]. A lateral release is performed for mild lateral patellar maltracking, whereas a full patellar subluxation or dislocation requires either a Grammont [54, 61] or a Langenskiöld procedure with a Grammont [54, 62, 63]. A knee flexion contracture should be treated with a release of the posterior capsule of the knee to achieve full extension if this is not achieved after shortening of the femur during the SUPERhip. Hemiepiphysiodesis of the medial distal femur may also be performed to correct frontal plane deformities. The ideal age for the preparatory procedures in patients with CFD is between ages 2 and 4 years old.

> **Box 29.5 Planning Surgery for the CFD Patient**
> - Determine the classification and total discrepancy of the deficiency to plan out a timeline of surgeries.
> - Have a low threshold to perform preparatory surgeries of the hip and knee to prevent subluxation or dislocation, which can be disastrous.
> - Do not lengthen until the femoral neck has ossified. BMP2 can be used off-label to promote ossification.
> - The fascia lata must be released or resected before lengthening.
> - The safe range of each lengthening is 5–8 cm.
> - The rule of 4: First lengthening at 4 years of age and then every 4 years thereafter as needed.
>
> Contralateral epiphysiodesis can be used to avoid one lengthening. The rationale behind the rule of 4 is that it takes 3–4 years to physically and psychologically recover from an external fixation lengthening. With the advent of implantable lengthening, recovery time is shorter and can be reduced to 2–3 years. Time between lengthening also minimizes the amount of childhood spent undergoing medical treatments.

SUPERhip 1 Surgical Technique

> **Box 29.6 The Evolution of the SUPERhip Procedure**
> Dror Paley, MD
>
> The SUPERhip name originally arose as a billing code to avoid writing down the multiple CPT codes that comprised this multistep conglomerate procedure. While there was no intention to call this operation the SUPERhip procedure, the name stuck. To avoid the name being misperceived the SUPER prefix was then made into an acronym: Systematic Utilitarian Procedure for Extremity Reconstruction. Other SUPER joint reconstructive procedures for congenital knee and ankle deformities developed by Paley were subsequently renamed the SUPERknee and SUPERankle procedures, usually by my former fellows with a sense of humor. Again the names stuck.
>
> My understanding of CFD began with my experience at the Hospital for Sick Children, Toronto, in 1984. I worked with Drs. Robert Gillespie and Ivan Krajbich, who treated the severe CFD cases by rotationplasty. In 1986 and 1987, I witnessed reconstructive options for these deformities in Kurgan, USSR. Drs. Popkov and Maltzev showed me how to do pelvic support osteotomy to bypass the tethered and deformed hip. The message of these experts was that the CFD-deformed hip did not lend itself to anatomic reconstruction.
>
> After beginning my practice in 1987 at the University of Maryland, I tried to find alternative reconstructive solutions to the CFD hip. I performed many valgus, extension, and internal rotation osteotomies on young children with this deformity. Initially, they had excellent bony correction with the reduction of the leg length difference since such osteotomy corrects the preexisting fixed pelvic obliquity. Gradually, I watched the deformity recur, presumably through the proximal femoral physis or unossified femoral neck. I realized that the reason for this recurrence was that I had not treated the hip flexion and abduction contractures that existed prior to the surgery. In 1996, I recognized that in order to succeed, I needed to untether the proximal femur from its extra-articular contractures and then realign the bone and joint to a neutral position. This was a radical concept, and I was left with the challenge of how to safely release the hip abductors. Borrowing from the concept of the Hardinge approach to the hip, which took down the anterior third of the hip abductors as a sleeve with the quadriceps muscle, I decided to take down the entire hip abductors with the vastus lateralis as one sleeve. In 1997, I performed the first such procedure.
>
> While the psoas, rectus, and TFL were all lengthened as they are today, treating the hip abductors by releasing the gluteus and vastus tendons off of the greater trochanter together turned out to be a bad idea. While this freed up the proximal femur to rotate into neutral by extension, adduction, and internal rotation of the hip joint, it also changed the muscle-tendon

length ratio, thus permanently weakening the hip abductors. This is discussed in more detail below. I initially fixed the femur using a Rush rod and a tension band wire (non-fixed-angle device, see ref. [15]). There was no fixation up the femoral neck. When this procedure was performed for a subtrochanteric type Paley 1b or for a Paley 1a, no recurrence of the deformity occurred since the delayed ossification part was resected. When it was performed for a neck type Paley 1b, the varus usually recurred and the neck did not ossify.

In 2001, I switched to using a fixed-angle plate. I used the 130° sliding hip screw (Smith and Nephew, Memphis, TN). Some of the cases ossified, but most did not. Some of the plates broke and the deformity recurred, while in others the plate began to cut through the head as the varus recurred. I decided that a blade plate would be the best implant to avoid cutout as well as to control flexion and extension forces. With the engineers at Smith and Nephew, I designed an infant and pediatric 130°-angle cannulated blade plate, to correspond to the normal neck-shaft angle. Since 2004, I have been using this new plate. This minimized recurrent deformities, but incomplete ossification of the femoral neck was the usual result.

It was apparent that while we could correct this complex deformity, we could not get the delayed ossification of the cartilage to ossify. To get some of these failed cases to ossify, I resorted to the insertion of BMP2 up the femoral neck into the non-ossified cartilage. The result was dramatic: the recalcitrant-delayed ossification cases ossified. Since BMP-2 (Infuse, Medtronic, Memphis, TN) was not FDA-approved for use in children, we were initially hesitant and reserved in its application. We only used it to salvage previously failed SUPERhips. With the unexpected success that we saw from such an application, I decided to apply it to new cases in 2006. The results were equally remarkable. All of the necks were ossified and there were almost no recurrent deformities. Clearly, we needed to combine a mechanical with a biologic solution to solve the CFD deformity puzzle. (Refer to the article in ref. [15] for more details on this.)

The soft-tissue part of the operation also went through an evolution to its present state. In the first 5 years, we not only employed the release of the conjoint tendon off of the greater trochanter to treat hip abduction contracture, but we also released the hip capsule off of the greater trochanter (superior-lateral capsule). This was done in an extra-articular fashion so that the joint was never opened. No initial consequence of this was observed. However, when we started to lengthen femurs that had previously had a SUPERhip procedure, we encountered two new complications: hip dislocation and slipped capital femoral epiphysis (SCFE). In retrospect, we realize that both were related to the release of the superior capsular ligament from the pelvis to the greater trochanter. Our selective release of the superior capsular ligament demonstrated the importance of this band. This superior capsular pelvic-trochanteric band is essential to prevent the femoral head from moving laterally relative to the acetabulum. After recognizing this, we stopped releasing this band and we no longer experienced frequent dislocations or slips following a SUPERhip.

After 10 years of performing the SUPERhip, we had solved the recurrent varus deformity problem, the delayed ossification problem, and the dislocation/SCFE problem. We noticed, however, that the children walked with a marked lurch or Trendelenburg gait. We attributed this to the abductor tendon release. By detaching the hip abductors from the greater trochanter, we had changed the muscle-tendon length ratio of the gluteus medius and minimus muscles, which was difficult to recover. Essentially, we had added tendon length to the glutei due to the quadriceps tendon moving proximally. To solve this problem in 2008, I began to perform the abductor muscle slide off of the ilium instead of the distal tendon lengthening. This preserved the muscle-to-tendon length ratio, keeping the muscle-tendon length and tension constant after surgery. The slide is achieved by shortening the height of the iliac crest. As an added benefit, the glutei are a peculiar group of muscles since they have a growth plate connected to them that grows in a direction that lengthens the muscles. After the repair of the abductor slide, the iliac apophysis can increase the tension and re-elevate the origin of this muscle. Since adding the abductor slide, patients do not have the previously noted lurch or Trendelenburg gait. The newest recognized problem is the coxa breva. Since these children lack a proximal femoral growth plate and since with the addition of BMP2, the femoral neck ossifies and closes any existing proximal femoral physis, the greater trochanter overgrows and the neck remains short. This can lead to impingement and can also contribute to lateral subluxation. It is remedied later in childhood by either a valgus proximal femur osteotomy or a relative neck lengthening with greater trochanteric transfer. This will be discussed later in this chapter.

SUPERhip 1 Surgical Technique (Figs. 29.9, 29.10, and 29.11)

1. *Positioning, Prepping, and Draping* (Fig. 29.9a). An epidural is placed by the anesthesia service with a catheter running up the back on the nonoperative side. A Foley catheter is placed and also routed to the nonoperative side. The patient should be moved to the edge and foot of the radiolucent table in a supine position. The ipsilateral arm should be appropriately padded and placed across the patient's chest. A radiolucent bump (usually a folded towel or sheet) is placed beneath the ipsilateral ischium to roll the pelvis 45° toward the opposite side. The bump should not be beneath the iliac crest or lower back. The entire side should be prepped and draped free from the nipple to the toes. The drapes should extend from the mid-buttocks to the scrotal/labial-thigh fold. The lower limb should be completely free of the drapes. The patella points anterior in the bumped position.

2. *Incision* (Fig. 29.9b). With the leg in maximum extension, a long mid-lateral incision is made from the top of the iliac crest to the tibial tuberosity. The incision is kept as straight as possible, passing over the proximal femo-

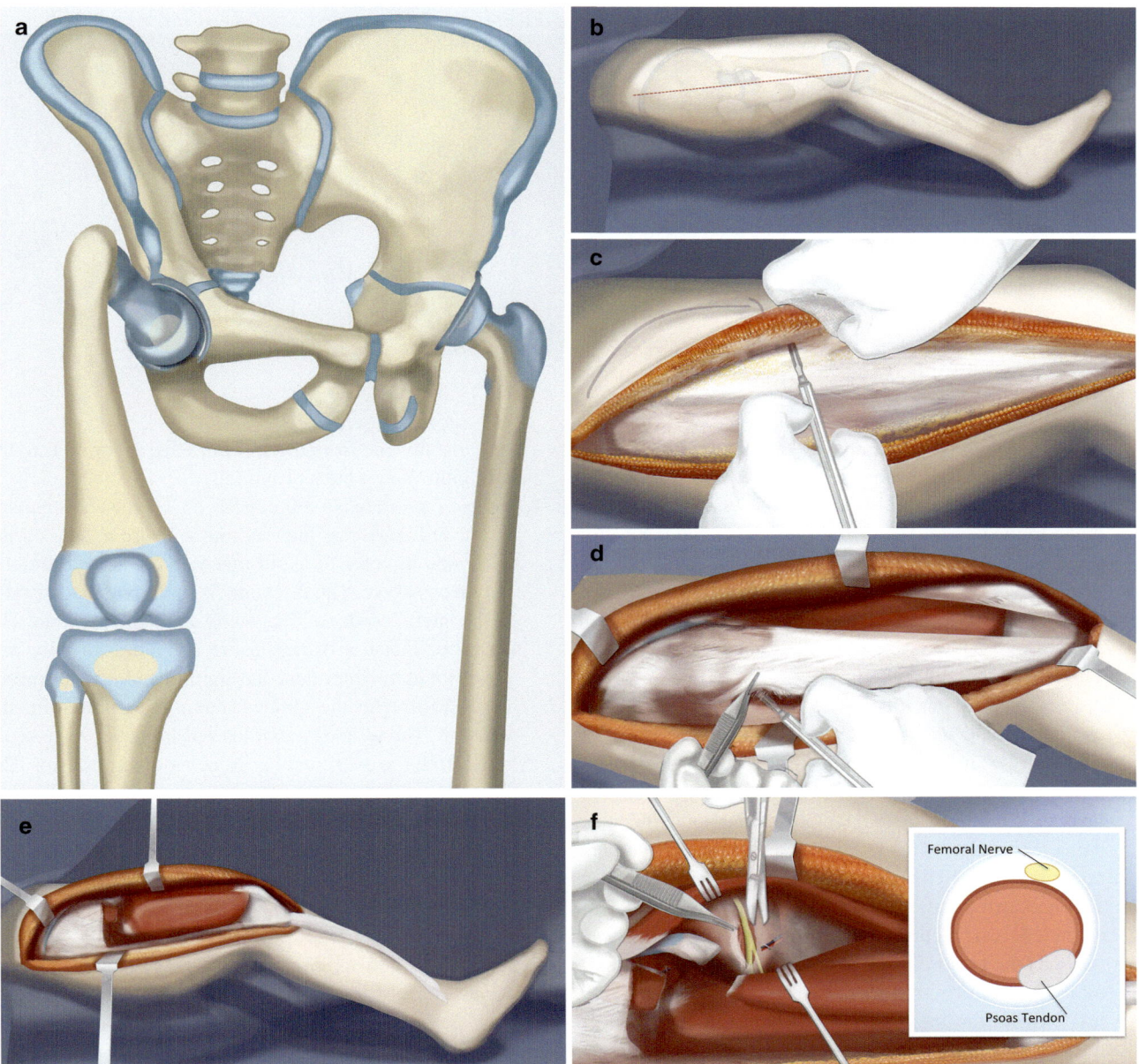

Fig. 29.9 (a–j) SUPERhip procedure: soft tissue releases (follow text for steps and captions) (Copyright: The Paley Foundation. Reproduced with permission. All rights reserved.)

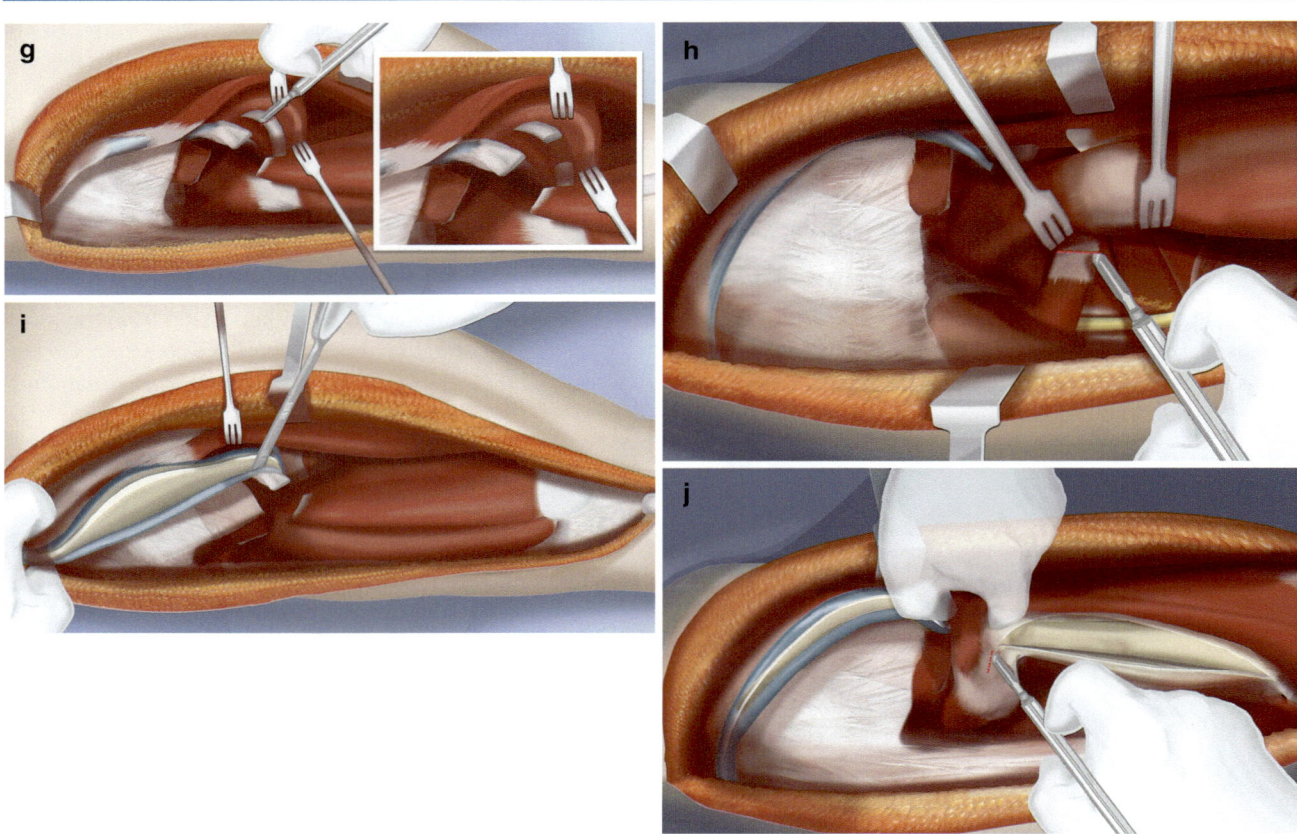

Fig. 29.9 (continued)

ral "bump" and continuing longitudinally toward Gerdy's tubercle crossing slightly anterior toward the distal aspect of the tibial tubercle. The incision is carried down to the depth of the underlying fascia lata and iliotibial band.

3. *Flap Elevation* (Fig. 29.9c). The subcutaneous tissues and skin are elevated as one large flap anteriorly and posteriorly off the fascia of the thigh and pelvic region. The fat is adherent to the fascia and should be dissected preferably with an electrocautery. The electrocautery should be held flat, parallel to the plane of dissection. This can be quite technically difficult until one learns how to separate the fat without perforating the fascial layer or leaving fat behind. It is important not to incise or damage the fascia if it is being used for knee ligament reconstruction (SUPERknee procedure). Dissection may also be carried out with scissors. Anteriorly, the flap is extended just medial to the Smith-Peterson interval between the tensor fascia lata (TFL) and sartorius proximally. Posteriorly, the subcutaneous flap is elevated to just beyond the intermuscular septum. Distally, reflect the flap to the lateral border of the patella if no ligament reconstruction is to be done and to the medial border of the patellar tendon if ligament reconstruction is needed. The fascia lata is now fully exposed from the patella to a couple of centimeters posterior to the intermuscular septum distally and from the anterior edge of the TFL to the mid gluteus maximus proximally.

4. *Fascia Lata Release* (Fig. 29.9d, e). The fascia is incised at the TFL-sartorius interval making sure to stay on the TFL side in order to avoid injury to the lateral femoral cutaneous nerve. The fascial incision is extended distally to the lateral border of the patella ending at the tibia. The posterior incision of the fascia lata starts distally and posterior at the intermuscular septum and extends proximally to overlie the gluteus maximus in line with the incision. The gluteus maximus (GMax) should be separated from the overlying fascia, remaining posterior. The fascia should be retracted anteriorly and away from the underlying muscle, while the GMax should be dissected off of the fascia and the intermuscular septum that separates it from the TFL. The GMax should not be split in line with the fascial incision to avoid denervating the muscle anterior to the split. It can now be reflected posteriorly to allow exposure of the greater trochanter, piriformis muscle, and sciatic nerve.

If knee ligamentous reconstruction is planned, the fascia lata is cut proximally and anteriorly at the musculotendinous junction. The proximal transverse fascial cut starts over the GMax and TFL muscles separating the fascia from the muscle and extends distally past the musculotendinous junction to merge with the iliotibial

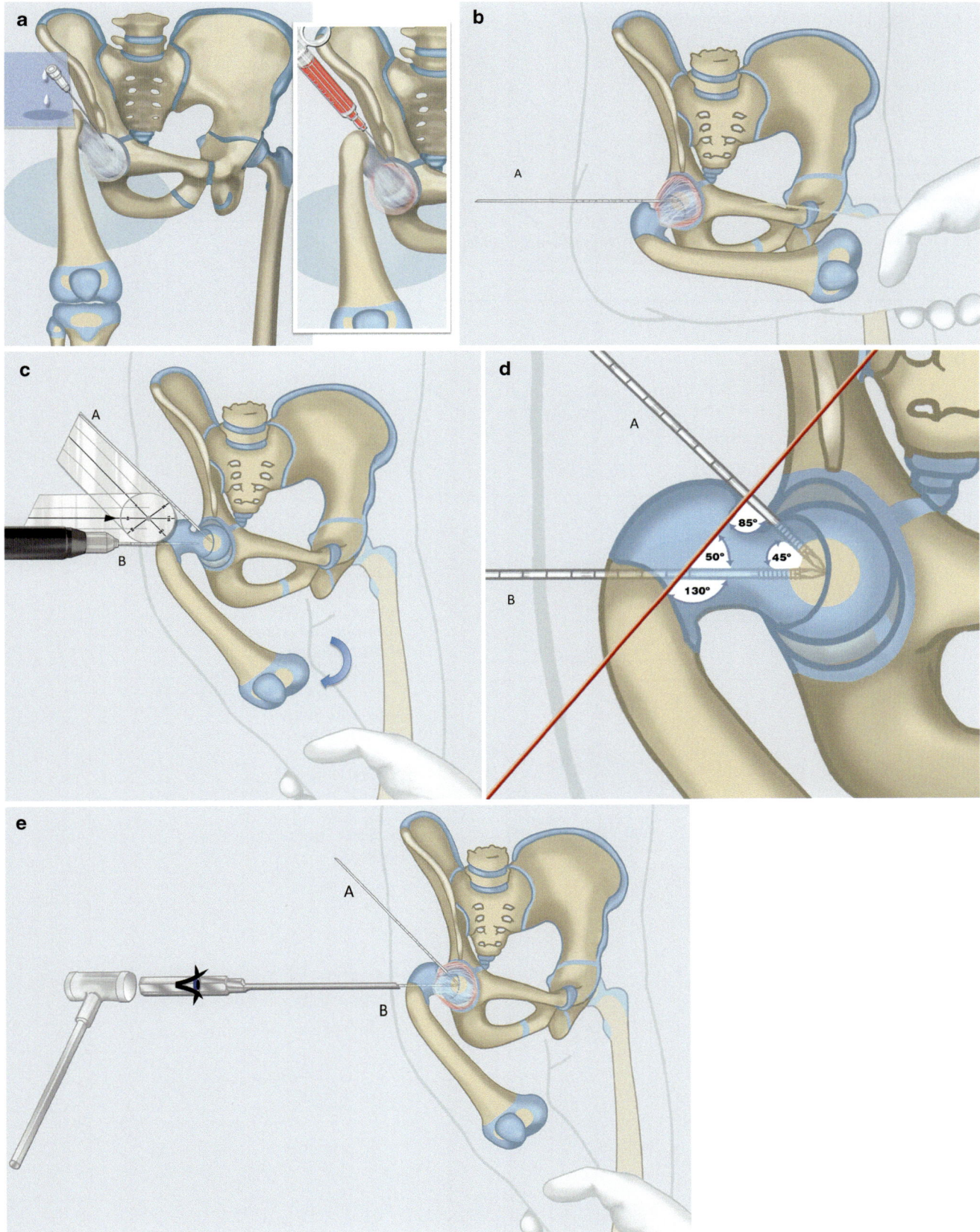

Fig. 29.10 (a–z) SUPERhip bony procedure (follow text for steps and captions) (Copyright: The Paley Foundation. Reproduced with permission. All rights reserved.)

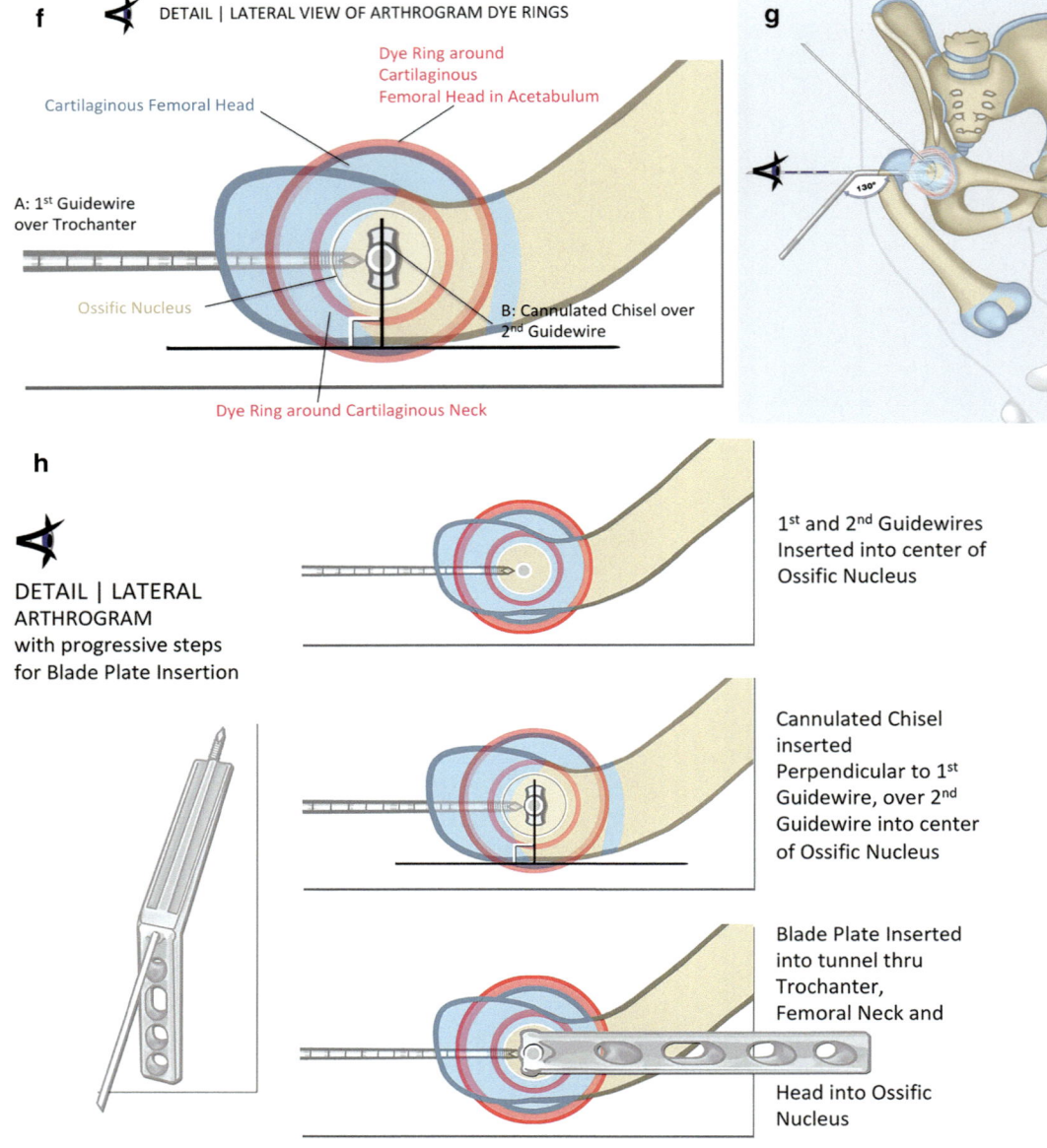

Fig. 29.10 (continued)

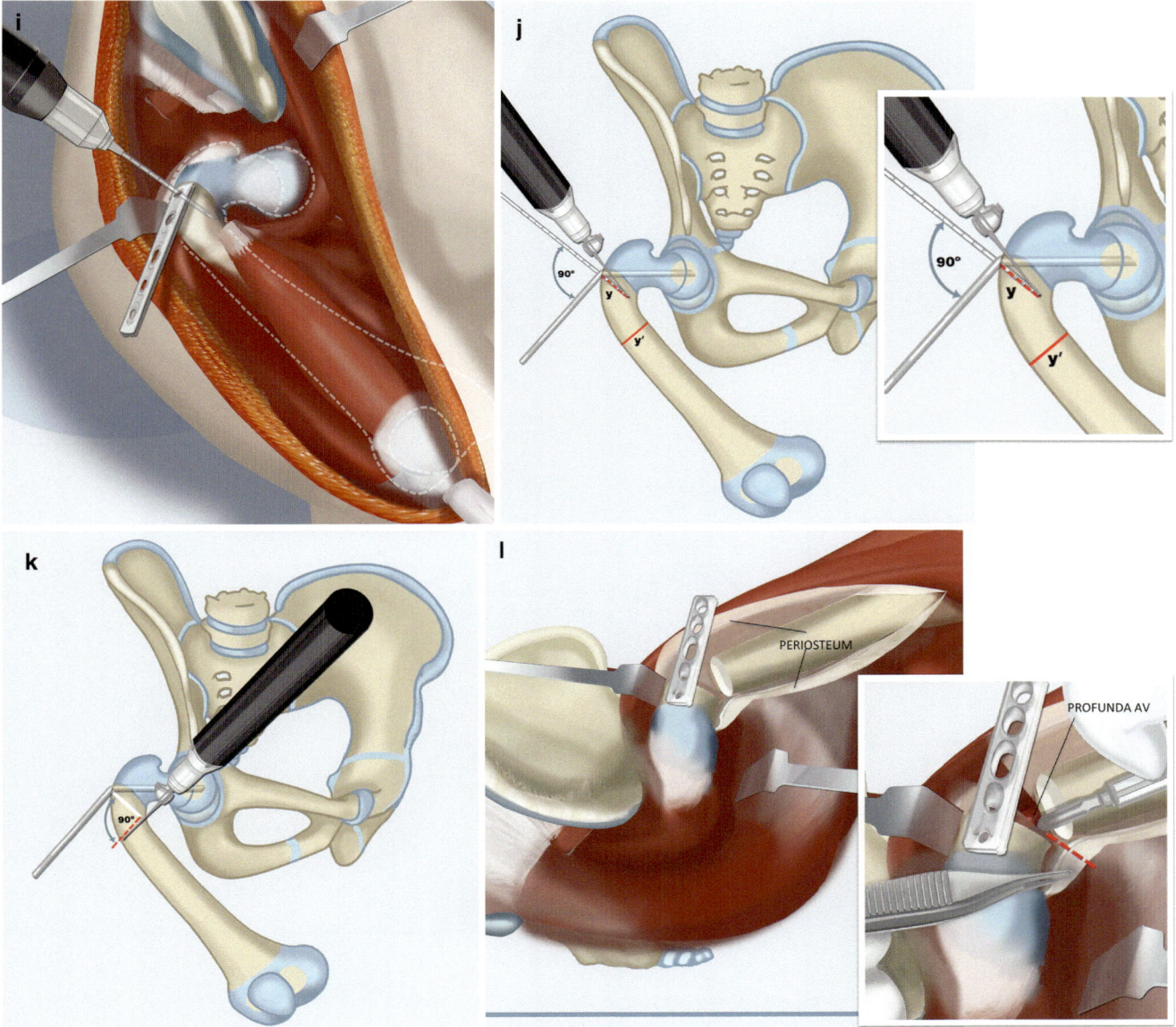

Fig. 29.10 (continued)

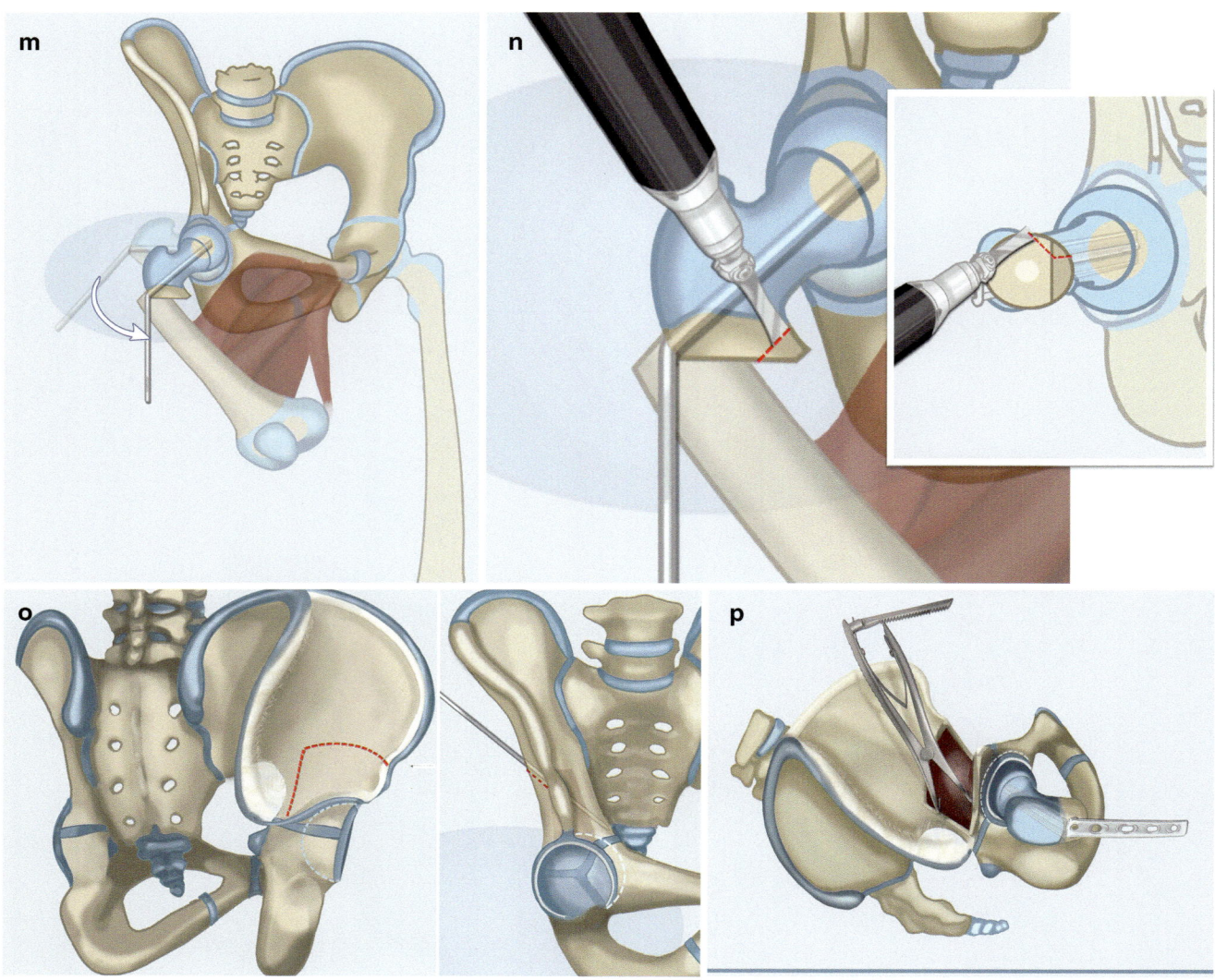

Fig. 29.10 (continued)

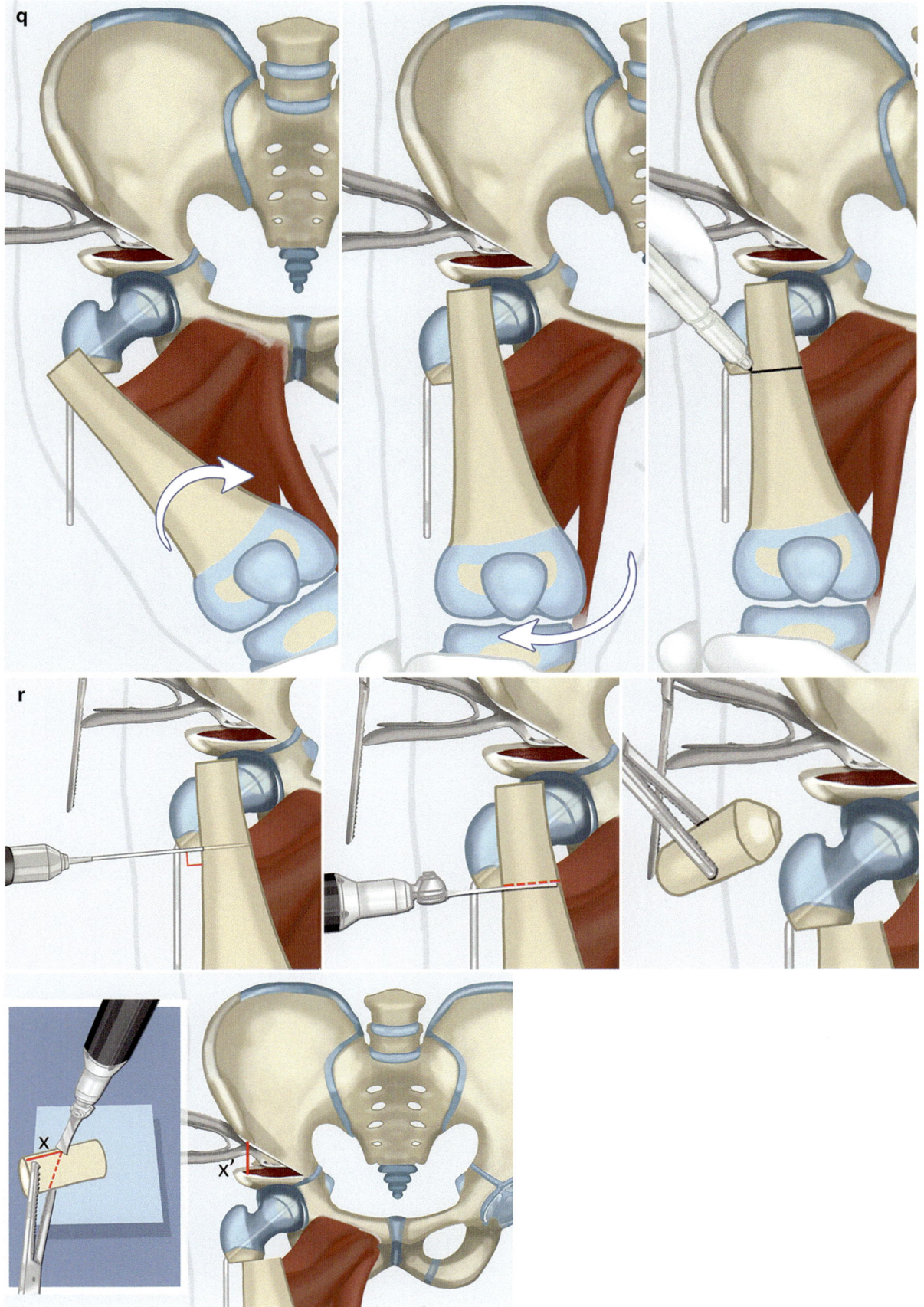

Fig. 29.10 (continued)

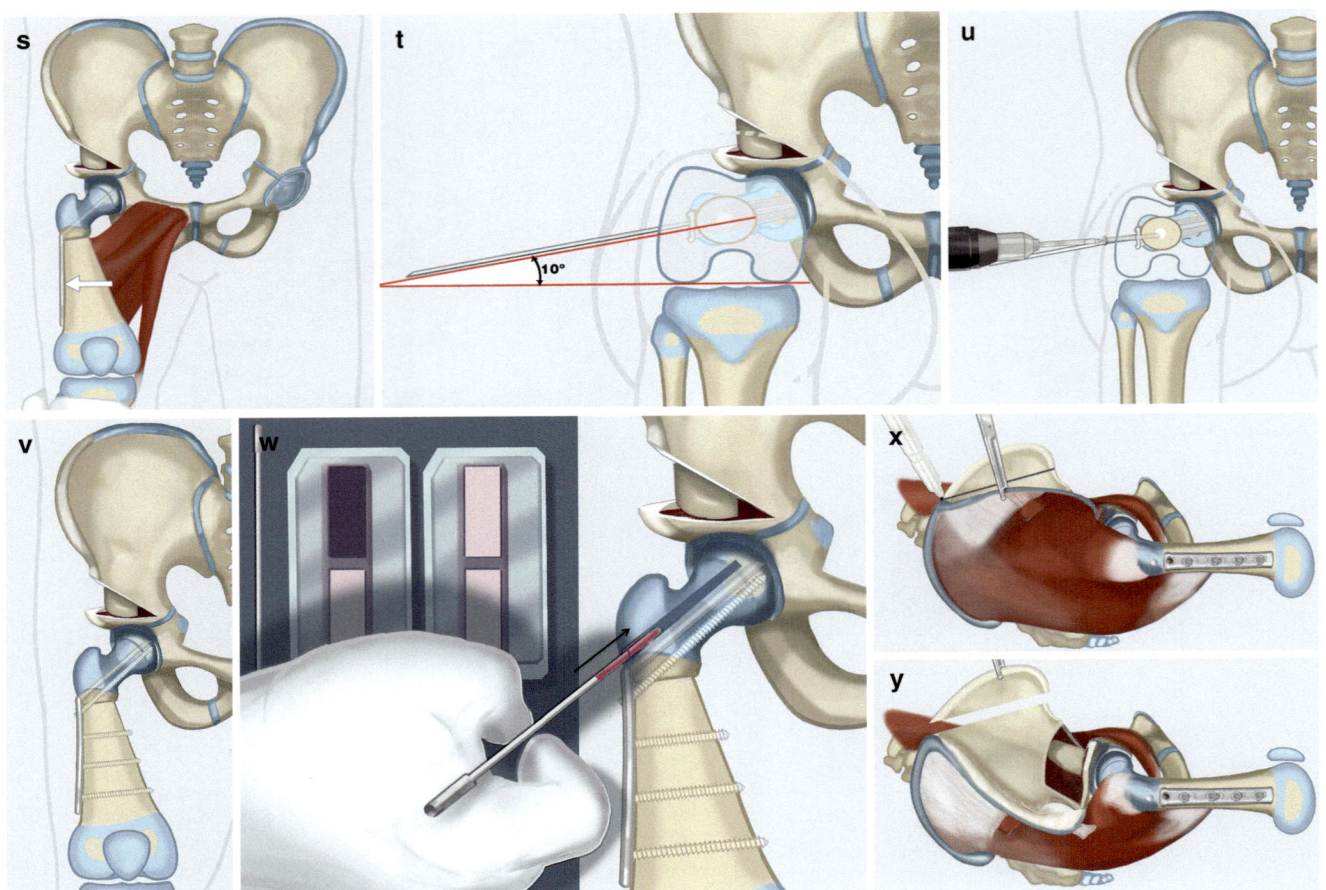

Fig. 29.10 (continued)

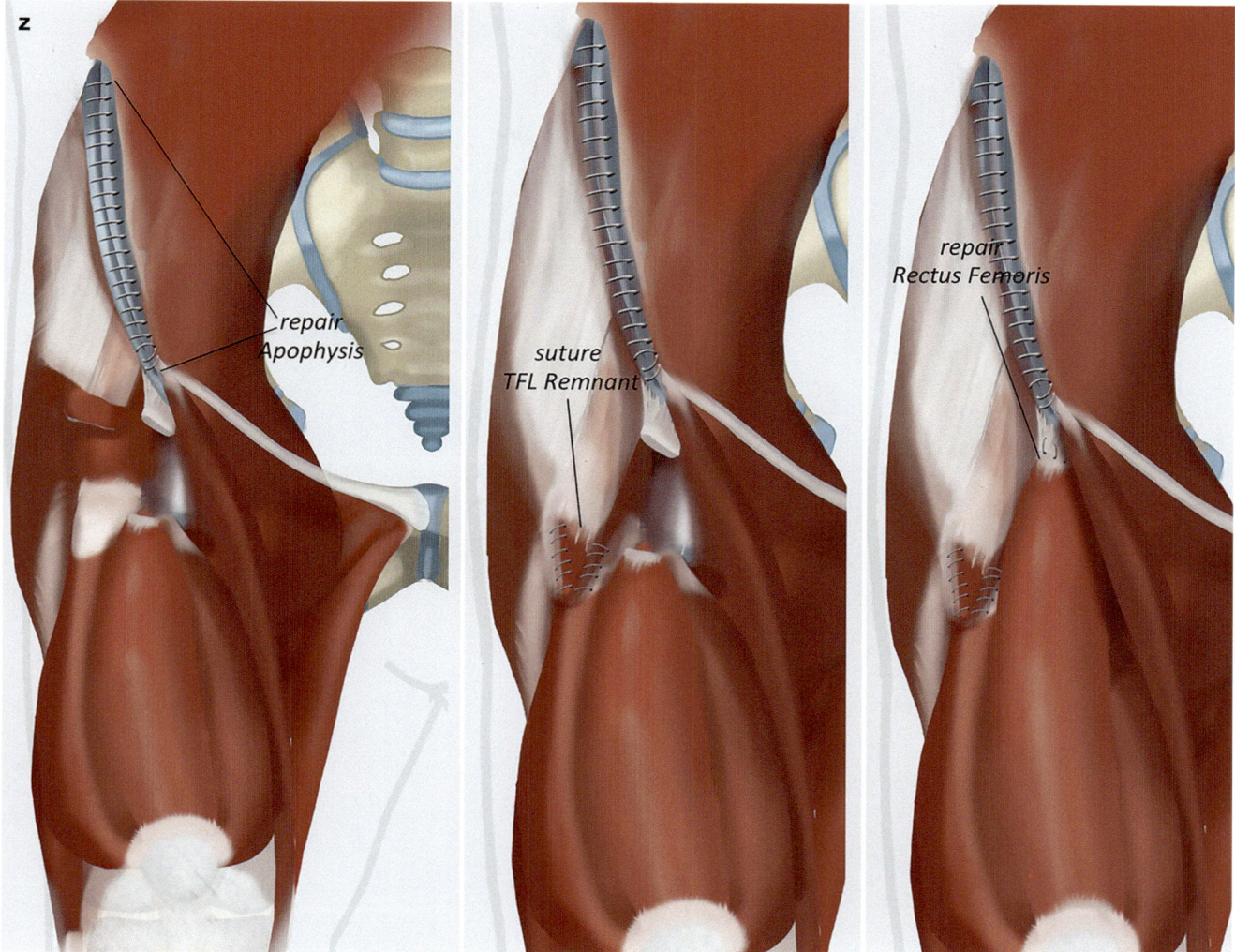

Fig. 29.10 (continued)

band. The fascia lata is reflected distally to merge with the knee capsule all the way to Gerdy's tubercle. It does not have to be separated from the underlying gluteus medius (GMed). The two muscles are often adherent to each other, and it may be difficult to differentiate the muscle fibers. The distinguishing feature is that the GMed fibers insert on the greater trochanter, while the TFL and GMax do not. The distal fascia lata becomes the iliotibial band and blends with the underlying lateral knee capsule, which may be partially reflected with the iliotibial band. The fascia should be mobilized all the way until Gerdy's tubercle. The fascia can then be divided into two halves using a straight pair of scissors. It should be kept moist while the rest of the surgery proceeds. The two limbs of the fascia are ready for later use in the SUPERknee procedure.

5. *Hip Flexion Contracture Releases* (Fig. 29.9f, g). The sartorius is retracted medially to find the rectus femoris tendon. The rectus femoris tendon insertion is identified at the anterior inferior iliac spine. In the more dysplastic and deformed cases, the entire femoral nerve may be lying immediately medial to the rectus femoris tendon especially if there is a lot of upward migration of the proximal femur. Before cutting the rectus femoris tendon, the femoral nerve should be identified and decompressed below the inguinal ligament. The constant ascending branch of the lateral femoral circumflex artery and vein is cauterized prior to cutting the tendon. The conjoint rectus femoris tendon (distal to the split into reflected and direct heads) is cut and allowed to retract distally. Care should be taken not to go too distal on the rectus femoris to avoid injury to its innervating branch

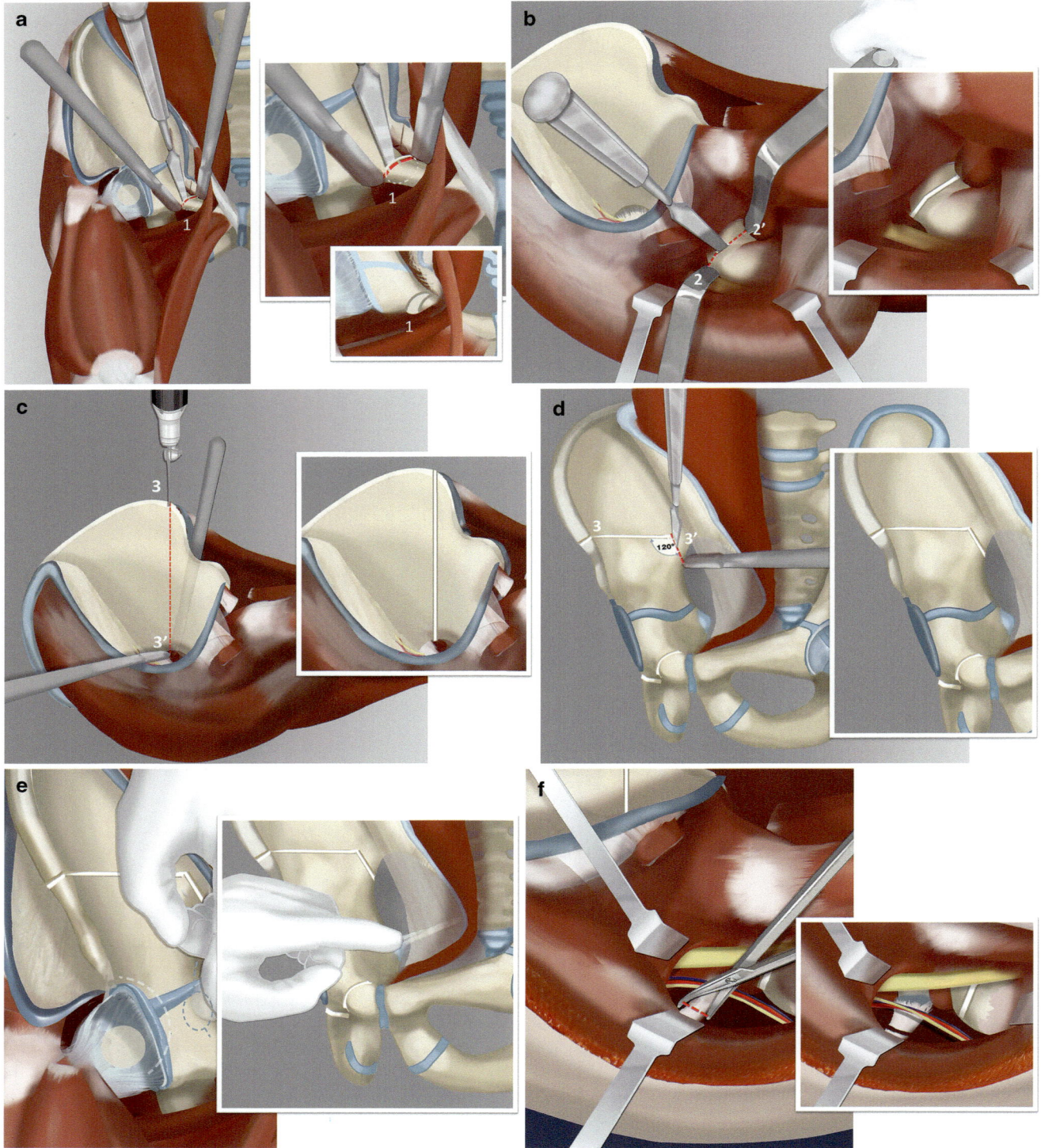

Fig. 29.11 (**a–p**) PATO procedure (follow text for steps and captions) (Copyright: The Paley Foundation. Reproduced with permission. All rights reserved.)

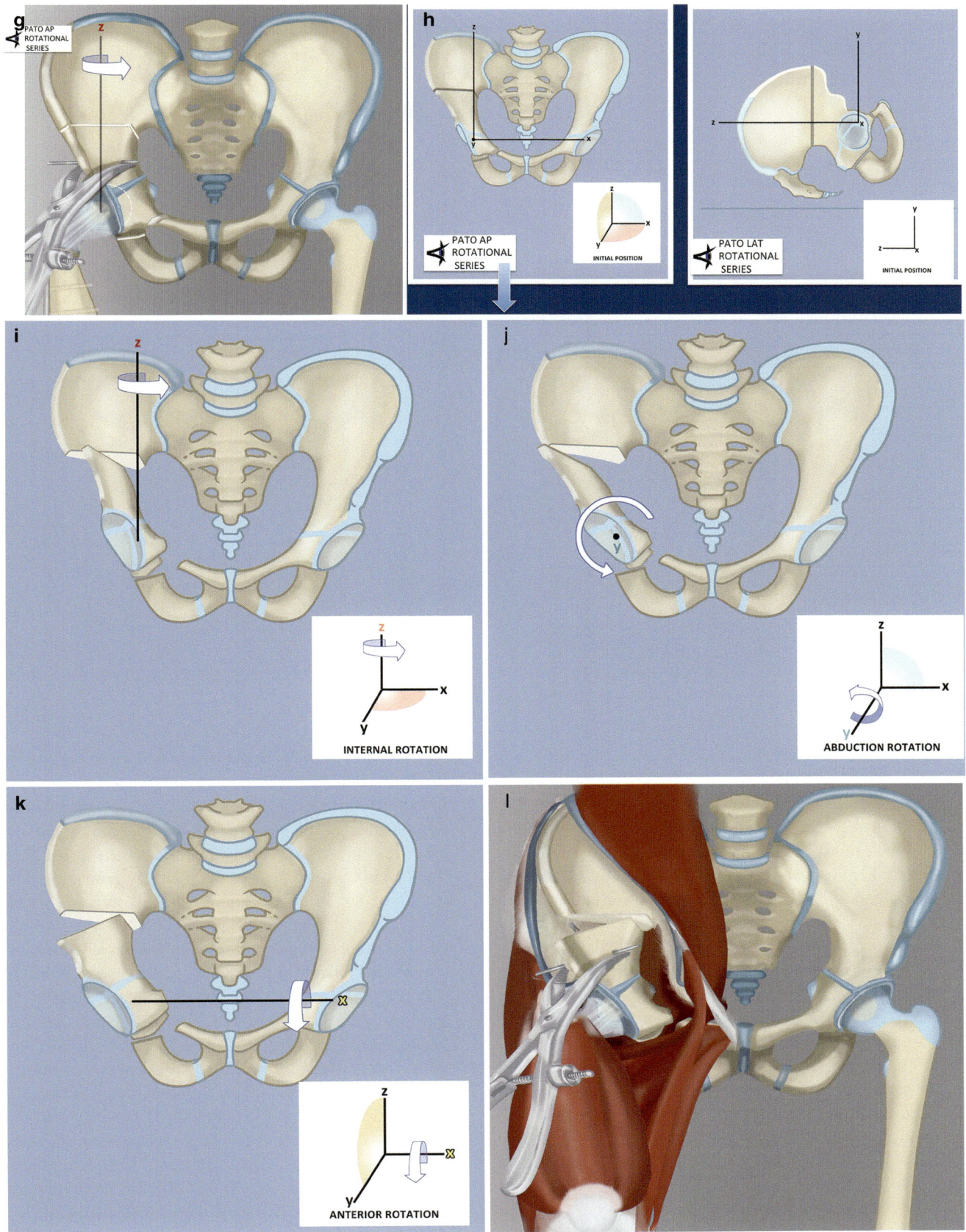

Fig. 29.11 (continued)

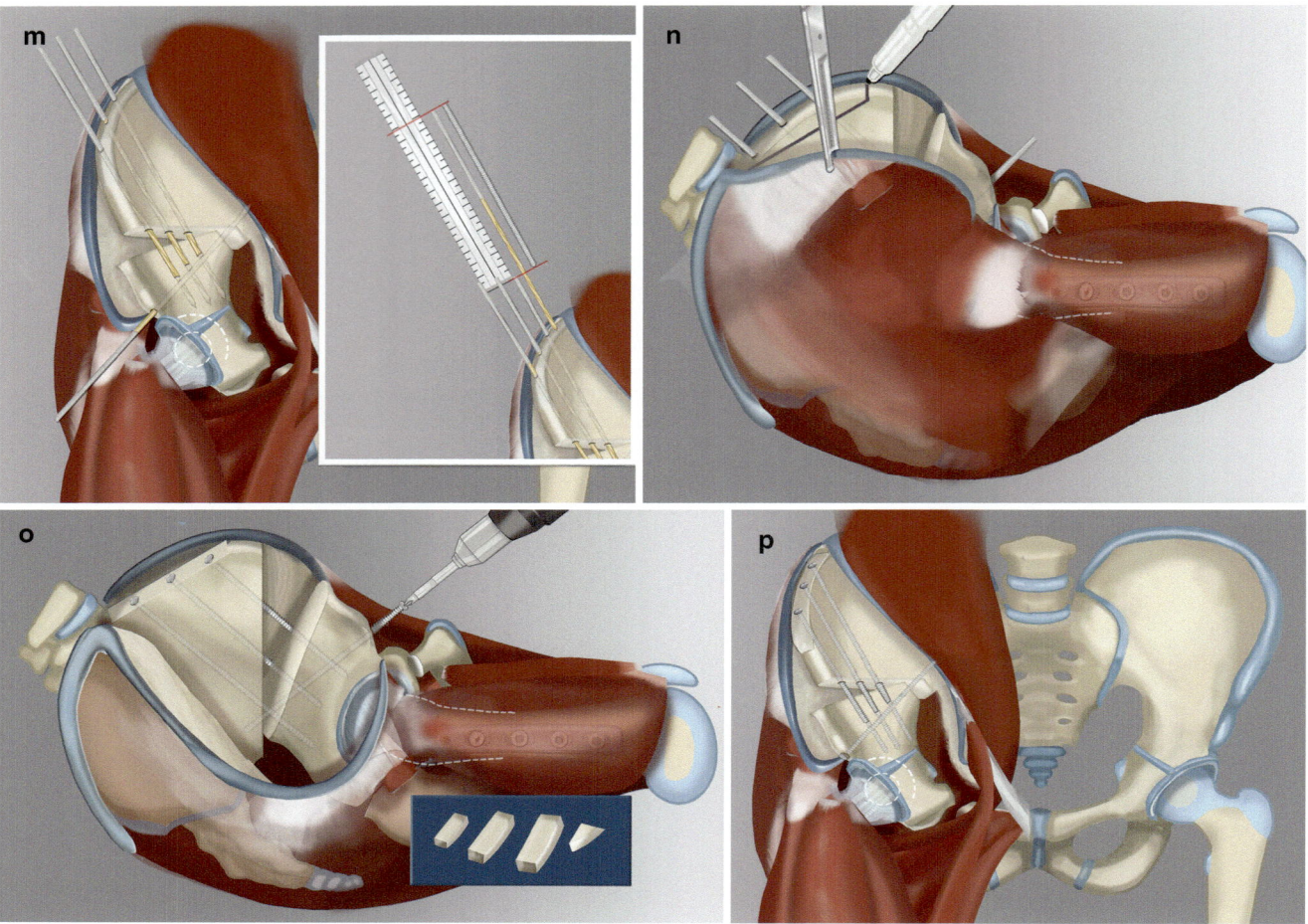

Fig. 29.11 (continued)

of the femoral nerve. Just medial to the rectus is the iliopsoas muscle. The iliocapsularis muscle (capsular origin head of iliopsoas muscles) can also be seen here. The femoral nerve lies on the anteromedial surface of the iliopsoas muscle. The posterior aspect of the iliopsoas muscle belly is now elevated from lateral to medial. The psoas tendon is located on the posteromedial surface in the substance of the muscle. The tendon is exposed and cut. Any remaining flexion contracture of the hip is due to the gluteus medius and minimus (the part of these muscles originating anterior to the center of rotation of the femoral head in the sagittal plane) and the anterior fascia of the thigh. The release of the gluteus medius and minimus muscles is accomplished by the abductor muscle slide technique (see step 7). If the anterior thigh or sartorius fascia are still tight, they can also be released, taking care not to injure the lateral femoral cutaneous nerve, which should be identified and decompressed under the inguinal ligament.

6. *External Rotation Contracture Release* (Fig. 29.9h). The piriformis tendon is contracted and prevents internal rotation of the hip. It should be released off of the greater trochanter. To gain access to see this tendon, the gluteus maximus muscle must be retracted posteriorly. It can be left attached at its distal insertion on the femur and can be swept posteriorly as a large sheet of muscle. The greater trochanter can be identified by palpation. The posterior border of the gluteus medius muscle is very distinct inserts on the greater trochanter. Deep to the medius is the gluteus minimus, and just distal to the minimus is the piriformis muscle. Its tendon can be palpated through its muscle. It may be difficult to identify the piriformis from the minimus. Care should be taken to avoid dissection at the distal border of the piriformis tendon. This is where the medial femoral circumflex branch anastomoses with the inferior gluteal artery branch. To get good visualization it is helpful to have an assistant lift up the patient (limb?) using a sharp Senn retractor (also known as a *cat's paw* retractor). The sharp end is inserted into the posterior edge of the bump on the femur, and the femur is pulled anteriorly, lifting the hip off of the table. The entire piriformis is transected about

1 cm from its insertion onto the trochanter. The sciatic nerve can be identified and if necessary decompressed. It is more posterior and medial to the trochanter and runs deep to the piriformis.

7. *Abductor Muscle Slide* (Fig. 29.9i). The abductors may not appear to be tight on first inspection because of the coxa vara. Adduction into a true AP of the hip, with the neck oriented normally in the acetabulum, is now restricted by the gluteus medius and minimus since the fascia lata has already been cut. Furthermore, the Dega osteotomy, which lengthens the height of the ilium, makes the abductors even tighter. The abductors should be detached at their origin and not their insertion. This avoids changing the muscle-tendon length ratio and avoids weakening the hip abductors, avoiding a lurch or Trendelenburg gait.

    The subcutaneous tissue flaps should be elevated to provide adequate exposure to the iliac crest apophysis. There is a tendency to have inadequate posterior exposure, and the flaps should be elevated just beyond the highest lateral point of the apophysis. The anterior extent is the anterior superior and inferior iliac spines, which has been exposed for the release of the rectus femoris tendon. The abdominal external oblique muscles are partially released off of the entire length of the apophysis. Split the cartilaginous apophysis from the anterior inferior iliac spine to the anterior superior iliac spine, and then, continue posteriorly splitting from anterior to posterior along the iliac crest. This should be done with a #15 blade. To know where to split, pinch the apophysis between thumb and index finger of the hand not holding the knife. Stay in the middle of the apophysis along its entire length, pushing down hard with the knife blade until one feels bone. Using a periosteal elevator, pop off the apophysis from the ilium. This should be done at multiple sites to get the entire apophysis to peel back as a unit from the ilium. The apophysis and lateral periosteum are reflected distally, thus relaxing the abductor muscles. The medial half of the apophysis is reflected medially with the iliacus muscle. Since some of the abductors act as flexors of the hip, the abductor slide helps eliminate any remaining flexion deformity of the hip. Furthermore, the iliacus muscle slide also relaxes any residual tension in the iliopsoas.

8. *Elevation of Quadriceps* (Fig. 29.9j). The quadriceps are now elevated off of the lateral femur in a subperiosteal fashion. Since the femur is so short, the exposure may extend as far as the distal femoral physis. The perforator vessels need to be cauterized as the quadriceps is detached from the linea aspera. Proximally, the vastus lateralis should be elevated off of part of the cartilage of the greater trochanteric apophysis by sharp dissection. Stay anterior to the gluteus maximus tendon which does not need to be dissected from the femur.

9. *Arthrogram* (Fig. 29.10a). A hip arthrogram is now performed using a 20-gauge spinal needle. With the trocar inside, the needle is placed into the hip joint from the anterolateral side. Traction of the femur may facilitate placement. Once the needle appears to be in the joint on the image intensifier, the trocar is removed and normal saline is injected. If the needle is in the joint the saline should go in with little pressure, and when the syringe is removed from the needle, the saline should drip back out. These signs confirm that the needle is in the joint space. The arthrographic dye can now be injected into the hip joint to outline the femoral head, acetabulum, and femoral neck. The reason for this two-step arthrogram is that if a false injection of dye occurs, it will obscure the visualization of the hip joint. The two-step method is a more secure way of confirming intra-articular needle placement.

10. *Guide Wire Insertion* (Fig. 29.10b–e). Since the abduction, flexion, and external rotation contractures have all been released, the femoral head and neck can now be placed in a neutral orientation to the pelvis by extending and maximally adducting the lower limb across the opposite leg. A guide wire should now be drilled up the center of the femoral neck to guide the insertion of a fixed-angle fixation device. Since the femoral neck is unossified and short, it is very difficult to drill a guide wire at the correct angle up the femoral neck. The goal is to create a 130° neck-shaft angle and a medial proximal femoral angle (MPFA) of 85° (Fig. 29.10e). In the normal femur, the angle between the neck-shaft line and the tip of the greater trochanter to the center of femoral headline is 45°.

    The first guide wire is inserted from the tip of the greater trochanter to the center of femoral head (Fig. 29.10b). Since the tip of the trochanter is cartilaginous in young children, it cannot be seen radiographically. The tip of the trochanter is located by palpation using the wire tip. From this point, the wire is then drilled toward the center of the femoral head as shown in the arthrogram. The image intensifier is placed into the lateral view, and the leg is rotated until a bull's eye of three concentric circles is seen. This is formed by the overlapping dye shadows: The outermost circle is the femoral head, the middle circle is the femoral neck, and the inner circle is the ossific nucleus of the femoral head. A second wire should be drilled into the center of the bull's-eye at a 45° angle to the first wire (Fig. 29.10c, d). Using a depth gauge or another wire of the same length as the second wire, measure the amount of wire inside the femoral neck by placing it alongside the second wire and measuring the difference in length between the two wires. This will be the length of the blade of the blade plate to be used. The position of the neck wire can also be confirmed by flexing the hip to 90° and looking at a frog-leg lateral of the neck.

11. *Blade Plate Insertion* (Fig. 29.10f–h). The cannulated chisel should be rotated until it is perpendicular to the posterior aspect of the greater trochanter. The chisel should now be hammered up the femoral neck guided by the second guide wire (Fig. 29.10f). Tap the chisel out of the femur, and reinsert the guide wire in its previous position. Insert the appropriate length 130° blade plate over this wire to the depth of the bend of the plate (Fig. 29.10g). Make sure on the image intensifier that the tip of the blade is not too deep into the femoral head. Check its position on AP and lateral planes, and use the approach-withdrawal technique with live fluoroscopy to ensure that the blade is not advanced too close to the articular surface of the femoral head. If the blade is suspected of being too long, then replace it with one with a shorter length. Furthermore, if plate placement is off-center, there is a greater risk of protrusion into the joint. The posterior edge of the plate should be parallel to the back of the greater trochanter. The femur diaphysis is usually flexed to the plate (Fig. 29.10h).

12. *Subtrochanteric Osteotomy* (Fig. 29.10i–k). Insert a wire perpendicular to the plate just below the bend in the plate. Using a saw, cut along this wire (Fig. 29.10j). Keep the plane of the saw blade perpendicular to the plate in all planes. A second subtrochanteric osteotomy should be made oriented 90° to the first osteotomy toward the base of the femoral neck (Fig. 29.10k).

13. *Periosteum Release* (Fig. 29.10l–n). After the second osteotomy extends to the medial cortex, the distal femur is easily stripped of its surrounding periosteum. Posteriorly, it is very thick and tethers stretching and correction of deformity. Cut the periosteum transversely around the femur, carefully separating it from the surrounding muscle (Fig. 29.10l). Be careful to avoid injury to the profunda femoris and its perforators, which pass immediately under the periosteum. Cutting the periosteum allows the thigh to stretch longitudinally, reducing the amount of shortening required of the femur. The hip adductors become the main tether to the length of the femur (Fig. 29.10m). The anteromedial corner of the femur should be resected to prevent impingement in flexion (Fig. 29.10n).

14. *Pelvic Osteotomy Option 1: Paley Unicortical Iliac Osteotomy* (Fig. 29.10o, p) [58, 64, 65]

    It is preferable to perform the pelvic osteotomy at this juncture since it can affect the amount of femoral shortening. The lateral iliac periosteum is reflected back to the edge of the acetabulum and to the sciatic notch. The periosteum should also be dissected off the anterior wall of the sciatic notch, feeling for the soft cartilage of the triradiate cartilage as it separates the ilium from the ischium. Using the image intensifier, a guide wire is drilled approximately 2 cm proximal to the lateral edge of the acetabulum toward the triradiate cartilage medially. Start the osteotomy posteriorly parallel to the sciatic notch anterior border. Start near the triradiate cartilage and continue proximally. Stay only a few millimeters anterior to the sciatic notch at the distal end of this limb of the cut. Continue in a straight line proximally to the level of the guide wire. Then, turn the osteotome 90° and head toward the guide wire and the space between the ASIS and AIIS. Incline this cut medially toward the triradiate parallel to the guide wire (Fig. 29.10o). The osteotomy remains unicortical except where it exits anteriorly. It is even unicortical as it heads toward the pubic eminence. The osteotomy is levered distally to bring the roof of the acetabulum down. A laminar spreader is used to distract the osteotomy (Fig. 29.10p). The posterior vertical limb of the osteotomy extending down to the triradiate cartilage at the ilioischial junction allows for greater bending and greater lateral coverage. This osteotomy is very different from the Dega osteotomy and its numerous variations. Dega described an osteotomy that went through both tables of the ilium and converged on the triradiate cartilage between the ilium and the pubis [66]. The Dega osteotomy also converged on the sciatic notch posteriorly. The Paley unicortical iliac osteotomy goes only through the outer table and converges on the triradiate cartilage between the ilium and the pubis, as well as the ilium and the ischium. It does not enter the sciatic notch. It truly hinges on the entire triradiate cartilage of the roof of the acetabulum. As with the Dega, San Diego, and Pemberton Osteotomies, the correction does not improve posterior coverage since the posterior lip is part of the ischium and not the ilium. The Dega, San Diego, Pemberton, and Paley osteotomies are only iliac. Because the Paley osteotomy is between the tables and extends more distally, it achieves more coverage than the Salter, Dega, San Diego, or Pemberton innominate osteotomies. The bump under the buttocks should be removed at this stage. This allows one to assess the coverage of the femoral head in the frontal plane with fluoroscopy. The laminar spreader can be distracted as needed to gain additional coverage and reorientation of the acetabular sourcil. The laminar spreader should be kept posterior to avoid increasing the anterior coverage and creating impingement. The dysplasia of the acetabulum in CFD cases is posterolateral. The Paley osteotomy can only provide lateral coverage and avoid anterior overcoverage by not distracting the anterior part. The laminar spreader is left in place. At this point, the femoral shortening should be carried out and the excised bone segment cut to fit the opening wedge gap of the pelvic osteotomy. Additional bone from the iliac crest, which is resected during the abductor slide, may be inserted to fill the remaining space.

Pelvic Osteotomy Option 2: Paley Periacetabular Triple Osteotomy (PATO)(Fig. 29.11) [58, 65, 67]

Pubis: The pubis is exposed subperiosteally by reflecting the medial iliac apophysis and periosteum more medially. The triradiate cartilage arm at the pubis is exposed, and the dissection is carried out just distal to it. The superior pubic ramus can be cut under direct vision under the protection of two Hohmann retractors with an osteotome (Fig. 29.11a). Ischium: The ischium is exposed by returning to the back of the femur and finding the sciatic nerve. The nerve is followed to the ischium. To avoid stretching the nerve, do not place a retractor between the nerve and the ischium. A Hohmann retractor can be placed anterior to the ischium. Subperiosteal elevation of the ischial periosteum is carried out. The ischium should be cut under direct vision near the junction where it forms the inferior wall of the acetabulum, distal to the triradiate cartilage (Fig. 29.11b). Ilium: The ilium is cut with a saw from the anterior superior iliac spine toward the junction of the true and false pelvis in line with the sciatic notch (Fig. 29.11c). As the cut reaches the junction of the true pelvis on the medial side, an osteotome is used to change the angle of the cut and break into the sciatic notch (Fig. 29.11d). This bend in the cut rounds off the medial corner of the distal segment and creates a posterior lip of bone on the proximal segment. This increases the surface area and creates a posterior buttress while making the distal segment rotate more easily with less distraction. This third bone cut completes the triple osteotomy. Sacrospinous ligament release: For large corrections, it is important to release the tether of the sacrospinous ligament. This ligament can be palpated after dissecting the medial iliac periosteum off of the quadrilateral plate inside the true pelvis (Fig. 29.11e). A finger can be placed on the tip of the ischial spine, and the ligament is then felt. The ligament can be palpated and seen from the lateral side. Make sure the sciatic nerve and pudendal nerve and vessels are out of the way. The ligament can be cut with a blunt pair of curved Mayo scissors from the lateral side, cutting directly onto one's own finger (Fig. 29.11f). Next, the triradiate cartilage at the pubic eminence should be temporarily pinned with a 1.8-mm smooth wire to avoid bending or fracture or the physis during manipulation of the acetabular segment as the second wire is inserted transversely before inserting a lion jaw clamp to manipulate the periacetabular osteotomies (Fig. 29.11g). Since CFD is associated with a hypoplastic acetabulum, there is usually posterior and lateral deficiency (Fig. 29.11h). To gain posterior and lateral coverage, the acetabular segment should first be rotated internally based on the long axis of the body (Fig. 29.11i). This increases the posterior coverage at the expense of the anterior coverage. It should then be rotated laterally (Fig. 29.11j). This gives lateral coverage without changing the posterior or anterior coverage. Finally, it also needs to be flexed to regain anterior coverage (Fig. 29.11k). To rotate internally, a lion jaw bone clamp is placed anteroposteriorly, superior to the acetabulum (Fig. 29.11l). It can also be placed around the pubis to lever the acetabulum laterally. If the acetabular fragment does not move sufficiently, then each osteotomy site should be checked for completeness. The ischial or pubis osteotomy is often the culprit, and the periosteum around the ischium and or pubis may need to be divided. Fixation of the triple osteotomy is achieved using long 2.7–3.5-mm screws from the ilium to the acetabular fragment depending on the age of the child. Four equal-length drill bits are used to fix the osteotomy, three antegrade and one retrograde. A samesized drill bit is used to compare lengths with the drill bits inside the bone to determine the screw lengths (Fig. 29.11m). Because of the abductor slide, the proximal part of the iliac wing must be resected prior to screw fixation (Fig. 29.11n). The level of iliac wing resection is determined by pulling up the apophysis with the femur held in a neutral position (Fig. 29.11n). The bone proximal to the level of the apophysis should be resected (Fig. 29.11o). One by one, the drill bits are removed and replaced with solid, non-cannulated screws, making sure that they do not enter the triradiate cartilage or the hip joint (Fig. 29.11p).

15. *Femoral Shortening* (Fig. 29.10q–s). The distal femur is now mobile and can be corrected into valgus and rotated internally. The distal femur is too long to fit end-to-end with the proximal femoral cut. The two ends should be overlapped, and a mark should be made at the point of overlap (Fig. 29.10q). The distal femur should be shortened at this level. A wire is drilled perpendicular to the femur at the level of the osteotomy and a saw is used to cut, using copious irrigation to prevent thermal necrosis (Fig. 29.10r). The segment of bone is kept moist on the back table for use as a bone graft to fill the opening wedge iliac osteotomy. This is usually a trapezoidshaped piece about 1–1.5 cm long (Fig. 29.10s).
16. *Bone Grafting Paley Unicortical Iliac Osteotomy* (Fig. 29.10r–t). The segment of bone from the femoral shortening is cut to the dimensions needed to support the opening wedge pelvic osteotomy (Fig. 29.10r). The dimension of the graft needed is measured from the size of the opening wedge base using a caliper. A trapezoidalshaped graft is then fashioned from the femoral shortening segment. It is inserted into the pelvic osteotomy to support and stabilize it (Fig. 29.10r, s).
17. *Distal Femur Fixation and Internal Rotation* (Fig. 29.10s–v). The femur is now brought to the plate

(Fig. 29.10s). The bone ends should oppose without tension. The femur is internally rotated to correct the external torsion deformity. To adjust the femur to the correct anteversion, the guide wire should be reinserted into the cannulation of the plate to show the orientation of the femoral neck. The knee should be flexed to 90°, and the angle between the wire and the frontal plane of the femur as judged by the perpendicular plane to knee flexion is observed (Fig. 29.10t). This wire should appear at least 10° anteverted, relative to the knee. The most distal hole in the plate can now be drilled with the femur held in this rotation (Fig. 29.10u). The drill hole should be made at the distal edge of the hole to compress the osteotomy with screw insertion. Two more screw holes are drilled and screws are inserted. The most proximal hole in the plate is designed to drill parallel to the blade of the plate and secures the plate to the proximal femur. The wire in the cannulated hole can be used to guide the drill bit. In type 1b cases, the blade of the plate and the oblique screw goes across the proximal physis and into the femoral head (Fig. 29.10v). In type 1a cases with a horizontally oriented growth plate, neither the blade nor the screw should cross the growth plate of the upper femur. In type 1a cases with a vertically oriented growth plate, the blade but not the screw should cross the physis.

18. *Bone Morphogenic Protein (BMP2) Insertion* (Fig. 29.10w) [25]. In type 1b neck cases, BMP2 should be inserted into the upper femur to induce ossification of the cartilaginous neck of the femur. A wire is drilled proximal and parallel to the guide wire in the cannulation of the plate. A 4.0-mm hole is then drilled over this guide wire. The drill hole should extend all the way to the ossific nucleus. BMP-2 (Infuse, Wright Medical) is then prepared on collagen sponges. The radiocontrast dye can also be applied to the collagen sponges. The sponges are loaded into a metal tube whose outer diameter is 4 mm (Craig needle biopsy set). This cannula is then inserted into the drill hole. Using a blunt trocar the sponge is pushed out of the tube inside the femoral neck. Using the image intensifier, it is possible to see the sponge in the unossified neck. It should be emphasized that such use of BMP (Infuse implant) is an off-label use of this product since the product is not FDA-cleared in children. Usually, two sponges are used in one drill hole. Bone wax is used to seal the lateral entry hole to prevent leakage of BMP and heterotopic ossification overtop of the blade plate.

19. *Iliac Wing Osteotomy* (Fig. 29.10x, y). After the pelvic osteotomy, the apophysis should be sutured back together. Due to the abductor muscle contracture, the lateral apophysis cannot reach the top of the iliac crest. Part of the crest has to be resected to allow repair of the apophysis. Putting traction on the lateral apophysis with the femur held in a neutral position, one can mark the level to which the apophysis can reach (Fig. 29.10x). A saw is used to cut and remove the proximal part of the iliac wing, effectively a shortening osteotomy of the ilium. The removed bone is used as a graft for the opening wedge Paley iliac osteotomy (Fig. 29.10y). It can also be used as a bone graft around the subtrochanteric femoral osteotomy. The apophysis is then repaired with a running #1 Vicryl suture. The medial and lateral halves of the apophysis should be well opposed to avoid a bifid iliac wing. The external abdominal muscles should be advanced and repaired over the apophysis as a separate layer to avoid an abdominal wall hernia (Fig. 29.10z).

20. *Muscle Repairs and Transfers* (Fig. 29.10z). The rectus femoris muscle is sutured to the TFL. This restores its pelvic origin while lengthening this muscle at the same time. The interval between the TFL and the sartorius is closed, carefully avoiding suturing the lateral femoral cutaneous nerve. The quadriceps is sutured to the region of the linea aspera. Finally, the gluteus maximus is advanced back to the posterior border of the TFL.

21. *Closure.* If no knee releases or reconstruction are required, the fascia lata should be resected from Gerdy's tubercle. The incision can now be closed. Since there is no fascia lata, the deepest layer is the subcutaneous fat layer, called the "underlayer." One medium-sized drain is placed, exiting anterosuperiorly. The drain is secured with a clear adhesive sterile dressing (e.g. Tegaderm, 3M, Minnesota). It is important to close the wound in a fashion that the opposite layers get sutured at the same level. The deep edges of the subcutaneous underlayer are brought together with a running #1 braided absorbable suture. The Scarpa's fascia is closed with a running 2-0 braided absorbable suture. The deep dermal layer is closed with a running 3-0 braided absorbable suture, and the skin is closed using a subcuticular 4-0 monofilament suture. Dermabond™ may be used, and sterile dressings are applied.

Final radiographs are taken: an AP pelvis and lateral knee, both including the femur. The patient is then placed into a one-legged spica cast. The operative limb should be placed in full hip and knee extension with the foot and ankle left free. The cast should be bivalved to allow for swelling, before leaving the operating room.

22. *Postoperative Course*: Parents are educated on cast care, hygiene, and how to transport the child in the cast. The bivalved spica cast can be converted into a removable cast after about one week. The patient can then start gentle passive flexion and extension of the hip from 0 to 90°, as well as passive abduction. The patient remains non-weight-bearing for six weeks. After that, the spica cast is discontinued. The patient has progressed to full weight-bearing. The end goal is to restore the child to normal function before they proceed with limb lengthening.

Case Examples (Figs. 29.12 and 29.13)

SUPERhip 1 for Paley Type 1b Subtrochanteric-Type Surgical Technique [58, 65]

The following steps are modified when treating a subtrochanteric type 1b. The deformity is often of greater magnitude and the bump more prominent. When elevating the quadriceps, open the interval between the quads and the gluteus medius. This allows the quadriceps to be lifted off of the sharp bump of the subtrochanteric region. The next difference is taking down the subtrochanteric delayed ossification site (which is like a stiff pseudarthrosis site. Instead of inserting the guide wires first, break up the stiff pseudarthrosis line and separate the bone ends. Allow the distal fragment to be freed from the periosteum. This untethers the proximal femoral segment, which now becomes more mobile. Since the femoral shaft has been removed from the proximal segment, the best way to manipulate it is to apply a clamp (e.g., lion jaw) to its distal end. The guide wires can now be inserted to find the center of the femoral neck and the cannulated chisel

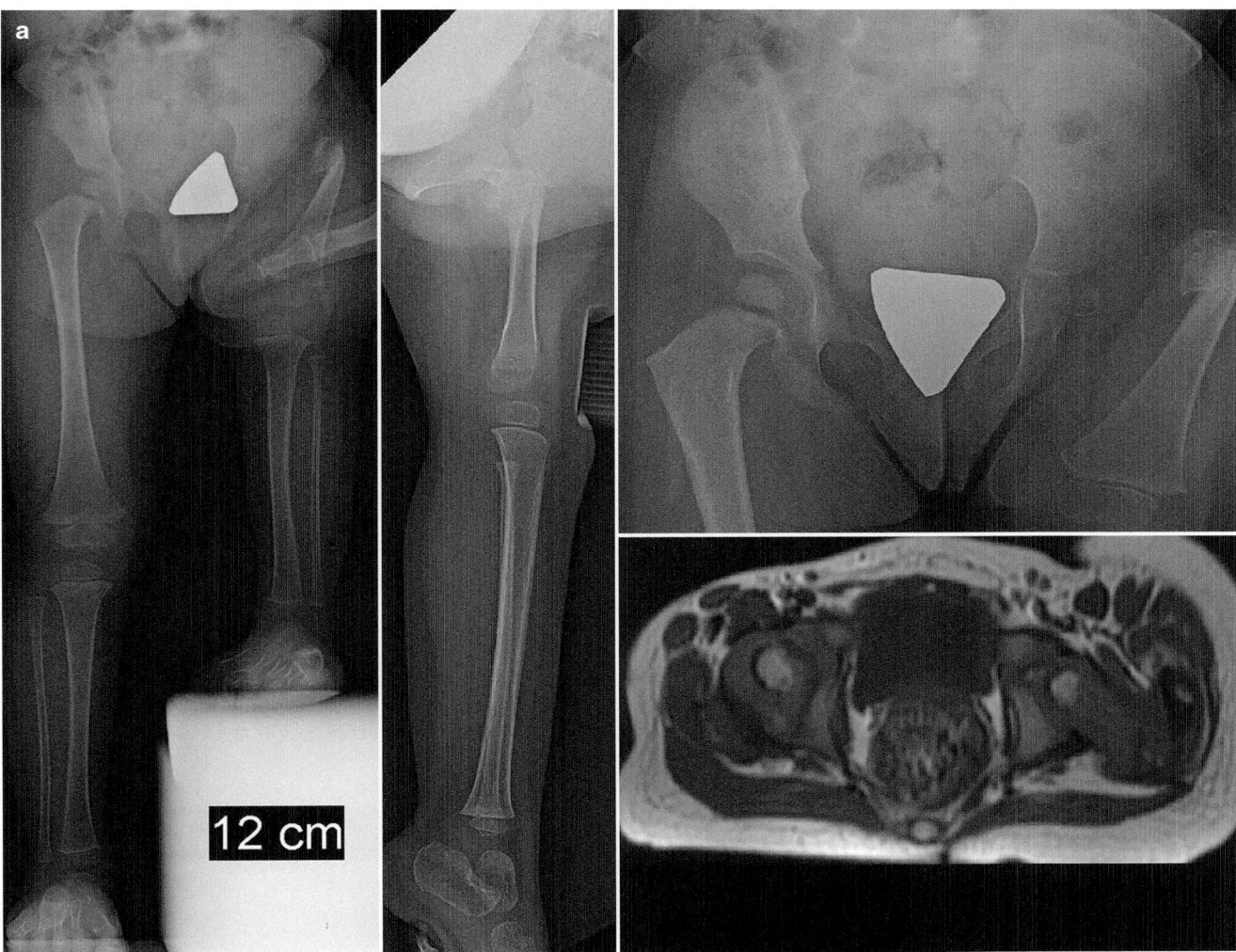

Fig. 29.12 (a) Preoperative EL (left), long lateral (middle), AP pelvis (right top), and axial MRI (right bottom) of a 2-year-old girl. The femoral head can be seen in the acetabulum radiographically and the femur sits quite lateral to the pelvis suggesting there is something keeping it lateral. The MRI confirms that there is an intact non-ossified femoral neck. Based on the MRI and the radiographs, this can now be classified as a Paley Type 1b3 (combined subtrochanteric-neck type). (b) Intraoperative fluoroscopy during SUPERhip procedure demonstrating drilling of the non-ossified femoral neck for insertion of BMP2. Note the small size of the femur that required the most distal screw hole in the plate be cut off. The end of the plate sits at the junction with the physis. (c) One-year follow-up EL (left) and long lateral (right) radiographs showing well-healed femur and pelvic osteotomy with excellent hip coverage. The distal femur has grown away from the bottom of the plate, and the femoral neck is now fully ossified. Compared to the opposite femur, there is evidence of growth stimulation (Copyright: The Paley Foundation. Reproduced with permission. All rights reserved.)

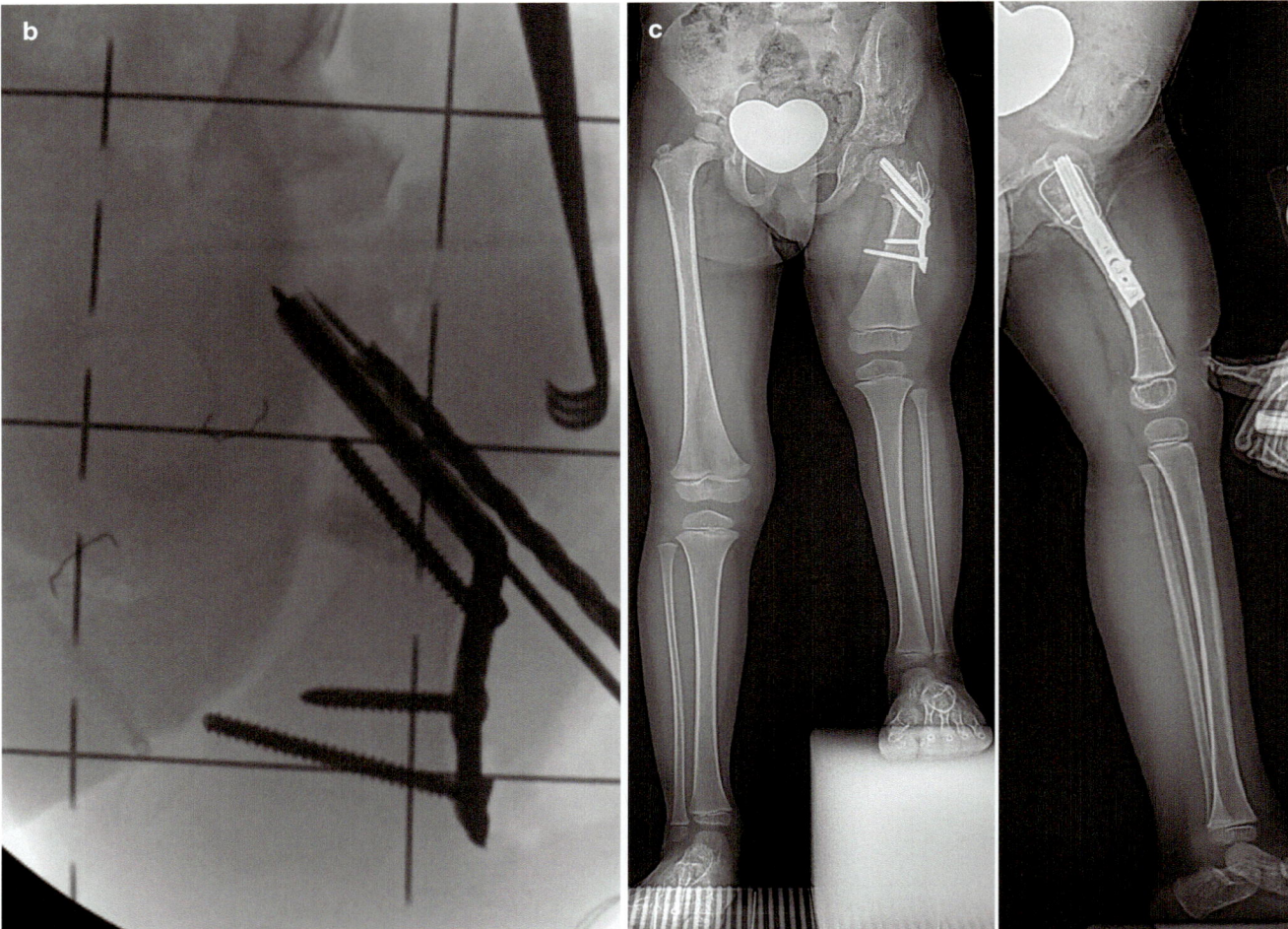

Fig. 29.12 (continued)

followed by the blade plate inserted. The proximal femur needs an osteotomy perpendicular to the plate to establish a proximal bone healing surface. The rest of the procedure is as for the neck type except that no BMP2 or neck drill holes are needed in these cases.

> **Box 29.7 SUPERhip Tips and Tricks**
> - Pay careful attention to soft-tissue handling, making sure that the subcutaneous flaps are cleanly dissected to preserve their integrity and prevent fat necrosis.
> - The lateral femoral cutaneous nerve is usually found just under the sartorius fascia and originates from deep to the inguinal ligament.
> - The femoral nerve lies on the anteromedial side of the iliopsoas muscle. The psoas tendon lies posteromedial.
> - Do not dissect distal or deep to the piriformis tendon to avoid interrupting the inferior gluteal anastomosis with the medial femoral circumflex artery.
> - The apophysis should be split with a single continuous cut, pushing hard down to the bone. Multiple passes will piecemeal the apophyseal cartilage.
> - Palpate the back of the greater trochanter while placing the chisel and blade plate to make sure that they stay perpendicular to its posterior border in the sagittal plane.
> - The extent of the flexion and adduction deformity should be fairly evident by the orientation of the blade plate to the uncut femur. Greater than 45° of flexion deformity and up to 90° of varus deformity are not uncommon.
> - Place the guide wire in the cannulated plate to help guide the rotational correction and BMP hole placement and determine femoral anteversion.

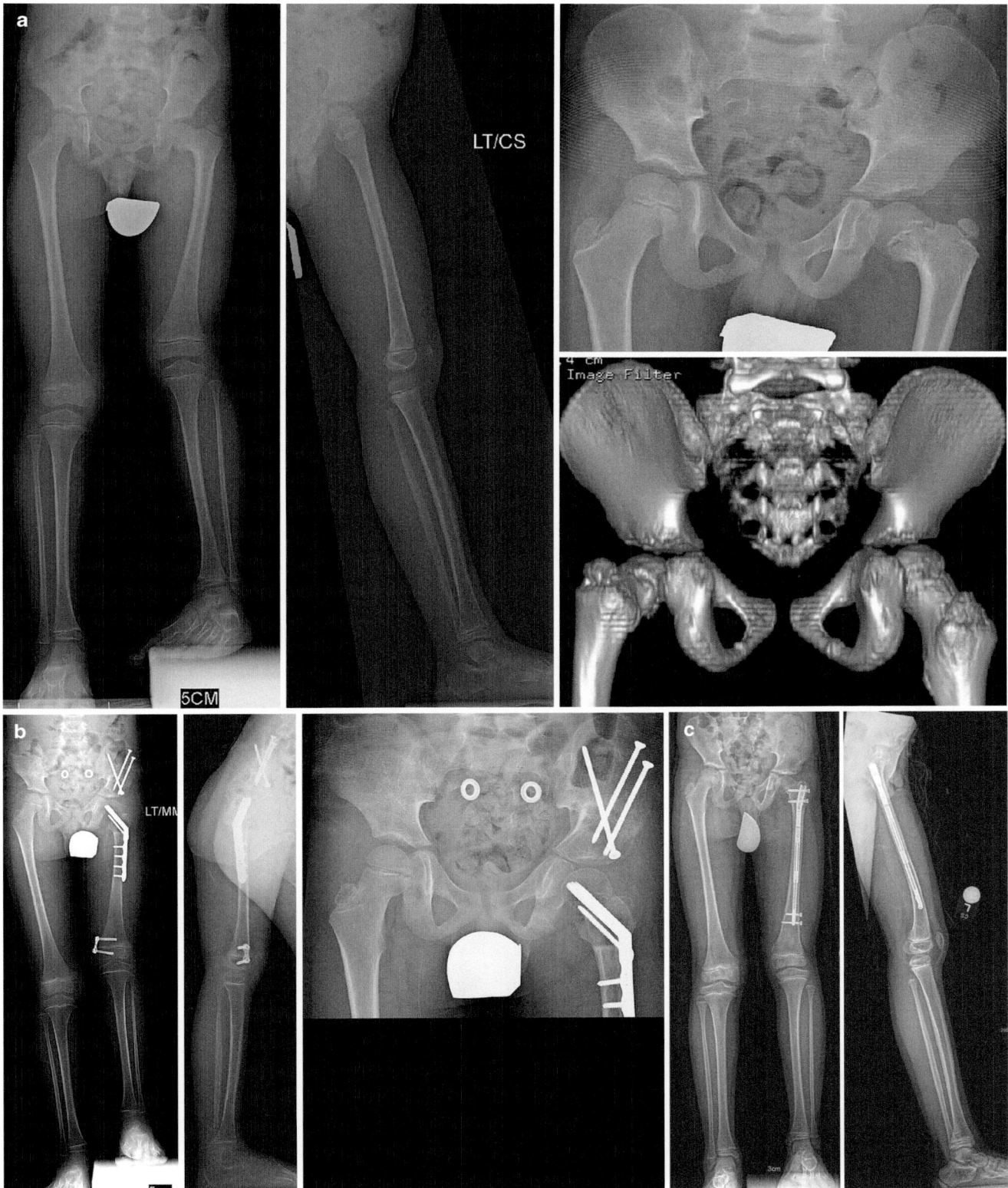

Fig. 29.13 (a) Preoperative EL (left), long lateral (middle), AP pelvis (right top), and 3D CT pelvis (right bottom) of a 5-year-old boy with Type 1a3 CFD. The 3D CT is rotated to a PA view and demonstrates decreased posterior coverage of the affected hip with upsloping roof of the acetabulum (left side) compared to the normal hip (right). (b) 6-month postoperative radiographs after the patient underwent SUPERhip with triple periacetabular osteotomy (TPAO). At the time of the SUPERhip surgery, a hemiepiphysiodesis plate was placed on the medial distal femur to correct genu valgum. (c) EL and long lateral X-ray taken 3 years later, after completing 5 cm of femoral lengthening with an intramedullary lengthening nail (Precice, NuVasive, San Diego) (Copyright: The Paley Foundation. Reproduced with permission. All rights reserved.)

Preparatory Surgery of the Knee

> **Box 29.8 History of SUPERknee Procedure**
> Dror Paley, MD
>
> The knee reconstruction that I developed in 1994 is called the SUPERknee procedure. The SUPERknee is a conglomerate procedure combining two or more of the following five procedures, three of which were previously described by other authors and two of which were developed by me: (1) the Langenskiöld procedure for congenital dislocation of the patella; (2) the MacIntosh procedure for ACL deficiency including extra and intra-articular ACL reconstruction using the fascia lata; (3) the Grammont procedure for recurrent dislocation of the patella; (4) the Paley procedure also referred to as the reverse MacIntosh to prevent external rotatory instability and to act as an extra-articular posterior cruciate ligament; and (5) the Paley approach to posterior capsulotomy of knee. Combinations of two or more of these five procedures are referred to as the SUPERknee procedure and can be performed at the same time as a pelvic osteotomy and/or SUPERhip procedure.
>
> The SUPERknee procedure is a combination of some or all of these components including extra- and intra-articular knee ligament reconstruction, patellar realignment, posterior capsulotomy, and knee flexor tendon releases. Typically, the SUPERknee consists of the MacIntosh extra- and intra-articular ACL reconstruction, the reverse MacIntosh (Paley) extra-articular PCL reconstruction, the Grammont patellar tendon realignment, lateral release of the patella, and in some cases the modified Langenskiöld (Paley) procedure for patellar reduction. If performed with a SUPERhip procedure, the incision is a distal extension of the SUPERhip incision. If performed as an isolated procedure, it can be done through one midline anterior incision or one medial and one lateral incision. If the SUPERknee is performed without the SUPERhip procedure, the entire surgery can be performed under tourniquet control. My personal preference is to use the Hemaclear tourniquet (HEMACLEAR, New Jersey) because of its narrow width. There is typically not enough room in a young patient with a congenital short femur for a pneumatic tourniquet to be placed proximal to the surgical incision. The release of the posterior capsule is performed only when there is a significant knee flexion contracture greater than 15°.
>
> David MacIntosh first described an extra-articular ligament reconstruction for the ACL-deficient knee and later a combined extra- and intra-articular reconstruction with the "over-the-top" technique. This method, although no longer used in sports medicine, is a very useful technique for congenitally deficient knees. In CFD, the instability pattern is different than in an isolated tear of the ACL. There is more of a rotary instability in CFD. Therefore, a purely intra-articular ligament reconstruction is insufficient and can lead to recurrent instability. Thus, the combination of extra- and intra-articular ACL ligament reconstruction is ideal. Having studied under MacIntosh and having learned this procedure directly from him, it was natural for me to think about its application in the CFD cruciate-deficient knee. I have modified this procedure slightly to adapt it to the skeletally immature knee. In my experience, it can now be safely done as young as 2 years of age.
>
> To prevent the tibia from rotating externally, which leads to subluxation of the patella and of the tibia on the femur posteriorly, a medial extra-articular ligament can be created using the anterior half of the fascia lata. This creates a strap going around the medial tibia tethering it to the medial distal femur. This is the opposite direction of the extra-articular ligament created with the posterior half of the fascia lata, which is described in the next step. This lateral extra-articular ligament was described by Dr. David MacIntosh for ACL reconstruction. In his honor and memory (he was one of my professors and mentors in Toronto in 1985) and in recognition of his idea of a lateral extra-articular ligament, I have referred to the medial extra-articular ligament procedure as the reverse MacIntosh or extra-articular PCL procedure.
>
> With more than 20-year follow-up on some of these, I noticed that the congenitally absent intercondylar notch in some cases pinches the ligament and eventually tears or attenuates it. As such I now combine the intra-articular ACL procedure with an open notchplasty through a small medial parapatellar tendon incision.

The knee in CFD may range from a normal, stable, normal morphology knee to a contracted, unstable, deformed, or even fused joint. The most common deformity of the knee is valgus, which is usually nonprogressive but tends to recur even after hemiepiphysiodesis treatment. Due to hypoplasia of the lateral femoral condyle, patients with CFD often have a variable degree of anteroposterior and rotatory instability of the knee related to absent or hypoplastic cruciate ligaments. Manner et al. related the radiographic appearance of the tibial spines to the degree of hypoplasia of the ACL [34].

The patella is usually hypoplastic and may maltrack laterally, but may also present with dislocation in flexion or have a fixed lateral dislocation. Finally, many cases of CFD have a fixed flexion deformity of the knee.

Isolated anteroposterior(AP) instability is not necessarily an indication of knee ligament reconstructive surgery in children with CFD. However, AP ligamentous instability with no endpoint on anterior and posterior drawer tests will usually become symptomatic as the child gets older and contribute to the risk of knee subluxation with future lengthening [68]. If the child is going to undergo a SUPERhip procedure prior to lengthening, the fascia lata can be used to reconstruct the knee ligaments. In some children, there is a catching, locking, or clunk sensation in the knee when going from extension to flexion. It may be painful and require a trick motion to release it. This is due to contracture of the iliotibial band, combined with aplasia of the ACL causing the femoral condyles to catch on or roll over the meniscus. In more severe cases, the tibia actually subluxates or dislocates anteriorly on the femur and reduces at about 30° of flexion. In older patients, the posterior aspect of the tibia may be rounded, contributing to anterior dislocation of the tibia on the femur. It is not clear whether this is a secondary change due to chronic dislocation or a primary deformity, since the tibia is not ossified posteriorly in infancy.

Patellar hypoplasia and instability are also very common. The patella frequently maltracks laterally with progressive knee flexion. In some cases, the patella may dislocate with knee flexion. This is due to a combination of factors: valgus distal femur, hypoplastic or absent patellar groove, contracture of the lateral retinaculum with the tight iliotibial band, and external rotatory instability of the tibia on the femur due to cruciate ligament deficiency, which lateralizes the patellar tendon insertion. These can lead to fixed lateral dislocation as well. Patellar maltracking or subluxation/dislocation should be corrected prior to limb lengthening.

Flexion contracture of the knee is another congenital deformity that may be present and should be corrected before proceeding with limb lengthening. When the femur is very short, the acute angle created by the posterior thigh muscles gives the clinical appearance of a flexion contracture which may be misleading. The definition of a flexion contracture is a flexed angle between the anterior cortical line of the distal femur and proximal tibia in maximum extension. When the contracture is 15° or greater, it should be corrected surgically prior to lengthening. Knee flexion deformity can be due to bony or soft-tissue causes. In CFD, it is usually a capsular contracture. There may be some extra-articular contribution due to contracture of the hamstring muscles and gastrocnemius muscle, but the release of these muscles alone does not correct the flexion deformity, while capsular release without complete hamstring release corrects the contracture. In some cases, there is a true bony flexion of the distal femur that may need to be corrected by osteotomy.

If significant knee instability is present, a SUPERknee procedure should be performed conjointly with the SUPERhip procedure. The SUPERknee procedure should be considered a congenital knee reconstruction used to treat congenital knee AP or rotatory instability and/or patellar maltracking, subluxation or dislocation, and/or knee fixed flexion contracture. Different parts of the procedure can be used depending on the knee pathology present.

SUPERknee Surgical Technique (Figs. 29.14 and 29.15)

1. *Incision and Dissection* (Fig. 29.14a, b). If performed independently, the same mid-lateral straight incision is used (Fig. 29.14a) distal to the tourniquet. The anterior and posterior margins of the fascia lata are incised longitudinally. The fascia lata is transected as proximally as possible (including the fascia overlying the tensor fascia lata muscle belly) and reflected distally until its insertion onto the tibia (Fig. 29.14b, c).
2. *Preparation of the Ligaments* (Fig. 29.14c, d). The fascia lata is split into two longitudinal strips to make two ligaments (Fig. 29.14c). The posterior half is twisted to tubularize the fascia. A Krackow whipstitch [69] is used to run a nonabsorbable suture from Gerdy's tubercle end toward the end of the ligament (Fig. 29.14d).
3. *Femoral Notchplasty* (Fig. 29.14e, f). Before doing an intra-articular ACL procedure, a notchplasty is performed. Most CFD knees lack an intercondylar notch. An incision is made on the medial side of the patellar tendon. A medial parapatellar tendon arthrotomy is made, and the fat pad is excised to expose the notch (Fig. 29.14e). An osteotome or gouge is used to create a round notchplasty under direct vision with care not to cross the distal femoral physis and not to remove the insertion of the PCL (Fig. 29.14f).
4. *Tibial Tunnel* (Fig. 29.14g–i). A wire is passed from the anteromedial to the patellar tendon to midway along the anteroposterior width of the tibia. This wire should be intra-epiphyseal (Fig. 29.14g, h). The tubularized fascia is sized for diameter, and then, an ACL reamer of the correct size is used to drill a hole in the epiphysis (Fig. 29.14i).
5. *Extra-articular PCL Reconstruction* (Fig. 29.14j–m). A medial incision is made to expose the adductor magnus tendon. The sartorius and saphenous nerves are moved out of the way. A tunnel is created under the magnus tendon, and a passing suture is inserted there. The anterior limb of the fascia lata is not tubularized. It is passed under the patellar tendon from lateral to medial (Fig. 29.14j) and then through a medial retinacular tunnel with the knee flexed (Fig. 29.14k, l). The graft is then passed

through a subperiosteal tunnel under the adductor magnus tendon. Finally, it is sutured to itself with absorbable suture with the knee flexed to 90° (Fig. 29.14m). This is also referred to as the reverse MacIntosh repair or extra-articular PCL reconstruction. It acts as a restraint to anterior drawer in knee flexion and a restraint to external rotation. The latter is a PCL function, ergo the name. However, it has properties of both ACL and PCL. This extra-articular ligament was first created and used by the senior author (DP) in 1994.

6. 6. *Extra-articular ACL Reconstruction* (Fig. 29.14n–q). The MacIntosh extra-articular ACL reconstruction is then performed. The lateral collateral ligament (LCL) is identified. The tubularized fascia is passed under the LCL (Fig. 29.14n). Then, a subperiosteal tunnel is made, from anterior and proximal to posterior and distal, over the lateral intramuscular septum of the femur (Fig. 29.14o). A hole is made in the posterior knee joint capsule by inserting a curved clamp from the "over-the-top" position. The fascial graft is passed over the top of the septum and through the subperiosteal tunnel through the hole in the tibia using a suture passer (Fig. 29.14p). The graft is passed and fixed with a bioabsorbable tenodesis screw to secure the graft, while the knee is held in full extension

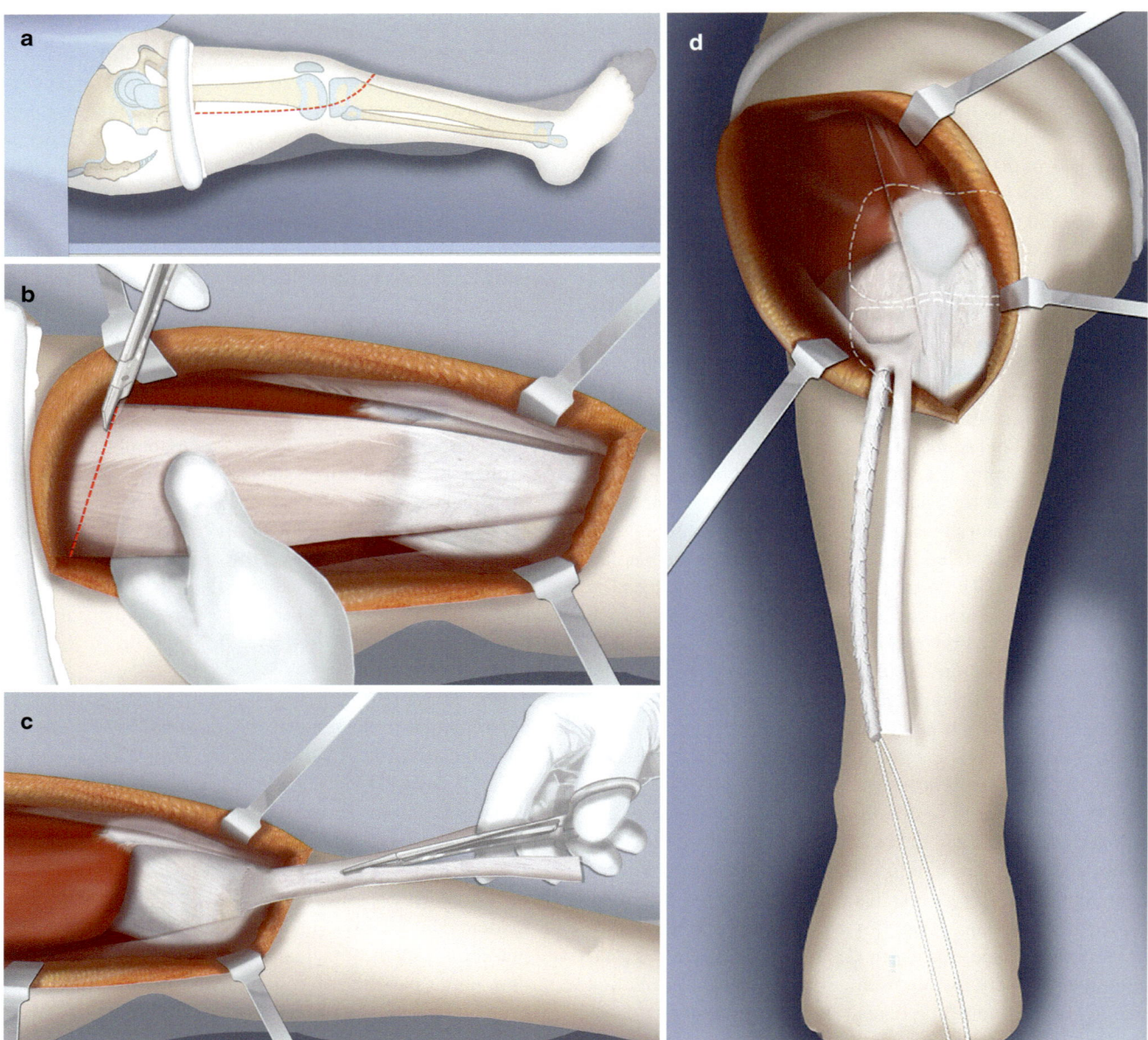

Fig. 29.14 (a–s) SUPERknee procedure (follow text for steps and captions) (Copyright: The Paley Foundation. Reproduced with permission. All rights reserved.)

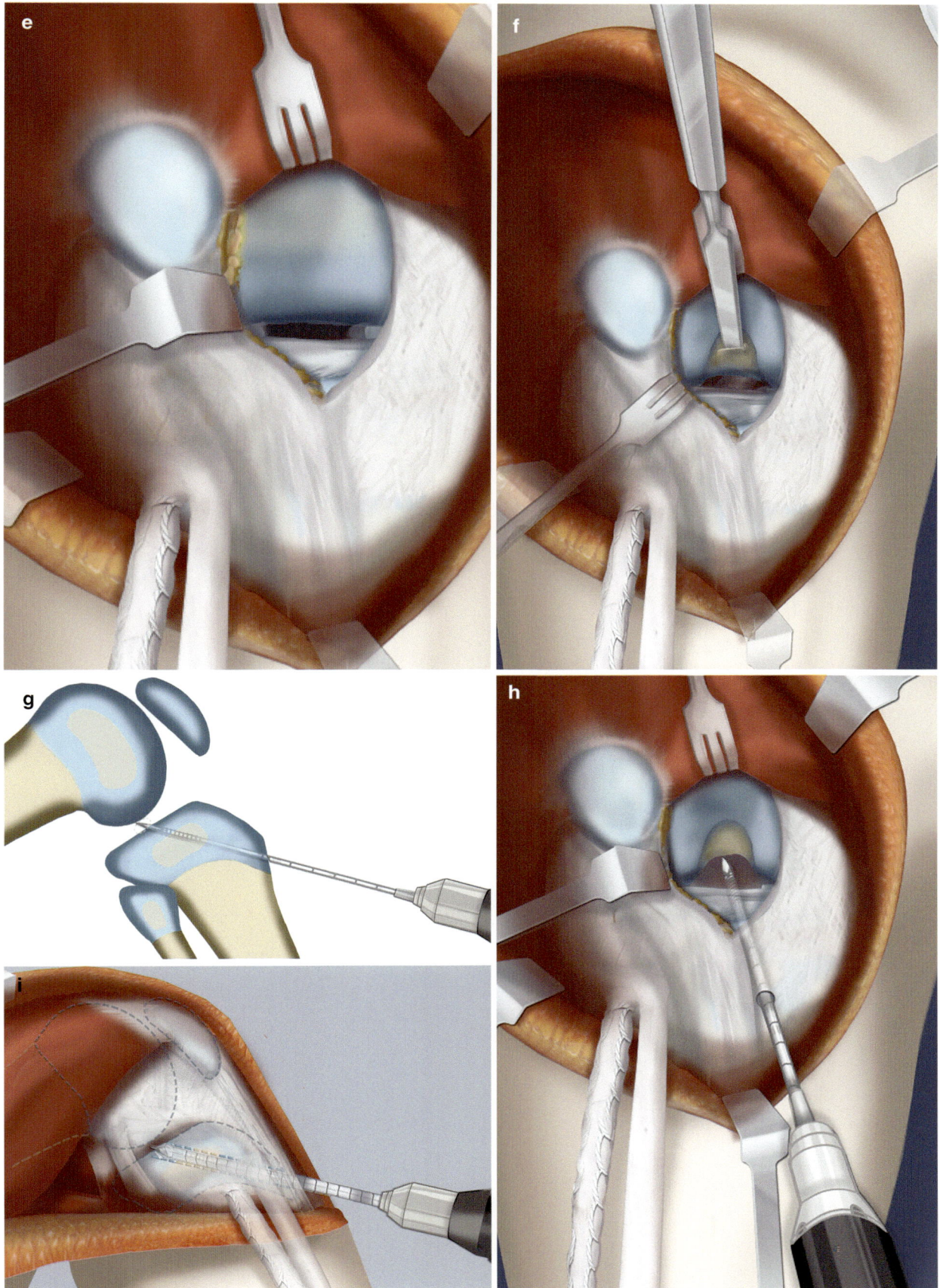

Fig. 29.14 (continued)

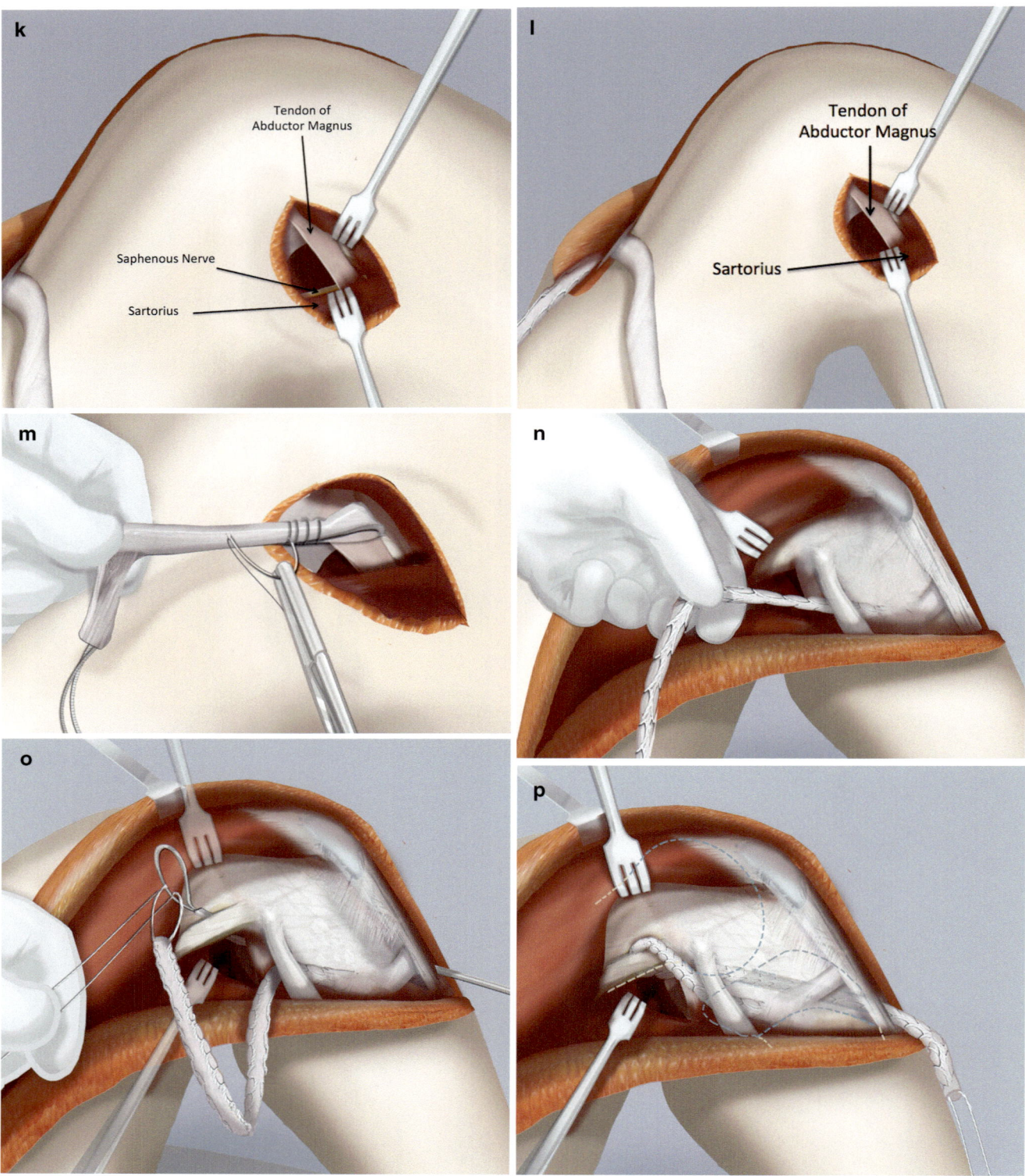

Fig. 29.14 (continued)

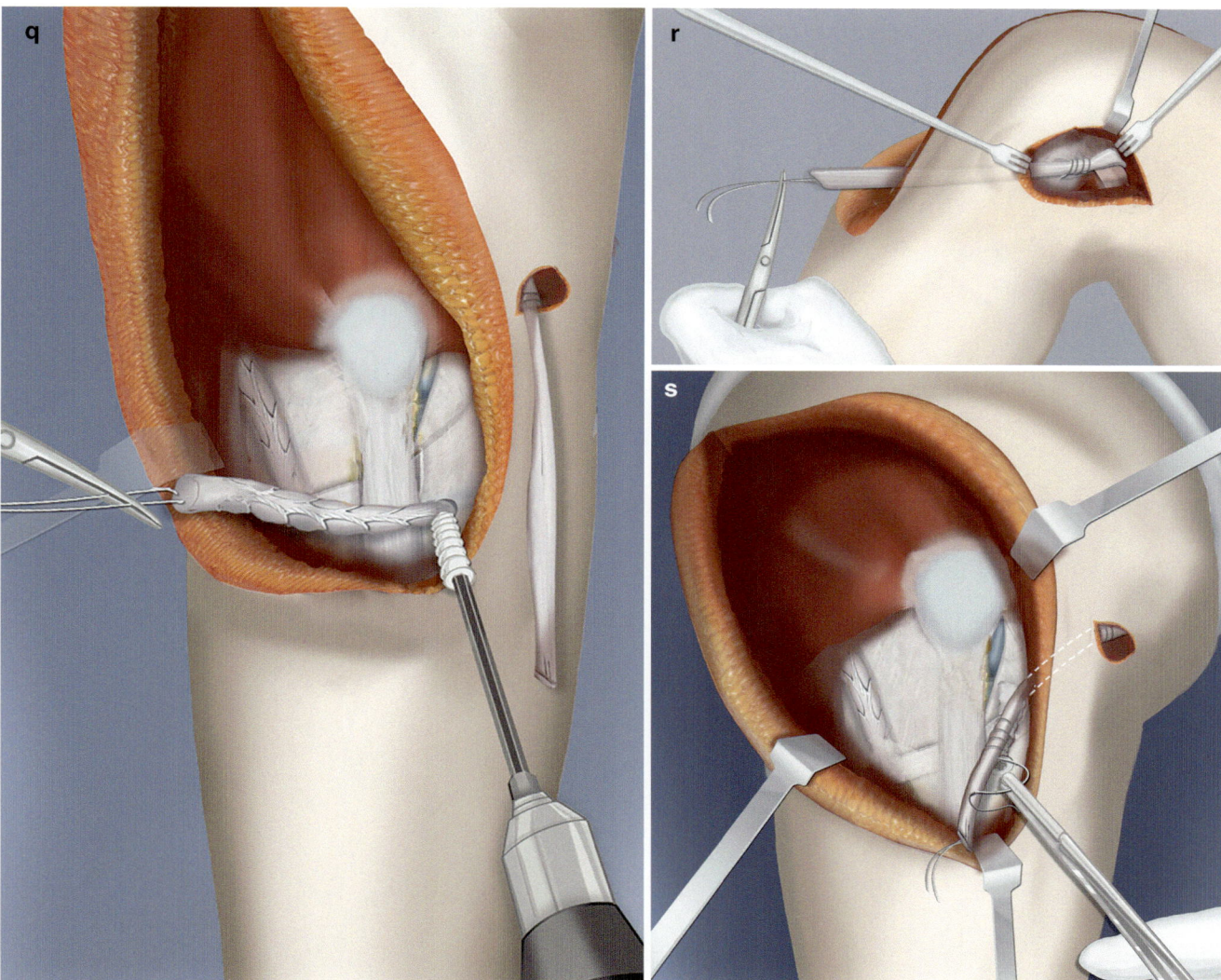

Fig. 29.14 (continued)

(Fig. 29.14q). If only an extra-articular ACL repair is needed, no drill hole or notchplasty is performed and the fascia lata is looped around the intermuscular septum and back to itself.

7. *Secure the Ends of the Ligaments* (Fig. 29.14r, s). Finally, the medial fascial graft is brought overtop the retinaculum (Fig. 29.14r) and sutured to the intra-articular ACL end of the lateral graft (Fig. 29.14s). This secures both grafts to each other (belt and suspenders).
8. *Intra-Articular PCL Reconstruction (not commonly needed)* (Fig. 29.15a–f). The peroneal nerve is identified, decompressed, and protected. The lateral head of the gastrocnemius muscle is then released from the femur. The posterior aspect of the proximal tibial epiphysis is identified as the midline. An anterior-to-posterior drill hole is made through the epiphysis from Gerdy's tubercle to the center of the proximal tibial epiphysis posteriorly (Fig. 29.15a). The fascia lata graft is passed from anterior to posterior, exiting near the midline posteriorly (Fig. 29.15b). Another drill hole that passes through the medial distal femoral epiphysis from anteromedial to posterolateral is made (Fig. 29.15c). The ligamentized fascia lata is pulled through the posterior capsule and into the notch and into the medial femoral epiphyseal tunnel using its leading suture (Fig. 29.15d). It is fixed in place in the femur with a bioabsorbable tenodesis screw after tensioning in flexion (Fig. 29.15e). If there is sufficient length of the graft, it can be brought under the medial retinaculum to the medial parapatellar region and sutured to the end of the intra-articular ACL (Fig. 29.15f). This adds an extra-articular PCL to the intra-articular PCL using one graft.

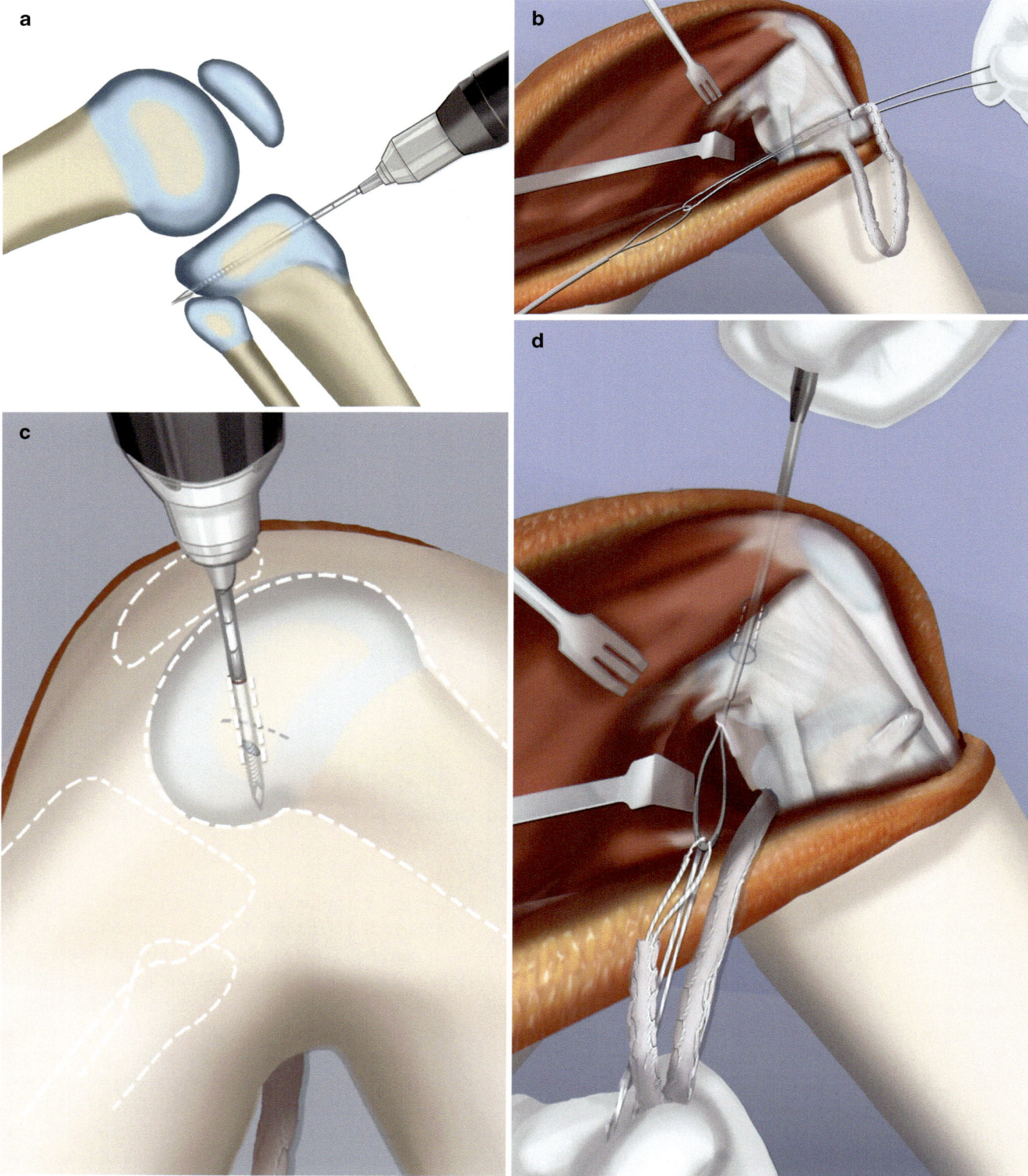

Fig. 29.15 (**a–f**) SUPERknee intra-articular PCL (follow text for steps and captions) (Copyright: The Paley Foundation. Reproduced with permission. All rights reserved.)

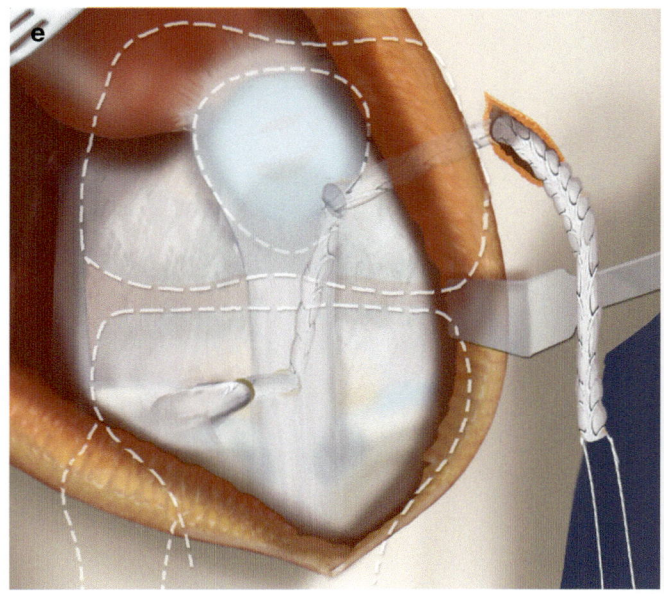
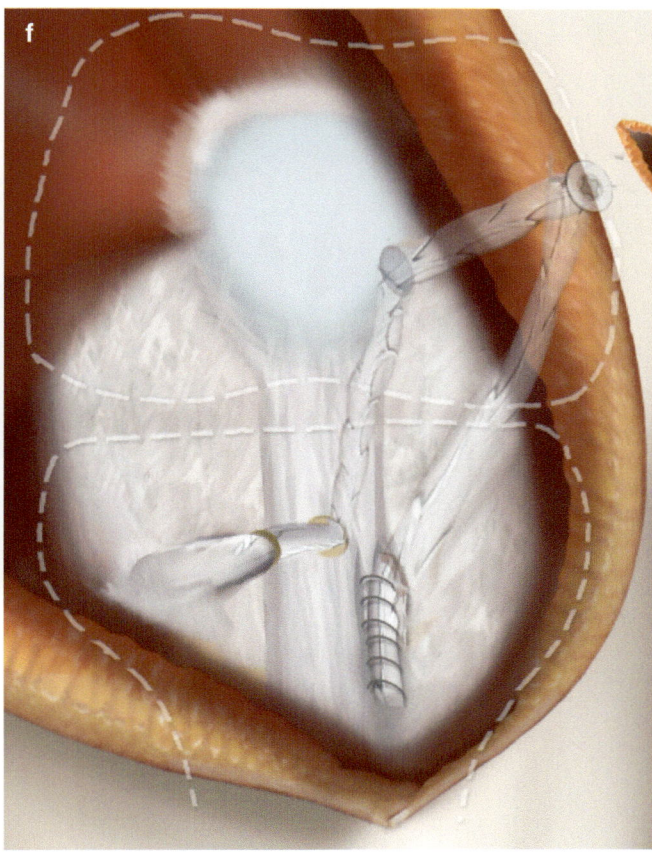

Fig. 29.15 (continued)

Patellar Realignment Surgical Techniques (Fig. 29.16)

Patellar instability can manifest as maltracking, subluxation, or dislocation. The thumb-in-notch sign is often present (ability to place a thumb into the intercondylar notch with the knee in flexion. Normally, the patella covers the notch and makes this impossible). Lengthening in the face of patellar maltracking, instability or dislocation will lead to worsening of the condition and can convert maltracking or subluxation to frank dislocation. Therefore, this must be recognized in advance of lengthening and procedures to realign the patella performed as preparatory procedures to lengthening. Patellar realignment procedures can be combined with other knee procedures such as ligament reconstruction as part of the SUPERknee procedure.

Surgery for maltracking only (Grammont procedure) (Fig. 29.16):

1. *Lateral Patellar Release* (Fig. 29.16a). A lateral release of the knee capsule, leaving the synovium intact, is performed if the patella is maltracking. The lateral release is extended distally to the lateral aspect of the patellar tendon.
2. *Grammont Procedure* (Fig. 29.16b, c). If the patella is subluxated (thumb-in-notch sign present), the patellar tendon is also sharply elevated off of the tibial apophysis with a strip of distal periosteum. (Grammont procedure [61]: pediatric equivalent of the Elmslie-Trillat procedure). The patellar tendon can be reattached more medially (Fig. 29.16c). A medial plication can also be added for additional stability.

Surgery for congenital patellar dislocation (modified Langenskiöld procedure) (Fig. 29.17):

1. *Capsular Separation* (Fig. 29.17a–d). The capsule is incised and separated from the patella and synovium both medially and laterally (Fig. 29.17a). On the medial side, the two layers are separated all the way to the medial gutter (Fig. 29.17b). The medial capsule is cut transversely at

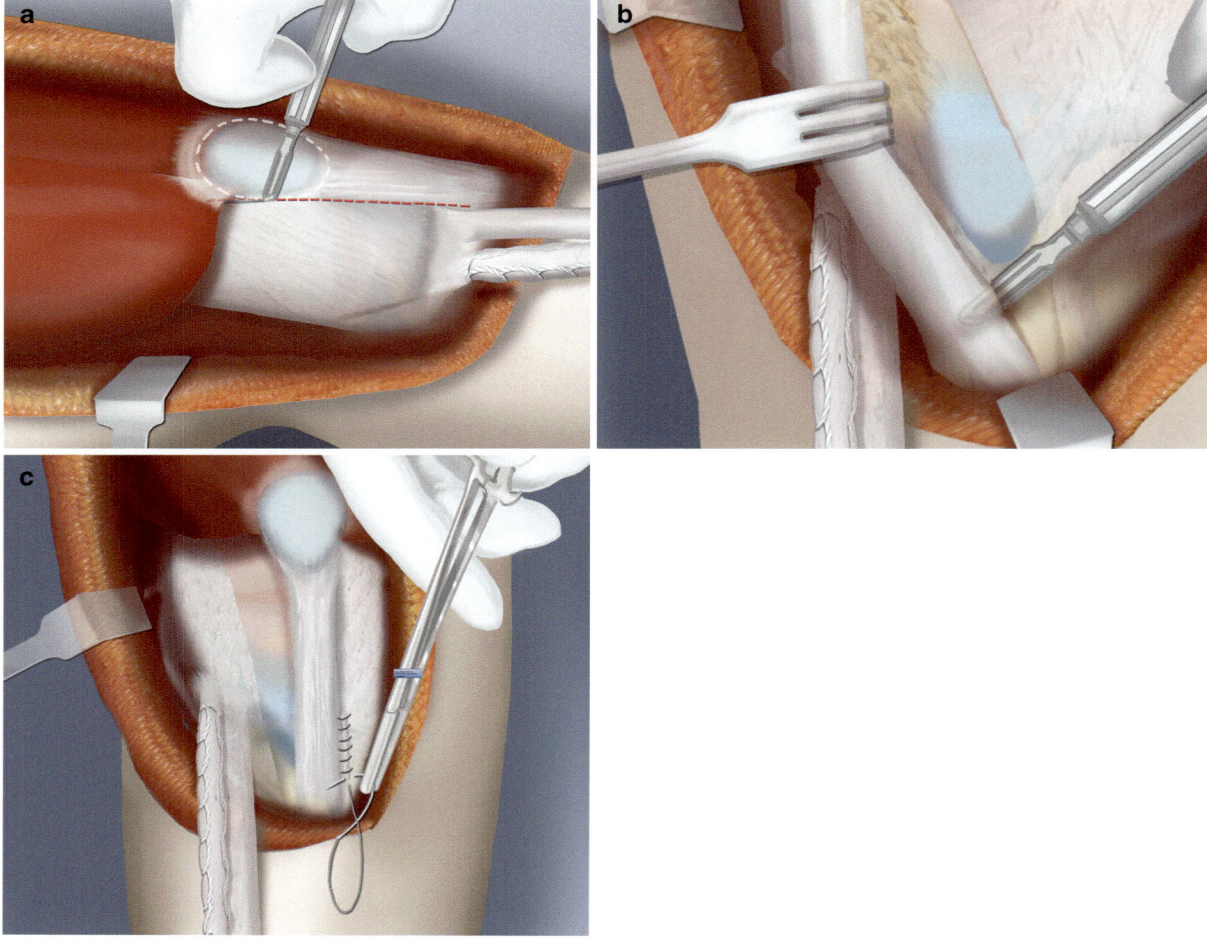

Fig. 29.16 (a–c) Grammont procedure for the treatment of patellar maltracking (follow text for steps and captions) (Copyright: The Paley Foundation. Reproduced with permission. All rights reserved.)

its distal end. The patellar tendon and the quadriceps are also separated from the synovium distally and proximally, respectively (Fig. 29.17c, d).

2. *Patellar Separation from Synovium* (Fig. 29.17 e–g). The synovium is now incised circumferentially around the patella, separating the patella from the synovium completely (Fig. 29.17e). The quadriceps tendon is left attached to the patella proximally, and the patellar tendon remains attached to the patella distally. The synovium is separated from these structures, leaving a patella-sized hole in it (Fig. 29.17f), which is sutured closed in a longitudinal direction (Fig. 29.17 g). This leaves the patella temporarily as an extra-articular structure.

3. *Patellar Tendon Mobilization* (Fig. 29.17h). The patellar tendon is elevated from the apophysis by sharp dissection after circumscribing a medial and lateral incision extending distally into periosteum (Grammont procedure). If the patient is skeletally mature, a tibial tubercle osteotomy can be performed in place of the Grammont. After the tendon is elevated, it is shifted medially at least a centimeter.

4. *Patellar Reimplantation into Synovium* (Fig. 29.17i–k). A new central incision in the synovium should be made. The level of the patella with the knee in extension is marked (Fig. 29.17j). A longitudinal incision is made in the synovium. The adhesions in the suprapatellar pouch are released (Fig. 29.17j). The center of the patella is inserted into this new hole, and the synovium is sutured to the patella circumferentially (Fig. 29.17k).

5. *Medial Capsular Advancement* (Fig. 29.17l–n). The medial capsule with the vastus medialis is now advanced over the top of the patella and stitched to its lateral border with the knee in flexion (Fig. 29.17l). The knee should be taken through a range of motion to ensure that the patella does not medially dislocate, as this reduction can be over-

powering. The tension of the vastus medialis can be adjusted to maintain central tracking of the patella. The lateral capsule is left open. If the reverse MacIntosh procedure is used, the extra-articular ligament reconstruction should not be fixed in place until after the Langenskiöld repair is completed (Fig. 29.17m, n).

Posterior Capsule Release of Knee Surgical Technique (Fig. 29.18)

A knee flexion deformity >15 after shortening of the femur can be treated by posterior capsular release. This is often done in combination with a SUPERhip procedure or one of the knee reconstruction procedures described above. The posterior capsule must be released prior to ligamentous reconstruction of the knee.

1. *Peroneal Nerve Decompression*(Fig. 29.18a, b). To avoid direct surgical and indirect stretch injury, the common peroneal nerve should be identified and decompressed at the neck of the fibula (first tunnel) (Fig. 29.18a) and the deep peroneal nerve decompressed at the intermuscular septum between the anterior and lateral compartments (second tunnel) (Fig. 29.18b).

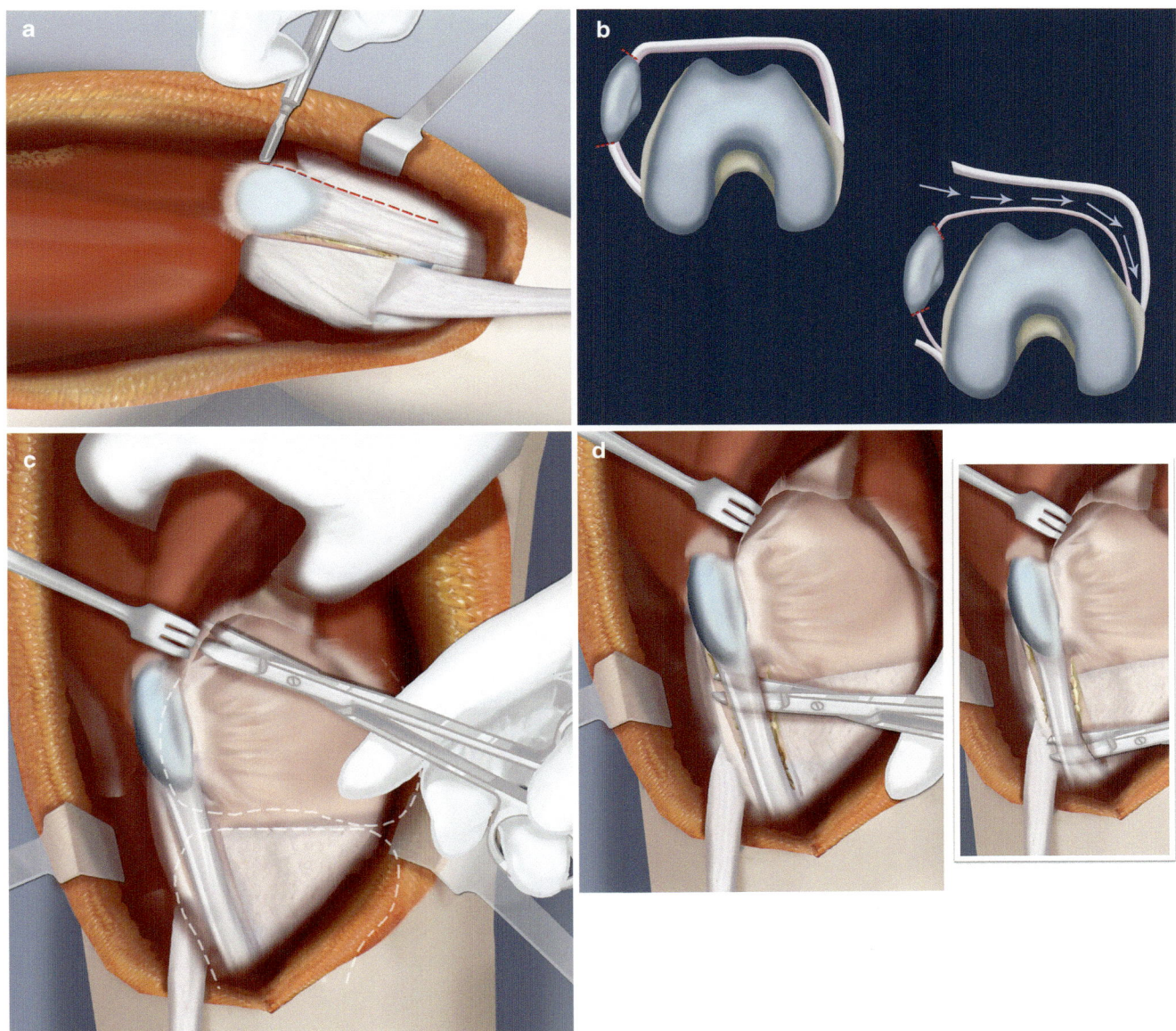

Fig. 29.17 (a–n) Treatment of patellar dislocation with modified Langenskiöld (follow text for steps and captions) (Copyright: The Paley Foundation. Reproduced with permission. All rights reserved.)

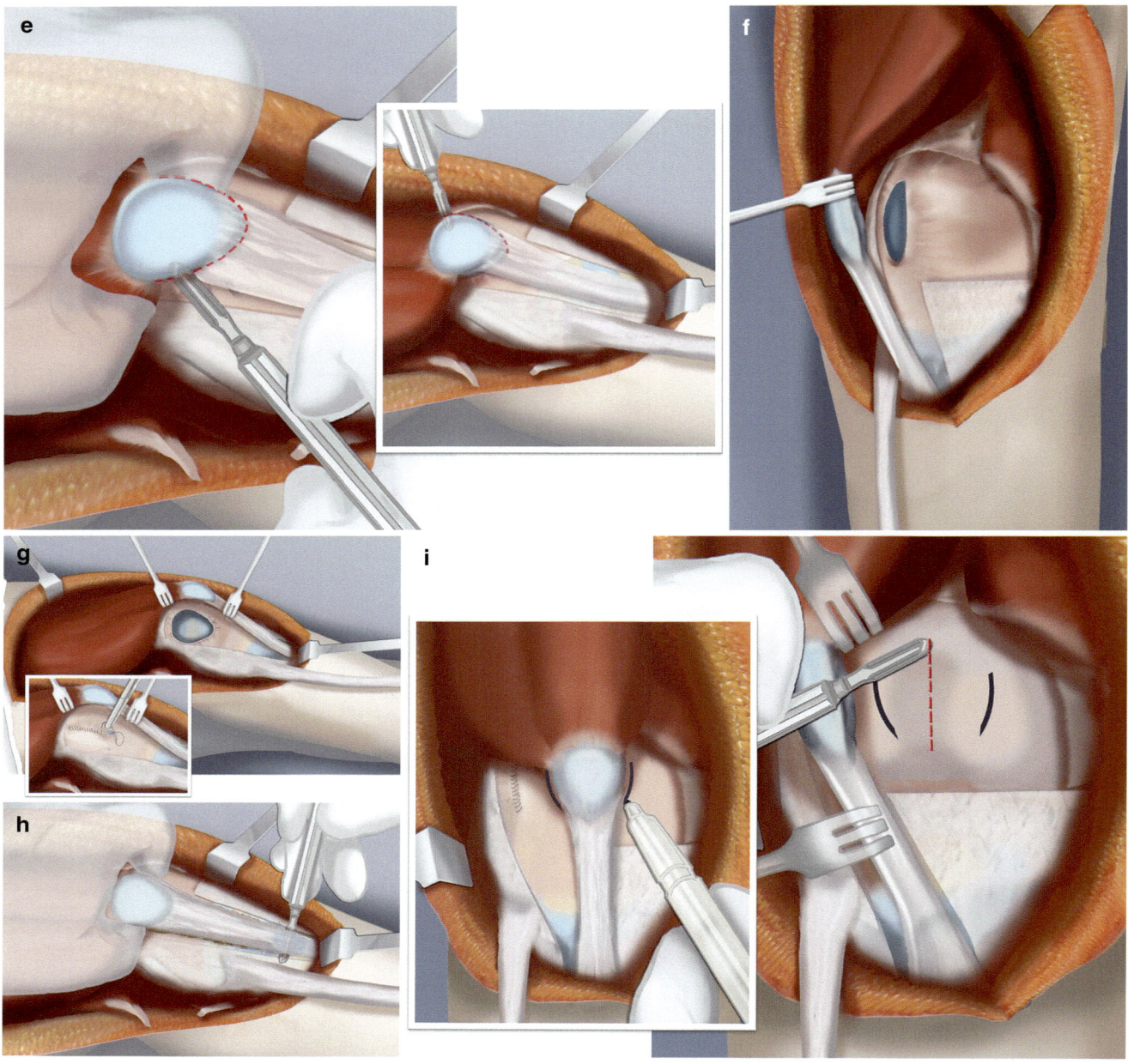

Fig. 29.17 (continued)

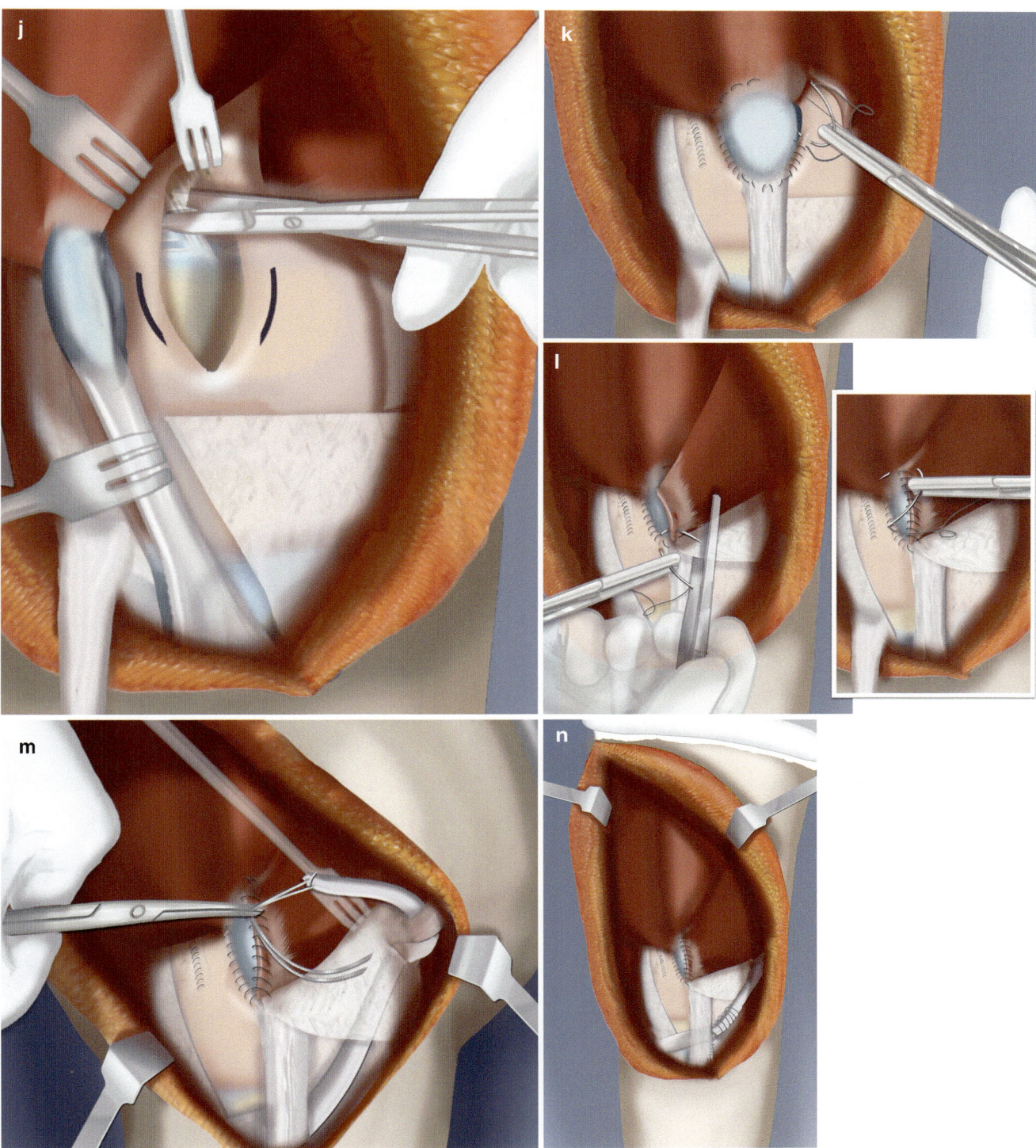

Fig. 29.17 (continued)

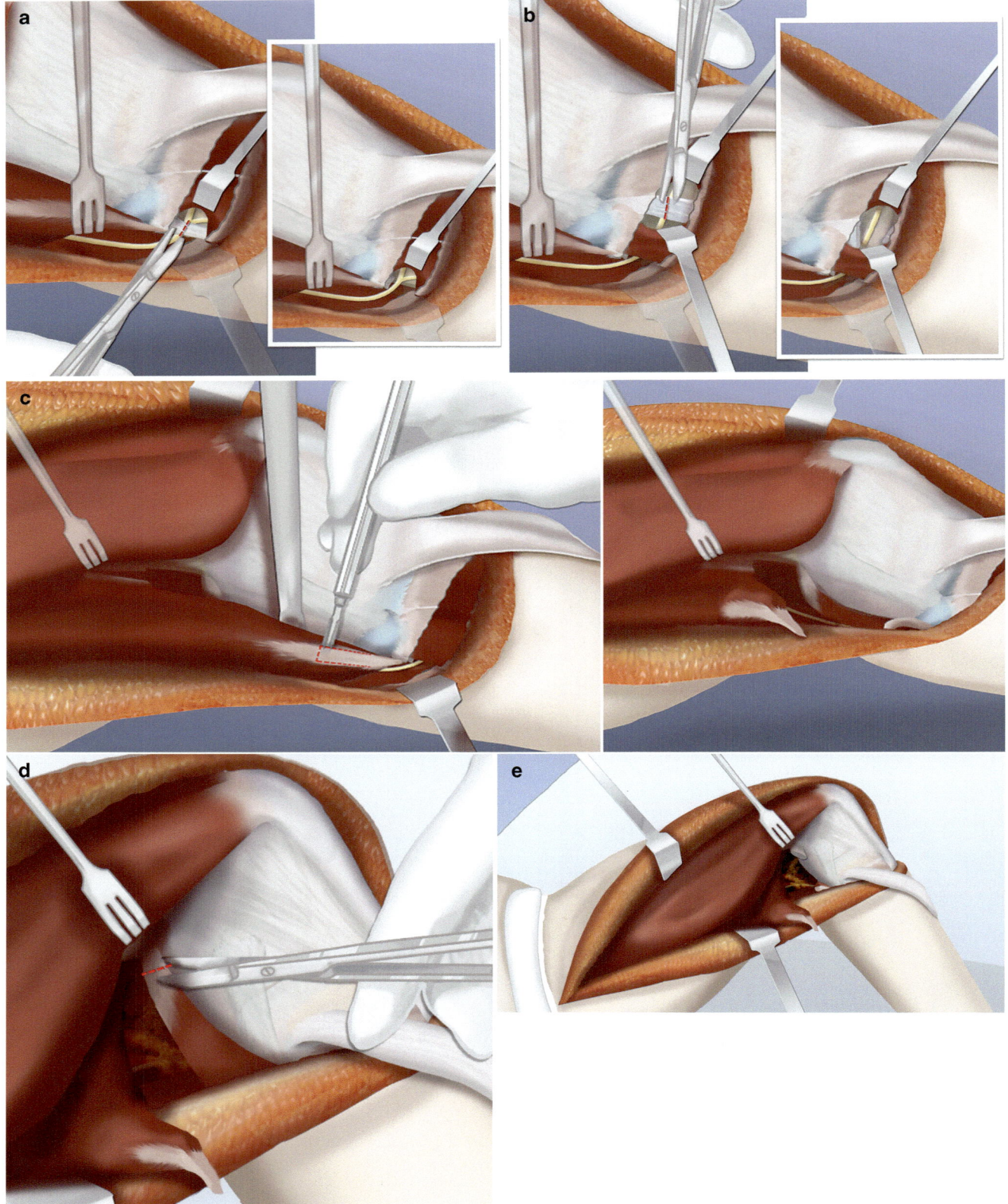

Fig. 29.18 (a–m) Posterior capsulotomy of the knee (follow text for steps and captions) (Copyright: The Paley Foundation. Reproduced with permission. All rights reserved.)

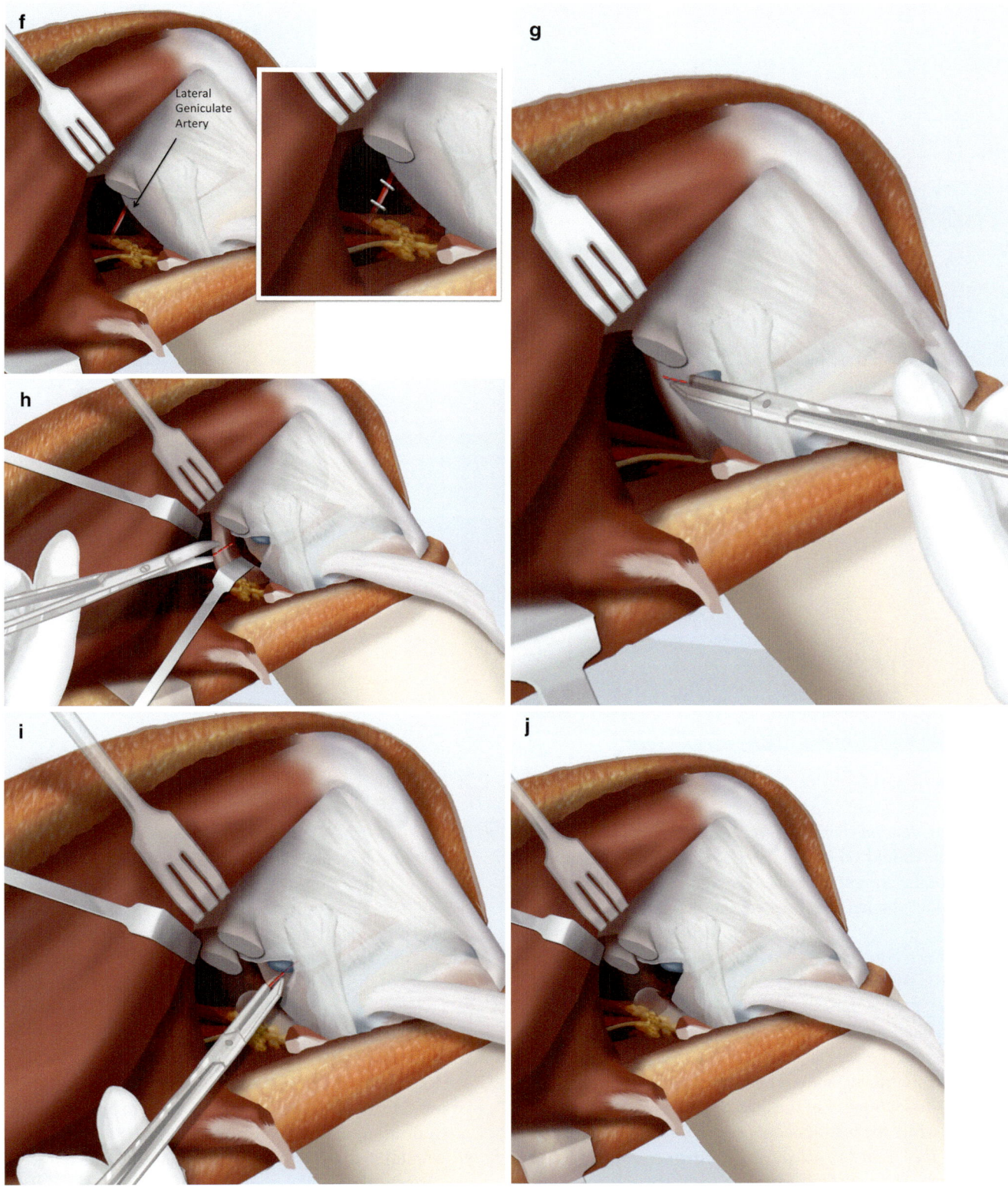

Fig. 29.18 (continued)

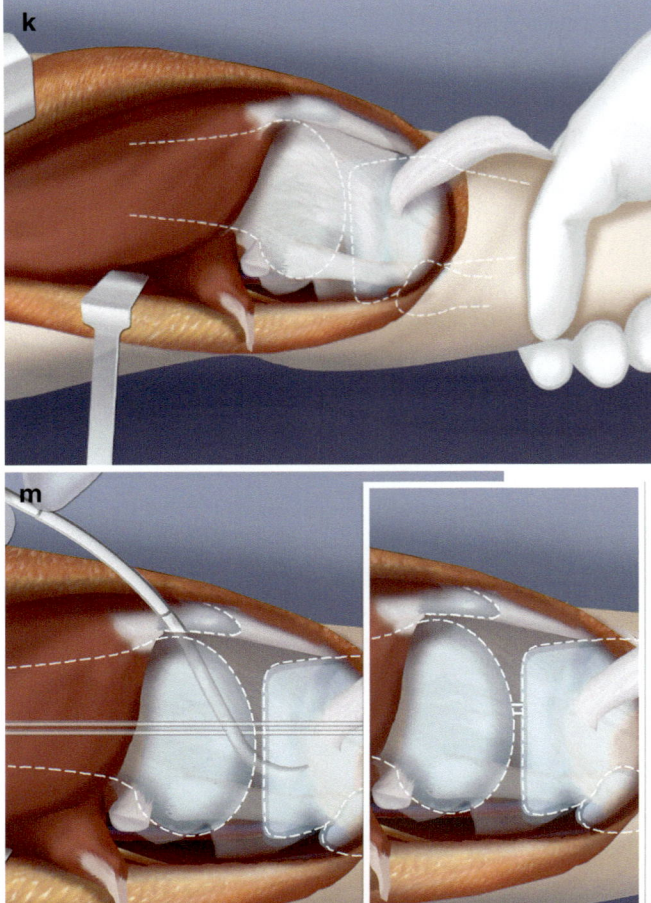

Fig. 29.18 (continued)

2. *Biceps Tendon Lengthening* (Fig. 29.18c). The biceps tendon should be Z-lengthened. Extend the decompression of the common peroneal nerve under the biceps muscle. With the nerve protected and visualized, Z-lengthen the biceps muscle and tendon. In congenital cases, there is little tendon and mostly muscle. The biceps muscle consists of two parts: the short and long heads. To avoid damage to this muscle, the short head should be dissected off of the periosteum of the femur. Try and keep as much of the muscle together and reflect this part proximally. Isolate as much of the central tendon as possible with sharp dissection off of the muscle and reflect this part distally, while the rest remains proximal (Fig. 29.18c).

3. *Cut the Lateral Head of Gastrocnemius Tendon* (Fig. 29.18d, e). The lateral head of the gastrocnemius should be released from the femur (Fig. 29.18d). It has a very broad insertion of muscle and tendon. This is the doorway to the posterior knee capsule (Fig. 29.18e)

4. *Exposure to the Posterior Knee Capsule* (Fig. 29.18f). The lateral capsule can now be identified. Dissect the contents of the popliteal fossa away from the posterior capsule. To confirm that it is the posterior capsule, incise it posterolaterally and enter the knee joint. With the knee flexed, the only vascular structures that one should see at the level of the knee joint are the central geniculate artery and vein (Fig. 29.18f). These can be dissected free and cauterized. Care should be taken to make sure that the dissection does not inadvertently go distal to the level of the knee joint. If the dissection is behind the tibia instead of the femur, the anterior tibial vessels may be encountered or injured. The rest of the popliteal soft tissues can be carefully dissected off of the capsule and retracted posteriorly all the way to the medial side.

5. *Cutting of the Posterior Knee Capsule* (Fig. 29.18g). The capsule can be cut under direct vision (Fig. 29.18g). A head lamp may be useful for this part of the procedure.

Once the posterior capsule is open, try and extend the knee joint. If there is still too much resistance, revisit the dissection and make sure the capsular release includes the entire posteromedial capsule.

6. *Cutting the Medial Head of Gastrocnemius Tendon* (Fig. 29.18h). The medial head of the gastrocnemius can now be visualized and cut under direct vision from the lateral side (Fig. 29.18h).
7. *Cutting the Posteromedial Capsule* (Fig. 29.18i). The posteromedial capsule is dissected free from the popliteal fossa to communicate with the lateral dissection. The posterior capsule can then be cut under direct vision from the lateral side (Fig. 29.18i, j). The knee should now be able to fully extend (Fig. 29.18k). If there is posterior subluxation with full extension, the knee should be reduced using a Hohmann elevator from the front (Fig. 29.18l) and temporarily fixed with either crossed or intramedullary wires to keep it fully reduced for six weeks while the capsule heals (Fig. 29.18m).
8. *Medial Hamstring Release.* If the medial hamstrings are felt to be tight after the capsulotomy, they can be lengthened with a tendon recession through a separate medial incision.

After doing the knee capsular release, the knee is examined for instability. If it is unstable, then the ligamentous reconstruction of the SUPERknee procedure is carried out as described above. If a large flexion contracture is released (>45°), the knee should be temporarily held in extension with k-wires for 6 weeks, as the small size of the leg will make it impossible to maintain the knee extension in a cast (Fig. 29.18m). Femoral shortening may be needed to prevent acute distraction injury to the nerves and vessels (Fig. 29.19). This shortening can be part of a SUPERhip osteotomy of the femur or as an independent femoral osteotomy of the upper femur in conjunction with a capsular release. Physical therapy to regain knee flexion can be started 6 weeks later after the wires are removed.

> **Box 29.9 SUPERknee Tips and Tricks**
> - The stability of the knee cannot be fully assessed until the fascia lata has been released.
> - Take a small portion of biceps fascia and intermuscular septum for a wider graft. If the graft is still narrow, bias the more important posterior limb of the graft to be larger.
> - Send the ACL reamer all the way into the knee to make sure that the tunnel is adequately drilled for passing the ACL graft.

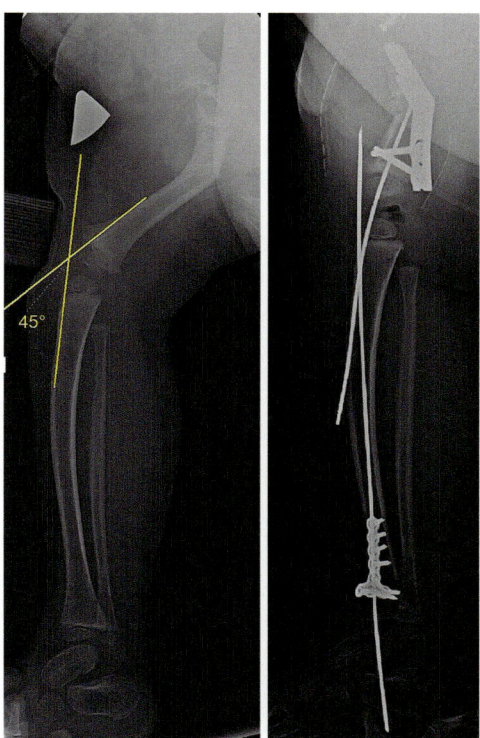

Fig. 29.19 Left: preoperative long lateral X-ray demonstrating a child with CFD type 1a with a knee flexion deformity of 45° as measured by anterior cortical lines (left). Postoperative long lateral radiograph after posterior capsulotomy of the knee in conjunction with SUPERhip and osteotomy of distal tibia (right). Note the temporary arthrodesis wires across the knee. The long wire is also temporarily crossing the ankle. (Copyright: The Paley Foundation. Reproduced with permission. All rights reserved.)

> - Tighten the reverse MacIntosh with the knee in flexion and the MacIntosh graft with the knee in extension.
> - Suture the ends of both limbs of the graft together at the end for additional fixation.
> - When cutting the posterior capsule, do not stray distal to the knee joint line to avoid injury to the anterior tibial vessels

Treatment for Paley Type 2 CFD

Paley type 2 CFD is characterized by the absence of a true femoral neck, having only a fibrous anlage extending from the base of the greater trochanter to the femoral head (Fig. 29.7). There may be a well-formed synovial joint present with a mobile femoral head (type 2a), partially formed synovial joint with a partial fusion of the femoral head to the acetabulum at one spot (type 2b), or an absent or circumferentially fused femoral head (type 2c). The defining anatomic feature that characterizes all three of these is the presence of a greater trochanteric apophysis, which is missing in Paley type 3 CFD. Radiographically, the apophysis can be recognized when the proximal end of the femur appears rounded, while in most Paley type 3 cases, the upper end of the femur appears sharp and pointed. An MRI makes this distinction much more definitive (Fig. 29.20).

There are three lengthening reconstruction approaches for the treatment of Paley type 2: (1) femoral sling procedure with serial lengthening and later pelvic support osteotomy, (2) SUPERhip 2 for selective cases of type 2a CFD, or (3) pelvic support osteotomy

Femoral Sling Surgical Technique (Fig. 29.21)

The femoral sling is indicated when the hip joint cannot be reconstructed due to a lack of femoral neck and an absent or fused femoral head. The proximal femur is proximally migrated and rests posterior to the iliac wing, preventing adduction and extension of the hip (Fig. 29.21a). This proce-

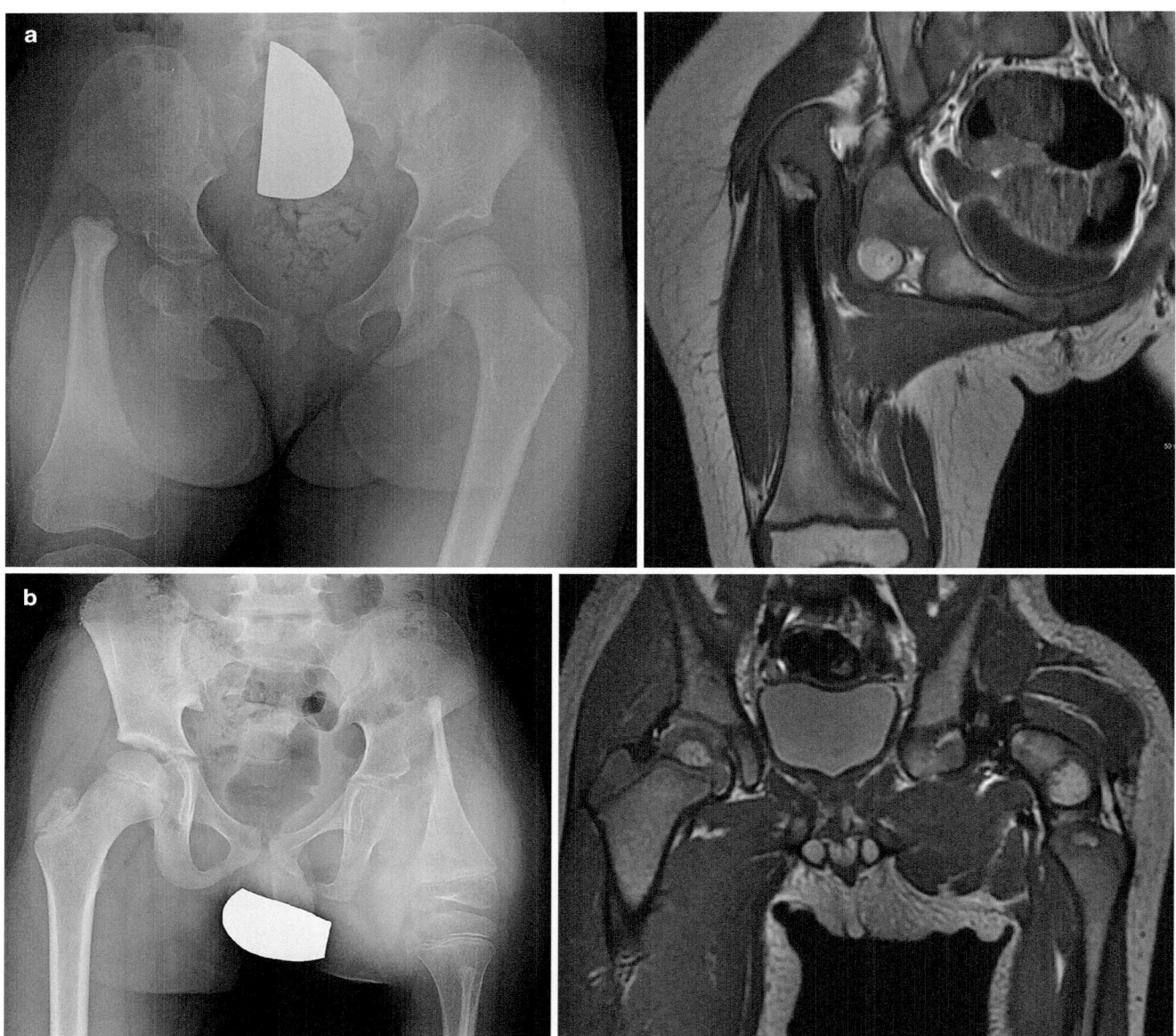

Fig. 29.20 (a) CFD type 2. AP pelvis radiograph showing the rounded appearance of the proximal femur, consistent with the presence of a trochanteric apophysis (left) and coronal MRI that visualizes the trochanteric apophysis with an absent femoral neck (right). (b) CFD type 3. AP pelvis radiograph showing the more pointed or sharp appearance of the upper femur, consistent with the lack of trochanteric apophysis (left) and coronal MRI that shows the absence of the greater trochanter apophysis and femoral neck. The femoral head can be seen in the acetabulum with a posterior fusion to the ischium. (Copyright: The Paley Foundation. Reproduced with permission. All rights reserved.)

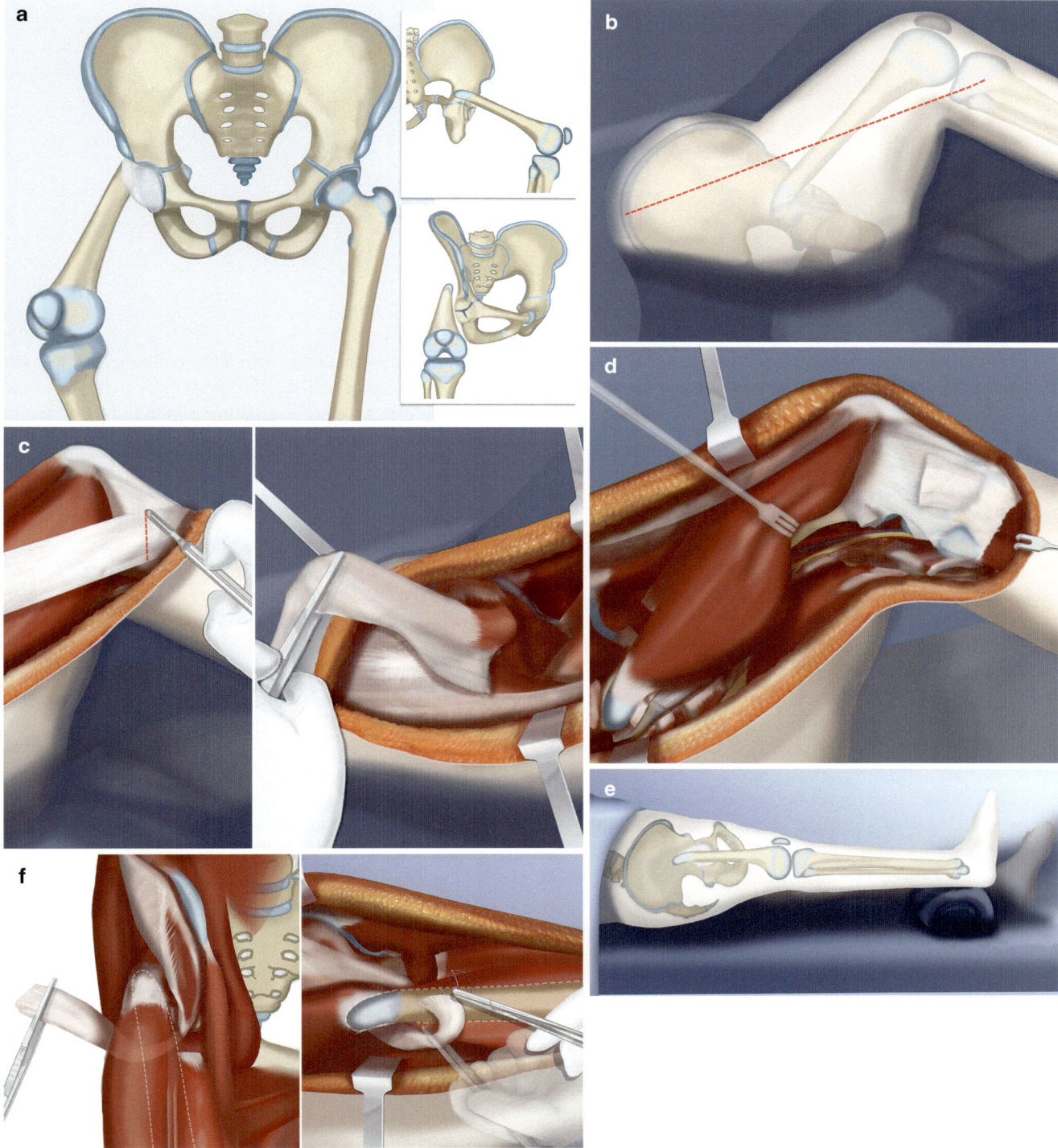

Fig. 29.21 (**a–h**) Femoral sling surgical technique (follow text for steps and captions) (Copyright: The Paley Foundation. Reproduced with permission. All rights reserved.)

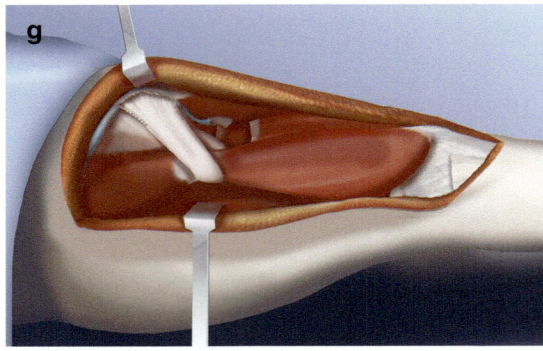 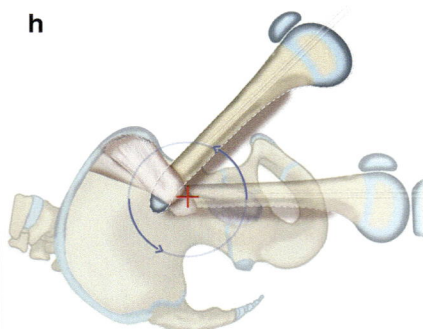

Fig. 29.21 (continued)

dure is most commonly used to treat Paley type 2 CFD; however, for families who wish to undergo lengthening reconstruction in type 3CFD and refuse other options, the sling may be indicated.

1. *Positioning, Prepping, and Draping.* An epidural may be placed by the anesthesia service with a catheter running up the back on the nonoperative side. A Foley catheter is placed and also routed to the nonoperative side. The patient should be moved to the edge and foot of the radiolucent table in a supine position. The ipsilateral arm should be appropriately padded and placed across the patient's chest. No bump is used under the patient. The entire side should be prepped and draped free from the nipple to the toes. The drapes should extend from the mid-buttocks to the scrotal/labial-thigh fold. The lower limb should be completely free of the drapes. A straight lateral incision is marked out from the top of the iliac crest to the tibial tubercle (Fig. 29.21b).
2. *Elevate the Flap.* The anterior thigh flap is elevated, and the fascia lata and ITB are exposed as in SUPERhip 1. The ITB is detached distally at the tibia and reflected proximally (Fig. 29.21c). If there is a contracture of the psoas or rectus femoris, it is released.
3. *Straighten the Knee.* If a knee flexion contracture is present, a posterior capsulotomy as in Fig. 29.18 is performed. The knee flexion contracture is addressed with a decompression of the peroneal nerve, Z-lengthening of the biceps femoris tendon, release gastrocnemius tendons, and a posterior capsulotomy of the knee (Fig. 29.21d). Temporary arthrodesis of the knee, in full extension, should be considered. After releasing the soft-tissue contractures, the leg should lie in full extension. A bump should be placed under the ankle to keep the leg in maximum extension for the femoral sling procedure (Fig. 29.21e).
4. *Create the Sling.* The ITB is passed from medial to lateral and from anterior to posterior around the proximal femur (Fig. 29.21f). The ITB is then tensioned to keep the femur in full extension and the free end of the is sewn to the anterior iliac apophysis, creating a "sling" for the femur (Fig. 29.21g). The new ITB "sling" prevents the proximal femur from returning to its original position stuck behind the pelvis. The sling allows the proximal femur to pivot in the flexion-extension arc as the patient uses their intact quadriceps and hamstrings (Fig. 29.21h).
5. *Closure.* The incision can now be closed. Since there is no fascia lata, the deepest layer is the subcutaneous fat layer. A drain is placed, exiting anterosuperiorly. The drain is secured with a clear adhesive sterile dressing (e.g., Tegaderm, 3M, Minnesota). It is important to close the wound in a fashion that the opposite layers get sutured at the same level.
6. *Lengthening.* Lengthening of the femur with a monolateral rail device that is articulated to the tibia and pelvis may be used to lengthen the femur in the same setting (Fig. 29.22). The surgical technique for monolateral rail lengthening is detailed later in the chapter.

SUPERhip 2 Surgical Technique (Figs. 29.23 and 29.24)

The SUPERhip 2 procedure converts type 2A CFD to type 1A. This procedure is indicated in the setting of a mobile femoral head (type 2a) or a minimally fused femoral head (type 2b), which can be confirmed on MRI.

1. *Incision and Initial Dissection.* Use the same anesthesia, preparation, positioning, and incision as for the SUPERhip procedure described previously. Create the same subcutaneous flap and exposure and resection of the fascia lata and iliotibial band. Release the rectus femoris tendon and decompress the femoral nerve as previously described.
2. *Rectus Tendon and Femoral Nerve.* Identify and dissect free the femoral nerve and release the rectus femoris tendon, but do not cut the psoas tendon. (Fig. 29.23a).

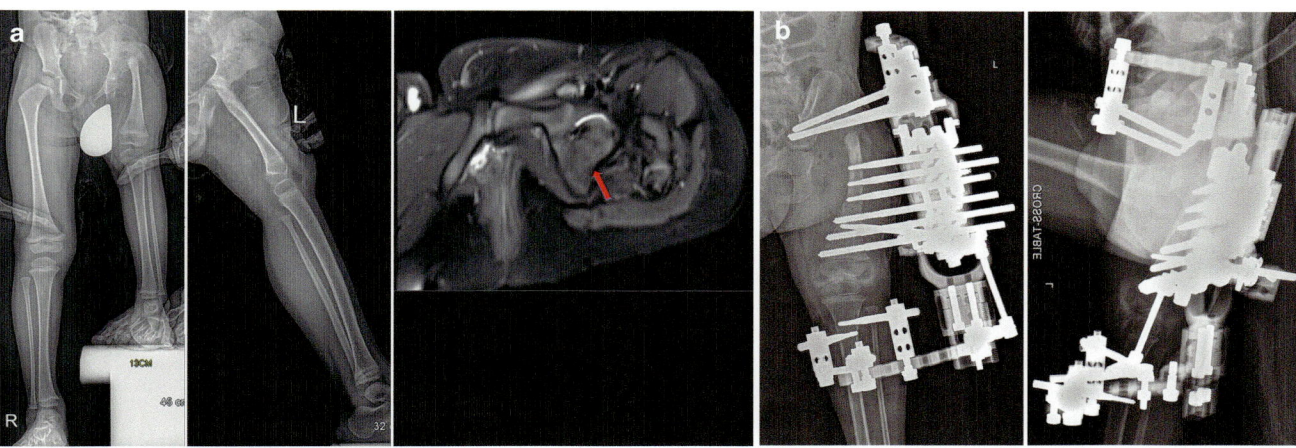

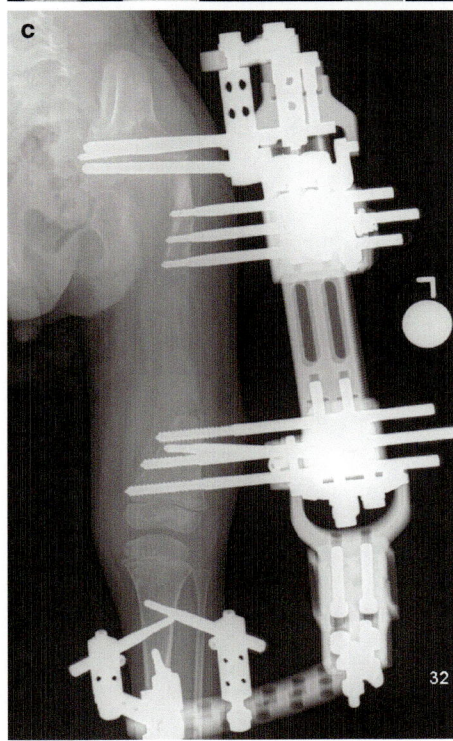

Fig. 29.22 (a) Preoperative EL (left) and long lateral (middle) radiographs of a 3-year-old boy with type 2b CFD. An axial MRI (right) shows the fused femoral head and intact trochanteric apophysis. (b) Immediate postoperative AP and lateral X-rays after he underwent a sling procedure and application of an external fixator for femoral lengthening. Note the full hip extension on the lateral. The monolateral fixator is bridged to the pelvis and to the tibia with hinges to allow motion. (c) AP X-ray after completing 8 cm of femoral lengthening (Copyright: The Paley Foundation. Reproduced with permission. All rights reserved.)

3. *Anterior Exposure*. Separate the vastus muscles from the hip abductors anteriorly to help expose the anterior hip capsule. The vastus muscle insertion is shaped like a Gothic arch (Fig. 29.23b).
4. *Gluteus Maximus and Abductor Muscle Slide*. Release the gluteus maximus tendon off of the femur, reflect this muscle posteriorly, split the iliac apophysis, and allow the abductors to slide distally (Fig. 29.23c).
5. *Sciatic Nerve Decompression and Release of External Rotators*. Identify and free the sciatic nerve. Release all of the external rotators off of the back of the femur. Also, release the piriformis tendon off of the greater trochanter (Fig. 29.23d)
6. *Psoas Tenotomy*. Follow the psoas tendon to its insertion on the back of the femur. Release this tendon off of the femur. Try and preserve the medial femoral circumflex vessel and its ascending branch. Tag the psoas tendon for later transfer (Fig. 29.23e).
7. *Femoral Neck Fibrous Anlage Release*. Identify the femoral neck anlage, which travels from the femoral head to

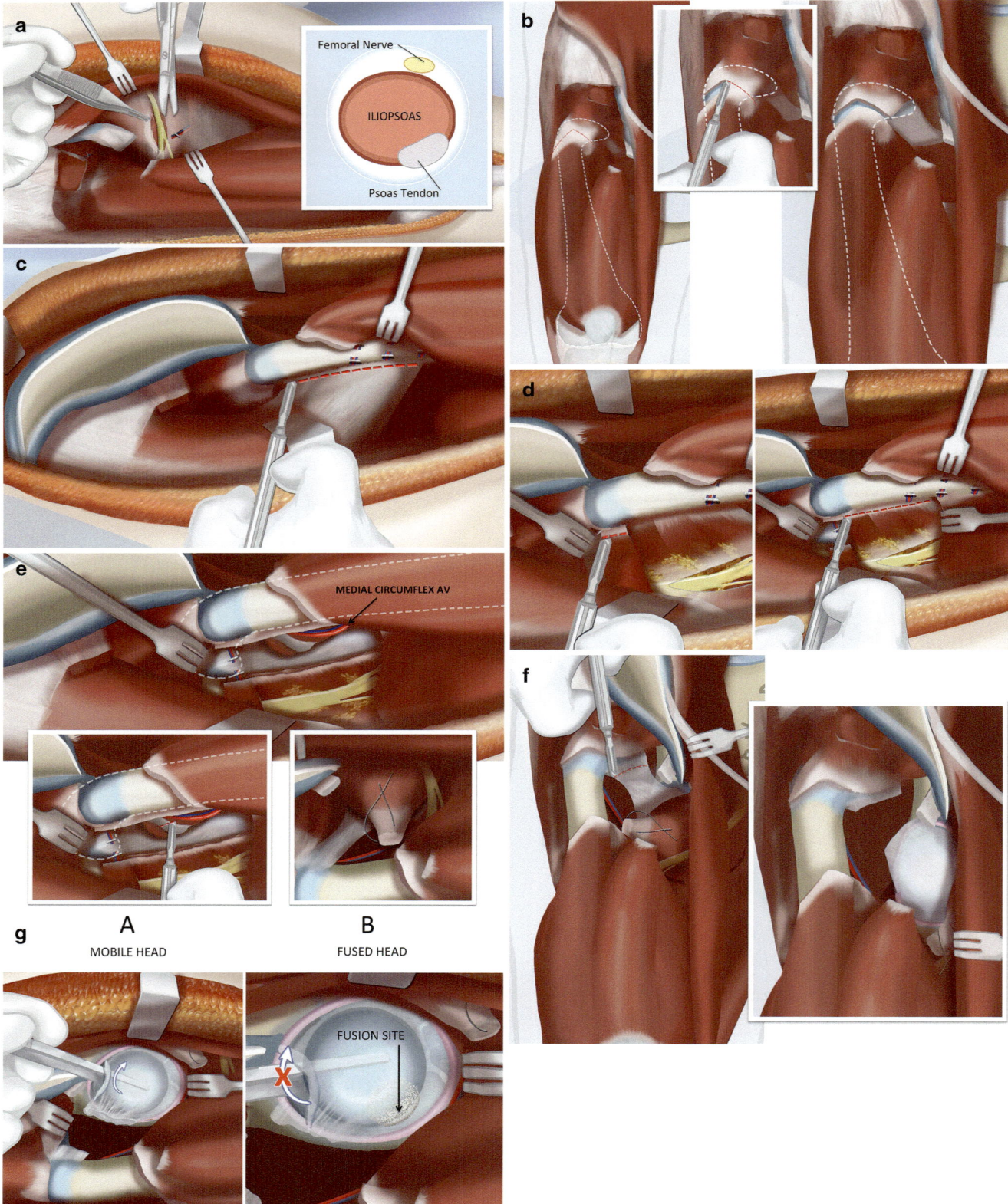

Fig. 29.23 (**a–s**) SUPERhip two surgical techniques (follow text for steps and captions) (Copyright: The Paley Foundation. Reproduced with permission. All rights reserved.)

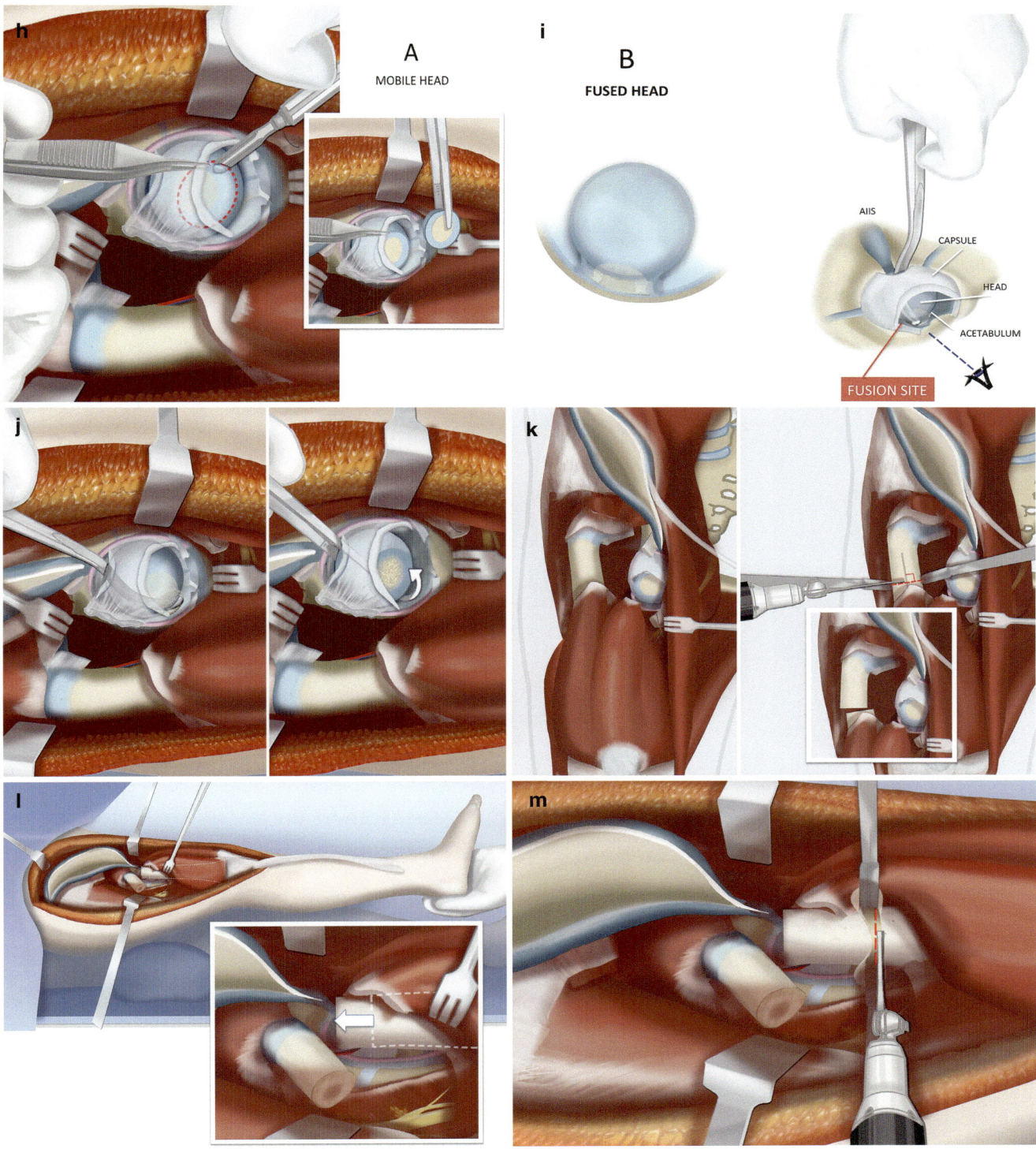

Fig. 29.23 (continued)

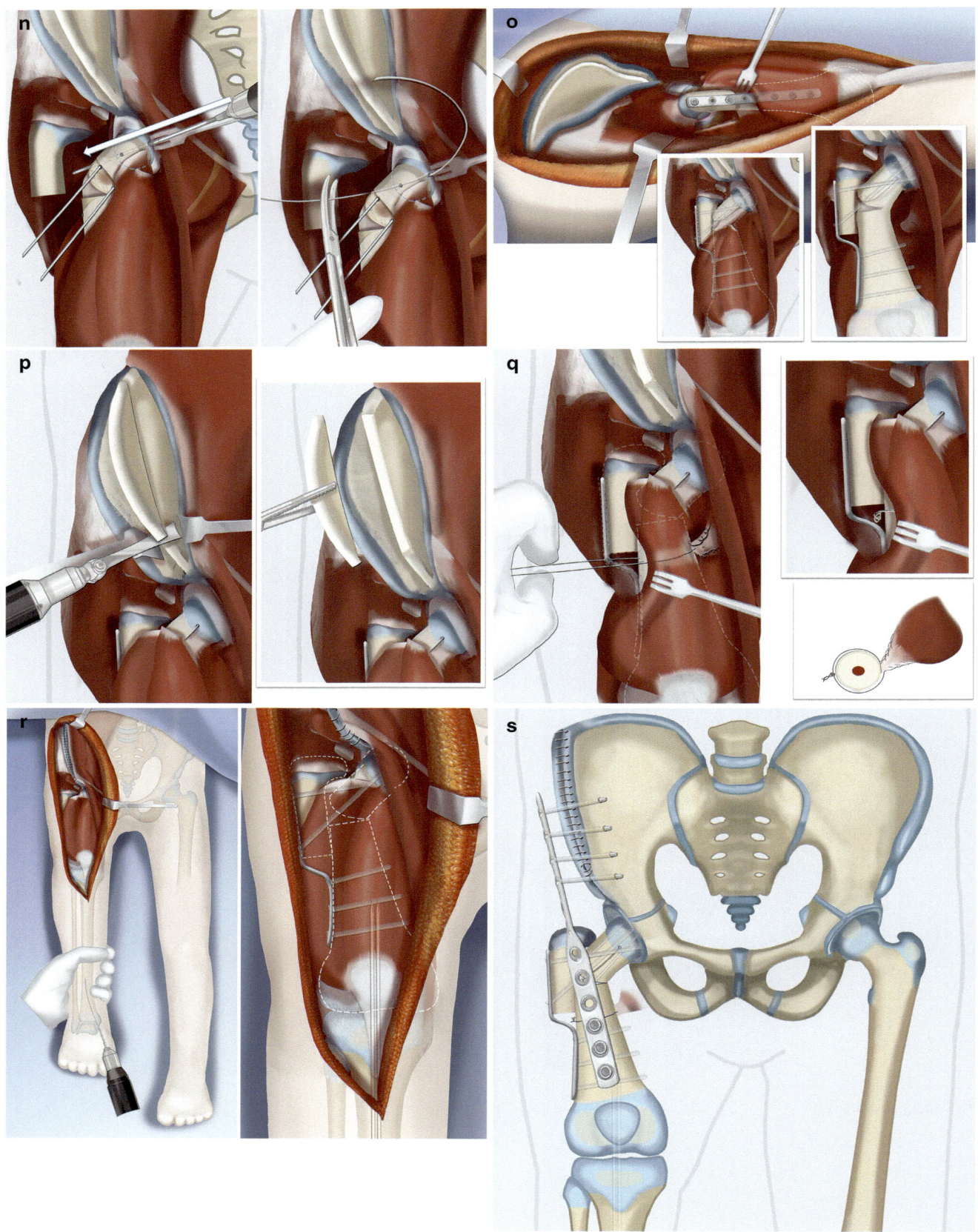

Fig. 29.23 (continued)

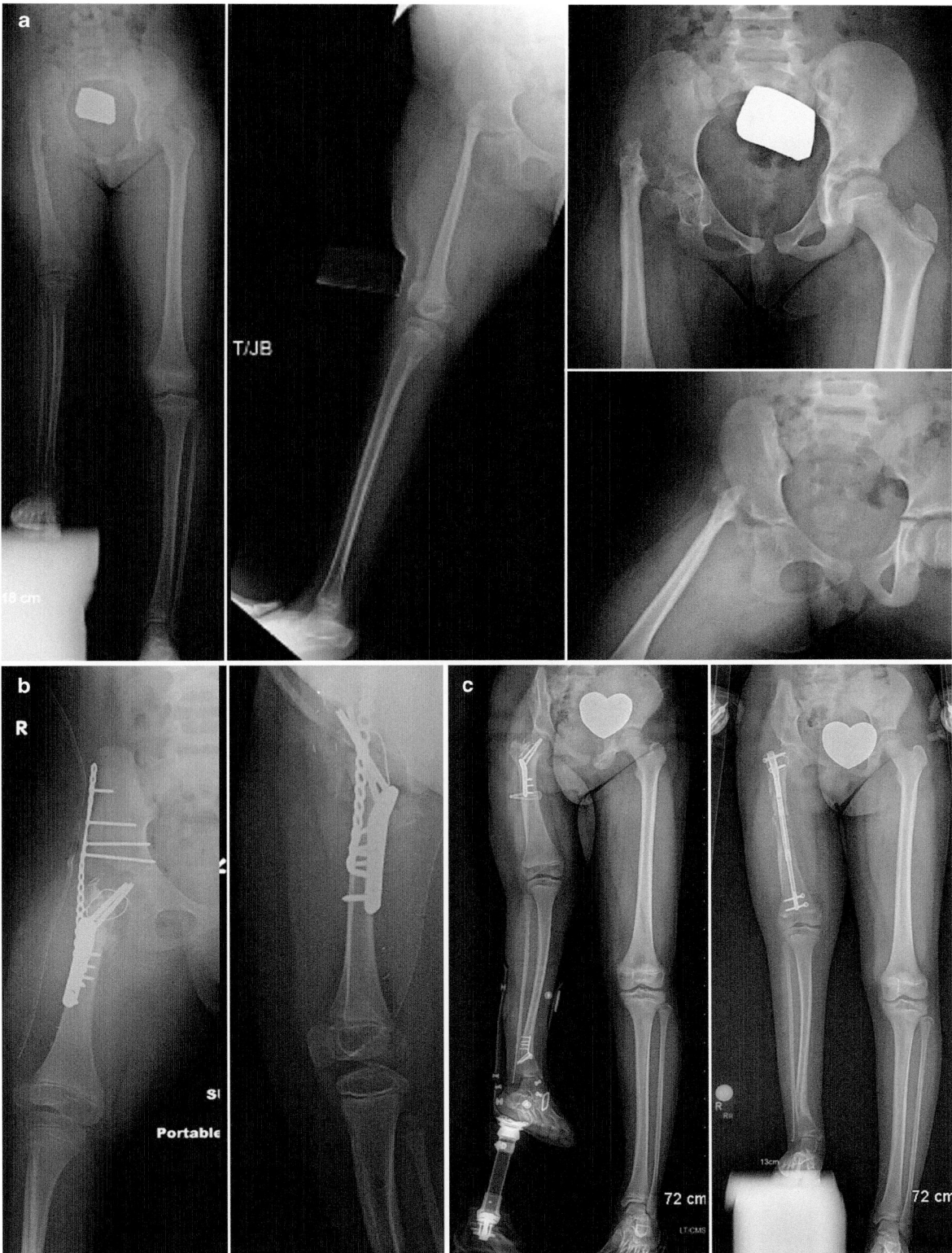

Fig. 29.24 (a)_EL (left), long lateral (middle), AP pelvis (right top), and AP pelvis with abduction (right bottom) radiographs of a 10-year-old girl with untreated CFD type 2a. (**b**) AP and lateral femur X-rays after SUPERhip2 procedure with temporary arthrodesis plate in place. (**c**) EL at age 11 with an intact femoral neck (left) prior to lengthening. The plate was removed and an implantable lengthening nail inserted and lengthening of 5 cm performed (Precice, NuVasive, San Diego) (Copyright: The Paley Foundation. Reproduced with permission. All rights reserved.)

the greater trochanter (Fig. 29.23f). Resect/release this thick structure.
8. *Hip Capsulotomy and Femoral Head Mobility.* Incise the superior capsule and confirm that the femoral head is either mobile or fused (Fig. 29.23g).
9. *Inferior Capsulotomy and Expose Ossific Nucleus.* Incise the inferior capsule, cut the transverse acetabular ligament, and cut through the cartilage to the ossific nucleus (see Fig. 29.23h).
10. *Break Fusion Site.* If the femoral head has a fusion site, identify the location of this site (opposite the ischium) and break this fusion using a small, curved instrument (Fig. 29.23i). Rotate the exposed bone of the femoral head outward, and expose it by cutting away some cartilage of the head (Fig. 29.23j).
11. *Base of Trochanter Osteotomy.* The greater trochanteric osteotomy is performed opposite of the femoral head so that the cut surface of the distal segment which is the new neck is at the correct level to fuse to the femoral head (Fig. 29.23k).
12. *Knee Flexion Contracture.* If the knee joint has a flexion contracture, a posterior capsulotomy with peroneal nerve decompression and biceps and gastrocnemius tendon releases is done. After the knee is fully straight, it is pinned to hold the knee straight. This affects the amount of femoral shortening needed. Shorten the femur further as needed so that the cut surface of the femur is opposite the femoral head. The proximal femur can be exposed extra-periosteally only on its lateral side with care not to strip any periosteum or muscle from the linea aspera or medial side (Fig. 29.23l)
13. *Osteotomy of Intercalary Neck Segment.* The periosteum is cut transversely on the lateral side at the level of the planned osteotomy, and the bone is then cut across (Fig. 29.23m)
14. *Fixation of the Femoral Neck to the Femoral Head.* The intercalary segment is bent approximately 45° into varus to create a 135° neck-shaft angle. Care is taken to preserve its periosteum and muscle attachments medially and posteriorly. It is fixed to the neck with k-wires and one or two cerclage wires that go through the femoral head (Fig. 29.23n)
15. *Fixation of the Greater Trochanter (GT) to the Femur.* The GT is fixed to the neck and shaft segments using a malleable locking plate which is bent into a Z-shape to hold all the segments together (Fig. 29.23o).
16. *Shortening Osteotomy of Ilium.* To allow closure of the apophysis, the iliac crest is shortened (Fig. 29.23p)
17. *Psoas Tendon Transfer.* The psoas tendon is transferred to the shaft of the femur and sutured in its new location (Fig. 29.23q).
18. *Repair All the Muscles in Place.* The apophysis is closed, and the quadriceps is sutured into place. The knee can be temporarily arthrodesed with retrograde wires to hold the knee straight for 12 weeks (braces and casts do not work very well to hold such a short femur knee straight (Fig. 29.23r)
19. *Temporary Arthrodesis of Hip with Internal Fixation.* Since the femoral neck has very limited fixation, it is useful to immobilize it with a spanning plate from the pelvis to the femur (Fig. 29.23s). This is removed three months later.
20. *Removal of Temporary Arthrodesis Fixation.* The temporary arthrodesis of the hip and knee are removed 12 weeks later.

Pelvic Support Osteotomy Surgical Technique (Fig. 29.25)

A pelvic support osteotomy (PSO) is used to treat type 2b and 2c in older children, combined with a distal femoral lengthening and realignment osteotomy This combination is called the *Ilizarov hip reconstruction* [70]. Pelvic support osteotomy is usually enough to prevent proximal migration of the femur during lengthening. In young children, the valgus proximal component of the pelvic support osteotomy will remodel straight, so this is more appropriately performed closer to skeletal maturity.

1. *Proximal Osteotomy Level.* The proximal osteotomy is performed at the level at which the proximal femur crosses the ischial tuberosity in maximum cross-legged adduction. The amount of valgus is equal to the total amount of adduction of the hip plus 15° of overcorrection. The proximal osteotomy should also be internally rotated and extended. The amount of rotation is judged by the position of the knee relative to the hip in maximum adduction. The amount of extension depends on the amount of hip fixed flexion deformity.
2. The level of the distal osteotomy is determined by the intersection of the proximal and distal mechanical axes. The proximal mechanical axis passes through the proximal femoral osteotomy site and is perpendicular to the horizontal line of the pelvis. The distal axis is from the center of the ankle to the center of the knee. Varus correction can be made through the distal osteotomy.
3. The pelvic support osteotomy can be fixed with an external fixator or with a plate proximally. If concurrent lengthening is planned, then the external fixator must be extended to the tibia with hinges (Fig. 29.25). If the patient's anatomy is amenable to internal lengthening, a retrograde intramedullary nail can be used in conjunction with a plate for the proximal osteotomy (Fig. 29.26).

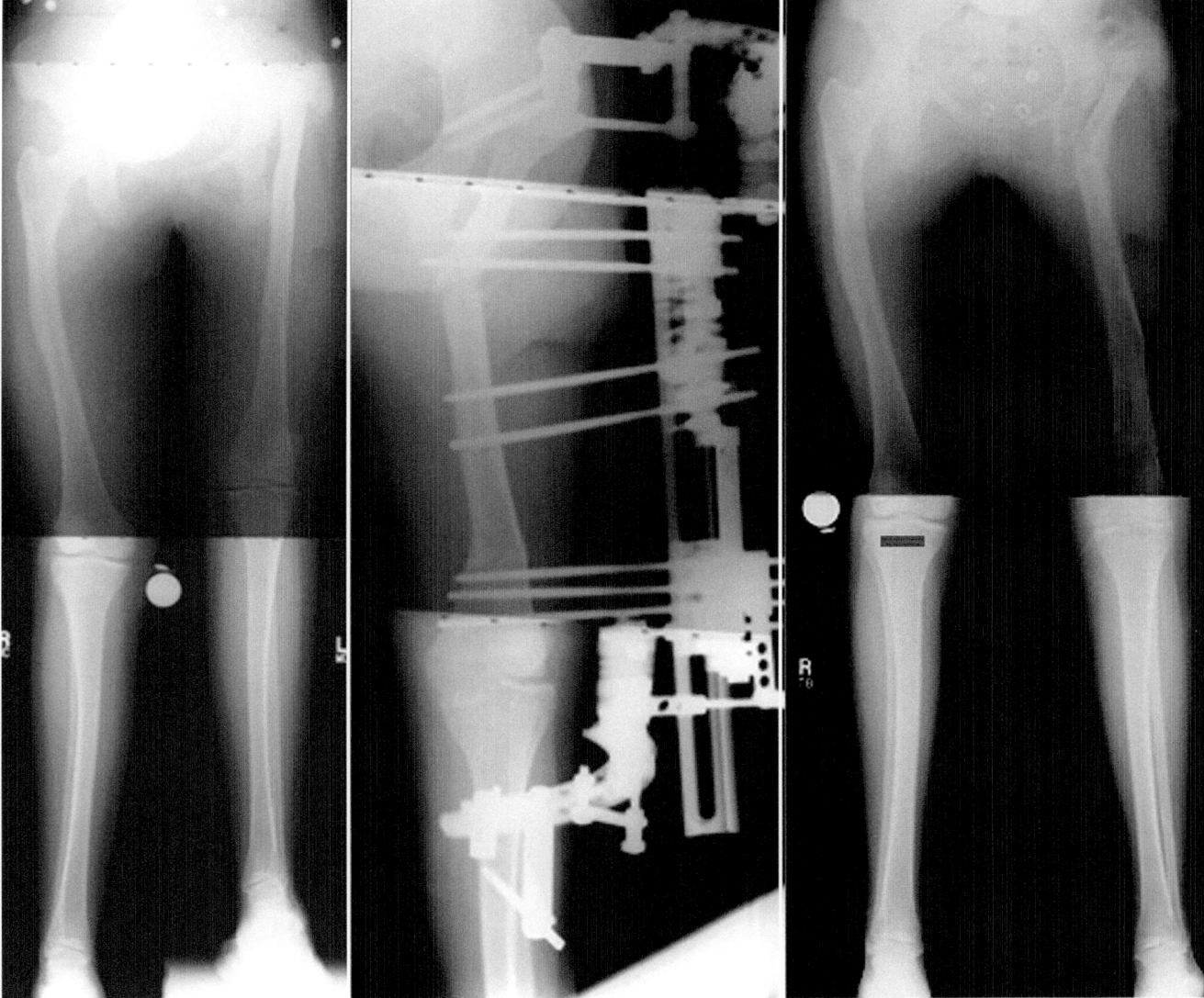

Fig. 29.25 EL radiograph of 15-year-old girl with type 2 CFD after prior lengthening of left femur by 13 cm. The remaining discrepancy of 10 cm (left). AP femur X-ray showing how she was treated with external fixation articulating to the pelvis and tibia with a pelvic support osteotomy proximally and a distal femoral osteotomy with realignment and lengthening distally (middle). Final EL radiograph (right) showing the pelvic support osteotomy and equal leg lengths. She is able to walk and run and has good hip and knee motion and almost no limp (Copyright: The Paley Foundation. Reproduced with permission. All rights reserved.)

Treatment for Type 3 CFD

Deficiency of the proximal femur with an absent femoral head, greater trochanter, and proximal femoral metaphysis results in a mobile pseudoarthrosis and a very short femoral remnant. The foot is frequently at the level of the contralateral knee. The type 3a CFD has a mobile knee with at least 45° of motion, usually with a 45° knee flexion deformity. Type 3b has a stiff knee with less than 45° of motion and usually has a greater flexion deformity. The most predictable and reliable treatment option in these cases remains prosthetic reconstruction surgery with rotationplasty [43, 71, 72]. Lengthening reconstruction surgery has a limited role in these cases to equalize LLD; however, the number of patients treated this way is small, so the ultimate functional result for these cases remains unpredictable.

Lengthening Reconstruction Surgery for Type 3

Limb reconstructive surgery and future lengthening are most applicable to Paley type 3a cases that have functional knee range of motion. The femoral sling procedure (Fig. 29.21) in combination with a posterior capsule release of the knee sta-

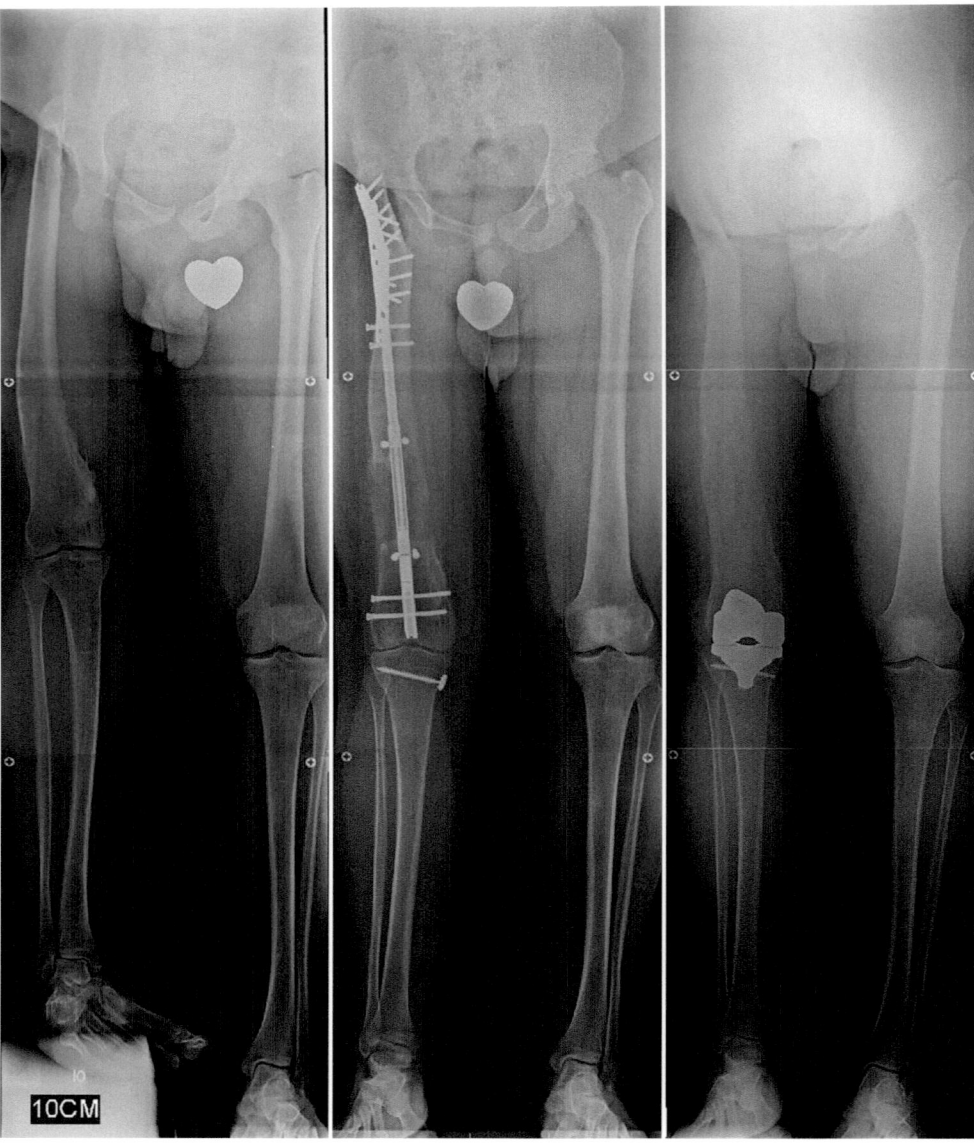

Fig. 29.26 EL radiograph of a 17-year-old boy with CFD (left). He underwent a pelvic support osteotomy with the insertion of a retrograde intramedullary lengthening nail and completed 8 cm of lengthening (middle). The patient subsequently underwent a right knee replacement with quadricepsplasty. Final EL shows the leg lengths are within 2 cm. The patient has pain-free hip motion, good ankle motion, and a 90-degree arc of motion of the knee (right) (Copyright: The Paley Foundation. Reproduced with permission. All rights reserved.)

bilizes the hip for weight-bearing and achieves full knee extension. A monolateral rail, bridged to the pelvis and tibia, for femoral lengthening can be applied to the femur in the same surgical setting if the femoral remnant is large enough to accommodate this. Up to 8 cm of lengthening can be achieved as long as the knee range of motion is maintained.

The rest of the treatment is the same as a type 2b: serial lengthenings and eventually a pelvic support osteotomy combined with a final lengthening (Fig. 29.27). Since the predicted discrepancy ranges between 30 and 40 cm, at least four lengthenings and an epiphysiodesis are required to equalize limb lengths.

Limb Lengthening Surgery

A prediction of total leg length discrepancy at skeletal maturity helps determine the approximate number of lengthening surgeries required. This can be done using the Paley multiplier method [33]. The majority of CFD cases will require at least two lengthenings. The goal of each lengthening depends on the total discrepancy at maturity. The safe amount of lengthening is 5 cm in most children, but up to 8 cm when performed with external fixation spanning the knee and/or the hip. This is predicated on having access to a daily specialized limb lengthening physical therapy program. This limit on the amount of lengthening should not be based on a percent of the length of the bone. The limit of lengthening is correlated to amount rather than percent [73, 74].

The first lengthening of the femur can be performed as early as 12 months after the preparatory surgery, assuming that the femoral neck has ossified. If the preparatory surgery is performed between the ages of 2 and 3 years, then the first lengthening can follow between the ages of 3 and 4

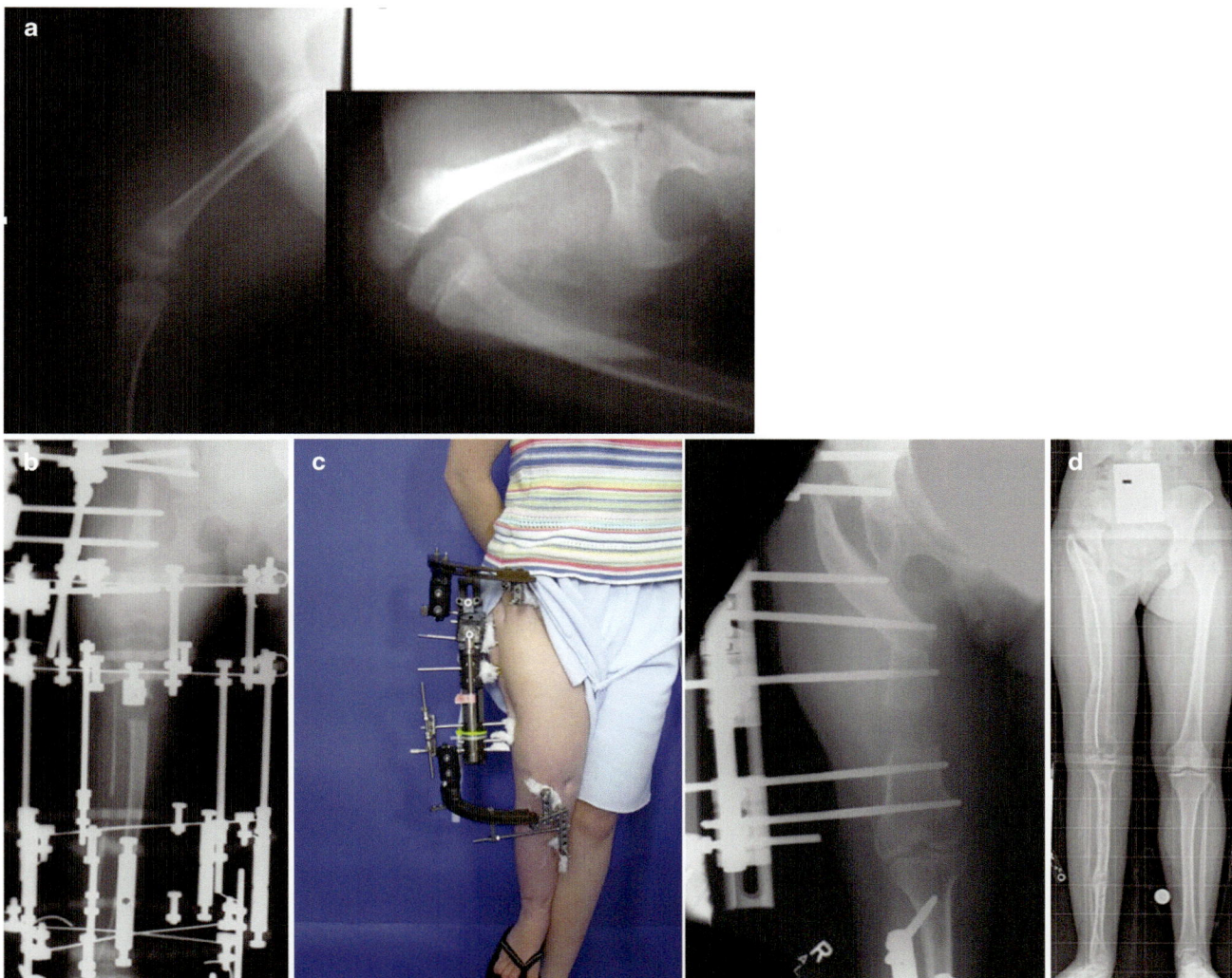

Fig. 29.27 (**a**) A child with CFD type 3a. Preoperative maximum knee extension (left) and flexion (right) demonstrate an arc of motion of 70°. The family chose to pursue lengthening reconstruction. (**b**) The child achieved 25 cm of lengthening with external fixation, 12.5 cm in the femur + tibia at age 7 and again at age 10. (**c**) At age 14, the child had a pelvic support osteotomy in combination with a 10 cm of femoral lengthening using an external fixator. (**d**) EL radiograph at age 18, after undergoing a total of 50 cm of lengthening in the femur and tibia combined. Her knee motion arc is maintained at 70°, and she has good hip and ankle motion, no pain, and walks with a minimal limp (Copyright: The Paley Foundation. Reproduced with permission. All rights reserved.)

years. By beginning lengthening at a young age, the level of prosthetic or orthotic need is reduced earlier in a child's life. In the senior author's experience, the complication rate for limb lengthening is no different for the younger age group [73] Lengthening of the femur in children younger than 6 years may be associated with sustained growth stimulation [74].

The frequency of lengthening should preferably be spread apart by 4 years or more. The rule of 4 is a good guiding strategy: one lengthening every 4 years starting by 4 years of age. Assuming that a preparatory surgery is done between ages 2 and 3 years, the first lengthening can be done between ages 3 and 4 years. The second lengthening would occur around age 8 years and a third lengthening, if needed, around age 12 years. Ideally, one should try and complete the lengthening program before the child starts high school education. This is simply to reduce disruption to education, sports, and socialization. If a fourth lengthening is required, it can be done around age 16 years. Patients may also have lengthenings performed later in life as an adult. If the tibia is also short, a combined femoral and tibial lengthening can allow for a greater total lengthening amount in a shorter time frame. Note that a combined lengthening will achieve greater total length gain but less per bone segment. In young children, growth inhibition of the tibia was noted with combined lengthening [74].

Aston et al. published a series of 27 patients with Paley type 1 CFD who underwent a total of 30 femoral lengthening procedures with multiplanar Ilizarov-type external fixator [75]. The mean gain in length was 5.8 cm (3.3–10.4 cm), 18.65% of the total length of the femur (9.7–48.8%). The mean time in the frame was 223 days (75–363) with a mean distraction index of 1.28 months per cm. The authors performed the first 17 osteotomies in the distal femur and then changed to a proximal osteotomy, noticing a significant increase in the mean range of knee motion from 98.1° to 124.2° ($p = 0.041$) and a trend toward a reduced requirement for quadricepsplasty, although this was not statistically significant ($p = 0.07$). The overall incidence of regenerate deformation or fracture requiring open reduction and internal fixation was similar in both osteotomy groups (56.7% and 53.8%, respectively). In the proximal osteotomy group, preplacement of a Rush nail reduced fractures from 100% without a nail to 0% ($p < 0.001$). When compared to a distal osteotomy, a proximal osteotomy with a Rush nail had a significant decrease in fracture rate from 58.8% to 0%, respectively ($p = 0.043$). This supports the recommendations of Paley and Herzenberg that CFD patients undergoing external fixation lengthening should be lengthened over a small-diameter solid rod or have a rod inserted at the time of frame removal to reduce the risk of regenerate bending or fracture [76].

Paley et al studied a group of 95 patients with CFD who underwent lengthening between the years 1988 and 2000 (Table 29.1). These patients did not undergo preparatory surgery (SUPERhip or SUPERknee) prior to lengthening. All femoral lengthenings were done with the Ilizarov device with hinged extension to the tibia. The postoperative result, based on scoring of knee and hip range of motion, gait, lengthening goal, alignment, pain, and activity level, was excellent and good in over 93% of all groups. The mean overall length achieved was 6.0 cm (range, 2.2–12.5). Complications included femur fracture, pin-site problems requiring surgery, premature consolidation, nerve irritation/palsy, delayed union, knee subluxation, and hip subluxation. The fracture rate in the older age group was significantly lower than the other groups, but it included several patients who were undergoing lengthening over nails. There was no significant difference in unplanned surgery rates between groups 1 and 2 (Table 29.1). The difference with group 3 was related to refractures. Prophylactic rodding was not performed at the time of fixator removal in this series of patients, but is now part of the standard treatment algorithm, given the high rate of fractures [73]. These results were also correlated by Abdelgawad et al., who showed that prophylactic rodding after external fixator removal reduced fracture rate from 34% to 18% ($p = 0.04$). The infection rate was 7% and all were treated with debridement and removal with no recurrent infection [77].

The result of femoral lengthening after a hip stabilization procedure has also been presented [78]. A retrospective review was performed of 35 patients with CFD, Paley types 1a and 1b, who underwent femoral lengthening with external fixation after a pelvic osteotomy, proximal femoral osteotomy, or a combination. Patients underwent a hip stabilization procedure at a mean age of 2.4 years (2–5.5). The mean age at first femoral lengthening was 3.7 years (3–10.7). The mean overall limb length difference prior to femoral lengthening was 64.8 mm (47–100), with a mean postoperative difference of 8.1 mm (−14 to 32). The average amount of time in the external fixator was 186.1 days (107–311) or 1.1 months/cm. Preoperatively, average knee ROM was 2°–131°, and hip ROM was −2° extension to 115° flexion. Follow-up at a mean of 14.4 months (5.6–45.2) showed a return to baseline ROM in the knee of 2°–119° and hip from −1° extension to 91° flexion. The overall rate of obstacles and complications was 37.1% and 32.4%, respectively [79].

Table 29.1 Limb lengthening results and complications in 95 patients

	Group 1 (<6 years)	Group 2 (6–13 years)	Group 3 (>13 years)
Number of patients (*n*)	30	40	25
Amount of length achieved			
Length (cm)	5.4 (2.8–8.5)	6.2 (2.5–11)	6.3 (2.2–12.5)
Relative (%)	39 (12–71)	24 (7–54)	20 (5–58)
Lengthening index (month/cm)	1.0 (0.5–1.8)	1.1 (0.5–2.2)	1.1 (0.5–2.2)
Good/excellent outcome score	28/30 (93%)	37/40 (93%)	24/25 (96%)
Problems, obstacles, and complications			
Femur fracture	13	14	4
Pin-site problems requiring surgery	4	3	1
Nerve irritation/palsy	3	3	1
Premature consolidation	0	3	3
Delayed union	2	4	3
Knee subluxation	5	5	3
Hip subluxation	3	3	1
Total unplanned surgery	21 (70%)	22 (55%)	9 (36%)

Leite et al. performed a systematic review of knee complications during lengthening for CFD. A total of 4 studies encompassing 120 patients with CFD undergoing femoral lengthening by various external fixation methods (Wagner-38, Ilizarov-38, monolateral external fixation-44) were assessed. A total of 54 patients demonstrated clinical AP instability. During lengthening, 57.4% of the unstable knees and 25.8% of the stable knees demonstrated subluxation. Articulation of the external fixator across the knee joint was successful in preventing and treating knee subluxation [68].

Paley et al first reported on the use of the PRECICE intramedullary nail (NuVasive Specialized Orthopedics, San Diego, CA). Twenty-three out of 48 patients were treated for congenital leg length discrepancy, including CFD. These patients had a mean gain in length of 4.5 cm, with a mean initial lengthening goal of 4.91 cm. All congenital femur lengthening patients were treated with postoperative HKAFO bracing to maintain knee extension. One patient developed soft-tissue contractures that required a return trip to the operating room, and one patient developed a knee subluxation while simultaneously lengthening both femur and tibia [80]. Szymczuk et al published a comparison of monolateral external fixation and magnetic motorized intramedullary nail, PRECICE (NuVasive Specialized Orthopedics, San Diego, CA). The cohort included 32 patients who had external fixation and 30 patients who had PRECICE. The mean gain in length was 5.6 cm and 4.8 cm, respectively ($p = 0.052$). No significant difference was found between distraction rate and consolidation time. Patients who underwent PRECICE lengthening had fewer problems, specifically related to lack of pin-site infections, and significantly improved knee range of motion at the end of distraction and once consolidation was achieved compared to the external fixation group [81].

The newest technique in the arsenal of limb lengthening is extramedullary internal limb lengthening (EMIL) [82–84]. In patients who have a femur that is too short for intramedullary implantation or is unable to accommodate an intramedullary implant due to diameter or anatomy, the lengthening nail can be affixed to the lateral side of the femur. Shannon and Paley published their results of 13 patients, 8 of whom had CFD, who underwent EMIL procedures. A supplementary small-diameter solid rod (SLIM, Pega Medical, Montreal, Qu) was inserted into the femur at the index surgery. The average length gained was 48.5 cm. All patients were treated with postoperative HKAFO to maintain knee extension. Two patients developed hip subluxation that was successfully treated with pelvic osteotomy [82]. Dahl et al published a report on 11 patients who underwent EMIL for congenital limb shortening. Nine of these patients had a diagnosis of CFD. The average gain in length was 32.3 cm. Preoperative knee instability was treated with a temporary spanning plate across the knee joint in full extension. No joint subluxations were reported [83]. Most recently, Iobst and Bafor published a series of five patients who underwent retrograde femur EMIL for femoral shortening. The average length gained was 3.5 cm, and no complications were noted. Two patients underwent simultaneous deformity correction of distal femoral valgus [84].

Monolateral External Fixator Technique (Fig. 29.28a–i)

A hinged external fixator is one technique used to lengthen the femur in patients with CFD. This is the preferred technique in young children with small femurs (less than 150 mm) as they cannot accommodate internal lengthening devices. External fixation should also be the lengthening method selected when there is the concern for instability of the hip or knee due to the devices ability to articulate across the knee and hip joints. The authors' preference is the Drive Rail (Orthopediatrics, Warsaw, IN), a monolateral articulated external fixator that was designed by the senior author specifically for CFD lengthening.

1. *Preparatory Surgery*. If there are no indications for hip or knee surgery, the fascia lata and rectus femoris proximally and the iliotibial band and biceps tendon distally should be released at the time of the lengthening surgery. If these tissues were released with a previous pelvic osteotomy, SUPERhip procedure, or SUPERknee procedure, there is no need to do any additional soft-tissue releases.
2. *Positioning, Prepping, and Draping*. The patient is positioned supine on a radiolucent table. The entire lower extremity including the hemi-pelvis should be draped out to ensure adequate access for fixator application. The ipsilateral arm is padded and secured across the chest.
3. *Position the Knee Hinge* (Fig. 29.28d). The knee hinge is placed first by performing an arthrogram of the involved knee under fluoroscopy. In the lateral view, the femoral condyles are rotated until they superimpose each other. This is considered a "true lateral of the knee" (note that this is not the patella-forward position—the patella will be externally rotated approximately 10° in this position). The center of knee rotation is identified. The center of rotation is the intersection of the posterior cortical line and the distal femoral physeal line with the posterior femoral condyles overlapped. A 2-mm Steinmann pin is inserted into the distal femoral physis at the center of rotation and parallel to the distal femoral joint line in the frontal plane.
4. *Apply the Femoral Fixator* (Fig. 29.28e, f). A half-pin is inserted into the femur at the proximal end parallel to this hinge axis pin. The pin should err posteriorly due to the bow of the femur. To accurately place the half-pin, use a cannulated drill technique (Fig. 29.28e): Insert a

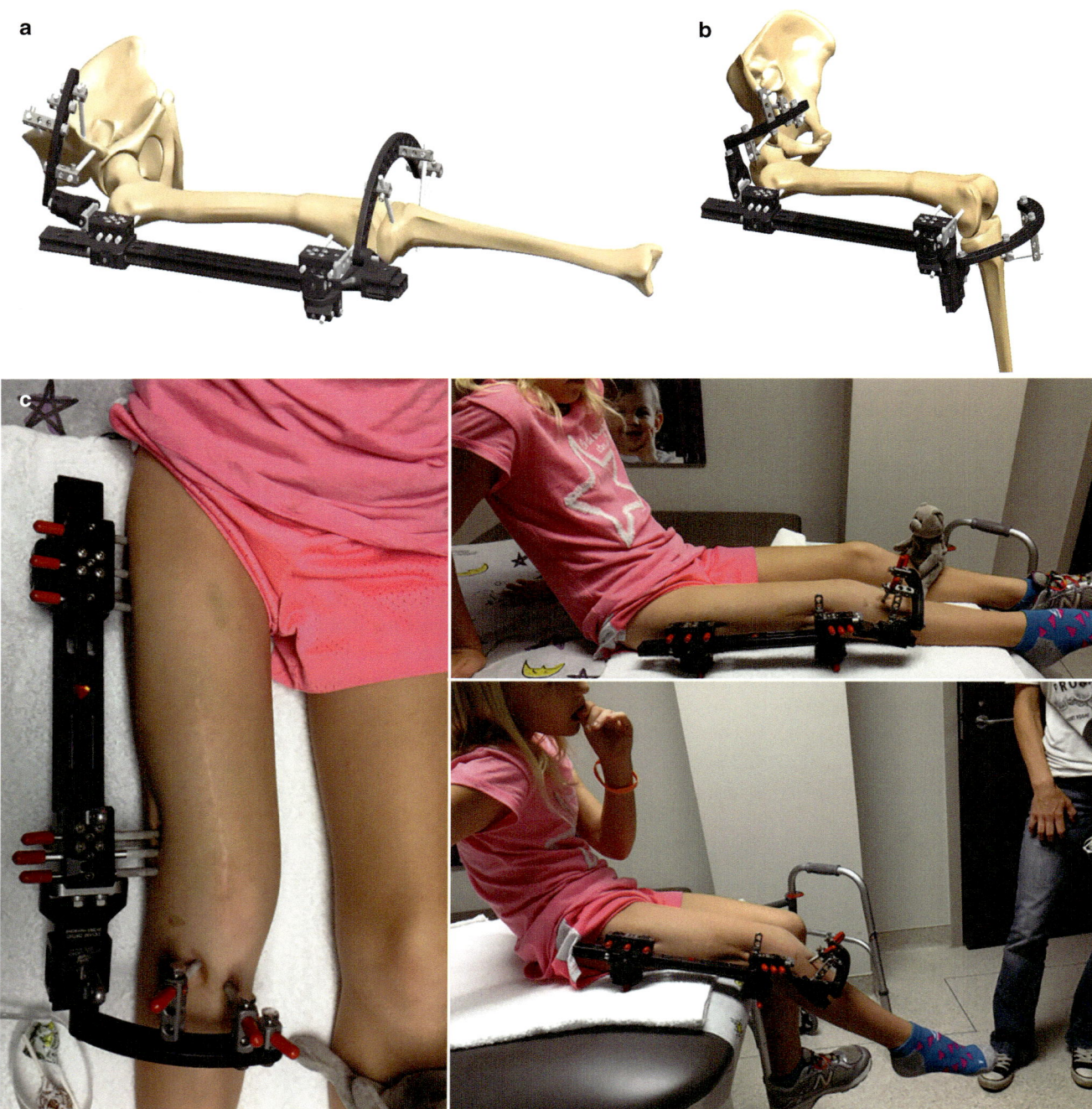

Fig. 29.28 (a) Drive Rail (Orthopediatrics, Warsaw, IN) device for femur lengthening shown articulated and spanning the hip and knee with both joints in extension. (b) Drive Rail device for femoral lengthening with hip and knee flexed. The hip and knee hinges are aligned to the centers of rotation of these joints. (c) Clinical example of patient with CFD lengthening with Drive Rail spanning the knee joint. (d) Intraoperative fluoroscopy demonstrating a lateral view of the knee after an arthrogram. A Steinmann pin is in the center of rotation of the knee. The posterior femoral condyles are aligned and the pin is at the posterior aspect of the physis, where it intersects with the posterior cortex of the femoral shaft. (e) The first half-pin is located in the proximal femur. A wire is inserted parallel to knee axis pin. Cannulated technique is used to insert the half-pin. (f) Intraoperative fluoroscopy lateral view showing three proximal and three distal half-pins in place. (g) AP (left) and lateral (right) femur showing Drive Rail in place with knee spanning to tibia. (h) Lateral fluoroscopy view of hip with center of rotation pin in place (left). AP fluoroscopy view with knee and hip center of rotation pins at slight varus angle (middle). The proximal and distal pins are placed perpendicular to each segment for correction of the varus deformity (right). The osteotomy is located just proximal to the distal pin cluster. (i) Preoperative EL of a child with left-side CFD with an unstable hip (left). Drive Rail application for lengthening of left femur 8 cm with spanning to pelvis and tibia (middle). The rail was removed and the femur rodded with a SLIM rod (Pega Medical, Montreal, Canada) (right) (Copyright: The Paley Foundation. Reproduced with permission. All rights reserved.)

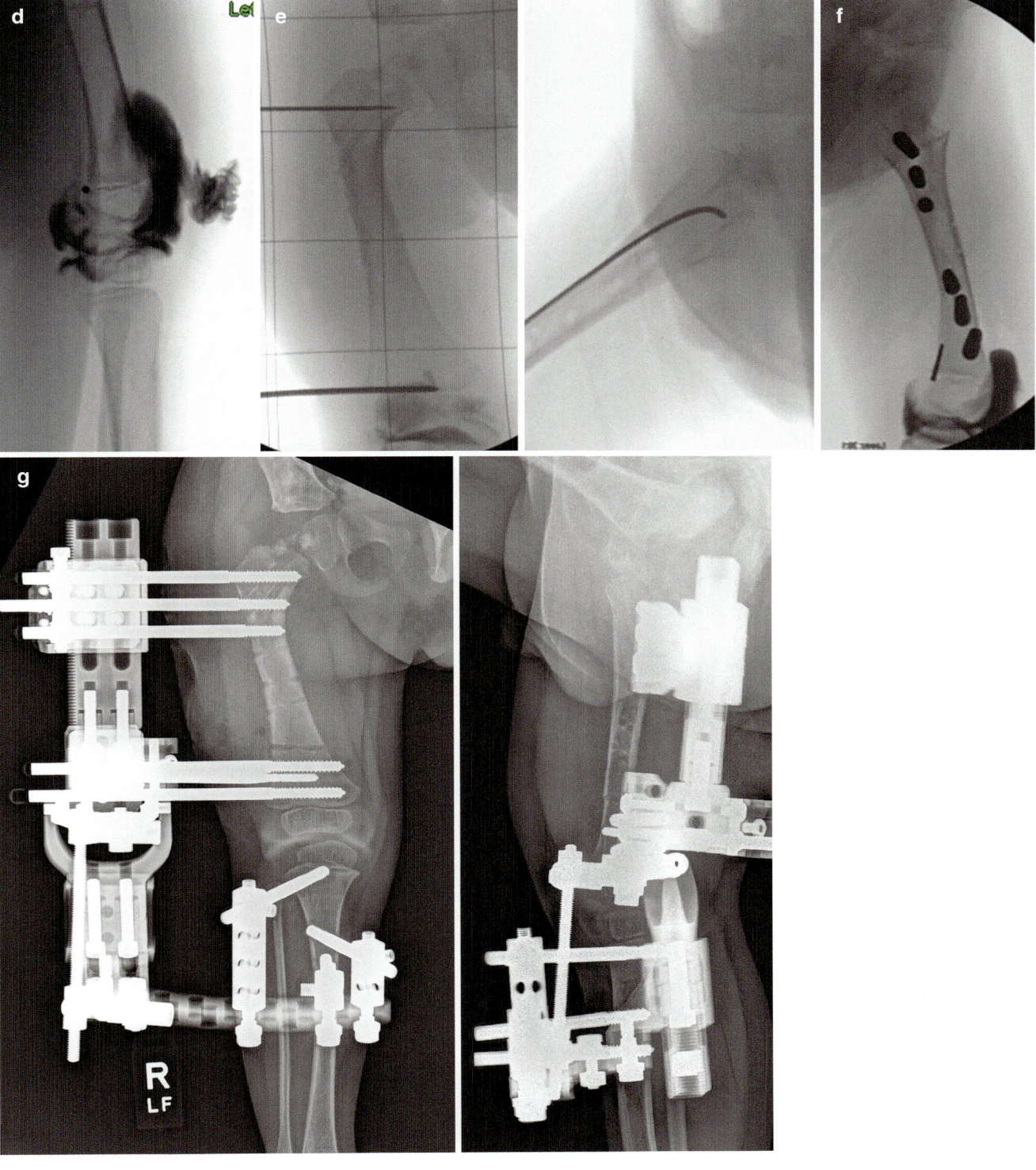

Fig. 29.28 (continued)

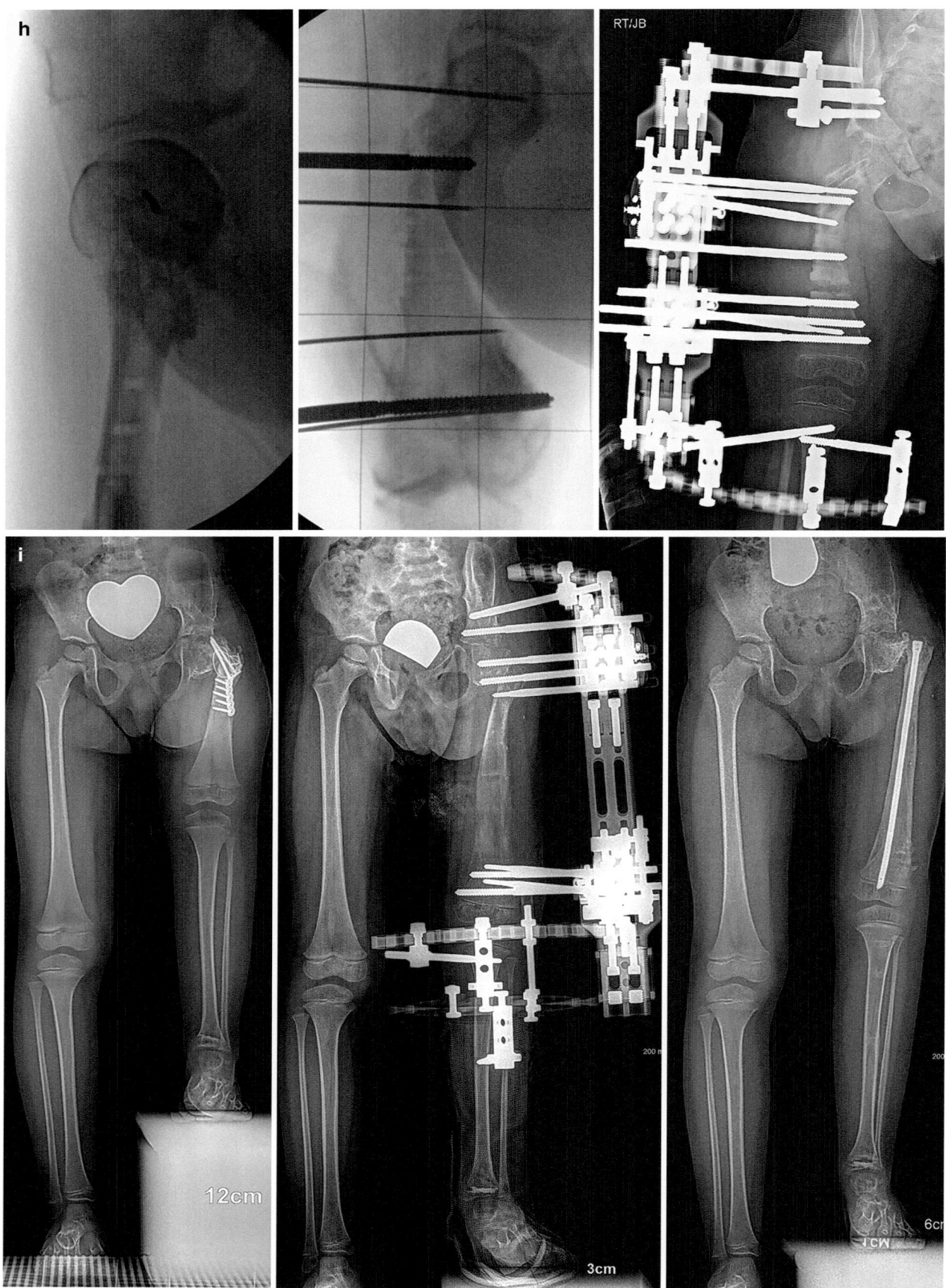

Fig. 29.28 (continued)

wire into the femur, and check it is in the correct location with the image intensifier. Then, overdrill the wire with a cannulated drill. The half-pin is then inserted in a perfect position. The preconstructed fixator is applied so that the Steinmann pin goes through the cannulated hinge bolt distally and the half-pin goes through the most proximal hole on the upper clamp. The most distal half-pin is placed one hole proximal and anterior to the knee axis reference wire. At this point, the position of the hinge axis is a fixed point to the initial distal half-pin. The additional half-pins are placed proximal and distal. Three frontal plane half-pins should be placed in each segment (Fig. 29.28f). In very small femurs, two frontal plane half-pins may be adequate which also keeps the osteotomy in the distal metaphysis. Caution is needed when placing the distal half-pins. If they are placed in the anterior half of the femoral diaphysis, this can result in a fracture either during the lengthening process or after frame removal due to the increased tendency to be a stress riser. If concurrent distal valgus deformity or rotation is being corrected, the proximal and distal pins are placed at the desired angle of correction to each other, and the osteotomy is performed after there are two proximal and two distal pins. The rail is only placed after the deformity is corrected. The deformity is corrected acutely, and the rest of the fixation is for the undeformed bone.

5. *Osteotomy*. The osteotomy is made immediately proximal to the distal pin group. This is done through a one cm lateral incision, followed by multiple drill holes, and completed with an osteotome. The preferred location is in the distal metaphysis where the bone is wide and preferably without previously violated periosteum. As noted in step 4, only two frontal plane half-pins may be necessary to avoid a more diaphyseal osteotomy (Fig. 29.28g).

6. *Complete the Femoral Fixation*. The external fixation is completed with insertion of one distal posterolateral oblique half-pin.

7. *Span the Knee*. A distal rail segment is used to suspend a floating arch. The tibial fixation is attached to this arch. A single-hole Ilizarov cube is placed on the arch, and an AP half-pin is placed in the proximal tibia. The knee should be in full extension and reduced. After the first half-pin is inserted into the tibia, the hinge is tested with gentle ROM of the knee. If the motion is smooth, a drop-leg test is performed. The drop-leg test consists of lifting the lower extremity off the bed and fully extending the knee. The thigh is supported, and the foot is dropped. If the knee flexes with no catching or friction, two additional half-pins are placed in the tibia. If there is friction during the drop-leg test, the connection to the pin needs to be adjusted (e.g., fix it in flexion first). After the adjustment, the drop-leg test is repeated until knee ROM is smooth, with no friction. The floating arch is not fixed on the rail, allowing it to slide. It therefore does not impede the growth of the distal femoral and proximal tibial physes.

8. *Knee Extension Bar*. A knee extension bar is built using Ilizarov parts between the fixed bracket on the femoral rail and the tibial arch. It should be parallel to the leg and the frame with the knee in full extension. This knee extension bar can be removed to allow knee motion. It should be used all night and part-time during the day to prevent knee flexion contracture.

9. *Span the Hip*. If hip stabilization is required, a hip hinge clamp is used. It is centered on the center of the femoral head. The Steinmann pin for the hip hinge should be placed after the knee hinge pin and before the femoral half-pins (Fig. 29.28h). Three pins are placed in the pelvis and fixed with an arch as the last step. The hip should be held in 10–15° of abduction and neutral rotation when fixed to the frame (Fig. 29.28i)

10. *Botox Application*. At the conclusion of the procedure, Botox, 10 units per kilogram of body weight, is injected into the proximal quadriceps using multiple injection sites. This is to reduce quadriceps muscle spasms and pain during knee flexion stretches.

Extramedullary Implantable Limb Lengthening Technique [58, 82] (Fig. 29.29a–f)

1. *Positioning, Prepping, and Draping*. The patient is positioned supine on a radiolucent table. The entire lower extremity including the hemi-pelvis should be draped out to ensure adequate access for nail insertion.

2. *SLIM Rod*. In order to guide the lengthening and neutralize the adduction and flexion forces, especially when using a nail with only one locking screw at each end, a SLIM rod (Pega Medical, Montreal, Canada) is inserted into the femur through a trochanteric starting point. If the SLIM is not available, a Rush rod or something similar may be used. A guide wire followed by a cannulated drill is used prior to insertion of the nail. The nail should span the entire length of the bone up to the distal growth plate. The SLIM rod is secured by screwing the proximal portion into the greater trochanter.

3. *Osteotomy*. Unlike intramedullary lengthening, the level of the osteotomy is not dependent on the length of the implant. The osteotomy should be made in an area where the periosteum has not been violated, such as the site of a prior plate removal. The proximal and middle thirds of the femur are the author's preferred osteotomy level for congenital cases to avoid stiffness and subluxation of the knee. A distal osteotomy can be considered, although the SLIM rod will be pulled out of the distal segment during

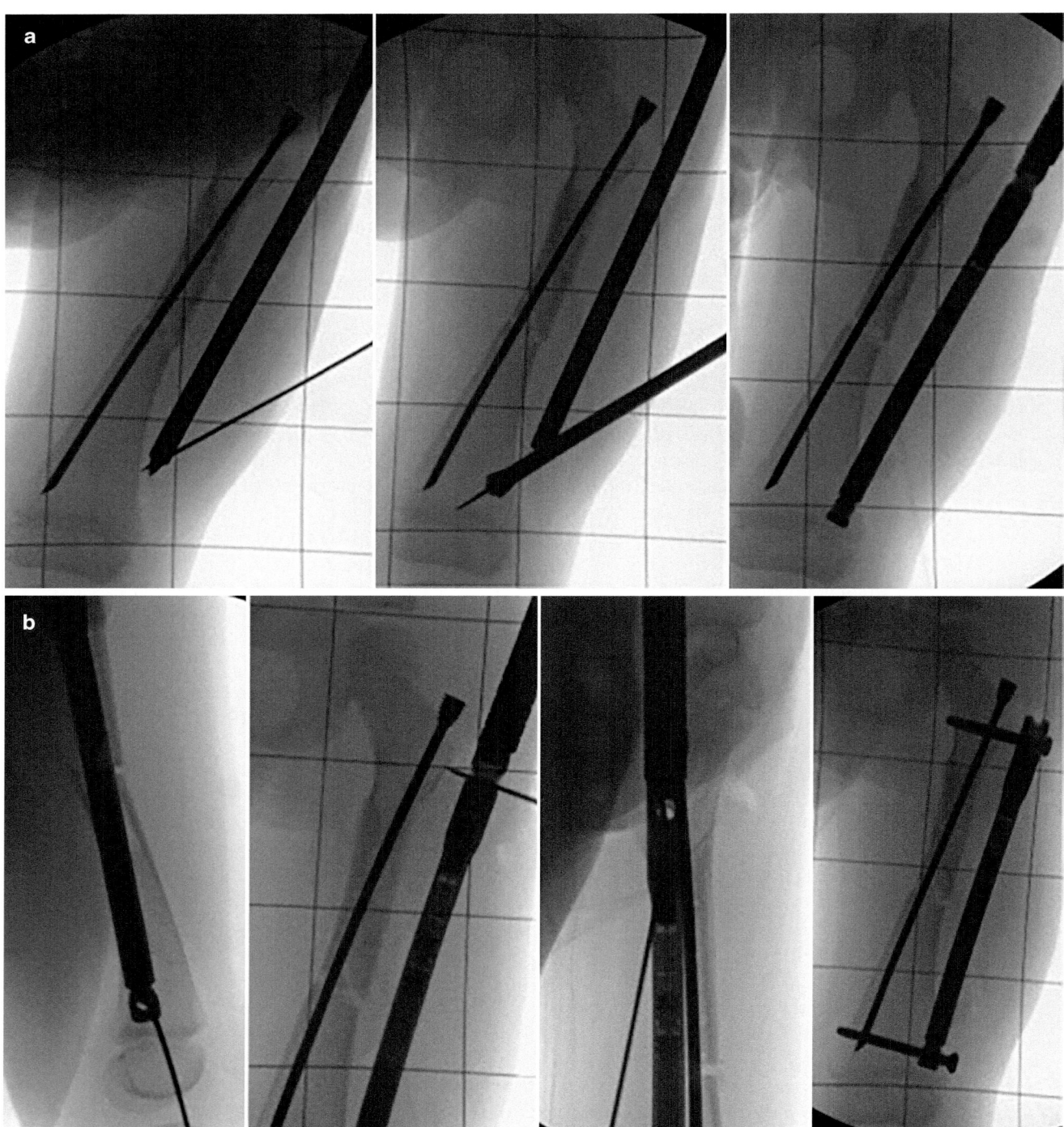

Fig. 29.29 (a) The long trocar can be used to dilate the submuscular space for nail insertion. The location where the tip of the trocar contacts the lateral femoral condyle is marked with a wire (left). An ACL reamer is passed over the wire to create a docking site for the nail in the bone (middle). The nail is inserted into this docking site distally. This improves the stability of the lengthening construct by reducing the distance of the nail from the bone (right). (b) The nail is affixed to the bone using perfect circle technique. Fully threaded screws are preferred. (c) Preoperative EL and long lateral radiographs of a 4-year-old child with CFD type 1a. (d) Postoperative AP and lateral radiographs showing 1 cm of distraction. (e) EL and long lateral radiographs after completion of 5 cm of femoral lengthening with full consolidation. (f) AP and lateral radiographs of the femur after removal of the extramedullary nail. The small intramedullary rod is left in place to protect the regenerated bone (Copyright: The Paley Foundation. Reproduced with permission. All rights reserved.)

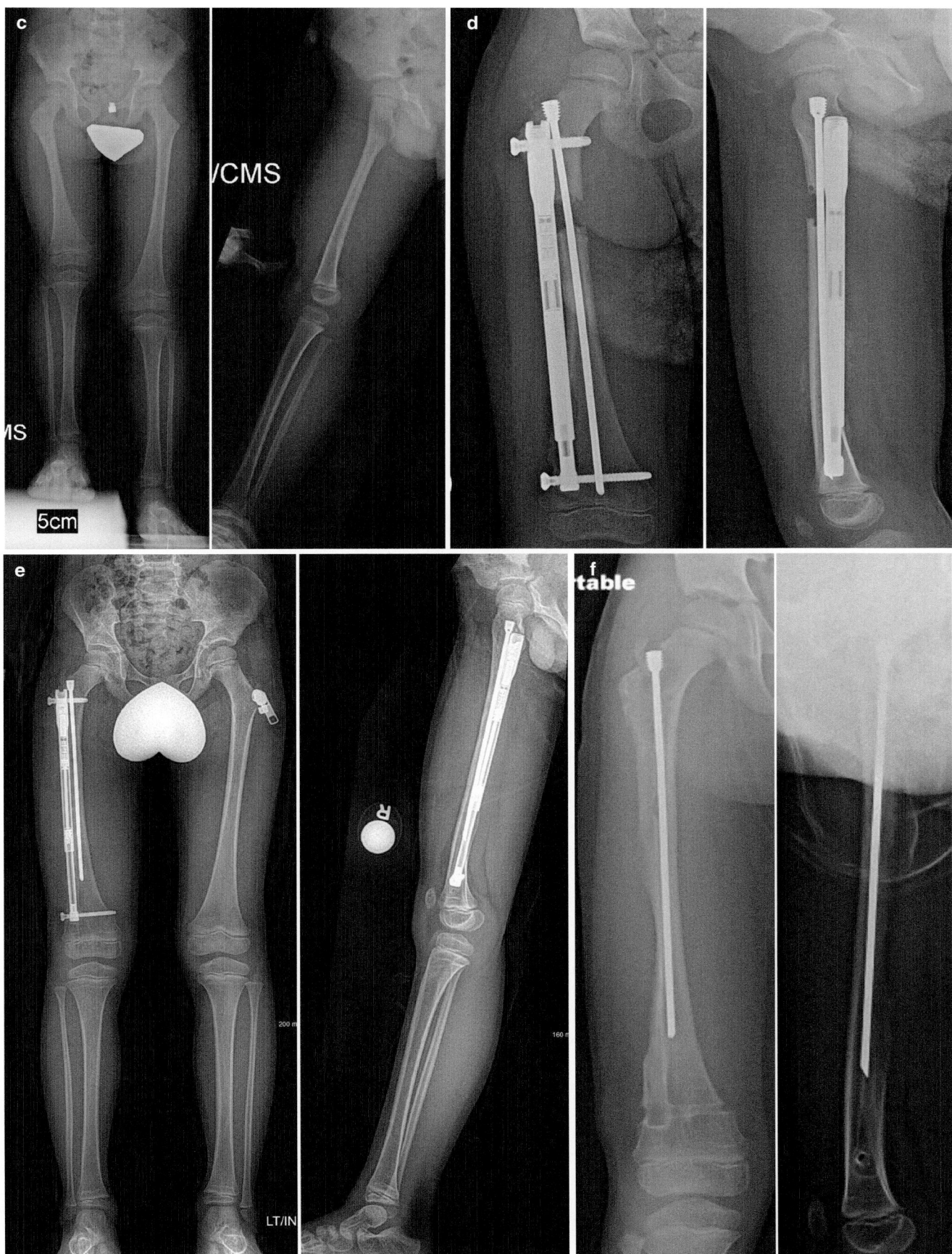

Fig. 29.29 (continued)

lengthening, no longer protecting the regeneration. In cases with a greater risk of hip subluxation, it is better to move the osteotomy level more distal. Conversely in cases with a greater risk of knee subluxation, it is preferable to make the osteotomy more proximal. Once a level is selected, the SLIM rod is backed out to the level of the intended osteotomy. A less than one cm incision is made in the skin, and multiple drill holes are made perpendicular to the femur using a drill or a 1.8-mm bayonet tip wire. The osteotomy is completed with an osteotome. The SLIM rod is advanced across the osteotomy and screwed back into the trochanter. Since most of the periosteum is intact, the osteotomy remains rotationally stable.

4. *Submuscular Nail Placement* (Fig. 29.29a). A lateral incision is made at the level of the greater trochanter. A submuscular path is created for the nail under the vastus lateralis along the lateral border of the femur. The drill sleeve and trocar can be used to dilate this space.

5. *Secure the Nail* (Fig. 29.29a, b). Create a docking hole in the lateral distal femoral metaphysis for the distal end of the nail. The closer the nail is positioned to the bone, the smaller the bending moment will be on the nail. Distally, the nail can be docked into the distal metaphysis by creating a hole in the metaphyseal flare. Through a separate lateral incision, a wire followed by an ACL reamer slightly larger than the diameter of the selected nail, such as a 10-mm reamer for an 8.5-mm nail, is used to create a 1–2-cm depth hole. The nail can now be advanced antegrade and nested into the distal hole. It is locked distally first and then proximally. The proximal locking guide remains on as a handle until a wire is inserted through the one proximal locking hole. The hole is drilled, and the wire is removed and replaced with a threaded screw. The proximal guide is removed to allow the nail to get pulled down to the bone by the lag effect of the threaded screw. If there are four interlocking holes, then the second pair are drilled and two more screws are added. After completing the locking, the incisions are closed.

6. *Locking Screw Choice*. It is important to use a threaded screw to prevent lateral migration of the implant; therefore, either the fully threaded Precice titanium screws or the partially threaded Stryde screws should be used. Both screws have a larger diameter threaded section near the head of the screw that was designed for fixation of the near cortex in intramedullary fixation. With extramedullary fixation, it does not fit into the locking hole and therefore makes the screw head prominent. This is more of a problem in the distal femur than in the proximal femur. To avoid significant screw head prominence, a metal cutting matchstick burr should be used to shave off the larger diameter threads near the screw head.

7. *Testing the Nail*. The nail should be tested with the ERC device to demonstrate that it is working. This is done by distracting one mm in the operating room after implantation. The location of the magnet should be marked on the patient's leg for later lengthening.

Intramedullary Implantable Limb (IMIL) Lengthening Technique (Fig. 29.30)

1. *Preoperative Planning*. The Precice nail comes in 8.5, 10.7, and 12.5 mm diameters. Precice nails have a much wider array of lengths, with one as short as 150 mm with only one locking screw at each end for a nail that can lengthen only 5 cm. Trochanteric entry nails are preferred in skeletally immature patients. The outer diameter of the femur is measured on AP and lateral views to determine if it can accommodate the nail. Since the femur is overreamed by 2 mm, the smallest outer diameter that can accommodate the 8.5-mm nail is 16.5 mm. Anything smaller than this should be treated by EMIL.

2. *Positioning, Prepping, and Draping*. Position the patient supine on radiolucent operating table and prep and drape up to the ribs and to the midline both anterior and posterior, with the leg free.

3. *Osteotomy-Level Selection*. The osteotomy should be made at a level that will ensure that the larger diameter of the nail (outer tube) remains engaged on the distal side of the osteotomy at the end of the lengthening. This level is calculated by marking the intended position of the upper end of the nail on the skin (Greater trochanter for skeletally immature patients, piriformis for skeletally mature patients). Based on the length of nail chosen, the lower end of the nail position is marked out as well. Measuring retrograde from the lower end of the nail, the most distal permissible level of the osteotomy is calculated as the sum of the total amount of desired lengthening + 2–3 cm of planned overlap + 3 cm (representing the amount of the male portion of the rod protruding from the end of the nail), e.g., 5 cm lengthening +2 cm overlap +3 cm end of rod = 10 cm from distal end of rod. The osteotomy may be made and any point proximal to this level (Fig. 29.30b).

4. *Osteotomy*. The osteotomy level is marked on the skin. Make a lateral stab wound at the level of planned osteotomy and use the 4-mm drill bit to make multiple drill holes at the osteotomy level. This will allow decompression of the canal during reaming to avoid fat embolism and will also allow the reamings to graft the osteotomy site.

5. *Nail Insertion*. Insert a Steinmann pin percutaneously into the proximal medial tip of the greater trochanter with

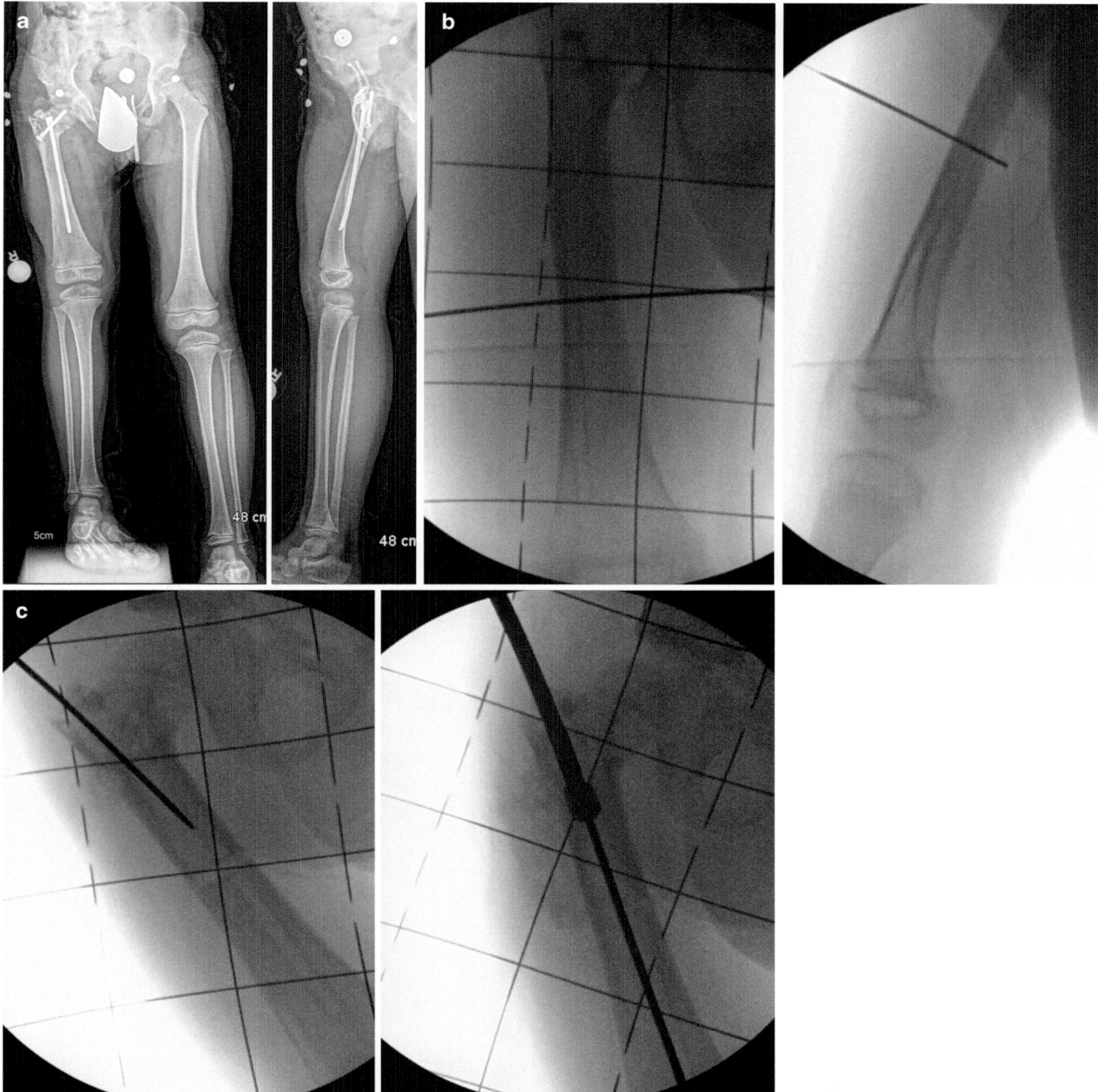

Fig. 29.30 (a) Preoperative EL and long lateral radiographs of a 6-year-old by with CFD type 1b3 who has previously undergone a SUPERhip procedure. (b) The osteotomy level is marked based on the preoperative measurements: desired lengthening + end of nail + overlap = minimum distance from tip of nail (e.g., 5 cm + 3 cm +2 cm= 10 cm from tip of nail). The osteotomy is then predrilled to vent the femoral canal. (c) A Steinman pin is used to obtain the starting point (left) and a ball tip guidewire is placed in the femoral canal. Reamers are then passed over the guide rod to a diameter 2 mm larger than the nail diameter (right). (d) The nail is inserted into the osteotomy level, and a osteotome is used to complete the osteotomy. The nail can then be fully seated in the bone. (e) AP and lateral radiographs after 1 cm of distraction. Note the single proximal and distal interlocking screws fixing a 150-mm length nail. (f) EL and long lateral radiographs after completing 5 cm of lengthening and consolidation of the regenerate (Copyright: The Paley Foundation. Reproduced with permission. All rights reserved.)

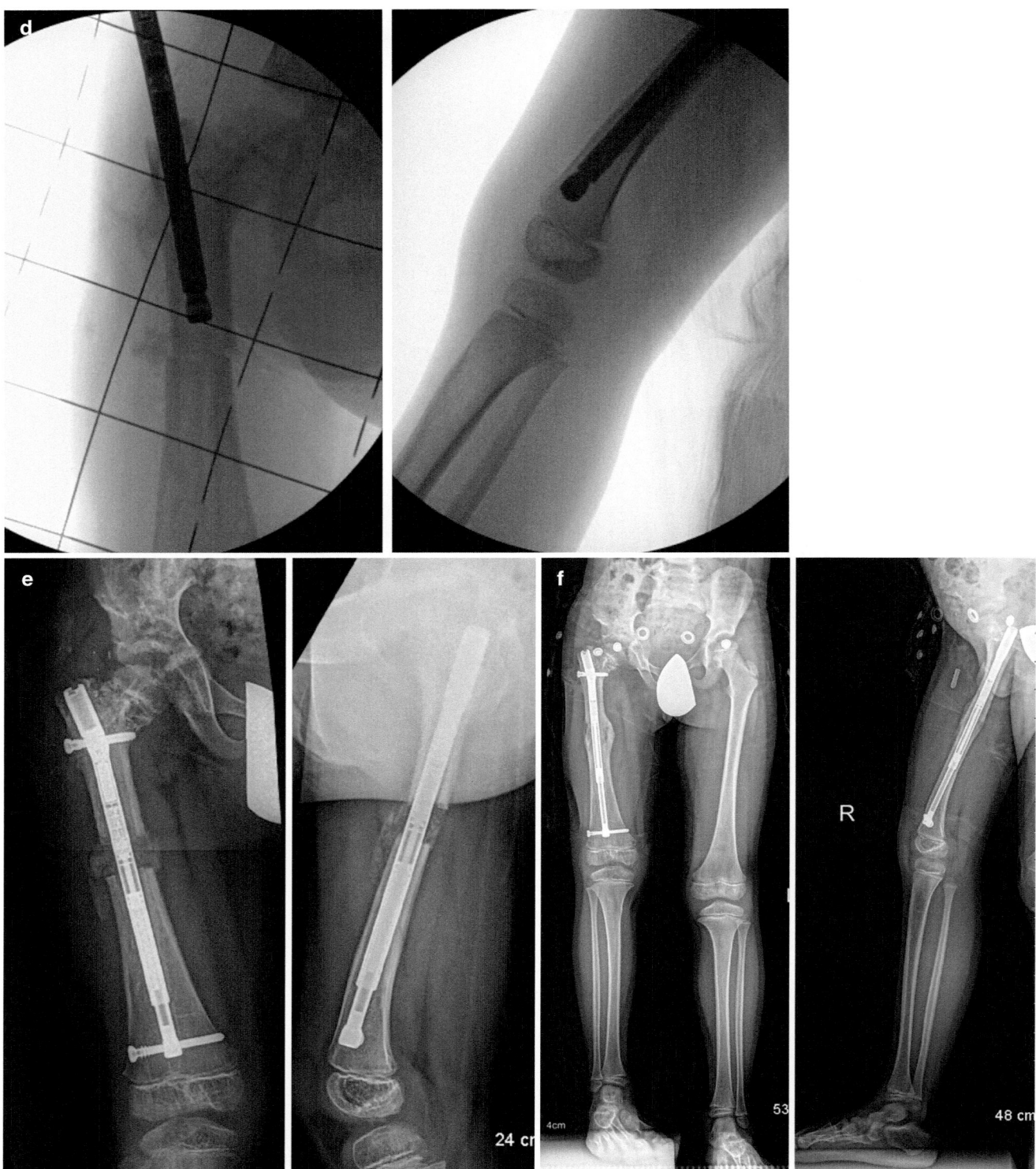

Fig. 29.30 (continued)

the leg adducted. Confirm with the image intensifier on AP and lateral views. Make a 15 mm incision around the pin and ream open the starting point with a 10-mm ACL reamer. Insert the beaded guide rod down the femur. Ream the femur in 1 mm increments until there is chatter, and then, reduce to half-mm increments. Ream 2 mm greater than the diameter of the nail to be used (Fig. 29.30c).

6. *Complete the Osteotomy.* Insert the selected lengthening nail down to the level of the planned osteotomy. Two assistants are needed to support the limb: One holds onto the foot and supports it in the air with traction and without rotating the foot. The leg should not touch anything that could give it support. The other holds the nail with its introducer and lifts toward the ceiling to create an extension moment arm. With the extension moment in place use an osteotome through the lateral incision to complete the osteotomy. No loss of rotation occurs since the anterior cortex of the bone is under compression from the extension moment and traction. The nail is advanced down the femur crossing the osteotomy site. Once it is safely on the other side, the assistant holding the leg lowers it down to rest on the table while maintaining traction. The nail is advanced until its upper end is at the level of the top of the piriformis fossa or seated in the greater trochanter (Fig. 29.30d).

7. *Lock the Nail.* Proximally, attach the locking screw insertion jig. Mark the skin with the drill sleeves for the proximal screw. If the nail has two screw holes, then make one skin incision that will be used for both drill holes. Drill the more distal upper screw first. This makes sure that you start on the greater trochanter and do not move down into the concavity at its base where it is more difficult to start. Drill both cortices and measure the screw length. Insert the screw using power on the ream setting. Now, drill the most proximal upper screw after drilling this hole. Distally, use a free-hand locking technique after obtaining perfect circles on the image intensifier in the lateral position. Insert a bayonet-tipped wire into the two distal holes. Use a cannulated drill for the first cortex, and then, drill the second cortex with a solid drill to avoid wire breakage. Insert the first lower locking screw, and then, repeat the process for the second one.

8. *Closure.* Curette out the reamings from the nail insertion site proximally. No blocking screws are needed except if the osteotomy is very proximal, above the level of the isthmus. If needed, insert a medial blocking screw using the Precice pegs. All the incisions are closed.

9. *Testing the Nail.* The nail should be tested with the ERC device to demonstrate that it is working. This is done by distracting one mm in the operating room after implantation. The location of the magnet should be marked on the patient's leg for later lengthening.

Rehabilitation and Follow-Up During Lengthening [54, 85]

Femoral lengthening requires close follow-up and intensive rehabilitation to identify problems and maintain a functional extremity. Clinically, the patient is assessed for hip and knee range of motion, nerve function, and pin-site problems if lengthening with external fixation. Radiographically, the distraction gap length, regenerated bone quality, limb alignment, and joint location are assessed. If the lengthening rate is 0.75 mm per day, then follow-up is usually every 2 weeks. If there is delayed healing of the regenerated bone, or if knee motion is decreasing, then the rate of lengthening is often decreased. If the lengthening rate is decreased to 0.5 mm per day, then the follow-up can be increased to 3 weeks. Rarely, if there is concern for premature consolidation and the lengthening rate is increased, then follow-up is more frequent.

Patients are allowed to weight-bear as tolerated with their external fixator. Internal devices have weight-bearing restrictions (50–75 lbs for intramedullary nails, 0–20 lbs for extramedullary devices). Physical therapy is begun within 1 or 2 days after surgery and continues daily throughout the distraction phase. In the authors' opinion, the amount of therapy is directly related to a better functional result and faster rehabilitation after removal. During distraction, patients have one to two formal physical therapy sessions daily (45–60 min each). In addition, at least two home sessions (60 min each) are recommended. Patients undergoing lengthening are at their best immediately after surgery and have difficulty with muscle tightness, and the range of motion only after lengthening has started. It is not until the consolidation phase that the usual orthopedic pattern of rehabilitation and recovery occurs. Thus, lengthening should be thought of as a prolonged procedure that lasts until the end of the distraction period and should not even be considered in the absence of adequate therapy.

The majority of therapy time for femoral lengthening is spent obtaining knee flexion and maintaining knee extension. Knee flexion should be maintained as close to 90° (or the patient's preoperative baseline) as possible. It is important to start pushing the extremes of passive knee flexion (especially prone) during the 1-week latency period after surgery. Once distraction begins, there is more resistance from muscle spasm. If knee flexion begins to diminish (<75°), then lengthening should be stopped or slowed to rehabilitate the knee better, sometimes waiting for improvement before resuming lengthening. Function should never be sacrificed for length, and preserving the knee joint and motion is paramount. For patients with external fixation, a knee extension bar is used at night and part-time during the day to prevent a knee flexion contracture. For patients with internal devices, a custom-made hip-knee-ankle-foot (HKAFO) orthosis is worn with the knee in full extension during sleep. Posterior subluxation can occur with a fixed flexion deformity and is suspected clinically based on a change in the shape of the front of the knee. The patella becomes very prominent and the tibia appears depressed (ski hill sign).

During the distraction phase, therapy is focused on passive range of motion exercises to maintain hip and knee range of motion. During the consolidation phase, the priority shifts to the active range of motion and strengthening to regain any motion lost during distraction. Hip abduction and extension exercises help prevent adduction and flexion contractures that can lead to hip subluxation.

After the lengthening regeneration is healed, recovery is limited by two factors: joint range of motion and muscle weakness. In most cases, joint motion is regained faster than muscle strength. The three antigravity muscles are the limiting factor to full recovery: the hip abductors, quadriceps, and gastro-soleus muscles. To minimize disability, these muscles should have resistance training throughout the lengthening program to prevent atrophy. Other modalities such as electrical stimulation or aquatic therapy may be helpful.

Fixator Removal and Rodding of Femur

If an external fixator was used, it can be removed once the regenerated bone is fully healed radiographically. The biggest risk after removal is fracture of the femur, which can manifest as painless bending of the femur or as a completely displaced fracture. The use of a spica cast does not reduce the fracture rate. A study performed by the author in 1999 showed a fracture rate of 34% after CFD lengthening, compared to 9% for other etiologies [86, 87]. These results have been confirmed by numerous other studies [76, 77] The regenerated bone should show no gaps, the interzone should be closed, and based on AP and lateral views, there should be evidence of corticalization on at least three sides of the lengthened regenerate. In order to prevent fracture, prophylactic rodding of the femur should be performed. The authors prefer to use a SLIM rod (Pega Medical Montreal, Can). The risk of infection was found to be 4% [76]. This is controlled by prescribing a 2-week course of oral antibiotics to prevent colonization of the new rod.

Surgical Technique for Prophylactic Rodding of Femur at Time of External Fixator Removal (Fig. 29.31)

1. The external fixator is removed under general anesthesia, ensuring that the patient is deeply asleep (to avoid involuntary muscle spasms which could lead to fracture of the regenerate at the time of removal). Slightly loosen all of the pins while they are still supported by the frame, which is especially important in hydroxyapatite-coated pins. Remove the middle pins, while the fixator is still on. The most distal and proximal pins are removed, while an assistant provides bimanual support of the thigh above and below the lengthening zone.
2. After prepping the thigh, curettage any loose granulation tissue from the pinholes. The pinholes in the bone are also curetted in the event of osteolysis or infection. Cover and seal the pinholes with an adherent plastic dressing (e.g., Tegaderm, 3M, Minneapolis, MN).
3. Prep and drape the lower limb free, being careful not to manipulate the leg. A bump may be placed under the ischium to raise the femur for lateral viewing on image-intensifier radiography.
4. Insert a guidewire for the SLIM rod at the tip of the greater trochanter (Fig. 29.31b). Advance the wire either with a drill or by tapping it with a mallet. A slight bend in the wire may be necessary to direct the wire. The wire is passed through the center of the intramedullary canal and regenerated bone, all the way to the distal femoral physis if possible. A second wire of equal length can then be used to subtraction measure the length of the canal.
5. Drill over the wire with respective size drill bit for the SLIM rod (Fig. 29.31c).
6. Insert an appropriate length SLIM rod (Fig. 29.31d). The SLIM rod can be locked with proprietary locking pegs (Fig. 29.31e) or k-wires at the proximal and distal ends for additional stability.
7. After rodding, the patient goes home with sterile, dry dressings covering the pin sites and a 2 week course of oral antibiotics, usually a first-generation cephalosporin. Weight-bearing and physical therapy are restricted for 1 month. A gentle range of motion of the knee is allowed at home.

Box 29.10 Fixator Removal Tips and Tricks

- Do not remove the fixator until the three sides have corticalized.
- Use a rush rod or intramedullary device to prevent fracture through the regenerated bone.
- Slightly turn or "crack" all the half-pins while in the fixator prior to removing the frame. The hydroxyapatite bond can be quite strong.
- Curettage out any hypertrophic granulation tissue. Loose pins warrant more thorough curettage of the bone.
- It may not be possible to direct a thin Ilizarov wire all the way down the femur. Drill just the proximal portion and then proceed to the Rush rod.
- If needed, put a small bend in the Rush rod in line with the bevel to augment guided insertion.
- Hold off on physical therapy for a month after fixator removal.

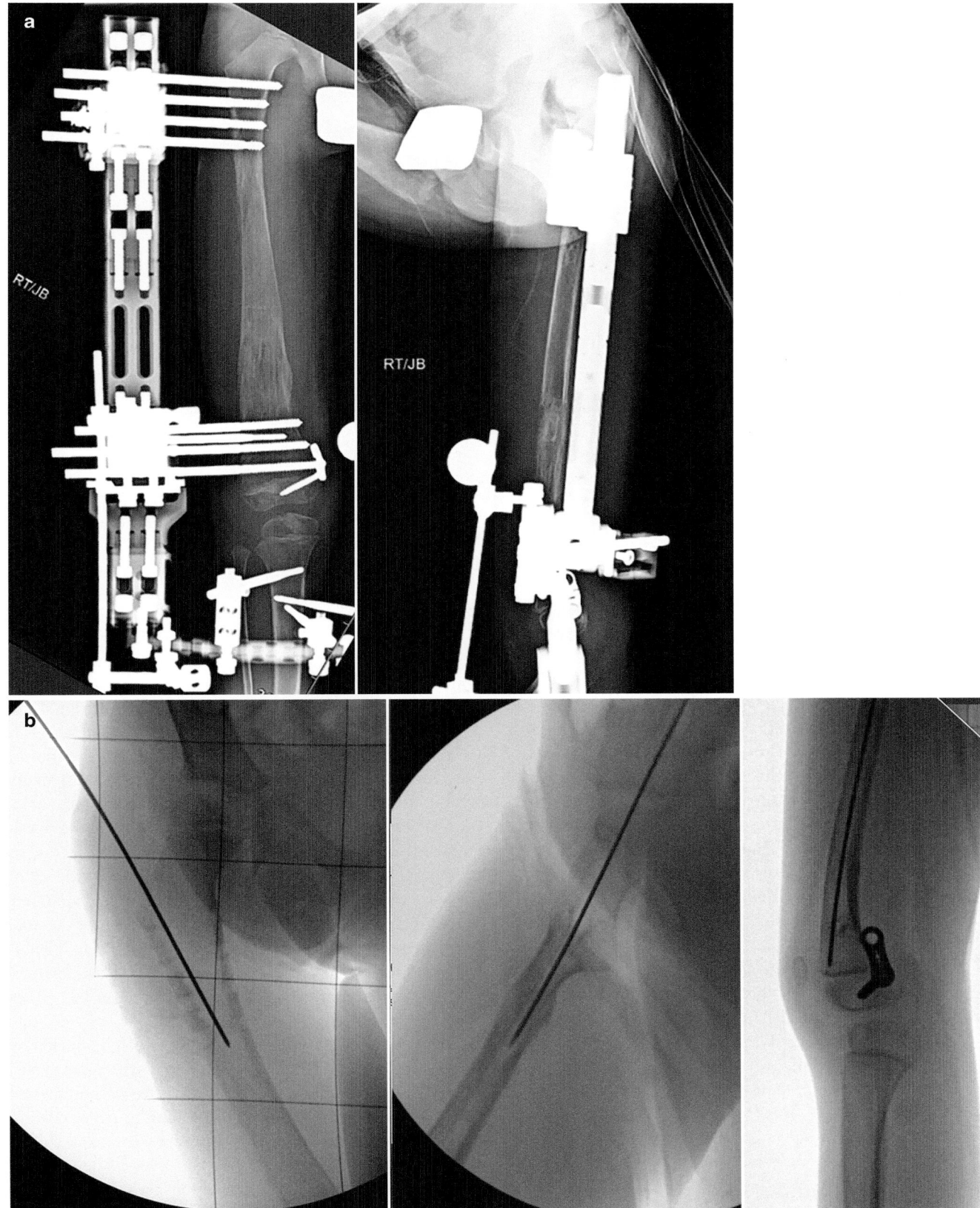

Fig. 29.31 (a–e) External fixator removal and femoral rodding (follow text for steps and captions) (Copyright: The Paley Foundation. Reproduced with permission. All rights reserved.)

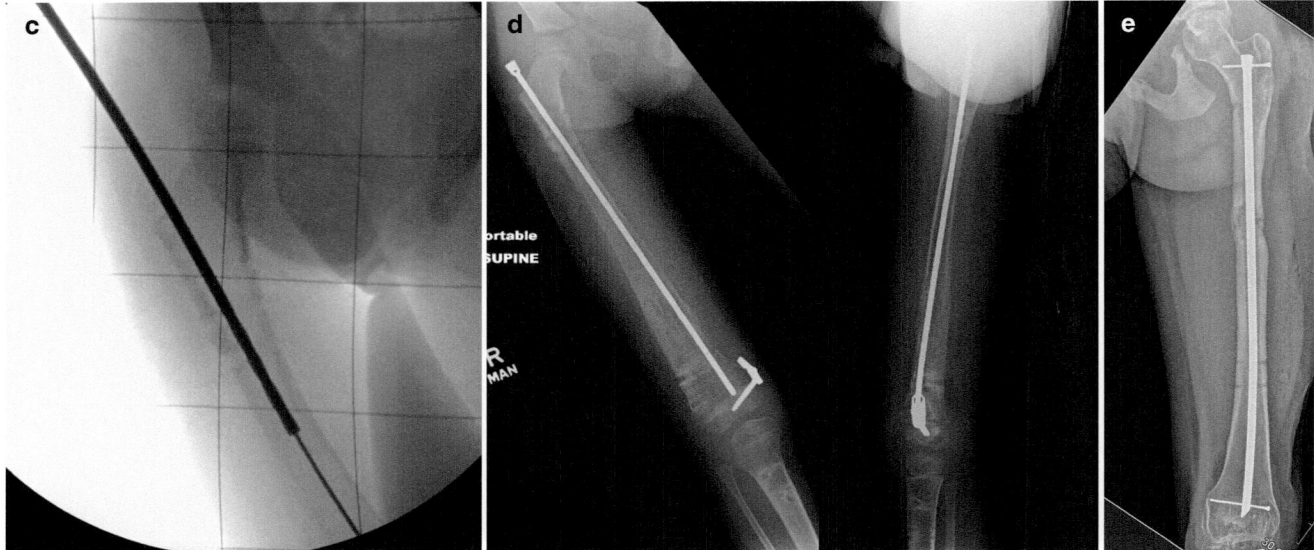

Fig. 29.31 (continued)

Epiphysiodesis and Hemi-epiphysiodesis

Contralateral epiphysiodesis around the knee is used as an adjuvant method to equalize LLD. Patients should be presented with this option, especially if it reduces the need for one lengthening surgery or reduces the need to lengthen in second bone. Parents are often reticent to agree to epiphysiodesis because they do not like the idea of operating on the normal leg. The advantages of epiphysiodesis are that it is a small outpatient procedure that most pediatric orthopedic surgeons can perform reliably and which requires little follow-up. The disadvantages of epiphysiodesis are twofold: (1) loss of height equivalent to the amount of correction and (2) unpredictability (inaccuracy), especially in children with premature or delayed maturation. The use of skeletal age instead of chronologic age should be considered to reduce this prediction error. Calculation of the timing of epiphysiodesis can be achieved quickly and with a 1 cm accuracy using the multiplier method [33, 88].

Ipsilateral hemiepiphysiodesis is very useful to correct the valgus deformity of the knee from distal femoral or proximal tibial origins. The plate and screw construct is a simple way to temporarily arrest the one side of physeal growth [89, 90]. While previously one of the advantages of external fixator lengthening was the simultaneous ability to correct distal femoral valgus, this can now be achieved by hemiepiphysiodesis. This makes the use of proximal lengthening with implantable nails more practical.

Complications and Their Treatment for Congenital Femoral Deficiency Lengthening

Nerve Injury

Nerve injury from surgery or distraction is unusual with femoral lengthening. To avoid peroneal nerve injury from the external fixator pins, the posterolateral pin should not enter posterior to the biceps tendon. During distraction, if the patient complains of pain in the dorsum of the foot or asks for frequent massage of the foot, this is most likely referred pain from stretch entrapment of the peroneal nerve. More advanced symptoms include dysesthesia in the distribution of the peroneal nerve or extensor hallucis longus weakness. A nerve conduction study may show evidence of nerve injury, but most cases will be negative since too many fibers are conducting normally. Quantitative sensory testing using the pressure-sensitive sensory device (PSSD), if available, is the most sensitive test to assess for nerve involvement [91]. Near-nerve conduction using very fine electrodes is also very accurate.

If a nerve problem is identified early, it can be treated by slowing the rate of distraction. However, if symptoms persist or motor signs develop, then peroneal nerve decompression should be performed [92, 93]. The timing of nerve decompression affects the rate of recovery of neuropraxia, and an early decompression leads to faster recovery. The peroneal nerve should be decompressed at the neck of the fibula, including transverse fasciotomy of the anterior and lateral compartment and release of the intermuscular septum between these compartments [94] (p10). When peroneal nerve decompression was performed on patients undergoing limb lengthening, intraoperative findings included hemorrhage, nerve flattening, narrowing of the nerve at the entrance of the fascial tunnel, and reduction of the perineural vascularization at the site of compression. These findings are typical of nerve entrapment and not of stretch injury. In addition, no relationship was found between nerve injury and the amount or percentage of lengthening.

Poor or Failed Bone Formation

Hypotrophic regenerate formation requires slowing of the distraction rate. The rate can be slowed to 0.75, 0.5, or 0.25 mm per day. If the regenerated bone does not improve, a decision needs to be made whether or not to continue lengthening. If the defect in the distraction gap does not fill, it will need bone grafting. Bisphosphonate infusion (e.g., zoledronic acid) can be used to prevent bone resorption while permitting bone formation [95, 96].

Complete failure of bone formation is very unusual. Partial defects, especially laterally, are common. Dynamization of the fixator or IM nail and bone growth stimulators (e.g., Exogen™) can be used. Resection of the fibrous tissue in these defects and cancellous bone grafting may become necessary if the bone fails to heal.

There are two methods of bone grafting the regenerate:

1. *Autogenous Cancellous Bone Grafting.* The distraction gap should be opened and the fibrous tissue excised, leaving behind any regenerated bone. Once all of the fibrous tissue has been removed, a cancellous autogenous bone graft can be harvested and inserted. In most children, this is obtained from the iliac crest. In young children, there may not be enough bone from the standard anterior iliac crest approach. More bone graft can be obtained by splitting the tables of the iliac crest and taking graft from both the anterior and posterior ilium if needed, referred to as decancellousization [97, 98]. This allows the harvesting of a large cache of bone that is normally not available for grafting, providing enough bone to fill the distraction gap.
2. *Cortical Allograft.* This technique is used when the distraction gap is very long and exceeds the available autogenous cancellous bone graft. The technique is credited to Wasserstein [99]. He described inserting a slotted allograft into a distraction gap to create early structure and bridging of the gap. A non-slotted allograft can be used instead, stabilized with an intramedullary nail. BMP-2 can be added for both cancellous and cortical grafts.

Incomplete Osteotomy and Premature Consolidation

If there is a lack of separation of the osteotomy site after a week of distraction, it may be due to an incomplete osteotomy or a periosteal hinge that will not separate. Continued distraction can lead to an acute separation of the bone ends, which is usually very painful and may have an audible pop. The pain will continue unabated until the bone is acutely shortened by a few millimeters. It is important to advise the patient of this possibility. If the bone does not separate or if the patient or parents wish to avoid a painful separation, a repeat osteotomy at the same site should be performed.

Overabundant bone formation may lead to premature consolidation. Watch for a mismatch between the distraction performed and the radiographic distraction. Increasing the distraction rate for a few days may prevent a premature consolidation in such cases. Patients should be checked weekly during this time. If premature consolidation occurs, a repeat osteotomy should be performed at a new location, as a repeat osteotomy through the original site is more likely to lead to failure of bone formation. Leave the fixator in tension, as the osteotomy will separate easier when cut under tension. After the osteotomy, the tension in the frame should be reduced to normal.

Hip Subluxation/Dislocation

There is often mild or moderate acetabular dysplasia in patients with CFD. The pattern is different than DDH; the femoral head is usually uncovered laterally rather than anterolaterally. If the CE angle is less than 20°, the hip joint is considered at risk for dislocation [59]. The orientation of the sourcil should also be horizontal. If it is inclined superiorly, then the hip joint is potentially unstable even with a normal CE angle. It is always safer to err on the side of performing a pelvic osteotomy prior to femoral lengthening than to end up with a hip subluxation, as this complication can be catastrophic to the function of the hip joint [100, 101]. Hip joint subluxation or dislocation during lengthening is diagnosed radiographically. The earliest sign is a break in Shenton's line or increased medial acetabular clear space. The hip usually has an adduction and flexion contracture and may also exhibit stiffness with flexion and extension.

Eidelman et al reviewed a series of 69 children with unilateral CFD Paley type 1a (43) and 1b (26), who underwent 91 femoral lengtheings. Hip subluxation/dislocation occurred in 15% (14/91) lengthenings. Factors that contributed to an increased risk of hip instability were having type 1b CFD, pre-lengthening hip uncoverage, proximal femoral osteotomy, and increased amount of total lifetime lengthening. Use of a monolateral external fixator was also found to be a risk factor; however, this was thought to be related to the proximal osteotomy that was performed with the fixator construct [102].

If hip subluxation occurs, distraction must stop. The patient should be taken to the operating room to reduce the hip. Release the adductor longus and gracilis, and the TFL and rectus femoris if needed. Abduction should reduce the hip subluxation. If not, the distraction gap should be shortened to loosen the hip joint. If using an external fixator, it should be extended to the pelvis with or without a flexion-extension hinge. Pelvic fixation consists of at least two anterolateral pins between the two tables above the anterior inferior iliac spine followed by two off-axis lateral pins. The femur should be in 15–20° of abduction to the pelvis to maintain the reduction. A hip extension bar should be added to prevent flexion contracture with a hinge. If using an internal device, a bilateral hip abduction brace with a rigid pelvic band can be used to maintain hip abduction. Lengthening should not be resumed at this time.

If a pelvic osteotomy is performed after lengthening, care must be taken not to force the hip into the acetabulum. Since the femoral head is osteoporotic, it can be easily crushed with attempts at reduction. A hip dislocation that occurs after frame removal or during IM nail consolidation should be treated with an open reduction, capsulorraphy, femoral shortening, and pelvic osteotomy. The femur should be osteotomized after the capsulotomy and the femoral head reduced into joint. The bone ends of the femur are overlapped to determine the amount of shortening required. It is essential to shorten it. There must be no tension on the femoral head if it is to remain in the acetabulum. It is important to preserve the superior capsule; if released, it will lead to recurrent dislocation. If the hip is difficult to stabilize despite all of these measures, it can be tethered in place using a suture anchor in the cotyloid notch, with the suture passing through the fovea and out the lateral neck. This creates a mobile tether that prevents dislocation while limiting motion. This technique was developed by the senior author and has been used since 2002 (Fig. 29.32).

Knee Subluxation/Dislocation

Most cases of CFD usually have hypoplastic or absent cruciate ligaments in the knee [34, 68]. The tendency toward flexion contracture during lengthening predisposes the tibia to posterior subluxation. Posterolateral or external rotatory subluxation may occur with a tight fascia lata and biceps. The anterior or anteromedial subluxation can result from extension contractures and patella alta.

A more proximal femoral lengthening is less likely to cause knee subluxation, but it often has narrower and less well-formed regenerated bone, leading to higher fracture risk [86].

To prevent knee subluxation, the distal fascia lata should be released. If using an external fixator, it should span the knee to include the tibia. The spanning fixator also protects the knee cartilage and physis from increased forces. An articulated hinge can be used to allow the patient to maintain knee range of motion. If using an internal lengthening device, a custom HKAFO is used to maintain the knee in full extension while still allowing a range of motion. Posterior or anterior subluxation can be monitored on a lateral knee radiograph in full extension [103]. If the knee begins to subluxate, the rate of lengthening may need to be decreased, as well as the addition of more intensive physical therapy for stretching.

If the knee subluxates or dislocates after removal of the external fixator or consolidation of the regenerate when using an internal device, it should initially be treated by aggressive physical therapy, traction, and splinting. Physical therapy measures include pulling the tibia forward or backward depending on the direction of subluxation and rotating it inward during knee extension and flexion range of motion. If the knee remains subluxated despite an adequate trial of several months of therapy, it requires a version of the SUPERknee procedure called a "rescue knee." This involves lengthening the biceps femoris and the iliotibial band if it is intact. In some cases, the Langenskiöld is done to reduce the patella into joint (Fig. 29.33). If there is a fixed flexion deformity, the femur must be shortened proximally to avoid creating a quadriceps lag. In the most severe cases, a posterior capsulotomy is required. If the knee also has an extension contracture, this can be combined with a Judet quadricepsplasty [104].

Limb Malalignment

Limb length equalization should be based on full-length standing radiographs. Limb alignment is assessed for the femur and tibia both separately and in combination. The joint orientation of the knee should be measured using the malalignment test [105].

Axial deviation from lengthening (procurvatum and valgus for distal femoral lengthening and procurvatum and varus for proximal lengthening) is identified and corrected at the end of the distraction phase, when the regenerated bone is still malleable. This is easiest to do when lengthening with an external fixator, but is still possible with internal lengthening methods. When there is malalignment of the femur and tibia, the femoral malalignment is corrected to a normal distal femoral joint orientation. The femur is not over- or undercorrected to compensate for the tibial deformity. The tibia should be corrected separately, either during the same treatment or at a later treatment. Residual malalignment can usually be addressed with hemiepiphysiodesis or repeat osteotomy.

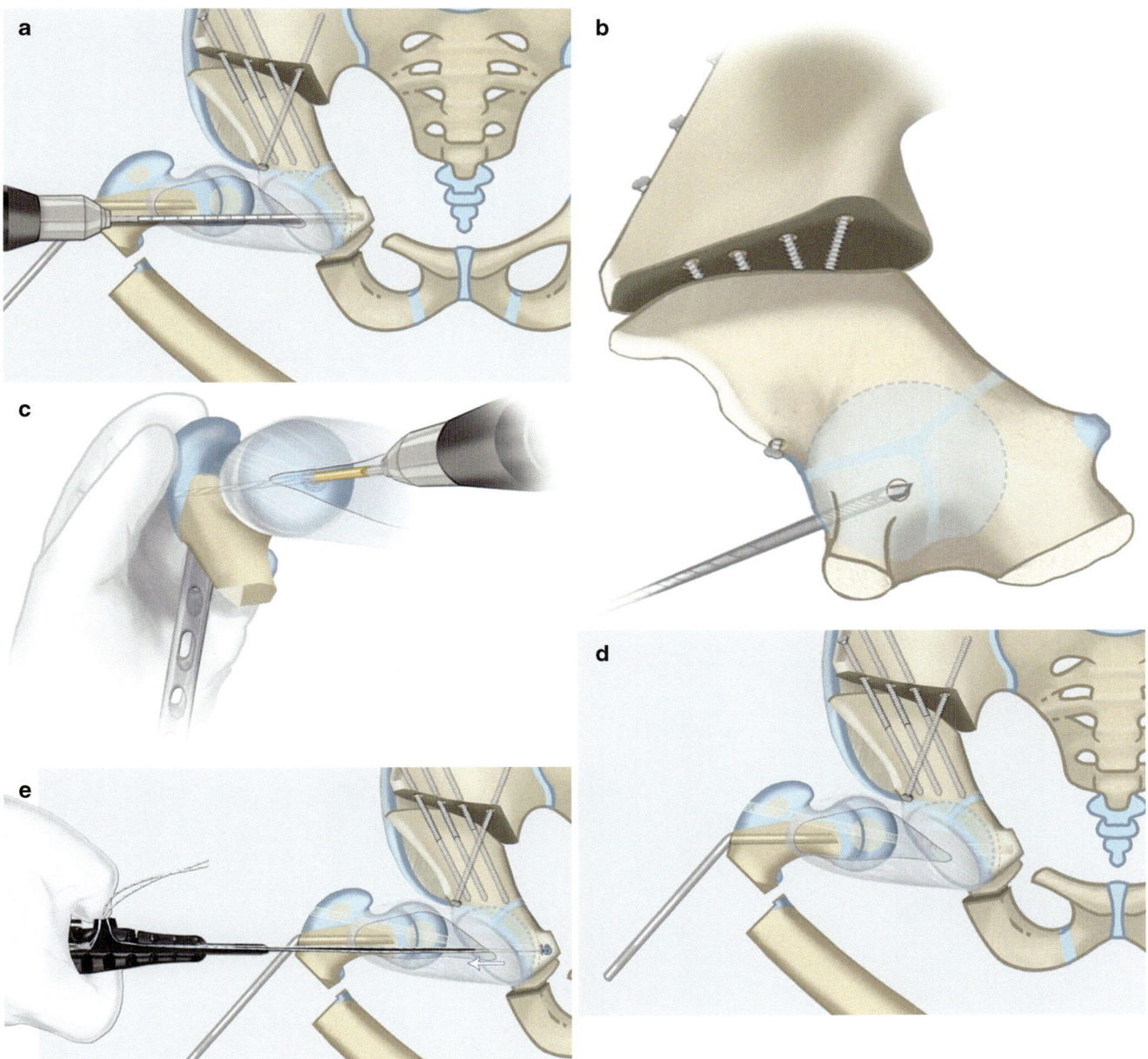

Fig. 29.32 (a) After the pelvic osteotomy is fixed, a guidewire for the suture anchor is inserted into the cotyloid notch and a cannulated drill is passed over the wire. (b) The suture anchor should sit medial and anterior to the triradiate cartilage. (c) A hole is then drilled in retrograde fashion, through the fovea of the femoral head, exiting at the base of the greater trochanter. (d) The hip should sit in slightly abducted position due to the trajectory of the tunnel. (e) The suture anchor is inserted into the cotyloid notch and secured. (f) Medial view of suture anchor position. (g) The sutures are passed through the femoral head tunnel. (h) The head is reduced, and the sutures are secured. (i) The femur ends can now be overlapped and the amount of shortening measured. (j) A second osteotomy is performed of the femoral shaft to remove the overlapping segment. The femur shaft can now be fixed to the plate (Copyright: The Paley Foundation. Reproduced with permission. All rights reserved.)

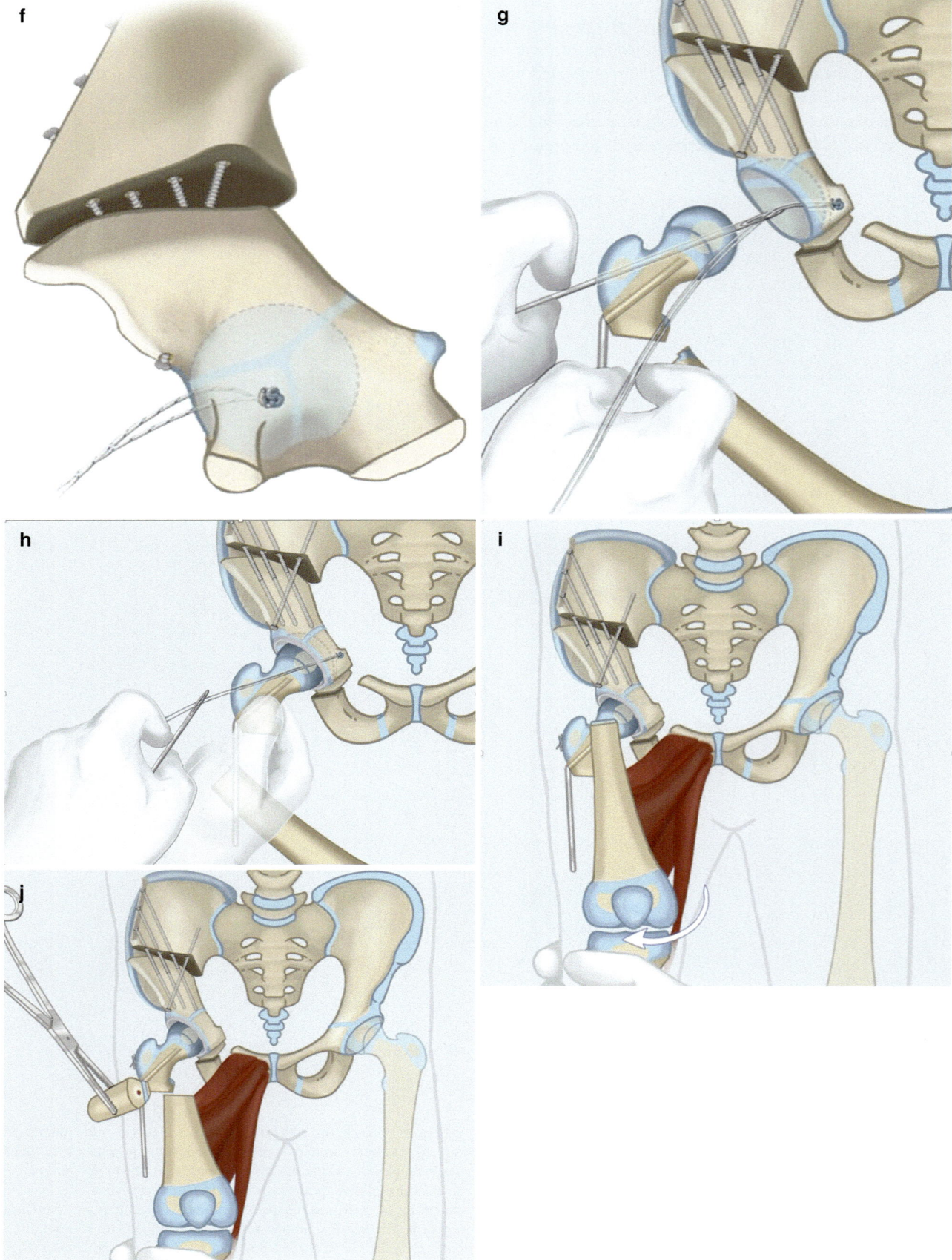

Fig. 29.32 (continued)

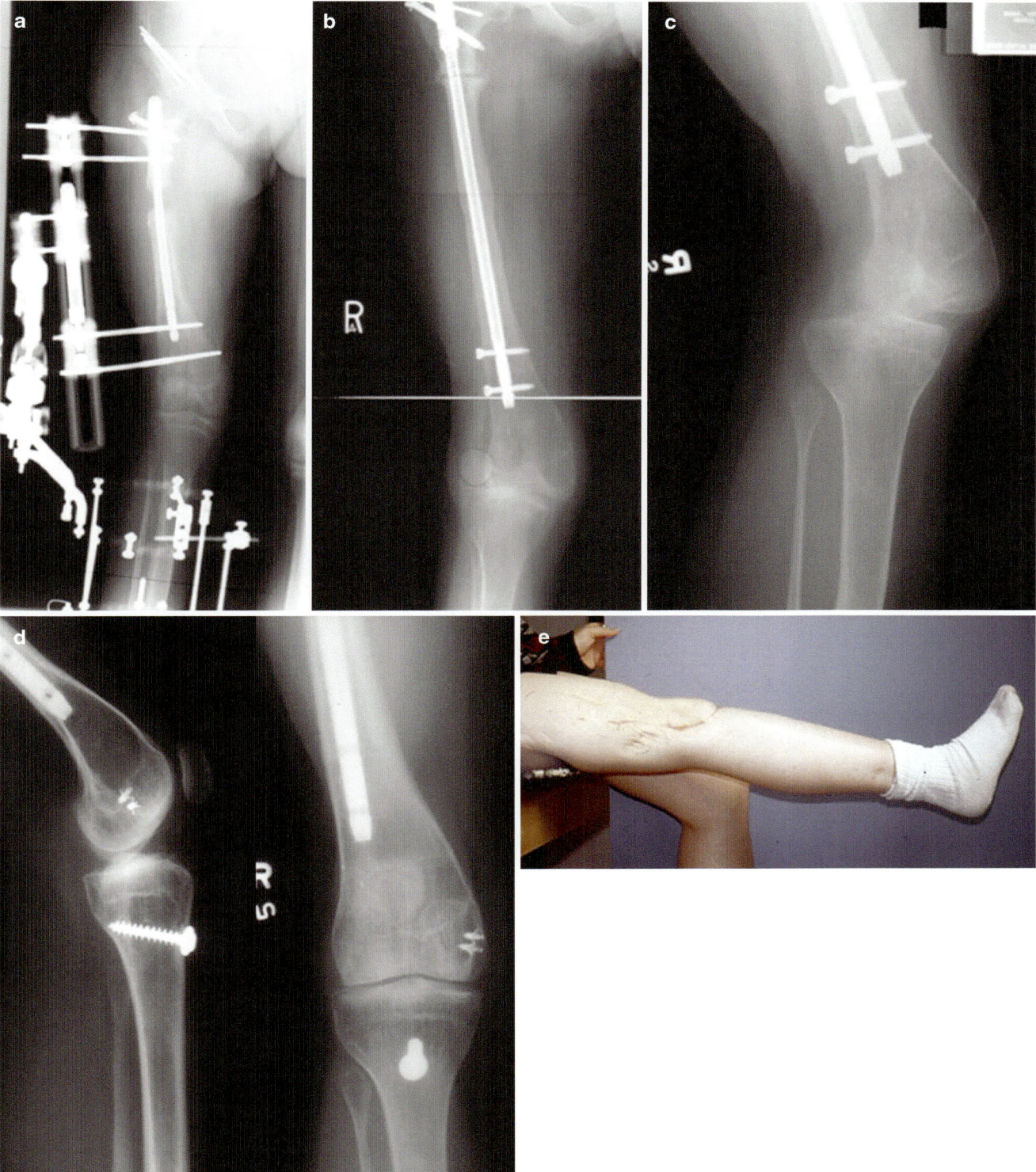

Fig. 29.33 (a) 13-year-old girl with CFD who underwent lengthening over a nail with a monolateral external fixator articulated across the knee. (b) After the nail was locked and the fixator removed, the knee developed an external rotatory subluxation with lateral patellar dislocation. (c) A true AP X-ray of the tibia that demonstrates an oblique view of the femur, which is internally rotated in relation to the tibia. (d) AP and lateral radiographs of the knee after undergoing a rescue knee procedure, including a reverse Macintosh, Elmslie-Trillat tubercle transfer, and Langenskiöld patellar realignment. The knee joint is now well reduced, and the patella tracking has been restored. (e) Clinical photographs 10 years after Rescue knee surgery demonstrating full knee extension and (f) full knee flexion (Copyright: The Paley Foundation. Reproduced with permission. All rights reserved.)

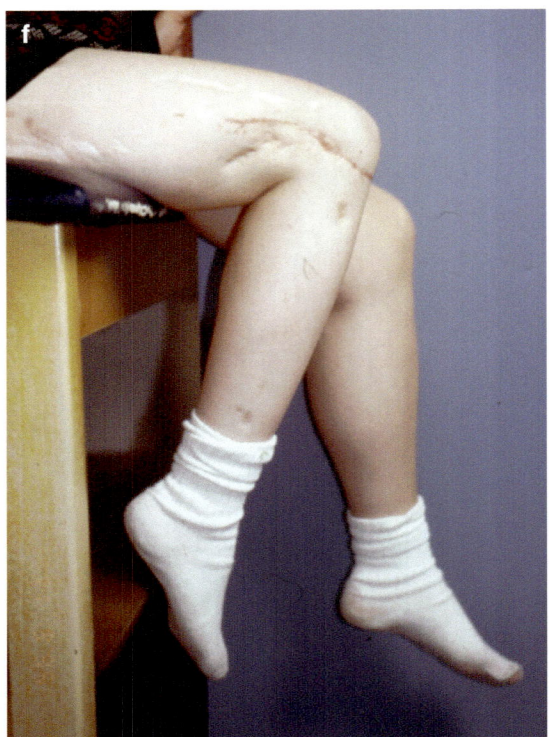

Fig. 29.33 (continued)

Fractures

Fractures associated with limb lengthening can occur throughout and after the lengthening process. Fractures can occur through pin or screw holes, at stress risers at the tip of intramedullary nails, or be pathologic secondary to disuse osteoporosis. A fall on a frame can cause a femoral neck fracture or a pinhole fracture, usually the second most proximal pin. Physical therapy manipulation can cause flexion buckle fractures of the proximal tibia or distal femur. An unexpected muscle spasm during frame removal can cause flexion failure of the femur through a pinhole or the regeneration. After frame removal, fractures can occur through pinholes or the regenerated bone, usually at the mid-regenerate area or host bone junction. The incidence of all these types of fractures associated with CFD lengthening was 34% compared to 9% for non-congenital femoral lengthening [86, 87, 106]. In many cases, this was despite the use of a spica cast after removal.

By prophylactically rodding the femur at the time of removal, the risk of refracture is much lower [76]. There is still a concern for intramedullary infection, so proper irrigation, debridement, and curettage before nail insertion are warranted. Patients are given intraoperative antibiotics and a 10-day course of oral antibiotics.

Prophylactic rodding permits the continuation of knee mobility after removal. To protect from osteoporotic stress fractures through the tibial pinholes, we hold formal physical therapy for a month but permit the patient a gentle range of

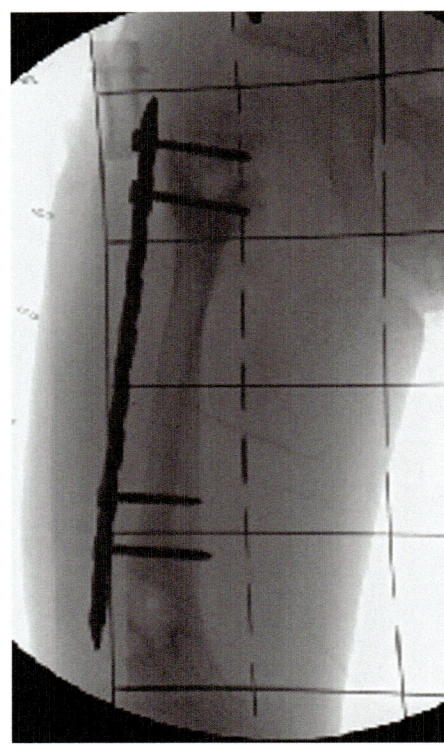

Fig. 29.34 Intraoperative fluoroscopy demonstrating submuscular plating after severely infected external fixator removal. Note that the screw locations are surrounding but not involving the infected pin sites in the femur (Copyright: The Paley Foundation. Reproduced with permission. All rights reserved.)

knee motion. Rodding also permits weight-bearing with a removable spica cast right after frame removal. Fractures may still occur after rodding if the rod is too small or too short. The appropriate diameter rod should be used in each case. In most small children, the 3.2- or 4-mm SLIM rod is used. In larger children, the 4.8-mm rod is preferable, and in older children, the 5.4- or 6.4-mm SLIM rod is chosen. In general, the SLIM rod is passed as distal as possible to the edge of the distal femoral physis.

Alternatively, a prophylactic submuscular plate can be used when the pin sites are too infected to allow safe rodding (Fig. 29.34).

Joint Stiffness and Contracture

The knee can develop both flexion and extension contractures during lengthening. Although transfixing pins or wires may contribute to difficulty in flexion, even lengthening with internal distractors may still lead to loss of knee flexion with increased length. However, stiffness of the knee is preventable. Surgical release and lengthening of specific soft tissues (fascia lata, rectus femoris) reduce the joint reactive forces on the knee due to lengthening. They can be done acutely with the index procedure, but the soft tissues may heal together prior to the end of distraction. A delayed release at about 6 weeks allows more soft-tissue distraction since the release occurs when the soft tissues are taut from lengthening.

Dynamic splinting can be done by using commercially available products or office-customized splints such as those developed by Bhave [107]. The custom knee device consists of two fiberglass casting material cuffs for the thigh and lower leg connected by cast brace hinges. The elastic forces are applied using elastic bandages anteriorly off of various towers suspended proximal and distal to the knee. This is a very efficient and inexpensive type of dynamic splinting.

Physical therapy is essential to successful CFD lengthening. This is especially true for the knee, and one should not consider lengthening a CFD case without adequate outpatient PT. If the knee gets stiff in flexion despite adequate rehabilitation, then a quadricepsplasty should be performed. Rozbruch recommends doing this at or shortly after frame removal [108]. He cuts the central tendon of the quadriceps while leaving the medial and lateral musculature intact. He claims that this does not lead to a quadriceps lag. Martin et al published a series of six patients who underwent a distal quadricepsplasty with an oblique transection of the extensor mechanism [109]. The senior author prefers to do a full Judet quadricepsplasty instead. With a concomitant flexion contracture, either an external fixator with gradual distraction or an open posterior capsule release can be performed.

Prosthetic Reconstruction Surgery for CFD

Rotationplasty

Rotationplasty has been a commonly accepted treatment for patients with CFD with significant proximal deficiency, which is deemed "unreconstructable" [71, 72, 110–112]. Popularized in 1950 by Van Nes for use in patients with CFD [110], the lower limb is rotated 180° to allow the ankle to function as a knee joint and a below-knee-type prosthesis can be fitted onto the foot. This original version left the hip floating free in relation to the pelvis and fused the knee in extension. Krajbich modified this method with the use of a long lateral S-shaped incision. The lack of anchor at the hip resulted in a tendency for the limb to derotate, decreasing the function of the rotationplasty [113].

Brown presented a new type of rotationplasty in the late 1990s that makes use of a circumferential incision to fuse the femoral remnant to the pelvis. This allowed the knee to contribute to hip flexion with the ankle. The anchoring of the femur to the pelvis also served to prevent the loss of rotation [72, 114] (Fig. 29.35a–f).

In 1997, the Paley-Brown rotationplasty was described by Paley. A Chiari osteotomy of the pelvis was added to allow the femoral remnant to be fused to the pelvis in a more ana-

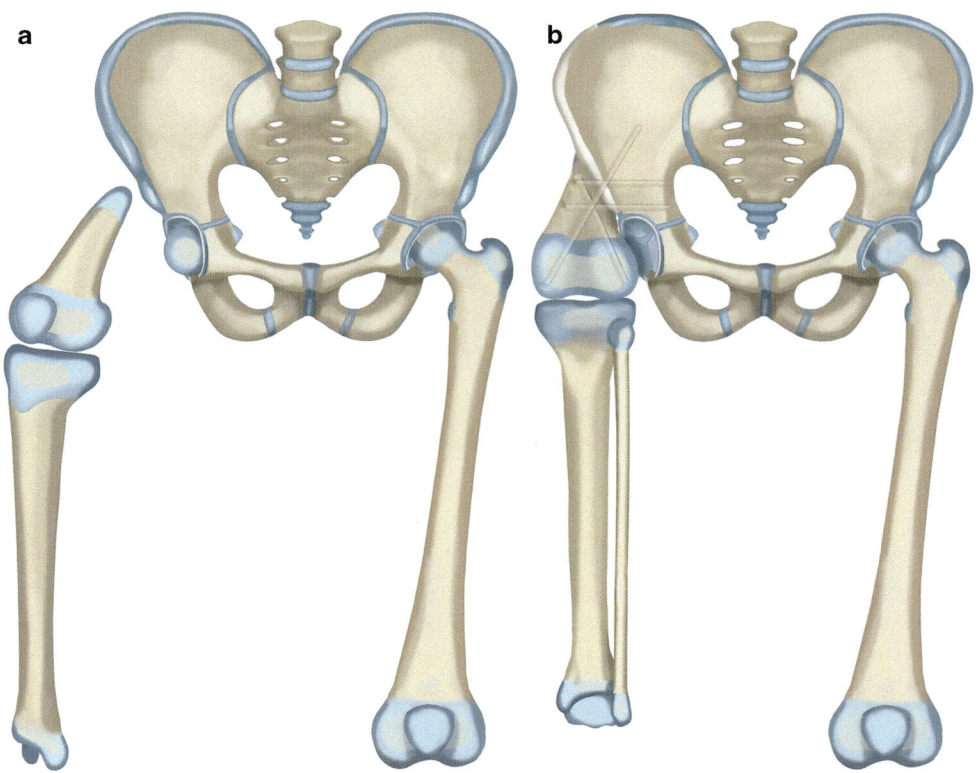

Fig. 29.35 (a) CFD Paley type 3 with an absent proximal femur. (b) Brown rotationplasty (RP) for type 3a or 3b CFD. (c) AP pelvis X-ray of a 14-year-old boy with Paley type 3b CFD. (d) Preoperative EL of the same boy. Note that the right ankle is at the level of opposite knee. (e) AP pelvis radiograph in the same boy 7 years after healed Brown RP. (f) EL radiograph wearing his prosthetic 7 years after Brown RP with supramalleolar osteotomy to improve ankle (knee) alignment. Clinically, he has excellent function (Copyright: The Paley Foundation. Reproduced with permission. All rights reserved.)

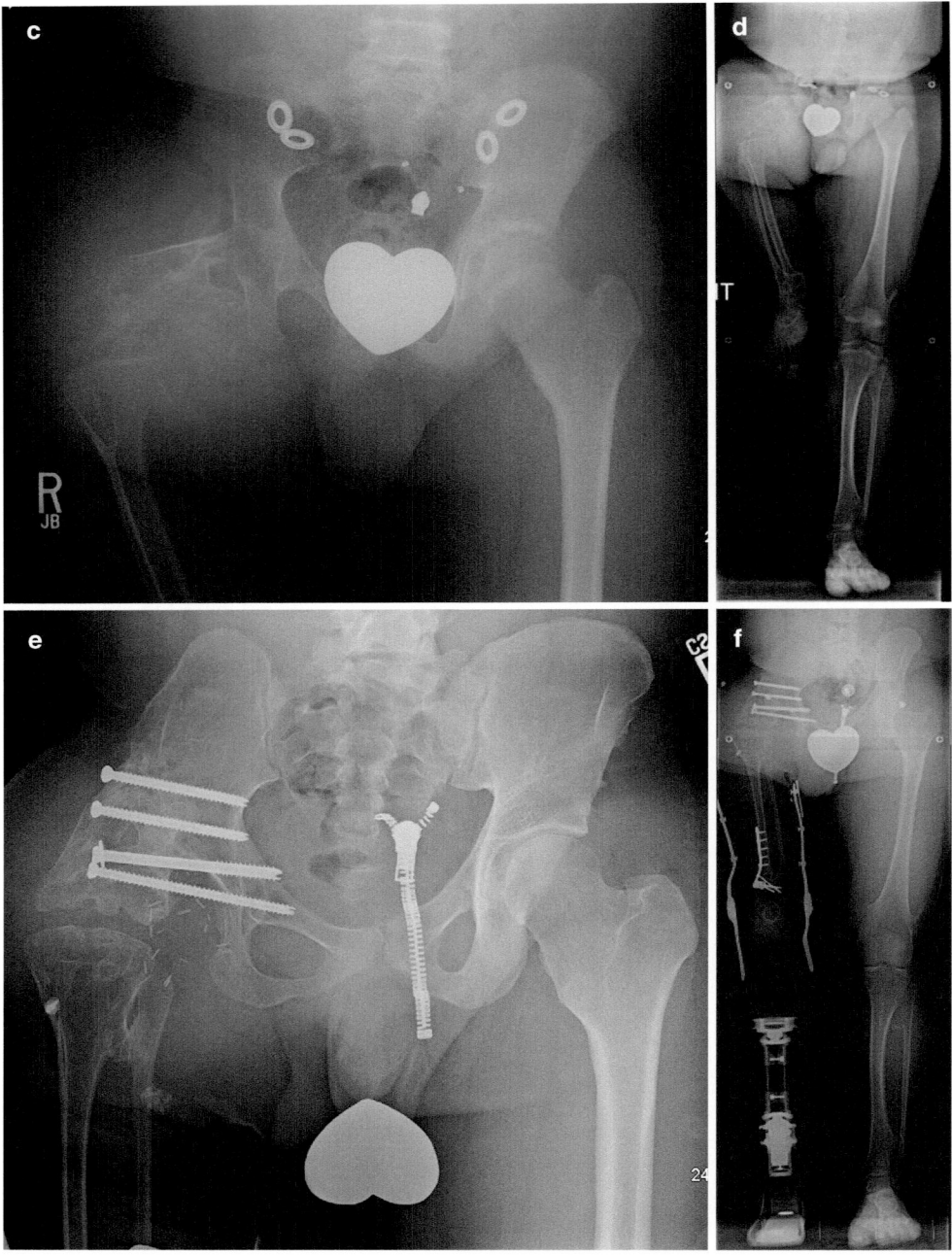

Fig. 29.35 (continued)

tomic alignment with medialization of the lower extremity. This improved the hip mechanics, as well as the cosmesis [43]. The detached muscles are not removed and are instead transferred distally as much as possible. Care is taken to appropriately shorten the knee muscles so that they can function adequately as hip flexors and extensors. The fascia lata connected to the gluteus maximus is reattached to the tibia to serve as a hip abductor. Posterior capsule release of the knee is performed as the knee is often contracted as much as 90°. The peroneal nerve is decompressed to prevent injury and allow greater rotation. A supramalleolar osteotomy may be performed to correct the internal rotation deformity of the tibia. Epiphysiodesis is done with the same screws used for fixation of the femur to the pelvis [43] (Fig. 29.36a–d).

In type 2a, 3a, or 3b CFD, where there is a mobile or minimally fused femoral head in the acetabulum, the Paley rotationplasty takes advantage of this and fuses the femoral remnant directly to the mobile femoral head. This preserves hip abduction and rotation, as well as hip flexion and extension [43] (Fig. 29.37a–e).

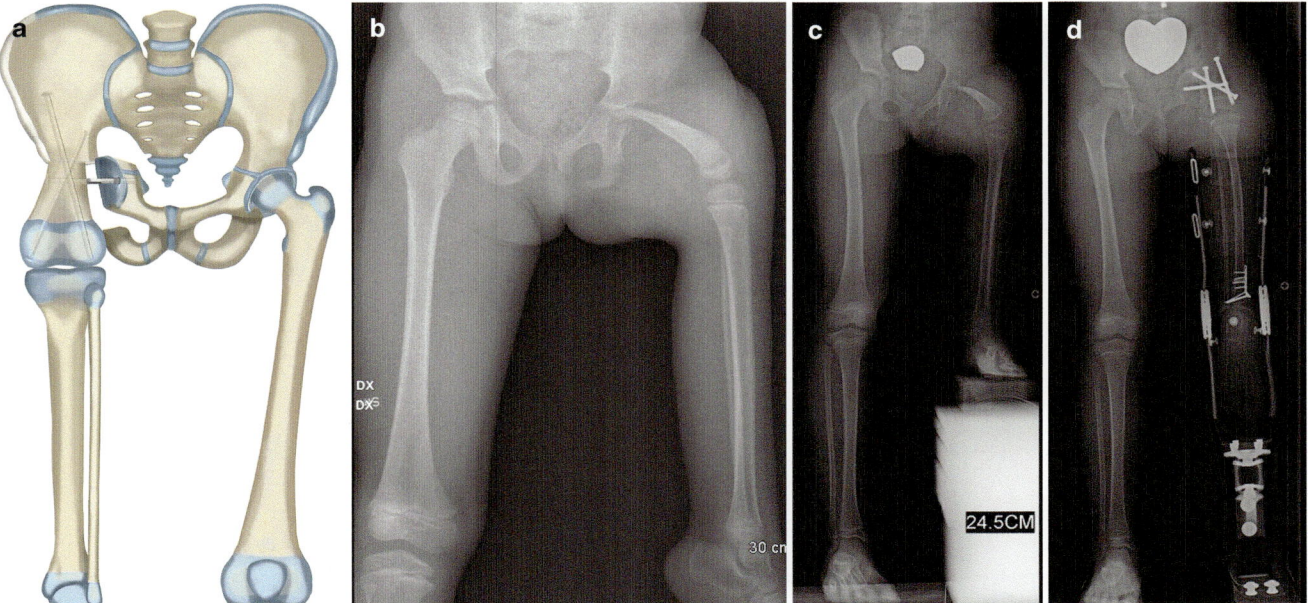

Fig. 29.36 (**a**) Paley-Brown Rotationplasty for Paley type 3a or 3b, (**b**) AP pelvis radiograph in a 3-year-old girl with Paley type 3a CFD, (**c**) standing long radiograph showing the left ankle is at the level of the right knee, and (**d**) standing long radiograph two years after Paley-Brown rotationplasty. The ankle is at the level of the opposite distal femoral physis (level of knee center of rotation) Clinically, she has excellent gait and function. (Copyright: The Paley Foundation. Reproduced with permission. All rights reserved.)

In the case of an ankylosed or absent knee joint, the above rotationplasty types are not indicated due to the inability to create hip motion. Winkelman described a version of the procedure that articulates the tibial plateau in the acetabulum in cases where a total femur resection was required for tumor resection. Paley modified this in 2014 for type 3c CFD (Paley-Winkelman rotationplasty). The fused femoral head was enucleated, and the small femoral remnant or tibial plateau was then articulated in the acetabulum with a suture tether device. Reattachment of the muscles allows preservation of hip flexion/extension [43] (Fig. 29.38a–g).

Rotationplasty may be indicated in CFD cases that have a severely deformed proximal femur, typical of Paley type 1a3 or 1b, as well as in patients with CFD-associated congenital knee fusion, who have severe leg length discrepancy. These patients can be treated with a long S-shaped incision with a modified Van Nes rotationplasty including knee fusion combined with one of the following two hip procedures: (1) SUPERhip procedure to treat the severely deformed proximal femur for types 1a3 or 1b CFD (PaleySUPERhip-Van Nes) (Fig. 29.39a–f) or (2) femoral sling procedure for type 2 or 3 CFD (PaleySling-Van Nes) when a congenital knee fusion is present (Fig. 29.40a–e). Both prevent derotation of the limb after the rotationplasty due to stabilization of the hip joint by either the SUPERhip or sling procedure. In cases of CFD with congenital knee fusion, rotationplasty is performed through the congenital knee fusion level.

In all cases, the ankle should be evaluated for alignment and stability after the limb has been rotated. If there is malorientation of the ankle plane of motion, a derotational supra-malleolar osteotomy can be performed to correct this. In cases where there is proximal migration of the distal fibula with valgus instability of the ankle, the rotationplasty can be combined with a shortening osteotomy realignment distal tibia (SHORDT) procedure to stabilize and realign the ankle [115, 116].

Fuller et al recently published the largest study of rotationplasty surgeries for CFD. This was a single surgeon series of 19 rotationplasty procedures performed over 10 years. The average age at the time of surgery was 8.6 years (2–36 years). The diagnoses included 1 type 1, 3 type 2, and 15 type 3 CFD. The series included ten Paley-Brown, five Paley, two Paley-Winkelman, one Brown, and one PaleySUPERhip-Van Nes rotationplasty. All patients achieved independent walking in a below-knee style prosthesis. The complication rate was high at 63%; however, the most common problem was related to healing of the skin flap (10/19). Other complications that required a return to the operating room included one patient who developed a compartment syndrome, one patient who developed a sciatic nerve palsy, one delayed union of a proximal tibial osteotomy, and two incomplete femur epiphysiodesis. Eleven elective surgeries were performed in the late follow-up period. These included five osteotomies to correct coronal plane deformity, three ankle realignment osteotomies, one

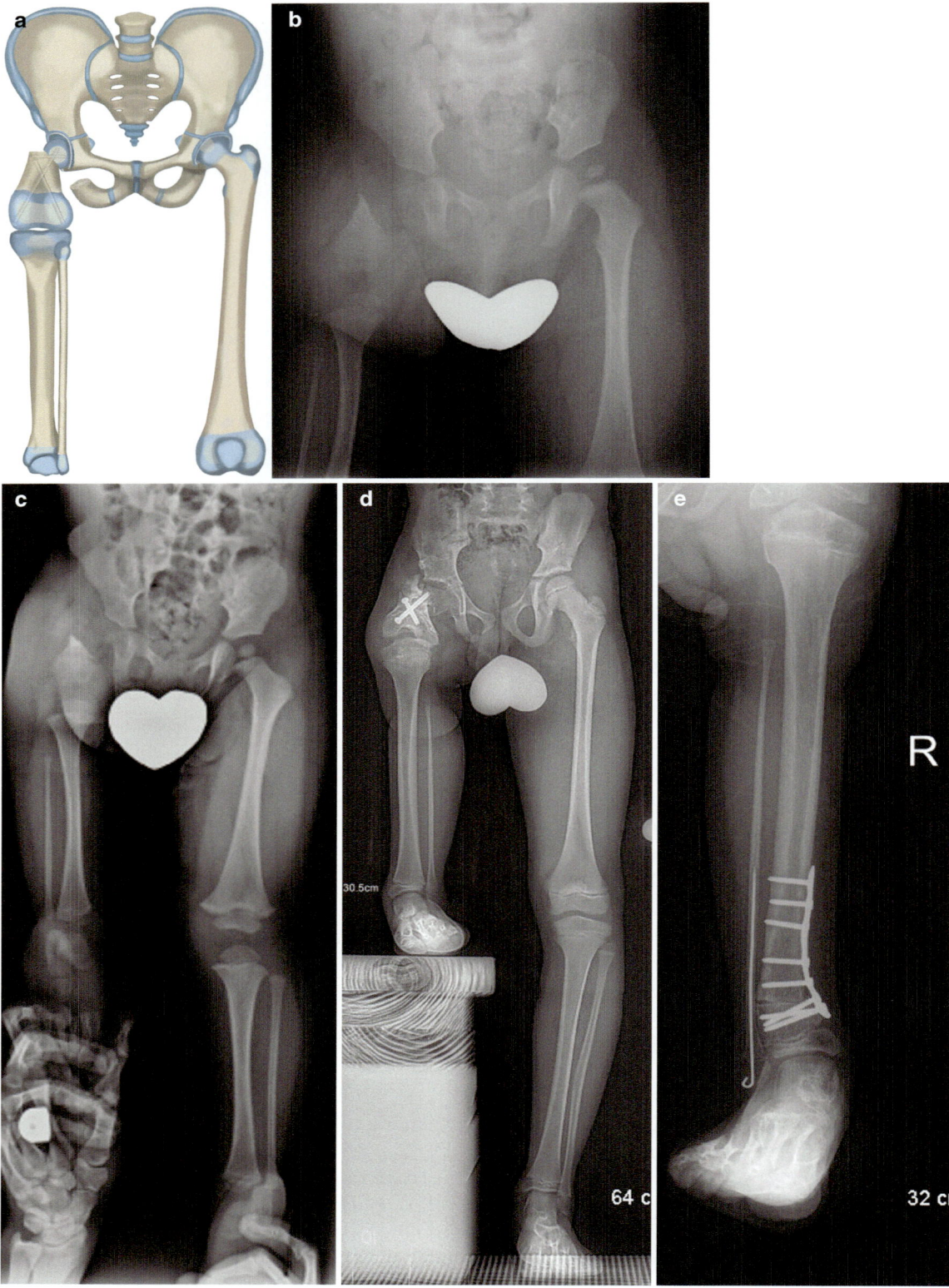

Fig. 29.37 (a) Paley rotationplasty for type 3a or 3b. (b) AP pelvis of 2-year-old boy with CFD Paley type 3a. (c) Standing radiographs in same boy before surgery showing ankle is at level of opposite knee. (d) The femoral head was mobile, so a Paley rotationplasty was performed. Standing long radiograph in same boy, 8 years after Paley rotationplasty. (e) To improve his prosthetic fitting, he had a varus derotation supramalleolar osteotomy performed 8 years after the original rotationplasty. Clinically, he is very sports-active and has excellent gait and function (Copyright: The Paley Foundation. Reproduced with permission. All rights reserved.)

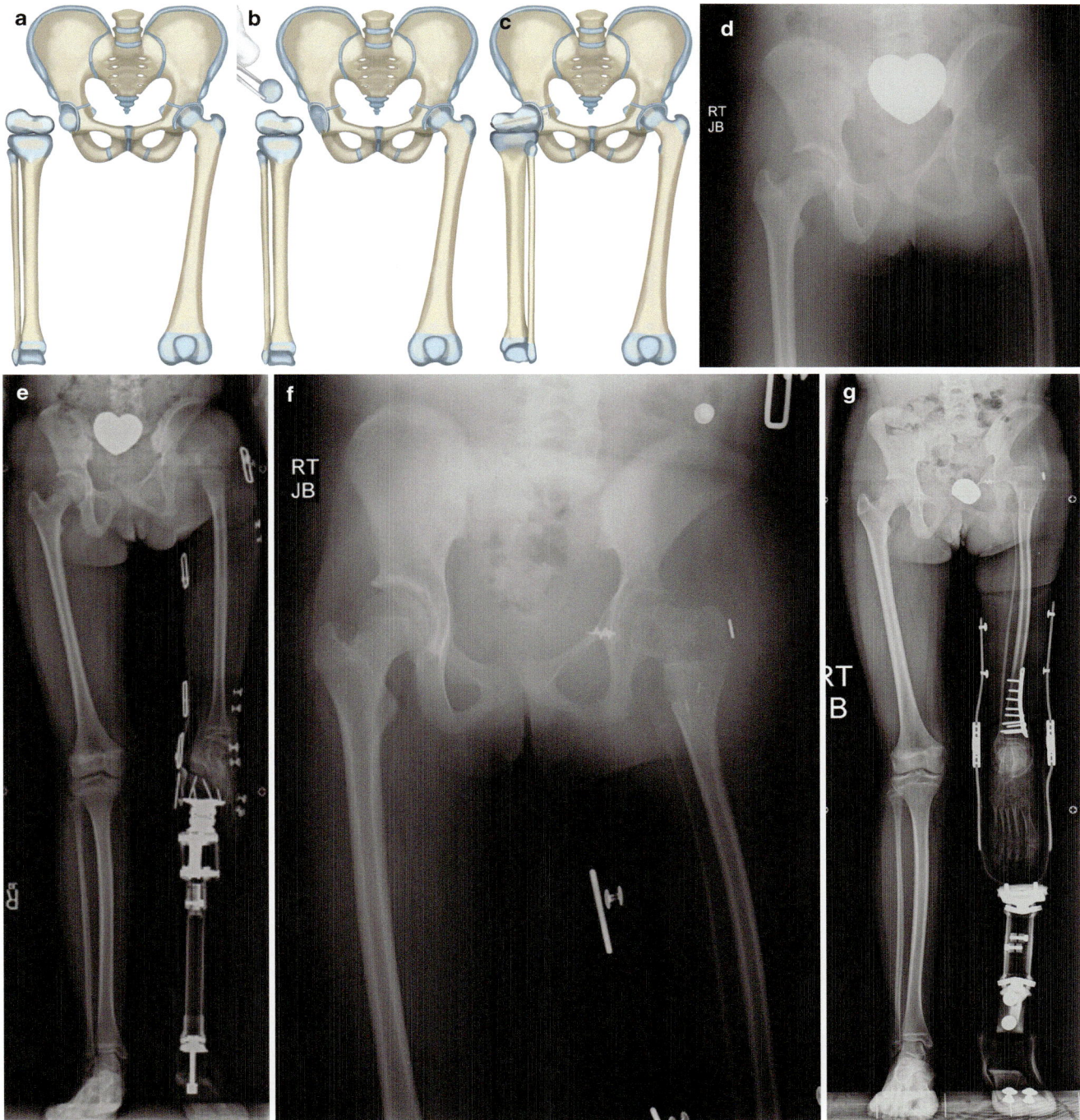

Fig. 29.38 (a) CFD type 3c. There is an ankylosed knee with a small distal femoral remnant. (b) Illustration showing the femoral head enucleated to make room for the femoral condyle or tibial plateau in the acetabulum. (c) Paley-Winkelmann RP illustration, inserting the femoral condyle remnant into the acetabulum secured with a hip tethering suture. (d) AP pelvis radiograph of a 12-year-old girl with CFD Paley type 3c. (e) Standing long radiograph of same RP with femoral condyle in the acetabulum. (f) The tethering suture anchor is seen at the left hip. (g) Standing radiograph of same girl 5 years after Paley-Winkelmann RP. She has excellent function of the new hip joint and can walk and run with minimal limp (Copyright: The Paley Foundation. Reproduced with permission. All rights reserved.)

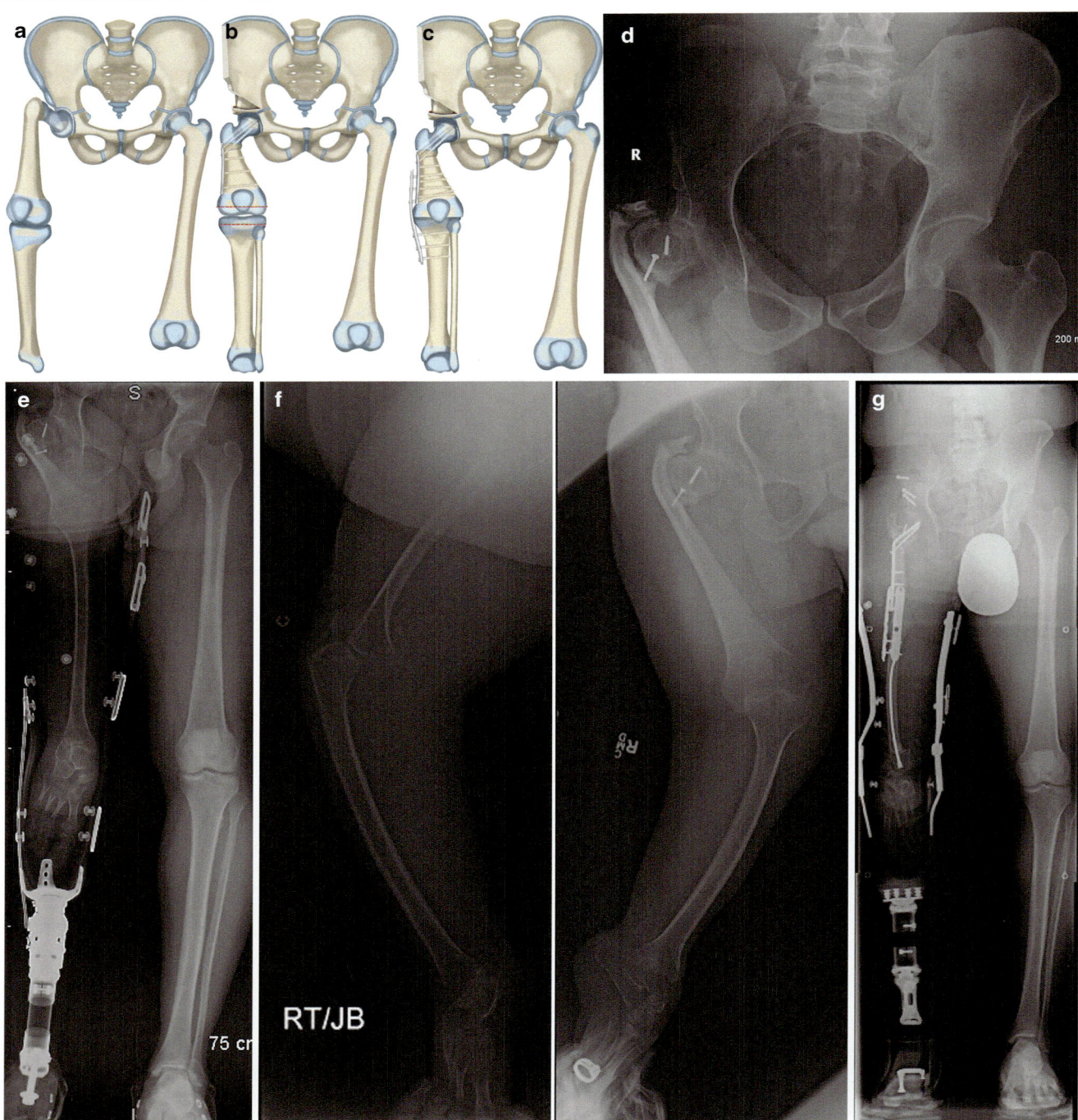

Fig. 29.39 (a) CFD type 1a3 or 1b. (b) Step 1—SUPERhip procedure with resection of knee joint. (c) Step 2—PaleySUPERhip-Van Nes rotationplasty at level of the knee fusion. (d) AP pelvis of a 36-year-old man with CFD type 1b who had undergone prior failed hip surgery. (e) EL radiograph showing that his ankle is at the level of his opposite knee joint. (f) Long lateral and AP radiographs showing the knee joint in the same patient was unstable, deformed, and subluxated. (g) Standing radiograph one year after PaleySUPERhip-Van Nes procedure including SUPERhip, knee fusion, and supramalleolar osteotomy, wearing rotationplasty prosthetic. Ankle is at level of opposite knee. This procedure greatly improved his quality and of life, gait, and function (Copyright: The Paley Foundation. Reproduced with permission. All rights reserved.)

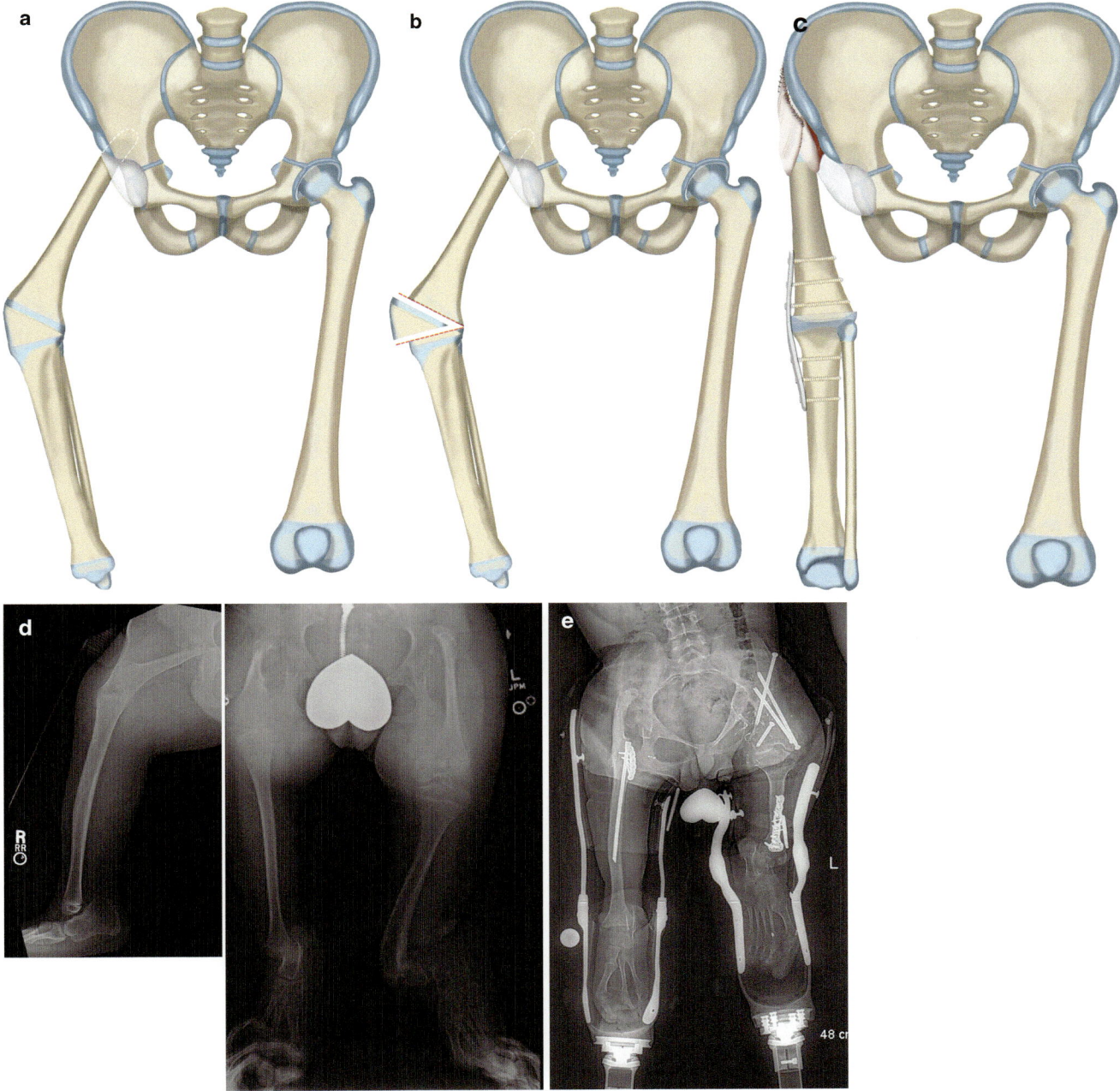

Fig. 29.40 (**a**) CFD type 2c with congenital knee fusion and knee flexion deformity. The fibrous femoral neck anlage tethers the upper femur from migrating proximally. (**b**) Step 1—the PaleySling-VanNes RP. The RP is performed through the knee fusion site. (**c**) Step 2—The proximal femur is stabilized using the fascia lata by creating a sling around the proximal femur. The sling and the fibrous neck anlage stabilize the upper femur from migrating proximally while preserving flexion and extension motion. (**d**) EL (right) of a 14-year-old boy with bilateral CFD. The right side is classified as type 2c and also has a congenital knee fusion as seen on the long lateral radiograph (left). The left side is classified as CFD type 3b, and the knee joint is present and functional. (**e**) EL one year after bilateral RP performed in two separate surgeries. On the right leg, the RP was performed through the congenital knee fusion site together with a sling for the hip (PaleySling-VanNes). On the left leg, a Paley-Brown RP was performed together with a supramalleolar osteotomy for realignment (Copyright: The Paley Foundation. Reproduced with permission. All rights reserved.)

gluteal advancement, and two hardware removals [43]. No patient developed derotation of the limb. The final average pelvo-lower extremity alignment was 94° from the horizontal plane of the pelvis.

Rotationplasty Surgical Technique

Steps for Paley-Brown and Paley Rotationplasty Surgical Procedures

1. Racket incision is made just proximal to the skin crease in the popliteal fossa with a longitudinal extension to this incision that extends to the anterior superior iliac spine and iliac crest (Fig. 29.41a). Posteriorly, a triangle is created for the purpose of adjusting the circumference of the flap at the time of closure (Fig. 29.41b).
2. Elevate full-thickness flaps with the superficial fascia to preserve blood supply to the skin (Fig. 29.41c).
3. Identify the saphenous vein medially, preserve it, and dissect the saphenous vein proximally to where it joins the femoral (Fig. 29.41c).
4. Dissect the femoral artery and vein from this point distally to the knee. Ligate, staple, or cauterize all side branches of the femoral artery and vein, including the profunda femoris and circumflex vessels. The femoral artery and vein need to end up as tubular conduits without tethering branches from the inguinal canal to where they divide at the popliteal fossa (Fig. 29.41d).
5. Dissect free the sartorius muscle, and release it distally from the tibia. Take care to preserve, and dissect free the saphenous nerve which lies adjacent to this muscle. Follow the saphenous nerve back to identify and protect the femoral nerve (Fig. 29.41e).
6. Release the hip adductor muscles off of the medial femur. Clip or cauterize the large number of vessels in this area (Fig. 29.41f).
7. Release the remaining medial hamstrings off of the tibia (Fig. 29.41g).
8. Go to the lateral side, and dissect free the fascia lata. Cut across the iliotibial band at the tibia, and reflect this structure proximally (Fig. 29.41h, i).
9. Identify the posterior border of the biceps femoris muscle, and then, find the common peroneal nerve (Fig. 29.41j).
10. Follow the common peroneal nerve distally to where it enters the peroneal fascia, and decompress it at this first tunnel. Make a transverse incision across the fascia of the lateral and anterior compartments. Find the intermuscular septum and release it to decompress the deep peroneal nerve at the second tunnel (Fig. 29.41k).
11. Now that the peroneal nerve is visible release the biceps tendon from the fibula (Fig. 29.41l).
12. Release the gluteus maximus from the femur (Fig. 29.41m), and identify and release the piriformis muscle (Fig. 29.41n). Follow the peroneal nerve proximally to where it is joined by the posterior tibial nerve and becomes the sciatic nerve (Fig. 29.41o).
13. Release the rest of the external rotators from the femur (Fig. 29.41p).
14. Decompress the sciatic nerve all the way to the sciatic notch. Release the hip abductors off of the proximal end of the femur (Fig. 29.41q).
15. Elevate the quadriceps muscles off of the femur extraperiosteally, starting from lateral to medial. Release the quadriceps distally either at the proximal end of the patella if it is present or at the level of the knee joint if there is no patella. Lift the quadriceps from distal to proximal off of the femur (Fig. 29.41q).
16. Release the rectus femoris tendon off of the anterior inferior iliac spine (Fig. 29.41r).
17. Find the psoas tendon, release it from the femur, and tag it so that it does not retract into the pelvis (Fig. 29.41r).
18. Release the fibrous anlage of the femoral neck off of the femur (Fig. 29.41s).
19. Open the superior capsule and examine if the femoral head is present, fused to the acetabulum, or mobile. In the latter case, consider doing a Paley type of rotationplasty instead of the Paley-Brown (Fig. 29.41t).
20. The proximal femur is now free to rotate since it is no longer tethered by any structures originating from the pelvis. On the lateral side, release the tendon of the lateral head of gastrocnemius off of the femur (Fig. 29.41u).
21. On the medial side, release the tendon of the medial head of the gastrocnemius off of the femur. Dissect the vessels free of the distal femur, but do not damage the branches to the two heads of the gastrocnemius (Fig. 29.41u).
22. Now, rotate the femur externally until the posterior aspect is facing anterior (Fig. 29.41v). If there is a flexion contracture of the knee joint (present in almost all cases), perform a posterior capsulotomy of the knee joint and straighten the knee into full extension (Fig. 29.41w).

Paley-Brown Rotationplasty

1. For the Paley-Brown, split the apophysis. For the Paley type, there is no need to split the apophysis (Fig. 29.41x).
2. Elevate the periosteum off of the medial and lateral walls of the ilium down to the sciatic notch. Laterally, elevate the periosteum off the anterior aspect of the notch to reach the ischium (Fig. 29.41x).
3. Return to the adductor muscles, and resect them from their origins. This requires dissection down to the pubic

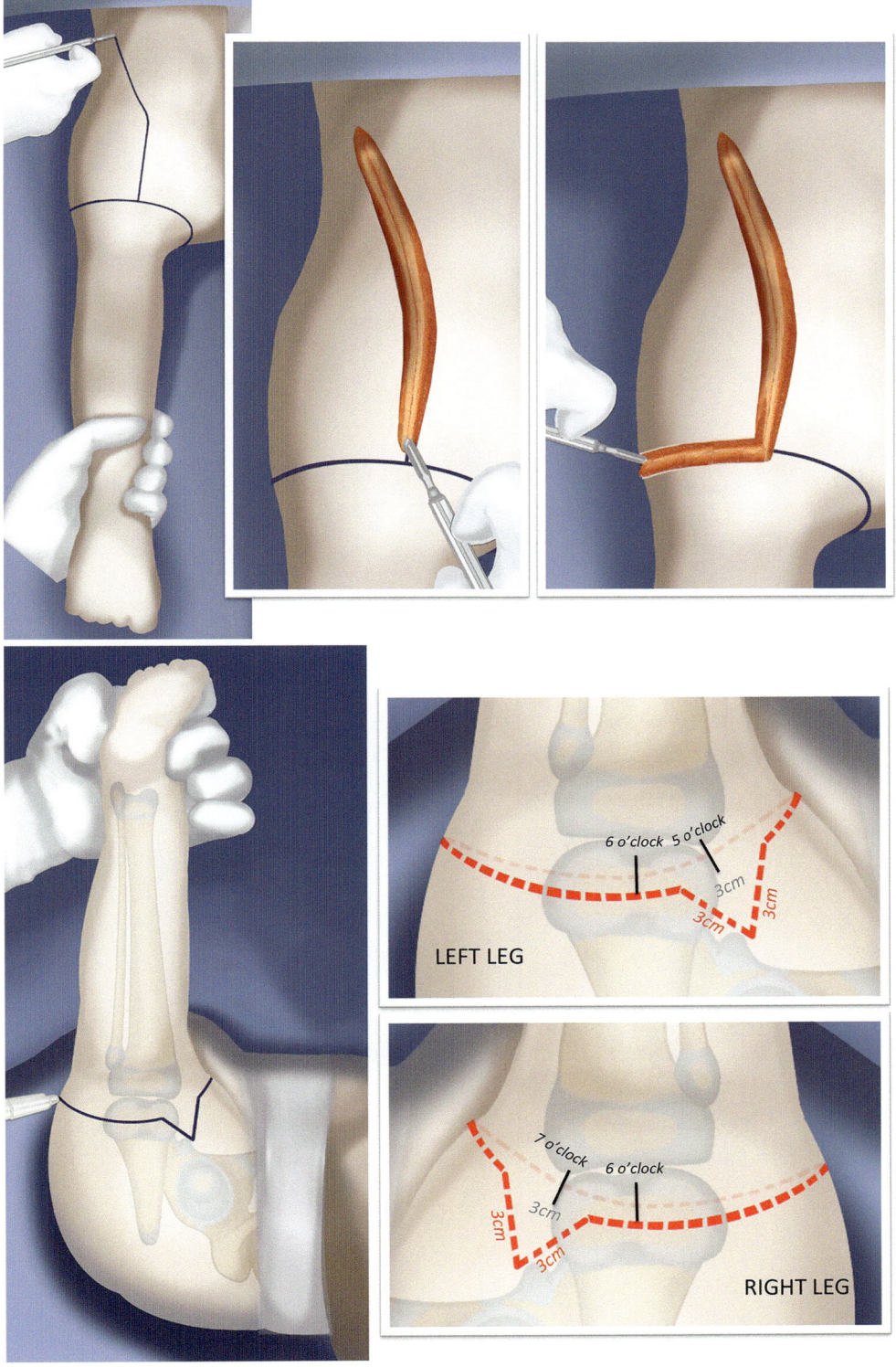

Fig. 29.41 Paley-Brown and Paley Rotationplasty procedures (follow text for steps and captions) (Copyright: The Paley Foundation. Reproduced with permission. All rights reserved.)

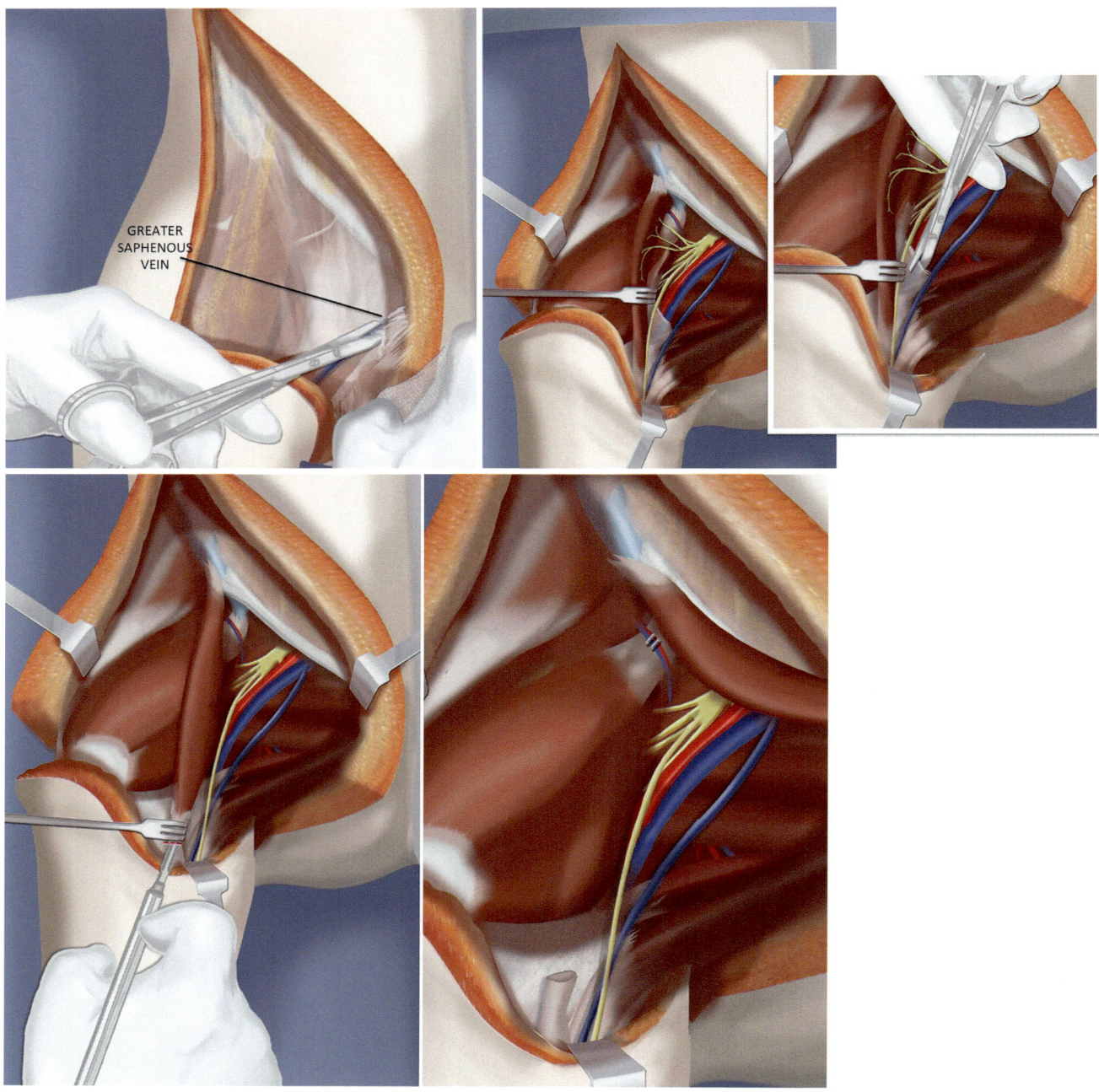

Fig. 29.41 (continued)

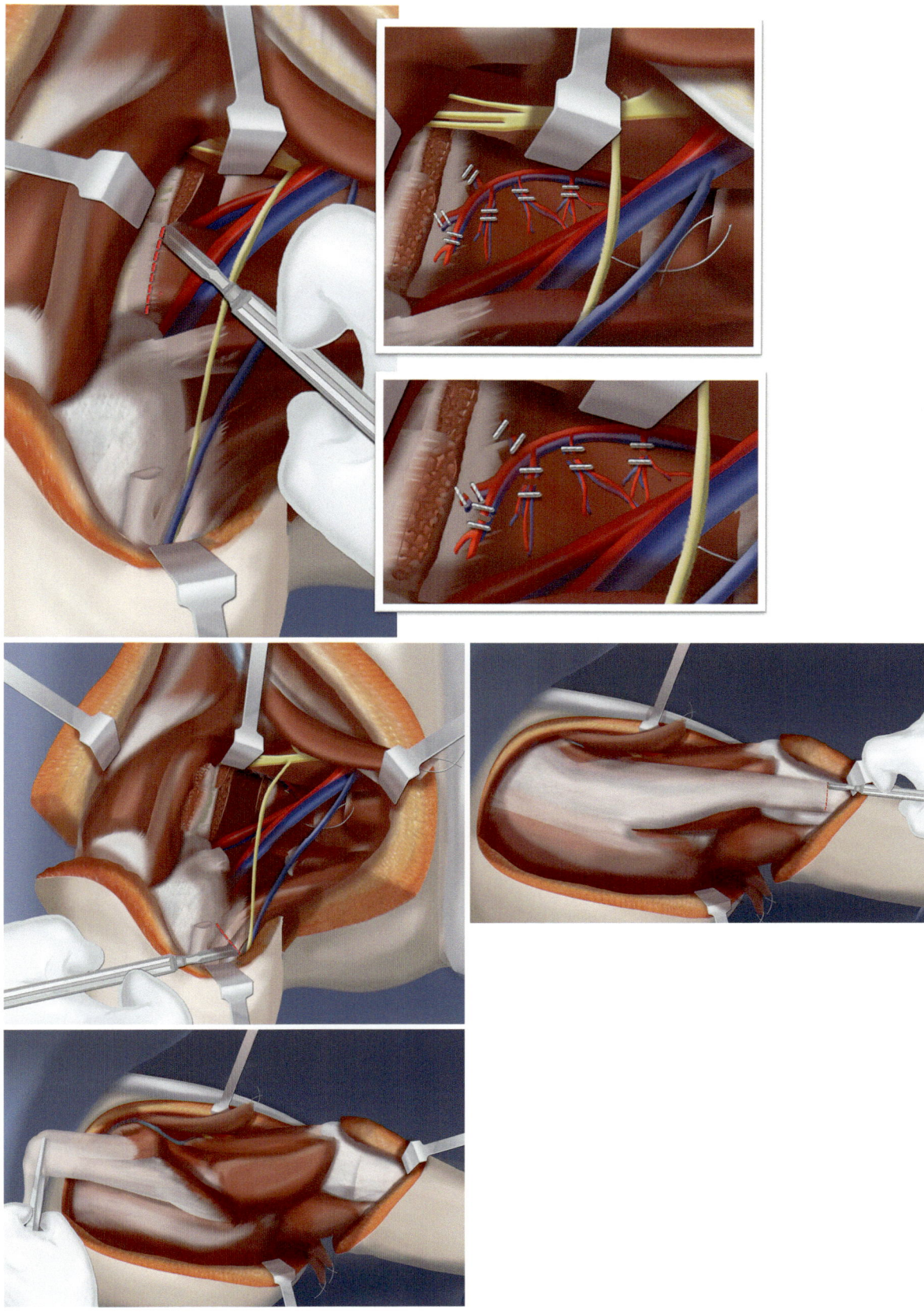

Fig. 29.41 (continued)

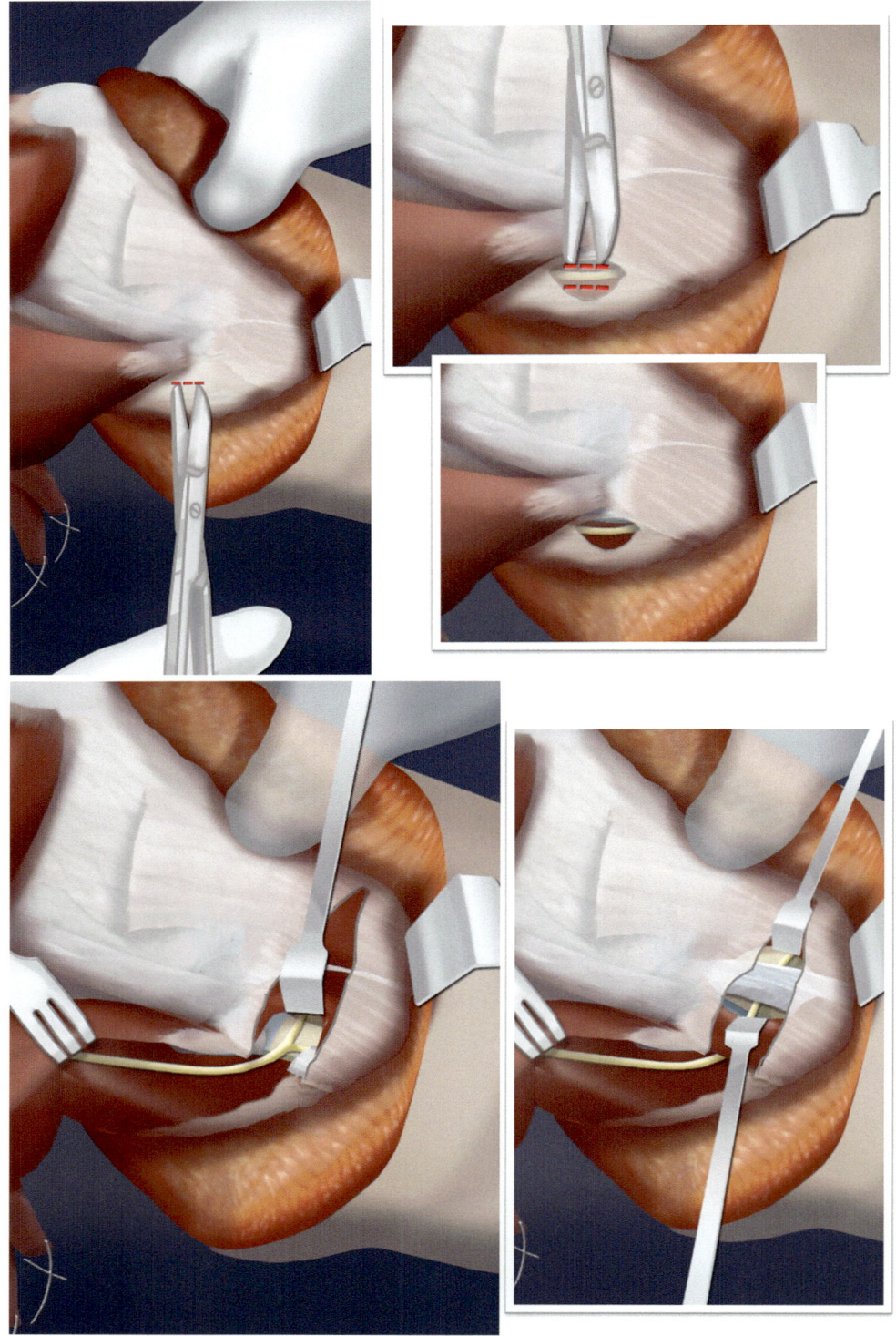

Fig. 29.41 (continued)

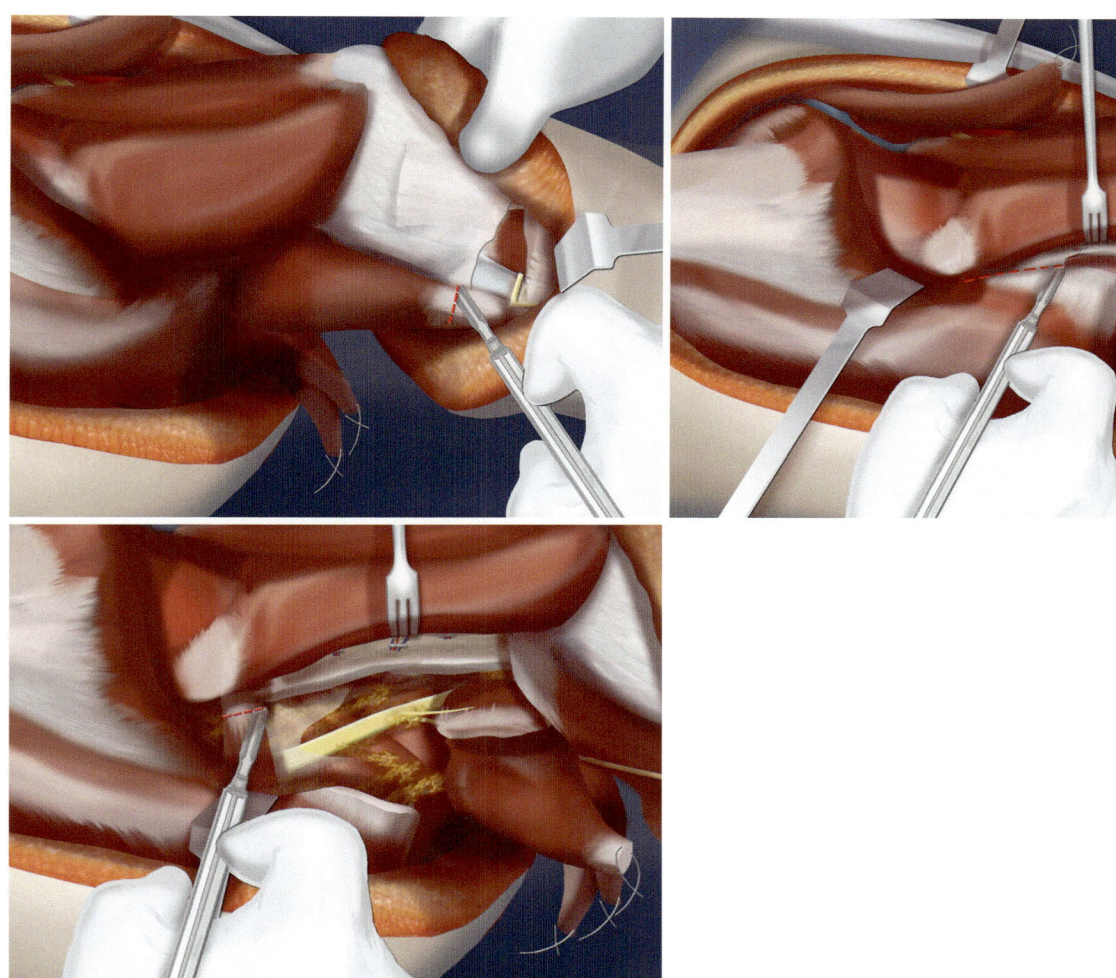

Fig. 29.41 (continued)

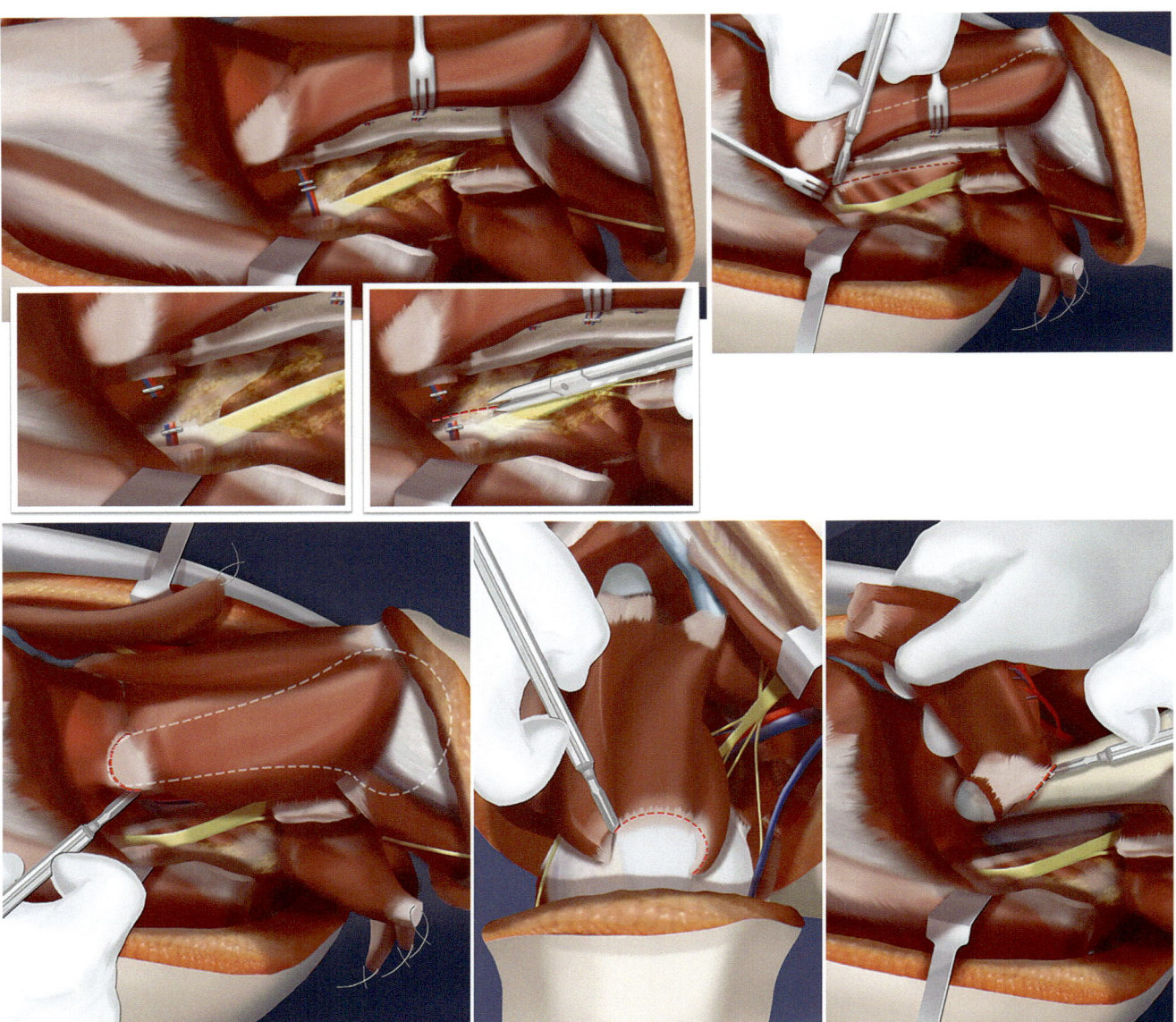

Fig. 29.41 (continued)

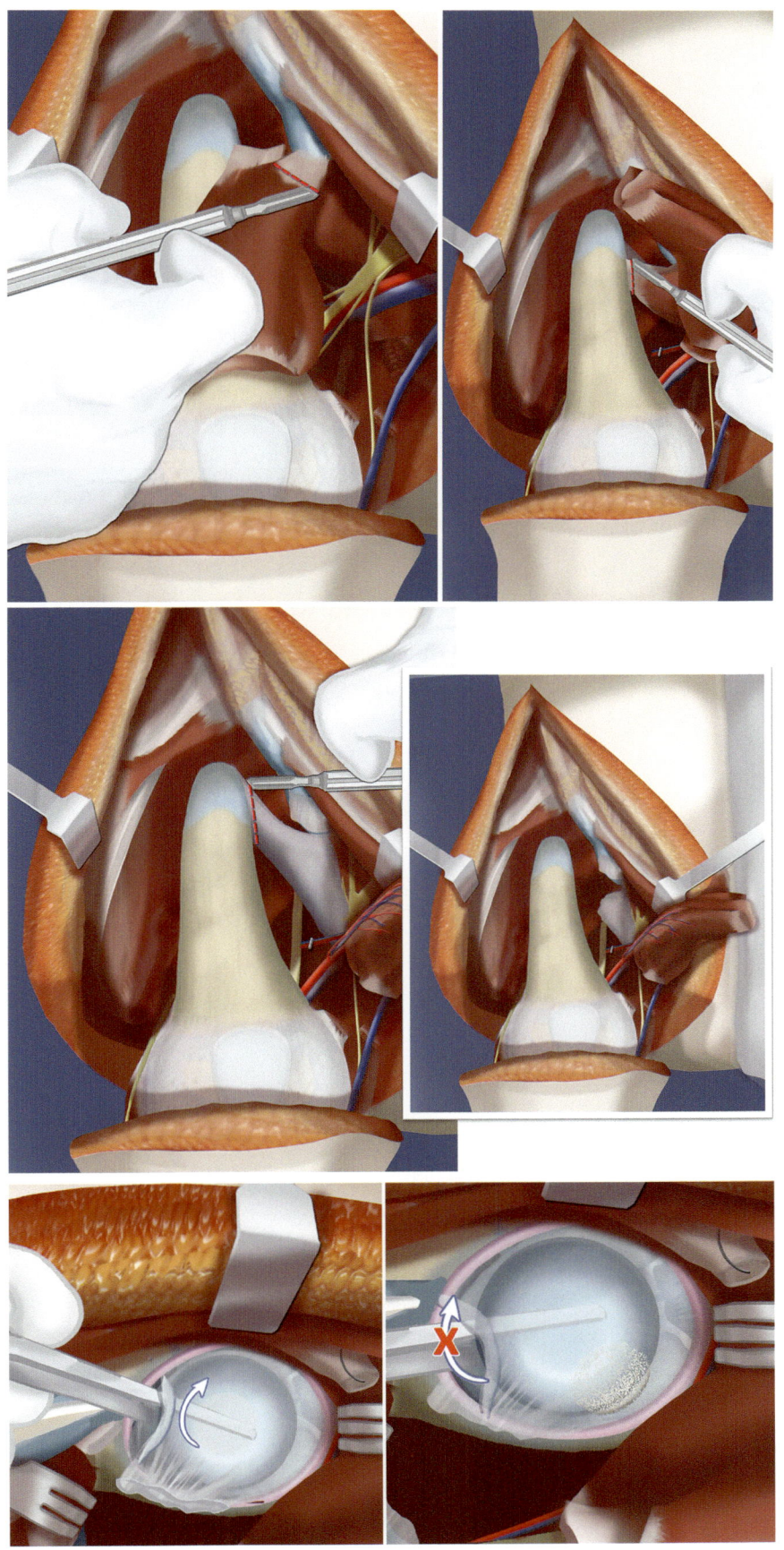

Fig. 29.41 (continued)

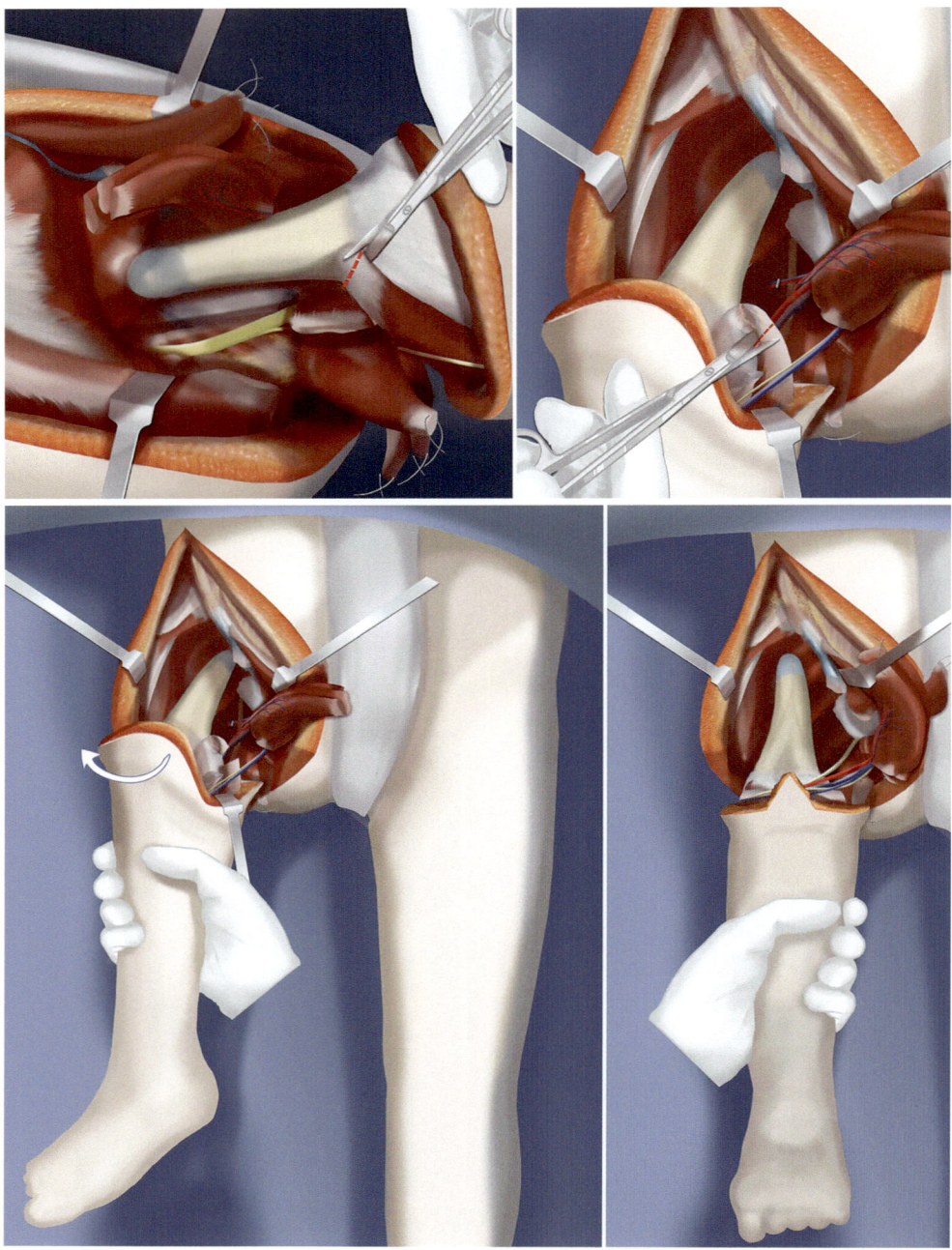

Fig. 29.41 (continued)

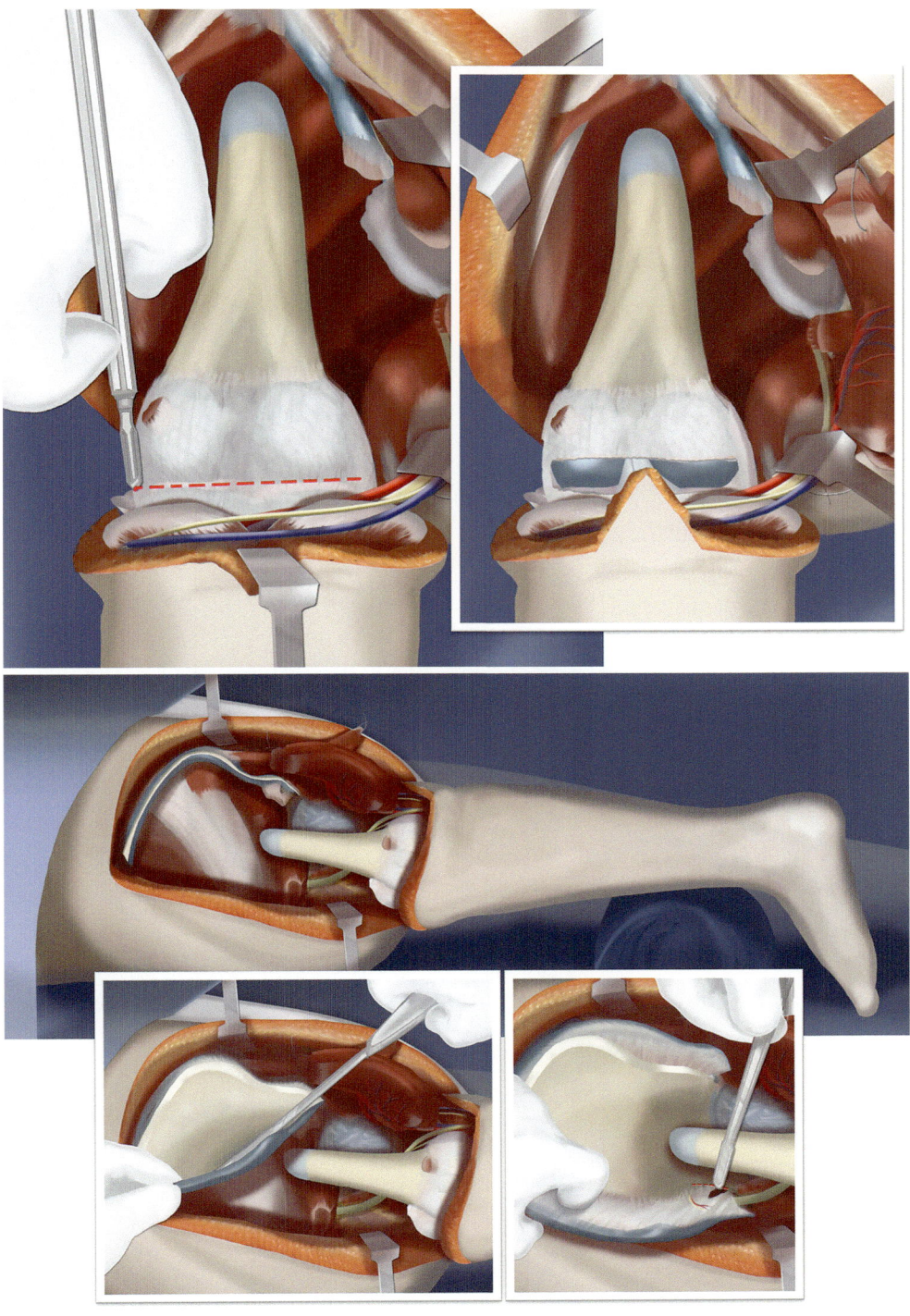

Fig. 29.41 (continued)

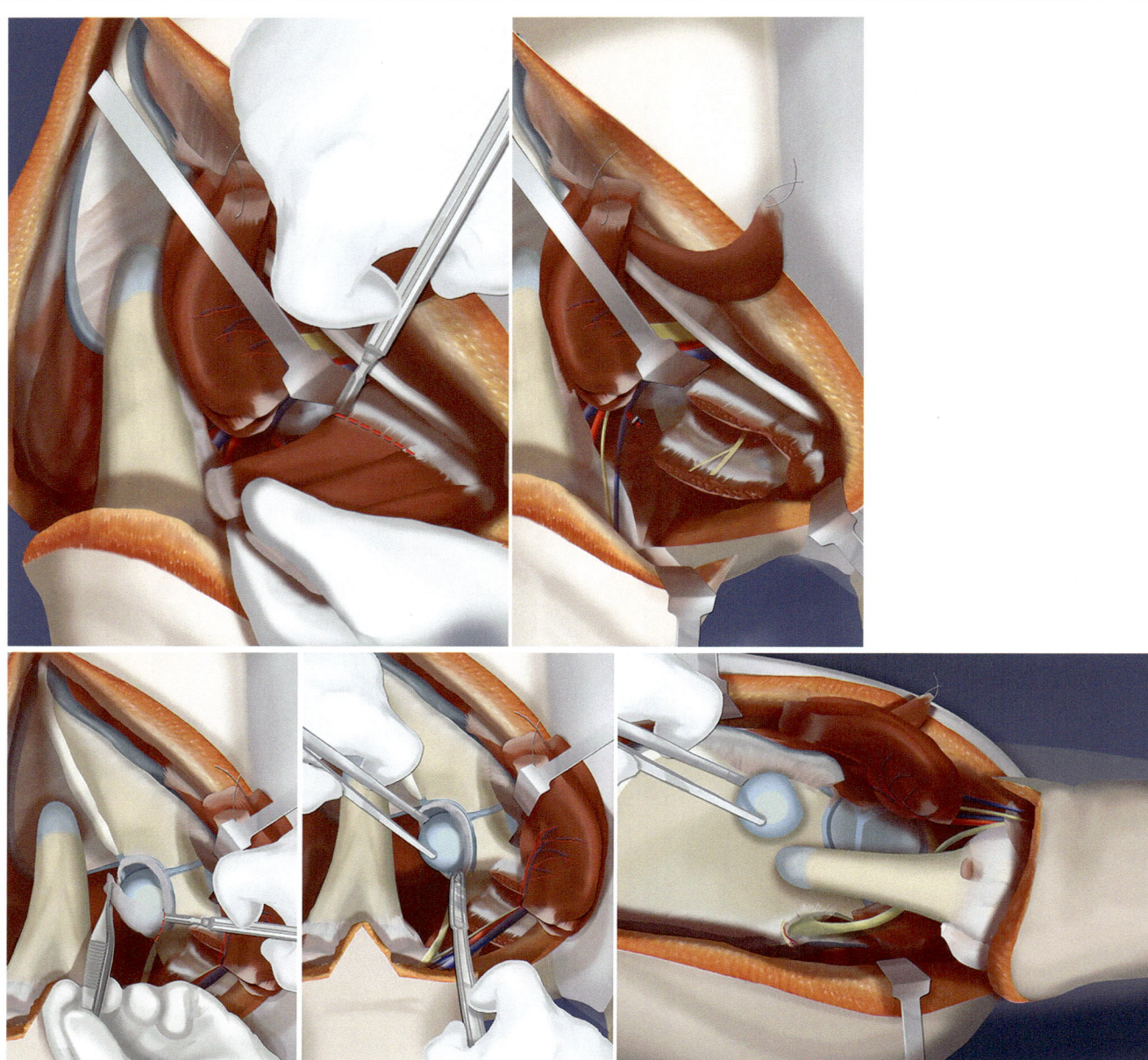

Fig. 29.41 (continued)

29 Congenital Femoral Deficiency Reconstruction and Lengthening Surgery

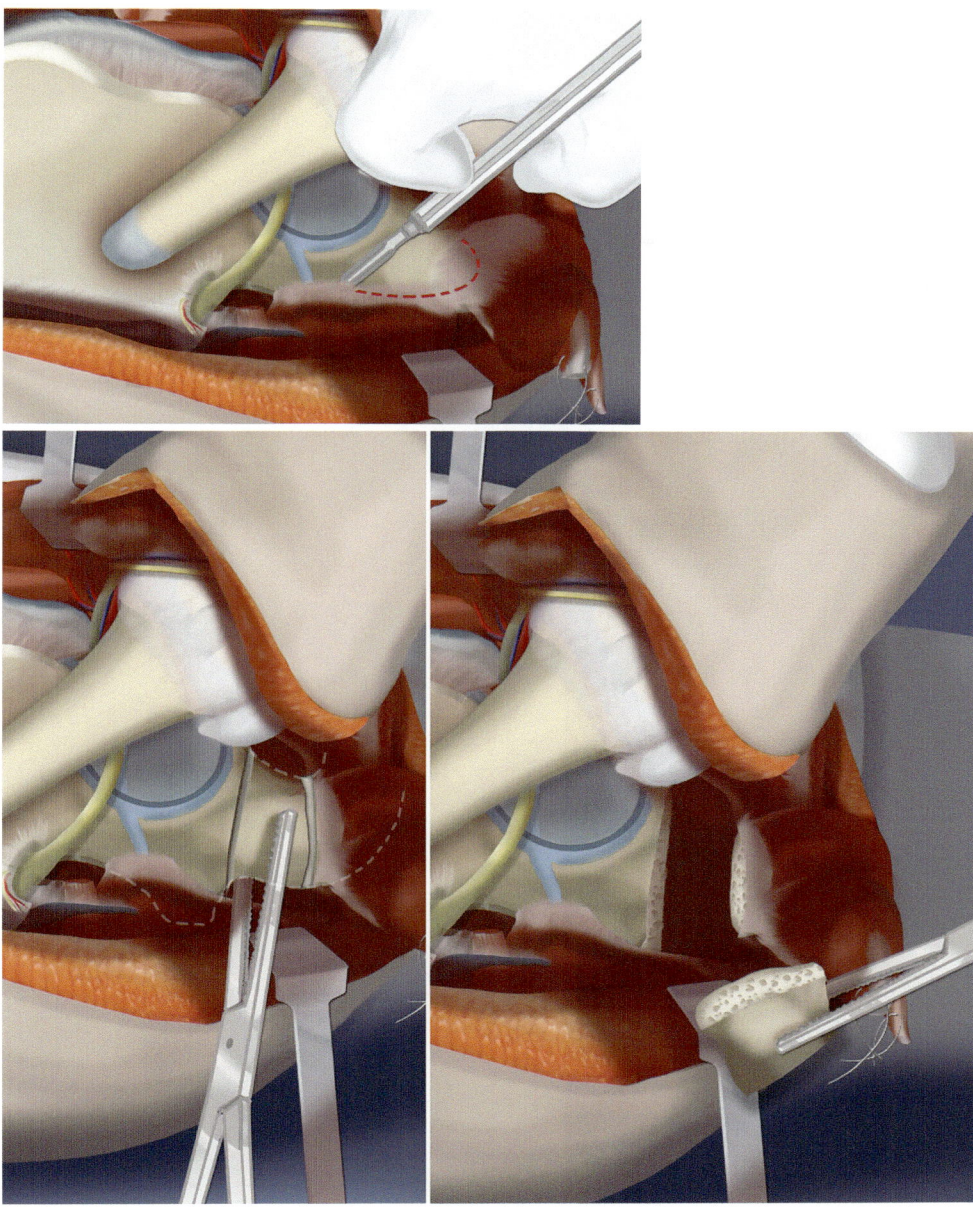

Fig. 29.41 (continued)

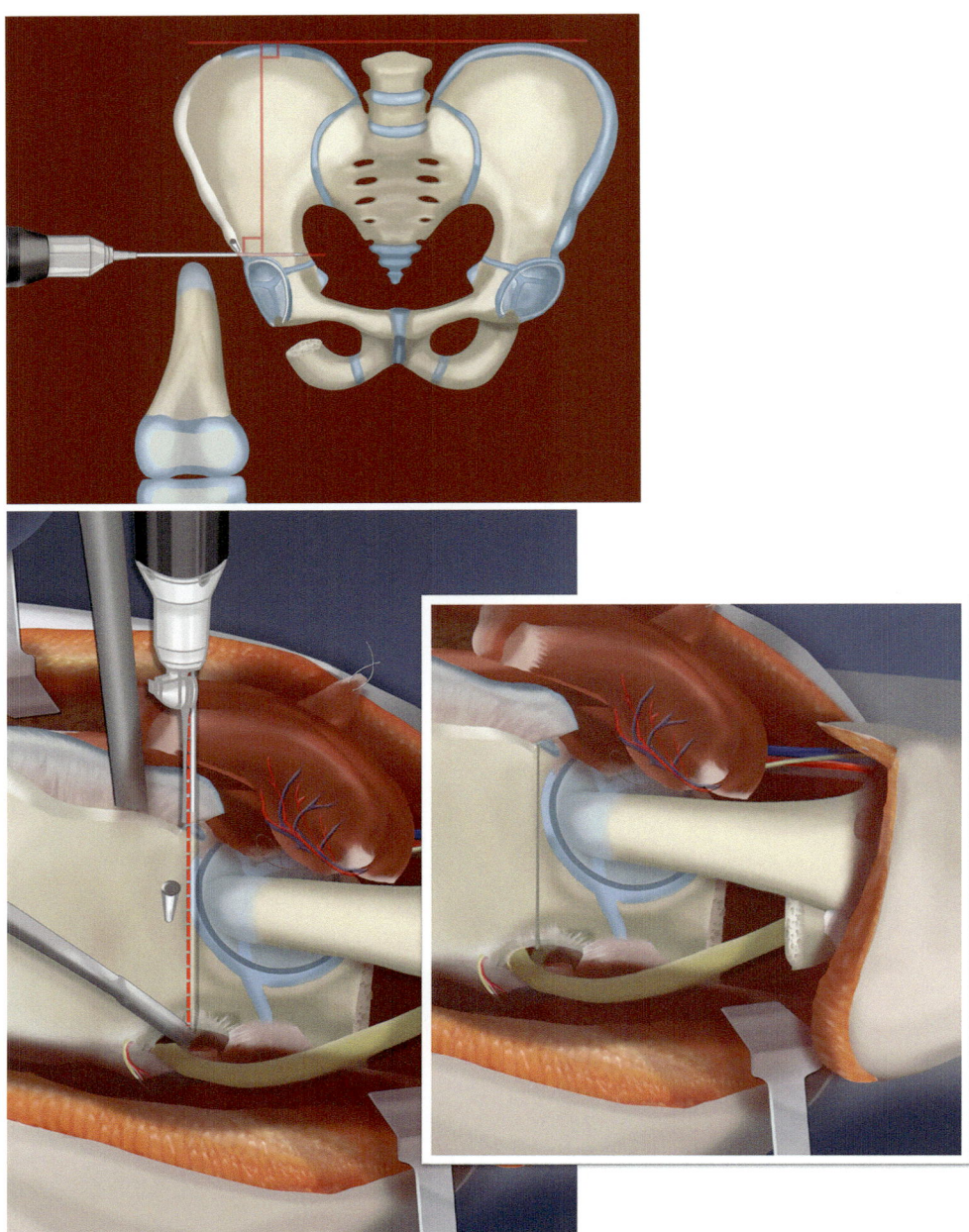

Fig. 29.41 (continued)

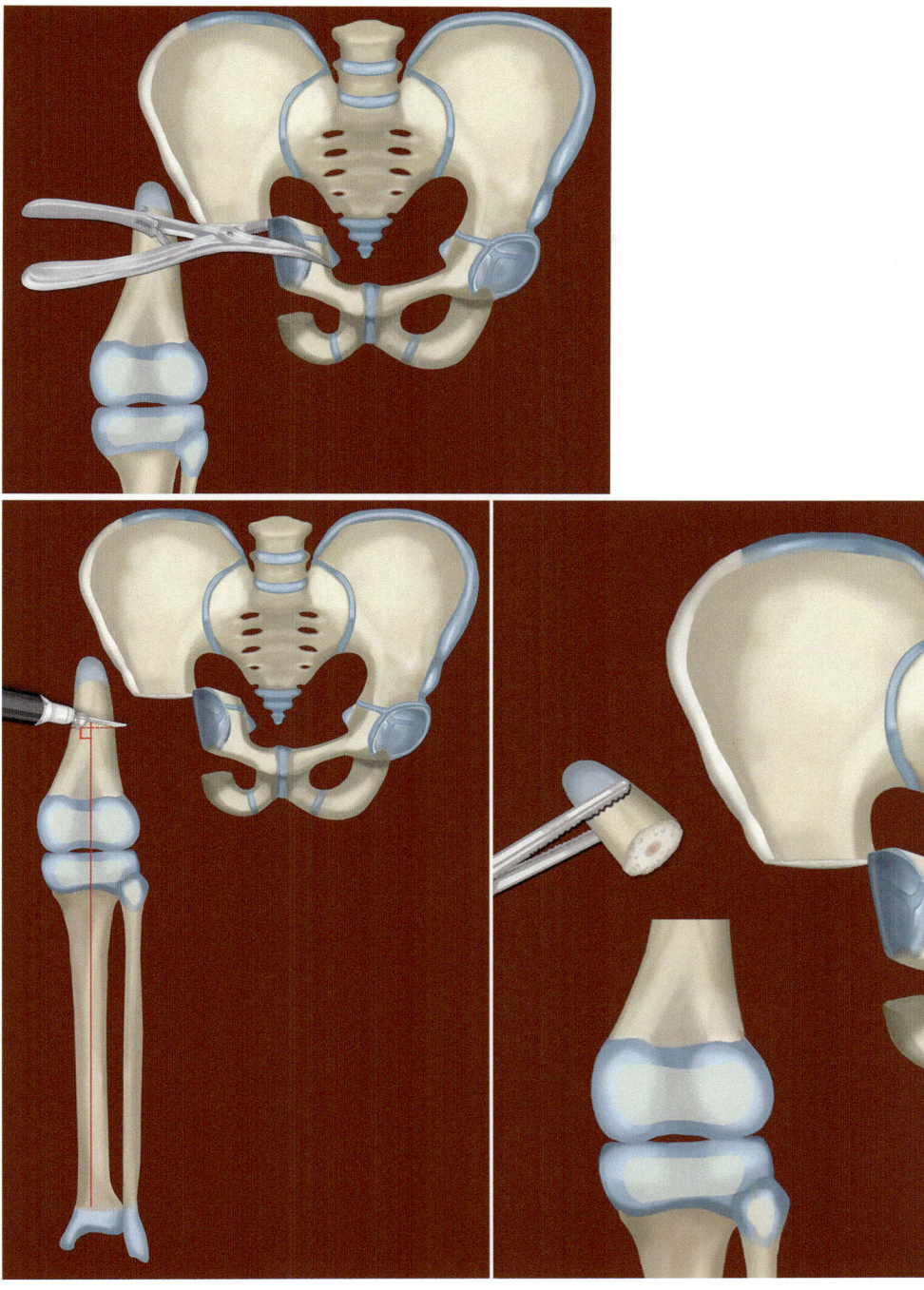

Fig. 29.41 (continued)

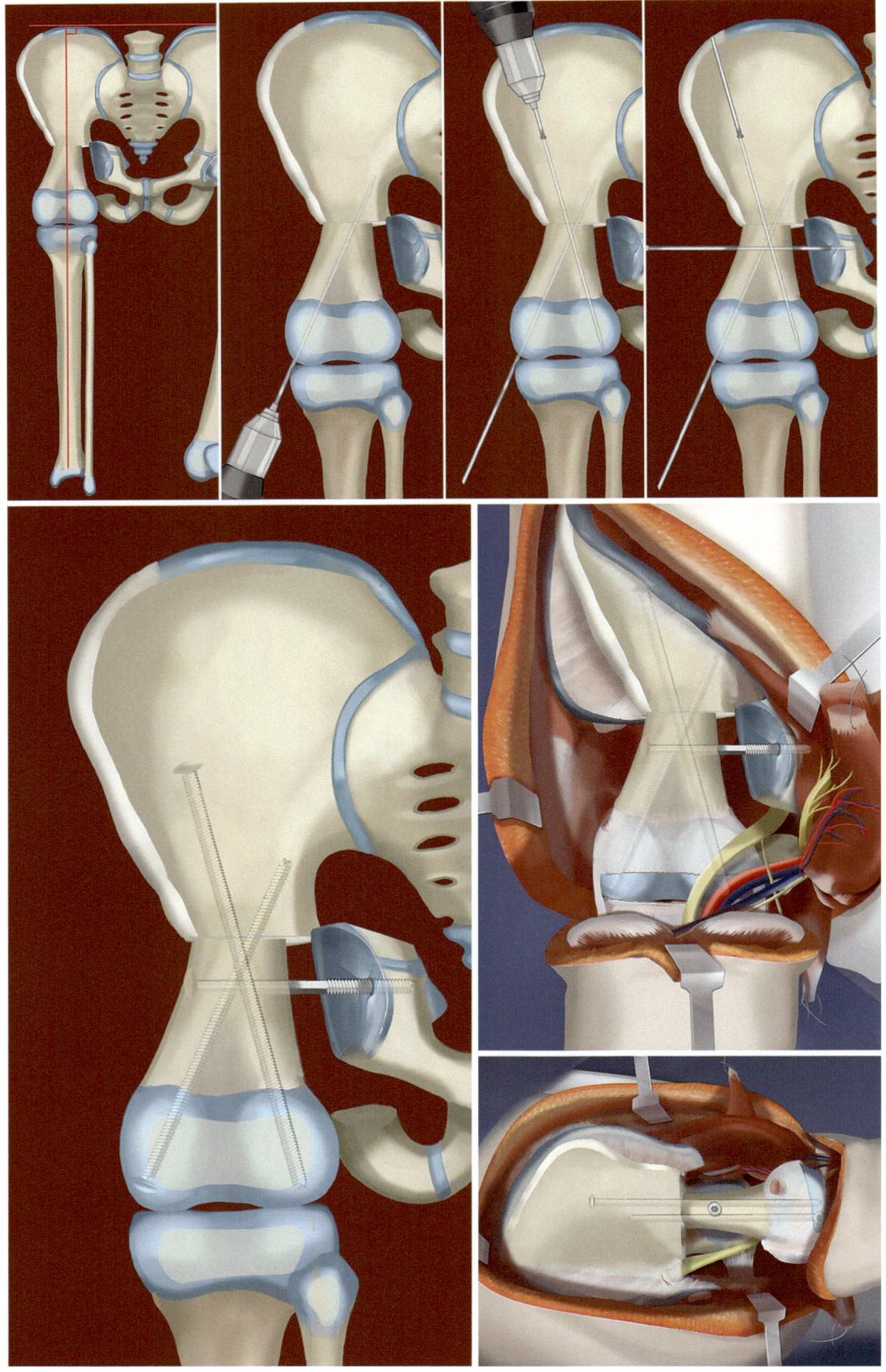

Fig. 29.41 (continued)

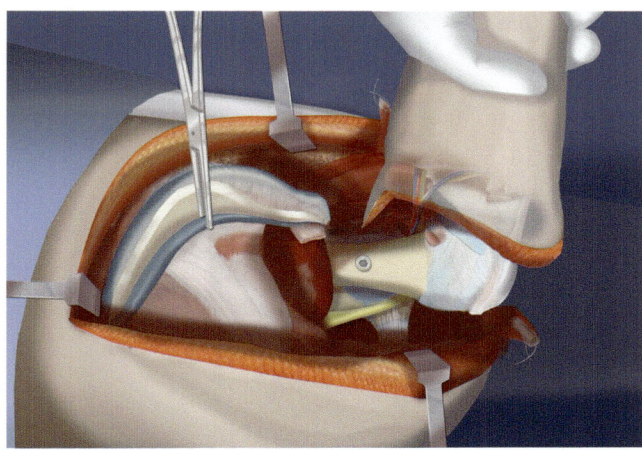

Fig. 29.41 (continued)

rami. The adductor muscles are completely resected in the Paley-Brown since they get in the way of medializing the femur. They also have no role since the new hip joint is a knee joint with no ability to abduct or adduct. Also, resect the sartorius muscle taking care not to injure the femoral nerve. For the Paley type, resect only some of the adductors, but leave some (Fig. 29.41y).
4. Enucleate the femoral head for the Paley-Brown (Fig. 29.41z).
5. Expose the ramus of the ischium for both Paley and Paley-Brown (Fig. 29.41za). The biceps origin must be released from the ischium. Resect a generous portion of the ischial ramus using a saw(Fig. 29.41zb). This allows the sciatic nerve to move medially into this space and avoid becoming entrapped by the femoral remnant when it is fused to the ilium or the femoral head. This step is essential in the Paley-Brown and is also preferred for the Paley type too. It is not necessary for the Brown type since the femur stays lateral.
6. Insert a frontal plane guide wire parallel to the line going across the tops of the iliac crests (Fig. 29.41zc). Make the Chiari osteotomy parallel to this line using a saw (Fig. 29.41zd).
7. Displace the acetabular segment medially to hook onto the inside of the ilium (Fig. 29.41ze).
8. Insert a guide wire into the femur perpendicular to the long axis of the tibia. Cut the femur along this wire. Depending on the length of the distal femur remnant, shorten the femur sufficiently to keep the knee joint as proximal as possible so that it is as close as possible to the anatomic hip joint level (Fig. 29.41zf).
9. With the femur rotated 180°, fix the distal femur with guide wires: one retrograde from the medial femoral condyle (lateral side) and one antegrade from inside the pelvis into the lateral femoral condyle (medial side). Make sure both of these cross the distal femoral growth plate to create an epiphysiodeses (this prevents the new hip joint from growing away from the pelvis). Add a third transverse wire to fix to the acetabulum proximal to the triradiate (Fig. 29.41zg).
10. Drill over each guide wire, and insert three 5.5 mm fully threaded screws (Fig. 29.41zh).
11. Test the rotation by flexing the knee (new hip) 90° (Fig. 29.41zi)

Paley Rotationplasty

1. Make an inferior capsulotomy, and expose the femoral head in the acetabulum.
2. Using a scalpel, remove cartilage in the inferolateral aspect of the femoral head until the ossific nucleus is identified (Fig. 29.42a).
3. Bevel the lateral proximal corner of the femur 45° (Fig. 29.42b).
4. Insert one guide wire transversely across the femur into the femoral head. Insert a second guide wire in a retrograde oblique angle from the medial femoral condyle (lateral side) to the femoral head. Replace both of these guide wires with 5.5-mm cannulated screws. Add a third guide wire antegrade from the medial proximal femur (lateral side) to cross the lateral side of the physis into the lateral femoral condyle (medial side). The two oblique cross screws create a distal femoral epiphysiodesis (Fig. 29.42c).
5. Add a temporary arthrodesis spanning plate to neutralize the forces on the hip joint (Fig. 29.42d).

Muscle Transfers and Closure for Both Paley and Paley-Brown

1. Suture the psoas tendon to the medial head of gastrocnemius tendon (lateral side). The lateral head of gastrocnemius is left free to avoid any pressure on the femoral vessels that cross it (Fig. 29.43a).
2. Suture the medial hamstrings (semimembranosus and semitendinosus) to the lateral anterior aspect of the tibia (posteromedial). The gracilis and sartorius are not transferred since they were resected (Fig. 29.43b).
3. With the knee in flexion, suture the biceps muscle to the mid-anterior tibia (now posterior).
4. In the Paley type, transfer the hip abductor muscles to the femur laterally. In the Paley-Brown, there is no need to transfer these muscles (Fig. 29.43c).
5. Close the apophysis, and then, advance the gluteus maximus and fascia lata-iliotibial band, to the patella if present or to the remnant of the distal quadricep (Fig. 29.43d, e). This repair is critical to create a good active extension of the hip.

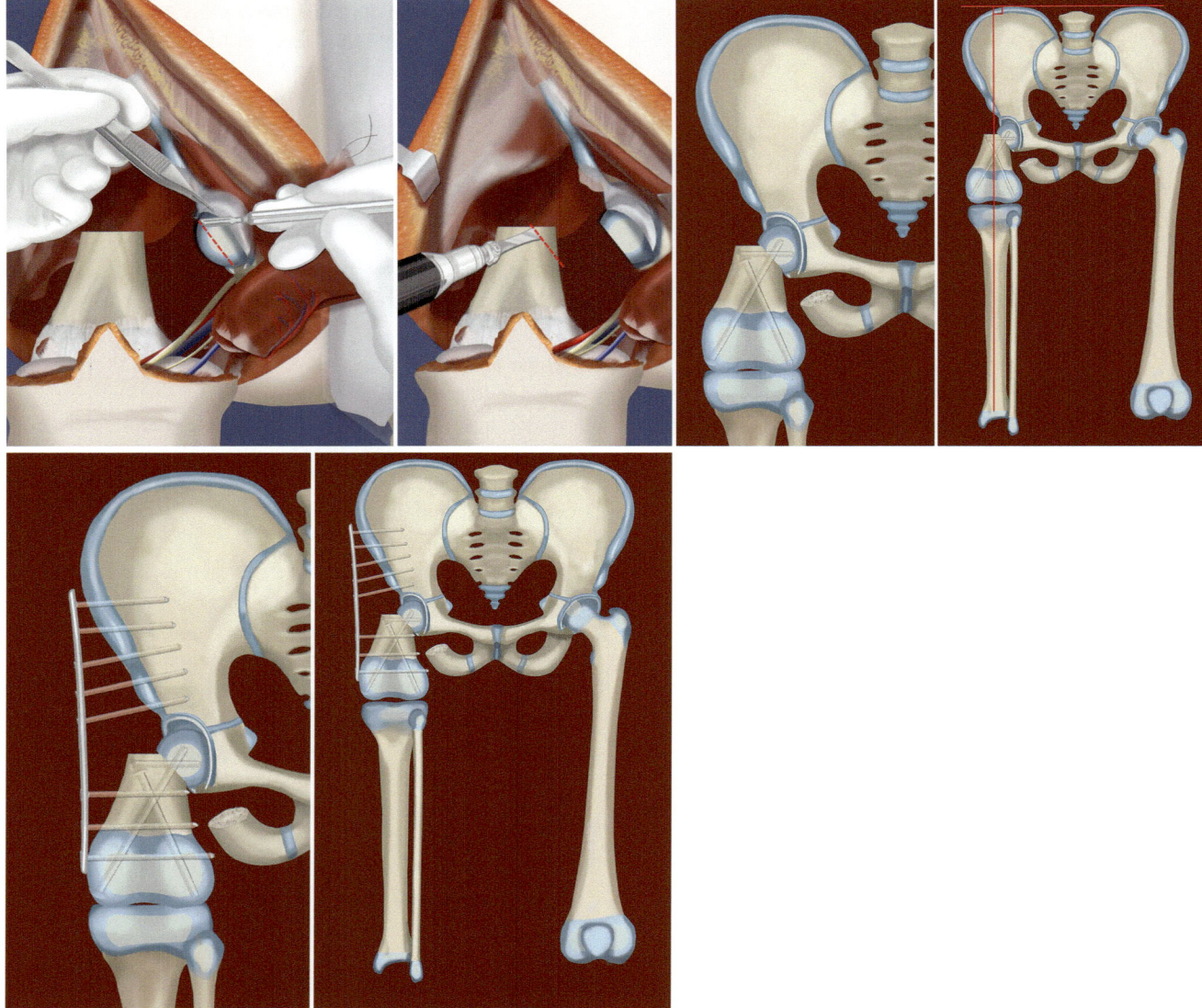

Fig. 29.42 Paley-Brown and Paley Rotationplasty procedures (follow text for steps and captions) (Copyright: The Paley Foundation. Reproduced with permission. All rights reserved.)

6. Suture the quadriceps to the anterior superior spine. Resect the vastus lateralis. Resect the sartorius. Suture the distal quadriceps to the fascia of the gastrocnemius muscles passing overtop the femoral and saphenous vessels (Fig. 29.43f, g).
7. Place two drains running in different directions around the femur (Fig. 29.43h).
8. A multiplanar closure is done to close the dead space (Fig. 29.43i). Skin edges are resected prior to closure, including to allow for the shortening and to facilitate closure. Most recently, the Pinsky incision and closure method has been used (ala Dr. Mark Pinsky). The authors' preference is to have a plastic surgeon close the incision. This serves several purposes. It allows for a meticulous closure to be done by a surgeon who is fresh and not tired from the long rotationplasty surgery and also is a surgeon who specializes in closure of skin flaps.

Supramalleolar Osteotomy or SHORDT for Rotationplasty

In the Paley-Brown or Brown, the distal femur is fixed to the pelvis. If there is any malrotation of the ankle joint, then the ankle which serves as the new knee will be malorientated for prosthetic fitting (Fig. 29.44a). Furthermore, there can be ankle valgus present which should be aligned for the same reason. When there is no fibula or when the fibula is present but is at the station (distal fibular physis at the level of tibial plafond), a supramalleolar osteotomy can be performed from the anatomic medial tibia for rotation and valgus correction. If there is also some equinus, the osteotomy is shortened to relax the Achilles tendon. The Achilles is never lengthened to avoid weakening the new quadriceps of the new knee. If the fibula is present but is hypoplastic so it is proximal to the station, the SHORDT procedure is per-

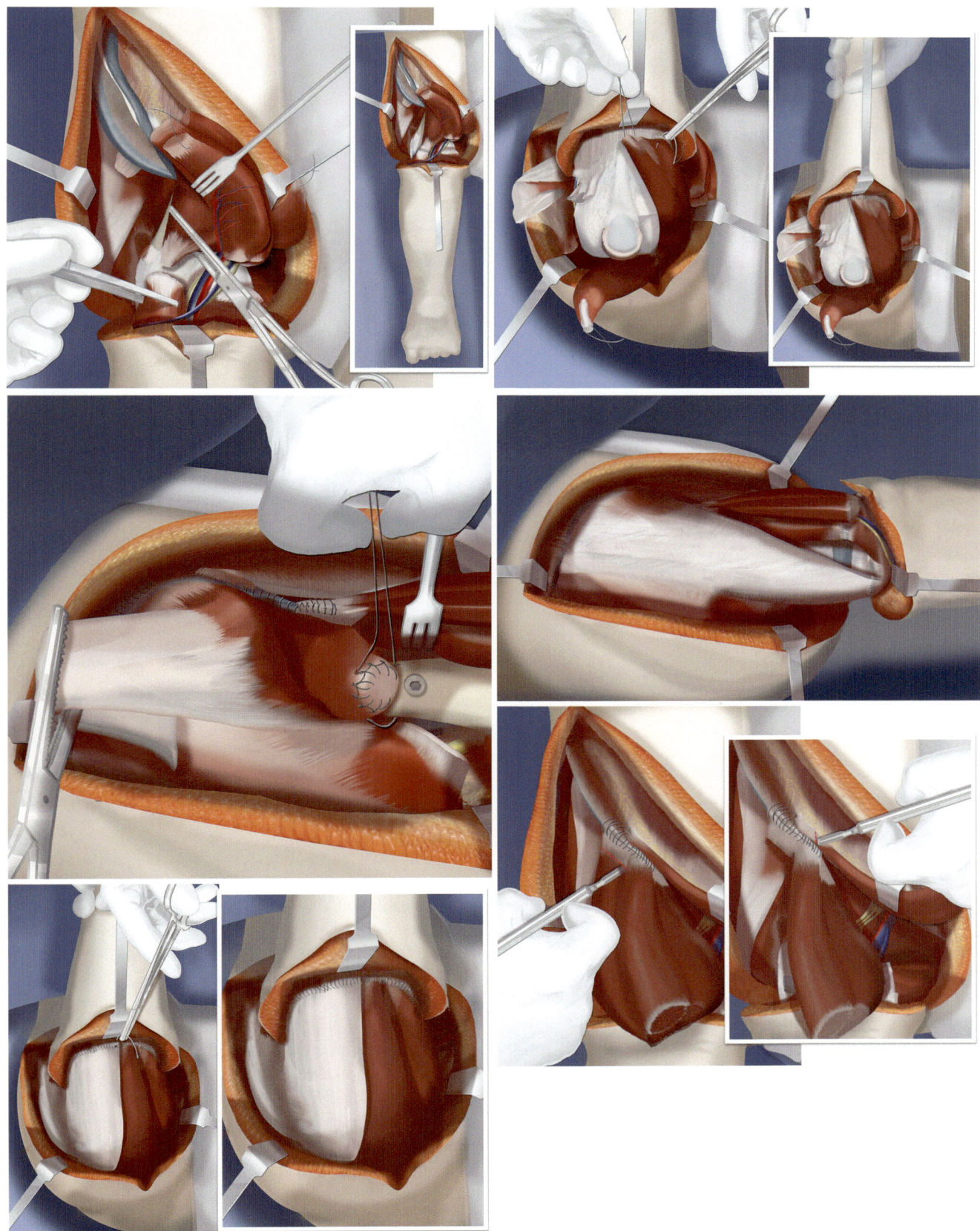

Fig. 29.43 Paley-Brown and Paley Rotationplasty procedures (follow text for steps and captions) (Copyright: The Paley Foundation. Reproduced with permission. All rights reserved.)

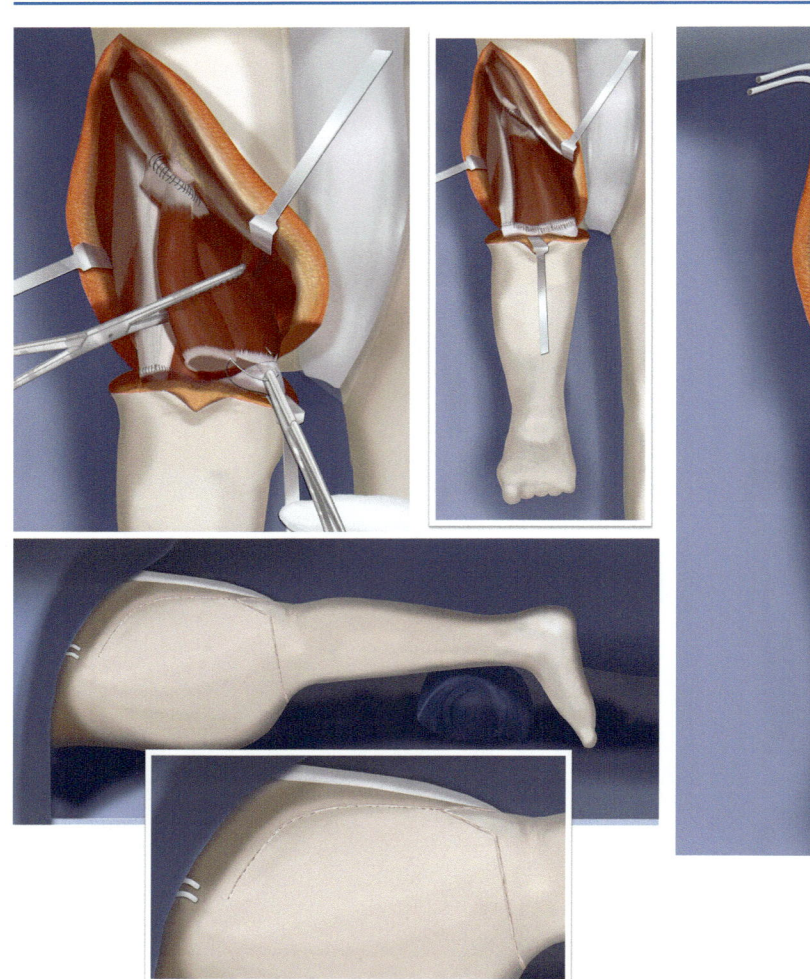
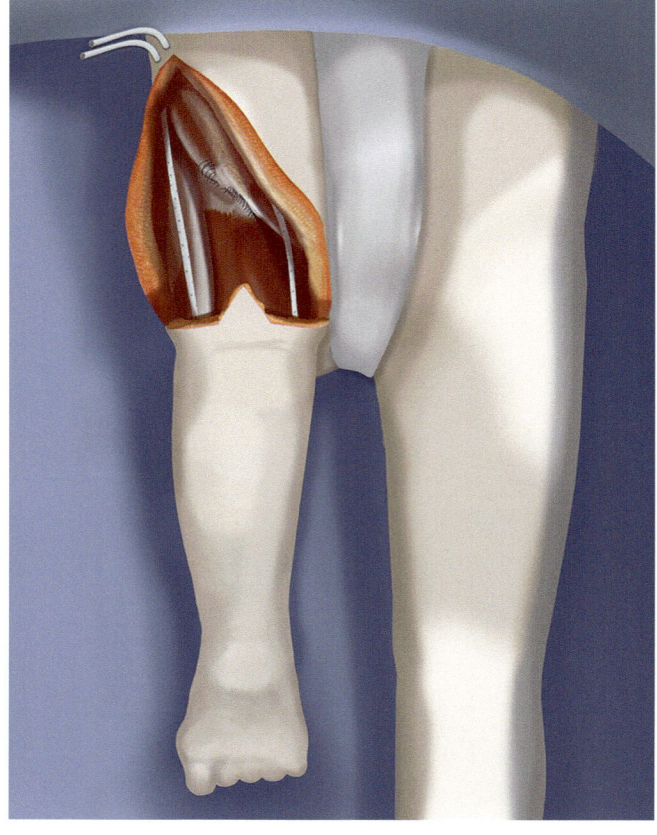

Fig. 29.43 (continued)

formed (Fig. 29.44b–d) (Shortening Osteotomy Realignment Distal Tibia) [115].

Postoperative Management

Patients are monitored for circulation in the ICU. Physical therapy for passive range of motion of the hip and knee (original knee and ankle) is started. Patient is kept non-weight-bearing 12 weeks until evidence of radiographic union. Patients are fitted with a rotationplasty prosthesis 12 weeks after the Paley-Brown rotationplasty. In the Paley rotationplasty, they are taken to the operating room to remove the temporary spanning (arthrodesis) plate or external fixator after 12 weeks. After that, they were fitted for a prosthetic device. After they receive their prosthetic, gait training with the prosthetic begins and lasts for several months.

Summary

CFD is a spectrum of congenital deficiency, deformity, and discrepancy of the femur that involves not only the osseous part of the femur, but also the surrounding musculature, ligaments, and joints. All of these components must be addressed if one is to be successful in the treatment of CFD. Though the definitive origin of CFD is still not known, it is a problem that can affect the function of a patient for his or her entire life. Depending on the severity, there are several treatment strategies, reconstructive surgeries, and prosthetic options, all of which can improve a patient's gait, function, and quality of life. As each deformity is different, so also is each patient and family, and therefore, treatment should be tailored to their individual needs and cultural expectations. Advances in surgical techniques, new biologic agents, and new technologies have

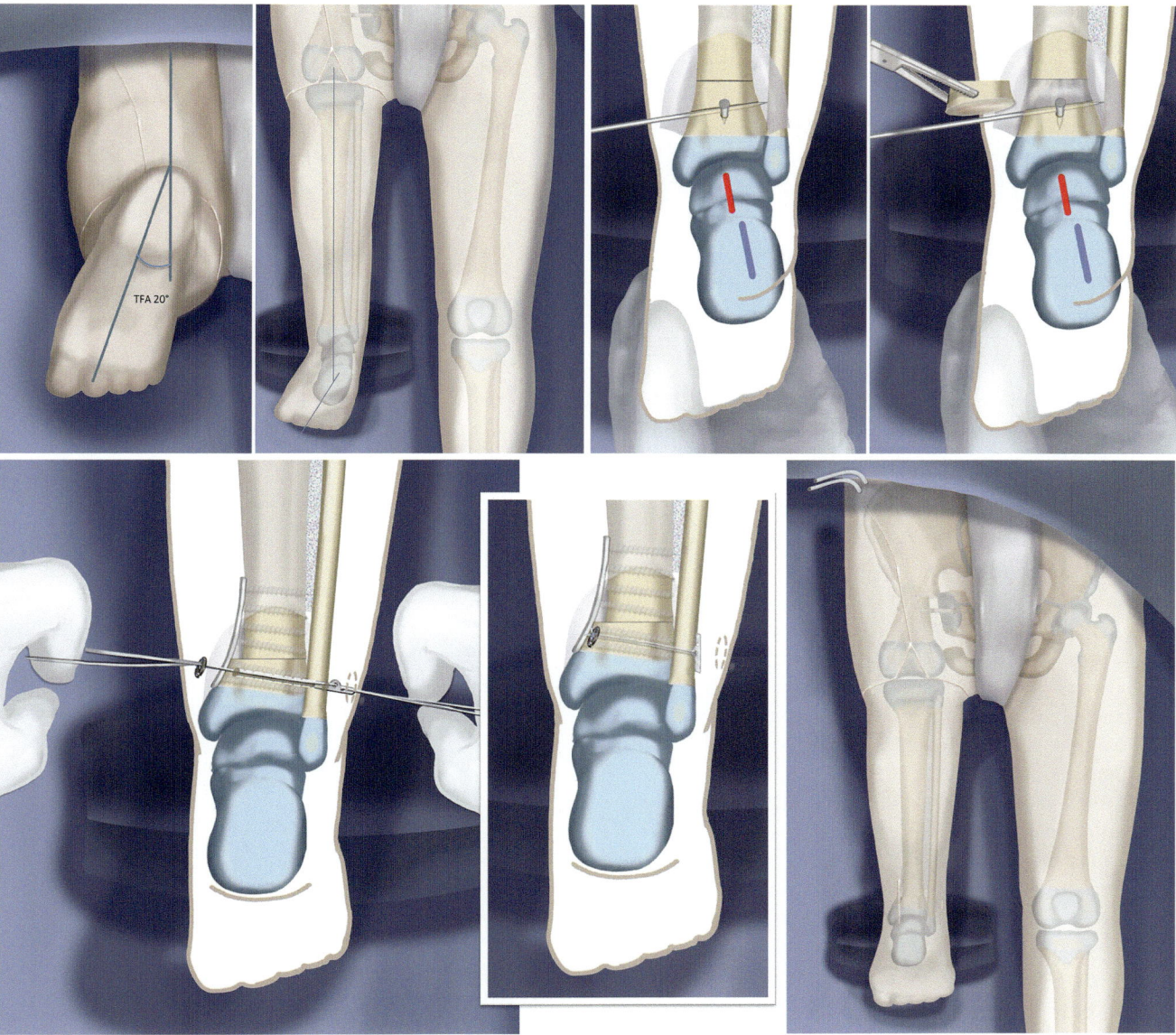

Fig. 29.44 (**a–d**) SHORDT. (**a**) The tibia is malrotated to the knee and has valgus. It is treated by a supramalleolar shortening osteotomy with correction of valgus and rotation. (**b**) The syndesmosis is disrupted between the distal tibia and fibula. Guidewires are placed into the tibia, and a wedge of bone is resected that will correct the tibial/hindfoot malalignment, as well as shorten the tibia to bring the fibula to station at the ankle. The foot can be rotated through this osteotomy as well. (**c**) Once the tibial osteotomy is fixed, a syndesmotic repair device (ZipTight, Zimmer Biomet, Warsaw, IN) is inserted to stabilize the distal tibiofibular joint. (**d**) The foot and ankle should now lie in neutral alignment to the flexion axis of the knee (hip) joint in extension (Copyright: The Paley Foundation. Reproduced with permission. All rights reserved.)

expanded the reconstructive indications and options in lieu of amputation. Though more research on newer treatments and their long-term outcomes is needed, there are now more options and hope for a brighter future for a child with CFD.

Acknowledgements The author would like to thank Pamela Boullier Ross who illustrated all of the figures in this manuscript. The author would also like to thank the Paley Foundation for funding the cost of making these illustrations and giving permission for their reproduction in Pediatric Lower Limb Deformities, Principles and Techniques of Management (Springer).

Commentary

Peter Calder
Peter.calder@nhs.net
The Royal National Orthopaedic Hospital, Stanmore,
London, UK

Epidemiology
- The commonest lower limb deficiency is fibular hemimelia (at a rate of 1–2/100,000 live births) and tibial deficiency is the rarest (1/1,000,000).
- The reported rate of femoral deficiency varies from 1/50,000 to a much rarer 1/200,000 live births. This may be explained by the difficulty in differentiating isolated femoral deficiency from whole limb involvement, for example, those included with fibula deficiency.

Etiology and Wide Spectrum of Anatomical Presentation
- Fetal limb development occurs between weeks 4 and 8 under the control of multiple different genes, with a resultant opportunity for defects to occur. Causes can be attributed to environmental, vascular anomalies, errors in genetic control, and amniotic band syndrome resulting in construction and amputation.
- Most congenital limb deformities are sporadic and non-transmissible. Nevertheless, parental genetic counseling may be needed for reassurance and in the case of a rare transmissible disease (especially those with autosomal recessive inheritance).
- Congenital femoral deficiency has both clinical heterogeneity, ranging from simple hypoplasia to complete absence of the proximal femur, and all modes of inheritance have been reported in the literature.

Bony Deformity and Soft-Tissue Abnormality
- The generic name of congenital femoral deficiency may be applied to simple hypoplasia of an anatomically normal femur, to a severe complex deformity of the femur, pelvis, and surrounding soft tissues and finally complete absence of the proximal femur including associated deformity of the pelvis.
- In general terms, the relatively constant deformity in proximal femoral focal deficiency consists of coxa vara, retroversion, and recurvatum, with associated acetabular dysplasia.
- Delay in proximal femoral ossification or discontinuity of the proximal femur to the femoral head leading to instability on loading may occur.
- Hypoplasia of the lateral femoral condyle will produce genu valgum.
- Associated soft-tissue anomalies include hypertrophy of the sartorius (Tailor's muscle) with resultant contracture of flexion, abduction, and external rotation, which produces the characteristic position of the bulbous, shortened thigh seen in severe congenital femoral deficiency.
- Cruciate ligament absence is to be expected, especially if there is hypoplasia of the tibial eminence seen radiographically. This highlights the risk of knee subluxation and dislocation during lengthening procedures.

Evaluation
- The clinical diagnosis of severe deficiency is usually straightforward with the classic appearance of a shortened bulbous thigh held in flexion, abduction, and external rotation.
- It is often difficult to measure accurately range of hip and knee movement in the very young child, due to a combination of soft-tissue contracture and small length of thigh segment. The fixed flexion (recurvatum of the proximal femur) also adds difficulty when measuring the leg lengths. Pistoning of the thigh segment may give an indication of hip stability.
- Look for features for fibula hemimelia and associated upper limb deficiencies or deformities. These may include absent lateral foot rays, hindfoot valgus and restricted inversion, and fibula absence or shortening in comparison to the medial malleolus.
- When assessing the radiographs, length may be underestimated due to the foreshortening of the thigh caused by flexion of the hip. This may lead to an overestimation of the ultimate leg length discrepancy using the multiplier method.
- MRI will confirm cartilage continuity between the proximal femur and femoral head in those cases of delayed ossification. In the young child, this investigation will almost always require a general anesthetic, and this offers an opportunity to perform a dynamic arthrogram at the same time, where hip stability can be assessed in real time.

Classification
- Early classification systems concentrated on radiological appearance with the aim of predicting femoral development and guiding management. Unfortunately, these have been proven to be unreli-

able in predicting the natural history of hip formation and stability.
- The Paley classification is the latest classification, which aims to group patients with similar anatomical features and offer a surgical plan for limb reconstruction. It is logical and reasonably straightforward to apply. In the literature most recently published, it appears to be the classification of choice to differentiate different groups.

Treatment and Complications
- A clear understanding of the diagnosis and natural history is given at the first consultation. Treatment options include correction of anatomical deformity, limb reconstruction, and the need for supportive orthosis or prosthetics, both temporary or definitive.
- Surgical goals need careful explanation with both goals and risk of complications described.
- Just because you can lengthen a large amount does not mean you should. Lengthening greater than 20% of the original bone length (or greater than 6 centimeters as a rule of thumb) is often associated with an exponential increase in complications. Multiple shorter lengthening procedures would require more surgical episodes but may be associated with a faster rehabilitation and overall less complications.

Hip Reconstruction
- The correction of the severe proximal femoral deformity involves a combination of bony correction and soft-tissue release. The deforming forces must be overcome; in this case, the sartorius, tensor fascia lata, psoas, straight head of rectus, and external rotators are released, and the shortened hamstrings can be overcome by a shortening of the femur, which seems counterintuitive as the femur is so small. By undertaking this, the blade plate may need to be shortened, due to the shortened femoral shaft. An available Midas Rex can be used intraoperatively to cut the plate.
- A fixed-angled plate should prevent the recurrence of the varus deformity. It may also be argued that performing hip reconstruction in the older patients further prevents the recurrence of deformity.
- Dega acetabuloplasty results in improved acetabular coverage, and the bone resected from the femoral shortening is used to maintain reduction. Trimming of the iliac crest to enable repair of the iliac apophysis with the optimum abductor muscle tension is a more elegant reconstruction technique compared to an abductor muscle slide.

Lengthening
- Lengthening in congenital femoral deficiency remains one of the most challenging operations for the limb reconstruction surgeon. An appreciation of the potential risks and complications is paramount before undertaking these procedures.
- Poor and delayed bone consolidation can be associated with regenerate deformity and fracture. Lengthening over an intramedullary implant is recommended to reduce risk.
- Joint subluxation or dislocation of both the hip and knee is arguably the most serious potential complications.
- Pre-lengthening correction of hip dysplasia and appropriate soft-tissue release (straight head of rectus) are recommended to ensure optimum hip stability.
- Bridging of the knee during lengthening with an external fixator and iliotibial band release helps reduce the risk of rotational knee subluxation. Patients often present with knee pain as the knee starts to sublux. When asked they will point directly over the patella. Stopping the lengthening process and immediately reversing by up to a centimeter often resolves the pain. Knee alignment should be assessed by a shoot-through lateral radiographs with the leg in full extension and perpendicular AP views. Patient education to ensure they are aware of the potential risks is once again paramount to ensure that they do not continue the lengthening process and cause further complication. They should be counseled to report these events immediately to the limb reconstruction team.
- When using intramedullary lengthening nails, splints to maintain knee extension can be used with removal for ROM exercises. After the length has been achieved, the splint is maintained for approximately one month. The lengthening rate may also be reduced to 1/3 mm twice per day which appears to be tolerated better by the soft tissues. An antegrade nail is preferred, with the nail ending between middle and distal thirds of the femur. If knee subluxation was to occur during lengthening, a bridging fixator can be applied over the knee, with fixation achievable in the distal third of the femur.

Prosthetic Fitting and Function
- It would appear logical to restore the proximal femoral deformity with the intention of improving hip function, even if a decision has been made not to consider further limb lengthening.

- Reduced hip extension can be compensated for by knee flexion in stance. The prosthesis ideally should be below knee to allow this movement and maintain a good step length.
- There remain questions over the surgical benefit of rotationplasty procedures and Syme disarticulation. Studies in favor of the Van Nes rotationplasty state an improved gait pattern and oxygen consumption. However, the end cosmetic result often results in parents not accepting this technique, and most recently, the improvement on the function has been challenged. Syme amputation may be performed for cosmetic reasons, or when combined with a knee fusion, to produce a single bone thigh segment.
- Furthermore, the surgical management in cases of severe proximal femoral focal deficiency, where the proximal femur is absent, remains a philosophical challenge. Any surgery performed has a goal of functional improvement, with a paucity of studies reporting small numbers, and an agreement of best practice will continue to be debated for the foreseeable future.

References

1. Rogala EJ, Wynne-Davies R, Littlejohn A, Gormley J. Congenital limb anomalies: frequency and aetiological factors: Data from the Edinburgh Register of the Newborn (1964-68). J Med Genet. 1974;11(3):221–33.
2. Oppenheim WL, Setoguchi Y, Fowler E. Overview and comparison of Syme's amputation and knee fusion with the van Nes rotationplasty procedure in proximal femoral focal deficiency. In: Herring J, Birch J, editors. The child with a limb deficiency. Chicago, IL: American Academy of Orthopaedic Surgeons; 1998.
3. Hill RE. How to make a zone of polarizing activity: Insights into limb development via the abnormality preaxial polydactyly. Dev Growth Differ. 2007;49(6):439–48. https://doi.org/10.1111/j.1440-169X.2007.00943.x.
4. Zhu X, Zhu H, Zhang L, et al. Wls-mediated Wnts differentially regulate distal limb patterning and tissue morphogenesis. Dev Biol. 2012;365(2):328–38. https://doi.org/10.1016/j.ydbio.2012.02.019.
5. Zhang Z, Yi D, Xie R, Hamilton JL, Kang QL, Chen D. Postaxial limb hypoplasia (PALH): the classification, clinical features, and related developmental biology. Ann N Y Acad Sci. 2017;1409(1):67–78. https://doi.org/10.1111/nyas.13440.
6. Mikic B, Battaglia TC, Taylor EA, Clark RT. The effect of growth/differentiation factor-5 deficiency on femoral composition and mechanical behavior in mice. Bone. 2002;30(5):733–7. https://doi.org/10.1016/S8756-3282(02)00699-3.
7. Zigman M, Laumann-Lipp N, Titus T, Postlethwait J, Moens CB. Hoxb1b controls oriented cell division, cell shape and microtubule dynamics in neural tube morphogenesis. Development. 2014;141(3):639–49. https://doi.org/10.1242/dev.098731.
8. Power SC, Lancman J, Smith SM. Retinoic acid is essential for shh/hoxd signaling during rat limb outgrowth but not for limb initiation. Dev Dyn. 1999;216(4/5):469–80. https://doi.org/10.1002/(SICI)1097-0177(199912)216:4/5<469::AID-DVDY15>3.0.CO;2-3.
9. Stratford T, Logan C, Zile M, Maden M. Abnormal anteroposterior and dorsoventral patterning of the limb bud in the absence of retinoids. Mech Dev. 1999;81(1–2):115–25. https://doi.org/10.1016/S0925-4773(98)00231-7.
10. Klopocki E, Kähler C, Foulds N, et al. Deletions in PITX1 cause a spectrum of lower-limb malformations including mirror-image polydactyly. Eur J Hum Genet. 2012;20(6):705–8. https://doi.org/10.1038/ejhg.2011.264.
11. Gupta DS, Gupta SK. Familial bilateral proximal femoral focal deficiency. Report of a kindred. JBJS. 1984;66(9):1470–2.
12. Sorge G, Ardito S, Genuardi M, et al. Proximal femoral focal deficiency (PFFD) and fibular a/hypoplasia (FA/H): A model of a developmental field defect. Am J Med Genet. 1995;55(4):427–32. https://doi.org/10.1002/ajmg.1320550409.
13. Bohring A, Oppermann HC. A further case of vertical transmission of proximal femoral focal deficiency? Am J Med Genet. 1997;71(2):194–6. https://doi.org/10.1002/(SICI)1096-8628(19970808)71:2<194::AID-AJMG14>3.0.CO;2-9.
14. Tan TY, Kilpatrick N, Farlie PG. Developmental and genetic perspectives on Pierre Robin sequence. Am J Med Genet C Semin Med Genet. 2013;163C(4):295–305. https://doi.org/10.1002/ajmg.c.31374.
15. Roberts J, Torres-Martinez W, Farrow E, et al. A case of Robin sequence, microgastria, radiohumeral synostosis, femoral deficiency, and other unusual findings: a newly recognized syndrome? Am J Med Genet A. 2014;164A(2):287–90. https://doi.org/10.1002/ajmg.a.36273.
16. Boden SD, Fallon MD, Davidson R, Mennuti MT, Kaplan FS. Proximal femoral focal deficiency. Evidence for a defect in proliferation and maturation of chondrocytes. JBJS. 1989;71(8):1119–29.
17. Paranjape M, Cziger A, Katz K. Ossification of Femoral Head: Normal Sonographic Standards. J Pediatr Orthop. 2002;22(2):217–8.
18. Hamanishi C. Congenital short femur. Clinical, genetic and epidemiological comparison of the naturally occurring condition with that caused by thalidomide. J Bone Joint Surg Br. 1980;62B(3):307–20. https://doi.org/10.1302/0301-620X.62B3.7410462.
19. Zhang Y, Wray AE, Ross AC. Perinatal exposure to vitamin A differentially regulates chondrocyte growth and the expression of aggrecan and matrix metalloprotein genes in the femur of neonatal rats. J Nutr. 2012;142(4):649–54. https://doi.org/10.3945/jn.111.152660.
20. Aitken G. Limb development and deformity: problems of evaluation and rehabilitation. In: Thomas CC, ed. PFFD - Definition, Classification, and Management; 1969. Accessed December 28, 2021. http://myplace.frontier.com/~pffdvsg1/med-nas69.htm
21. Herring J, Birth J. The Child with a Limb Deficiency. AAOS; 1998.
22. Camera G, Dodero D, Parodi M, Zucchinetti P, Camera A. Antenatal ultrasonographic diagnosis of a proximal femoral focal deficiency. J Clin Ultrasound JCU. 1993;21(7):475–9. https://doi.org/10.1002/jcu.1870210714.
23. Dora C, Bühler M, Stover MD, Mahomed MN, Ganz R. Morphologic characteristics of acetabular dysplasia in proximal femoral focal deficiency. J Pediatr Orthop Part B. 2004;13(2):81–7. https://doi.org/10.1097/00009957-200403000-00004.
24. Sanpera I, Sparks LT. Proximal femoral focal deficiency: does a radiologic classification exist? J Pediatr Orthop. 1994;14(1):34–8. https://doi.org/10.1097/01241398-199401000-00008.

25. Paley D, Shannon CE, Nogueira M, Chiari C, Harris M. Can adding BMP2 improve outcomes in patients undergoing the SUPERhip procedure? Children. 2021;8(6):495. https://doi.org/10.3390/children8060495.
26. Musielak BJ, Shadi M, Kubicka AM, et al. Is acetabular dysplasia and pelvic deformity properly interpreted in patients with congenital femoral deficiency? A 3D analysis of pelvic computed tomography. J Child Orthop. 2020;14(5):364–71. https://doi.org/10.1302/1863-2548.14.200065.
27. Amstutuz H. The morphology, natural history, and treatment of proximal femoral focal deficiencies. In: PFFD: A congenital anomaly. National Academy of Sciences; 1969. Accessed December 28, 2021. http://myplace.frontier.com/~pffdvsg1/medamstutz69.htm
28. Ring PA. Congenital short femur; simple femoral hypoplasia. J Bone Joint Surg Br. 1959;41-B(1):73–9. https://doi.org/10.1302/0301-620X.41B1.73.
29. Westin GW, Sakai DN, Wood WL. Congenital longitudinal deficiency of the fibula: follow-up of treatment by Syme amputation. J Bone Joint Surg Am. 1976;58(4):492–6.
30. Hootnick D, Boyd NA, Fixsen JA, Lloyd-Roberts GC. The natural history and management of congenital short tibia with dysplasia or absence of the fibula. J Bone Joint Surg Br. 1977;59(3):267–71. https://doi.org/10.1302/0301-620X.59B3.893503.
31. Shapiro F. Developmental patterns in lower-extremity length discrepancies. J Bone Jt Surg. 1982;64(5):639–51. https://doi.org/10.2106/00004623-198264050-00001.
32. Aguilar JA, Paley D, Paley J, et al. Clinical validation of the multiplier method for predicting limb length at maturity, part I. J Pediatr Orthop. 2005;25(2):186–91. https://doi.org/10.1097/01.bpo.0000150809.28171.12.
33. Paley D, Bhave A, Herzenberg JE, Bowen JR. Multiplier method for predicting limb-length discrepancy. JBJS. 2000;82(10):1432.
34. Manner HM. Dysplasia of the cruciate ligaments: radiographic assessment and classification. J Bone Jt Surg Am. 2006;88(1):130. https://doi.org/10.2106/JBJS.E.00146.
35. Johansson E, Aparisi T. Missing cruciate ligament in congenital short femur. J Bone Joint Surg Am. 1983;65(8):1109–15.
36. Chomiak J, Podškubka A, Dungl P, Ošt'ádal M, Frydrychová M. Cruciate ligaments in proximal femoral focal deficiency: arthroscopic assessment. J Pediatr Orthop. 2012;32(1):21–8. https://doi.org/10.1097/BPO.0b013e31823d34db.
37. Pirani S, Beauchamp RD, Li D, Sawatzky B. Soft tissue anatomy of proximal femoral focal deficiency. J Pediatr Orthop. 1991;11(5):563–70.
38. Panting AL, Williams PF. Proximal femoral focal deficiency. J Bone Joint Surg Br. 1978;60(1):46–52. https://doi.org/10.1302/0301-620X.60B1.627578.
39. Biko DM, Davidson R, Pena A, Jaramillo D. Proximal focal femoral deficiency: evaluation by MR imaging. Pediatr Radiol. 2012;42(1):50–6. https://doi.org/10.1007/s00247-011-2203-3.
40. Senior HD. An interpretation of the recorded arterial anomalies of the human leg and foot. J Anat. 1919;53(Pt 2–3):130–71.
41. Chomiak J, Horák M, Masek M, Frydrychová M, Dungl P. Computed tomographic angiography in proximal femoral focal deficiency. J Bone Joint Surg Am. 2009;91(8):1954–64. https://doi.org/10.2106/JBJS.H.00902.
42. Senior HD. An interpretation of the recorded arterial anomalies of the human pelvis and thigh. Am J Anat. 1925;36(1):1–46. https://doi.org/10.1002/aja.1000360102.
43. Fuller CB, Lichtblau CH, Paley D. Rotationplasty for severe congenital femoral deficiency. Children. 2021;8(6):462. https://doi.org/10.3390/children8060462.
44. Paley J, Gelman A, Paley D, Herzenberg JE. The prenatal multiplier method for prediction of limb length discrepancy. Prenat Diagn Publ Affil Int Soc Prenat Diagn. 2005;25(6):435–8.
45. Aitken G. Amputation as a treatment for certain lower-extremity congenital abnormalities. J Bone Joint Surg Am. 1959;41-A:1267–85.
46. Fixsen JA, Lloyd-Roberts GC. The natural history and early treatment of proximal femoral dysplasia. J Bone Joint Surg Br. 1974;56(1):86–95.
47. Pappas AM. Congenital abnormalities of the femur and related lower extremity malformations: classification and treatment. J Pediatr Orthop. 1983;3(1):45–60. https://doi.org/10.1097/01241398-198302000-00009.
48. Gillespie R, Torode IP. Classification and management of congenital abnormalities of the femur. J Bone Joint Surg Br. 1983;65(5):557–68. https://doi.org/10.1302/0301-620X.65B5.6643558.
49. Kalamchi A, Cowell HR, Kim KI. Congenital deficiency of the femur. J Pediatr Orthop. 1985;5(2):129–34.
50. Paley D. Lengthening reconstruction surgery for congenital femoral deficiency. In: Herring J, Birch J, editors. The child with a limb deficiency. AAOS; 1998. p. 113–32.
51. Maldjian C, Patel TY, Klein RM, Smith RC. Efficacy of MRI in classifying proximal focal femoral deficiency. Skeletal Radiol. 2007;36(3):215–20. https://doi.org/10.1007/s00256-006-0218-x.
52. Herring JA. Disorders of the leg. In: Herring JA, editor. Tachdjian's pediatric orthopaedics. 5th ed. Elsevier Health Sciences; 2013. p. 713–58.
53. Paley D, Chong DY, Prince DE. Congenital femoral deficiency reconstruction and lengthening surgery. In: Sabharwal S, editor. Pediatric lower limb deformities: principles and techniques of management. Springer; 2016. p. 361–425.
54. Paley D, Guardo F. Lengthening reconstruction surgery for congenital femoral deficiency. In: Kocaoglu M, editor. Advanced techniques in limb reconstruction surgery. Springer; 2014. p. 245–99.
55. Paley D, Shannon C. Treatment of congenital femoral deficiency. In: Flynn J, editor. Operative techniques in pediatric orthopaedic surgery. 3rd ed. Lippincott Williams & Wilkins; 2021.
56. Herring JA. Tachdjian's pediatric orthopaedics. 6th ed. Elsevier Health Sciences; 2020.
57. Paley D. Treatment of congenital femoral deficiency. In: Wiesel SW, editor. Operative techniques in orthopaedic surgery. 2nd ed. Lippincott Williams & Wilkins; 2015. p. 1532–51.
58. Paley D, Shannon C. Treatment of congenital femoral deficiency. In: Wiesel SW, editor. Operative techniques in orthopaedic surgery. Lippincott Williams & Wilkins; 2021. chapter 37 In Press.
59. Suzuki S, Kasahara Y, Seto Y, Futami T, Furukawa K, Nishino Y. Dislocation and subluxation during femoral lengthening. J Pediatr Orthop. 1994;14(3):343–6. https://doi.org/10.1097/01241398-199405000-00013.
60. Bowen JR, Kumar SJ, Orellana CA, Andreacchio A, Cardona JI. Factors leading to hip subluxation and dislocation in femoral lengthening of unilateral congenital short femur. J Pediatr Orthop. 2001;21(3):354–9. https://doi.org/10.1097/00004694-200105000-00018.
61. Grammont PM, Latune D, Lammaire IP. Treatment of subluxation and dislocation of the patella in the child. Elmslie technic with movable soft tissue pedicle (8 year review). Orthopade. 1985;14(4):229–38.
62. Langenskiöld A, Ritsilä V. Congenital dislocation of the patella and its operative treatment. J Pediatr Orthop. 1992;12(3):315–23. https://doi.org/10.1097/01241398-199205000-00007.
63. Ramos O, Burke C, Lewis M, Morrison MJ, Paley D, Nelson SC. Modified Langenskiöld procedure for chronic, recurrent, and congenital patellar dislocation. J Child Orthop. 2020;14(4):318–29. https://doi.org/10.1302/1863-2548.14.200044.
64. Bor N, Dujovny E, Rozen N, Rubin G. The Paley ilioischial limb modification of the Dega osteotomy. World J

Pediatr Surg. 2020;3(4):e000143. https://doi.org/10.1136/wjps-2020-000143.
65. Paley D. SUPERhip and SUPERhip2 procedures for congenital femoral deficiency. In: Hamdy R, editor. Pediatric pelvic and proximal femorla osteotomies. Springer; 2018. p. 287–35.
66. Grudziak JS, Ward WT. Dega osteotomy for the treatment of congenital dysplasia of the hip. J Bone Joint Surg Am. 2001;83(6):845–54. https://doi.org/10.2106/00004623-200106000-00005.
67. Grigoryan G, Korcek L, Eidelman M, Paley D, Nelson S. Direct lateral approach for triple pelvic osteotomy. J Am Acad Orthop Surg. 2020;28(2):e64–70. https://doi.org/10.5435/JAAOS-D-16-00918.
68. Leite CBG, Grangeiro PM, Munhoz DU, Giglio PN, Camanho GL, Gobbi RG. The knee in congenital femoral deficiency and its implication in limb lengthening: a systematic review. EFORT Open Rev. 2021;6(7):565–71. https://doi.org/10.1302/2058-5241.6.200075.
69. Krackow KA, Thomas SC, Jones LC. A new stitch for ligament-tendon fixation. Brief note. JBJS. 1986;68(5):764–6.
70. Rozbruch SR, Paley D, Bhave A, Herzenberg JE. Ilizarov hip reconstruction for the late sequelae of infantile hip infection. J Bone Joint Surg Am. 2005;87(5):1007–18. https://doi.org/10.2106/JBJS.C.00713.
71. Ackman J, Altiok H, Flanagan A, et al. Long-term follow-up of Van Nes rotationplasty in patients with congenital proximal focal femoral deficiency. Bone Jt J. 2013;95-B(2):192–8. https://doi.org/10.1302/0301-620X.95B2.30853.
72. Brown KLB. Resection, rotationplasty, and femoropelvic arthrodesis in severe congenital femoral deficiency : a report of the surgical technique and three cases. JBJS. 2001;83(1):78.
73. Paley D, Saghieh S, Kocaogulu M, Herzenberg J. Lengthening for congenital femoral deficiency: results according to age of treatment. Presented at: Pediatric Orthopedic Society of North America annual meeting; May 3, 2002; Salt Lake City, Utah.
74. Sabharwal S, Paley D, Bhave A, Herzenberg JE. Growth patterns after lengthening of congenitally short lower limbs in young children. J Pediatr Orthop. 2000;20(2):137–45.
75. Aston WJS, Calder PR, Baker D, Hartley J, Hill RA. Lengthening of the congenital short femur using the Ilizarov technique: a single-surgeon series. J Bone Joint Surg Br. 2009;91(7):962–7. https://doi.org/10.1302/0301-620X.91B7.21304.
76. Herzenberg JE, Branfoot T, Paley D, Violante FH. Femoral nailing to treat fractures after lengthening for congenital femoral deficiency in young children. J Pediatr Orthop Part B. 2010;19(2):150–4. https://doi.org/10.1097/BPB.0b013e32833033ac.
77. Abdelgawad AA, Jauregui JJ, Standard SC, Paley D, Herzenberg JE. Prophylactic intramedullary rodding following femoral lengthening in congenital deficiency of the femur. J Pediatr Orthop. 2017;37(6):416–23. https://doi.org/10.1097/BPO.0000000000000694.
78. Prince D, Standard S, Herzenberg J, Paley D. First femoral lengthening for congenital femoral deficiency. In: LLRS annual meeting; 2010.
79. Paley D. Problems, obstacles, and complications of limb lengthening by the Ilizarov technique. Clin Orthop. 1990;250:81–104.
80. Paley D, Harris M, Debiparshad K, Prince D. Limb Lengthening by Implantable Limb Lengthening Devices. Tech Orthop. 2014;29(2):72–85. https://doi.org/10.1097/BTO.0000000000000072.
81. Szymczuk VL, Hammouda AI, Gesheff MG, Standard SC, Herzenberg JE. Lengthening With monolateral external fixation versus magnetically motorized intramedullary nail in congenital femoral deficiency. J Pediatr Orthop. 2019;39(9):458–65. https://doi.org/10.1097/BPO.0000000000001047.
82. Shannon C, Paley D. Extramedullary internal limb lengthening. Tech Orthop. 2020;35(3):195–200. https://doi.org/10.1097/BTO.0000000000000466.
83. Dahl MT, Morrison SG, Laine JC, Novotny SA, Georgiadis AG. Extramedullary motorized lengthening of the femur in young children. J Pediatr Orthop. 2020;40(10):e978–83. https://doi.org/10.1097/BPO.0000000000001593.
84. Iobst CA, Bafor A. Retrograde extramedullary lengthening of the femur using the PRECICE nail: technique and results. J Pediatr Orthop. 2021;41(6):356–61. https://doi.org/10.1097/BPO.0000000000001831.
85. Bhave A, Shabtai L, Woelber E, Apelyan A, Paley D, Herzenberg JE. Muscle strength and knee range of motion after femoral lengthening: 2- to 5-year follow-up. Acta Orthop. 2017;88(2):179–84. https://doi.org/10.1080/17453674.2016.1262678.
86. O'Carrigan T, Paley D, Herzenberg JE. Obstacles in limb lengthening: fractures. In: Limb lengthening and reconstruction surgery. New York, NY: Informa Healthcare; 2007:675-679.
87. O'Carrigan T, Herzenberg J, Paley D. Fractures during and after limb lengthening. In: 70th Annual meeting of the American Academy of Orthopedic Surgery; 2003:Paper 212.
88. Aguilar JA, Paley D, Paley J, et al. Clinical Validation of the Multiplier Method for Predicting Limb Length Discrepancy and Outcome of Epiphysiodesis, Part II. J Pediatr Orthop. 2005;25(2):192–6. https://doi.org/10.1097/01.bpo.0000150808.90052.7c.
89. Stevens PM. Guided growth for angular correction: a preliminary series using a tension band plate. J Pediatr Orthop. 2007;27(3):253–9. https://doi.org/10.1097/BPO.0b013e31803433a1.
90. Burghardt RD, Herzenberg JE, Standard SC, Paley D. Temporary hemiepiphyseal arrest using a screw and plate device to treat knee and ankle deformities in children: a preliminary report. J Child Orthop. 2008;2(3):187–97. https://doi.org/10.1007/s11832-008-0096-y.
91. Nogueira MP, Paley D, Bhave A, Herbert A, Nocente C, Herzenberg JE. Nerve lesions associated with limb-lengthening. JBJS. 2003;85(8):1502–10.
92. Nogueira MP, Paley D. Prophylactic and therapeutic peroneal nerve decompression for deformity correction and lengthening. Oper Tech Orthop. 2011;21(2):180–3. https://doi.org/10.1053/j.oto.2011.01.001.
93. Fabre T, Piton C, Andre D, Lasseur E, Durandeau A. Peroneal nerve entrapment. J Bone Joint Surg Am. 1998;80(1):47–53. https://doi.org/10.2106/00004623-199801000-00009.
94. Paley D. Chapter 10: Lengthening considerations: gradual versus acute correction of deformities. In: Principles of deformity correction. 1st ed. Springer; 2002. p. 269–89.
95. Bosemark P, Isaksson H, McDonald MM, Little DG, Tägil M. Augmentation of autologous bone graft by a combination of bone morphogenic protein and bisphosphonate increased both callus volume and strength. Acta Orthop. 2013;84(1):106–11. https://doi.org/10.3109/17453674.2013.773123.
96. Kiely P, Ward K, Bellemore CM, Briody J, Cowell CT, Little DG. Bisphosphonate rescue in distraction osteogenesis: a case series. J Pediatr Orthop. 2007;27(4):467–71. https://doi.org/10.1097/01.bpb.0000271326.41363.d1.
97. Paley D. Congenital pseudarthrosis of the tibia: biological and biomechanical considerations to achieve union and prevent refracture. J Child Orthop. 2019;13(2):120–33. https://doi.org/10.1302/1863-2548.13.180147.
98. Paley D. Paley Cross-Union Protocol for Treatment of Congenital Pseudarthrosis of the Tibia. Oper Tech Orthop. 2021;31(2) https://doi.org/10.1016/j.oto.2021.100881.
99. Wasserstein I. Twenty-five years' experience with lengthening of shortened lower extremities using cylindrical allografts. Clin Orthop. 1990;250:150–3.
100. Dahl MT, Gulli B, Berg T. Complications of limb lengthening. A learning curve. Clin Orthop. 1994;301:10–8.
101. Dhawale AA, Johari AN, Nemade A. Hip dislocation during lengthening of congenital short femur. J Pediatr

Orthop B. 2012;21(3):240–7. https://doi.org/10.1097/BPB.0b013e32834f2524.
102. Eidelman M, Jauregui JJ, Standard SC, Paley D, Herzenberg JE. Hip stability during lengthening in children with congenital femoral deficiency. Int Orthop. 2016;40(12):2619–25. https://doi.org/10.1007/s00264-016-3289-x.
103. Paley D. Chapter 3: Radiographic assessment of lower limb deformities. In: Principles of deformity correction. 1st ed. Springer; 2002. p. 31–60.
104. Judet R. Mobilization of the stiff knee. J Bone Jt Surg Br. 1959;41:856–7.
105. Paley D. Chapter 2: Malalignment and malorientation in the Frontal Plane. In: Principles of deformity correction. 1st ed. Springer; 2002. p. 19–30.
106. Simpson AH, Kenwright J. Fracture after distraction osteogenesis. J Bone Joint Surg Br. 2000;82(5):659–65. https://doi.org/10.1302/0301-620x.82b5.9945.
107. McGrath MS, Mont MA, Siddiqui JA, Baker E, Bhave A. Evaluation of a custom device for the treatment of flexion contractures after total knee arthroplasty. Clin Orthop. 2009;467(6):1485–92. https://doi.org/10.1007/s11999-009-0804-z.
108. Khakharia S, Fragomen AT, Rozbruch SR. Limited quadricepsplasty for contracture during femoral lengthening. Clin Orthop. 2009;467(11):2911–7. https://doi.org/10.1007/s11999-009-0951-2.
109. Martin BD, Cherkashin AM, Tulchin K, Samchukov M, Birch JG. Treatment of femoral lengthening-related knee stiffness with a novel quadricepsplasty. J Pediatr Orthop. 2013;33(4):446–52. https://doi.org/10.1097/BPO.0b013e3182784e5d.
110. Van Nes CP. Rotation-plasty for congenital defects of the femur. J Bone Joint Surg Br. 1950;32-B(1):12–6. https://doi.org/10.1302/0301-620X.32B1.12.
111. Kostuik JP, Gillespie R, Hall JE, Hubbard S. Van Nes rotational osteotomy for treatment of proximal femoral focal deficiency and congenital short femur. J Bone Joint Surg Am. 1975;57(8):1039–46.
112. Hamel J, Winkelmann W, Becker W. A new modification of rotationplasty in a patient with proximal femoral focal deficiency Pappas type II. J Pediatr Orthop Part B. 1999;8(3):200–2. https://doi.org/10.1097/01202412-199907000-00012.
113. Krajbich JI. Modified van nes rotationplasty in the treatment of malignant neoplasms in the lower extremities of children. Clin Orthop Relat Res. 1991;262:74–7.
114. Brown KL. Rotationplasty with hip stabilization in congenital femoral deficiency. In: Herring J, Birch J, editors. The child with a limb deficiency; 1998. p. 103–9.
115. Paley D. Surgical reconstruction for fibular hemimelia. J Child Orthop. 2016;10(6):557–83. https://doi.org/10.1007/s11832-016-0790-0.
116. Fuller CB, Shannon CE, Paley D. Lengthening reconstruction surgery for fibular hemimelia: a review. Children. 2021;8(6):467. https://doi.org/10.3390/children8060467.

Fibular Hemimelia in the Pediatric Patient

Philip K. McClure, John E. Herzenberg, and Shawn C. Standard

Introduction

The etiology of lower extremity deficiencies remains elusive, and is therefore categorized by the predominant long bone deficiency. Occasional heritable groupings have been reported but have not led to a consensus understanding of cause or spectrum of disease. Fibular hemimelia (FH) is the most common congenital long bone deficiency, and the incidence in the USA is between 7.4 to 20 cases per million live births (up to 1 per 50,000 live births) [1–3]. It is primarily associated with lower extremity anomalies such as femoral shortening, hypoplastic lateral femoral condyle, genu valgum, anteromedial bowing of the tibia, limb length discrepancy (LLD), absent or deficient anterior cruciate ligament (ACL) or posterior cruciate ligament (PCL), ball-and-socket ankle joint, equinovarus or equinovalgus foot, tarsal coalition, and absence of foot rays (Fig. 30.1). The fibula is generally the most striking variance in FH; it can vary from mild shortening to complete absence.

Stevens et al suggested that FH is a manifestation of "postaxial" hypoplasia, existing along with congenital femoral deficiency (CFD) in many cases, with one component generally dominant. There are certainly a plenty of clinical examples to support this concept, as it is typical to find components of both FH and CFD in individual patients [4]. The "postaxial" moniker however may be in need of some revision. Birch et al reported radiographic analysis of the foot in their series of patients, noting that the deficiencies were predominantly central rays, with the cuboid/5th metatarsal complex present in the majority of cases [5]. More recently, Hootnick and Levinsohn reinforced this concept in embryologic studies [6]. Upper extremity manifestations may include syndactyly and ulnar hemimelia [7–9]. Rodriguez-Ramirez et al examined the prevalence of associated congenital osseous anomalies in patients with FH and found that lateral femoral condyle hypoplasia was the most common associated anomaly (93%), followed by ball-and-socket ankle joint (80%), congenital femoral deficiency (72%), tarsal coalition (51%), and forefoot ray deletion (44%) [7]. Equinovalgus is much more common than equinovarus. Roux and Carlioz demonstrated absence of the anterior cruciate ligament in 95% of the cases [8]. Components of FH are present in various genetic syndromes that affect multiple organ systems; hence a thorough examination is required to determine if referral to genetics is indicated. A broad phenotypic spectrum of presentation may occur (Fig. 30.1)

Because of FH's broad spectrum of severity, there is a wide range of treatments, from observation in patients with nearly normal anatomy and minimal LLD to comprehensive treatment strategies for severe limb anomalies and massive LLD. The common alternative to extensive lengthening is amputation and prosthetic rehabilitation [5, 9–17]. The challenge in limb lengthening is to achieve normal limb alignment and length with a functional, painless, shoeable, and plantigrade foot. This undertaking is often characterized by repeated surgical procedures and a high rate of complications and sequelae such as pin tract infections, residual LLD, delayed union, ankle and knee stiffness, re-fracture, knee subluxation, and residual/recurrent foot deformities. Deciding which treatment to apply (lengthening versus amputation) can be challenging for the surgeon and the family [9–13]. Regardless of treatment path, surgeons need to be well-versed in the entire spectrum of disease and advanced treatment options for the knee—even when amputation is the chosen method. Knee instability, genu valgum, tibial deformity, and hip pathology remain the significant causes of difficulty for patients who have selected the "one-and-done" treatment approach.

P. K. McClure · J. E. Herzenberg (✉) · S. C. Standard
International Center for Limb Lengthening, Rubin Institute for Advanced Orthopedics, Sinai Hospital of Baltimore, Baltimore, MD, USA
e-mail: pmcclure@lifebridgehealth.org; jherzenberg@lifebridgehealth.org; sstandar@lifebridgehealth.org

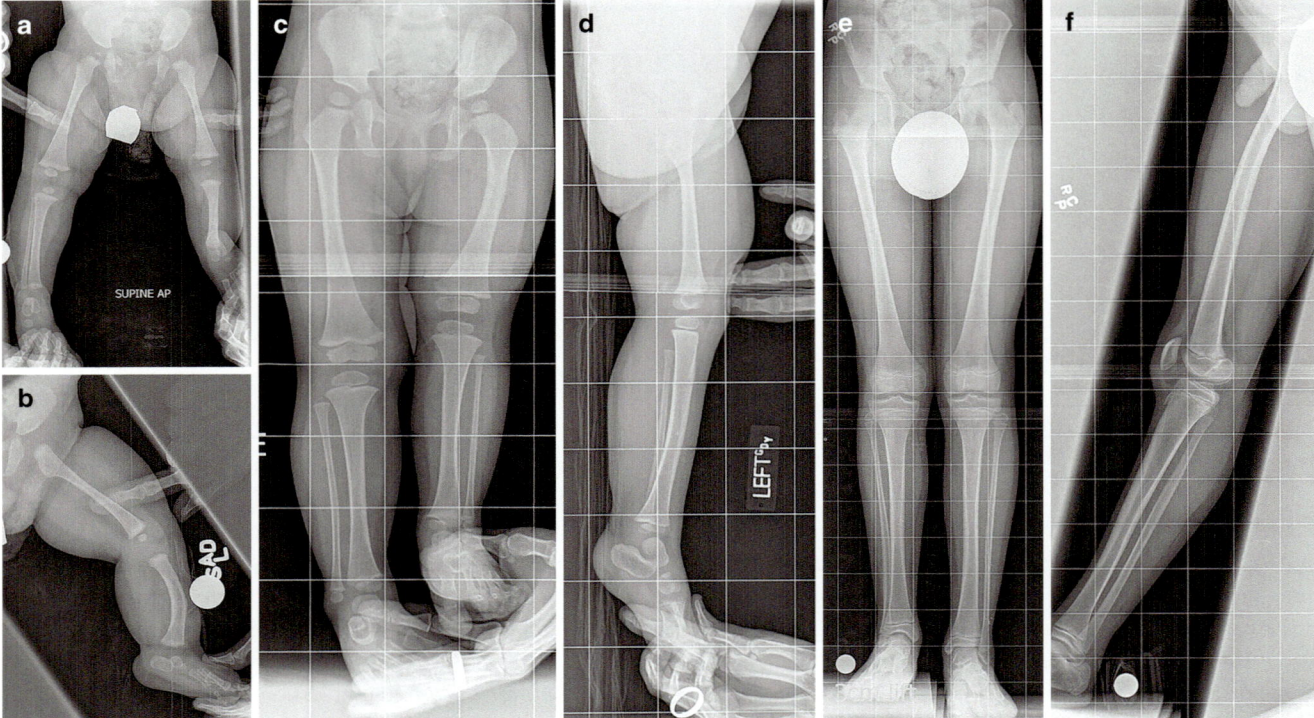

Fig. 30.1 AP (**a**) and lateral (**b**) view radiographs show a 10-month-old infant with fibular hemimelia, concurrent congenital femoral deficiency, a typical anterior bow of the tibia, and equinovalgus foot deformity. AP (**c**) and lateral (**d**) view radiographs show a 2-year-old child with fibular hemimelia and congenital femoral deficiency as well as mild genu valgus and ankle valgus. AP (**e**) and lateral (**f**) view radiographs of a 12-year-old patient with fibular hemimelia who has genu valgus, mild leg length discrepancy, a ball-and-socket ankle joint, and talocalcaneal coalition. Reprinted with permission from the Rubin Institute for Advanced Orthopedics, Sinai Hospital of Baltimore

Parents must be aware of all the options and associated potential complications before making treatment decisions. Though surgical treatment is generally not indicated in the first year of life, much input is required from the conscientious surgeon. Parents often have a knee-jerk reaction toward or away from amputation depending on cultural, religious, or other influences. The surgeon must take the primary role in counseling families during the decision process regarding treatment options and their implications. This often requires multiple meetings with the family and is a marked deviation from typical orthopedic clinic flow. Initial and follow-up encounters often require an hour or more to be sure that the family understands the process adequately. This often is true even when amputation is chosen for more severe cases, as prosthetic fitting, follow-up care, and surgical treatments for associated pathology of the limb are often present.

The aim of this chapter is to discuss in detail the principles and techniques of management of lengthening and reconstruction for FH by understanding and addressing each deformity in this complex, multifaceted disorder. A detailed description of the amputation options (Syme or Boyd) is covered in the amputation chapter (Chap. 19) by J.A. Herring. Interestingly, Calder et al recently found that the foot in severe FH can be left on (not amputated) and accommodated with an extension prosthesis, though long-term outcome scores favored foot amputation [18]. They also found that the common diaphyseal anteromedial bow in FH does not need to be corrected with amputation, and that it may help with socket suspension.

Typical Deformities Associated with FH

Tibial shortening
- Equinovalgus foot
- Missing all or part of the fibula
- Missing one or more central or lateral rays
- Talocalcaneal coalition—can also include mid foot coalitions/deletions
- Anteromedial bowing of the tibia
- Cruciate ligament insufficiency
- Genu valgum
- Hypoplasia of lateral femoral condyle
- Limb length difference
- Congenital femoral deficiency
- Hip dysplasia
- Syndactyly
- Ball-and-socket ankle joint
- Cup-and-saucer knee joint
- Equinovarus foot

Classification

Several classifications exist for FH. The earliest published classification is the Coventry and Johnson classification from 1952 (Fig. 30.2) [19]. They divide patients with FH into three types:

Type I: Partial unilateral absence of the fibula; normal or slight bowing of the tibia with some shortening of the limb; the foot is normal or slightly deformed.
Type II: The fibula is completely or almost absent; anterior bowing of the tibia with skin dimpling; deformed ankle joint; deformed foot with absent rays.
Type III: Includes type I or type II but is associated with other congenital deformities or bilateral involvement.

The Achterman and Kalamchi classification from 1979 is the most used (Fig. 30.3) [20]. They divide the patients into two groups with one subdivision:

Type I: Incomplete fibular deficiency; type I is subdivided into: type I-A: The proximal fibular epiphysis is distal to the level of the upper tibial growth plate and the distal fibular growth plate is proximal to the dome of the talus; and type I-B: 30 to 50% fibular shortening and the fibula does not articulate with the talus.
Type II: Complete fibular deficiency, with or without a small distal fibular remnant.

The Stanitski classification from 2003 (Fig. 30.4) is a morphologic description that divides FH into four categories primarily based on radiographic presentation [21]:

1. Fibula: Normal, partially absent, or completely absent
2. Ankle joint: According to the morphology of the tibiotalar joint: horizontal, valgus, or ball-and-socket joint
3. Tarsal bones: Tarsal coalition present or absent
4. Foot: Numbers of rays.

Birch et al presented a new classification system in 1998, based on the clinical status of the foot and the magnitude of limb shortening as a percentage of the contralateral limb on radiographs, to anticipate the extent of deformity at maturity and recommend the appropriate treatment required (Fig. 30.5) [22]. Birch et al later modified the proposed treatment for fewer amputations and more reconstruction procedures [5, 23]. Cases are divided into two categories:

Type 1: Functional foot, in which the foot has at least three rays and can provide a stable weightbearing platform. Type 1 is divided into four subtypes according to the percentage of total limb shortening compared with the contralateral side:
Type 1A: <6% leg length inequality; the treatment is orthosis or contralateral epiphysiodesis.
Type 1B: 6 to 10% leg length inequality; the treatment is epiphysiodesis ± lengthening.
Type 1C: 11 to 30% leg length inequality; the treatment is one or two lengthening procedures ± epiphysiodesis or extension orthosis.
Type 1D: >30% leg length inequality; the treatment proposed is more than two lengthening procedures or amputation or extension orthosis.

Fig. 30.2 Coventry and Johnson classification of FH: Type I: partial unilateral absence of fibula, normal or slight bowing of the tibia with some shortening of the limb, and the foot is normal or slightly deformed. Type II: the fibula is completely or almost entirely absent, anterior bowing of the tibia with skin dimpling, deformed ankle joint, and deformed foot with absent rays. Type III: includes type I or II associated with other congenital deformities or bilateral involvement. Reprinted with permission from the Rubin Institute for Advanced Orthopedics, Sinai Hospital of Baltimore

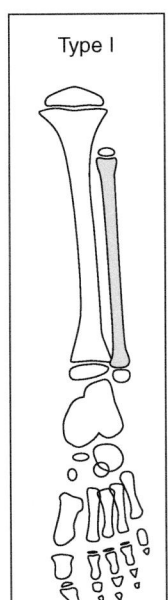
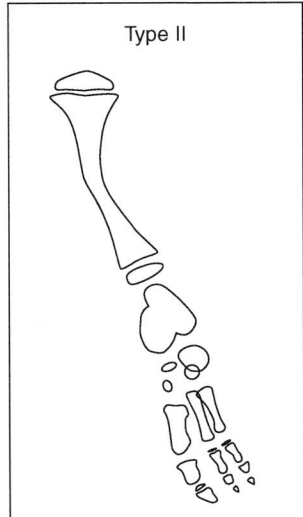
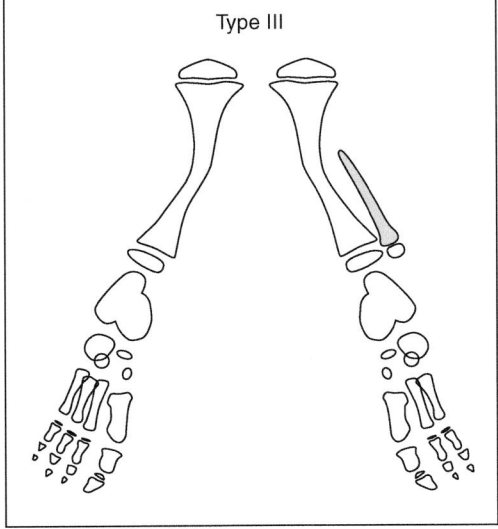

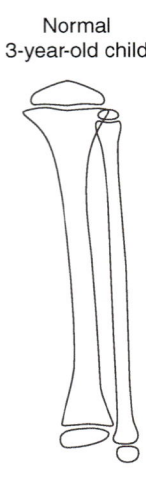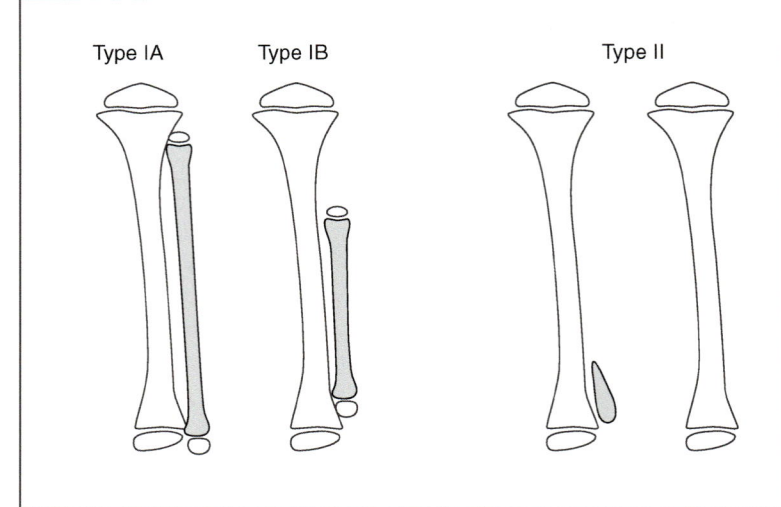

Fig. 30.3 Achterman and Kalamchi classification of FH: Type I: incomplete fibular deficiency, subdivided into I-A and I-B. Type I-A: proximal fibular epiphysis is distal to the level of the tibial growth plate, distal fibular growth plate is proximal to the dome of the talus. Type I-B: 30–50 % partial fibular absence, fibula does not articulate with the talus. Type II: complete fibular deficiency, with or without a tiny distal fibular remnant. Reprinted with permission from the Rubin Institute for Advanced Orthopedics, Sinai Hospital of Baltimore

Type 2: Non-functional foot. Type 2 is subdivided into types 2A and 2B according to the functionality of the upper extremity:

> Type 2A: Upper extremities are functional; therefore, the treatment proposed is early amputation.
>
> Type 2B: Upper extremities are non-functional, and so foot amputation is contraindicated, as the foot must act as a replacement for the upper extremity.

These classifications serve to draw attention to various components of the pathology present in FH. In the authors' opinion, the Birch classification is highly valuable, as it focuses the surgeon's assessment and thought process on the function of the joints, and the patient's needs for the use of the limb. Failure on the part of the surgeon to consider the patient's likely result and functional needs is a severe failure indeed.

Classification Schemes Used in the USA for FH

Coventry and Johnson
  Achterman and Kalamchi
  Stanitski
  Birch
  Paley

A 2003 classification proposed by Paley presumes reconstruction, rather than amputation. Each type has its own reconstruction protocol. (Fig. 30.6) [17]. This system classifies FH into four types, based on the ankle pathology:

Type 1: Stable normal ankle.
Type 2: Dynamic valgus ankle.
Type 3: Fixed equinovalgus ankle. Type 3 is divided into four subtypes according to the location of the valgus deformity:

  Type 3a: Ankle type
  Type 3b: Subtalar type
  Type 3c: Combined ankle and subtalar type
  Type 3d: Talar body type.
Type 4: Fixed equinovarus ankle (clubfoot).

This system was slightly modified in 2016, to subdivide type 3B into 3b1 (lateral malleolus present, albeit proximally migrated) and 3b2 (absent fibula) [24]. For type 1, tibial lengthening is recommended, along with tendo Achilles lengthening. For type 2, tibial lengthening is recommended, along with tendo Achilles lengthening and a supramalleolar reorientation osteotomy. For type 3, soft tissue lengthening (peroneal tendons and tendo Achilles), resection of the fibrous anlage and interosseous membrane, and a reorientation osteotomy is recommended. This has been nicknamed the "SUPER (Systematic Utilitarian Procedure for Extremity Reconstruction) ankle" procedure and will be described later in the chapter. The osteotomy site varies according to whether the deformity is classified as type 3a, 3b, 3c, or 3d. Type 3a needs a supramalleolar osteotomy, type 3b needs a subtalar osteotomy, type 3c needs both supramalleolar and subtalar osteotomy, and type 3d—which is very rare—may be treated with an opening wedge osteotomy of the body of the talus. Type 4 (clubfoot type) is treated initially by applying Ponseti casts and performing an Achilles tenotomy followed by a SUPERankle procedure at age 12 to 24 months. The casting treatment typically converts the foot position from equinovarus to equinovalgus, which can then be addressed with the SUPERankle procedure. In some cases, surgical treatment of the ankle becomes unnecessary after the Ponseti treatment of the associated club foot deformity.

Fig. 30.4 Stanitski classification of FH according to four parameters: *1.* Fibula: normal, partially absent, or completely absent. *2.* Ankle joint: according to the morphology of the tibiotalar joint: horizontal, valgus, or spherical (ball-and-socket joint). *3.* Tarsal bones: tarsal coalition present or absent. *4.* Foot: numbers of rays. Reprinted with permission from the Rubin Institute for Advanced Orthopedics, Sinai Hospital of Baltimore

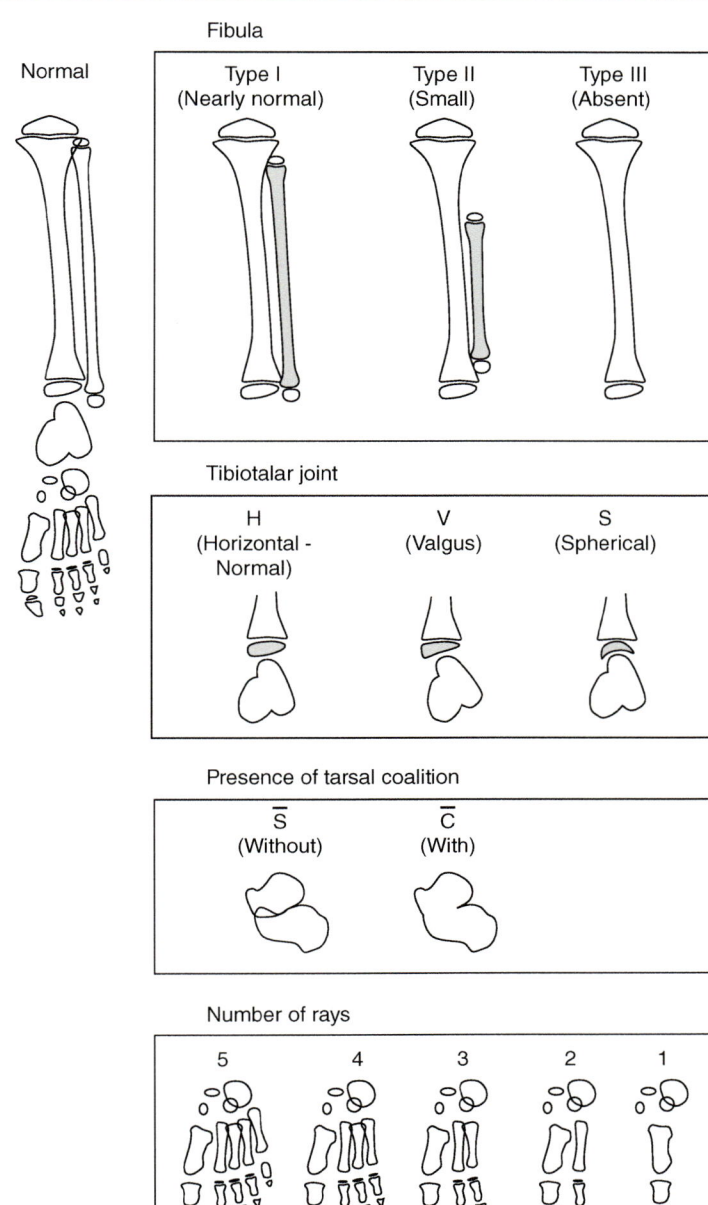

While the more severe type 3 cases should also be considered candidates for amputation, Paley's classification is geared towards reconstruction, with the subtype designation dictating the specific reconstructive procedure. The Paley classification, like other systems, does not draw the surgeon's attention to potential knee deficiencies that may require care-specific treatment, regardless of treatment approach. The specific knee deformities have been cataloged by Manner et al. [25].

Paley Classification of FH

Type 1: Normal ankle
Type 2: Dynamic valgus ankle
 Type 3a: Fixed equinovalgus ankle, supramalleolar type
 Type 3b: Fixed equinovalgus ankle, subtalar type
 Type 3c: Fixed equinovalgus ankle, combined supramalleolar/subtalar type
 Type 3d: Fixed equinovalgus ankle, talar body type
Type 4: Equinovarus type (clubfoot)

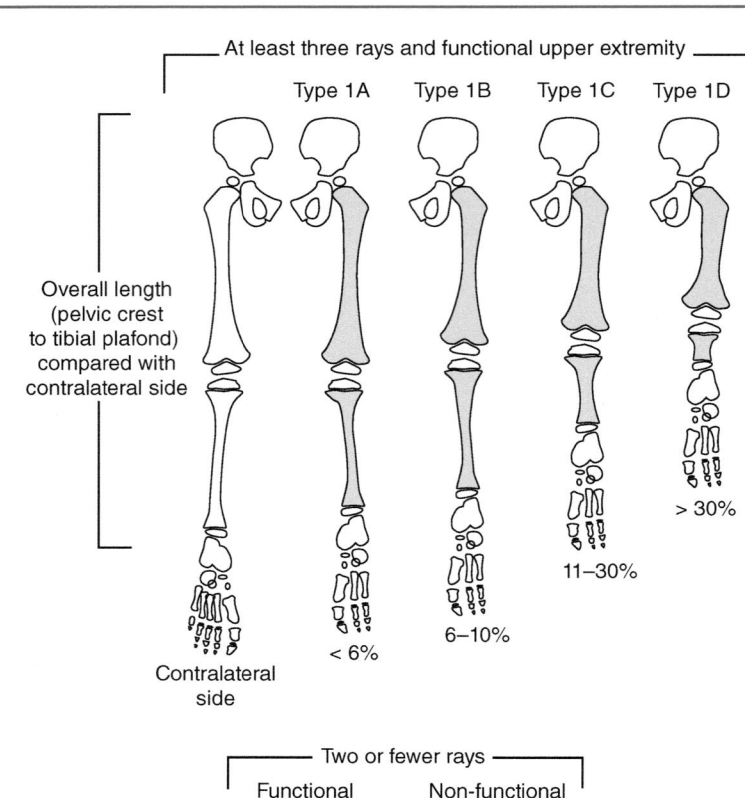
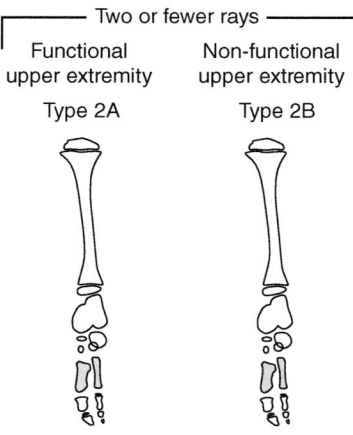

Fig. 30.5 Birch classification of FH. Type 1: Functional foot, foot with at least three rays that can provide a stable weight-bearing surface. Type 1 is divided into four subtypes according to the limb length difference compared with the normal side. Type 1A: <6% limb length inequality; Type 1B: 6–10% limb length inequality; Type 1C: 11–30% limb length inequality; Type 1D: >30% limb length inequality. Type 2: Nonfunctional foot (fewer than three rays). Type 2 is subdivided into Types 2A and 2B according to the functionality of the upper extremity. Type 2A: Functional upper extremity; Type 2B: Nonfunctional upper extremity. Reprinted with permission from the Rubin Institute for Advanced Orthopedics, Sinai Hospital of Baltimore

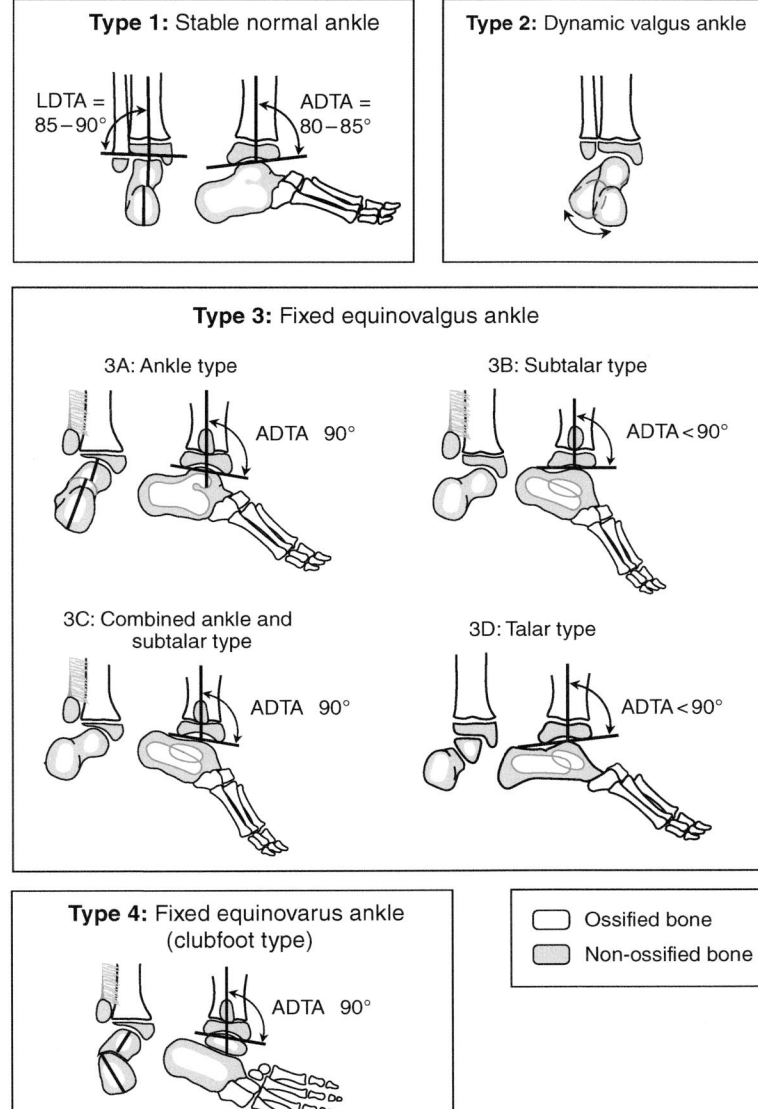

Fig. 30.6 Paley classification of FH. Type 1: Stable normal ankle. Type 2: Dynamic valgus ankle. Type 3: Fixed equinovalgus ankle. Type 3 is further subdivided according to the etiology of the valgus into 3A (ankle), 3B (subtalar), 3C (combined ankle and subtalar), and 3D (talar). Type 4: Fixed equinovarus ankle (clubfoot). Reprinted with permission from the Rubin Institute for Advanced Orthopedics, Sinai Hospital of Baltimore

Clinical Assessment

The initial clinical exam should include a complete orthopedic examination of the child, checking for associated anomalies. In the lower extremity, the number of rays and position of the foot and ankle are noted. Specifically, the ankle is examined to determine if it is mobile and well-aligned or contracted into equinovalgus or equinovarus. The range of motion and stability of the hip, knee, and ankle are assessed. The knee joint is often somewhat unstable (ACL or PCL deficiency) and may be in excessive valgus alignment.

If the involvement of the hip and knee are severe (as in combined FH and CFD), then the overall reconstruction plan is either concurrent hip/knee reconstruction or sequential reconstruction. Most commonly, the significantly involved hip and knee would be addressed first between the ages of 18 and 24 months (this is discussed at length in Chap. 28). The ankle reconstruction would then typically occur 6 to 12 months after the hip and knee reconstruction, although in certain cases, it may be feasible to perform simultaneous hip, knee, and ankle reconstruction (SUPERhip, SUPERknee, and SUPERankle procedures).

Even if the femur is not involved or minimally involved, there still may be instability of the knee due to an absent ACL. The degree of laxity that is best addressed with prophylactic ligament reconstruction remains a topic of some uncertainty and may vary from surgeon to surgeon. However, severe cases are not uncommon, with one to two centimeters of translation of the tibia on the femoral condyles on clinical examination. In such cases, the preoperative full-length standing lateral view radiograph may show anterior subluxation of the tibia on the femur. Consideration should be given to perform an ACL substitution procedure prior to tibial lengthening. If the PCL is also deficient, then an extra-articular PCL reconstruction should be performed at the same time.

Radiographic Assessment

In our practice, a patient with FH is usually seen during the first year of life. In fewer than one-third of cases, the diagnosis has already been made using prenatal ultrasonography [26]. During the initial visit, supine anteroposterior (AP) and lateral view radiographs of the legs are obtained. This is done to evaluate the exact configuration of the skeletal anatomy of the lower legs, determine the amount of LLD, and look for concurrent deformities such as CFD.

The initial radiographic assessment should include plain films: full-length AP radiograph depicting both legs with a lift under the short leg (Fig. 30.7), and a full-length lateral view of the affected leg with the knee in maximum extension

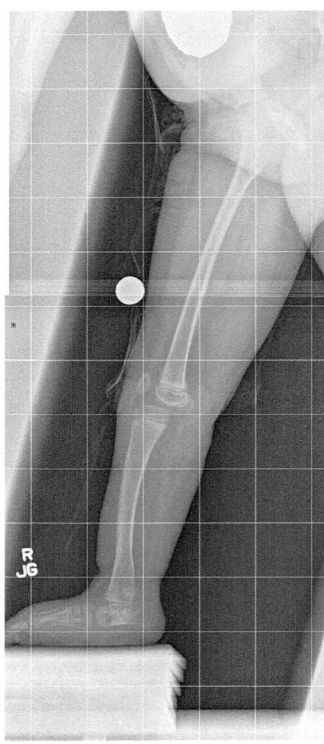

Fig. 30.8 Full-length standing lateral view radiograph shows a typical child with FH who has an apex anterior bow of the tibia and congenital instability of the knee due to the lack of functional intra-articular ligaments (ACL/PCL). Reprinted with permission from the Rubin Institute for Advanced Orthopedics, Sinai Hospital of Baltimore

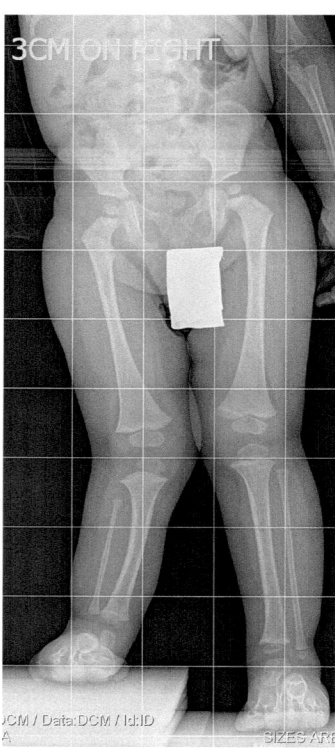

Fig. 30.7 Full-length standing AP view radiograph shows a typical child with FH who has knee valgus and tibial valgus bow. Reprinted with permission from the Rubin Institute for Advanced Orthopedics, Sinai Hospital of Baltimore

(Fig. 30.8). These are initially obtained supine but should be done standing once patients are able to do so. Given the number of images obtained for these patients throughout their childhood, consideration should be given to transitioning to low-dose slot scanners such as the EOSedge, as soon as feasible (EOS Imaging, SA, Paris, France).

The typical appearance in severe cases is a mild valgus deformity of the knee secondary to a hypoplastic lateral femoral condyle. This creates a mechanical lateral distal femoral angle (mLDFA) of <85°. Additional valgus may come from the periphyseal region of the tibia or an apex anteromedial bow in the diaphyseal tibia. A dimple on the skin is usually visible over the apex of this bow (Fig. 30.9). Metaphyseal deformity of the distal tibia also is relatively common. A lateral view radiograph of the foot may show overlap of the talus and calcaneus or a talo-calcaneal tarsal coalition. If the talus and calcaneus are on top of one another, the ankle valgus is typically from a tilt in the distal tibial plafond. The talus and calcaneus may be stacked on top of each other on the lateral view, which points toward the ankle as the source of valgus (Fig. 30.10). If the talus and calcaneus are overlapped on the lateral view (Fig. 30.11) or side-by-side on the AP

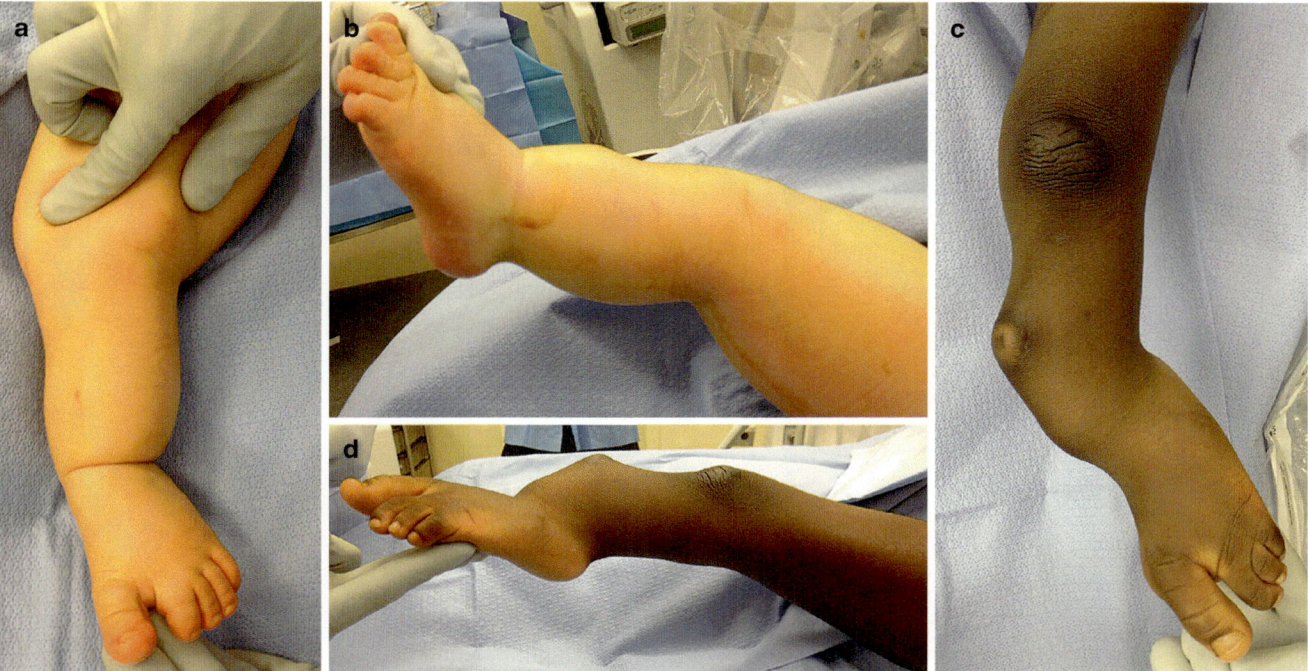

Fig. 30.9 (**a, b**) Clinical photos show a child with moderate deformity secondary to FH. The typical anteromedial bow, equinovalgus foot, and dimple at the apex of the tibial bow are shown. (**c, d**) Clinical photos show a severe deformity secondary to FH. Reprinted with permission from the Rubin Institute for Advanced Orthopedics, Sinai Hospital of Baltimore.

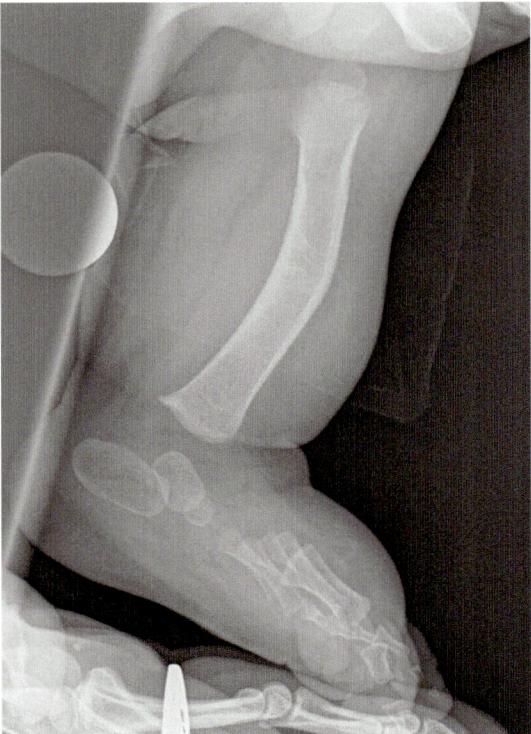

Fig. 30.10 Lateral view radiograph of the foot shows the talus and calcaneus stacked on top of each other, suggesting the hindfoot valgus is supramalleolar in origin. Reprinted with permission from the Rubin Institute for Advanced Orthopedics, Sinai Hospital of Baltimore

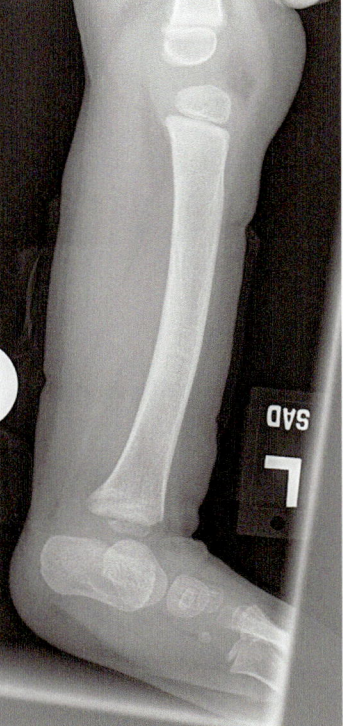

Fig. 30.11 Lateral view radiograph of the foot shows the talus and calcaneus overlapped on top of each other, suggesting the hindfoot valgus is subtalar in origin. Reprinted with permission from the Rubin Institute for Advanced Orthopedics, Sinai Hospital of Baltimore

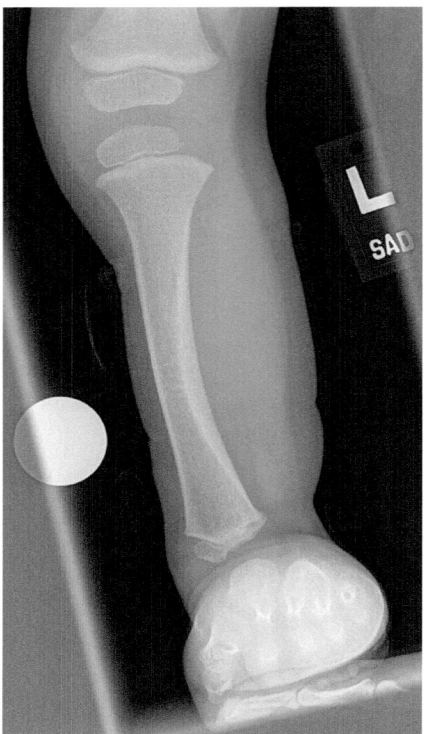

Fig. 30.12 AP view ankle radiograph shows the talus and calcaneus side by side, suggesting the hindfoot valgus is subtalar in origin. Reprinted with permission from the Rubin Institute for Advanced Orthopedics, Sinai Hospital of Baltimore

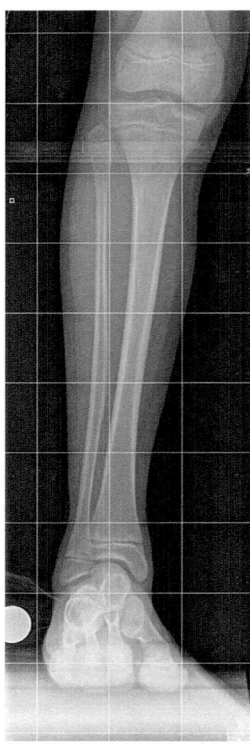

Fig. 30.13 AP view radiograph of the tibia, ankle, and foot in a typical child with FH shows a ball-and-socket ankle with a talocalcaneal coalition. As an infant, the talocalcaneal block is cartilaginous, but the talocalcaneal coalition becomes more radiographically evident as the child ages and the bones ossify. Reprinted with permission from the Rubin Institute for Advanced Orthopedics, Sinai Hospital of Baltimore

ankle (Fig. 30.12) view resembling a double-barreled shotgun, then the valgus component is more likely subtalar in origin. Most patients with FH have a talo-calcaneal coalition, which may not be evident on the initial radiographs obtained during infancy but becomes more obvious as the coalition ossifies with age (Figs. 30.13 and 30.14).

In addition to plain films for cases of Paley type 3 FH, it can be useful to obtain a magnetic resonance imaging (MRI) evaluation of the foot and ankle just prior to performing the SUPERankle procedure. Since much of the hindfoot and distal tibia is unossified during the first two years of life, it can be difficult to accurately classify the exact Paley type 3 subtype. In such cases, an MRI can help differentiate between type 3a, b, and c, thus allowing better preoperative planning (Figs. 30.15 and 30.16). The utility of the MRI must be weighed against the risk and cost of sedation required to get adequate studies for young children. An intraoperative arthrogram of the ankle joint can help delineate the valgus orientation at the ankle joint (Fig. 30.17).

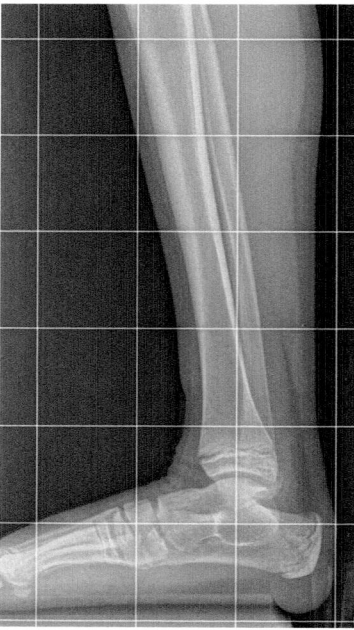

Fig. 30.14 Lateral view radiograph (the same child depicted in Fig. 30.13) shows the classic "C" sign of the talocalcaneal coalition and a concurrent talonavicular coalition. Reprinted with permission from the Rubin Institute for Advanced Orthopedics, Sinai Hospital of Baltimore

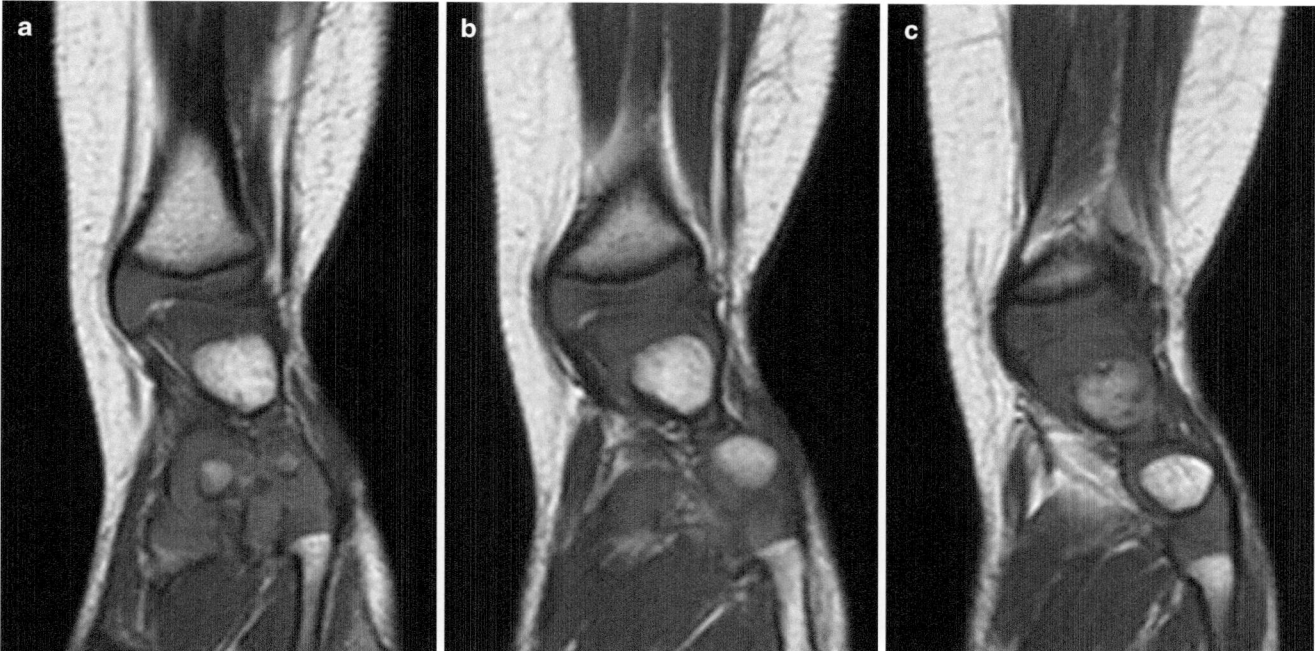

Fig. 30.15 (a–c) Sequential MRI scans of the left lower extremity in a patient with fibular hemimelia show that the valgus originates in the supramalleolar region (Paley Type 3A—ankle type). Reprinted with permission from the Rubin Institute for Advanced Orthopedics, Sinai Hospital of Baltimore

Fig. 30.16 MRI scan of the right lower extremity in a patient with fibular hemimelia shows that the hindfoot valgus originates in the subtalar joint (Paley Type 3B). Reprinted with permission from the Rubin Institute for Advanced Orthopedics, Sinai Hospital of Baltimore

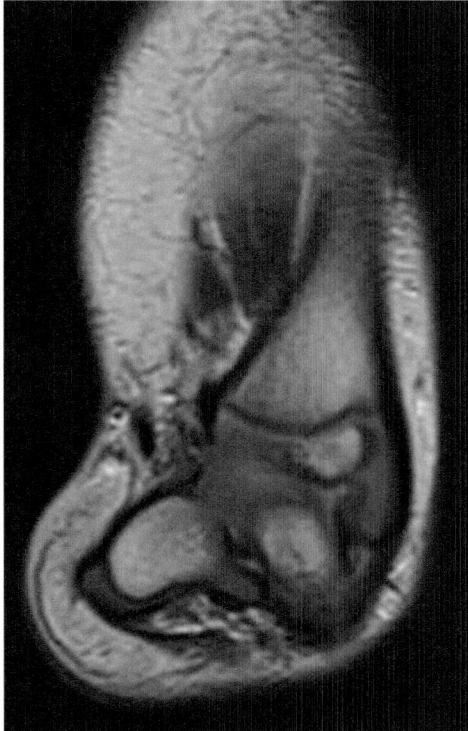

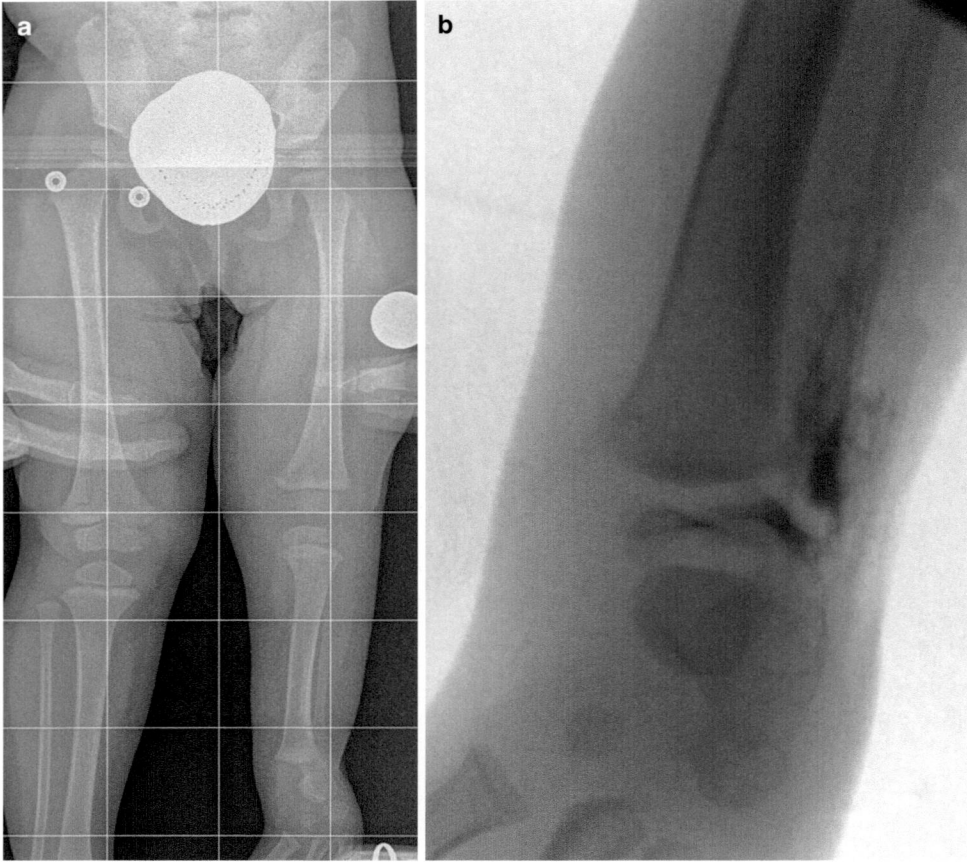

Fig. 30.17 (a) Supine full-length radiograph of an 18-month-old girl with left fibular hemimelia shows typical equinovalgus of the foot and ankle. (b) Intraoperative AP ankle arthrogram of the same patient shows the distal tibia as the source of the ankle valgus. Reprinted with permission from the Rubin Institute for Advanced Orthopedics, Sinai Hospital of Baltimore

Prediction of Height and Limb Length Discrepancy at Maturity

Based on the measured radiographic LLD (or the clinically measured LLD), the ultimate LLD at maturity can be predicted. We use the multiplier method to predict the ultimate LLD and height (based on the long leg) at skeletal maturity [27, 28]. This is easily done with the Multiplier mobile app (free for Apple iOS and Android devices). Recently, the Multiplier app has been demonstrated to be somewhat inaccurate for prediction of LLD when epiphysiodesis is the treatment approach [19, 29]. It remains useful, however, for prediction of total LLD and the creation of a treatment plan. The weaknesses are mitigated by performing the final lengthening after skeletal maturity has been reached.

These two predictions (LLD and height) allow for formulation of a multi-stage treatment plan for the family. The family should leave the first visit with a clear picture of pros and cons of the two main treatment styles: amputation versus reconstruction. Knowing the predicted height and LLD at skeletal maturity allows the surgeon to propose various treatment strategies. For example, if the multiplier method predicts an adult height for a boy to be 5'7" with an LLD of 6 cm, then most families would choose limb lengthening rather than epiphysiodesis. However, if the same boy had a predicted height of 6'2" with an LLD of 6 cm, then epiphysiodesis may be a more attractive option. Concerning the reconstruction option, the family needs to be told if it will be necessary to perform foot/ankle reconstruction, as well as how many lengthening procedures are anticipated.

Principles of Treatment

External fixation is the mainstay of lengthening in young children with FH [23]. Initial trials of a promising internal lengthening plate were somewhat disappointing, particularly in comparison to results obtained with external fixators. The plate has subsequently been withdrawn from market, with hope for redesign and re-release. In skeletally mature patients, it is often possible to use newer magnetic telescopic intramedullary (IM) nails for tibial lengthening [30]. Combinations of lengthening and epiphysiodesis can also be done to minimize the amount of lengthening procedures required [31].

Initial reconstruction is a very complex set of procedures that is unique for each child. The deformity related to FH is the combination of contracted soft tissues, unstable joints, and abnormally oriented joints of the ankle and foot. Treatment should address several issues such as limb shortening, lower leg deformity, and an abnormally positioned foot with or without absence of foot rays. The goals of treatment are to create a lower limb with a stable hip, knee, and ankle by:

1. Correcting the foot (usually equinovalgus) into a plantigrade position
2. Equalizing lower limb lengths by skeletal maturity
3. Restoration of neutral lower limb alignment.

In many of the more severe cases, it may not be possible to improve the limited ankle mobility. Furthermore, the treatment itself (multiple lengthening procedures or SUPERankle reconstruction plus multiple lengthening procedures) may result in further loss of ankle motion compared to the amount present initially. The success of reconstruction is not determined necessarily by final ankle motion. The amount of final ankle motion usually is predetermined by the amount of motion initially present at the ankle joint, and it does not improve with lengthening.

The amount of LLD predicted by the end of growth does not necessarily determine whether successful reconstruction is possible. However, the overall predicted LLD does help when estimating the number of lengthening treatments that will be needed to equalize the limb lengths before skeletal maturity. Dividing the amount of lengthening into smaller amounts might be less traumatic for the muscles, nerves, and adjacent joints than trying to perform a heroic lengthening during one treatment. For example, if the predicted discrepancy is 15 cm, this may be addressed better with three 5-cm lengthening treatments instead of two 7.5-cm lengthening treatments. Better yet, two 5-cm lengthening treatments combined with one 5-cm epiphysiodesis may yield the optimum outcome if the family and patient are willing to allow intervention on the "normal" leg [31].

For children with Paley type 3 (fixed equinovalgus deformity), the decision to lengthen during the first reconstructive surgery is determined by the amount of ankle motion present in combination with the anticipated LLD. If the ankle is intrinsically stiff and the overall lengthening goal will require three or more lengthening procedures, then a 4 to 5 cm lengthening may be performed at the same surgical setting as the SUPERankle procedure. If the ankle is relatively mobile, then another option is for the initial surgery to concentrate on positioning the foot and ankle in a stable or corrected position while concurrently correcting the bowing in the lower leg. This can be done with internal means while lengthening can be left for a later date, after the ankle has recovered from soft tissue dissection. With severe bows, Ilizarov-style external fixators are often the best choice, as the associated shortening required for closed deformity correction can leave patients with minimal tibia remaining.

The number of subsequent lengthening treatments is determined by the overall predicted lengthening goal. The subsequent lengthening treatments are performed at the intervals of four to six years apart for a total of up to three or even four lengthening treatments for the most severe grades of FH. The first lengthening usually achieves a 5 cm gain in length. Subsequent lengthenings can achieve between 5 and 7 cm of length each.

The amount of length gained during a single lengthening treatment is determined by the rate and quality of regenerate bone formation and by motion and stability of the joints above and below the lengthening site. In patients younger than six years of age, the maximum length typically gained during a single lengthening is 5 cm. The total amount of lengthening in a younger patient is limited to avoid extreme pressure on the growth plates that can cause premature closure of the growth plates and loss of potential natural growth. Older patients can often tolerate gaining more length in a single treatment (between 5 and 7 cm).

Bone formation is better in the proximal metaphysis rather than in the diaphysis. This is another reason why it may be preferable not to perform a large amount of lengthening through the diaphyseal bow, at the time of the initial SUPERankle procedure. Development of a knee flexion contracture or subluxation during lengthening may dictate the need to stop further lengthening. The knee must be splinted in full extension during the tibial lengthening to prevent contracture/subluxation.

FH Treatment Options

Amputation
 Lengthening with external fixator
 Lengthening over nails
 Lengthening with internal telescopic nails
 Foot/ankle reconstruction for dynamic valgus
 SUPERankle for rigid equinovalgus
 Shortening for Deformity Correction (SHORDT) in place of SUPERankle

Surgical Techniques

Lengthening for Paley Type 1

Mild cases of FH may be lengthened using standard limb lengthening methodology, which is described in Chap. 9. All patients with FH have a certain degree of tightness in the

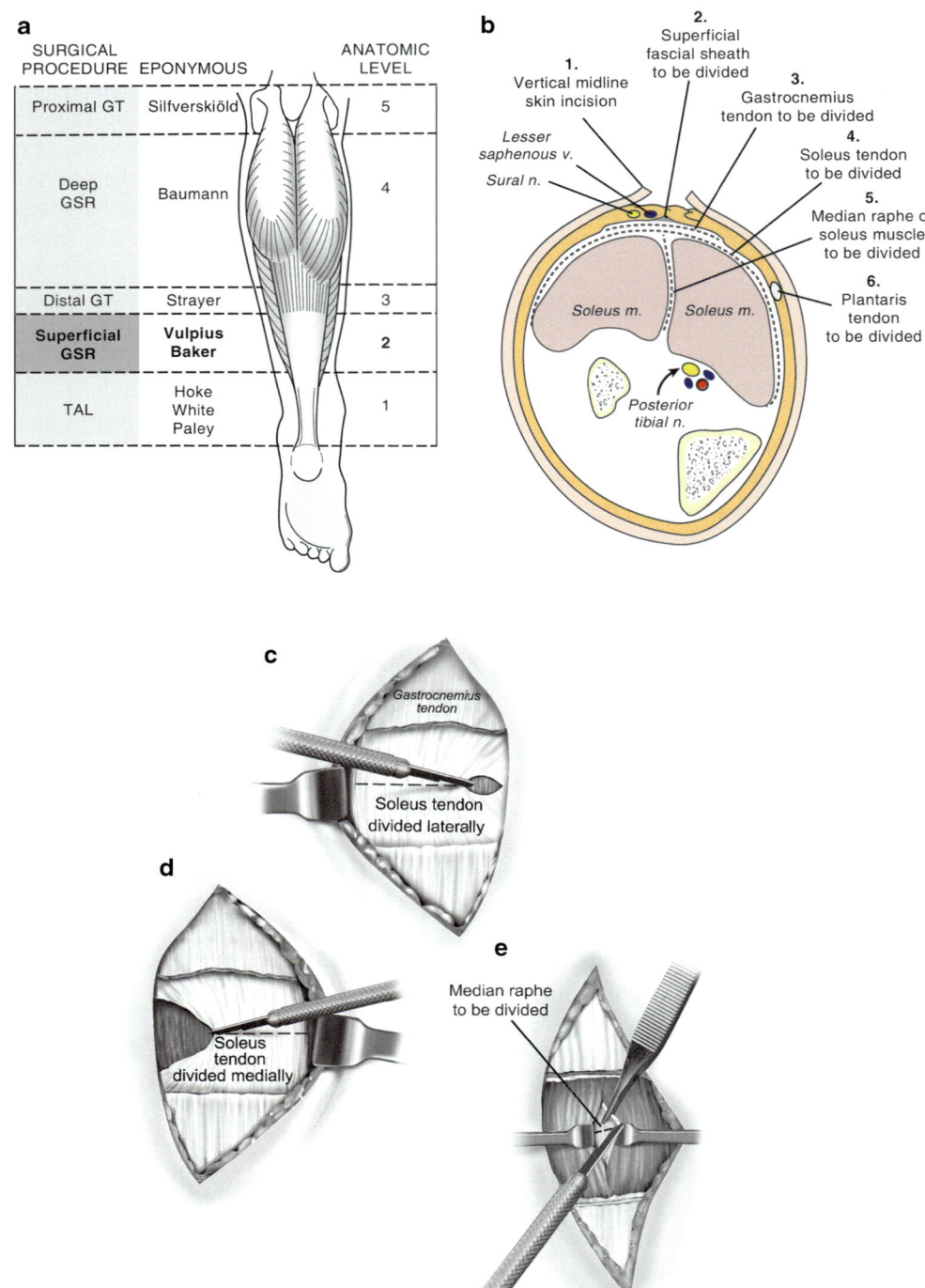

Fig. 30.18 Open Vulpius procedure is recommended for all Paley Type 1 and 2 FH lengthening procedures. (**a**) Posterior leg can be divided into five anatomic levels. (**b**) Cross-sectional view of anatomic level 2 with steps to perform gastrocnemius–soleus recession numbered sequentially. The *broken lines* represent the tendon portion of the gastrocnemius and soleus muscles and the median raphe of the soleus muscle. (**c**) After midline vertical incision, vertical division of the superficial fascia, and horizontal release of the gastrocnemius tendon, then the soleus tendon is released. (**d**) Soleus tendon is also released horizontally to the opposite edge (medially) of the tendon using deep retraction. (**e**) The median raphe (central tendon) of the soleus muscle is located and released. *GSR* gastrocnemius–soleus recession, *GT* gastrocnemius tenotomy, *m* muscle, *n* nerve, *TAL* tendo Achilles lengthening, *v* vein. Figure and legend reprinted with permission from the American Podiatric Medical Association. Lamm BM, Paley D, Herzenberg JE. Gastrocnemius soleus recession: a simpler, more limited approach. J Am Podiatr Med Assoc 2005; 95:18–25

Achilles tendon, which will be made worse with limb lengthening. Therefore, we recommend performing a triceps surae lengthening procedure at the time of tibial lengthening. We recommend an open Vulpius procedure (Fig. 30.18) and a prophylactic anterior compartment fasciotomy (Fig. 30.19). In FH, the posterior tibial neurovascular bundle is often closely applied to the edge of the Achilles, so this must be done carefully. The fasciotomy decreases the risk of compartment syndrome (a known complication of tibial osteotomy). An additional benefit of anterior compartment fasciotomy (especially if the longitudinal incision in the fascia is combined with a short cruciate incision [transverse]) is that it allows the anterior compartment musculature to bulge out, thus creating the impression of a larger diameter calf. This is desirable, as all patients with FH have a smaller ipsilateral calf due to combined bone and soft tissue hypoplasia.

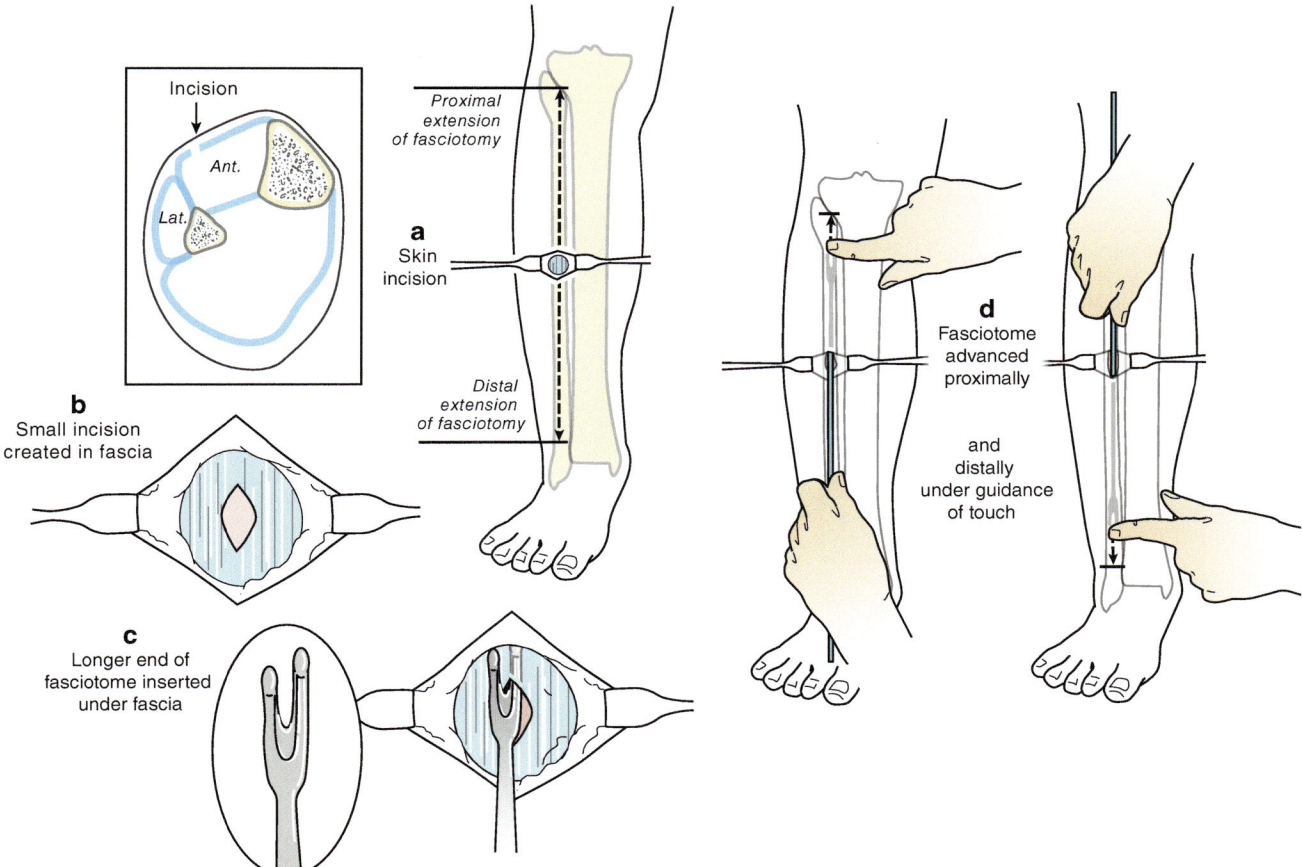

Fig. 30.19 Prophylactic anterior compartment fasciotomy is recommended for all FH lengthenings. This decreases the risk of post-osteotomy compartment syndrome and also causes a bulge of the anterior compartment musculature, increasing the circumference of the calf (a positive effect for a hypotrophic calf). (**a**) Small midline anterior longitudinal incision is made just lateral to the tibial crest. (**b**) Fascia is exposed using blunt dissection, and a small incision is created. (**c**) Fasciotome is then inserted under the fascia. (**d**) Fasciotome is advanced proximally, and care is taken not to invade the muscle. Note that the opposite index finger follows the leading edge of the fasciotome. *Ant.* anterior compartment, *Lat.* lateral compartment. Figure and legend reprinted with permission from the Rubin Institute for Advanced Orthopedics, Sinai Hospital of Baltimore

The fixator should be extended and include the foot to prevent equinus deformation of the ankle during lengthening. Once the lengthening is complete, the foot frame may be removed if there is no flexion contracture of the knee. We favor circular external fixators over monolateral external fixators for their superior ability to correct deviations that may occur during lengthening (typically procurvatum and valgus) and for the ability to insert fixation pins and wires from multiple directions, creating a more stable construct. Circular frames are generally well tolerated in the tibia and are easy to bridge across the ankle to the foot. Figure 30.20 shows a standard FH lengthening with external fixation. In pure external fixation cases, it is typical to use three pins/wires proximally, use two pins/wires in the distal segment, and include foot fixation. A wide space should be left between the proximal and distal rings to allow for better recruitment of soft tissue into the lengthening.

For skeletally mature patients in whom there is no longer a viable proximal tibial growth plate, it is attractive to use IM nails, either via the lengthening over nail (LON) technique or in the form of implantable IM telescopic nails. This telescopic nail is able to be controlled accurately and can go both forward and in reverse (in case of over lengthening or in case of poor bone formation).

With the LON technique, a standard trauma nail (8.5 to 10 mm diameter) is inserted and over-reamed by 2 mm to allow the bone to slide over the nail. The nail is locked proximally. The osteotomy must be proximal enough (and the nail long enough), so that at the end of lengthening, there is at least 5 cm of nail distal to the osteotomy (for stability). An

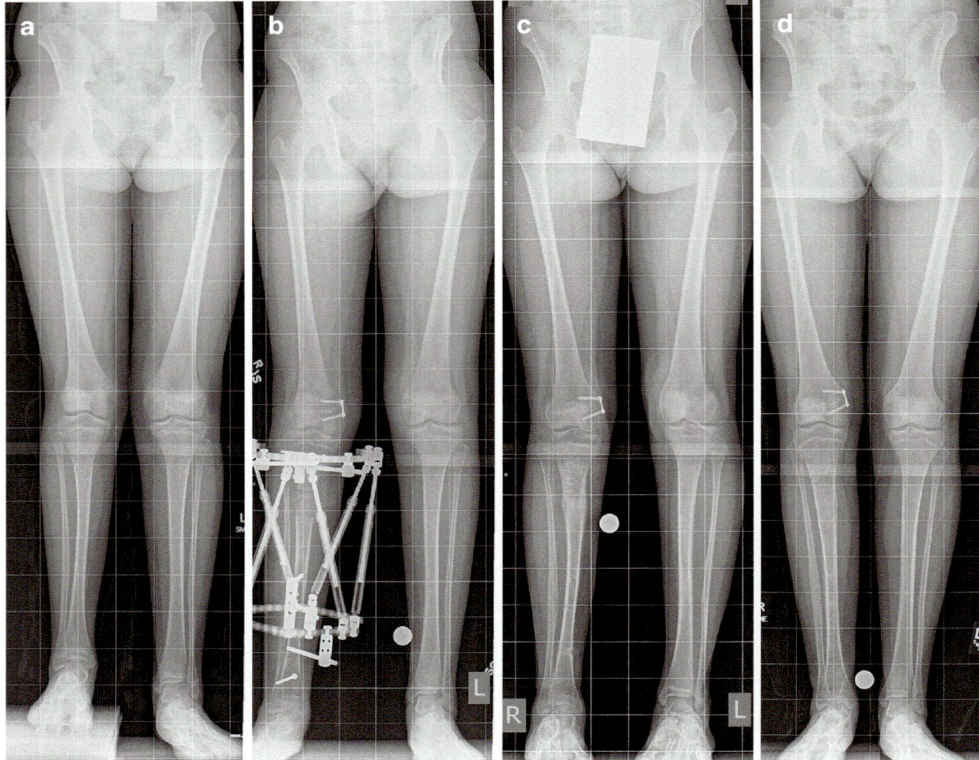

Fig. 30.20 Full-length standing AP view radiographs of a 12-year-old girl with FH before treatment (**a**), after distal femoral hemiepiphysiodesis and application of circular external fixation for lengthening (**b**), after removal of external fixation once lengthening and consolidation were achieved (**c**), and after full correction of distal femoral valgus with a normalized mechanical axis (**d**). Reprinted with permission from the Rubin Institute for Advanced Orthopedics, Sinai Hospital of Baltimore

important technical point is to drill holes in the anterior aspect of the tibia prior to reaming to vent the canal and to encourage the reamings to exit anteriorly to stimulate new bone formation at the lengthening site. The external fixator that is applied for the LON technique can be simple, with two points of fixation at either end. The rate of lengthening is adjusted according to bone formation. At the end of lengthening, the patient returns to the operating room for distal locking and frame removal (in that order, to prevent shortening). The bulk of the consolidation then takes place under the protection of the nail, without need for an external fixator. To control the foot during IM lengthening or LON, a temporary extra-articular ankle arthrodesis screw may be inserted from the back of the calcaneus into the distal tibia [32]. This screw is removed at the end of lengthening to allow mobilization of the ankle. Figure 30.21 shows an FH LON to decrease the duration of treatment time with the external fixator.

The technique for self-lengthening telescopic nails is similar to that described above for LON, except that the nail is locked proximally and distally, and no external fixator is needed. Blocking screws (Poller screws) can be used to prevent mechanical axis deviations during lengthening. Figure 30.22 shows an FH lengthening with a Precice IM lengthening nail, including the extra-articular screw technique to stabilize the ankle.

> **Lengthening for Moderate FH**
> Lengthen Achilles/Vulpius
>   Anterior compartment fasciotomy
>   Transfix foot during lengthening
>   Options: External fixation, LON, telescopic nails

Lengthening Plus Ankle Realignment for Paley Type 2

In this subset of patients, the recommendations for lengthening are largely identical to those described for type 1. However, in type 2 cases, the ankle has a dynamic valgus deformity. This will worsen with limb lengthening as the peroneal tendons tighten. For such cases, in older patients, we recommend intramuscular lengthening of the peroneal tendons and bony focal dome realignment of the ankle (Fig. 30.23). Figure 30.24 illustrates an example of a supramalleolar dome osteotomy in an adult with FH, who had symptomatic valgus/pronation, shown before (Saltzman view) and after (AP lat views).

For younger children with more remodeling potential, we have used Paley's SHORDT (Shortening Osteotomy

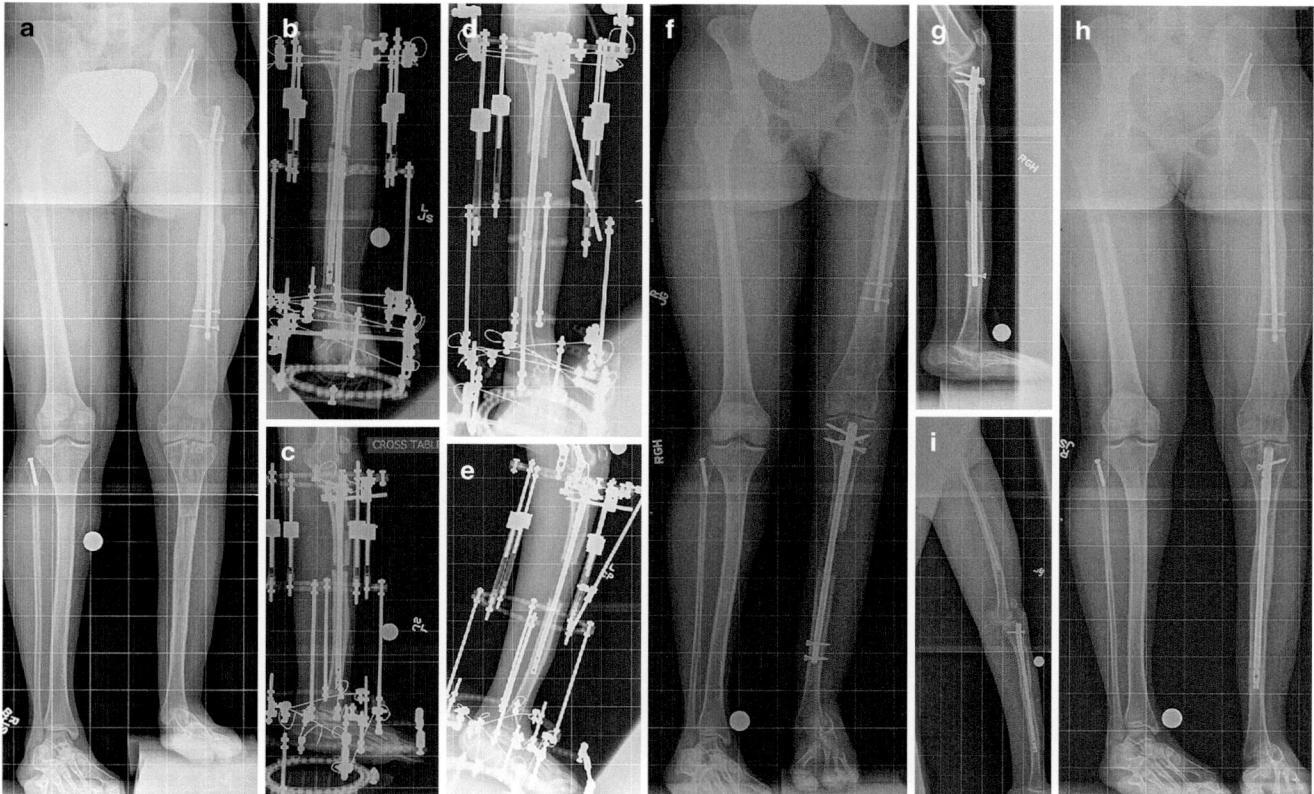

Fig. 30.21 (a) Preoperative full-length standing AP view radiograph shows a 16-year-old girl with left congenital femoral deficiency and fibular hemimelia prior to tibial lengthening with lengthening over nail (LON) technique. (**b**, **c**) One week postoperative AP (**b**) and lateral (**c**) view radiographs of the left tibia show the LON technique using an intramedullary tibial nail and concurrent classic Ilizarov circular external fixation device. (**d**, **e**) AP (**d**) and lateral (**e**) view radiographs of the left tibia after completion of the distraction phase and prior to external fixation removal. (**f**, **g**) Full-length standing AP view radiograph (**f**) and lateral view tibial radiograph (**g**) after locking of the intramedullary nail and removal of the external fixation device for the consolidation phase. (**h**, **i**) Final full-length standing AP (**h**) and lateral (**i**) view radiographs show complete healing of the tibial lengthening segment. After three of the four cortices had healed, the distal locking screws were removed for dynamization to improve the anterior cortical thickness. Reprinted with permission from the Rubin Institute for Advanced Orthopedics, Sinai Hospital of Baltimore

Realignment Distal Tibia) procedure [24]. This is indicated in cases of dynamic valgus and a relatively short fibula. It is essentially an anteromedial closing wedge osteotomy of the distal tibia, after first separating the distal tibial-fibular syndesmotic ligaments. The fibula stays stationary, and the tibia is repositioned proximally to restore the normal mortice relationship. There is typically no need to lengthen the peroneals or the gastrocsoleus. The fibula acts a buttress to prevent valgus (Fig. 30.25). While it could, in theory, be used more broadly, we limit its use in our practice to patients with intact distal fibulas and relatively mild overall disease burden. We find it difficult to justify medial shortening (which disrupts the optimal length-function curves of the medial structures, while further tensioning the already tight lateral structures), in more severe cases and prefer to use the above described SUPERankle technique.

Figure 30.26 shows a clinical example of a SHORDT in a four-year-old boy with type 2 FH and a dynamic equinovalgus ankle. While the postoperative radiographs show an improved anatomic alignment of the mortice, the long term durability of the SHORDT procedure is unknown.

Lengthening Plus SUPERankle Reconstruction for Paley Type 3

For the rigid equinovalgus type of FH, we use a modified Paley SUPERankle approach. This surgery can be performed when a child is as young as one or two years of age. The goal is to realign the foot relative to the distal tibia and make it plantigrade. It is an extra-articular reconstruction, as the ankle joint and its ligaments are not opened.

Fig. 30.22 Case example of a 14-year-old girl with fibular hemimelia and congenital femoral deficiency who underwent lengthening with the PRECICE. (**a, b**) Preoperative full-length standing AP (**a**) and lateral (**b**) view radiographs show that the child had an 8-cm limb length discrepancy and concurrent genu valgus. (**c, d**) Full-length standing AP (**c**) and lateral (**d**) view radiographs depict lengthening with the PRECICE magnetic intramedullary telescopic nail. This device contains a small magnet, which will gradually lengthen when activated by an externally applied magnetic field. The PRECICE is also reversible and controllable to a very accurate degree. (**e, f**) Full-length standing AP (**e**) and lateral (**f**) view radiographs obtained at the completion of lengthening. (**g, h**) Final full-length standing AP (**g**) and lateral (**h**) view radiographs obtained after nail removal. Note the equal limb lengths and the correction of the mechanical axis. Reprinted with permission from the Rubin Institute for Advanced Orthopedics, Sinai Hospital of Baltimore

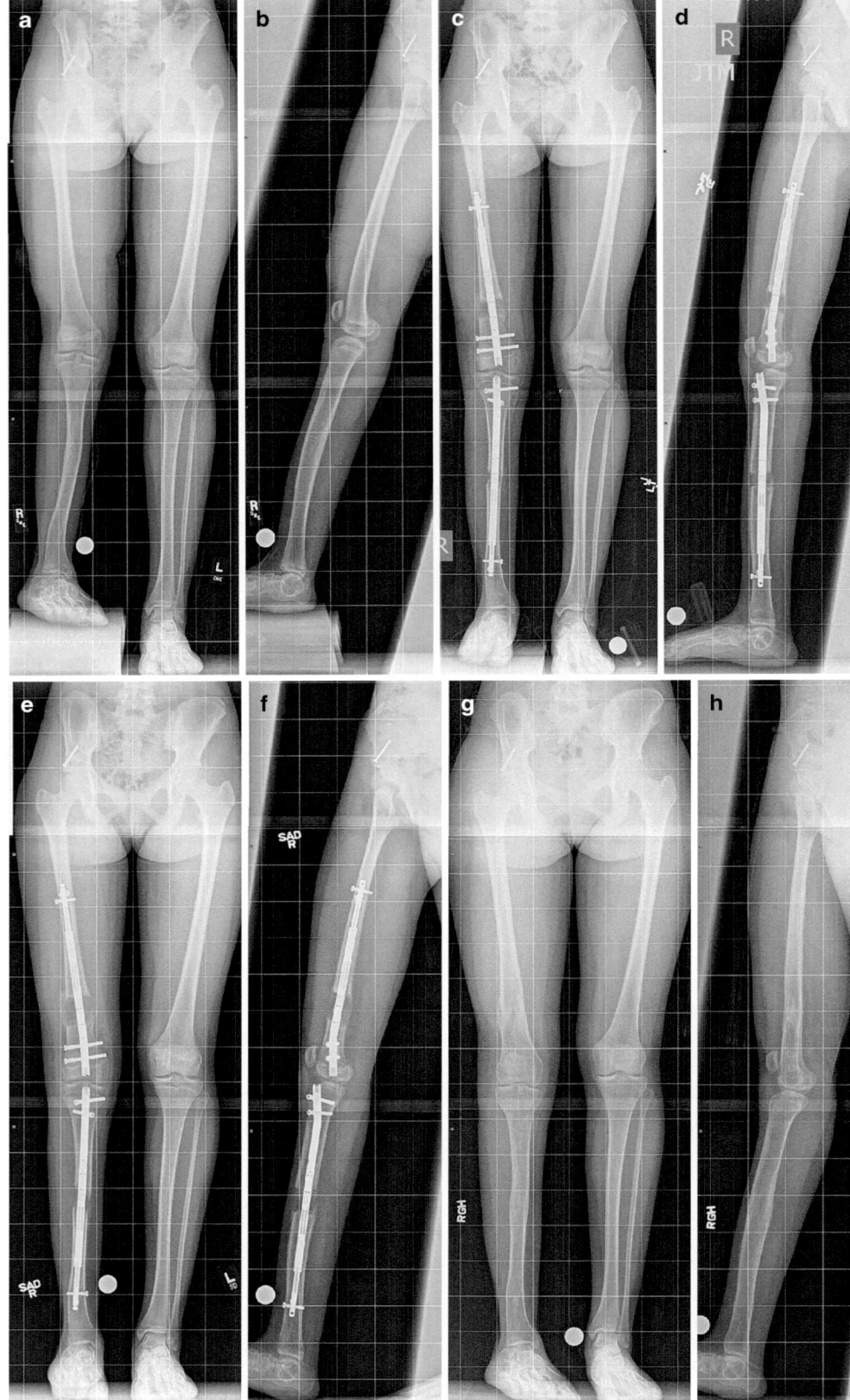

30 Fibular Hemimelia in the Pediatric Patient

Fig. 30.23 Illustration shows bony realignment of the valgus ankle for cases of Paley Type 2. Reprinted with permission from the Rubin Institute for Advanced Orthopedics, Sinai Hospital of Baltimore

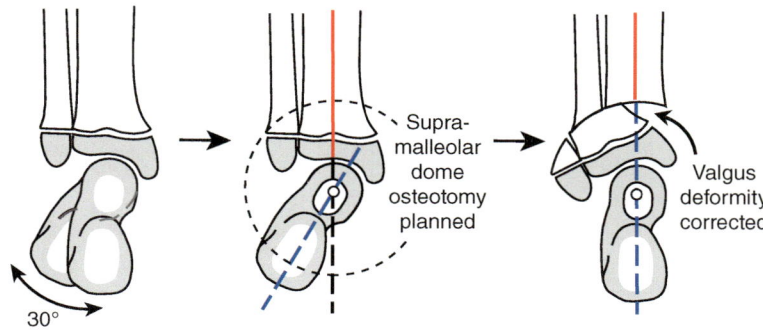

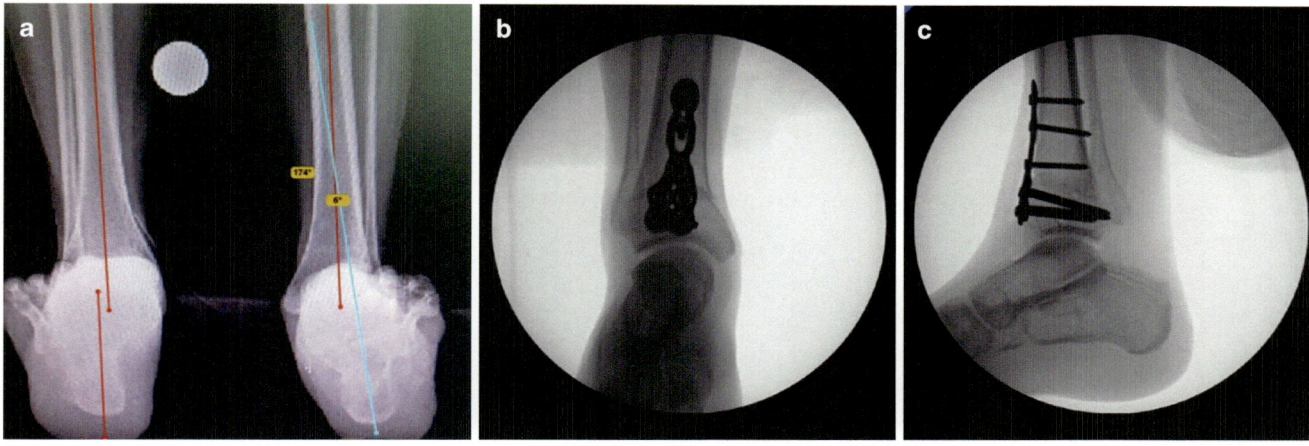

Fig. 30.24 Radiographs of a supramalleolar dome osteotomy in an adult with FH who had symptomatic valgus/pronation. (**a**) Preoperative Saltzman view. (**b, c**) Postoperative AP and lateral views. Reprinted with permission from the Rubin Institute for Advance Orthopedics, Sinai Hospital of Baltimore.

Fig. 30.25 (**a–c**) Illustration of SHORDT procedure with separation of distal tibial-fibular syndesmotic ligaments, anteromedial closing wedge osteotomy of the distal tibia, and fibular aiding in prevention of valgus. Reprinted with permission from the Rubin Institute for Advance Orthopedics, Sinai Hospital of Baltimore.

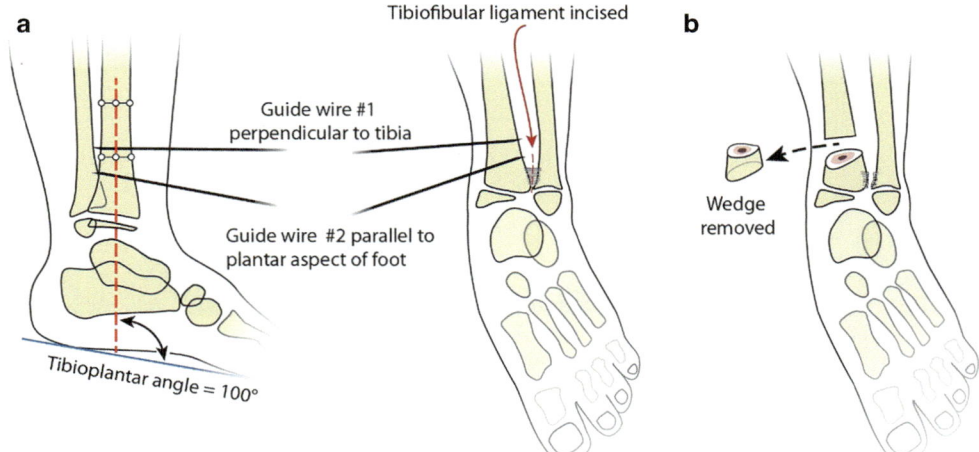

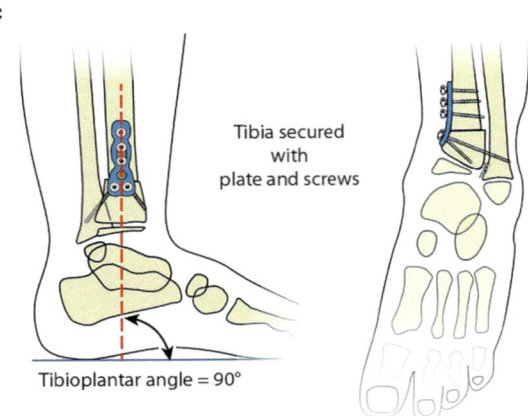

Fig. 30.25 (continued)

Surgical Technique for Paley Type 3a (Figs. 30.27 and 30.28)

Positioning
Supine position, bump under the ipsilateral sacrum, and tourniquet control.

Surgical Approach
Longitudinal (straight) incision starts laterally at the mid-calf and ends just above the sole of the foot. Peroneal tendons (sometimes only one is present) are cut with a Z-technique and later repaired in the lengthened configuration. If two are present, it may be desirable to lengthen only the brevis and to leave the longus intact to prevent forefoot supination. The very distal tip of the anlage of the fibula, if present, may be

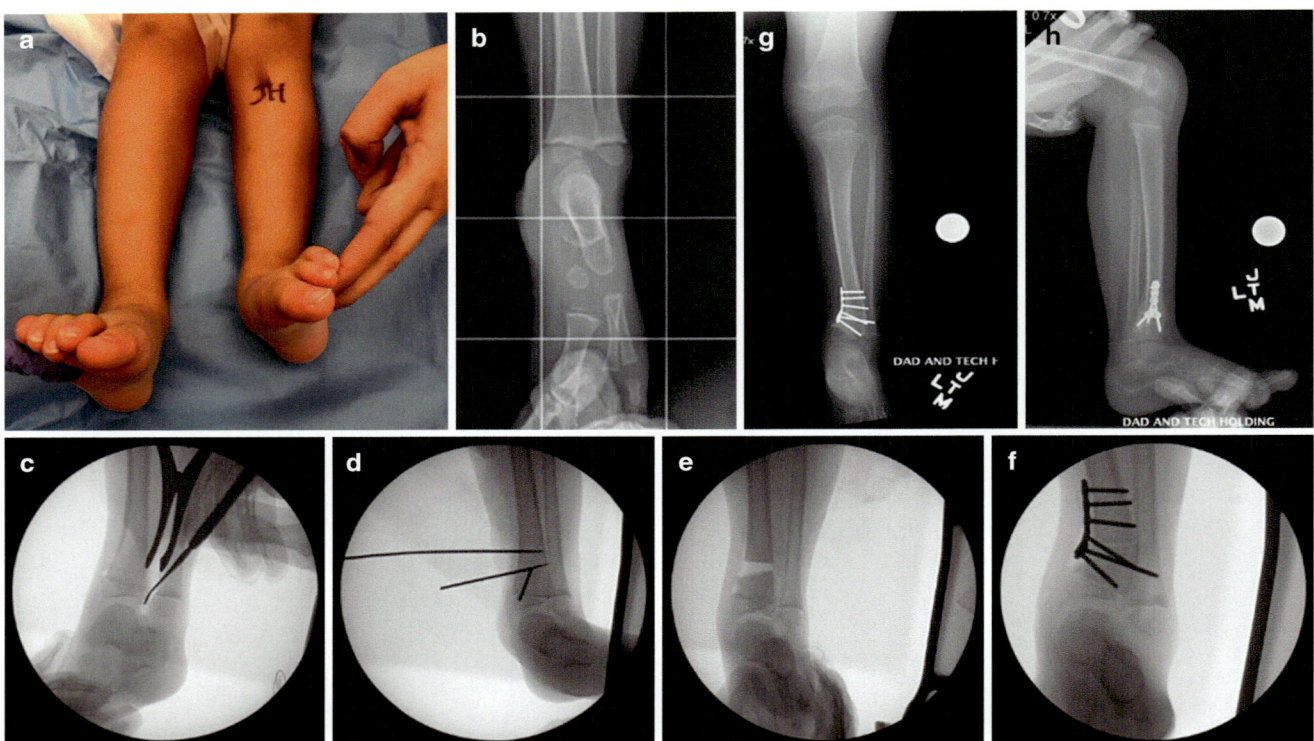

Fig. 30.26 (**a, b**) Preoperative clinical photograph and AP radiograph of a 4-year-old male patient with Paley type 2 FH and a dynamic equinovalgus ankle. (**c–f**) Intraoperative fluoroscopy views during SHORDT procedure. (**g, h**) Postoperative AP and lateral plain radiograph views. Reprinted with permission from the Rubin Institute for Advance Orthopedics, Sinai Hospital of Baltimore

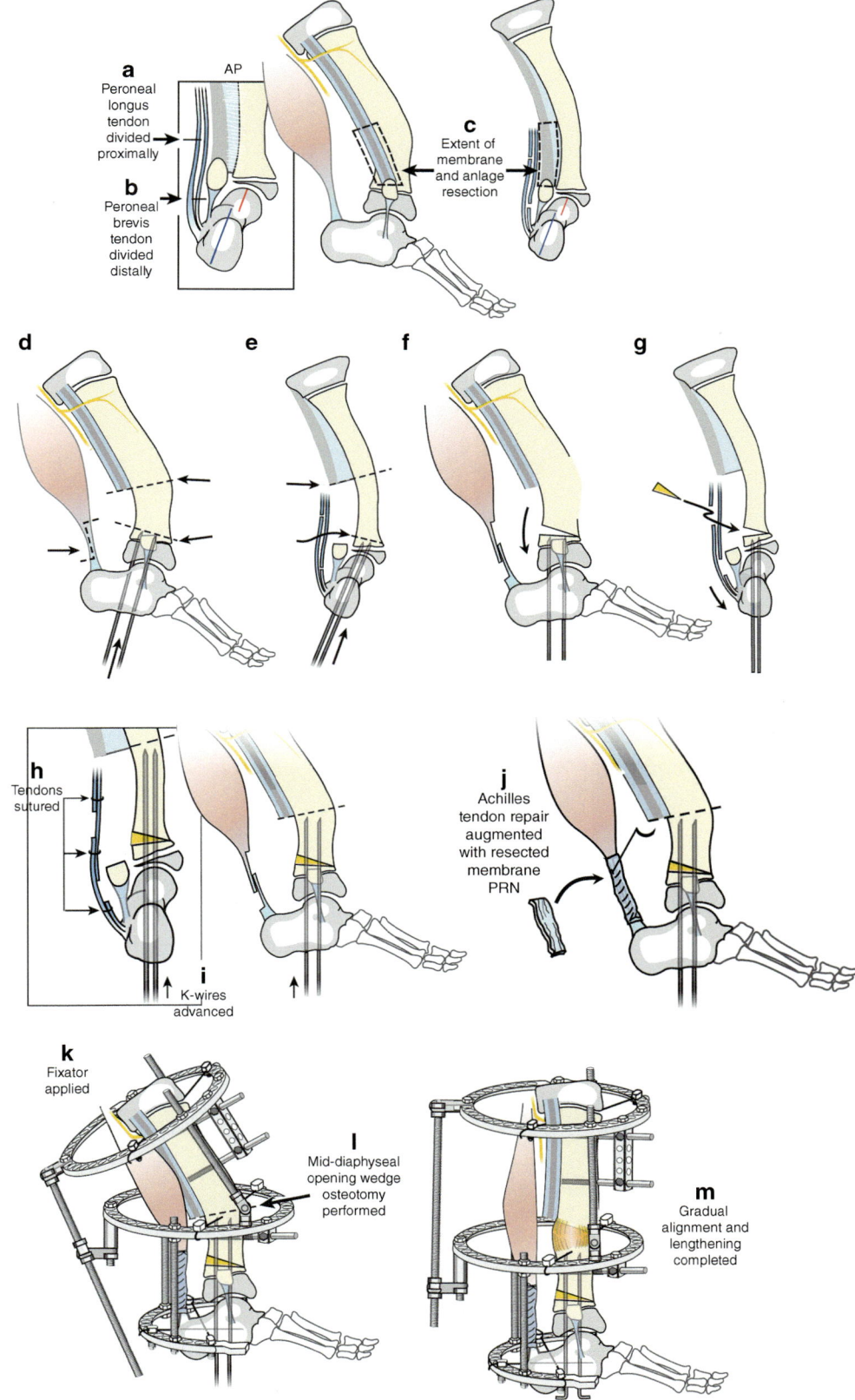

Fig. 30.27 (a–m) SUPERankle surgical technique used to treat supramalleolar type fibular hemimelia (Paley Type 3A—ankle type). Reprinted with permission from the Rubin Institute for Advanced Orthopedics, Sinai Hospital of Baltimore

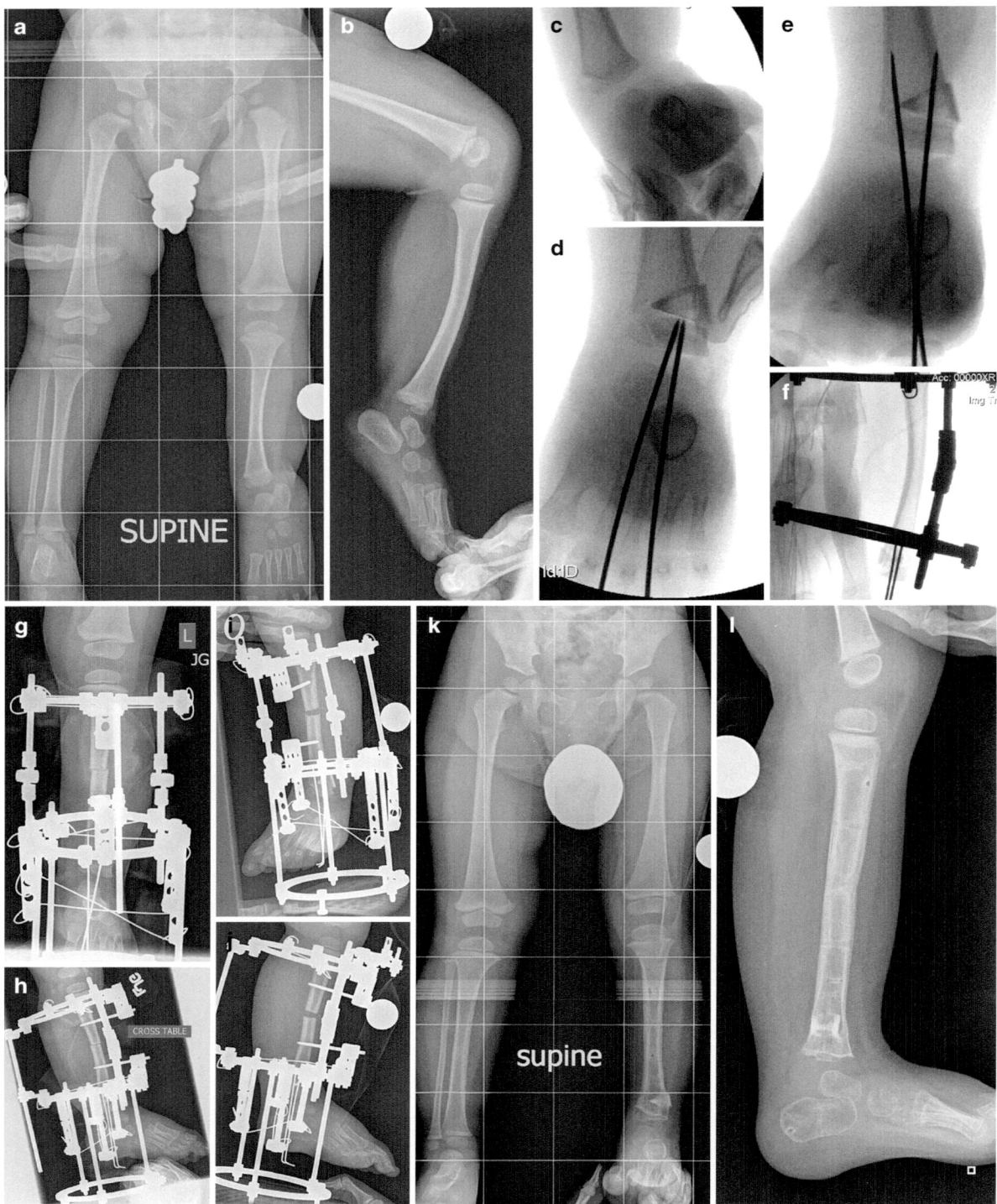

Fig. 30.28 Case example of an 18-month-old boy with Paley Type 3A fibular hemimelia. (**a**, **b**) Preoperative AP (**a**) and lateral (**b**) view radiographs depict the typical equinovalgus foot and ankle deformity along with the anterior tibial bow. (**c**–**e**) Intraoperative fluoroscopic images show the distal tibial osteotomy portion of the SUPERankle procedure (comprehensive reconstruction). (**f**) Intraoperative fluoroscopic image shows the application of the pediatric Ilizarov external fixator with the hinges positioned at the apex of the deformity on the convex side to produce both straightening and lengthening. (**g**, **h**) Immediate postoperative radiographs obtained after the completion of the SUPERankle procedure. (**i**, **j**) Postoperative radiographs obtained 2 weeks after SUPERankle procedure show correction of the midshaft tibial deformity along with limited bone lengthening. (**k**, **l**) AP (**k**) and lateral (**l**) view radiographs obtained at the time of external fixation removal (3 months after SUPERankle procedure). Note the complete correction of the tibia and the ankle. Reprinted with permission from the Rubin Institute for Advanced Orthopedics, Sinai Hospital of Baltimore

left in place. Anterior compartment fasciotomy is performed, and the superficial peroneal nerve is protected. The anterior compartment muscles are dissected off the cartilage anlage of the fibula and off the intermuscular septum.

The intermuscular septum is resected from the ankle proximally up to the mid portion of the tibia at the apex of the anteromedial bow. This resected intermuscular septum should be placed in a sterile specimen cup and covered with saline, as it may be recycled for repair and elongation of the Achilles tendon as needed. It should be noted that Paley's original technique described resection of the anlage all the way up to the proximal tibia and decompression of the common peroneal nerve through a separate proximal incision; we feel that this step is unnecessary.

Next, the sural nerve is identified and protected. The Achilles tendon and posterior tibial neurovascular bundle are identified through this posterolateral approach. Be careful not to damage the posterior tibial nerve, which is juxtaposed to the Achilles tendon. The flexor hallucis longus is identified as a guide to the anatomy of the posterolateral corner. The posterior tibial nerve is decompressed as far as can be seen into the tarsal tunnel distally through this posterolateral approach. The Achilles tendon is very short and can be made longer for purposes of Z-lengthening by scraping the distal muscle belly proximally to expose more of the tendon. Despite this, it is often necessary to fashion a tendon graft (from the resected intermuscular septum) to obtain sufficient elongation of the Achilles tendon. The foot is then placed into the maximum equinus and valgus position, and two 1.8-mm diameter Kirschner wires (K-wires) are inserted from the plantar surface of the heel, across the calcaneus and talus, and across the ankle joint and just past the distal physis, about 5 mm. This pins the ankle in the maximum valgus/equinus position.

Osteotomy

Next, a subperiosteal dissection of the distal tibia is performed, being careful not to damage the perichondrial ring of the growth plate. Mini-Hohmann retractors are placed anteriorly and posteriorly. An oscillating saw is used to make an oblique cut from posterolateral to anteromedial, but the anteromedial cortex is left intact. The osteotomy is levered open from the posterolateral direction with an osteotome or laminar spreader. This maneuver corrects the equinovalgus position of the hindfoot. The osteotomy is held open with a cortical allograft (a small piece of fibular allograft works well). Next, the two K-wires are passed across the osteotomy and up into the distal half of the tibia, stopping just short of the anteromedial bow in the apex of the diaphysis. The K-wires are bent outside the skin of the heel and can be incorporated into the frame (to be applied shortly). If the plan is to apply a cast, then these two wires are simply bent and left outside the skin. The foot is now corrected and plantigrade relative to the distal half of the tibia. The tourniquet can be let down for the closure. The Achilles and peroneal tendons are repaired in their lengthened configuration, and the incision is closed over a small drain, to prevent hematoma and compartment syndrome. The operation can conclude at this point if desired, and a long leg cast can be applied. The cast and pins are removed in 6 weeks, and then the patient can receive physical therapy for the ankle.

Frame Application

Six months after the initial procedure, the tibia can be lengthened with an Ilizarov external fixator through an osteotomy made at the apex of the anteromedial bow. Alternatively, the Ilizarov frame may be applied immediately and used to correct the apex anteromedial bow with minimal lengthening (1 to 2 cm). This frame is removed after healing of the diaphyseal corticotomy is complete, and a long leg cast is applied for 3 to 4 weeks. This is followed by mobilization and rehabilitation of the ankle to try to regain as much motion as possible.

Surgical Technique for Paley Type 3b (Figs. 30.29 and 30.30)

Positioning and Surgical Approach

The positioning and approach are identical to what is described previously for type 3a.

Osteotomy

An oblique slightly U-shaped osteotomy of the subtalar region is performed, rather than a supramalleolar osteotomy. It exits posteriorly between the talus and the Achilles insertion (tuberosity) and anteriorly in the sinus tarsi by the talonavicular joint. The cartilaginous anlage is discarded, divided, or dissected around. After the osteotomy is complete and the hindfoot can be fully mobilized, temporary antegrade K-wires are inserted across the ankle with the foot held in maximum eversion, to stabilize the tibia to the talus. One comes from superomedial and the other from superolateral. This keeps the talus anatomically positioned in the mortice and prevents correction through the joint, instead focusing the varus correction in the subtalar osteotomy. Two additional K-wires are then inserted in the calcaneus perpendicular to the plantar surface of the foot with the hindfoot in the maximally uncorrected position (equinus and valgus). Next, the distal half of the calcaneus and foot is translated medially and angulated into varus so these two plantar K-wires now face directly upwards toward the talus. This reduces the valgus lateral translation of the foot, which is dorsiflexed to create an open wedge posteriorly, if possible, for bone graft placement to correct the equinus position of the calcaneus. The smooth wires are driven across the osteotomy into the talus. In some cases, sufficient purchase is available in the talus, but for very young children, the wires should be driven across the ankle joint into the distal tibia for better purchase. At this point, the

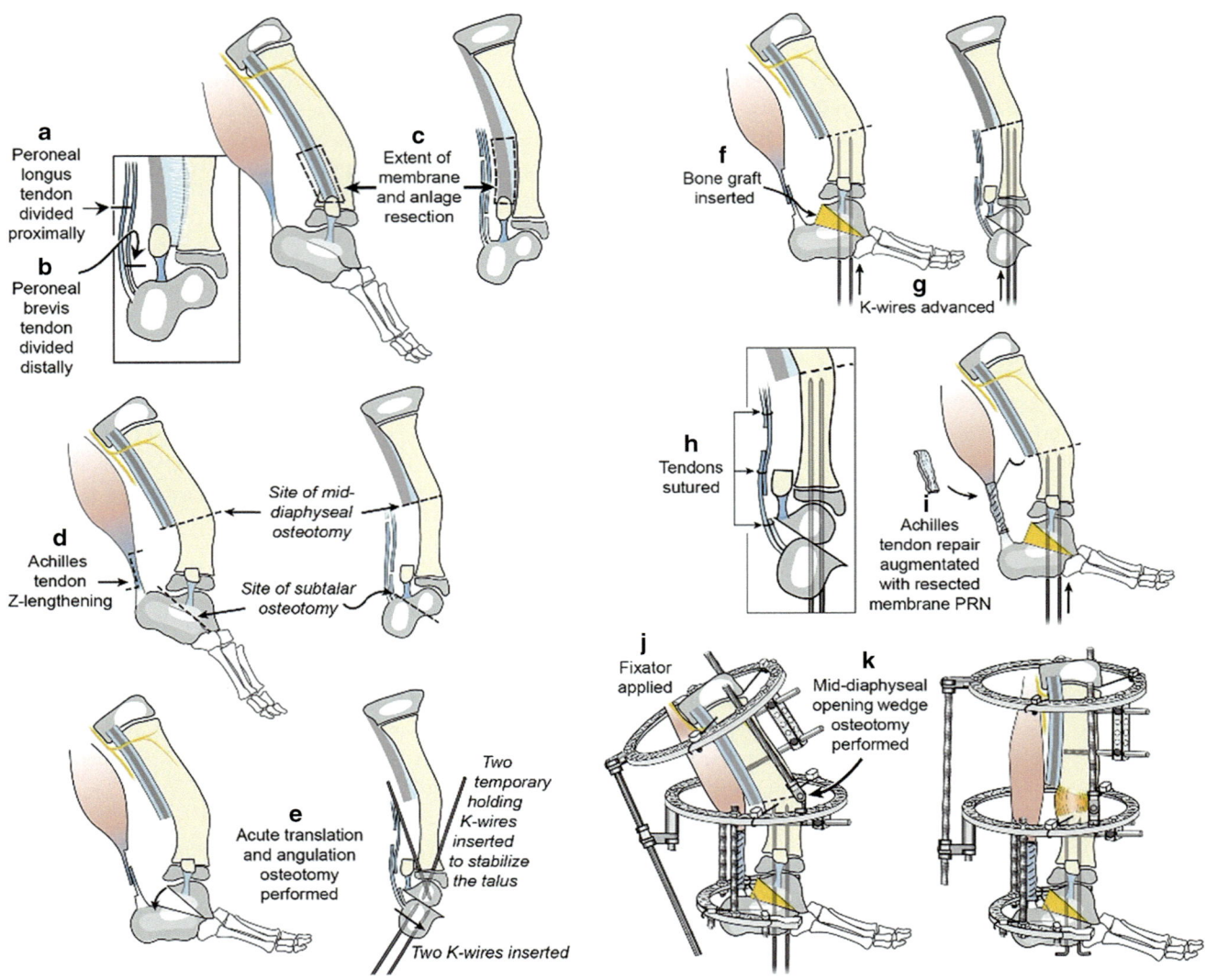

Fig. 30.29 (a–k) SUPERankle surgical technique used to treat subtalar type FH (Paley type 3B). Reprinted with permission from the Rubin Institute for Advance Orthopedics, Sinai Hospital of Baltimore

tourniquet is let down, and the closure proceeds as described above, including external fixator application and corticotomy of the mid-diaphyseal deformity.

Surgical Technique for Paley Type 3c (Fig. 30.31)

Positioning and Surgical Approach

The positioning and approach are identical to what is described previously for type 3a.

Osteotomy

This is essentially a combination of the technique for type 3a and 3b. Both a supramalleolar osteotomy and a hindfoot subtalar coalition osteotomy are performed, opened (supramalleolar), translated, angulated (subtalar), and held open with bone graft and transfixion K-wires. The subtalar osteotomy is done first, followed by the supramalleolar osteotomy. Intraoperative arthrography of the ankle joint helps to determine the degree of ankle valgus and whether it needs to be corrected or if only a subtalar osteotomy is sufficient.

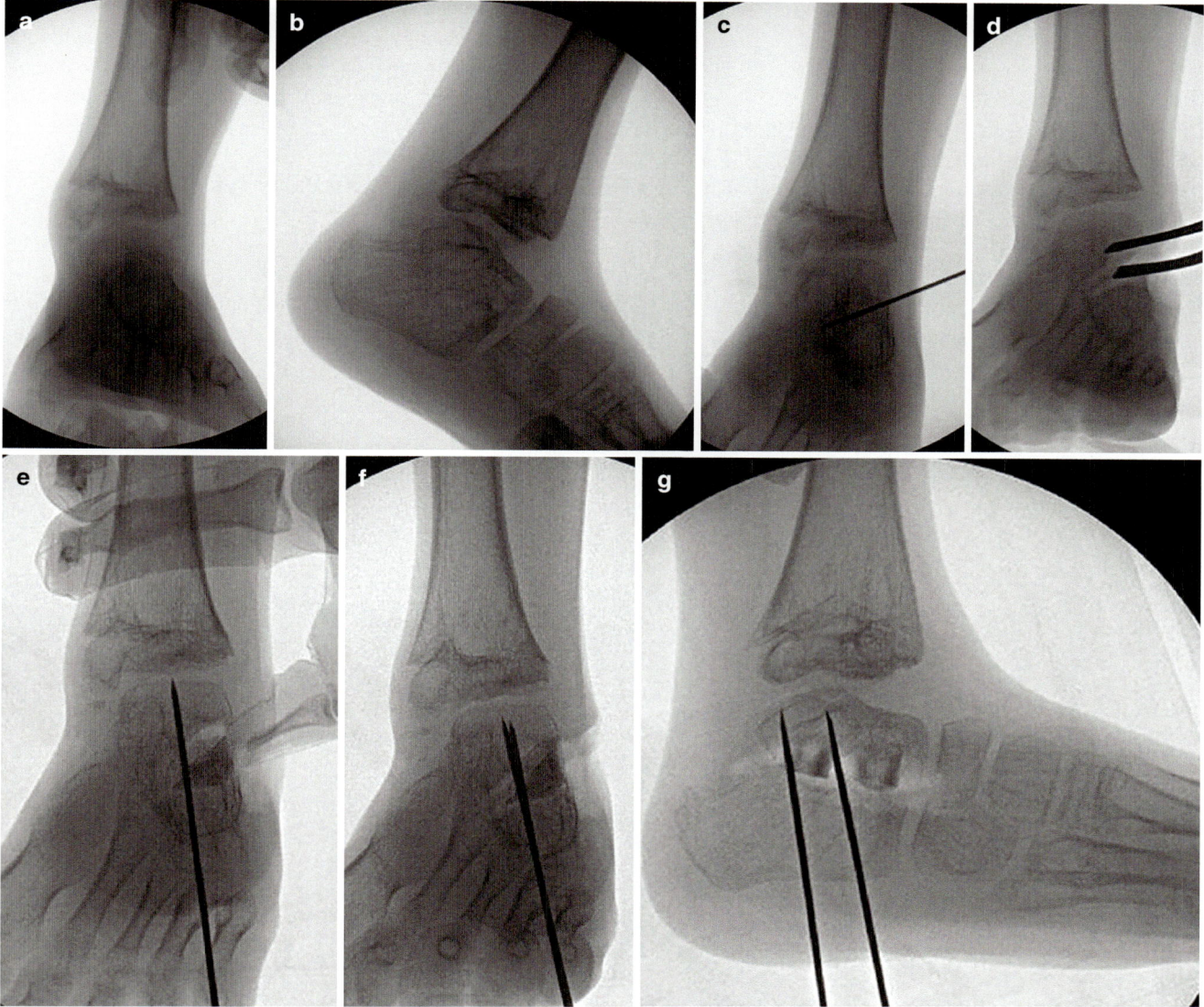

Fig. 30.30 Case example of a 6-year-old boy with left fibular hemimelia and residual hindfoot valgus secondary to a deformity in the subtalar region (Paley Type 3B). The osteotomy is performed through the talocalcaneal coalition. (**a**, **b**) AP (**a**) and lateral (**b**) view fluoroscopic images show residual hindfoot valgus after a previous supramalleolar osteotomy at 2 years of age. (**c**) Fluoroscopic image shows a guidewire inserted into the region of the subtalar coalition demonstrating the oblique osteotomy. (**d**) The subtalar osteotomy is completed with an osteotome and translated medially with concurrent varus angulation with a laminar spreader instrument. (**e**) Fluoroscopic image of fibular allograft wedge position with the surgeon's thumb maintaining medial translation of the calcaneal fragment and initial wire fixation. (**f**, **g**) Final fluoroscopic views of the subtalar osteotomy with medial translation and varus angulation of the calcaneal fragment stabilized with fibular allograft wedges and percutaneous wire fixation. Reprinted with permission from the Rubin Institute for Advanced Orthopedics, Sinai Hospital of Baltimore

---

SUPERankle Procedure for Paley Types 3a, b, and c

Lengthen peroneal tendons (Primarily peroneus brevis, but longus if needed)
  Lengthen Achilles
  Resect anlage and intermuscular septum
  Osteotomy: supramalleolar or subtalar or both
  Transfixion wires from the sole of the foot into the tibia
  External fixator to correct diaphyseal anteromedial tibial bow

Surgical Technique for Paley Type 3d (Fig. 30.32)

Diagnosing Type 3d
This subtype is extremely unusual and can be recognized in younger children through MRI evaluation or in older children through computed tomography. The hallmark of this deformity is a wedge shaped talar body.

Positioning and Surgical Approach
The positioning and approach are identical to what is described previously for type 3a.

Osteotomy
The opening wedge procedure is similar to the technique described for the type 3b (subtalar type), except the osteotomy does not pass completely through the medial side.

Surgical Technique for Paley Type 4 (Clubfoot Type)

Initial Nonsurgical Treatment
This subtype represents less than approximately 15% of FH cases; therefore, treatment must be individualized. In the

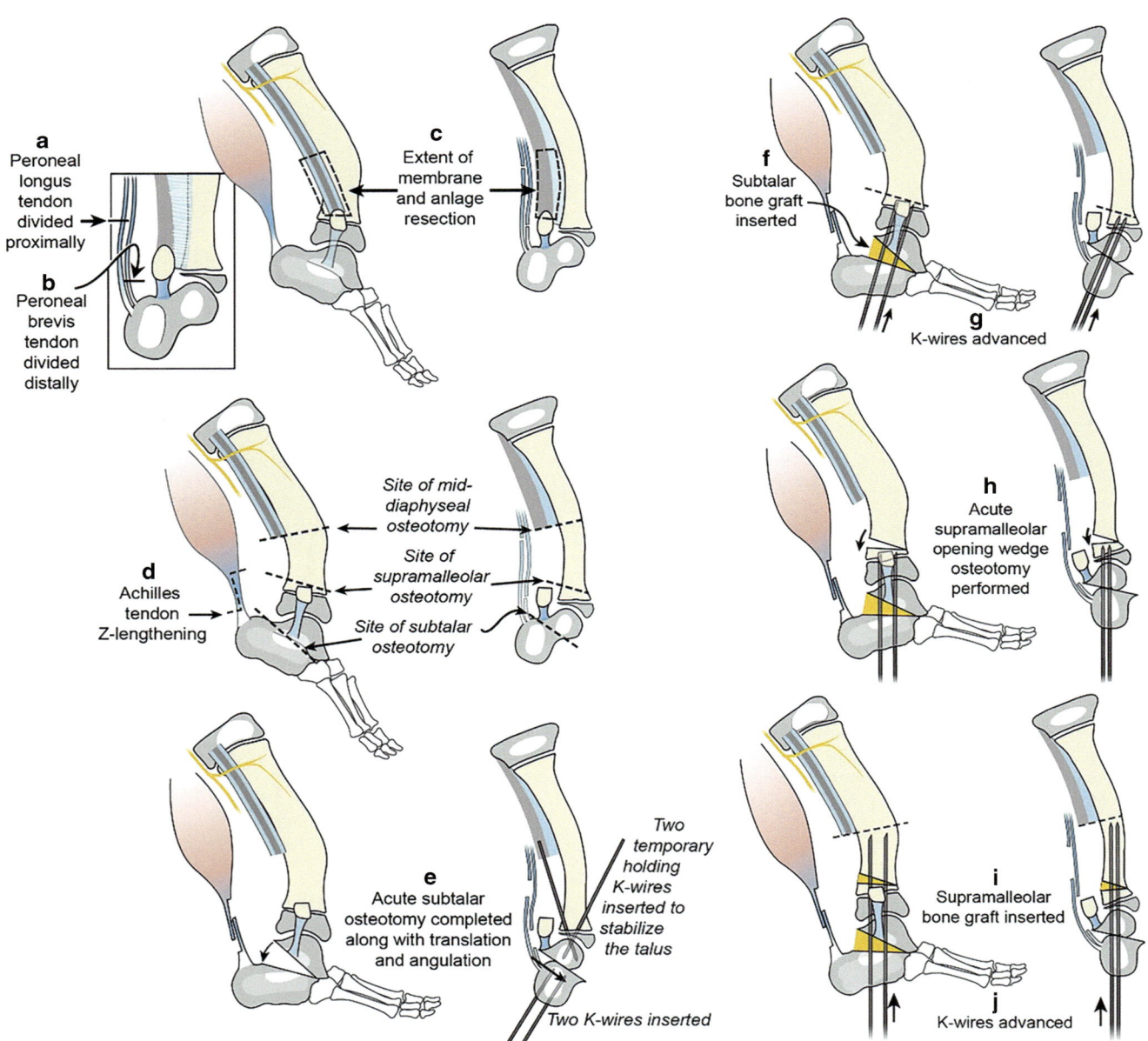

Fig. 30.31 (a–o) SUPERankle surgical technique used to treat combined ankle/subtalar type FH (Paley type 3C). Reprinted with permission from the Rubin Institute for Advance Orthopedics, Sinai Hospital of Baltimore

Fig. 30.31 (continued)

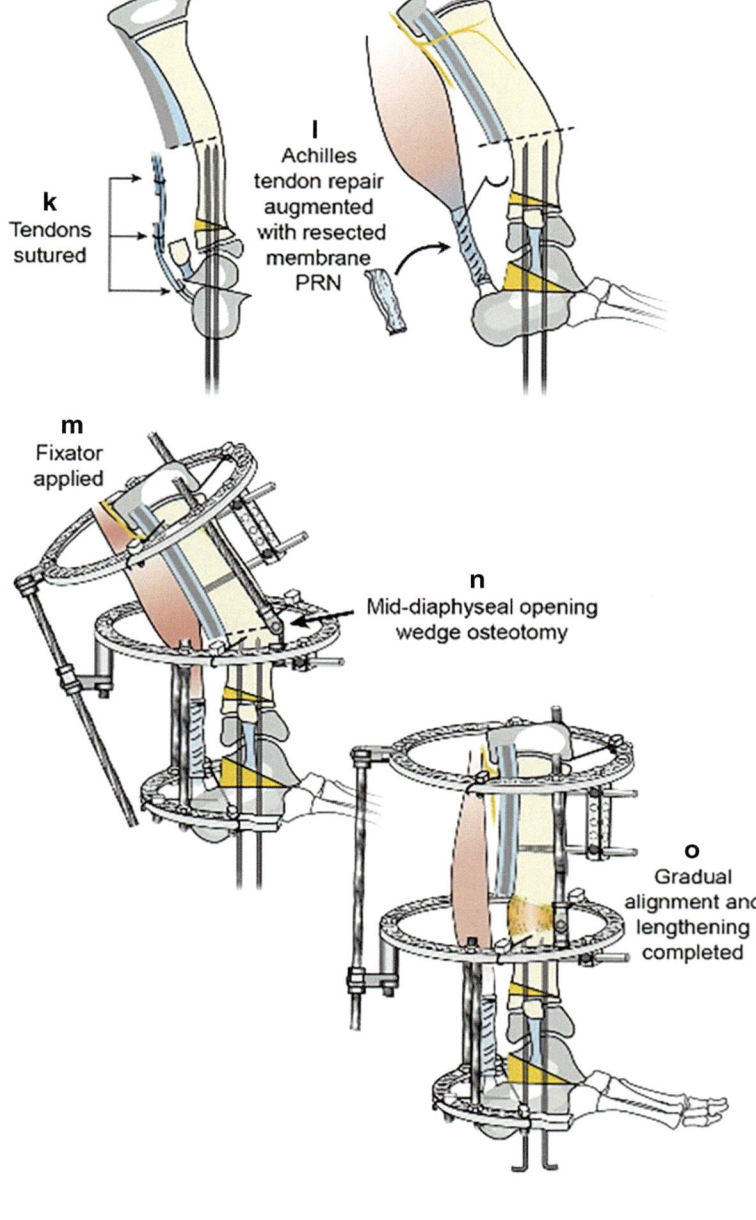

Fig. 30.32 Surgical technique used to treat talar body type fibular hemimelia (Paley Type 3D). Reprinted with permission from the Rubin Institute for Advanced Orthopedics, Sinai Hospital of Baltimore

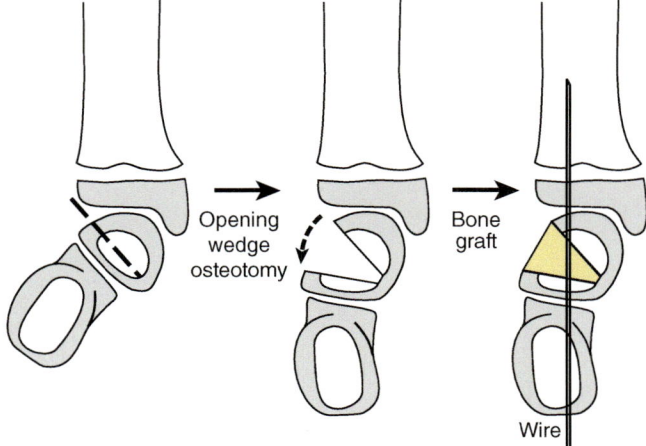

authors' experience, the initial treatment is nonsurgical, following the Ponseti principles. It is unclear why the Ponseti method is effective in correcting the varus deformity, as the Ponseti technique in idiopathic clubfoot works through the subtalar joint. In our experience, essentially all of these children have a coalition of the subtalar joint. After casting and tenotomy, the deformity is converted to a more typical equinovalgus type, which can then be corrected using the SUPERankle approaches described above. However, we have seen children treated elsewhere with preliminary open posteromedial release for type 4 FH.

Additional Procedures

During tibial lengthening, valgus deformity of the diaphysis, if present, should be corrected. Distal femoral valgus can be corrected with screw-plate devices for growth modulation, which is discussed in greater detail in Chap. 6. Once corrected, the screw-plate devices are removed, but rebound valgus is commonly observed (Fig. 30.33). After tibial lengthening, the valgus position of the lower extremity can recur due to abnormal growth at the physis of the distal femur and/or the proximal tibia. This progressive valgus deformity in FH may be attributed to hypoplasia of the lateral femoral condyle and/or to the tethering effect of the residual scar-like fibular band called the fibular anlage, if present. After lengthening, the Cozen phenomenon may also account for some of the rebound valgus that can be seen post-tibial lengthening (Fig. 30.34).

We have observed cases of relapse of ankle valgus several years after the SUPERankle procedure. After the initial correction of the foot and ankle with the SUPERankle procedure, the valgus deformity can recur with the appearance that the child is walking on the medial malleolus. This recurrence can be addressed with a revision surgery that includes acute osteotomy of the distal tibia and/or the hindfoot bones. Usually, the leg is placed in a cast for 4 to 6 weeks for healing, and then the child is allowed to wear regular shoes. Growth modulation of the medial malleolus is another potential option for the treatment of recurrent ankle valgus with open growth plates, although the distal tibial physis in some cases of FH is not robust enough to respond to guided growth.

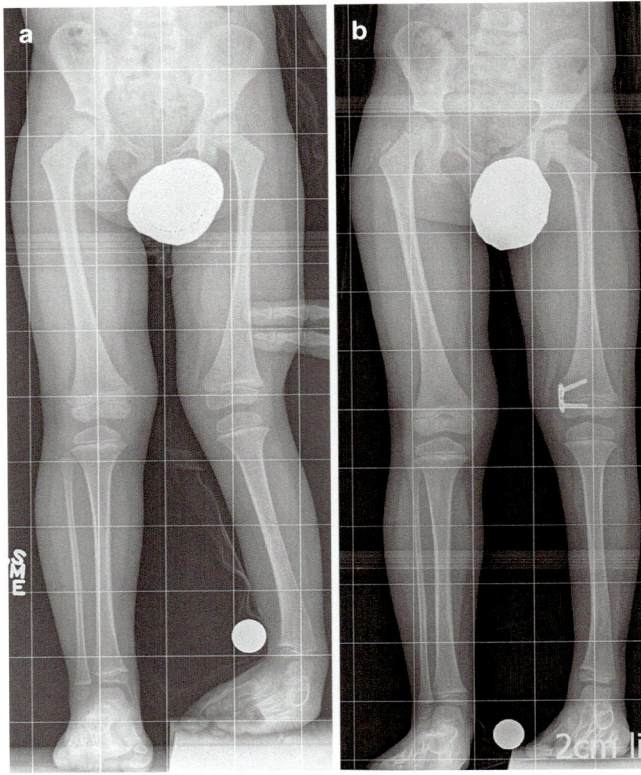

Fig. 30.33 (a) Full-length standing AP view radiograph of the same child shown in Fig. 30.28 at 3-year follow-up with genu valgus secondary to hypoplasia of the lateral femoral condyle and supination deformity of the forefoot. (b) Full-length standing AP view radiograph of the patient 10 months after distal femoral hemiepiphysiodesis and tibialis anterior tendon transfer to the dorsum of the foot. Reprinted with permission from the Rubin Institute for Advanced Orthopedics, Sinai Hospital of Baltimore

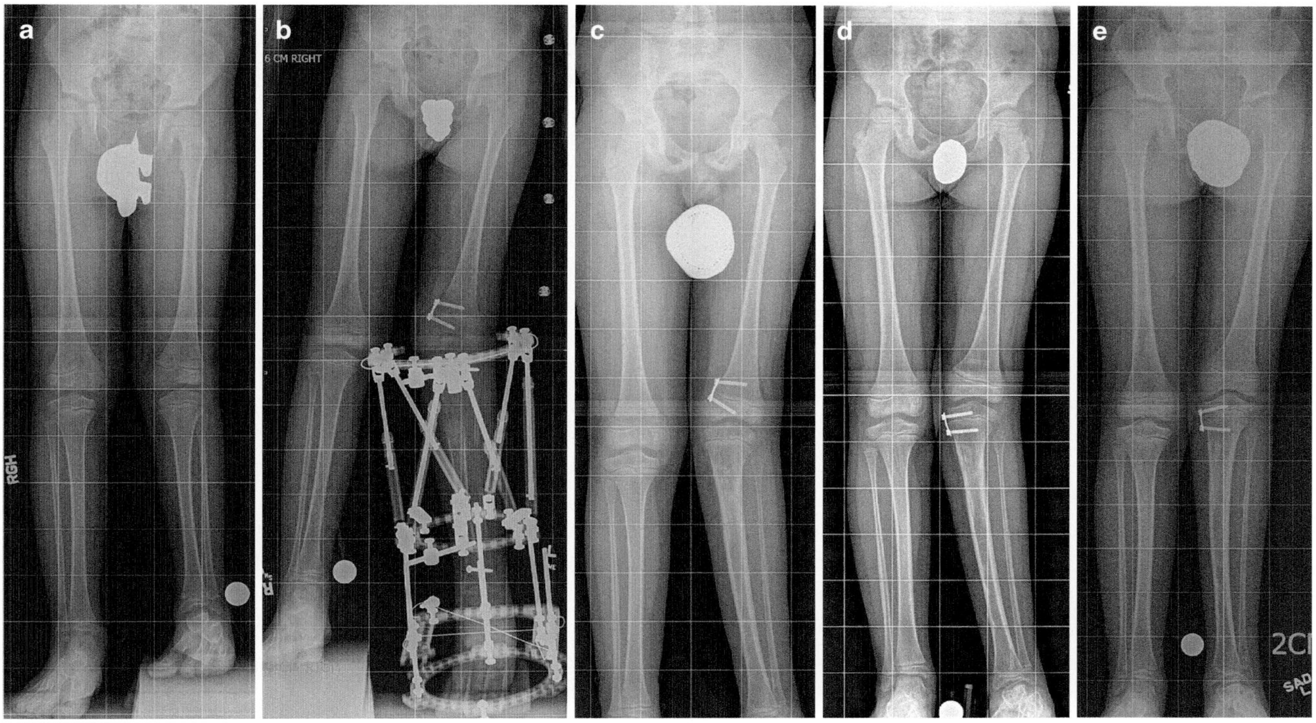

Fig. 30.34 (a) Full-length standing AP view radiograph of a 6-year-old boy obtained before he underwent tibial/fibular lengthening and distal femoral hemiepiphysiodesis. (b) Full-length standing AP view radiograph after 6 cm of lengthening. Note the mild knee flexion contracture but normalized medial proximal tibial angle. (c) Full-length standing AP view radiograph obtained 6 months after external fixation removal. Note the correction of the distal femur and the normalized lateral distal femoral angle. However, progressive recurrent genu valgus from the proximal tibia is also evident, possibly from a Cozen-type phenomenon. (d) Full-length standing AP view radiograph obtained after distal femoral guided growth plate removal and hemiepiphysiodesis of the proximal tibia. (e) Full-length standing AP view radiograph obtained 8 months after proximal tibial hemiepiphysiodesis shows continued correction of the recurrent valgus. Reprinted with permission from the Rubin Institute for Advanced Orthopedics, Sinai Hospital of Baltimore

Post-surgical Care

Lengthening and deformity correction of the tibia begins 7 days after the surgery at a rate of 0.25 mm three times daily. Physical therapy is the most important aspect of the lengthening process. Without proper physical therapy, the lengthening goals will not be achieved, and major complications will occur. Therefore, physical therapy requirements are very strict. The patient undergoing tibial lengthening must attend physical therapy sessions 5 days per week while at the same time performing an exercise and stretching program at home. Normally, the foot is included in the frame, so all physical therapy efforts are directed towards the knee and the toes. The knee tends to develop a flexion contracture, which can be prevented by diligent extension splinting. The toes also tend to develop flexion contractures. Night splints for the toes can be fabricated by the occupational therapists as a forefoot splint to support the toes. The physical therapy continues at this level of intensity for the duration of the distraction phase (2 to 3 months depending on the planned amount of lengthening). Younger patients can put as much weight as they can tolerate on the operated leg. Older and larger patients are kept at 50% weightbearing during the lengthening phase.

Normally, we include the foot in the tibial frame, so there is initially no physical therapy for the ankle. Once the lengthening is completed (provided the knee is not contracted), it is recommended that the foot wires be removed to allow rehabilitation of the ankle. During the lengthening with the foot included in the frame, the therapist may direct all efforts to preventing knee flexion contracture. Nighttime splinting in extension is also helpful. If despite best efforts, the patient develops a knee flexion contracture, then it is possible to extend the tibial frame to the femur in the form of a cast brace and use that as leverage to stretch the knee contracture. This can be done by building a thigh cuff using waterproof cast padding and incorporating a ring into the thigh cuff, which is then linked to the proximal tibial ring with two hinges at the knee joint and a posterior distraction rod to stretch out the knee flexion contracture. Please refer to Chap. 18 for more details regarding physical therapy for limb lengthening.

Outcomes

The treatment of FH remains a challenge. The goal is to achieve normal limb alignment and length with a functional plantigrade foot. This undertaking is often accompanied by repeated surgical procedures and a high rate of complications such as pin tract infections, residual LLD, delayed union, ankle and knee stiffness, refractures, knee subluxation, residual foot deformities, and even mild to severe depression.

McCarthy et al compared the final outcomes after reconstruction and amputation and found that children after early amputation were more active, had less pain, and were more satisfied with the results of treatment [9]. These children also had fewer procedures with fewer complications. The reconstruction group had a total of 21 complications and each patient underwent a mean of 7 procedures. In this study, the children in the lengthening group were older and therefore treated later, making treatment more difficult. Also 50% of the children were treated with the Wagner method, which is associated with more complications [33, 34].

Before 2000, there are several papers with similar poor outcomes, in which the authors [13, 33, 35] suggested that amputation is a more effective method of management than limb lengthening in severe FH cases. During the last decade, there was a tendency toward a reconstruction and lengthening treatment even for more severe cases with more favorable results.

Catagni et al treated 32 patients with type III FH according to the modified Dalmonte classification [11, 36]. In this study, the mean number of surgical procedures was six and the complication rate was 82% but most of the complications resolved except for two patients who ultimately underwent amputation. The outcomes were satisfactory in 17 of 32 patients.

Changulani et al reported the results of eight patients, in which each patient underwent an average of three surgical procedures [10]. All patients developed minor complications such as pin-tract infections. At last follow-up (average 15 years), all patients were ambulatory and mobile with acceptable limb lengths and limb alignment.

Oberc and Sulko published a study of 31 patients [14]. Only nine (29%) were treated with the elongation method. In these 9 patients, there were 12 elongation and 39 surgical procedures in total. The complication rate was 78%, and there were satisfactory results in five of nine patients.

El-Sayed et al reported the results of 157 patients with Achterman and Kalamchi type-II FH [15]. All patients underwent elongation, and 12 patients underwent concomitant femoral lengthening (average 13.6 cm). There were 107 minor complications, which were treated without to change the final outcomes and 19 major complications in which the desired lengthening was not achieved.

El-Tayeby and Ahmed performed ankle reconstruction prior to elongation in 13 patients [37]. All patients had a stable ankle without valgus deformity or subluxation after a mean follow-up of 18.6 months and showed good alignment in all cases.

Zarzycki et al treated ten patients with FH type II according to the Achterman and Kalamchi classification [38]. The mean lengthening was 23% of the preoperative length. Equal limb length and functional foot positioning were achieved in four patients, and the complication rate was 87.5%.

Başbozkurt et al reported his experience treating FH in five patients [39]. At last follow-up, three of five patients had plantigrade feet and two patients had equinus deformity. The other patients had minor complications (pain and pin-tract infection).

A recent comparison between amputation and reconstruction published by Birch et al. reviewed the outcomes of amputation-mediated treatment and reconstructive surgery for FH [40]. Both institutions involved were highly specialized: one with an on-site prosthetics department and the other with a very high concentration of surgical experience with congenital pathology. Minor differences were identified but felt to be clinically insignificant between the outcomes of each approach. Self-selected walking speed was 1.13 m/s in the reconstruction group versus 1.20 m/s in the amputation group. Both differed significantly from control patients at 1.25 m/s. This difference, though statistically significant, was not felt to be of clinical importance.

Paired with the evidence by Pate et al that the gap between treated patients with FH and control subjects narrows with age, this is a very positive indication for the long-term health of patients affected by FH [41]. Based on data presented by Birch et al, fears regarding the long-term impact of multiple procedures on quality of life for children may need to be reexamined, as reported mental health outcomes in both groups were equivalent [40]. Whether these results can be reproduced outside of highly specialized centers is not clear based on available evidence.

A meta-analysis by Elmherig et al showed that, overall, there was better satisfaction and less surgery/complications in the amputation versus reconstruction strategies [42].

There is still a major debate amongst pediatric orthopedic practitioners regarding the relative value of lengthening versus amputation for higher grades of FH. Regardless of the outcome of this debate, there will always be families that refuse amputation; therefore, reconstructive lengthening techniques should be available. For cases with more normal function of the foot and ankle and with at least four rays, the results of reconstruction should be predictable and the need for amputation in these moderately involved patients may be minimized. Further research and evaluation are necessary to determine the optimal treatment methodologies, as well as which patients are best suited for each treatment pathway.

Acknowledgments The authors thank the prior edition's co-author, Lior Shabtai, MD, for his enduring contributions to this work. The authors also thank their medical illustrator, Joy Marlowe, MA, CMI, and medical editor, Robert P. Farley, BS, for their invaluable assistance with this chapter.

Commentary

Christof Radler
Christof.Radler@oss.at

FH presents with hypoplasia or aplasia of the fibula, with shortening and malalignment of the tibia, joint and ligament anomalies at the knee and ankle joint, and ray deficiencies. While mild cases show only minor joint involvement and can be well managed with one lengthening or epiphysiodesis, more severe cases might need multiple surgeries including joint stabilization and reconstruction procedures to achieve a satisfying functional outcome.

The approach to FH has changed substantially in the last 10–15 years. Syme and Boyd amputation were classically the most recommended treatment options for medium to severe cases. Better understanding of multiple manifestations has allowed to improve and develop surgical approaches correcting associated deformities, important for the functional outcome. The experience gained in limb lengthening combined with better hardware in terms of external fixators and lengthening nails has reduced the rate of complications.

Those complications have been the main reason for poor functional outcome and/or late amputation after attempts at reconstruction. In the beginning of modern limb lengthening, at the end of the last century, lengthening was often performed without considering hip and/or knee joint instability. Patients ended up with dislocated hips, dislocated knees, or painful ankles in severe equinus and valgus, or any combination of the above. This resulted in long but nonfunctional limbs, often painful, which compared poorly to amputation and prosthetic fitting.

One factor that largely improved functional outcome was establishing specialized centers, and the understanding that those rare deformities should only be treated at those centers gathering high numbers of cases allowing for a short learning curve and expertise.

This chapter provides a balanced and comprehensive description of the treatment approach to FH based on decades of experience and an enormous case collection.

Success in treating FH is based on understanding the deformity, proper planning, and experience, but also reflection on the personal skill level. Things can be achieved in different ways; however, certain basic rules apply. One of the major functional problems in FH is the ankle joint. In mild and moderately severe cases, maintaining or restoring a mobile ankle joint with the heel in good alignment is the major goal. Mild cases may only need one lengthening toward the end of growth and can potentially be treated with a lengthening nail, if available. However, patient selection is important to ensure good engagement in physical therapy and compliance with bracing, if applied. In other cases, an external fixation frame spanning the foot and ankle might be preferable.

In some moderately severe cases (Paley type 2), the ankle joint might need a distal tibial realignment with a relative lengthening of the fibula by shortening of the tibia (SHORDT - Shortening Osteotomy Realignment Distal Tibia). This realignment of the ankle mortice works best if there is some remodeling possible - well before skeletal maturity.

In the severe ankle and subtalar type valgus cases (Paley type 3), the SUPER ankle allows to achieve a functional ankle and foot position. However, in some of cases remodeling with recurrent valgus might occur. Also, subsequent lengthening can lead to recurrence of some valgus and equinus deformities. In those severe cases, a realistic goal is to provide a plantigrade foot during childhood. Some of those cases as well as cases not previously corrected with the above-mentioned techniques might need an arthrodesis near or at skeletal maturity. If done correctly, this can result in a well functional limb, as the foot is usually short and allows proper propulsion during gait even with a stiff ankle.

Extreme care must be taken to protect the knee joint. Unstable knees can benefit from a SUPER knee procedure prior to limb lengthening. Although this surgery has the potential to substantially improve stability, stability might still not be comparable to a normal knee, which must be considered during subsequent lengthening. The recent recommendation to add a notch-plasty might protect the intraarticular portion of the reconstructed ligament from wear and tear and possible loss of fixation.

Notably, FH is never only FH, but almost always comes with some extent of CFD. Mild distal femoral valgus due to hypoplasia of the lateral condyle might be the only sign of CFD, but usually some femoral shortening is present. If shortening is around 2-3 cm, it can be addressed with an appropriately timed contralateral epiphysiodesis. More severe CFD must be included into the overall treatment plan and might alter the order and number of procedures.

The advances in reconstructive treatment of congenital deficiencies in the last 20 years were driven by a small number of pioneers, and others following and sometimes modifying or combining their techniques. New techniques only evolve if some are pushing the barriers—this must be done with the best interest of our patients in mind and by surgeons experienced enough to know where those barriers are. New technologies and techniques like lengthening plates and extramedullary nail lengthening might further improve patient comfort but must be used considering the safety of the adjacent joints. Studies in years to come will have to show how the new techniques and approaches we are using today improve the functional outcome.

References

1. Boakes JL, Stevens PM, Moseley RF. Treatment of genu valgus deformity in congenital absence of the fibula. J Pediatr Orthop. 1991;11(6):721–4.
2. Froster UG, Baird PA. Congenital defects of lower limbs and associated malformations: a population based study. Am J Med Genet. 1993;45(1):60–4.
3. Rogala EJ, Wynne-Davies R, Littlejohn A, Gormley J. Congenital limb anomalies: frequency and aetiological factors. Data from the Edinburgh Register of the Newborn (1964-68). J Med Genet. 1974;11(3):221–33.
4. Stevens PM, Arms D. Postaxial hypoplasia of the lower extremity. J Pediatr Orthop. 2000;20(2):166–72.
5. Birch JG, Lincoln TL, Mack PW, Birch CM. Congenital fibular deficiency: a review of thirty years' experience at one institution and a proposed classification system based on clinical deformity. J Bone Joint Surg Am. 2011;93(12):1144–51.
6. Hootnick DR, Levinsohn EM. Embryology of the lower limb demonstrates that congenital absent fibula is a radiologic misnomer. Anat Rec (Hoboken). 2022;305(1):8–17.
7. Rodriguez-Ramirez A, Thacker MM, Becerra LC, Riddle EC, Mackenzie WG. Limb length discrepancy and congenital limb anomalies in fibular hemimelia. J Pediatr Orthop B. 2010;19(5):436–40.
8. Roux MO, Carlioz H. Clinical examination and investigation of the cruciate ligaments in children with fibular hemimelia. J Pediatr Orthop. 1999;19(2):247–51.
9. McCarthy JJ, Glancy GL, Chnag FM, Eilert RE. Fibular hemimelia: comparison of outcome measurements after amputation and lengthening. J Bone Joint Surg Am. 2000;82(12):1732–5.
10. Changulani M, Ali F, Mulgrew E, Day JB, Zenios M. Outcome of limb lengthening in fibular hemimelia and a functional foot. J Child Orthop. 2010;4(6):519–24.
11. Catagni MA, Radwan M, Lovisetti L, Guerreschi F, Elmoghazy NA. Limb lengthening and deformity correction by the Ilizarov technique in type III fibular hemimelia: an alternative to amputation. Clin Orthop Relat Res. 2011;469(4):1175–80.
12. Patel M, Paley D, Herzenberg JE. Limb-lengthening versus amputation for fibular hemimelia. J Bone Joint Surg Am. 2002;84(2):317–9.
13. Naudie D, Hamdy RC, Fassier F, Morin B, Duhaime M. Management of fibular hemimelia: amputation or limb lengthening. J Bone Joint Surg Br. 1997;79(1):58–65.
14. Oberc A, Sułko J. Fibular hemimelia—diagnostic management, principles, and results of treatment. J Pediatr Orthop B. 2013;22(5):450–6.
15. El-Sayed MM, Correll J, Pohlig K. Limb sparing reconstructive surgery and Ilizarov lengthening in fibular hemimelia of Achterman-Kalamchi type II patients. J Pediatr Orthop B. 2010;19(1):55–60.
16. Das S, Ganesh GS, Pradhan S, Mohanty RN. Outcome of eight-plate hemiepiphysiodesis on genu valgum and height correction in bilateral fibular hemimelia. J Pediatr Orthop B. 2014;23(1):67–72.
17. Herzenberg JE, Paley D, Gillespie R. Limb deficiency. In: Staheli LT, editor. Pediatric orthopaedic secrets. 2nd ed. Philadelphia, PA: Hanley & Belfus Inc; 2003. p. 406–16.
18. Calder P, Shaw S, Roberts A, Tennant S, Sedki I, Hanspal R, Eastwood D. A comparison of functional outcome between amputation and extension prosthesis in the treatment of congenital absence of the fibula with severe limb deformity. J Child Orthop. 2017;11(4):318–25.
19. Makarov MR, Jackson TJ, Smith CM, Jo CH, Birch JG. Timing of epiphysiodesis to correct leg-length discrepancy: a comparison of prediction methods. J Bone Joint Surg Am. 2018;100(14):1217–22.
20. Achterman C, Kalamchi A. Congenital deficiency of the fibula. J Bone Joint Surg Br. 1979;61(2):133–7.
21. Stanitski DF, Stanitski CL. Fibular hemimelia: a new classification system. J Pediatr Orthop. 2003;23(1):30–4.
22. Birch JG, Lincoln TL, Mack PW. Functional classification of fibular deficiency. In: Herring JA, Birch JG, editors. The child with a Limb deficiency. Rosemont, IL: American Academy of Orthopaedic Surgeons; 1998. p. 161–70.
23. Hamdy RC, Makhdom AM, Saran N, Birch J. Congenital fibular deficiency. J Am Acad Orthop Surg. 2014;22(4):246–55.
24. Paley D. Surgical reconstruction for fibular hemimelia. J Chil Orthop. 2016;10(6):557–83.
25. Manner HM, Radler C, Ganger R, Grill F. Knee deformity in congenital longitudinal deficiencies of the lower extremity. Clin Orthop. 2006;448:185–92.
26. Radler C, Myers AK, Hunter RJ, Arrabal PP, Herzenberg JE. Prenatal diagnosis of congenital femoral deficiency and fibular hemimelia. Prenat Diagn. 2014;34(10):940–5.
27. Paley D, Bhave A, Herzenberg JE, Bowen JR. Multiplier method for predicting limb-length discrepancy. J Bone Joint Surg Am. 2000;82(10):1432–46.
28. Paley J, Talor J, Levin A, Bhave A, Paley D, Herzenberg JE. The multiplier method for prediction of adult height. J Pediatr Orthop. 2004;24(6):732–7.
29. Birch JG, Makarov MR, Sanders JO, Podeszwa DA, Honcharuk EM, Esparza M, Tran EY, Jo CH, Rodgers JA. Lower-extremity segment-length prediction accuracy of the Sanders multiplier, Paley multiplier, and White-Menelaus formula. J Bone Joint Surg Am. 2021;103(18):1713–7.

30. Shabtai L, Specht SC, Standard SC, Herzenberg JE. Internal lengthening device for congenital femoral deficiency and fibular hemimelia. Clin Orthop Relat Res. 2014;472(12):3860–8.
31. McClure PK, Herzenberg JE. Epiphysiodesis: not just for equalization. J Limb Lengthen Reconstr. 2022;8:1–2.
32. Belthur MV, Paley D, Jindal G, Burghardt RD, Specht SC, Herzenberg JE. Tibial lengthening: extraarticular calcaneotibial screw to prevent ankle equinus. Clin Orthop Relat Res. 2008;466(12):3003–10.
33. Choi IH, Kumar SJ, Bowen JR. Amputation or limb-lengthening for partial or total absence of the fibula. J Bone Joint Surg Am. 1990;72(9):1391–9.
34. Dahl MT, Fischer DA. Lower extremity lengthening by Wagner's method and by callus distraction. Orthop Clin North Am. 1991;22(4):643–9.
35. Cheng JC, Cheung KW, Ng BK. Severe progressive deformities after limb lengthening in type-II fibular hemimelia. J Bone Joint Surg Br. 1998;80(5):772–6.
36. Catagni MA, Bolano L, Cattaneo R. Management of fibular hemimelia using the Ilizarov method. Orthop Clin North Am. 1991;22(4):715–22.
37. El-Tayeby HM, Ahmed AA. Ankle reconstruction in type II fibular hemimelia. Strategies Trauma Limb Reconstr. 2012;7(1):23–6.
38. Zarzycki D, Jasiewicz B, Kacki W, Koniarski A, Kasprzyk M, Zarzycka M, Tesiorowski M. Limb lengthening in fibular hemimelia type II: can it be an alternative to amputation? J Pediatr Orthop B. 2006;15(2):147–53.
39. Başbozkurt M, Yildiz C, Kömürcü M, Demiralp B, Kürklü M, Ateşalp AS. Management of fibular hemimelia with the Ilizarov circular external fixator [in Turkish]. Acta Orthop Traumatol Turc. 2005;39(1):46–53.
40. Birch JG, Paley D, Herzenberg JE, Morton A, Ward S, Riddle R, Specht S, Cummings D, Tulchin-Francis K. Amputation versus staged reconstruction for severe fibular hemimelia: assessment of psychosocial and quality-of life status and physical functioning in childhood. JBJS Open Access. 2019;4(2):e0053.
41. Pate JW, Hancock MJ, Tofts L, Epps A, Baldwin JN, McKay MJ, Burns J, Morris E, Pacey V. Longitudinal fibular deficiency: a cross-sectional study comparing lower limb function of children and young people with that of unaffected peers. Children (Basel). 2019;6(3):45.
42. Elmherig A, Ahmed AF, Hegazy A, Herzenberg JE, Ibrahim T. Amputation versus limb reconstruction for fibular hemimelia: a meta-analysis. J Pediatr Orthop. 2020;40(8):425–30.

Tibial Hemimelia

Dror Paley, Katherine Miller, and David Y. Chong

Introduction

The first case of tibial hemimelia was reported in 1841 by Otto [1] in the German literature. He incorrectly described it as fibular hemimelia, and Burckhardt later recognized this mistake in 1880 [2, 3]. Thus, the first correctly reported case of tibial hemimelia is credited to Billroth in 1861 [4, 5].

The presentation of tibial hemimelia can be variable, but the classic appearance of a shortened leg, flexed knee, and severe equinovarus foot position is easily recognized on clinical examination and can be diagnosed on prenatal ultrasound as early as 16 weeks of gestation [6]. Most often, there is a knee flexion contracture and the lower leg is in an adducted position. Multidirectional knee instability may be present due to a lack of ligaments. A patella and quadriceps mechanism may be present or absent. The quadriceps may terminate proximal to the knee and have limited function if present. Typical skin manifestations include a dimple over the knee or head of the fibula. When a partial tibia is present, its distal end may be covered by a pouch of skin, with a crease formed where the skin is tethered along the length of the fibula. The tibia may be shortened, dysplastic, partially or completely absent. Parts or all of the tibia may be unossified at birth and in infancy. The fibula can be normal or dysplastic, straight or bowed. The fibular head may be overgrown relative to the tibia at the proximal end. The fibula may be autocentralized to the femur or lateral to it with proximal migration. The tibial plafond, if present, is dysplastic (flat, round, or in varus). The foot is usually in equinovarus (club foot position). The forefoot is often adducted and supinated. The medial side of the foot may have a hypoplastic great toe and first ray. Toes and metatarsals are often duplicated or absent. Tibial hemimelia has many associated duplications or deficiencies including of the toes, metatarsals, tarsals, fibula, and femur.

The deficiency in tibial hemimelia is a spectrum of pathology, ranging from a congenitally short tibia with relative fibular overgrowth to complete absence of the tibia. It is to be distinguished from fibular hemimelia, where there is a progressive deficiency of the fibula, ranging from a congenitally short tibia with relative fibular hypoplasia to complete absence of the fibula. An important distinction between these two conditions is that the foot and ankle are always in varus with tibial hemimelia and almost always in valgus with fibular hemimelia. The progression of deficiency of the tibia is from distal to proximal in tibial hemimelia, contrary to fibular hemimelia, where the progression of fibular deficiency is from proximal to distal. Tibial hemimelia should be distinguished from TAR (thrombocytopenia absent radius) syndrome-associated deficiency or dysplasia of the knee joint. TAR deficiency of the knee ranges from simple genu varum to ball-and-socket-shaped, complete absence, or congenital fusion of the knee joint. Therefore, in order to prevent confusion, tibial hemimelia should be classified as an incremental deficiency of the tibia from distal to proximal.

Genetics

Tibial hemimelia is extremely rare with a reported incidence of one in one million live births [7, 8]. In 1941, there were 79 published cases [9], and since then there have been several hundred more reported. It is estimated that 30% of cases are bilateral [10], and it favors the right side for unknown reasons. Spiegel noted that all 11 of his unilateral cases affected the right side, and in his review, about 72% of unilateral cases in the literature affected the right side [11]. Tibial hemimelia has also been associated with multiple congenital

D. Paley (✉) · K. Miller
St. Mary's Medical Center, Paley Orthopedic and Spine Institute, West Palm Beach, FL, USA
e-mail: dpaley@paleyinstitute.org; kmiller@paleyinstitute.org

D. Y. Chong
Department of Orthopedic Surgery, University of Oklahoma Health Sciences Center, Oklahoma City, OK, USA
e-mail: david-chong@ouhsc.edu

anomalies. In Schoenecker's case series of 57 patients, 34 (60%) had associated anomalies [12]. Similarly, Launois and Kuss found that 24/41 (59%) of their cases had associated anomalies [13].

Tibial deficiency can be isolated or syndromic, and it can occur sporadically or with a known family history. The defect is thought to be mesodermal in origin, with known genetic mutations affecting the complex signalling pathways necessary for limb bud patterning and development [14]. There have been many studies on the genetic inheritance of tibial hemimelia. Multiple reports describe parent to child transmission (Nutt [9], Jones [15]) as well as families with multiple siblings affected (Aitken [16], Emami [17]). Autosomal dominant inheritance has been implicated by Clark [18], Cowell [19], and Lenz [20, 21]. Autosomal recessive inheritance has also been described (Fried [22], Mahloudji [23], and McKay [24]). Consanguinity has been linked to a high prevalence of tibial hemimelia in different regions [25, 26]. Variable penetrance and phenotypic presentations have been demonstrated in cases of monozygotic twins where one twin is either unaffected or has a distinct presentation [27, 28]. An interesting breeding trial of Galloway cattle with tibial hemimelia concluded that it was caused by homozygosity of a single autosomal recessive gene with variable expressivity and pleiotropic effects on various body systems [29].

Tibial hemimelia is associated with several syndromes. Werner mesomelic syndrome (WMS) (Fig. 31.1) or tibial hemimelia–polysyndactyly–triphalangeal thumb syndrome [30] (THPTTS) is an autosomal dominant disorder associated with bilateral tibial hemimelia. It is now thought to be one of a spectrum of disorders including triphalangeal thumb-polysyndactyly syndrome (TPTPS) [31–33]. Genetic studies have mapped both to mutations involving the ZRS gene on chromosome 7q, which regulates sonic hedgehog (SHH) expression in the zone of polarizing activity of the limb bud [33–35].

Langer-Giedion syndrome, or type II tricho-rhino-phalangeal syndrome (TRPS II), is responsible for another form of bilateral tibial hemimelia. It is caused by a deletion on chromosome 8q resulting in loss of function copies of TRPS1 and EXT1 genes and has features of both TRPS I and multiple hereditary exostosis [36, 37]. The combination of femoral bifurcation and tibial aplasia with or without ectrodactyly is known as the Gollop-Wolfgang complex (Fig. 31.2) and can be accompanied by other anomalies such as congenital heart defects, cleft lip or palate, and tracheoesophageal fistula [38–40].

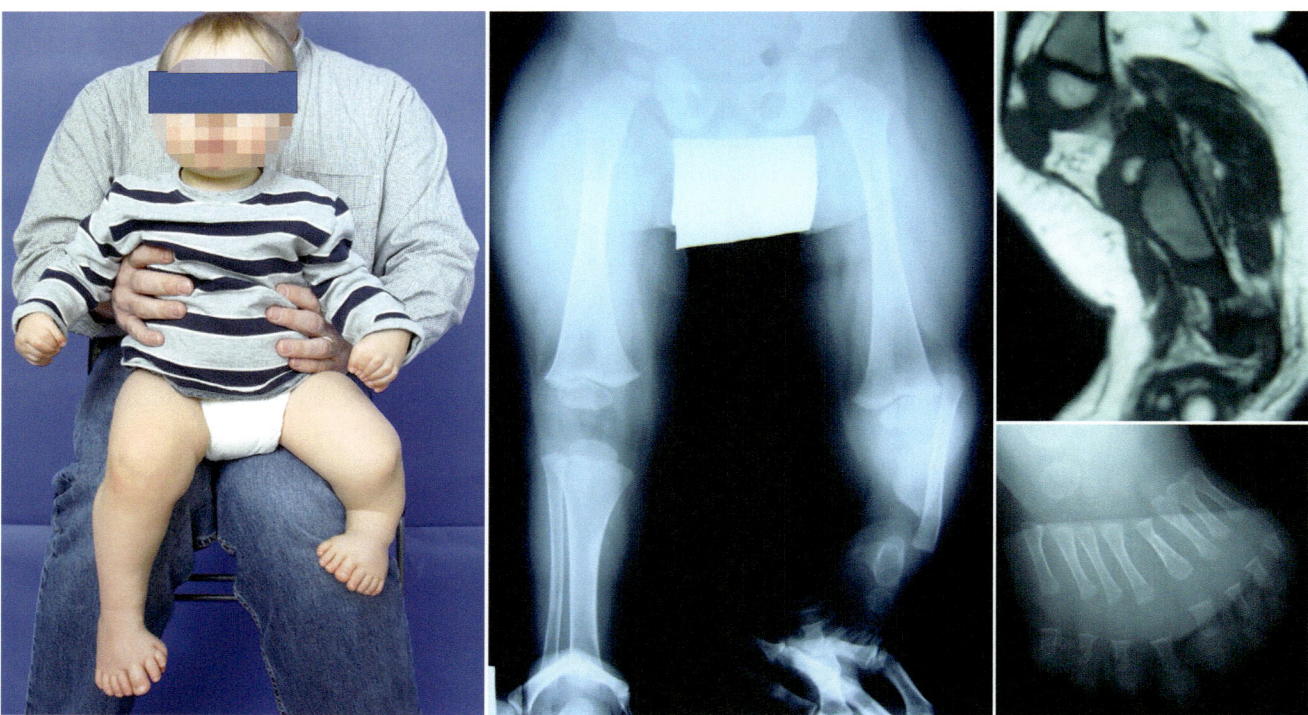

Fig. 31.1 Clinical photograph (left) of a patient with Werner syndrome. This child has bilateral tibial hemimelia (Paley type 2b left, Paley type 1 right +3 rays/toes bilateral), and the patient's mother and grandmother had the same autosomal dominant genetic condition. There is mirror polysyndactyly of the hands and feet. AP radiograph (middle) of this patient's lower limbs demonstrating a delta tibia on the left, which is commonly seen in tibial hemimelia associated with Werner's. MRI (top right) showing the delta tibia. AP foot radiograph (bottom right) of the left foot showing 8 metatarsals and toes mirrored around the great toe. This case is not classifiable by the Jones classification. (Copyright The Paley Foundation. Reproduced with permission. All rights reserved)

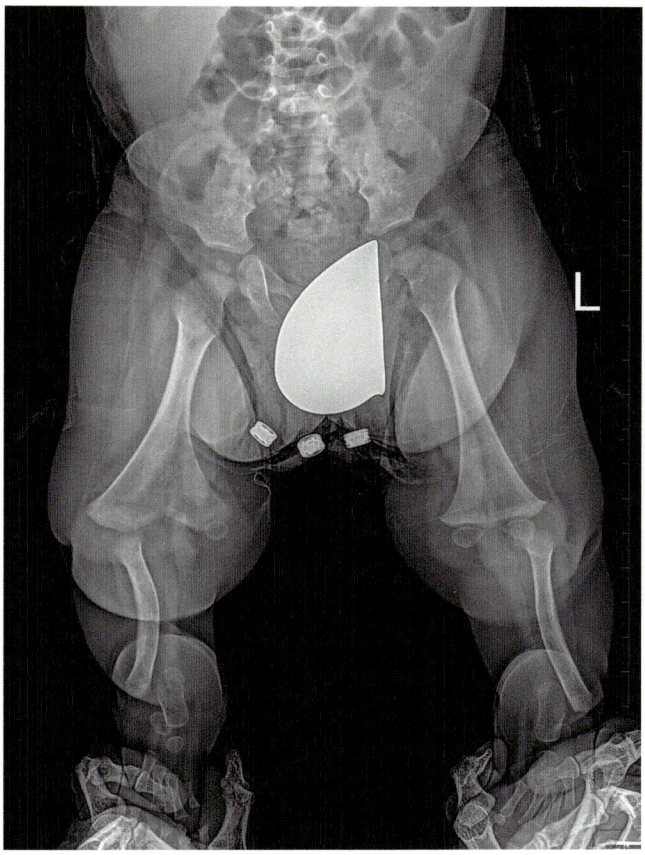

Fig. 31.2 Radiograph demonstrating classic findings associated with Gollop-Wolfgang complex, note the femoral bifurcation and complete tibial aplasia. On the right side, there were two distinct femoral condyles, while on the left side there was a more normal shaped distal femur with two ossific nuclei. Both sides had a patella with quadriceps muscle attached. These would be classified as Paley type 5a + femoral condyle duplication bilateral. This case is not classifiable by the Jones classification. (Copyright The Paley Foundation. Reproduced with permission. All rights reserved)

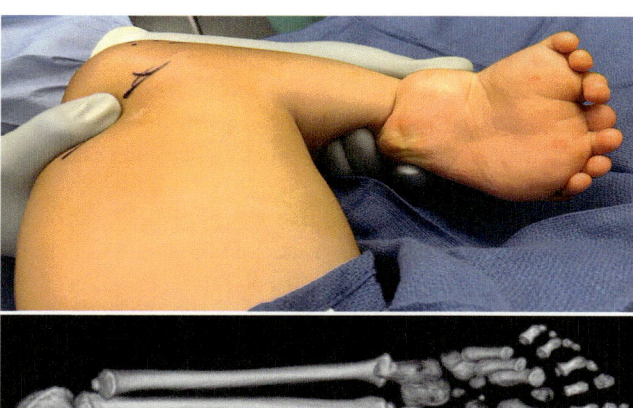

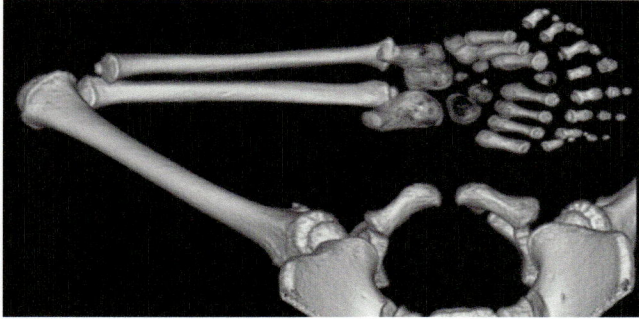

Fig. 31.3 Clinical photograph of tibial hemimelia-diplopodia syndrome (top). 3D CT of the lower extremity (bottom). There is duplication of the fibula, calcaneus, tarsal bones, metatarsals, and toes (mirror foot deformity) with an 8-ray foot. Interestingly there was only one talus. There was also duplication of the Achilles tendon and gastrocnemius muscles. Note the severe flexion contracture of the knee. There was no patella present. This case would be classified as Paley type 5c +fibula, calcaneus, tarsals, metatarsals, and toes. This case is not classifiable by the Jones classification. (Copyright The Paley Foundation. Reproduced with permission. All rights reserved)

Case reports have linked tibial hemimelia and other limb anomalies to CHARGE syndrome, a pattern of congenital anomalies including eye, nose, ear, heart, and genital defects [41–43]. Most cases of CHARGE syndrome are due to a mutation of the CHD7 gene (chromodomain helicase DNA-binding protein 7) located on chromosome 8q, which is expressed by the developing limb bud mesenchyme [44, 45]. Several other rare associations have been documented including tibial hemimelia–micromelia–trigonal brachycephaly syndrome [46]. Various presentations of tibial hemimelia-diplopodia syndrome [47, 48] (Fig. 31.3) include mirror foot as well as duplications of the fibula and/or tarsal bones while tibial hemimelia–split hand and foot syndrome is characterized by bilateral tibial aplasia and ectrodactyly of the hands or feet [49].

In the ipsilateral limb, additional deformities may be suppressive or duplicative. Associated anomalies of the lower extremity have been documented in numerous cases and can include congenital femoral deficiency, bifid femur, hip dysplasia or dislocation, coxa valga, missing patella or quadriceps, knee hyperextension or flexion, and duplicated fibula. Foot deformities include clubfoot, missing toes, syndactyly, supernumerary or duplicated great toe, ectrodactyly, and mirror foot or diplopodia [50–55]. Reported anomalies of the upper extremity include radial dysplasia, ectrodactyly, syndactyly, polydactyly, triphalangism, and missing fingers. Abnormalities of the spine such as hemivertebrae and myelomeningocele can also coexist [56–60]. Non-orthopedic abnormalities include deafness, cleft palate, pseudohermaphroditism, cryptorchidism, and hypospadias [10].

Pathoanatomy

Evans and Smith [57], in an anatomic examination of the leg in tibial hemimelia, described the deep fascia as thin and poorly developed and plantar fascia as ill-defined while the peroneal retinaculum was clearly distinguishable. They found that the quadriceps tendon was thin and expansive, blending with the knee capsule and that other tendons of the thigh were frequently absent or inserted directly onto the knee capsule or fibrocartilaginous remnant of the proximal tibia. They documented absence and duplication as well as aberrant pathways of many of the muscle-tendon units of the leg, some being essentially functionless, attaching to a single bone without crossing a joint. They postulated a mesoblast origin and not likely a mechanical or traumatic source, confirming what Hovelacque and Noel had found in mouse embryos in 1909 [61].

Turker et al. [62] dissected five Jones type Ia specimens. They found ipsilateral toe anomalies in most cases, ranging from four to eight digits. The affected leg had smaller girth, and a dimple was consistently found where the skin was tethered over the fibula. They found intact saphenous and lesser saphenous veins as well as sural and superficial peroneal nerves in the subcutaneous tissues. The deep peroneal and posterior tibial arteries were found associated with their respective nerves, but the posterior tibial bundle was found to be short and acting as a tether. Lateral and superficial posterior compartment muscles were generally intact with normal insertions. Gastrocnemius and soleus muscles had a confluent Achilles tendon which was inserted on the medial side of the calcaneal tubercle. The anterior and deep posterior compartments did not have a discrete boundary. Tendons had anomalous courses and sometimes split. No identifiable posterior tibial or anterior tibial muscle belly was found, but all specimens had a tendon inserting medially on the midfoot that tethered the foot in supination. Three specimens had an anomalous tendon inserting onto the neck of the talus. In addition, all specimens had a flat cable of tendon-like structures on the anterior border of the fibula with minimal muscle associated proximally. This unknown structure was wrapped around and inserted on the posterior capsule of the ankle. Abductor hallucis muscles were found in all specimens, even in feet without medial rays. No discrete plantar fascia was found. All specimens had subtalar coalitions, and some had midfoot coalitions. The talus articulated with the distal medial fibula on its posterolateral side with a vertical and sagittal orientation with only one plane of rotation.

> **Box 31.1 Introduction to Tibial Hemimelia**
> - Incidence is approximately one in one million.
> - Autosomal dominant and recessive inheritance has been reported, with variable expression.
> - Defects on chromosome 7q and 8q have been implicated, as well as the CHD7 gene.
> - Common associated deformities: congenital femoral deficiency, bifid femur, absent patella, mirrored foot, and polydactyly.
> - A dimple is often seen on the proximal fibula.
> - Anterior and deep posterior compartments of the leg are most deficient, with tendon remnants still attached to the foot.
> - The talus tends to follow the fibula in the deformity.

Classification

Frantz and O'Rahilly described a classification system for congenital skeletal limb deficiencies in 1961 [15, 63], dividing them into amelia, hemimelia, phocomelia, and other limb deficiencies. Hemimelia was further described as being complete, partial, or paraxial. They are then divided into terminal (distal) and intercalary (middle) deficiencies, and further subdivided into transverse and longitudinal deficiencies.

The Jones classification (Fig. 31.4), proposed in 1978, divided tibial hemimelia into four types based on radiographic criteria. The classification is arranged from most to least deficient. Type I deficiencies have no radiographically visible tibia; Ia has a hypoplastic distal femoral epiphysis and no tibial remnant; and Ib has normal ossification of the distal femoral epiphysis, and the presence of a non-ossified proximal tibial epiphysis. Type II has a radiographically visible proximal tibia with distal tibial aplasia. Type III has a radiographically visible distal tibia with proximal tibial aplasia. Type IV has distal tibiofibular diastasis [15].

Kalamchi and Dawe, in their study of 21 cases in 1985, reported their treatment results according to a modified version of the Jones classification which eliminated Jones type III and moved Jones type 1b into type II [64]. Kalamachi type I deficiencies were defined as a total absence of the tibia. This group had knee flexion contractures greater than 45° and no active quadriceps function. The fibular head is proximally migrated with hypoplasia of the distal femur. Type II deficiencies have a proximal tibia with distal tibial aplasia, active quadriceps function, and a knee flexion contracture between 25° and 45°. The width and epiphyseal ossification of the distal femur is normal, indicating the presence of a proximal tibial anlage. There is less proximal migration of the fibula. Type III deficiencies have distal tibia aplasia with diastasis of the tibiofibular syndesmosis. The knee joint is normal with good quadriceps function. The talus is subluxated proximally with a prominent distal fibula.

Weber introduced a new classification which takes into account the cartilaginous anlage, if present, using ultrasound, MRI, and intraoperative findings [65]. His classification describes 7 types of increasing severity with 12 subtypes, including a few types that were previously unclassifiable by previous schemes [66]. Subgroups are based on whether the cartilage anlage is present (a) or not (b). Weber type I is characterized by a fully formed but hypoplastic tibia with intact knee and ankle joints; type II by distal diastasis of the tibia and fibula; type III by distal tibial aplasia; type IV by proximal tibial aplasia; type V by bifocal (proximal and distal) tibial aplasia; type VI by complete tibial agenesis with duplicated fibula; type VII by complete tibial agenesis with a single fibula. A score is then assigned to quantify overall function of the limb, with higher scores indicating less impairment. The tibia (0–22 points) and presence of an

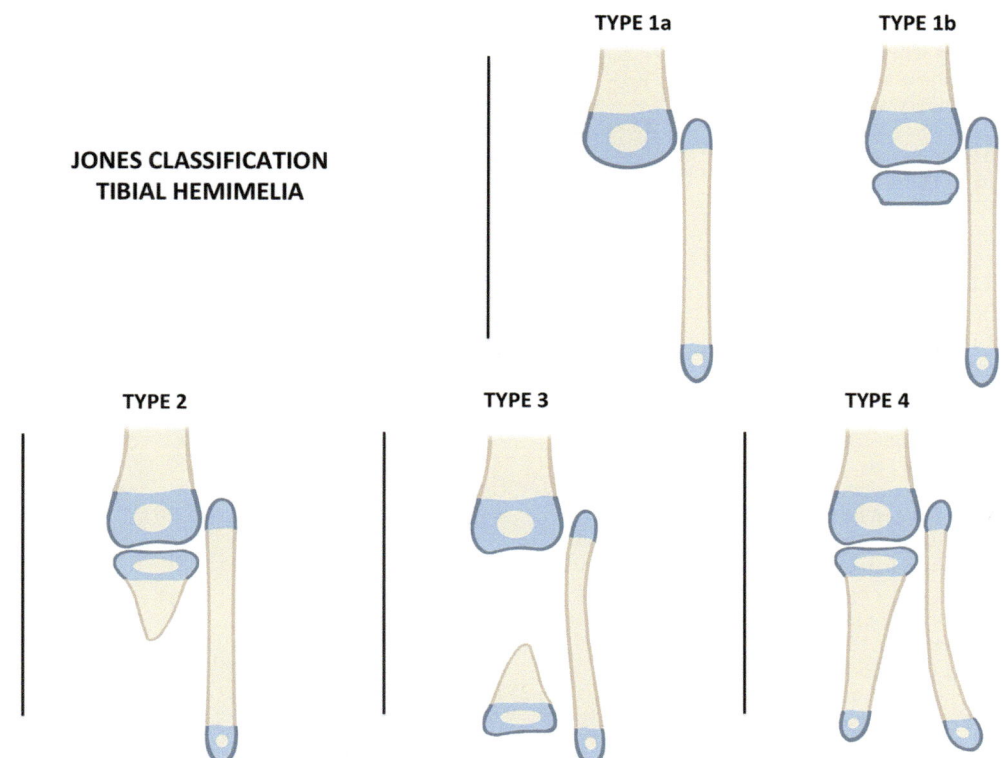

Fig. 31.4 Jones classification of tibial hemimelia (Copyright: The Paley Foundation. Reproduced with permission. All rights reserved)

anlage (+10 points) are weighed highest in importance, and the patella (0–3 points) is given slightly extra weight. The rest of the limb is scored from 0 to 2 points and included the hip joint, distal femur, fibula, foot, and muscle function of the hip, knee, and ankle joints. Five classes are defined based on the score indicating the degree of deficiency and difficulty of reconstruction.

Most widely used classifications in orthopedics organize pathology from the least to the most severe (e.g., Garden classification of hip fractures [67], Berndt and Harty classification of talar dome osteochondral fractures [68], Herring and Catterall classifications of Perthes [69, 70], and Kalamchi classification for fibular hemimelia [64]). The Paley classifications [71] for congenital femoral deficiency and fibular hemimelia (FH) follow a similar format. Some well-accepted published classifications follow the opposite format, starting with the most severe or deficient cases (e.g., Pappas classification for CFD [72], Kalamchi [64] and Jones [15] classification for tibial hemimelia). The Jones classification for tibial hemimelia has been the most widely used. The complete absence of the proximal tibia in Jones III makes its treatment similar to Jones Ia because the proximal tibia, and therefore the knee joint, is absent in both. The treatment at the knee still depends on the presence or absence of the patella and whether the fibula is autocentralized or not. The treatment of the foot does not change since the foot is in severe equinovarus as if this remnant of distal tibia was not present (Fig. 31.5). Along similar lines, Jones type 1b is more similar to Jones II given the presence of a proximal tibial anlage (which is why the Kalamchi classification lumps Jones 1b with Jones 2 together as Kalamchi type 2). Finally, the Jones classification lacks a description for several types of tibial deficiency that involve both the proximal and distal physes, such as the Delta tibia type [73] or types that have a normal appearing tibia beside a longer fibula. The Jones classification also does not consider the presence or absence of a patella, which is critical in determining treatment strategy.

The Weber Classification (Fig. 31.6) [65, 74] changed the order back to increasing severity of deficiency. It also included types with a proximal deficiency (type 3). Similar to the Pappas classification, it splits tibial hemimelia into a large number of types (total of 7). The Weber also subdivides into types that will eventually ossify and change into other types (types 3, 4, 5, 6, 7). The Weber scoring system, combined with the large number of subdivisions, makes this classification challenging for practical use.

Dissatisfied with the existing classifications and prior to Weber's publication, Paley proposed a new classification in 2003 [75]. It was modified in 2016 to ensure that the level of deficiency was accurately organized from least to most deficient and to include previously unrecognized forms of tibial hemimelia [75, 76]. Each type and subtype has a different surgical treatment, and the classification assumes that tibial hemimelia is a progressive spectrum of deficiency from distal to proximal. When comparing the Jones, Weber, and

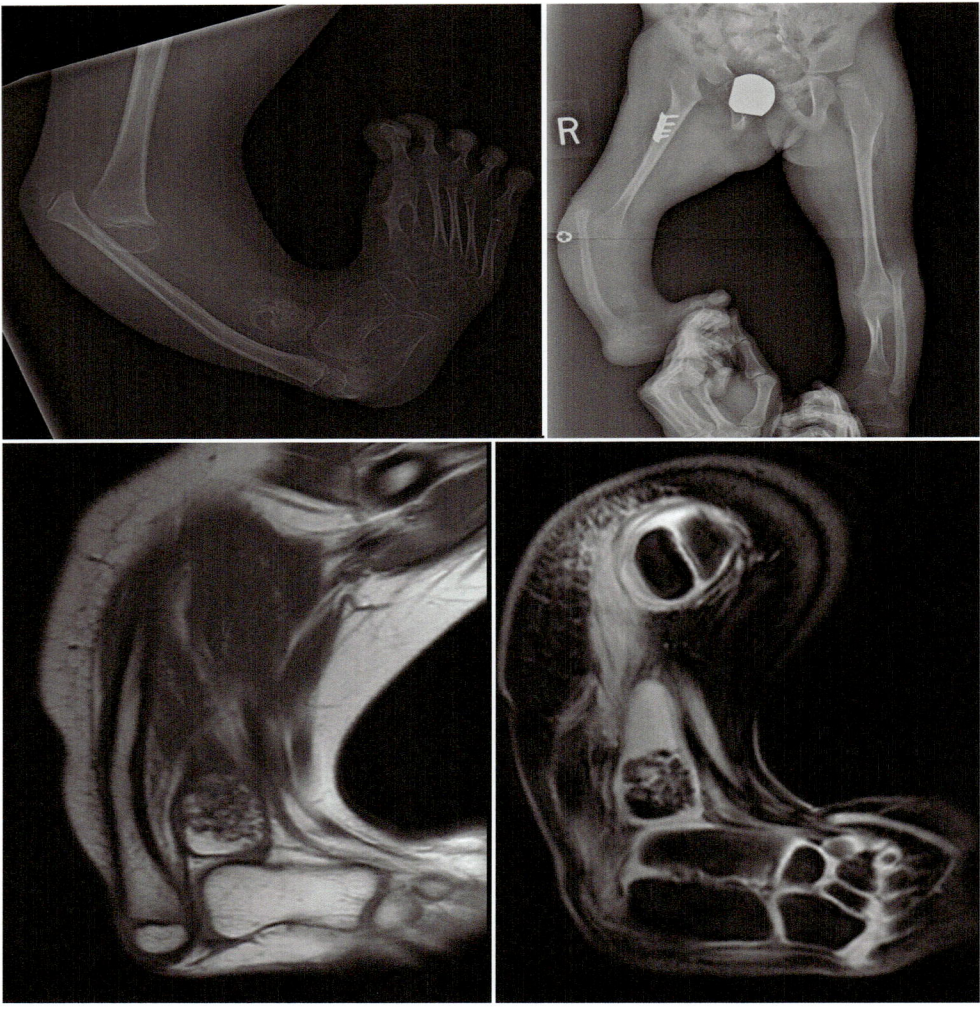

Fig. 31.5 AP radiograph (right) Jones type III tibial hemimelia (top left). This would be classified and treated as a Paley type 5c despite the remnant of distal tibia. The determining factor in treatment is the absence of the upper tibia which would be the same as a Jones type 1a. Therefore, the Jones type 3 is not a relevant distinction vs a Jones 1a. Long X-ray of both legs (top right) showing the bilateral nature of this rare type. The left leg is a Paley type 2a −quadriceps. The left side cannot be classified using the Jones classification. Magnetic resonance imaging (MRI) confirming that there is no cartilaginous proximal tibia (bottom right), but that a distal tibial remnant is present (bottom left). (Copyright The Paley Foundation. Reproduced with permission. All rights reserved)

Paley classifications, the latter was the only one that was able to classify all types of tibial hemimelia in a series of 113 cases [76]. The Paley classification (Fig. 31.7) is unique in that it was developed in direct relationship to treatment and prognosis. It consists of 5 types and 11 subtypes (Fig. 31.7; Table 31.1).

There is so much phenotypic variability with tibial hemimelia due to the associated duplications and deficiencies of bones, joints, and muscles that no classification based on different subtypes can give an accurate picture. To reconcile this problem, Paley added +/− modifiers. This is listed as plus (+) or minus (-) signs for toes, metatarsals, tarsals, fibula, distal tibial remnant, femoral condyle, femur, quadriceps, etc. The wide spectrum of pathology in tibial hemimelia lends itself to unique variants which continue to be identified to this day [77–79]. Cases that did not previously fit into a classification scheme can easily be described using the plus and minus modifiers with any of the Paley types or subtypes (Fig. 31.8).

> **Box 31.2 Jones Classification**
> - Type I: No visible tibia
>   - Ia: Hypoplastic distal femoral epiphysis
>   - Ib: Normal distal femoral epiphysis ossification (possible cartilaginous proximal tibia)
> - Type II: Distal tibia deficiency
> - Type III: Proximal tibia deficiency
> - Type IV: Shortened tibia with distal tibia-fibula diastasis

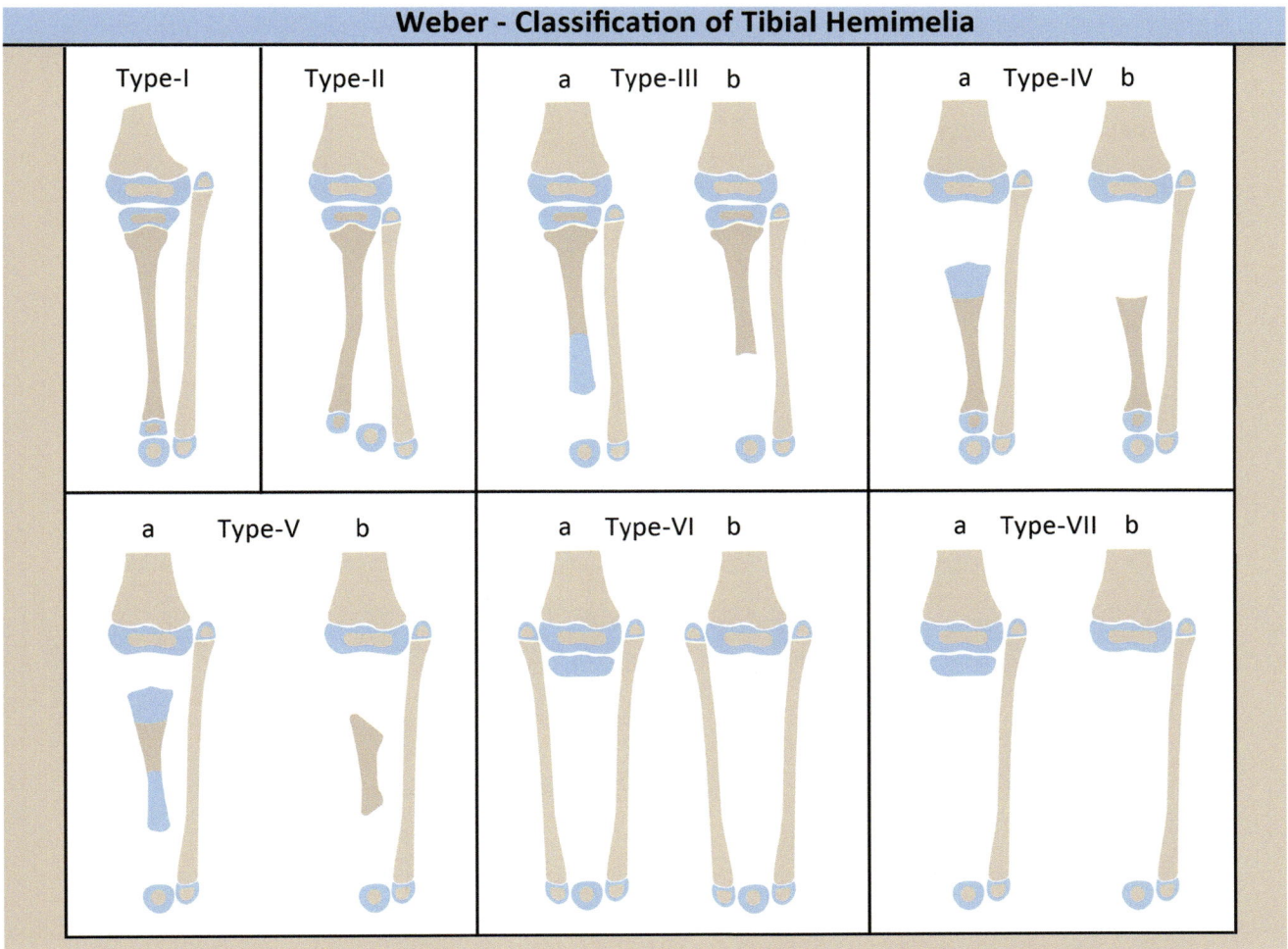

Fig. 31.6 Weber classification of tibial hemimelia. (Copyright The Paley Foundation. Reproduced with permission. All rights reserved)

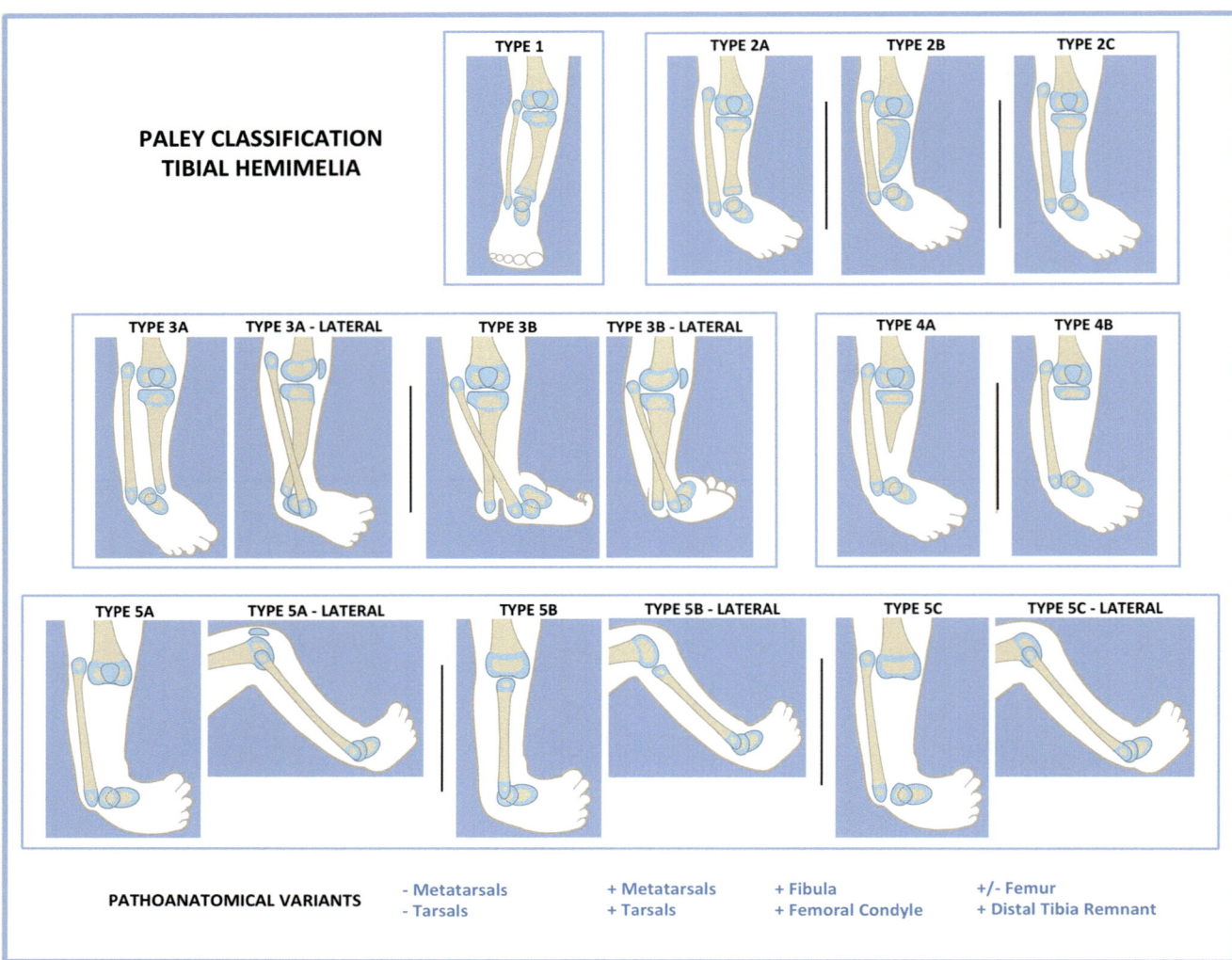

Fig. 31.7 Paley classification of tibial hemimelia: Note that the + or − symbols are added after the type to describe the associated duplication or deficiency of bones, joints, and muscles. (Copyright The Paley Foundation. Reproduced with permission. All rights reserved)

Table 31.1 Paley classification

	Knee Joint	Proximal Tibia	Tibial Shaft	Distal Tibia	Ankle Joint
Type 1	Normal	Normal or valgus	Shortened	Normal	Normal
Type 2	Normal	Normal or mild dysplasia (pagoda shaped)	Shortened	Variable	
2A				Well-formed	Dysplastic
2B				Delta tibia	
2C				Cartilage anlage	
Type 3	Normal	Normal	Varus, procurvatum	Absent Plafond	Tibiofibular diastasis; fibula internally rotated around tibia, foot follows fibula
3A					
3B					Skin cleft between tibia and fibula
Type 4	Normal	Present	Variable		
4A		Normal, physis present	Absent at level of diaphysis	Absent	Absent
4B		Non-ossified epiphysis, absent physis	Absent		
Type 5	Flexion contracture	Complete aplasia	Absent	Absent	Absent
5A	(+)Quad (+)Patella				
5B	(+)Quad (−)Patella	Auto-centralized fibula			
5C	(−)Quad (−)Patella	No knee capsule			

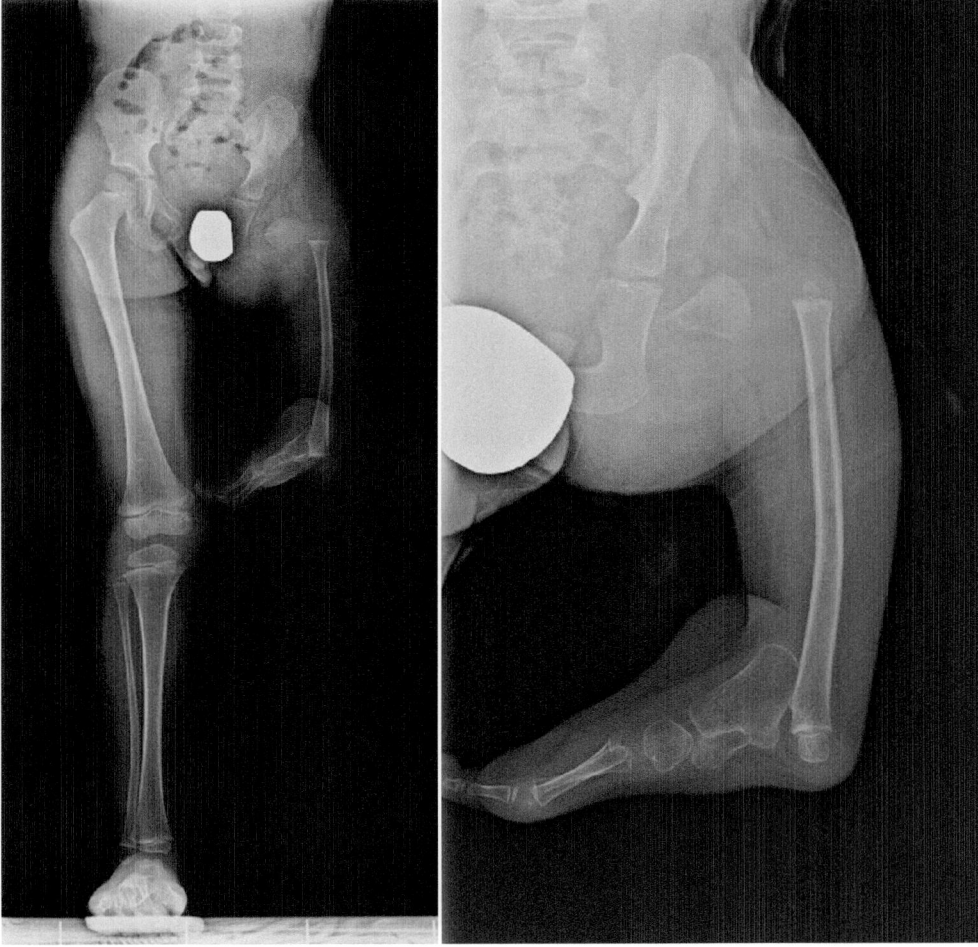

Fig. 31.8 AP radiographs of case of tibial hemimelia with congenital femoral deficiency. The Paley +/−modifiers can be used to classify this rare variant of tibial hemimelia as Paley type 5c, −proximal femur, −metatarsals. (Copyright The Paley Foundation. Reproduced with permission. All rights reserved)

History of Treatment

This section will be divided into historical treatments with published results and the author's preferred newer methods of treatment, which currently have limited published results.

Early Treatments

In 1877, Albert first published about the centralization of the fibula, fusing the femur and fibula [80]. In 1905, Myers [81] proposed a fibula-femoral arthroplasty, which was further developed by Brown in 1965. In the case of a partial absence of the tibia, there are early published reports of attempted synostosis between the tibial remnant and fibula, either side-to-side or end-to-end (Bade [56], Nove-Josserand [82]). Fraser and Robarts in 1914 reported a case with an intercalary defect in which they transplanted the contralateral fibula with reported success [83]. In 1929, Putti [84] was one of the first to give directives on treatment, describing different approaches to eight different cases: fusing the fibula to the talus in extreme equinus to increase the leg length, transfer of the proximal fibula to the intercondylar notch, and side-to-side synostosis of the fibula to the tibia both proximally and distally. Sulamaa and Ryoeppy [60] performed side-to-side opposition and recommended knee disarticulation for Jones type I deformity.

The treatment of choice for tibial hemimelia has historically been biased towards amputation. In some communities, however, the option of amputation is not accepted culturally, and patient families wish to pursue limb salvage. Notably, only one out of 24 patients in a single-center study out of India opted for amputation, despite the severity of their deformity, with authors attributing this to low cultural acceptance [85]. Another study out of India treated patients with Jones type I tibial hemimelia who either refused amputation or had no access to good prosthetic care with femoro-fibulo-clacaneal arthrodesis. This limb salvage technique enabled their patients to function independently, without the use of a prosthesis for ambulation [86]. With complete absence of the tibia (Jones type Ia), most current literature still points towards amputation [12, 50, 58, 64, 87, 88]. Reconstructive limb salvage options are available, though more severe deformity typically requires more complex surgery [89–91]. The presence of a tibia anlage, patella, and active quadriceps mechanism is an important factor when considering reconstructive options. In a patient with a fixed flexion deformity and no palpable patella, it is unlikely that a strong quadriceps mechanism exists [92]. The patella and cartilaginous tibial anlage can be difficult to identify clinically and radiographically; therefore, MRI and ultrasound are useful to determine their presence before deciding on a treatment strategy [93, 94]. Treatment and prevention of knee flexion contractures are imperative to avoid significant gait impairment with reconstruction [92].

Brown Procedure (Fibular Centralization)

Brown first published his surgical procedure of fibular transfer and centralization under the femur in 1965 [95]. This procedure was done for patients with complete absence of the tibia (Jones type I). He also recommended a Syme-type amputation of the foot. In 1972, Brown published his 15-year follow-up, in which 40 of 56 patients were available for review [96]. Eighteen required secondary surgery due to a knee flexion deformity. Of the remaining 22, one was nonambulatory and all but two were brace-dependent ambulators. He recommended attachment of the patellar ligament to the fibula, preoperative traction, as well as femoral shortening and soft tissue releases as needed to gain extension. He also recommended surgery before one year of age for maximal ambulatory and fibular remodelling potential. Inferior results were noted in patients with absent quadriceps function.

Jayakumar and Eilert [97] reported six cases treated with the Brown procedure. All patients received either a Boyd or Syme amputation. A good clinical outcome was defined as a knee with active motion of at least 10–80°, <5° varus/valgus instability, and no flexion contracture. Only two patients achieved these criteria, and they both had 3+/5 quadriceps strength. One patient had ipsilateral congenital femoral deficiency and underwent a femoral-fibula arthrodesis. Three patients had "poor" results from knee flexion contractures and two went on to knee disarticulations. The authors concluded that strong active quadriceps function was necessary for Brown reconstruction to have superior results to amputation.

Loder and Herring [87] reported nine cases of Jones type I deficiencies treated with the Brown procedure. All had preoperative knee flexion contractures. Initially, five of nine had good results with active range of motion and no flexion contractures. However, only one patient maintained quadriceps strength, and all progressively developed knee flexion contractures. Despite secondary procedures, outcomes were also considered poor due to knee instability and limited range of motion. At final follow-up, five had knee disarticulations and the remaining cases had poor range of knee motion (10–45°).

Epps and Schneider [98] published three cases of Brown procedures and noted that their results deteriorated over time, requiring secondary procedures due to progressive knee flexion contractures. In 1991, Epps et al. [88] reported on 14 patients (20 knees) who underwent centralization of the fibula for Jones type I tibial hemimelia. All patients developed progressive knee flexion contractures and needed multiple secondary procedures. This led the authors to recommend early knee disarticulation and prosthetic fitting as the treatment of choice. Results were considered to be failures due to the knee flexion deformities.

Simmons et al. [99] revisited the Brown procedure, publishing results on five patients and seven limbs. All cases were classified as Jones type Ia deformities, though one was later found to be 1b at the time of surgery and the rudimentary proximal tibia was utilized for fixation. All patients had equinovarus deformities of the foot and underwent Syme amputations. An anterolateral knee incision was used, and the biceps tendon and distal insertion of the patellar tendon released. Femoral or fibular shortening was performed as needed along with peroneal nerve decompression. The fibula was centralized underneath the femoral condyles and the knee stabilized in extension with a Steinmann pin. The patellar tendon was reattached to the fibula and a long leg spica cast was applied. Subsequent procedures included split thickness skin grafting, heel pad release for the Syme amputation, and one quadricepsplasty for lack of knee flexion. All ambulated with a patella-tendon-bearing socket with thigh extension. Average range of knee motion was 57° and only two patients achieved 10–80° of knee flexion. Despite limited knee motion, all patients were satisfied and none went on to knee disarticulation. They recommended narrowing indications for reconstruction to those patients with grade 3+/5 quadriceps strength, age younger than 1 year, no fibular bowing, and ambulatory potential.

Wada et al. [100] published nine cases of limb reconstruction in Jones type I and II cases. They performed four tibiofibular synostosis and five Brown procedures with concurrent foot centralization procedures and subsequent lengthening as needed. The tibia-fibular fusion patients had good results with preserved knee function. Of the Brown procedures, four had poor quadriceps function and one had persistent knee instability. All five had unsatisfactory functional results based on Jayakumar's criteria [97]; however, they were all household ambulators with only one patient requiring an orthosis.

Hosny [101] published a case series of 6 patients with tibial hemimelia in Egypt. Amputation was not accepted in his community and patients presented at an older age (3.5–13 years). Jones type I cases were treated with gradual distraction of the fibula with an external fixator followed by a Brown procedure 1 month later. Type II cases were treated with gradual distraction followed by fixation of the proximal fibula to the proximal tibia. Fibular lengthening was subsequently performed, but had limitations due to knee flexion contractures that resulted. Femoral lengthening was performed at a later stage. Hosny reported that all patients' families were satisfied with the outcome. All type II patients ambulated independently with minimal (<5°) knee flexion contractures and active ROM greater than 90°. The type I patients could walk with a knee-ankle-foot orthosis (KAFO) and walker and had limited ROM (10–35/40°), but could perform ADLs at home without pain.

Overall, most authors did not report good outcomes with the Brown procedure and recommended knee disarticulation rather than reconstruction as the best option for total absence of the tibia. Many of the poor outcomes were due to progressive knee flexion contractures, knee instability, and poor range of motion, as previously defined by Jayakumar [97]. However, for some patients in whom amputation is not an option or in countries where obtaining a prosthetic may be limited or impossible, a limb that is weight bearing, sensate, and functional is better than no limb.

As will be discussed, the presence of a quadriceps, patella, and proximal tibia may favor reconstruction with some of the newer methods such as patellar arthroplasty for Jones 1a (Paley 5a) and fibula to tibia transfer in Jones 1b or 2 (Paley type 4a,b). In addition, the use of gradual distraction with an external fixator prior to reconstruction can help overcome soft tissue contractures.

Amputation

Knee disarticulation has been described for treatment and remains a salvage option for failed Brown procedures as seen in many of the studies above. Kalamachi [64] treated three children with the Brown procedure, and all went on to subsequent knee disarticulations. These failures were attributed to knee flexion contractures and lack of quadriceps function, leading the authors to recommend early disarticulation of the knee without attempting reconstruction. Alternatively, if the femur was severely hypoplastic, a femoro-fibular arthrodesis was performed to effectively lengthen the femur, creating a longer lever arm for improved prosthetic fitting.

Similar results and conclusions were drawn by Schoenecker et al. [12]. In a series of 57 patients and 71 limbs, 86% of limbs eventually had some type of an amputation. Brown procedures were performed on 14 Jones type Ia limbs. Ten required secondary procedures due to knee instability or flexion contractures. Based on their results, they recommended evaluation for a proximal tibial anlage to differentiate between Jones types 1a and 1b. Type Ia were then treated with knee disarticulation due to their unsatisfactory results with the Brown procedure, while type 1b were candidates for fibula to tibia transfer.

Fernandez et al. [52] were also proponents of early amputation. Twenty-two cases of tibial hemimelia were reported, and the families of 17 patients elected to proceed with surgical management. All ten Jones type I cases underwent knee disarticulation. Three Jones type II and III cases had distal amputations. Only the remaining four Jones type IV cases had nonoperative treatment. The author recommended early amputation so that the patient would treat it as a "congenital amputation," allowing for better adaptation to their prosthesis and rehabilitation. For many of these patients, their socioeconomic status influenced their decision, necessitating a quicker and more definitive treatment option.

Spiegel et al. [11] described potential complications and sequelae of amputation in patients with tibial hemimelia. They treated nine Jones type I deficiencies with knee disarticulation without subsequent complications. Five type II deficiencies were initially treated with distal amputation (Chopart or Syme). They developed prosthetic irritation at the proximal fibula from the varus malalignment and prominent fibular head. Three patients subsequently underwent tibiofibular synostosis. One patient had progressive varus deformity and difficulty with prosthetic fitting that improved after hemiepiphysiodesis. Overall, the authors felt unsure about the best course of action for type II deficiencies. Four type III deficiencies were treated with Syme or Chopart amputations and did well.

In patients with symptomatic knee instability, one study found significantly better outcomes in patients who underwent amputation, leading them to recommend this treatment over reconstruction [102]. When amputation is the chosen treatment, most surgeons will opt for a through-knee amputation for Jones type 1, a through or below-knee amputation for Jones type 2, and a Syme's amputation for Jones type 4. The argument is that with modern prosthetics, amputation leads to good functional results and is likely the most reliable and predictable method for treatment. This dictum is currently being challenged by newer more successful methods of reconstruction, discussed later in this chapter.

Tibiofibular Synostosis

In the presence of a tibial anlage (Jones type Ib, Paley type 4b) or a proximal tibia (Jones type II, Paley type 4a), many authors have reported good results with tibiofibular synostosis. Kalamachi [64] reported ten patients with Jones type II tibial hemimelia who were treated with tibia and fibula synostosis. Three of these utilized a modified Brown procedure, fusing the fibula with the cartilaginous tibial anlage. They found good stability and adequate range of motion with only mild (20–30°) flexion contractures. Due to leg length discrepancies and foot deformities, half had concurrent Boyd amputations and prosthetic fitting.

Schoenecker [12] reported 8 of 15 Jones type II limbs successfully treated with tibiofibular synostosis. Twelve were treated with a Syme amputation and were functional below-knee amputees; one had a knee disarticulation, one was treated nonoperatively, and only one patient, who also had a tibiofibular synostosis, retained the foot. They recommended tibiofibular synostosis for Jones Ib and II with concurrent distal Syme or Boyd amputations.

Distal Tibia and Ankle Stabilization

For Jones type II deficiencies, distal tibia aplasia leads to an unstable ankle and a severe clubfoot deformity. These have historically been treated by distal fusion with some type of foot amputation. In Kalamachi's [77] series, three cases were treated with calcaneo-fibular fusions and Boyd amputation. Schoenecker [12] treated seven Jones type II limbs with Syme or Chopart amputations to function as below-knee amputee. Only two also had tibiofibular synostosis.

Jones type IV deficiencies have a normal knee joint, shortened tibia with distal tibia and fibula diastasis due to lack of a tibial plafond, and proximal migration of the talus between the two bones. The foot was often in some equinovarus and both malleoli were low to the ground and prominent. Tokmakova et al. [103] evaluated 11 patients with Jones type IV deficiencies, 7 of which were treated with Boyd or Syme amputation and 3 with ankle reconstruction. They recommended ankle reconstruction as the treatment of choice as these patients were independent ambulators with stable, pain free ankles and plantigrade feet.

In Schoenecker's series of ten Jones type IV limbs, one limb had a Syme amputation and nine limbs had ankle joint reconstruction and salvage of the foot. Of these nine, five had a Syme amputation within 3 years due to leg length discrepancy. He recommended ankle reconstruction and leg length equalization, similar to Fernandez [52].

Ernat et al. reported on two cases of Jones type IV tibial hemimelia. Both patients refused amputation and were therefore offered staged reconstruction. In the first stage, a Z-lengthening of the Achilles tendon was performed and the foot was distracted to the end of the distal tibia using an Ilizarov-type circular fixator. Once the foot was sufficiently distracted, patients underwent fibula osteotomy and open distal tibial epiphyseal-talar fusion with acute external rotation of the foot and preservation of the distal tibial physis. One patient underwent subsequent tibial lengthening for leg length discrepancy and fibular epiphysiodesis to prevent recurrent overgrowth. The second patient later underwent contralateral proximal tibia and fibula epiphysiodesis and declined any further limb length equalization procedures. At maturity, both patients ambulated without pain, functional limitation, or need for a prosthesis [104].

Limb Lengthening

Limb lengthening is also an option and commonly needed as an adjunct to reconstructive treatment due to significant shortening of the tibia and fibula [66, 105, 106]. Hootnick et al. [107] followed the natural history of tibial hemimelia and found that the leg length discrepancy remained proportional over time. They were therefore able to calculate a final predicted leg length discrepancy to help a family decide on lengthening versus Syme amputation. They recommended amputation for predicted discrepancies greater than 8.7 cm. However, with newer technology and a better understanding of the biology, staged reconstruction and limb lengthening may allow the trained surgeon to address more severe cases of congenital tibial hemimelia-related discrepancy than what has been reported previously.

Desanctis et al. [105] published three cases of Jones type II deficiencies treated with staged reconstruction. They corrected the foot deformity with serial casting and posteromedial soft tissue release followed by tibiofibular diaphyseal reconstruction, alignment of axis of the foot and leg, and limb lengthening using the Ilizarov technique. Javid [108] reported on a lengthening after centralization of the fibula in a Jones IIb deformity. They found that the fibula had delayed new bone formation, and compression-distraction technique with an Ilizarov device had to be utilized to promote osteogenesis. Devitt reported good results with differential lengthening of two cases of Weber type I deficiency [66].

Eidelman et al. [109] described a case of Jones type IV tibial hemimelia treated with staged reconstruction and lengthening. In the first stage, simultaneous correction of foot alignment, fibular shortening, temporary epiphysiodesis of the proximal tibia and fibula, and gradual tibial lengthening were performed. The patient underwent two subsequent lengthenings (one with an intramedullary device) and a contralateral epiphysiodesis of the distal femur and proximal tibia. At skeletal maturity, the patient had near normal ankle and foot function with equal leg lengths.

Weber Patellar Arthroplasty (Patelloplasty)

The Weber patelloplasty was published in 2002 [110] and describes a complex procedure in which the patella is converted into a tibial plateau. The knee contracture is gradually distracted with an external fixator to avoid the need to shorten the femur or fibula. The patella is brought down acutely with crossing "capsular visor" flaps and is chondrodesed to a centralized fibula. A Z-plasty of the quadriceps tendon is used to gain length and a hinged external ring fixator is used to stabilize while allowing knee range of motion and weight bearing. A second procedure is done later to achieve chondrodesis between the distal fibula and the talus. To our knowledge, there have been no publications of results of this procedure, though Weber did further describe and refine his procedure in 2006 [74]. Laufer et al. reported on 2 patients treated with a modified Weber patelloplasty after external fixator distraction with 2- and 8-year follow-up [111]. Both patients had significant coronal instability and required the use of a KAFO for ambulation at final follow-up. One patient had a 40 degree knee flexion contracture and the other had a knee extension contracture. They concluded that in families where amputation is not an acceptable option, reconstruction can provide a weight bearing limb with the use of an orthosis.

> **Box 31.3 Treatment Options**
> - Outcomes for the Brown procedure (centralization of the fibula) depend on the presence of a quadriceps mechanism and a mobile knee without flexion contractures.
> - Progressive knee flexion contractures and knee instability are common reasons for failure of the Brown procedure.
> - The presence of a proximal tibia or its anlage has had good results from synostosis with the fibula.
> - For some parents, a quicker and more definitive knee disarticulation may be a more attractive option, allowing a child to adapt early to a prosthesis.
> - Distal tibia deficiencies can be treated with distal fusion or synostosis or Syme-type amputation.
> - Advances in limb lengthening allow for limb length equalization.
> - The Weber patelloplasty converts an existing patella into a proximal tibia.

Limb Reconstruction Surgery (Senior Author's Preferred Techniques)

Since Brown introduced centralization of the fibula, many attempts to reconstruct the knee in the most severe types (Jones Ia, Paley 5) have been made. These have met with poor results, as previously discussed. Furthermore, knee reconstruction with the Brown procedure was always combined with foot amputation and prosthetic fitting. Knee reconstruction with foot and ankle reconstruction was not even considered prior to modern distraction methods [101]. Similarly, poor results of reconstruction for Jones types II and IV, Paley types 2, 3, and 4 have led most surgeons to conclude that through-knee amputation for Jones type I, through- or below-knee amputation for Jones type II, and Syme's amputation for Jones type IV are the best treatment for each type of tibial hemimelia. In light of modern prosthetic advancement, this is a logical and reasonable option that should be considered as the most tried and proven methods of treatment. More recently, advances in the treatment of all types of tibial hemimelia offer new options with excellent functional results as an alternative to amputation. The rest of this manuscript will focus on the reconstructive options for tibial hemimelia according to Paley type and subtype.

Paley Type 1 (Fig. 31.9)

These patients can have unilateral or bilateral involvement. The latter are usually familial with autosomal dominant inheritance. They have a hypoplastic but nondeficient tibia with intact, stable knees and ankles. The proximal fibula is overgrown and may articulate with the side of the femur. The tibia is short and genu valgum is often present. The valgus is usually from the proximal tibia, but can also originate from the distal femur. If treated when the physes are open, valgus can be corrected using temporary hemiepiphysiodesis and can be combined with epiphysiodesis of the proximal fibula to address the relative overgrowth. If bilateral, the biggest complaint patients have is mesomelic disproportion and short stature. When unilateral, there is a leg length discrepancy. If small, this discrepancy can be addressed with contralateral epiphysiodesis if desired. In bilateral cases, only the valgus deformity may need to be corrected if leg lengths are equal. Gradual deformity correction and lengthening can be considered in unilateral cases to equalize leg lengths or bilateral cases for correction of disproportionate short stature. In regard to the overgrown proximal end of the fibula, which often articulates with the side of the femur, it is preferable to leave it alone and not distract it distally. This avoids the problem of a knee flexion contracture that can result from transporting the fibula distally. If the proximal fibula is producing a noticeable bump that is bothersome to the patient, the tibia can be lengthened without cutting the fibula, transporting the fibula distally, but there is some risk of knee flexion contracture developing during distraction.

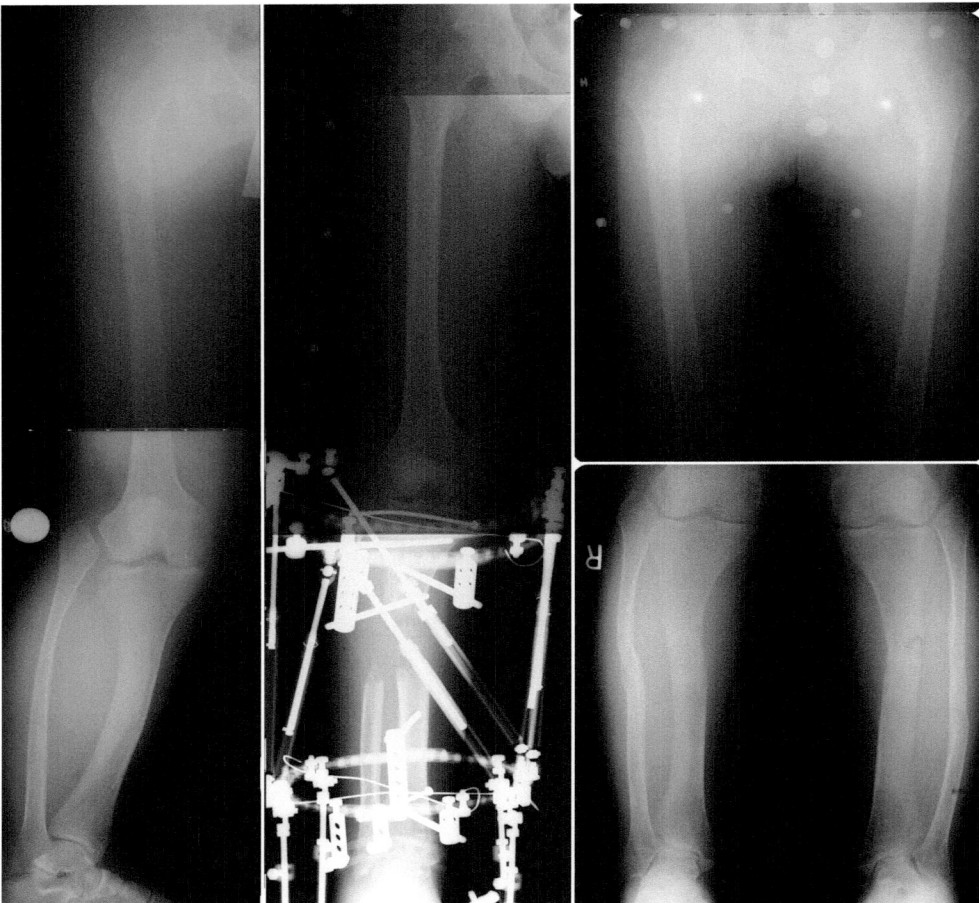

Fig. 31.9 Standing orthoroentgenogram of left lower limb preoperatively (left). This shows overgrowth of the fibula whose head is articulating with the lateral femur. The knee and ankle joint are stable and well formed. This is a mild type of tibial hemimelia classified as Paley type 1. It can be unilateral or bilateral as in this patient. The primary clinical problem is the genu valgum and the mesomelic disproportion. The patient underwent lengthening with realignment of the tibial valgus using a computer-dependent hexapodal external fixator (middle radiograph). The proximal fibula was fixed to the upper ring to prevent distal migration which can cause flexion contracture. Standing orthoroentgenogram both lower limbs (right) after healing bilateral lengthening and realignment tibia. The mesomelic disproportion was normalized. The fibular head position was not changed. (Copyright The Paley Foundation. Reproduced with permission. All rights reserved)

Paley Type 2

Patients with type 2 tibial hemimelia have a proximal and distal tibial epiphysis articulating as the knee and ankle. The knee is mobile but often unstable due to absence of cruciate ligaments and depression or deficiency of part of the tibial plateau. The distal tibial plafond is present but often dysplastic and thus the ankle does not have much motion. The presence of a plafond differentiates type 2 from type 3. Ankle diastasis is not typical, but some degree may be present depending on the severity of dysplastic changes of the tibial plafond. The foot is usually in equinovarus.

Paley Type 2a (Figs. 31.10 and 31.11)

There is a well-formed distal tibial physis that is separate from the proximal tibial physis. The tibial plafond is present but dysplastic. The foot is in marked equinovarus and is internally rotated relative to the knee. If the foot equinovarus deformity exceeds the malorientation of the tibial plafond, which is due to bony deformity, the ankle should first be distracted with an external fixator to correct the soft tissue contracture. The circular external fixator extends from the tibia to the foot, and the ankle is distracted out of equinovarus. In a second stage, an osteotomy of the tibia is performed, and

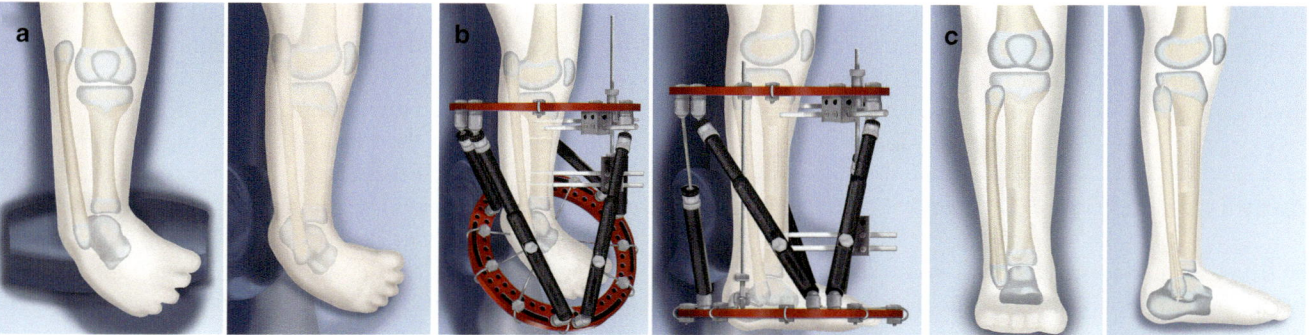

Fig. 31.10 Treatment of Paley type 2A. (**a**) Typical deformity with shortened tibia and equinovarus foot and overgrown proximal fibula (left AP, right lateral). (**b**) Application of external fixator for staged correction of foot equinovarus, distal fibular transport, and finally lengthening of the tibia. (left before distraction, right after distraction) (**c**) Final result after tibial lengthening with distal fibular screw epiphysiodesis (left AP, right lateral). (Copyright The Paley Foundation. Reproduced with permission. All rights reserved)

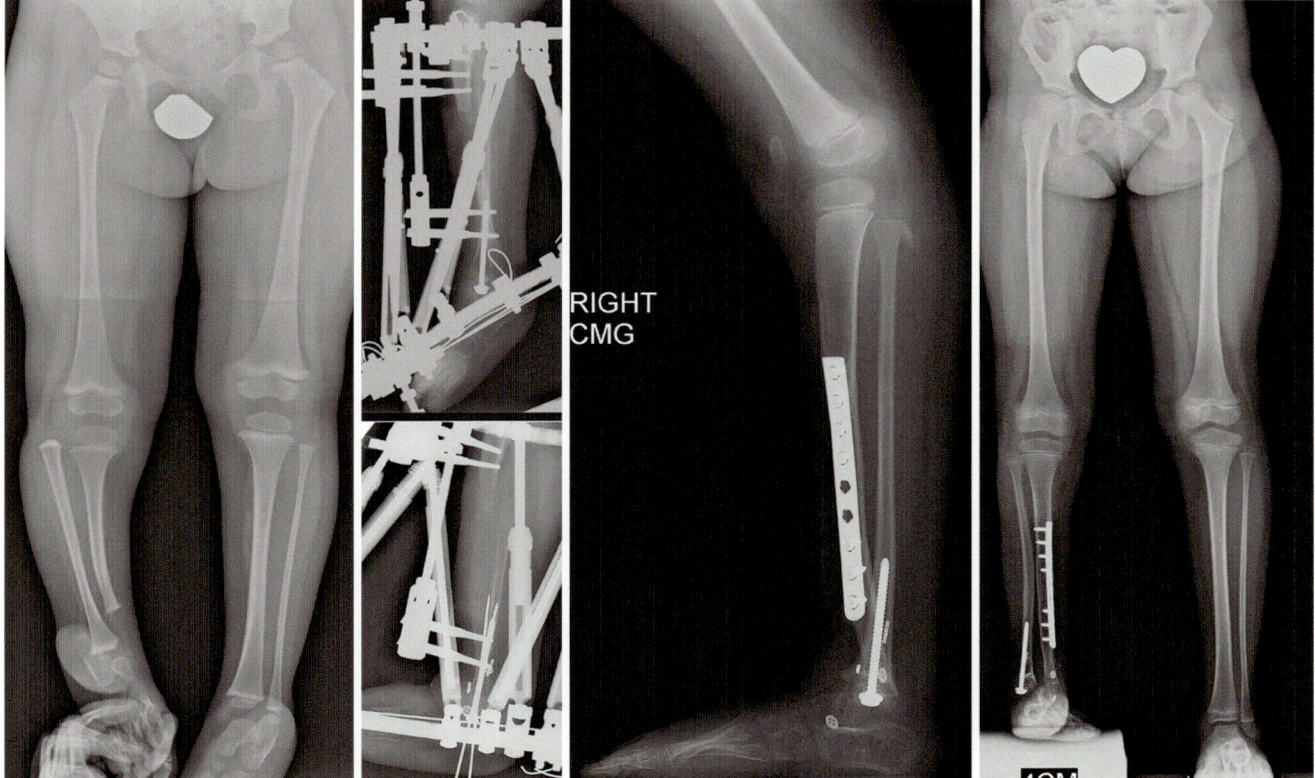

Fig. 31.11 Orthoroentgenogram of a 2-year-old girl with Paley type 2a unilateral tibial hemimelia, with equinovarus deformity of the foot and varus and varus deformity of the tibial diaphysis and proximal overgrowth of fibula. There is no diastasis of the distal tibiofibular joint. The ankle joint is present and dysplastic, a distal tibial epiphysis is present (left). Lateral radiographs showing computer dependent hexapod external fixator applied to the foot and leg (top left middle) with gradual correction of foot deformity (bottom left middle) and lengthening of tibia with distal transport of fibula. Final radiographs of tibia (right middle and right) showing consolidation of the regenerate bone (plate application was used to prevent refracture) and distal fibular screw epiphysiodesis to prevent fibular overgrowth. The foot is plantigrade, and the knee alignment is neutral. There is a 4cm leg length discrepancy (LLD) that will need future lengthening surgery. (Copyright The Paley Foundation. Reproduced with permission. All rights reserved)

the fibula is fixed to the distal ring. This allows the tibia to be lengthened simultaneously with distal fibular transport to bring the fibula to station proximally. The distal fibula is epiphysiodesed to prevent overgrowth.

Paley Type 2b (Figs. 31.12 and 31.13)

This type is often associated with syndromes (e.g., Werner's dysplasia). There is usually duplication of toes. The proximal and distal tibial physes are connected through a bracket epiphysis with malorientation of the knee and ankle joints. The bracket epiphysis can be oriented in any direction and does not always correspond to the deformity seen. The fibula is much longer than the tibia. The treatment in these cases requires consideration of the location of the bracket. To interrupt the bracket, the cartilage of the epiphysis and physis is resected and a tibial osteotomy is performed through the bone at the same level for acute or gradual correction. For acute correction, an opening wedge on the side of the bracket is performed along with a fibular shortening osteotomy to correct the varus deformity. Fixation is obtained with axial retrograde wires entering through the foot. This is followed by gradual lengthening at a separate time. For gradual correction, the external fixator is applied to the femur and extends down to attach to the upper tibia. Angular correction and lengthening are then performed simultaneously.

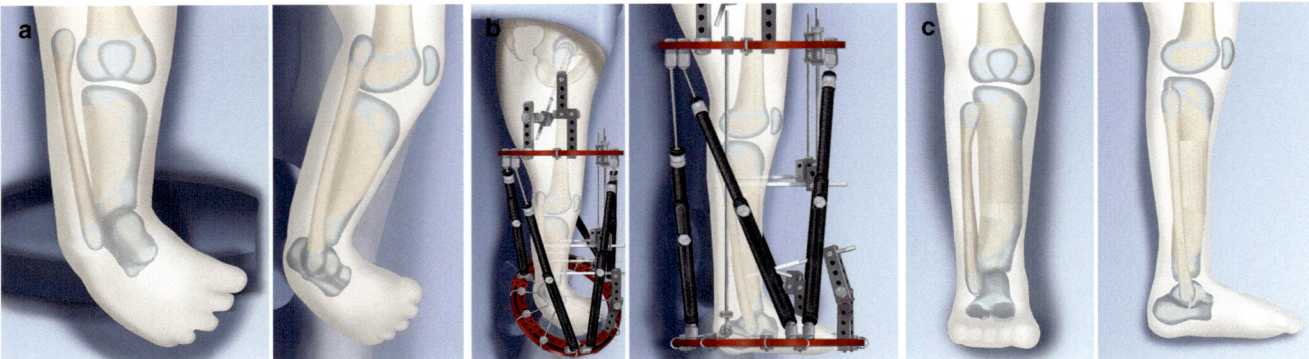

Fig. 31.12 Treatment of Paley type 2B. (**a**) Bracket epiphysis deformity of tibia AP (left), lateral (right). (**b**) Application of external fixator after excision of bracket (left), with staged gradual foot correction, distal fibular transport, and tibial lengthening (right). (**c**) Final result: foot plantigrade; fibula at station with a distal epiphysiodesis; tibia to fibula lengths restored (AP, left; lateral, right). (Copyright The Paley Foundation. Reproduced with permission. All rights reserved)

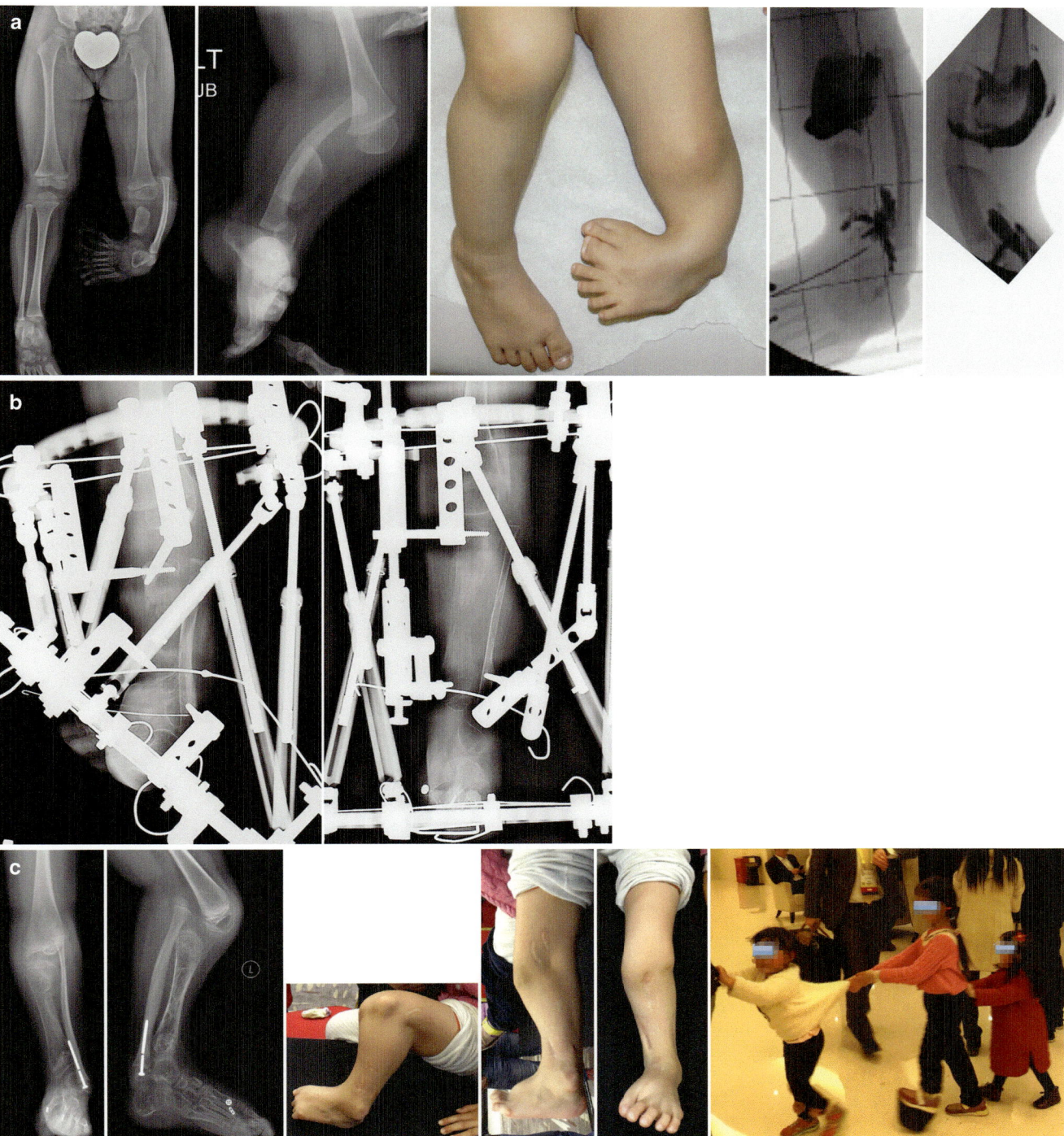

Fig. 31.13 (**a**) AP and lateral radiographs (left) and photograph (middle) of a 3-year-old girl with left side Paley type 2b tibial hemimelia +3metatarsals and toes. Intraoperative arthrogram AP and lateral of the knee and ankle (right), showing the recurvatum deformity of both joints and the flat dysplastic appearance of the ankle joint on the lateral view. On the AP view, the ankle is in varus and has a ball and socket appearance. (**b**) AP radiograph of tibia showing the external fixation during lengthening and before the foot correction (left). AP radiograph of tibia at the end of 8cm of lengthening, fibular transport, and foot correction (right). (**c**) Radiographs of the tibia 2 years after external fixator removal, showing a plantigrade foot and a recurvatum of the upper tibia and recurrence of proximal fibular overgrowth despite the screw epiphysiodesis of the distal fibula (left). Photographs showing knee range of motion (0–90°), mild knee valgus and a plantigrade foot with some forefoot supination typical of TH (middle). This girl remains very active and keeps up with her peers. She is shown playing with two other girls. She is the tall girl in the middle walking with a shoe lift. (Copyright The Paley Foundation. Reproduced with permission. All rights reserved)

Paley Type 2c (Figs. 31.14 and 31.15)

The distinguishing feature in this type of tibial hemimelia is delayed ossification of the distal tibial anlage. The distal tibial physis is absent. MRI is useful to confirm the presence of the anlage and to characterize the articulation between the tibia and the talus. Based on this imaging, a decision can be made as to whether the tibial deformity needs to be corrected to reorient the ankle to the knee. The ankle joint, while present in these cases, is not functional, and the goal is to create a plantigrade foot with a stable ankle. This usually requires distraction of the foot through the ankle joint, followed by an osteotomy in a second stage for deformity correction and lengthening, similar to the treatment for type 2a. Because the fibula is significantly longer than the tibia, two options can be considered to address the fibula: (1) resection of the mid-diaphysis of the fibula in an attempt to create a fibular nonunion and prevent recurrent fibular overgrowth, or (2) lengthening of the tibia without fixation of the fibula, which pulls the fibula down to its correct station at the knee and ankle.

Untreated, the unossified portion of the tibia will eventually ossify after many years which is why it is referred to as delayed ossification. To accelerate this process, bone morphogenic protein 2 (BMP-2) can be inserted into the cartilage. The use of BMP-2 in children is still considered off-label, and it may cause localized swelling but has had few directly attributable complications [112]. The basis of its use in tibial hemimelia is the author's experience using BMP-2 in delayed ossification of the femoral neck to promote ossification in congenital femoral deficiency [113]. Ossification of the tibia facilitates lengthening and deformity correction of the tibia through bone. If sufficient parts of the tibia are bony, an osteotomy can be made through the bony portion and pins placed in the bony portion. If an insufficient portion of the tibia is ossified to allow for external fixation, open surgery is performed to acutely realign the foot with a tibial osteotomy along with a fibular shortening osteotomy. BMP-2 is inserted into drill holes in the cartilage of the non-ossified portion of the tibia either at the time of acute osteotomy or the lengthening osteotomy. Stabilization of an acute osteotomy is achieved with retrograde axial wires through the foot and up the tibia. In most cases, ossification of the anlage is seen by 3 months after BMP-2 implantation. After acute correction, lengthening is typically done one year later when ossification of the anlage is complete.

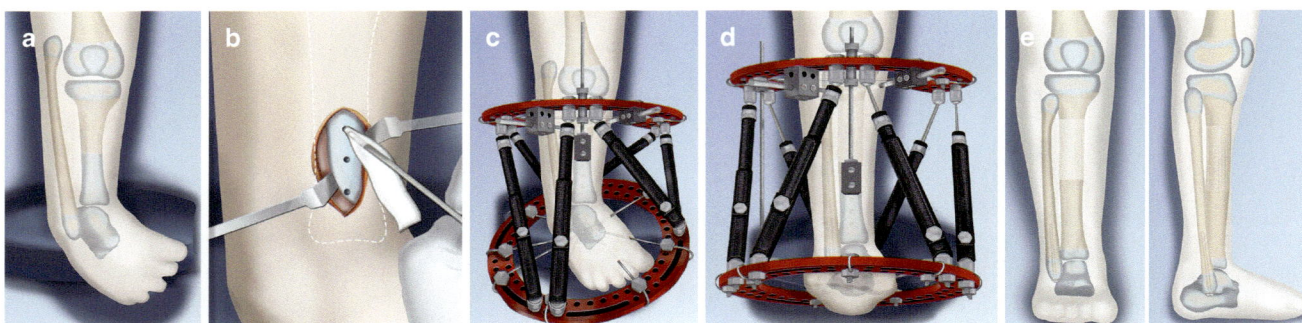

Fig. 31.14 Treatment of Paley type 2C. (**a**) Distal tibia cartilaginous anlage with no physis. (**b**) Insertion of bone morphogenic protein (BMP2) into tibial anlage. (**c**) External fixator for correction of foot deformity and distal fibular transport. (**d**) Tibial osteotomy and lengthening with fixator. (**e**) Final results after tibial lengthening with fibula at station and foot plantigrade. The distal tibia is now ossified secondary to the BMP2. (Copyright The Paley Foundation. Reproduced with permission. All rights reserved)

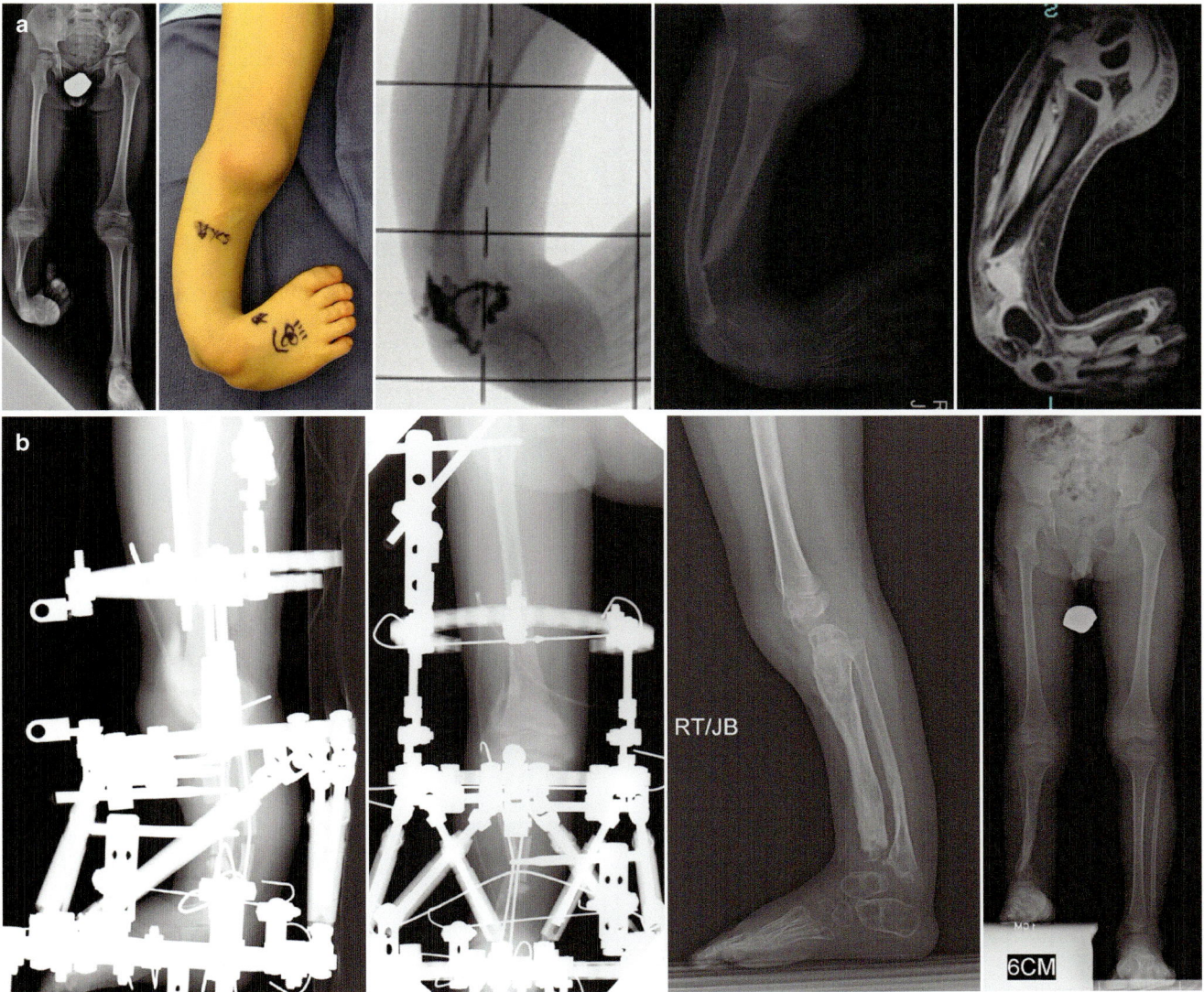

Fig. 31.15 (a) Radiograph (left) and clinical photograph (second to left) showing the severe equinovarus deformity of the foot and leg length discrepancy. Arthrogram showing the dysplastic ankle joint which is ball and socket and has varus malorientation (middle). AP radiograph shows the unossified region at the end of the tibia (second to right). This area is confirmed to be filled with unossified cartilage on the MRI (right). (b) Lateral and AP radiographs of tibia and femur (left), showing a hinged frame stabilizing the knee joint and a computer dependent hexapod external fixator on the tibia being used for foot correction and lengthening and distal fibular transport. Lateral and AP final radiographs (right) showing a plantigrade foot and an ossified distal tibia. (Copyright The Paley Foundation. Reproduced with permission. All rights reserved)

Paley Type 3a (Figs. 31.16 and 31.17)

Type 3 tibial hemimelia is characterized by distal tibiofibular diastasis and absence of the tibial plafond. The medial and lateral malleoli are present, and the talus is often located between the tibia and fibula due to absence of the plafond. The talus is proximally migrated relative to the distal tibia, but remains at the correct level relative to the distal fibula. The tibia may have a varus bow of its distal diaphysis. The foot is in an equinovarus position, internally rotated around the tibia and always remains with the fibula.

Since the ankle joint is to be reconstructed, the Achilles tendon is not cut, but a gastrosoleus recession may be performed. The foot is repositioned by gradual distraction using a circular ring external fixator. To prevent epiphysiolysis of the proximal and distal fibula, a 1.5-mm wire is drilled retrograde into the fibula and up the fibular diaphysis to exit through the proximal fibular epiphysis. The wire is

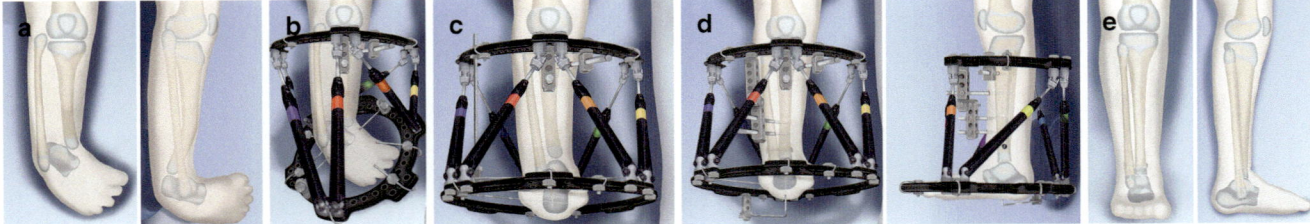

Fig. 31.16 Treatment of Paley type 3A. (**a**) Distal tibia-fibula diastasis AP and lateral views. The tibial plafond is absent and the end of the tibia is what normally would have been a medial malleolus; foot and fibula internally rotated around tibia. (**b**) Application of external fixator for gradual correction of foot and fibula position. (**c**) After distraction foot centralized under end of tibia, ready for tibiotalar arthroplasty. (**d**) Distal tibia reshaping to talus and stabilization of distal tibia and fibula diastasis and osteotomy of tibia for diaphyseal straightening. (**e**) Final result after hardware removal with plantigrade foot and distal fibula screw epiphysiodesis. (Copyright The Paley Foundation. Reproduced with permission. All rights reserved)

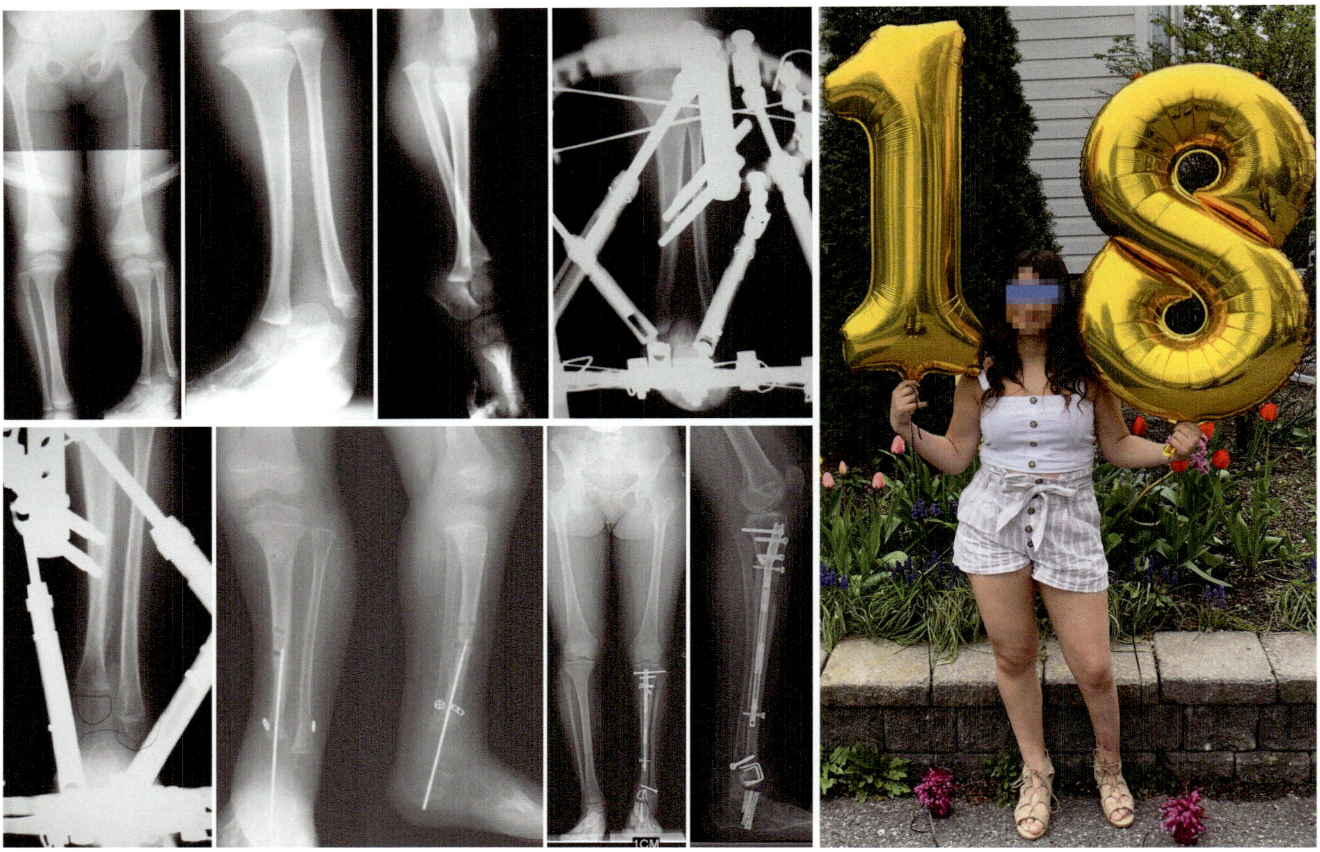

Fig. 31.17 Orthoroentgenogram, and AP and lateral tibial radiographs of Paley type 3a tibial hemimelia. There is an obvious distal tibiofibular diastasis with proximal herniation of the talus in the gap. The lateral radiograph shows the fibula and foot crossing anteriorly to the distal tibia. This appearance is due to the internal rotation of the tibia and foot around the tibia (top left). A computer-dependent hexapod external fixator is attached to the tibia and foot for gradual correction of the deformities (top middle). The order of correction is external rotation and distal fibular transport of the tibia and foot to bring the talus distal to the level of the distal tibial malleolus, followed by gradual correction of equinovarus foot deformity (bottom left). Ankle arthrotomy combined with biologic arthroplasty of the tibiotalar articulation combined with syndesmotic reconstruction using a suture-washer compression system is performed (bottom left middle). This girl underwent three lengthening procedures, the last of which was with a precice nail. This last procedure was combined with a supramalleolar osteotomy and a subtalar osteotomy for foot ankle realignment and stability (bottom right middle) resulting in a painless, mobile, plantigrade foot, and equal leg lengths. She is shown here at her 18th birthday wearing fashionable shoes, leading a normal life, including her passion of dance and drama. (Copyright The Paley Foundation. Reproduced with permission. All rights reserved)

brought through the skin proximally and then bent backwards on itself to form a hook. A small proximal incision is made and the wire is pulled back into the fibular head to lock into the proximal epiphysis. Distally, the wire is also bent 180°, then shortened and buried under the skin. This creates a temporary epiphysiodesis of the proximal and distal fibula.

One ring is applied to the proximal tibia with one wire and two half pins. The second ring is applied to the foot with three calcaneal wires and one talar wire. The equinovarus deformity is corrected by gradual distraction, with repositioning the talus under the distal tibial epiphysis. Since the fibula is overgrown relative to the tibia, it does not need to be fixed to the distal ring. Its association with the talus and calcaneus causes it to follow the foot distally. This moves the fibula from its relatively overgrown proximal position down to the normal station.

Once the foot is located under the distal tibial epiphysis, a planned second-stage surgery can be carried out. Under general anesthesia, the distal ring and wires are removed. The pin sites are covered by an occlusive dressing and the leg is prepped and draped free. A transverse incision is made on the medial side at the level of the tip of the medial malleolus. The tibiotalar joint is opened, and the distal tibia and proximal talus are exposed. The tibialis posterior tendon is often found dislocated between the tibia and fibula, where the plafond should have been located. It is moved out of this location and retracted posteromedial to the tibia to allow the fibula and tibia to come together. The distal end of the tibial cartilage is carved with a knife to the concavity of the tibial plafond, matching the convexity of the dome of the talus, creating a biologic arthroplasty. A retrograde axial wire, perpendicular to the sole of the foot, is passed through the dome of the talus, through the epiphysis of the distal tibia, and continues proximally into the tibial diaphysis. If the tibia has a varus diaphyseal bow to it, a percutaneous osteotomy should be made at the apex of this bow with an acute angular correction, straightening the tibia. The wire is advanced up the tibia to stabilize this osteotomy.

The tibiofibular diastasis is treated next. This is fixed by using a syndesmotic suture system such as the Arthrex-Tightrope™ or the Biomet-Ziptite™. The syndesmotic suture with its two washers is used to reduce and compress across the diastasis. The incision is then closed and the foot ring is reapplied with three new wires. This helps ensure that the foot remains in a plantigrade position.

The external fixator is left in place for 3 more months. The fibular wire and the transarticular tibial wire should be left in place even after fixator removal. The transarticular wire can be advanced into the calcaneus to allow for weight bearing. The author prefers to leave both of these in place for 6 more months. This serves several purposes: prevention of fracture of the now osteoporotic tibia and fibula, stabilization of the ankle joint to prevent recurrence of equinus, and retardation of the faster-growing fibula to prevent recurrent relative overgrowth. Six months later, both wires should be surgically removed. A solid ankle-foot orthosis (AFO) is used until the wires are removed, after which the patient is placed into an articulated AFO with a plantarflexion stop. Physical therapy is initiated after the transarticular ankle wire is removed.

> **Box 31.4 Surgical Tips**
> - Due to often aberrant anatomy, we recommend a mini-open incision for the Achilles tenotomy.
> - A single 1.5-mm intramedullary wire protects the fibular physes at both ends and prevents epiphysiolysis.
> - After the ankle arthroplasty, pass the wire antegrade through the center of the dome of the talus, then pass it retrograde through the distal tibia.
> - A syndesmotic suture-washer implant can be used to close the diastasis between the tibia and fibula.

Paley Type 3b (Figs. 31.18 and 31.19)

In this type of tibial hemimelia, there is a cleft between the tibia and fibula in addition to the diastasis. The first stage of treatment is the same as for type 3A. The talus is corrected out of equinovarus and brought down below the level of the distal tibial epiphysis. The second stage of surgery includes syndesmotic repair between the tibia and fibula, biologic arthroplasty of the tibiotalar joint, and closure of the skin cleft.

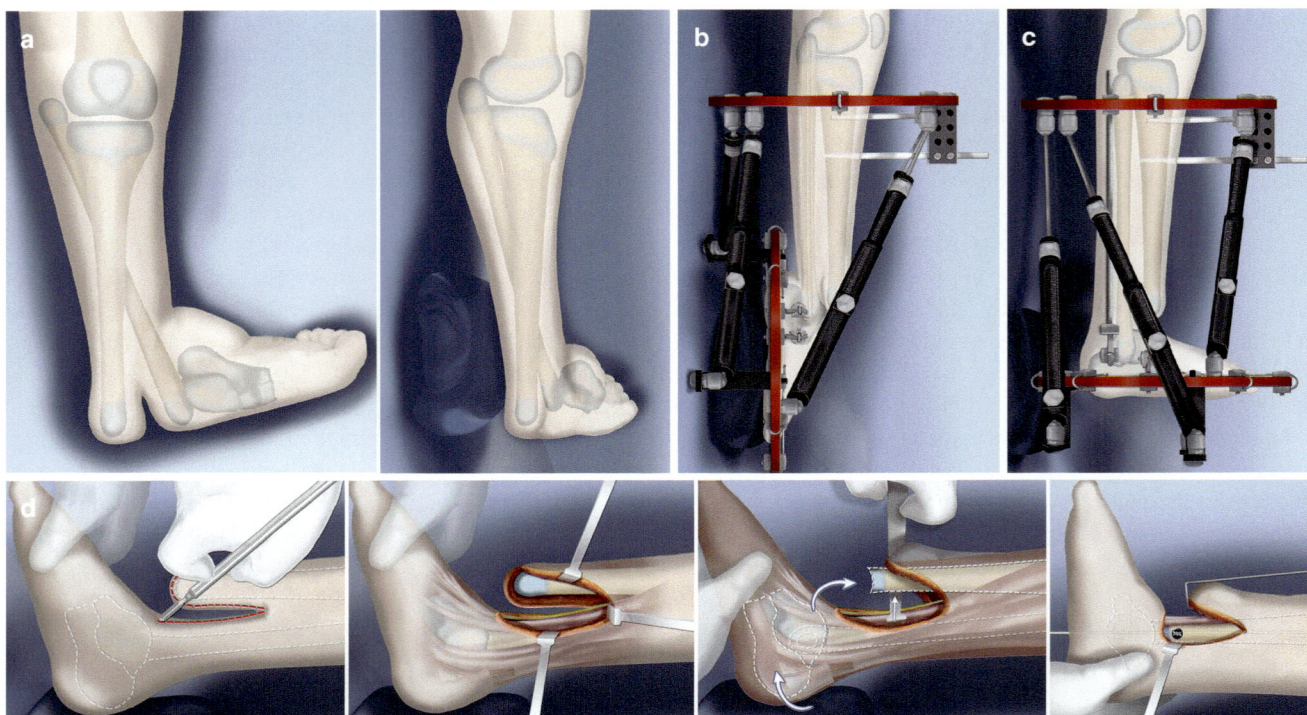

Fig. 31.18 Treatment of Paley type 3B. (**a**) Distal tibia and fibula diastasis with skin cleft. Fibula is associated with talus and foot (AP left, Lateral right). (**b**) Application of external fixator for distraction and gradual correction. (**c**) After distraction fibula is now at station and foot is in plantigrade position with the talus beneath the tibial epiphysis. (**d**) Excision and closure of skin cleft performed at same time as tibiofibular diastasis closure and tibiotalar biologic arthroplasty as in type 3A. (Copyright The Paley Foundation. Reproduced with permission. All rights reserved)

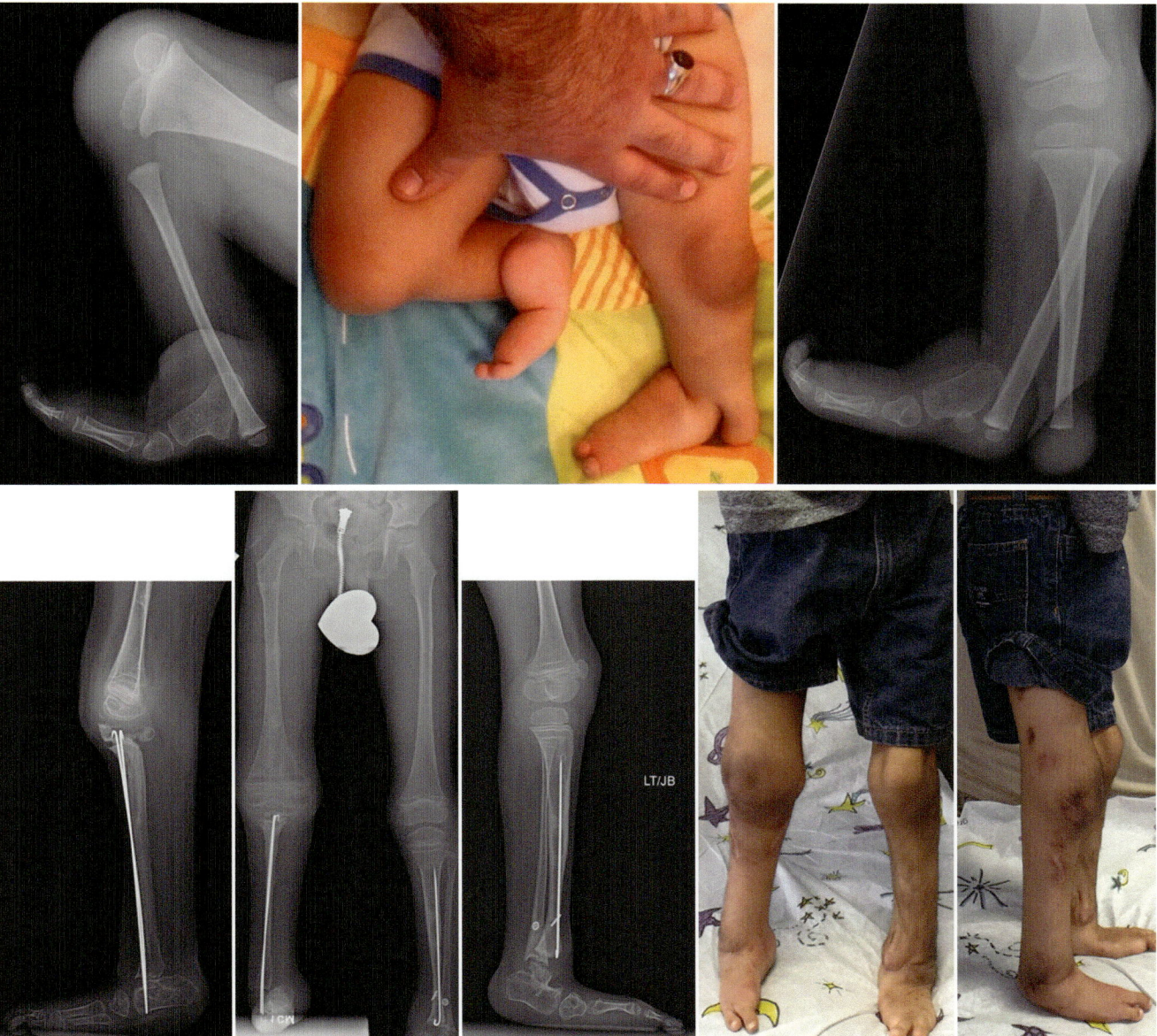

Fig. 31.19 Preoperative radiographs and photograph of bilateral tibial hemimelia, Paley type 5a on right and Paley type 3b on left (top row). AP and lateral standing radiographs following Paley-Weber patelloplasty on the right and diastasis-cleft reconstruction with biologic ankle arthroplasty on the left (bottom left). This resulted in full knee extension and plantigrade feet and functional knees bilaterally (bottom right). (Copyright The Paley Foundation. Reproduced with permission. All rights reserved)

Paley Type 4

In this type, the degree of deficiency of the proximal tibia varies, but the knee joint is present and functional with preservation of the proximal tibial epiphysis. The foot is in very severe equinovarus. The lack of a distal tibia makes creating a mobile ankle joint impossible. To reestablish integrity of the tibia, the fibula is transferred to the tibia at the level of agenesis. Articulating the talus with the distal fibula in a biologic arthroplasty has met with recurrent deformity and failure; therefore, fusion of the talus to the distal fibular epiphysis remains the best reconstructive option.

Type 4a (Figs. 31.20 and 31.21)

This is the most common type 4 seen. The proximal tibial epiphysis, physis, and metaphysis are well formed, a patella is present, and active and passive knee motions are present through a normal range. There is absence of the distal tibia

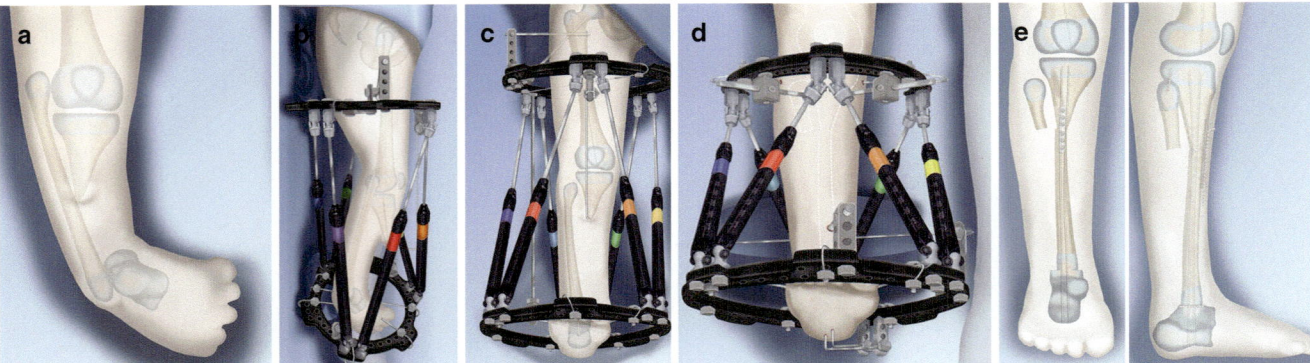

Fig. 31.20 Treatment of Paley type 4A. (**a**) Well-formed proximal tibia and knee with distal tibia aplasia. (**b**) External fixator used to gradually correct equinovarus foot position and distally transport fibular head. (**c**) Fibula brought down to station and foot plantigrade. (**d**) Fibular osteotomy performed with transfer to proximal tibia. Distal fibula epiphysis is fused to talus without damaging the distal fibular physis. External fixator remains in place 3 months to complete ankle fusion. (**e**) Intramedullary wires are left in place to allow the fibula to hypertrophy. (Copyright The Paley Foundation. Reproduced with permission. All rights reserved)

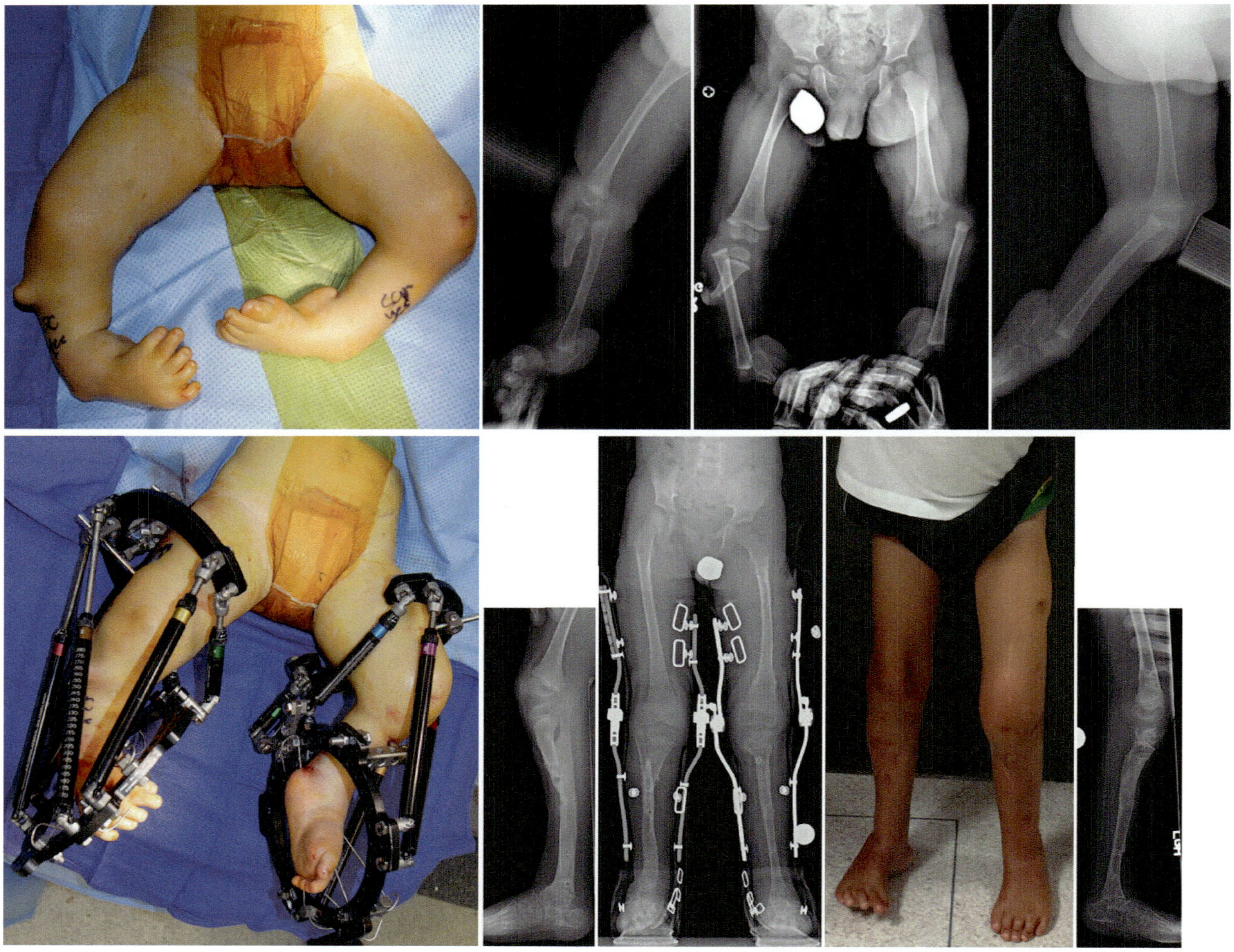

Fig. 31.21 Clinical photograph and radiographs of bilateral tibial hemimelia with Paley type 4a on the right and Paley type 4b on the left (top row). Both patellas are present. The left side appears like a Paley type 5a. MRI and clinical exam showed the presence of a proximal tibial cartilaginous anlage. Both feet are dislocated to the fibula and are in severe equinovarus. Bilateral computer-dependent hexapodal external fixators were applied for gradual distal fibular transport, distraction of the talus under the distal fibula, and correction of equinovarus foot deformity (bottom left). Staged transfer of the fibula to the tibial remnants was performed bilaterally, and both ankles had fibular epiphysis to talar fusions. This is seen in the AP and lateral radiographs and the clinical photograph (bottom right). BMP was used to ossify the left proximal tibial remnant. The right knee range of motion is 0–130°, and the left knee motion is 0–80°. He walks runs, jumps, and plays sports and is currently 12 years old. (Copyright The Paley Foundation. Reproduced with permission. All rights reserved)

from the level of the diaphysis with a pointed bone end often covered by a separate skin pouch. The fibula is overgrown and proximally migrated and the foot is in extreme equinovarus. The cruciate knee ligaments may be absent leading to instability. The goal of treatment is to correct the foot deformity, fuse the talus to the end of the fibular epiphysis distally, and transfer the fibular diaphysis to the distal end of the tibia proximally. This creates a one-bone leg. While this can be accomplished in one stage, it is safer, easier, and more length-preserving to do this in two stages.

The first stage involves an Achilles tenotomy followed by application of a circular external fixator to the femur, tibia, and foot. Two wires are inserted into the fibula and hooked around both ends of the fibula to prevent physiolysis during distraction. These are considered temporary epiphysiodesis wires. At the distal end of the fibula, one of these wires is bent at 90 degrees to be fixed to the distal tibial ring for distal transport of the fibula. A computer-dependent circular external fixator with one ring on the femur and one ring on the tibia is applied. The knee is locked in extension by inserting an axial wire through the distal tip of the tibia up to the level of the knee joint. This tibial wire is then bent at 90 degrees to connect to the femoral ring and hold the tibia in full extension. The femoral fixation includes two half-pins, one at the femoral neck and one at lesser trochanter, and one olive wire or a third half-pin at the level of the ring. There are no half-pins in the tibia; this avoids having a contaminated pin site in the operative field at the time of the second-stage surgery. The distal ring is fixed to three calcaneal wires and one transverse talar wire. Six struts are connected between the rings and computer planning is carried out.

Gradual distraction is done in two steps. In the first step, the proximal fibula is realigned to correct varus-flexion deformity at the knee and transported distally to bring the fibular head down to station next to the tibia. The temporary epiphysiodesis wires inside the fibula that are hooked around the head of the fibula prevent physiolysis during this distraction. It can take 6–12 weeks to complete this first step. The second step is to gradually correct the foot equinovarus. This is done by redoing the computer planning without any surgery. Prior to starting this second correction schedule, the fibular wire is disconnected from the distal ring and connected via a long threaded rod to the proximal ring. This holds the fibula at station, while the foot is corrected out of its deformed position and then distracted to bring the talus below the distal fibular epiphysis. The foot correction usually takes another 6–12 weeks, depending on the degree of equinovarus and the amount of lengthening required to transport the talus beneath the fibular epiphysis.

Once the foot is plantigrade and the talus is under the fibula, a second surgery to fuse the ankle and transfer the fibula to the tibia is performed. A few days before this surgery, the only tibial wire is removed to allow its pin site to heal prior to surgery. The first step is to remove the foot ring and wires and cover the pin sites with an occlusive dressing to minimize contamination during surgery. After the leg is prepped and draped free, a transverse lateral incision is made over the distal tip of the fibula. The distal epiphysis of the fibula and the dome of the talus are exposed. The capsular connections between them are cut to mobilize both bones relative to each other. A small incision is made proximally over the fibular wire. The fibular epiphysiodesis wires are cut proximally and pulled out distally. Two new wires are immediately inserted in the same track to protect the fibula from fracture. The fibula is often osteoporotic at this stage, and without an intramedullary wire, it can easily break upon manipulation of the foot or leg. The new wires are brought out proximally through the small incision made over the head of the fibula. The cartilage at the end of the fibula is cut back until the ossific nucleus of the fibula is reached. If there is no ossific nucleus, then BMP-2 can be inserted to promote ossification of the epiphysis. The ossific nucleus of the talus is exposed by cutting across the talar dome, parallel to the sole of the foot. The two ossific nuclei are then aligned, and the fibular wires are advanced from the proximal end through the talus and sole of the foot to hold the foot plantigrade to the fibula.

A Z-shaped incision is made around the accessory skin pouch at the end of the tibia. The proximal longitudinal limb of the Z is medial to the tip of the tibia, the transverse part is in the crease below the tip, and the longitudinal distal limb is lateral to the tibia. Fasciotomy of the anterior compartment is carried out. The distal tip of the tibia is uncovered. The anterior compartment muscles are elevated off the lateral aspect of the tibia, and an extra-periosteal path is dissected to the fibula along the interosseous membrane. The fibula is exposed subperiosteally. The tibia is osteotomized near its tip to create a fresh surface for union to the transferred fibula. The wires in the fibula are pulled back to the level of the planned osteotomy. The fibula osteotomy is made at the level of the tibial cut. The fibula is then shifted over to the tibia under the muscles. The fibula is fixed to the tibia by first advancing the intramedullary wires, then plating the two bones using a mini locking plate and screws. All of the incisions are now closed in layers. The external fixation wires in the foot are reinserted, fixed, and tensioned to a ring. Struts are now connected between the upper femoral ring and the distal foot ring. The external fixator maintains the alignment of the foot and knee to achieve fusion of the tibia and fibula proximally and of the fibula and talus distally. A transverse fibular wire is added to compress the ankle fusion site. Fusion usually takes 3 months. After that, the external fixator is removed, leaving one wire buried in the foot and fibula to protect the fibula from fracture. The knee motion is restored with physical therapy. In the future, lengthening of the one-bone leg can be carried out without crossing the knee joint. If symptomatic instability of the knee arises from the congenital absence of cruciate ligaments, the knee joint ligaments can be reconstructed prior to lengthening.

Type 4b (Figs. 31.21 and 31.22)

In this type, there is only a proximal tibial epiphysis and no proximal tibial physis. The proximal tibial epiphysis is often unossified at an early age. The foot is in severe equinovarus, and the fibula is relatively overgrown and proximally migrated at the knee. The treatment preferred is also a two-stage surgery, similar to that described for type 4a. There is often a knee flexion contracture present in these cases, which is also treated by distraction of the knee and foot with the same external fixator. Since the tibial epiphysis is so small, it needs to be fixed to the proximal femoral ring with an axial wire and/or a transverse tibial epiphysis wire to prevent the tibial epiphysis from being transported distally during the distal transport of the fibula. There are two options for fibular transport. The first option is to bring it down to station and then osteotomize as described for type 4a. The second option is to distract the fibular head below the level of the proximal tibial epiphysis. In this case, the proximal tibial epiphysis is fused to the proximal fibular epiphysis (Fig. 31.10 JCO, left leg). This has the advantage of preserving and transferring the proximal fibular physis to become the proximal tibial physis, thus reducing leg length discrepancy from the absence of a proximal tibial physis.

Since the proximal tibial epiphysis is too small for plating, intramedullary hooked wires as shown for Paley type 5a tibial hemimelia can be used instead (similar to Fig. 31.12h, i JCO). Cerclage wires between the tibial epiphysis and fibula can also create compression. If the proximal tibial epiphysis is unossified, then BMP-2 is inserted into drill holes in the epiphyseal cartilage. The fixator (similar to Fig. 31.12i JCO) remains in place for approximately 2–4 months until the proximal fibula fuses to the tibial epiphysis proximally and the distal fibular epiphysis fuses to the talus distally. After fixator removal, a cast is used for 1 month, followed by a knee-ankle-foot orthotic (KAFO). Knee range of motion is restored with physical therapy, including active and passive range of motion exercises.

> **Box 31.5 Synostosis and Ankle Fusion Tips**
> - The Paley type 4 lacks a distal tibia, and the goal is to obtain a fusion of the upper tibial remnant and the fibular diaphysis proximally, and a fusion of the distal fibular epiphysis and talar ossific nucleus distally.
> - The femoral ring is kept relatively high on the femur to stay out of the surgical field for subsequent surgeries.
> - Protect the fibula from physiolysis with an intramedullary temporary epiphysiodesis wire.
> - Once the proximal fibula is brought in line with the proximal tibia, switch the transverse wires in the fibula from the distal ring to the proximal ring. Then reprogram the computer-dependant external fixator to correct the foot deformity and to bring the talus under the fibular epiphysis.
> - Remove the tibial wire several days prior to the second surgery to minimize infection risk.
> - In the second surgery, cut the fibula as high as possible and transfer it to the tibia.
> - BMP-2 can be used to promote ossification of cartilage if there is no ossific nucleus in the distal fibula or talus.
> - Exchange the intramedullary wires in the fibula and maintain in place during the fibular osteotomy and ankle fusion to prevent a fracture from occurring in the now osteoporotic fibula at the time of the second surgery.
> - Use the external fixator and intramedullary wires to provide stability and maintain correction until fusion is achieved.
> - An arch wire can help provide compression to the talo-fibular fusion.

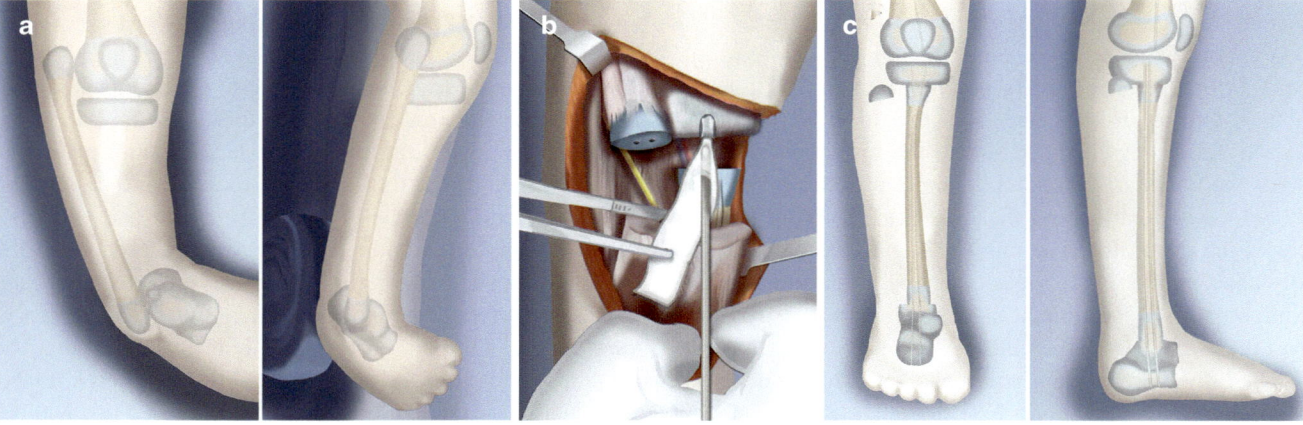

Fig. 31.22 Treatment of Paley type 4B. (**a**) Unossified proximal tibial anlage with no physis. Initial treatment the same as 4A, with fibula distraction and foot correction. (**b**) Insertion of BMP2 into proximal tibia anlage. (**c**) Fixator removal following healing from physeal sparing proximal fibula osteotomy and transfer to proximal tibia. Physeal sparing fibula-talar fusion. (Copyright The Paley Foundation. Reproduced with permission. All rights reserved)

Paley Type 5

Type 5 is characterized by tibial aplasia with a flexion contracture of the knee. Complete absence of the tibia presents the biggest challenge for reconstruction because there is no knee joint. While ankle fusion gives good function with little disability, knee fusion leads to significant disability for sitting and climbing stairs. It is preferable to avoid a knee fusion. Even if active knee motion cannot be achieved, a mobile knee joint supported by a brace is preferable to a knee fusion. This is not dissimilar to a paralytic knee from polio. Therefore, the following two methods have been developed to reconstruct the knee.

Paley Type 5a (Figs. 31.23, 31.24, 31.25, and 31.26)

Type 5a is characterized by presence of a patella and quadriceps muscle. If a patella is present, it can be converted to a tibial plateau. This original idea was first published by Michael Weber [74, 110]. The patella is moved on a vascular pedicle (visor capsular flaps) from its normal position, anterior to the femur, to the distal end of the femur. The fibula is centralized to the patella and its epiphysis fused to the patella. This procedure is referred to as the Weber patellar arthroplasty (patelloplasty) or Weber procedure.

Weber recommended performing the patellar arthroplasty as the index procedure combined with gradual correction of the remaining knee flexion contracture and foot equinovarus using a circular external fixator. Weber performed the patellar arthroplasty procedure through a longitudinal anterior incision. Fusion of the patella to the fibula was achieved using chondroplasty by suturing perichondral flaps of the patella and fibula together. A biologic arthroplasty of the ankle was carried out to stabilize the foot.

Paley modified the Weber procedure [76]. This Paley-Weber modification involves seven major changes to the original Weber procedure: (1) applying a computer-dependent external fixator to the femur, fibula, and foot, to sequentially and gradually reposition the fibula under the femur and the talus under the fibula; (2) protecting the fibula during this distraction with temporary epiphysiodesis wires to prevent fibular physiolysis; (3) using a transverse anterior incision across the knee joint to minimize wound complications; (4) dividing the upper pole of the patella when creating the upper visor flap to allow a patella to regenerate; (5) using hooked wires for stabilization of the patella-fibular fusion site; (6) ossifying the unossified patella in patients under age 4 by inserting BMP2 between the patella and the fibula to achieve an synostosis, not a chondrodesis; (7) fusion of the distal fibular epiphysis to the talus through a transverse lateral incision at the ankle.

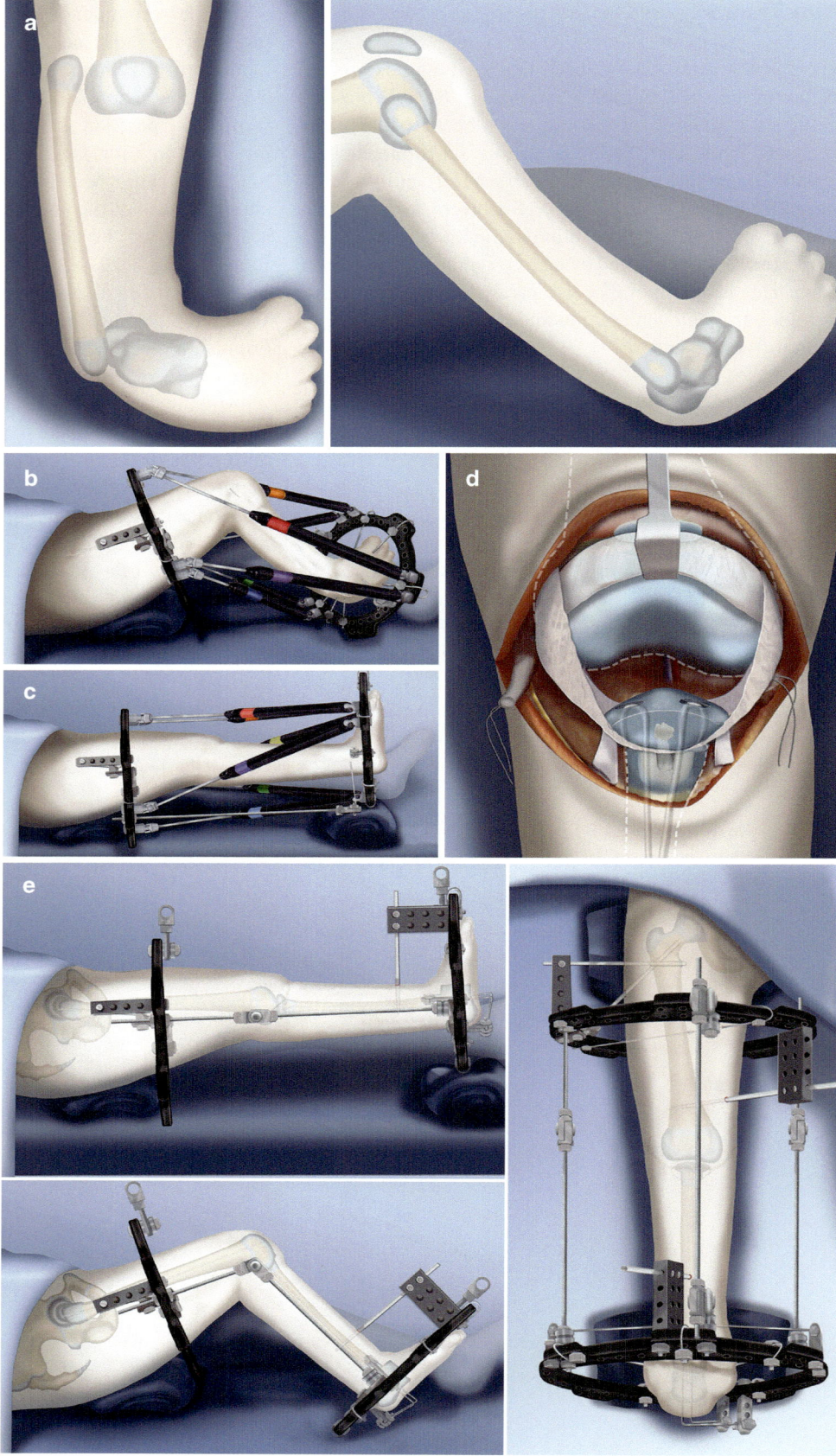

Fig. 31.23 Treatment of Paley type 5A. (**a**) Complete aplasia of tibia, but patella and quadriceps are present (AP left, lateral right). (**b**) External fixator placement for gradual fibula distraction and foot correction. (**c**) Knee flexion contracture corrected to straight position, preparing for physeal sparing patellar arthroplasty and physeal sparing talofibular fusion. (**d**) Paley-Weber patelloplasty converting the patella into a tibial plateau. (**e**) Hinged external fixator to protect arthroplasty but allow knee motion. (Copyright The Paley Foundation. Reproduced with permission. All rights reserved)

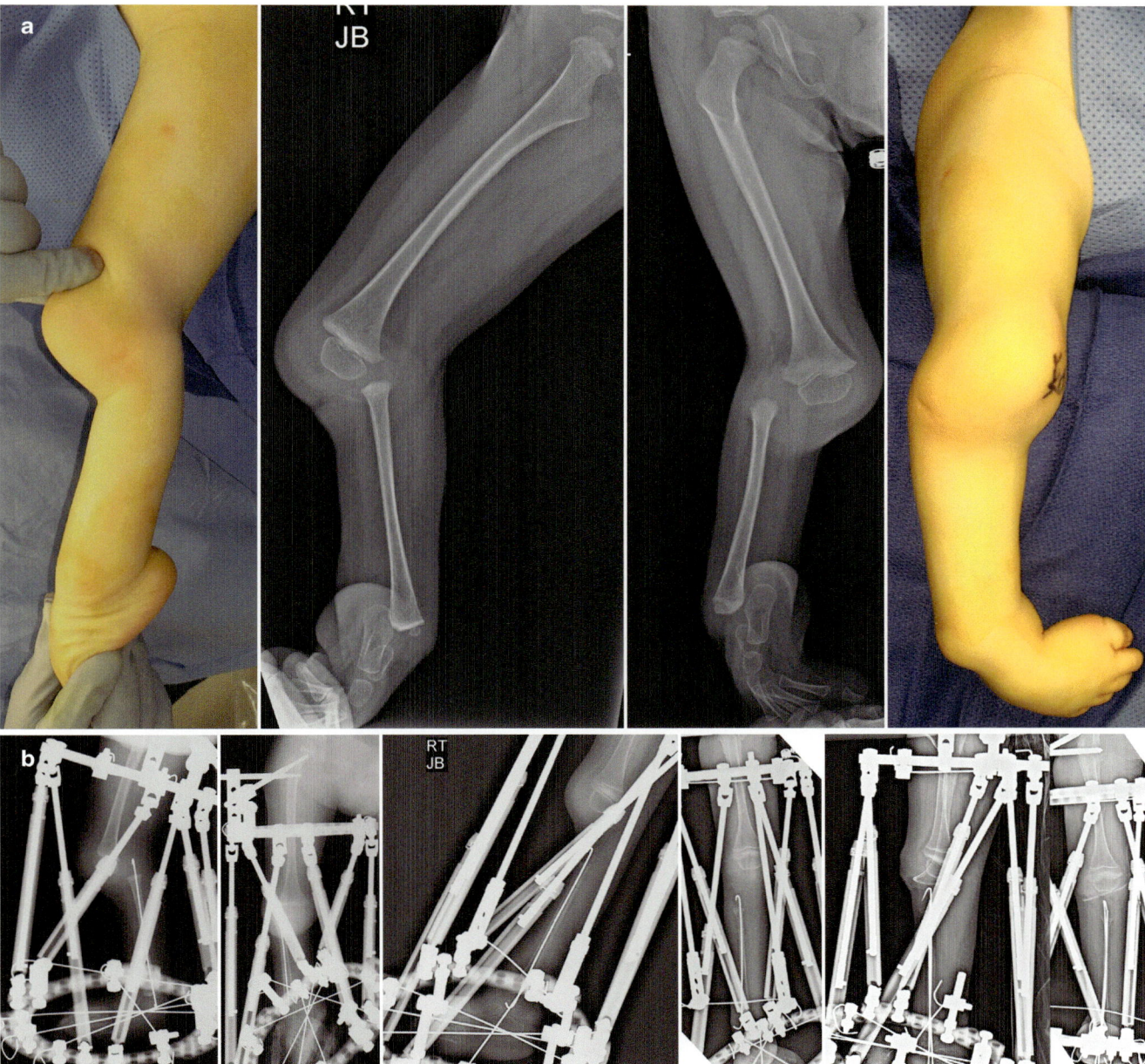

Fig. 31.24 (a) Lateral (left and center left) and AP (right and center right) photographs and radiographs of the right leg of a 2-year-old boy with bilateral tibial hemimelia. Only the right side is shown. The right side has Paley type 5A tibial hemimelia and the left side Paley type 4A. Note the flexion contracture of the right knee and the equino-varus-adductus foot deformity. (b) Lateral (left) and AP (right) radiographs showing the external fixator in place with femoral and foot rings. The fibula is secured to the foot ring with a transverse wire. Note the temporary epiphysiodesis wire in the fibula hooked at both ends. Also note the wire across the neck of the talus (left). Lateral (left) and AP (right) radiographs at the end of gradual distraction. The fibular head is centered under the end of the femur. The foot position has not changed, and the transverse fibular wires remain connected to the foot ring (middle). Intraoperative lateral (left) and AP (right) radiographs after the Paley-Weber patelloplasty with ankle fusion surgery. Note the Hemovac drain can be seen at the knee. BMP2 was inserted into a drill hole in the patella and proximal fibula lead to ossification and fusion of both the patella and fibular epiphysis. A transverse distal fibular wire is arced to the foot ring to apply compression across the fusion site (right). (c) Radiographs showing the patella and proximal fibular epiphysis are ossified and fused together with preservation of the proximal fibula physis (right). The patella now serves as a tibial plateau. The talus has also fused to the distal fibula but the distal fibular physis has closed. Clinical photographs, showing 90° of knee flexion (left) and full extension (middle). (Copyright The Paley Foundation. Reproduced with permission. All rights reserved)

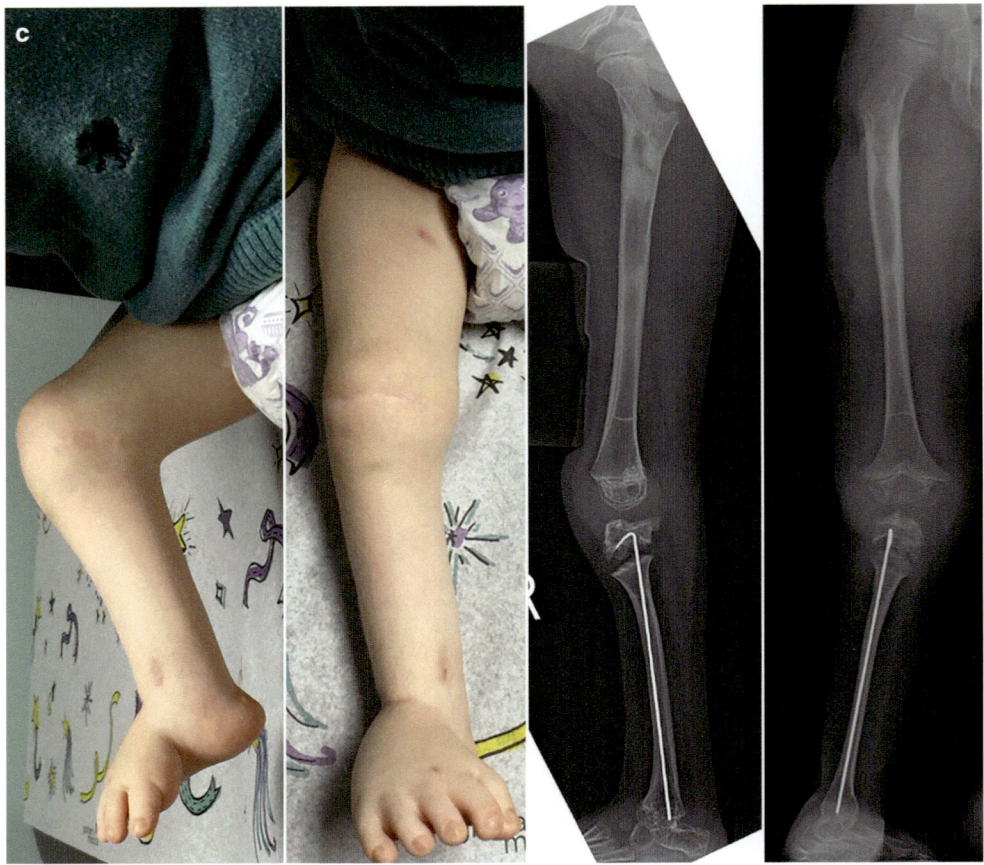

Fig. 31.24 (continued)

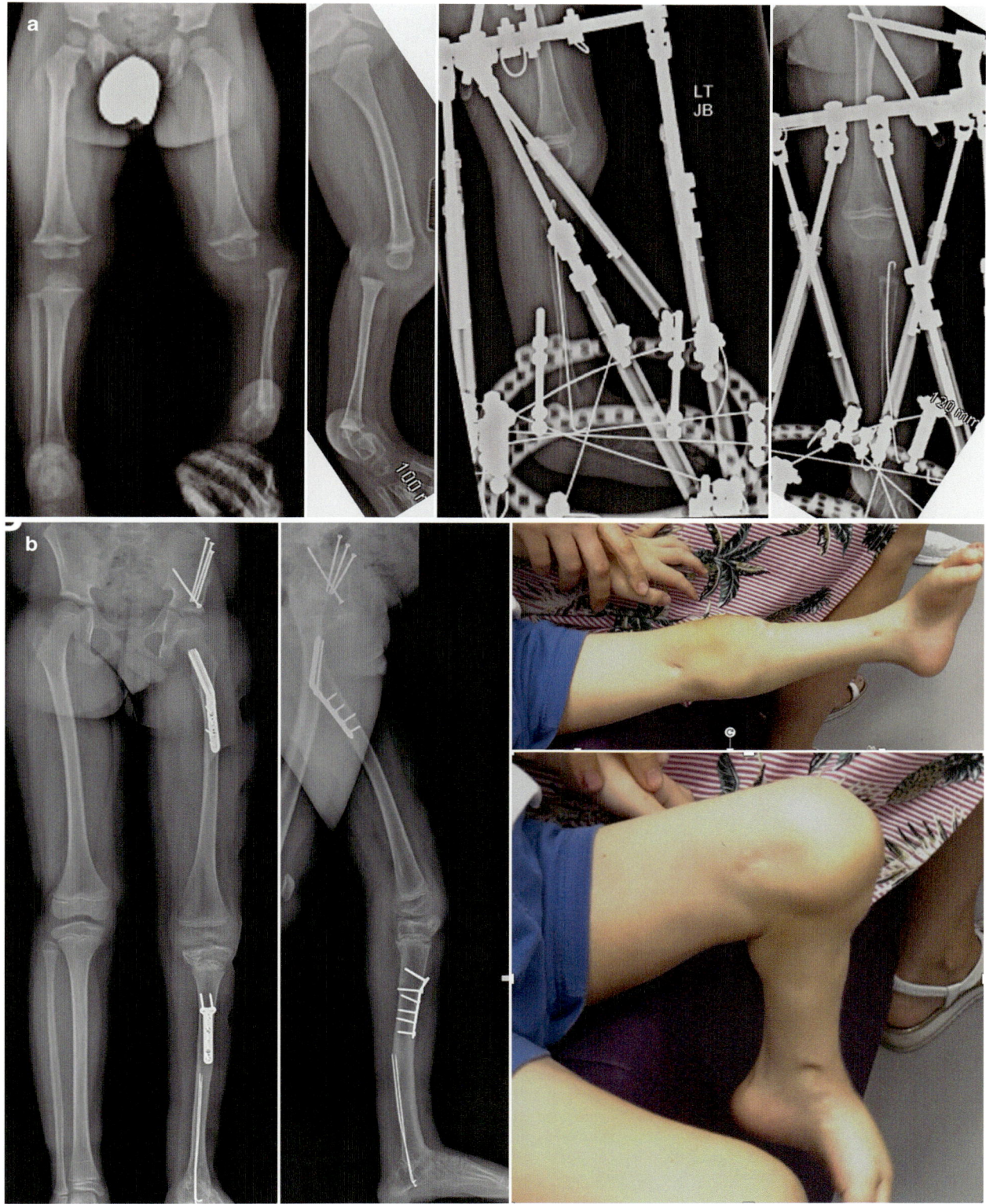

Fig. 31.25 (**a**) AP and lateral radiograph of an 18-month-old boy with left Paley type 5a tibial hemimelia (left 2). Radiographs shown after computer-dependent hexapod external fixator used with staged reconstruction according to Paley-Weber technique. Note the hooked wire holding the patella to the fibular head with BMP2 used to ossify the junction (right 2). (**b**) Radiographs at age 9 following one lengthening surgery and prior patelloplasty and ankle fusion and pelvic osteotomy (left 2). Note that the tibial plateau looks like a normal plateau and that the proximal fibular growth plate is still patent. The distal fibular growth plate is closed. Clinical photos showing active knee motion against gravity with a range of 0–100° (right 2). The knee is stable. (Copyright The Paley Foundation. Reproduced with permission. All rights reserved)

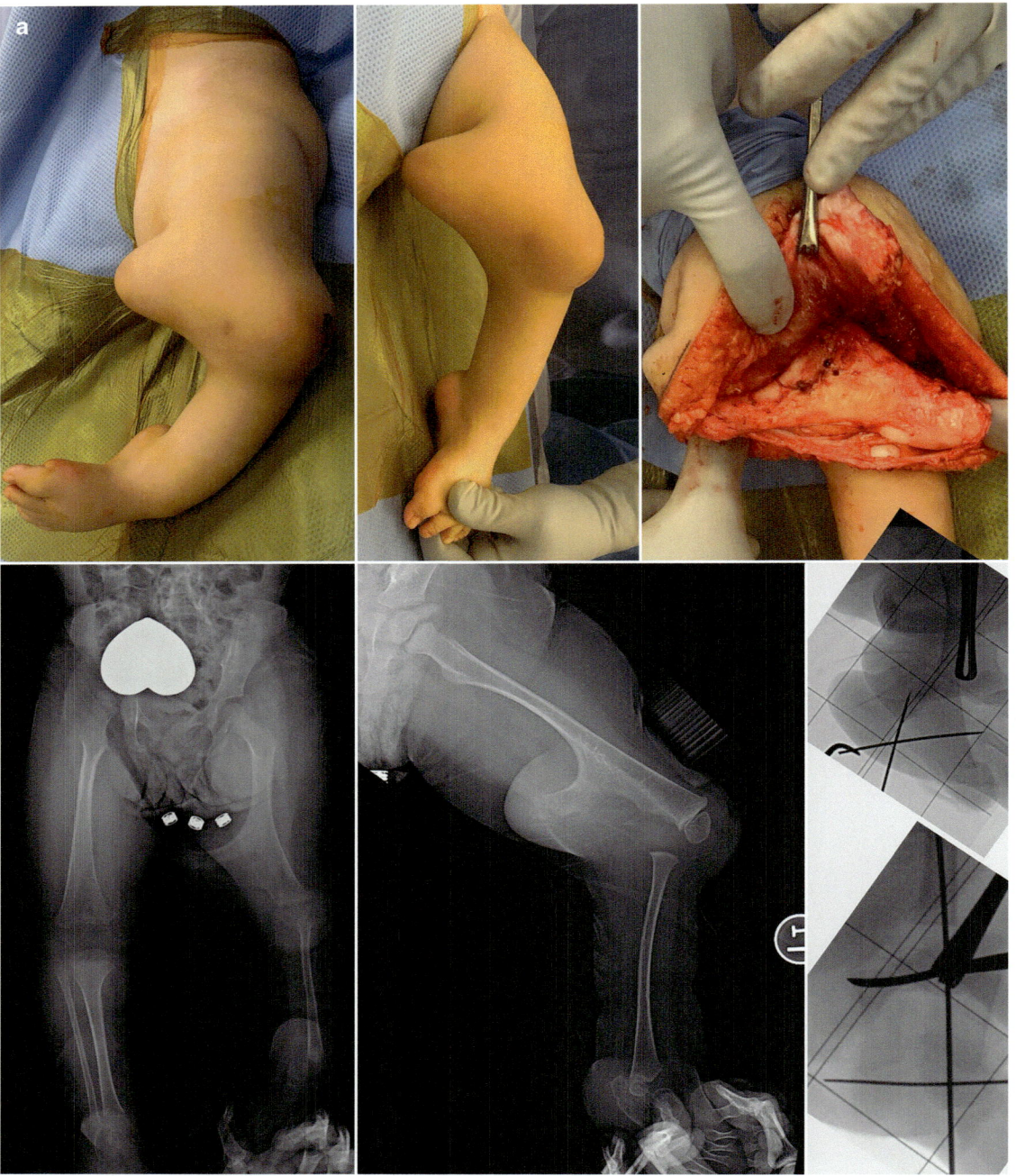

Fig. 31.26 (a) Gallop-Wolfgang syndrome with duplicated left femoral condyles. Clinical photographs (top left and middle) and radiographs (bottom left and middle). This classified as Paley type 5a +femoral condyle. Note the hypoplastic patella in the intercondylar region (top right). The femoral condyles were osteotomized along the lines marked by the two wires in the fluoro shot (top row of bottom right). The condyles were placed beside each other and fixed across their epiphyses (bottom row of bottom right). (b) Olecranization of the patella to the fibula was carried out at the same time as centralization of the fibula. Radiograph showing a hinged external fixator was mounted to hold the foot plantigrade at the ankle fusion site and to allow knee motion at the centralized fibula site (left). AP and lateral radiographs showing the olecranized fibula sits perfectly centralized on the femur (middle and left). (c) Two-year follow-up radiographs show hypertrophy of the centralized fibula which is able to bend 90° at the knee joint. The knee is stable due to the olecranization of the patella. The condyles of the femur are growing together (left and middle). An enlarged view of the lateral shows the patella is starting to ossify anterior to the femoral condyles. It has a chondrodesis to the proximal fibular epiphysis. BMP was not used. (d) Illustration of bifid femur (left) with patella present. To realign the condyles, perpendicular cuts are made to each segment and some shortening (middle). The condyles can be brought together and fixed as shown (right). The patella sits over the space between the condyles. (e) Olecranization is performed attaching the patella to the anterior aspect of the fibular head. A chondrodesis is created. Axial wires used for the ankle fusion can be extended to secure the patella (left and right). A cerclage non-absorbable suture can be used as a tension band (center). (f) The patella is elevated with the quadriceps muscle off of the femur. Lateral flaps are created attached to the two femoral condyles (left and middle left). The lateral flaps secure the patella on the femur and help it track with stability. The tracking of the knee can be seen in flexion and extension (right middle and right). (Copyright The Paley Foundation. Reproduced with permission. All rights reserved)

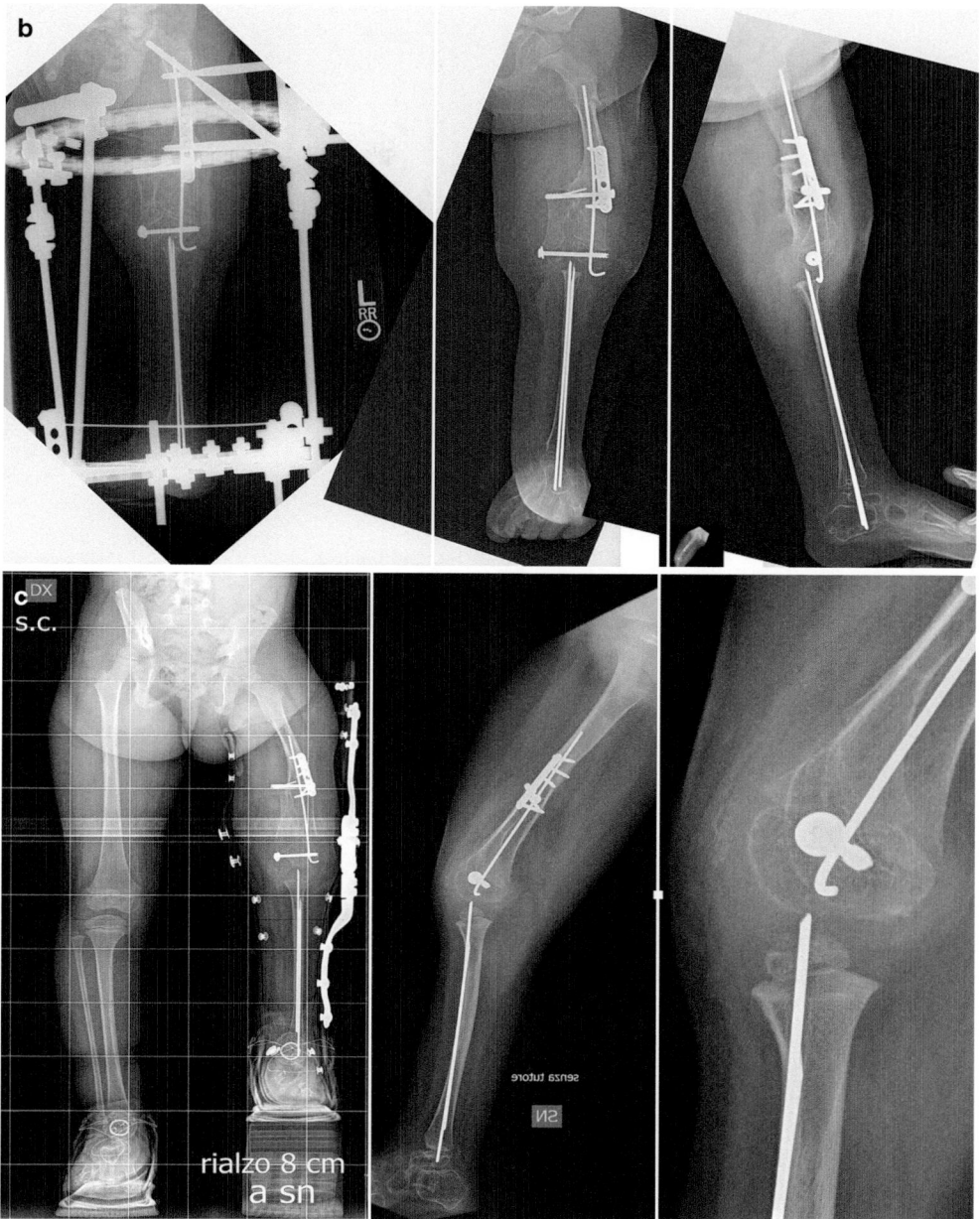

Fig. 31.26 (continued)

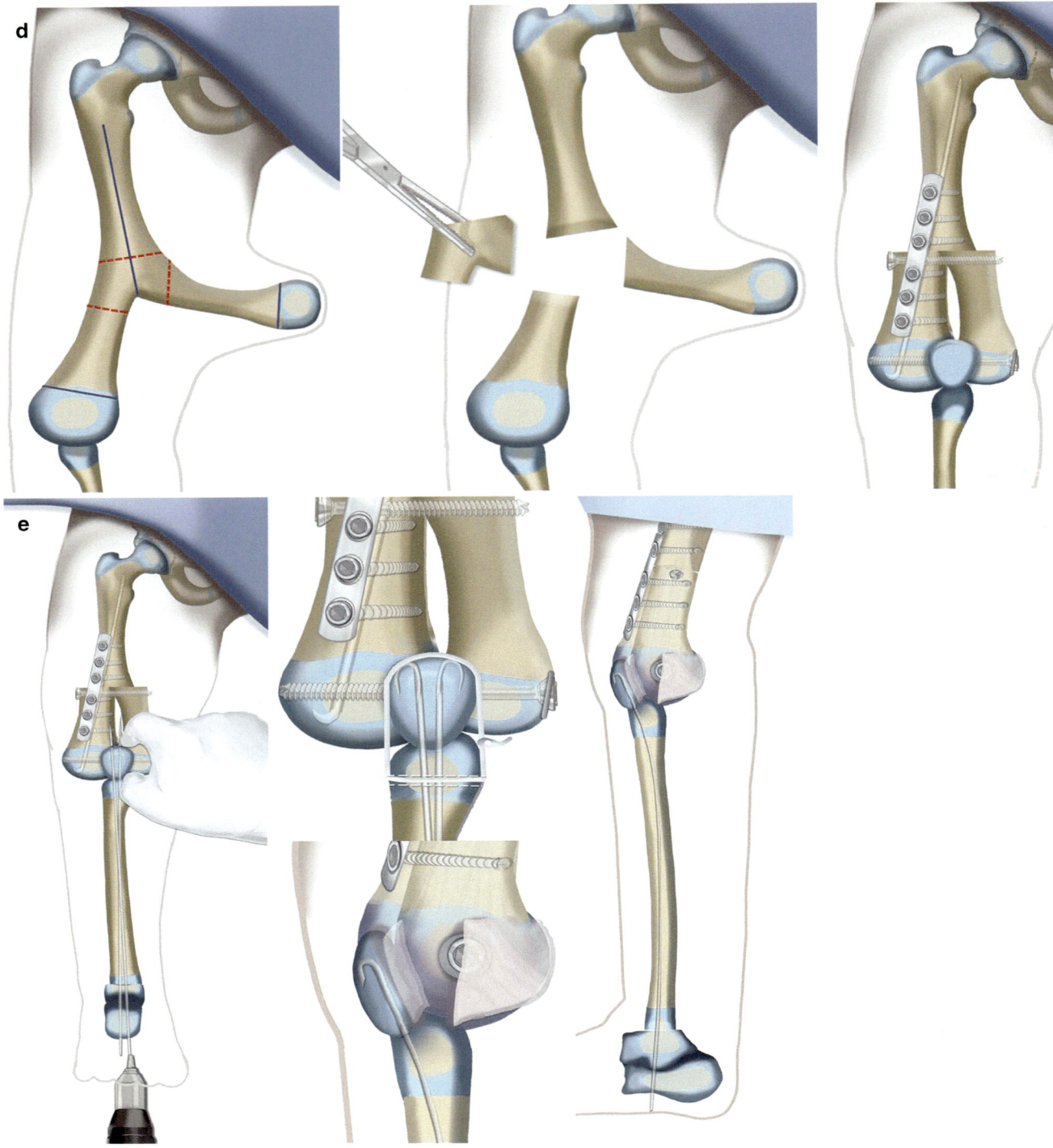

Fig. 31.26 (continued)

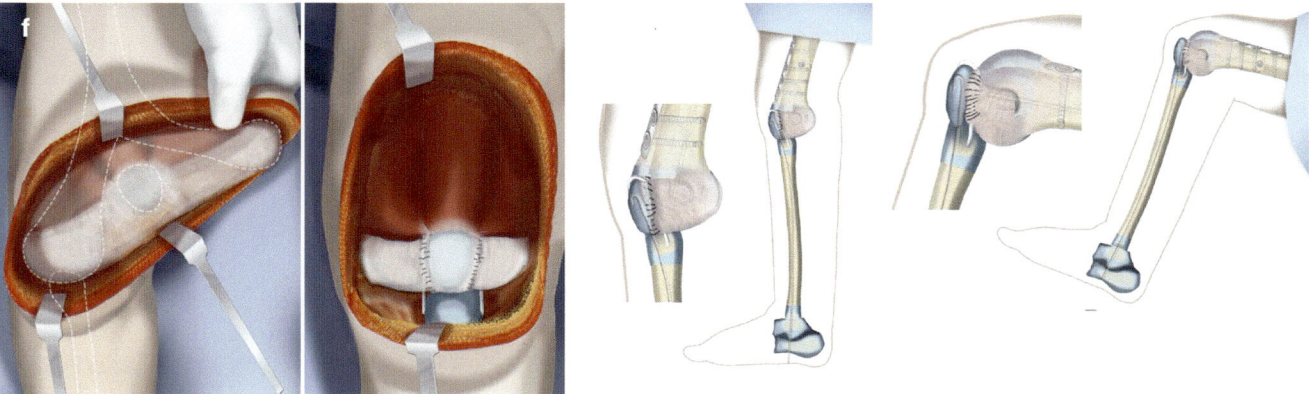

Fig. 31.26 (continued)

Paley-Weber Patellar Arthroplasty

Surgery 1: A hexapod external fixator is applied to the femur-fibula-foot in the same manner as for type 4. The fibula is distracted from the femur to correct the knee contracture, distalize the head to the level of the end of the femur, and align the femur to the fibula. The knee contracture is gradually corrected over the course of many weeks.

Surgery 2: The rings of the external fixator are removed including the foot wires. The fibular wires are prepped in the field. A Z-shaped incision is made with the proximal limb mid-lateral and the distal limb mid medial. The transverse part of the Z is across the knee joint. The fibula, patella, and distal femur are exposed. Three lines outlining two capsular visor flaps (like the visor on a motorcycle helmet) are marked. At the medial and lateral ends, the pedicle for each visor is kept as wide as possible. The proximal visor flap contains the patella. The distal visor flap is all capsular. In the Paley modification, the quadriceps muscle remains attached to the superior pole of the patella. This allows a new patella to form anterior to the femur. The proximal two visor incisions are made. The most inferior one is made after first detaching the biceps tendon laterally and the semitendinosis and gracilis tendons medially. The medial head of the gastrocnemius muscle is identified. Dissection is carried out along the lateral border of the medial head of this muscle to identify and protect the popliteal vessels which lie immediately lateral to the gastrocnemius medial head. Once the vessels are protected, the inferior visor capsular incision is made. The perichondrium on the anterior surface of the patella is incised like the capital letter H, creating two flaps of perichondrium. The superior visor flap is brought under the inferior one to move it distally. The quadriceps muscle is elevated off the anterior femur extraperiosteally as a quadricepsplasty. The femur is shortened approximately 3cm to allow advancement of the quadriceps muscle distally. An axial wire is inserted retrograde up the femur to replace the one that is already there and to act as a prophylactic wire to prevent femur fracture. The anterior femur is plated with a small locking plate. The medial aspect of the anterior compartment is dissected off the fibula. Care should be taken not to injure the posterior tibial artery and also the anterior tibial artery. If the patella is unossified, it is drilled centrally on its dorsal surface to make room for BMP-2. The proximal fibular wires are exposed. The distal fibular wires are then exposed through a transverse incision at the tip of the distal fibular epiphysis. The dome of the talus and the distal fibula is exposed with the wires in place. The wires from the fibula are unbent and removed. New wires are immediately inserted. It is important to keep intramedullary wires in the fibula to prevent inadvertent fracture of the now osteoporotic fibula. The wires are retracted distally, and the proximal epiphysis is cut across with a knife. The two wires exiting the foot are now advanced in a retrograde fashion through the patella, and the wires protruding on the patellar articular surface are bent 180 degrees into a hook. The hook is advanced into the substance of the patella to pull the patella down to the fibula. These two wires need to be pulled below the articular surface to prevent their protrusion into the knee joint. A single BMP-2 sponge is inserted between the fibula and the patella. A small gauge dental wire can be inserted into the patella and fibula and twisted to compress the patella to the fibular epiphysis. The visor flaps can now be sewn across to each other. The inferior visor flap is flipped upwards and sewn to the distal edge of the quadriceps muscle. The Internal Joint Stabilizer (IJS) from Skeletal Dynamics is applied with an axis pin in the distal femur epiphysis and the plate onto the fibula. The knee is now stable to varus valgus stress, but can flex and extend 90°. The biceps and semitendinosus tendons are sutured to the lateral and medial aspects of the fibula, respectively. The external fixator is remounted. The proximal ring is reattached to the proximal pins. A middle ring is added, connected to the proximal ring by medial and lateral hinges that are aligned to the IJS axis. This ring is fixed to the distal fibular wire which is bent at 90° twice. This supports the fibula so that it can be extended. One additional transverse wire can be added in the mid fibula. The distal foot ring is reapplied after first inserting new foot wires. The middle and distal rings are connected with 6 struts. Finally, a removable knee extension bar is created. This newer construct, compared to the one previously published, prioritizes knee motion by getting the reconstructed knee earlier and only then starting to distract the foot. In this way, physical therapy can begin exercising the knee during the entire time of the foot distraction in order to prevent knee stiffness. The foot distraction is aimed at correcting the equinovarus foot deformity and bringing the talus distal to the fibular epiphysis. Once the talus is centralized, a third surgery is performed to fuse the distal fibula to the talus.

Surgery 3: The distal ring and foot wires are removed. A transverse distal incision is made at the tip of the lateral malleolus. The tip of the fibula is exposed with the fibular wires left in place. The top of the talus is exposed. The cartilage of the fibula is cut transversely to expose the ossific nucleus. The top of the talus is cut with a knife to and through its ossific nucleus. The two ossific nuclei are lined up, and two new retrograde wires are inserted through the sole of the foot, through the ossific nucleus of the talus, into the ossific nucleus of the fibula, and into the fibular shaft. The two existing fibular wires are cut off so that they no longer protrude from the end of the fibula. The incision is closed, new foot wires are inserted, and the foot ring reapplied. New struts are applied to compress the ankle fusion site. An arched wire is inserted transversely in the fibula to compress the ankle fusion site. The external fixator remains in place for three more months until ankle fusion is achieved. Physical therapy to the knee continues all throughout this time.

Surgery 4: The external fixator is removed as an outpatient procedure. The hooked patellar wires are retracted with pliers and mallet until they unhook and remain lodged in the fibula to prevent fracture. These wires are cut and buried inside the calcaneus. A hip-knee-ankle-foot orthosis (HKAFO) is used. Immediate physical therapy is resumed to work on active and passive knee motion and gait training.

> **Box 31.6 Weber Patelloplasty Tips**
> - Correct knee flexion contractures as much as possible with frame distraction before surgery. A posterior capsulotomy may be necessary.
> - Find and protect the peroneal nerves and the posterior tibial neurovascular bundle.
> - Transfer the medial and lateral hamstrings to the fibula after the patelloplasty
> - Keep the visor flap pedicles as wide as possible. Deepen the cuts just enough to allow the mobility to slide them around each other. The upper patella flap goes underneath.
> - Patellas can be present in various shapes. A vertical patella can be easily split, such that a small remnant is translated superiorly with the visor flap and forms a new patella.
> - Cut down into the cartilage of the patella and proximal fibula until reaching the ossific nucleus. If these are not present, then consider placing BMP-2 to promote ossification.
> - Use hooked intramedullary wires and a tension band wire for fixation
> - Shorten the femur to allow the new tibial plateau to flex to 90°
> - Augment the stability by adding an IJS device
> - Reapply the external fixator with a hinge at the knee and a hexapod fixator for gradual ankle/foot distraction
> - Fuse the ankle at the next stage
> - Remove the fixator 3 months after the ankle fusion surgery and apply an HKAFO and start PT
> - Maintain intramedullary wires in the fibula

Olecranization of Patella (Fig. 31.26)

Another way to use the patella is called olecranization. In this option, the patella is fused to the fibula in situ. No visor flap is required. The patella, which sits anterior to the femur, is fused directly to the anterior proximal fibular epiphysis. The fibular intramedullary wires are driven directly into the patella and through to its proximal end. The wires are then hooked over the patella proximal border. A tension-band suture or fine wire is added to compress the patella to the fibular epiphysis. The head of the fibula articulates with the distal femur. The goal is to give the proximal fibula an olecranon, which will keep it centered in the intercondylar notch of the femur and prevent it from subluxating posteriorly. This concept was called olecranization by Lord and Musy [114] in a procedure designed for the hyperextension deformity associated with polio, and since then it has been adapted for temporary treatment of posterior cruciate ligament instability [115].

The rest of the procedure is carried out with the same technique as patelloplasty. BMP-2 can be added externally, but great care must be taken to avoid leakage into the joint. The external fixator is articulated at the knee. The IJS device can be added for additional temporary stability with mobility. This technique is especially useful for the patella in Gollop-Wolfgang complex (Fig. 31.2). In these bifid femoral condylar cases, the patella sits in the sulcus between the two femoral condyles and does not lend itself to the Weber patellar arthroplasty. Olecranization is a better option in such cases (Fig. 31.26). Interestingly, the fibula is often autocentralized to one of the femoral condyles in these cases (similar to type 5b).

Type 5b (Fig. 31.27)

When there is no patella but the fibula is autocentralized, then there is usually a quadriceps muscle in continuity to the fibula with a capsule present. The distal femur is usually less dysplastic in these cases. The knee still presents with a fixed flexion contracture, and the foot presents similar to Paley type 5a tibial hemimelia, dislocated and in extreme equinovarus. The treatment is to distract the knee contracture until the fibula and femur are collinear. The foot should also be distracted relative to the fibula to centralize it under the distal end of the fibula. This is also accomplished with a computer-dependent circular external fixator. Once the distraction correction at both the knee and ankle are completed, a second-stage surgery is performed to reconstruct collateral ligaments at the knee and to advance the quadriceps muscles onto the fibula. Local tissue or allograft tendon may be used. An ankle fusion as previously described is performed. The after-treatment is with an HKAFO as described above. If any duplicated bones are to be excised, then olecranization of the bone to be excised (e.g., phalanx, metatarsal, etc.) can be performed to add greater stability to the knee joint.

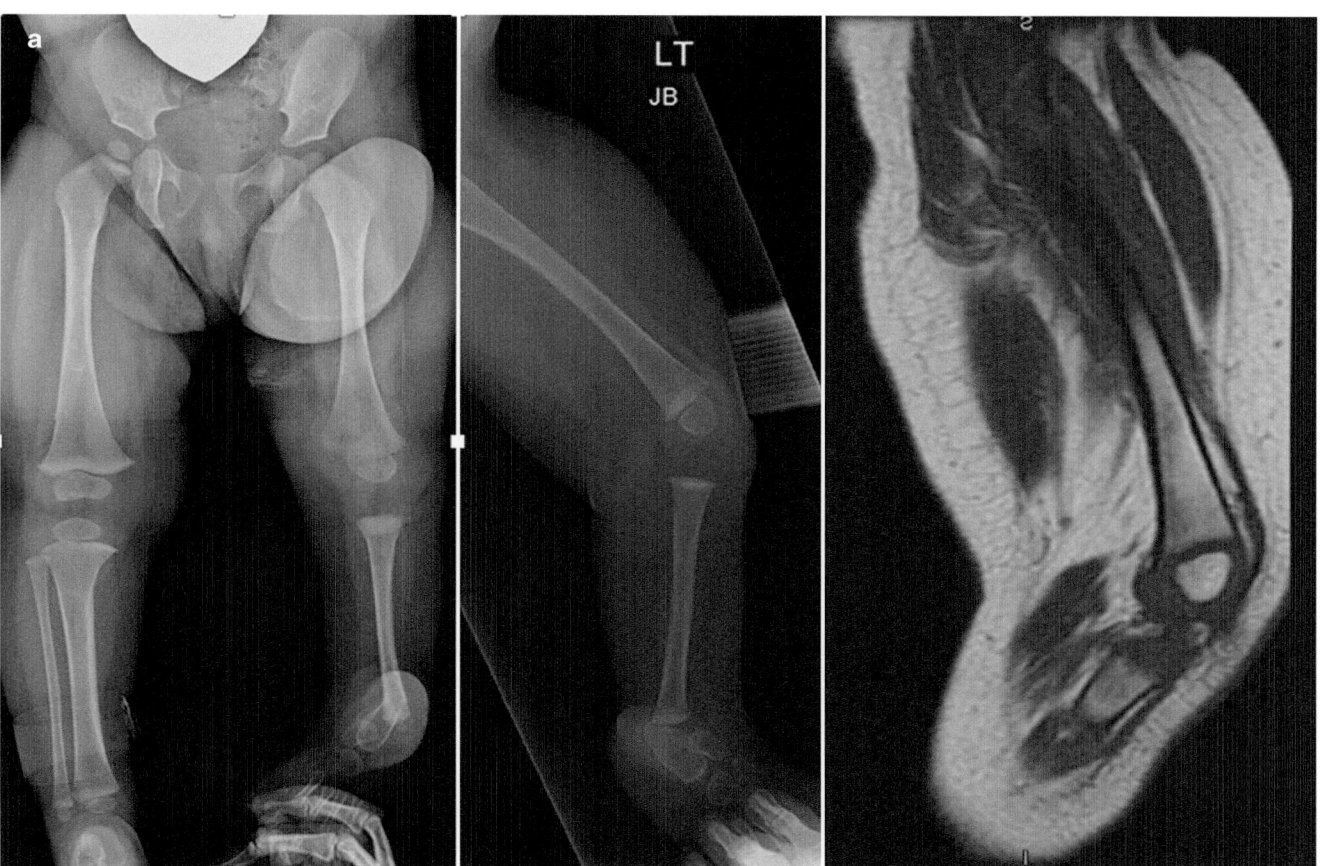

Fig. 31.27 (**a**) AP and lateral radiographs showing autocentralized fibula with auto-hypertrophy of the fibula (left and middle). MRI shows a quadriceps mechanism with a joint formed between fibula and femur. No patella is present. (**b**) Knee reconstruction supported with hinge distraction treatment of knee joint and hexapod gradual correction of equinovarus foot deformity (left). Radiographs after external fixator removal show a good articulation of the centralized fibula to the femur. There is a slight knee flexion deformity (middle 2). This child is able to ice skate and play hockey using a skate with a shoe lift (right). Clearly a very functional extremity. (Copyright The Paley Foundation. Reproduced with permission. All rights reserved)

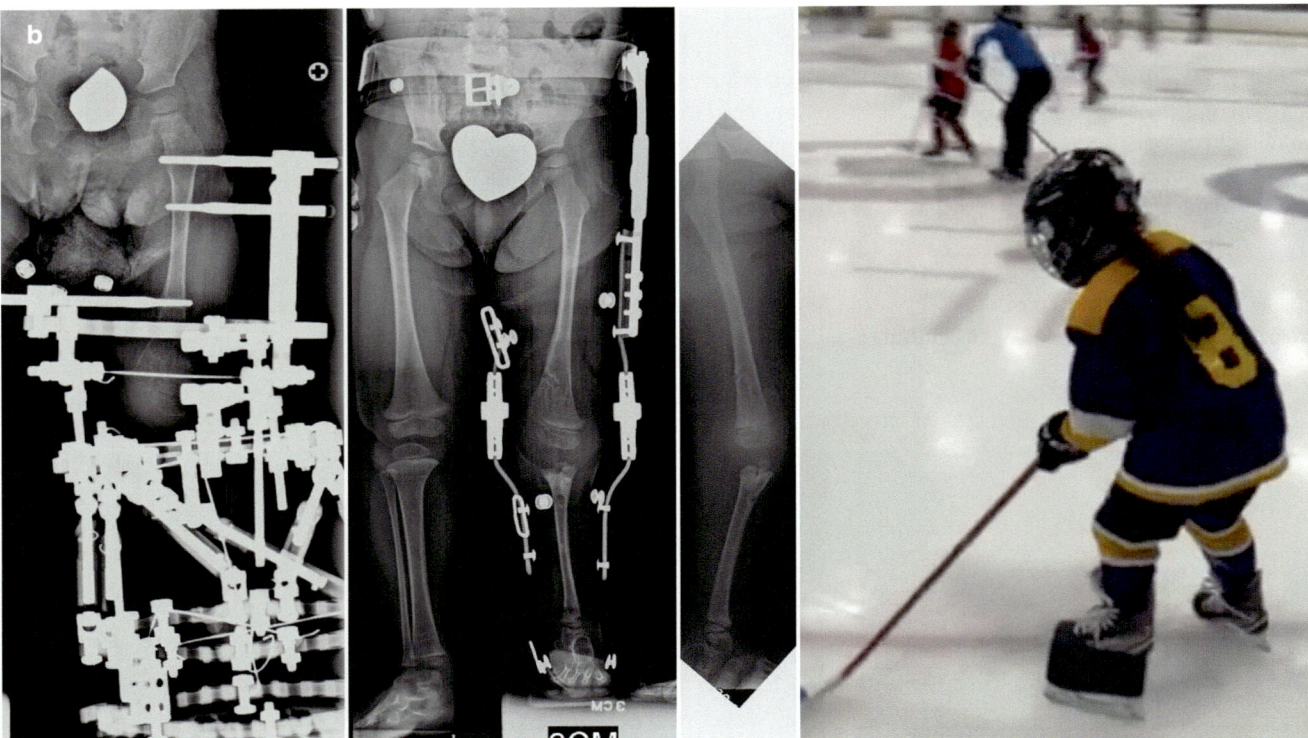

Fig. 31.27 (continued)

Type 5c (Figs. 31.28 and 31.29)

In type 5c, there is no patella, and the fibula is lateral and proximally migrated. If a quadriceps muscle is present, it ends on the distal femur. When the fibula is dislocated, it can be centralized by distraction as described for type 5a.

It may take up to 5–6 months to centralize the knee and ankle, such that the contractures at the knee and ankle are eliminated, the proximal fibula is centered under the femur, and the talus is centered under the fibula. Once this is accomplished, the patient returns to the operating room. The rings and foot wires are removed, and the leg is prepped and draped free. An occlusive dressing is placed over the wire sites at the foot, and the upper femoral pins are prepped and covered with a surgical towel to prevent contact with the more sterile operative field. A Z-shaped incision as for the Paley-Weber patelloplasty is made. The peroneal nerve is liberated and decompressed from the fibula. The biceps tendon is detached from the fibula laterally, and the semitendinosus muscle is dissected free medially. The tensor fascia lata and its iliotibial band are also detached and mobilized.

If the quadriceps muscle is attached distally to the femur, it can be mobilized extraperiosteally similar to a quadricepsplasty. The femur is shortened to allow the quadriceps to move distally. The medial fibula is exposed between the anterior and posterior compartment muscles. The IJS device is applied to stabilize the fibula to the femur in its centralized position. This allows the fibula to flex and extend 90° while maintaining varus-valgus stability. The quadriceps are attached to the head of the fibula. The fascia lata is used to create a lateral collateral ligament. The medial and lateral hamstrings are attached to the fibula. This procedure for reconstruction of the type 5c knee is referred to as the Paley type reconstruction.

Amputation remains the gold standard for treatment of Paley type 5c cases. Paley knee reconstruction should be recommended for those patients who refuse amputation, or to treat one side of bilateral type 5c cases. Knee fusion is the other alternative to amputation. To save length, knee fusion can be performed instead of the Paley knee reconstruction technique described above. The proximal fibular epiphysis should be fused to the distal femoral epiphysis in a way so as not to damage the adjacent physes of these two bones. This is achieved by minimizing dissection of the epiphyses to avoid devascularizing them and by cutting across to the ossific nuclei of both bones. The ossific nuclei can be held in apposition to each other using the external fixator and an intramedullary wire until the knee is fused.

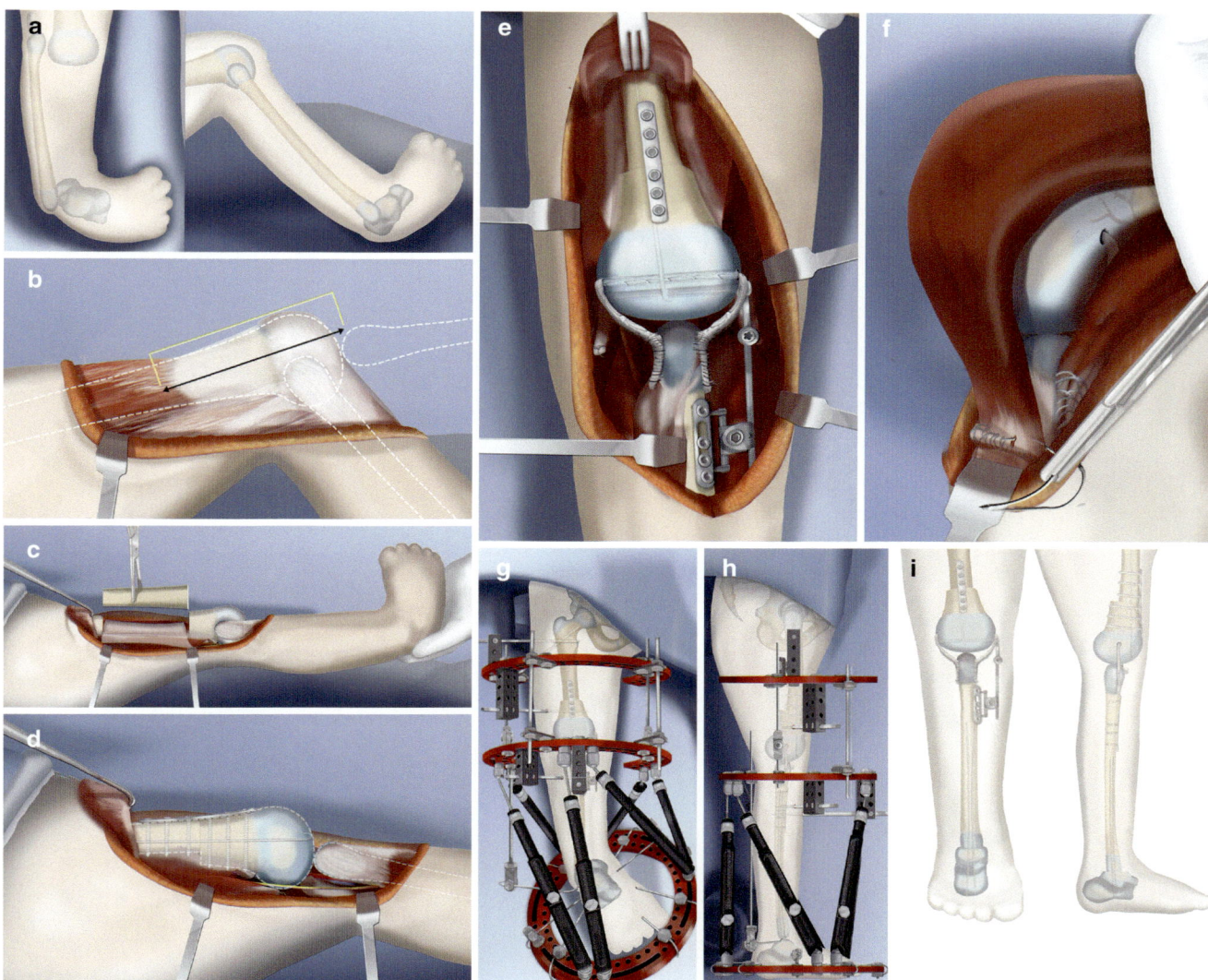

Fig. 31.28 Treatment of Paley type 5C. (**a**) Complete aplasia of tibia with no patella. (**b**) Quadriceps are distally absent and end in distal femur. Femur needs to be shortened significantly to be able to bring the quadriceps to the level of the knee joint. (**c**) Femoral shortening osteotomy. (**d**) Plate fixation and intramedullary pinning of femoral osteotomy and distalization and centralization of fibula. (**e**) Knee stabilized with IJS internal articulated joint distractor. Collateral ligaments made from autograft. Reconstruction of collateral ligaments and placement of internal joint distraction system. (**f**) After quadricepsplasty, quadriceps muscle is advanced and sutured to the fibula head. (**g**) Placement of two-level external fixator: upper two rings with hinges for articulated stabilization of knee; lower two rings for gradual foot distraction. (**h**) Once talus is beneath the fibula and foot at 90°, physeal sparing fusion of distal fibular epiphysis to talus is carried out. (**i**) Final results after fixator removal. The IJS (Skeletal Dynamics) device side arm is disconnected 6 months later to allow for proximal fibular growth. (Copyright The Paley Foundation. Reproduced with permission. All rights reserved)

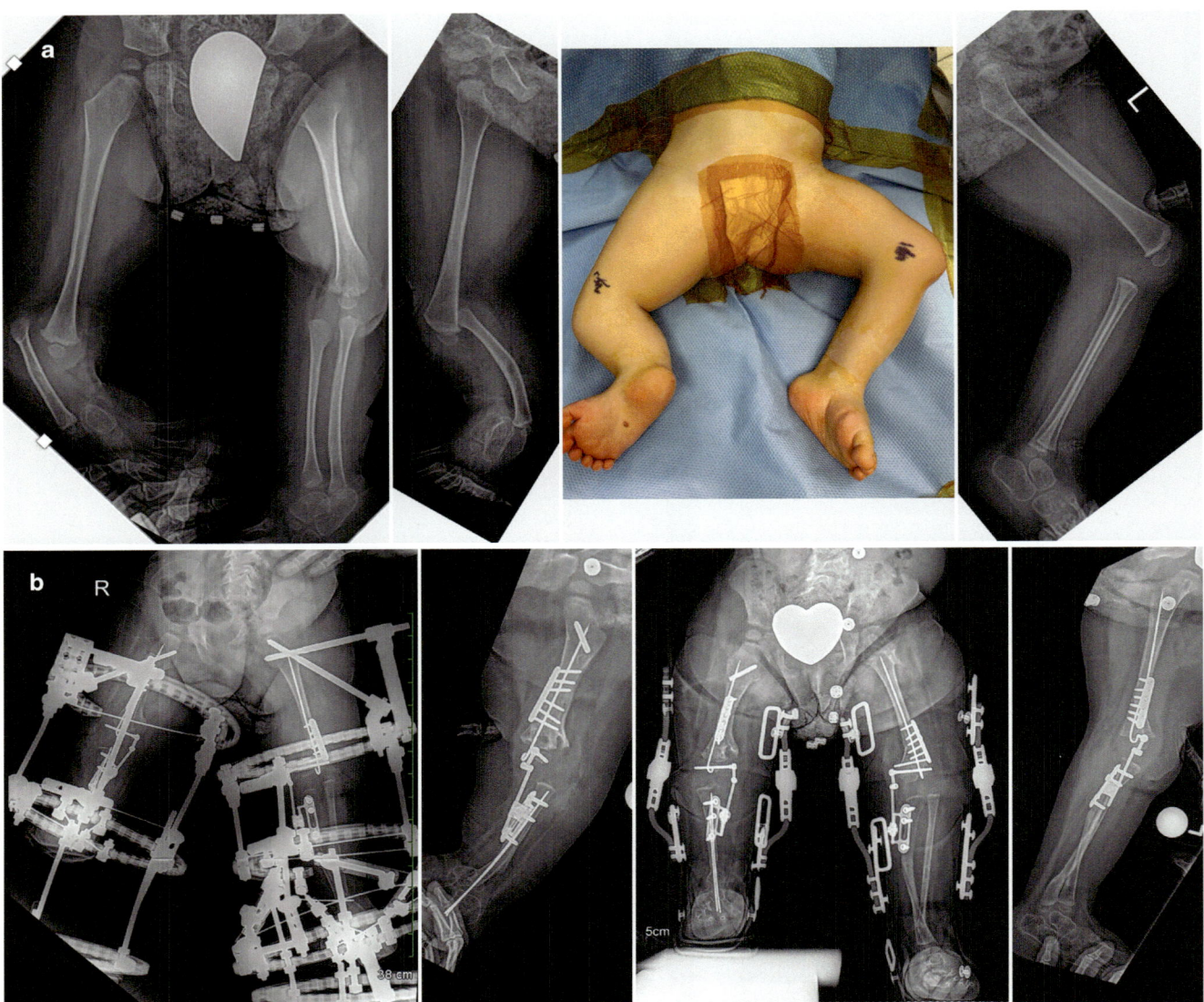

Fig. 31.29 (a) AP and lateral radiographs and photograph of 3-year-old girl with syndromic bilateral tibial hemimelia classified as Paley type 5c +metatarsal and toe on right and Paley type 5c +fibula on the left. The right foot was in equinovarus but the left foot was almost plantigrade. (b) After gradual distraction knee reconstruction was performed bilaterally including femoral shortening, quadricepsplasty, centralization of fibula, application of IJS internal hinge distractor, and ankle fusion on the right and left. A new external fixator was applied with a hinge to allow knee motion and with compression of the ankle fusion site below the knee (left). Radiographs at 1-year follow-up demonstrate excellent alignment and good position of the fibula relative to the femur with IJS in place. Knee motion was 90° bilaterally. (Copyright The Paley Foundation. Reproduced with permission. All rights reserved)

Summary

Through-knee amputation remains the best recommendation for unilateral complete tibial aplasia without a patella. It is certainly a reliable option that can be carried out by most orthopedic surgeons. In bilateral cases of Paley type 5c, complete tibial aplasia reconstruction by one of the techniques described above should be considered since the oxygen consumption of bilateral through knee amputation is very high. Leaving one sensate, braceable leg, especially if passive knee motion can be preserved, is advantageous over bilateral through-knee amputation. When a patella with quadriceps mechanism is present, consideration should be given to a patelloplasty or olecranization by a surgeon experienced in such surgery. Amputation is certainly overused in Paley type 2, 3, and 4 tibial hemimelia. In the senior author's experience, reconstructive results for these types are reliable and successful in achieving a functional lower extremity.

The reconstructive options for tibial hemimelia have improved greatly over the past two decades. With continued success and improvements, they may one day overtake the amputation option. Other anatomic variants of tibial hemimelia, including duplication of fibula, tarsals, metatarsals and toes, and secondary femoral condyles, have not been discussed. They are referred to in the classification by adding +/− modifiers. For example, a duplicated fibula with complete tibial absence and no patella is classified as type 5c +fibula. Its treatment is either a through-knee amputation or a Paley knee reconstruction. Duplicated foot bones and toes require resection. Duplicated femur requires resection of the extra part of the femur. An absent proximal femur becomes more of a problem of congenital femoral deficiency and is beyond the scope of this chapter. The presence of distal tibia with absent proximal tibia is treated the same as a type 5. The significance of these variants must be evaluated individually on a case by case basis, using the above treatment algorithms as a foundation for treatment strategies and options.

Acknowledgments The author would like to thank Pamela Boullier Ross, who illustrated all of the figures in this manuscript. The author would also like to thank the Paley Foundation for funding the cost of making these illustrations and giving permission for their reproduction in Pediatric Lower Limb Deformities, Principles, and Techniques of Management (Springer).

Commentary

J. Eric Gordon
gordone@wustl.edu

Patients with tibial hemimelia can pose some of the most challenging reconstructive issues for surgeons. Anatomic problems include dysfunction of the extensor mechanism of the knee, length issues of the lower extremity, and instability of the ankle and foot. Significant advances have been made over the last several years in improving patient function through limb reconstruction. Goals in reconstruction of patients with tibial hemimelia involve first preserving and improving the knee extensor mechanism, secondly correcting the limb length discrepancy, and finally providing a stable ankle with a plantigrade foot to allow weight bearing.

Reconstruction and lengthening must always be considered in light of the functional goals that can be achieved by amputation and by weighing the risks and benefits to both the family and the patient. When the extensor mechanism of the knee cannot be adequately reconstructed, the tibia almost inevitably falls into a flexed position despite bracing and therapy and often the reconstruction is unstable as well, making normal ambulation extremely difficult. Only in situations where the societal implications of amputations are extremely severe should such reconstructions be undertaken. In contrast, when a stable active knee can be achieved, the advantages to the patient are so significant in potential activities and energy savings during gait that families should almost always be strongly encouraged to pursue the reconstruction.

Options for providing limb length can be thought of as falling into one of two general categories. When an intact tibia spans the area between the knee and ankle and both joints are either stable or can be adequately reconstructed, lengthening of the tibia is the preferred approach. When only a portion of the tibia is present (most often the proximal tibia), the fibula can be employed to create a stable ankle and to functionally make the tibia longer through synostosis with the tibia with subsequent lengthening as needed.

Limb length and a stable ankle with a plantigrade foot are advantageous but the advantages in activity and energy savings are not as dramatic as those seen when preserving an active knee. Some families, because of inadequate resources or inability to comply with treatment, may choose ablation. When an active knee is present, a Syme amputation allows early prosthetic fitting and activity with the prosthesis providing both length and a functional ankle and foot mechanism. When considering advances in prosthetic function over the last 20 years, the standards for the function of reconstructed limbs have become much higher.

In spite of the excellent function of below knee prosthetics, the gold standard for function and the preference for most families remain retaining a functional, sensate foot with a mobile ankle and equal limb lengths. This obviates the need for repeated prosthetic expenses for the patient as they mature as well as for continued prosthetic fitting and replacement in adulthood, particularly when the patient is active. With modern reconstructive and lengthening techniques, repeated lengthening of a limb to correct even large discrepancies is well tolerated. Embarking on reconstruction in patients with tibial hemimelia with large discrepancies and unstable joints is probably better reserved for surgeons who have significant experience in limb reconstruction and who practice at centers where the complications and difficulties can be expeditiously managed.

References

1. Otto AW. Monstrorum sexcentorum descriptio anatomica. Sumptibus Ferdinandi Hirt; 1841.
2. Burckhardt L. Beitrage zur Diagnostik und Therapie koiigenitaler Knochendefekte.
3. Young JK. Double congenital deformity of the tibia. Am J Med Sci. 1888;XCV:145–50.
4. Billroth T. Ueber einige durch Knochendefecte bedingte Krümmungen des Fusses. Arch Klin Chir. 1861;1:252–68.
5. Dankmeijer J. Congenital absence of the tibia. Anat Rec. 1935;62:179–94.
6. Ramirez M, Hecht JT, Taylor S, Wilkins I. Tibial hemimelia syndrome: prenatal diagnosis by real-time ultrasound. Prenat Diagn. 1994;14(3):167–71. https://doi.org/10.1002/pd.1970140304.
7. Brown FW. The brown operation for total hemimelia tibia. In: Aitken GT, editor. Selected lower-limb anomalies. National Academy of Sciences; 1971. p. 20–8.
8. Weber M, Schroeder S, Berdel P, Niethard FU. Register zur bundesweiten Erfassung angeborener Gliedmaßenfehlbildungen. Z Orthop. 2005;143:1–5.
9. Nutt J, Smith E. Total congenital absence of the tibia. Am J Roentgen. 1941;46:841.
10. Aitken GT, Bose K, Brown F. Tibial Hemimelia. In: Canale ST, editor. Campbell's operative orthopaedics. 9th ed. Mosby; 1998. p. 937–1003.
11. Spiegel DA, Loder RT, Crandall RC. Congenital longitudinal deficiency of the tibia. Int Orthop. 2003;27(6):338–42. https://doi.org/10.1007/s00264-003-0490-5.
12. Schoenecker PL, Capelli AM, Millar EA, et al. Congenital longitudinal deficiency of the tibia. J Bone Joint Surg Am. 1989;71(2):278–87.
13. PaKG L. Rev D'Orthop. 1901:327–411.
14. Deimling S, Sotiropoulos C, Lau K, et al. Tibial hemimelia associated with GLI3 truncation. J Hum Genet. 2016;61(5):443–6. https://doi.org/10.1038/jhg.2015.161.
15. Jones D, Barnes J, Lloyd-Roberts GC. Congenital aplasia and dysplasia of the tibia with intact fibula. Classification and management. J Bone Joint Surg Br. 1978;60(1):31–9. https://doi.org/10.1302/0301-620X.60B1.627576.
16. Aitken GT, National Research Council (U.S.). Subcommittee on Child Prosthetics Problems. Selected lower-limb anomalies: surgical and prosthetics management; a symposium held in Washington, D.C. May 8-9, 1969. Natl Acad Sci; 1971:vii, 72 p.
17. Emami-Ahari Z, Mahloudji M. Bilateral absence of the tibias in three sibs. Birth Defects Orig Artic Ser. 1974;10(5):197–200.
18. Clark MW. Autosomal dominant inheritance of tibial meromelia. Report of a kindred. J Bone Joint Surg Am. 1975;57(2):262–4.
19. Cowell H. Jayakumar 1978.
20. Lenz W. Genetics and limb deficiencies. Clin Orthop Relat Res. 1980;148:9–17.
21. Lenz W. Genetic causes of malformations in man. Verhandl Dtsch Gesellsch Pathol. 1982;66:16–24.
22. Fried K, Goldberg MD, Mundel G, Reif R. Severe lower limb malformation associated with other deformities and death in infancy in two brothers. J Med Genet. 1977;14(5):352–4. https://doi.org/10.1136/jmg.14.5.352.
23. Mahloudji M, Farpour H. An unusual limb deformity in an inbred community. Birth Defects Orig Artic Ser. 1974;10(5):75–80.
24. McKay M, Clarren SK, Zorn R. Isolated tibial hemimelia in sibs: an autosomal-recessive disorder? Am J Med Genet. 1984;17(3):603–7. https://doi.org/10.1002/ajmg.1320170308.
25. Naveed M, Al-Ali MT, Murthy SK, et al. Ectrodactyly with aplasia of long bones (OMIM; 119100) in a large inbred Arab family with an apparent autosomal dominant inheritance and reduced penetrance: clinical and genetic analysis. Am J Med Genet A. 2006;140(13):1440–6. https://doi.org/10.1002/ajmg.a.31239.
26. Taleb H, Afshar A, Abdi Rad I, Tabrizi A, Ghazani RB, Bateni A. A high prevalence rate of Tibia Hemimelia in a subregion of West Azarbaijan, Iran. J Pediatr Genet. 2019;8(3):137–41. https://doi.org/10.1055/s-0039-1692971.
27. Dayer R, Ceroni D, Bottani A, Kaelin A. Tibial aplasia-hypoplasia and ectrodactyly in monozygotic twins with a discordant phenotype. J Pediatr Orthop. 2007;27(3):266–9. https://doi.org/10.1097/BPO.0b013e3180340d6c.
28. Leite JA, Lima LC, Sampaio ML. Tibial hemimelia in one of the identical twins. J Pediatr Orthop. 2010;30(7):742–5. https://doi.org/10.1097/BPO.0b013e3181edba12.
29. Ojo SA, Guffy MM, Saperstein G, Leipold HW. Tibial hemimelia in Galloway calves. J Am Vet Med Assoc. 1974;165(6):548–50.
30. Werner P. Ueber einen seltenen Fall von Zwergwuchs. Arch Gynaekol. 1915;104:278–300.
31. Kantaputra PN, Chalidapong P. Are triphalangeal thumb-polysyndactyly syndrome (TPTPS) and tibial hemimelia-polysyndactyly-triphalangeal thumb syndrome (THPTTS) identical? A father with TPTPS and his daughter with THPTTS in a Thai family. Am J Med Genet. 2000;93(2):126–31. https://doi.org/10.1002/1096-8628(20000717)93:2<126::aid-ajmg9>3.0.co;2-s.
32. Balci S, Demirtas M, Civelek B, Piskin M, Sensoz O, Akarsu AN. Phenotypic variability of triphalangeal thumb-polysyndactyly syndrome linked to chromosome 7q36. Am J Med Genet. 1999;87(5):399–406.
33. Norbnop P, Srichomthong C, Suphapeetiporn K, Shotelersuk V. ZRS 406A>G mutation in patients with tibial hypoplasia, polydactyly and triphalangeal first fingers. J Hum Genet. 2014;59(8):467–70. https://doi.org/10.1038/jhg.2014.50.
34. Cho TJ, Baek GH, Lee HR, Moon HJ, Yoo WJ, Choi IH. Tibial hemimelia-polydactyly-five-fingered hand syndrome associated with a 404 G>A mutation in a distant sonic hedgehog cis-regulator (ZRS): a case report. J Pediatr Orthop B. 2013;22(3):219–21. https://doi.org/10.1097/BPB.0b013e32835106b2.
35. Wieczorek D, Pawlik B, Li Y, et al. A specific mutation in the distant sonic hedgehog (SHH) cis-regulator (ZRS) causes Werner mesomelic syndrome (WMS) while complete ZRS duplications underlie Haas type polysyndactyly and preaxial polydactyly (PPD) with or without triphalangeal thumb. Hum Mutat. 2010;31(1):81–9. https://doi.org/10.1002/humu.21142.
36. Carvalho DR, Santos SC, Oliveira MD, Speck-Martins CE. Tibial hemimelia in Langer-Giedion syndrome with 8q23.1-q24.12 interstitial deletion. Am J Med Genet A. 2011;155A(11):2784–7. https://doi.org/10.1002/ajmg.a.34233.
37. Stevens CA, Moore CA. Tibial hemimelia in Langer-Giedion syndrome-possible gene location for tibial hemimelia at 8q. Am J Med Genet. 1999;85(4):409–12. https://doi.org/10.1002/(sici)1096-8628(19990806)85:4<409::aid-ajmg19>3.0.co;2-6.
38. Erickson RP. Agenesis of tibia with bifid femur, congenital heart disease, and cleft lip with cleft palate or tracheoesophageal fistula: possible variants of Gollop-Wolfgang complex. Am J Med Genet A. 2005;134(3):315–7. https://doi.org/10.1002/ajmg.a.30636.
39. van de Kamp JM, van der Smagt JJ, Bos CF, van Haeringen A, Hogendoorn PC, Breuning MH. Bifurcation of the femur with tibial agenesis and additional anomalies. Am J Med Genet A. 2005;138(1):45–50. https://doi.org/10.1002/ajmg.a.30918.
40. Nlandu A, Docquier PL. Gollop-Wolfgang complex: an alternative to amputation. Acta Orthop Belg. 2013;79(2):239–42.
41. Alazami AM, Alzahrani F, Alkuraya FS. Expanding the "E" in CHARGE. Am J Med Genet A. 2008;146A(14):1890–2. https://doi.org/10.1002/ajmg.a.32376.
42. Prasad C, Quackenbush EJ, Whiteman D, Korf B. Limb anomalies in DiGeorge and CHARGE syndromes. Am J

43. Aukema SM, de Geus CM, Robben SGF, et al. Tibia hemimelia in a patient with CHARGE syndrome: a rare but recurrent phenomenon. Am J Med Genet A. 2021; https://doi.org/10.1002/ajmg.a.62600.
44. Hsu P, Ma A, Wilson M, et al. CHARGE syndrome: a review. J Paediatr Child Health. 2014;50(7):504–11. https://doi.org/10.1111/jpc.12497.
45. Sanlaville D, Etchevers HC, Gonzales M, et al. Phenotypic spectrum of CHARGE syndrome in fetuses with CHD7 truncating mutations correlates with expression during human development. J Med Genet. 2006;43(3):211–7. https://doi.org/10.1136/jmg.2005.036160.
46. Wiedemann HR, Opitz JM. Brief clinical report: unilateral partial tibia defect with preaxial polydactyly, general micromelia, and trigonomacrocephaly with a note on "developmental resistance". Am J Med Genet. 1983;14(3):467–71. https://doi.org/10.1002/ajmg.1320140310.
47. Verghese R, Shah H, Rebello G, Joseph B. Pre-axial mirror polydactyly associated with tibial deficiency: a study of the patterns of skeletal anomalies of the foot and leg. J Child Orthop. 2007;1(1):49–54. https://doi.org/10.1007/s11832-006-0001-5.
48. Laurin CA, Favreau JC, Labelle P. Bilateral absence of the Radius and Tibia with bilateral reduplication of the Ulna and Fibula. A case report. J Bone Joint Surg Am. 1964;46:137–42.
49. Majewski F, Kuster W, ter Haar B, Goecke T. Aplasia of tibia with split-hand/split-foot deformity. Report of six families with 35 cases and considerations about variability and penetrance. Hum Genet. 1985;70(2):136–47. https://doi.org/10.1007/BF00273072.
50. Granite G, Herzenberg JE, Wade R. Rare case of tibial hemimelia, preaxial polydactyly, and club foot. World J Clin Cases. 2016;4(12):401–8. https://doi.org/10.12998/wjcc.v4.i12.401.
51. Chinnakkannan S, Das RR, Rughmini K, Ahmed S. A case of bilateral tibial hemimelia type VIIa. Indian J Hum Genet. 2013;19(1):108–10. https://doi.org/10.4103/0971-6866.112924.
52. Fernandez-Palazzi F, Bendahan J, Rivas S. Congenital deficiency of the tibia: a report on 22 cases. J Pediatr Orthop B. 1998;7(4):298–302. https://doi.org/10.1097/01202412-199810000-00008.
53. Jose RM, Kamath AK, Vijayaraghavan S, Varghese S, Nair SR, Nanadakumar UR. Tibial hemimelia with 'mirror foot'. Eur J Plast Surg. 2004;27:39–41.
54. Orimolade EA, Ikem IC, Oginni LM, Odunsi AO. Femoral bifurcation with ipsilateral tibia hemimelia: early outcome of ablation and prosthetic fitting. Niger J Clin Pract. 2011;14(4):492–4. https://doi.org/10.4103/1119-3077.91764.
55. Yetkin H, Cila E, Bilgin Guzel V, Kanatli U. Femoral bifurcation associated with tibial hemimelia. Orthopedics. 2001;24(4):389–90.
56. Bade P. Zur Pathologie und Therapie des Tibiadefektes. Z Orthop Chir. 1906;16:150–66.
57. Evans EL, Smith NR. Congenital absence of Tibia. Arch Dis Child. 1926;1(4):194–229. https://doi.org/10.1136/adc.1.4.194.
58. Fujii H, Doi K, Baliarsing AS. Transtibial amputation with plantar flap for congenital deficiency of the tibia. Clin Orthop Relat Res. 2002;403:186–90. https://doi.org/10.1097/00003086-200210000-00027.
59. Salinas-Torres VM, Barajas-Barajas LO, Perez-Garcia N, Perez-Garcia G. Bilateral tibial hemimelia type 1 (1a and 1b) with T9 and T10 hemivertebrae: a novel association. Sao Paulo Med J. 2013;131(4):275–8. https://doi.org/10.1590/1516-3180.2013.1314494.
60. Sulamaa M, Ryoeppy S. Congenital absence of the Tibia. Acta Orthop Scand. 1964;34:337–48. https://doi.org/10.3109/17453676408989329.
61. Hovelacque A, Noel R. Processus embryologique de l'absence congenitale du tibia. C R Soc Biol Paris. 1923;88:577–8.
62. Turker R, Mendelson S, Ackman J, Lubicky JP. Anatomic considerations of the foot and leg in tibial hemimelia. J Pediatr Orthop. 1996;16(4):445–9. https://doi.org/10.1097/00004694-199607000-00005.
63. Frantz CH, O'Rahilly R. Congenital skeletal limb deficiencies. J Bone Jt Surg Am. 1961;43:1202–24.
64. Kalamchi A, Dawe RV. Congenital deficiency of the tibia. J Bone Joint Surg Br. 1985;67(4):581–4. https://doi.org/10.1302/0301-620X.67B4.4030854.
65. Weber M. New classification and score for tibial hemimelia. J Child Orthop. 2008;2(3):169–75. https://doi.org/10.1007/s11832-008-0081-5.
66. Devitt AT, O'Donnell T, Fogarty EE, Dowling FE, Moore DP. Tibial hemimelia of a different class. J Pediatr Orthop. 2000;20(5):616–22. https://doi.org/10.1097/00004694-200009000-00013.
67. Garden RS. Low-angle fixation in fracdtures of the femoral neck. J Bone Jt Surg Br. 1961;43-B:647–63.
68. Berndt AL, Harty M. Transchondral fractures (osteochondritis dissecans) of the talus. J Bone Joint Surg Am. 1959;41-A:988–1020.
69. Catterall A. The natural history of Perthes' disease. J Bone Joint Surg Br. 1971;53(1):37–53.
70. Herring JA, Neustadt JB, Williams JJ, Early JS, Browne RH. The lateral pillar classification of Legg-Calve-Perthes disease. J Pediatr Orthop. 1992;12(2):143–50. https://doi.org/10.1097/01241398-199203000-00001.
71. Paley D. Principles of deformity correction, vol. xxv. Springer; 2002. 806 p
72. Pappas AM. Congenital abnormalities of the femur and related lower extremity malformations: classification and treatment. J Pediatr Orthop. 1983;3(1):45–60. https://doi.org/10.1097/01241398-198302000-00009.
73. Currarino G, Herring JA, Johnston CE Jr, Birch JG. An unusual form of congenital anterolateral tibial angulation-the delta tibia. Pediatr Radiol. 2003;33(5):346–53. https://doi.org/10.1007/s00247-002-0856-7.
74. Weber M. Congenital leg deformities: tibial hemimelia. In: Rozbruch SR, Ilizarov S, editors. Limb lengthening and reconstruction surgery. Informa Healthcare USA Inc.; 2007.
75. Paley D, Herzenberg JE, Gillespie R. Limb deficiency. In: Staheli LT, editor. Pediatric orthopaedic secrets. Hanley & Belfus; 2003. p. 455–81.
76. Paley D. Tibial hemimelia: new classification and reconstructive options. J Child Orthop. 2016;10(6):529–55. https://doi.org/10.1007/s11832-016-0785-x.
77. Senthil V, Kottamttavide IV, Shah H. Unclassified tibial hemimelia. BMJ Case Rep. 2016; https://doi.org/10.1136/bcr-2016-215305.
78. Shah K, Shah H. Tibial hypoplasia with a bifid tibia: an unclassified tibial hemimelia. BMJ Case Rep. 2016; https://doi.org/10.1136/bcr-2016-216622.
79. Shrivastava S, Nawghare S, Dulani R, Singh P, Jain S. A rare variant of tibial hemimelia and its treatment. J Pediatr Orthop B. 2009;18(5):220–4. https://doi.org/10.1097/BPB.0b013e32832e4737.
80. Albert E. Wein Med Presse. 1877:111.
81. Myers H. Congenital absence of tibia: transplantation of head of fibula: arthrodesis at the ankle-joint. J Bone Jt Surg Am. 1905;2:72–85.
82. Nove-Josserand G. Bull Soc Chir Lyon. 1899:259.
83. Fraser J, Robarts H. Congenital deficiency of the radius and a homologous condition in the leg. Lancet. 1914;183:1606–8.
84. Putti V. The treatment of congenital absence of the tibia or fibula. Chir Org Mov. 1929;7:513.
85. Kumar Sahoo P, Sahu MM, Prasad DS. Clinical spectrum of congenital tibial hemimelia in 35 limbs of 24 patients: a sin-

gle center observational study from India. Eur J Med Genet. 2019;62(7):103666. https://doi.org/10.1016/j.ejmg.2019.05.005.
86. Yadav SS. Type-I tibial Hemimelia: a Limb-Salvage and Lengthening technique. JB JS Open Access. 2019;4(1):e0029. https://doi.org/10.2106/JBJS.OA.18.00029.
87. Loder RT, Herring JA. Fibular transfer for congenital absence of the tibia: a reassessment. J Pediatr Orthop. 1987;7(1):8–13. https://doi.org/10.1097/01241398-198701000-00002.
88. Epps CH Jr, Tooms RE, Edholm CD, Kruger LM, Bryant DD 3rd. Failure of centralization of the fibula for congenital longitudinal deficiency of the tibia. J Bone Joint Surg Am. 1991;73(6):858–67.
89. Khalifa NM, Ghaly NA. Surgical treatment of type II congenital dysplasia of the tibia. J Orthop Trauma. 2004;8:129–34.
90. Sharma S, Mir S, Sharma V, Dar I. Congenital absence of the Tibia. JK Sci. 2002;4:213–4.
91. Wehbe MA, Weinstein SL, Ponseti IV. Tibial agenesis. J Pediatr Orthop. 1981;1(4):395–9. https://doi.org/10.1097/01241398-198112000-00007.
92. Christini D, Levy EJ, Facanha FA, Kumar SJ. Fibular transfer for congenital absence of the tibia. J Pediatr Orthop. 1993;13(3):378–81. https://doi.org/10.1097/01241398-199305000-00020.
93. Kaplan-List K, Klionsky NB, Sanders JO, Katz ME. Systematic radiographic evaluation of tibial hemimelia with orthopedic implications. Pediatr Radiol. 2017;47(4):473–83. https://doi.org/10.1007/s00247-016-3730-8.
94. Grissom LE, Harcke HT, Kumar SJ. Sonography in the management of tibial hemimelia. Clin Orthop Relat Res. 1990;251:266–70.
95. Brown FW. Construction of a knee joint in congenital total absence of the Tibia (Paraxial Hemimelia Tibia): a preliminary report. J Bone Joint Surg Am. 1965;47:695–704.
96. Brown F. Construction of a knee joint in meromelia tibia (congenital absence of the tibia): a 15 year follow-up study. J Bone Jt Surg Am. 1972;54:1333.
97. Jayakumar SS, Eilert RE. Fibular transfer for congenital absence of the tibia. Clin Orthop Relat Res. 1979;139:97–101.
98. Epps CH Jr, Schneider PL. Treatment of hemimelias of the lower extremity. Long-term results. J Bone Joint Surg Am. 1989;71(2):273–7.
99. Simmons ED Jr, Ginsburg GM, Hall JE. Brown's procedure for congenital absence of the tibia revisited. J Pediatr Orthop. 1996;16(1):85–9. https://doi.org/10.1097/00004694-199601000-00017.
100. Wada A, Fujii T, Takamura K, Yanagida H, Urano N, Yamaguchi T. Limb salvage treatment for congenital deficiency of the tibia. J Pediatr Orthop. 2006;26(2):226–32. https://doi.org/10.1097/01.bpo.0000218529.21115.9d.
101. Hosny GA. Treatment of tibial hemimelia without amputation: preliminary report. J Pediatric Orthop B. 2005;14:250–5.
102. Balci HI, Saglam Y, Bilgili F, Sen C, Kocaoglu M, Eralp L. Preliminary report on amputation versus reconstruction in treatment of tibial hemimelia. Acta Orthop Traumatol Turc. 2015;49(6):627–33. https://doi.org/10.3944/AOTT.2015.15.0005.
103. Tokmakova K, Riddle EC, Kumar SJ. Type IV congenital deficiency of the tibia. J Pediatr Orthop. 2003;23(5):649–53. https://doi.org/10.1097/00004694-200309000-00014.
104. Ernat JJ, Wimberly L, Samchukov ML, Cherkaskin AM, Birch JG. Staged reconstruction for type IV tibial deficiency (distal tibiofibular diastasis): a report of 2 cases. JBJS Case Connect. 2019;9(4):e0088. https://doi.org/10.2106/JBJS.CC.19.00088.
105. de Sanctis N, Razzano E, Scognamiglio R, Rega AN. Tibial agenesis: a new rationale in management of type II--report of three cases with long-term follow-up. J Pediatr Orthop. 1990;10(2):198–201.
106. Brdar R, Petronic I, Abramovic D, et al. Type III longitudinal deficiency of the tibia and outcome of reconstructive surgery in a female patient. Medicina (Kaunas). 2010;46(2):125–8.
107. Hootnick D, Boyd NA, Fixsen JA, Lloyd-Roberts GC. The natural history and management of congenital short tibia with dysplasia or absence of the fibula. J Bone Joint Surg Br. 1977;59(3):267–71. https://doi.org/10.1302/0301-620X.59B3.893503.
108. Javid M, Shahcheraghi GH, Nooraie H. Ilizarov lengthening in centralized fibula. J Pediatr Orthop. 2000;20(2):160–2.
109. Eidelman MKP. Treatment of tibial hemimelia jones type 4 by ankle-sparing reconstruction (from birth to skeletal maturity). J Limb Lengthen Reconstr. 2021;7(1):52–6.
110. Weber M. A new knee arthroplasty versus Brown procedure in congenital total absence of the tibia: a preliminary report. J Pediatr Orthop B. 2002;11(1):53–9. https://doi.org/10.1097/00009957-200201000-00009.
111. Laufer A, Frommer A, Gosheger G, et al. Femoro-pedal distraction in staged reconstructive treatment of tibial aplasia. Bone Joint J. 2020;102-B(9):1248–55. https://doi.org/10.1302/0301-620X.102B9.BJJ-2019-1484.R1.
112. Oetgen ME, Richards BS. Complications associated with the use of bone morphogenetic protein in pediatric patients. J Pediatr Orthop. 2010;30(2):192–8. https://doi.org/10.1097/BPO.0b013e3181d075ab.
113. Paley D, Shannon CE, Nogueira M, Chiari C, Harris M. Can adding BMP2 improve outcomes in patients undergoing the SUPERhip procedure? Children (Basel). 2021;8(6) https://doi.org/10.3390/children8060495.
114. Lord G, Musy G. Treatment of severe recurvation of the knee in poliomyelitis. Role of olecranization of the patella. Rev Chir Orthop Reparatrice Appar Mot. 1975;61(2):135–40. Traitement du recurvatum grave du genou poliomyelitique. Place de l'olecranisation de la rotule
115. Rungee JL, Fay MJ, Deberardino TM. Olecranization of the patella. Orthopedics. 1995;18(1):27–34.

Treatment of Congenital Pseudarthrosis of the Tibia

Claire E. Shannon and Dror Paley

Introduction

Congenital pseudarthrosis of the tibia (CPT) is a rare condition with an incidence of between 1:140,000 and 1:250,000 live births [1]. It is commonly associated with neurofibromatosis (NF), fibrous dysplasia, or osteofibrous dysplasia. It presents as anterolateral bowing of the tibia with or without fracture of the tibia and/or fibula. When it presents without fracture of the tibia, the standard of care is to prevent fracture by bracing. Fracture of the tibia has been treated by a wide variety of surgical techniques despite a high failure at obtaining and maintaining union. The rate of union without refracture, reported from meta-analysis of the literature or multicenter studies, is approximately 50% [2–5]. Failure to obtain union is accepted as part of the natural history of this condition. Failure to maintain union, even when union is initially achieved, leads to repeated surgeries and secondary changes. These secondary changes include calcaneo-cavo-valgus foot deformity with foot length discrepancy, leg length discrepancy, recurvatum valgus proximal tibial deformity, coxa valga, and hip dysplasia [5, 6]. Repeated surgeries due to failures of treatment or for treatment for secondary changes lead to interruptions of childhood and prolonged repeated disability, and in some cases, a recommendation for amputation as a primary or secondary treatment [7, 8].

Until recently, no single treatment has emerged that is based on an understanding of the pathobiology and pathomechanics of CPT. No single treatment has stood out as superior to all of the rest. To achieve this status, a treatment would have to demonstrate safety, reliability, and reproducibility in obtaining and maintaining union.

The Paley Cross-Union Protocol has been reported to achieve union in 100% of cases and reduce the refracture rate to 0% [5].

Classification of CPT

There have been several different classifications of CPT (Anderson [9], Boyd [10], Crawford [11], El-Rossasy-Paley [12]). More recently, Choi et al. classified the fibula in CPT [13]. The goal of a classification is to guide treatment and to categorize cases for comparison. The Anderson, Boyd, and Crawford classifications are all descriptive and emphasize the presence of sclerosis, cystic changes, and dysplasia of the tibia. These changes, however, do not necessarily impact treatment or prognosis. The El-Rossasy-Paley classification factored in the stability and width of the bone ends in the pseudarthrosis (mobile vs. stiff, narrow atrophic vs. wide hypertrophic) similar to what is done in adult nonunion [12]. This is based on the principle that mobile-atrophic-narrow bone ends require open treatment, while stiff-hypertrophic-wide bone ends are amenable to gradual distraction based on anticipated dense fibrocartilaginous tissue between the bone ends. The mobile-narrow bone ends type was divided into two groups; without previous surgery vs. with previous surgery with the assumption that those with previous surgery had a bone defect or dead bone which after resection would produce a bone defect. These would be treated with bone grafting in the absence of a bone defect or bone transport vs. acute shortening when a bone defect was present. The El-Rossasy-Paley classification was the first classification where the type was related to the treatment algorithm. The Choi et al. classification of the fibula was the first to factor in the important consideration of proximal fibular migration [13], although they did not recommend any treatment for this. The Paley classification [5], introduced by one of the authors (DP) to help guide treatment, factors in (1) the integrity of the tibia and fibula; (2)

C. E. Shannon (✉) · D. Paley
Paley Orthopedic and Spine Institute, West Palm Beach, FL, USA
e-mail: cshannon@paleyinstitute.org; dpaley@paleyinstitute.org

the presence or absence of proximal migration of the distal fibula; and (3) the presence of a significant bone defect. These three factors affect the treatment protocol. Other factors such as the presence or absence of NF or Fibrous Dysplasia, prior surgery, atrophic or hypertrophic and stiff or mobile bone ends, and age are not considered in the classification.

Paley Classification of Congenital Pseudarthrosis of the Tibia (Fig. 32.1)

Type 1: Intact tibia and fibula with anterolateral bowing (Fig. 32.2)
Type 2a: Intact tibia with fibula fracture without proximal migration distal fibula (Fig. 32.3)
Type 2b: Intact tibia with fibula fracture with proximal migration distal fibula
Type 3: Fractured tibia with intact fibula (Fig. 32.4)
Type 4a: Fractured tibia and fibula without proximal migration distal fibula
Type 4b: Fractured tibia and fibula with proximal migration distal fibula (Fig. 32.5)
Type 4c: Fractured tibia and fibula with bone defect and proximal migration distal fibula (Fig. 32.6)

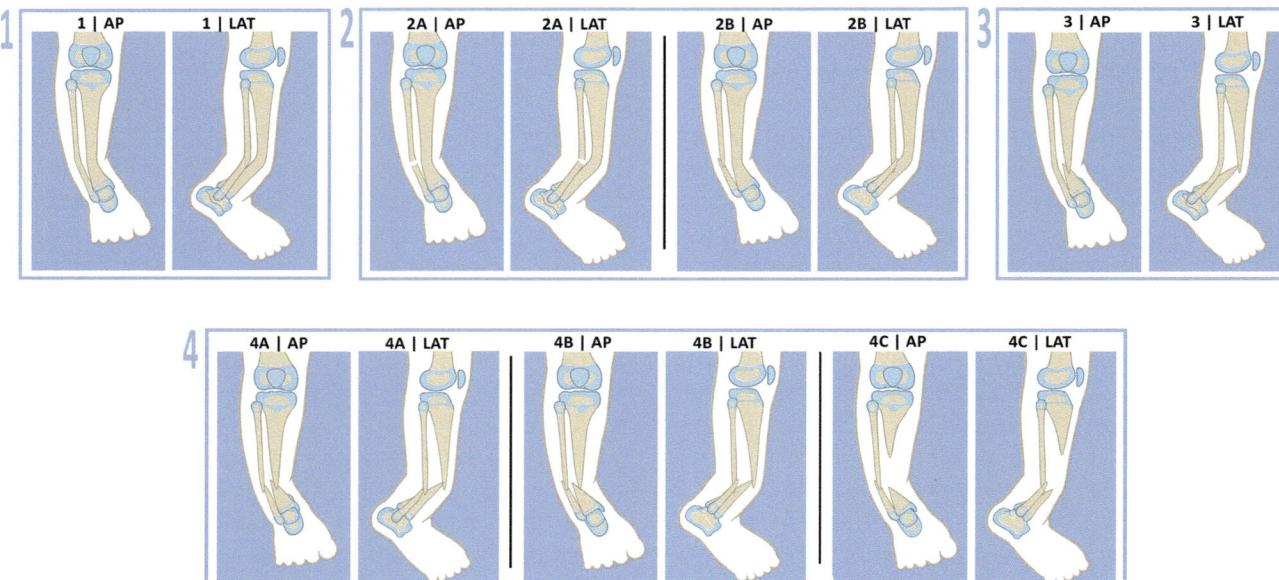

Fig. 32.1 Paley Classification of CPT (reproduced with permission of the Paley Foundation). (Copyright The Paley Foundation. Reproduced with permission. All rights reserved)

Fig. 32.2 (a) Paley type 1 pre-CPT, AP, and lateral radiographs of tibia in seven-year-old girl with NF1. Anterolateral bowing is seen without facture. She complains of pain and is limited in activities. (Copyright The Paley Foundation. Reproduced with permission. All rights reserved.) (b) AP and lateral radiographs one year after CPT cross-union protocol. The tibia is aligned and growing normally. (Copyright The Paley Foundation. Reproduced with permission. All rights reserved)

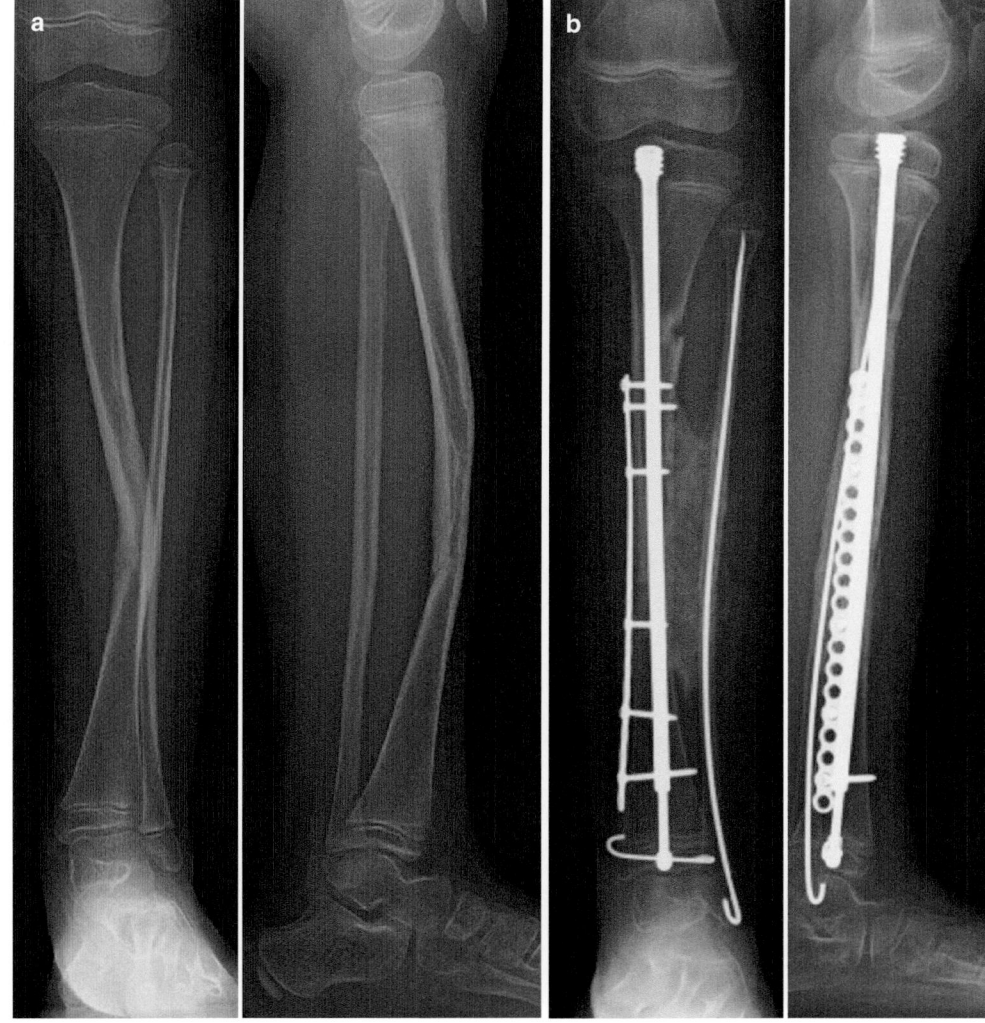

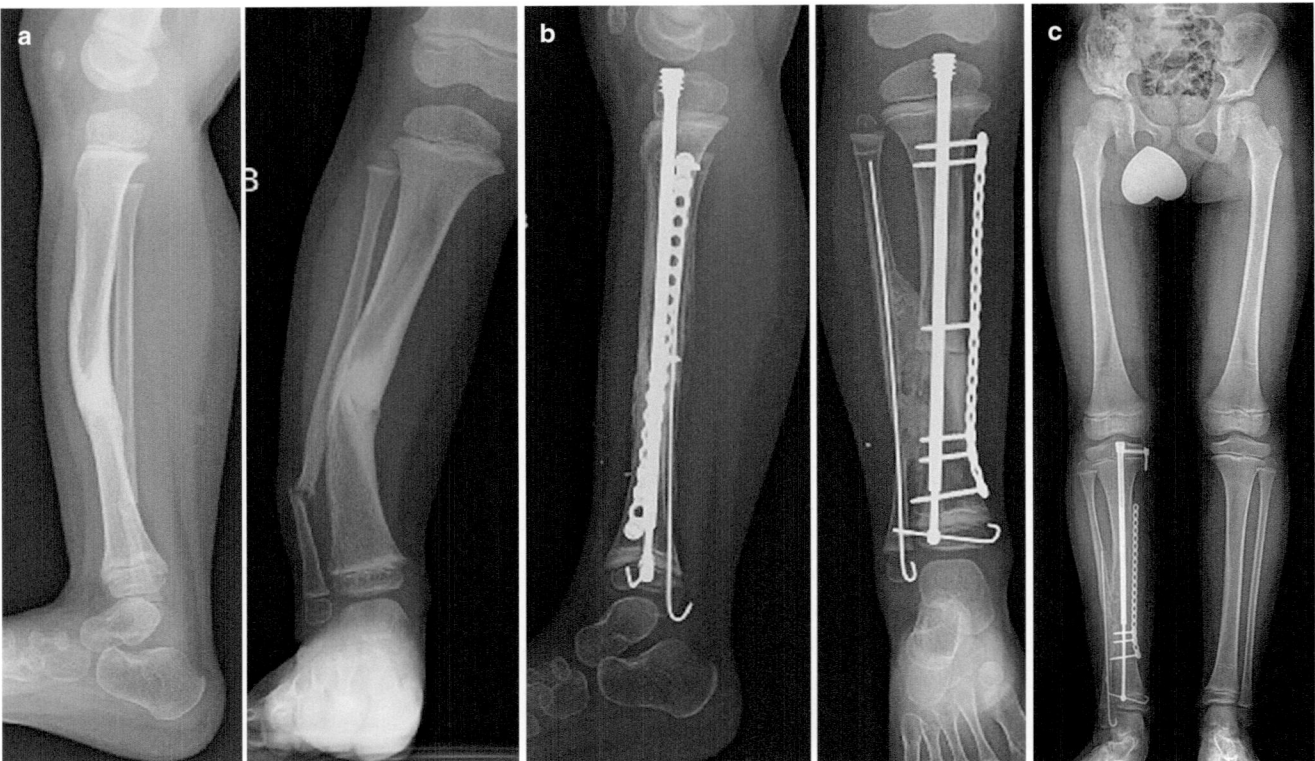

Fig. 32.3 (a) Paley type 2a CPT, AP, and lateral radiographs of tibia in a 3-year-old boy, tibia intact and fibula broken. (Copyright The Paley Foundation. Reproduced with permission. All rights reserved.) (b) 3 months after cross-union protocol surgery AP and lateral radiographs. Union and cross-union achieved. (Copyright The Paley Foundation. Reproduced with permission. All rights reserved.) (c) Two years after cross-union surgery, AP and lateral radiograph. There is significant growth post-surgery and the rod has telescoped and also pulled out of distal epiphysis. Hemiepiphysiodesis was done and released for correction of knee valgus. Rod exchange will be the next step. Note leg lengths are equal and the pelvis and hip appear normal after previous decancellousization of ilium. (Copyright The Paley Foundation. Reproduced with permission. All rights reserved)

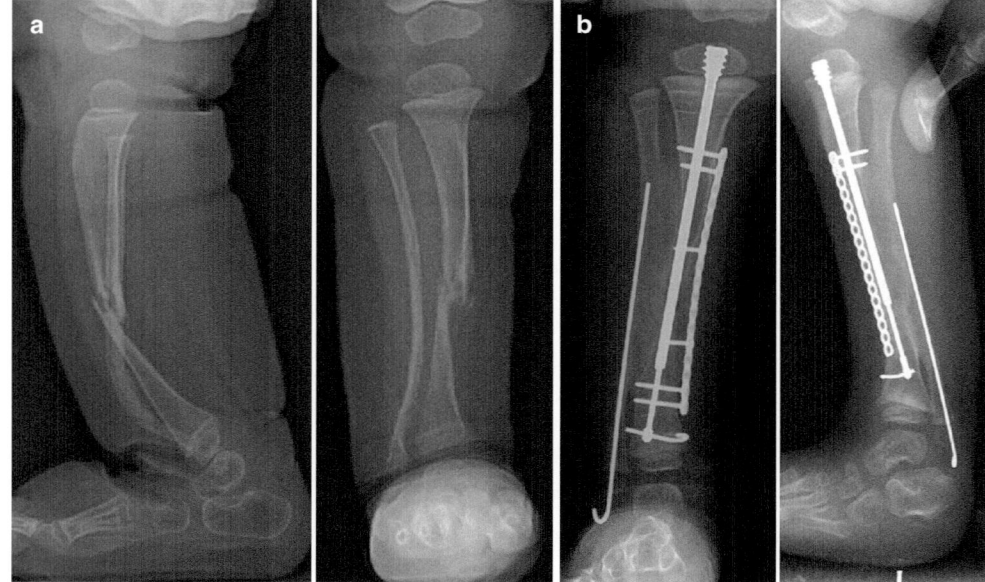

Fig. 32.4 (a) Paley type 3 CPT, AP, and lateral radiographs of tibia in a 13 mo. old girl. (Copyright The Paley Foundation. Reproduced with permission. All rights reserved.) (b) AP radiograph (left) 1 year later showing mature cross-union extending between tibia and fibula above and below the healed CPT site. Internal oblique lateral radiograph a few days later after removing the lower screws to dynamize the fixation. Again, note the mature cross-union between the tibia and fibula. (Copyright The Paley Foundation. Reproduced with permission. All rights reserved)

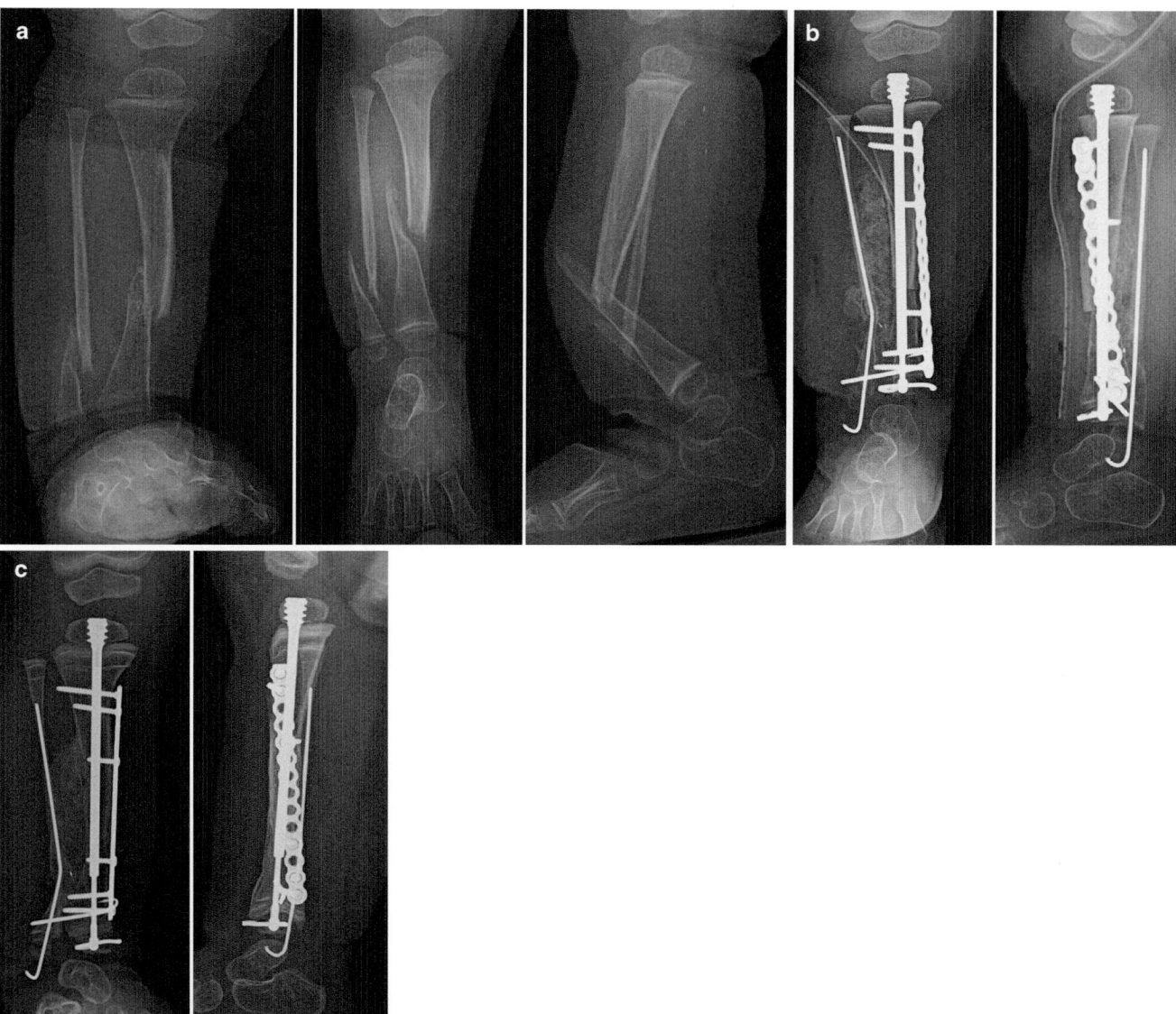

Fig. 32.5 (a) Paley type 4b CPT, AP (left), maximum plantar flexion AP (middle), and lateral (right) radiographs. Note the proximal migration of the fibula, seen best in the plantarflexion AP which is in plane with the ankle joint. (Copyright The Paley Foundation. Reproduced with permission. All rights reserved.) (b) AP and lateral immediate postoperative radiographs from day of surgery show a large area of bone graft between the tibia and fibula, as well as reduction of the fibula to station. This is held with a wire between the two bones (Copyright The Paley Foundation. Reproduced with permission. All rights reserved.) (c) AP and lateral radiographs of the tibia 6 months after surgery, showing maintained reduction of the fibula and a mature crossunion. (Copyright The Paley Foundation. Reproduced with permission. All rights reserved)

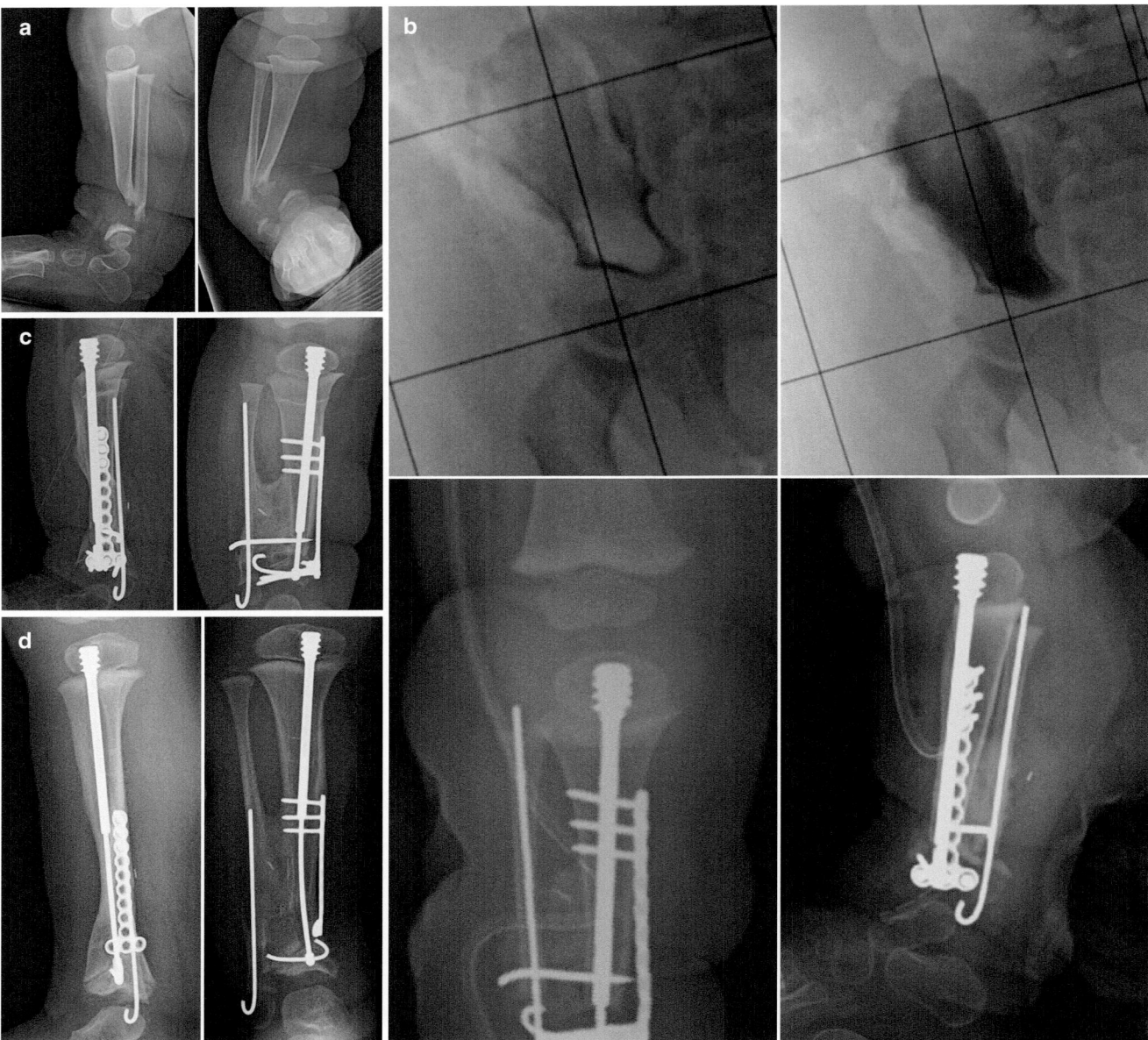

Fig. 32.6 (a) Paley type 4c CPT, AP, and lateral radiographs of tibia in a 12-month-old girl. This is a very distal CPT with very little tibia remaining proximal to the growth plate. The fibula is proximally migrated such that the distal fibular physis is no longer opposite the level of the ankle joint line. (Copyright The Paley Foundation. Reproduced with permission. All rights reserved.) (b) Immediate postoperative radiographs from date of cross-union surgery. The decancellousization of the ilium is seen (top left) compared to the ilium after filling with calcium phosphate bone filler (top right). The fixation with FD rod and plate is seen with drain in place after surgery. The bone graft fills the space between tibia and fibula and the CPT site is well opposed. Note the transverse k-wire fixation to hold the fibula at station after it was surgically reduced (bottom left and right). A T-plate was used instead of a straight plate in order to gain fixation in the distal tibial epiphysis since there is no bone available for fixation proximal to the epiphysis. (Copyright The Paley Foundation. Reproduced with permission. All rights reserved.) (c) Cross-union is mature after three months from surgery. (d) The epiphyseal screws were removed after 3 months. The distal tibial physis continued to grow normally as evidenced by the migration of the plate away from the distal tibial physis. The fibula remains at station. (Copyright The Paley Foundation. Reproduced with permission. All rights reserved.) (e) AP and lateral radiographs 3 years after cross-union surgery. The FD rod was replaced and the plate removed. The distal end of the rod pulled through the distal epiphysis. The distal tibial physis is still growing normally and the fibula remains at station. (Copyright The Paley Foundation. Reproduced with permission. All rights reserved)

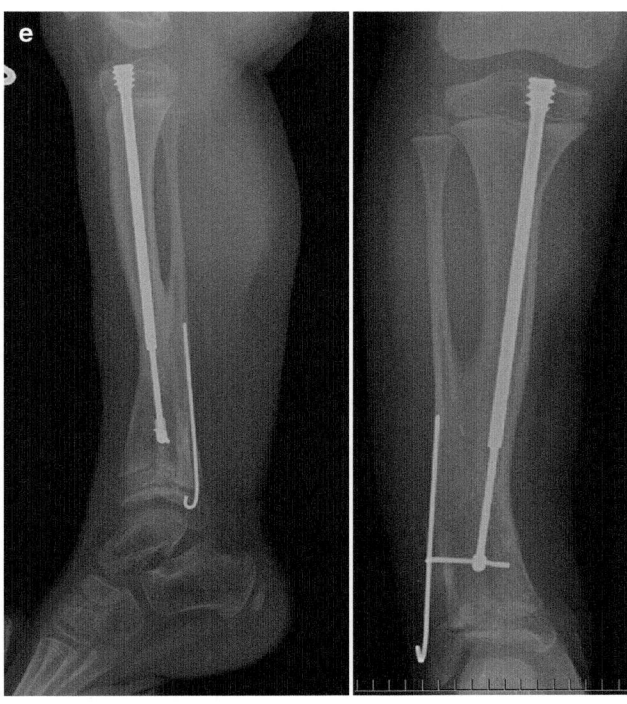

Fig. 32.6 (continued)

Pathobiology and Pathomechanics

The pathobiology of CPT starts with a fibrous hamartoma replacing the healthy periosteum [14]. This tissue has been shown to be very osteoclastic resulting in osteolysis of the tibia [5, 15, 16]. The hamartoma may also cause vascular constriction of the bone, which may lead to sclerosis of the bone and obliteration of the medullary canal [17]. In addition, the osteocytes in NF and CPT have been shown to produce lower levels of bone morphogenic protein (BMP) [18], resulting in a decreased osteoblastic response of the periosteum and bone cells [19]. This demonstrates that CPT is primarily a disorder of the soft tissues that surround the bone, rather than the bone itself, which remains viable despite the osteolysis, atrophy, and hamartomatous constriction.

The pathomechanics that weaken the bone are related to geometric changes in the tibia and fibula. The diaphyseal deformity (anterolateral bow) creates a large stress concentration at the apex of angulation. The osteolysis reduces the cross-sectional area at the apex of angulation, greatly reducing the yield strength of the bone, leading to a stress fracture. Both osteopenic and osteosclerosis changes make the bone more brittle. Fracture of the fibula increases stresses on the tibia. Fracture of the fibula is also followed by proximal migration and valgus deformity at the ankle adding additional mechanical stresses to the tibia and fibula [5].

Primary vs. Secondary Changes in CPT

The primary changes in CPT are (1) anterolateral bowing, (2) nonhealing fracture (pseudarthrosis) of tibia and/or fibula, and (3) proximal migration of the fibula. As a consequence of these three primary conditions, a myriad of secondary deformities can develop. Most of the secondary conditions are due to the effect of the primary condition on the surrounding soft tissues and joints and the secondary effects on the growth and development of the lower limb. The anterolateral bowing relaxes the posterior muscles leading to decreased tension on the Achilles tendon. This leads to atrophy and thinning of the calf muscles and eventually to a calcaneo-cavus deformity of the foot with a pistol grip heel. The anterior bow of the tibia causes the foot to assume a dorsiflexed position. The anterior soft tissues fail to elongate, and the anterior capsule is never stretched into plantarflexion. This leads to a dorsiflexion contracture of the ankle (calcaneus deformity of the foot). The proximal migration of the fibula causes the talus to follow the fibula. This leads to lateral subluxation of the ankle joint and valgus instability of the ankle. The distal tibial plafond becomes wedge-shaped relative to the distal tibial physis. The wedging of the distal tibial epiphysis produces a valgus plafond orientation. The ankle valgus serves to compensate for the lateral bowing, which in effect is a varus distal tibial deformity. Similarly, the proximal tibial physis grows into recurvatum and valgus to compensate for the procurvatum-varus diaphyseal deformity. A recent publication by Deng et al. demonstrated that persistent pseudarthrosis of the fibula and shortening of the fibula, even in the setting of tibial union, resulted in a statistically significant ankle and knee valgus compared to patients who had an intact fibula that maintained station [20]. The lack of loading on the tibia and the altered muscle forces, as well as the proximity of the pseudarthrosis to the distal tibial physis, lead to the slowing of the growth of the distal tibial and fibular physes and leg length discrepancy. In response to the altered forces in the lower leg, the proximal femur responds by growing into coxa valga [21]. The coxa valga may explain the overgrowth of the femur despite the undergrowth of the tibia. CPT is one of the few conditions with developmental leg length discrepancy (LLD) that compensates for overgrowth in the femur. In some cases, the coxa valga can be so extreme that it leads to hip dysplasia. The LLD, foot, ankle, knee, femur, and hip deformities are all secondary problems associated with CPT.

Fixing the primary problems in patients with CPT is the primary goal of treatment. The secondary problems are usually only addressed if the primary nonunion and angular deformity of the tibia can be successfully treated. Therefore, the primary objectives of treatment for patients with CPT are to: (1) straighten the anterolateral bowing at the CPT site; (2)

obtain and maintain the union of the tibia at the CPT site; (3) obtain union of the fibula to prevent or treat proximal fibular migration. The secondary objectives are to prevent or treat the secondary deformities of the ankle and foot and the leg length discrepancy.

Treatment Methods

There have been many surgical techniques used to treat patients with CPT. In the past 30 years, the most common methods have been: free vascularized fibular grafting (FVFG), intramedullary (IM) nailing with bone grafting, Ilizarov external fixation (EF), combined Ilizarov and bone grafting, and amputation [7, 10, 15, 22–41]. In all of these treatments, the primary union rates range from 61% to 100% [4]. Refracture occurs 21 to 68% of the time, and up to 24% of patients were treated with amputation. Failure of treatment is best represented by the rate of failure to achieve union combined with the refracture rate. Stated differently, the success rate is defined as the number of patients achieving union with the index procedure who did not refracture.

Ilizarov External Fixation

Paley et al. [26] reported on 15 patients who had 16 tibiae with congenital pseudarthrosis. The mean patient age was 8 years, the rate of union was 94% in 15 patients with Ilizarov frames, refracture occurred in five tibiae (31%), and the mean follow-up duration was 4 years.

Boero et al. [27] reported on 21 patients with NF treated with Ilizarov frames. The mean patient age was 8.8 years. The primary union rate was achieved in 17 of 21 (81%) patients. Refracture occurred in four of the 17 patients (19%), and the minimum follow-up duration was 2 years.

The European Pediatric Orthopaedic Society (EPOS) multicenter study [22] of 340 patients with CPT reported a 75% healing rate achieved with Ilizarov external fixation and recommended the use of prophylactic IM rodding to prevent refracture.

In a series of 17 tibiae with CPT treated by Paley and Herzenberg [28], the mean patient age was 8 years, CPT union was obtained in 100% of the patients, and refracture occurred in 68% when the Ilizarov device without IM rodding was used. When IM rodding was combined with external fixation, the refracture rate dropped to 29%.

Ohnishi et al. [29] reported 73 cases that were treated with different treatment protocols: 26 with Ilizarov fixation, 25 with vascularized fibular grafting, 7 with the combination of the previous two techniques, 6 with IM rodding combined with free bone grafting, 5 with plating and grafting, and the remaining 4 with different treatment protocols. The average patient age was 5 years. CPT union was achieved in all patients treated with Ilizarov fixation (four experienced refracture), 22 of 25 (88%) patients treated with free vascularized fibular grafting (one experienced refracture), and all patients treated with both fibular grafting and Ilizarov fixation.

Intramedullary Rodding

IM rodding has been a commonly used treatment option to achieve and maintain union in patients with CPT, although the reported results are variable. Joseph and Mathew [30] reported 14 skeletally immature patients treated with IM rodding and double onlay autogenous bone grafting from the contralateral tibia. The mean patient age was 4.5 years. The union rate was 86% and the mean follow-up was 3 years with a refracture rate of 21% (3 of 14).

Johnston [31] reported on 23 patients treated with different techniques of IM rodding and grafting. The mean patient age was 2 years 4 months, the mean follow-up duration was 9 years, the primary union rate was 87%, and 13% had persistent nonunion and poor outcomes. The author identified that two factors associated with the best outcomes were perfect limb alignment and the use of IM rods to achieve union, prevent refracture, and maintain alignment.

Kim and Weinstein [32] reported on 11 patients with 12 tibiae with congenital pseudarthrosis treated with IM rodding and free bone grafting. The mean patient age at index operation was 2.5 years. Four of the 11 patients healed after the primary index operation. Two of the four experienced refracture. The other seven did not heal after the index operation. Four of them achieved healing after undergoing multiple surgical procedures (1 free vascularized fibular grafting, 3 repeat IM rodding and grafting). Healing could not be achieved in the other three patients (2 underwent below-knee amputation, and 1 persistent nonunion at the latest follow-up). Kim concluded that IM rodding provides more predictable results in cases of late-onset pseudarthrosis [32].

Dobbs et al. [23] reported the long-term follow-up (mean 14.2 years) of 21 patients with CPT (mean age 5.1 years) treated with IM rodding and bone grafting. The primary union rate was 86% (18 patients), and three patients required additional bone grafting to achieve union. Twelve patients (57%) experienced refracture, and five (24%) required amputation.

Vascularized Fibular Grafting

Free vascularized fibular grafting had been described by several authors as a good option for achieving union in patients with CPT, although it can be associated with many drawbacks, including nonunion, refracture, and recurrent nonunion at one site of the graft end [33–38]. Angular deformity of the affected tibia (valgus or anterior bowing) has been reported. The deformities usually are progressive and require further treatment

[36–38]. Donor site morbidity, such as progressive ankle valgus with proximal migration of the distal fibula, is another problem associated with FVFG [36–38]. The tibiofibular synostosis can only delay but not prevent ankle valgus [38].

Weiland et al. [35] reported a 95% union rate in 19 patients treated by FVFG. Initial failure to achieve union occurred in 26% and those patients required secondary procedures to achieve union (4 healed and 1 underwent amputation).

Gilbert [33] reported the long-term follow-up of 29 patients who had CPT treated with FVFG, all of whom had reached skeletal maturity. The union rate was 94%, with a mean healing time of 6 months. The mean patient age at the time of the index operation was 5.5 years, the refracture rate was 14%, and the recurrence rate was 7%. Donor site morbidity occurred in 24%, tibial deformity on the affected side (valgus and anterior bowing) occurred in 24%, progressive LLD occurred in 7%, and no amputation was recorded.

The EPOS study [36, 37] reported a healing rate of 61% (19 of 31 patients) for FVFG. Seven of the 19 healed patients required additional procedures. The remaining 12 healed after the primary treatment. Three patients (10%) required amputation, seven (23%) had not healed, and five (16%) experienced a fracture of the transferred fibula.

Toh et al. [38] reported seven cases of CPT treated with FVFG, with a mean follow-up duration of 12.1 years. Casting or monolateral external fixation was used initially; an Ilizarov fixator was used as for postoperative immobilization in one case. The author concluded that combined FVFG and postoperative Ilizarov external fixation would provide the best outcome.

El-Gamal et al. [25] reported three cases of CPT treated with FVFG combined with Ilizarov fixation to distract the fibular graft to correct LLD with a single operation. They called it 'telescoping vascularized fibular graft.' The mean patient age was 9 years, and the mean follow-up duration was 2 years. Union was achieved in all cases. One patient experienced refracture, and another patient experienced ankle valgus of the affected site.

Adjunct Treatment

Pharmacotherapeutic adjunctive treatment has also been employed as part of the treatment of CPT, including the use of BMP2, BMP7, and/or bisphosphonate therapy, most commonly with Zoledronic Acid (ZA) [39, 40]. Studies of the tissue in CPT and NF have demonstrated that the hamartoma has increased numbers of osteoclasts that induce osteolysis and decreased endogenous BMP production by osteoblasts causing limited osteogenesis [18, 19, 42]. The combined use of BMP to upregulate osteogenesis and ZA to downregulate osteoclastic activity combats both of these factors to increase the chances of achieving union in CPT.

Lee et al. [39] reported on 5 CPTs treated with BMP7 combined with allograft, IM rodding, and external fixation. The mean age was 6 years, and the mean follow-up was 14 months. They concluded that the use of recombinant human BMP7 was not enough to overcome the poor healing environment associated with CPT. Birke et al. [41] used ZA for patients with CPT to control the activity of osteoclasts to promote a union. The bisphosphonate was given after bone graft harvest, and therefore was not present in the bone graft to minimize the chance of resorption.

Thabet, Paley et al. [43] reviewed 20 patients with CPT who were treated with periosteal grafting, autogenous bone grafting, IM rodding of the tibia and fibula, and circular EF. The mean age was 4.2 years. Eleven patients (55%) had NF. Union was achieved in all patients (100%). The mean time spent in external fixation was 5.2 months (range, 3–12 months). Limb lengthening (mean 2.5 cm, range 0–7 cm) was simultaneously carried out in 12 patients. Refracture occurred in 8 patients: 1 refracture in 6 patients and 2 refractures in 2 patients. Six of the 8 patients with refracture had fibular pseudarthrosis. The mean time between the original surgery and refracture was 2.3 years (1–5.8 years), and the mean time to second refracture was 4.7 years. All the refractures were united with additional surgery.

Amputation

Amputation is either a primary or a last resort option in cases of CPT [7, 8]. The incidence varies from series to series. Foot condition, number of operations, and severity of LLD are the factors considered in making the decision for amputation [7].

Treatment Results

A meta-analysis of CPT treatment performed by Paley [5] evaluated union, refracture, and success rates (union without refracture) of 25 published studies between 1990 and 2018. The studies were divided into four treatment groups: (1) rodding (10 studies, 196 patients); (2) Ilizarov (6 studies, 115 patients); (3) Ilizarov plus rodding (5 studies, 152 patients); (4) FVFG (4 studies, 84 patients). Primary union was achieved in 61% of the rodding group, 93.5% of the Ilizarov group, 72% of the Ilizarov plus rodding group, and 66% of the FVFG group. The refracture rate was 24% in the rodding group, 41% in the Ilizarov group, 17% in the Ilizarov plus rodding group, and 11% in the FVFG group. Multiplying the union rate by one minus the refracture rate yields the success probability of achieving union without refracture, which is the ultimate goal of surgery. The success probability was 40% for the rodding group, 57% for the Ilizarov group, 58% for the Ilizarov plus rodding group, and 58% for the FVFG group. The average success probability of the combined 25 studies was 50.7%.

This conclusion is further supported by a number of recent studies. Shah et al. [3] reported a long-term follow-up retrospective multicenter study of patients with CPT. Patients were treated with a variety of methods, including Williams rods, Ilizarov fixation, bone grafting, and FVFG. Union was achieved after the index procedure in 102/119 (86%). Amputation was performed in 11/17 that failed primary union. Data regarding refracture were available on 94 of the primary union cases. Forty of these sustained a refracture (42.5%). The probability of union without refracture was 49.5%. The mean age at primary union was 5.6, and the mean age at refracture was 8 years. The refractured cases underwent 53 surgeries. At skeletal maturity, 82/119 were united (69%). A strong union was associated with no surgery on the fibula, the use of cortical bone graft, and either IM nailing or Ilizarov treatment. The combination of Ilizarov and IM nailing had a high rate of a weak union. The use of BMP was associated with a poorer outcome. Transfixation of the ankle was shown to improve the chance of obtaining union.

Kesireddy et al. [2] did a meta-analysis reporting on 33 published studies that encompassed 401 cases of CPT. The mean age was 5.2 years, and NF1 was present in 262 (65%). The mean follow-up was 8 years. The mean rate of primary union was 75%, and the rate of refracture was 35%. The probability of union without refracture was 49%.

Laufer et al. [44] reported on 26 patients treated for CPT between 1997 and 2019. Six (Group A) were treated by resection of pseudarthrosis and bone transport with grafting of the docking site. Fifteen (Group B) were treated by resection of pseudarthrosis, acute shortening of the bone defect with grafting and lengthening of the tibia. Five (Group C) were treated by resection of the pseudarthrosis, acute shortening of the bone ends with grafting, and rodding with no lengthening. Group A had a 50% union rate with no refractures. Group B had an 80% union rate with a 33% refracture rate. Group C had a 60% union rate with no refractures. In total, 18/26 patients (69%) achieved union with a 22% refracture rate. These authors came with the first publication to apply Paley's success probability to a clinical study. They reported that the long-term success probability of union without refracture in their series was 53.8%.

The success probability of these recently published studies was 49.5%, 49%, and 53.8% respectively, which is very similar to Paley's meta-analysis result of 50.7%. There appears to be a glass ceiling of success probability of approximately 50% with current methods of treatment.

Rastogi and Agarwal [4] performed a systematic review of cross-union versus the more traditional treatment methods for CPT; rodding, ilizarov, combined ilizarov with rodding, and vascularized fibular graft. Fifty-seven studies were included that encompassed 1227 patients. Nineteen studies (339 patients) were on rodding, 11 on Ilizarov (182 patients), 15 on combined rodding with Ilizarov (366 patients), 16 on FVFG (248 patients), and 5 on cross-union (92 patients). Cross-union demonstrated shorter time to healing (4.5 m), higher primary union rate (100%), and the lowest refracture rate (22.7%) of any method. One of the cross-union series was noted to be an outlier with all of the refractures occurring in only this patient group. This review shows that the data in support of cross-union are promising, despite relatively short follow-up, compared to other traditional treatment methods that cannot surpass the 50% success probability ceiling.

Most studies report union and refracture rates, but few studies have examined functional outcomes after surgical treatment for CPT. Karol et al. published that patients had 68% reduced push-off strength if they had been treated with transarticular rodding across the ankle joint compared to 36% reduced strength when the rod did not cross the ankle joint [45]. Seo et al. reported that ankle function was well preserved after successful Ilizarov treatment of CPT [46], where no rod transfixed the ankle joint. Therefore, techniques that leave a rod across the ankle and subtalar joints are less desirable.

Evolution of the Paley Cross-Union Protocol

Paley first published a report on CPT in 1992 [26], including 16 patients treated for CPT with the Ilizarov method. Long-term follow-up of this cohort and subsequently treated cases of CPT demonstrated a high refracture and retreatment rate [28]. The initial treatment was resection of the hamartoma and bone grafting of the CPT site with Ilizarov fixation. The healing rate was nearly 100%, but the refracture rate was over 50%. In some cases, an intramedullary rod (flexible titanium or Rush rod) was added and the refracture rate dropped. Clearly, the Ilizarov fixation method was excellent at obtaining union but failed to maintain union. The IM rod was excellent at maintaining union and decreasing refracture. The same conclusion was found in a multicenter EPOS study by Weintraub and Grill [22]. The efficacy of the IM rod was also increased by rodding both bones in the leg rather than just one.

The El Rosasy, Paley et al. study [12, 28] also identified two other factors that decreased refracture: (1) increasing the cross-sectional area of union and (2) eliminating angular deformity at the CPT site. Paley combined all of these principles as well as adding a periosteal graft at the CPT site and these results were reported in 2008 [43]. Treatment involved resection of the hamartoma, iliac crest bone and periosteal grafting of the CPT site, and rodding of the tibia and fibula. Union was achieved in 100%. Refracture occurred in 8/20 (40%).

The achievement of mechanical stability and biologically favorable conditions was reliably producing union but still demonstrating refracture. A review of the cases that did not refracture in the Thabet, Paley et al. study demonstrated the development of a cross-union between the tibia and fibula [14, 43]. This was thought to be a result of the large amount of bone graft obtained using the decancellousization method of bone graft harvest [5]. After resection of tibial and fibular hamartomas, the two bones were bone-grafted circumferentially, but with no intention to create a cross-union. This unintentionally generated a cross-union in several of those patients.

To prevent bone graft resorption, in 2004 the author started infusing zoledronic acid (ZA) two weeks prior to surgery. This allows this third-generation bisphosphonate to be taken up by the cancellous bone of the ilium and downregulate the osteoclast activity, to prevent resorption of the transplanted bone graft. It also protects the native bone of the tibia from further osteoclastic resorption.

Finally, to boost the osteogenic response of the graft and native bone, BMP2 was added. The synergistic use of ZA to downregulate bone resorption and BMP to upregulate bone formation leads to an optimal biologic environment for bone healing [18, 19, 42].

Prior Treatment Lessons [5]

1. Hamartoma resection should be comprehensive, back to normal fat planes
2. The medullary canal should be reestablished
3. All tissue at the CPT site including bone and soft tissues should be considered alive
4. Autogenous cancellous bone graft is superior to autogenous cortical or allograft bone and provides more stem cells
5. Cancellous bone graft can be rapidly resorbed
6. Intramedullary fixation helps prevent refracture
7. Stable fixation of the CPT site is critical for healing
8. Exogenous BMP augments the lower BMP levels produced by the bone cells at the CPT site
9. Bisphosphonate (e.g., Zoledronic Acid) reduces osteoclasis at the CPT site
10. Zoledronic acid given prior to bone graft harvest prevents bone graft resorption after surgery
11. Angular correction at the CPT site is critical for mechanical stability
12. Periosteal grafting can help with the healing of the CPT site and avoid a new hamartoma
13. Larger cross-sectional area of healing at the CPT site has a lower risk of fracture due to mechanical strength
14. Cases with accidental cross-union between the tibia and fibula do not refracture
15. Union rates are not age-dependent

The author used all of these considerations to construct a treatment protocol that is based on biology, biomechanics, and more than a century of cumulated knowledge about CPT.

In 2007, Paley first combined all of these techniques to create an intentional cross-union between the tibia and the fibula [14]. The treatment protocol was: presurgical infusion of ZA; hamartoma resection around tibia and fibula; tibial and fibular rodding; decancellousization of the ilium to harvest a large cancellous bone graft; harvest of a periosteal graft from the underside of the iliacus muscle; apply a 3-layer graft composed of periosteum around the CPT; cancellous bone between and around the tibia and fibula; BMP2 posterior and anterior to the bone graft covered by soft tissues. The last step was application of the Ilizarov apparatus. The Ilizarov apparatus was used to compress the CPT site and to give rotational stability. The smooth non-locking telescopic rod only gives angular support but does not prevent the bone ends pulling apart or rotating to each other. More recently (since 2014) the author replaced the external fixator with an internal fixator (locking plate) [5].

Paley Cross-Union Protocol Surgical Technique [47, 48] (Figs. 32.7, 32.8, 32.9, 32.10, 32.11, 32.12, 32.13, 32.14, 32.15, and 32.16)

Step 1: Preoperative Bisphosphonate Infusion: one to two weeks prior to the surgery the patient is given a zoledronic acid infusion intravenously (0.02 mg/kg) over 30 min. One hour later calcium gluconate 60 mg/kg is given intravenously over the course of 1 h. The patient is given 1200 mg calcium daily for 14 days and 1000IU Vitamin D_3 daily 14 days after the infusion.

Step 2: Prep and Incision: The patient is placed supine, with a bump under the ipsilateral buttock, on a radiolucent table. The entire lower extremity and hemipelvis are prepped and draped free. The leg is exsanguinated, and tourniquet applied. The pseudarthrosis site is approached through an anterior longitudinal incision (Fig. 32.7a).

Step 3: Anterior Fasciotomy: The anterior compartment fascia is incised, and the fasciotomy is extended proximally and distally (Fig. 32.7b).

Step 4: The medial skin and subcutaneous tissues are elevated together with the superficial fascia off of the subcutaneous border of the tibia. It may be necessary to take the most superficial layer of the hamartoma with the skin to ensure that the fascia is connected to the medial flap. The dissection continues until the posteromedial border of the tibia (Fig. 32.7c).

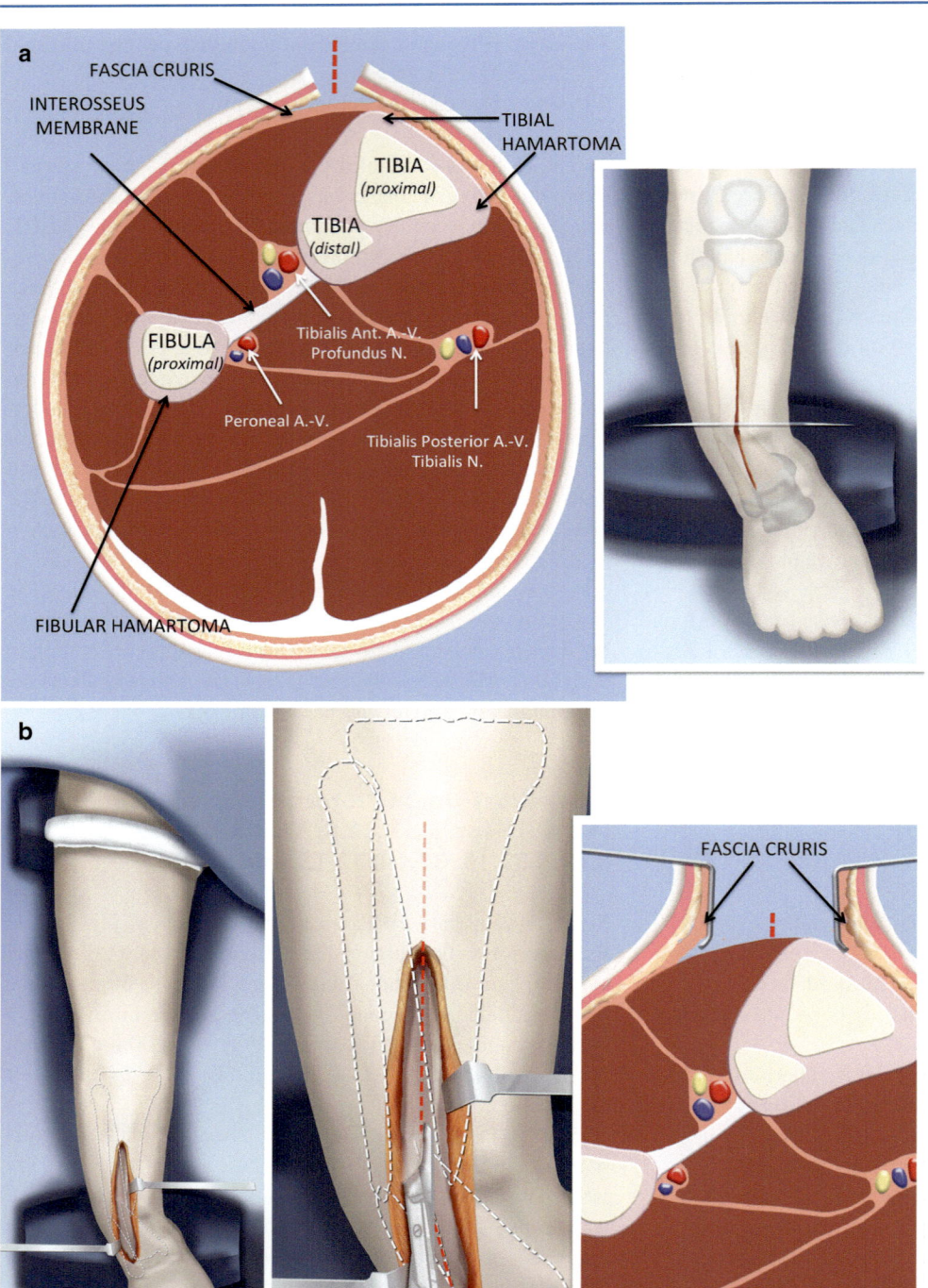

Fig. 32.7 (**a–k**) Reproduced with permission from the Paley Foundation (Copyright The Paley Foundation. Reproduced with permission. All rights reserved.) (**a**) Incision (anterior view right and cross-section view right). Note the circumferential hamartoma surrounding the tibia and fibula labelled on the cross-section view. The anterior tibial and peroneal neurovascular bundles lie very close to this tissue and can be adherent to it. (Copyright The Paley Foundation. Reproduced with permission. All rights reserved.) (**b**) Anterior compartment fasciotomy (Copyright The Paley Foundation. Reproduced with permission. All rights reserved.) (**c**) Dissection between anterior fascia adherent to skin and medial tibial hamartoma. (Copyright The Paley Foundation. Reproduced with permission. All rights reserved.) (**d**) Elevation of anterior compartment off tibia, interosseous membrane, and fibula. (Copyright The Paley Foundation. Reproduced with permission. All rights reserved.) (**e**) Deep posterior compartment exposure and fasciotomy (Copyright The Paley Foundation. Reproduced with permission. All rights reserved.) (**f**) Deep posterior compartment muscle elevation off posterior tibia (AP view left, cross-section view right). (Copyright The Paley Foundation. Reproduced with permission. All rights reserved.) (**g**) Excision of interosseous membrane (cross-section view left and AP view right). Care is taken to avoid injury to the peroneal vessels, which lie posterolateral to the membrane. These vessels perforate the membrane distally to pass anterior to the membrane. (Copyright The Paley Foundation. Reproduced with permission. All rights reserved.) (**h**) Incision of tibial hamartoma (left). Dashed red lines show the anterior longitudinal incision for both the tibial and fibular hamartomas and the radial incision lines at the limits of resection (right). (Copyright The Paley Foundation. Reproduced with permission. All rights reserved.) (**i**) Circumferential excision of the tibial hamartoma (top to bottom left then bottom right). The proximal and distal radial cuts are made to circumferentially excise the hamartoma. (Copyright The Paley Foundation. Reproduced with permission. All rights reserved.) (**j**) Anterior and radial incision of fibular hamartoma with complete removal of this tumor (left to right). Cross-section view showing that both the tibial and fibular hamartomas have been excised circumferentially (right). The dissection does not extend to the distal tibiofibular syndesmosis since the fibula is not proximally migrated. (Copyright The Paley Foundation. Reproduced with permission. All rights reserved.) (**k**) When the fibula is proximally migrated, the dissection should be extended distally to expose the tibiofibular syndesmosis. The peroneal vessels run over this area (left) and should be mobilized and retracted out of the way (second to left). The anterior tibiofibular ligament is cut (middle) and then by separating the bones, the posterior tibiofibular ligament is visualized (second to right) and cut (right). This frees up the fibula to be reduced to station when the fibula is proximally migrated. (Copyright The Paley Foundation. Reproduced with permission. All rights reserved)

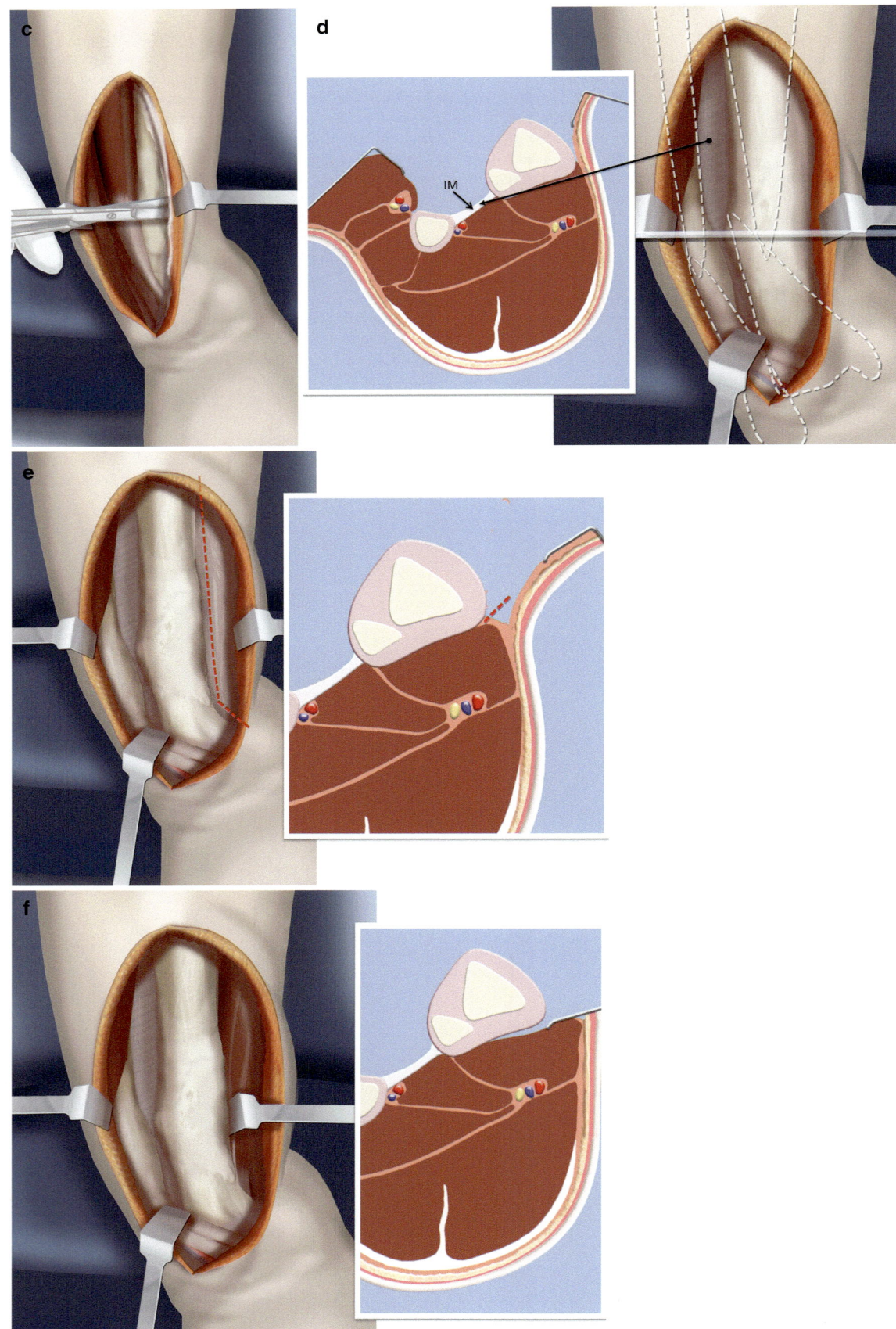

Fig. 32.7 (continued)

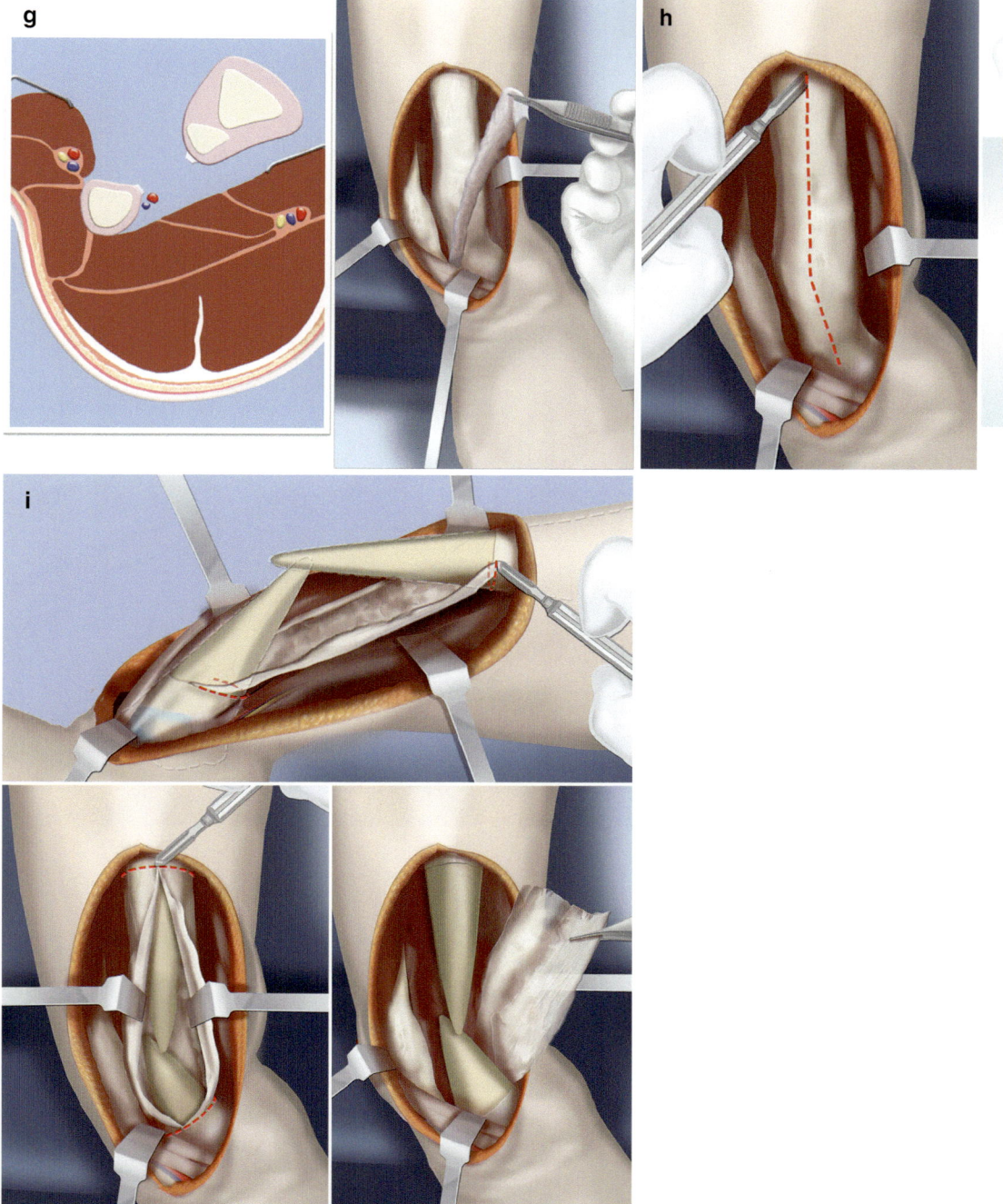

Fig. 32.7 (continued)

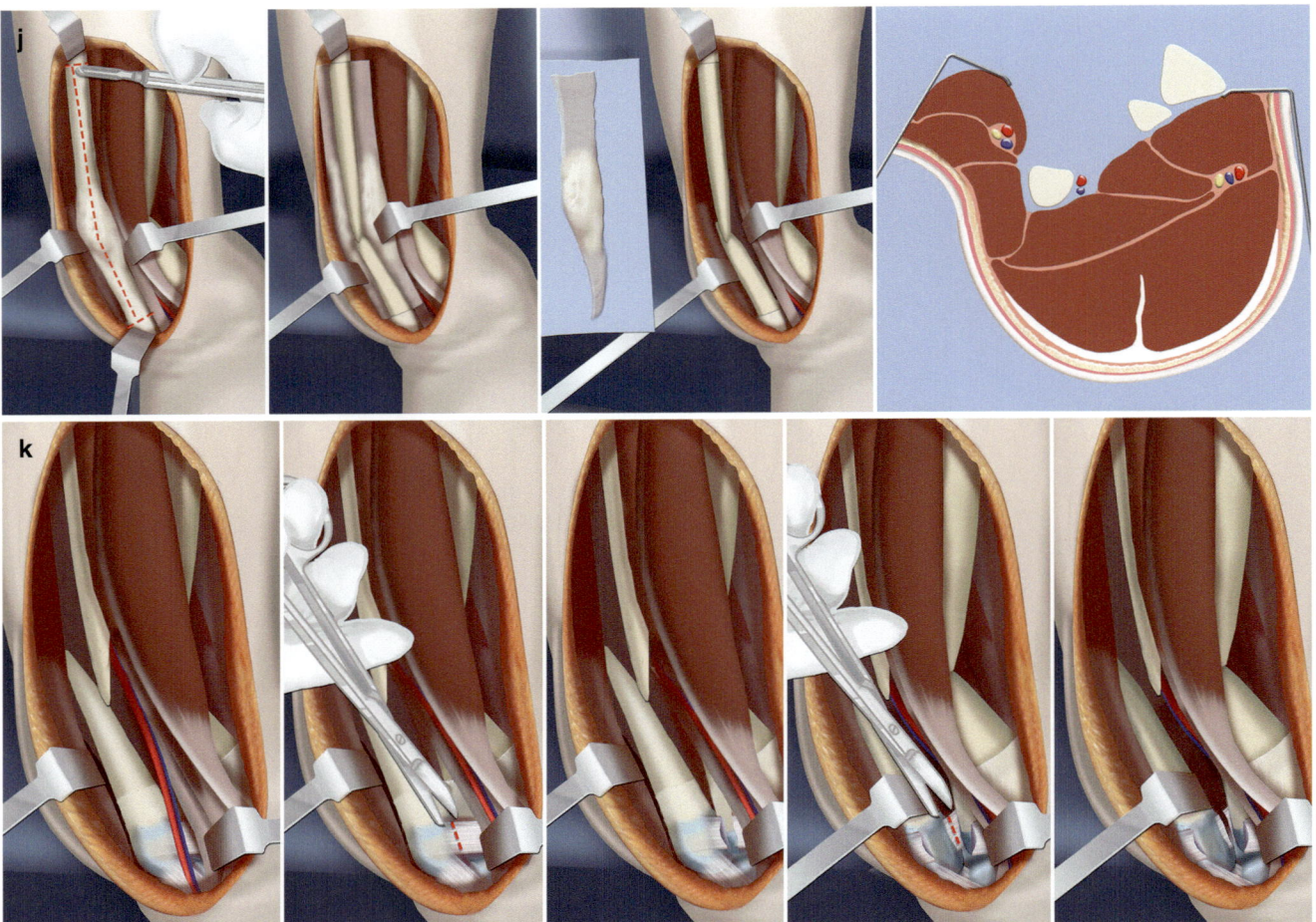

Fig. 32.7 (continued)

Step 5: Anterior Compartment Muscle Elevation: The anterior compartment muscles including the anterior tibial vessels and deep peroneal nerve are gently elevated off of the lateral border of the tibia and off of the interosseous membrane until the medial wall of the fibula is exposed (Fig. 32.7d).

Step 6: Deep Posterior Compartment Fasciotomy: The deep posterior compartment fascia is incised longitudinally (Fig. 32.7e).

Step 7: Posterior Compartment Muscle Elevation: The deep posterior compartment muscles are gently dissected off the posterior hamartoma/periosteum around the back of the tibia and off the interosseous membrane (Fig. 32.7f).

Step 8: Interosseous Membrane Excision: Incise the interosseous membrane on its tibial and fibular borders from anterior to posterior avoiding injury to the peroneal vessels. Excise the membrane in the entire region planned for the cross-union. Dissect around the fibular hamartoma circumferentially. Be careful to avoid injury to the peroneal artery as it passes from posterior to the membrane to anterior to the membrane at the distal end of the interosseous space (Fig. 32.7g).

Step 9: Hamartoma Incision: Longitudinally incise the hamartoma of the tibia anteriorly for the entire length of planned resection. Make sure that the incision of this tissue exceeds the region of thickened periosteum (Fig. 32.7h).

Step 10: Circumferential Excision of Hamartoma: Radially incise the periosteum proximally and distally to resect the hamartoma from the tibia (Fig. 32.7i).

Step 11a: Excise Hamartoma from Fibula but do not release syndesmosis if Fibula at station (Type 1, 2a, 3, 4a). (Distal fibular physis at level of ankle mortis): Longitudinally and radially incise the periosteum of the fibula and excise the fibular hamartoma at the same levels as the tibial hamartoma excision (Fig. 32.7j). Do not disrupt the syndesmotic ligaments.

Step 11b: Release Syndesmotic Ligaments if Fibula proximally migrated/not at station (Type 2b, 4b). (Distal fibular physis proximal to level of ankle mortis): Expose the anterior tibiofibular syndesmotic ligament. If necessary, extend the

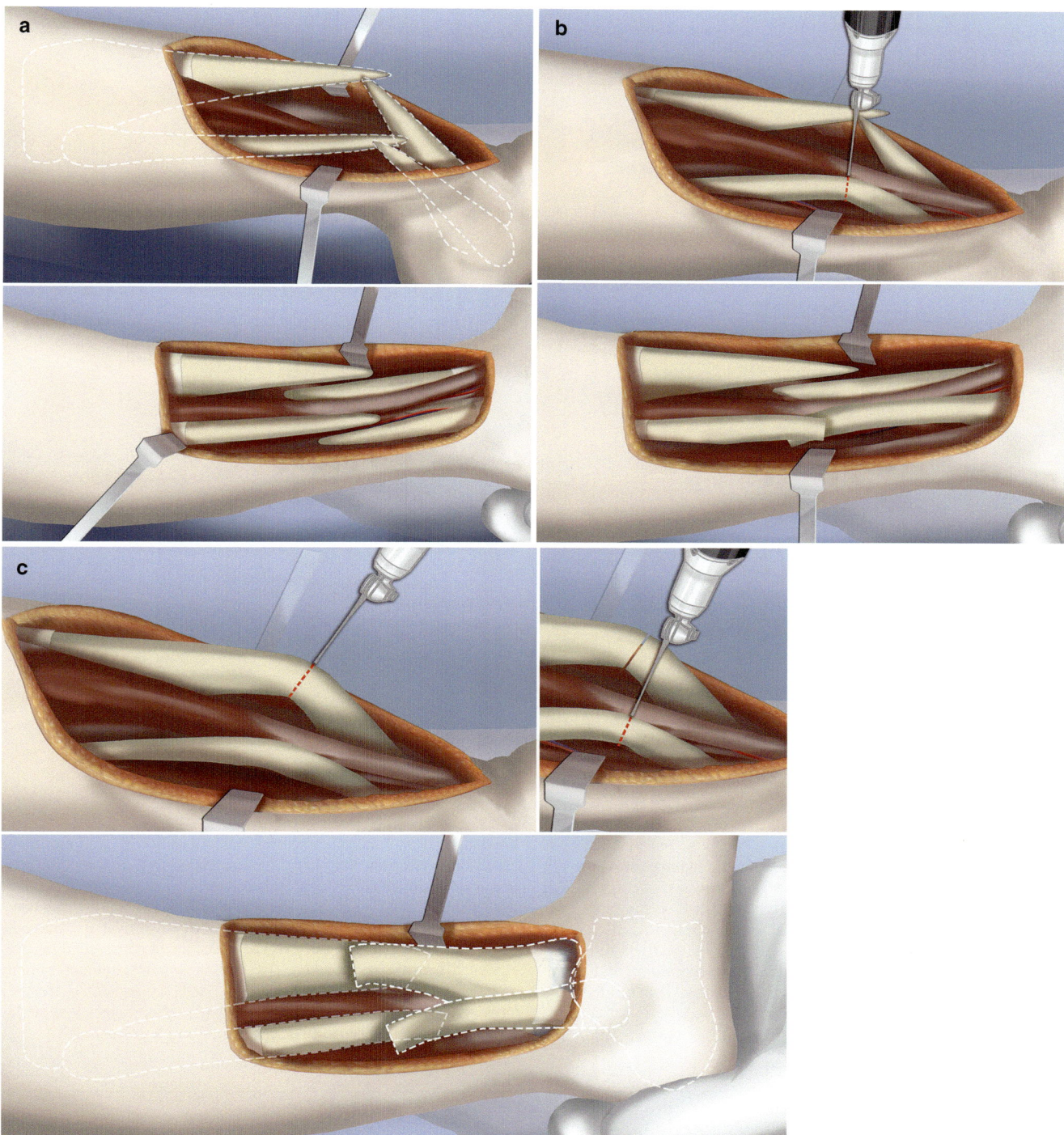

Fig. 32.8 (**a–c**) Reproduced with permission by the Paley Foundation. (Copyright The Paley Foundation. Reproduced with permission. All rights reserved.) (**a**) The anterolateral bowing of the CPT (top) can now be straightened by allowing the bone ends to shorten (overlap) relative to each other (bottom). (Copyright The Paley Foundation. Reproduced with permission. All rights reserved.) (**b**) If the fibula is intact with a CPT of the tibia, the fibula must first be osteotomized (top) before the anterolateral bowing can be straightened (bottom) allowing for overlap of the bone ends. (Copyright The Paley Foundation. Reproduced with permission. All rights reserved.) (**c**) If the tibia and fibula are both intact with anterolateral bowing, the tibia (top left) and fibula (top right) must first be osteotomized before the anterolateral bowing can be straightened (bottom) allowing for overlap of the bone ends. (Copyright The Paley Foundation. Reproduced with permission. All rights reserved)

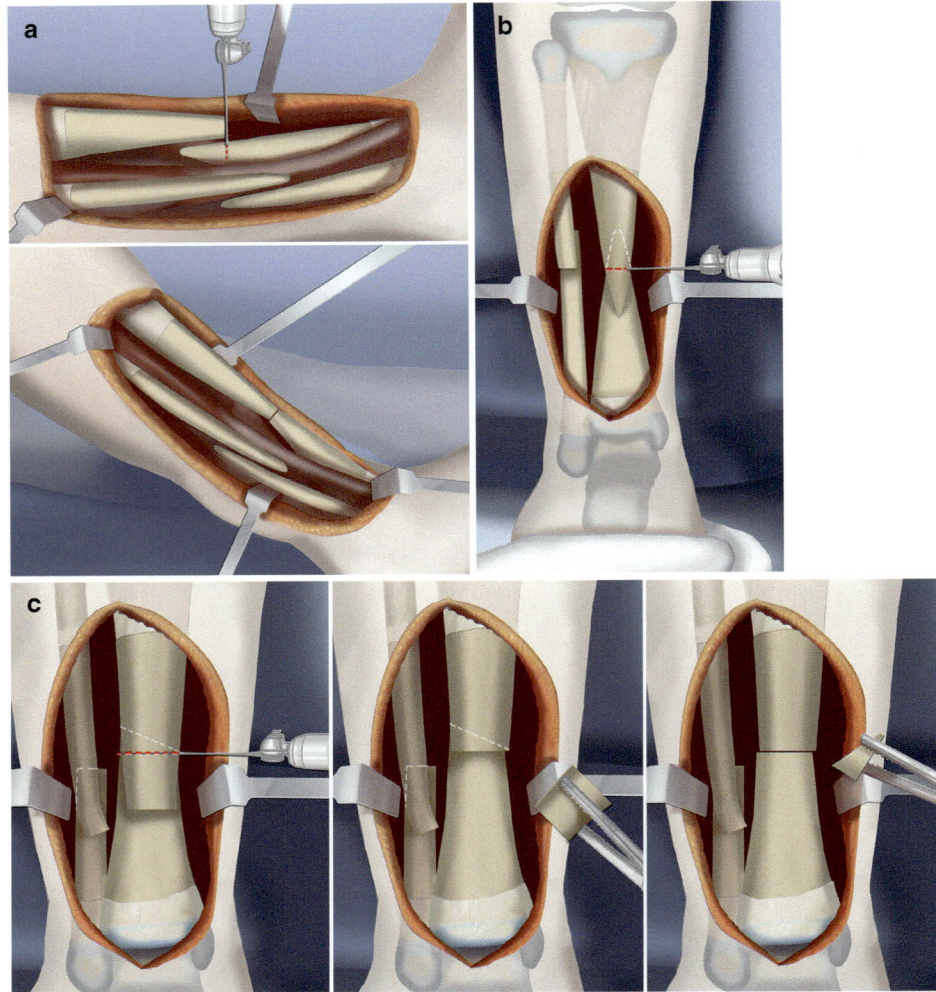

Fig. 32.9 (**a–c**) Reproduced with permission by the Paley Foundation. (Copyright The Paley Foundation. Reproduced with permission. All rights reserved.) (**a**) The tibial bone ends are cut at the level that will maximize the cross-sectional area of contact between the bone ends when the tibia is reduced. The fibula is not cut at this time. (Copyright The Paley Foundation. Reproduced with permission. All rights reserved.) (**b**) In the case of an intact fibula, the tibial bone ends are cut at the level that will maximize the cross-sectional area of contact between the bone ends when the tibia is reduced. The fibula which was previously osteotomized does not have its bone ends cut yet. (Copyright The Paley Foundation. Reproduced with permission. All rights reserved.) (**c**) In the case of an intact tibia and fibula: The tibial bone ends are cut at the level that will maximize the cross-sectional area of contact between the bone ends when the tibia is reduced. The fibula which was osteotomized is not cut further at this time and its ends are allowed to overlap. Since the distal tibia is shorter than the proximal tibia, the larger resection is usually taken from the proximal end (left) and the minimal amount from the distal end (middle). At the end, the bone ends are square so that they have good alignment and contact(right). (Copyright The Paley Foundation. Reproduced with permission. All rights reserved)

Fig. 32.10 (**a–f**) Reproduced with permission by the Paley Foundation. (Copyright The Paley Foundation. Reproduced with permission. All rights reserved.) (**a**) A 1.8 mm guide wire is drilled retrograde through the proximal fragment to exit anteriorly in the tibia and patella. It is necessary to flex the knee maximally to pass this wire. Distally there may be no medullary canal. The wire should be drilled to recreate this canal. (Copyright The Paley Foundation. Reproduced with permission. All rights reserved.) (**b**) A cannulated drill from the Fassier-Duval set is used to ream open the canal of the proximal tibia. These drill bits are slightly larger than the diameter of the corresponding nail. The smallest diameter nail is 3.2 mm. (Copyright The Paley Foundation. Reproduced with permission. All rights reserved.) (**c**) A wire is drilled antegrade into the distal tibia. It is important to center this wire in the distal tibial epiphysis as much as possible. (Copyright The Paley Foundation. Reproduced with permission. All rights reserved.) (**d**) A cannulated drill from the Fassier-Duval set is used to ream open the distal medullary canal. (Copyright The Paley Foundation. Reproduced with permission. All rights reserved.) (**e**) A small diameter wire (1, 1.5, or 1.8 mm) is used to drill open the medullary canal of both ends of the fibula. If the fibular end is too thin or sclerotic, try drilling the wire from the epiphyseal end to exit the bone in the diaphysis. Even if the exit point is not the very tip of the fibula, the wire hole can be used later in an "in – out – in pathway. After completing this, back the wire out the distal end and leave it in the distal fragment. (Copyright The Paley Foundation. Reproduced with permission. All rights reserved.) (**f**) Insert a 1.8 mm k-wire down the tibia exiting out the upper end. This wire should span the entire length of the reduced tibia (left). Insert a second wire of the same length down the tibia to perch on the tibial plateau joint surface. Measure the difference in length between these two wires to determine the total length of the nail needed. (Copyright The Paley Foundation. Reproduced with permission. All rights reserved)

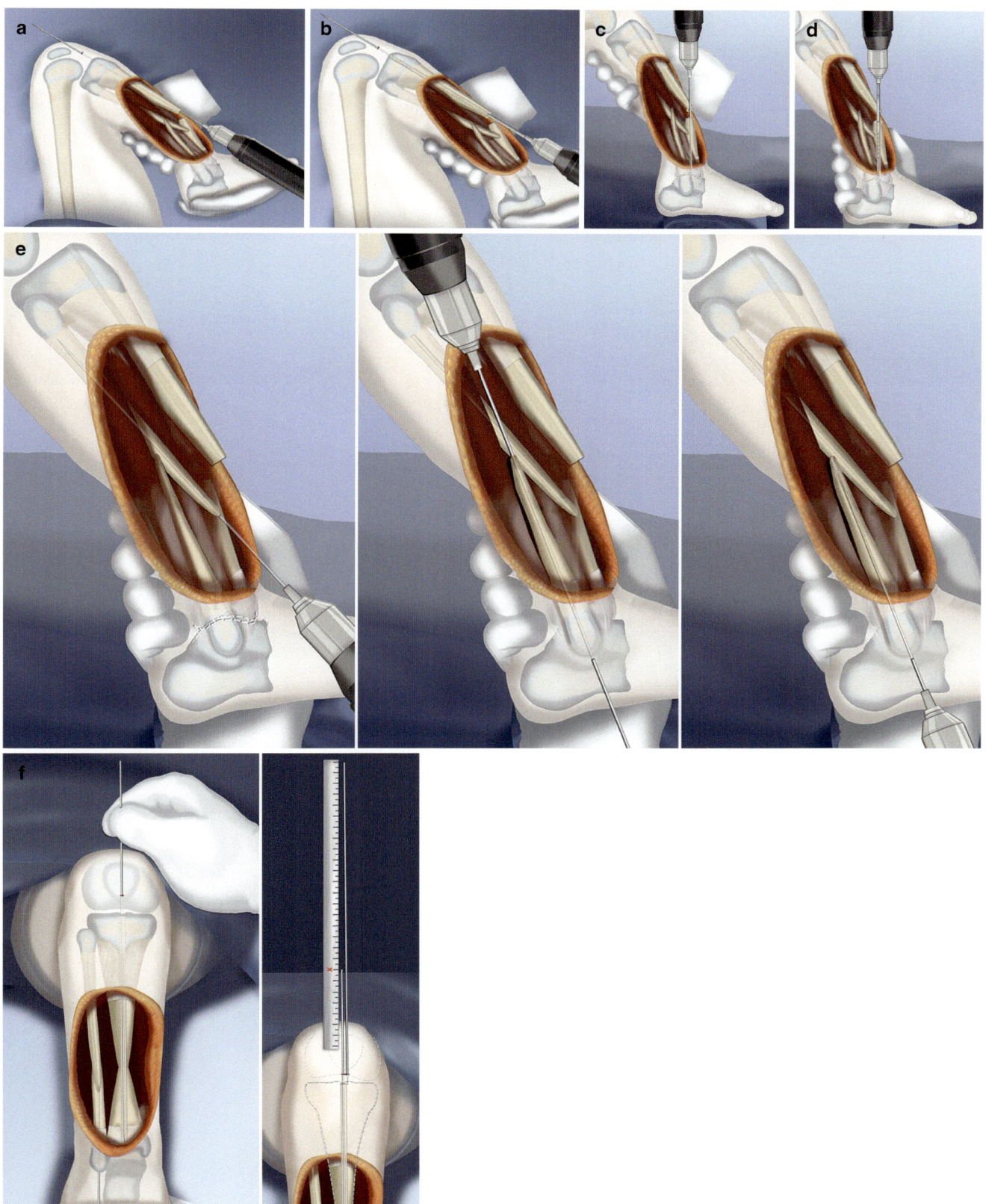

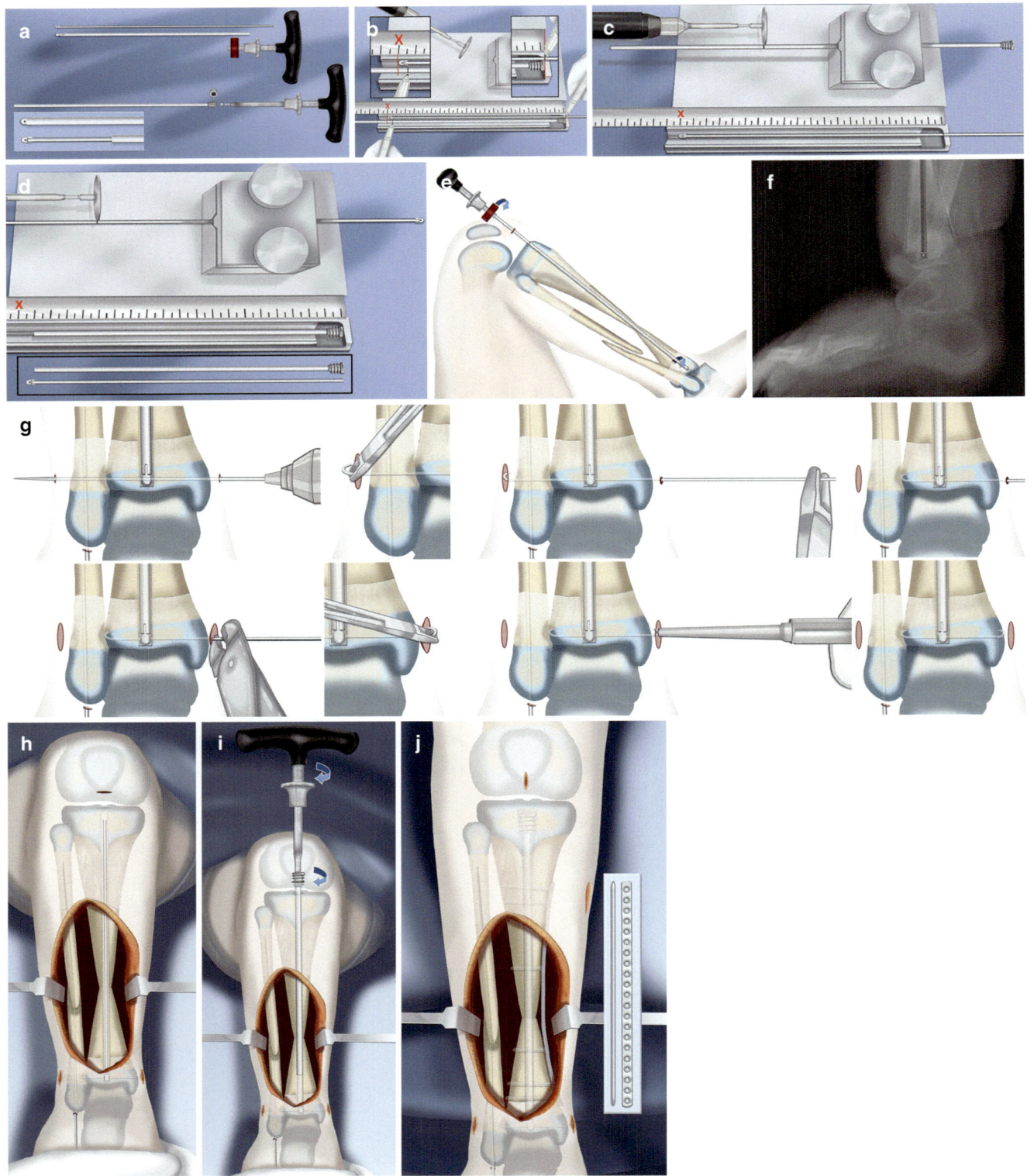

Fig. 32.11 (**a–j**) Reproduced with permission by the Paley Foundation. (Copyright The Paley Foundation. Reproduced with permission. All rights reserved.) (**a**) Fassier-Duval equipment: Top: Male rod with introducer. The introducer is slotted to control rotation of the male component that has a fin that fits in the slot at its distal end. Bottom: Female end and its wrench. The female rod slides over the male rod. Note that the male rod has a locking hole at its end and not a screw end (the screw end is used for osteogenesis imperfect but not for CPT). This locking male end is the preferred type for CPT due to the small size of the distal tibial epiphysis. (Copyright The Paley Foundation. Reproduced with permission. All rights reserved.) (**b**) The uncut male and female ends are measured relative to each other on a cutting jig, and relative to the total length of the nail 'x' measured determined in Fig. 32.10f. Both rods are marked. (Copyright The Paley Foundation. Reproduced with permission. All rights reserved.) (**c**) The female end is fixed in a vice. A high-speed diamond-tipped metal cutting wheel is used to cut the female end at the correct length. (Copyright The Paley Foundation. Reproduced with permission. All rights reserved.) (**d**) A high-speed diamond wheel metal cutting wheel is used to cut the male end at the correct length (top). The male end is fixed in a vice. The customized male and female ends are measured to ensure they are the desired lengths (bottom). (Copyright The Paley Foundation. Reproduced with permission. All rights reserved.) (**e**) The male introducer inserts the male rod through the canal of the tibia to the distal epiphysis. The hole in the nail is rotated so its opening is medial-lateral. (Copyright The Paley Foundation. Reproduced with permission. All rights reserved.) (**f**) Using the image intensifier, the end of the nail is visualized and the image is magnified. (Copyright The Paley Foundation. Reproduced with permission. All rights reserved.) (**g**) The hole in the rod is 1.6 mm diameter for 3.2 mm FD rods and larger for larger size rods. For the 3.2 mm rod, a 1.5 mm k-wire is drilled from the medial side through the hole in the nail and out the lateral side (top left). The wire is then bent 180° (top left center) and pulled to the bone (top right center and top right). The wire is then cut short (bottom left) and bent 180° (bottom left center) and then impacted into the bone, so it is completely flat under the thin skin on the medial side of the tibia (bottom right center). The wire is left flush to bone on the medial side (bottom right). (Copyright The Paley Foundation. Reproduced with permission. All rights reserved.) (**h**) The male rod is inside the tibia and is distally locked. (Copyright The Paley Foundation. Reproduced with permission. All rights reserved.) (**i**) The female rod is introduced overtop the male rod and advanced until its threaded head is screwed into the proximal tibial epiphysis. (Copyright The Paley Foundation. Reproduced with permission. All rights reserved.) (**j**) To control axial rotation and length, a small diameter locking plate is used on the medial side of the tibia. One screw is placed at either end and then the additional screws added. The screws pass either anterior or posterior to the rod. It is important that they do not impinge on the rod since both ends of the rod need to slide within the bone in response to growth from the physes at each end. The plate is shown in profile and face on. The author's preference is the Smith and Nephew EVOS plate with its very small screws. It is important not to use screws bigger than 2 or 2.7 mm in diameter. (Copyright The Paley Foundation. Reproduced with permission. All rights reserved)

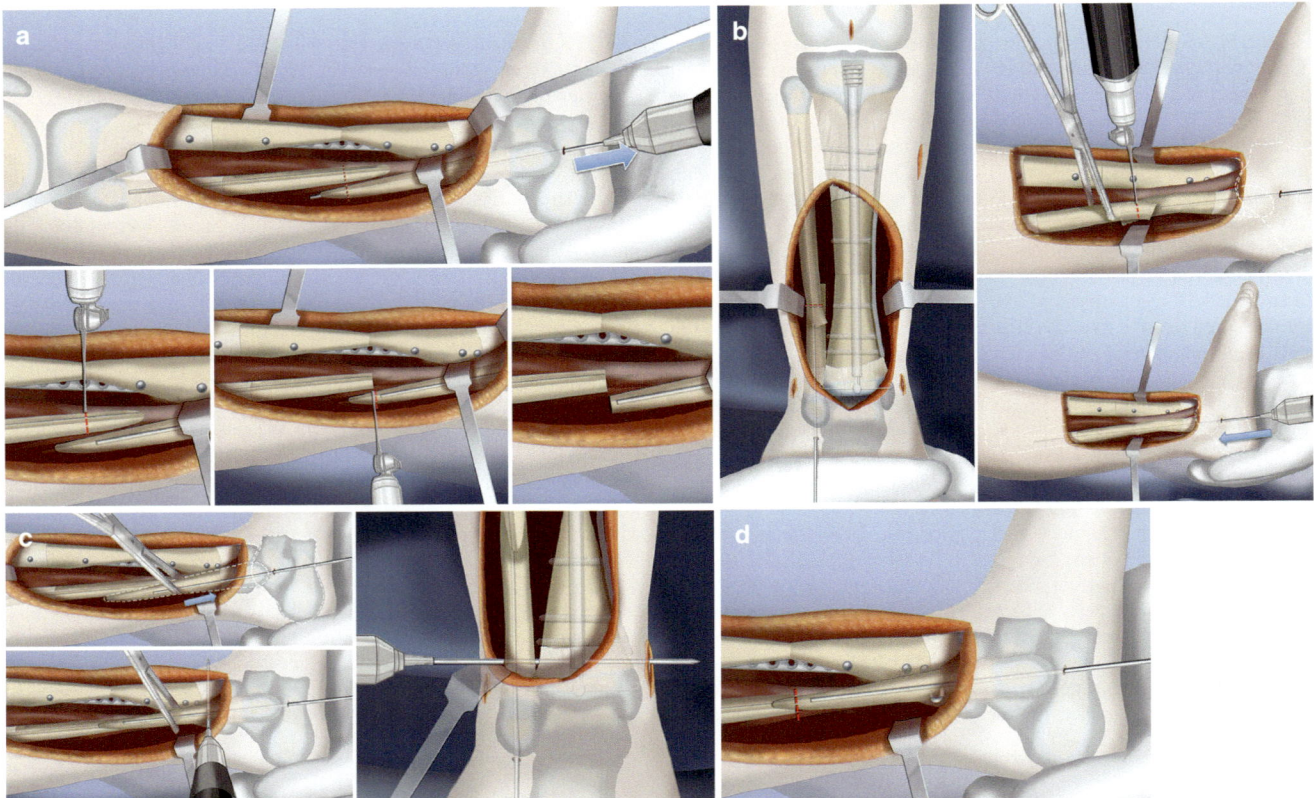

Fig. 32.12 (**a–d**) Reproduced with permission by the Paley Foundation. (Copyright The Paley Foundation. Reproduced with permission. All rights reserved.) (**a**) Lateral view of the tibia with fibula at station, showing the screws of the plate posterior to the nail (top). The fibular bone ends are overlapping. The fibula is cut to maximize the diameter of contact (bottom left). It is better to cut the bone 1 mm too long (bottom middle and right) so that the bone ends are under compression when reduced. (Copyright The Paley Foundation. Reproduced with permission. All rights reserved.) (**b**) If the fibula was osteotomized as in Fig. 32.9b or c, the ends of the fibula need to be cut square (left and top right) and then reduced and the wire advanced across the fibula to stabilize it (bottom right). (Copyright The Paley Foundation. Reproduced with permission. All rights reserved.) (**c**) If the fibula has migrated proximally (top left) as in Fig. 32.7k, the fibula should be acutely transported distally (bottom right). When it is restored to the correct station (distal fibular physis at level of ankle joint), the fibula should be transfixed with a wire to the tibia to hold it reduced at station (bottom left and right). (Copyright The Paley Foundation. Reproduced with permission. All rights reserved.) (**d**) For the example in Fig. 32.12c, the fibula can now be cut. (Copyright The Paley Foundation. Reproduced with permission. All rights reserved)

skin incision distally, to allow for direct exposure of the tibiofibular syndesmosis. Retract the peroneal artery and vein to see the ligament. Cut the anterior ligament and then separate the bones and under direct vision cut the posterior ligament (Fig. 32.7k).

Step 12a: Bone End Separation (Type 4a: Tibia and fibula CPT present): Separate the tibia and fibula CPT bone ends from each other and allow the bone ends to overlap (shorten) as the deformity is straightened (Fig. 32.8a).

Step 12b: Bone End Separation (Type 3: Tibia CPT present, Fibula intact): Osteotomize the fibula at the apex of its deformity. If the fibula has no angulation, osteotomize it at the level of the tibial CPT. Separate the fibular bone ends and allow the tibia and fibula bone ends to overlap, as the deformity is acutely corrected (Fig. 32.8b).

Step 12c: Bone End Separation (Type 1: Tibia and Fibula intact): Osteotomize the tibia at the apex of its deformity. Osteotomize the fibula at the apex of its deformity. If the fibula has no angulation, osteotomize it at the level of the tibial osteotomy. Separate the tibial and fibular bone ends and allow the tibia and fibula bone ends to overlap, as the deformity is acutely corrected (Fig. 32.8c).

Step 13a: Square Off Tibial Bone Ends (Type 4: Tibia and fibula CPT present): Mark the level where to cut the two ends of the tibia proximally and distally. Square them off using a saw and irrigation. Try and make the cuts so that the most sclerotic and atrophic parts of the tibia are resected. Try and minimize the resection. The intention is not to resect the CPT. The cuts are simply to bring two ends of the tibia together in a straight alignment position with the minimum amount removed. The intention is to also make the tibial cuts at a level that is as wide as possible to maximize the bone-to-bone contact area (Fig. 32.9a).

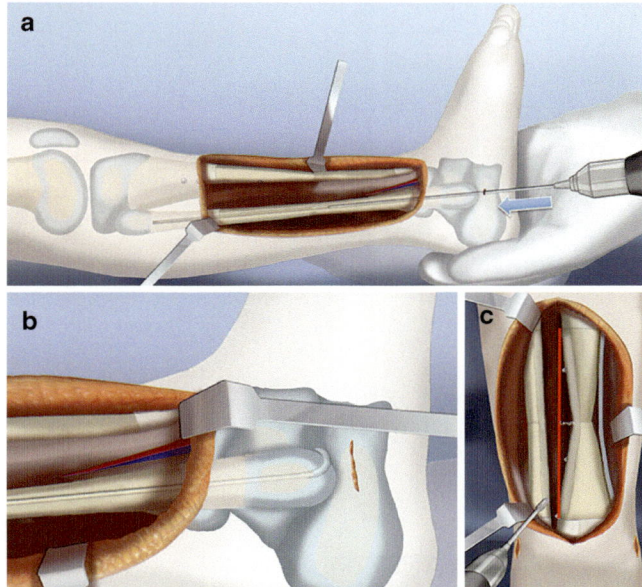

Fig. 32.13 (a–c) Reproduced with permission by the Paley Foundation. (Copyright The Paley Foundation. Reproduced with permission. All rights reserved.) (**a**) Advance the fibular wire from distal to proximal into the predrilled hole in the proximal fibula. (Copyright The Paley Foundation. Reproduced with permission. All rights reserved.) (**b**) Cut, curl, and bury the end of the wire. It is important to make sure this wire is not prominent since it will stay buried until skeletal maturity. (Copyright The Paley Foundation. Reproduced with permission. All rights reserved.) (**c**) Using a high-speed burr and irrigation, burr the facing sides of the tibia and fibula. This will help the cross-union to develop. The tourniquet is removed after this step. (Copyright The Paley Foundation. Reproduced with permission. All rights reserved)

Step 13b: Square Off Tibial Bone Ends (Type 3: Tibia CPT present, Fibula intact): Follow the same instructions as in Step 13a (Fig. 32.9b).

Step 13c: Square Off Tibial Bone Ends (Tibia and Fibula intact): Follow the same instructions as in Step 13a (Fig. 32.9c).

Step 14: Proximal Guide Wire: Drill a retrograde proximal tibial guide wire. Make sure this guide wire enters at the distal medullary canal and exits through the proximal epiphysis in the anterior half of the tibia in the sagittal plane and midline in the frontal plane (Fig. 32.10a).

Step 15: Proximal Tibial Reaming: Drill the proximal tibia with a cannulated drill overtop the guide wire. Use the diameter of drill corresponding to the diameter of nail planned for fixation (Fig. 32.10b).

Step 16: Distal Guide Wire: Drill an antegrade distal tibial guide wire. Make sure this guide wire enters at the proximal medullary canal and ends in the mid-distal epiphysis (Fig. 32.10c).

Step 17: Distal Tibial Reaming: Drill the distal tibia with a cannulated drill overtop the guide wire. Use the diameter of drill corresponding to the diameter of nail planned for fixation (Fig. 32.10d).

Step 18: Drill the Fibula with a Wire: Use a wire to drill the two ends of the fibula from the level of the CPT or osteotomy. Distally, it should come out the lateral malleolus. At the distal end, leave the wire protruding out the lateral malleolus (Fig. 32.10e).

Step 19: Measure Intramedullary Length: Measure the length of the reamed track of the intramedullary canal of the proximal and distal tibia combined by inserting a guide wire down the entire track. Measure the length of this wire protruding proximally by inserting a second equal length wire down to the proximal surface of the tibial epiphysis (Fig. 32.10f).

Step 20: Fassier-Duval Telescopic Nail Preparation: The Fassier-Duval Telescopic Nail (Pega Medical, Montreal, Canada) is used. It consists of a male and female portions that fit together passively, by sliding the thinner male end into the larger diameter female part (lower picture). The male end has a hole at its end for locking into the distal epiphysis. The female part has a threaded head to screw into the proximal epiphysis. A T-handle with introducer is used to insert the male end (top upper picture), and a hexagonal driver is used for the female end (bottom lower picture) (Fig. 32.11a).

A special measuring jig is used to mark where to cut the male and female ends (Fig. 32.11b).

Use a metal cutting saw to cut the female (Fig. 32.11c) and male (Fig. 32.11d) Fassier-Duval nails to the measured length while they are held in a special vice.

Step 21: Male Component Insertion: Insert the male portion of the Fassier-Duval (FD) with the locking hole end into the epiphysis. Use the introducer to control the insertion. It is preferable to use what is known as the Paley modification or LON version of the male FD nail. The screw-tipped male FD nail used for osteogenesis imperfecta does not fit well into the small distal tibial epiphysis. Use the lockable male end, which uses a transverse wire for locking (Fig. 32.11e).

Step 22: Distal Locking: Using the handle of the introducer, rotate the male component so that the hole faces medial-lateral. Center the hole on the image intensifier screen and magnify it maximally (Fig. 32.11f). Now use the largest diameter K-wire that fits through the hole and drill it from the medial side of the epiphysis centered on the hole. Drill it across the epiphysis and exit out the lateral side. Make a small incision on the lateral side and after bending the tip of the wire 180°, pull it back into the distal epiphysis. Do the same on the medial side. Cut the wire short and bend it using a small needle driver. Use a tamp (punch) to push the bent wire into the bone from medial to lateral, so it is not prominent on the medial side (Fig. 32.11g). Now remove the introducer (Fig. 32.11h).

Step 23: Insert the Female Component: Insert the precut female FD nail, capturing the male end in its cannulation. Screw the female end into the upper tibial epiphysis (Fig. 32.11i). Take care to use the fully threaded female end

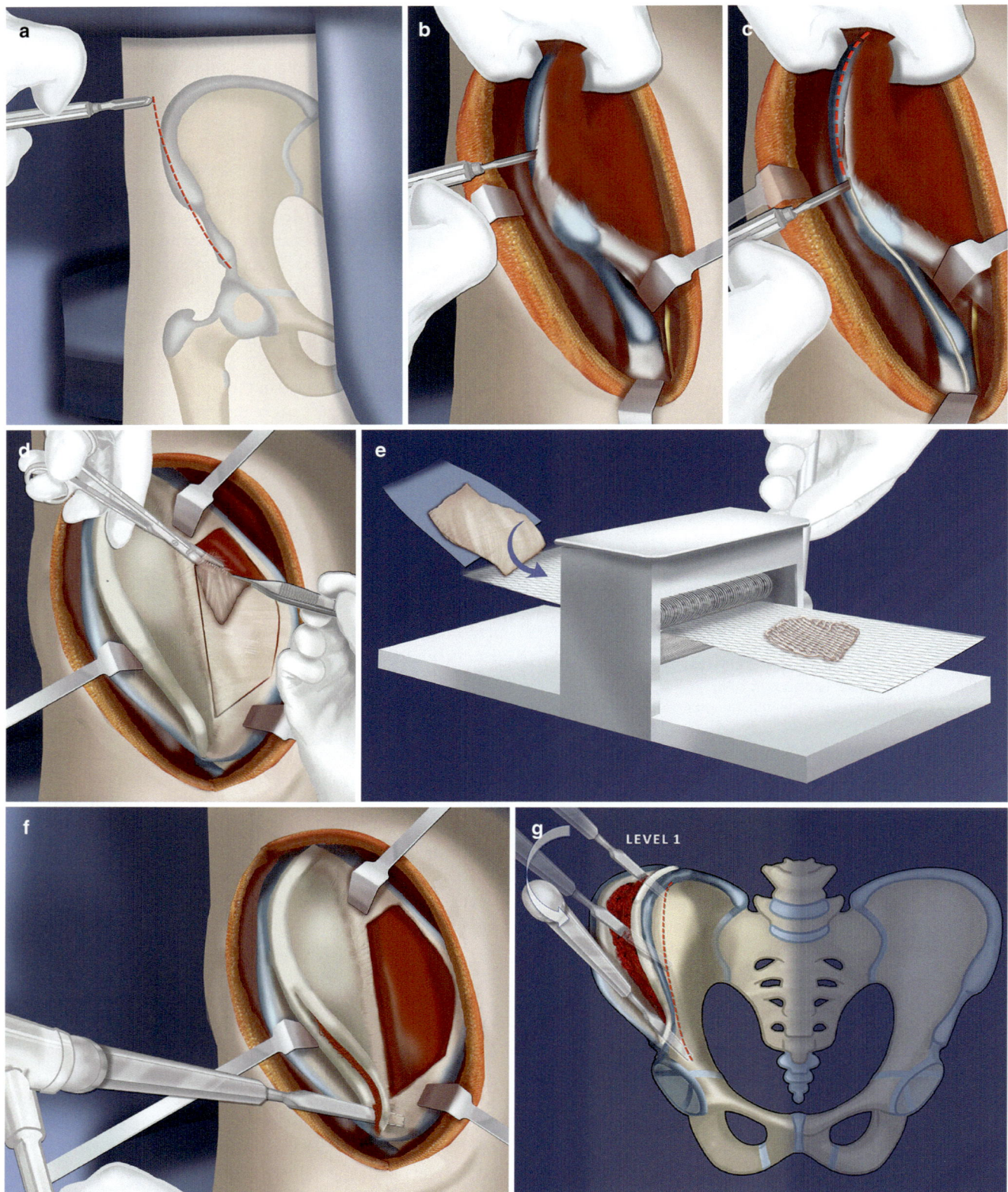

Fig. 32.14 (a–o) Reproduced with permission by the Paley Foundation. (Copyright The Paley Foundation. Reproduced with permission. All rights reserved.) (**a**) Make a long bikini incision along the ipsilateral iliac crest. (Copyright The Paley Foundation. Reproduced with permission. All rights reserved.) (**b**) Find and decompress the lateral femoral cutaneous nerve and protect it. Expose the cartilage of the iliac apophysis by raising some of the external oblique muscle from lateral to medial. (Copyright The Paley Foundation. Reproduced with permission. All rights reserved.) (**c**) Split the apophysis from the anterior inferior iliac spine (AIIS) to the anterior superior iliac spine (ASIS) to the crest of the tibia from anterior to posterior. Split the crest as far as possible all the way to the posterior iliac crest. This is much farther than normally done for a pelvic osteotomy. (Copyright The Paley Foundation. Reproduced with permission. All rights reserved.) (**d**) Reflect back the medial apophysis and periosteum off the ilium. Incise the periosteum to excise a large rectangular window of periosteum from the undersurface of the iliacus muscle. (Copyright The Paley Foundation. Reproduced with permission. All rights reserved.) (**e**) The periosteum immediately shrinks to one quarter its area. Use a skin graft mesher to mesh the periosteum so that it can be enlarged again. (Copyright The Paley Foundation. Reproduced with permission. All rights reserved.) (**f**) Use a very thin, sharp osteotome to split the tables of the ilium. Start by separating the cortices between the AIIS and ASIS. (Copyright The Paley Foundation. Reproduced with permission. All rights reserved.) (**g, h, i**) Split the iliac tables apart by going from anterior to posterior and only penetrating a cm at a time. Do not advance too far at any one spot. Work back and forth from front to back penetrating ever deeper into the ilium and avoiding exiting the cortical bone. If accidentally the osteotome exits, try and find a way to reenter the bone at that level. It is possible to split even the thinnest part of the ilium with a thin sharp osteotome. Guide the osteotome with the image intensifier to avoid entering the hip or sacroiliac joints or the triradiate cartilage. It is essential to reach these structures as well as the roof of the sciatic notch. Please note that the split goes all the way back to the posterior iliac crest. It is not difficult to reach there from this incision and from the front. It is important to follow the round contour of the iliac wing to avoid perforating the bone. This step is the hardest part of the entire procedure. Once the split is complete, you can lever the medial wall away from the lateral wall using the osteotome. Do not do this prematurely and do not lever the lateral wall away from the medial. Make sure to split the apophysis from the inside all the way to the back. (Copyright The Paley Foundation. Reproduced with permission. All rights reserved.) (**j**) The ilium will now open like a book exposing its entire cache of cancellous bone. Use straight and angled curettes to remove the spongiosa bone. Do not remove cortical bone. (**k**) Curette out layer by layer of bone from superficial to deep. The entire posterior iliac crest cancellous bone can be retrieved by this approach. (Copyright The Paley Foundation. Reproduced with permission. All rights reserved.) (**l**) The biggest trove of bone is above the dome of the acetabulum and extending to the triradiate cartilage. All of this bone should be removed without perforating these structures. (**m**) At the end there is no more cancellous bone in the ilium. This is why this is called decancellousization of the ilium. The cup should contain at least 15 to 20 cm of bone or more depending on the age and size of the patient. (Copyright The Paley Foundation. Reproduced with permission. All rights reserved.) (**n**) The space created by the curettage can either be left to fill in on its own or can be back filled with a bone void filler. The author recommends a calcium phosphate cement that can be injected and then harden in place. It will slowly be replaced with normal cancellous bone. (Copyright The Paley Foundation. Reproduced with permission. All rights reserved.) (**o**) Suture closed the apophysis and also suture the external oblique muscle to avoid creating an abdominal hernia. Take care not to inadvertently catch the lateral femoral cutaneous nerve in the suture line. (Copyright The Paley Foundation. Reproduced with permission. All rights reserved)

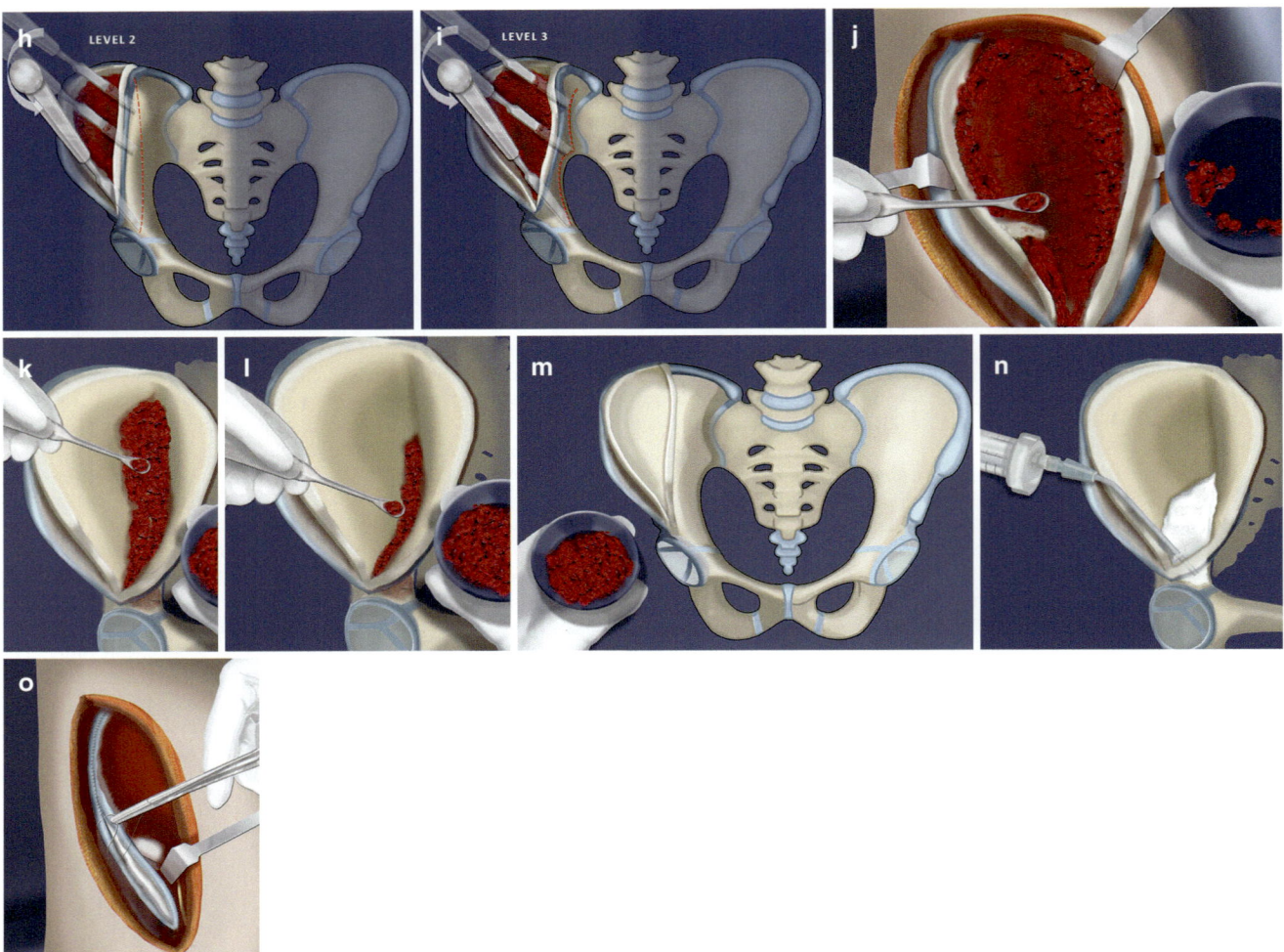

Fig. 32.14 (continued)

Fig. 32.15 (**a–h**) Reproduced with permission by the Paley Foundation. (Copyright The Paley Foundation. Reproduced with permission. All rights reserved.) (**a**) Twenty minutes prior to completion of the bone graft harvest, add the BMP to the collagen sponges. Approximately four sponges (medium size Infuse implant, Medtronics) should be prepared. The periosteum and bone graft are also ready, and the surgical site should be irrigated and dried. (Copyright The Paley Foundation. Reproduced with permission. All rights reserved.) (**b**) Apply two BMP collagen sponges posterior to the tibia and fibula on the surface of the posterior muscles. (Copyright The Paley Foundation. Reproduced with permission. All rights reserved.) (**c**) Apply the periosteal graft cambium layer down on the CPT site. Tuck it under the plate to anchor it and wrap it around the lateral and posterior tibia. (Copyright The Paley Foundation. Reproduced with permission. All rights reserved.) (**d**) Pack layer by layer of the cancellous bone graft between the tibia and fibula. (Copyright The Paley Foundation. Reproduced with permission. All rights reserved.) (**e**) Extend the bone graft to the entire length of the area where the hamartoma was removed. There should be enough bone graft to create a long cross-union. Lay some of the graft anteriorly over the CPT site. The length and width of the bone graft is marked. (Copyright The Paley Foundation. Reproduced with permission. All rights reserved.) (**f**) Apply two more BMP collagen sponges anterior to the bone graft. (Copyright The Paley Foundation. Reproduced with permission. All rights reserved.) (**g**) Suture the tibialis anterior muscle to the fascia underlying the medial skin incision. The muscle will cover the anterior aspect of the tibia (left). A cross-section showing the BMP sandwich with the bone graft in the middle (right). Note that the BMP should be in contact with muscle so that it can recruit and induce cells from the muscle to form bone. The anterior and posterior tibial muscles lie on the surface of the anterior and posterior BMP sponges, respectively. Note the location of the periosteal graft. It is critical that an adequate fasciotomy was performed since the anterior muscles have been displaced anteriorly. The width and height of the bone graft are marked. (Copyright The Paley Foundation. Reproduced with permission. All rights reserved.) (**h**) The wound is seen prior to closure with the anterior muscles overlying most of the bone. A hemovac drain should be placed between the muscle and the subcutaneous tissue. It should not be in contact with the BMP sponges. The wound is closed in layers at this time. (Copyright The Paley Foundation. Reproduced with permission. All rights reserved)

a
b
c
d
e
f
g
TIBIALIS
ANTERIOR
SUTURE
FASCIA
CRURIS
Width
Height

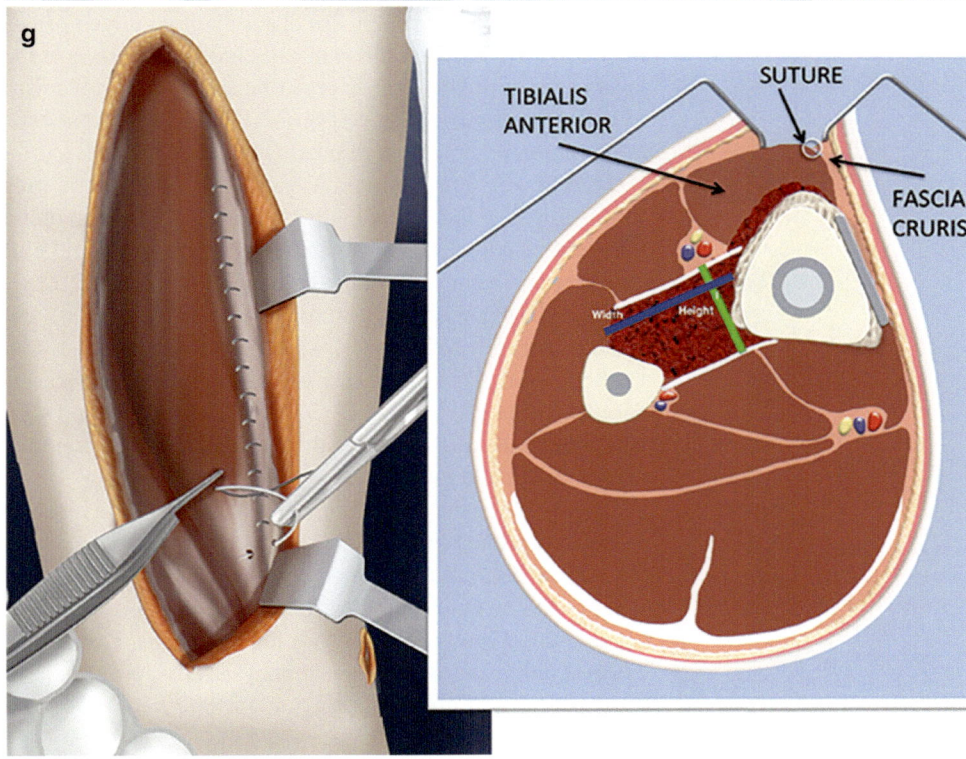

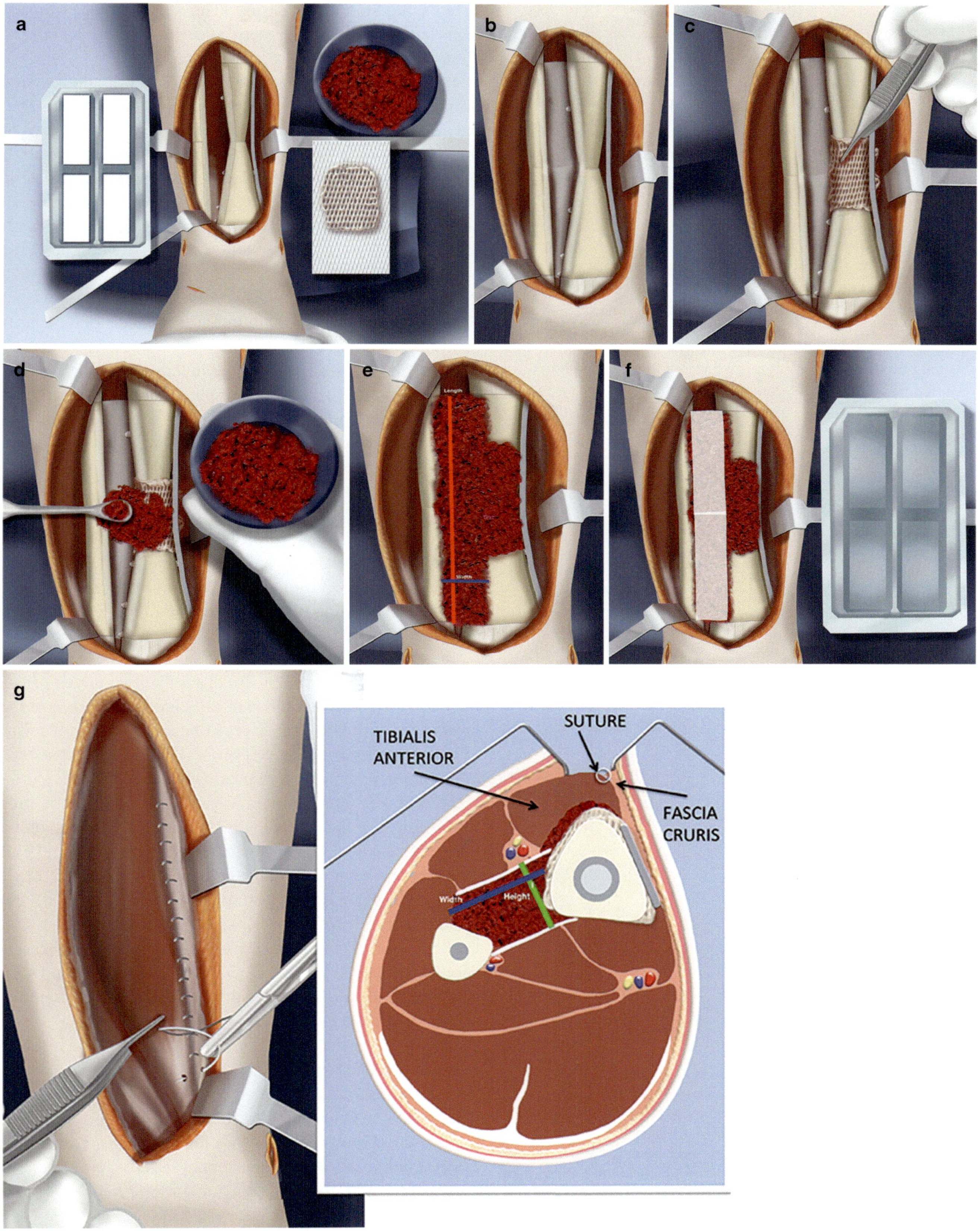

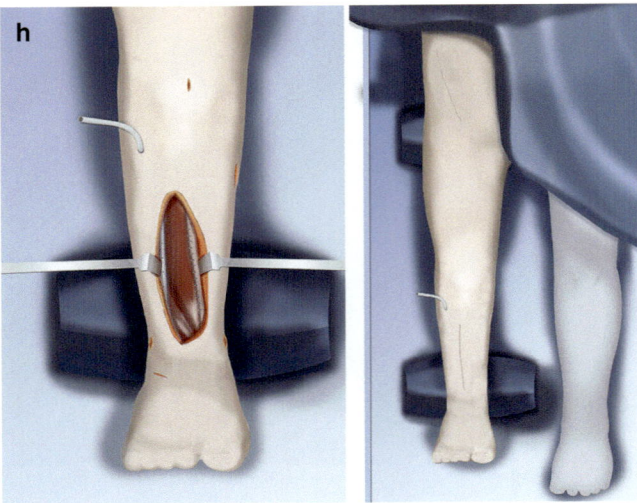

Fig. 32.15 (continued)

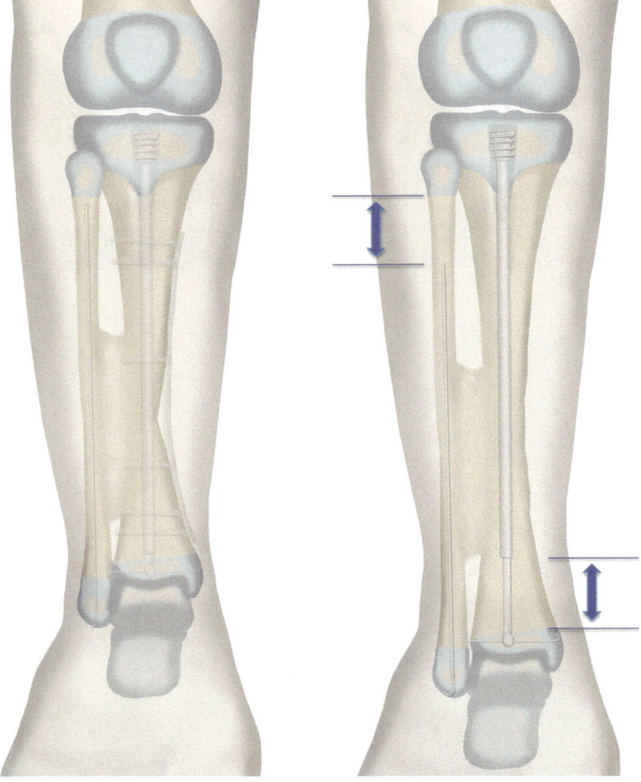

Fig. 32.16 By three months after surgery, a robust cross-union exists between the tibia and fibula (left) The CPT of the tibia and fibula are usually healed by this time. Growth can proceed with telescoping of the Fassier-Duval nail (right). The plate does not impede bone. A second dose of Zoledronic Acid is given at three months after surgery. (Reproduced with permission by the Paley Foundation.) (Copyright The Paley Foundation. Reproduced with permission. All rights reserved)

without the smooth extension. The newer female components have a hole through them, allowing for wire locking of the female component.

Step 24: Locking Plate: The locking plate should be a low profile thin long straight plate that extends from the distal to the proximal tibia. Stabilize the tibial osteotomy with two to three screws on either side of the CPT with compression of the pseudarthrosis (Fig. 32.11j). Author's preferred plate is the Smith and Nephew™ EVOS plate. This may require an additional medial incision for the proximal screws. Use manual compression to compress the bone ends. To compress the bone using the plate, first fix the two end screws. Then add the two more central screws and have these pull the straight plate down to bone. This deformation of the plate causes compression at the CPT site.

Step 25a: Cut the Ends of the Fibula when there is a CPF (If fibula at station- distal fibular physis opposite ankle joint line): The overlapping ends of the fibula can now be cut. It is best to err on cutting too little than too much. This way, there is compression of the ends of the fibula when the two ends are brought together (Fig. 32.12a).

Step 25b: Cut the Ends of the Fibula when the Fibula was Intact and was Osteotomized (Types 1, 2a, 3, 4a; fibula at station): The overlapping ends of the fibula can now be cut. It is best to err on cutting too little than too much. This way, there is compression of the ends of the fibula when the two ends are brought together (Fig. 32.12b).

Step 25b: Cut the Ends of the Fibula after Moving Distal Fibula to Station (Types 2b, 4b; distal fibula migrated proximally): Move the distal fibula distally until its physis is at the level of the joint line. Transfix the fibula and tibia with a wire to hold the fibula at station (Fig. 32.12c). Now cut the ends of the fibula relative to each other (Fig. 32.12d).

Step 26: Fibular Nailing: Advance the wire that is protruding through the lateral malleolus into the proximal fibula up to the proximal fibular physis (Fig. 32.13a). Cut and curl this wire and bury it into the lateral malleolus (Fig. 32.13b).

Step 27: Burr the Opposing Surfaces of the Tibia and Fibula: Burr all the surfaces, which will be in contact with the bone graft. These are especially the opposing surfaces of the distal tibia and fibula (Fig. 32.13c). Pack the wound with wet gauze and wrap the leg with an elastic bandage. Remove and/or deflate the tourniquet.

Step 28: Incision at the Iliac Crest: Make a bikini incision at the iliac crest (Fig. 32.14a).

Step 29: Expose the Iliac Apophysis: Cut through the fascia over the sartorius and identify and decompress the lateral femoral cutaneous nerve. Expose the apophysis. Dissect the external oblique muscle off the apophysis. Dissect and expose the apophysis from the superior to inferior iliac spine (Fig. 32.14b).

Step 30: Split the Apophysis: Use a #15 blade, to cut through the apophysis from the inferior to superior spine and then across the iliac crest from anterior to posterior (Fig. 32.14c).

Step 31: Periosteal Graft Harvest and Meshing: Peel the periosteum off the medial side of the ilium. Incise the periosteum on the undersurface of the iliacus muscle. Incise it in a rectangular pattern removing as large a piece as possible (Fig. 32.14d). Dissect this periosteum from the muscle and then lay it on the plastic sheet used for meshing a skin graft. Mesh the periosteum in order to expand it (Fig. 32.14e).

Step 32: Split Iliac Bone: Use a thin osteotome to split the two cortices of the ilium. Start by splitting the cortices between the superior and inferior iliac spines (Fig. 32.14f). Then go from anterior to posterior splitting the cortices to the same depth. The osteotome is advanced one cm at each place along the crest and then repeated one cm deeper (Fig. 32.14g, h, i). This avoids splintering the crest, especially posteriorly. It is very easy to perforate the cortices as one moves into the very thin region between the anterior and posterior crests. Advance the osteotome deeper at each level until one reaches the dome of the acetabulum and the triradiate cartilage anteriorly; the sciatic notch in the middle; and the sacroiliac joint posteriorly. When the split is deep enough, we start to lever the medial crest medially. Never lever the lateral crest laterally. This levering with the osteotome will gradually open the ilium like a book. It will hinge on the deepest cortex. Do not start the cancellous bone harvest until the two tables of the ilium are fully separated.

Step 33: Iliac Bone Decancellousization: Curette the cancellous bone off the two tables of the ilium. Do not harvest or break off segments of cortical bone. There is a large amount of cancellous bone in the supra-acetabular, triradiate, sacroiliac notch and sacroiliac/posterior iliac crest, and spine regions. Gradually, curette the areas until they are devoid of cancellous bone (Fig. 32.14j, k, l). Use the image intensifier to prevent penetrating or damaging the hip, triradiate, or sacroiliac regions. The harvested cancellous bone totals between 20 and 45cc in most children even as young as 12 months of age (Fig. 32.14m).

Step 34: Backfill Iliac Crest: Backfill the iliac crest with a synthetic bone void filler such as a calcium phosphate (Fig. 32.14n). Suture closed the iliac apophysis including securing the external oblique muscles (Fig. 32.14o). This step may be done after first bone grafting the CPT (Steps 35–40).

Step 35: Preparation of Periosteum, BMP2, and Bone Graft: The periosteal graft was already harvested and should be stored in saline to prevent drying. At least 15 min prior to completing the bone graft harvest, a medium BMP2 (Infuse Implant, Medtronics) with its 4 collagen sponges should be soaked with BMP2 solution. This needs to soak for 15 min to allow the BMP2 protein to bond to the collagen sponge. The bed for the bone graft is dried and soft tissues retracted prior to insertion of the periosteum and BMP. To minimize bone graft time out of the body (cold time) and maximize the viability of the bone graft, the bone graft harvest is timed to be ready for insertion only after all the bone graft bed has been fully prepared (Fig. 32.15a).

Step 36: Insert BMP2 Posteriorly: Insert two of the BMP2 collagen sponges behind the tibia and fibula spanning the space between them. The BMP2 collagen sponges lie on the surface of the deep posterior muscles (Fig. 32.15b).

Step 37: Periosteal Grafting: Apply the periosteal graft, cambium layer down, overtop the CPT site. Since the plate is on the medial side, the periosteum is mostly on the lateral, anterior, and posterior sides. If possible, tuck the periosteum under the plate to anchor it and wrap it around the lateral and posterior sides (Fig. 32.15c). The last two more central screws in the plate can be loosened and then retightened after tucking the periosteal graft under the plate.

Step 38: Insert the Cancellous Bone: Insert the cancellous bone in layers between the tibia and fibula (Fig. 32.15d). Pack it into this interosseous space and then layer some anterior to the tibia. Do not place any medially to avoid having the plate become covered by bone (Fig. 32.15e). Check the location of the bone graft with the image intensifier to ensure that it covers the areas above and below the CPT of the tibia and fibula as desired.

Step 39: Insert BMP Anteriorly: Insert two of the BMP2 sponges anterior to the tibia and fibula spanning the space between them and overlying the cancellous bone graft (Fig. 32.15f).

Step 40: Anterior Muscle Placement: The anterior compartment muscles are moved to lie over the BMP2 sponges and tibia. To maintain them there, the medial edge of the muscle is sutured to the subcutaneous fascia under the medial skin. The muscle forms an important layer overtop the bone, bringing new blood supply to this healing area. The cancellous bone is sandwiched between two layers of BMP2 sponges, which are sandwiched between the anterior and posterior muscles (Fig. 32.15g).

Step 41: Leg Incisions Closure: Insert a drain between the muscle and subcutaneous tissues to help manage the dead space and prevent hematoma (Fig. 32.15h). Close the skin in layers and apply sterile dressings. Also close all the smaller leg incisions.

Step 42: Iliac Incision Closure: Close this incision in multiple layers. Take care to avoid entrapping the lateral femoral cutaneous nerve with the fascial closure. A drain is not needed.

Step 43: Final Radiographs: Obtain and AP and Lateral Radiograph of the tibia.

Postoperative Management: The leg is elevated for the first few days and ice is used for edema management. Only splinting is needed initially since the internal fixation is sufficiently stable. One to two weeks after surgery, a long leg cast is applied. The leg is kept non-weightbearing for the first six weeks to protect the hip. After six weeks, an articulated ankle-foot-orthosis (AFO) is made. Full weight-bearing is permitted, and the patient can start some physical therapy. The cross-union may be evident by 6 weeks and is usually well established by 12 weeks. The patient is allowed to resume all activities with the brace. The brace does not need to be worn in the pool or in bed or inside the house. No activity restrictions are placed.

Three months after the surgery, a second zoledronic acid infusion should be done. The FD rod should be changed after there is sufficient growth where the female part of the rod is at the level of the original CPT (Fig. 32.16). This keeps the larger diameter of the rod crossing the CPT site to help maintain union. Since the length of the bone doubles from age 3 in girls and age 4 in boys until skeletal maturity, the telescopic rod has to be changed, at least once before maturity. Hemiepiphysiodesis is also performed if a valgus ankle or knee is present. The presence of the rod does not impede the use of a hemiepiphysiodesis screw plate device.

Cross-Union Results

Choi et al. [49] recommended the creation of a cross-union between the tibia and fibula for CPT only in cases where the fibula was broken but minimally proximally migrated. The two fibula bone ends were converged towards the tibia bone ends in what they called a "4-in-1 Osteosynthesis." A corticocancellous sheet of the outer wall of the ilium combined with cancellous bone chips was used to achieve the cross-union. They did not recommend this method when the fibula was intact or when the fibula was significantly proximally migrated. Eight patients treated at a mean age of 6.3 years demonstrated 100% union with a cross-union to the fibula. There were no refractures at an average of 7.4 years follow-up (2.7–12.4 years). They compared this to a group of 5 patients who had end-to-end repair of the tibia without cross-union. All 5 united and then refractured and required further treatment for the CPT. Choi et al. attributed the large cross-section of the bone at the level of the cross-union as the reason for no refractures. To quantitate this, Choi et al. measured what they called the relative cross-sectional area (rCSA = area at the CPT site after union divided by area at the upper tibial physis). The rCSA was significantly lower in the non-cross-union group than in the cross-union group; 0.13 vs. 0.27 [49].

Paley [14] reported preliminary results dating back to 2007, using combined pharmacological and surgical management with cross-union. Fixation was with an intramedullary Fassier-Duval (FD) rod for the tibia, intramedullary wire for the fibula, and circular external fixator to compress the bone ends over the rods and to control rotation. The author subsequently reported a larger study of the cross-union protocol with external fixation (EF) [50, 51]. Primary union and cross-union with the index procedure were achieved in 17/17 (100%). The total EF time was an average of 4 months (3–5). The mean radiographic union time was 4 months (1.5–6 months). No refractures occurred in any of these patients. The calculated probability of union without refracture with this method was 100%, which is the same as in the Choi et al. series [49]. Unpublished further follow-up of these 17 tibias shows no deterioration or refracture with up to 14 years (mean 7 years, range 6–14 years) follow-up. The rCSA in the Paley study was a mean of 0.46 ± 0.14 [50]. This rCSA is much higher than 0.27 reported by Choi et al. [13]. This is not surprising since the fibula and tibia in the Paley protocol are not converged as in the '4 in 1' Choi et al. technique. To evaluate whether decancellousization of the ilium has any effect on hip development, the center-edge angle (CEA) and acetabular index (AI) were measured on the harvested versus unharvested side. There were no significant differences in CEA and AI between sides.

In a study by Hell et al. [5], 18 cases of CPT treated by Paley cross-union protocol with external fixation (EF) were compared to 18 cases of CPT treated by Paley cross-union protocol with plate internal fixation (P). The mean age at treatment was 5.6 years (1 to 13) EF and 3.5 years (1 to 5) P, and 4.6 years combined group (EF + P = C). The mean follow-up was: 5.3 years EF (3 to 11) and 1.7 years P (1 to 4) and 3.5 years C. Neurofibromatosis was present in 67% EF, 83% P, and 75% C. Fibrous dysplasia was present in 11% EF, 6% P, and 8% C. Failed previous CPT surgery occurred in 33% EF and 17% P. Unequivocal radiographic CPT union and tibiofibular cross-union were achieved in all 36 tibias. The radiographic time to union was a mean of 16 weeks EF (6 to 24), 12 weeks P (6 to 18), and 14 weeks C. There were no refractures. Three very distal fibular pseudarthroses remained ununited but stable due to the cross-union of the proximal fibula to the tibia across the CPT site. The percent of cross-union length relative to total length of the tibia at seven, 28, and 70 months was 32%, 22%, and 17%, respectively. The telescopic rod was pulled out of the epiphysis distally or proximally in 17% of cases (6 EF, 0 P). There were two wound complications treated by debridement and closure (1 EF, 1 P); three pin infections (EF) and 2 cases of cellulitis (1 EF, 1 P) treated with antibiotics. In conclusion, identical results were achieved whether the Paley cross-union protocol was performed using circular external fixation or locking plate internal fixation. Both devices serve to compress the CPT site and to control rotation. Using the internal fixation eliminates the risk of pin infections and eliminates one surgical procedure as the plate can be removed at the time of a future rod exchange. The authors now exclusively use the plate.

Two additional reports of cross-union treatment for CPT using modifications of the Paley and Choi methods show similar results: Vaidya et al. [52] reported 10/10 patients healed with no refracture (100%), and Liu et al. [53] reported on 17/17 patients healed with no refracture (100%) at 4-year follow-up. In addition, an as-of yet unpublished study (personal communication) by Dr. Bo Ning from Fudan University, Shanghai, China, reports on 18 patients with CPT treated by Paley cross-union protocol using all internal fixation, with 18/18 achieving CPT union with 0% refracture during a mean follow-up of 4.3 years (range 1.5–6.3 years) [54]. Longer-term follow-up and more corroboration of these results are expected.

More recently, Shannon et al. [55] published a retrospective study on 39 cases of CPT all treated by Paley cross-union protocol using plate fixation. Neurofibromatosis was present in 25/39 (64%). Mean age at the time of surgery was 3.3 years (range 1–13.5 years). Seven of 36 (19%) had undergone previous failed surgery. There were 13 unbroken tibias (5 type 1, 8 type 3). The mean follow-up was 35 months (range 24–85 months). All 39 (100%) achieved union of the CPT and cross-union between the tibia and fibula. All but two achieved union of the fibula. Fourteen had subsequent surgery for leg lengthening or deformity correction.

There were 5 postoperative complications. One patient developed skin necrosis requiring debridement and skin grafting. There were 4 complications related to the FD rod: one proximal end backed out into the knee joint requiring reinsertion; three procedures were needed to revise the distal locking wire due to prominence or backing out.

Intraoperative transfusion of packed red blood cells was required in 24 of 36 patients. This was related to blood loss from the decancellousization of the ilium. No adverse outcomes related to the transfusion were noted. Subsequent modifications to the protocol were made, based on this observation, to include tranexamic acid (TXA) prior to the start of the surgery, the use of autogenous blood salvage (Cell Saver, Haemonetics Corporation, Braintree, MA, USA), infusion of Venofer (intravenous iron), and a lower threshold for transfusion (<Hgb = 6). Eighteen subsequent patients who underwent cross-union protocol surgery but were excluded due to less than 2 year follow-up were evaluated and found to have only a 17% (3/18) transfusion rate. All patients achieved union without refracture. Seventeen (94%) of these patients received TXA, and 16 (89%) received an immediate postoperative Venofer (iron) infusion. The decrease in transfusion rate from 67% to 17% clearly demonstrates that the decancellousization does not have to lead to such a high transfusion rate.

Proximal migration of the distal fibula is a common problem seen in patients with CPT. Migration of the fibula is related to fibular fracture and the development of valgus of the ankle plafond [20, 56, 57]. This subsequently leads to deformity, instability, and degeneration of the ankle joint. Choi classified the fibular migration separately [13]. Paley incorporated fibular migration into his CPT classification, designated with a-or-b modifier after the type number [5], as well as recommending to restore the fibular station at the time of cross-union surgery. Interestingly, the b-type fibulas that were distalized at the time of cross-union maintained their corrected fibular station 83% of the time. This demonstrates that moving the fibula distally in 2b and 4b cases is effective. On the contrary, in a-type CPT, 35% of fibulas were proximally migrated at final follow-up with an average proximal change of 3.7 mm. Studies of post-traumatic cross-union of the tibia and fibula have demonstrated proximal migration of the fibula due to the differential growth rate of the tibia and fibula [58, 59]. The distal tibial physis grows faster than the distal fibular physis. Accordingly, one would expect that all type-a fibulas would migrate proximally.

The biomechanical success of the cross-union to resist fracture is explained by the increased cross-sectional diameter of the bone in the area of pseudarthrosis. The torsional rigidity of a bone is proportional to the radius to the 4th power, and the bending strength of a hollow cylinder is proportional to the radius to the 3rd power [60]. Both of these numbers, and therefore, the strength of the bone to resist torsion and bending, are dramatically increased as the diameter of the bone increases. The cross-union achieves this increase in diameter by linking the two bones together, with additional stability provided by the use of intramedullary rodding. With a rod filling the canal of both the tibia and fibula, the bending strength of the cross-union can now be calculated as a solid cylinder, which is proportional to the radius to the 4th power. The exponential increase in the leg's structural stability leads directly to a decreased risk of fracture, as demonstrated by the complete lack of refractures.

Even in very short tibial segments, the plate fixation can extend with screws into the distal tibial epiphysis using a T-plate to temporarily span the distal tibial physis (Fig. 32.6). The epiphyseal screws are removed 6–12 weeks later. The only failure experienced in achieving union in this study was at the fibula in two cases. This was also previously reported by Paley in 8% of cases [5]. This complication is likely related to the lack of preparing and filling of the interosseous space in very distal fibular pseudarthrosis cases. To prevent persistent fibular nonunion, the periosteum between the two bones should be removed on the opposing surfaces of both bones down to the level just proximal to the distal tibial physis. It is important to pack autogenous grafts into this interspace.

In the cross-union protocol, the goal of grafting is to fill the space between the tibia and fibula opposing surfaces without specifically grafting around the pseudarthrosis sites of each bone. The volume of bone required to achieve this can be calculated simply from AP, lateral and mortis view

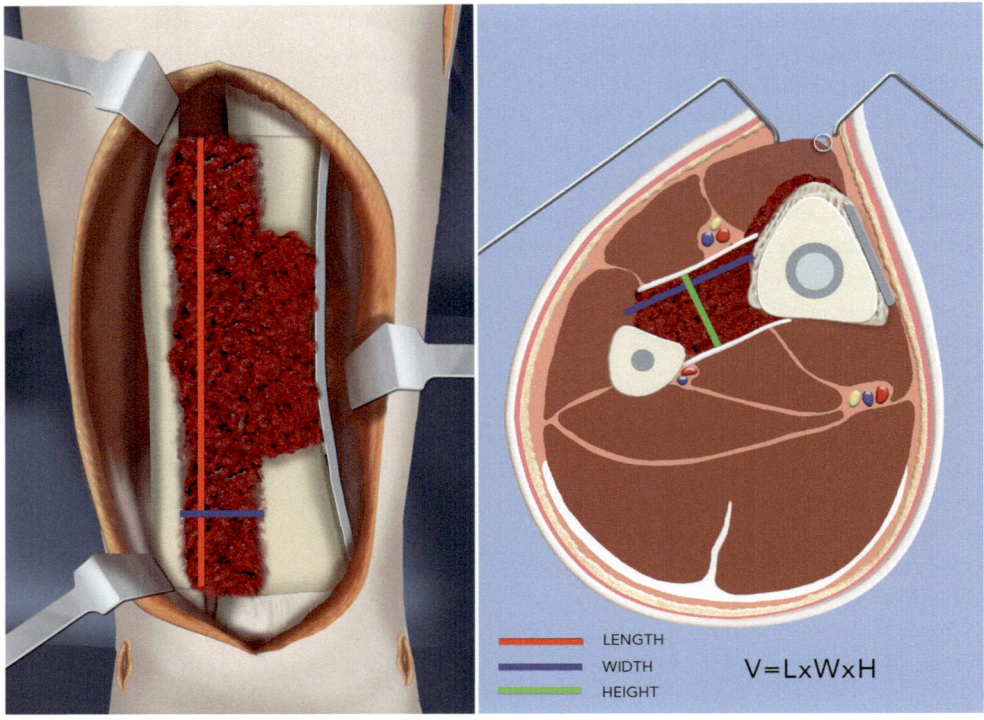

Fig. 32.17 The volume of bone required can be approximately calculated by multiplying the length by the width and by the height as shown in these illustrations. (Reproduced with permission by the Paley Foundation.) (Copyright The Paley Foundation. Reproduced with permission. All rights reserved)

radiographs by measuring the length of the planned cross-union (X) from the AP view (Fig. 32.14e), the width between the two bones (Y) (Fig. 32.14e, g) from a mortis view, and the height of the space between the bones (Z) from a lateral view (Fig. 32.14g). Although a more accurate way might involve obtaining a CT scan or MRI, the added radiation or need to sedate the child is not indicated for this approximate calculation, which is used to guide the bone graft harvest. The volume (V) of bone graft needed is $V = X \times Y \times Z$ (Fig. 32.17) (e.g., in an 18-month-old child where the length = 6 cm, width = 1.5 cm, and height = 1.5 cm, the volume of graft required is $6 \times 1.5 \times 1.5 = 13.5$ cc).

Postoperative Considerations

FD Rod Pull Out

Although a telescopic rod offers many advantages in the growing child, there are also potential problems with this implant. The most common problem is pulling out of the epiphysis with distal migration of the proximal end and proximal migration of the distal end. In Shannon et al.'s [55] work, out of a total of 39 rods placed at the index procedure, 9 rods migrated distally at the proximal end, 1 rod migrated proximally at the proximal end, and 15 rods migrated proximally at the distal end. Two tibias had the rod migrate at both ends. Five rods redeveloped migration after the initial rod exchange. Two of the rods pulled out at the distal end, and 3 rods pulled out at both ends.

FD Rod Exchange

Planned FD rod exchange occurred once in 22 tibias and twice in one tibia in the study by Shannon et al. [55]. The timing of rod exchange ranged from 7 to 35 months following the index surgery. The average interval to rod exchange in 1–2 year-olds ($n = 8$) was 19 months vs. 29 months in 2–4 year-olds ($n = 10$) vs. 20 months in the over 4 year-olds ($n = 4$).

Hemiepiphysiodesis

Guided growth can be used to correct angular deformities that develop in the tibia or femur. This can be done with success with a telescopic rod in place. Most patients can have this timed with a planned rod exchange to minimize additional procedures.

Leg Length Discrepancy

Limb length differences (LLD) are often present in patients with CPT. The affected leg can be shorter due to atrophic bone ends and overlap with significant bowing, or longer due to femoral overgrowth. After cross-union surgery, the affected leg is often noted to grow at an accelerated rate for a period of time. Many patients self-resolve their LLD as a result of this phenomenon. If a true LLD remains, lengthening can be undertaken but requires special considerations beyond the scope of this chapter.

Calcaneo-Valgus Foot Deformity

Valgus of the ankle joint is not an uncommon developmental deformity of CPT [5, 10, 20, 23, 61, 62]. It is related to proximal migration of the fibula and wedging of the distal tibial epiphysis [20]. The proximal fibular migration can be recognized and treated at the time of the cross-union procedure. Notwithstanding this, recurrent proximal migration, possibly due to differential growth of the distal tibia and fibula, may occur [58]. One option to correct this is to perform a shortening osteotomy of the distal tibia relative to the fibula (SHORDT: Shortening Osteotomy Realignment Distal Tibia [63]). This will correct the problem, but requires a repeat osteotomy of the distal tibia which has high risk of pseudarthrosis. In order to prevent a nonunion, the SHORDT should be accompanied by preoperative zoledronic acid infusion and cancellous bone grafting, even cross-union to fibula, at the level of osteotomy (Fig. 32.18). Another option is to perform a lengthening of the distal fibula. This can be carried out with a mini external fixator (Fig. 32.19). Isolated distal tibial valgus can be addressed with hemiepiphysiodesis of the medial distal tibia (Fig. 32.18).

The calcaneus deformity of the foot is a secondary consequence of the anterior bow of the tibia. The longer this bow remains uncorrected, the more likely a dorsiflexion contracture will develop at the ankle joint. Furthermore, the anterior bow relaxes the gastrosoleus muscles, effectively weakening them and allowing the foot to dorsiflex further. This leads to increased calcaneal pitch, or a 'pistol grip' deformity of the heel (calcaneo-cavus) [64, 65] (Fig. 32.20). This may need to be treated by reducing the calcaneal pitch with a calcaneal osteotomy (Fig. 32.20). Residual distal tibial procurvatum deformity can also result in an ankle dorsiflexion contracture. The net outcome is restricted

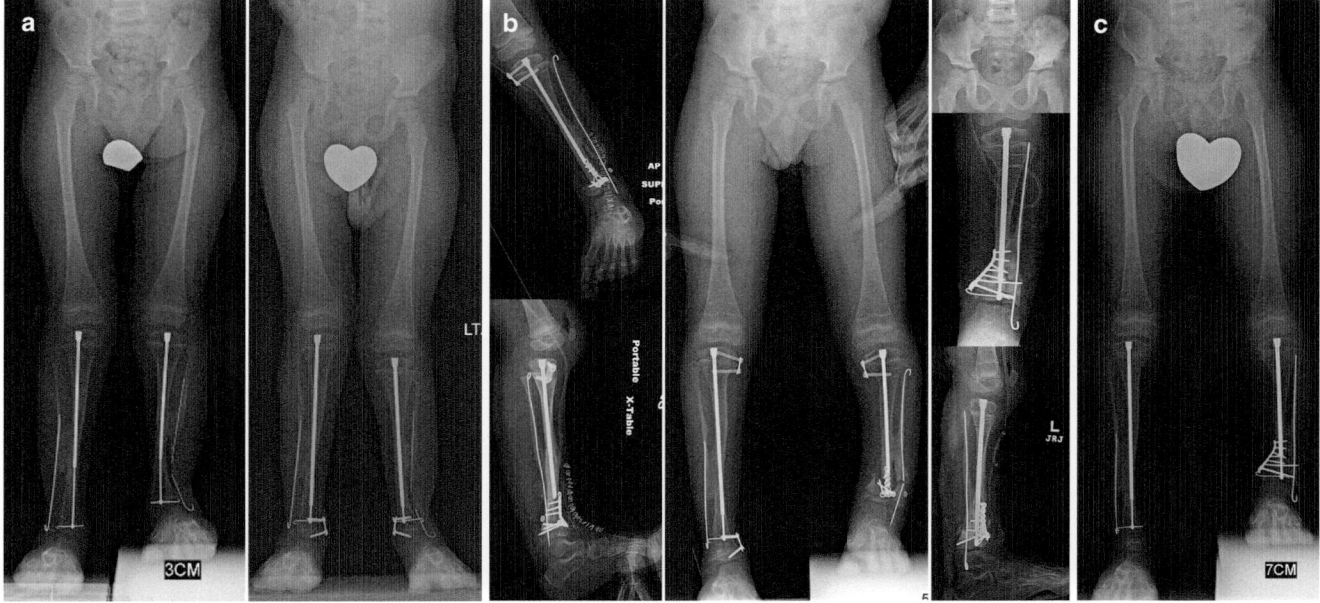

Fig. 32.18 (a) Left: Standing radiograph after undergoing bilateral cross-union. Both of the ankles are in valgus and there is a 3 cm leg length discrepancy on the left. Right: Standing radiograph of the same patient after undergoing hemiepiphysiodesis of the bilateral medial distal tibia. The right side is correcting, but the left foot side remains in significant valgus. (Copyright The Paley Foundation. Reproduced with permission. All rights reserved.) (b) Left: Immediate postoperative AP and lateral radiographs of the left tibia after undergoing a SHORDT procedure and proximal tibial hemipiphysiodesis. The alignment of the distal tibia and station of the fibula is now restored. Middle: Standing radiograph 1-year post-op demonstrating failure of healing of the distal tibial and fibular osteotomies on the left. On the right leg, the hemiepiphysiodesis has completely corrected the ankle valgus. Right: AP and lateral radiographs of the left tibia after undergoing revision of the SHORDT with iliac crest bone grafting and BMP placement to achieve a cross-union at the osteotomy site. AP pelvis radiograph demonstrates the amount of bone graft taken with backfilling of the crest with calcium phosphate bone void filler. Of note is that this was a reharvest of the same iliac crest used for the original cross-union. The bone had completely regenerated and was even more ample than before due to increased age and widening of the tables. The lesson learned was that the SHORDT should not be done without simultaneously expanding the cross-union around the supramalleolar osteotomy. The bone resected from the distal tibia in the SHORDT is usually ample enough to use for the bone grafting. (Copyright The Paley Foundation. Reproduced with permission. All rights reserved.) (c) Standing radiograph 1-year after left side revision SHORDT with bone grafting. The tibia and fibula are united and the distal tibial alignment is maintained. The right ankle remains well aligned after removal of the hemiepiphysiodesis plate. (Copyright The Paley Foundation. Reproduced with permission. All rights reserved)

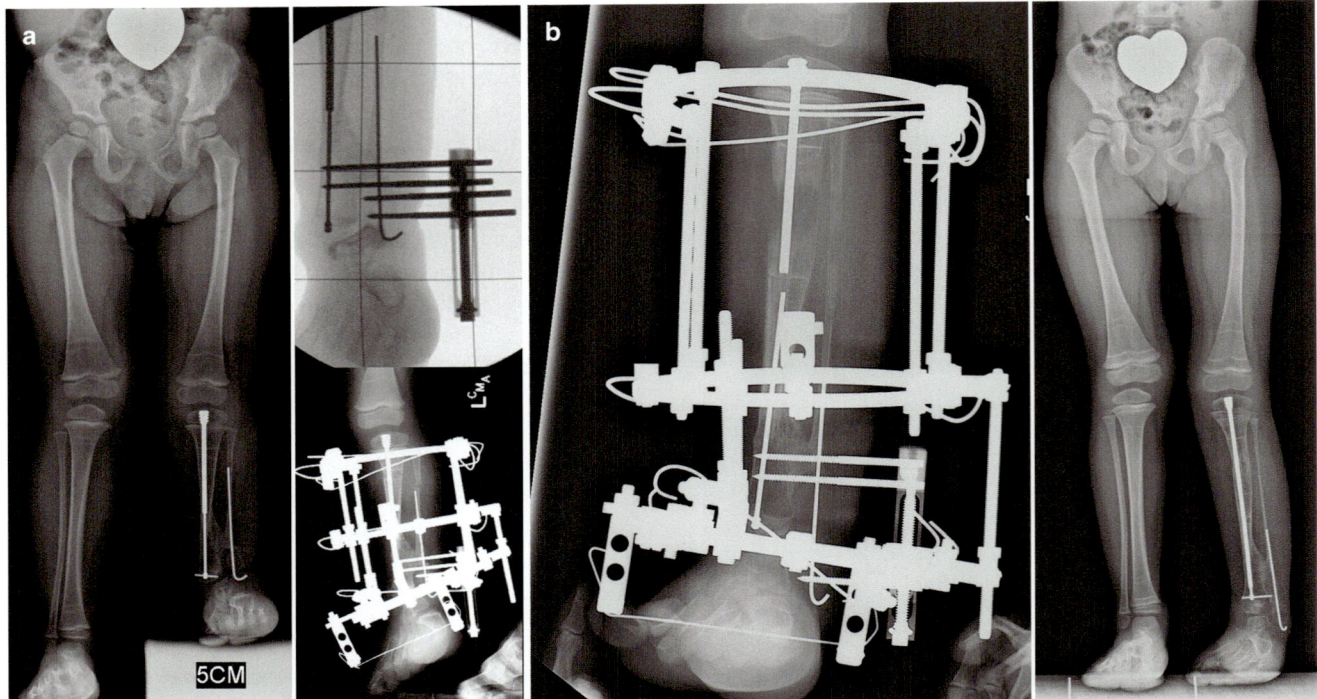

Fig. 32.19 (**a**) Left: Standing radiograph of a patient who underwent a left cross-union. The ankle is in valgus due to proximal migration of the fibula with lateral wedging of the distal tibial epiphysis. There is a 5 cm leg length discrepancy(LLD). Right: Intraoperative fluoroscopy demonstrating the application of a mini-fixator to the fibula for isolated distraction of the distal fibula to station at the ankle. An arthrogram of the ankle highlights the distal tibial wedging (Top). Immediate postoperative AP radiograph demonstrating the mini-fixator for the fibula incorporated into a tibial external fixator for proximal tibia and fibula lengthening to correct the LLD (Bottom). (Copyright The Paley Foundation. Reproduced with permission. All rights reserved.) (**b**) Left: AP radiograph showing the completed distraction of the distal fibula, restoring the ankle mortise. Note the ankle is no longer in valgus. Proximally, the patient completed 5 cm of tibial lengthening. Right: Standing radiograph 2 years after distraction. The ankle remains in proper alignment and the leg lengths are symmetric. (Copyright The Paley Foundation. Reproduced with permission. All rights reserved)

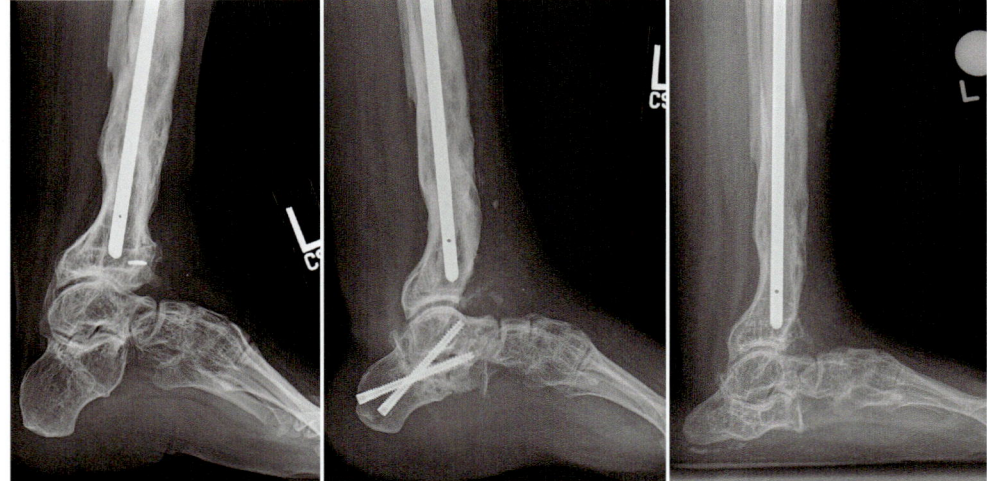

Fig. 32.20 Left: preoperative lateral X-ray of a patient with a "pistol grip" deformity of the hindfoot (calcaneo-cavus). Middle: postoperative lateral X-ray showing correction of the calcaneal pitch with a dome type osteotomy and subtalar fusion. Right: Lateral X-ray of the same patient 3 years after surgery. A bumpectomy of the plantar aspect of the calcaneus served to both eliminate the prominence of the heel bone and to release the attached plantar fascia. Note that the foot is very flat after this surgery. (Copyright The Paley Foundation. Reproduced with permission. All rights reserved)

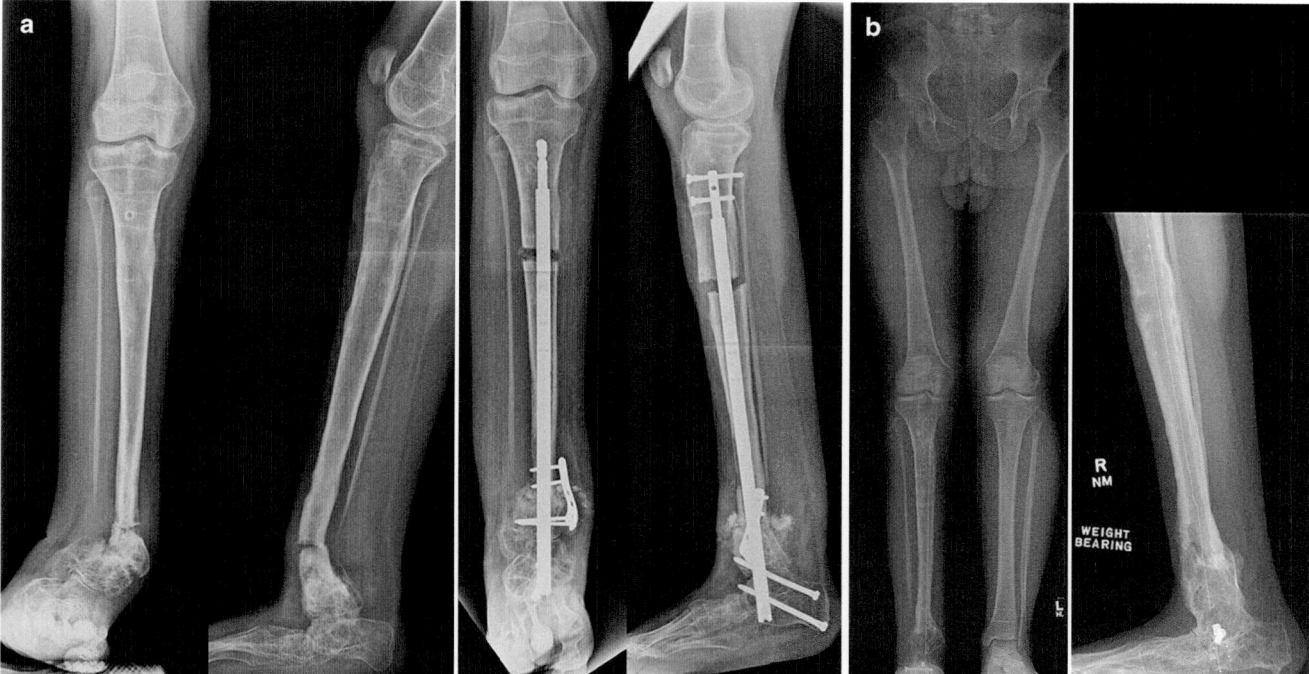

Fig. 32.21 (a) Left: AP and lateral X-rays of a skeletally mature patient who presented with longstanding right distal CPT with failed union. The ankle is severely deformed with degenerative changes and the right leg is shorter than the left. Right: Postoperative AP and lateral X-rays demonstrating correction of the ankle malalignment, bone grafting, and plating of distal tibial pseudarthrosis and ankle fusion performed with a retrograde lengthening nail. The lengthening is performed via a separate osteotomy of the upper tibia. (Copyright The Paley Foundation. Reproduced with permission. All rights reserved.) (b) Standing long AP and lateral X-rays of the same patient 6 years after ankle fusion and lengthening. The foot is plantigrade and in neutral coronal alignment, and the leg lengths are equal. The patient is an avid bowler and reports no pain as of follow-up in 2022. (Copyright The Paley Foundation. Reproduced with permission. All rights reserved)

plantarflexion of the ankle, despite the procurvatum deformity of the distal tibia. Eventually, this can lead to stiffness and arthritic degeneration of the ankle joint. In cases of long-standing deformity with significant joint damage, ankle fusion is a reasonable solution (Fig. 32.21).

Alternatively, if the deformity and contracture are identified early, this can be treated by distal tibial and foot osteotomies combined with soft tissue releases of the anterior compartment muscles (soft tissue slide and tendon lengthening) (Fig. 32.22).

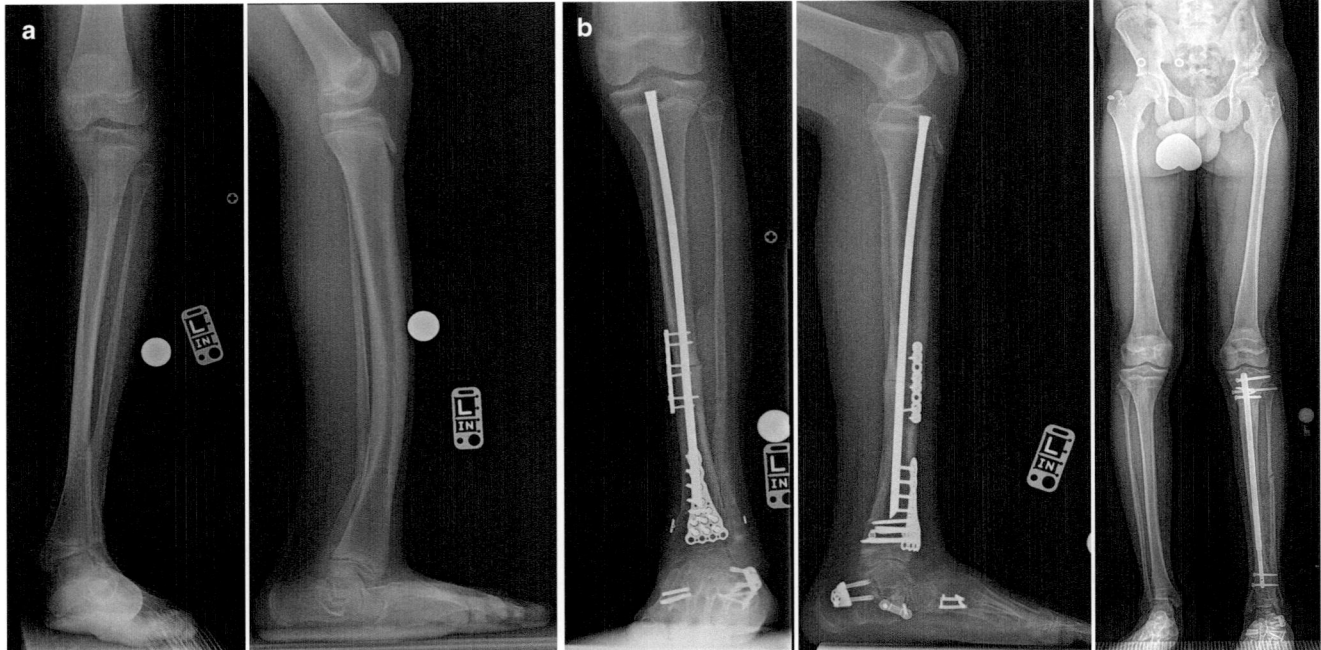

Fig. 32.22 (**a**) AP and lateral radiographs of a 13-year old boy with left Paley type 1 CPT with significant residual bowing deformity, proximal fibular migration with pes planovalgus, and anterior ankle contracture. The leg is also shorter than the right. No previous fracture occurred. (Copyright The Paley Foundation. Reproduced with permission. All rights reserved.) (**b**) Left: AP and lateral X-rays of the left tibia and foot after undergoing a SHORDT, modified Evans, medial calcaneal shift, midfoot osteotomy, anterior ankle release, diaphyseal tibial osteotomy to straighten tibia with cross-union. Right: Standing long AP of the same patient 3 years after cross-union surgery and subsequent left tibial lengthening using Precice nail. His leg lengths are equal and his ankle alignment is maintained with no pain. (Copyright The Paley Foundation. Reproduced with permission. All rights reserved)

Pre-CPT (Paley Type 1 and 2)

The treatment of patients with pre-CPT (Paley type 1 and 2) by the cross-union protocol is controversial. The conventional treatment for pre-CPT cases has been to brace them as long as possible to prevent fracture. Nonoperative treatment likely does not prevent the development of secondary changes of atrophy, leg length discrepancy, fibular migration, ankle valgus and calcaneus, cavus foot, coxa valga, etc. Since straightening the tibia in pre-CPT puts the tibia at risk of developing a pseudarthrosis of the osteotomy site, the treatment of pre-CPT has been nonoperative until the tibia fractures, despite the development of secondary changes. Laufer et al. treated 4/26 patients with pre-CPT (Paley 1 in three and Paley 2a in 1) and all four obtained union and one refractured [44]. With the cross-union protocol showing 100% success probability, it is reasonable to perform the cross-union protocol in pre-CPT. Hell et al. [5, 66] demonstrated that 6 intact tibias achieved union after osteotomy for cross-union. The results from Shannon et al. [55] demonstrated the union was achieved in all five type 1 and eight type 2 CPT cases. Therefore, it is reasonable to treat intact CPT by the cross-union protocol once a surgeon is proficient in its use in fractured CPT cases

Recently, guided growth was proposed as a treatment method in young patients with intact anterolateral bowing to prevent the development of fracture and pseudarthrosis and to correct deformity early [67]. The preliminary results appear promising, with all ten patients in the series avoiding any tibial fracture and obtaining a significant improvement in the bony alignment. Further follow-up is needed to determine if fracture and secondary changes of leg length difference, ankle, and foot deformity will be prevented with this technique. The guided growth method is certainly appealing since it is minimally invasive compared with performing cross-union and does not prevent a cross-union from being performed in the future should it be required.

Conclusions

Radiographic success in treatment of CPT is defined as union without refracture. More than 100 years of results of various surgical procedures designed to treat CPT have resulted in a glass ceiling success rate not greater than 50% union without refracture [2–5]. Adding intentional cross-union of the tibia to the fibula has increased that success rate by a factor of 2. Given the large differential in success rate from 50% to 100% [5, 28–31, 35–37], the cross-union protocol should be considered the new standard for treatment of CPT. Based on our experience, older less successful methods to obtain and maintain union in this condition should be retired and abandoned.

Acknowledgments The author would also like to thank Pamela Boullier Ross who illustrated all of the figures in this manuscript and the Paley Foundation for funding the cost of making these illustrations and giving permission for their reproduction.

Commentary

In Ho Choi
inhoc1@caumc.or.kr

Anterolateral bowing of the tibia with congenital dysplasia, often called somewhat inaccurately as congenital pseudarthrosis of the tibia (CPT), poses one of the most challenging treatment problems in pediatric orthopedics. It is a heterogeneous disease entity with a wide spectrum of disease ranging from pre-pseudarthrosis to established pseudarthrosis. CPT should be considered as a 'soft bone disease' or 'fragile bone disease' because of inherent poor mineralization, thin cortex, and poor remodeling. Fibrous hamartoma (FH) tissue, originating from aberrant periosteal growth, is regarded to a central feature of the pathology. This tissue is found at pseudarthrosis sites of the affected tibia and/or fibula and is continuous with abnormally thickened periosteum in the adjacent bone segments. There are some reports suggesting that FH cells do not undergo osteoblastic differentiation in response to bone morphogenetic protein (BMP) and are more osteoclastogenic than normal periosteal cells. Once pseudarthrosis is established, osteosynthesis becomes very difficult because of increased osteoclastic activity, poor local blood supply, and poor osteoinductive and remodeling capacity of the lesion.

Despite successful primary osteosynthesis, subsequent problems or residual sequelae such as refracture, residual tibial deformity, ankle stiffness and foot deformity, shortening, and atrophied lower-limb are frequently encountered and perplexing, which might necessitate unwanted multiple surgeries. Of these, refracture is a big concern, which is often associated with residual ankle valgus. Sometimes, residual problems can jeopardize function of the affected extremity. Hence, to obtain a stable, functional extremity at the completion of treatment, most efficacious, safe, and practical 'one shot one kill' approach should be set before jumping to surgery. This should aim to accomplish multi-targeted goals, including osteosynthesis without axial or rotational malalignment, stabilization and early mobilization of the ankle mortise for foot and ankle in order to preserve function, and limb-length equalization.

In very young children who present in the prepseudarthrosis stage, the initial goal is fracture prevention, usually with prophylactic bracing. It is recommended to delay any definite surgical intervention until after walking age. Prophylactic bypass grafting and guided growth modulation might be selectively indicated alone, or in combination for treatment of prepseudarthrosis of the tibia with severe anterolateral bowing.

Treatment approaches are varied once the tibia has fractured; these include intramedullary (IM) fixation, vascularized fibular grafting, circular external fixation (EF), cement-membrane-induced osteogenesis technique, Choi "4-in-1 osteosynthesis" or Paley "cross-union", or a combination of approaches. Cross-union technique has seemingly become a game changer in the management of atrophic-type CPT, providing near 100% of primary bone healing with no or little risk of refracture. Cross-union technique provides not only mechanical, but also biologic advantages. It affords maximization of cross-sectional area of healing at the level of pseudarthrosis and adjacent dystrophic bone by linking the tibia and fibula together. When considering the four cortices united as one mass as seen on AP view, with or without additional stability with use of intramedullary nailing, the strength of the bone to resist torsion and bending will be dramatically increased. This will certainly increase the chance of successful osteosynthesis. It also enables early ankle stabilization with prevention of proximal migration of distal segment of fibula causing ankle valgus, with which ankle mobility can be preserved. One concern lies in the fact that cross-union might disturb ankle kinetics and kinematics by hindering normal growth and development of the fibula as well as blocking normal up- and down movement during walking and running. However, in our study (Seo and Choi et al. Foot and ankle Function at maturity after Ilizarov treatment for atrophic-type congenital pseudarthrosis of the tibia: A comprehensive outcome comparison with normal controls JBJS Am. 2016;98:490-8), no significant difference in terms of clinical outcomes scores and most biomechanical gait parameters was found between the tibiofibular cross-union group and the intact-fibular group in children with atrophic-type CPT treated by the Ilizarov treatment. Residual ankle valgus deformity caused by short fibula can be corrected with various surgical techniques including medial hemiepiphysiodesis of the distal tibia, lengthening of the distal fibula at just below the cross-union site, supramalleolar osteotomy, and shortening osteotomy realignment distal tibia.

In summary, a timely, well-performed cross-union technique should be considered as one of the 'one shot one kill' surgical options for atrophic-type CPT that ensures osteosynthesis, while leaving the ankle mobile to help build up ankle plantarflexion muscle power, and consequently, lead to an improved gait. The combination of surgical and biological approaches is justified to breakthrough the challenges related to CPT. Further in-depth investigation on the role of periosteal graft, adjuvant bisphosphonate treatment, recombinant biologics, and genotype-phenotype correlation of NF-1 is warranted in patients with CPT with high heterogeneity.

References

1. Hefti F, Bollini G, Dungl P, et al. Congenital pseudarthrosis of the tibia: history, etiology, classification, and epidemiologic data. J Pediatr Orthop B. 2000;9(1):11–5. https://doi.org/10.1097/01202412-200001000-00003.
2. Kesireddy N, Kheireldin RK, Lu A, Cooper J, Liu J, Ebraheim NA. Current treatment of congenital pseudarthrosis of the tibia: a systematic review and meta-analysis. J Pediatr Orthop Part B. 2018;27(6):541–50. https://doi.org/10.1097/BPB.0000000000000524.
3. Shah H, Joseph B, Nair BVS, et al. What factors influence union and refracture of congenital pseudarthrosis of the tibia? A multicenter long-term study. J Pediatr Orthop. 2018;38(6):e332–7. https://doi.org/10.1097/BPO.0000000000001172.
4. Rastogi A, Agarwal A. Surgical treatment options for congenital pseudarthrosis of tibia in children: cross-union versus other options: a systematic review. J Pediatr Orthop Part B. 2022;31(2):139–49. https://doi.org/10.1097/BPB.0000000000000924.
5. Paley D. Congenital pseudarthrosis of the tibia: biological and biomechanical considerations to achieve union and prevent refracture. J Child Orthop. 2019;13(2):120–33. https://doi.org/10.1302/1863-2548.13.180147.
6. Herring JA. Disorders of the leg. In: Herring JA, editor. Tachdjian's pediatric orthopaedics. 5th ed. Elsevier Health Sciences; 2013. p. 713–58.
7. McCarthy RE. Amputation for congenital pseudarthrosis of the tibia. Indications and techniques. Clin Orthop. 1982;166:58–61.
8. Guille JT, Kumar SJ, Shah A. Spontaneous union of a congenital pseudarthrosis of the tibia after Syme amputation. Clin Orthop. 1998;351:180–5.
9. Andersen KS. Radiological classification of congenital pseudarthrosis of the tibia. Acta Orthop Scand. 1973;44(6):719–27. https://doi.org/10.3109/17453677308989112.
10. Boyd HB, Sage FP. Congenital pseudarthrosis of the tibia. JBJS. 1958;40(6):1245–379.
11. Crawford AH, Bagamery N. Osseous manifestations of neurofibromatosis in childhood. J Pediatr Orthop. 1986;6(1):72–88. https://doi.org/10.1097/01241398-198601000-00015.
12. El-Rosasy M, Paley D, Herzenberg J. Congenital pseudarthrosis of the tibia. In: Rozbruch S, Ilizarov S, editors. Limb lengthening and reconstruction surgery. Informa Healthcare; 2007. p. 485–93.
13. Choi IH, Cho TJ, Moon HJ. Ilizarov treatment of congenital pseudarthrosis of the tibia: a multi-targeted approach using the Ilizarov technique. Clin Orthop Surg. 2011;3(1):1. https://doi.org/10.4055/cios.2011.3.1.1.
14. Paley D. Congenital pseudarthrosis of the tibia: combined pharmacologic and surgical treatment using biphosphonate intravenous infusion and bone morphogenic protein with periosteal and cancellous autogenous bone grafting, tibio-fibular cross union, intramedullary. In: Zorzi A, editor. Bone grafting. InTech; 2012. https://doi.org/10.5772/31149.
15. McElvenny RT. Congenital pseudo-arthrosis of the tibia; the findings in one case and a suggestion as to possible etiology and treatment. Q Bull Northwest Univ Med Sch. 1949;23(4):413–23.
16. Boyd HB. Pathology and natural history of congenital pseudarthrosis of the tibia. Clin Orthop. 1982;166:5–13.
17. Hermanns-Sachweh B, Senderek J, Alfer J, et al. Vascular changes in the periosteum of congenital pseudarthrosis of the tibia. Pathol Res Pract. 2005;201(4):305–12. https://doi.org/10.1016/j.prp.2004.09.013.
18. Schindeler A, Ramachandran M, Godfrey C, et al. Modeling bone morphogenetic protein and bisphosphonate combination therapy in wild-type and *Nf1* haploinsufficient mice: BMP and bisphosphonate combination therapy. J Orthop Res. 2008;26(1):65–74. https://doi.org/10.1002/jor.20481.
19. Schindeler A, Birke O, Yu NYC, et al. Distal tibial fracture repair in a neurofibromatosis type 1-deficient mouse treated with recombinant bone morphogenetic protein and a bisphosphonate. J Bone Joint Surg Br. 2011;93-B(8):1134–9. https://doi.org/10.1302/0301-620X.93B8.25940.
20. Deng H, Mei H, Wang E, et al. The association between fibular status and frontal plane tibial alignment post-union in congenital pseudarthrosis of the tibia. J Child Orthop. 2021;15(3):261–9. https://doi.org/10.1302/1863-2548.15.200255.
21. Song MH, Park MS, Yoo WJ, Cho TJ, Choi IH. Femoral overgrowth in children with congenital pseudarthrosis of the tibia. BMC Musculoskelet Disord. 2016;17(1):274. https://doi.org/10.1186/s12891-016-1157-x.
22. Grill F, Bollini G, Dungl P, et al. Treatment approaches for congenital pseudarthrosis of tibia: results of the EPOS multicenter study. J Pediatr Orthop B. 2000;9(2):75–89. https://doi.org/10.1097/01202412-200004000-00002.
23. Dobbs MB, Rich MM, Gordon JE, Szymanski DA, Schoenecker PL. Use of an intramedullary rod for treatment of congenital pseudarthrosis of the tibia. A long-term follow-up study. J Bone Joint Surg Am. 2004;86(6):1186–97. https://doi.org/10.2106/00004623-200406000-00010.
24. Dormans JP, Krajbich JI, Zuker R, Demuynk M. Congenital pseudarthrosis of the tibia: treatment with free vascularized fibular grafts. J Pediatr Orthop. 1990;10(5):623–8. https://doi.org/10.1097/01241398-199009000-00010.

25. El-Gammal TA, El-Sayed A, Kotb MM. Telescoping vascularized fibular graft: a new method for treatment of congenital tibial pseudarthrosis with severe shortening. J Pediatr Orthop B. 2004;13(1):48–56. https://doi.org/10.1097/00009957-200401000-00010.
26. Paley D, Catagni M, Argnani F, Prevot J, Bell D, Armstrong P. Treatment of congenital pseudoarthrosis of the tibia using the Ilizarov technique. Clin Orthop. 1992;280:81–93.
27. Boero S, Catagni M, Donzelli O, Facchini R, Frediani PV. Congenital pseudarthrosis of the tibia associated with neurofibromatosis-1: treatment with Ilizarov's device. J Pediatr Orthop. 1997;17(5):675–84. https://doi.org/10.1097/00004694-199709000-00019.
28. El-Rosasy M, Paley D, Herzenberg J. Ilizarov techniques for the management of congenital pseudarthrosis of the tibia. Presented at: 2001; Tanta University, Egypt.
29. Ohnishi I, Sato W, Matsuyama J, et al. Treatment of congenital pseudarthrosis of the tibia: a multicenter study in Japan. J Pediatr Orthop. 2005;25(2):219–24. https://doi.org/10.1097/01.bpo.0000151054.54732.0b.
30. Joseph B, Mathew G. Management of congenital pseudarthrosis of the tibia by excision of the pseudarthrosis, onlay grafting, and intramedullary nailing. J Pediatr Orthop Part B. 2000;9(1):16–23. https://doi.org/10.1097/01202412-200001000-00004.
31. Johnston CE. Congenital pseudarthrosis of the tibia: results of technical variations in the charnley-williams procedure. J Bone Joint Surg Am. 2002;84(10):1799–810.
32. Kim HW, Weinstein SL. Intramedullary fixation and bone grafting for congenital pseudarthrosis of the tibia. Clin Orthop. 2002;405:250–7. https://doi.org/10.1097/00003086-200212000-00032.
33. Gilbert A, Brockman R. Congenital pseudarthrosis of the tibia. Long-term followup of 29 cases treated by microvascular bone transfer. Clin Orthop. 1995;314:37–44.
34. Kanaya F, Tsai TM, Harkess J. Vascularized bone grafts for congenital pseudarthrosis of the tibia. Microsurgery. 1996;17(8):459–69.; discussion 470–471. https://doi.org/10.1002/(SICI)1098-2752(1996)17:8<459::AID-MICR9>3.0.CO;2-9.
35. Weiland AJ, Weiss AP, Moore JR, Tolo VT. Vascularized fibular grafts in the treatment of congenital pseudarthrosis of the tibia. J Bone Joint Surg Am. 1990;72(5):654–62.
36. Keret D, Bollini G, Dungl P, et al. The fibula in congenital pseudoarthrosis of the tibia: the EPOS multicenter study. J Pediatr Orthop B. 2000;9(2):69–74. https://doi.org/10.1097/01202412-200004000-00001.
37. Romanus B, Bollini G, Dungl P, et al. Free vascular fibular transfer in congenital pseudoarthrosis of the tibia: results of the EPOS multicenter study. European Paediatric Orthopaedic Society (EPOS). J Pediatr Orthop Part B. 2000;9(2):90–3. https://doi.org/10.1097/01202412-200004000-00003.
38. Toh S, Harata S, Tsubo K, Inoue S, Narita S. Combining free vascularized fibula graft and the Ilizarov external fixator: recent approaches to congenital pseudarthrosis of the tibia. J Reconstr Microsurg. 2001;17(7):497–508.; discussion 509. https://doi.org/10.1055/s-2001-17752.
39. Lee FYI, Sinicropi SM, Lee FS, Vitale MG, Roye DP, Choi IH. Treatment of congenital pseudarthrosis of the tibia with recombinant human bone morphogenetic protein-7 (rhBMP-7). A report of five cases. J Bone Joint Surg Am. 2006;88(3):627–33. https://doi.org/10.2106/JBJS.D.02201.
40. Högler W, Yap F, Little D, Ambler G, McQuade M, Cowell CT. Short-term safety assessment in the use of intravenous zoledronic acid in children. J Pediatr. 2004;145(5):701–4. https://doi.org/10.1016/j.jpeds.2004.06.066.
41. Birke O, Schindeler A, Ramachandran M, et al. Preliminary experience with the combined use of recombinant bone morphogenetic protein and bisphosphonates in the treatment of congenital pseudarthrosis of the tibia. J Child Orthop. 2010;4(6):507–17. https://doi.org/10.1007/s11832-010-0293-3.
42. Cho TJ, Seo JB, Lee HR, Yoo WJ, Chung CY, Choi IH. Biologic characteristics of fibrous hamartoma from congenital pseudarthrosis of the tibia associated with neurofibromatosis type 1: J Bone Jt Surg-Am 2008;90(12):2735-2744. doi:10.2106/JBJS.H.00014
43. Thabet AM, Paley D, Kocaoglu M, Eralp L, Herzenberg JE, Ergin ON. Periosteal grafting for congenital pseudarthrosis of the tibia: a preliminary report. Clin Orthop. 2008;466(12):2981–94. https://doi.org/10.1007/s11999-008-0556-1.
44. Laufer A, Frommer A, Gosheger G, et al. Reconstructive approaches in surgical management of congenital pseudarthrosis of the tibia. J Clin Med. 2020;9(12) https://doi.org/10.3390/jcm9124132.
45. Karol LA, Haideri NF, Halliday SE, Smitherman TB, Johnston CE. Gait analysis and muscle strength in children with congenital pseudarthrosis of the tibia: the effect of treatment. J Pediatr Orthop. 1998;18(3):381–6.
46. Seo SG, Lee DY, Kim YS, Yoo WJ, Cho TJ, Choi IH. Foot and Ankle function at maturity after Ilizarov Treatment for atrophic-type congenital pseudarthrosis of the tibia: a comprehensive outcome comparison with normal controls. J Bone Jt Surg. 2016;98(6):490–8. https://doi.org/10.2106/JBJS.15.00964.
47. Paley D. Supplement to: congenital pseudarthrosis of the tibia: biological and biomechanical considerations to achieve union and prevent refracture. J Child Orthop. 2019;13(2):14.
48. Paley D. Paley cross-union protocol for treatment of congenital pseudarthrosis of the tibia. Oper Tech Orthop. 2021;31(2) https://doi.org/10.1016/j.oto.2021.100881.
49. Choi IH, Lee SJ, Moon HJ, et al. "4-in-1 Osteosynthesis" for atrophic-type congenital pseudarthrosis of the tibia. J Pediatr Orthop. 2011;31(6):697–704. https://doi.org/10.1097/BPO.0b013e318221ebce.
50. Paley D. Congenital pseudarthrosis of the tibia. In: Johari A, Waddell J, editors. Current progress in orthopaedics. Tree Life Media, Kothari Medical Subscription Services Pvt Ltd; 2017. p. 318–48.
51. Packer D, Robb J, Liu R, Robbins C, Paley D. Combined pharmacologic and biological treatment of congenital pseudarthrosis of the tibia; 100% union; no re-fractures! J Child Orthop. 2016;10:S19–20.
52. Vaidya SV, Aroojis A, Mehta R, et al. Short term results of a new comprehensive protocol for the management of congenital pseudarthrosis of the tibia. Indian J Orthop. 2019;53(6):736–44. https://doi.org/10.4103/ortho.IJOrtho_155_19.
53. Liu Y, Yang G, Liu K, et al. Combined surgery with 3-in-1 osteosynthesis in congenital pseudarthrosis of the tibia with intact fibula. Orphanet J Rare Dis. 2020;15(1):62. https://doi.org/10.1186/s13023-020-1330-z.
54. Ning B. Combination treatment by cross fusion of the tibia and fibula, autogenic iliac bone grafting, reliable fixation and bone morphogenetic proteins for the treatment of refractory congenital pseudarthrosis of the tibia (Personal communication). Published online April 25, 2021.
55. Shannon CE, Huser AJ, Paley D. Cross-union surgery for congenital pseudarthrosis of the tibia. Children. 2021;8(7):547. https://doi.org/10.3390/children8070547.
56. Malhotra D, Puri R, Owen R. Valgus deformity of the ankle in children with spina bifida aperta. J Bone Joint Surg Br. 1984;66(3):381–5.
57. Yablon G, Heller FG, Shouse L. The key role of the lateral malleolus in displaced fractures of the ankle. J Bone Jt Surg. 1977:59–169.
58. Frick SL, Shoemaker S, Mubarak SJ. Altered fibular growth patterns after tibiofibular synostosis in children. JBJS. 2001;83(2):247.
59. Jung ST, Wang SI, Moon YJ, Mubarak SJ, Kim JR. Posttraumatic tibiofibular synostosis after treatment of distal tibiofibular fractures in children. J Pediatr Orthop. 2017;37(8):532–6. https://doi.org/10.1097/BPO.0000000000000708.
60. Rodríguez-González FÁ. Biomaterials in orthopaedic surgery. ASM Press; 2009.

61. Lovell W, Weinstein S, Flynn J. Lovell and winter's pediatric orthopaedics. 7th ed. Wolters Kluwer Health/Lippincott Williams & Wilkins; 2014.
62. Eisenberg KA, Vuillermin CB. Management of congenital pseudoarthrosis of the tibia and fibula. Curr Rev Musculoskelet Med. 2019;22:356–68. https://doi.org/10.1007/s12178-019-09566-2.
63. Paley D. Surgical reconstruction for fibular hemimelia. J Child Orthop. 2016;10(6):557–83. https://doi.org/10.1007/s11832-016-0790-0.
64. Bradley GW, Coleman SS. Treatment of the calcaneocavus foot deformity. J Bone Joint Surg Am. 1981;63(7):1159–66.
65. Schwend RM, Drennan JC. Cavus foot deformity in children. J Am Acad Orthop Surg. 2003;11(3):201–11. https://doi.org/10.5435/00124635-200305000-00007.
66. Lippross S, Tsaknakis K, Lorenz HM, Hell AK. Cross (X)-Union-Technik zur Behandlung der kongenitalen Tibiapseudarthrose (CPT). Unfallchirurg. 2021;124(9):768–73. https://doi.org/10.1007/s00113-021-01057-9.
67. Laine JC, Novotny SA, Weber EW, Georgiadis AG, Dahl MT. Distal tibial guided growth for anterolateral bowing of the tibia: fracture may be prevented. J Bone Jt Surg. 2020;102(23):2077–86. https://doi.org/10.2106/JBJS.20.00657.

Congenital Posteromedial Bowing of the Tibia

Benjamin Joseph, Hitesh Shah, and N. D. Siddesh

Introduction

Congenital posteromedial bowing of the tibia is a relatively uncommon condition. It is one among a group of congenital bowing deformities of the tibia that include anteromedial, anterolateral, and posteromedial bowing. In the past, these three deformities were arbitrarily grouped together and referred to as congenital kyphoscoliotic tibia [1]. It is well recognized that the clinical features, natural history, and long-term prognosis of posteromedial bowing of the tibia are distinctly different from the more sinister anterolateral bowing associated with neurofibromatosis and congenital pseudarthrosis and anteromedial bowing associated with fibular deficiency [2–5]. Though a diagnosis may be made in the antenatal period during routine ultrasound evaluation of pregnancy [6, 7], in the majority of instances the diagnosis is made at birth.

Incidence

The exact incidence of congenital posteromedial bowing of the tibia is unknown though hospital-based reports suggest that it is an uncommon condition. Pappas [5] reported a series of 33 patients gathered over a 36-year period; Hoffman and Wenger [8] reported 13 patients seen over a 14-year period; Johari et al. saw 31 children in an 18-year period [9] and we reported 20 patients seen over a 19-year period [10]. These four reports, all based on retrospective data from tertiary care centers, suggest that most of such centers would probably encounter one or two new cases of congenital posteromedial bowing per year. These hospital-based estimates, however, are prone to several biases and hence are, at best, rough indicators of the magnitude of the problem. In 2008, we put in place a registry for congenital posteromedial bowing of the tibia and have been prospectively following up all new cases. In these last 13 years, we documented 69 new cases. This suggests that the condition is much more common than previously estimated from retrospective studies. The greater frequency of cases noted over the last 13 years is likely to be a reflection of more reliable nature of data generated prospectively rather than an increase in the incidence.

Demographic Features

Bilateral involvement is rare; we encountered one bilateral case among 69 cases. There is an unexplained predilection for the left limb to be affected; left-sided involvement is almost twice as frequent as the right [10]. Boys and girls appear to be equally affected.

Etiology

Dawson attributed the deformity to malunion of an intrauterine fracture, though he provided no real evidence to support this hypothesis [11]. De Maio et al. [7] had the unique opportunity of having performed an autopsy on a fetus with posteromedial bowing aborted at 24 weeks of gestation. They noted evidence of amniotic rupture and attributed this as the possible underlying cause of the deformity in that fetus.

B. Joseph (✉)
Kasturba Medical College, Manipal, Karnataka, India

H. Shah
Department of Paediatric Orthopedics, Kasturba Medical College, Kasturba Hospital, Manipal Academy of Higher Education, Manipal, Karnataka, India

N. D. Siddesh
Department of Orthopaedics, Dubai Hospital, Dubai Health Authority, Dubai, United Arab Emirates

Deformities

The Tibia

The tibia is bowed posteriorly and medially (Fig. 33.1a–d); in the newborn the posterior bow is usually more pronounced than the medial bow, though the medial bow may exceed the posterior bow in some instances [10]. The degree of posterior angulation in the newborn may be as high as 90° (see Fig. 33.1b). The site of the primary deformity is characteristically at the junction of the middle and lower thirds of the leg. It is important to be aware that there may be compensatory deformities above and below the diaphyseal bowing. Consequently, simply correcting through the diaphysis may leave unexpected residual deformity.

A skin dimple may be seen at the apex of the bow. The tibia is invariably shorter than the unaffected side and the degree of shortening is proportionate to the severity of bowing (Fig. 33.2a, b).

Though the degree of shortening frequently is in the order of 15 or 20%, up to 40% of shortening has been recorded [10]. Occasionally, there may be an associated torsional deformity of the tibia (see Fig. 33.2b).

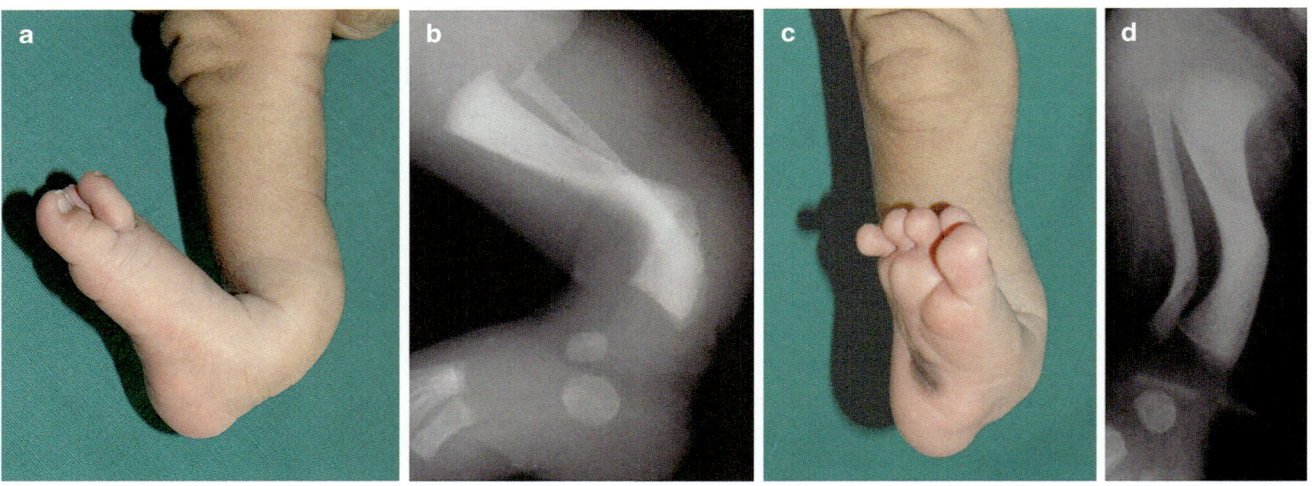

Fig. 33.1 Congenital posteromedial bowing of the tibia in a newborn. The clinical and radiographic appearances of the posterior bow (**a**, **b**) and the medial bow (**c**, **d**) are clearly seen. A delay in the ossification of the proximal tibial epiphysis and the cuboid is evident

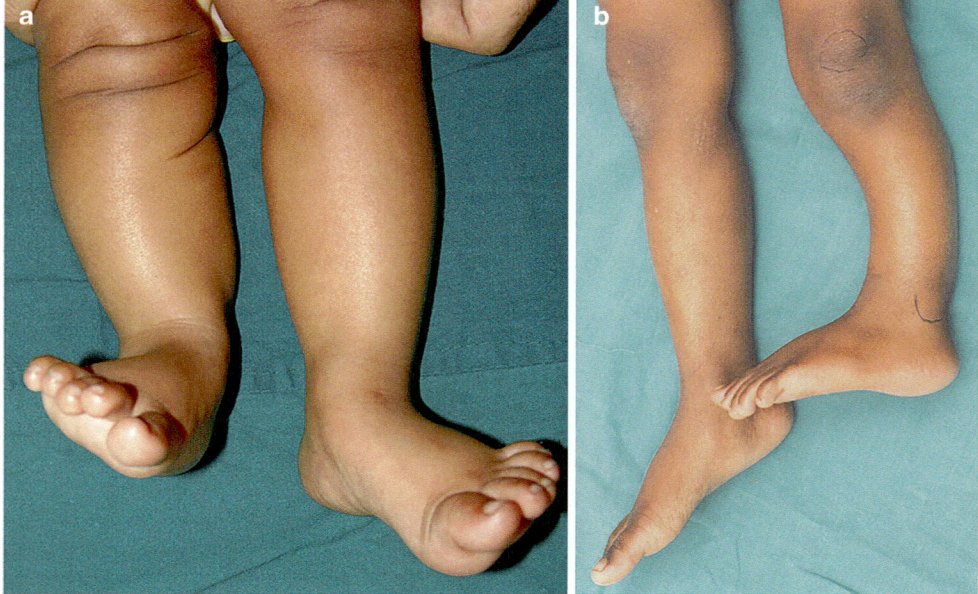

Fig. 33.2 Examples of a short tibia associated with congenital posteromedial bowing. The shortening is mild when the bowing is mild (**a**) and greater when the bowing is more severe. Occasionally, a torsional deformity may also be present (**b**). The patella and lateral malleolus have been marked to demonstrate the torsional deformity

33 Congenital Posteromedial Bowing of the Tibia

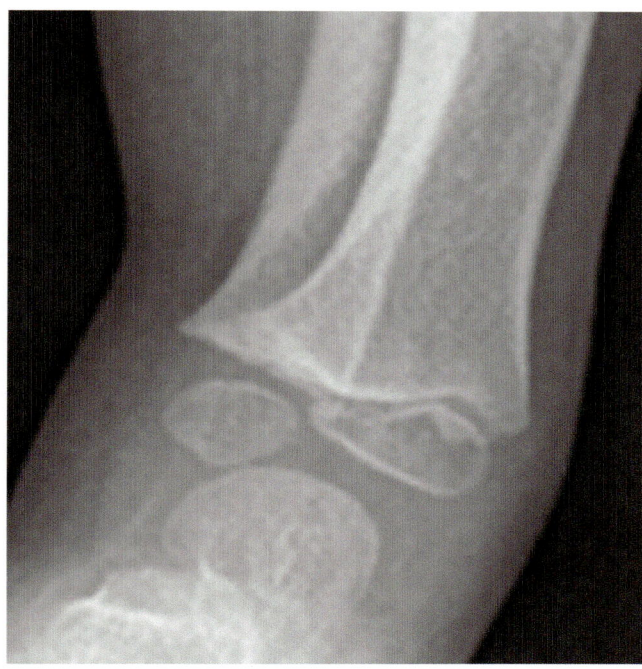

Fig. 33.3 The fibular physis is at a higher level than normal (at the level of the ankle joint)

> **Box 33.1 The Deformity**
> - Posteromedial bowing at the junction of the middle and lower thirds of the tibia and fibula.
> - Posterior bow is usually more severe than medial bow.
> - Shortening is proportionate to severity of bowing.
> - Always associated with a calcaneo-valgus deformity of the foot.
> - Valgus deformity of the ankle may develop later due to growth abnormalities of the distal tibia and fibula.

The Fibula

The fibula is also bowed and the degree of deformity parallels the tibial deformity. The distal fibula physis is often at a higher level than normal, suggesting that there is a relative growth retardation of the fibula as compared to the affected tibia (Fig. 33.3).

The Ankle and Foot

The tibial deformity is invariably associated with a calcaneo-valgus deformity which may be very severe at birth with the dorsum of the foot lying almost in contact with the shin (Fig. 33.4). The deformity of the foot chould be differentiated from congeital vertical talus (convex pes valgus) which is a rigid deformity characterized by reversal of the medial longitudinal arch that does not improve when the foot is passively plantarflexed. The distal tibial epiphysis may appear late, and when it does appear, it may be eccentrically positioned towards the medial side (Fig. 33.5a) [10]. The epiphysis may then develop asym-

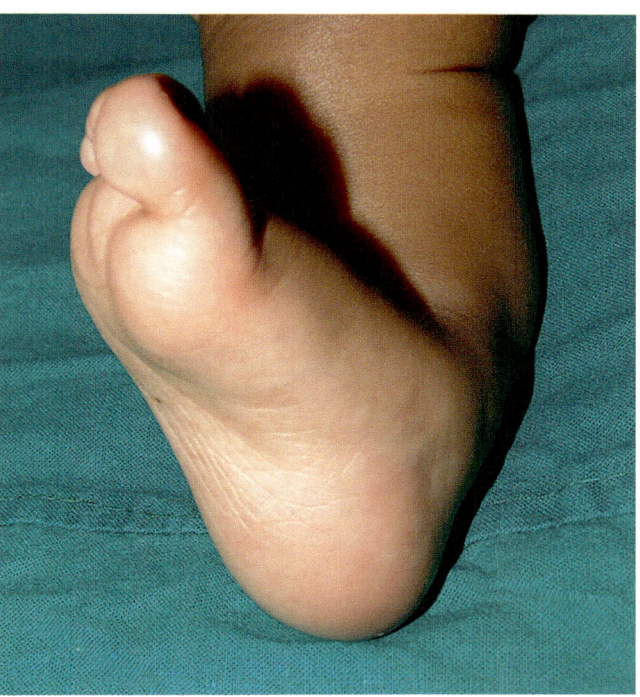

Fig. 33.4 Calcaneo-valgus deformity seen in association with congenital posteromedial bowing of the tibia

metrically into a wedge-shaped epiphysis (see Fig. 33.5b), resulting in a valgus tilt of the ankle mortise [10]. The growth delay of the fibula with a high lateral malleolus referred to above also contributes to ankle valgus (see Fig. 33.5c).

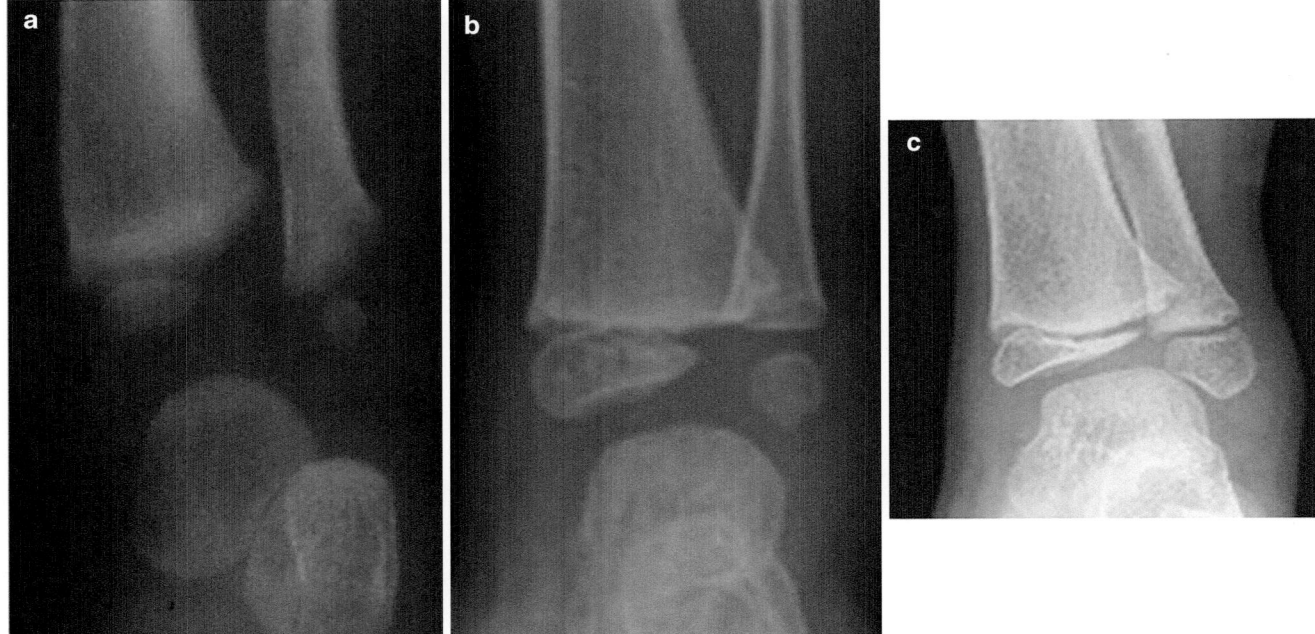

Fig. 33.5 Eccentric ossification of the distal tibial epiphysis in a toddler with congenital posteromedial bowing of the tibia (**a**) and a *wedge-shaped* distal tibial epiphysis in an older child with congenital posteromedial bowing of the tibia (**b**). The valgus tilt of the ankle becomes more evident as the child grows older (**c**)

The Natural History

Rate and Pattern of Spontaneous Remodeling

The posteromedial bowing deformities of the tibia and fibula tend to improve spontaneously over time. The resolution of the bony deformity occurs by two distinct mechanisms; one entails resorption of bone from the convex surface and new bone deposition on the concavity of the bow in accordance with Wolff's law [10]. De Maio et al. demonstrated that this pattern of remodeling begins in utero [7]. At 24 weeks of gestation, an abundance of osteoclasts was present at the apex of the deformity, while an osteoblastic response was seen in the concavity. As this process of remodeling progresses, the angular deformity decreases and the angulation between the proximal and distal segments of the bone diminishes. The second mechanism of spontaneous correction of the deformity involves realignment of the proximal and distal growth plates. Physeal reorientation occurs at a faster rate than remodeling at the site of the deformity [10]. Remodeling of the deformity by both these mechanisms occurs at a rapid rate during the first year of life, and thereafter, the rate of remodeling decreases quite substantially dropping to half the initial rate (Fig. 33.6) [10]. Di Gennaro et al. studied the pattern of spontaneous resolution of the tibial deformity in two planes over time and suggested that the resolution of the tibial deformity does not follow a linear pattern, but a log-linear pattern of spontaneous correction of the medial bow and an exponential pattern for correction of the posterior bow [12].

Residual Deformities, Shortening, and Functional Problems

Complete resolution of the diaphyseal deformity does not occur in a proportion of children and residual deformity that is clinically discernable may be seen in children older than 4 or 5 years of age (Fig. 33.7a, b) [10].

Shortening of the limb increases with growth [8] and the limb length discrepancy at skeletal maturity may frequently be of a magnitude to warrant treatment. Pappas noted a median shortening of 4.1 cm at skeletal maturity with a range between 3.3 and 6.9 cm [5]. The foot length of the affected limb is often less than the normal foot [5, 8, 13].

Limitation of ankle motion may persist; limitation of both plantar flexion and dorsiflexion has been reported [8, 10].

Weakness of plantar flexion (Fig. 33.8) has been observed in some children, even though the bony deformity may have remodeled almost completely [10]. On occasion, the weakness of the gastrocsoleus may be severe enough to result in a calcaneal hitch and a visible gait abnormality requiring surgical intervention [10]; we have encountered two such children.

Fig. 33.6 The rate of spontaneous resolution of bowing is rapid in the first year of life, slows down thereafter, and reaches a plateau by 4–5 years of age

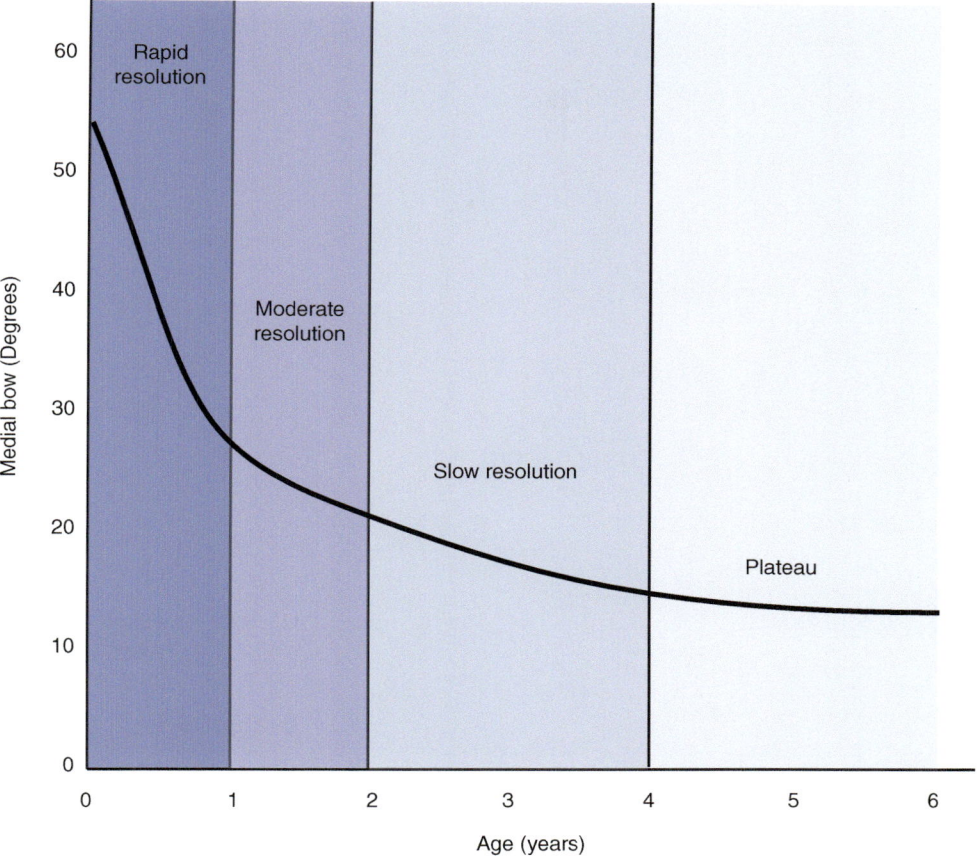

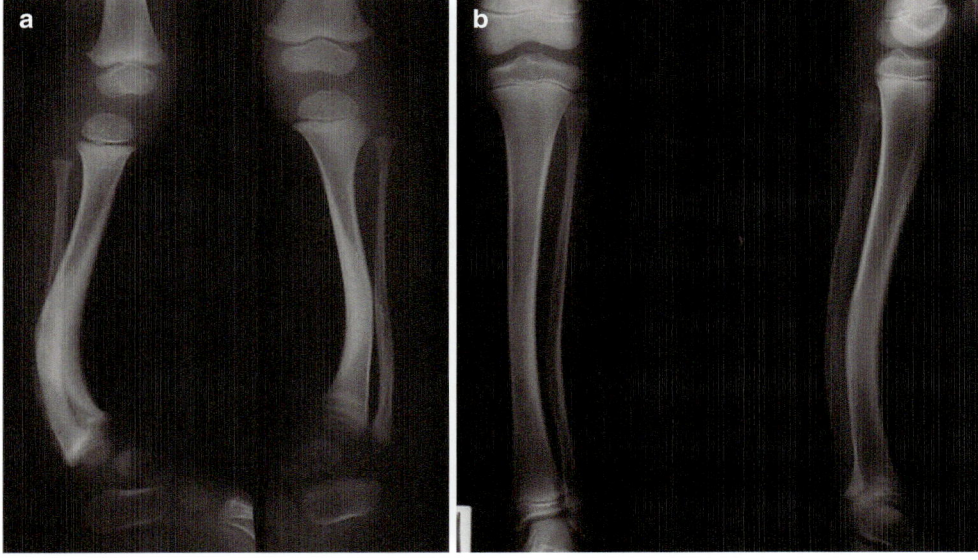

Fig. 33.7 Residual posterior bowing of both tibiae in a child aged 4 years with bilateral posteromedial bowing of the tibia (**a**) and residual bowing at 8 years in another child (**b**). The AP radiograph shows that the distal tibial articular surface is not parallel to the plane of the knee joint, even though the medial bow has remodeled to a very large extent

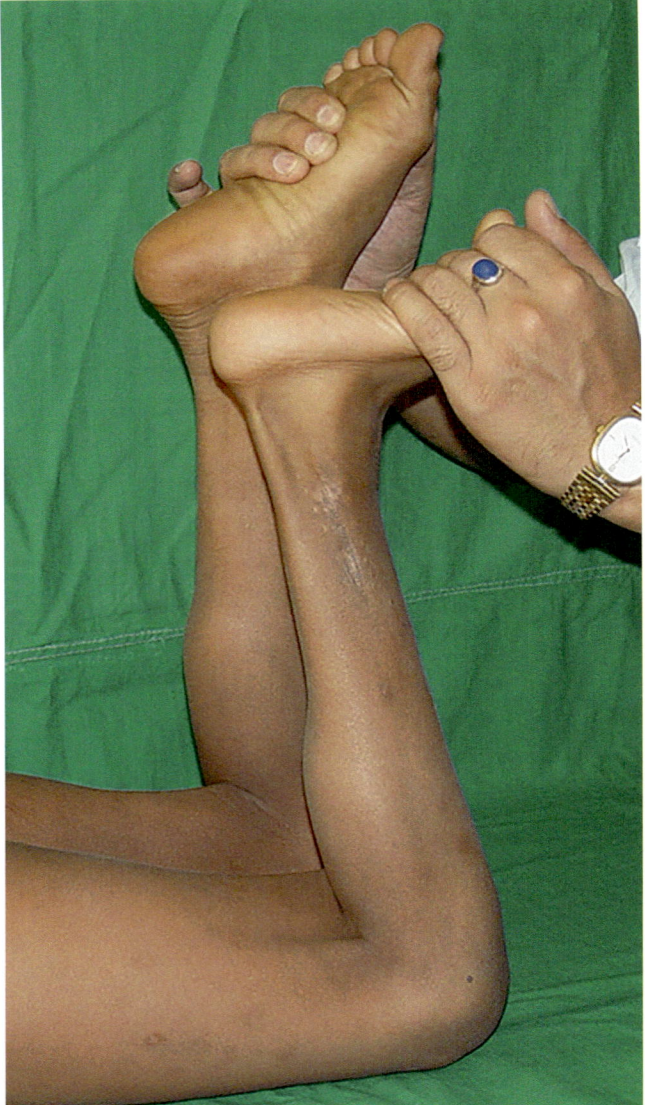

Fig. 33.8 The power of plantar flexion is being tested in a boy with congenital posteromedial bowing of the tibia. Weakness of plantar flexion on the affected side is clearly evident. This weakness that was present before he underwent corrective osteotomy for residual deformity still persists

---

Box 33.2 Spontaneous Resolution of Bowing
- Occurs by local remodeling and by physeal realignment.
- Occurs rapidly in the first year of life.
- Little remodeling occurs after 4–5 years of age.
- Complete resolution may not occur.

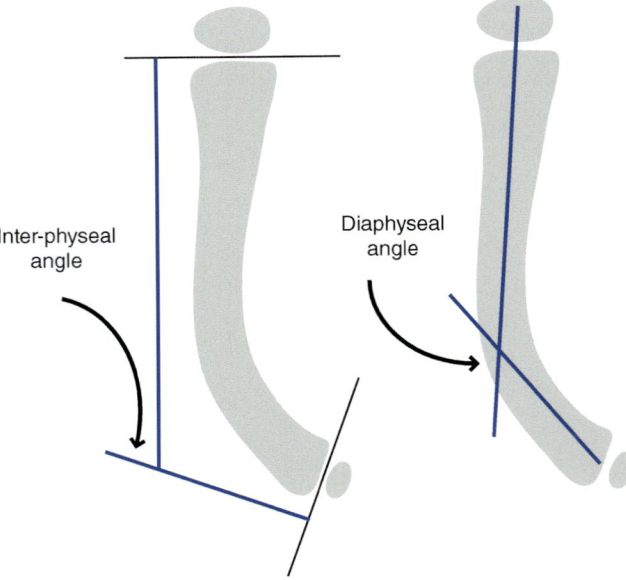

Fig. 33.9 The diaphyseal bow and the inter-physeal angles can be measured on the anteroposterior and lateral radiographs

Evaluation

Establishing the diagnosis in the newborn is not difficult once the plane of the deformity is clear. The evaluation should include a careful documentation of the clinical estimate of the severity of the diaphyseal deformity in the coronal and sagittal planes. The foot should be passively plantar flexed and inverted to assess the rigidity of the calcaneo-valgus deformity. Anteroposterior and lateral full-length plain radiographs of both tibias and a scanogram should be taken to facilitate accurate estimation of the angulation and shortening. The degree of shortening of the tibia should be documented and expressed both as a percent of the normal tibial length and in centimeters. The extent of bowing should be estimated by measuring the diaphyseal angle and the inter-physeal angles on the radiographs (Fig. 33.9). The parents should be counselled and reassured that the deformity will reduce spontaneously, but they need to be warned that complete resolution may not occur. They should also be instructed to perform passive stretching exercises of the foot into plantar flexion and inversion and encouraged to do it at least twice a day.

The child should be reexamined at 6 months of age to evaluate the extent of correction of the calcaneo-valgus deformity and the tibial bowing. If sufficient resolution of the foot deformity has not occurred, casting should be considered. The child should be seen again at 1 year of age to plan the extent of shoe raise that may be required to facilitate more normal walking. The child should then be followed up annually for the next 4 years at which time a decision should be taken regarding intervention for residual deformities and shortening.

The child should be reviewed finally at skeletal maturity to document if limb lengths have been equalized and if there are any residual deformities or functional limitations.

Treatment

Indications

1. Treatment is indicated for any deformity of the leg, ankle, or foot that is cosmetically unacceptable, provided adequate time has been given for spontaneous resolution of the deformities.
2. Treatment should be recommended if, by the age of 6 years, sufficient resolution of the deformity has not occurred to make the articular surface of the distal tibia parallel or almost parallel (<5°) to the knee joint on the anteroposterior radiograph of the tibia.
3. Treatment should be recommended for any functional deficit that may affect normal gait.

Aims of Treatment

- Correct the calcaneo-valgus deformity of the foot in the infant.
- Correct residual coronal, sagittal, and transverse plane (torsional) deformities of the tibia and fibula in the older child.
- Restore the normal alignment of the ankle to restore a horizontal tibial plafond.
- Equalize limb lengths.
- Improve the power of ankle plantar flexion if there is severe weakness of the gastrocsoleus.

Treatment Options

Correction of the Calcaneo-Valgus Foot Deformity

Passive stretching: The mild degree of calcaneo-valgus deformity responds to gentle passive stretching similar to the response seen in idiopathic congenital calcaneo-valgus deformities not associated with posteromedial bowing of the tibia.

Serial casting: The more severe degrees usually respond to serial manipulation and cast application; very rarely, anterior soft tissue release may be required [14].

Correction of Sagittal, Coronal, or Torsional Deformities of the Tibia and Fibula

Acute correction: Acute correction by performing an osteotomy at the site of the deformity is a simple and attractive option particularly when the residual deformity is in a single plane and when the extent of limb length discrepancy does not warrant formal limb lengthening. Fixation of the osteotomy may be with either internal or external fixation.

Gradual correction: Gradual correction with an external fixator may be the more appropriate option when there are deformities in two or three planes and if concomitant limb lengthening is required.

Correction of the Valgus Ankle

Physeal manipulation (guided growth): Valgus deformity of the ankle due to abnormal distal tibial physeal and epiphyseal growth is best addressed by modulating physeal growth such that the growth of the medial part of the physis is restrained using either an extra-periosteal plate and screw device or a single transphyseal screw. The latter option is simpler and the authors' preferred option (Fig. 33.10).

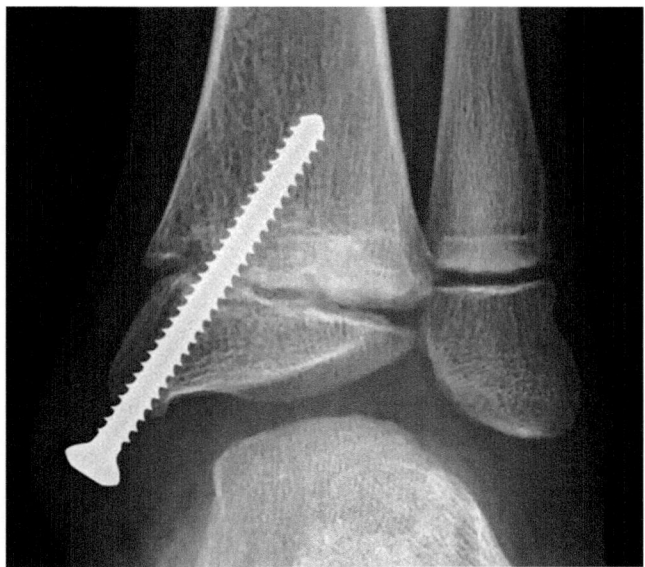

Fig. 33.10 A medial screw epiphysiodesis has been performed to correct ankle valgus. The wedge-shaped distal tibial epiphysis and the abnormal proximal location of the distal fibular physis are seen

Supramalleolar osteotomy: If the distal tibial epiphysis is normal in shape and the relative lengths of the tibia and fibula are normal, a valgus deformity of the distal tibia should be corrected by a supramalleolar osteotomy.

Correction of Limb Length Inequality

Contralateral epiphysiodesis: In many instances, the projected limb length discrepancy at skeletal maturity is less than 5 cm. An acceptable option is to perform a contralateral proximal tibial and fibular epiphysiodesis at the appropriate time based on the anticipated correction estimated from a growth chart. This option is particularly attractive when the shortening is in the order of 2–3 cm and there are no residual deformities to be addressed.

Limb lengthening: Gradual lengthening of the tibia is typically needed when the limb length discrepancy at skeletal maturity is likely to exceed 5 cm. Lengthening may also be considered for smaller degrees of discrepancy when deformity correction is also required. In such situations, both these problems can be addressed by a single procedure [15]. However, the lengthening cannot usually be performed through the osteotomy site used for correcting the tibial deformity as the apex of the tibial diaphyseal deformity tends to be too far distal; a second osteotomy in the proximal tibia is typically required for more reliable new bone formation during limb lengthening. If a circular fixator is used, gradual correction of the deformity at the distal osteotomy site can be undertaken while distraction for limb length equalization proceeds at the proximal osteotomy site. Limb lengthening through an osteotomy in the proximal tibia can also be undertaken with a monolateral frame once acute correction of the biplanar deformity is achieved at the site of bowing in the same sitting (Fig. 33.11a, b).

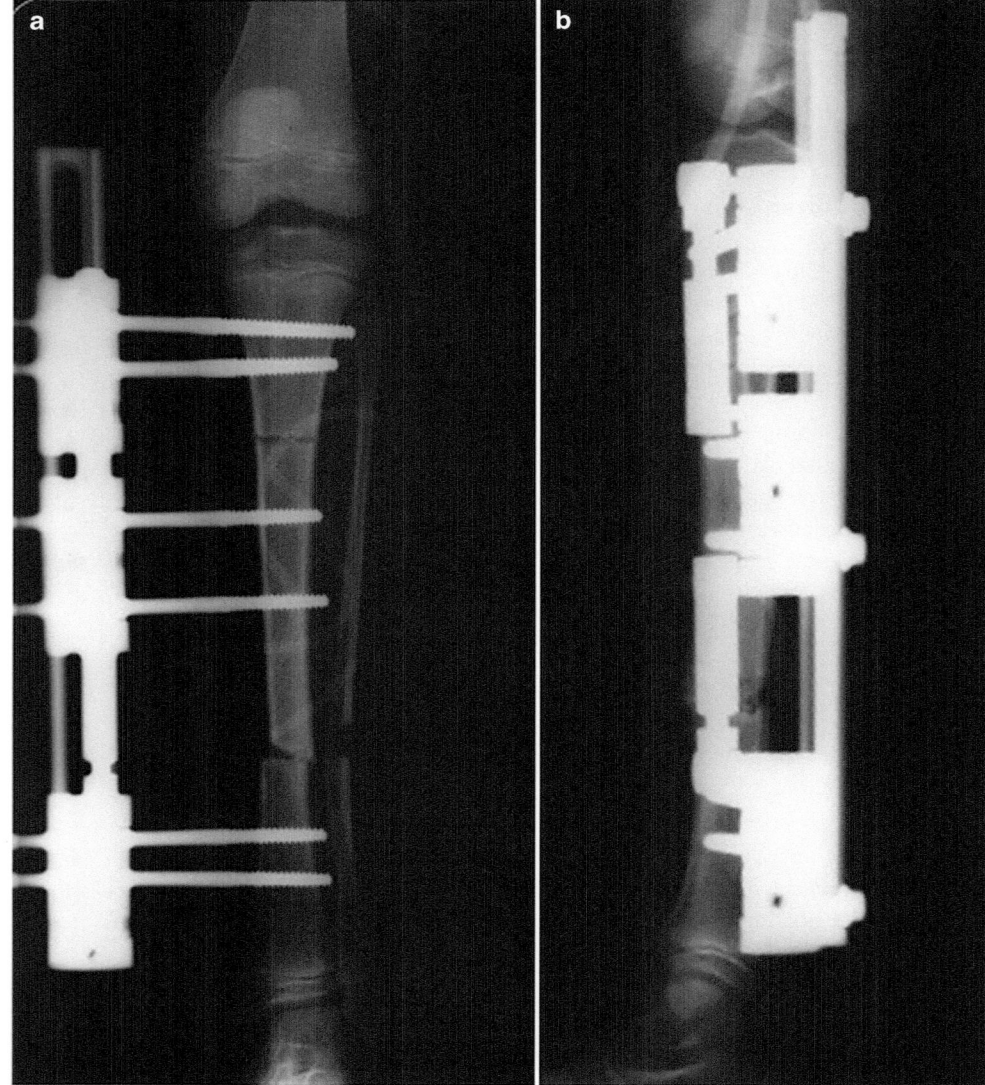

Fig. 33.11 Corrective osteotomy for correction of residual bowing combined with a more proximal osteotomy for limb lengthening has been performed. Acute correction of the posterior (**b**) and medial (**a**) bow was first performed through the distal osteotomy and the fixator was applied taking care to ensure that the normal alignment of the tibia was restored in both planes. The proximal osteotomy for the limb lengthening was then performed

Correction of Muscle Imbalance Across the Ankle

Tendon transfer: Tendon transfers are seldom effective in restoring powerful push-off if the gastrocsoleus is completely paralyzed [16], but may be effective in posteromedial bowing of the tibia where the gastrocsoleus is weak with some residual muscle function. We prefer to perform a peroneal translocation in which the peroneus longus tendon is rerouted behind the calcaneum under tension (without dividing and reattaching the tendon as in a tendon classic transfer) to augment the gastrocsoleus in this situation (Fig. 33.12) [17].

> **Box 33.3 Treatment**
> - Nonoperative correction of calcaneo-valgus foot deformity in infancy.
> - Surgical correction of residual deformities of the tibia and fibula after 6 years of age
> - Equalization of limb lengths
> - Correction of valgus ankle
> - Correction of weak plantar flexion

Decision Making

The factors to be taken into consideration while planning treatment are [18–22]:

- The degree of spontaneous resolution of the tibial deformity in a child over 4 years of age
- The extent of anticipated limb length inequality at skeletal maturity
- The site of ankle deformity, if present

The outline of treatment is shown in Table 33.1.

Recent reports have highlighted the need for surgery in many children with posteromedial bowing of the tibia to address residual deformity and limb length inequality [19–22]. However, there is no agreement regarding the timing of surgery. Though surgery has been done in very young children [22], we see no benefit of intervening before the age of 5 years when potential for spontaneous resolution of the deformity is still present. Recurrence of shortening has also been observed in children who underwent lengthening of the tibia under the age of 10 years [20]. For this reason, limb lengthening is best done closer to skeletal maturity [18, 20].

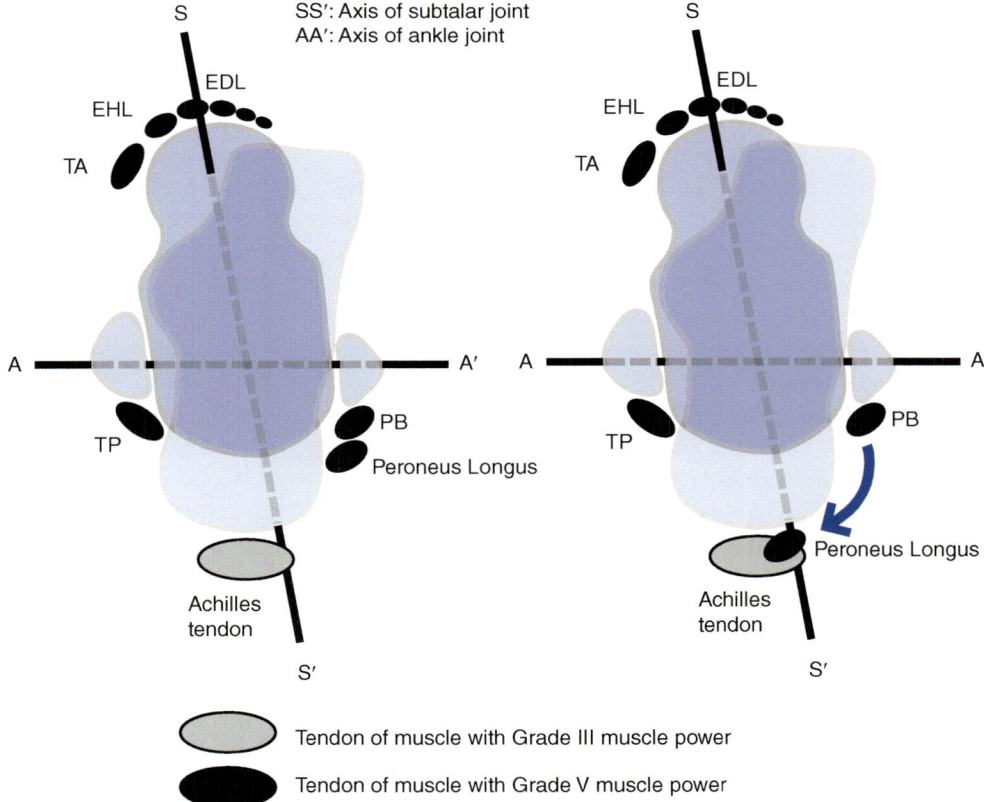

Fig. 33.12 Diagrammatic representation of how the muscle balance is restored across the axis of the ankle joint by performing a peroneal translocation operation

Table 33.1 Outline of management of congenital posteromedial bowing of the tibia[a]

Indication	Treatment recommendation
Anticipated limb length discrepancy at skeletal maturity < 2 cm Near-complete resolution of tibial deformities in all planes No ankle deformity	No intervention
Anticipated limb length discrepancy at skeletal maturity 2–4 cm Near-complete resolution of tibial deformities in all planes No ankle deformity	Contralateral epiphysiodesis of the proximal tibia and fibula at appropriate time so as to equalize limb lengths by skeletal maturity
Anticipated limb length discrepancy at skeletal maturity >4 cm Near-complete resolution of tibial deformities in all planes No ankle deformity	Proximal tibial lengthening to equalize limb lengths close to skeletal maturity
Anticipated limb length discrepancy at skeletal maturity >2 cm Unacceptable residual tibial deformity No ankle deformity	Tibial metaphyseal lengthening with diaphyseal osteotomy to correct tibial deformity
Ankle valgus at supramalleolar level (no wedging of distal tibial epiphysis)	Supramalleolar osteotomy (in addition to treatment outlined in rows 1, 2, 3, or 4)
Ankle valgus at physeal level with wedging of the distal tibial epiphysis	Medial screw epiphysiodesis of the distal tibia (in addition to treatment outlined in rows 1, 2, 3, or 4)

[a]Modified from [18]

Pitfalls in Diagnosis and Treatment

Pitfalls in the diagnosis and management of posteromedial bowing can be prevented by careful observation of the site and the plane of the deformities. An erroneous diagnosis of congenital pseudarthrosis of the tibia can be avoided by noting that the direction of tibial bowing is diametrically opposite to anterolateral bowing of pseudarthrosis.

Before embarking on treatment of ankle valgus, it is imperative that the site of the deformity is clearly identified. An abnormal wedge-shaped distal tibial epiphysis with an inclined distal tibial articular surface should be treated by medial hemiepiphysiodesis, while ankle valgus caused by distal tibial angulation should be treated by a supramalleolar osteotomy.

Commentary

Simon P. Kelley
simon.kelley@sickkids.ca

Given the striking deformity seen in neonates with this condition, caregiver anxiety can be high. Serial photographs of the neonate's lower limbs taken by the caregivers can be very helpful for reassurance to the family in the early months after birth confirming the rapid early resolution of the deformity.

Resist the temptation of surgical intervention in the first 5 years of life. Significant remodelling is expected to occur; only after this time can the true extent of residual deformity and functional limitations be identified.

Always perform a comprehensive deformity analysis prior to establishing a surgical treatment plan as, despite the eye being drawn to the obvious diaphyseal tibial deformity, there are always multiple sites of deformity. These can include the proximal tibial physis, the distal tibial physis, and epiphysis.

The mechanical axis test is extremely important in assessment. If the axis passes close to the centre of the knee with a noticeable diaphyseal deformity, look for the other sites of primary and secondary deformities!

Always consider that not all residual tibial diaphyseal deformities need surgical correction. A mild residual bow with appropriate proximal tibial physeal remodelling can leave the limb very nicely aligned. A contralateral epiphysiodesis for a modest limb length discrepancy may be all that is required for an excellent clinical outcome at maturity.

Acute bony correction of the diaphyseal deformity of the tibia is harder than it looks! Given the coronal, sagittal, and axial planar elements of this complex deformity, gradual correction using a circular fixator is often a better choice as it is more accurate and reliable in this situation. Furthermore, a circular fixator can also be used to simultaneously lengthen the limb, either through the apex of the deformity or using a double-level approach with lengthening at a more proximal site.

> In more severe cases, a combined comprehensive approach in the skeletally immature individual is typically necessary and may include guided growth at both the distal and proximal tibial physes along with gradual diaphyseal deformity correction and lengthening at the apex of the deformity.

References

1. Badgley CE, O'Connor SJ, Kudner DF. Congenital kyphoscoliotic tibia. J Bone Joint Surg Am. 1952;34:349–494.
2. Heyman CH, Herndon CH. Congenital posterior angulation of the tibia. J Bone Joint Surg Am. 1949;31:571–80.
3. Miller BF. Congenital posterior bowing of the tibia with calcaneovalgus. J Bone Joint Surg Br. 1951;33B:50–5.
4. Heyman CH, HerndonCH CH, Heiple KG. Congenital posterior angulation of the tibia with talipes calcaneus: a long-term report of eleven patients. J Bone Joint Surg Am. 1959;41:476–88.
5. Pappas AM. Congenital posteromedial bowing of the tibia and fibula. J Pediatr Orthop. 1984;4–5:525–31.
6. Zollinger PE, Wessels MW, Wladimiroff JW, Diepstraten AFM. Prenatal ultrasonographic diagnosis of posteromedial bowing of the leg: two case reports. Ultrasound Obstet Gynecol. 2000;15:150–3.
7. De Maio F, Corsi A, Roggini M, Riminucci M, Bianco P, Ippolito E. Congenital unilateral posteromedial bowing of the tibia and fibula: insights regarding pathogenesis from prenatal pathology. A case report. J Bone Joint Surg Am. 2005;87(7):1601–5.
8. Hofmann A, Wenger DR. Posteromedial bowing of the tibia. Progression of discrepancy in leg lengths. J Bone Joint Surg Am. 1981;63(3):384–8.
9. Johari AN, Dhawale AA, Salaskar A, Aroojis AJ. Congenital postero-medial bowing of the tibia and fibula: Is early surgery worthwhile? J Pediatr Orthop B. 2010;19(6):479–86.
10. Shah HH, Doddabasappa SN, Joseph B. Congenital posteromedial bowing of the tibia: a retrospective analysis of growth abnormalities in the leg. J Pediatr Orthop B. 2009;18(3):120–8.
11. Dawson GR. Intra-uterine fractures of the tibia and fibula. Report of a case with correction by osteotomy and plating. J Bone Joint Surg Am. 1949;31A:406–8.
12. Di Gennaro GL, Gallone G, Martinez Vazquez EA, et al. Deformity progression in congenital posteromedial bowing of the tibia: a report of 44 cases. BMC Musculoskelet Disord. 2020;21(1):430.
13. Grimes JB, Blair VP 3rd, Gilula LA. Roentgen rounds #81. Posteromedial bowing of the tibia. Orthop Rev. 1986;15(4):249–55.
14. Yadav SS, Thomas S. Congenital posteromedial bowing of the tibia. Acta Orthop Scand. 1980;51(2):311–3.
15. Kaufman SD, Fagg JA, Jones S, Bell MJ, Saleh M, Fernandes JA. Limb lengthening in congenital posteromedial bow of the tibia. Strategies Trauma Limb Reconstr. 2012;7(3):147–53.
16. Joseph B. The paralysed foot and ankle. In: Joseph B, Nayagam S, Loder RT, Torode I, editors. Paediatric orthopaedics—a system of decision-making. 2nd ed. CRC Press Taylor & Francis Group; 2016. p. 461–73.
17. Makin M, Yossipovitch Z. Translocation of the peroneus longus tendon in the treatment of paralytic pes calcaneus. A follow-up study of thirty-three cases. J Bone Joint Surg Am. 1966;48:1541–7.
18. Joseph B. Posteromedial bowing of the tibia. In: Joseph B, Nayagam S, Loder RT, Torode I, editors. Paediatric orthopaedics—a system of decision-making. 2nd ed. CRC Press. Taylor & Francis Group; 2016. p. 81–4.
19. Ariyawatkul T, Kaewpornsawan K, Chotigavanichaya C, Eamsobhana P. The results of lengthening in congenital posteromedial angulation of tibia. J Med Assoc Thail. 2016;99(10):1137–41.
20. Wright J, Hill RA, Eastwood DM, Hashemi-Nejad A, Calder P, Tennant S. Posteromedial bowing of the tibia: a benign condition or a case for limb reconstruction? J Child Orthop. 2018;12(2):187–96.
21. Gordon JE, Schoenecker PL, Lewis TR, Miller ML. Limb lengthening in the treatment of posteromedial bowing of the tibia. J Child Orthop. 2020;14(5):480–7. https://doi.org/10.1302/1863-2548.14.20011.
22. Sagade B, Jagani N, Chaudhary I, Chaudhary M. Congenital posteromedial bowing of tibia: comparison of early and late lengthening. J Pediatr Orthop. 2021;41(9):e816–22.

Controversies in Blount's Disease

David A. Podeszwa and John G. Birch

Introduction

Much has been written about Blount's disease since its presumed earliest description by Erlacher [1], including early "definitive" (and classic) works of Blount [2] (for whom many have adopted his name to describe the condition) and Langenskiöld [3] (who described the classic radiographic classification of the infantile form of the disease). Blount and Langenskiöld both described two forms of the disorder: occurring in a younger population with generally greater epiphyseal and physeal distortion (infantile Blount's disease) and that occurring in older patients with generally less pronounced epiphyseal and physeal distortion (adolescent Blount's disease). Despite having been described so long ago, this disorder can be aptly described as an arena of controversy: controversy as to name, classification (by age and radiographic type), etiology, and treatment of all types. In this chapter, we review these controversies as well as what is known, and unknown, about Blount's disease.

Terminology

Usually progressive proximal tibial varus deformity in an otherwise healthy child or adolescent was termed osteochondrosis deformans tibiae by Blount and tibia vara by Langenskiöld. Tibia vara (infantile or adolescent) is commonly used in the literature, while some authors prefer to refer to both forms as "Blount's disease."

Classification

Separation of Blount's disease into two distinct forms, infantile and adolescent, is generally accepted. The infantile form typically onsets as an evolution or persistence of physiologic varus, with (usually) progressive clinical and radiographic deformity. The Langenskiöld classification of infantile Blount's is frequently cited (Fig. 34.1). He described six presumably progressive radiographic stages, the mildest form characterized by mild medial epiphyseal and physeal irregularity, with progressively severe distortion, culminating in Stage VI. Stage VI is characterized by complete medial physeal arrest.

Lamont et al. modified the Langenskiöld classification into a 3-stage classification: Type A has a partially lucent medial metaphyseal defect, with or without "beaking"; Type B has a downward sloping curvature of the lateral and inferior rim of a completely lucent metaphyseal defect, which then has an upslope at the medial rim, resembling a ski-jump, with no epiphyseal downward slope; Type C has vertical, downsloping deformity of both the epiphysis and metaphysis, with no upward curvature projecting medially at the inferior extent, while the epiphysis slopes downward into the metaphyseal defect. Patients with Type C deformity have a poor prognosis for successful correction by high tibial osteotomy alone or in combination with an epiphysiolysis. The utility of this classification for predicting success of growth modulation of infantile Blount's disease has not yet been established [4].

Adolescent Blount's disease (Fig. 34.2a) is characterized by later onset, with more subtle physeal and much less epiphyseal distortion. Interestingly, there are neither radiographic classifications nor descriptions of the natural history of adolescent Blount's disease during remaining growth: steady progression of varus deformity once onset during the remainder of growth is assumed.

There is some controversy as to the existence of an intermediate form of Blount's disease (called "juvenile" by Thompson) [5, 6]. This form is characterized as intermediate

D. A. Podeszwa (✉) · J. G. Birch
Department of Orthopedics, Scottish Rite for Children, Dallas, TX, USA
e-mail: david.podeszwa@tsrh.org; john.birch@tsrh.org

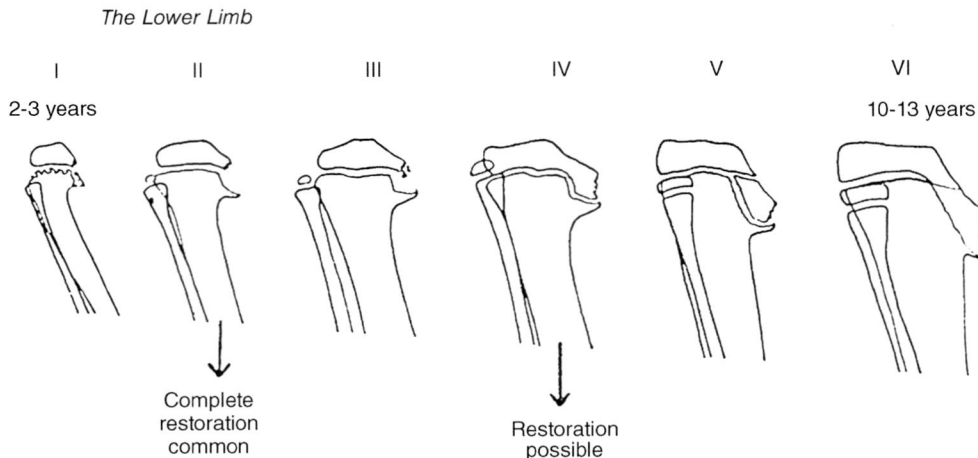

Fig. 34.1 Langenskiöld radiographic classification of infantile Blount's disease. Langenskiöld described six presumably progressive radiographic stages of deformity in infantile Blount's disease. Stage I is often difficult to distinguish from persistent physiologic varus. Langenskiöld noted that spontaneous correction was possible despite radiographic severity as advanced as Stage IV. Stage VI is characterized by complete medial proximal tibial physeal closure (bar). (Reprinted from Langenskiöld A. Tibia vara. Acta Chir Scand 1952; 103:9, with permission from John Wiley & Sons)

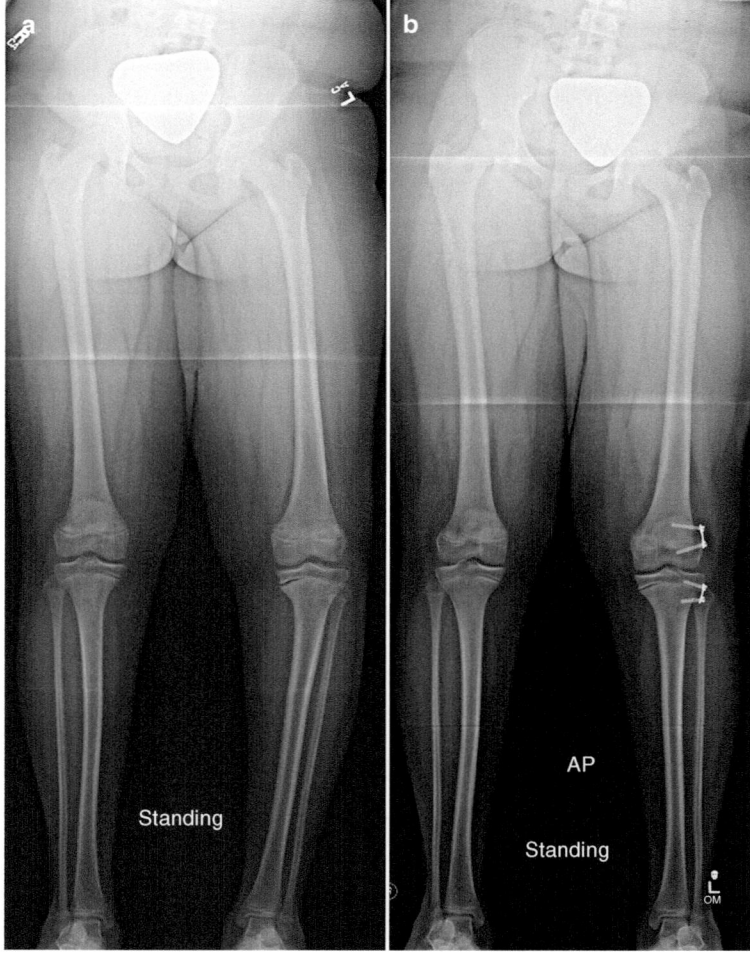

Fig. 34.2 Radiographic appearance of adolescent Blount's disease. (**a**) The characteristic radiographic features of Adolescent Blount Disease include varus deformity of the proximal tibia and medial proximal tibial physeal widening. Distal femoral varus deformity (accentuating the varus deformity) and presumably secondary distal tibial valgus deformity may be present. (**b**) Radiographic appearance after growth modulation of lateral distal femur, lateral proximal tibia, and proximal fibular epiphysiodesis. Note the residual leg length inequality

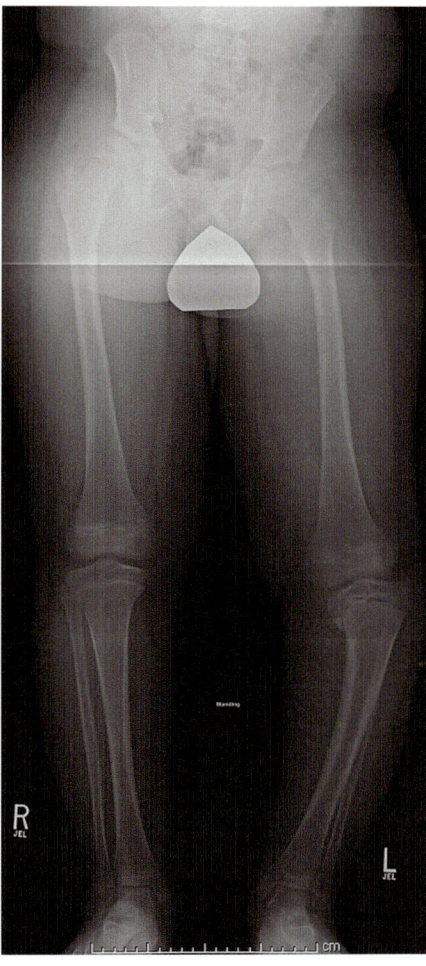

Fig. 34.3 Nine-year-old boy presenting with progressive varus deformity of the left tibia. Note the "intermediate" nature of the patient by presenting age and radiographic epiphyseal/metaphyseal distortion (between "infantile" and "adolescent" Blount's disease). Note the irregularity of the entire proximal tibial physis. Some authors refer to such intermediate cases as "juvenile Blount's disease"

Differential Diagnosis

The most difficult differential diagnosis for infantile Blount's disease is the distinction between persistent physiologic varus and early infantile Blount's disease. Some authors report the efficacy of the metaphyseal–diaphyseal angle in providing this distinction [7–10]. The problem is compounded by the opportunity for true infantile Blount's disease to resolve spontaneously (as reported originally by Langenskiöld [3]) and for presumably true persistent physiologic varus to progress to infantile Blount's disease (Box 34.1).

> **Box 34.1 Differential Diagnosis of (Progressive) Varus Deformity in Children**
> - Persistent physiologic varus
> - True infantile Blount's disease (resolving or progressive)
> - Renal-metabolic disorders (vitamin D deficiency, renal osteodystrophy)
> - Vitamin D-resistant rickets (VDRR)
> - Thromocytopenia absent radius (TAR) syndrome
> - Focal fibrocartilaginous dysplasia of the proximal tibia
> - Epiphyseal dysplasias (multiple; spondyloepiphyseal; metaphyseal dysostosis)

Other disorders to consider are epiphyseal dysplasias, dwarfing syndromes, thrombocytopenia-absent-radius (TAR) syndrome, metabolic bone disease, including true vitamin D deficiency and vitamin D-resistant (hypophosphatemic) rickets, and the mimicking metaphyseal dysostoses (Schmidt and Jansen types) (Figs. 34.4 and 34.5).

in age of onset and radiographic severity of epiphyseal and physeal distortion. At best, this form is much less common than either infantile or adolescent Blount's disease. Some cases have been described as having an appearance of a "slipped proximal tibial epiphysis" with diffuse widening and irregularity of the physis and the impression of medial displacement of a relatively intact epiphysis to produce the varus deformity [6] (Fig. 34.3).

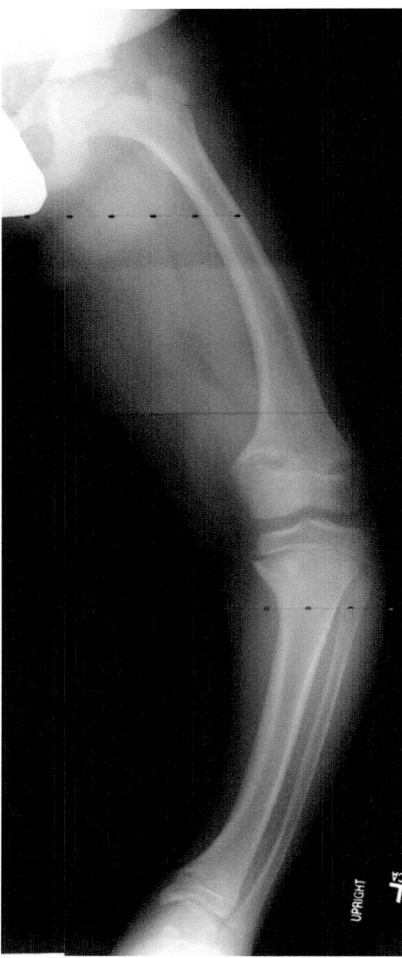

Fig. 34.4 Anteroposterior radiograph of the left lower extremity of a 13-year-old male with poorly controlled vitamin D-resistant rickets (VDRR). Note significant varus deformity of the distal femur, proximal tibia, and distal tibial as well as widening and irregularity of all physes

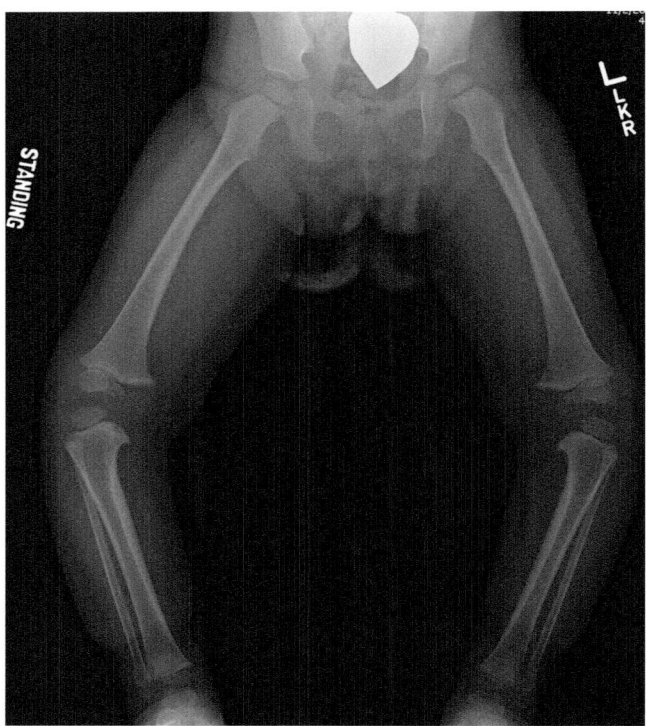

Fig. 34.5 Anteroposterior radiograph of a 3-year-old girl with thrombocytopenia-absent-radius (TAR) syndrome. Note the apparent medial proximal tibial epiphyseal defect and severe resulting varus deformity of the legs. The patient has no thumb or radius

Natural History

Langenskiöld reported that spontaneous correction can occur in infantile Blount's disease, even occasionally in advanced stages [3]. While this certainly seems to be true in milder stages, our experience has been less fortunate in later stages. Thus, the short-term natural history for infantile Blount's disease may be to progress or resolve. The long-term natural history is towards premature intra-articular pathology or early degenerative joint disease, even when angular deformity has been addressed, presumably because of the associated epiphyseal distortion [11, 12].

Interestingly, the short-term natural history of adolescent Blount's disease is not known: no documentation of radiographic changes during growth has been reported. In general, patients appear to have a more benign long-term natural history with respect to degenerative arthritis [11, 13]. However, the association of adolescent Blount's disease with morbid obesity and the recent reports of the failure of deformity correction to impact body mass index portend poorly for the general health and longevity of patients with associated obesity [14–19].

Treatment

Controversies in the Treatment of Infantile Blount's Disease

Does Bracing Work?

There are several studies that address the question of efficacy of bracing in the prevention of progression, or more importantly, the resolution of deformity in infantile Blount's disease [20–22]. Unfortunately, these studies are retrospective and lack the ability to address fundamental questions such as patient compliance with treatment protocols. Furthermore, wear protocols (day, night, or day-and-night) also vary among published studies. It is not surprising then that authors have arrived at different conclusions, that is, "bracing is effective" (in specific cases) or "bracing is ineffective". We still typically prescribe long-leg, anti-varus braces in patients who are age three or less and have radiographic Langenskiöld stage II or less infantile Blount's disease, based on our intra-institutional anecdotal and retrospective experience. We are skeptical about the efficacy of bracing in patients with bilateral infantile Blount's disease, although we may prescribe them even in such cases from time to time, if the clinical picture (e.g., family expectations, resistance to surgery, or similar scenarios) seems to warrant a trial of bracing.

Growth Modulation

Whether identifiable in the published literature or not, it is likely that any experienced pediatric surgeon approaches high tibial osteotomy with trepidation, based on some previous bitter or frightening experience with the major acute complications of that surgery, specifically, compartment syndrome, deep infection, or peroneal nerve injury (never mind skin irritation, challenging fixation/casting scenarios, and recurrent deformity). In that context, the wise surgeon always seeks a more benign treatment and will generally recommend a trial of the same, if there is any hope of effectiveness. This is the current state of temporary hemiepiphysiodesis, or "growth modulation," in infantile Blount's disease [23–27]. The concept is tantalizing: implant one of the commercially available 2-hole (or more) tension band plates, staples, or staple-like implants on the proximal lateral tibia spanning the physis, for the purpose of temporarily tethering growth in that area, thereby avoiding the significant complication risks associated with high tibial and fibular osteotomy, hoping to effect gradual correction of deformity with further growth.

Peer-reviewed data confirming the efficacy of such treatment are currently limited, but relatively favorable. Scott et al. [25] reported 89% success rate in 18 affected limbs. Danino et al. analyzed 55 limbs in 45 patients in three groups, infantile (11 limbs), juvenile (12 limbs), and adolescent (32 limbs) [28]. At final follow-up (average 24.5 months), the normalization of the mechanical medial proximal tibial angle (mMPTA 85°–90°) for the infantile, juvenile, and adolescent groups was 63.6%, 66.7%, and 87.5%, respectively. For the entire study group, the average rate of correction was 1° per month. Complications included three limbs (5.5%) with growth plate closure and two with a broken cannulated screw. The likelihood of recurrence of deformity after correction and removal of a growth modulation device in infantile tibia vara is not clear. Leveille et al. reviewed a cohort of 67 limbs in 45 patients with heterogeneous diagnoses, including 10 limbs of varying age with Blount's disease [29]. Of all diagnoses, Blount's disease had the lowest mean rebound in the hip–knee–ankle angle (HKA). The patients with the highest risk of rebound overall were those undergoing growth modulation at a young age (girls <10 years, boys < than 12 years) and those with initial HKA >20°. However, rebound did not occur in all patients and overcorrection only into a clinically acceptable alignment should be considered. More esoteric questions such as lateral tether due to perichondral ring damage by disruption of appositional epiphyseal/physeal growth by the implant in the very young patient or by direct surgical injury, indications for concomitant epiphysiodesis of the relatively overgrown fibula, or management of the often-associated internal tibial torsion and proximal tibial flexion deformities (Fig. 34.6) remain to be clarified in the era of growth modulation. It is clear that such devices, particularly but not exclusively cannulated titanium screws, are at risk for fracture [25]. At a minimum, solid, stainless steel screw devices are preferred for growth modulation in Blount's disease. The use of more robust "H" or similar 4 hole plates is at the surgeon's discretion, but we typically reserve them for morbidly obese patients with severe deformity and less than 2 years of growth remaining. The surgeon and family must contract to regular longitudinal follow-up to monitor growth and intervene as needed, and the family should be educated as to the possibility of implant breakage and failure of this surgical modality, even in the presence of good radiographic indications and apparently technically adequate implant insertion.

Risks of High Tibial Osteotomy and Acute Deformity Correction

High tibial (below the tibial tubercle) osteotomy of the tibia with concomitant osteotomy of the fibula to "overcorrect" the varus deformity is the presumptive "gold standard" management of infantile Blount's disease [30–33]. Typically, the

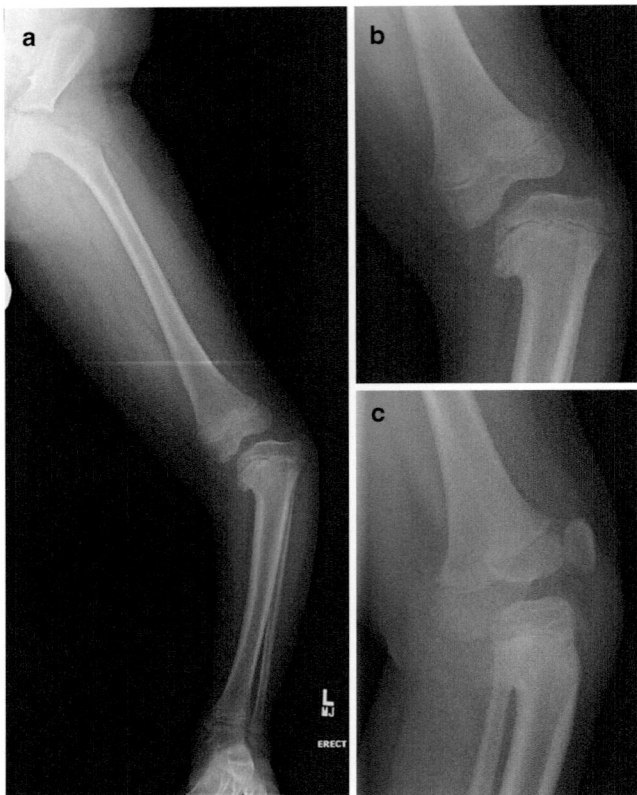

Fig. 34.6 Radiographic appearance of infantile Blount's disease. (**a**) Radiographic appearance of left lower extremity. Note the epiphyseal distortion and varus deformity of the proximal tibia, and mild compensatory valgus deformity of the distal femur and distal tibia. (**b**) Radiographic appearance of the left knee, same patient. (**c**) Lateral radiograph of the knee. Note the procurvatum deformity of the proximal tibia, and the rotational deformity of the limb

distal fragment is externally rotated as well (Fig. 34.7a, b). This operation has serious risks, the most important of which are compartment syndrome and direct or indirect injury to the peroneal nerve from manipulation, traction, or entrapment within fascial planes during manipulation of the fragments (Fig. 34.8). Soft tissue irritation, deep infection, and recurrent deformity are also not inconsequential risks. There are several important considerations the surgeon must assess before proceeding:

1. Is the physis still "open" medially, i.e., is the extent of medial physeal involvement less than Langenskiöld stage VI? If the patient has progressed to Langenskiöld stage VI, recurrent deformity is inevitable, and an alternative or adjunct procedure (e.g., completion of epiphysiodesis effect and management of limb length inequality) selected.
2. What is the current leg length discrepancy, and what's the plan to manage it?
3. What are the concomitant deformities, where are they, and how severe are they? Typically, concomitant deformities include distal femoral valgus (variable), proximal tibial "procurvatum" (flexion deformity), and internal tibial torsion. Typically, all of these should be addressed by at least full correction (some argue for "overcorrection" in the skeletally mature patient) to unload the medial proximal tibial epiphyseal load-bearing [33].

The surgeon has to decide on the geometry and type of osteotomy: opening wedge, closing wedge, and oblique osteotomies have all be described [30–33]. In contradistinction to adolescent Blount's, there has been no argument for leaving the fibula intact, presumably because the magnitude of deformity, the desire to overcorrect the varus (coronal plane) deformity, and the need to externally rotate the distal fragment more or less mandate that the fibula be divided to allow full correction. Next to be decided is fixation: cast only, cast and (one or two pins), and external fixation have all been used. Finally, should prophylactic anterior compartment fasciotomy be performed? Some authors support performing a limited anterior compartment fasciotomy in conjunction with tibial osteotomy, while others make no recommendation [30–33]. At a minimum, careful and continuous evaluation of the patient for the presence of compartment syndrome (untoward pain despite adequate release of constrictive splints or casts, or inability to dorsiflex the foot) is essential. In our experience, partial prophylactic anterior compartment fasciotomy neither absolutely protects against the development of compartment syndrome, nor is it an entirely innocuous procedure: patients may complain of muscle herniation, discomfort, weakness, or suffer cutaneous nerve injury. The surgeon must carefully weigh his or her strategy in the context of these risks.

Effectiveness of Physeal Arrest Resection

Studies have demonstrated that at least in some cases of infantile Blount's disease, medial proximal tibial physeal growth may be restored by a variation of Langenskiöld's physeal arrest resection surgery [34, 35], often combined with high (below the physis) osteotomy. Manchanda et al. reported a series of 40 cases (26 females average age 7.2, 14 males average age 7.9) of Blount's disease that underwent isolated physeal arrest resection [36]. 14 (35%) demonstrated continued growth for at least 2 years postoperatively, while an additional 5 (12.5%) demonstrating growth for at least 6 months but less than 2 years. Of those 19 cases, only one continued to grow until skeletal maturity. 15 (79%) of those with continued growth and all resection failures (21

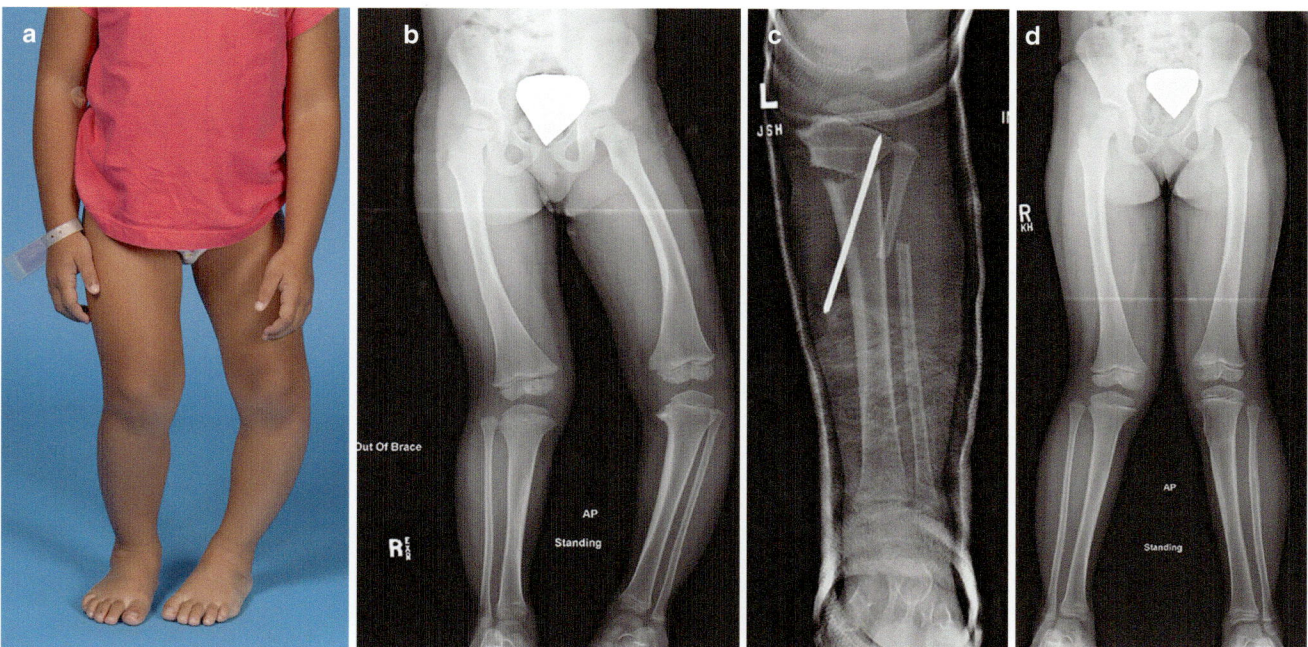

Fig. 34.7 Three-year-old girl with progressive infantile Blount's disease of the left leg, Langenskiöld stage III, who failed conservative treatment with an anti-varus brace. (**a**) Preoperative clinical appearance. (**b**) Preoperative radiographic appearance. (**c**) Postoperative radiographic appearance. Note the lateral translation of the distal fragment to effect restoration of the tibial mechanical axis. The distal fragment is manipulated to correct both varus and internal rotational deformities associated with infantile Blount's disease. (**d**) Radiographic results 2 years postoperatively, age 5 years. Patient has symmetric valgus deformity, with improvement of epiphyseal distortion of the left proximal tibia

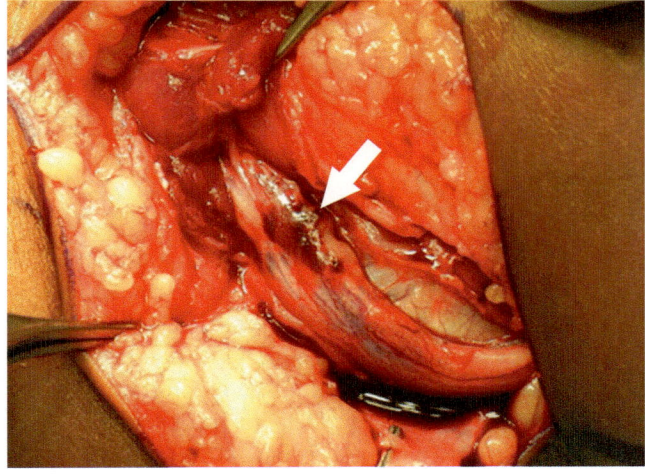

Fig. 34.8 Peroneal nerve compression detected and released in the immediate postoperative period. The patient developed peroneal nerve palsy shortly after surgery. Her compartments were soft. At exploration, the nerve was found to be compressed under a fascial band as it passed into the deep anterior compartment. *Arrow* indicates contused peroneal nerve after release of the fascial band. Same patient as Fig. 34.7

cases) went on to at least one subsequent surgery (average 1.5–2.4 additional procedures). This procedure is neither universally accepted nor successful. Patients with Blount's disease typically have an advanced bone age [37]. The wise surgeon will assess the patient's bone age and the adage of "average" proximal tibial physeal growth of 6 mm per year in the healthy proximal tibial physis to determine if adequate growth remains to warrant an effort at this procedure. A minimum of 4 years of growth remaining would seem to be a reasonable threshold criterion for consideration of physeal bar resection as potentially indicated. Our experience is that even patients who experience resumption of growth will subsequently develop late deceleration/cessation of that growth. Embedding metallic markers or some other method of exact determination of growth persisting is important to allow prompt recognition of secondary cessation of growth (Fig. 34.9a, b). Completion of the epiphysiodesis at that time can save the patient from the development of recurrent deformity requiring an additional osteotomy and appropriate management of any associated leg length inequality.

Utility of Physeal Arrest Resection Surgery in the Absence of a Bony Physeal Arrest

Andrade and Johnston [38] have recommended "physeal bar resection" surgery in patients with advanced infantile Blount's disease, but at Langenskiöld stage less than VI, i.e.,

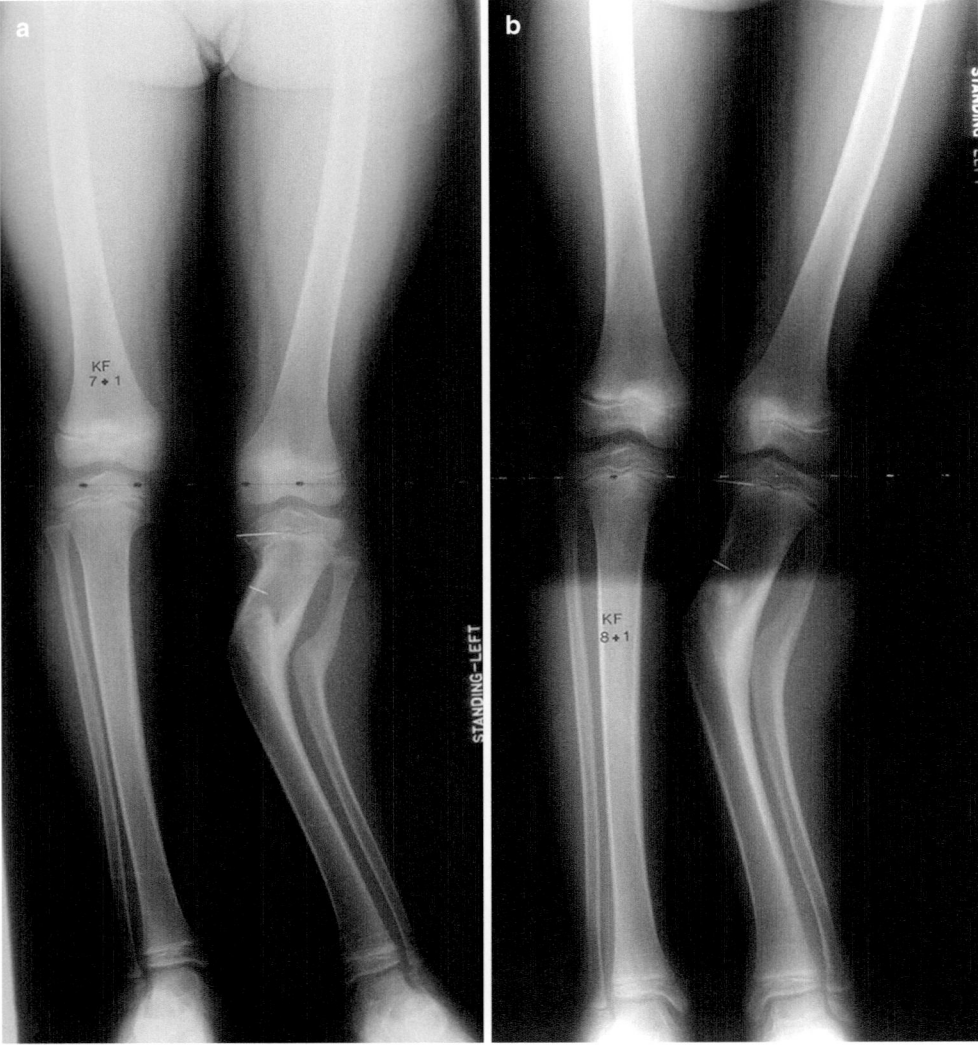

Fig. 34.9 This 6-year, 9-month old girl underwent third-time repeat height tibial osteotomy, combined with partial physeal bar excision for recurrent infantile Blount's disease of the left tibia. (**a**) Four months postoperatively, the patient has persistent iatrogenic valgus deformity at the osteotomy site. Note the metallic markers in the proximal medial tibial epiphysis and metaphysis. (**b**) Sixteen months postoperatively (1 year after radiograph in part **a**), the patient has persistent valgus deformity. The markers have been separated by approximately 20 mm

without demonstrable frank physeal bony bar formation on advanced imaging. They report good (>80% successful in preventing recurrence of varus deformity, in patients less than 7 years of age) results, but there is not a comparable group treated by high tibial osteotomy alone to confirm the relative efficacy of this procedure.

What to Do with the "Failed" Case?

Usually, the surgeon is faced with many things to consider, when the patient has undergone previous high tibial osteotomy with recurrent deformity. These include: the extent of lower extremity scarring, recurrent (potentially complex) deformity, including variable amount of varus, procurvatum, and internal tibial torsion, leg length inequality in unilateral cases, and potential continued asymmetric growth in the skeletally immature patient (both within the tibia due to the medial arrest, and between the affected and unaffected legs).

There can be no "cookbook" strategy in such cases (Fig. 34.10). The surgeon must individualize the correction plan with careful consideration of all these parameters in the development of a treatment strategy suitable and acceptable to the family and their circumstances. External fixation, with either acute or gradual correction, provides the surgeon with an excellent tool to manage all of these deformities during one treatment stage, if acceptable to the patient and family.

The surgeon must always keep in mind the fact that patients with infantile Blount's disease may have premature or "atraumatic" meniscal tears or other degenerative changes, even in the presence of presumably adequate angular and rotational deformity correction [10, 39]. This risk is presumably the result from the epiphyseal distortion that is unique to infantile Blount's disease and which distinguishes it from adolescent Blount's disease. Thus, if the patient has significant intra-articular complaints or abnormalities on physical examination, appropriate pursuit of the potential for these structural abnormalities (MRI or arthroscopy) should be carried out.

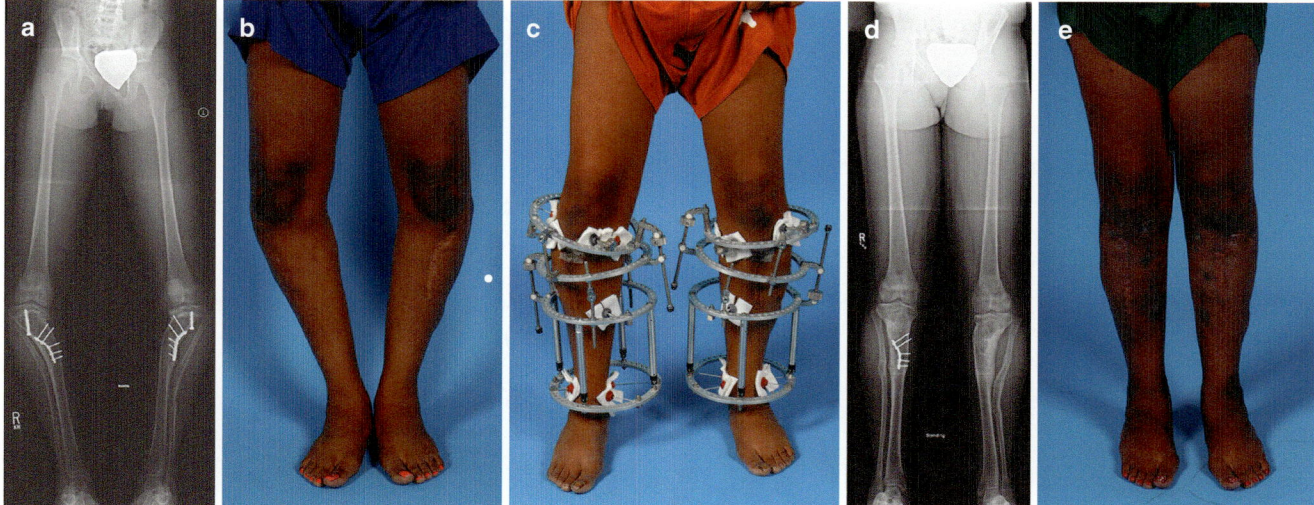

Fig. 34.10 Patient with failed previous treatment of infantile Blount's disease. (**a**) Radiographic appearance. The patient has had several prior surgical procedures, including high tibial osteotomies and attempted lateral proximal tibial physeal arrest with retained implants, recurrent varus deformity, and postsurgical proximal metaphyseal valgus deformity. Note the medial translation of the patient's mechanical axis caused by a failure to lateralize the distal fragment in conjunction with the previous valgus-producing osteotomy. (**b**) Clinical appearance. (**c**) Clinical appearance during staged treatment. The patient was managed by staged surgical procedures, including (partial) implant removal and two-level osteotomies of the tibiae with gradual correction of the varus and valgus deformities using a circular external fixator. (**d**) Final postoperative radiographic appearance. (**e**) Final clinical appearance

Is There a Role of "Hemi-Plateau Elevation"?

Radiographs in the advanced stage of infantile Blount's leave the observer with the distinct impression of a "sagging" or "depressed" medial tibial plateau. This perception (or reality) has led a number of authors to describe "hemi-plateau elevation" [40–42] (in effect, an intra-articular fracture with restoration of the transverse condylar relationships [unless the surgeon is fortunate enough to effect cartilaginous deformation of the articular surface without fracture]). It should be noted that some other authors dispute at least the universal presence of a true depression of the medial plateau and confirmed the presence of a cartilaginous medial tibial plateau by knee arthrogram [43], or more recently, MRI [39, 44]. The procedure of hemi-plateau elevation has been described in isolation or in conjunction with a second osteotomy of the tibia to correct coexisting varus deformity. Maré et al. reported excellent outcomes (1°–11° residual valgus) in 51% and good outcomes (<9° residual varus) in 24% of 64 limbs undergoing medial plateau elevation with concomitant proximal tibial epiphysiodesis [45]. The poor outcomes were those with significant residual varus (20%) or valgus (5%). Fifty (78%) underwent simultaneous dome osteotomy below the tibial tubercle to correct residual varus, procurvatum, and internal rotation after the plateau elevation. In spite of the concomitant epiphysiodesis, 19% of the deformities recurred. Similar procedures, including medial plateau elevation with concomitant dome osteotomy proximal to the tubercle and medial plateau with a lateral shortening closing wedge osteotomy, have been described with comparable outcomes [46, 47]. We have not, in our institutional experience, used these procedures to manage even the most severe cases of infantile Blount's disease (Box 34.2).

> **Box 34.2 Controversies in Infantile Blount's Disease**
> - Etiology, including obesity
> - Differentiation between persistent physiologic varus and true infantile Blount's disease
> - Efficacy of lower extremity bracing
> - Efficacy, timing, and time-to-removal of growth modulation plates for surgical correction

Adolescent Blount's Disease

While adolescent Blount's disease was described by both Langenskiöld and Blount in their original series, side by side with infantile Blount's disease, it is clear that adolescent Blount's disease is a completely distinct disorder. Not only do infantile and adolescent Blount's diseases affect an entirely different age group, the radiographic features, nature and location of concomitant ipsilateral limb deformities, incidence of intra-articular abnormalities, and published long-term premature degenerative arthritis prevalence are all distinctly different as well [10, 12, 13]. Furthermore, while obesity seems to be a risk factor for both conditions, obesity seems to be more specifically related to adolescent Blount's disease [14–17, 19].

> **Box 34.3 Controversies in Adolescent Blount's Disease**
> - Etiology, including obesity
> - Role of growth modulation in surgical armamentarium
> - Indications for correction of associated deformities (distal femoral varus, distal tibial valgus)
> - Gradual versus acute correction by high tibial osteotomy, with or without external fixation

No specific useful radiographic classification exists for adolescent Blount's disease, either for morphological characterization or prognostic purposes. The "classic" deformity consists of proximal tibial varus deformity of the affected extremity with a medial proximal tibial physeal widening or "zone of injury" on radiographs (see Fig. 34.2). Biopsy specimens from this area of radiographic physeal lucency show disorganized microscopic physeal architecture and/or replacement of normal physis by fibrous tissue. It is assumed that some patient risk factors (familial, persistent mild physiologic varus, subclinical metabolic abnormality) with or without obesity results increased compressive forces across the physis with disruption of normal function and deceleration of growth [5, 48, 49]. There are no short-term natural history reports to confirm the presumption of progressive worsening varus deformity or radiographic abnormality in untreated patients during the remainder of growth. Setting aside general health issues related to obesity, with or without persistent varus deformity of the leg, published reports suggest a more benign natural history with respect to degenerative arthritis of the knee in patients with adolescent Blount's disease compared to infantile Blount's disease [10, 12, 13].

Treatment Considerations in Adolescent Blount's Disease

Role of Obesity and Impact of Treatment on Obesity

It is well recognized that obesity in the general population is increasing and represents a significant health problem. Sadly, that increased incidence is extending into the adolescent and now pediatric population [15–17, 50–52] with significant implications for long-term health consequences. It has been long noted that patients with adolescent Blount's disease are frequently (but not universally) obese or morbidly obese, and obesity, rightly or wrongly, is considered a risk factor for the development of adolescent Blount's disease. Interestingly, there are no reliable population surveys that confirm an increased incidence of adolescent Blount's disease in association with the increased prevalence of adolescent obesity in the general population. Soberingly, Sabharwal et al. [18] have noted that correction of angular deformity (both of infantile and adolescent Blount's disease) is NOT associated with subsequent reduction in BMI in their study population, thus calling into question the myth or circular argument that leg deformity begets pain and exercise intolerance, with the implicit expectation of surgeon and patient that deformity correction will result in increased physical activity and subsequent weight reduction (Fig. 34.11). This calls into ques-

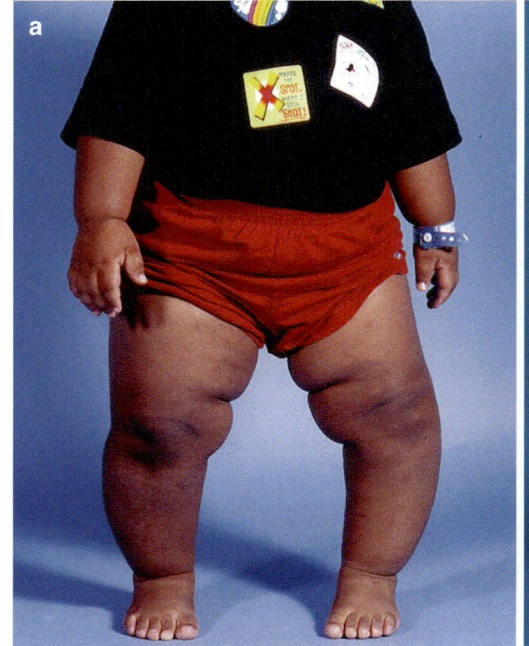 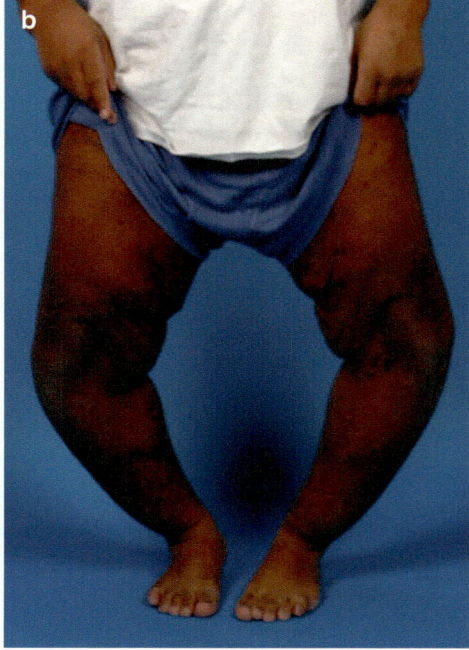

Fig. 34.11 Recurrent infantile Blount's disease in an obese child. (**a**) At age 8, this patient had progressive, recurrent infantile Blount's disease associated with obesity. (**b**) At age 15, the patient's deformities have recurred after high tibial osteotomy, but through a self-directed program of diet and exercise, the patient lost weight despite the leg deformities, and at this time, weighs less than he did at age 8

tion what our responsibility as surgeons should be: while we console ourselves that deformity correction will open the door to a healthier lifestyle and thus represents a noble pursuit on behalf of the patient, it warrants tolerance of myriad increased challenges and complications associated with performing angular deformity correction in patients with morbid obesity (anesthesia risks, sleep apnea, wound complications, deep infection, fixation challenges, and greater difficulty affecting complete deformity correction). Furthermore, there is no clear evidence that correcting angular deformity associated with Blount's disease increases the longevity of the knee in affected extremities. Thus, as patient health advocates, we must seriously question the merit of surgical treatment for adolescent Blount's disease until an effective weight management program has been embraced by the patient.

In the overall picture, probably the most important associated abnormality in patients with adolescent Blount's disease is morbid obesity, because not only is it a threat to the patient's overall health, its presence results in specific potential for sleep apnea, type II diabetes, and increased risks of delayed wound healing, deep infection, and myriad soft tissue challenges in the perioperative period. In addition, patients with obesity will mask significant varus deformity (indeed, the "fat-thigh syndrome" as described by Davids [53] is a potential cause of adolescent Blount's: the need to stand with the legs separated to accommodate fat thighs results in the skeletally immature secondary adaption of medialization of the lower leg to bring the feet closer to the midline) (Fig. 34.12). One of the consequences is that "full" correction of the varus deformity will typically make the patient appear to have valgus deformity (Fig. 34.13), which is usually cosmetically displeasing to the family/patient. This puts the surgeon in a vexing situation of either inadvertently or deliberately undercorrecting varus deformity, or justifying the production of deformity in the patient's perception. There is no easy answer here, but we usually prefer to correct the deformity anatomically (as best we can), explaining the outcome and its rationale in advance and in the (perhaps unlikely) hopes that the patient will lose weight in the future. The surgeon should educate the patient and the family regarding the presence of associated deformities and be prepared to address them, should the need arise.

Associated Deformities

In contradistinction to infantile Blount's disease, ipsilateral deformities of the distal femur and distal tibia are frequent (see Figs. 34.2a and 34.13) [54–57]. Interestingly, the most common associated deformity of the distal femur is an accentuating varus, seen in patients of all ages with Blount's disease [58]. In some cases of infantile Blount's disease and

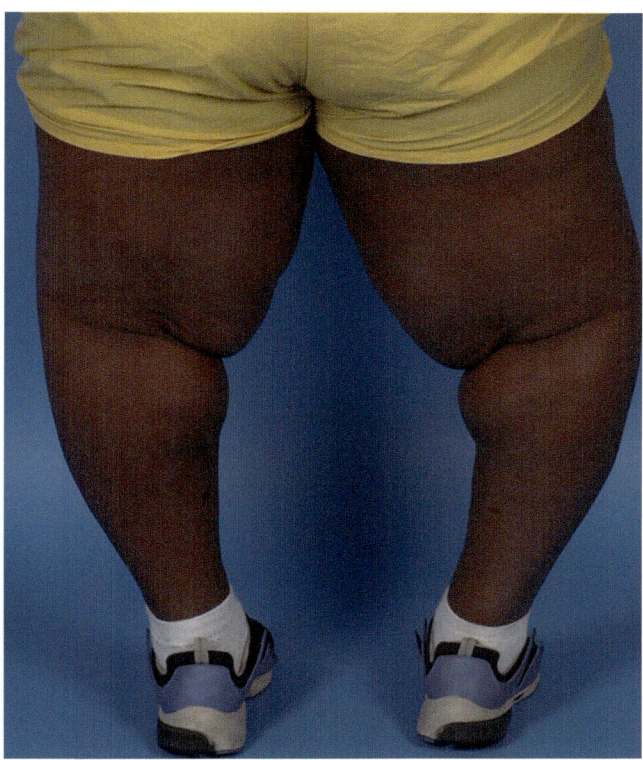

Fig. 34.12 Patient with adolescent Blount's disease and morbid obesity. The "fat thighs" require the patient to stand with the legs relatively abducted. Some conjecture that this posture in an adolescent may be the cause of adolescent Blount's disease, at least in some patients

many traumatic physeal growth disturbances, a partial compensating reverse deformity at the adjacent femoral physes may develop. This suggests a more global etiology (rather than simple deceleration of growth of the medial proximal tibial physes) or unrecognized endocrinopathy as the underlying cause or at least accelerant of adolescent Blount's disease.

Along those lines, interestingly, several patients we have treated have developed a contralateral valgus deformity (i.e., "windswept" appearance) during the course of treatment for presumptive adolescent Blount's disease (Fig. 34.14), in the absence of an identifiable metabolic disorder or endocrinopathy. This too would suggest a systemic component to the etiology of adolescent tibia vara, at least in some patients.

Distal tibial valgus (which would seem to be a more intuitively logical consequence of proximal varus deformity) is often noted in patients with adolescent Blount's disease. "Comprehensive correction" strategies [54] describe surgical correction of this deformity. However, it has been our experience that patients rarely complain of ankle pain or deformity and only rarely has primary or secondary correction of this deformity been necessary in our patient population.

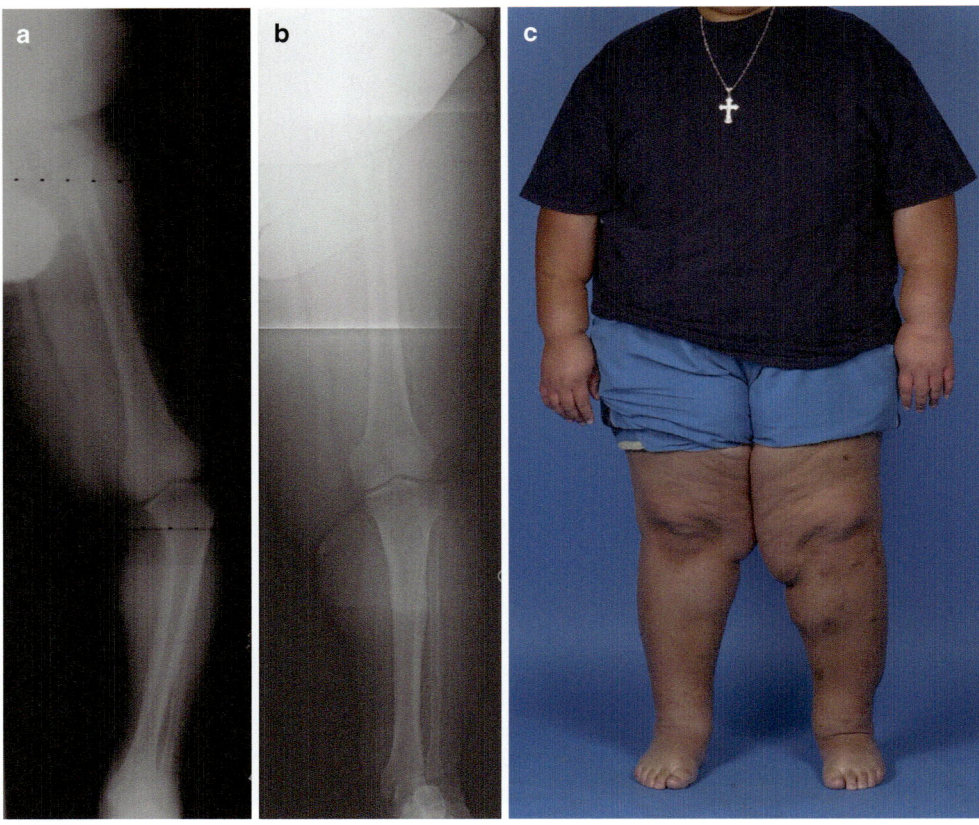

Fig. 34.13 Apparent valgus "deformity" after correction of adolescent Blount's disease varus deformity in the left leg of an obese patient. (**a**) Preoperative radiographic appearance. (**b**) Postoperative radiographic appearance. Note the incomplete correction of the varus deformity. (**c**) Postoperative clinical appearance. Note that despite incomplete correction of the varus deformity radiographically, the patient appears to have valgus deformity clinically

Finally, similarly to infantile Blount's disease, patients will usually be noted to have an internal tibial torsional deformity on clinical examination, and on careful radiographic assessment, "procurvatum" (flexion deformity) of the proximal tibia [57]. The severity of these deformities must be taken into consideration in determining the best surgical treatment strategy for individual patients.

Growth Modulation

Open hemiepiphysiodesis of the lateral proximal tibia, with or without concomitant epiphysiodesis of the proximal fibula and/or lateral femur, was the first described method of "growth modulation" of this deformity [59]. It is interesting to note that in at least some cases, this procedure is effective despite the persistence of presumed "causative roles" of deformity and obesity in the disruption/deceleration of normal medial proximal tibial physeal growth. Considering this procedure with acceptance of an uncertain outcome is almost universally motivated by the challenges and risks created by osteotomy, particularly in the obese patient. Open hemiepiphysiodesis has been replaced by staple, tension band plate, or percutaneous transphyseal screw (PETS) growth modulation methods [26, 60–63] (see Fig. 34.2b). Enthusiasm for the original "8" plate (titanium cannulated screws and 2-hole plate) has waned in favor of stronger non-cannulated stainless steel screws, and/or more robust "H" or similar plates (i.e., two screws on either side of the physis) due to reports of screw fracture with the original device [23, 24], an event which seems to be nearly unique to the metaphyseal screws in Blount's patients (particularly adolescent type). Reported rates of successful restoration of the mechanical axis and/or the mMPTA range from 34 to 87.5% [28, 64, 65]. In a series of 64 limbs in 45 patients with the majority having moderate to severe deformity, McIntosh et al. identified age >14, BMI ≥45 kg/m^2, and a mMPTA <76° as significant risk factors for failure of correction. PETS, as described by Metaizeau, has become increasingly popular, with its perceived advantages of a smaller incision, lower risk of hematoma, and minimal postoperative activity limitation [64]. Murphy et al. analyzed 14 limbs in 9 patients (average age 10.4 years) and demonstrated a significant improvement in the average MAD and mMPTA with no implant failure, need for revision surgery, or subsequent corrective osteotomy [62]. Braga et al. followed 20 limbs in 13 patients for an average of 65 months and, similarly, reported a significant improvement in MAD and mMPTA. However, they also reported rebound in 2 limbs after screw removal and 2 other limbs that required corrective osteotomy [63]. Both the surgeon and patient must accept that even apparently technically adequate implant placement and retention do not

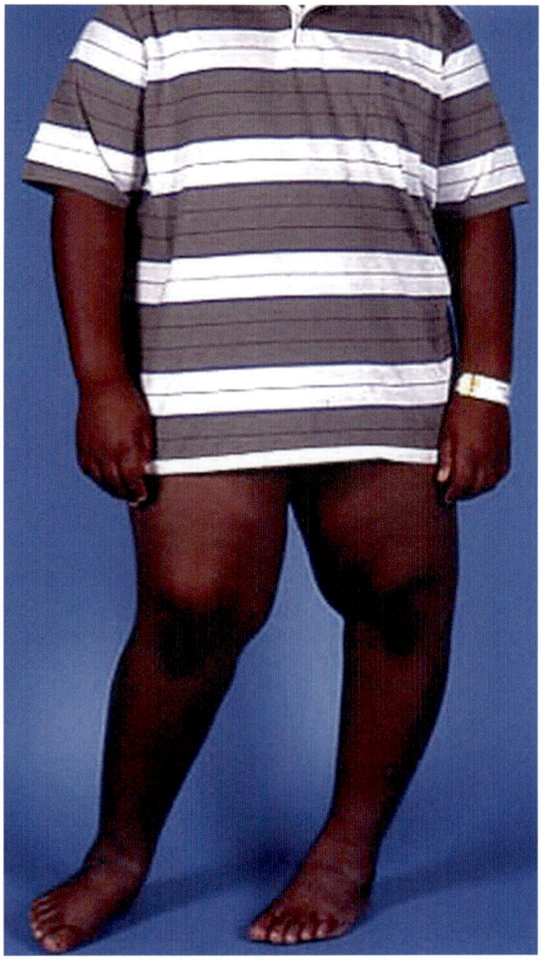

Fig. 34.14 Apparently healthy adolescent with left-sided varus deformity typical of adolescent Blount's disease developed apparently idiopathic contralateral valgus deformity ("windswept" deformity). There was no identifiable endocrine or skeletal dysplasia abnormality in this patient

guarantee effective correction of the angular deformity. For this reason, and for the happy possibility of correction prior to skeletal maturity, both the patient and surgeon must commit to regular longitudinal follow-up to prevent overcorrection and manage failure to correct appropriately.

Acute Correction with Internal Fixation

High tibial osteotomy (either above or below the tibial tubercle, at the surgeon's preference, because the patient is nearly skeletally mature) can be opening wedge, closing wedge, or a combination at surgeon's preference. Due to the average patient's age, size, weight, and body habitus, rarely are pin fixation and cast immobilization practical or effective. The surgeon is therefore left with the decision of internal fixation or external fixation, the latter of course then subjecting all to the inconvenience, pin care, and increased soft tissue irritation of such patients. Internal fixation is typically of some plate device. Some authors have noted that fibular osteotomy is not necessary if modest opening-wedge correction strategy is used [66].

The patient is at risk for wound dehiscence, deep wound infection, delayed union, nonunion, implant failure, compartment syndrome, inadequate correction, and the inability to adjust correction postoperatively (without revision surgery); some of these complications are inherent to tibial osteotomy and the patient's body habitus, and some are risks associated with acute correction and internal fixation strategy: the surgeon and patient should be cognizant of these risks and deem them acceptable in context. We reserve acute correction for patients with less than 15° of proximal tibial deformity coronal plane deformity, minimal proximal tibial procurvatum deformity, and a leg length and rotational profile that is acceptable to the patient and family, as neither is corrected as part of the procedure.

Correction with External Fixation (Acute or Gradual) (with 6-Strut Fixators/Others)

Gradual correction of adolescent tibia vara [66–75] offers several theoretical and practical advantages: there is presumably a lower risk of compartment syndrome and deep infection, greater deformities can be addressed more precisely, lengthening can be achieved, it is easier by fragment translation to effect a truly anatomic restoration of limb alignment, and the complex deformity (with procurvatum, internal tibial torsion, with or without shortening) can be addressed, either acutely, gradually, or sequentially. For smaller deformities with minimal lengthening required, the fibula may remain intact and unfixed (at least proximally). Six-strut (hexapod) frames are particularly valuable for this deformity, although traditional circular fixators or monolateral fixators are preferred by some authors.

The flexibility of external fixation devices and strategy, however, have to be weighed against the generally more prolonged postoperative recovery and management of the device and the patient in the device, particularly with the increased soft tissue irritation in this specific patient population [75].

Adolescent Blount's Disease Summary

Patients with adolescent Blount's represent a significant challenge to the clinician because of the complex nature of the deformity itself, the frequent coexistence of other ipsilateral deformities, and the frequent occurrence of large size and/or obesity. The surgeon must carefully assess the overall health status, commitment and expectations of the patient, the presence and severity of concomitant deformities, and existing and projected leg length inequality before adopting a well-reasoned treatment strategy for the patient. Epiphysiodesis, growth modulation, acute correction with internal or external fixation, and gradual correction with external fixation are options that may in any combination represent excellent strategy in individual cases.

Does Juvenile Blount's Disease Exist?

Some authors [5, 6] noted a third, intermediate type of Blount's disease, intermediate in time of onset (between infancy and adolescence) and radiographic deformity (having less epiphyseal distortion typical of infantile Blount's, but more extensive physeal changes than seen in classical adolescent Blount's). We have a few cases which fit this description, and some which do not neatly fit either "traditional" category, and thus it is believed that this is a separate entity. Treatment decisions, however, remain the same as for either condition, except that conservative treatment (observation or bracing) would seem to be unhelpful modalities. There are no reports or personal experience with growth modulation strategies in such patients to our knowledge.

Summary

Infantile and adolescent Blount's diseases must be considered separate and distinct entities, occurring in a dissimilar patient population, at different ages, with entirely different radiographic features, concomitant deformities, and likely natural history. What they share are a lack of our understanding as to their etiology and (presumably) progressive, complex varus deformity of the tibia, which challenge the surgeon to create an effective treatment plan. Gradual correction of these deformities by growth modulation or by osteotomy and external fixation, with or without lengthening, is an important and valuable surgical correction technique that should be in the surgeon's armamentarium. Many aspects of infantile and adolescent Blount's disease warrant attention by further research, including identification of their etiologies, favorably influencing childhood obesity, unequivocally determining the effectiveness of bracing in the infantile form, developing an effective growth modulation method of correcting the associated internal tibial torsional deformity, and determining an appropriate threshold for correcting concomitant deformities of the distal femur and distal tibia.

Commentary

Controversies in Blount's Disease

R. E. Christopher Rose

The exact cause of Blount's Disease is still unknown. What we do know is that compressive forces inhibit growth, and that the growth inhibition can result in varying degrees of retardation of growth at the proximal medial tibial plateau. What is also known is that the growth plate is "sick", not "dead". The Langenskiold Classification of Blount's Disease continues to be widely used despite significant interobserver variability. There are two clinically and radiologically distinct types of Blount's Disease—Infantile and Adolescent. Full-length anteroposterior radiograph of both lower limbs with patellae facing forwards is the workhorse imaging modality. It allows a complete frontal plane analysis of the limb deformities.

The treatment instituted must be individualized, and it depends on the age, the degree of deformity or deformities, limb length discrepancies, and where in the world the surgeon resides and practices. Since the end point of treatment is when the child reaches skeletal maturity, it is important that the surgical procedures embarked upon result in normal limb alignment, normal joint orientation, and equal limb lengths at skeletal maturity.

There are many reasons for the controversies in Blount's Disease, and the following are but a few:

- Unpredictability as to when the medial physis would close.
- We still do not know what causes the unhealthy medial physis.

- No agreement as to whether the mechanical axis should be normalized or placed in slight valgus and the degree of valgus at the time of surgical correction.
- Accurate acute realignment of the mechanical axis on the operating table may not be possible in patients with ligamentous laxity.
- Accurate postoperative alignment is difficult due to the bulky frame, the tendency of the operated limb to be held in external rotation, and slight knee flexion.
- No consensus as to whether medial hemi-plateau elevation is necessary.
- No long-term studies comparing the onset and severity of symptoms of osteoarthritis in the Black population who had received surgical treatment for Blount's, versus an untreated group, versus a group without Blount's.
- More attention should be paid to the valgus deformity of the ankle and the plano valgus foot in the Blount patient.

Bracing/Orthoses

In the English-speaking Caribbean where I practice, the cost of the orthosis, the compliance of the parent, who in many households is a single mother with other children to care for, and the effectiveness of the orthosis in the treatment of early Infantile Blount are factors to be considered. The cost of the orthosis for many of the single mothers is prohibitive; there is usually poor compliance, and to date there is no conclusive evidence that bracing works. The reported successes of bracing may have been in some cases of physiological bow legs.

Bracing/orthosis is not routinely used for managing a child with Blount's disease in my practice, and a similar approach is used by other colleagues in the English-Speaking Caribbean.

Guided Growth

Temporary hemiepiphysiodesis by tension band plating has for some time been the accepted treatment of choice for coronal deformities around the knee in children with Infantile Blount's, who have at least 2 years of growth remaining in the proximal medial tibial physis, a limb length discrepancy not greater than 1 cm, and a Body Mass Index (BMI) of less than 40.

The use of staples has been largely abandoned due to the early "backing out" of the staples. Although the guided growth plate is available to us, and is used, in some cases a simple proximal tibial osteotomy alone is performed between the ages of 3 and 4 years. The osteotomy corrects the varus angulation, the internal tibial torsion, and off-loads the medial compartment immediately. Temporary hemiepiphysiodesis by tension band plating is a simple and relatively safe procedure, but it is not without risks. However, tension band plating does not always fully correct internal tibial torsion.

In our setting, the increased the risk of implant failure in the obese child, the lack of compliance with follow-up, and the cost of the guided growth implants, make the osteotomy the preferred treatment in my current practice.

There is no consensus as to the timing for removal of the guided growth plate once full correction has been achieved. Some authors advocate removal of the metaphyseal screw, while maintaining the plate and the epiphyseal screw, thus allowing reinsertion of another metaphyseal screw in the event of recurrence. However, there is risk of development of a bony bar and growth arrest should the plate and epiphyseal screw be maintained after correction.

The incidence of recurrence is significantly reduced if surgery is performed before age 4 years. Should there be a recurrence, a medial physeal bar is suspected and investigation with either an MRI scan (no radiation) or CT scan is performed.

Acute Deformity Correction

It allows complete correction of internal tibial torsion, varus angulation, procurvatum, and restoration of the mechanical axis of the tibia in one surgical procedure. Nothing further is required of the patient, except care of the pin-sites.

There are many complications, and in some cases serious ones, following acute deformity correction for significant varus angulation and internal tibial torsion.

In our setting (Public Hospitals), the following are our challenges when gradual corrections were undertaken—inadequate supervision at home with respect to regular and correct turnings; inconsistent follow-up due to lack of funds for weekly transportation; and inability to obtain time-off from work by the parent and other time constraints of the parent.

I therefore perform acute corrections to avoid these challenges. To date, the following are my results on 20 patients with Infantile Blount's, and who were older than 6 years at the time of surgery: no compartment syndrome; one foot-drop, three cases of postoperative temporary weakness of the extensor hallucis longus; one case of skin breakdown at the proximal osteotomy site that required plastic surgery intervention; and no vascular compromises.

Complications were minimized by adhering to the following:

1. Peroneal nerve issues can be significantly reduced by making the skin incision for the fibula osteotomy at the junction of the proximal 2/3 and distal 1/3 of the fibula. The fibula is approached along its posterolateral aspect and the periosteum is reflected. Lanes retractors are positioned between the periosteum and the bone. A segment of fibula is removed. The fascia is not closed.
2. Proximal osteotomy is performed and I prefer a dome-like osteotomy, although the types of osteotomies which are utilized may not affect the outcome. What is important is to restore the mechanical axis. The correction is undertaken in the following manner—external rotation of the distal fragment, lateral translation since the osteotomy is not at the apex of deformity, and the last correction is that of the varus and procurvatum. To correct the procurvatum acutely, a small piece of bone is removed from either the anterior aspect of the proximal or distal fragment. The periosteum is elevated along the medial aspect of the tibia, and this assists in correction of the varus deformity. Temporary fixation is achieved by placing a Steinmann pin across the osteotomy site. Alignment is checked by using the bovie cord and screening from the center of the femoral head to the center of the ankle joint. Correct alignment is achieved when the bovie passes through the center of the knee. As a general rule, I do not overcorrect the mechanical axis.

To ensure that there is adequate blood flow in the limb post the acute correction, a pulse oximeter is placed on the hallux of the operated leg. Usually after 1–2 min, the readings of the pulse oximeter are normal. This is because the tibial artery can go into spasm following the acute correction. The Ilizarov frame is then applied. The fascia is never closed.

In the case of unilateral Blount's, any residual limb length discrepancy (approximately 2 cm) can easily be corrected by limb lengthening. In the case of bilateral Blount's corrections, no lengthening is usually required.

Should there be closure of the medial proximal tibial physis, a lateral hemiepiphysiodesis is performed at the time of the acute correction to prevent further angular deformity.

Is There a Role For Hemi-Plateau Medial Elevation

One of the goals of treatment of Blount's Disease is restoration of normal joint orientation at skeletal maturity. In Langenskiold Stages V and VI, there is depression of the medial tibial plateau, the full extent of which cannot be ascertained on plain radiographs.

The benefits of medial hemi-plateau elevation include immediate stability of the knee joint; reduction or elimination of medial knee pain; possible reduction in the severity of early osteoarthritis; and a technically easier total knee arthroplasty surgery, should it be needed in the future.

Either an MRI scan prior to surgery or an arthrogram at surgery should be performed to evaluate the thick unossified cartilage on the medial side and also the degree of thickness and width of the posteromedial aspect of the medial meniscus. Following elevation of the medial plateau, whether complete or not, the medial plateau is held in place with wires that are tensioned. A fibular strut is inserted to provide support to the posteromedial aspect of the medial plateau. The multiplanar deformities of the limb, if present, are then corrected via a proximal tibial osteotomy. In order to reduce the risk of recurrence, I perform a hemiepiphysiodesis of the proximal lateral tibial physis and proximal fibular physis at the time of frame removal.

Adolescent Blount's Disease

Although it is referred to as Blount's Disease, Adolescent Blount's is a distinct disorder from Infantile Blount's—physeal irregularity is less severe than the infantile type; it occurs in children older than 10 years; and affected adolescent children often have a higher Body Mass Index (BMI) with associated varus of the distal femur and proximal tibia.

With regard to the treatment of Adolescent Blount's, if the Mechanical Axis Deviation is abnormal, look for the deformities in the distal femur, proximal tibia, and the joint.

With a varus distal femur and open physis, guided growth is the treatment of choice. In case of a varus distal femur with closed physis, osteotomy of the distal femur should be performed. A multiplane deformity of the proximal tibia should be treated with a high tibial osteotomy.

Summary

There is much that we do not know and understand about Blount's Disease. The treatment of complex Blount's deformities can be very challenging. The surgeon must have in his armamentarium the knowledge to accurately perform preoperative planning, the decision-making skills to choose the appropriate surgical procedure or procedures for each individual patient, and the expertise required to achieve a successful outcome at skeletal maturity.

References

1. Erlacher P. Deformierende prozesse der epiphysengegend bei kindern. Arch Orthop Unfallchir. 1922;20:81.
2. Blount W. Tibia vara: osteochondrosis deformans tibiae. J Bone Jt Surg. 1937;29:1–29.
3. Langenskiold A. Tibia vara; (osteochondrosis deformans tibiae); a survey of 23 cases. Acta Chir Scand. 1952;103(1):1–22.
4. LaMont LE, McIntosh AL, Jo CH, Birch JG, Johnston CE. Recurrence after surgical intervention for infantile tibia vara: assessment of a new modified classification. J Pediatr Orthop. 2019;39(2):65–70.
5. Thompson GH, Carter JR, Smith CW. Late-onset tibia vara: a comparative analysis. J Pediatr Orthop. 1984;4(2):185–94.
6. Sanghrajka AP, Hill RA, Murnaghan CF, Simpson AH, Bellemore MC. Slipped upper tibial epiphysis in infantile tibia vara: three cases. J Bone Jt Surg Br. 2012;94(9):1288–91.
7. Levine AM, Drennan JC. Physiological bowing and tibia vara. The metaphyseal–diaphyseal angle in the measurement of bowleg deformities. J Bone Jt Surg Am. 1982;64(8):1158–63.
8. Auerbach JD, Radomisli TE, Simoncini J, Ulin RI. Variability of the metaphyseal–diaphyseal angle in tibia vara: a comparison of two methods. J Pediatr Orthop. 2004;24(1):75–8.
9. Davids JR, Blackhurst DW, Allen BL Jr. Radiographic evaluation of bowed legs in children. J Pediatr Orthop. 2001;21(2):257–63.
10. Feldman MD, Schoenecker PL. Use of the metaphyseal–diaphyseal angle in the evaluation of bowed legs. J Bone Jt Surg Am. 1993;75(11):1602–9.
11. Hofmann A, Jones RE, Herring JA. Blount's disease after skeletal maturity. J Bone Jt Surg Am. 1982;64(7):1004–9.
12. Ingvarsson T, Hagglund G, Ramgren B, Jonsson K, Zayer M. Long-term results after infantile Blount's disease. J Pediatr Orthop B. 1998;7(3):226–9.
13. Ingvarsson T, Hagglund G, Ramgren B, Jonsson K, Zayer M. Long-term results after adolescent Blount's disease. J Pediatr Orthop B. 1997;6(2):153–6.
14. Guven A, Hancili S, Kuru LI. Obesity and increasing rate of infantile Blount disease. Clin Pediatr (Phila). 2014;53(6):539–43.
15. Montgomery CO, Young KL, Austen M, Jo CH, Blasier RD, Ilyas M. Increased risk of Blount disease in obese children and adolescents with vitamin D deficiency. J Pediatr Orthop. 2010;30(8):879–82.
16. Pirpiris M, Jackson KR, Farng E, Bowen RE, Otsuka NY. Body mass index and Blount disease. J Pediatr Orthop. 2006;26(5):659–63.
17. Sabharwal S, Zhao C, McClemens E. Correlation of body mass index and radiographic deformities in children with Blount disease. J Bone Jt Surg Am. 2007;89(6):1275–83.
18. Sabharwal S, Zhao C, Sakamoto SM, McClemens E. Do children with Blount disease have lower body mass index after lower limb realignment? J Pediatr Orthop. 2014;34(2):213–8.
19. Scott AC, Kelly CH, Sullivan E. Body mass index as a prognostic factor in development of infantile Blount disease. J Pediatr Orthop. 2007;27(8):921–5.
20. Loder RT, Johnston CE 2nd. Infantile tibia vara. J Pediatr Orthop. 1987;7(6):639–46.
21. Richards BS, Katz DE, Sims JB. Effectiveness of brace treatment in early infantile Blount's disease. J Pediatr Orthop. 1998;18(3):374–80.
22. Zionts LE, Shean CJ. Brace treatment of early infantile tibia vara. J Pediatr Orthop. 1998;18(1):102–9.
23. Burghardt RD, Specht SC, Herzenberg JE. Mechanical failures of eight-plateguided growth system for temporary hemiepiphysiodesis. J Pediatr Orthop. 2010;30(6):594–7.
24. Schroerlucke S, Bertrand S, Clapp J, Bundy J, Gregg FO. Failure of Orthofix eight-plate for the treatment of Blount disease. J Pediatr Orthop. 2009;29(1):57–60.
25. Scott AC. Treatment of infantile Blount disease with lateral tension band plating. J Pediatr Orthop. 2012;32(1):29–34.
26. Stevens PM. Guided growth for angular correction: a preliminary series using a tension band plate. J Pediatr Orthop. 2007;27(3):253–9.
27. Wiemann JM 4th, Tryon C, Szalay EA. Physeal stapling versus 8-plate hemiepiphysiodesis for guided correction of angular deformity about the knee. J Pediatr Orthop. 2009;29(5):481–5.
28. Danino B, Rodl R, Herzenberg JE, Shabtai L, Grill F, Narayanan U, et al. The efficacy of guided growth as an initial strategy for Blount disease treatment. J Child Orthop. 2020;14(4):312–7.

29. Leveille LA, Razi O, Johnston CE. Rebound deformity after growth modulation in patients with coronal plane angular deformities about the knee: who gets it and how much? J Pediatr Orthop. 2019;39(7):353–8.
30. Black BE. Tibial opening greenstick osteotomy for Blount's disease. J South Orthop Assoc. 1997;6(3):204–9.
31. Ferriter P, Shapiro F. Infantile tibia vara: factors affecting outcome following proximal tibial osteotomy. J Pediatr Orthop. 1987;7(1):1–7.
32. Hayek S, Segev E, Ezra E, Lokiec F, Wientroub S. Serrated W/M osteotomy. Results using a new technique for the correction of infantile tibia vara. J Bone Jt Surg Br. 2000;82(7):1026–9.
33. Johnston CE 2nd. Infantile tibia vara. Clin Orthop Relat Res. 1990;255:13–23.
34. Langenskiold A. An operation for partial closure of an epiphysial plate in children, and its experimental basis. J Bone Jt Surg Br. 1975;57(3):325–30.
35. Langenskiold A. Surgical treatment of partial closure of the growth plate. J Pediatr Orthop. 1981;1(1):3–11.
36. Manchanda K, Rodgers J, Kanaan Y, Chan-Hee J, Podeszwa D, Birch JG. Results of lower extremity physeal bar resection. Iran J Orthop Surg. 2019;17(4):132–41.
37. Sabharwal S, Sakamoto SM, Zhao C. Advanced bone age in children with Blount disease: a case-control study. J Pediatr Orthop. 2013;33(5):551–7.
38. Andrade N, Johnston CE. Medial epiphysiolysis in severe infantile tibia vara. J Pediatr Orthop. 2006;26(5):652–8.
39. Sabharwal S, Wenokor C, Mehta A, Zhao C. Intra-articular morphology of the knee joint in children with Blount disease: a case-control study using MRI. J Bone Jt Surg Am. 2012;94(10):883–90.
40. McCarthy JJ, MacIntyre NR 3rd, Hooks B, Davidson RS. Double osteotomy for the treatment of severe Blount disease. J Pediatr Orthop. 2009;29(2):115–9.
41. Schoenecker PL, Johnston R, Rich MM, Capelli AM. Elevation of the medical plateau of the tibia in the treatment of Blount disease. J Bone Jt Surg Am. 1992;74(3):351–8.
42. Gkiokas A, Brilakis E. Management of neglected Blount disease using double corrective tibia osteotomy and medial plateau elevation. J Child Orthop. 2012;6(5):411–8.
43. Stanitski DF, Stanitski CL, Trumble S. Depression of the medial tibial plateau in early-onset Blount disease: myth or reality? J Pediatr Orthop. 1999;19(2):265–9.
44. Ho-Fung V, Jaimes C, Delgado J, Davidson RS, Jaramillo D. MRI evaluation of the knee in children with infantile Blount disease: tibial and extra-tibial findings. Pediatr Radiol. 2013;43(10):1316–26.
45. Mare PH, Thompson DM, Marais LC. The medial elevation osteotomy for late-presenting and recurrent infantile Blount disease. J Pediatr Orthop. 2021;41(2):67–76.
46. Abraham E, Toby D, Welborn MC, Helder CW, Murphy A. New single-stage double osteotomy for late-presenting infantile tibia vara: a comprehensive approach. J Pediatr Orthop. 2019;39(5):247–56.
47. Nada AA, Hammad ME, Eltanahy AF, Gazar AA, Khalifa AM, El-Sayed MH. Acute correction and plate fixation for the management of severe infantile Blount's disease: short-term results. Strateg Trauma Limb Reconstr. 2021;16(2):78–85.
48. Carter JR, Leeson MC, Thompson GH, Kalamchi A, Kelly CM, Makley JT. Late-onset tibia vara: a histopathologic analysis. A comparative evaluation with infantile tibia vara and slipped capital femoral epiphysis. J Pediatr Orthop. 1988;8(2):187–95.
49. Wenger DR, Mickelson M, Maynard JA. The evolution and histopathology of adolescent tibia vara. J Pediatr Orthop. 1984;4(1):78–88.
50. Dietz WH. Health consequences of obesity in youth: childhood predictors of adult disease. Pediatrics. 1998;101(3 Pt 2):518–25.
51. Gordon JE, Hughes MS, Shepherd K, Szymanski DA, Schoenecker PL, Parker L, et al. Obstructive sleep apnoea syndrome in morbidly obese children with tibia vara. J Bone Jt Surg Br. 2006;88(1):100–3.
52. Henderson RC. Tibia vara: a complication of adolescent obesity. J Pediatr. 1992;121(3):482–6.
53. Davids JR, Huskamp M, Bagley AM. A dynamic biomechanical analysis of the etiology of adolescent tibia vara. J Pediatr Orthop. 1996;16(4):461–8.
54. Gordon JE, Heidenreich FP, Carpenter CJ, Kelly-Hahn J, Schoenecker PL. Comprehensive treatment of late-onset tibia vara. J Bone Jt Surg Am. 2005;87(7):1561–70.
55. Henderson RC, Kemp GJ. Assessment of the mechanical axis in adolescent tibia vara. Orthopedics. 1991;14(3):313–6.
56. Myers TG, Fishman MK, McCarthy JJ, Davidson RS, Gaughan J. Incidence of distal femoral and distal tibial deformities in infantile and adolescent Blount disease. J Pediatr Orthop. 2005;25(2):215–8.
57. Sabharwal S, Lee J Jr, Zhao C. Multiplanar deformity analysis of untreated Blount disease. J Pediatr Orthop. 2007;27(3):260–5.
58. Firth GB, Ngcakani A, Ramguthy Y, Izu A, Robertson A. The femoral deformity in Blount's disease: a comparative study of infantile, juvenile and adolescent Blount's disease. J Pediatr Orthop B. 2020;29(4):317–22.
59. Henderson RC, Kemp GJ Jr, Greene WB. Adolescent tibia vara: alternatives for operative treatment. J Bone Jt Surg Am. 1992;74(3):342–50.
60. Park SS, Gordon JE, Luhmann SJ, Dobbs MB, Schoenecker PL. Outcome of hemiepiphyseal stapling for late-onset tibia vara. J Bone Jt Surg Am. 2005;87(10):2259–66.
61. Westberry DE, Davids JR, Pugh LI, Blackhurst D. Tibia vara: results of hemiepiphyseodesis. J Pediatr Orthop B. 2004;13(6):374–8.
62. Murphy RF, Pacult MA, Barfield WR, Mooney JF 3rd. Hemiepiphyseodesis for juvenile and adolescent tibia vara utilizing percutaneous transphyseal screws. J Pediatr Orthop. 2020;40(1):17–22.
63. Braga SR, Akkari M, Waisberg G, Sutton CH, Gama NF, Santili C. Percutaneous hemiepiphysiodesis using transphyseal screws for adolescent tibia vara. J Pediatr Orthop B. 2022;31(2):127–33.
64. McIntosh AL, Hanson CM, Rathjen KE. Treatment of adolescent tibia vara with hemiepiphysiodesis: risk factors for failure. J Bone Jt Surg Am. 2009;91(12):2873–9.
65. Funk SS, Mignemi ME, Schoenecker JG, Lovejoy SA, Mencio GA, Martus JE. Hemiepiphysiodesis implants for late-onset tibia vara: a comparison of cost, surgical success, and implant failure. J Pediatr Orthop. 2016;36(1):29–35.
66. Eidelman M, Bialik V, Katzman A. The use of the Taylor spatial frame in adolescent Blount's disease: is fibular osteotomy necessary? J Child Orthop. 2008;2(3):199–204.
67. Clarke SE, McCarthy JJ, Davidson RS. Treatment of Blount disease: a comparison between the multiaxial correction system and other external fixators. J Pediatr Orthop. 2009;29(2):103–9.
68. Coogan PG, Fox JA, Fitch RD. Treatment of adolescent Blount disease with the circular external fixation device and distraction osteogenesis. J Pediatr Orthop. 1996;16(4):450–4.
69. Feldman DS, Madan SS, Koval KJ, van Bosse HJ, Bazzi J, Lehman WB. Correction of tibia vara with six-axis deformity analysis and the Taylor spatial frame. J Pediatr Orthop. 2003;23(3):387–91.
70. Feldman DS, Madan SS, Ruchelsman DE, Sala DA, Lehman WB. Accuracy of correction of tibia vara: acute versus gradual correction. J Pediatr Orthop. 2006;26(6):794–8.
71. Gaudinez R, Adar U. Use of Orthofix T-Garche fixator in late-onset tibia vara. J Pediatr Orthop. 1996;16(4):455–60.
72. Gilbody J, Thomas G, Ho K. Acute versus gradual correction of idiopathic tibia vara in children: a systematic review. J Pediatr Orthop. 2009;29(2):110–4.
73. Price CT, Scott DS, Greenberg DA. Dynamic axial external fixation in the surgical treatment of tibia vara. J Pediatr Orthop. 1995;15(2):236–43.
74. Rozbruch SR, Blyakher A, Haas SB, Hotchkiss R. Correction of large bilateral tibia vara with the Ilizarov method. J Knee Surg. 2003;16(1):34–7.
75. Wilson NA, Scherl SA, Cramer KE. Complications of high tibial osteotomy with external fixation in adolescent Blount's disease. Orthopedics. 2007;30(10):848–52.

Part V

Sequelae and Complications

Methods to Enhance Bone Formation in Distraction Osteogenesis

Hae-Ryong Song, Dong-Hoon Lee, Young-Hwan Park, and Ashok Kumar Ramanathan

Introduction

Regeneration of bone defects resulting from conditions including trauma and congenital deformity correction by distraction osteogenesis (DO) is one of the most interesting issues in the field of regenerative medicine [1]. DO is an increasingly popular technique used to stimulate new bone formation to treat orthopedic disorders resulting from bone defects and deficits [2]. However, the long treatment period with various complications [3] and the potential for nonunion under some circumstances remain major limitations of current treatment procedures. Regeneration of bone in the presence of rigid fixation and maintenance of the osteogenic tissue (marrow, endosteum, nutrient artery, and periosteum) require many factors for stimulation of bone regeneration [4]. Therefore, the development of procedures to accelerate the formation and maturation of regenerate is clearly desirable.

To regenerate the bone defects, autologous and allogenic bone grafting are the most widely used methods. However, these methods are associated with a number of drawbacks, including donor site morbidity and blood loss. To overcome these drawbacks, tissue engineering strategies have demonstrated a potential role in developing bone graft substitutes. Different mechanical and biophysical stimuli could provide effective augmentation of bone regenerate maturation. These include biologic stimulation such as bone morphogenetic proteins (BMP), platelet-rich plasma (PRP), stem cells, parathyroid hormone, and growth hormone [5, 6]. In addition, physical stimulation such as ultrasound, mechanical, and electromagnetic stimulation has been used [7–10]. Even though a bone defect during DO possesses the intrinsic capacity to heal spontaneously following surgery, beyond a certain critical size the defect in bone may not heal adequately by itself and further intervention is often required (Box 35.1).

> **Box 35.1 Quantitative Methods to Monitor the Regenerate Bone**
> - Quantitative ultrasound
> - Dual-energy X-ray absorptiometry
> - Quantitative computed tomography
> - Pixel value ratio method

Monitoring of Regenerate Bone

Various methods have been proposed for the monitoring of the regenerate bone [11] quantitatively and qualitatively. Indirect quantitative methods, including ultrasound, dual-energy X-ray absorptiometry (DEXA), and quantitative computed tomography, have already been found to be sensitive [12–14]. However, owing to their high cost, inability to detect soft tissue changes, and poor measurements in the presence of artifacts, the routine use of such modalities in clinical practice is not popular. An image analysis method is also proposed for the monitoring of the regeneration of the bone. Radiographic investigation is one of the most important methods because it is the simplest; it provides continuous information and it can be easily interpreted. A recent approach that is being used to determine callus stiffness is to evaluate the pixel value ratio (PVR) using a picture archiving

H.-R. Song (✉) · Y.-H. Park
Department of Orthopedic Surgery, Korea University Medical Center, Guro Hospital, Seoul, Republic of Korea
e-mail: songhae@korea.ac.kr

D.-H. Lee
Department of Orthopedic Surgery, Severance Children's Hospital, Seoul, Republic of Korea

A. K. Ramanathan
Department of Orthopedic Surgery, Madurai Medical College, Madurai, Tamil Nadu, India

and communication system (PACS). The PVR is the ratio of the proximal segment to that of the regenerate, and it correlates well with the bone mineral density (BMD) [15, 16]. Shim et al. [17] analyzed serial pixel values of different cortices in both femoral and tibial lengthening and demonstrated that pixel values for distraction callus conformed to a sigmoidal curve. Song et al. [18] reported that BMD measurement can thus function as an effective adjunct to measure callus stiffness, along with PVR, using digital radiographs, especially in situations where callus maturation and stiffness are doubtful.

Many studies [19–21] have been published in an attempt to find a relation between the callus pattern and the prognosis of the limb lengthening procedure because such a system or classification can help the surgeon to quantitatively assess the progress of the distraction callus and to predict the chance of callus fracture and can thus impact the clinical outcome of the procedure. Devmurari et al. [22] reported that the Ru Li classification [23] is an effective method for the evaluation of the chance of callus fracture and a lucent pathway was seen in all fracture cases with concave, lateral, and other shapes (Fig. 35.1). Early removal of the fixator may lead to fracture of the regenerate, whereas prolonged use leads to joint stiffness, pin-site infection, and discomfort to the patient, as well as delayed complications like subsidence and angulation [24, 25]. Recently, Blázquez-Carmona et al. [26] introduced real-

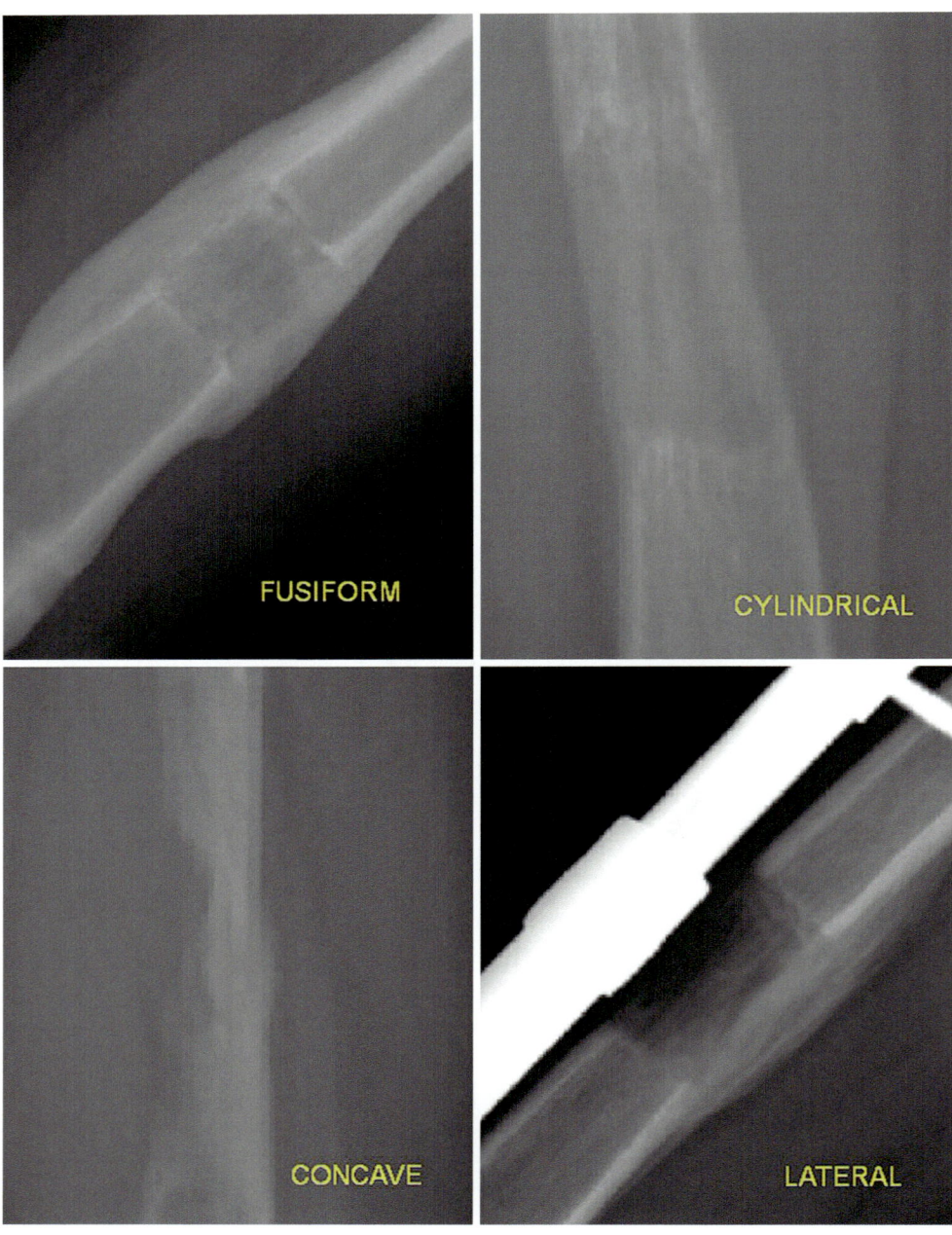

Fig. 35.1 Callus patterns

time wireless platform that allows the in vivo mechanical characterization of the bone callus. Research is in progress to define callus maturation and corticalization and hence to identify the ideal time for removal of the fixator.

Physical Stimulation

Mechanical Stimulation

Controlled mechanical stimulation is considered to be an important stimulus for the regenerate in DO. There are preclinical and clinical evidences that physiologic weight bearing stimulates new bone formation and consolidation of new bone in DO [27–30]. Controlled compressive but not shear force has been shown to affect the biologic nature of the healing response by early expression of BMP 2/4 and the messengers for collagen 1 and osteocalcin [31] and increase the size and strength of the regenerate [30, 32].

"Pumping" of the regenerate (also referred to as the accordion maneuver)—the procedure of alternative compression and distraction—is a well-known method to stimulate new bone formation in the clinical situation of poor regenerate [33, 34]. But, from the literature review, we found that it is still a conflicting issue. Mofid et al. [34], in an animal model of mandibular distraction, performed daily alternative compression and distraction at an amplitude of 1 mm/day for 3 weeks and observed improved bone healing in terms of cortical thickness, cortical:cancellous bone ratio, and mineral apposition. In contrast, Greenwald et al. [33], in an animal model of mandibular distraction, distracted to a length of 2.5 mm (at a rate of 0.25 mm twice daily) for 5 days, then compressed 1.0 mm for a 2-day period, and redistracted to a length of 5 mm. They demonstrated no significant differences between experimental ("pumping") and control group in radiological and histological parameter. The timing of oscillating motion is also a conflicting issue. Kassis et al. [35] showed that the effect of axial micromotion is evident only after the end of elongation rather than during active distraction. Further investigations are necessary to establish the effect and the optimal protocol for "pumping" including the timing, amplitude of sequential movement, and frequency.

Rhythm of distraction is another conflicting issue for enhancing bone regenerate. Ilizarov in an animal model demonstrated better callus in motorized distraction group (1/60 mm, 60 times/day) compared with the standard rhythm (1/4 mm, 4 times/day) [36, 37]. Mizuta proved that an increase in the distraction frequency (eight steps vs. four steps) in open-wedge osteotomies of the proximal tibia with hemicallotasis provides better bone formation, resulting in a shorter external fixation period [38]. Meanwhile, there have been reports that the rhythm of distraction does not significantly influence bone healing [39, 40]. Lengthening procedure is not confined to the bone and soft tissues are also important. Makarov et al. demonstrated in a goat model that a more fractionated rhythm of distraction was associated with enhanced preservation of muscle fibers and greater regenerative activity of the muscle [41]. Further investigation is necessary to clarify the benefit of the more fractionated distraction and the optimal rhythm.

Low-Intensity Pulsed Ultrasound

Low-intensity pulsed ultrasound (LIPUS) is a form of mechanical stimulation that is delivered as high-frequency acoustic pressure waves. The physical process through which LIPUS stimulates bone healing remains unclear. It is speculated that ultrasound enhances fracture healing by inducing low-level mechanical forces at the fracture site, reproducing the effect of functional loading [42]. The mechanisms through which the mechanical signal is translated into a biochemical signal have not been fully understood, but ultrasound seems to influence certain cellular reactions involved in each phase of the healing process such as inflammatory reaction, angiogenesis, chondrogenesis, intramembranous ossification, endochondral ossification, and bone remodeling [42, 43]. LIPUS is one of the best studied treatment modalities in DO, but the results from preclinical experiments are still conflicting regarding its efficacy [44, 45]. There are well-designed clinical studies for the acute fracture healing, suggesting that LIPUS can be beneficial in the treatment of certain nonoperatively treated fractures by shortening the time to radiological and clinical union [46–48]. Most successful reports with LIPUS are in the treatment of conservatively managed acute fractures. There are only limited reports in the literature involving surgically treated fractures and most of them reported disappointing results [49–51]. Emami et al. [49] concluded that low-intensity ultrasound treatment did not shorten healing time in acute tibial fractures treated with a reamed and statically locked intramedullary nail. In addition, Simpson et al. [52] performed multicentre double-blind randomized control trial to assess the effect of LIPUS and concluded that LIPUS does not influence the rate of bone healing in patients who undergo DO. On the other hand, Song et al. [53] retrospectively analyzed the application of LIPUS for the DO of the tibial lengthening over intramedullary nail procedure and found that LIPUS enhances callus consolidation. In a meta-analysis of randomized clinical trials performed by Raza et al. [54], it was found that LIPUS may provide a reduction in the overall treatment time for tibial DO. However, the authors cautioned that the risk of bias was moderate to high in all five studies included in the analysis.

The effect of LIPUS on DO is not conclusive especially regarding the timing of application [44, 45, 55, 56]. Among patients undergoing DO, neither the treatment time nor the risk of complications could be reduced by LIPUS therapy [57]. Further well-designed studies are required to clarify the role of LIPUS in humans undergoing DO.

Pulsed Electromagnetic Field

Most of the available studies regarding pulsed electromagnetic field (PEMF) are related to its effect on the treatment of acute fractures [58–60] and suggest that PEMF may be beneficial in the treatment of certain nonoperatively treated fractures. However, there are only few studies that investigated its effect on DO [10, 60–62]. Therefore, despite the fact that some studies have reported a supportive effect on enhancing callus healing [62, 63], additional high-level studies in human subjects are necessary before we can recommend PEMF as a valid treatment option (Box 35.2).

Box 35.2 Biologic Stimulants
- Local application
  - BMP
  - BMAC/PRP
  - Stem cells
  - Experimental—TP508, ED71, FGF-2
- Systemic application
  - Parathyroid hormone
  - Growth hormone
  - Experimental—hyperbaric oxygen, androgens

Biologic Stimulation

Local Application-Bone Morphogenetic Protein

The BMPs are known to have a strong osteoinductive potential [64–66]. There are several preclinical studies on the effect of BMPs on DO [67–71]. Mizumoto et al. [71] used a single injection of rhBMP-7 into osteotomy gap on the day of surgery in a rat DO model and observed a larger amount of new bone throughout the distraction phase. Hamdy et al. showed that application of OP-1 early during the distraction phase in rabbit tibiae accelerated new bone formation by densitometry and micro-CT analysis [68, 70]. Also, Yang et al. [67] demonstrated enhanced bone formation by injection of BMP-2 at the end of distraction in rat femora. Several clinical studies have been reported using BMP-2 or BMP-7/OP-1 for open tibial fractures and spinal fusion [72, 73], but not for DO so far. There are conflicting issues about the risk of cancer by using rhBMP-2 [74–79]. TGF-beta ligand is known to have the ability to alter cell signaling that can lead to tumor promotion, and certain BMPs are expressed during the growth of some types of cancer [74, 75, 77, 79–82]. TGF-beta/BMP plays a fundamental role in the regulation of bone organogenesis through the activation of receptor serine/threonine kinases [83]. Through the TGF-beta signaling pathway, panax notoginseng saponin promotes bone regeneration in DO [84]. Recent systematic review for the application of the rhBMPs for bone regeneration, onlay block grafting, and DO demonstrated clinical differences in the analyzed results, but verification of the statistically significant difference was failed [85]. Therefore, further investigations for optimal dose, optimal timing, and potential risk of various BMPs are required before they can be recommended for clinical use.

Bone Marrow Cells/Platelet-Rich Plasma

Osteogenic differentiation from bone marrow-derived mesenchymal stem cells (MSC) has several advantages when compared to the differentiation of other mesenchyme tissues [86]. First, bone marrow cells (BMCs) have abundant mononuclear cells. Second, the differentiation of osteoblasts from BMCs is well described and standardized. Third, due to its autogenous delivery properties, the complications such as infection, immunogenic reactions, and disease transmissions can be minimized. Fourth, the harvesting process of bone marrow cells using a Jamshidi vacuum aspiration is minimally invasive and has low donor-site morbidity. Lastly, we are not aware of any reports of malignant transformation of autologous BMCs in the literature [86]. Local administration of allogeneic or autologous bone marrow-derived MSC was found to enhance early bone consolidation in DO model [87–89]. Though a lot of animal studies using bone marrow transplant have shown that bone marrow has enriched osteoblast progenitor cells and it is a valuable bone graft in bone defect, there have been only limited investigations on its clinical application in DO [90–92].

The PRP is abundant in various growth factors released from platelets, which have been known to increase vascular ingrowth and mitogenic effects on bone-forming cells [93–96]. Kawasumi et al. [95] observed that a high platelet concentration combined with osteoblastic cells in PRP accelerated new bone formation during DO in a rat model. In contrast to these findings, Arpornmaeklong et al. [97] noted an inhibitory effect of PRP on osteogenic differentiation of marrow-derived pre-osteoblasts.

There have been few clinical studies using PRP in human subjects [98–100]. Latalski et al. [98] reported a shorter healing index in the PRP group in a retrospective human DO study with a small sample size. The role of PRP in bone regeneration is still a controversial issue and its mechanism is not yet fully understood [97, 98, 101–111]. BMCs and PRP have been used simultaneously showing favorable clinical results. Kitoh et al. [90, 112] studied transplantation of culture-expanded bone marrow cells combined with PRP that accelerated new bone formation during the DO, especially in the femur. Tonogai et al. histologically analyzed the muscle belly of the gastrocnemius in mice tibial DO and reported PRP did not significantly reduce skeletal muscle fibrosis caused by DO [113].

Lee et al. [99] showed that the combined injection of bone marrow aspirate concentrate (BMAC) and PRP during surgery enhanced bone regeneration in human tibial DO (Fig. 35.2). The difference in the abovementioned studies conducted by Kitoh et al. and Lee et al. lies in how to process BMC-culture expansion or concentration. Jäger et al. [86] described the strength of the concentration compared with culture-expanded method. An immediate autologous transplantation of bone marrow concentrate can prevent complications related to the reduced quality of the transplanted cells such as pre-aging due to telomere shortening, reduced viability, or dedifferentiation/reprogramming that is associated with in vitro cultivation. The risk of infection is reduced by decreasing the ex vivo time period; and injection can be performed by single-stage surgery. Although there is only limited clinical evidence, BMAC and/or PRP seems to be a promising treatment option. Though all these studies show a favorable prophylactic role of BMAC/PRP in enhancing the regenerate in DO, their role in established delayed/nonunion after DO is uncertain and warrants further studies.

Well-designed preclinical and clinical studies are necessary, especially to evaluate whether BMAC or PRP contributes more to bone formation—or if the effect is synergistic, the optimal timing of injections and the optimal concentrations and cell counts.

Stem Cells

There have been many debates about using biotechnology on fracture healing, but there is little scientific evidence about the positive effect of tissue engineering on osteogenesis. Tissue engineering combines osteogenic bone marrow mesenchymal stem cells, synthetic scaffolds, and growth factors in order to form hybrid constructs. Stem cells have been used for other indications including the treatment of long bone defects [114], fracture healing [115], and avascular necrosis [116] apart from enhancing the regenerate in DO.

Stem cells can be of two types:

1. Bone marrow-derived mesenchymal stem cells (MSC)
2. Osteogenic differentiated progenitor cells

Bone marrow-derived MSC can be directed towards the osteogenic lineage if cultured with osteogenic supplements like dexamethasone, β-glycerophosphate, and ascorbic acid phosphate [117]. In a study done by Peters et al. [118] in rats using histomorphometric analysis, it has been shown that

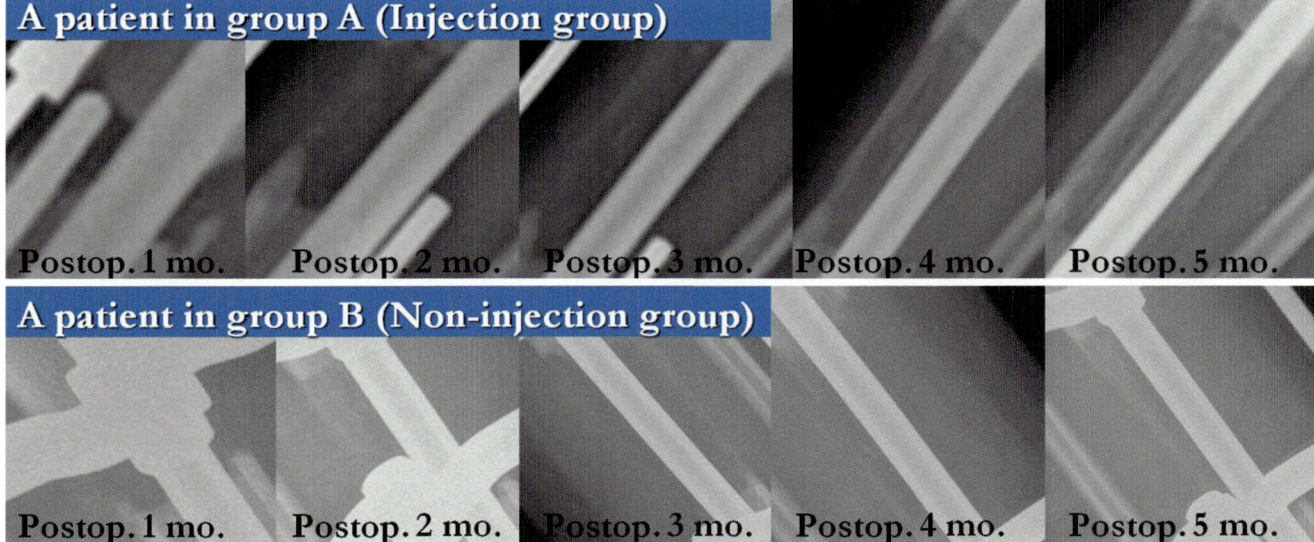

Fig. 35.2 Serial anteroposterior plain radiographs (postoperative 1–5 months, monthly) of the tibia in a patient undergoing lengthening over nail. More callus regeneration was seen in the injection group (group A). Images in group A were obtained from a patient in an injection group, showing postoperative 1–5-month states with an increment of 1 month. Images in group B (non-injection group) were from a patient in a control group with the same postoperative months above

locally applied osteogenic differentiated progenitor cells are more effective than mesenchymal stem cells in enhancing bone healing.

Growth Factors

Growth factors may be added to improve the results of stem cell therapy. There are several osteoinductive growth factors including platelet-derived growth factor, insulin-like growth factor, and transforming growth factors. PRP contains all these growth factors [119]. PRP can also be a suitable carrier for cell transplantation because it coagulates immediately by an addition of thrombin and calcium. Combination of stem cells and PRP accelerates bone healing and the bone remodeling process by stimulating angiogenesis [120].

In a study conducted by Kitoh et al. [112] in 46 patients of skeletal dysplasia and limb length discrepancy, the group that received transplantation of osteogenic differentiated stem cells (approx. 2.3×10^7 cells) and PRP around 3 weeks after the lengthening surgery had a shorter healing index of approx. 31 days/cm compared with the control group which had an average healing index of 55 days/cm and also had reduced associated complications.

Scaffolds

Stem cells may need a scaffold for osteoconduction. The 3-D structure of a scaffold determines the extent of cell migration and differentiation, bone ingrowth, vascularization, and mass transfer between the cells and the environment. All of these processes benefit from increased scaffold porosity, interconnected pore networks, large surface area-to-volume ratio, and increased surface roughness [121]. Bioactive scaffolds aid in bone bonding. It is important for scaffolds to interact with surrounding tissues to induce specific cellular responses [122] (Box 35.3).

> **Box 35.3 Properties of an Ideal Scaffold**
> - Increased and interconnected porosity
> - Large surface area-to-volume ratio
> - Same mechanical strength as bone
> - Bioactive
> - Biocompatible
> - Biodegradable
> - Optimal release profile

One method to achieve this goal is to construct the scaffold with biomaterial that can stimulate platelets to release growth factors. For instance, collagen is known to be as effective as thrombin in activating platelets [123]. The activated platelets would then release growth factors, which will enhance tissue regeneration, proliferation, and differentiation. Therefore, a scaffold made with collagen type 1 will likely be effective in bone formation and bonding.

The mechanical strength of a scaffold should approximate that of bone. Weaker scaffolds cannot support the skeleton, whereas stiffer scaffolds lead to stress shielding. The carrier should be biocompatible to minimize interference with bone induction. It must be biodegradable to minimize the effects on the biomechanical properties of the regenerate, and yet it must persist in vivo long enough to maintain bioactive elements at the site of implantation and optimize their release [124].

Scaffolds available for use with stem cells include PRP gel carrier, collagen, hydroxyapatite (HA) ceramic scaffold, resorbable polylactide membrane, and polycaprolactone (PCL). Collagen scaffold seems to be a good delivery vehicle for other graft materials [124]. Maracci et al. [114] have demonstrated that extensive long bone defects in human subjects treated with stem cell-seeded HA scaffolds have healed and integrated well with the host bone. Even after a 7-year follow-up, the durability of the regenerated bone was good and there were no long-term complications noted. Ren et al. [125] found that the use of rhBMP-2/7 heterodimer and RADA16 hydrogel scaffold significantly promoted mandibular DO. Ma et al. [126] concluded that the incorporation of osteogenic bone marrow-derived MSC sheets into HA particles greatly promoted bone regeneration, which offers therapeutic alternatives for DO. In addition, Zhao et al. [127] investigated the influence of the scaffold pore size on periosteal DO of a rabbit skull using 3-D-printed poly-L-lactic acid scaffolds. The results showed that distractors with larger pore sizes were more favorable for new bone regeneration.

Other Uses of Stem Cells

A case of avascular necrosis of femoral head being treated effectively by stem cells has been reported by Kim et al. [116]. Lee et al. [128] have reported successful reconstruction of 15-cm segmental defects by bone marrow stem cells and autogenous bone graft in central hemangioma of the mandible. Trials are also being carried out by using stem cells in osteoporotic fractures [129]. "Osteogenic matrix coating," a method to prevent loosening of joint prostheses by coating them with osteogenic cells or their precursors, has been proposed by Ohgushi and Caplan [130].

Osteogenic Progenitor Stem Cell Culture Technique

Our technique for procuring and processing the bone marrow aspirate and culture of osteogenic progenitor stem cells is explained below [115].

Approximately 3–5 mL of bone marrow is collected from the anterosuperior iliac spine and added to a container filled with 30 mL of 10% FBS-α MEM and 350 units of heparin (Fig. 35.3). The mixture is then taken to the lab and centrifuged at 4 °C for 10 min, after which the supernatant was discarded and 20 mL of culture medium was added to the remaining pellets. The mixture is then filtered, 10 mL of the medium is added per T-75 culture flask, and the culture is initiated. The incubator is maintained at 37 °C with 5% CO_2. The next day, 50 μg L-ascorbic acid/10 mL and dexamethasone 10^{-7} M are added to facilitate cell differentiation into osteoblasts. The cell culture condition is evaluated using a light microscope, and the culture medium is changed on the fifth day of culture, after which the culture medium is changed every 3 days with the subsequent addition of L-ascorbic acid. On the 14th day of culture, nitro blue tetrazolium chloride 5-bromo-4-chloro-3-indolyl phosphate (NBTBCIP) staining was performed to confirm activation of the alkaline phosphatase. Twenty-four days after beginning the culture, Alizarin red staining is performed to detect newly produced calcium, and thus confirming that most of the cultured cells are osteoblasts. One vial (0.4 mL) contains over 12 million autologous cultured osteoblasts. Every patient may need 1–6 vials (12–72 million cells).

Injection Technique (Fig. 35.4)

In the non-sterile area, transfer whole amount of the cell suspension in two vials into the mixing vial using an 18-G needle. In the sterile area, transfer only 0.1–0.2 mL of thrombin into the mixing vial and discard the rest of thrombin. Mix stem cell and thrombin in a mixing vial and transfer 1 mL

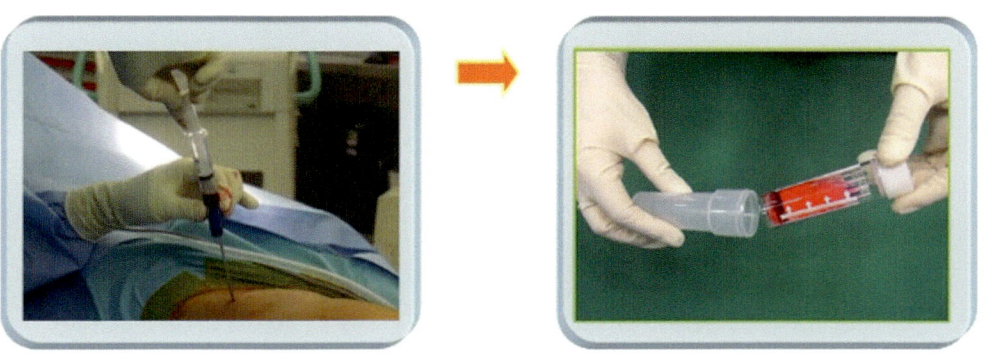

Fig. 35.3 Collection of bone marrow

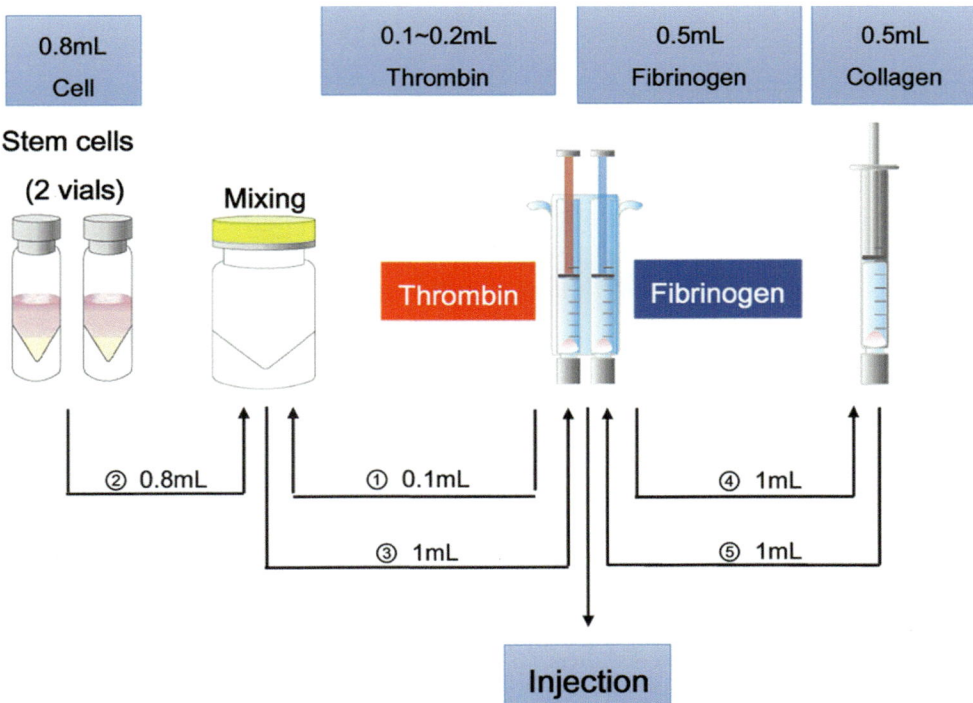

Fig. 35.4 Flowchart depicting the preparation of stem cell mixture

into red (thrombin) syringe. Mix 1 mL of collagen and 1 mL of fibrinogen with two 3-mL syringes using a three-way connector (Fig. 35.5). Transfer 1 mL of mixed collagen and fibrinogen into blue (fibrinogen) syringe. Install the red syringe and blue syringe into Y-piece and implant stem cells with injector and spinal needle by checking the defect site through C-arm (Fig. 35.6). After injection, this becomes a gel within 3–5 min.

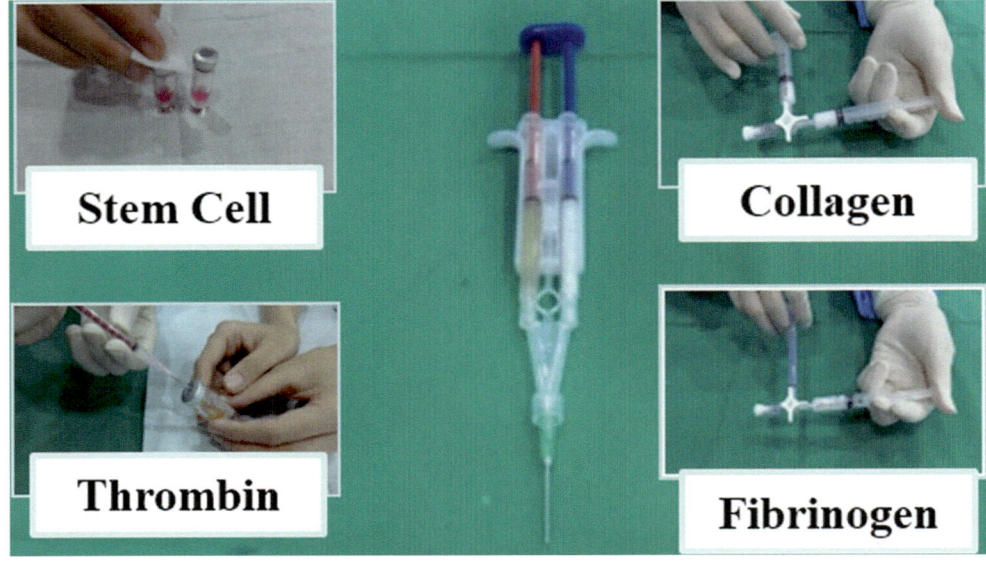

Fig. 35.5 Using a three-way connector, stem cell and thrombin are mixed in a red syringe. Similarly, collagen and fibrinogen are mixed in a blue syringe. Then both of these are attached to the Y-piece

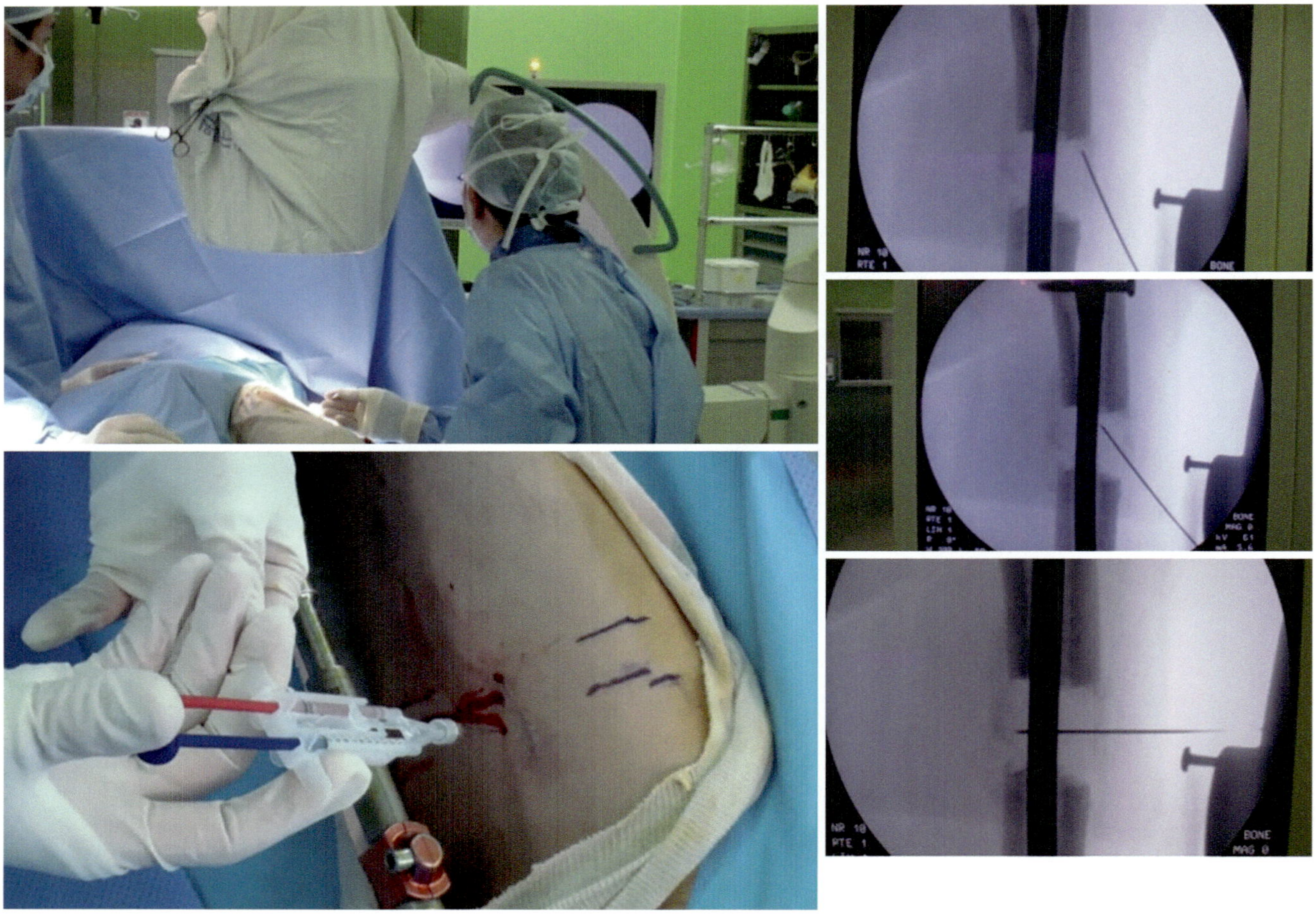

Fig. 35.6 Injection of the stem cell preparation under C-arm control

Although the initial results are encouraging, further studies are necessary to assess the safety and efficacy of stem cells in DO.

Other Experimental Local Stimuli

Osteogenic peptides are cheaper to produce as they are synthetic. They are less likely to lose their bioactivity during storage and delivery because of their short, linear structure.

TP508

One of these osteogenic peptides is TP508, which includes a 23-amino acid peptide that is the non-proteolytic receptor-binding domain of human thrombin. The effects of TP508 include changes in the inflammatory response, improvements in cell recruitment, and angiogenesis [131]. The doses of TP508 used in the experimental studies vary from 0.1 to 300 µg, and results differ depending on the dose. The animals given the higher dose had a larger area of newly formed bone [132–134].

ED-71

Yamamoto [135] reported that administration of 2-β-(3-hydroxypropoxy)-1α, 25-dihydroxyvitamin D3 (ED-71), an analog of synthetic vitamin D3, increased the bone mineral content (BMC) at the lengthened callus. According to Yamane et al. [136], ED-71 promoted both bone matrix formation and mineralization of the callus at 1 week after completion of lengthening, during which BMC increased markedly and may be effective for shortening the duration of therapy in callus distraction.

FGF-2

Fibroblast growth factor-2 (FGF-2 or basic FGF) is recognized as a potent mitogen for a variety of mesenchymal cells. In skeletal tissues, FGF-2 is produced by cells of osteoblastic lineage, accumulated in bone matrix, and acts as an autocrine/paracrine factor for bone cells [137]. FGF-2 shows variable regulations of proliferation and differentiation of cells of osteoblastic lineage and modulates bone formation. Aronson [138] has reported that the age-related deficits of endosteal bone formation were reversed by administering exogenous rhFGF-2 in an animal study. In another study, Okazaki et al. [137] have reported that a single local injection of FGF-2 at the center of distracted callus facilitated the consolidation during bone lengthening in rabbit tibiae even under strenuous conditions of rapid and long distraction. In a study conducted by Jiang et al. [139], osteodistraction was applied in craniofacial bone of rabbits to observe the effects of MSCs with or without bFGF gene transfected on bone regeneration. They noted that excellent bone formation and highest BMD and BMC were achieved in the bFGF gene transfected group.

CO_2

Kumabe et al. [140] investigated the effect of transcutaneous CO_2 during DO in rabbits. A DO rabbit tibia model was created and distraction was performed at 1 mm per day for 10 days. Beginning the day after the osteotomy, a 20-min transcutaneous application of CO_2 on the operated leg using a CO_2 absorption-enhancing hydrogel was performed five times per week and callus parameters were measured with micro-CT to assess callus microstructure. The results showed that transcutaneous application of CO_2 accelerated bone generation in a DO model of rabbit tibias. They concluded that CO_2 treatment might affect bone regeneration in DO by promoting angiogenesis, blood flow, and endochondral ossification.

Optimal Timing of Biologic Stimulants

There is no clear evidence to guide us in terms of the timing of injection to achieve better bone regeneration. Angiogenesis has been shown to be of vital importance and intricately involved in the inflammatory response, soft callus formation, and transition from cartilaginous callus to bone [141, 142]. Proangiogenic factors such as vascular endothelial growth factor (VEGF) are especially important during early phase of distraction, when their expression is significantly higher than in later periods [143]. So, administration of growth factors during the early phases may stimulate neoangiogenesis and/or enhance the formation of regenerate bone. Several preclinical studies showed enhanced new bone formation by applying BMPs on the day of the surgery [71, 144, 145] and immunohistochemical analysis has shown high expression of growth factor receptors during the distraction phase [95, 143, 146–149]. In a randomized controlled trial, Lee et al. [99] clinically demonstrated that injection of BMAC and PRP on the day of surgery enhanced new bone formation (Fig. 35.7).

Hamdy and Rauch et al. [68, 150] observed high levels of expression of BMP-2, 4 and OP-1 during the distraction phase, with a rapid decline thereafter. They hypothesized that the best time for exogenous injection of BMPs would be at the end of the distraction phase, when the endogenous expression of BMPs is decreasing. But, they could not

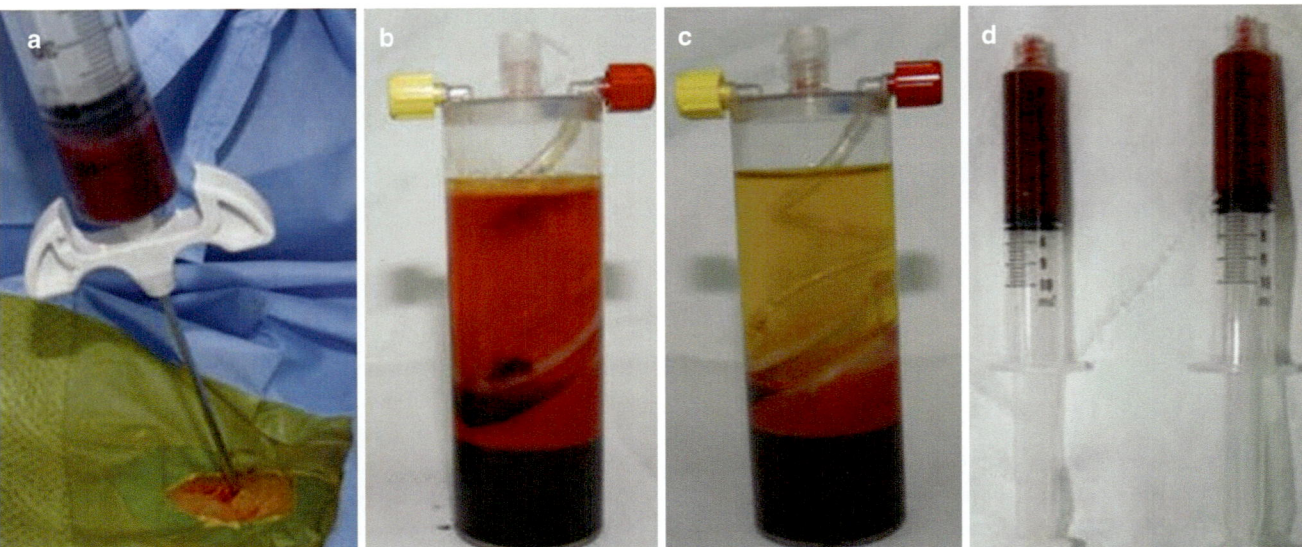

Fig. 35.7 BMAC and PRP are prepared in the operation room at the end of index surgery: 60 mL of bone marrow is aspirated at the iliac crest (**a**) and 60 mL of peripheral blood is obtained. Bone marrow and peripheral blood are centrifuged to make BMAC (**b**) and PRP (**c**). Six milliliters of the aspirate sampled from the mid-layer are prepared for the injection (**d**)

observe enhanced bone healing when OP-1 is injected at the end of distraction, but found twofold increase in bone volume when injected during early phase of distraction [68, 70]. There are also several reports of enhanced healing when applied at the end of distraction [98, 151, 152]. The optimal timing of the injection of the biological stimulants is an important but still unresolved issue. Hence, further well-designed investigations are required.

Biological Stimulation: Systemic Application

Parathyroid Hormone

Parathyroid hormone (PTH) is one of the most promising therapeutic agents for osteoporosis. Human and animal studies have demonstrated that daily systemic injection of parathyroid hormone increases BMD [153–156]. PTH stimulates bone formation and resorption and can increase or decrease bone mass, depending on the mode of administration. Continuous infusions and daily subcutaneous injections of PTH stimulate bone formation similarly, but have different effects on bone resorption and bone mass [157, 158]. It has been reported that the combination of systemic and local parathyroid hormone led to higher BMD, BMC, and bone area, a trend for greater radiographic-detected bone area and higher expression of osteocalcin in osteotomy sites when compared with the individual treatment or control groups [159]. Skripitz et al. [160] conjectured that since PTH seemed to have a greater effect on new bone formation than on normal bone remodeling, it might become useful for improving the incorporation of orthopedic implants and stimulating fracture repair. Neer et al. [161] reported that the clinical benefits of PTH reflect its ability to stimulate bone formation and thereby increase bone mass and strength. Ye et al. [162] concluded that low-dose intermittent rhPTH administration not only enhances new bone formation, but also can prevent fixator-related osteoporosis of surrounding segments after rapid mandibular DO in rabbits. Leiblein et al. [163] suggested that perioperative treatment of complex and/or osteoporotic fractures with PTH (1–34) and raloxifen might be useful as a stimulator of bone formation and mineralization to shorten the consolidation time in humans. As a clinical trial, Wagner et al. [164] performed a randomized prospective study investigating the effect of rhPTH (1–34) (Teriparatide) on bone formation in patients undergoing tibia bone transport. BMD of the regenerate was measured at the time of docking, 8 weeks after docking, and 16 weeks after docking. The results showed that Teriparatide treatment during the consolidation phase of distraction osteogenesis doubled the mineralization rate of the regenerate when compared to no treatment. Given the enhancement of bone formation by the local stimulator such as BMP and the systemic application of PTH, combination therapies may be beneficial for bone tissue engineering.

The mechanism of this anabolic effect, however, has not been well established. It is widely believed that the anabolic effect of PTH may be due to increased osteoblast differentiation. Other report indicated that prevention of osteoblast apoptosis is a crucial mechanism for the anabolic effects of PTH on bone [165].

Growth Hormone

Systemic administration of recombinant homologous growth hormone (GH) has been reported to greatly accelerate ossification of bone regenerate in DO [166]. GH administration increases bone turnover by enhancing both bone formation and resorption [167]. Correspondingly, an increase in the mechanical strength of the whole bone occurs, whereas the mechanical quality of the osseous tissue is equivalent in GH-injected animals and controls [6]. Various studies demonstrate that systemic administration of GH is able to enhance bone regeneration and mechanical strength of healing critical size bone defects in animal models [168–170].

Other Experimental Systemic Stimuli

Hyperbaric oxygen therapy has been used to treat a variety of diseases and has been described as helping patients who have delayed healing or bone defects [171]. This technology consists of intermittently administering 100% oxygen at pressures greater than 1 atm. absolute entirely enclosed in a pressure chamber [171]. However, one systematic review [172] performed recently failed to locate any relevant clinical evidence to support or refute the effectiveness of hyperbaric oxygen therapy for the management of delayed union or established nonunion of bony fractures. Good-quality clinical trials are needed to define its role in DO.

Androgens such as testosterone are also known to have proliferative effects on osteoblasts and increase fracture healing by systemic and local stimulation of bone formation [173]. In clinical application, androgens may be a possibility to increase bone formation, especially in elderly patients. Furthermore, it may be possible to shorten postoperative rehabilitation because of the effects of androgens on muscles [174].

Roseren et al. [175] performed systemic administration of the granulocyte colony-stimulating factor (G-CSF) to determine the effects of the G-CSF on a rat model of DO. Their results indicate that G-CSF accelerates bone regeneration and modulates mobilization of progenitor cells during DO.

Anticatabolic Therapy: Systemic Application

Bisphosphonate

The potential anabolic effect of bisphosphonates has been reported [176, 177]. Recent advances in the pharmacological treatment of osteoporosis with bisphosphonates [178–180] have encouraged surgeons to explore their use in limb lengthening. In general, bisphosphonates have been considered antiresorptive agents with limited effect on osteoblasts [181].

The anabolic effect of bisphosphonates has been questioned as they are not internalized by osteoblasts, and therefore, they may not exert a direct effect on osteoblast activity. However, there is evidence to support that there is an effect of bisphosphonates on the osteoblast side not directly on mature osteoblasts, but more likely on osteoblast precursors in the bone marrow. First, only nanomolar concentrations of bisphosphonates are needed to stimulate the production of osteoclast inhibitory factor, which is mostly secreted by osteoblast precursors [182]. Second, bisphosphonates have shown to stimulate fibroblastic colony formation by murine and human bone marrow both in in vitro and ex vivo cultures [183].

The use of external fixators or any form of fixation may be associated with stress shielding of the spanned bone interval in this case, the regenerate and the surrounding bone, resulting in osteopenia. Eyres et al. [14] noted a mean decrease in BMD of 44% in the tibia and 61% in the femur distal to the regenerate in children undergoing limb lengthening. Maffulli et al. [184] noted that the BMC adjacent to the regenerate decreased to less than 40% of its original value in 6 of 11 patients. There was a reversal of osteopenia, increased regenerate volume, and increased mechanical strength of the bone when bisphosphonates were administered. However, healing index remained very prolonged [185].

Im et al. [186] have shown that both risedronate and alendronate could increase osteoblast and osteoblast progenitor numbers in primary human trabecular cultures with enhanced expression of BMP-2, type I collagen, and osteocalcin. Akbulut et al. [187] evaluated the effects of the systemic zoledronic acid application on new bone genesis in a DO model of rat femurs and found that new bone formation of the zoledronic acid group in consolidation period in DO was higher compared with the control group. These effects are not limited to osteoblastogenesis but also to the promotion of osteoblast survival as per their efficacy as antiapoptotic agents [188]. Furthermore, bisphosphonates were reported to enhance bone marrow mesenchymal stem cell osteogenic differentiation [189] and facilitate human adipose-derived stem cell osteogenesis for bone regeneration [190]. Not only bone formation but also bone resorption are highly activated in the regenerated bone, implying high bone turnover. Sufficient nitrogen-containing bisphosphonate (N-BP) causes a notable modulation in morphological properties of the regenerated bone through inhibition of highly activated bone resorption and eventually increased mechanical properties [191]. The main effects of N-BP are at the lumbar spine and proximal femur, where they stop bone loss, reduce fracture risk, and increase BMD [192]. In addition, N-BP are prescribed for the treatment of bone diseases such as osteoporosis, multiple myeloma, cancer metastases, and Paget's disease.

However, the conventional systemic way of administration of bisphosphonates may have some undesirable side effects such as gastrointestinal ulceration and jaw osteonecrosis [192, 193]. Recent studies have indicated that local administration of a low dose of bisphosphonates was able to enhance bone regeneration in vivo [194–196]. Alp et al. [197] applied 0.75 µg/kg of alendronate local injections into the distraction gap of the rabbit mandible and found a significant increase in mean bone mineral density. However, in comparative study of zoledronic acid in mandibular DO, systemic application was found more effective compared with local application [198].

Other Experimental Anticatabolic Therapies

The influence of calcitonin on various stages of bone formation has been investigated [199]. Weiss et al. [200] reported that when calcitonin is administered during the initial phases of bone formation, it increases bone formation due to a stimulation of proliferation of cartilage and bone precursor cells. In humans, serum calcitonin rises during pregnancy, growth, and lactation [201]. It is during these periods of calcium stress that a tonic antiresorptive hormone will best exert its effect to limit skeletal loss. This may be the primary role of calcitonin in skeletal conservation [202]. There is considerable support for the thesis that, in addition to its inhibitory effects on bone resorption, calcitonin enhances osteoblastic bone formation both in vitro and in vivo [203]. The putative anabolic osteoblastic effect of calcitonin may be of clinical importance in sustaining the bone formation rate despite inhibition of bone resorption.

Summary

Insufficient bone regeneration is an unpredictable and unsolved issue in DO. Avoiding the detrimental factors is also important, but there are unavoidable factors like host-related causes including smoking, diabetes, and systemic illness. Biologic stimulation is more promising because it can be used proactively rather than as a treatment after poor bone regeneration is observed. Efforts to improve regenerate bone formation are still in progress. The efficacy, safety, optimal dose, timing and route of administration, and cost-effectiveness of each of the agents that can enhance bone formation in DO should be studied further by well-designed investigations.

Commentary

Methods to Enhance Bone Formation in Distraction Osteogenesis

Reggie C. Hamdy
rhamdy@shriners.mcgill.ca

Distraction osteogenesis (DO) is a surgical technique where gradual and controlled distraction of two bony fragments following an osteotomy leads to the induction of new bone formation in the distracted gap. Either external or internal distraction devices, or a combination of both, could be used for the stabilization of the proximal and distal ends of the bone during the distraction and the consolidation phases. When the desired length of regenerate bone is reached (distraction phase), distraction is stopped and the distraction device is kept on until the newly formed bone is mechanically strong enough to allow removal of the fixator (consolidation phase). DO is considered a type of in vivo tissue engineering and is widely used worldwide in the management of limb length discrepancies by lengthening the short bones, gradual correction of severe bony or soft tissue deformities, and the replacement of bone loss secondary to infection, trauma, or post-resection of tumors. DO is superior to many other techniques of bone regeneration (such as autografts or allografts, bone graft substitutes, Masquelet technique) as it allows for the spontaneous formation of large amounts of de novo native bone without the need for bone grafts or substitutes. It also allows the simultaneous regeneration of soft tissues.

Although DO usually gives satisfactory results in most cases, one major **drawback of this procedure** is the prolonged period of time for the new bone to be regenerated in the distracted gap, whether an external or internal fixator is being used. Usually, under optimal conditions of DO, it takes about 1 month fixator time for every centimeter lengthening for a satisfactory regenerate to develop. However, under certain conditions, this consolidation time may be prolonged beyond 1 month and this requires the fixator device to be kept even longer. This prolonged period of time for which the fixator has to be kept on until the regenerate consolidates may lead to numerous medical, psychosocial, and financial problems to the patient, family, and health care institutions. Two questions then arise: the first, how to stay out of trouble by preventing a poor regenerate from developing, and the second, how to get out of trouble once a poor regenerate develops.

How to stay out of trouble can be addressed by a comprehensive preoperative preparation and planning. This usually requires a multidisciplinary team that includes surgeons, physicians, nurses, physiotherapists and psychologists. The indication for surgery is reviewed to ensure that it is the right indication; host-related risk factors such as obesity, smoking, diabetes, and other systemic disorders should be taken into consideration; psychosocial issues are of paramount importance and could be of significance as DO is a prolonged procedure with major rehabilitation involvement. The availability of proper type of instrument (external or internal) and various sizes should be preoperatively planned. Intraoperative strict adherence to the Ilizarov principles cannot be overemphasized, including choosing the appropriate site and technique of the osteotomy, preservation of the periosteum, rate and rhythm of distraction, stability of the fixation, and functional use of the limb and importance of extensive physiotherapy.

Monitoring of the regenerate bone during the entire process of distraction osteogenesis, specifically the distraction and consolidation phases, is of paramount importance for early detection of a poor regenerate and hence deal with this problem as soon as it is identified. It is very important to realize that the methods used to enhance bone formation in the regenerate may vary according to the phase of DO in which the poor regenerate is first detected (distraction versus consolidation) and whether the targeted amount of lengthening or correction was reached or not. Despite extensive research in that area, plain radiography remains the uniformly accepted standard for monitoring regenerate bone formation, as this method is easily accessible and available worldwide, is cost effective, and is reproducible. Other techniques include DEXA (Dual Energy X-ray absorptiometry) and pixel value ratio (PVR). Frequent radiological monitoring of the regenerate has special value in deciding when to remove the fixator.

Once a poor regenerate is identified, then the second question arises: **how to get out of trouble** and still try to attain the desired goal of DO, with no or minimal effect on the final outcome. The last decades have seen an explosion of research in that area and the development of many new products related to bone stimulation. However, despite remarkable advances, *autogenous and allogenic bone grafts* still remain the gold standard in the management of poor regenerate. Autogenous cancellous bone graft possesses all three qualities required for a perfect bone graft: it is osteoconductive, osteoinductive, and osteogeneic. The iliac crest remains the preferred donor site. Bone marrow aspiration and injection in areas of poor regenerate is also a very popular technique that is not expensive and can be easily performed without complications. However, questions remain as to the inconsistency of the number of osteogenic stem cells present in the aspirate. Most recently, the discovery that adipose tissue constitutes the largest reservoir of mesenchymal stem cells with osteogenic potential in the body led to a revolution in the field of stem cells and their potential use in bone regeneration. Advantages of adipose tissue over the standard bone marrow aspiration as a source of osteogenic mesenchymal stem cells include its easy accessibility and availability in huge amounts and minimal morbidity as a donor site. Furthermore, adipose-derived mesenchymal cells have been shown to possess superior osteogenic potential than bone marrow-derived stem cells. The use of adipose tissue-derived stem cells may well be the ideal candidate for bone regeneration in the near future.

Allogenic bone grafts (allografts) provide both osteoconduction and osteoinduction, but have no osteogenic properties. They are commonly available in various types (powder, granules, blocs), various sizes and shapes (e.g., triangular, squares), and even as various separate bones (such as fibular and femoral head allografts). Demineralized bone matrix (DBM) is another type of allograft commonly used.

Mechanical methods are the easiest methods to use and are noninvasive. It is well known that physiological weight bearing and controlled compression stimulate bone formation. The application of alternating compression and distraction forces during the process of DO—the Accordion technique—has been described to enhance bone formation in DO; however, the exact details of this technique are poorly described in the literature.

Outside application techniques include LIPUS (low-intensity pulsed ultrasound), pulse electromagnetic field, and extra corporeal vibration. These techniques may help in enhancing bone formation; however, inconsistent results have been reported with their use in the context of DO and are not commonly used.

Systemic application of pharmacological agents includes PTH (parathyroid hormone), growth hormone, calcitonin, and anti-sclerostin. However, because of the potential problems that may develop with systemic administration, the use of most of these substances still remains experimental in DO. The use of bisphosphonates as a systemic anti-catabolic agent has been well described in the context of osteoporosis and in the management of children with Osteogenesis Imperfecta and is used worldwide as a standard treatment for these conditions, either oral or intravenous administration. However, although systemic and local use of bisphosphonates has been reported in the context of DO, it is not considered a standard approach to address a poor regenerate.

Local application of biologics, specifically osteogenic growth factors, either in isolation or in combination, has been extensively investigated. The most studied of these growth factors are BMPs (bone morphogenetic proteins—specifically BMP2 and BMP7). Although the BMPs have been shown to be powerful anabolic agents, they have several disadvantages: first and most important, huge doses of these factors need to be applied in order to obtain a significant biologic response, and these large doses may lead to potential problems. Furthermore, BMPs are very expensive which also limit their use. Numerous other growth factors have been reported to enhance bone formation such as Fibroblast Growth Factors; however, to date none of them is commonly used in DO. Plasma-derived growth factor (PDGF) is a potent activator of cells of mesenchymal origin and, as a biologic, is often used to stimulate new bone formation.

Bone graft substitutes include an array of artificial bone grafts such as TCP (Tricalcium Phosphate). All these are commercially available. The most important disadvantage of these bone graft substitutes is that none of them possesses osteoinductive or osteogenic potential. They are only osteoconductive and could provide excellent scaffolds.

Tissue engineering is a new approach to address bone poor or no bone formation and is gaining in popularity. It is considered a form of polytherapy where a combination of more than one method of bone stimulation (for example, scaffolds with stem cells) is used.

What does the future bring us? Since its discovery more than 70 years ago by Gavriil Ilizarov, the "Magician of Kurgan", the surgical technique of DO, has stood the test of time as a most powerful tool in our armamentarium for the successful management of patients afflicted with bone deformities and bone loss. DO remains the only available technique that can regenerate large amounts of native, fully vascularized bone of the same micro and macrostructure, physical properties, and geometry as the host bone. Furthermore, no other known technique can simultaneously regenerate soft tissues. However, poor regenerate bone formation still remains a major drawback of this technique. Despite the numerous advances that have been made over the years to address poor bone formation, much more research efforts are needed in that area. The ideal method to enhance bone formation in DO still remains elusive.

References

1. Jimi E, Hirata S, Osawa K, Terashita M, Kitamura C, Fukushima H. The current and future therapies of bone regeneration to repair bone defects. Int J Dent. 2012;2012:148261.
2. Iobst C. Limb lengthening combined with deformity correction in children with the Taylor spatial frame. J Pediatr Orthop B. 2010;19(6):529–34.
3. Kim SJ, Balce GC, Agashe MV, Song SH, Song HR. Is bilateral lower limb lengthening appropriate for achondroplasia? Midterm analysis of the complications and quality of life. Clin Orthop Relat Res. 2012;470(2):616–21.
4. Merloz P. Bone regeneration and limb lengthening. Osteoporos Int. 2011;22(6):2033–6.
5. Li G, Bouxsein ML, Luppen C, et al. Bone consolidation is enhanced by rhBMP-2 in a rabbit model of distraction osteogenesis. J Orthop Res. 2002;20(4):779–88.
6. Andreassen TT, Jorgensen PH, Flyvbjerg A, Orskov H, Oxlund H. Growth hormone stimulates bone formation and strength of cortical bone in aged rats. J Bone Miner Res. 1995;10(7):1057–67.
7. Claes L, Willie B. The enhancement of bone regeneration by ultrasound. Prog Biophys Mol Biol. 2007;93(1–3):384–98.
8. Pomini KT, Andreo JC, Rodrigues Ade C, et al. Effect of low-intensity pulsed ultrasound on bone regeneration: biochemical and radiologic analyses. J Ultrasound Med. 2014;33(4):713–7.
9. Jiang X, Yang J, Chai Z, Song J, Deng F, Wang Z. Low intensity pulsed ultrasound irradiating combined with guided bone regeneration for promoting the repair effect of periodontal bone defect. Hua Xi Kou Qiang Yi Xue Za Zhi. 2012;30(5):487–92.
10. Luna Gonzalez F, Lopez Arevalo R, Meschian Coretti S, Urbano Labajos V, Delgado RB. Pulsed electromagnetic stimulation of regenerate bone in lengthening procedures. Acta Orthop Belg. 2005;71(5):571–6.
11. Windhagen H, Kolbeck S, Bail H, Schmeling A, Raschke M. Quantitative assessment of in vivo bone regeneration consolidation in distraction osteogenesis. J Orthop Res. 2000;18(6):912–9.
12. Romanowski CA, Underwood AC, Sprigg A. Reduction of radiation doses in leg lengthening procedures by means of audit and computed tomography scanogram techniques. Br J Radiol. 1994;67(803):1103–7.
13. Eyres KS, Bell MJ, Kanis JA. Methods of assessing new bone formation during limb lengthening. Ultrasonography, dual energy X-ray absorptiometry and radiography compared. J Bone Jt Surg Br. 1993;75(3):358–64.
14. Eyres KS, Bell MJ, Kanis JA. New bone formation during leg lengthening. Evaluated by dual energy X-ray absorptiometry. J Bone Jt Surg Br. 1993;75(1):96–106.
15. Song SH, Sinha S, Kim TY, Park YE, Kim SJ, Song HR. Analysis of corticalization using the pixel value ratio for fixator removal in tibial lengthening. J Orthop Sci. 2011;16(2):177–83.
16. Hazra S, Song HR, Biswal S, et al. Quantitative assessment of mineralization in distraction osteogenesis. Skelet Radiol. 2008;37(9):843–7.
17. Shim JS, Chung KH, Ahn JM. Value of measuring bone density serial changes on a picture archiving and communication systems (PACS) monitor in distraction osteogenesis. Orthopedics. 2002;25(11):1269–72.
18. Song SH, Agashe M, Kim TY, et al. Serial bone mineral density ratio measurement for fixator removal in tibia distraction osteogenesis and need of a supportive method using the pixel value ratio. J Pediatr Orthop B. 2012;21(2):137–45.
19. Hamanishi C, Yasuwaki Y, Kikuchi H, Tanaka S, Tamura K. Classification of the callus in limb lengthening. Radiographic study of 35 limbs. Acta Orthop Scand. 1992;63(4):430–3.
20. Donnan LT, Saleh M, Rigby AS, McAndrew A. Radiographic assessment of bone formation in tibia during distraction osteogenesis. J Pediatr Orthop. 2002;22(5):645–51.

21. Minty I, Maffulli N, Hughes TH, Shaw DG, Fixsen JA. Radiographic features of limb lengthening in children. Acta Radiol. 1994;35(6):555–9.
22. Devmurari KN, Song HR, Modi HN, Venkatesh KP, Ju KS, Song SH. Callus features of regenerate fracture cases in femoral lengthening in achondroplasia. Skelet Radiol. 2010;39(9):897–903.
23. Li R, Saleh M, Yang L, Coulton L. Radiographic classification of osteogenesis during bone distraction. J Orthop Res. 2006;24(3):339–47.
24. Noonan KJ, Price CT, Sproul JT, Bright RW. Acute correction and distraction osteogenesis for the malaligned and shortened lower extremity. J Pediatr Orthop. 1998;18(2):178–86.
25. Shyam AK, Singh SU, Modi HN, Song HR, Lee SH, An H. Leg lengthening by distraction osteogenesis using the Ilizarov apparatus: a novel concept of tibia callus subsidence and its influencing factors. Int Orthop. 2009;33(6):1753–9.
26. Blazquez-Carmona P, Sanchez-Raya M, Mora-Macias J, Gomez-Galan JA, Dominguez J, Reina-Romo E. Real-time wireless platform for in vivo monitoring of bone regeneration. Sensors (Basel). 2020;20(16):4591.
27. Brighton CT, Hunt RM. Early histological and ultrastructural changes in medullary fracture callus. J Bone Jt Surg Am. 1991;73(6):832–47.
28. Choi IH, Ahn JH, Chung CY, Cho TJ. Vascular proliferation and blood supply during distraction osteogenesis: a scanning electron microscopic observation. J Orthop Res. 2000;18(5):698–705.
29. Moore DC, Leblanc CW, Muller R, Crisco JJ 3rd, Ehrlich MG. Physiologic weight-bearing increases new vessel formation during distraction osteogenesis: a micro-tomographic imaging study. J Orthop Res. 2003;21(3):489–96.
30. Pacicca DM, Moore DC, Ehrlich MG. Physiologic weight-bearing and consolidation of new bone in a rat model of distraction osteogenesis. J Pediatr Orthop. 2002;22(5):652–9.
31. Fink B, Krieger M, Schneider T, Menkhaus S, Fischer J, Ruther W. Factors affecting bone regeneration in Ilizarov callus distraction. Unfallchirurg. 1995;98(12):633–9.
32. Kassis B, Glorion C, Tabib W, Blanchard O, Pouliquen JC. Callus response to micromovement after elongation in the rabbit. J Pediatr Orthop. 1996;16(4):480–3.
33. Greenwald JA, Luchs JS, Mehrara BJ, et al. "Pumping the regenerate": an evaluation of oscillating distraction osteogenesis in the rodent mandible. Ann Plast Surg. 2000;44(5):516–21.
34. Mofid MM, Inoue N, Atabey A, et al. Callus stimulation in distraction osteogenesis. Plast Reconstr Surg. 2002;109(5):1621–9.
35. Kassis B, Glorion C, Tabib W, Blanchard O, Pouliquen JC. Callus response to micromovement during elongation in the rabbit. J Pediatr Orthop. 1998;18(5):586–8.
36. Ilizarov GA. The tension-stress effect on the genesis and growth of tissues: part II. The influence of the rate and frequency of distraction. Clin Orthop Relat Res. 1989;239:263–85.
37. Ilizarov GA, Green SA. The transosseous osteosynthesis: theoretical and clinical aspects of the regeneration and growth of tissue. Berlin: Springer; 1992. p. 800.
38. Mizuta H, Nakamura E, Kudo S, Maeda T, Takagi K. Greater frequency of distraction accelerates bone formation in open-wedge proximal tibial osteotomy with hemicallotasis. Acta Orthop Scand. 2004;75(5):588–93.
39. Bright AS, Herzenberg JE, Paley D, Weiner I, Burghardt RD. Preliminary experience with motorized distraction for tibial lengthening. Strateg Trauma Limb Reconstr. 2014;9(2):97–100.
40. Welch RD, Birch JG, Makarov MR, Samchukov ML. Histomorphometry of distraction osteogenesis in a caprine tibial lengthening model. J Bone Miner Res. 1998;13(1):1–9.
41. Makarov MR, Kochutina LN, Samchukov ML, Birch JG, Welch RD. Effect of rhythm and level of distraction on muscle structure: an animal study. Clin Orthop Relat Res. 2001;384:250–64.
42. Griffin XL, Costello I, Costa ML. The role of low intensity pulsed ultrasound therapy in the management of acute fractures: a systematic review. J Trauma. 2008;65(6):1446–52.
43. Azuma Y, Ito M, Harada Y, Takagi H, Ohta T, Jingushi S. Low-intensity pulsed ultrasound accelerates rat femoral fracture healing by acting on the various cellular reactions in the fracture callus. J Bone Miner Res. 2001;16(4):671–80.
44. Shimazaki A, Inui K, Azuma Y, Nishimura N, Yamano Y. Low-intensity pulsed ultrasound accelerates bone maturation in distraction osteogenesis in rabbits. J Bone Jt Surg Br. 2000;82(7):1077–82.
45. Tis JE, Meffert CR, Inoue N, et al. The effect of low intensity pulsed ultrasound applied to rabbit tibiae during the consolidation phase of distraction osteogenesis. J Orthop Res. 2002;20(4):793–800.
46. Hannemann PF, Mommers EH, Schots JP, Brink PR, Poeze M. The effects of low-intensity pulsed ultrasound and pulsed electromagnetic fields bone growth stimulation in acute fractures: a systematic review and meta-analysis of randomized controlled trials. Arch Orthop Trauma Surg. 2014;134(8):1093–106.
47. Heckman JD, Ryaby JP, McCabe J, Frey JJ, Kilcoyne RF. Acceleration of tibial fracture-healing by non-invasive, low-intensity pulsed ultrasound. J Bone Jt Surg Am. 1994;76(1):26–34.
48. Kristiansen TK, Ryaby JP, McCabe J, Frey JJ, Roe LR. Accelerated healing of distal radial fractures with the use of specific, low-intensity ultrasound. A multicenter, prospective, randomized, double-blind, placebo-controlled study. J Bone Jt Surg Am. 1997;79(7):961–73.
49. Emami A, Petren-Mallmin M, Larsson S. No effect of low-intensity ultrasound on healing time of intramedullary fixed tibial fractures. J Orthop Trauma. 1999;13(4):252–7.
50. Handolin L, Kiljunen V, Arnala I, et al. No long-term effects of ultrasound therapy on bioabsorbable screw-fixed lateral malleolar fracture. Scand J Surg. 2005;94(3):239–42.
51. Handolin L, Kiljunen V, Arnala I, et al. Effect of ultrasound therapy on bone healing of lateral malleolar fractures of the ankle joint fixed with bioabsorbable screws. J Orthop Sci. 2005;10(4):391–5.
52. Simpson AH, Keenan G, Nayagam S, Atkins RM, Marsh D, Clement ND. Low-intensity pulsed ultrasound does not influence bone healing by distraction osteogenesis: a multicentre double-blind randomised control trial. Bone Jt J. 2017;99-B(4):494–502.
53. Song MH, Kim TJ, Kang SH, Song HR. Low-intensity pulsed ultrasound enhances callus consolidation in distraction osteogenesis of the tibia by the technique of lengthening over the nail procedure. BMC Musculoskelet Disord. 2019;20(1):108.
54. Raza H, Saltaji H, Kaur H, Flores-Mir C, El-Bialy T. Effect of low-intensity pulsed ultrasound on distraction osteogenesis treatment time: a meta-analysis of randomized clinical trials. J Ultrasound Med. 2016;35(2):349–58.
55. Sakurakichi K, Tsuchiya H, Uehara K, Yamashiro T, Tomita K, Azuma Y. Effects of timing of low-intensity pulsed ultrasound on distraction osteogenesis. J Orthop Res. 2004;22(2):395–403.
56. Taylor KF, Rafiee B, Tis JE, Inoue N. Low-intensity pulsed ultrasound does not enhance distraction callus in a rabbit model. Clin Orthop Relat Res. 2007;459:237–45.
57. Lou S, Lv H, Li Z, Tang P, Wang Y. Effect of low-intensity pulsed ultrasound on distraction osteogenesis: a systematic review and meta-analysis of randomized controlled trials. J Orthop Surg Res. 2018;13(1):205.
58. Adie S, Harris IA, Naylor JM, et al. Pulsed electromagnetic field stimulation for acute tibial shaft fractures: a multicenter, double-blind, randomized trial. J Bone Jt Surg Am. 2011;93(17):1569–76.
59. Bassett CA, Mitchell SN, Gaston SR. Treatment of ununited tibial diaphyseal fractures with pulsing electromagnetic fields. J Bone Jt Surg Am. 1981;63(4):511–23.
60. Hannemann PF, Gottgens KW, van Wely BJ, et al. The clinical and radiological outcome of pulsed electromagnetic field treatment for acute scaphoid fractures: a randomised double-

blind placebo-controlled multicentre trial. J Bone Jt Surg Br. 2012;94(10):1403–8.
61. Fredericks DC, Piehl DJ, Baker JT, Abbott J, Nepola JV. Effects of pulsed electromagnetic field stimulation on distraction osteogenesis in the rabbit tibial leg lengthening model. J Pediatr Orthop. 2003;23(4):478–83.
62. Taylor KF, Inoue N, Rafiee B, Tis JE, McHale KA, Chao EY. Effect of pulsed electromagnetic fields on maturation of regenerate bone in a rabbit limb lengthening model. J Orthop Res. 2006;24(1):2–10.
63. Jauregui JJ, Ventimiglia AV, Grieco PW, Frumberg DB, Herzenberg JE. Regenerate bone stimulation following limb lengthening: a meta-analysis. BMC Musculoskelet Disord. 2016;17(1):407.
64. Lane JM. Bone morphogenic protein science and studies. J Orthop Trauma. 2005;19(10 Suppl):S17–22.
65. Schmidmaier G, Schwabe P, Wildemann B, Haas NP. Use of bone morphogenetic proteins for treatment of non-unions and future perspectives. Injury. 2007;38(Suppl 4):S35–41.
66. Schmidmaier G, Wildemann B, Cromme F, Kandziora F, Haas NP, Raschke M. Bone morphogenetic protein-2 coating of titanium implants increases biomechanical strength and accelerates bone remodeling in fracture treatment: a biomechanical and histological study in rats. Bone. 2002;30(6):816–22.
67. Yang JH, Kim HJ, Kim SE, et al. The effect of bone morphogenic protein-2-coated tri-calcium phosphate/hydroxyapatite on new bone formation in a rat model of femoral distraction osteogenesis. Cytotherapy. 2012;14(3):315–26.
68. Hamdy RC, Amako M, Beckman L, et al. Effects of osteogenic protein-1 on distraction osteogenesis in rabbits. Bone. 2003;33(2):248–55.
69. Janicki P, Schmidmaier G. What should be the characteristics of the ideal bone graft substitute? Combining scaffolds with growth factors and/or stem cells. Injury. 2011;42(Suppl 2):S77–81.
70. Mandu-Hrit M, Haque T, Lauzier D, et al. Early injection of OP-1 during distraction osteogenesis accelerates new bone formation in rabbits. Growth Factors. 2006;24(3):172–83.
71. Mizumoto Y, Moseley T, Drews M, Cooper VN 3rd, Reddi AH. Acceleration of regenerate ossification during distraction osteogenesis with recombinant human bone morphogenetic protein-7. J Bone Jt Surg Am. 2003;85-A(Suppl 3):124–30.
72. Friedlaender GE, Perry CR, Cole JD, et al. Osteogenic protein-1 (bone morphogenetic protein-7) in the treatment of tibial nonunions. J Bone Jt Surg Am. 2001;83-A(Suppl 1(Pt 2)):S151–8.
73. Govender S, Csimma C, Genant HK, et al. Recombinant human bone morphogenetic protein-2 for treatment of open tibial fractures: a prospective, controlled, randomized study of four hundred and fifty patients. J Bone Jt Surg Am. 2002;84(12):2123–34.
74. Bokobza SM, Ye L, Jiang WG. When BMP signalling goes wrong: the intracellular and molecular mechanisms of BMP signalling in cancer. Curr Signal Transduct Ther. 2009;4(3):174–95.
75. Carragee EJ, Chu G, Rohatgi R, Hurwitz EL, Weiner BK, Yoon ST, et al. Cancer risk after use of recombinant bone morphogenetic protein-2 for spinal arthrodesis. J Bone Jt Surg Am. 2013;95(17):1537–45.
76. Cooper GS, Kou TD. Risk of cancer after lumbar fusion surgery with recombinant human bone morphogenic protein-2 (rhBMP-2). Spine (Phila Pa 1976). 2013;38(21):1862–8.
77. Kokorina NA, Lewis JS Jr, Zakharkin SO, Krebsbach PH, Nussenbaum B. rhBMP-2 has adverse effects on human oral carcinoma cell lines in vivo. Laryngoscope. 2012;122(1):95–102.
78. Poynton AR, Lane JM. Safety profile for the clinical use of bone morphogenetic proteins in the spine. Spine. 2002;27(16 Suppl 1):S40–8.
79. Rothhammer T, Poser I, Soncin F, Bataille F, Moser M, Bosserhoff AK. Bone morphogenic proteins are overexpressed in malignant melanoma and promote cell invasion and migration. Cancer Res. 2005;65(2):448–56.
80. Bierie B, Moses HL. Tumour microenvironment: TGFbeta: the molecular Jekyll and Hyde of cancer. Nat Rev Cancer. 2006;6(7):506–20.
81. Fu R, Selph S, McDonagh M, et al. Effectiveness and harms of recombinant human bone morphogenetic protein-2 in spine fusion: a systematic review and meta-analysis. Ann Intern Med. 2013;158(12):890–902.
82. Shweikeh F, Hanna G, Bloom L, Sayegh ET, Liu J, Acosta FL, et al. Assessment of outcome following the use of recombinant human bone morphogenetic protein-2 for spinal fusion in the elderly population. J Neurosurg Sci. 2014;60(2):256–71.
83. Rahman MS, Akhtar N, Jamil HM, Banik RS, Asaduzzaman SM. TGF-beta/BMP signaling and other molecular events: regulation of osteoblastogenesis and bone formation. Bone Res. 2015;3:15005.
84. Liu D, Zhao Z, Jiang W, et al. *Panax notoginseng* saponin promotes bone regeneration in distraction osteogenesis via the TGF-beta1 signaling pathway. Evid Based Complement Alternat Med. 2021;2021:2895659.
85. Cicciu M, Fiorillo L, Cervino G, Habal MB. Bone morphogenetic protein application as grafting materials for bone regeneration in craniofacial surgery: current application and future directions. J Craniofac Surg. 2021;32(2):787–93.
86. Jager M, Jelinek EM, Wess KM, et al. Bone marrow concentrate: a novel strategy for bone defect treatment. Curr Stem Cell Res Ther. 2009;4(1):34–43.
87. Yang Y, Pan Q, Zou K, et al. Administration of allogeneic mesenchymal stem cells in lengthening phase accelerates early bone consolidation in rat distraction osteogenesis model. Stem Cell Res Ther. 2020;11(1):129.
88. Pan Q, Li Y, Li Y, et al. Local administration of allogeneic or autologous bone marrow-derived mesenchymal stromal cells enhances bone formation similarly in distraction osteogenesis. Cytotherapy. 2021;23(7):590–8.
89. Montes-Medina L, Hernandez-Fernandez A, Gutierrez-Rivera A, et al. Effect of bone marrow stromal cells in combination with biomaterials in early phases of distraction osteogenesis: an experimental study in a rabbit femur model. Injury. 2018;49(11):1979–86.
90. Kitoh H, Kitakoji T, Tsuchiya H, Katoh M, Ishiguro N. Distraction osteogenesis of the lower extremity in patients with achondroplasia/hypochondroplasia treated with transplantation of culture-expanded bone marrow cells and platelet-rich plasma. J Pediatr Orthop. 2007;27(6):629–34.
91. Takamine Y, Tsuchiya H, Kitakoji T, et al. Distraction osteogenesis enhanced by osteoblastlike cells and collagen gel. Clin Orthop Relat Res. 2002;399:240–6.
92. Lim HJ, Lee EM, Kim WK, Kim HJ, Kim BC, Lee J. Application of autologous human bone marrow-derived mesenchymal stem cells in distraction osteogenesis for the treatment of bilateral mandibular hypoplasia. J Craniofac Surg. 2018;29(6):1629–32.
93. Arora NS, Ramanayake T, Ren YF, Romanos GE. Platelet-rich plasma in sinus augmentation procedures: a systematic literature review: part II. Implant Dent. 2010;19(2):145–57.
94. Dallari D, Fini M, Stagni C, et al. In vivo study on the healing of bone defects treated with bone marrow stromal cells, platelet-rich plasma, and freeze-dried bone allografts, alone and in combination. J Orthop Res. 2006;24(5):877–88.
95. Kawasumi M, Kitoh H, Siwicka KA, Ishiguro N. The effect of the platelet concentration in platelet-rich plasma gel on the regeneration of bone. J Bone Jt Surg Br. 2008;90(7):966–72.
96. Thor A, Wannfors K, Sennerby L, Rasmusson L. Reconstruction of the severely resorbed maxilla with autogenous bone, platelet-rich plasma, and implants: 1-year results of a controlled prospective 5-year study. Clin Implant Dent Relat Res. 2005;7(4):209–20.

97. Arpornmaeklong P, Kochel M, Depprich R, Kubler NR, Wurzler KK. Influence of platelet-rich plasma (PRP) on osteogenic differentiation of rat bone marrow stromal cells. An in vitro study. Int J Oral Maxillofac Surg. 2004;33(1):60–70.
98. Latalski M, Elbatrawy YA, Thabet AM, Gregosiewicz A, Raganowicz T, Fatyga M. Enhancing bone healing during distraction osteogenesis with platelet-rich plasma. Injury. 2011;42(8):821–4.
99. Lee DH, Ryu KJ, Kim JW, Kang KC, Choi YR. Bone marrow aspirate concentrate and platelet-rich plasma enhanced bone healing in distraction osteogenesis of the tibia. Clin Orthop Relat Res. 2014;472(12):3789–97.
100. Sauerbier S, Rickert D, Gutwald R, et al. Bone marrow concentrate and bovine bone mineral for sinus floor augmentation: a controlled, randomized, single-blinded clinical and histological trial—per-protocol analysis. Tissue Eng Part A. 2011;17(17–18):2187–97.
101. Aghaloo TL, Moy PK, Freymiller EG. Investigation of platelet-rich plasma in rabbit cranial defects: a pilot study. J Oral Maxillofac Surg. 2002;60(10):1176–81.
102. Anitua E. Plasma rich in growth factors: preliminary results of use in the preparation of future sites for implants. Int J Oral Maxillofac Implants. 1999;14(4):529–35.
103. Anitua E, Andia I, Ardanza B, Nurden P, Nurden AT. Autologous platelets as a source of proteins for healing and tissue regeneration. Thromb Haemost. 2004;91(1):4–15.
104. Fang TD, Salim A, Xia W, et al. Angiogenesis is required for successful bone induction during distraction osteogenesis. J Bone Miner Res. 2005;20(7):1114–24.
105. Gandhi A, Doumas C, O'Connor JP, Parsons JR, Lin SS. The effects of local platelet rich plasma delivery on diabetic fracture healing. Bone. 2006;38(4):540–6.
106. Gruber R, Karreth F, Fischer MB, Watzek G. Platelet-released supernatants stimulate formation of osteoclast-like cells through a prostaglandin/RANKL-dependent mechanism. Bone. 2002;30(5):726–32.
107. Hernandez-Fernandez A, Velez R, Soldado F, Saenz-Rios JC, Barber I, Aguirre-Canyadell M. Effect of administration of platelet-rich plasma in early phases of distraction osteogenesis: an experimental study in an ovine femur model. Injury. 2013;44(7):901–7.
108. Kanno T, Takahashi T, Tsujisawa T, Ariyoshi W, Nishihara T. Platelet-rich plasma enhances human osteoblast-like cell proliferation and differentiation. J Oral Maxillofac Surg. 2005;63(3):362–9.
109. Kilian O, Flesch I, Wenisch S, et al. Effects of platelet growth factors on human mesenchymal stem cells and human endothelial cells in vitro. Eur J Med Res. 2004;9(7):337–44.
110. Marx RE. Platelet-rich plasma (PRP): what is PRP and what is not PRP? Implant Dent. 2001;10(4):225–8.
111. Shanaman R, Filstein MR, Danesh-Meyer MJ. Localized ridge augmentation using GBR and platelet-rich plasma: case reports. Int J Periodontics Restorative Dent. 2001;21(4):345–55.
112. Kitoh H, Kitakoji T, Tsuchiya H, Katoh M, Ishiguro N. Transplantation of culture expanded bone marrow cells and platelet rich plasma in distraction osteogenesis of the long bones. Bone. 2007;40(2):522–8.
113. Tonogai I, Hayashi F, Iwame T, Takasago T, Matsuura T, Sairyo K. Platelet-rich plasma does not reduce skeletal muscle fibrosis after distraction osteogenesis. J Exp Orthop. 2018;5(1):26.
114. Marcacci M, Kon E, Moukhachev V, et al. Stem cells associated with macroporous bioceramics for long bone repair: 6–7-year outcome of a pilot clinical study. Tissue Eng. 2007;13(5):947–55.
115. Kim SJ, Shin YW, Yang KH, et al. A multi-center, randomized, clinical study to compare the effect and safety of autologous cultured osteoblast(Ossron) injection to treat fractures. BMC Musculoskelet Disord. 2009;10:20.
116. Kim SJ, Bahk WJ, Chang CH, Jang JD, Suhl KH. Treatment of osteonecrosis of the femoral head using autologous cultured osteoblasts: a case report. J Med Case Rep. 2008;2:58.
117. Pittenger MF, Mackay AM, Beck SC, et al. Multilineage potential of adult human mesenchymal stem cells. Science. 1999;284(5411):143–7.
118. Peters A, Toben D, Lienau J, et al. Locally applied osteogenic predifferentiated progenitor cells are more effective than undifferentiated mesenchymal stem cells in the treatment of delayed bone healing. Tissue Eng Part A. 2009;15(10):2947–54.
119. Marx RE, Carlson ER, Eichstaedt RM, Schimmele SR, Strauss JE, Georgeff KR. Platelet-rich plasma: growth factor enhancement for bone grafts. Oral Surg Oral Med Oral Pathol Oral Radiol Endod. 1998;85(6):638–46.
120. Lucarelli E, Fini M, Beccheroni A, et al. Stromal stem cells and platelet-rich plasma improve bone allograft integration. Clin Orthop Relat Res. 2005;435:62–8.
121. Bueno EM, Glowacki J. Cell-free and cell-based approaches for bone regeneration. Nat Rev Rheumatol. 2009;5(12):685–97.
122. Cen L, Liu W, Cui L, Zhang W, Cao Y. Collagen tissue engineering: development of novel biomaterials and applications. Pediatr Res. 2008;63(5):492–6.
123. Fufa D, Shealy B, Jacobson M, Kevy S, Murray MM. Activation of platelet-rich plasma using soluble type I collagen. J Oral Maxillofac Surg. 2008;66(4):684–90.
124. Vaccaro AR. The role of the osteoconductive scaffold in synthetic bone graft. Orthopedics. 2002;25(5 Suppl):s571–8.
125. Ren LF, Shi GS, Tong YQ, Jiang SY, Zhang F. Effects of rhBMP-2/7 heterodimer and RADA16 hydrogel scaffold on bone formation during rabbit mandibular distraction. J Oral Maxillofac Surg. 2018;76(5):1092 e1–e10.
126. Ma G, Zhao JL, Mao M, Chen J, Dong ZW, Liu YP. Scaffold-based delivery of bone marrow mesenchymal stem cell sheet fragments enhances new bone formation in vivo. J Oral Maxillofac Surg. 2017;75(1):92–104.
127. Zhao D, Jiang W, Wang Y, et al. Three-dimensional-printed poly-L-lactic acid scaffolds with different pore sizes influence periosteal distraction osteogenesis of a rabbit skull. Biomed Res Int. 2020;2020:7381391.
128. Lee J, Sung HM, Jang JD, Park YW, Min SK, Kim EC. Successful reconstruction of 15-cm segmental defects by bone marrow stem cells and resected autogenous bone graft in central hemangioma. J Oral Maxillofac Surg. 2010;68(1):188–94.
129. Antebi B, Pelled G, Gazit D. Stem cell therapy for osteoporosis. Curr Osteoporos Rep. 2014;12(1):41–7.
130. Ohgushi H, Caplan AI. Stem cell technology and bioceramics: from cell to gene engineering. J Biomed Mater Res. 1999;48(6):913–27.
131. Fife C, Mader JT, Stone J, et al. Thrombin peptide Chrysalin stimulates healing of diabetic foot ulcers in a placebo-controlled phase I/II study. Wound Repair Regen. 2007;15(1):23–34.
132. Cakarer S, Olgac V, Aksakalli N, Tang A, Keskin C. Acceleration of consolidation period by thrombin peptide 508 in tibial distraction osteogenesis in rats. Br J Oral Maxillofac Surg. 2010;48(8):633–6.
133. Hanratty BM, Ryaby JT, Pan XH, Li G. Thrombin related peptide TP508 promoted fracture repair in a mouse high energy fracture model. J Orthop Surg Res. 2009;4:1.
134. Wang H, Li X, Tomin E, et al. Thrombin peptide (TP508) promotes fracture repair by up-regulating inflammatory mediators, early growth factors, and increasing angiogenesis. J Orthop Res. 2005;23(3):671–9.
135. Yamamoto S. The effect of 2 beta-(3-hydroxypropoxy)-1 alpha, 25-dihydroxyvitamin D3 (ED-71) on callotasis in rabbit. Nihon Seikeigeka Gakkai Zasshi. 1995;69(4):209–21.

136. Yamane K, Okano T, Kishimoto H, Hagino H. Effect of ED-71 on modeling of bone in distraction osteogenesis. Bone. 1999;24(3):187–93.
137. Okazaki H, Kurokawa T, Nakamura K, Matsushita T, Mamada K, Kawaguchi H. Stimulation of bone formation by recombinant fibroblast growth factor-2 in callotasis bone lengthening of rabbits. Calcif Tissue Int. 1999;64(6):542–6.
138. Aronson J. Modulation of distraction osteogenesis in the aged rat by fibroblast growth factor. Clin Orthop Relat Res. 2004;425:264–83.
139. Jiang X, Zou S, Ye B, Zhu S, Liu Y, Hu J. bFGF-modified BMMSCs enhance bone regeneration following distraction osteogenesis in rabbits. Bone. 2010;46(4):1156–61.
140. Kumabe Y, Fukui T, Takahara S, et al. Percutaneous CO_2 treatment accelerates bone generation during distraction osteogenesis in rabbits. Clin Orthop Relat Res. 2020;478(8):1922–35.
141. Maes C, Coenegrachts L, Stockmans I, et al. Placental growth factor mediates mesenchymal cell development, cartilage turnover, and bone remodeling during fracture repair. J Clin Invest. 2006;116(5):1230–42.
142. Street J, Bao M, deGuzman L, et al. Vascular endothelial growth factor stimulates bone repair by promoting angiogenesis and bone turnover. Proc Natl Acad Sci USA. 2002;99(15):9656–61.
143. Weiss S, Zimmermann G, Baumgart R, Kasten P, Bidlingmaier M, Henle P. Systemic regulation of angiogenesis and matrix degradation in bone regeneration—distraction osteogenesis compared to rigid fracture healing. Bone. 2005;37(6):781–90.
144. Nunotani Y, Abe M, Shirai H, Otsuka H. Efficacy of rhBMP-2 during distraction osteogenesis. J Orthop Sci. 2005;10(5):529–33.
145. Sailhan F, Gleyzolle B, Parot R, Guerini H, Viguier E. Rh-BMP-2 in distraction osteogenesis: dose effect and premature consolidation. Injury. 2010;41(7):680–6.
146. Haque T, Amako M, Nakada S, Lauzier D, Hamdy RC. An immunohistochemical analysis of the temporal and spatial expression of growth factors FGF 1, 2 and 18, IGF 1 and 2, and TGFbeta1 during distraction osteogenesis. Histol Histopathol. 2007;22(2):119–28.
147. Jacobsen KA, Al-Aql ZS, Wan C, Fitch JL, Stapleton SN, Mason ZD, et al. Bone formation during distraction osteogenesis is dependent on both VEGFR1 and VEGFR2 signaling. J Bone Miner Res. 2008;23(5):596–609.
148. Siwicka KA, Kitoh H, Kawasumi M, Ishiguro N. Spatial and temporal distribution of growth factors receptors in the callus: implications for improvement of distraction osteogenesis. Nagoya J Med Sci. 2011;73(3–4):117–27.
149. Tavakoli K, Yu Y, Shahidi S, Bonar F, Walsh WR, Poole MD. Expression of growth factors in the mandibular distraction zone: a sheep study. Br J Plast Surg. 1999;52(6):434–9.
150. Rauch F, Lauzier D, Croteau S, Travers R, Glorieux FH, Hamdy R. Temporal and spatial expression of bone morphogenetic protein-2, -4, and -7 during distraction osteogenesis in rabbits. Bone. 2000;26(6):611–7.
151. Lesaichot V, Leperlier D, Viateau V, Richarme D, Petite H, Sailhan F. The influence of bone morphogenic protein-2 on the consolidation phase in a distraction osteogenesis model. Injury. 2011;42(12):1460–6.
152. Park HW, Yang KH, Lee KS, Joo SY, Kwak YH, Kim HW. Tibial lengthening over an intramedullary nail with use of the Ilizarov external fixator for idiopathic short stature. J Bone Jt Surg Am. 2008;90(9):1970–8.
153. Dempster DW, Cosman F, Parisien M, Shen V, Lindsay R. Anabolic actions of parathyroid hormone on bone. Endocr Rev. 1993;14(6):690–709.
154. Reeve J, Hesp R, Williams D, et al. Anabolic effect of low doses of a fragment of human parathyroid hormone on the skeleton in postmenopausal osteoporosis. Lancet. 1976;1(7968):1035–8.
155. Andreassen TT, Cacciafesta V. Intermittent parathyroid hormone treatment enhances guided bone regeneration in rat calvarial bone defects. J Craniofac Surg. 2004;15(3):424–7.
156. Tam CS, Heersche JN, Murray TM, Parsons JA. Parathyroid hormone stimulates the bone apposition rate independently of its resorptive action: differential effects of intermittent and continuous administration. Endocrinology. 1982;110(2):506–12.
157. Hock JM, Gera I. Effects of continuous and intermittent administration and inhibition of resorption on the anabolic response of bone to parathyroid hormone. J Bone Miner Res. 1992;7(1):65–72.
158. Podbesek R, Edouard C, Meunier PJ, et al. Effects of two treatment regimes with synthetic human parathyroid hormone fragment on bone formation and the tissue balance of trabecular bone in greyhounds. Endocrinology. 1983;112(3):1000–6.
159. Chen H, Frankenburg EP, Goldstein SA, McCauley LK. Combination of local and systemic parathyroid hormone enhances bone regeneration. Clin Orthop Relat Res. 2003;416:291–302.
160. Skripitz R, Andreassen TT, Aspenberg P. Strong effect of PTH (1–34) on regenerating bone: a time sequence study in rats. Acta Orthop Scand. 2000;71(6):619–24.
161. Neer RM, Arnaud CD, Zanchetta JR, et al. Effect of parathyroid hormone (1–34) on fractures and bone mineral density in postmenopausal women with osteoporosis. N Engl J Med. 2001;344(19):1434–41.
162. Ye B, Li Y, Zhu S, Sun S, Hu J, Zou S. Effects of intermittent low-dose parathyroid hormone treatment on rapid mandibular distraction osteogenesis in rabbits. J Oral Maxillofac Surg. 2017;75(8):1722–31.
163. Leiblein M, Henrich D, Fervers F, Kontradowitz K, Marzi I, Seebach C. Do antiosteoporotic drugs improve bone regeneration in vivo? Eur J Trauma Emerg Surg. 2020;46(2):287–99.
164. Wagner F, Vach W, Augat P, et al. Daily subcutaneous Teriparatide injection increased bone mineral density of newly formed bone after tibia distraction osteogenesis, a randomized study. Injury. 2019;50(8):1478–82.
165. Jilka RL, Weinstein RS, Bellido T, Roberson P, Parfitt AM, Manolagas SC. Increased bone formation by prevention of osteoblast apoptosis with parathyroid hormone. J Clin Invest. 1999;104(4):439–46.
166. Raschke MJ, Bail H, Windhagen HJ, et al. Recombinant growth hormone accelerates bone regenerate consolidation in distraction osteogenesis. Bone. 1999;24(2):81–8.
167. Ohlsson C, Bengtsson BA, Isaksson OG, Andreassen TT, Slootweg MC. Growth hormone and bone. Endocr Rev. 1998;19(1):55–79.
168. Cacciafesta V, Dalstra M, Bosch C, Melsen B, Andreassen TT. Growth hormone treatment promotes guided bone regeneration in rat calvarial defects. Eur J Orthod. 2001;23(6):733–40.
169. Bak B, Andreassen TT. The effect of growth hormone on fracture healing in old rats. Bone. 1991;12(3):151–4.
170. Bak B, Jorgensen PH, Andreassen TT. The stimulating effect of growth hormone on fracture healing is dependent on onset and duration of administration. Clin Orthop Relat Res. 1991;264:295–301.
171. Sirin Y, Olgac V, Dogru-Abbasoglu S, Tapul L, Aktas S, Soley S. The influence of hyperbaric oxygen treatment on the healing of experimental defects filled with different bone graft substitutes. Int J Med Sci. 2011;8(2):114–25.
172. Bennett MH, Stanford R, Turner R. Hyperbaric oxygen therapy for promoting fracture healing and treating fracture non-union. Cochrane Database Syst Rev. 2005;1:CD004712.
173. Notelovitz M. Androgen effects on bone and muscle. Fertil Steril. 2002;77(Suppl 4):S34–41.
174. Maus U, Andereya S, Schmidt H, et al. Therapy effects of testosterone on the recovery of bone defects. Z Orthop Unfall. 2008;146(1):59–63.

175. Roseren F, Pithioux M, Robert S, et al. Systemic administration of G-CSF accelerates bone regeneration and modulates mobilization of progenitor cells in a rat model of distraction osteogenesis. Int J Mol Sci. 2021;22(7):3505.
176. Yun YP, Kim SJ, Lim YM, et al. The effect of alendronate-loaded polycaprolactone nanofibrous scaffolds on osteogenic differentiation of adipose-derived stem cells in bone tissue regeneration. J Biomed Nanotechnol. 2014;10(6):1080–90.
177. von Knoch F, Eckhardt C, Alabre CI, Schneider E, Rubash HE, Shanbhag AS. Anabolic effects of bisphosphonates on peri-implant bone stock. Biomaterials. 2007;28(24):3549–59.
178. Allgrove J. Use of bisphosphonates in children and adolescents. J Pediatr Endocrinol Metab. 2002;15(Suppl 3):921–8.
179. Licata AA. Bisphosphonate therapy. Am J Med Sci. 1997;313(1):17–22.
180. Fleisch H. New bisphosphonates in osteoporosis. Osteoporos Int. 1993;3(Suppl 2):S15–22.
181. Russell RG. Bisphosphonates: from bench to bedside. Ann N Y Acad Sci. 2006;1068:367–401.
182. Kavanagh KL, Guo K, Dunford JE, Wu X, Knapp S, Ebetino FH, et al. The molecular mechanism of nitrogen-containing bisphosphonates as antiosteoporosis drugs. Proc Natl Acad Sci U S A. 2006;103(20):7829–34.
183. Giuliani N, Pedrazzoni M, Negri G, Passeri G, Impicciatore M, Girasole G. Bisphosphonates stimulate formation of osteoblast precursors and mineralized nodules in murine and human bone marrow cultures in vitro and promote early osteoblastogenesis in young and aged mice in vivo. Bone. 1998;22(5):455–61.
184. Maffulli N, Cheng JC, Sher A, Lam TP. Dual-energy X-ray absorptiometry predicts bone formation in lower limb callotasis lengthening. Ann R Coll Surg Engl. 1997;79(4):250–6.
185. Kiely P, Ward K, Bellemore CM, Briody J, Cowell CT, Little DG. Bisphosphonate rescue in distraction osteogenesis: a case series. J Pediatr Orthop. 2007;27(4):467–71.
186. Im GI, Qureshi SA, Kenney J, Rubash HE, Shanbhag AS. Osteoblast proliferation and maturation by bisphosphonates. Biomaterials. 2004;25(18):4105–15.
187. Akbulut Y, Gul M, Dundar S, et al. Evaluation of effects of systemic zoledronic acid application on bone maturation in the consolidation period in distraction osteogenesis. J Craniofac Surg. 2021;32(8):2901–5.
188. Plotkin LI, Weinstein RS, Parfitt AM, Roberson PK, Manolagas SC, Bellido T. Prevention of osteocyte and osteoblast apoptosis by bisphosphonates and calcitonin. J Clin Invest. 1999;104(10):1363–74.
189. Duque G, Rivas D. Alendronate has an anabolic effect on bone through the differentiation of mesenchymal stem cells. J Bone Miner Res. 2007;22(10):1603–11.
190. Wang CZ, Chen SM, Chen CH, et al. The effect of the local delivery of alendronate on human adipose-derived stem cell-based bone regeneration. Biomaterials. 2010;31(33):8674–83.
191. Takahashi M, Yukata K, Matsui Y, Abbaspour A, Takata S, Yasui N. Bisphosphonate modulates morphological and mechanical properties in distraction osteogenesis through inhibition of bone resorption. Bone. 2006;39(3):573–81.
192. Yoshiga D, Yamashita Y, Nakamichi I, et al. Weekly teriparatide injections successfully treated advanced bisphosphonate-related osteonecrosis of the jaws. Osteoporos Int. 2013;24(8):2365–9.
193. Curi MM, Cossolin GS, Koga DH, Zardetto C, Christianini S, Feher O, et al. Bisphosphonate-related osteonecrosis of the jaws—an initial case series report of treatment combining partial bone resection and autologous platelet-rich plasma. J Oral Maxillofac Surg. 2011;69(9):2465–72.
194. Srisubut S, Teerakapong A, Vattraphodes T, Taweechaisupapong S. Effect of local delivery of alendronate on bone formation in bioactive glass grafting in rats. Oral Surg Oral Med Oral Pathol Oral Radiol Endod. 2007;104(4):e11–6.
195. Omi H, Kusumi T, Kijima H, Toh S. Locally administered low-dose alendronate increases bone mineral density during distraction osteogenesis in a rabbit model. J Bone Jt Surg Br. 2007;89(7):984–8.
196. Kucuk D, Ay S, Kara MI, Avunduk MC, Gumus C. Comparison of local and systemic alendronate on distraction osteogenesis. Int J Oral Maxillofac Surg. 2011;40(12):1395–400.
197. Alp YE, Taskaldiran A, Onder ME, et al. Effects of local low-dose alendronate injections into the distraction gap on new bone formation and distraction rate on distraction osteogenesis. J Craniofac Surg. 2017;28(8):2174–8.
198. Dundar S, Artas G, Acikan I, et al. Comparison of the effects of local and systemic zoledronic acid application on mandibular distraction osteogenesis. J Craniofac Surg. 2017;28(7):e621–e5.
199. Ziegler R, Delling G. Effect of calcitonin on the regeneration of a circumscribed bone defect (bored hole in the rat tibia). Acta Endocrinol. 1972;69(3):497–506.
200. Weiss RE, Singer FR, Gorn AH, Hofer DP, Nimni ME. Calcitonin stimulates bone formation when administered prior to initiation of osteogenesis. J Clin Invest. 1981;68(3):815–8.
201. Whitehead M, Lane G, Young O, et al. Interrelations of calcium-regulating hormones during normal pregnancy. Br Med J (Clin Res Ed). 1981;283(6283):10–2.
202. Hoff AO, Catala-Lehnen P, Thomas PM, et al. Increased bone mass is an unexpected phenotype associated with deletion of the calcitonin gene. J Clin Invest. 2002;110(12):1849–57.
203. Wallach S, Farley JR, Baylink DJ, Brenner-Gati L. Effects of calcitonin on bone quality and osteoblastic function. Calcif Tissue Int. 1993;52(5):335–9.

Residual Deformities of the Hip

Shawn C. Standard and Daniel K. Ruggles

Introduction: Defining Hip Deformity

Hip deformity in children may be caused by numerous etiologies and encompasses deformities that involve both the acetabulum and proximal femur. The three-dimensional configuration of the hip requires specific terminology to categorize these deformities (Box 36.1).

Coxa breva is defined as shortening and widening of the femoral neck. It is typically caused by growth disturbance of the proximal femoral physis, which alters the relationship of the tip of the greater trochanter to the center of the femoral head (Fig. 36.1). A mechanical disadvantage is created by diminishing the lever arm of the hip through decreasing the distance between the origin and insertion points of the gluteus medius muscle [1, 2]. Common causes of coxa breva are avascular necrosis (AVN) of the proximal femoral epiphysis, osteomyelitis of the proximal femur, and deformity associated with skeletal dysplasias.

Box 36.1 Anatomical classification of Hip Deformities

Deformity	Plane of deformity	Radiographic indicator example
Coxa breva	Axial deformity of femoral neck	Asymmetric/decreased tip of greater trochanter to center of femoral head distance (Fig. 36.1)
Coxa vara/Valga	Coronal deformity of femoral neck	NSA (neck shaft angle) <124°,>136° aMPFA (anatomic medial proximal femoral angle) <80°,>89° (Fig. 36.1a, b)
Coxa magna	Multiplanar deformity of femoral head	Increased/asymmetric femoral head width Loss of sphericity of femoral head (Fig. 36.4)
Acetabular anteversion/retroversion	Rotational deformity of acetabulum	Crossover sign
Femoral anteversion/retroversion	Rotational deformity of femoral neck	Southwick angle
Acetabular dysplasia	Multiplanar deformity of acetabulum	AI (acetabular index) <30° CEA (center edge angle) <20° Flattened/upsloped sourcil

---

S. C. Standard (✉)
International Center for Limb Lengthening, Rubin Institute for Advanced Orthopedics, Sinai Hospital of Baltimore, Baltimore, MD, USA
e-mail: sstandar@lifebridgehealth.org

D. K. Ruggles
Department of Orthopedic Surgery, Nicklaus Children's Hospital, Miami, FL, USA

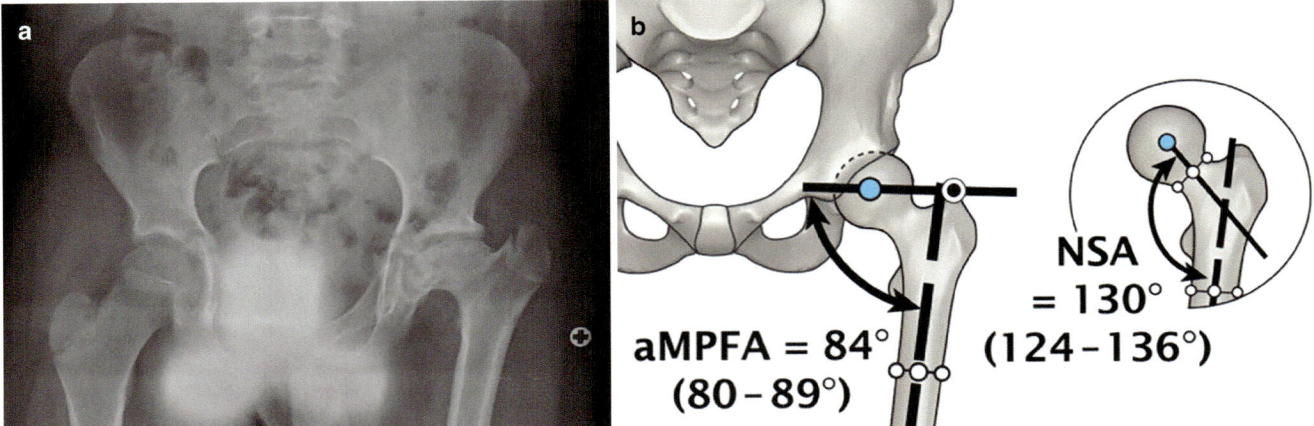

Fig. 36.1 (a) A 11-year-old patient with history of remote left septic hip presents with coxa breva and a Trendelenburg type gait of his left hip. Decreased neck length, decreased working length of the gluteus medius, and relative decreased anatomic medial proximal femoral angle (aMPFA) create a suboptimal biomechanical scenario for ambulation. (b) Anatomic norms for the sagittal plane of the proximal femur. Reprinted with the permission of Daniel Ruggles, DO and the Rubin Institute for Advanced Orthopedics, Sinai Hospital of Baltimore

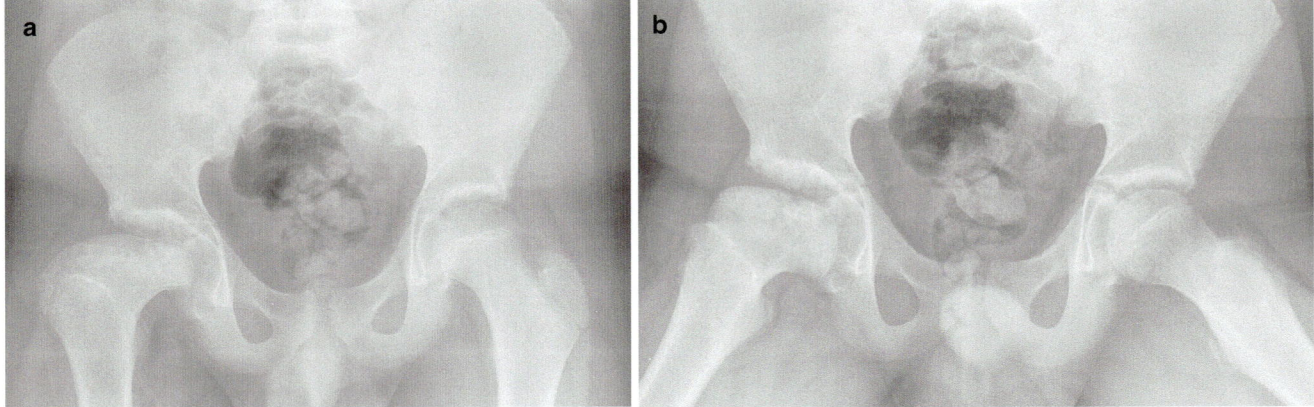

Fig. 36.2 A 12-year-old patient with severe coxa magna resulting from Perthes disease of the right hip as demonstrated on the AP (a) and lateral (b) views. Reprinted with permission from the Rubin Institute for Advanced Orthopedics, Sinai Hospital of Baltimore

Coxa magna is defined as an enlargement with the deformation of the femoral head. It is most commonly associated with a history of AVN. Collapse of the proximal femoral epiphysis and abnormal joint pressures alter the normal circumferential growth of the femoral head cartilage, resulting in irregular femoral head morphology [3]. Coxa magna can cause loss of congruency between the femoral head and acetabulum leading to femoral-acetabular impingement (FAI) (Fig. 36.2a, b). Sequelae of severe coxa magna includes chronic inflammation, loss of motion, labral pathology, chondromalacia, and eventual joint degeneration [4–7]. The differential diagnosis of pediatric hip AVN includes Legg–Calvé–Perthes disease, infection, sickle cell disease, chronic steroid use, trauma, and iatrogenic injury of the proximal femoral blood supply [8].

Acetabular deformity is typically termed "dysplasia" with abnormal anatomical characteristics of decrease depth, increased circumference, and increased slope in relation to the horizontal pelvic line [9]. This deformity results in an oblong-shaped, or "capacious" acetabulum, that allows lateral and proximal migration of the femoral head (Fig. 36.3). This abnormal position reduces coverage and total contact surface between the articular cartilage of the femoral head and acetabulum. Consequently, there are increased and concentrated contact forces that ultimately increase wear rate of the articular cartilage. The etiologies of acetabular dysplasia include developmental dysplasia of the hip (DDH), conditions of chronic joint laxity/instability (e.g., Down's syndrome), and joint contractures associated with neuromuscular disease [10, 11].

Hip deformity can also be described by rotational deformity, namely, anteversion and retroversion. Acetabular anteversion and retroversion are anterolateral and posterolateral directional deformities, respectively. The "cross-over" sign is a typical radiographic marker used to identify acetabular retroversion which is associated with FAI. Femoral anteversion and retroversion manifest clinically as intoeing or outtoeing, and can be attributed to rotational deformity of the femoral head (e.g., SCFE), femoral neck (e.g., congenital femoral deficiency), or the femoral shaft (e.g., physiologic femoral anteversion).

Because residual hip deformity often involves both acetabular dysplasia and femoral head deformity, surgeons must appreciate the concept of hip congruity. Developmental deformities in younger patients with remodelling potential may ultimately create a dysplastic, yet congruent, acetabulum that "matches" an abnormal femoral head (Fig. 36.4). This scenario may produce a relatively functional, mobile, and asymptomatic hip joint. However, potential impingement problems and early degenerative changes must be appreciated in terms of long-term prognosis.

This chapter will concentrate on treatment of residual hip deformities resulting from common pediatric hip pathology including DDH, slipped capital femoral epiphysis, and Legg–Calvé–Perthes disease. Innovative treatment strategies are presented with detailed surgical techniques of seven innovative procedures: open reduction and acetabuloplasty, triple pelvic osteotomy, modified Dunn procedure, modified Southwick intertrochanteric osteotomy, Morscher femoral neck lengthening osteotomy, femoral head reduction osteotomy, and hip distraction with a hinged external fixator.

Residual Hip Deformities Secondary to Developmental Dysplasia

The early postnatal examination and screening for congenital dislocation of the hip has substantially decreased the incidence of patients presenting with late dislocations of the hip joint during infancy and early childhood [12, 13]. However, the stable hip with mild to moderate hip dysplasia that is silent during the early developmental years remains a challenge to detect with clinical exam alone. Infants and children under the age of 2 years are able to be treated with nonoperative or minimally-invasive procedures [14] (Box 36.2).

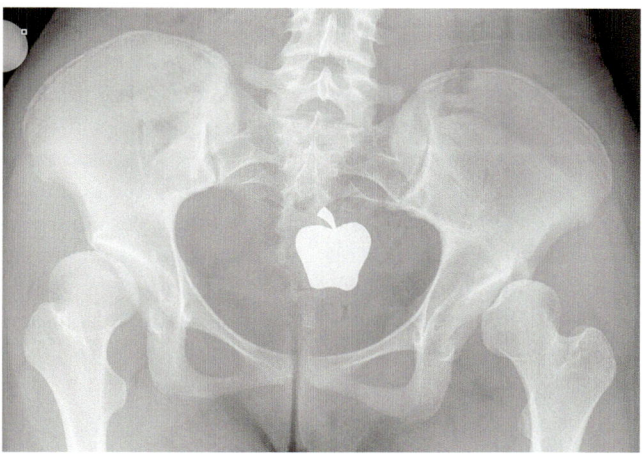

Fig. 36.3 A 14-year-old female with Down's syndrome and bilateral acetabular dysplasia noted by the enlarged, oblong, and shallow acetabulum and concurrent femoral head migration. Reprinted with permission from the Rubin Institute for Advanced Orthopedics, Sinai Hospital of Baltimore

Box 36.2 Treatment of DDH in Children <2 Years Old

Age	Treatment
< 6 months	Pavlik harness or abduction bracing
>6–18 months	Dysplasia: Abduction bracing Dislocation: Closed/open reduction and spica casting ± adductor tenotomy

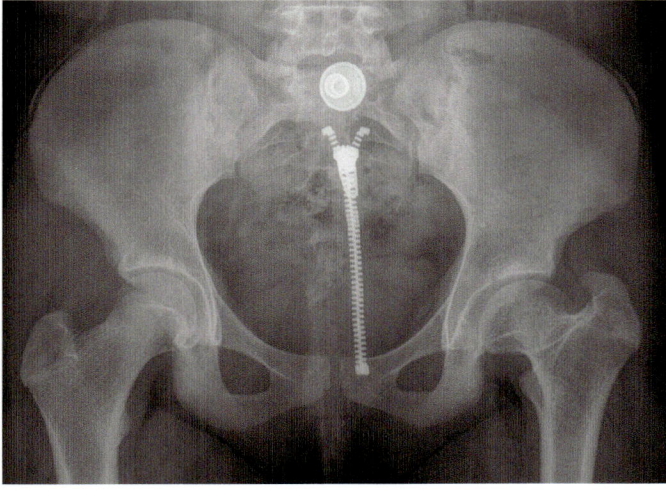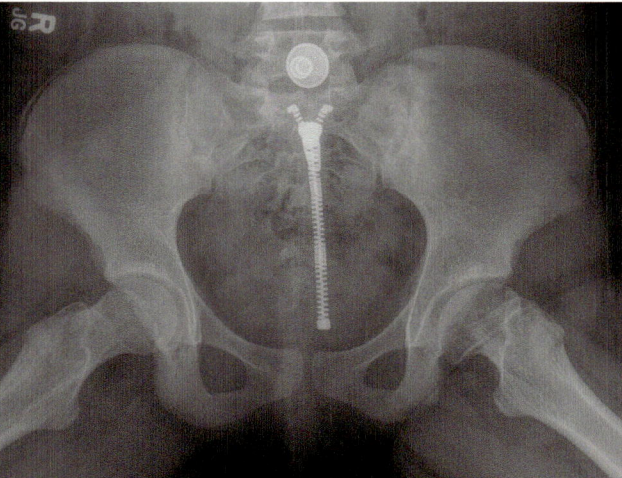

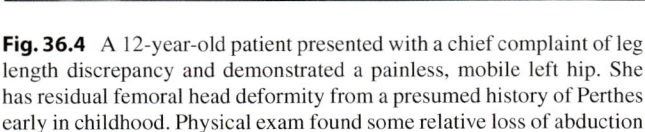

Fig. 36.4 A 12-year-old patient presented with a chief complaint of leg length discrepancy and demonstrated a painless, mobile left hip. She has residual femoral head deformity from a presumed history of Perthes early in childhood. Physical exam found some relative loss of abduction and rotation but within a functional range of overall motion. Radiographically, the hip joint shows excellent congruency and coverage despite the relative acetabular dysplasia and coxa magna. Reprinted with the permission of Daniel Ruggles, DO

The diagnosis of hip dysplasia for the older infant, toddler, and young child is radiographically defined by an acetabular index (AI) measurement >30° [15, 16]. For the older child, preadolescent, or adolescent, hip dysplasia can be designated by a center edge angle (CEA) of <20° [17]. Other radiographic signs of acetabular dysplasia are an abnormal sourcil, decreased femoral head coverage, and lateral/proximal migration of the femoral head [18].

> **Box 36.3 Radiographic Parameters of Acetabular Dysplasia**
>
> - Acetabular index >30°.
> - Center edge angle <20°.
> - Flattened/upsloped sourcil.

Treatment of Residual Hip Dysplasia in the Skeletally Immature Child

Establishing the goal of resolving acetabular dysplasia early in childhood (age 2–4 years) may ensure normal hip development as a child progresses through maturity. Surgeons may consider taking an aggressive approach to residual dysplasia to prevent residual hip deformity. Weinstein published a 40+ year follow-up study comparing closed reduction versus open reduction and Salter osteotomy for children with DDH from ages 18 months to 5 years. By reviewing 58 cases, he found hip survival rates of 50% and 69%, and estimated eventual failure rates of 91% and 55%, respectively, for closed reduction and spica casting versus open reduction and pelvic osteotomy, indicating the advantage of surgical reconstruction to treat residual dysplasia in young children [19].

Two types of pelvic osteotomies have been classically described to treat residual hip dysplasia in skeletally immature children: innominate osteotomy (Salter) and pericapsular acetabuloplasty (Dega, Pemberton). Robert Salter first described his osteotomy technique in 1961 and has since documented 45-year follow-up data [20, 21]. The original publication stated the indication as "instability of reduction in congenital dislocation and subluxation of the hip in children over the age of 18 months." The Salter osteotomy consists of a osteotomy from just above the anterior inferior iliac spine to the sciatic notch, including both inner and outer tables of the ilium. The Salter is a re-directional osteotomy that hinges on the flexible symphysis pubis. The complete osteotomy allows significant acetabular movement and correction; however, it requires internal fixation due to the amount of inherent instability. The osteotomy may provide excellent anterolateral coverage, but it is a relative contraindication when there is associated posterior acetabular insuf-

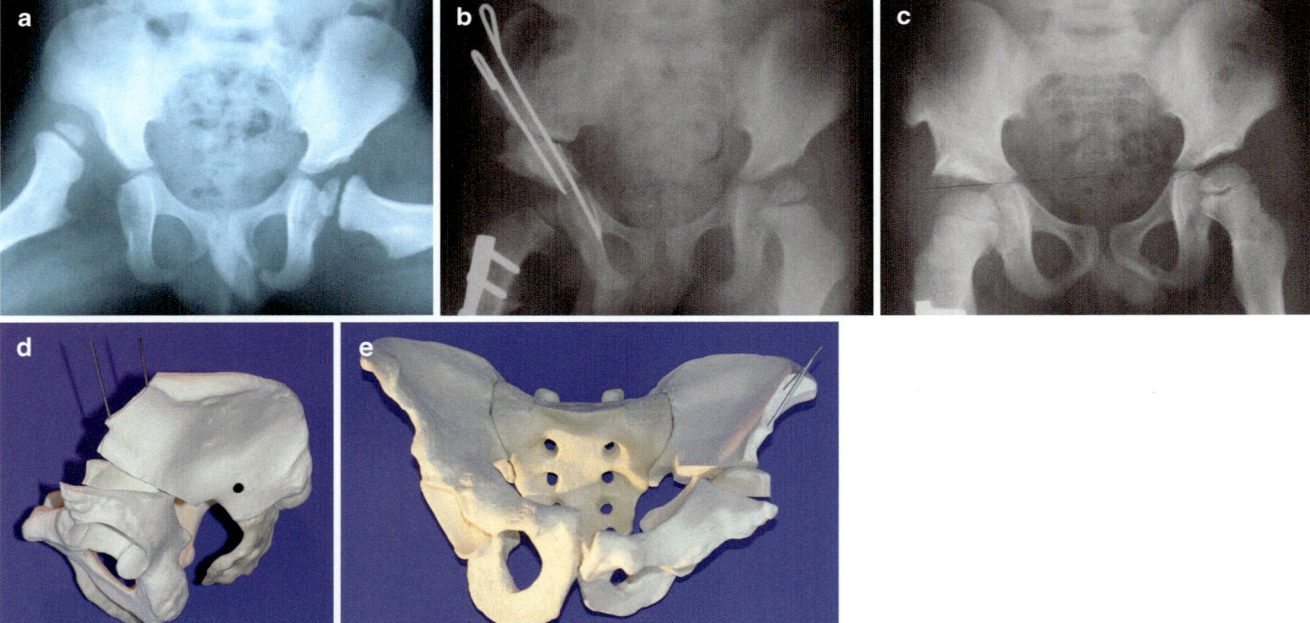

Fig. 36.5 (**a**) A 5-year-old male with R DDH. (**b**) Status-post open reduction, capsulorraphy, femoral shortening derotational osteotomy, and Salter innominate osteotomy. (**c**) Healed osteotomy with complete restoration of normal acetabular index, center-edge angle, and Shenton's line. (**d–e**) Bone models representing the Salter osteotomy. Reprinted with permission from Scott Nelson, MD

ficiency as it can further uncover the femoral head leading to posterior instability (Fig. 36.5a–e).

Pericapsular acetabuloplasties are incomplete osteotomies that hinge on the intact sciatic notch and bend through the triradiate cartilage creating a volume-reducing effect on the acetabulum (Fig. 36.6a–c). These curvilinear osteotomies may be fashioned by the surgeon to address the direction and severity of the acetabular deficiency in a particular case. An advantage of the single-cut acetabuloplasty is that they are inherently stable and typically do not require fixation. Wedges of bone graft (autograft harvested from the iliac crest or from the proximal femur when a shortening is performed, versus allograft bone) can strategically be placed in the osteotomy site to provide a combination of increased anterior and/or lateral coverage.

Pemberton first described his pericapsular osteotomy in 1965 with a cut through the inner and outer table of the ilium in an anterior to posterior direction, creating an opening anterior wedge that can provide increased anterolateral coverage for the congenital subluxed or dislocated hip [22]. Dega first reported his pelvic osteotomy technique in 1969. His technique involves cutting the outer table from a lateral to medial direction, leaving the inner table intact [23, 24]. Although still hinging on the triradiate cartilage, it creates a more laterally directed correction. The "San Diego" modification of the Dega involves using a Kerrison rongeur to resect the edge of the sciatic notch. This allows more coverage directed laterally without sacrificing posterior coverage, and was originally described for hip dysplasia associated with neuromuscular disease, which typically is characterized by posterior acetabular deficiency [25].

> **Box 36.4 Acetabuloplasties in the Skeletally Immature**
> For choosing your osteotomy, the following points must be remembered:
>
> - Planning your osteotomy is determined by acetabular deficiencies specific to underlying etiologies (i.e., DDH = anterolateral, congenital femoral deficiency = lateral, neuromuscular = posterolateral).
> - The Salter osteotomy can provide significant deformity correction, but requires internal fixation for stability.
> - The Dega, San Diegoplasty, and Pemberton osteotomies do not require fixation routinely.
> - Bone graft wedges can strategically be placed in a Dega osteotomy to provide more anterior, posterior, or lateral coverage.

The upper age limit to consider surgical reduction of a developmentally dislocated hip is controversial. There is a paucity in the literature providing evidence for or against hip reduction versus benign neglect in older children. The authors of a review article in 2016 stated their general consensus to be "the upper age limit for attempting the standard treatment of idiopathic DDH is approximately 6 years." [26]. However, we believe chronically dislocated hips in otherwise healthy children, especially in unilateral cases, can be considered to be reduced up to the age of 8 years and older with appropriate surgical planning and execution (Fig. 36.7).

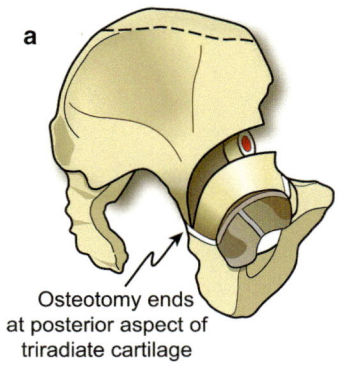 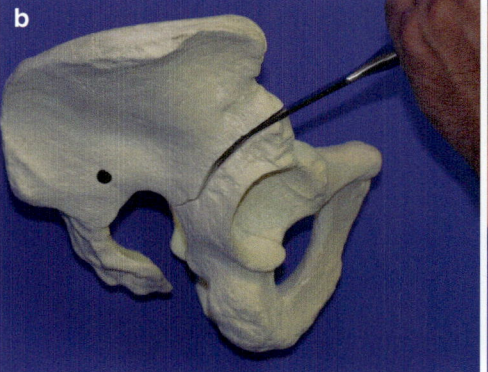 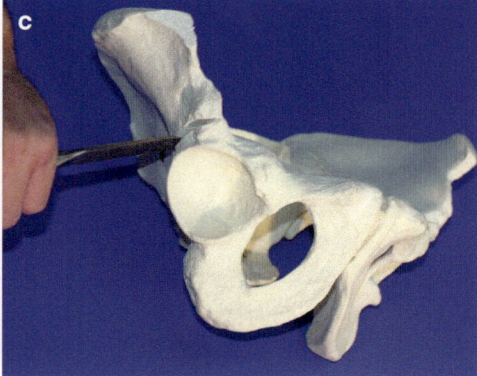

Fig. 36.6 (a) The pericapsular acetabuloplasty curves from the anterior inferior iliac spine to the triradiate cartilage posteriorly hinging on both the inner iliac table and the triradiate cartilage. (b–c) Bone models of pericapsular osteotomy techniques. In a Pemberton, the osteotome is directed from anterior to posterior, cutting both the inner and outer table. The Dega directs the osteotome from lateral to medial, leaving the inner table intact to create a more medial hinge. Reprinted with permission from the Rubin Institute for Advanced Orthopedics, Sinai Hospital of Baltimore

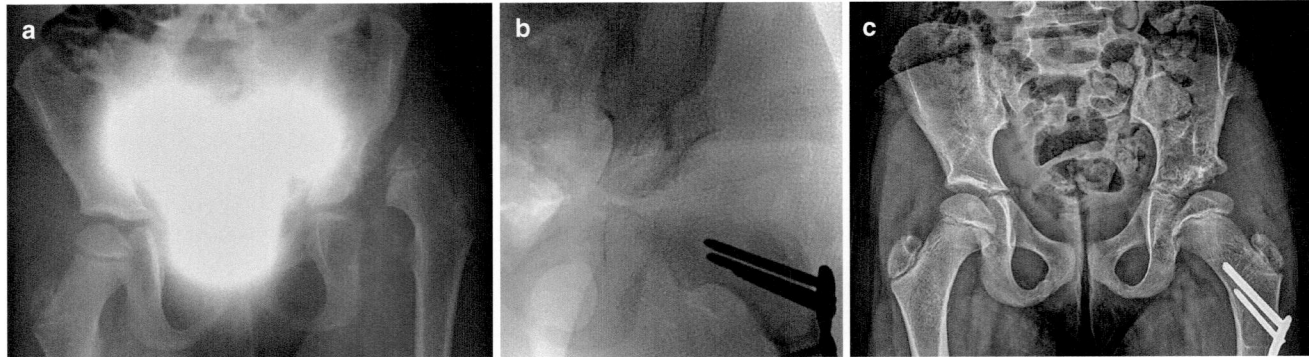

Fig. 36.7 (a) 6+3-year-old female presented with a chief complaint of asymptomatic unilateral toe-walking. AP pelvis radiograph revealed a chronic hip dislocation with pseudoacetabulum. (b) Fluoroscopic images after open reduction, capsulorraphy, proximal femoral shortening/derotation, and pelvic osteotomy. Femoral shortening of 1.8 cm was utilized as a bone graft for an aggressive pericapsular acetabuloplasty. (c) Weightbearing radiograph 2-years post-op, finds the hip well reduced with normalized Shenton's line and coverage, an AI of 19° and progressively ossifying and improving lateral sourcil. No indication of AVN. Patient had no pain, hip motion within normal limits, and residual LLD of 1 cm

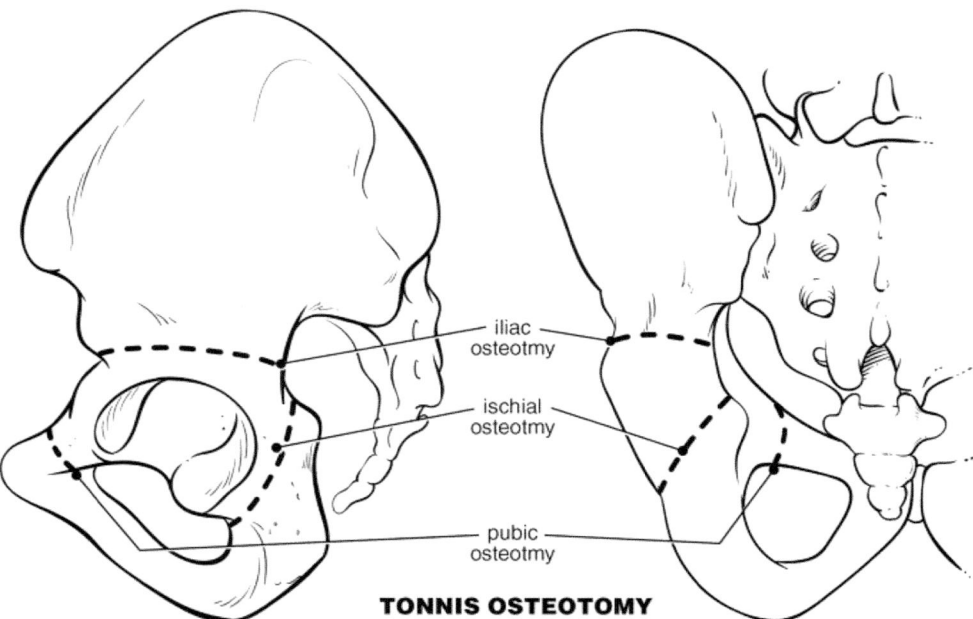

Fig. 36.8 Schematic view of ischial osteotomy for the Tönnis triple osteotomy

Treatment of Residual Hip Dysplasia for Patients After Closure of the Triradiate Growth Plate

As the patient becomes older, the treatment for hip dysplasia becomes more complicated and invasive. However, unlike the asymptomatic younger child who is usually diagnosed incidentally and treated prophylactically, the older patient typically presents with mild to moderate pain associated with activity. Therefore, the treatment goals in this age group are often alleviation of pain, improved joint function, and prevention of early degenerative joint disease of the hip.

In the authors' practice, the preferred method of treatment for symptomatic residual hip dysplasia in the young patient after the closure of the triradiate cartilage is the periacetabular triple osteotomy (Box 36.5). The triple is a redirectional osteotomy including ischial, pubis, and supra-acetabular innominate bone cuts. An early technique described by Steel has continued to evolve [27]. Tonnis modified the procedure by performing the ischial cut in closer proximity to the acetabulum (Fig. 36.8), facilitating acetabular fragment mobility and greater correction of severe acetabular dysplasia [28]. Originally described as a two-incision procedure, further modifications of the triple osteotomy utilize an one-incision technique [29]. A brief description of the technique will follow, highlighting certain technical tips.

The Ganz periacetabular osteotomy is another very popular type of pelvic osteotomy [30]. This particular osteotomy

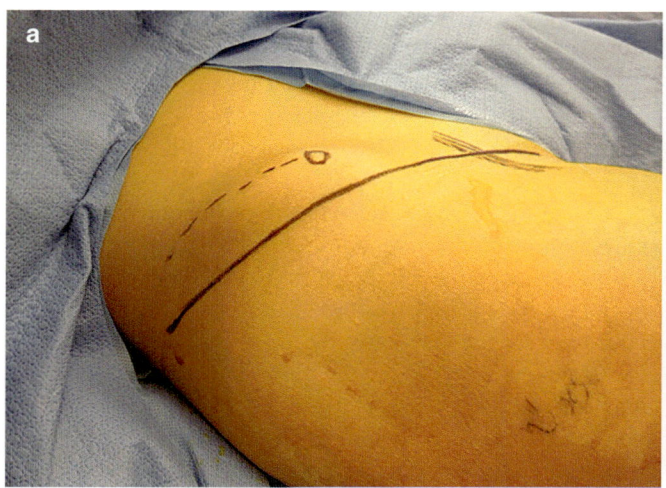 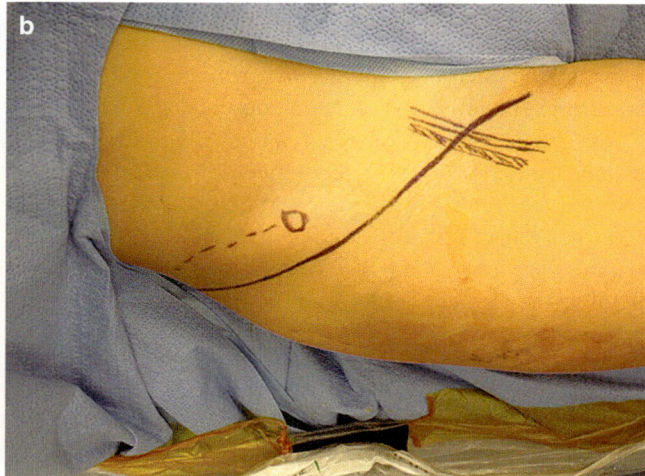

Fig. 36.9 (**a**, **b**) The single incision technique is depicted from an anterior and lateral view. The iliac crest is marked with the *dashed line* ending at the ASIS. The *longitudinal marked structures* are the palpable neurovascular bundle. Reprinted with permission from the Rubin Institute for Advanced Orthopedics, Sinai Hospital of Baltimore

maintains the integrity of the posterior column by performing a bone cut connecting the iliac osteotomy to the partial ischial osteotomy. This osteotomy travels through a very narrow column of bone in the young patient. Therefore, the author prefers the periacetabular triple technique for adolescent and smaller adult patients.

Periacetabular Triple Osteotomy of the Pelvis: Operative Technique

Positioning and Exposure

The patient is placed supine on the operating table with no bumps placed under the pelvis. The entire lower extremity includes the groin, gluteal region, and subcostal area are prepared and isolated into the sterile field. A single incision is performed in the flexion crease of the hip joint, approximately 1 cm below the anterior superior iliac spine. This incision starts just medial to the palpable neurovascular bundle and extends 6–8 cm lateral to the anterior superior iliac spine (Fig. 36.9).

The entire operation is performed through this single anterior incision. The interval between the sartorius and tensor fascia lata muscles is defined in the typical fashion protecting the lateral femoral cutaneous nerve. The rectus femoris tendon is identified and released, tagging the insertional portion of tendon. Next, the iliac crest is exposed. Both the inner and the outer tables are subperiosteally dissected to the sciatic notch. Surgical gauze and/or bone wax may be used to control bleeding from the iliac wing. The dissection of the medial structures is subsequently performed. The fascia overlying the sartorius and iliopsoas muscles is divided. The iliopsoas tendon is identified (typically on the posterior aspect of the muscle) and fractionally lengthened within the muscle belly. Gentle retraction of the

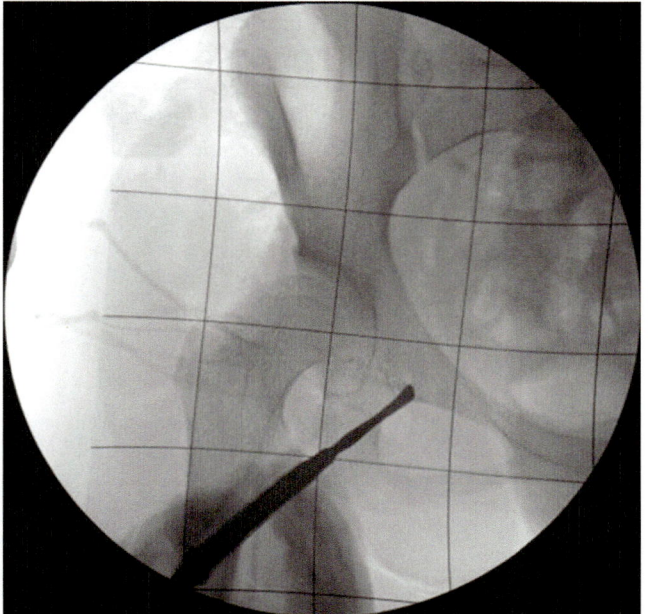

Fig. 36.10 A 4-year-old female undergoing a triple osteotomy for right hip dysplasia. Intraoperative fluoroscopic image demonstrating the position for the superior pubic ramus cut. This position is usually directly behind or medial to the neurovascular bundle. Reprinted with permission from the Rubin Institute for Advanced Orthopedics, Sinai Hospital of Baltimore

iliopsoas muscle belly brings the femoral nerve into the operative field. The femoral nerve should be identified prior to the division of the iliopsoas tendon. The femoral nerve, artery, and vein are carefully identified and exposed with individual small vessel loops placed around each structure. Fluoroscopic visualization of the superior pubic ramus is performed to confirm the osteotomy position just medial to the pubic eminence (Fig. 36.10). It is always surprising how medial the dissection must be carried out in order to place the superior pubic ramus osteotomy in the correct position. Typically, the osteotomy site lies between the femoral nerve and artery. However, with smaller patients, the osteotomy position can be medial to the femoral vein. The interval between the femoral nerve and artery is exposed down to the periosteum of the superior pubic ramus. Great care must be used when retracting the neurovascular bundle. If the interval for the exposure of the superior pubic ramus is performed lateral to the femoral nerve, then the tension placed on the neurovascular structures will be substantially increased in order to reach the proper osteotomy position.

Osteotomies

After the exposure of the correct interval for the pubic ramus osteotomy is completed, the overlying periosteum is divided. Multiple drill holes are created in the superior pubic ramus using a smooth wire of 1.8 mm to 2.0 mm in length. The osteotomy is completed with an osteotome. The interval for the ischial osteotomy is then created. This interval lies between the medial aspect of the hip capsule and the iliopsoas muscle. The interval is carefully created with gentle blunt dissection using a large curved Mayo scissor. The interval is opened and widened by gentle spreading of the blunt tipped scissor. A small Cobb elevator is placed into the interval to palpate the superior portion of the ischium, just below the acetabulum (Fig. 36.11). A Cobb elevator is advanced on both the medial and lateral sides of the ischium to push the soft tissues away and prepare a path for the Ganz osteotome (Fig. 36.12d, e).

The Ganz osteotome is inserted into the prepared interval and positioned just under the acetabulum. It is critical to have adequate fluoroscopic visualization for this osteotomy. The osteotome is aimed approximately 45–55° proximally in order to direct the osteotomy above the ischial spine (Fig. 36.12).

This osteotomy is visualized with an oblique fluoroscopic view, similar to an obturator Judet view (C-arm is rotated toward the operative hip between 30° and 50° from the AP position). Again, fluoroscopic visualization of the acetabulum, ischium, and ischial spine is essential in this oblique view in order to complete the periacetabular ischial osteotomy successfully. Another critical technical tip is the protection of the femoral nerve while completing the ischial osteotomy. During this osteotomy, the hip must be flexed 15–20° to prevent stretch of the femoral nerve as the Ganz osteotome handle is levered distally in order to aim the osteotomy above the ischial spine. Before the final osteotomy of the ilium, two reference half pins are inserted into the acetabular fragment. These two reference half pins enhance the accuracy of the bony correction and help prevent secondary deformities (Fig. 36.13).

The first half pin is placed from the anterior to posterior direction, just lateral to the superior pubic ramus osteotomy. This anterior reference half pin marks the acetabular version. The second half pin is inserted from lateral to medial in the supra-acetabular region, parallel to the roof or sourcil of the acetabulum. This lateral reference half pin marks the dysplastic acetabular roof. After the reference half pins are placed, the final osteotomy of the ilium is performed. A Gigli saw is carefully passed through the sciatic notch. The final osteotomy is completed with the Gigli saw from the sciatic

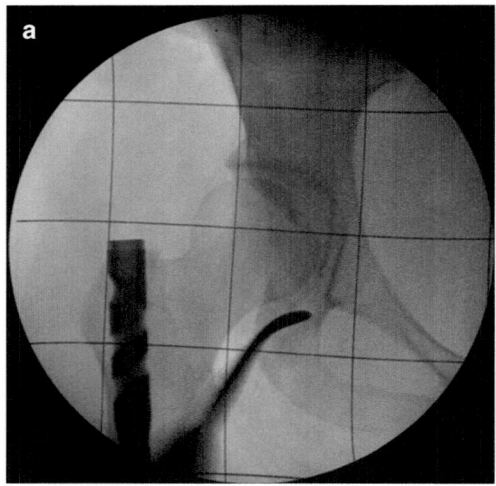
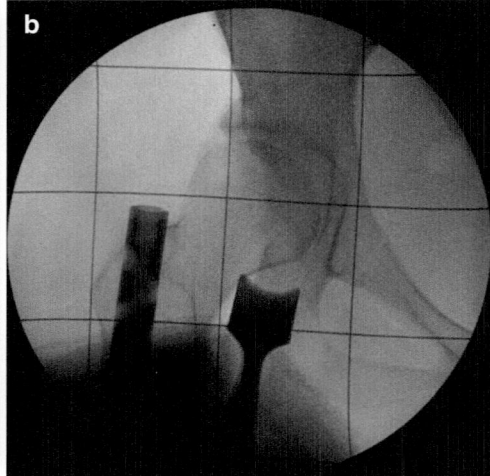

Fig. 36.11 A 16-year-old female undergoing a triple pelvic osteotomy for retroversion of the right hip. (**a**) Intraoperative fluoroscopic image of a Cobb instrument palpating the superior portion of the ischium just beneath the acetabulum. (**b**) Image demonstrating the placement of the Ganz osteotomy at the same location as identified by the Cobb instrument. Reprinted with permission from the Rubin Institute for Advanced Orthopedics, Sinai Hospital of Baltimore

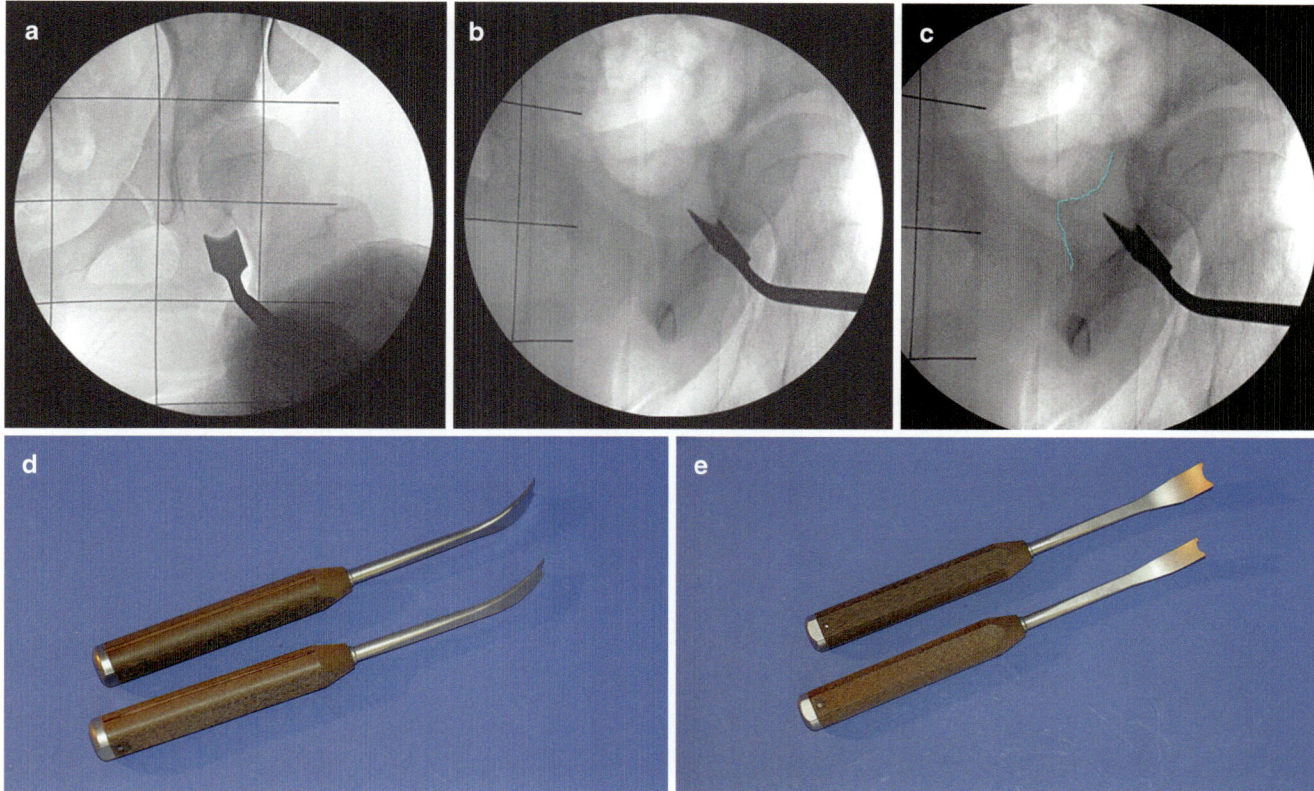

Fig. 36.12 (**a**) Fluoroscopic view denoting the position of the Ganz osteotome in the AP view preparing to perform the lateral cortical cut of the ischium. (**b**) Fluoroscopic view in the oblique position to confirm placement of the Ganz osteotome under the acetabulum and directed above the ischial spine. (**c**) Same fluoroscopic view as Fig. 36.12b with the ischial spine highlighted. (**d**, **e**) Clinical pictures of the specialized Ganz osteotomes. Reprinted with permission from the Rubin Institute for Advanced Orthopedics, Sinai Hospital of Baltimore

notch to the anterior aspect of the ilium, just above the anterior inferior iliac spine.

Deformity Correction and Fixation

The acetabular fragment should become freely mobile after the third bone cut. If the fragment does not easily move, then the pubic ramus osteotomy and ischial osteotomy are revisited with a repeat passage of the osteotome. After mobilizing the acetabular fragment, the reference half pins are used to reorient the acetabulum and temporary fixation is performed (Fig. 36.14a). The anterior half pin should still be pointed in a straight anterior to posterior direction if the version of the acetabulum was planned to remain the same. If anteversion is needed, then the anterior half pin should be internally rotated. Similarly, if the anterior half pin is externally rotated, then the retroversion has been imparted to the new acetabular position. The temporary fixation consists of three separate 1.8-mm Ilizarov or similar sized smooth k-wires. After adequate correction and repositioning of the acetabulum is completed and confirmed under fluoroscopy, the wires are sequentially overdrilled with a cannulated 3.2-mm drill bit

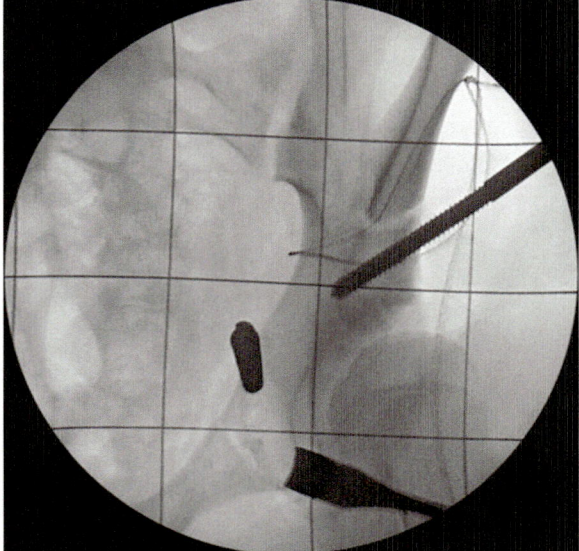

Fig. 36.13 Fluoroscopic view demonstrating the placement of the two reference half pins prior to the completion of the iliac osteotomy. The AP half pin marks the acetabular version whereas the lateral to the medial half pin marks the slope of the acetabular roof. Reprinted with permission from the Rubin Institute for Advanced Orthopedics, Sinai Hospital of Baltimore

and solid 4.5-mm screws are inserted for final stabilization (Fig. 36.14b).

The following figures are case examples of the triple pelvic osteotomy (Figs. 36.14, 36.15, and 36.16).

Closure proceeds with repair of the iliacus fascia to the gluteus medius fascia to cover the exposed iliac crest, repair of the rectus femoris tendon, and a layered closure of the subcutaneous tissues and skin over a drain.

Postoperative Care

The patient is placed into a hip abduction pillow prior to leaving the operative suite and converted to a single leg hip abduction brace before discharge from the hospital. Toe-touch weight bearing is allowed with crutches or a walker for 6 weeks. After radiographic confirmation of healing, the patient is advanced to full weight bearing and physiotherapy.

Two-Incision Tönnis Triple Technique

An alternative to the single incision technique for the Tönnis triple is the two-incision technique. The two-incision technique consists of the previously described anterior incision with an additional lateral incision. The ischial cut is performed under direct visualization from the sciatic notch to the obturator foramen. The indications for the two-incision

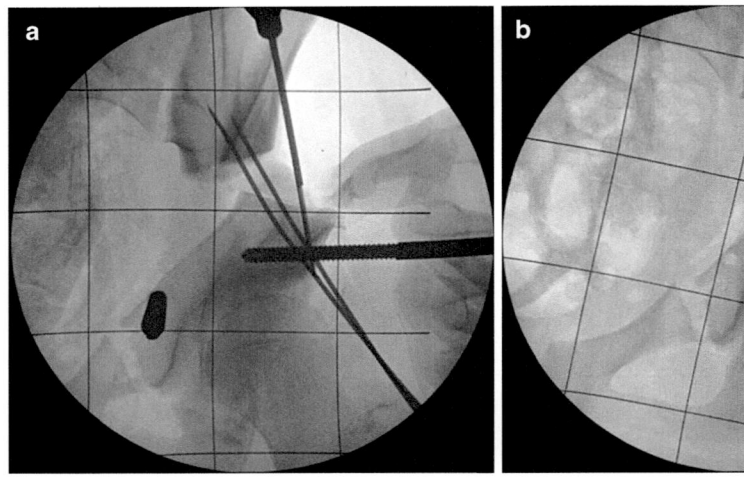

Fig. 36.14 (**a**) After the acetabular fragment is reduced into the corrected position, temporary fixation is achieved with smooth wires. (**b**) The smooth wires are sequentially overdrilled with a 3.2-mm cannulated drill and 4.5-mm solid screws are inserted. This is the same patient as Fig. 36.14. Reprinted with permission from the Rubin Institute for Advanced Orthopedics, Sinai Hospital of Baltimore

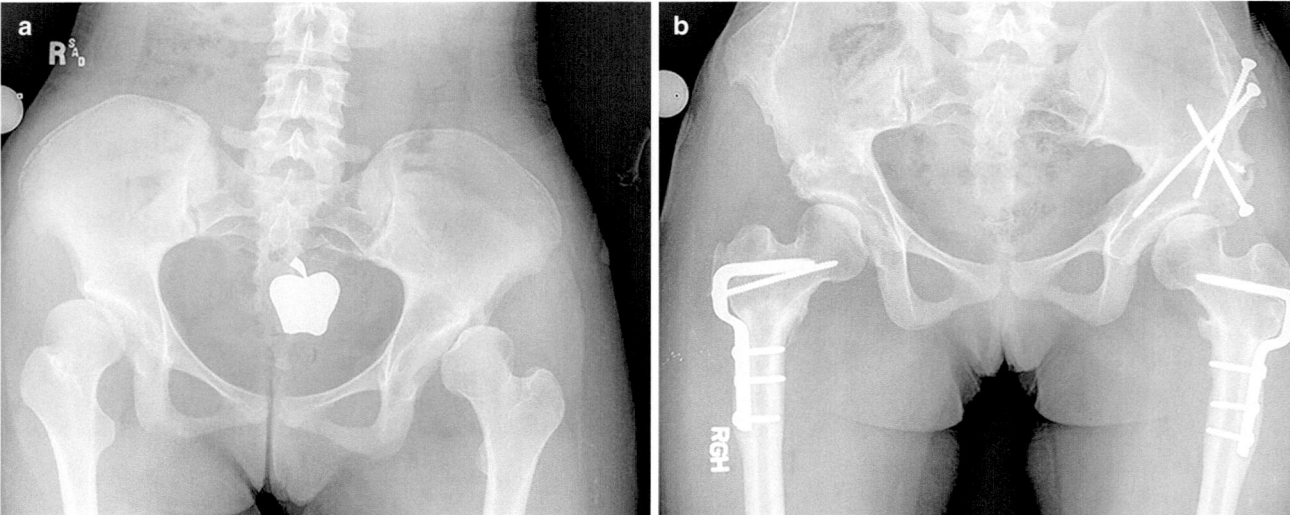

Fig. 36.15 (**a**) A 14-year-old female with Down's syndrome and concurrent severe coxa valga and acetabular dysplasia. (**b**) Left hip corrected with proximal varus osteotomy of the femur with periacetabular triple osteotomy. Reprinted with permission from the Rubin Institute for Advanced Orthopedics, Sinai Hospital of Baltimore

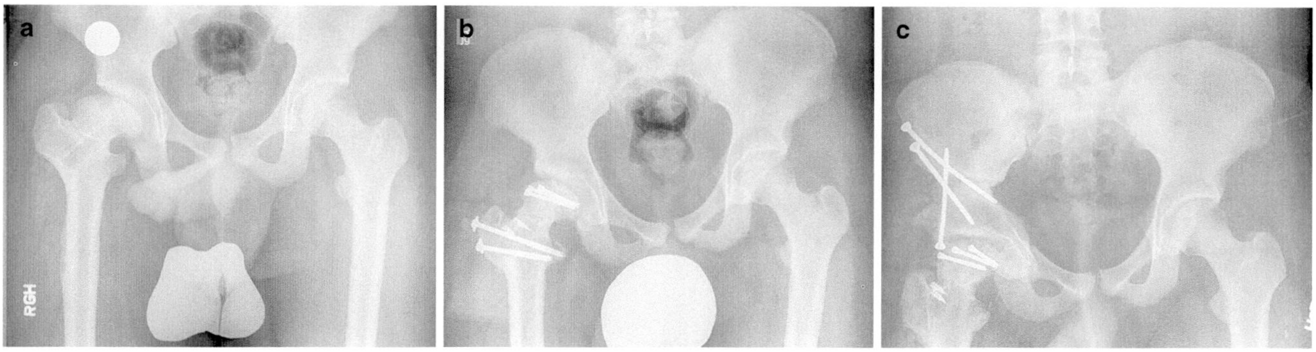

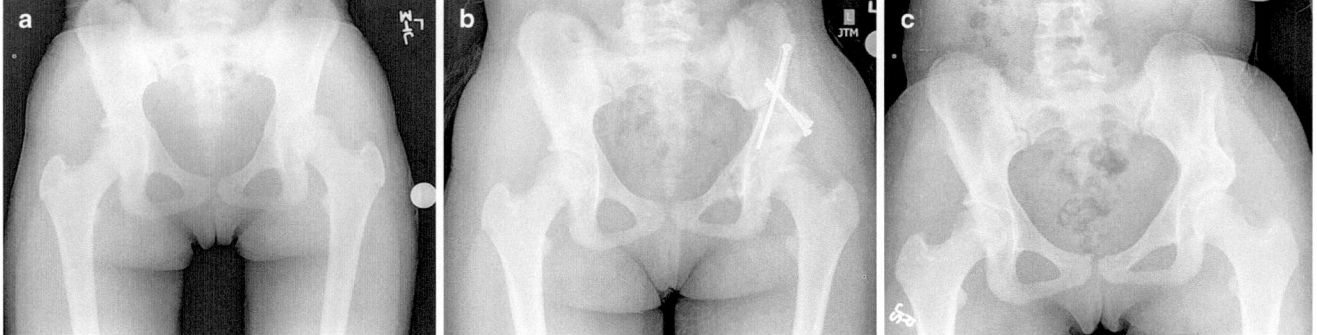

Fig. 36.16 (**a**) An 18-year-old male with history of Perthes disease of the right hip who had previously undergone approximal femoral valgus osteotomy with residual impingement pain and gluteus medius weakness. (**b**) Same patient after Ganz femoral head reduction surgery and relative femoral neck lengthening with greater trochanter transfer. (**c**) Subsequent triple pelvic osteotomy in the same patient to address residual hip pain due to decrease contact area between newly shaped femoral head and oblong acetabulum. Reprinted with permission from the Rubin Institute for Advanced Orthopedics, Sinai Hospital of Baltimore

Fig. 36.17 A 13-year-old female basketball player presents with new-onset left hip pain with radiographs depicting underlying acetabular dysplasia (**a**), radiographs after triple osteotomy with improvement of femoral head position and coverage and normalization of the center edge angle (**b**). (**c**) Radiographic appearance of pelvis after hardware removal with excellent left hip configuration and no compromise of the pelvic outlet for future childbearing. This is the same patient shown in Figs. 36.12, 36.13, and 36.14. Reprinted with permission from the Rubin Institute for Advanced Orthopedics, Sinai Hospital of Baltimore

technique include patients undergoing simultaneous surgical hip dislocation, proximal femoral osteotomies, or trochanteric advancement. Additionally, patients that have undergone previous limb lengthening should be approached with the two-incision technique. This approach allows for direct visualization and decompression of the sciatic nerve.

Technique

The patient is initially placed in the lateral decubitus position, and the entire extremity to include the hip, iliac crest, and gluteal region is prepped and draped. A 15–25 cm incision is created on the lateral thigh. If the only goal is to decompress the sciatic nerve and perform the ischial osteotomy, then a 15 cm incision starting at the base of the greater trochanter and extended proximally is usually adequate. For additional proximal femoral procedures, a larger incision will be needed. The skin and subcutaneous tissues are sharply divided to the deep fascia. The fascia is then divided in line with the incision, and the plane between the gluteus maximus and gluteus medius muscles is developed. A Charnley retractor is utilized to retract the fascia anteriorly and the gluteus maximus muscle posteriorly. The hip is placed into a full extended position using a padded mayo stand for leg support. This maneuver provides wide exposure to the posterior aspect of the hip (Fig. 36.18a). The sciatic nerve is identified and decompressed for the entire length of the incision. Two vessel loops are placed around the nerve to assist in identification and gentle retraction (Fig. 36.18b). With the sciatic nerve gently retracted posteriorly, the ischial tuberosity is easily palpated. A freer elevator is inserted into the sciatic notch under the superior gemellus and piriformis muscles. A small homan retractor replaces the freer elevator. The freer elevator is then inserted into the superior portion of the obturator foramen under the inferior gemellus and quadratus femoris muscles. A second homan retractor replaced the freer elevator. The obturator internus muscle is bluntly divided and the tendon is released. An osteotomy using a straight small/medium osteotome is then performed between

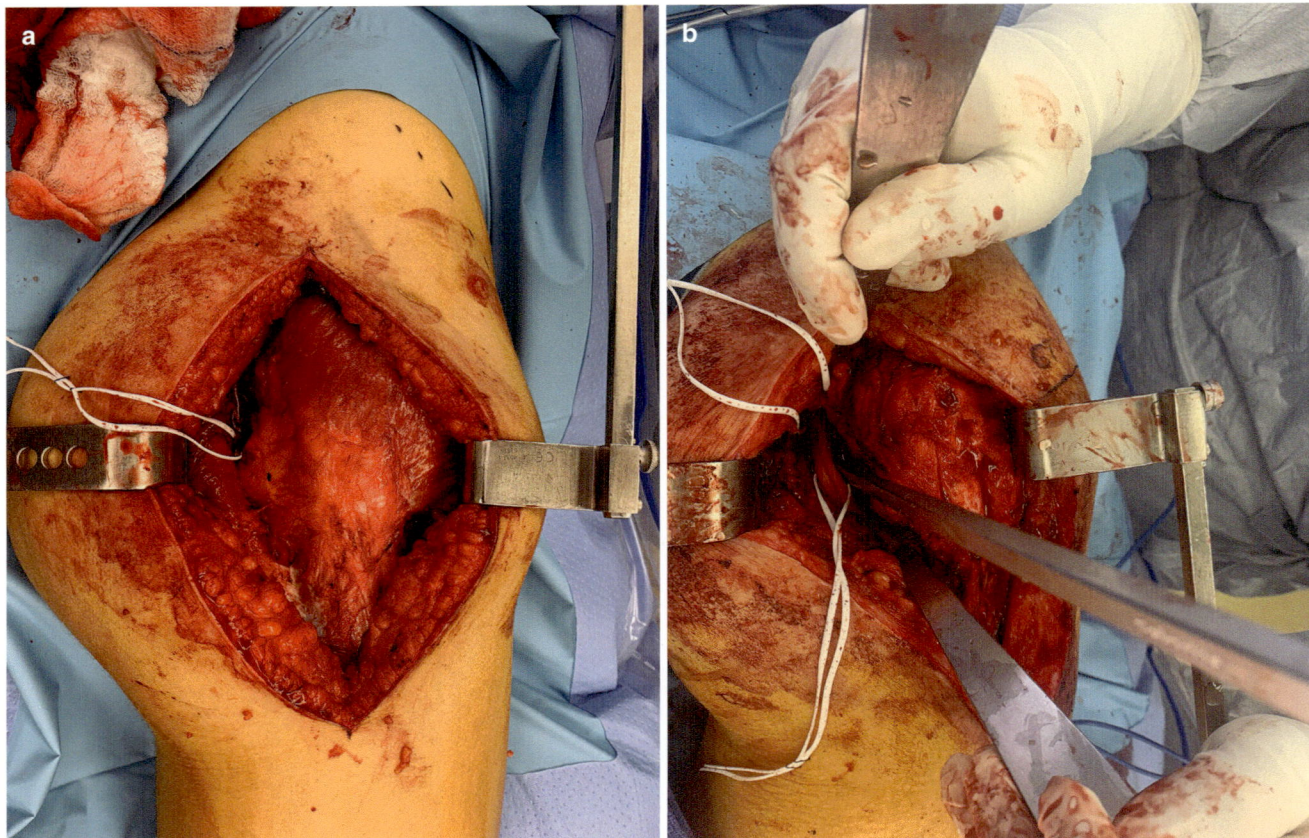

Fig. 36.18 (a) Hip extension provides wide exposure and access to the ischium. (b) The sciatic nerve is identified with vessel loops. The picture demonstrates the proximity of the osteotome performing the ischial osteotomy to the sciatic nerve. Great care is needed to perform this osteotomy safely

the two homan retractors posterior to the acetabulum. With the patient in the lateral decubitus position, the direction of the osteotome is straight anterior to posterior. The angulation of the osteotome in an anterior direction will risk violation of the hip joint. It is very important to ensure the retractors are in the proper position with fluoroscopy prior to the osteotomy. It is easy to mistake the lesser sciatic notch for the greater sciatic notch. This will result in an osteotomy that creates an ischial fragment distal to the sacral spine. This intact sacrospinous ligament attached to the acetabular fragment will decrease the acetabulum's ability to mobilize. This osteotomy is performed by tactile and auditory confirmation. The osteotomy is carefully driven to the second cortex, and the pitch changes as the osteotome completes the cut. It is imperative to carefully advance the osteotome and not to plunge. As the osteotomy progresses from proximal to distal, each pass can be checked for completion by gently probing the site with a blunt freer elevator. Once the osteotomy is complete, the osteotomy site will be easily mobile. At this point, the vessel loops are left in place and the skin is temporarily closed with skin staples. The incision is then isolated with ioban dressing. The operative drapes are removed, and the patient is then placed into a supine position. The entire leg/hip is prepped and draped for the second time. The lateral incision is reopened by removing the skin staples, and the vessel loops are located.

The remainder of the procedure is the same as described for the single incision triple osteotomy technique. As the acetabular fragment is mobilized, the sciatic nerve is monitored to insure that no overt tension is created. If the nerve is found to be under significant tension, then the proximal segment of the iliac osteotomy should be recessed to allow slight shortening of 0.5–1.0 cm. This maneuver will relax the sciatic nerve. The incisions should be closed over hemovac drains. The post-operative care is the same for both techniques.

> **Box 36.5 Modified Triple Osteotomy**
> The technical tips are given as follows:
>
> - Can be performed with a single anterior ilioinguinal incision.
> - Identify, isolate with a vessel loop, and protect the femoral nerve, artery, and vein prior to iliopsoas tenotomy as well as during the superior ramus and ischial bone cut.
> - Adequate medial exposure must be achieved for the superior rami bone cut.
> - The superior rami osteotomy site usually lies directly behind the neurovascular bundle.
> - A multiple-drill hole technique, Ganz osteotome, and Gigli saw are utilized for the pubic rami, ischial, and ileal bone cuts, respectively.
> - Proper oblique fluoroscopic views are critical to perform the ischial osteotomy.
> - The Ganz osteotomy must be directed above the ischial spine for the correct ischial osteotomy.
> - It is critical to flex the hip 15–20° while levering the Ganz osteotome distally to achieve the proper osteotomy direction; this position protects the femoral nerve from a tension injury.
> - Two half-pins are used as anatomical reference points and for controlled mobilization of the fragment.
> - Three to four large fragment screws (4.5 mm) are adequate for fixation.

Residual Deformities of the Hip Joint Secondary to Slipped Capital Femoral Epiphysis

The residual deformities that result from a previous slipped capital femoral epiphysis (SCFE) are typically varus, extension, external femoral rotation, leg length discrepancy, and anterolateral femoral acetabular impingement (FAI) [31, 32]. The clinical relevance of each of these deformities depends on the severity of the SCFE and the prior treatment. Some patients will present with a long-standing SCFE with severe deformity that has never been diagnosed previously.

The typical treatment of in situ screw fixation for minimal or mild SCFE has proven effective with long-term success [33]. However, the same strategy for moderate or severe magnitude of SCFE often results in unacceptable residual deformities and is associated with pain, gait abnormality, and joint dysfunction [34, 35]. There is no absolute criterion for the amount of deformity that requires immediate or eventual reconstruction. However, surgeons are increasingly managing even milder deformity associated with FAI in order to prevent poor long-term outcomes [36, 37]. The decision to perform a corrective osteotomy should be based on the patient's function and symptoms, as well as the magnitude of deformity. If conservative observation is the treatment strategy, then the physician should follow the patient well into young adulthood to monitor the presence of early degenerative joint disease or impingement that would require a more aggressive treatment plan.

The recommended treatment strategy for residual hip deformities secondary to SCFE consists of either a modified Southwick intertrochanteric osteotomy or a modified Dunn procedure for femoral head reorientation. The osteotomy elected may depend on whether the proximal femoral growth plate is open or closed. If the physis remains open, then the author's treatment of choice is the modified Dunn procedure via a surgical hip dislocation described by Ganz [38]. Once the physis has closed, the proximal femoral periarticular retinaculum becomes very thin, resulting in a higher risk of AVN for the modified Dunn procedure. In the face of a significant proximal femoral deformity with a closed capital femoral physis, a modified Southwick intertrochanteric osteotomy is recommended.

Performing a subcapital osteotomy versus an intertrochanteric osteotomy for a chronic SCFE deformity remains controversial. Several studies of the modified Dunn procedure have reported favorable results with significantly low rates of AVN; however, there exists inconsistent reports on the incidence of AVN associated with subcapital osteotomies [38–44]. The decision may be surgeon dependent and related to experience with surgical hip dislocation and the modified Dunn procedure. Surgeons may elect to stage treatment of a skeletally immature, chronic stable SCFE by first performing in situ screw fixation, and then following with a planned intertrochanteric osteotomy after physeal closure. An open or arthroscopic osteoplasty, or "bumpectomy," of the femoral neck deformity can also be performed in combination with this approach to avoid FAI.

The Modified Dunn Procedure for Residual Deformities of the Proximal Femur Secondary to SCFE: Operative Technique

The modified Dunn procedure has been described multiple times in the current literature. H. Huber et al. provided an excellent description of this procedure in 2009 [41].

Positioning and Exposure

The modified Dunn procedure is performed with the patient in the lateral decubitus position. The incision is centered on the greater trochanter with approximately 5–8 cm distal and 5–8 cm proximal (Fig. 36.19).

The interval between the tensor fascia lata and gluteus maximus muscles is used to gain access to the level of the vastus lateralis and gluteus medius muscles. The posterior border of the vastus lateralis muscle is identified at the level of the vastus ridge. The posterior border of the gluteus medius muscle is identified along with the piriformis tendon and the sciatic nerve. A greater trochanteric osteotomy is performed with an oscillating saw that connects the posterior border of the vastus lateralis muscle to the posterior border of the gluteus medius muscle. The greater trochanteric fragment should be approximately 1–1.5 cm thick for adequate fixation at the end of the procedure. The digastric muscle flap to include the vastus lateralis muscle, the greater trochanteric fragment, and gluteus medius muscle is flipped medially allowing exposure of the gluteus minimus muscle and underlying hip joint capsule (Fig. 36.20a–c).

Surgical Hip Dislocation

The next step in the procedure is the exposure of the hip capsule and the Z capsulotomy. A small Cobb elevator is used to lift the gluteus minimus muscle off of the capsule and provide an interval for a Taylor retractor to be inserted onto the outer table of the ilium. The surgeon will note a prominence in the hip capsule caused by the superior ridge of the femoral neck that was "left" behind as the femoral head progressively slipped in a posterior and medial direction. The Z-capsulotomy is performed with the longitudinal limb in the midline of the capsule. The anterior limb of the capsulotomy is performed at the base of the femoral neck while the posterior limb is extended along the posterior rim of the acetabulum (Fig. 36.21).

The critical step at this point in the procedure is the creation of the retinacular soft tissue flap that will contain the blood vessels to the femoral head. Careful removal of bone from the base of the greater trochanter will create this flap that consists of the proximal femoral periosteum, pericapsular retinaculum, and short external rotator muscles. The creation of this flap is accomplished by removing 5–8 mm of bone from the posterior aspect of the greater trochanteric base by the "inside out technique"(Fig. 36.22). It is critical to minimize soft tissue tension and stretch while excising the bone.

Similarly, the proximal aspect of the greater trochanter base is removed to create a surface that is flush with the superior portion of the femoral neck. This will result in the "relative" femoral neck lengthening after the greater trochanteric fragment is advanced distally during the closure.

If the femoral head has not been previously secured with prior screw fixation, then temporary fixation with a stout

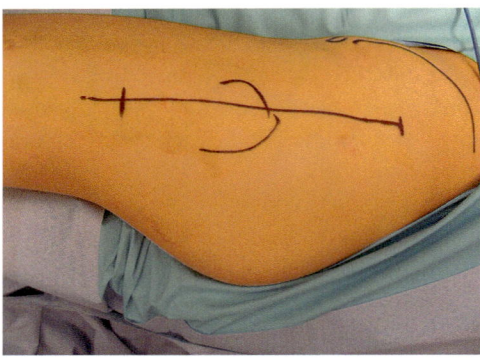

Fig. 36.19 The incision is centered on the greater trochanter for a total length of 15–20 cm. The clinical photograph depicts the outline of the iliac crest, the ASIS, the greater trochanter, and the longitudinal incision centered on the greater trochanter. Reprinted with permission from the Rubin Institute for Advanced Orthopedics, Sinai Hospital of Baltimore

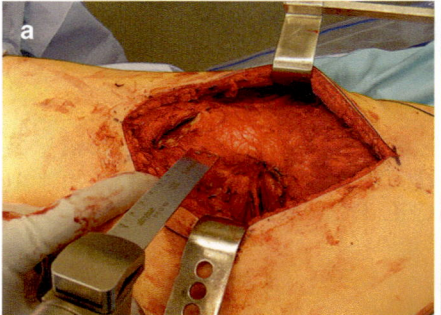 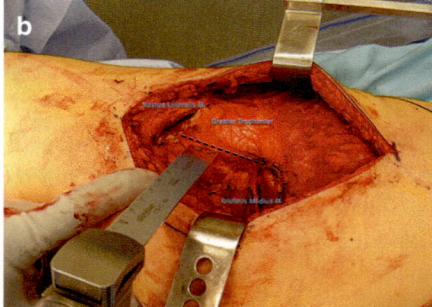 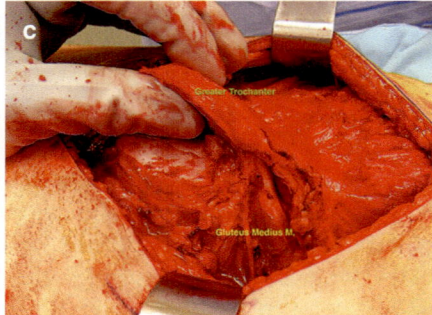

Fig. 36.20 (**a**, **b**) The greater trochanteric osteotomy begins at the posterior border of the vastus lateralis muscle and extends to the posterior border of the gluteus medius muscle. (**c**) The greater trochanteric fragment should be approximately 1.0–1.5 cm in thickness. Reprinted with permission from the Rubin Institute for Advanced Orthopedics, Sinai Hospital of Baltimore

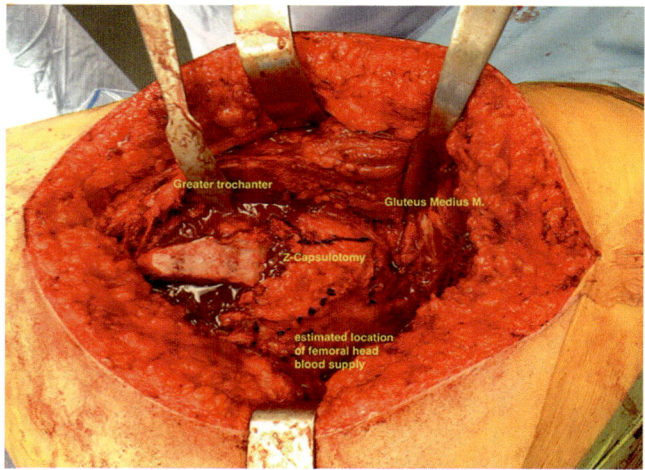

Fig. 36.21 The Z-capsulotomy is created with a longitudinal incision in the capsule in line with the femoral neck. The anterior limb of the capsulotomy is performed anterior at the base of the femoral neck. The posterior limb of the capsulotomy is directed along the posterior border of the acetabulum. Reprinted with permission from the Rubin Institute for Advanced Orthopedics, Sinai Hospital of Baltimore

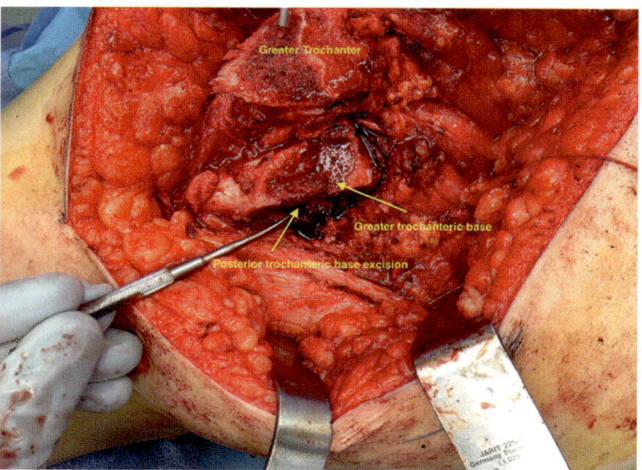

Fig. 36.22 The posterior aspect of the base of the greater trochanter is excised to create the soft tissue vascular sleeve to the femoral head. The excision of 5–8 mm of bone produces soft tissue redundancy that allows greater mobility of the femoral head during the realignment procedure. Reprinted with permission from the Rubin Institute for Advanced Orthopedics, Sinai Hospital of Baltimore

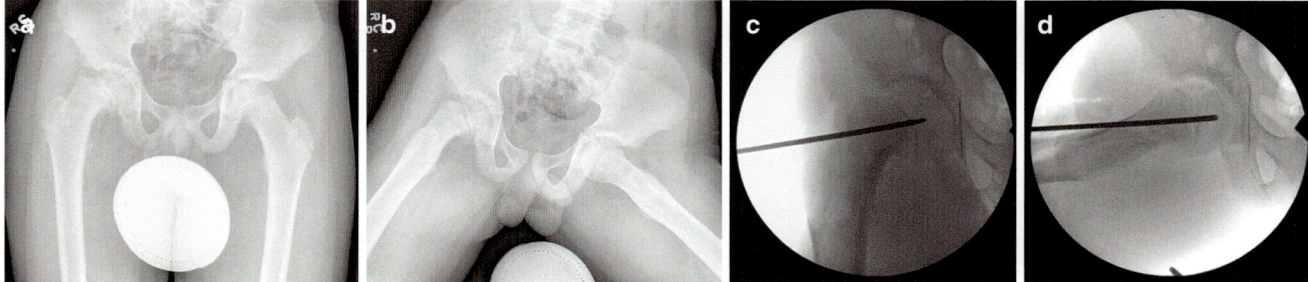

Fig. 36.23 (**a**, **b**) A 14-year-old male who presented with an acute slipped capital femoral epiphysis (**c**, **d**) Intraoperative fluoroscopic views depicting temporary head fixation to allow for surgical dislocation of the hip without compromising the vascular supply to the femoral head. Reprinted with permission from the Rubin Institute for Advanced Orthopedics, Sinai Hospital of Baltimore

single threaded K-wire is performed (Fig. 36.23). The hip is gently dislocated with release of the ligamentum teres from the fovea capitis. After the femoral head is delivered out of the joint, the acetabulum and labrum are inspected for any detrimental changes. Next, the periosteum and retinaculum of the femoral neck is carefully peeled from anterior to the midline both medially and laterally. The lateral aspect of this dissection is critical, and the continuity of the soft tissue flap to the femoral head must be maintained.

Deformity Correction and Fixation

Following dislocation, the femoral head fixation is removed and a curved osteotome is inserted into the physis. Gentle levering of the curved osteotome is performed to allow the femoral head to gradually detach from the femoral neck. While the femoral head is carefully being levered off the neck, the retinacular soft tissue flap should be visualized to prevent any tearing or stretching. If the final posterior portion of the physis is difficult to detach, then the osteotome is carefully directed slightly distally, removing a small portion of the posterolateral femoral neck with the femoral head in order to protect the blood supply. The femoral head along with the soft tissue vascular flap is allowed to fall back into the acetabulum and the femoral neck is lifted into the operative field for inspection (Fig. 36.24).

The femoral neck is trimmed of excess bone and shortened to eliminate any tension of the vascular leash with femoral head reduction. The shortening does not have to be excessive, approximately 1 cm, as long as no tension of the blood supply is evident when the femoral head is reduced.

The femoral head is carefully retrieved from the acetabulum and reduced to the "new" femoral neck. The vascular retinacular leash is inspected to ensure no tension is present after which temporary K-wire fixation is performed. The hip joint is reduced and its position is confirmed under fluoroscopy. The fixation is finalized via 4.5-mm screws, 3.5-mm screws, or threaded K-wires. The size of the fixation depends on the size of the femoral head and balancing stable fixation while minimizing the amount of area of the femoral head violated to prevent devascularization. The capsule is repaired with care not to over tighten the posterior capsule, which could stretch the blood supply to the femoral head. The greater trochanter is advanced distally and repaired with two 4.5 mm solid screws or two 5.5-mm cannulated screws. The goal of the greater trochanteric transfer is to advance the proximal tip of the greater trochanter below the newly established center of the femoral head (Fig. 36.25). The remainder of the closure is performed in the typical fashion over a drain.

> **Box 36.6 Modified Dunn Procedure**
>
> The technical tips are given as follows:
>
> - Adequate thickness of the greater trochanter osteotomy must be maintained for later fixation (1–1.5 cm width).
> - The most critical aspect of the exposure is creating and maintaining the posterior retinacular soft tissue sleeve.
> - The femoral head must be temporarily stabilized before the hip is dislocated to insure the vascular leash is not torn.
> - Removing 5–8 mm of bone from the posterior margin and the base of the greater trochanter as well as shortening the neck up to 1 cm will aid in relieving tension on the vascular flap.
> - Fixation of the femoral head can be done with 4.5 mm screws, 3.5 mm screws, or threaded Steinman pins.
> - The hip capsule should be repaired with minimal tension to avoid stretch of the vascular supply to the femoral head.
> - The greater trochanter should be advanced until the proximal tip is at or below the center of the femoral head.
> - The greater trochanter is repaired with two 4.5-mm or 5.5-mm screws with washers.

Postoperative Care

The patient is placed into the hip abduction pillow prior to leaving the operative room and converted to a single leg hip abduction brace before discharge from the hospital. The patient remains toe touch weight bearing for 12 weeks with gentle and limited passive range of motion of the hip. The initial 6-week postoperative range of motion is performed with a CPM (continuous passive motion) device. The second

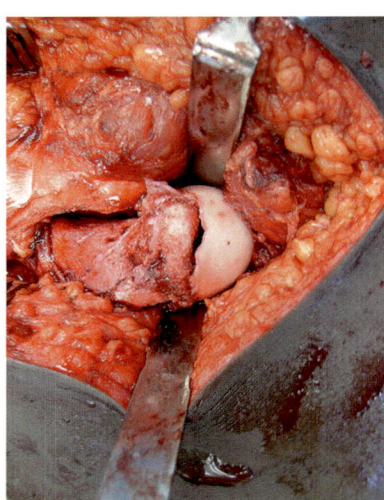

Fig. 36.24 The femoral head is allowed to fall back into the acetabulum after gently levering the femoral head off of the neck through the pathological physis. Reprinted with permission from the Rubin Institute for Advanced Orthopedics, Sinai Hospital of Baltimore

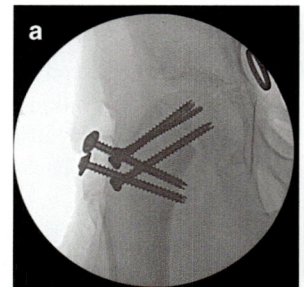 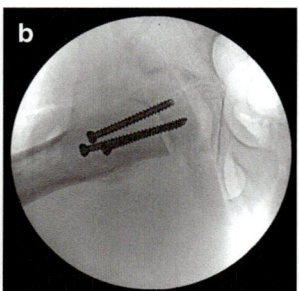 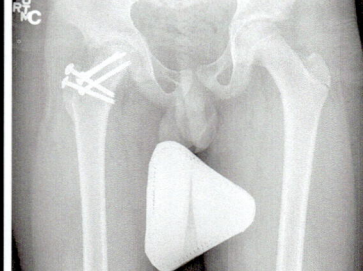 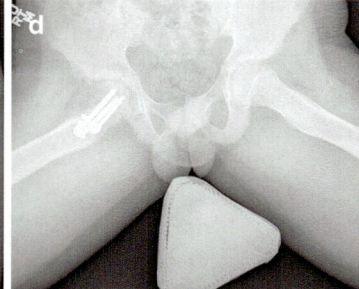

Fig. 36.25 (**a**, **b**) Demonstrating the same patient as in Fig. 36.23 with intraoperative fluoroscopic views of the final femoral head alignment after reduction of the slipped capital femoral epiphysis. (**c**, **d**) AP and frog pelvis radiographs at 8-month postoperative follow-up. Reprinted with permission from the Rubin Institute for Advanced Orthopedics, Sinai Hospital of Baltimore

6-week period therapy protocol consists of gentle, limited passive hip range of motion and CPM. At the 12-week postoperative mark, the patient begins gradual advance to full weight bearing, hip joint range of motion, and hip muscle strengthening.

The Modified Southwick Osteotomy for Residual Deformities of the Proximal Femur Secondary to SCFE: Operative Technique

The Southwick osteotomy has been described in very complicated terms in the past, such as a biplanar or a triplanar osteotomy [45]. In actuality, the osteotomy can be a simple transverse osteotomy stabilized with either an internal blade plate fixation or a simple Ilizarov external fixation. The femoral neck deformity can be described as being in a single oblique plane in the anterolateral direction. This oblique plane deformity is seen as a varus deformity in the coronal view and an extension deformity in the sagittal view. A true second plane of deformity in a residual SCFE exists in the axial plane with retroversion of the hip, or external femoral torsion. However, with proper execution, the Southwick osteotomy can correct both the oblique plane deformity and the external femoral torsion deformity. The one legitimate criticism of the Southwick osteotomy is the inability to resolve the anterolateral prominence at the femoral head-neck junction that causes the FAI (Fig. 36.26).

The simple modification to the original Southwick procedure is an addition of an anterior approach to the hip with a capsulotomy and excision of the impinging prominence (Fig. 36.27) (Box 36.7). The Southwick osteotomy can be performed with either internal or external fixation. The authors' internal fixation implant of choice is a 130° cannulated locking blade plate. The external fixation of choice can be either a ring fixation device or lower profile external fixator as described by Sabharwal [46].

Positioning and Exposure

The operative technique for the Southwick osteotomy using a 130° blade plate begins with the patient placed on the operating table in the supine position. The entire lower extremity to include the groin, gluteal region, and iliac crest is sterilely prepared and draped. A lateral longitudinal incision is performed starting at the base of the greater trochanter and extended distally for approximately 10–15 cm. A typical lateral approach to the proximal femur is performed. This is

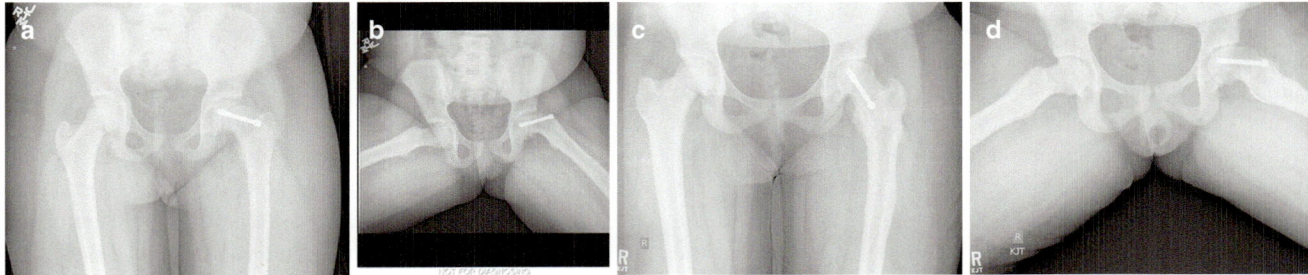

Fig. 36.26 (**a, b**) A 13-year-old female AP and frog pelvis radiographs demonstrating residual deformity after slipped capital femoral epiphysis of the left hip treated with in situ screw fixation. (**c, d**) AP and frog pelvis radiographs after proximal femoral Southwick realignment osteotomy with residual anterior deformity resulting in femoral acetabular impingement (FAI). Reprinted with permission from the Rubin Institute for Advanced Orthopedics, Sinai Hospital of Baltimore

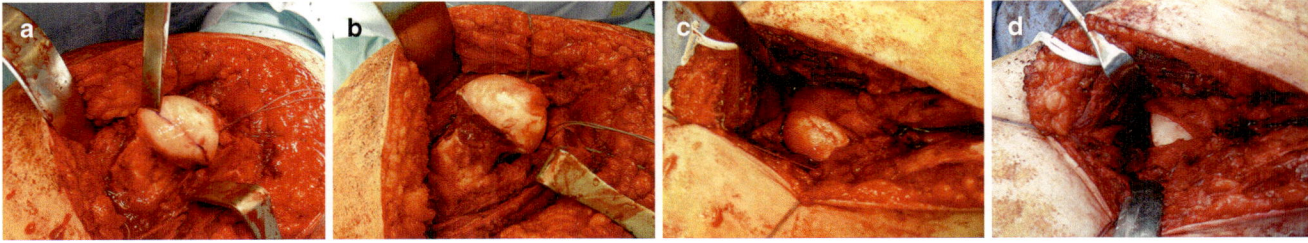

Fig. 36.27 (**a**) An example of anterolateral impingement as seen from a surgical dislocation approach; this impingement is similar to that seen after realigning the residual deformity from a SCFE with an intertrochanteric osteotomy. (**b**) The same femoral head as shown in Fig. 36.25a after bony impingement resection. (**c, d**) A similar bony resection accomplished through an anterior approach without the need for complete dislocation of the hip joint. Reprinted with permission from the Rubin Institute for Advanced Orthopedics, Sinai Hospital of Baltimore

accomplished by splitting the tensor fascia lata and retracting the vastus lateralis muscle anteriorly. The lower extremity can be extended, adducted, and internally rotated to visualize the normal profile of the femoral head within the acetabulum. This position can only be obtained by allowing the leg to hang off the side of the operating table. This is accomplished by raising the operative table and allowing the leg to extend off the side of the table on a sterile padded Mayo stand. The position of the leg denotes the deformity that must be corrected.

Deformity Correction and Fixation

A threaded guide pin is inserted into the center of the femoral head under fluoroscopic guidance in both the coronal and sagittal planes. The guide pin is first measured to determine the length of the blade, and then the appropriate-sized chisel is placed over the guide pin. The position of the guide pin determines the correction of the varus deformity, whereas, the rotation of the chisel will determine the deformity correction in the sagittal plane. In order to correct the extension deformity caused by the posteriorly slipped epiphysis, the chisel is rotated the number of degrees towards the ceiling equal to the amount of sagittal plane deformity. After the correct chisel track has been created, a transverse osteotomy in the intertrochanteric zone is performed with an oscillating saw. The chisel is withdrawn and the appropriately sized cannulated 130° blade plate is inserted over the original guide pin. An ideal 130° blade plate design has no medial offset. The distal femoral fragment is first rotated internally to correct the external femoral torsion and then reduced and secured to the plate with cortical screws, correcting the varus and extension deformities. The osteotomy is distal to the center, or apex, of the deformity, which lies at the level of the previous physis, creating an obligatory translation of the distal fragment best visualized in the sagittal plane.

Femoral Neck Osteoplasty

After completing the intertrochanteric osteotomy, all components of the SCFE have been corrected except the anterolateral impingement. An anterior approach is performed through a "bikini" type incision made in the flexion crease of the hip. The incision is approximately 2 cm below the anterior superior iliac spine and measures 6–8 cm centered over the interval between the sartorius muscle and the tensor fascia lata muscle. A typical anterior approach is performed by elevating the sartorius and tensor fascia lata muscles off of the iliac crest and releasing the rectus femoris tendon. The anterior hip capsule is identified, and a T or Z capsulotomy is performed. The anterolateral bony prominence is identified and removed with osteotomes and/or rongeurs completing the femoral neck osteoplasty (Fig. 36.28). Anteriorly, the rectus femoris tendon is repaired along with the insertions of the sartorius and tensor fascia lata muscles. Laterally, the vastus lateralis muscle is repaired to the vastus ridge and the fascia lata sutured longitudinally. The superficial tissues and skin are closed in a layered fashion over a drain.

Postoperative Care

Postoperatively, the patient is placed in a hip abduction pillow and converted to a single leg hip abduction brace before being discharged from the hospital. The patient remains with toe touch weight bearing for approximately 6 weeks and then advanced to full weight bearing after radiographic confirmation of healing at the proximal femoral osteotomy site.

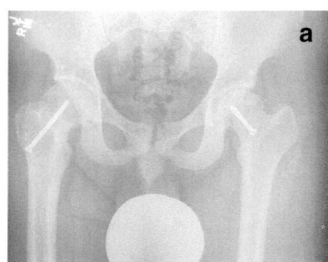 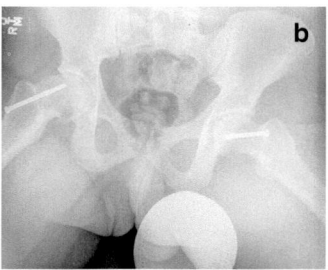 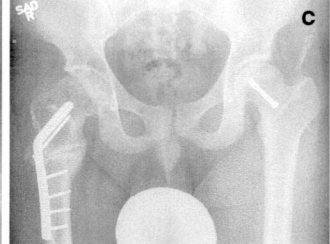 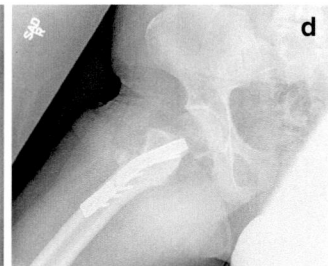

Fig. 36.28 (**a**, **b**) AP and frog pelvis radiographs of 18-year-old male with residual proximal femoral retroversion and external torsion from a previous SCFE treated at an outside facility at the age of 13 years. Preoperatively, the patient had hip flexion to 80° with significant impingement and concurrent external foot progression angle during gait. (**c**, **d**) AP pelvis and lateral hip radiographs demonstrating the results after a Southwick osteotomy with concurrent open anterior femoral acetabular impingement resection. Postoperatively, the patient attained hip flexion to 110° with no clinical impingement and a neutral foot progression angle during gait. Reprinted with permission from the Rubin Institute for Advanced Orthopedics, Sinai Hospital of Baltimore

Alternative Technique: Percutaneous Osteotomy and External Fixation

The Southwick osteotomy stabilized with an external fixation device is similar in concept, but it is performed in a percutaneous fashion. The initial proximal half pin is placed parallel to a proximal reference wire inserted from the tip of the greater trochanter to the center of the femoral head. This half pin is placed directly lateral to medial at the base of the greater trochanter. A femoral arch is attached to the initial half pin and rotated the number of degrees towards the ceiling equal to the amount of sagittal plane deformity. This is the similar technique to the chisel position described above. After the proximal femoral arch is placed in the perfect position mimicking the deformity, a second half pin is inserted from an anterolateral to posteromedial direction stabilizing the proximal construct. A distal femoral arch is mounted via two transverse half pins placed perpendicular to the anatomic axis of the proximal third of the femur. A third half pin is added to both the proximal and distal arches completing and strengthening the final construct. A multiple drill hole percutaneous osteotomy is performed through a lateral 1-cm incision in the intertrochanteric region. The two femoral arches are grasped like handles, and the fragments are manipulated correcting the deformity. The sequence of correction is rotation, translation, and then angulation. The two arches should be parallel or nearly parallel once the deformity is corrected. The two arches are now connected via three to four threaded rods with conical washers (Fig. 36.29). The anterior impingement excision is performed as previously described. Postoperatively, the patient with external fixation is allowed 50% weight bearing immediately with concurrent physiotherapy for a range of motion of the hip. Radiographs are performed every 4 weeks to determine complete consolidation of the osteotomy and eventual external fixation removal.

> **Box 36.7 Modified Southwick Osteotomy**
> The technical tips are given as follows:
>
> - A 130°, zero-offset, cannulated blade plate is an ideal implant for the procedure.
> - Directing the blade plate chisel in an appropriate oblique plane is critical for correcting varus and flexion deformities.
> - The lower extremity can be extended, adducted, and internally rotated to achieve a correct AP position of the proximal femur—this is achieved by allowing the lower extremity to come off and slightly under the OR table on a sterile padded Mayo stand; this position allows for accurate insertion of the chisel for the blade plate.
> - To minimize the risk of impingement, the surgeon should consider performing an anterior approach with anterior capsulotomy to remove the anterolateral "bump" at the neck-epiphyseal junction.
> - A percutaneous intertrochanteric osteotomy with the application of an Ilizarov external frame is a proven, alternative technique.

Residual Deformities of the Hip Joint Secondary to Legg–Calvé–Perthes Disease

Idiopathic osteonecrosis of the epiphysis in the immature hip, better known as Legg–Calvé–Perthes disease or the abbreviated Perthes disease, almost always leaves a mark or

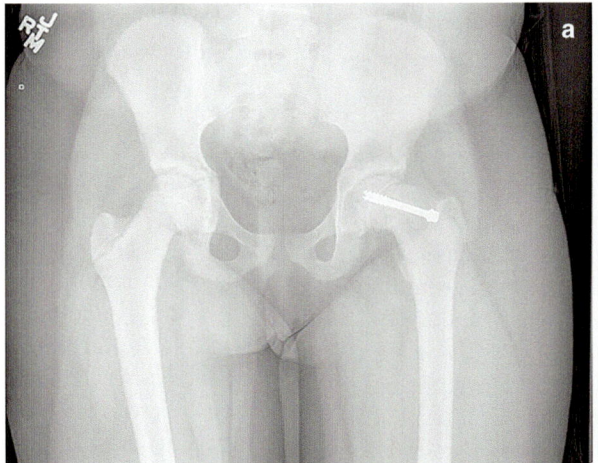 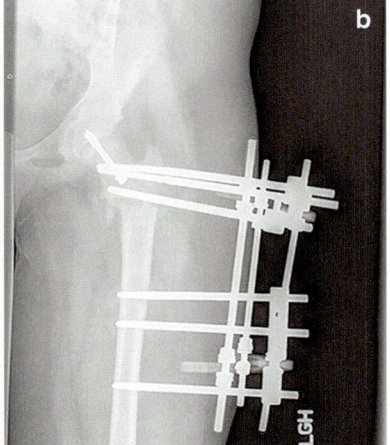

Fig. 36.29 (a, b) A 13-year-old female as previously depicted in Fig. 36.26 demonstrating the preoperative and postoperative radiographs of a proximal femoral Southwick osteotomy using an Ilizarov external fixation device. Reprinted with permission from the Rubin Institute for Advanced Orthopedics, Sinai Hospital of Baltimore

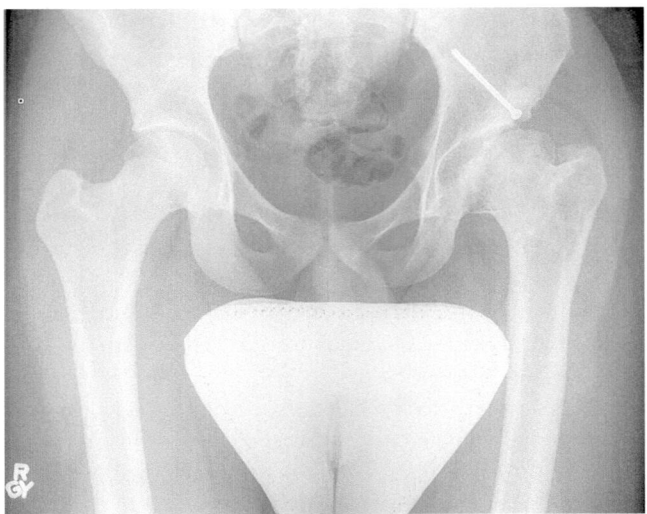

Fig. 36.30 A 16-year-old male with a history of left hip Perthes disease with residual coxa magna and coxa breva. Reprinted with permission from the Rubin Institute for Advanced Orthopedics, Sinai Hospital of Baltimore

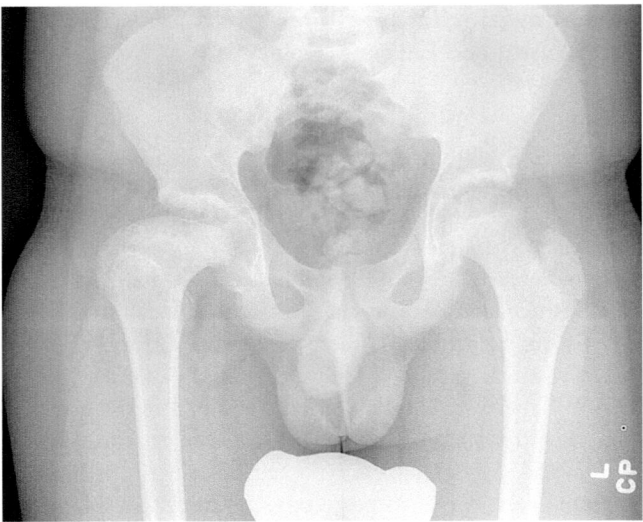

Fig. 36.31 A 12-year-old male with severe right hip residual deformity after conservative treatment for late onset Perthes disease. Reprinted with permission from the Rubin Institute for Advanced Orthopedics, Sinai Hospital of Baltimore

"foot print" on the involved hip even after the resolution of the process. The evolution of the deformity and final head morphology depends on the age of the patient and degree of vascular insult [47, 48]. The vast majority of younger patients (onset of symptoms <6 years) with Perthes disease progress through the natural healing process with good clinical outcome [49]. However, even in the case of a successful outcome with Perthes disease, residual changes or deformities of the hip can still be present. A multicentered, long-term study indicated patients with Perthes disease treated nonoperatively leads to pain, FAI, poor subjective function, and a higher incidence of osteoarthritis than previous reports [50].

The most common residual deformities are coxa breva and coxa magna (Fig. 36.30).

In the older child or in the face of an unsuccessful previous treatment, the deformities can be more severe with substantial effects on patient comfort and function. These types of residual deformities also include coxa breva and coxa magna, but severe femoral head deformity, residual proximal and lateral displacement of the femoral head, and concurrent joint contractures are also present (Fig. 36.31).

Leg length discrepancy is another residual effect of Perthes disease. Paradoxically, the younger patient with Perthes disease has a better prognosis for natural resolution of femoral head deformity, but it has a higher incidence of a clinically significant leg length discrepancy (>2.0 cm) [51]. These young patients tend to be <4 years of age at the onset of symptoms. The older patient (onset >7 years) has a worse prognosis for natural resolution, but often does not develop a clinically significant leg length discrepancy. In the authors' opinion, this is due to the fact that the femoral neck has established the majority of its natural length by this age. The more common cause of leg length discrepancy in Perthes disease is iatrogenic in nature. The proximal femur varus osteotomy is a common treatment for Perthes disease. However, an overly aggressive varus osteotomy can result in a significant coxa vara, limb shortening, and a decreased articulo-trochanteric distance, which is associated with a mechanically weak hip abductor mechanism causing a long lasting limp [52–55]. Furthermore, the "containment" afforded by the varus osteotomy does not unload the hip or guarantee maintenance of this containment in the postoperative period. Therefore, the author does not recommend the varus osteotomy as the treatment of choice for Perthes disease. Instead, for Perthes disease that has failed conservative management in the younger age group or in late onset Perthes disease, the author recommends articulated hip distraction via open soft tissue releases and external fixation placement. Details of this technique are described later in the chapter.

Coxa Breva

As previously stated, coxa breva is defined as shortening and widening of the femoral neck, which alters the relationship of the tip of the greater trochanter to the center of the femoral head [2]. This creates a mechanical disadvantage of the hip joint by decreasing the lever arm of the hip and decreasing the distance between the origin and insertion points of the gluteus medius muscle. The radiographic presence of coxa breva is not a definitive indication for surgical correction. In reality, coxa breva is ubiquitous in the post-Perthes patient, but very few actually require surgical reconstruction. The indication for surgical reconstruction is based on the patient's function, gait, and leg length discrepancy. Coxa breva in the presence of a persistent Trendelenburg gait, hip fatigue, and hip pain with prolonged activity requires surgical reconstruction. Surgical treatments described for coxa breva include greater trochanteric epiphysiodesis, and greater trochanter transfer (i.e., relative neck lengthening), but ideal treatment remains ill-defined [1, 56].

The author's preferred method of correction of coxa breva is a femoral neck lengthening osteotomy with concurrent greater trochanteric transfer, originally described by Edwin Morscher in 1980 [57] (Box 36.8). The Morscher osteotomy improves the lever arm length of the hip joint by lengthening the femoral neck, corrects a leg length discrepancy up to 1.5–2.0 cm, and reestablishes the center of the femoral head to the tip of the greater trochanteric relationship through distal transfer of the greater trochanter. The greater trochanteric transfer not only increases the distance between the origin and insertion of the gluteus medius muscle, but it also adds lateral distance to the mechanical lever arm of the hip joint, which imparts greater mechanical advantage to the gluteus medius muscle. For the Morscher osteotomy to be successful, the hip joint should be congruent with full range of motion with no evidence of FAI. The following is a brief description of the author's preferred technique for the Morscher osteotomy.

The Morscher Osteotomy for Coxa Breva Secondary to Perthes Disease: Operative Technique

Positioning and Exposure

The operative technique for the Morscher osteotomy begins with the patient placed on the operating table in the supine position. The entire lower extremity to include the groin, gluteal region, and iliac crest is sterilely prepared and draped (Fig. 36.32).

A lateral longitudinal incision is performed starting approximately 5 cm above the tip of the greater trochanter and extending distally for approximately 10 cm. A lateral approach to the proximal femur is performed by splitting the tensor fascia lata and lifting the vastus lateralis muscle anteriorly. Proximally, the gluteus maximus muscle fibers should be dissected away from the tensor fascia allowing the gluteus maximus to fall posteriorly. This allows for better visualization of the gluteus medius muscle and easier dissection of the greater trochanteric fragment-gluteus medius muscle complex later in the procedure.

Deformity Correction and Fixation

The internal fixation of choice is a 130° cannulated blade plate. After exposure of the lateral aspect of the proximal femur, a central threaded guide pin is inserted up the femoral neck and into the femoral head. This guide wire represents the eventual path of the blade plate and the new femoral neck orientation. Three additional guide wires are inserted parallel to the initial guide wire. The second guide wire is inserted at the level of the superior base of the femoral head, which represents the new level of the superior border of the femoral neck. The third wire is inserted approximately 1 cm above the second wire. This represents the new base of the greater trochanter (Fig. 36.33).

The interval bone segment between the second and third wire will be removed and used as a bone graft. The final guide wire is inserted at the level of the inferior border of the femoral neck. This final guide wire represents the sliding osteotomy surface that will result in femoral neck lengthening as well as lower extremity lengthening. Again, it is important that the guide wires are inserted in a parallel or near parallel fashion. Next, the appropriately sized blade plate chisel is

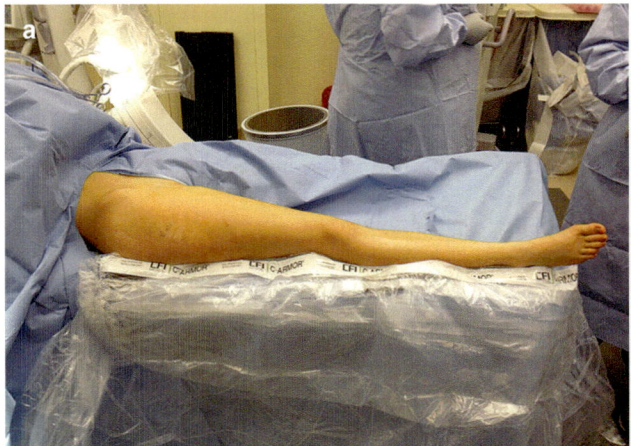
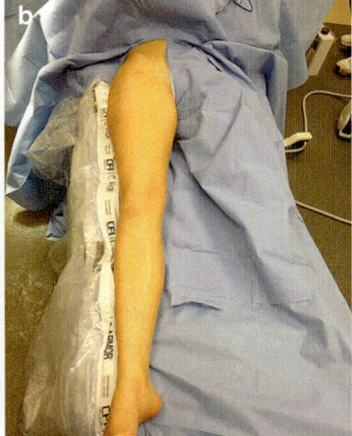

Fig. 36.32 (a, b) Clinical pictures depicting the typical patient position and draping for the Morscher osteotomy. Reprinted with permission from the Rubin Institute for Advanced Orthopedics, Sinai Hospital of Baltimore

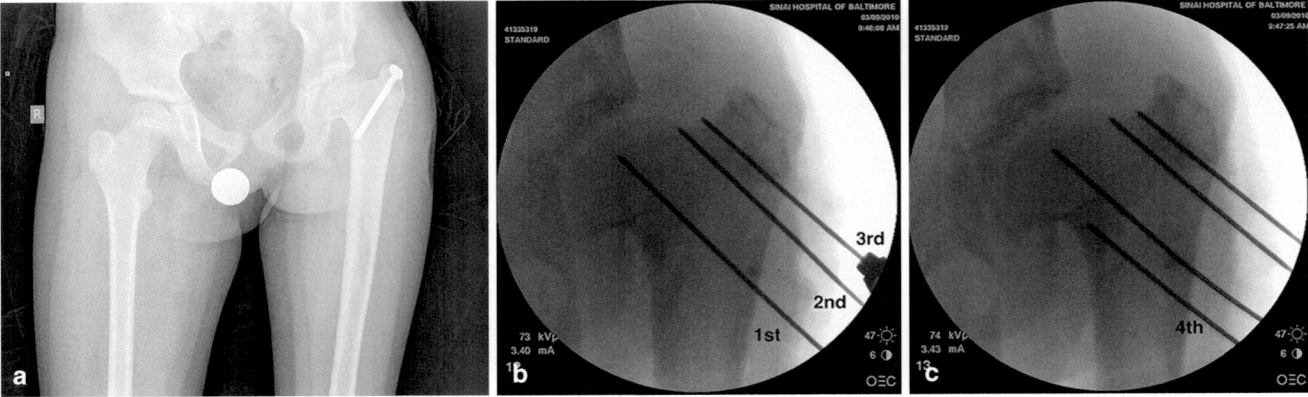

Fig. 36.33 (a) AP pelvis radiography demonstrating severe coxa breva of the left hip. (b, c) The same patient undergoing left hip Morscher osteotomy with intraoperative fluoroscopic views demonstrating the placement of the guide wires. The first guide wire is inserted at an angle of 130° and marks the path for the blade plate; the second wire marks the superior border of the new femoral neck; the third wire marks the trochanteric osteotomy site; and the fourth wire marks the inferior border of the new femoral neck. Reprinted with permission from the Rubin Institute for Advanced Orthopedics, Sinai Hospital of Baltimore

driven over the central guide wire. The chisel should be held in neutral rotation in the sagittal plane to prevent secondary flexion or extension of the osteotomy that would result in minimal contact between the proximal and distal fragments. Once the chisel is fully seated, the appropriate blade length is calculated by adding an additional 1–1.5 cm of length to the chisel length. An oscillating saw is used to cut the bone along the two proximal and the distal most guide wires. The first cut is the most proximal osteotomy that is used to mobilize the greater trochanteric fragment along with the gluteus medius muscle. The second cut creates the new superior border of the femoral neck allowing for mobilization and removal of the interval bone segment (Fig. 36.34).

This bone should be placed into a moist sponge for later use. The final osteotomy creates the distal border of the femoral neck that separates the proximal femoral segment from the distal femoral shaft. After the osteotomies are completed, the chisel is removed and the selected blade plate is inserted over the initial threaded guide wire. The blade should be driven to a level that leaves approximately 1–1.5 cm of blade exposed laterally (Fig. 36.35).

The distal fragment is then reduced to the plate with bone holding forceps. This maneuver causes the distal fragment to slide down the oblique osteotomy, accomplishing femoral neck lengthening, as well as lower extremity lengthening (Fig. 36.36).

The previously removed bone fragment is now notched and placed over the exposed end of the blade plate at the 130° bend.

The final step of the procedure is the mobilization and advancement of the greater trochanter both laterally and distally. The appropriate level of the greater trochanteric transfer is accomplished when the tip of the greater trochanter is at or below the level of the center of the femoral head. This position is obtained by carefully mobilizing the gluteus medius muscle and abducting the hip 10–15° before fixation. The greater trochanteric fragment is stabilized with a cannulated 5.5-mm screw and washer, tension band wiring, or a combination of both techniques (Fig. 36.37).

The operative incision is closed as previously described in a layered fashion over a drain.

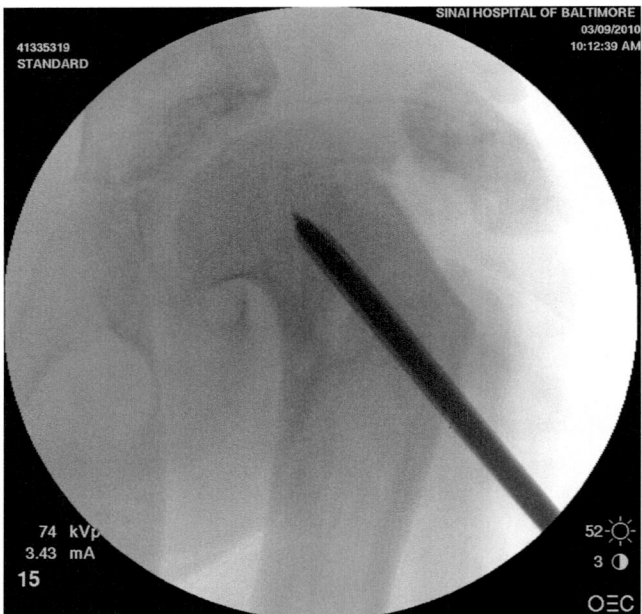

Fig. 36.34 A fluoroscopic image demonstrating the completion of the first two osteotomy cuts allowing for mobilization of the greater trochanter, removal of interval bone segment, and the creation of the new superior border of the femoral neck. Reprinted with permission from the Rubin Institute for Advanced Orthopedics, Sinai Hospital of Baltimore

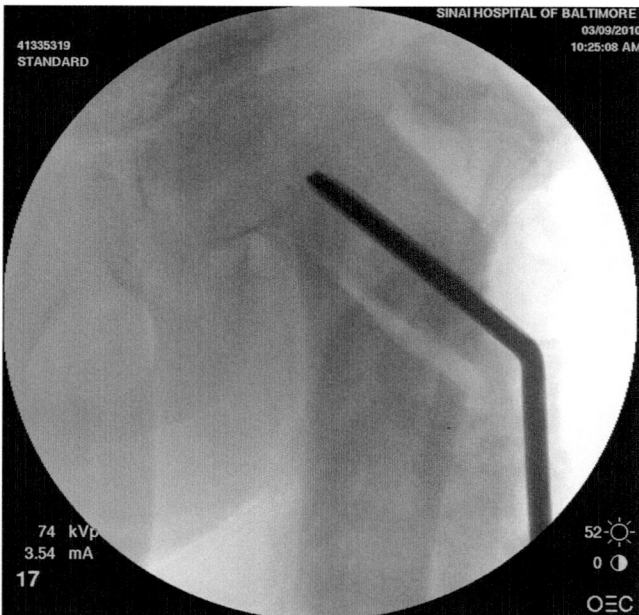

Fig. 36.35 Fluoroscopic image demonstrating the final osteotomy cut that creates the inferior border of the new femoral neck and the insertion of the 130° blade plate. Reprinted with permission from the Rubin Institute for Advanced Orthopedics, Sinai Hospital of Baltimore

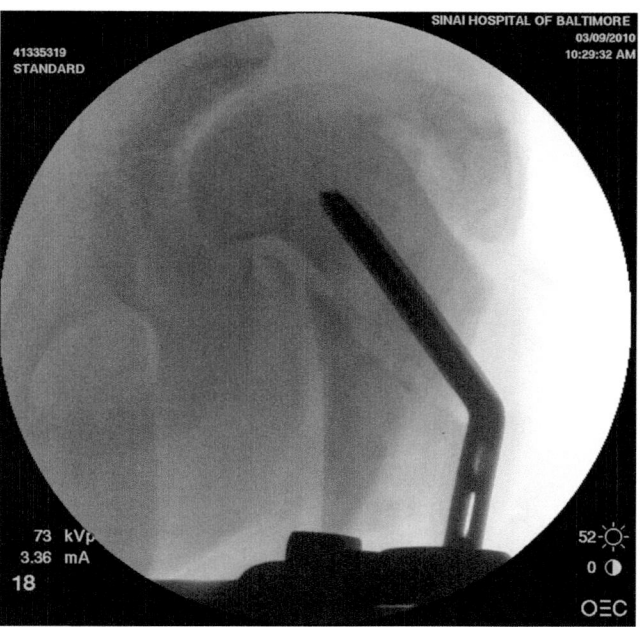

Fig. 36.36 Fluoroscopic image showing the reduction of the distal femoral segment reduced to the blade plate that extended out of the proximal segment by 1.0–1.5 cm, which results in a lengthened femoral neck. Reprinted with permission from the Rubin Institute for Advanced Orthopedics, Sinai Hospital of Baltimore

Fig. 36.37 (a, b) Fluoroscopic images demonstrating the advancement of the greater trochanter with temporary wire fixation and final fixation with a cannulated screw and tension wire. Reprinted with permission from the Rubin Institute for Advanced Orthopedics, Sinai Hospital of Baltimore

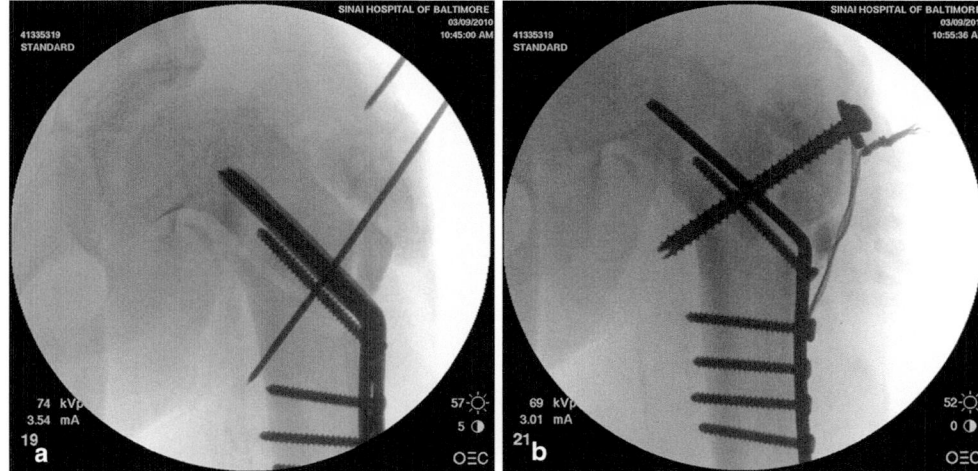

Postoperative Care

The patient is placed in a hip abduction pillow immediately and converted to a single leg hip abduction brace before discharge from the hospital. The patient is maintained a at toe touch weight bearing status and full time brace wear for the initial 6 weeks. After 6 weeks, the brace is used at night for an additional 6 weeks and gradual advancement of weight bearing, hip range of motion, and hip strengthening begins under the supervision of a physiotherapist.

Two key tips for the Morscher osteotomy are the amount of lateral displacement of the distal fragment and the initial position of the chisel in the sagittal plane. First, the distal femoral fragment should not be translated laterally more than 50% of the original diameter of the proximal femur. If the bone-to-bone contact is less than 50% of the original diameter, then there is a significant increase in implant failure. Second, the chisel position in the sagittal plane should be shifted slightly anterior or posterior to allow enough space for the eventual trochanteric cannulated screw to pass without difficulty (Figs. 36.38 and 36.39).

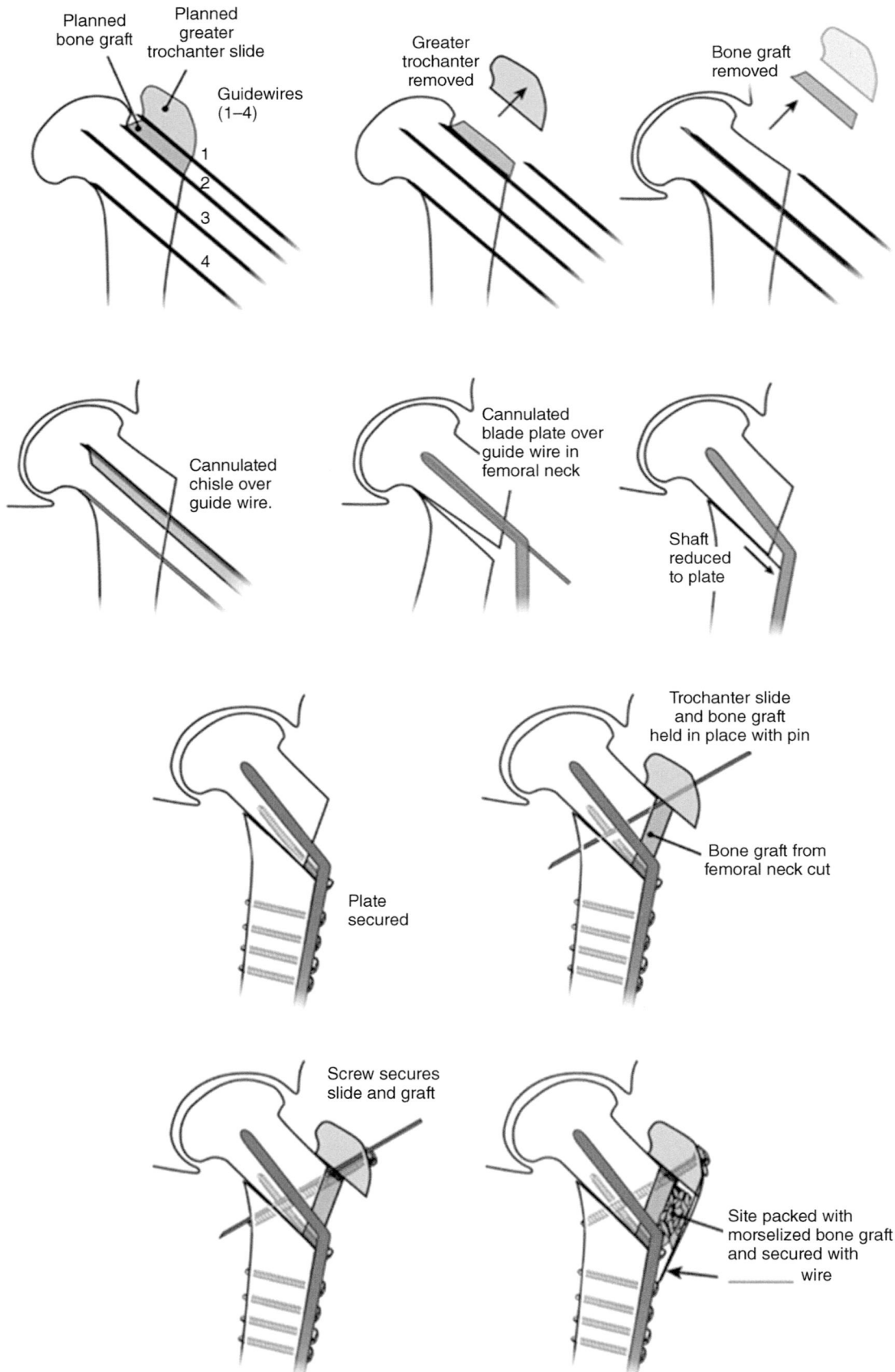

Fig. 36.38 Step-by-step schematic summary of the Morscher osteotomy. Reprinted with permission from the Rubin Institute for Advanced Orthopedics, Sinai Hospital of Baltimore

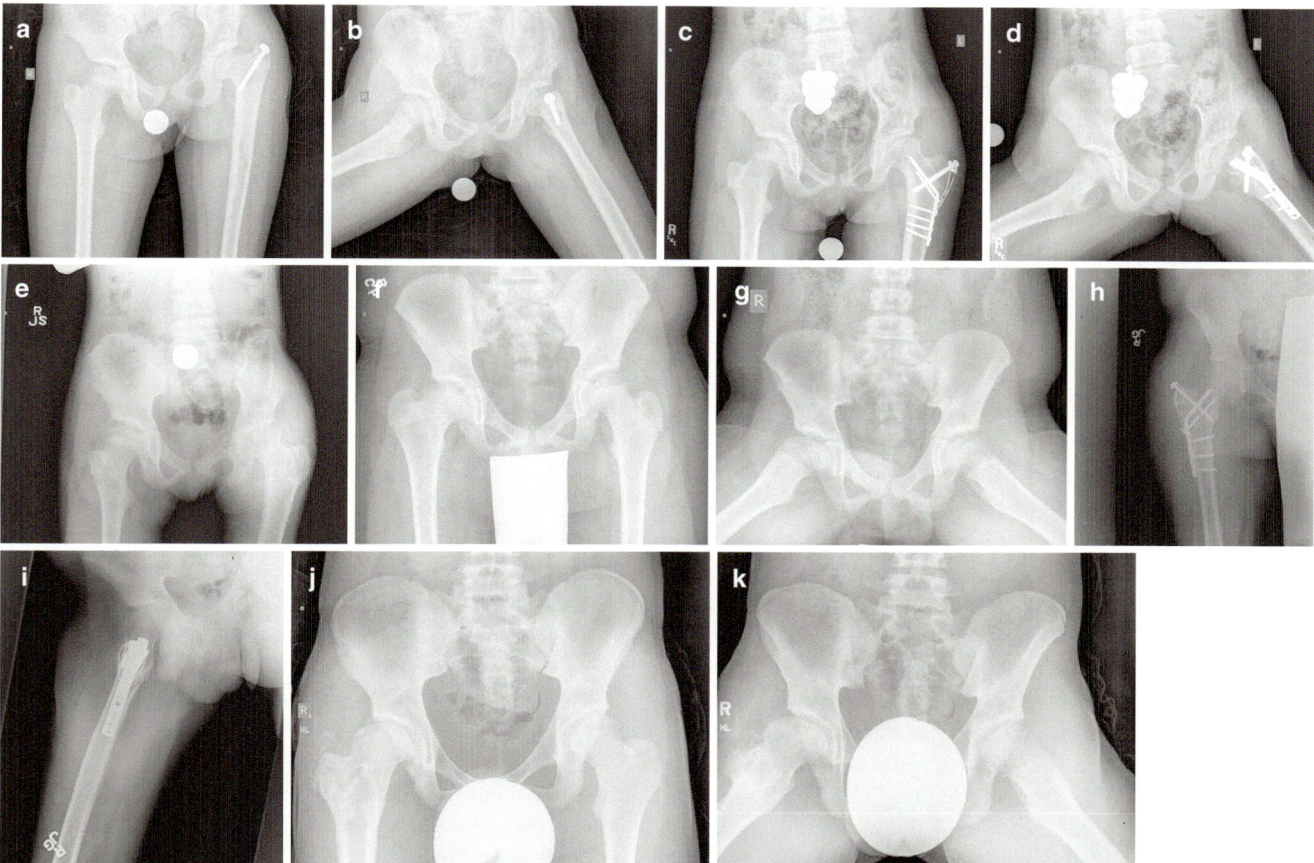

Fig. 36.39 (**a**, **b**) A 12-year-old female with severe left hip coxa breva from previous AVN. This is the same patient depicted in Figs. 36.33, 36.34, 36.35, 36.36, and 36.37. (**c**, **d**) One year post-reconstruction of the left hip using the Morscher osteotomy technique. (**e**) Three years post-reconstruction AP pelvis radiograph after internal implant removal. (**f**, **g**) Another example of coxa breva demonstrated by AP and frog pelvis of a 13-year-old male with residual right hip deformity from Perthes disease. (**h**, **i**) Immediate postoperative AP and lateral radiographs of the right hip after Morscher osteotomy. (**j**, **k**) Five-year follow-up of the same patient after internal implant removal. Reprinted with permission from the Rubin Institute for Advanced Orthopedics, Sinai Hospital of Baltimore

---

Box 36.8 Morscher Osteotomy for Coxa Breva
The technical tips are given as follows:

- The initial guide wire is inserted at an angle of 130°. This is the angulation of the new femoral neck.
- A 130°, zero-offset, cannulated blade plate is an ideal implant for the procedure.
- The length of the blade plate is determined by measuring the initial guide wire inserted up the femoral neck and adding 10–15 mm to this measurement.
- When the blade plate is inserted, the plate is left away from the lateral cortex by 10–15 mm; this will allow the distal fragment to shift laterally, lengthening the femoral neck.
- It is critical not to translate the distal segment more than 50% of the original diameter of the subtrochanteric width of the femur. If greater than a 50% translation is performed, then inadequate bone contact will be present and an increased risk for implant failure will occur.
- The trochanteric fragment must be carefully mobilized without compromising the innervation of the gluteus medius muscle.
- The interval bone segment removed from the superior femoral neck osteotomy should be saved for femoral neck bone grafting around the proximal bend of the 130° blade plate.
- The greater trochanter should be advanced until the proximal tip is at or below the center of the femoral head.

Coxa Magna

As previously stated, coxa magna is a common residual deformity of Perthes disease. Coxa magna is defined as the enlargement and deformation of the femoral head. This deformity can result in the loss of congruency between the femoral head and acetabulum resulting in FAI. Severe coxa magna causes pain, loss of motion, labral and cartilage degeneration, and eventual osteoarthritis [3–6]. Coxa magna is caused by a combination of the collapse of the proximal femoral epiphysis and altered growth of the articular cartilage (Fig. 36.40).

The coxa magna deformity begins as the femoral head settles after the initial subchondral collapse of the epiphysis. This results in a decreased height and an increased width of the femoral head, similar to applying downward pressure on a water balloon. The amount of continued collapse appears to be related to the amount of epiphyseal involvement and the age of the patient. However, there is a significant variation to the pattern of collapse between individual patients, and an exact method for predicting the amount of eventual collapse has not been developed. The second variable in the development of coxa magna is the abnormal articular cartilage growth. This abnormal growth is caused by asymmetric pressure applied to the growing femoral head. The cause of the abnormal femoral head growth and deformation is directly related to the loss of hip joint motion and the presence of a significant hip joint contracture. In the stiff hip that has lost significant range of motion, the joint pressures are asymmetric over the femoral head. The zone of contact between the femoral head and the superior articular surface of the acetabulum and acetabular rim represents areas of increased pressure, whereas the portions of the femoral head that are anterior and lateral to the acetabular rim and medial within the acetabular fossa are areas of decreased pressure. The areas of increased pressure obviously expedite any collapse as the underlying epiphysis loses structural integrity. Furthermore, this pressure also compresses and slows the articular cartilage growth. Conversely, the areas of decreased pressure allow the articular cartilage to grow into the "unweighted" zones, thereby exacerbating the femoral head deformation and coxa magna formation.

Another crucial variable in the evaluation of the coxa magna deformity is the adaptive remodeling changes of the acetabulum. In young patient (<6 years) with Perthes disease, full collapse of the epiphysis can occur with coxa magna formation, but the femoral head remains spherical and the hip joint congruent. It is the author's experience and opinion that this outcome is directly related to the maintenance of adequate hip range of motion during the entire healing process of the femoral head. The only true method to maintain "containment" of the femoral head is to maintain an adequate hip range of motion. The adequate hip range of motion is defined by the author as hip motion that is >50% of the contralateral normal hip. Even in the face of an enlarged and oblong femoral head, adequate range of motion of the hip joint allows the acetabulum to remodel into a larger and oblong congruent joint. This situation can provide a pain-free functional hip joint for several decades with excellent quality of life (Fig. 36.41).

However, in males more than 12 years of age and females more than 10 years of age, even with successful maintenance of hip range of motion and a relatively spherical femoral head, the amount of acetabular remodeling is minimal in the author's experience. Even mild changes to the overall diameter or shape of the femoral head are not tolerated in this age group. Although these patients have initial good results, the mild to moderate incongruence of the hip joint will eventually lead to FAI and the need for hip reconstruction to avoid early degenerative changes.

The treatment of choice for significant coxa magna deformity of the femoral head is the femoral head reduction osteotomy, also known as the "head splitting" or "head reshaping" osteotomy, initially described by Ganz [58]. This technique utilizes Ganz's well-described surgical hip dislocation approach and has shown promising early results [58–60]. The following is a brief description of the opera-

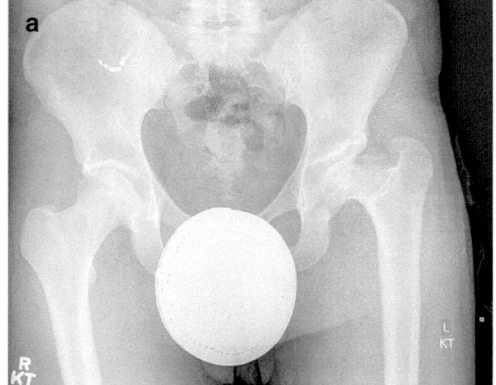 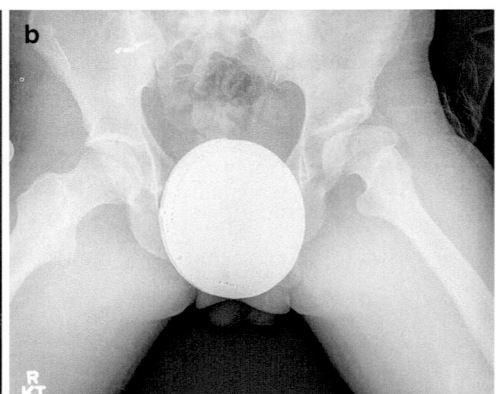

Fig. 36.40 (a, b) Radiographic example of a coxa magna deformity resulting in loss of congruency of the hip joint and femoral acetabular impingement. Reprinted with permission from the Rubin Institute for Advanced Orthopedics, Sinai Hospital of Baltimore

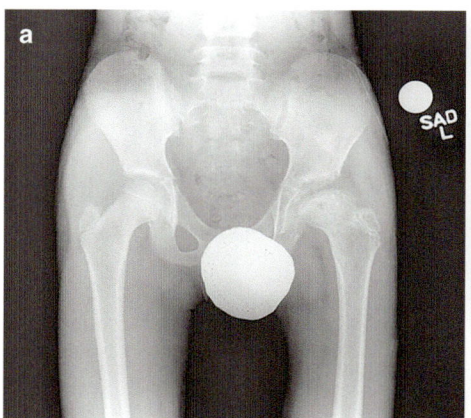
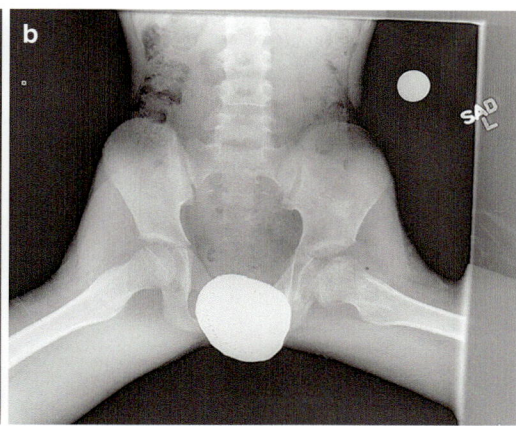

Fig. 36.41 (**a, b**) AP and frog pelvis radiographs demonstrating a congruent coxa magna and oblong acetabulum in a patient after late-onset Perthes disease. Reprinted with permission from the Rubin Institute for Advanced Orthopedics, Sinai Hospital of Baltimore

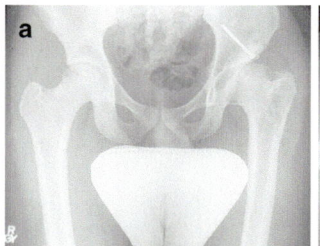
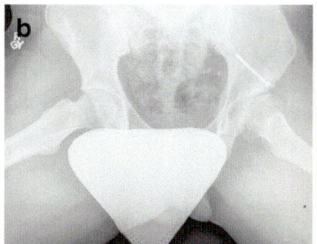
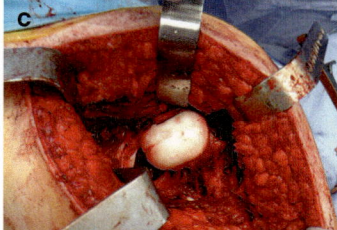
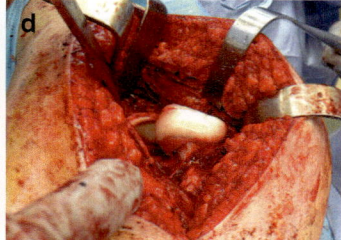

Fig. 36.42 (**a, b**) AP and frog pelvis radiographs depicting the same patient in Fig. 36.30, a 16-year-old male with coxa magna, coxa breva, and concurrent FAI. (**c, d**) Clinical appearance of the femoral head of the same patient after surgical dislocation. It is the author's experience that the true three-dimensional shape of the femoral head does not consistently correlate with various imaging studies; therefore, MRI and CT scans are rarely indicated or performed. Reprinted with permission from the Rubin Institute for Advanced Orthopedics, Sinai Hospital of Baltimore

tive technique for the femoral head reduction osteotomy (Box 36.9).

The Femoral Head Reduction Osteotomy for Coxa Magna Secondary to Perthes Disease: Operative Technique

Positioning and Exposure

The patient positioning and operative approach are identical to the surgical hip dislocation as described above for the modified Dunn procedure. After the capsulotomy and gentle dislocation of the hip, the acetabulum and labrum are inspected for any pathological changes. With the femoral head dislocated, the posterolateral soft tissue leash is inspected for any undue tension and the exact three-dimensional head shape is visualized for planning the osteotomy (Fig. 36.42).

Any cartilage softening and depressed areas are noted as the femoral head is inspected. These areas need to be included in the segmental resection of the mid portion of the femoral head. Femoral head sizing templates, surgical experience, and three-dimensional awareness are used to determine the exact position of the femoral head cuts (Fig. 36.43).

Deformity Correction and Fixation

The femoral head cut is rarely in a pure anterior to posterior direction. Usually, the cut is from an anterolateral to a posteromedial direction. The greater the amount of the sagittal plane deformity, the more lateral the starting point for the osteotomy needs to be placed. The planned resection of the bone can be in a shape of a wafer or a wedge depending on the deformity to be corrected. The greater the sagittal plane deformity present, the more likely a wedge shape is needed to completely correct the oblique plane deformity. Two K-wires are inserted to represent the two longitudinal cuts (Fig. 36.44).

The most medial cut is performed first with great care to leave greater than a third of the original diameter of the femoral neck intact. Rotating the saw blade in a counterclockwise direction allows a greater segment of the medial neck to remain intact for stability of the medial head fragment. The second osteotomy is now performed. This bone cut is the

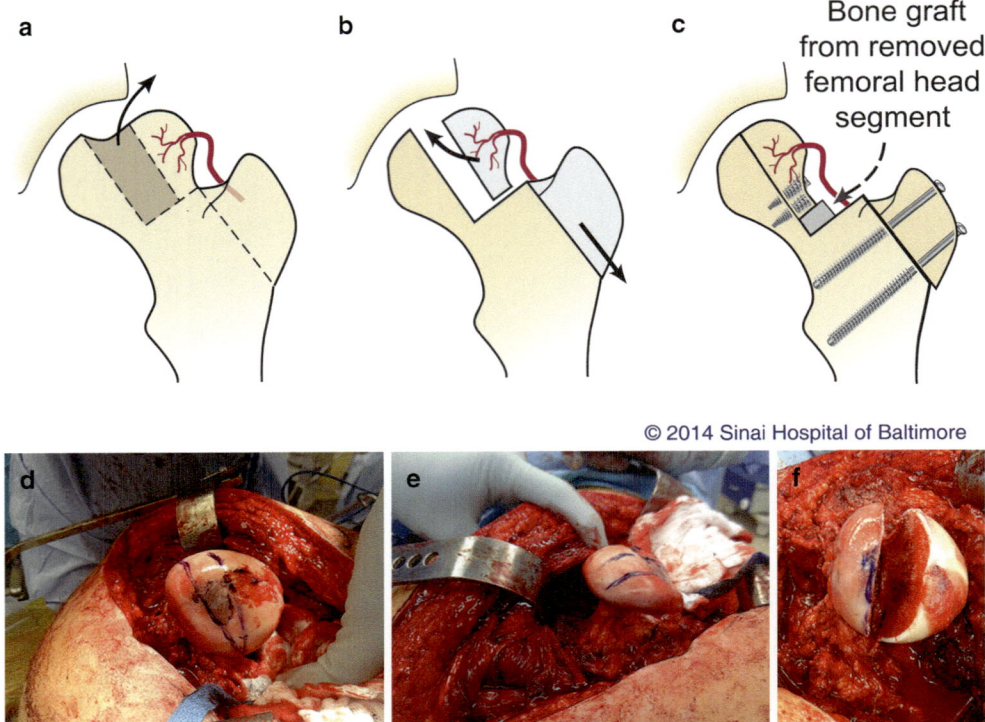

Fig. 36.43 (**a–c**) Schematic representation of the femoral head reduction/reshaping osteotomy depicting the creation of a spherical femoral head by excising an interval deformed section of bone. (**d–f**) Clinical pictures of another case demonstrating the femoral head osteotomy planning lines that resolves a three-dimensional puzzle into two separate pieces that can be placed together to form a spherical object. Reprinted with permission from the Rubin Institute for Advanced Orthopedics, Sinai Hospital of Baltimore

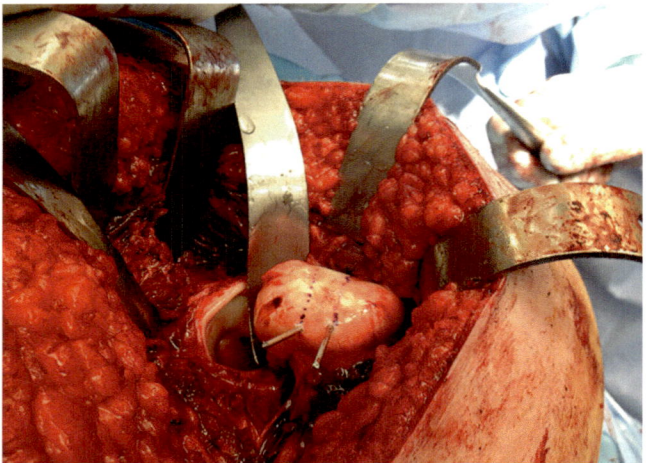

Fig. 36.44 Two guide wires are placed at the planned longitudinal osteotomy sites. Reprinted with permission from the Rubin Institute for Advanced Orthopedics, Sinai Hospital of Baltimore

closest to the posterolateral segment containing the blood supply; and so, great care is needed to avoid the retinacular vessels entering in the lateral femoral head segment. The final transverse bone cut is performed at the base of the femoral neck, connecting the first two vertical bone cut (Fig. 36.45).

Again, this transverse cut must be performed with great care to avoid the intact medial neck and the posterolateral head-neck junction where the blood supply is entering the lateral femoral head segment. This final cut creates separation of the central free fragment from the medial head fragment that is still attached to the intact medial femoral neck, and the lateral mobile femoral head segment attached via the soft tissue vascular leash. The middle segment is carefully removed and the lateral fragment is mobilized (Fig. 36.46).

The lateral fragment is reduced to the stable medial head fragment and held with pointed bone reduction forceps. The lateral femoral head fragment usually requires proximal advancement along with the medial translation. The vascular leash is inspected for tension or tenting over the residual base of neck. If a significant medial translation or closing wedge is needed, then the posterolateral base of the femoral neck must be reduced in size to prevent impingement and tension on the vascular leash. After the femoral head is reduced and vascular supply is inspected, three transverse headless screws are inserted to secure the femoral head osteotomy (Fig. 36.47a, b).

The gap between the base of the lateral femoral head fragment and the femoral neck is filled with a bone graft obtained from the removed femoral head fragment. The femoral head is gently reduced into the acetabulum and joint motion is assessed. Any residual impinging bone of the anterior femoral head or neck is excised. The capsule is repaired with absorbable heavy suture and suture anchors at the base of the femoral neck as needed. It is crucial not to over tighten the capsular repair that can place undue tension on the posterior capsule and thereby on the vascular leash.

After the femoral head has been reduced, the acetabular coverage should be assessed. If a triple osteotomy is determined to be needed either preoperatively or after the femoral head osteotomy has been completed, then the previously

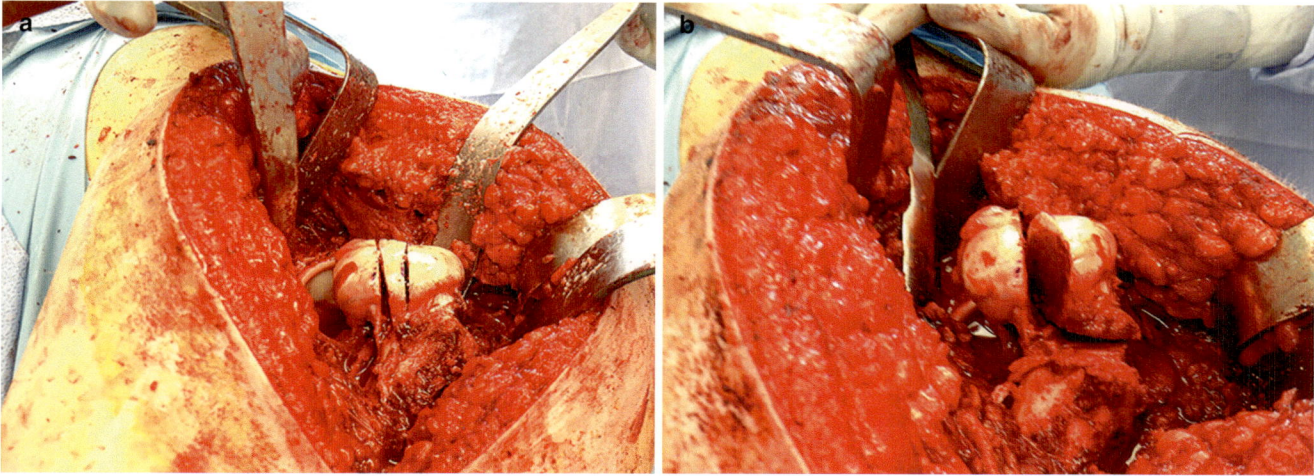

Fig. 36.45 Clinical pictures denoting the two longitudinal cuts (**a**) and the transverse cut (**b**) that create the mobile lateral femoral head fragment attached via the vascular leash. Reprinted with permission from the Rubin Institute for Advanced Orthopedics, Sinai Hospital of Baltimore

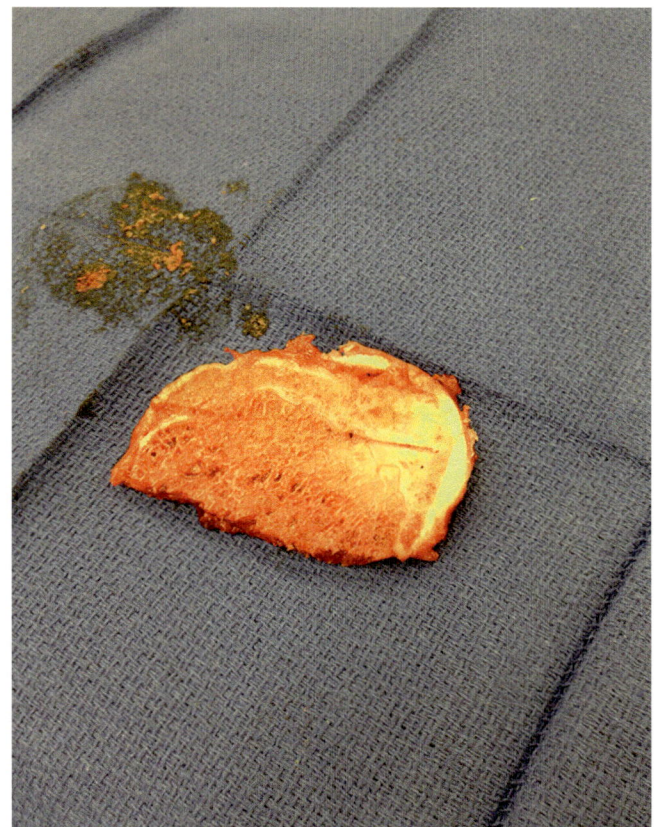

Fig. 36.46 Clinical picture of the excised middle segment. The bone at the base of the cut can be utilized as bone graft in the femoral neck. Reprinted with permission from the Rubin Institute for Advanced Orthopedics, Sinai Hospital of Baltimore

described two incision Tönnis triple pelvic osteotomy techniques should be performed (Fig. 36.48a and b—X-ray example of combined femoral head osteotomy and Tonnis triple osteotomy).

The hip is placed in mild abduction, and the greater trochanter is advanced distally until the tip of the greater trochanter is equal to or below the center of the newly shaped femoral head. The greater trochanter is secured via two 5.5-mm cannulated screws. It is crucial to direct the screws away from the medial femoral neck base to prevent propagation of a fracture from the screw hole to the medial femoral neck which will result in destabilization of the medial head fragment (Fig. 36.47c, d).

The incision is closed in a routine layered fashion with the tensor fascia lata, subcutaneous tissues, and skin closed over a drain. The patient is gently placed into a supine position with an abduction pillow and a final radiography is performed (Fig. 36.49).

Postoperative Care

Postoperatively, the patient is placed in a single-leg abduction brace full time except when using a CPM machine for hip flexion and extension. The CPM machine is used 2–4 h during the day and all night for the first 6 weeks. Alternatively, the patient may use the CPM for a greater time during the day and utilize the hip abduction brace at night. The protocol can be adjusted per the patient's preference. Physical therapy consists of simple passive range of motion of the hip not to exceed the following parameters: 75° of hip flexion, 30–40° of hip abduction, full hip extension, zero hip adduction, and 30° of internal rotation and 30° of external rotation. Active sitting and CPM motion can be maximized, increasing the hip flexion to the patient's tolerance. The CPM and daytime bracing are discontinued 6 weeks postoperatively. Toe touch weight bearing is mandated for 3 months to ensure complete healing of the femoral head (Figs. 36.50 and 36.51).

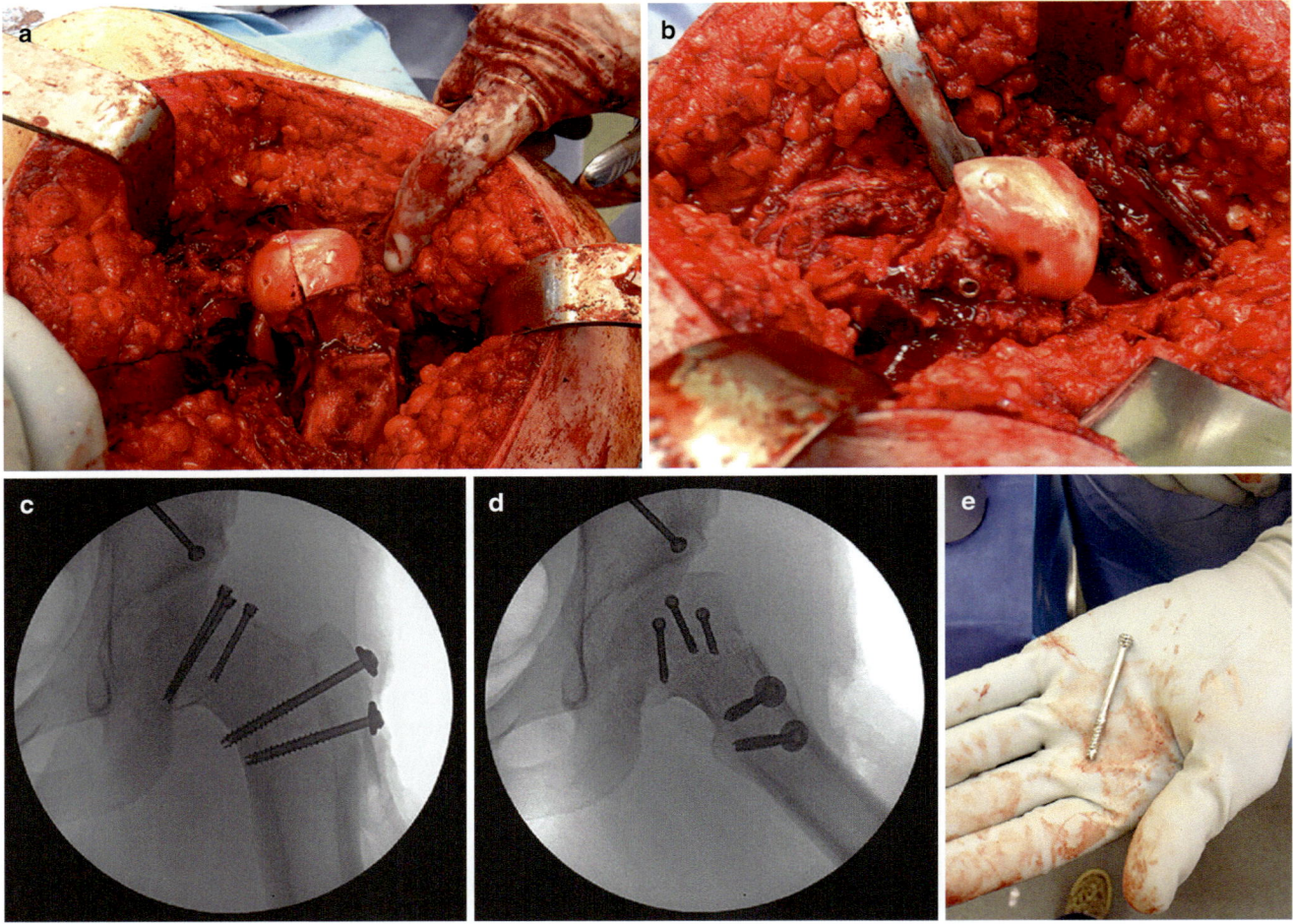

Fig. 36.47 (**a**, **b**) Clinical pictures of the final configuration of the femoral head after fixation of the medial and lateral head fragments with three transverse headless screws. (**c**, **d**) Fluoroscopic images of the final femoral head fixation, hip reduction, and greater trochanter fixation. (**e**) Typical headless screw is used to fix the femoral head osteotomy. Reprinted with permission from the Rubin Institute for Advanced Orthopedics, Sinai Hospital of Baltimore

Box 36.9 Femoral Head Reduction Osteotomy

The technical tips are given as follows:

- Adequate thickness of the greater trochanter osteotomy must be maintained for later fixation (1–1.5 cm width).
- The most critical aspect of the exposure is creating and maintaining the posterior retinacular soft tissue sleeve to the lateral femoral head segment.
- Removing 5–8 mm of bone from the posterior margin and the base of the greater trochanter will aid in relieving tension on the vascular flap.
- The determination of the medial and lateral head fragments is performed with femoral head sizing templates and intra-operative three-dimensional analysis.
- The medial longitudinal femoral head osteotomy should leave at least 1/3 of the femoral neck intact.
- The lateral longitudinal femoral head osteotomy should be placed to remove all interval damaged/deformed femoral head; the goal is to reduce the femoral head to a size that is completely contained within the acetabulum.
- The transverse femoral neck osteotomy that creates the free interval and lateral femoral head fragments should not violate the medial femoral neck.
- If the residual femoral neck is less than 1/3 the original diameter, then a retrograde 4.5-mm screw should be inserted from the proximal femoral metaphysis into the medial femoral head fragment.
- The femoral head osteotomy is stabilized with three to four 3.0 mm/4.3 mm headless screws.
- The mobile, lateral femoral head fragment is advanced proximally and medially to the stable medial femoral head fragment; the excised bone

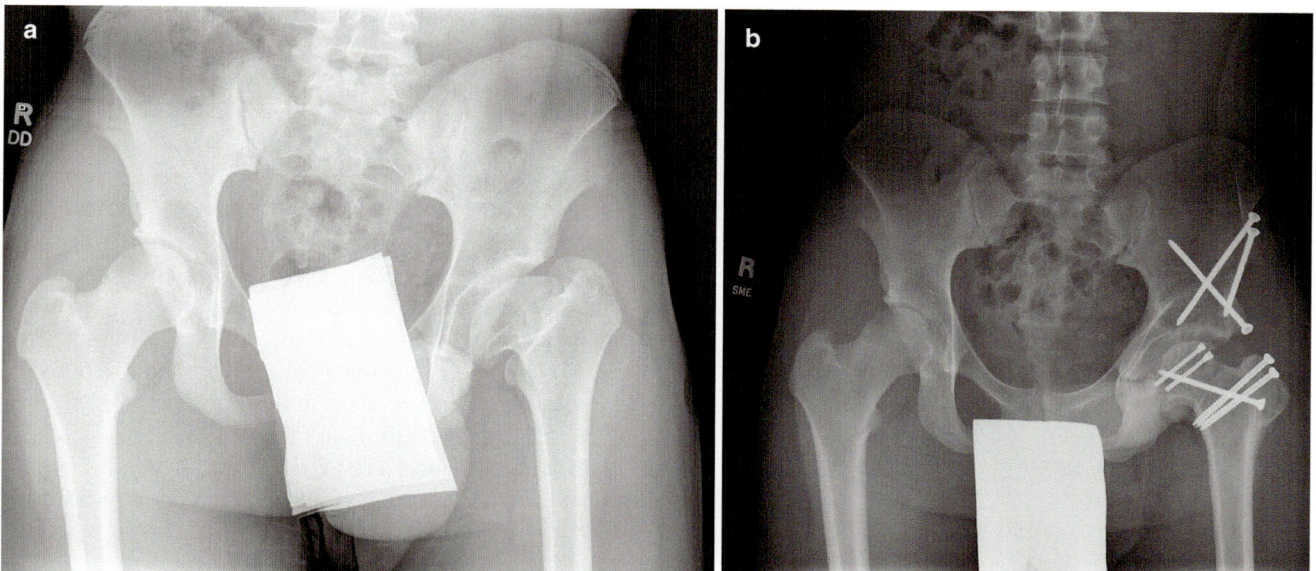

Fig. 36.48 (**a** and **b**) Pre- and 1-year post-op radiograph of patient with residual deformity from Perthes disease. The radiographs demonstrate significant coxa breva and coxa magna with concurrent acetabular dysplasia. The patient was treated with femoral head reduction osteotomy and Tönnis triple osteotomy

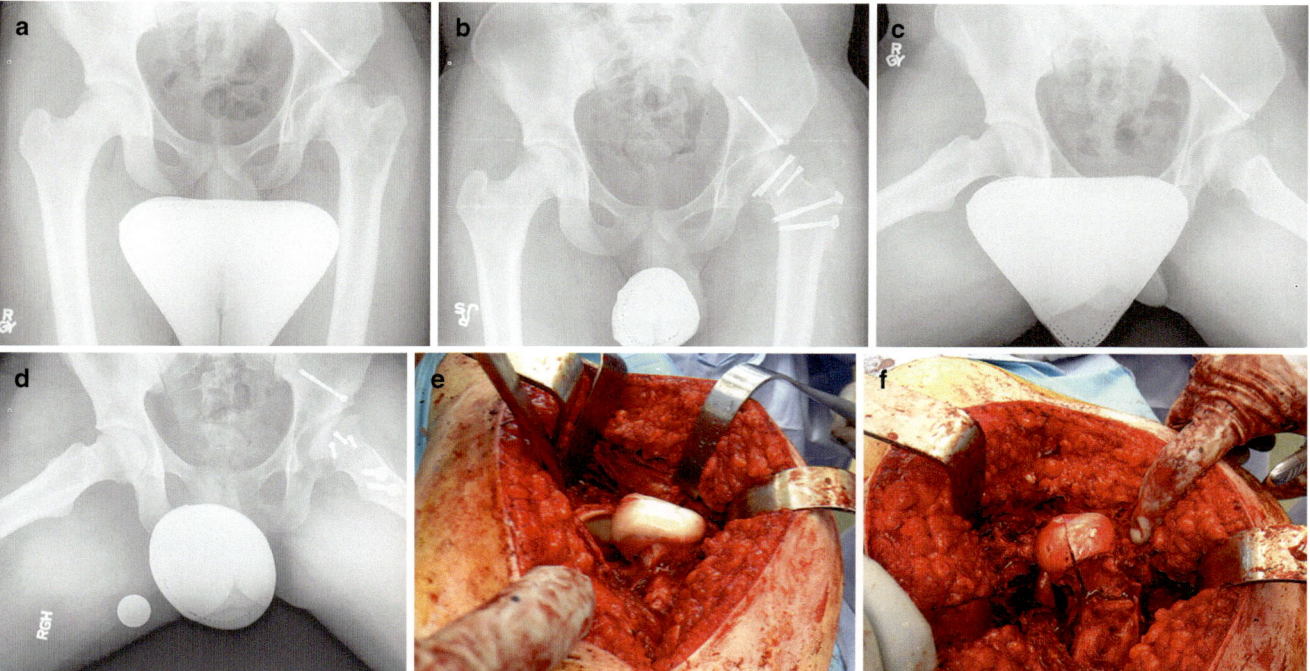

Fig. 36.49 (**a, b**) Preoperative and postoperative AP pelvis radiographs after surgical dislocation of the hip with femoral head reduction and transfer of the greater trochanter. (**c, d**) Preoperative and postoperative frog pelvis radiographs. (**e, f**) Preoperative and postoperative clinical pictures. Reprinted with permission from the Rubin Institute for Advanced Orthopedics, Sinai Hospital of Baltimore

should be used as a bone graft under the lateral femoral head fragment.
- The hip capsule should be repaired with minimal tension to avoid stretch of the vascular supply to the femoral head.
- The greater trochanter should be advanced until the proximal tip is at or below the center of the femoral head.
- The greater trochanter is repaired with two 4.5-mm or 5.5-mm screws with washers.
- It is critical that the fixation screws for the greater trochanter are directed distal away from the residual medial intact femoral neck to prevent postoperative femoral neck fracture.

Residual Femoral Head Subluxation

Residual femoral head subluxation or migration can result from untreated or unsuccessful treatment of Perthes disease. The residual femoral head subluxation is truly a migration or "settling" of the joint as the femoral head deforms from both internal collapse and abnormal femoral head cartilage growth. This migrated joint position is exacerbated by concurrent soft tissue contractures, typically hip flexion and hip adduction contractures. If this abnormal joint position is prolonged, then the permanent femoral head deformity will result. The femoral head that demonstrates significant residual deformity after the reconstitution or healing phase can only be corrected with the femoral head reduction osteotomy described above. However, if the femoral head is still within the active phase of Perthes (fragmentation or early reconsti-

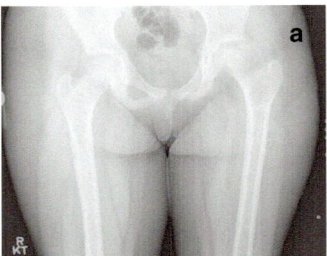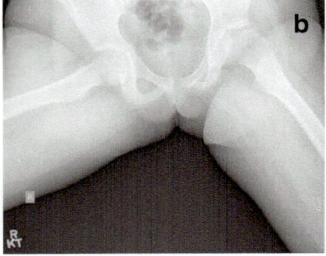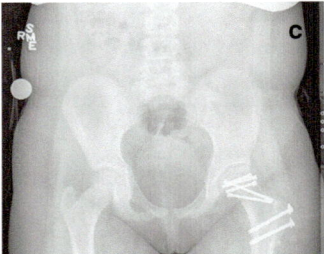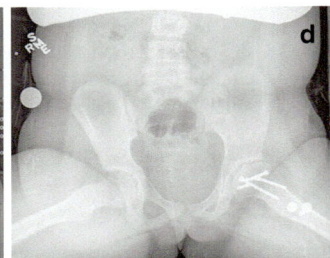

Fig. 36.50 (**a, b**) Radiographic example of a 12-year-old female with severe impingement secondary to residual deformity of the femoral head after late-onset Perthes disease of the left hip. (**c, d**) Same patient after left hip reconstruction with surgical dislocation, femoral head reduction and reshaping, and greater trochanter transfer. Reprinted with permission from the Rubin Institute for Advanced Orthopedics, Sinai Hospital of Baltimore

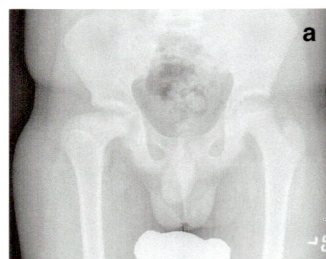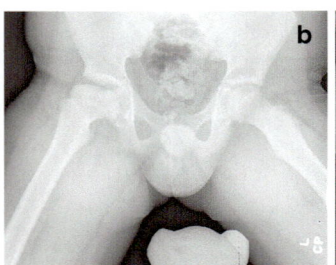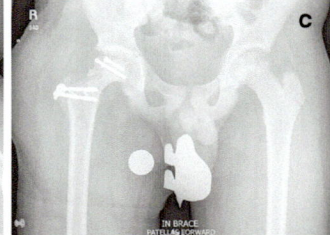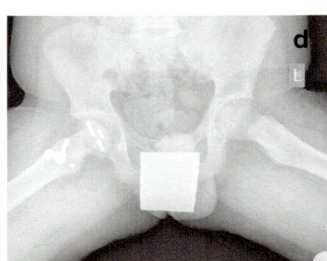

Fig. 36.51 (**a, b**) A 12-year-old male with residual right coxa magna resulting in an incongruent hip and FAI secondary to Perthes disease. (**c, d**) Radiographs of the same patient after right hip reconstruction via a femoral head reduction osteotomy and greater trochanter transfer. Reprinted with permission from the Rubin Institute for Advanced Orthopedics, Sinai Hospital of Baltimore

tution) and the hip joint is contracted with residual femoral head migration, then a specialized treatment exists that can salvage this situation. This treatment consists of a hip distraction protocol that consists of arthrodiastasis of the hip joint using a hinged external fixation device and selective soft tissue releases. Although there is limited prospective data on hip arthrodiastasis, the concept of using articulating hip distraction as an ideal means to reduce deforming joint pressures, and also maintain range-of-motion, has been described [61, 62]. Adjunctive procedures include a multiple small diameter core decompression and autogenous bone stem cell graft injection. The author has achieved a high rate of success for the most severe late onset Perthes patients after failed previous treatment, and thus, it utilizes this protocol for primary treatment of Perthes patients in high-risk groups and those that have failed early conservative treatment methods (Box 36.10).

Hip Distraction Treatment for Residual Femoral Head Subluxation Secondary to Perthes Disease: Operative Technique

Patient Positioning

The patient is placed supine on the operating room table after an epidural catheter is inserted. There are no bumps placed under the patient's hip or sacrum. The involved extremity is sterilely prepared to include the entire lower extremity, gluteal region, and iliac crest as proximal as the subcostal margin. A sterile Mayo stand with a pillow is prepared to allow for positioning the leg in adduction during pertinent parts of the procedure.

Core Decompression

The first step of the procedure consists of small diameter core decompression of the femoral head in order to stimulate a healing response within the epiphysis. A 1.8-mm wire is inserted percutaneously from the lateral thigh and driven up the femoral neck under fluoroscopic guidance into the femoral epiphysis (Fig. 36.52).

This is repeated five to six times in order to cover all affected zones of the epiphysis.

Stem Cell Injection

The second surgical step begins with harvesting bone marrow aspirate from the iliac crest. A 3-mm trephine needle is used to aspirate approximately 60 cc of bone marrow, followed by centrifuge preparation to separate the bone stem cells. Next, a 1.5-mm wire is driven into the anterolateral portion of the femoral epiphysis. Via a small stab incision, the 1.5-mm wire is overdrilled with a 3.2-mm cannulated drill. A fenestrated cannula is inserted into the bony channel and manually pushed, or carefully tapped with a mallet, into the epiphysis.

The bone stem cell graft is then injected into the femoral epiphysis via the fenestrated cannula. Prior to injection, the bone stem cell graft is diluted with 1 cc of radiopaque dye to allow visualization of the graft distribution under fluoroscopy (Fig. 36.53).

If dye is seen diluting into the joint, then the cannula is readjusted as necessary and the injection commences.

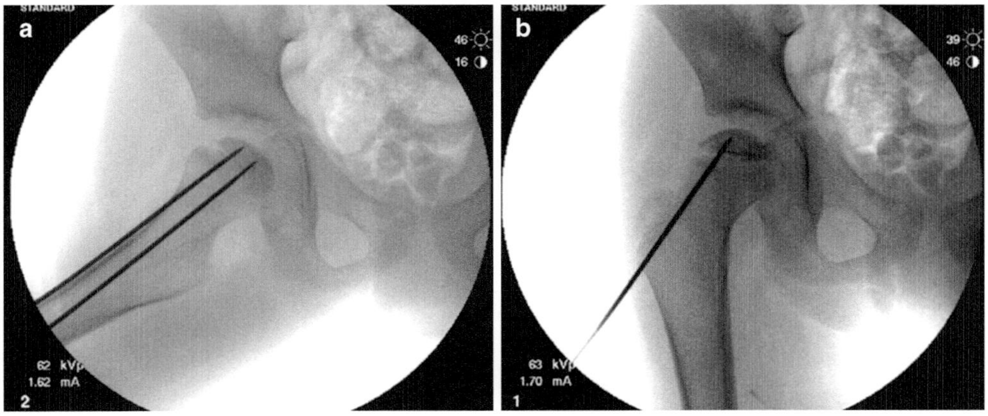

Fig. 36.52 Fluoroscopic views (**a** and **b**) of a small-diameter core decompression. Reprinted with permission from the Rubin Institute for Advanced Orthopedics, Sinai Hospital of Baltimore

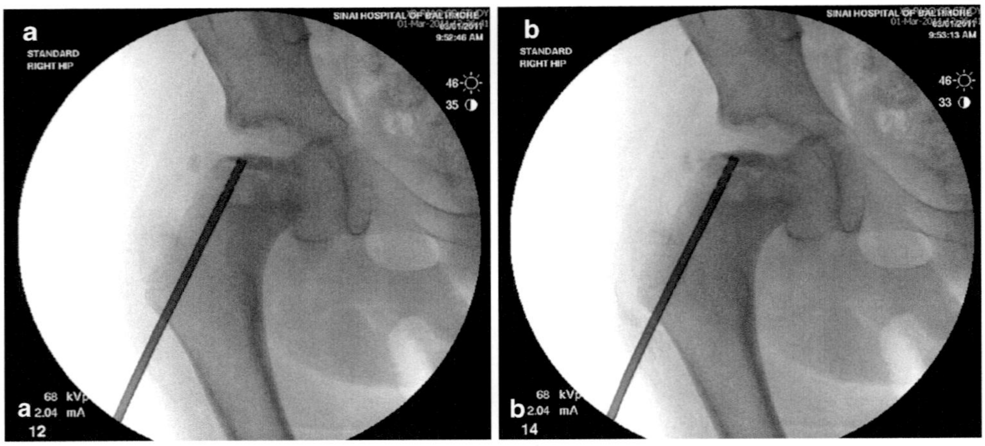

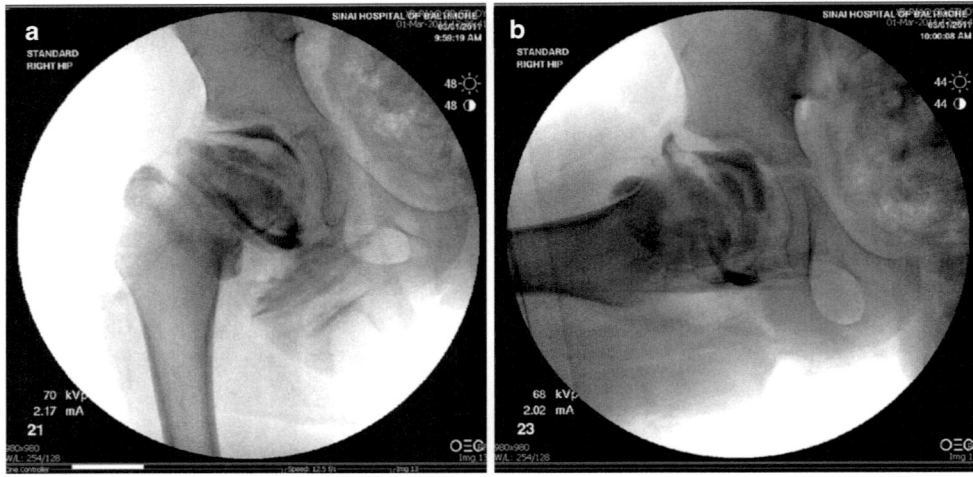

Fig. 36.53 Intraoperative fluoroscopic image (**a** and **b**) demonstrating the insertion of the fenestrated cannula into the femoral epiphysis with an injection of bone stem graft. The bone stem cell graft is visualized by adding a small amount of dye, which appears as the darkened epiphysis. Reprinted with permission from the Rubin Institute for Advanced Orthopedics, Sinai Hospital of Baltimore

Fig. 36.54 Intraoperative fluoroscopic views (**a** and **b**) of the right hip after intra-articular injection of dye. The actual femoral head deformity can be visualized and documented. Reprinted with permission from the Rubin Institute for Advanced Orthopedics, Sinai Hospital of Baltimore

Soft Tissue Releases

The leg is placed into a "frog leg" position, and an adductor tenotomy is performed through a small stab incision. The adductor longus muscle and gracilis muscle are released during this percutaneous tenotomy. The adductor longus muscle is released with the hip and knee flexed, whereas the gracilis muscle is released with the hip flexed but the knee extended. In a heavier patient, the physician may alternatively make a 2–3 cm mini-open approach to perform adductor releases under direct visualization.

Following adductor releases, the leg is placed back into a neutral supine position and a 3-cm anterior oblique incision is performed in the flexion crease of the groin approximately 2 cm below the anterior superior iliac spine. The incision starts medially at the point of the palpable femoral artery and extends laterally. The interval between the sartorius muscle and tensor fascia lata muscle is palpated and the fascia overlying the sartorius muscle is opened. This fascia is divided from lateral to medial until the septum separating the sartorius muscle and iliopsoas muscle is identified. The fascia overlying the iliopsoas muscle is divided and the muscle is carefully retracted laterally. By gently pulling the iliopsoas muscle laterally, the femoral nerve comes into the operative field and is easily identified. The fascia overlying the femoral nerve is divided, and the medial and lateral borders of the nerve are dissected. The overlying fascia proximal and distal along the nerve is released, allowing the nerve to mobilize. The femoral nerve is retracted medially, and the iliopsoas muscle is retracted laterally and everted exposing the iliopsoas tendon. The tendon is lifted into the operative field with a right angle clamp and sharply released under direct visualization. The incisions are closed in a typical layered fashion, and an arthrogram of the hip is performed. The hip is examined under fluoroscopy to determine the exact shape of the femoral head, position of the labrum, and containment of the femoral head with 20° of hip abduction (Fig. 36.54).

Hip Distractor Application

The hinged external fixation device (Orthofix articulated hip distractor) is placed by inserting half pins into the pelvis and

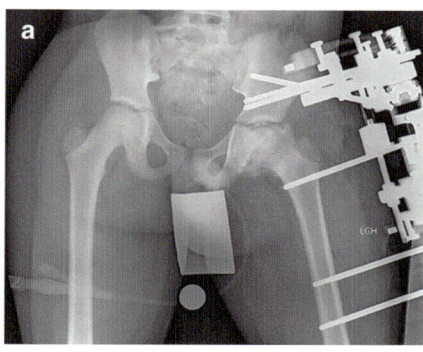 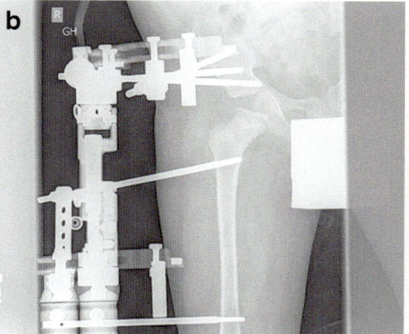 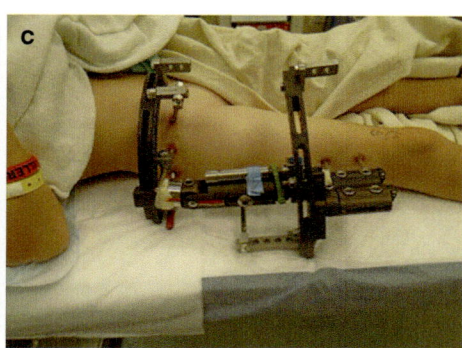

Fig. 36.55 (a) An AP pelvis radiography demonstrating a typical articulated hip external fixation device application for arthrodiastasis. (b) Another example of articulated hip distraction demonstrating an adequate distraction gap of 8–10 mm. (c) Clinical picture of the articulated hip distracting external fixation (Orthofix). Reprinted with permission from the Rubin Institute for Advanced Orthopedics, Sinai Hospital of Baltimore

into the middle third of the femoral shaft. The leg is positioned on the prepared mayo stand with the hip in full extension, neutral rotation, and 20° of abduction. A 3/32 Steinman pin is inserted perpendicular to the anatomic axis of the femoral shaft 8–10 mm below the center of the femoral head, and serves as the temporary hinge guide pin. In the sagittal view, the position of the guide pin is confirmed to be in the center of the femoral head. The hinged external fixation device is placed over the hinge guide pin. The proximal arch is secured to the pelvis by two supra-acetabular half pins. The distal pin clamp is utilized for the placement of two half pins into the femoral shaft. Avoid placing the distal half pin anteriorly near the cortex, as this places the patient at risk for femoral shaft fracture. After securing the device to the half pins, a second arch is secured to the distal half pins. The hinge pin may now be removed and fluidity of the articulation checked by passive hip flexion and extension to ensure a properly applied frame. The final femoral fixation point is placed at the level of the lesser trochanter built off the posterolateral distal arch. The final pelvic fixation point is inserted from an oblique anterior to posterior direction under fluoroscopic control down the posterior column of the pelvis (Fig. 36.55).

After completing external fixator application, the hip is acutely distracted 8–10 mm. A modular, removable anterior hip extension bar is attached to the anterior portion of the proximal and distal arches.

Postoperative Care

The postoperative protocol consists of continued gradual distraction at the rate of 0.5 mm per day for 7–10 days if needed. The goal of distraction is to over reduce Shenton's line by 5–10 mm. In smaller patients, the acute intra-operative distraction is all that is needed. Physical therapy is employed to maintain hip flexion and extension and mobilization with 50% partial weight bearing. The anterior extension bar is used for 2–3 h during the day and all night for the duration of the external fixation. The external fixation device is maintained for 4 months. Frame removal is performed under general anesthesia with a repeat arthrogram and Botox injection into the adductor longus and gracilis muscles. The dosage of Botox is typically 10 units per kilogram of weight, with a max dose of 200 units. The post-frame removal protocol consists of abduction hip bracing with a Scottish Rite brace and hip mobilization with physiotherapy and home exercises (Fig. 36.56).

The previously described technique of hip distraction for the treatment of late onset Perthes disease is modified for adolescent AVN. Male patients over 13 years of age and female patients over 10 years of age require a more aggressive form of bone grafting. The femoral head is accessed via the femoral neck with a 9 mm bone channel. The femoral head is debrided utilizing the X-ream femoral head reamer (Wright Medical). The femoral head is then back filled with a combination of autograft, allograft, BMP, and synthetic bone void filler such as Cerament (Bone Support) or MG (Wishbone). The soft tissue releases, and the external fixation application is the same as previously described. The external fixation device is maintained for 3 months followed by 3 months of modified weightbearing (Fig. 36.48 example of adolescent AVN).

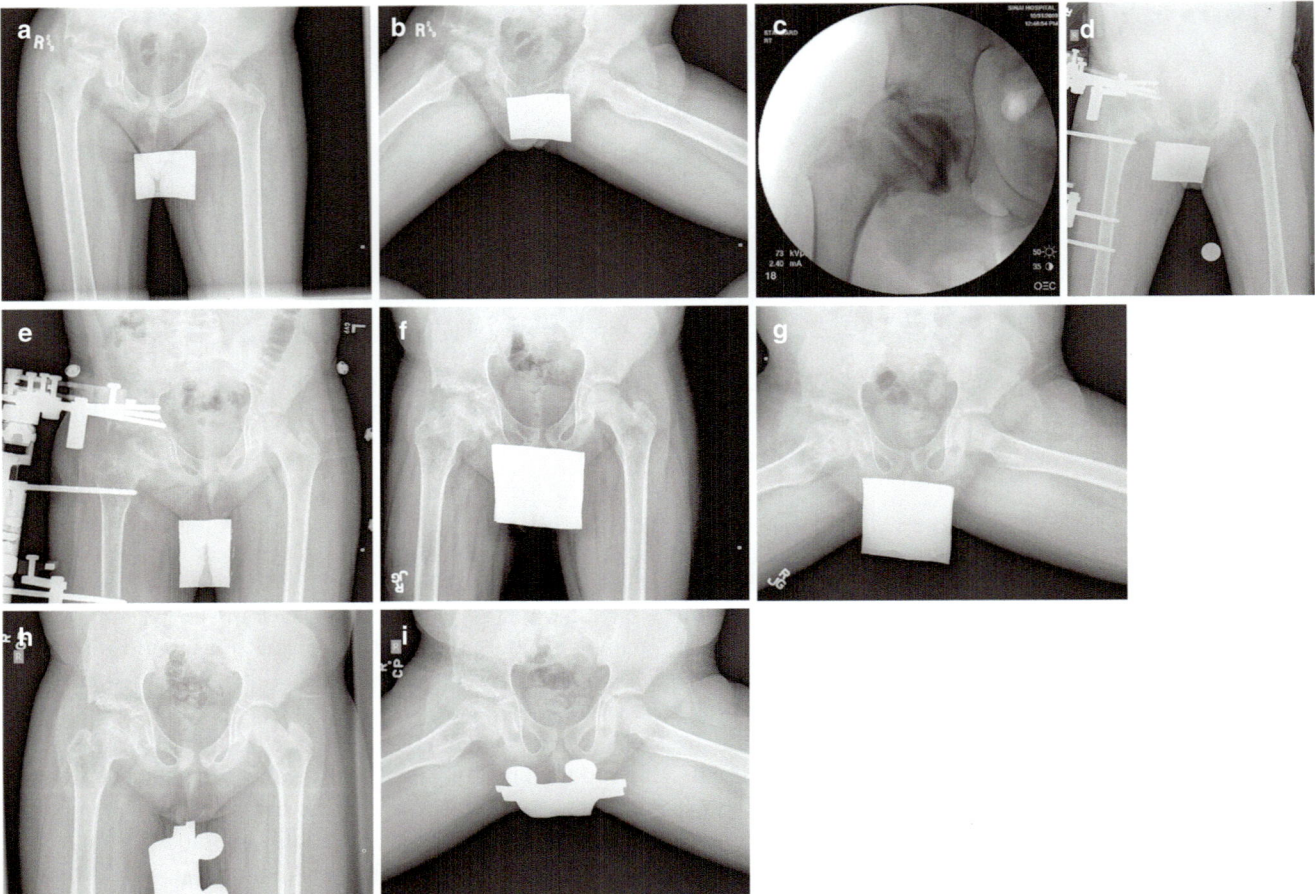

Fig. 36.56 (**a, b**) An 11-year-old male with severe residual deformity in the late fragmentation stage of Perthes disease; the patient had failed a previous shelf arthroplasty at an outside institution. (**c**) Intraoperative arthrogram demonstrating lateral and proximal migration of the femoral head and true "hinge abduction." (**d**) Radiograph 6 weeks following core decompression, open iliopsoas muscle release, percutaneous hip adductor tenotomy, and articulated hip distraction with full reduction of the hip joint and early reossification. (**e**) AP pelvis radiograph after 4 months of joint distraction prior to removal of external fixation; the radiography demonstrates significant reossification of the femoral head. (**f, g**) One-year postoperative AP and frog pelvis radiographs demonstrating excellent healing and sphericity of the femoral head with concurrent excellent congruency of the hip joint. (**h, i**) Three-year follow-up with excellent right hip healing and congruency; the patient continues to be pain free and participates in all activities. Reprinted with permission from the Rubin Institute for Advanced Orthopedics, Sinai Hospital of Baltimore

---

Box 36.10 Hip Distraction with a Hinged External Frame
The technical tips are given as follows:

- Arthrodiastasis is best performed simultaneously with adjunctive procedures: soft tissue contracture releases, core decompression, and autograft bone stem cell injection.
- Six multiplanar 6-mm half-pins are used to stabilize the fixator: two supra-acetabular pins, one oblique posterior column pin, two femoral shaft pins, and one posterolateral pin at the lesser trochanter.
- Acutely distract the hip 8–10 mm, followed for gradual distraction as needed to achieve a distraction gap of 5–10 mm.
- A removable, modular extension bar will help prevent hip flexion contracture; the hip extension bar is inserted for 1–2 h during the day and all night.
- Postoperative physiotherapy both prior to and after fame removal is paramount to optimizing outcome.
- After the external fixation is removed, the adductor muscles are injected with Botox, a Scottish Rite hip abduction orthosis is placed, and immediate mobilization with "Perthes exercises" is performed.

Summary

Residual hip deformities may present in any pediatric age group as a result of persistent, recurrent, iatrogenic, or neglected disease. The complex, multiplanar nature of these deformities is challenging for the treating surgeon.

Acetabuloplasty techniques continue to be modified to provide better outcomes for DDH, but emphasis must also be placed on improving screening and early, less invasive treatment with the hope of preventing residual dysplasia. A modernized triple osteotomy is an ideal procedure to reorient a dysplastic acetabulum and regain adequate femoral head coverage in a child approaching or following closure of the triradiate cartilage.

Residual deformity from moderate and severe slipped capital femoral epiphysis leads to both short-term and long-term sequelae ranging from pain, functional deficit, impingement, and eventual degenerative arthritis. Improvements in surgical approach have led to more aggressive surgical treatment to correct associated femoral neck deformity through the modified Dunn procedure. Long-term studies may emerge in the future to provide surgeons more guidance on whether subcapital or intertrochanteric osteotomies are the ideal treatment of a chronic slipped capital deformity.

Achieving consistent excellent results in treating AVN of the immature femoral head continues to elude the pediatric orthopedic community. Surgical intervention during the early fragmentation stage of Perthes may be crucial to preserving femoral head morphology and improving long-term outcome. Currently, an appropriately applied hip distraction protocol may be the only treatment method that simultaneously provides containment as well as relief from deforming joint pressures, while allowing maintenance of range-of-motion. Further investigation is needed into hip arthrodiastasis and adjunctive treatments such as core decompression and stem cell injection to optimize the treatment protocol described in this chapter.

AVN of the femoral head leads to proximal femur deformities, namely, coxa breva and coxa magna. Coxa breva negatively alters proximal femur biomechanics, and it is associated with hip abductor weakness, limb length discrepancy, and limping. In contrast to a relative neck lengthening procedure, the Morscher osteotomy is a true neck lengthening osteotomy and directly addresses the femoral neck deficiency. Intracapsular femoral head reshaping osteotomies are technically demanding, but provide the only reconstructive option for a symptomatic coxa magna in the severely deformed and incongruent femoral head.

Commentary

Commentary on Residual Hip Deformity Chapter

Oliver Birke
oliver.birke@health.nsw.gov.au

Residual hip deformities in pediatric patients are complex three-dimensional "puzzles" to be solved by the treating orthopedic surgeon. This commentary represents my personal opinion and experience and it is not intended to be comprehensive, but rather to highlight some key points and my train of thought when I try to tackle these complex cases. Often the deformities involve both the acetabular and femoral side, and therefore, I try to break them down into "bite-sized" puzzle pieces. And even more importantly, each patient is unique and should be assessed and managed on an individual basis. This includes considering their functional limitations (now vs future?), their anatomical deformity, their socio-economic background, as well as their behavioral health history which will influence their ability to deal with potentially repeated major surgery, prolonged periods of hospitalization, immobilization, and/or external fixation. Also, in the absence of clear long-term outcome data for the more advanced operative techniques, our reconstructive efforts should aim at improving hip function, but never alter the hip anatomy to an extent that precludes our patients from having an uncomplicated primary total hip replacement (THR) down the road — "the most successful orthopedic operation."

In younger children, residual acetabular dysplasia (often a consequence of delayed treatment of DDH) is usually addressed with a pelvic osteotomy. In my experience, in children with a wide-open triradiate, a reshaping acetabuloplasty is often more powerful than the redirectional innominate Salter osteotomy, as the latter hinges at the symphysis pubis which is a long way away from the acetabulum and also has the inherent risk of inadvertently retroverting the acetabulum.

This example shows a Pemberton/Dega-type pelvic osteotomy in a 6-year-old girl where the lateral placement of the graft achieved sufficient correction and near normal post-operative coverage. In children from about 4 years of age, a single screw can hold the graft in place and a hip spica cast can be avoided, which greatly simplifies post-operative care.

Complex hip deformities in older children are usually either the consequence of a SCFE (slipped capital femoral epiphysis) or the sequelae of growth-disturbances following infection, AVN (avascular necrosis) or Perthes. While some types of growth disturbances are more common, each case is different and needs careful assessment of both the acetabular and femoral side. The aim should be to reconstruct both the acetabular coverage and proximal femoral anatomy as close to normal as possible.

Reinhold Ganz and his team have revolutionized our reconstructive tool box with the development of the periacetabular osteotomy (PAO) and probably, even more importantly, with the safe surgical hip dislocation technique with its concept of the retinacular soft tissue flap which preserves the femoral head vascularity during reconstructive procedures. This trochanter flip approach to the hip, if performed correctly, allows us to practically "do anything" without compromising the blood supply of the femoral head. Depending on the extent and complexity of the reconstruction, it may not be necessary to develop the retinacular soft tissue flap completely — the principle is rather obvious: wherever we want to do osteotomies, the vessel needs to be protected.

In an aim to address all components of this three-dimensional puzzle, I like to separate the proximal femur into three pieces and try to get them all into the right place and relationship to each other:

- Femoral head and neck.
- Femoral shaft offset.
- Greater trochanter (GT).

When utilizing the trochanter flip approach with the development of the retinacular soft tissue flap, each of these pieces can be safely put into the correct relationship to each other. The femoral head/neck should be in an appropriate valgus alignment, and an inter—or sub-trochanteric osteotomy may be required to achieve this goal. As a guide for the femoral shaft offset, I use a line dropped down from the lateral acetabular edge which should line up with the medial femoral shaft. Typically, the shaft needs to be medialized for varusing osteotomies and lateralized for valgusing osteotomies. At the end, the GT should be fixed back in a lateral position with the tip at the level of the center of the femoral head for optimal abductor function. I routinely use two small fragment 3.5 mm cortex screws for refixation of the trochanteric flip.

Additional acetabular dysplasia or pathological acetabular version can then be addressed with a pelvic osteotomy (usually, a PAO once the tri-radiate cartilage is closing/closed).

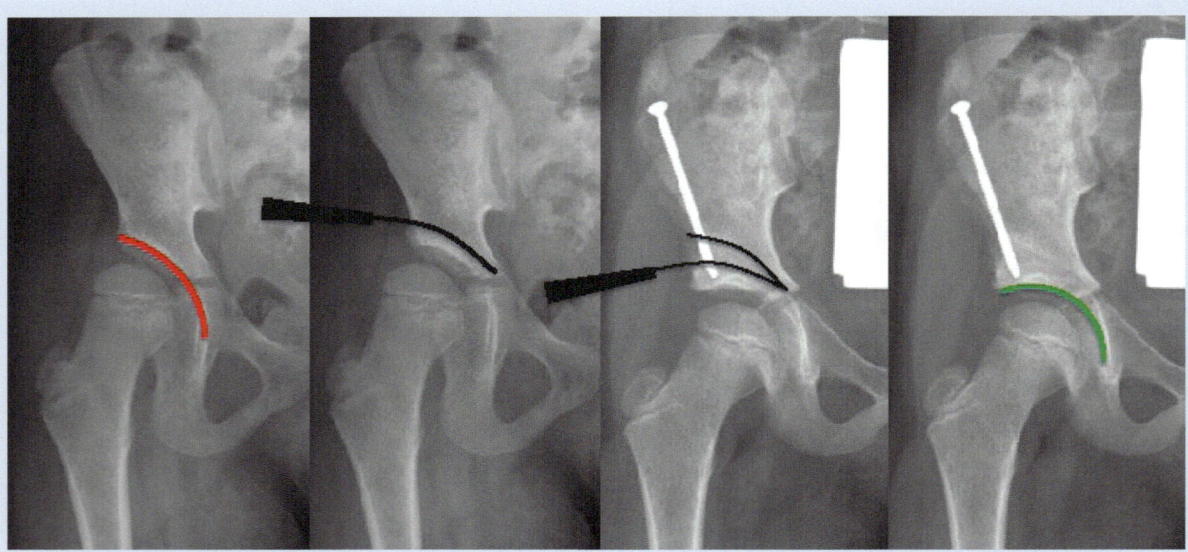

Some thoughts and examples from personal experience with the trochanter flip approach reconstructions in order to increase complexity are given as follows:

- Relative neck lengthening (RNL)

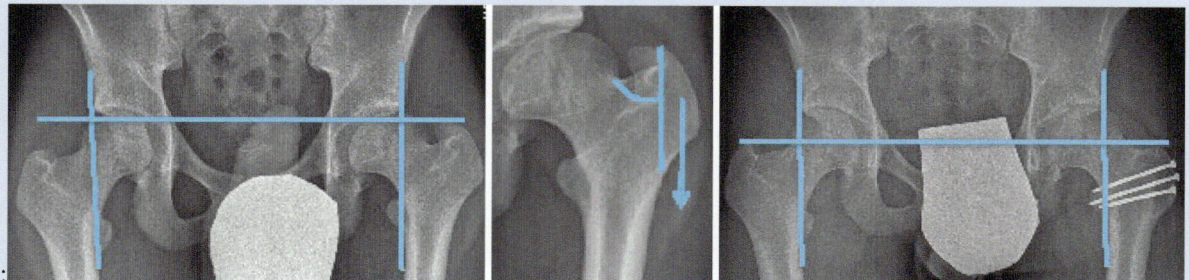

In cases with sufficient acetabular coverage and femoral shaft offset, a relative neck lengthening (RNL) may suffice to reshape the femoral neck and reconstruct the abductor lever arm with the tip of the GT at the level of the center of the femoral head.

- Relative neck lengthening (RNL) combined with PAO:

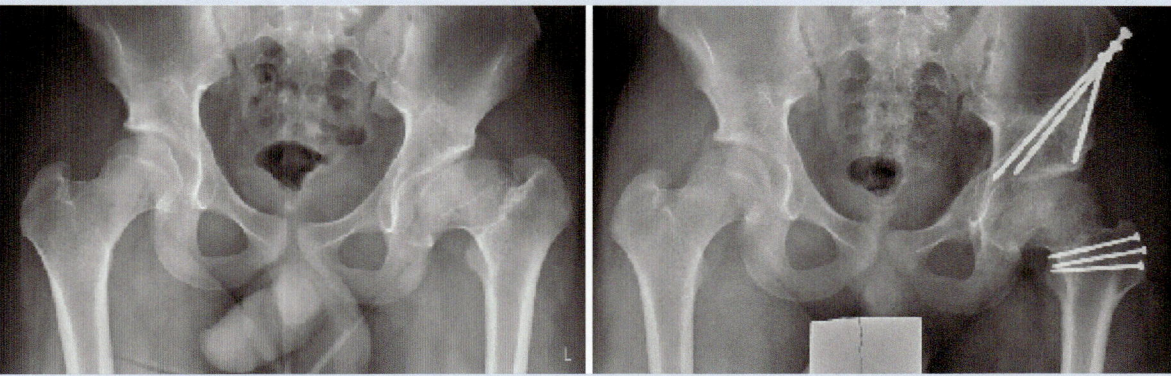

If additional acetabular coverage or change of version is desired, then a RNL can be safely combined with a PAO; however, the RNL needs to be performed first in order to create sufficient space for the redirection of the acetabulum.

- True femoral neck lengthening: Trochanter flip modified Morscher osteotomy

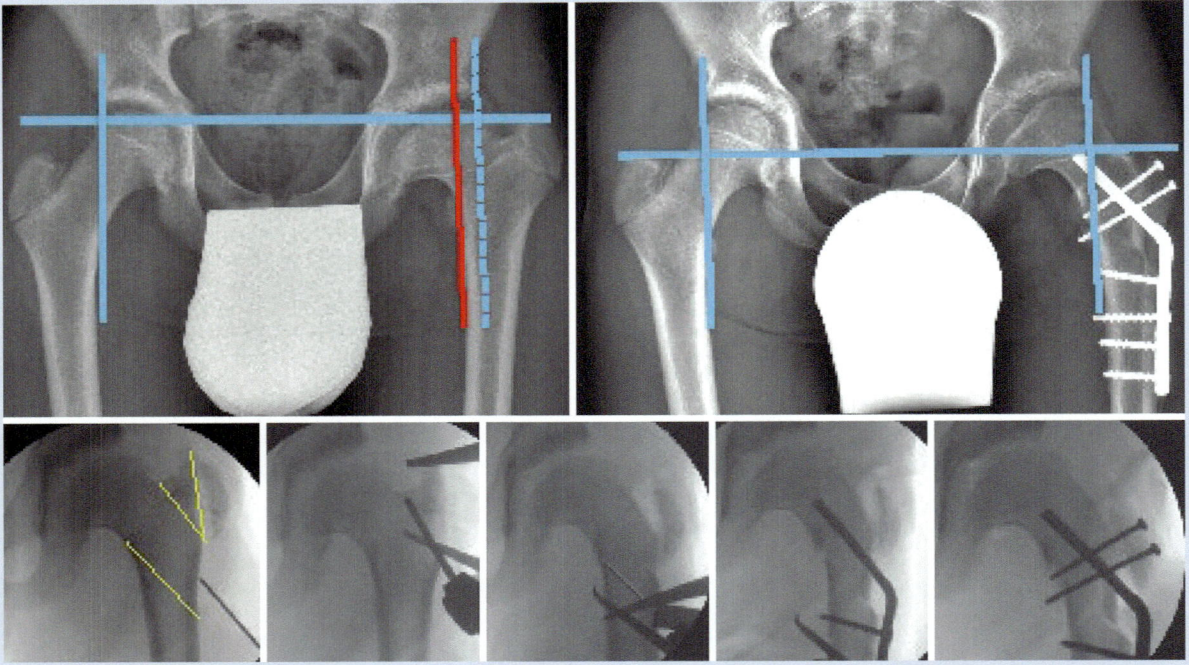

If severe coxa breva reduces the femoral shaft offset, then a true femoral neck lengthening may be required, for which I modified the Morscher osteotomy to be performed via the trochanter flip approach and with the development of the retinacular soft tissue flap. This allows the superior neck and GT osteotomy cuts to be performed safely, also in patients with open proximal femoral physes where the femoral head blood supply solely relies on the circumflex artery along the postero-lateral femoral neck, which is where these femoral neck osteotomies are performed.
- Varusing osteotomy with RNL and trochanter distalization for Perthes:

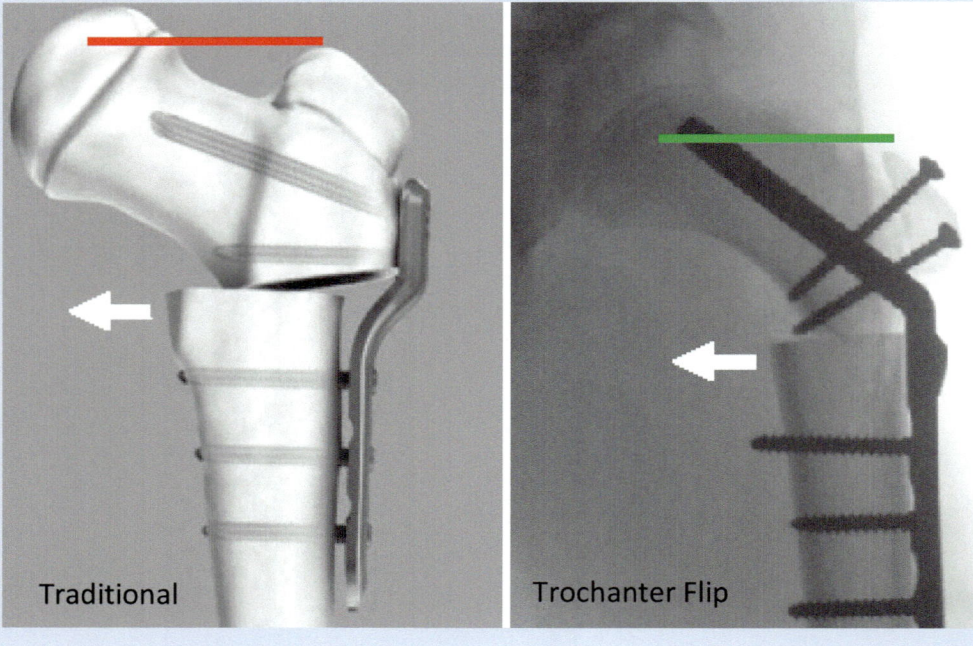

In Perthes, one may consider a varusation for containment. However, on top of the inherent growth disturbance, a traditional varus osteotomy would further weaken the abductors. To enable a varusation and at the same time, distalization of the GT to the level of the center of the femoral head, I like to perform this varusing osteotomy via the trochanter flip approach. I utilize a 130° cannulated blade plate and modified osteotomy with a lateral "release cut" to incorporate the offset of the traditional varus osteotomy plates into the osteotomy and allow medialization of the shaft and an appropriate surface area for re-fixation of the distalized GT.

- Modified Dunn procedure for moderate to severe SCFE with open physis:

The most complex of the trochanter flip approach procedures probably is the modified Dunn procedure for moderate to severe SCFEs. It is the most powerful corrective SCFE procedure as it corrects through the slipped physis. Complete and meticulous preparation of the retinacular soft tissue flap and resection of the posterior callus are crucial to safely take off and then reposition the femoral head (fixation with 2 × 6.5 mm fully threaded cannulated screws). We found our protocol with a modified capsulotomy that allows stable anterior capsular closure without any tension on the reticular soft tissue flap and intra-operative monitoring of the femoral head perfusion to be safe without causing AVN in over 100 stable SCFEs (Birke et al., JCO 2021).

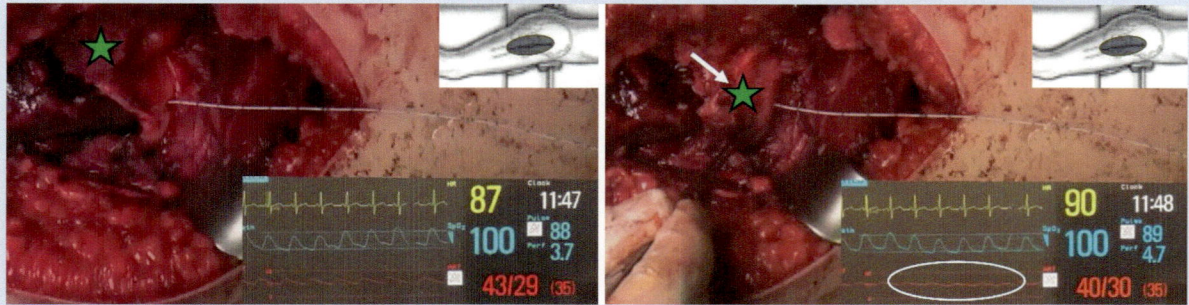

Even gentle tension on the postero-superior capsular flap of the original Z-shaped capsulotomy like shown here intra-operatively with a forceps (arrow) can flatten the waveform of the epiphyseal blood flow on Codman monitoring. We therefore modified the capsulotomy. (This figure is reproduced with permission from Birke O, George JSt, Gibbons PJ, Little DG. The modified Dunn procedure can be performed safely in stable slipped capital femoral epiphysis but does not alter avascular necrosis rates in unstable cases: A large single-centre cohort study. *Journal of Children's Orthopaedics*. 2021;15(5):479–487. doi:https://doi.org/10.1302/1863-2548.15.210106).

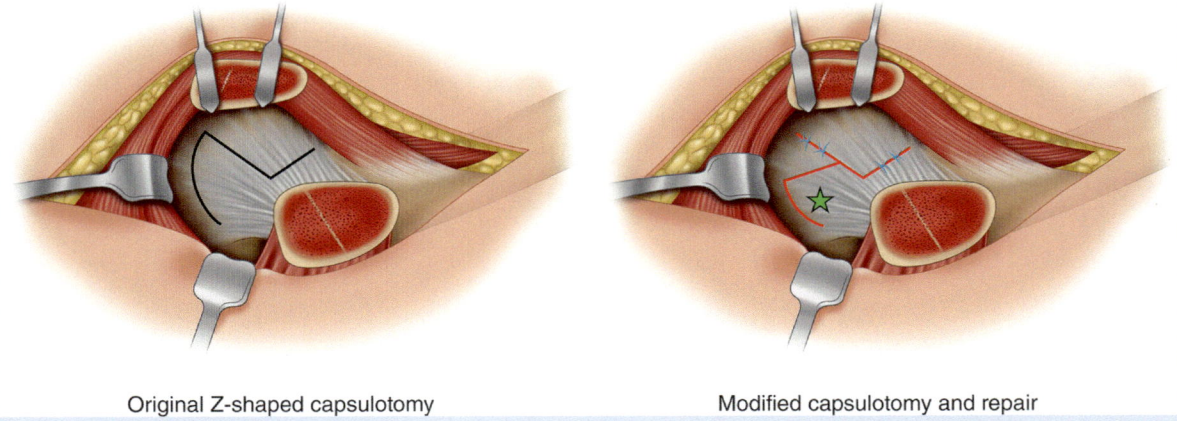

Original Z-shaped capsulotomy   Modified capsulotomy and repair

Modified capsulotomy and repair: We have changed the central limb of the original Z-shaped capsulotomy from a straight incision to one that is Y-shaped. This creates a V-shaped superior flap that facilitates a stable anterior closure and avoids tension on the vessel posteriorly. (This figure is reproduced with permission from Birke O, George

JSt, Gibbons PJ, Little DG. The modified Dunn procedure can be performed safely in stable slipped capital femoral epiphysis but does not alter avascular necrosis rates in unstable cases: A large single-centre cohort study. *Journal of Children's Orthopaedics.* 2021;15(5):479–487. doi:https://doi.org/10.1302/1863-2548.15.210106).

- Flexion-Valgus osteotomy with bumpectomy and RNL for chronic severe SCFE with closed physis:

When the capital physis closes, the blood supply to the femoral head changes and the AVN risk increases for a subcapital realignment with the modified Dunn procedure. The CORA of the SCFE deformity however is at the level of the physis, and therefore, any subtrochanteric corrective osteotomy will introduce translation at the osteotomy site and limit the amount of correction, As a consequence, a severe SCFE cannot be fully corrected with a subtrochanteric osteotomy. The traditional Southwick osteotomy moves both femoral head/neck and GT at the same time, which may leave the one and/or the other in a suboptimal position. Even if appropriate valgus and/or flexion is achieved, the GT is often rotated back and out of its optimal position for abductor function. Also, potential intra-articular pathology cannot be addressed or requires an additional anterior approach to the joint.

Furthermore, a subtrochanteric osteotomy with a large flexion component may create an iatrogenic femoral deformity ("zig-zag pattern") that could preclude a primary THR down the road.

Therefore, I prefer to utilize the trochanter flip approach and due to the size and weight of most of our SCFE patients, a DHS plate provides the most solid fixation of the osteotomy (blade plates or locking hip plates have failed or did break in our patient population).

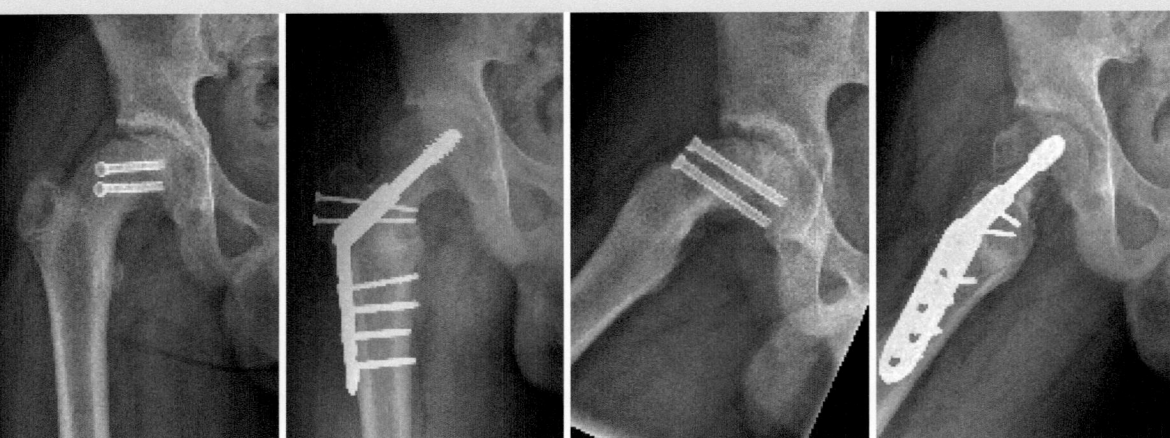

After the trochanter flip, the femoral neck guide wire is placed from an anterior entry point aimed posteriorly towards the femoral head and in an appropriate position for the valgus component of the osteotomy. The flexion correction then translates the posterior corner of the proximal fragment posteriorly, but this posterior corner can be resected and used as an anterior graft and more importantly, the anterior entry point leaves the "new femoral neck" in line with both femoral head and femoral shaft and reconstructs an anatomy that allows a primary THR down the road. In addition, any intra-articular pathology can be addressed, and in this case, a bumpectomy was performed, and at the end, the GT can be repositioned laterally in appropriate rotation and with its tip at the center of the femoral head.

Summary

In my view and experience, reconstructing near normal acetabular coverage, proximal femoral anatomy, and abductor function will usually bring functional benefits for motivated patients. However, without clear long-term evidence for most of our complex reconstructive procedures, we have to carefully compare potential risks and benefits on an individual basis, and we should thrive to not alter the proximal femoral anatomy in a way that precludes our patients from an uncomplicated primary THR—just because we think we need to do "something" does not mean we should try in every case.

References

1. Stevens PM, Coleman SS. Coxa breva: its pathogenesis and a rationale for its management. J Pediatr Orthop. 1985;5(5):515–21.
2. Standard SC. Treatment of coxa brevis. Orthop Clin North Am. 2011;42(3):373–87.
3. Siffert RS. Patterns of deformity of the developing hip. Clin Orthop Relat Res. 1981;160:14–29.
4. Stulberg SD, Cooperman DR, Wallensten R. The natural history of Legg-Calvé-Perthes disease. J Bone Joint Surg Am. 1981;63(7):1095–108.
5. Ross JR, Nepple JJ, Baca G, Schoenecker PL, Clohisy JC. Intraarticular abnormalities in residual Perthes and Perthes-like hip deformities. Clin Orthop Relat Res. 2012;470(11):2968–77.
6. Maranho DA, Nogueira-Barbosa MH, Zamarioli A, Volpon JB. MRI abnormalities of the acetabular labrum and articular cartilage are common in healed Legg-Calvé-Perthes disease with residual deformities of the hip. J Bone Joint Surg Am. 2013;95(3):256–65.
7. Rowe SM, Moon ES, Song EK, Seol JY, Seon JK, Kim SS. The correlation between coxa magna and final outcome in Legg-calve-Perthes disease. J Pediatr Orthop. 2005;25(1):22–7.
8. McCarthy RE. Avascular necrosis of the femoral head in children. Instr Course Lect. 1988;37:59–65.
9. Vitale MG, Skaggs DL. Developmental dysplasia of the hip from six months to four years of age. J Am Acad Orthop Surg. 2001;9(6):401–11.
10. Gillingham BL, Sanchez AA, Wenger DR. Pelvic osteotomies for the treatment of hip dysplasia in children and young adults. J Am Acad Orthop Surg. 1999;7(5):325–37.
11. Sankar WN, Millis MB, Kim YJ. Instability of the hip in patients with down syndrome: improved results with complete redirectional acetabular osteotomy. J Bone Joint Surg Am. 2011;93(20):1924–33.
12. Shorter D, Hong T, Osborn DA. Cochrane review: screening programmes for developmental dysplasia of the hip in newborn infants. Evid Based Child Health. 2013;8(1):11–54.
13. Shipman SA, Helfand M, Moyer VA, Yawn BP. Screening for developmental dysplasia of the hip: a systematic literature review for the US preventive services task force. Pediatrics. 2006;117(3):e557–76.
14. Guille JT, Pizzutillo PD, MacEwen GD. Development dysplasia of the hip from birth to six months. J Am Acad Orthop Surg. 2000;8(4):232–42.
15. Sharp IK. Acetabular dysplasia: the acetabular angle. J Bone Joint Surg Br. 1961;43:268–72.
16. Scoles PV, Boyd A, Jones PK. Roentgenographic parameters of the normal infant hip. J Pediatr Orthop. 1987;7(6):656–63.
17. Wisberg G. Studies on dysplastic acetabula and congenital subluxation of the hip joint: with special reference to the complication of osteoarthritis. Acta Chir Scand Suppl. 1939;58:7–135.
18. Murphy SB, Ganz R, Müller ME. The prognosis in untreated dysplasia of the hip. A study of radiographic factors that predict the outcome. J Bone Joint Surg Am. 1995;77(7):985–9.
19. Scott EJ, Dolan LA, Weinstein SL. Closed vs. Open reduction/Salter innominate osteotomy for developmental hip dislocation after age 18 months: comparative survival at 45-year follow-up. J Bone Joint Surg Am. 2020;102(15):1351–7.
20. Salter RB. Innominate osteotomy in the treatment of congenital dislocation and subluxation of the hip. J Bone Joint Surg Br. 1961;43(3):518–39.
21. Thomas SR, Wedge JH, Salter RB. Outcome at forty-five years after open reduction and innominate osteotomy for late-presenting developmental dislocation of the hip. J Bone Joint Surg Am. 2007;89(11):2341–50.
22. Pemberton PA. Pericapsular osteotomy of the ilium for treatment of congenital dysplasia of the hip. J Bone Joint Surg Am. 1965;47:65–86.
23. Dega W. Selection of surgical methods in the treatment of congenital dislocation of the hip in children. Chir Narzadow Ruchu Ortop Pol. 1969;34(3):357–66.
24. Grudziak JS, Ward WT. Dega osteotomy for the treatment of congenital dysplasia of the hip. J Bone Joint Surg Am. 2001;83-A(6):845–54.
25. McNerney NP, Mubarak SJ, Wenger DR. One-stage correction of the dysplastic hip in cerebral palsy with the San Diego acetabuloplasty: results and complications in 104 hips. J Pediatr Orthop. 2000;20(1):93–103.
26. Murphy RF, Kim YJ. Surgical Management of Pediatric Developmental Dysplasia of the hip. J Am Acad Orthop Surg. 2016 Sep;24(9):615–24.
27. Steel HH. Triple osteotomy of the innominate bone. J Bone Joint Surg. 1973;55:343–50.
28. Tönnis D, Behrens K, Tscharani F. A modified technique Z of the triple pelvic osteotomy: early results. J Ped Orthop. 1981;1:241–9.
29. Conroy E, Sheehan E, O'Connor P, Connolly P, McCormack D. Triple pelvic osteotomy in Legg-calve-Perthes disease using a single anterolateral incision: a 4-year review. J Pediatr Orthop B. 2010;19(4):323–6.
30. Ganz R, Klaue K, Vinh TS, Mast JW. A new periacetabular osteotomy for the treatment of hip dysplasias. Technique and preliminary results. Clin Orthop Relat Res. 1988;232:26–36.
31. Aronsson DD, Loder RT, Breur GJ, Weinstein SL. Slipped capital femoral epiphysis: current concepts. J Am Acad Orthop Surg. 2006;14(12):666–79.
32. Ganz R, Parvizi J, Beck M, Leunig M, Nötzli H, Siebenrock KA. Femoroacetabular impingement: a cause for osteoarthritis of the hip. Clin Orthop Relat Res. 2003;417:112–20.
33. Loder RT, Aronsson DD, Weinstein SL, Breur GJ, Ganz R, Leunig M. Slipped capital femoral epiphysis. Instr Course Lect. 2008;57:473–98.
34. Millis MB, Novais EN. In situ fixation for slipped capital femoral epiphysis: perspectives in 2011. J Bone Joint Surg Am. 2011;93(Suppl 2):46–51.
35. Carney BT, Weinstein SL. Natural history of untreated chronic slipped capital femoral epiphysis. Clin Orthop Relat Res. 1996;322:43–7.
36. Kuzyk PR, Kim YJ, Millis MB. Surgical management of healed slipped capital femoral epiphysis. J Am Acad Orthop Surg. 2011;19(11):667–77.
37. Larson AN, Sierra RJ, Yu EM, Trousdale RT, Stans AA. Outcomes of slipped capital femoral epiphysis treated with in situ pinning. J Pediatr Orthop. 2012;32(2):125–30.
38. Ganz R, Huff TW, Leunig M. Extended retinacular soft-tissue flap for intra-articular hip surgery: surgical technique, indications, and results of application. Instr Course Lect. 2009;58:241–55.
39. Ziebarth K, Zilkens C, Spencer S, Leunig M, Ganz R, Kim YJ. Capital realignment for moderate and severe SCFE using a modified Dunn procedure. Clin Orthop Relat Res. 2009;467(3):704–16.
40. Slongo T, Kakaty D, Krause F, Ziebarth K. Treatment of slipped capital femoral epiphysis with a modified Dunn procedure. J Bone Joint Surg Am. 2010;92(18):2898–908.
41. Huber H, Dora C, Ramseier LE, Buck F, Dierauer S. Adolescent slipped capital femoral epiphysis treated by a modified Dunn osteotomy with surgical hip dislocation. J Bone Joint Surg Br. 2011;93(6):833–8.
42. Sankar WN, Vanderhave KL, Matheney T, Herrera-Soto JA, Karlen JW. The modified Dunn procedure for unstable slipped capital femoral epiphysis: a multicenter perspective. J Bone Joint Surg Am. 2013;95(7):585–91.
43. Souder CD, Bomar JD, Wenger DR. The role of capital realignment versus in situ stabilization for the treatment of slipped capital femoral epiphysis. J Pediatr Orthop. 2014;34(8):791–8.

44. Upasani VV, Matheney TH, Spencer SA, Kim YJ, Millis MB, Kasser JR. Complications after modified Dunn osteotomy for the treatment of adolescent slipped capital femoral epiphysis. J Pediatr Orthop. 2014;34(7):661–7.
45. Southwick WO. Osteotomy through the lesser trochanter for slipped capital femoral epiphysis. J Bone Joint Surg Am. 1967;49(5):807–35.
46. Sabharwal S, Mittal R, Zhao C. Percutaneous osteotomy for deformity correction in adolescents with severe slipped capital femoral epiphysis. J Pediatr Orthop B. 2006;15(6):396–403.
47. Herring JA, Williams JJ, Neustadt JN, Early JS. Evolution of femoral head deformity during the healing phase of Legg-Calvé-Perthes disease. J Pediatr Orthop. 1993;13(1):41–5.
48. Joseph B. Natural history of early onset and late-onset Legg-calve-Perthes disease. J Pediatr Orthop. 2011;31(2 Suppl):S152–5.
49. Rosenfeld SB, Herring JA, Chao JC. Legg-calve-Perthes disease: a review of cases with onset before six years of age. J Bone Joint Surg Am. 2007;89(12):2712–22.
50. Larson AN, Sucato DJ, Herring JA, Adolfsen SE, Kelly DM, Martus JE, Lovejoy JF, Browne R, Delarocha A. A prospective multicenter study of Legg-Calvé-Perthes disease: functional and radiographic outcomes of nonoperative treatment at a mean follow-up of twenty years. J Bone Joint Surg Am. 2012;94(7):584–92.
51. Grzegorzewski A, Synder M, Kozłowski P, Szymczak W, Bowen RJ. Leg length discrepancy in Legg-calve-Perthes disease. J Pediatr Orthop. 2005;25(2):206–9.
52. Sponseller PD, Desai SS, Millis MB. Comparison of femoral and innominate osteotomies for the treatment of Legg-Calvé-Perthes disease. J Bone Joint Surg Am. 1988;70(8):1131–9.
53. Castañeda P, Haynes R, Mijares J, Quevedo H, Cassis N. Varus-producing osteotomy for patients with lateral pillar type B and C Legg-Calvé-Perthes disease followed to skeletal maturity. J Child Orthop. 2008;2(5):373–9.
54. Karpinski MR, Newton G, Henry AP. The results and morbidity of varus osteotomy for Perthes' disease. Clin Orthop Relat Res. 1986;209:30–40.
55. Leitch JM, Paterson DC, Foster BK. Growth disturbance in Legg-Calvé-Perthes disease and the consequences of surgical treatment. Clin Orthop Relat Res. 1991;262:178–84.
56. Eilert RE, Hill K, Bach J. Greater trochanteric transfer for the treatment of coxa brevis. Clin Orthop Relat Res. 2005;434:92–101.
57. Buess P, Morscher E. Osteotomy to lengthen the femur neck with distal adjustment of the trochanter major in coxa vara after hip dislocation. Orthopade. 1988;17(6):485–90.
58. Leunig M, Ganz R. Relative neck lengthening and intracapital osteotomy for severe Perthes and Perthes-like deformities. Bull NYU Hosp Jt Dis. 2011;69(Suppl 1):S62–7.
59. Siebenrock KA, Anwander H, Zurmühle CA, Tannast M, Slongo T, Steppacher SD. Head reduction osteotomy with additional containment surgery improves sphericity and containment and reduces pain in Legg-Calvé-Perthes disease. Clin Orthop Relat Res. 2014;437(4):1274–83.
60. Paley D. The treatment of femoral head deformity and coxa magna by the Ganz femoral head reduction osteotomy. Orthop Clin North Am. 2011;42(3):389–99.
61. Gomez JA, Matsumoto H, Roye DP Jr, Vitale MG, Hyman JE, van Bosse HJ, et al. Articulated hip distraction: a treatment option for femoral head avascular necrosis in adolescence. J Pediatr Orthop. 2009;29(2):163–9.
62. Thacker MM, Feldman DS, Madan SS, Straight JJ, Scher DM. Hinged distraction of the adolescent arthritic hip. J Pediatr Orthop. 2005;25(2):178–82.

37. Posttraumatic Lower Limb Deformities in Children

Ashok N. Johari, Sandeep A. Patwardhan, and Taral Vishanji Nagda

Introduction

Posttraumatic deformities in children are unique. They are different from deformities that are congenital or secondary to other causes since the skeletal and soft tissue anatomy and physiology are often normal to start with. Hence, reparative mechanisms, natural history, and many management principles differ in these patients.

Posttraumatic deformities in children are different from adults. Children have the potential to influence future growth due to the possibility of substantial remodeling of a malunited fracture. Such remodeling can occur from different sources including the adjacent physis and differential periosteal growth of the affected diaphysis (Fig. 37.1). On the other hand, injury to a portion of the growth plate can lead to asymmetric growth of the physis with progressive deformities in children.

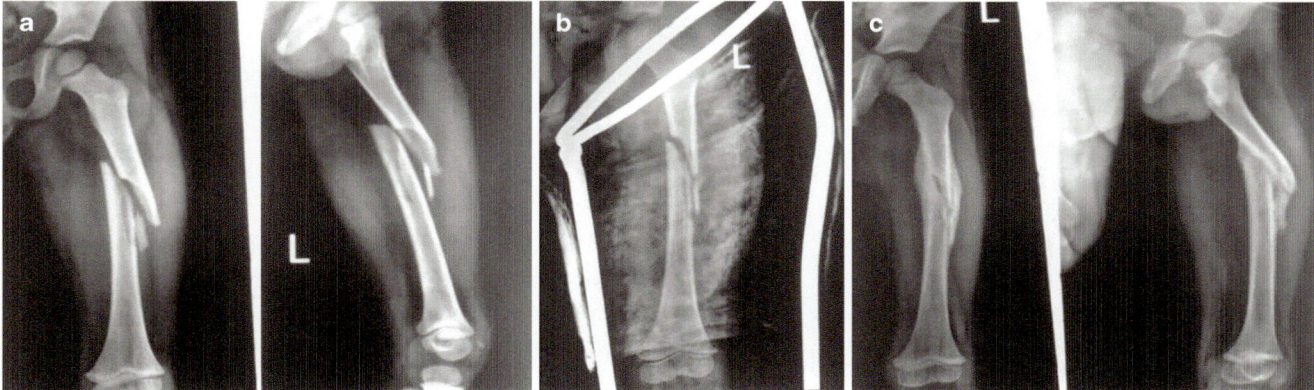

Fig. 37.1 Four-year-old child with femur fracture treated by traction in a Thomas' splint. (**a**) Injury film. (**b**) X-ray in Thomas's splint. (**c**) At 2 months, fracture united with 40° angulation and 3 cm shortening. The malunion is due to muscle forces that were not effectively managed

A. N. Johari (✉)
Department of Paediatric Orthopaedics, Children's Orthopaedic Centre, Mumbai, Maharashtra, India

S. A. Patwardhan
Department of Pediatric Orthopedics, Sancheti Institute for Orthopedics and Rehabilitation, Pune, Maharashtra, India

T. V. Nagda
Department of Pediatric Orthopedics, SRCC Children's Hospital Mumbai, Mumbai, Maharashtra, India

Deformities following trauma to the extremities are not uncommon and not always dependent on the level of care provided. While some deformities are inevitable due to high-energy trauma and damage to the growing area of long bones, other deformities occur because of malalignment allowing the limb to be positioned abnormally or allowing certain muscles to shorten and create a secondary deformity.

Deformities that are not clinically significant or have the potential for substantial remodeling to an acceptable level can be observed. In general, when the residual axial malalignment of a lower extremity long bone exceeds 10°, correction may be warranted.

Causation and Etiological Factors

A posttraumatic deformity can result from the initial soft tissue and skeletal injury, its management, or complications. In order to accurately identify the cause and anticipate the natural progression of the deformity, it is important to ascertain the mechanism of injury, initial soft tissue and bony injury, specifics of the treatment given—conservative and operative, postoperative care, complications and course of the deformity thus far (Box 37.1).

> **Box 37.1 Factors Related to Development of Posttraumatic Deformities**
> - Injury-related factors are as follows:
>   – Soft tissue
>   Skin and soft tissue loss.
>   Tendon and muscle injury.
>   Nerve injury.
>   Vascular injury.
>   – Skeletal
>   Type of fracture, fracture geometry, and comminution.
>   Growth plate injury.
>   Bone loss.
>   Intra-articular injury.
> - Treatment-related factors are as follows:
>   – Missed diagnosis of a fracture.
>   – Delayed presentation and management.
>   – Incorrect treatment choice.
>   – Suboptimal management.
>   – Overtreatment.
>   – Iatrogenic problems.
> - Complication-related factors are as follows:
>   – Infection.
>   – Loss of reduction.
>   – Compartment syndrome.
>   – Postoperative stiffness.
>   – Avascular necrosis.
> - Patient-related factors are as follows:
>   – Preexisting skeletal problems like dysplasia, syndromes.
>   – Neuromuscular problems like cerebral palsy, poliomyelitis, and muscular dystrophy.
>   – Altered bone physiology due to osteogenesis imperfecta, metabolic bone disease.
>   – Pathological fracture with underlying tumor, osteomyelitis.
>   – Immunocompromise.
>   – Malnutrition.

Deformities can be caused by one or more of the following etiological factors (Box 37.2):

> **Box 37.2 Etiological Mechanisms for Posttraumatic Deformities are as follows**
> - Postural or positional.
> - Muscle forces.
> - Neural and vascular injury.
> - Poor skeletal stabilization/inappropriate implant.
> - Damage to the growing area of bone.
> - Infection.

1. Postural or positional: Lack of immobilization or faulty immobilization may cause a deformity, often related to contracture of the adjacent soft tissues. Examples are an equinus deformity of the foot or a knee flexion deformity because of contracture of the gastro-soleus or the hamstrings, respectively.
2. Muscle forces: Varus deformity of the upper femur following a fracture is a classic example of muscle forces at work. The flexor-adductor predominance over the abductor-extensor forces causes this deformity (e.g., Fig. 37.2).
3. Neural or vascular injury: Neural injury can create deformity because of the imbalance of muscle forces or by muscle paralysis causing a postural deformity. Vascular injury may give rise to infarction of muscle followed by its fibrosis and eventually a contracture. Volkmann's ischaemic contracture is a typical example of such an etiology.
4. Poor skeletal stabilization, loss of reduction, and loss of fixation can all give rise to posttraumatic deformities.

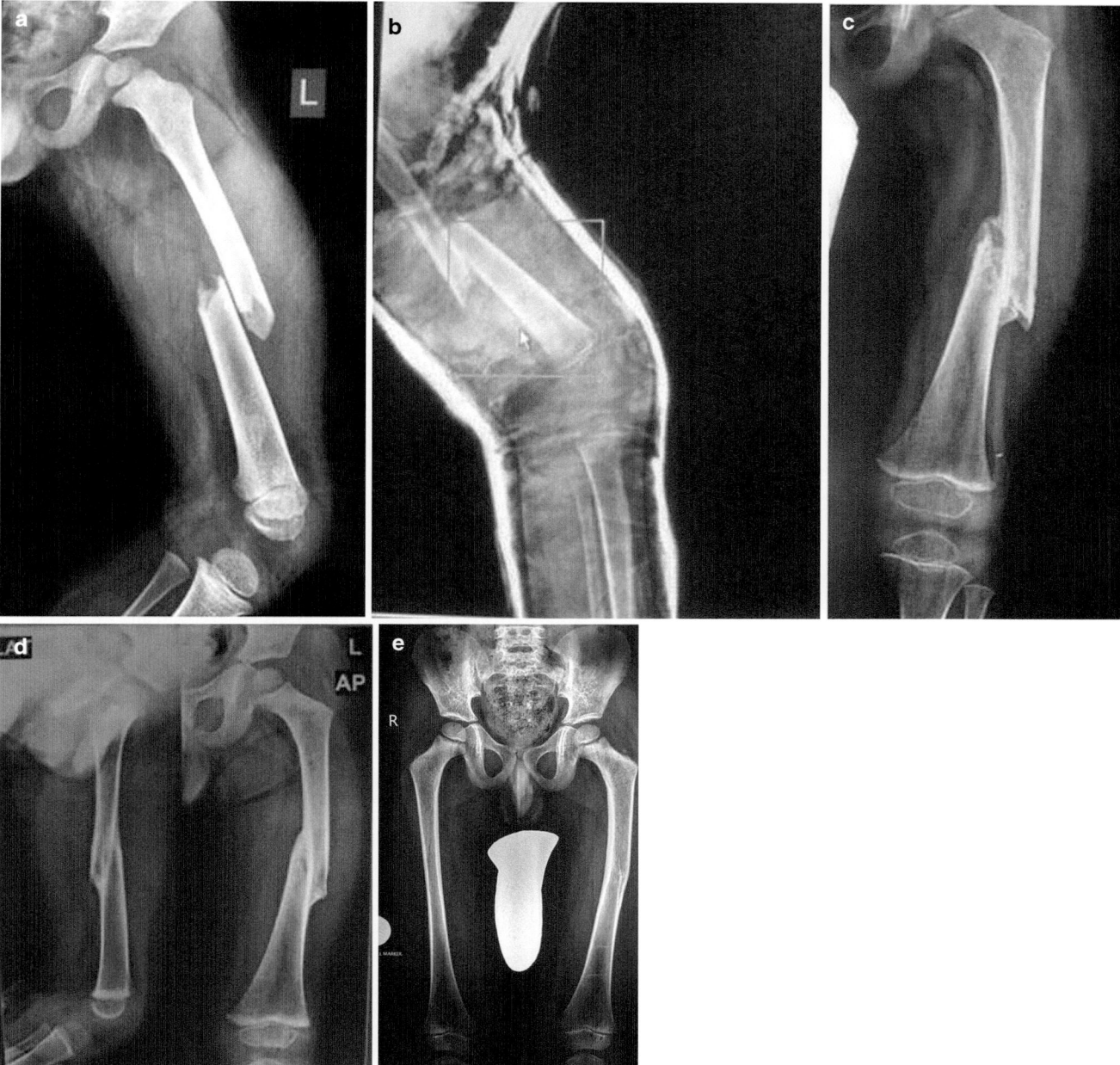

Fig. 37.2 Effect of remodeling and growth: Fracture shaft femur in a 4-year-old child. (**a**) Injury film. (**b**) Position in plaster after immediate spica showing shortening and recurvatum. (**c**) At 6 weeks, uniting with 20° varus and 2.5 cm shortening. (**d**) At 3 months, united with persistent shortening. (**e**) After 2 years, correction of deformity with equal limb lengths

Factors such as poor bone quality, traumatic bone loss, and fracture comminution may contribute to inadequate skeletal stabilization (e.g., Fig. 37.9).

5. Damage to the growing area of bone: Classic examples of these are partial physeal injuries with growth arrest giving rise to various angular deformities (e.g., Fig. 37.7). Symmetric physeal damage would give rise to limb shortening. Damage to the growing area may be a consequence of the mode of injury or may occur because of its poor management. Salter–Harris type 6 injury is a perichondrial ring injury presenting with a normal X-ray. This is an example of the mode of injury giving rise to deformity (e.g., Fig. 37.10).

6. Infection: Open skeletal injuries or iatrogenic issues can be complicated by infection which works by damaging bone and cartilage, causing bone lysis and loss, growth plate damage and its sequelae, as well as joint ankylosis and deformity.

7. Loss of soft tissue or bone: An open fracture or ischaemia can give rise to loss of soft tissue cover or bone loss giving rise to soft tissue contracture or bony deformity or bone gap.

Classification

Posttraumatic deformities can be classified in different ways to fully understand the current problems as well as potential issues that may arise in the future. Such classification helps in formulating the management plan for the individual patient (Box 37.3).

Box 37.3 Classification of Posttraumatic Deformities in Children

The following are related to the area of affected bone:

- Diaphyseal.
- Metaphyseal.
- Physeal.
- Epiphyseal.

The following are related to the anatomical effect:

- Angulation.
- Rotation.
- Limb length.
- Nonunion.
- Restriction of movement.
- Muscle weakness.

The following are related to the tissue affected:

- Soft tissue.
- Skin, fascia, muscle, capsule, or ligaments.
- Skeletal.
- Diaphyseal, growth plate, articular.

The following are related to the progression:

- Progressive: Improving: Partial or complete.
- Progressive: Improving, then progressive.

Clinical Manifestations

Fixed deformity of the joint, joint stiffness and ankylosis, shortening, angular and torsional deformities, and axial malalignment are all potential clinical manifestations in a posttraumatic situation. Meticulous clinical assessment may point to the static or progressive nature of the deformity. Presence or absence of infection is to be noted as it is an important consideration in management. Examination for neural injury is important and can be challenging in young children, especially in the presence of fixed contractures.

Radiographic Imaging

Besides plain X-rays, MRI and CT scans may be useful in some patients.

Plain X-rays are the simplest ways of monitoring bony deformity. In addition to standard views, one may need X-rays in the plane of the deformity. Full-length standing radiographs and scanograms are useful for monitoring limb length.

MRI can give a lot of information about the growth plate (e.g., Fig. 37.7f, g) and articular cartilage, periarticular ligamentous injury, osteochondral fractures, and articular alignment.

CT scans help define the fracture geometry, area of growth arrest, and presence of a bony bar. It is also a useful tool to quantify torsional deformities.

Occasionally, specialized scans like the radioisotope scans may be required to detect infection. Hematologic tests including a white cell count, sedimentation rate, and C-reactive protein are helpful in such a situation. A more comprehensive metabolic panel may be required in patients with underlying metabolic bone diseases such as various forms of rickets.

Remodeling of Bony Deformities

Remodeling may impact decision-making for correcting any bone deformity. The patient's functional capacity and the surgeon's experience should also be factors in determining whether to depend on the remodeling capacity of the specific fracture or to consider performing a more aggressive, invasive technique to achieve a satisfactory result [1].

In the typical long bone, 75% of the remodeling occurs by reorientation of the physis while appositional remodeling of the diaphysis can only be expected to contribute 25% to the remodeling process.

Important factors influencing remodeling are as follows (Box 37.4):

1. Age of the patient: The older the child, the less is the remodeling potential. In general, remodeling of posttraumatic deformities occurs more effectively in children younger than 10 years.
2. Location of the malunion: Metaphyseal fractures remodel better than diaphyseal fractures. Fractures near the fast-growing physes such as lower femur and upper tibia and lower radius and upper humerus remodel better than their counterparts.
3. The plane of the deformity: Angulation in the plane of the joint axis corrects better. Rotations do not correct for all practical purposes. In some fractures, overgrowth phenomenon gives rise to correction of limb shortening.
4. Magnitude of angulation and translation.

> **Box 37.4 Factors Affecting remodeling of Fractures in Children**
> - Age.
> - Location.
> - Plane of deformity.
> - Degree of deformity.

Some guidelines on acceptability of fracture reduction and remodeling are given at the end of this chapter (Appendix A Acceptability Criteria for Reduction in Lower Limb Fractures).

Case Study (Fig. 37.2)

Clinical Summary

A 4-year-old child was treated for fracture shaft femur by immediate spica. He had 2-cm shortening and varus deformity 3 months post fracture. Over a period of 2 years, the deformity corrected and child had equal leg lengths.

Philosophy of Treatment

Fracture healing can stimulate bone growth in certain femoral shaft fractures. The amount of overgrowth varies in different reports from 0.4 to 2.7 cm. Overgrowth in femoral fractures appears to be independent of age, fracture level, and position of the fracture at the time of healing. The effect of growth stimulation may continue for up to 3 years following the fracture.

Case Study (Fig. 37.3)

Clinical Summary

A 6-year-old girl presented 4 months after an open fracture of the tibial tuberosity with patellar tendon tear which was debrided, repaired, and casted. She developed a stiff knee for which the original surgeon did a manipulation under anaesthesia. However, the local swelling and deformity increased. A Salter–Harris type 1 injury was diagnosed at presentation. An MRI revealed a posterior displacement of the distal femoral epiphysis with loculated fluid collection along the posterior border.

Different options of management were considered but it was decided to leave her alone in view of the good possibility of remodeling. For the stiff knee, physical therapy with range of motion exercises was started. The sequential X-rays show the excellent remodeling (Table 37.1). She regained nearly full knee movement 2 years after the injury.

Philosophy of Management

The distal femoral epiphysis is one of the fastest growing physes with rapid remodeling in children. Undisplaced Salter–Harris type 1 injuries need not be fixed, as long as they are immobilized with restricted weight bearing and closely followed with serial radiographs. The ones with displacement may need a gentle reduction and fixation. We prefer that pins not be introduced from the knee level upwards but rather in a reverse fashion from the metaphysis into the epiphysis as recommended by Wall [2]. It is important not to leave pins sticking out of the skin if placed in a retrograde manner. If placed in this fashion, they should be buried under the skin for later removal.

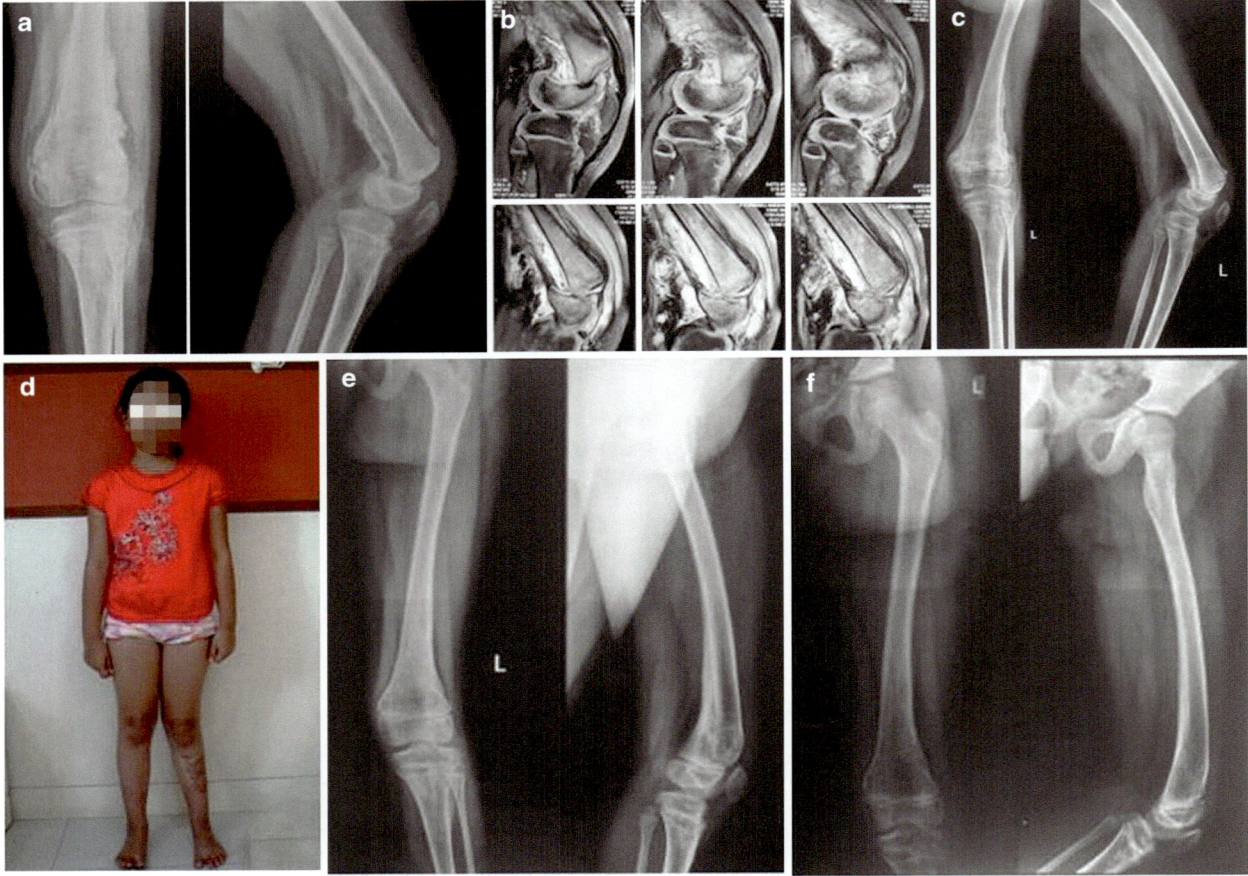

Fig. 37.3 A 6-year-old with malunited type 1 SH fracture. (**a**) Four months from injury, Feb 2011. (**b**) MRI showing posterior displacement of the physis. (**c**, **d**) X-ray and clinical picture 5 months postinjury. (**e**) X-rays 10 months postinjury showing remodeling and correction of angulation and translation. (**f**) Complete remodeling at 1.5 years postinjury in 2012

Table 37.1 Diaphyseal-epiphyseal angle

Feb 2011	38°
Mar 2011	42°
May 2011	54°
Aug 2011	70°
Nov 2011	82°
Apr 2012	90°

Management

Decision-making in posttraumatic deformity situations is based on a number of factors such as:

- Age of the patient.
- Location of the deformity.
- Morphological status of bone, soft tissue, and cartilage.
- Functional loss and impairment.
- Abnormal mechanical loading with risk of joint degeneration.
- Cosmetic aspect.

Table 37.2 presents a general schema of the types of interventions.

Table 37.2 General schema of the types of interventions

Type of deformity	Nature of intervention
Joint contractures	Manipulation
	Splintage
	Serial plasters
	Soft tissue release
	External fixation
	Osteotomy
	Arthrodesis
Muscle imbalance	Splintage
	Tendon transfer
	Arthrodesis
Angular and rotational bony deformities	Osteotomy
	Growth modulation
	Physeal bar excision
Shortening	Shoe raise
	Limb lengthening
	Contralateral epiphysiodesis
	Limb shortening
Bone loss and nonunion	Bone grafting
	Bone transport

Important Posttraumatic Deformities: Lower Limb

In this section, we briefly discuss some unique posttraumatic lower limb deformities in children and demonstrate a variety of treatment strategies. However, as noted earlier, the decision-making should be individualized based on patient, surgeon, and environmental factors.

Posttraumatic Chondrolysis of the Hip and Avascular Necrosis

Acetabular injuries may be complicated by chondrolysis of the hip, and this may give rise to a fixed flexion and adduction deformity. Likewise, hip dislocations and fractures of the femoral neck may be complicated by avascular necrosis. Avascular necrosis may follow the commonly described patterns in the classifications of Kalamchi and MacEwen [3] or Bucholz and Ogden [4] and management would follow the lines described for such conditions.

Arthrodiatasis [5, 6] is a useful modality for managing posttraumatic chondrolysis and stiffness of the hip, and an example is presented here.

Case Study (Fig. 37.4)

Clinical Summary

A 15-year-old boy sustained a motor cycle accident in 1999. He suffered a fracture of the medial wall of the acetabulum which was managed conservatively by traction. He gradually developed a fixed flexion and adduction deformity of the hip along with stiffness and awkward gait. He presented 2 years later for this problem having tried all conservative measures and physiotherapy. X-rays revealed narrowing of the right hip joint space, and MRI was not suggestive of infection or inflammation.

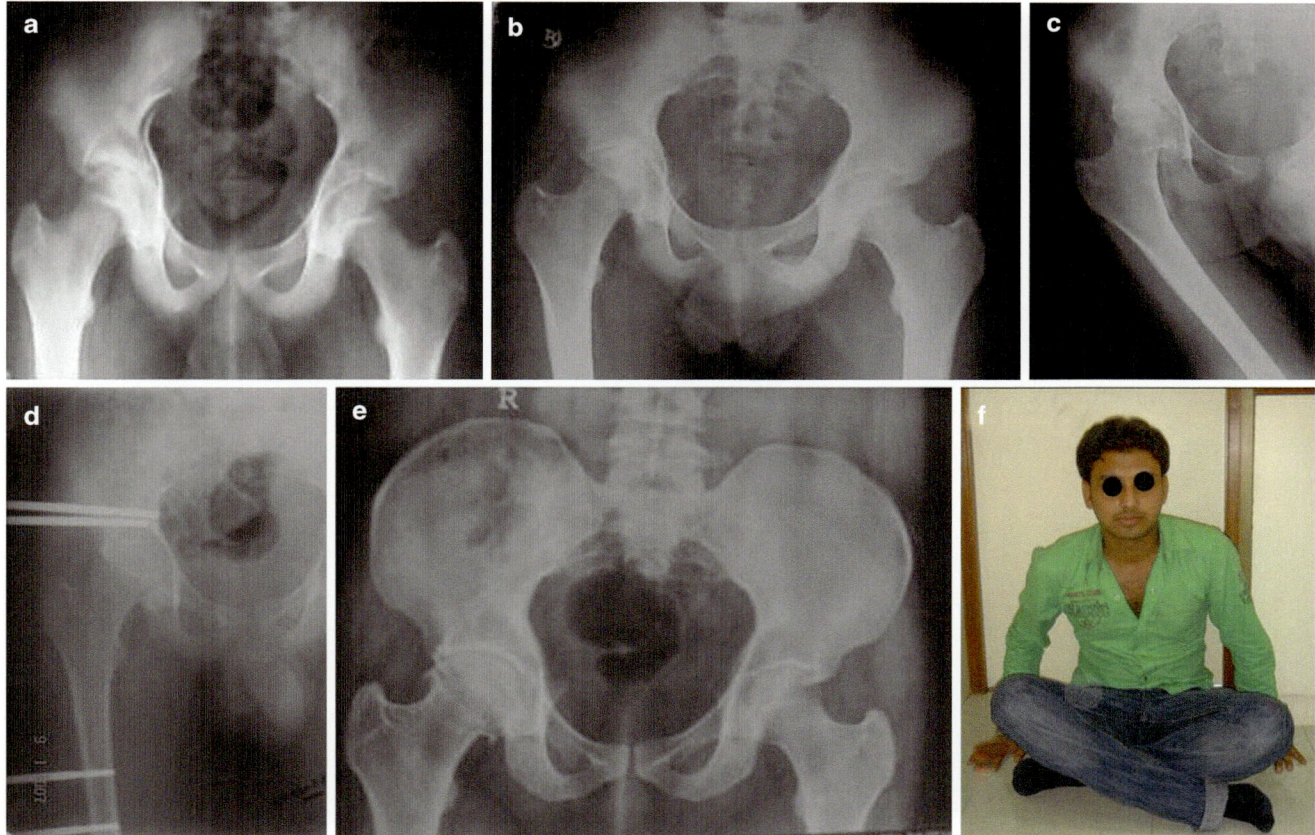

Fig. 37.4 Hip deformity due to posttraumatic chondrolysis in a 15-year-old child. (**a**) Injury film showing acetabular fracture. (**b**) X-ray showing healed fracture 2 months later. (**c**) The marked adduction of the hip and loss of joint space shown 1.5 years later. (**d**) Following arthrodiatasis with an adductor release nearly 2 years post accident. (**e**) X-rays 8 years post injury. (**f**) Clinical picture at this time

Philosophy of Treatment

He was managed by an adductor release and hip distraction. The flexion adduction deformity improved, and he gradually regained his hip motion. The hinged distractor was in place for 3 months and physiotherapy continued. On follow-up 8 years later, he still retained excellent motion at the hip and was able to squat and sit cross legged.

Posttraumatic Coxa Vara

Posttraumatic coxa vara may be caused by a malunion or even a nonunion of the proximal femur. Shear forces at the fracture site caused by the body weight and muscle forces may be responsible for the mal—or nonunion.

Restoration of the normal neck–shaft angle is important biomechanically and this would require correction of the malunion by a valgus osteotomy. A nonunion osteosynthesis may include internal fixation with or without bone grafting and a valgus osteotomy.

Case Study (Fig. 37.5)

Clinical Summary

Case of basicervical fracture of the femur in an 8-year-old child treated conservatively who presented with a limp related to a coxa vara deformity: The deformity was nonprogressive and uniplanar with the apex at the neck of femur.

Philosophy of Treatment

Both deformity correction and nonunion of femur neck fracture were treated with a valgus osteotomy performed at the subtrochanteric level and fixation with a plate.

Malunited Shaft Femur or Pseudarthrosis with Deformity

Either situation will demand skeletal realignment and stabilization by some form of internal or external fixation with or without bone grafting depending on the nature of the pseudarthrosis.

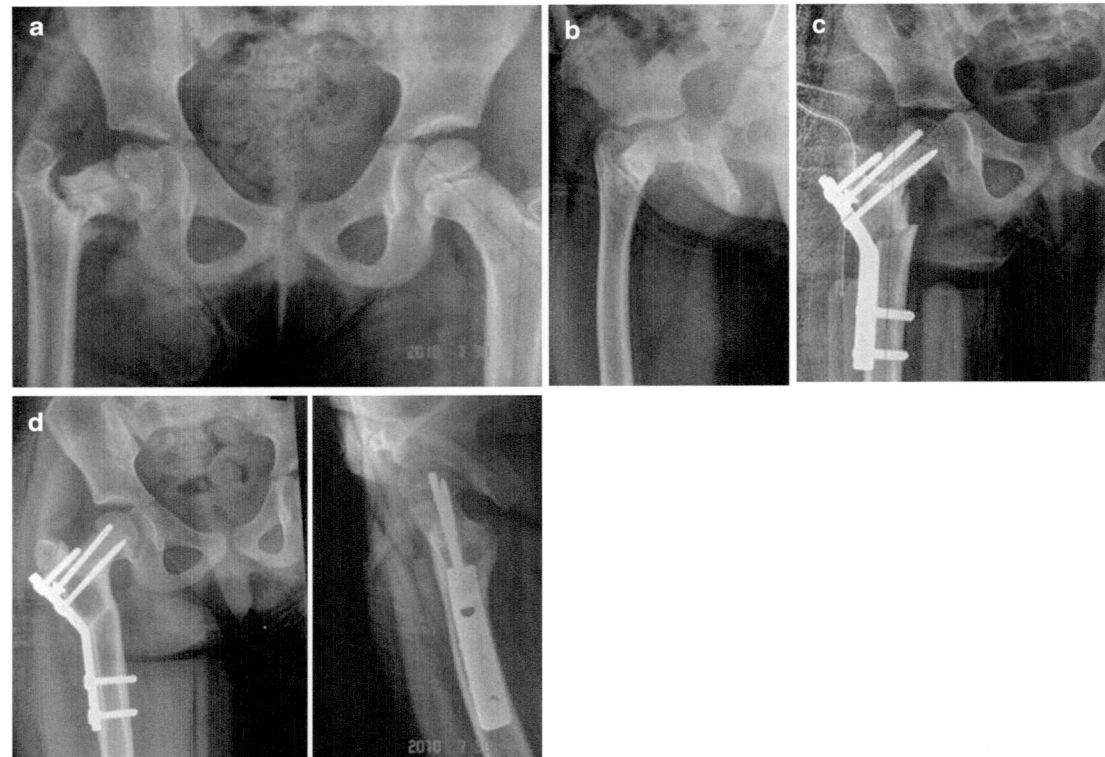

Fig. 37.5 Posttraumatic coxa vara due to fracture neck femur treated in spica. (**a**) Fibrous nonunion in varus with a neck–shaft angle of 100°. (**b**) Lateral X-ray showing ununited fracture line. (**c**) In situ fixation of nonunion with subtrochanteric valgus osteotomy. (**d**) Healing of fracture as well as osteotomy in 3.5 months

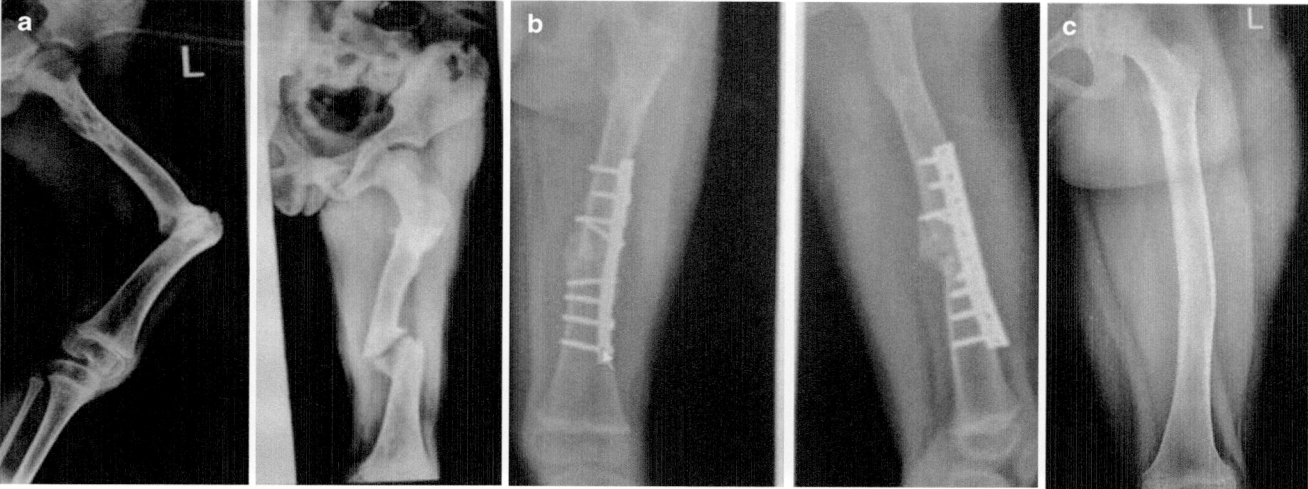

Fig. 37.6 Maluniting fracture shaft femur. (**a**) Fibrous nonunion shaft of femur with triplanar deformation. (**b**) Excision of fibrous tissue, deformity correction at apex, and plating without bone grafting. (**c**) Final healing after plate removal at 1 year

Case Study (Fig. 37.6)

Clinical Summary

Fracture of the femoral shaft which was treated conservatively presented with fibrous nonunion with unacceptable deformity at the fracture level.

The deformity was a triplanar deformity with malrotation of the femur, procurvatum of 90° and translation of about 1 cm, and valgus angulation at the fracture site.

Philosophy of Treatment

Fibrous nonunion of shaft of femur was treated with resection and freshening of the edges and fixation along with bone grafting. A corrective osteotomy was performed at the apex of deformity, i.e., at the fracture site, and fixation was done by a plate.

Case Study (Fig. 37.7)

Clinical Summary

A 7-year-old child with middle one-third comminuted fracture shaft femur with a butterfly fragment was treated with immediate hip spica. The spica was removed after 6 weeks. The child presented with limp with shortening and intoeing gait. The X-ray showed varus deformity of 30° with shortening of 3.5 cm with clinical evaluation showing internal rotation deformity of 50°. At 2 years follow-up, there was residual varus with persistent shortening and rotational deformity with gait issues.

Philosophy of Treatment

The child was treated with osteotomy at the fracture site with acute correction of varus and rotation with fixation with Rush nail and application of external fixator. The shortening was corrected with gradual distraction. The fixator was removed after consolidation of regenerate.

Case Study (Fig. 37.8)

Clinical Summary

Inadequate or inappropriate fixation leading to instability and implant failure is a common cause of deformity with fibrous or hypertrophic non-union especially in the femur.

A 12-year-old male child presented with pain, inability to weight bear, and an anterolateral thigh deformity with a stiff knee. He had been treated for a middle third shaft femur fracture with open Ender nailing 3 months ago.

X-rays revealed fixation with two Ender' nails from lateral entry. Serial X-rays showed bending of nails with hypertrophic non-union.

The child was operated with removal of nails, open plate fixation with osteoclasis for deformity correction with local osteoperiosteal flaps. Pre-operatively, the patient had only 10° of knee flexion, Therefore, the knee was gently manipulated and 90° of flexion was achieved.

Serial X-rays showed progressive healing in excellent alignment after plating.

Treatment Philosophy

Restoration of stability by plating with appropriate local bone grafting and deformity correction resulted in excellent result.

The inadequate stability created by the different size nails plus a very low entry resulted in the complication of stiffness, deformity, and non-union.

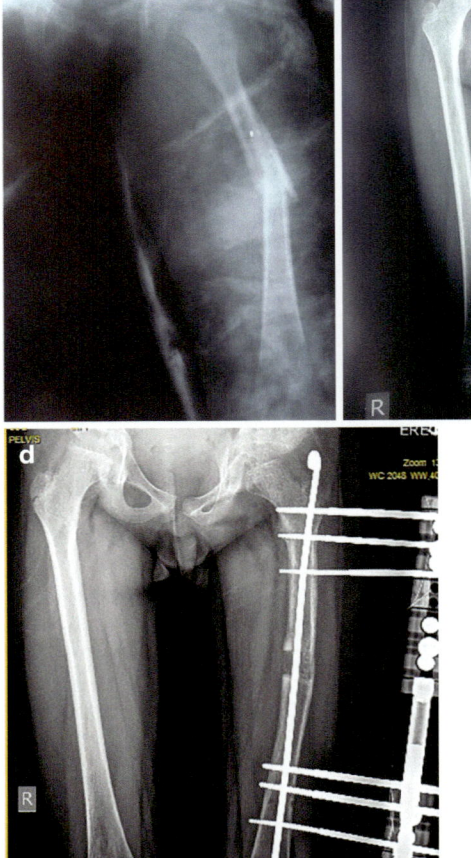

Fig. 37.7 Malunited fracture left shaft femur with shortening varus and rotational deformity. (**a**) Film through spica showing the middle one-third fracture with butterfly. (**b**) 6 months post injury showing varus deformity with shortening. (**c**) The clinical photo showing increased internal rotation on left hip suggestive of internal rotation deformity of 50°. (**d**) Treated with femoral osteotomy with acute correction of varus and rotation with gradual lengthening over Rush nail with uniplanar external fixator

Distal Femoral Deformity Following Iatrogenic Physeal Injury

The growth plate can be injured during insertion of elastic nails for a femoral shaft fracture or during implant removal. To avoid this problem, it is recommended that the entry point should be at least 2.5 cm s from the growth plate. Damage to the peripheral growth plate and a resultant bar can give rise to progressive angular deformity.

Excision of a physeal bar should be considered if there is at least 2-year growth left and area of the bar is less than 30% of total physeal area. The success of the surgery depends on the age of the patient, etiology, area of the bar, the bone involved, and the location of the bar [7] (central or peripheral). The deformities, if more than 30°, are treated by osteotomy but if the deformities are less than 30°, it can often be treated by simultaneous growth modulation surgery.

Case Study (Fig. 37.9)

Clinical Summary

A 11-year-old girl with progressive post-traumatic genu valgum: She had sustained a femoral shaft fracture at the age of 9 years which was treated elsewhere with a retrograde Rush nail.

A progressive deformity was noted after removal of the nail. X-rays revealed a lateral growth arrest. MRI showed peripheral physeal arrest with area less than 20%.

Philosophy of Treatment

As she had more than 2 years of growth available and area of the bar was less than 30% of the underlying physis, she was treated with excision of physeal bar and fat interposition. At the same time, she underwent growth modulation by plate hemiepiphysiodesis on medial side.

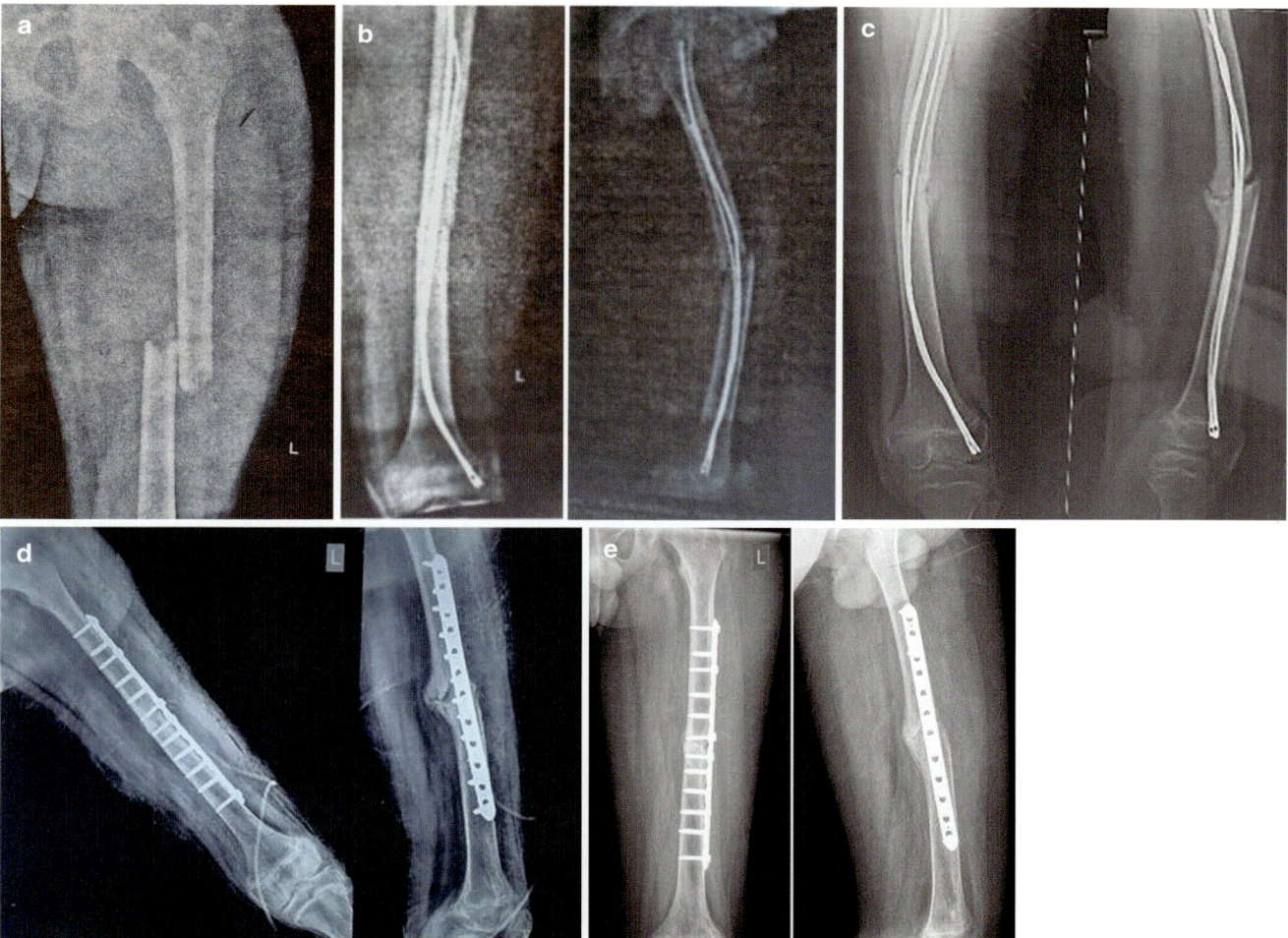

Fig. 37.8 Femoral deformity in fracture shaft femur due to poor fixation causing non-union. (a) Fracture shaft femur in a 12 years old. (b) Fixation with Ender' nails from lateral entry. (c) AP and lateral X-rays at 6 months post injury showing hypertrophic nonunion with valgus deformity. (d) Treated by removal of nail with plating and grafting. € 3 months post-surgery X-ray shows union

The medial hemiepiphysiodesis corrected the growth with restoration of lateral growth by physeal bar excision. At 1 year, the restoration of growth was evident by diverging screws of hemiepiphysiodesis plate and increase in the distance between markers.

Physeal Injury of the Distal Femur with Angular Deformity

Physeal injuries of the distal femur are notorious for the production of deformity. The incidence of angular deformity in such cases is 18–51% in different series, and the risk of shortening is 36–68% [7–10]. The risk of growth arrest has been reported to be between 40% and 52% [11, 12]. Salter–Harris (SH) 1 injuries had the lowest incidence of growth disturbance (36%), SH 2, 58%, and SH 3, 49%, whereas SH 4 injuries had the highest rate of growth disturbance at 64% [11].

Physeal injuries require very accurate repositioning of the growth plate and restoration of the articular alignment as growth disturbances can result in significant angular deformity. Intra-articular injuries should be open reduced and stabilized, and patients with physeal injuries should undergo rapid mobilization of the adjacent joints, generally by the fourth week postinjury, unless the fracture is very comminuted. Both SH classification and displacement of the fracture are significant predictors of the final outcome. The treatment method may influence the final outcome [13]. In relation to Salter–Harris type 2 injuries, Ilharreborde and colleagues stated that those with comminution and displacement had a greater risk of growth arrest (75%) compared with those without these risk factors (38%) [14].

In a post-trauma situation, angular deformities in children are usually caused by a physeal injury. Such deformities can be addressed by a hemiepiphysiodesis procedure utilizing

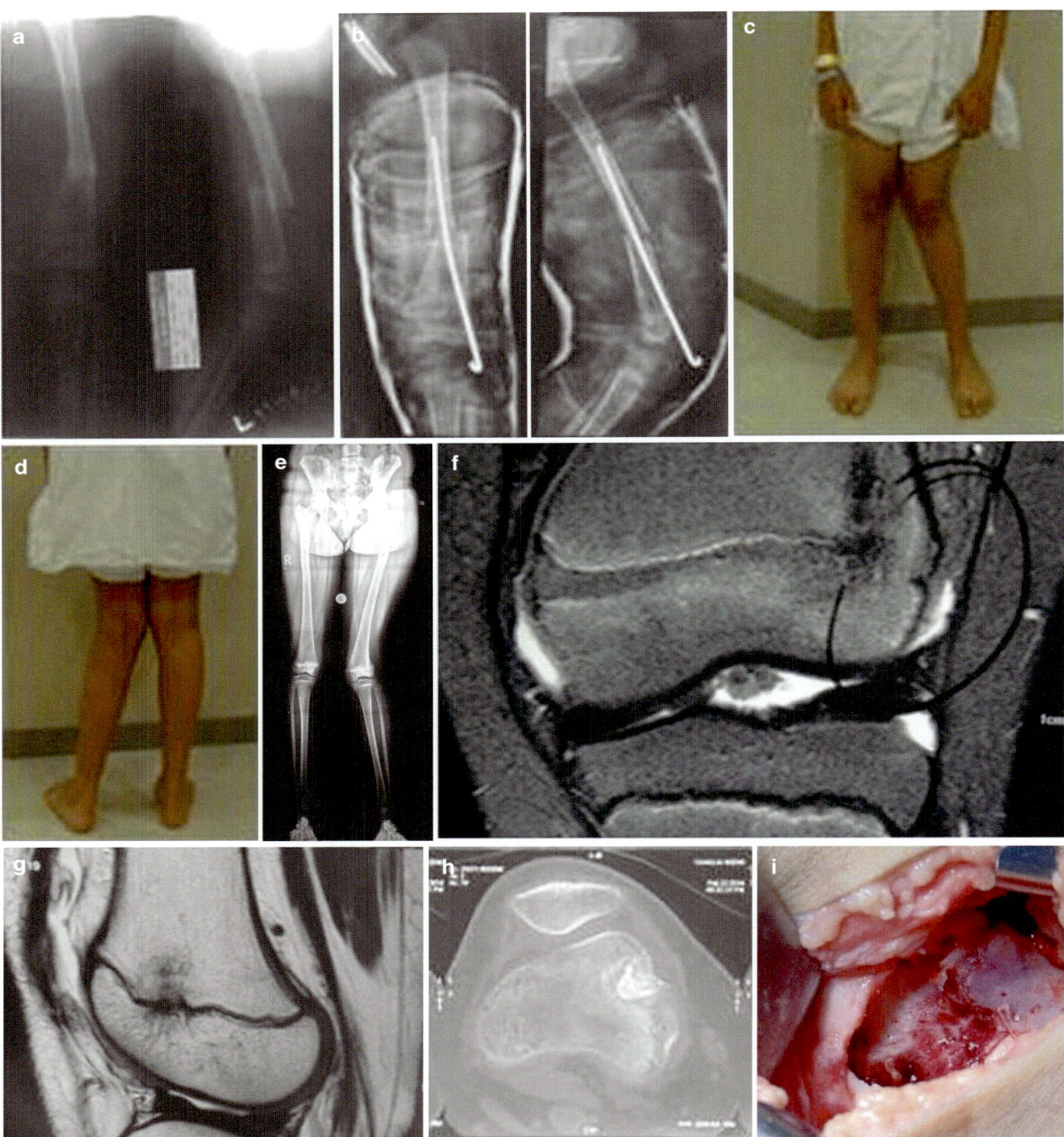

Fig. 37.9 A 11-year-old with a femoral shaft fracture treated by an intramedullary nail with physeal injury of lower femur and genu valgum. (**a**) Injury film. (**b**) X-rays showing fixation with a single intramedullary nail from lateral aspect. (**c–e**) Clinical photos and X-ray scanogram showing the deformity. (**f, g**) Gradient echo fat suppression MRI image showing lateral growth arrest due to physeal bar. (**h**) Mapping of the physeal arrest using a CT scan. (**i**) Intraoperative photo showing the excision of bony bar using a burr. (**j**) Interposition of the defect with subcutaneous gluteal fat. (**k**) Intraoperative image to confirm adequacy of the bar excision. (**l**) Postoperative X-ray showing hemiepiphysiodesis plate and markers. (**m, n**) Nine months postoperative clinical photo and X-rays showing resumption of growth and correction of deformity

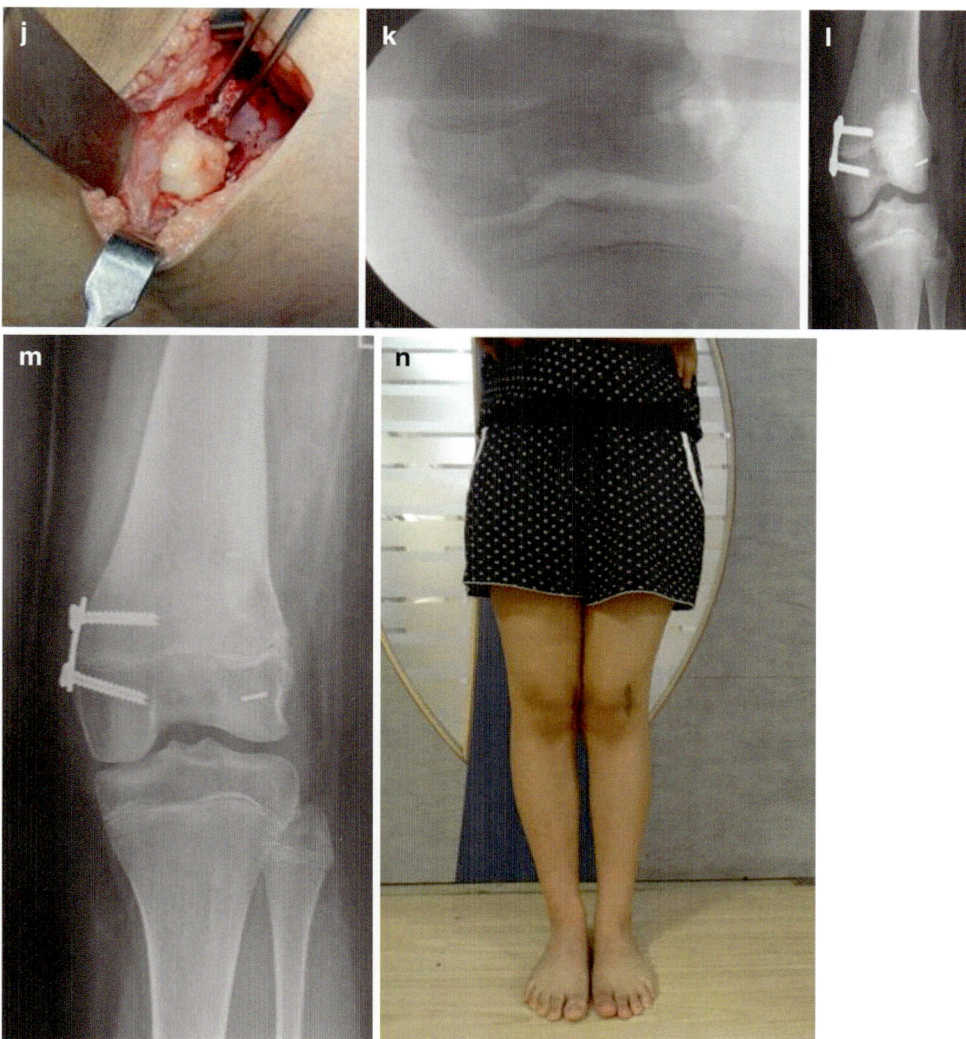

Fig. 37.9 (continued)

staples, transphyseal screws, or extra-periosteal tension band plates in combination with a bar resection where the deformity is deemed to be correctible with growth modulation. Appropriate selection of the age for intervention and time for removal of growth modulation devices is important. It is important to avoid repeat corrections via multiple osteotomies and hold the deformity constant in a progressive situation by epiphyseodesis. Final correction of deformity and limb length discrepancy can be done at skeletal maturity.

Case Study (Fig. 37.10)

Clinical Summary

This male patient had an open Salter–Harris type 2 injury of the left distal femur at 1.5 years age. The injury was debrided, open reduced, and fixed with a cancellous screw. Eight months later, a valgus deformity of the knee was noted that was gradually progressive. At 10 years from injury, the deformity was progressive and very noticeable. A CT scan revealed the growth disturbance at the distal femur.

Philosophy of Management

An extra-periosteal tension band plate medial hemiepiphysiodesis was done to prevent further angulation. The deformity remained unchanged until skeletal maturity but a residual shortening of 7 cm resulted. Realignment was done by a distal femoral osteotomy. The marked shortening was addressed by a simultaneous gradual lengthening of the femur using external fixation.

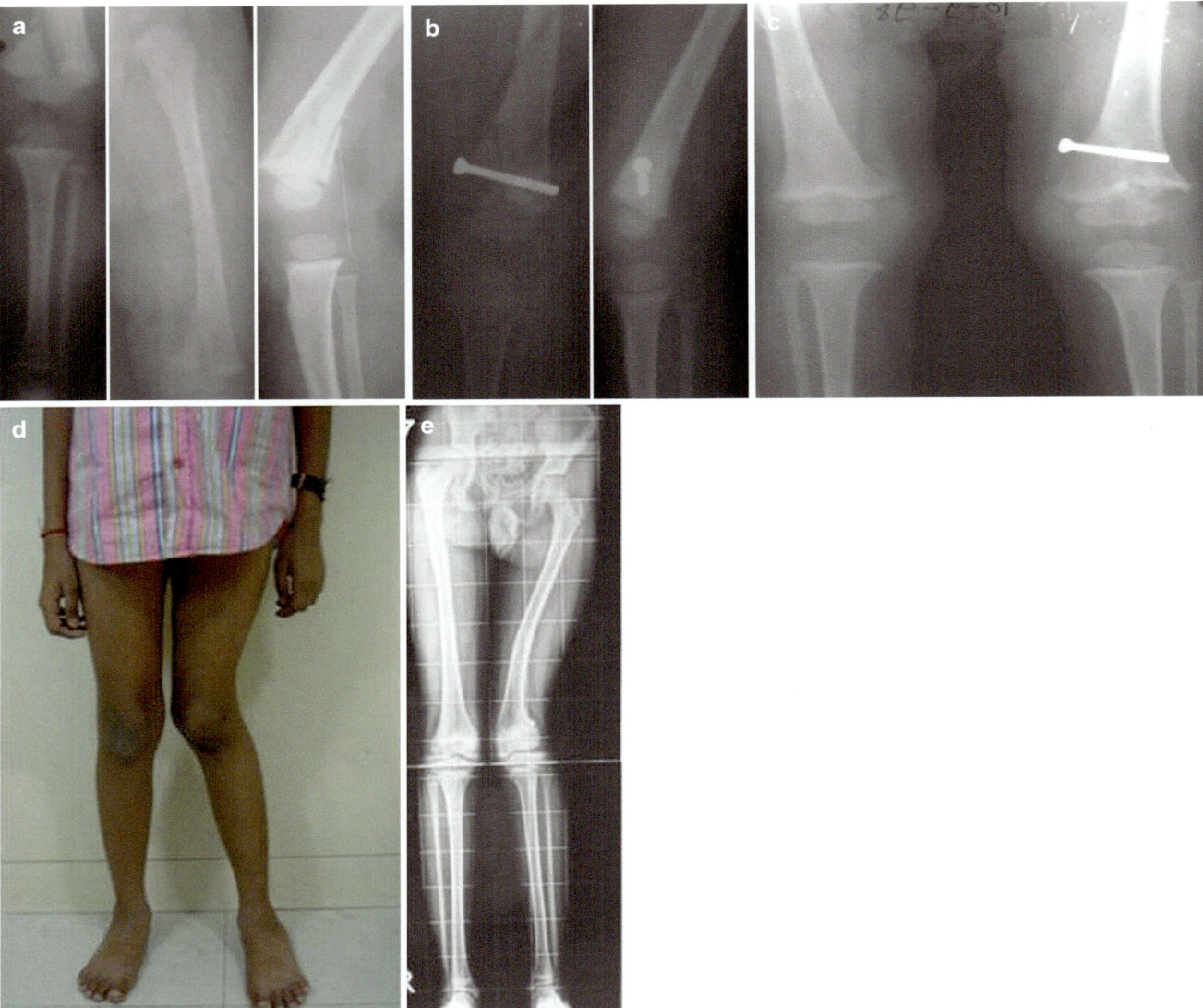

Fig. 37.10 Posttraumatic genu valgum and femoral shortening due to type 2 SH physeal injury of lower femur. (**a**) Injury film 1998. (**b**) Postoperative X-ray showing fixation with screw. (**c**) X-ray taken 6 months post op showing valgus deformity. (**d**, **e**) Clinical photo and X-ray in 2007, 9 years post injury showing progressive genu valgum. (**f**) CT shows extensive lateral physeal arrest involving more than 50% of the growth plate. (**g**) Hemiepiphysiodesis in 2007 using an 8 plate. This prevented progression of deformity holding the LDFA to 66° over 4 years. (**h**) Clinical picture, 2010. (**i**) Underwent medial closing-wedge distal femoral corrective osteotomy with limb lengthening proximally using external fixation. (**j**, **k**) X-ray at the end of lengthening after consolidation of the regenerate. (**l**, **m**) Follow-up in 2014, i.e., 16 years after injury showing correction of limb lengths and deformity. (**n**) 23 years later, scanogram and clinical picture

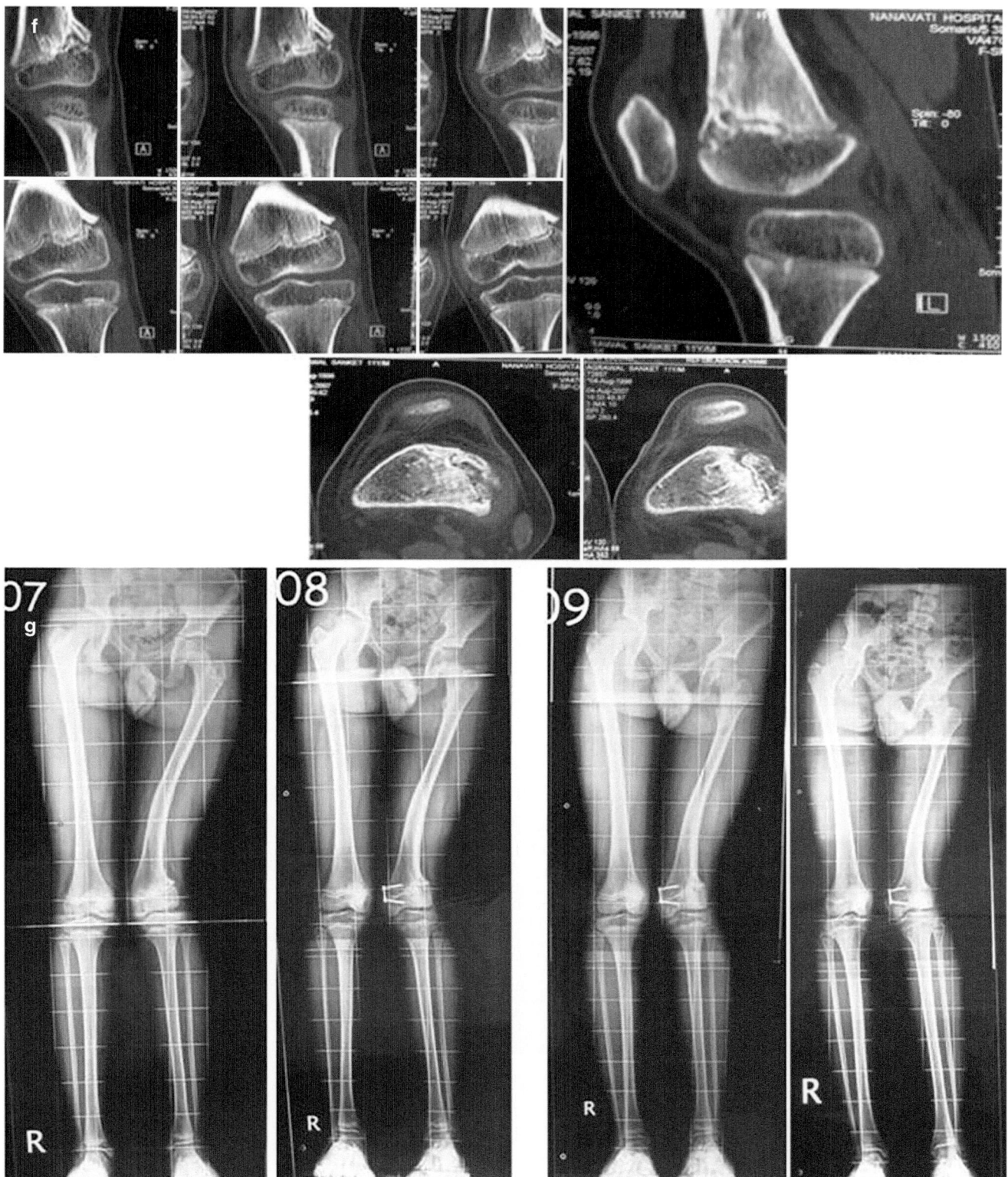

Fig. 37.10 (continued)

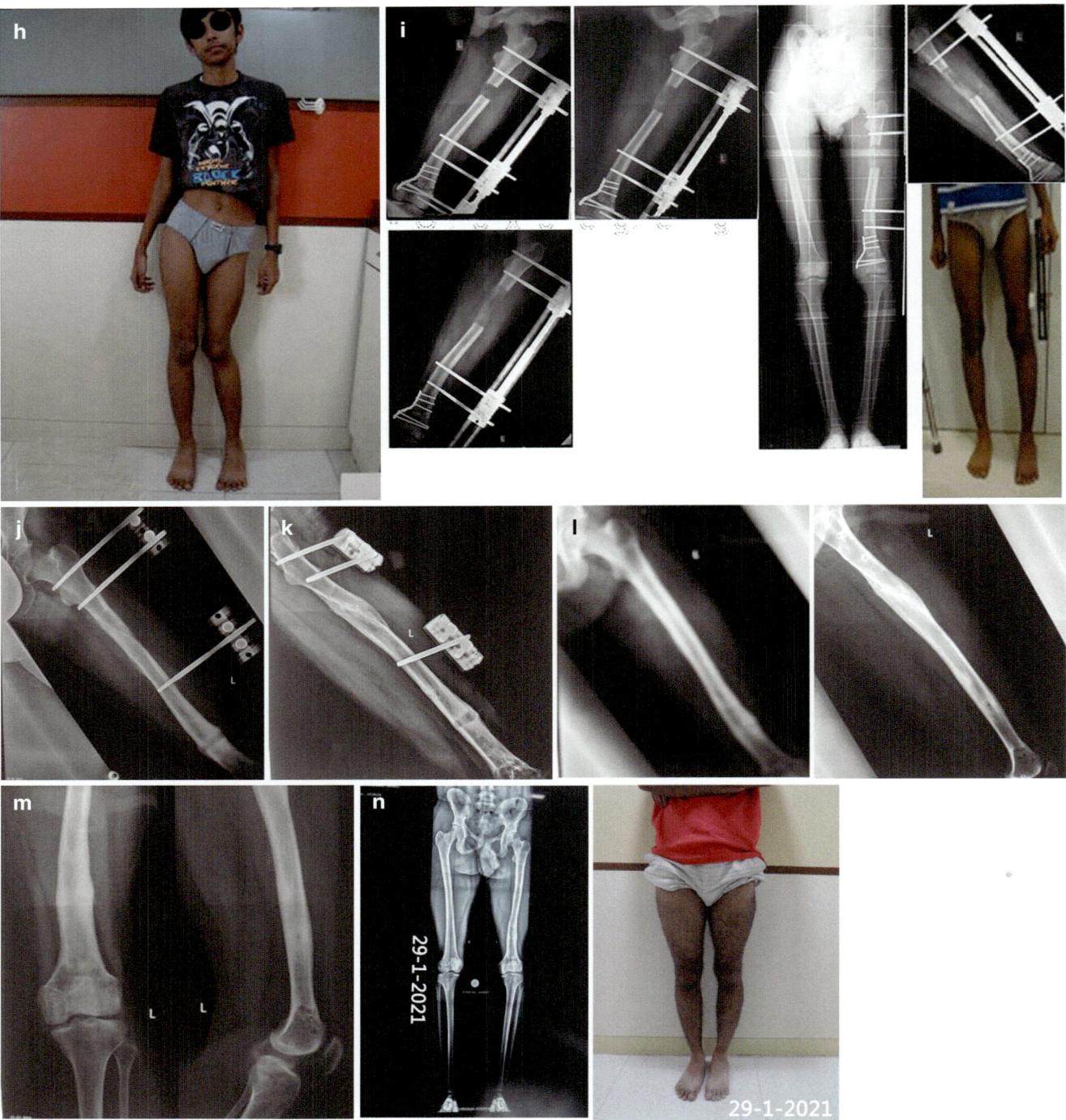

Fig. 37.10 (continued)

Malunited Intra-Articular Fractures

If presenting early, maluniting fractures can be addressed with open reduction and the osteochondral fragments repositioned to restore articular and physeal alignment. Late presentations may be fraught with the risks of poor results as articular congruity may be difficult to restore.

Case Study (Fig. 37.11)

A 17-year-old boy sustained a comminuted fracture of the upper tibia. This was treated by internal fixation. The reduction and fixation was unsatisfactory. The fracture malunited, and he presented after implant removal for deformity and loss of motion of the left knee. At this stage, management options such as arthrodesis and defor-

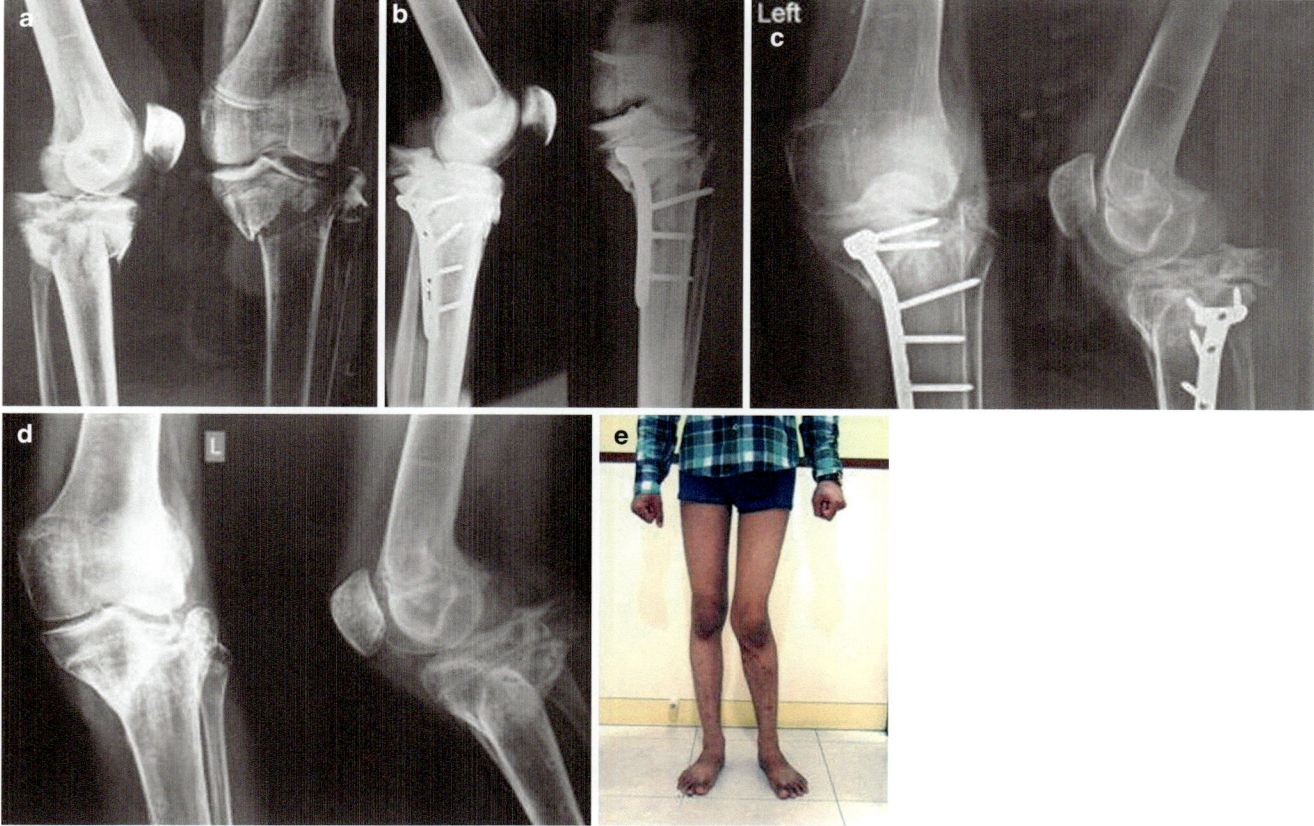

Fig. 37.11 Genu valgum due to malunited upper tibial fracture. (**a**) Injury film. (**b**) Postoperative X-ray. (**c**) Implant failure and malunion. (**d**, **e**) X-rays and clinical picture after implant removal

mity correction were discussed but the family refused further treatment.

Physeal Injury to Proximal Tibia

Injury to proximal tibial physis is less common than the distal femur but can produce progressive deformities as it is also a fast-growing physis. The management options include excision of the physeal bar coupled with osteotomy or growth modulation. In cases where growth cannot be restored, acute angular correction with an osteotomy combined with an epiphysiodesis (to prevent recurrent deformity with future growth) or limb lengthening at a later date can be utilized.

Case Study (Fig. 37.12)

Clinical Summary

A 11-year-old child with progressive tibial varus presented with blunt vehicular trauma with normal X-rays 2 years earlier.

He developed progressive tibial varus due to probably a Salter–Harris type 6 medial proximal tibial physeal injury indicating injury to perichondrial ring.

Philosophy of Treatment

The echogradient fat suppression MRI showed that the area of the bar was less than 25% of the surface area of the underlying physis. He was 11 years and had more than 2 years of active growth remaining. As he fulfilled the criteria for growth restoration, he was treated with physeal bar excision and interposition of bone cement in the defect to prevent reformation of the bar. Growth modulation was added on the lateral side with hemiepiphysiodesis plate to correct the deformity.

Case Study (Fig. 37.13)

Clinical Summary

The case of a 17-year-old boy who had a fracture of the upper end of tibia at the age of 10 years for which he was treated with above knee cast is discussed: He probably had an anterolateral proximal tibial physeal arrest which was undiagnosed. It resulted in progressive recurvatum and valgus deformity.

At 2 years after the injury, the patient presented with a deformity of genu recurvatum which was progressive in nature. There was anteroposterior instability of the knee with partial subluxation of the joint. Radiological examination showed anterior physeal arrest of the proximal tibial physis.

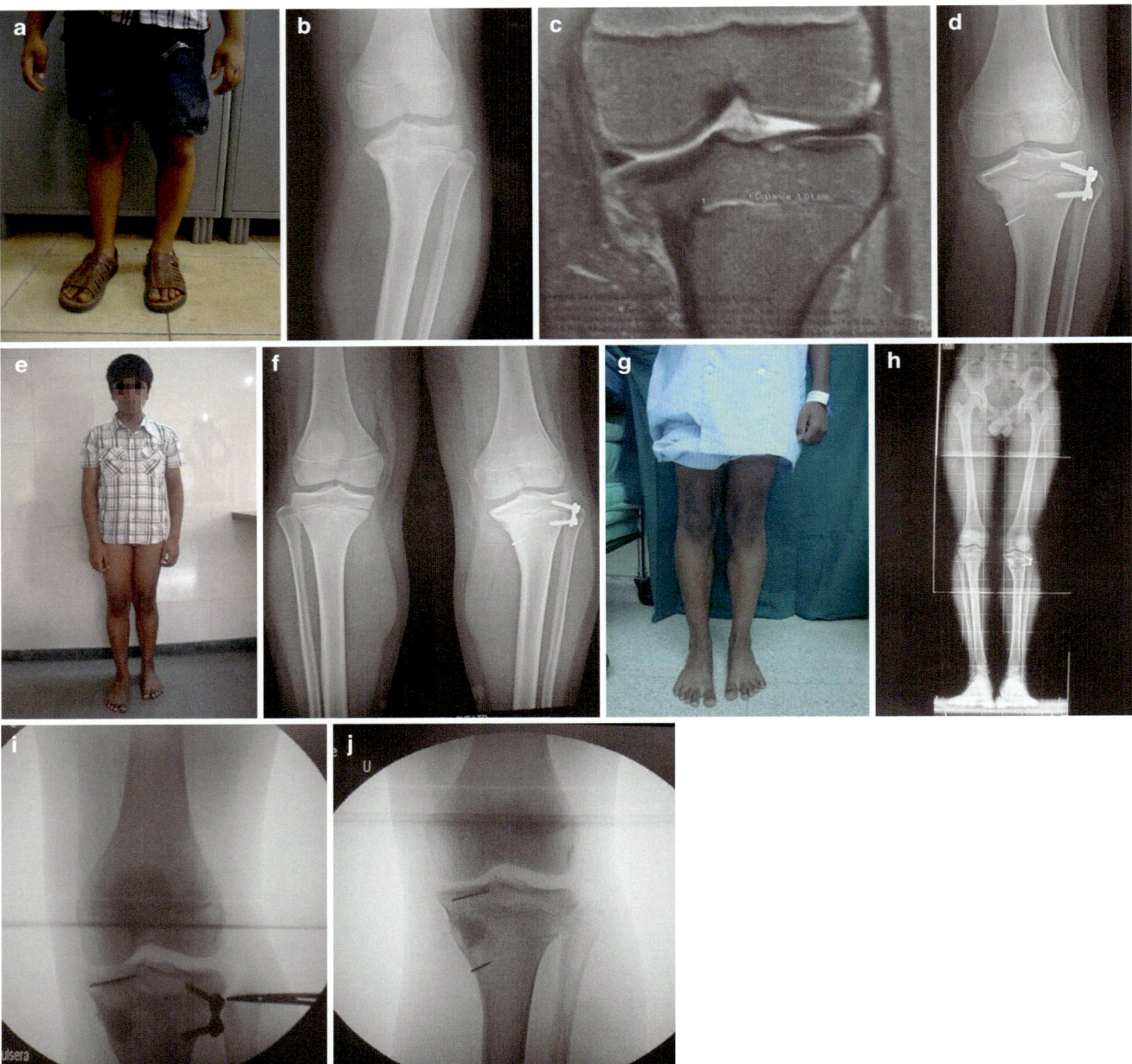

Fig. 37.12 Type 6 Salter–Harris injury to upper tibial physis perichondrial ring with resultant varus deformity. The child was treated with bar excision and growth modulation. (**a, b**) Clinical picture and X-ray 2 years following the injury showing varus deformity upper tibia. (**c**) Gradient echo fat suppression image showing perichondrial ring injury (*white arrow*) with the formation of bony bar (*red arrow*). (**d**) Postoperative X-ray showing bone cement used for interposition after excising bony bar, markers, and hemiepiphysiodesis plate. (**e, f**) Clinical picture and X-rays 6 months after surgery. (**g, h**) Clinical picture and scanogram 13 months postoperatively showing correction of deformity and restoration of growth. (**i, j**) Intraoperative images before and after removal of the plate. Note the divergence of the screws

The apex of the deformity was located at the upper end of the tibia.

Philosophy of Treatment

Perform a high tibial open-wedge osteotomy at the apex to correct the deformity and fill the defect with bone graft: The deformity correction was done acutely with an anterior open-wedge osteotomy at the upper end of the tibia. The osteotomy was stabilized with a plate. Tricortical iliac crest graft which was appropriately shaped was used. Additional tricalcium phosphate interposition material was used.

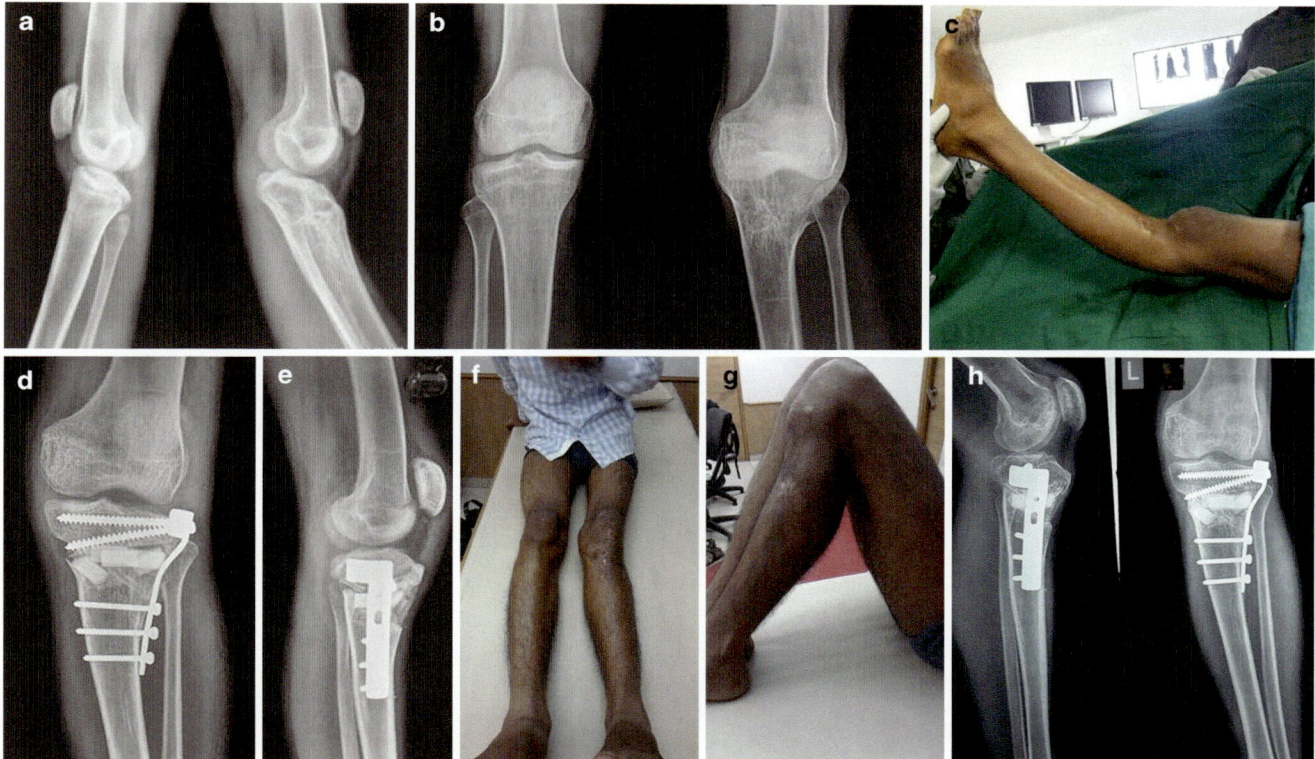

Fig. 37.13 A 17-year-old child with injury to upper tibial growth plate with recurvatum and varus deformity. (**a**, **b**) Anteroposterior X-rays showing the deformity. (**c**) Preoperative picture showing the extent of deformity. (**d**, **e**) Postoperative X-rays showing correction of deformity with osteotomy. (**f**–**h**) Six-month follow-up showing deformity correction and function with X-ray

Case Study (Fig. 37.14)

Clinical Summary

Case of posttraumatic tibia vara deformity secondary to fracture of upper end of tibia in a young child: The deformity was progressive and was biplanar with apex at the upper end of tibia. There was severe tibia vara with mild procurvatum of the tibia.

Philosophy of Treatment

Complex deformity in a post-physeal arrest tibia vara with progressive deformity was treated with staged gradual correction with oblique osteotomy through apex and distractors applied for gradual correction. Later, a fibular osteotomy was done and the same graft was used to fill the osteotomy defect site, which healed and acted like an epiphysiodesis.

Post-Traumatic Tibia Valga

An unusual complication of fractures of the upper tibia in children is progressive tibial valgus. There has been a lot of discussion on the mechanism of this valgus and a number of authors have advanced their hypotheses [15, 16].

Operative findings have disclosed soft tissue interposition in the form of periosteum, pes anserinus, or medial collateral ligament. A consequence of this interposition is loss of periosteal regulation of linear growth on the medial side of the tibia with consequent valgus.

Treatment of this condition is primarily watchful observation. Many authors have shown spontaneous resolution of the valgus with time. If the deformity does not resolve, any of the growth modulation techniques can be used. Late presentation may need an osteotomy [16].

Case Study (Fig. 37.15)

A 3-year-old boy was seen in the outpatient clinic with a deformity of the right leg. He had sustained a fracture of the right proximal tibial metaphysis at the age of 1 year and 10 months. He had had a cast treatment, and there was no history of manipulation at that time. The deformity was apparent a few months after the cast was removed.

Progressive deformity was noted that gradually increased to the current magnitude.

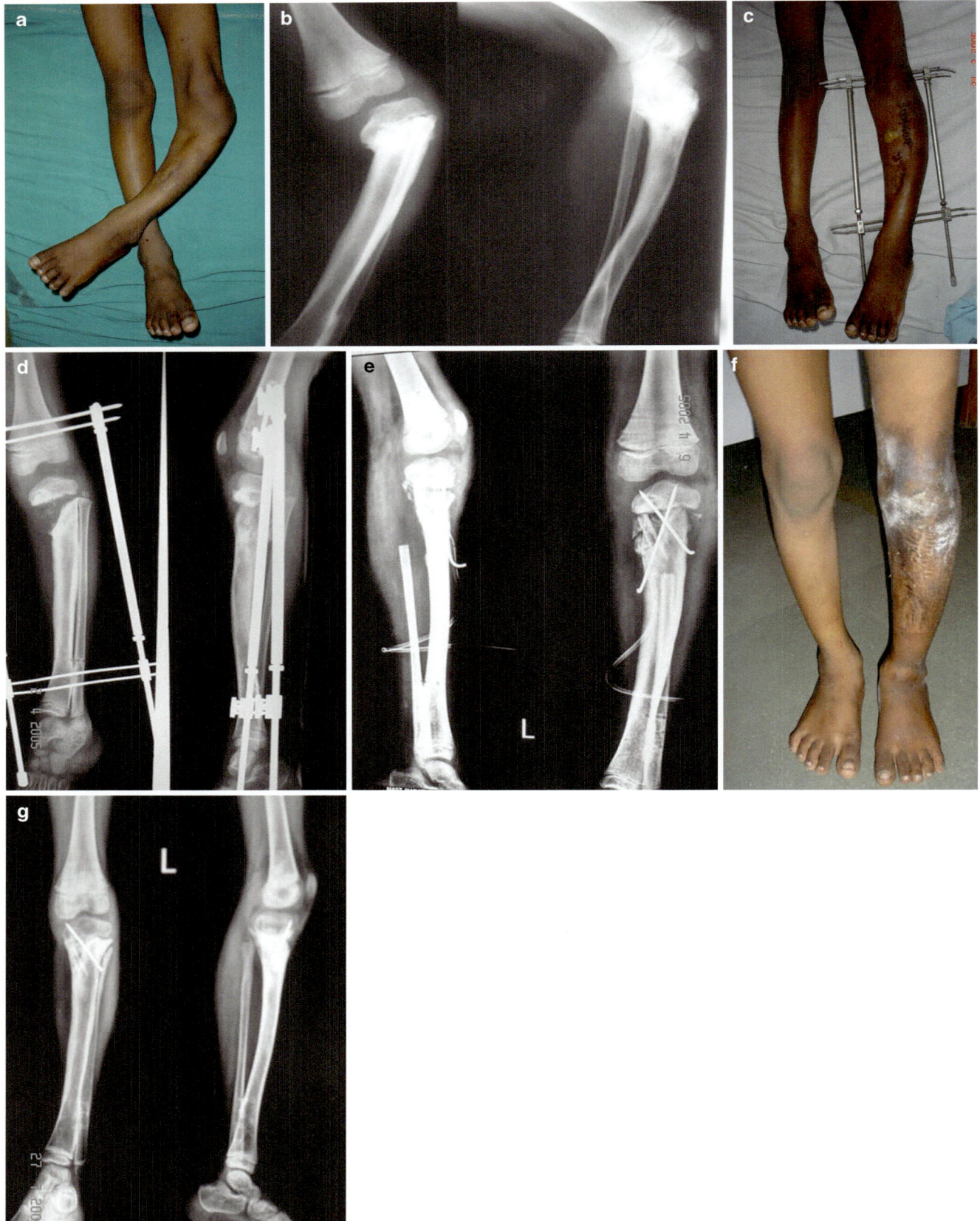

Fig. 37.14 Severe posttraumatic tibia vara secondary to upper tibial physeal arrest. (**a**, **b**) Preoperative clinical picture and X-ray. (**c**, **d**) After differential distraction by a minifixator. (**e**) After osteotomy and grafting. (**f**, **g**) Clinical picture and X-ray on healing

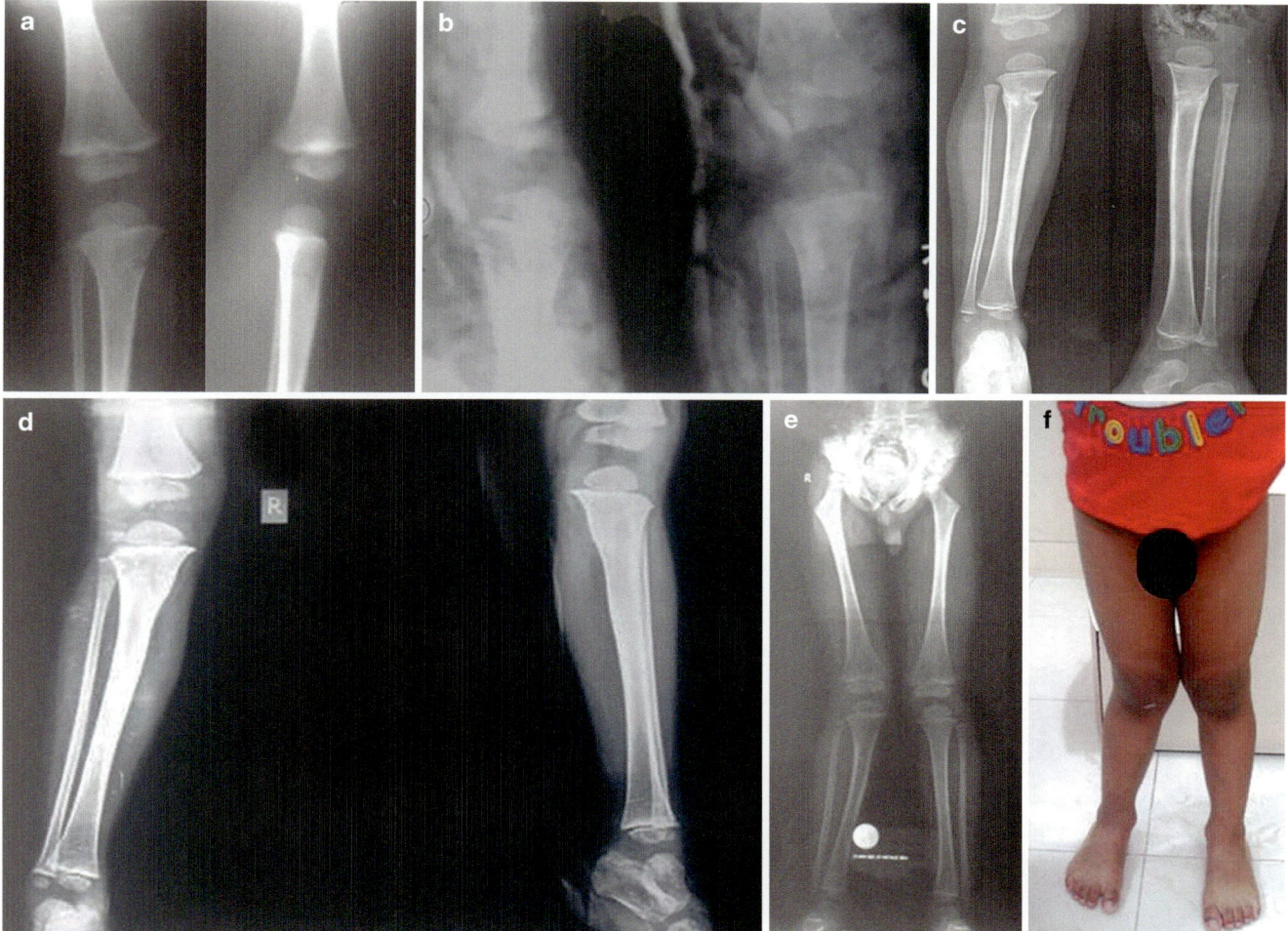

Fig. 37.15 Posttraumatic tibia valga following upper tibial metaphyseal fracture. (**a**) At trauma, May 2013, 1 year and 10 months of age. (**b**) X-ray in plaster cast. (**c**) At 1 year, 11 months of age, June 2013, after cast removal. (**d**) February 2014 at age 2 years, 6 months. (**e, f**) X-ray and clinical photo at presentation at 3 years of age, July 2014, MPTA 102°, TFA 18°

Physeal Injury Ankle with Malunion

The so-called MacFarland fracture is a Salter–Harris type 3 or 4 fracture of the lower tibia, and these fractures are associated with a high incidence of growth arrest and deformity. Accurate repositioning of these fractures and accurate restoration of the physeal plate and the joint surface are critical in reducing the incidence of growth arrest. Radiological observation and investigative scans are necessary to determine the progression and location of the physeal arrest.

Case Study (Fig. 37.16)

Clinical Summary
A patient with fracture of distal end of tibia treated conservatively presented with progressive varus deformity at the ankle joint and shortening: The apex of the deformity was present in the distal tibial physis. On radiological examination, there was a physeal bar present in the center of the distal tibial physis which was tenting it.

Philosophy of Treatment
An intrafocal osteotomy was done at the distal end of tibia and excision of the bar was done followed by fat graft. A corrective osteotomy was done at the distal end of tibia superior to the previous osteotomy and an external fixator was applied along with an above knee slab.

At present, the patient walks well with no recurrence of deformity and equal limb length at 5-year follow-up.

Case Study (Fig. 37.17)

Clinical Summary
A 12-year-old male with trauma to ankle treated with cast immobilization presenting with progressive valgus deformity within 1 year of the original injury: MRI showed distal fibular growth arrest with damage to lateral part of distal tibial physis.

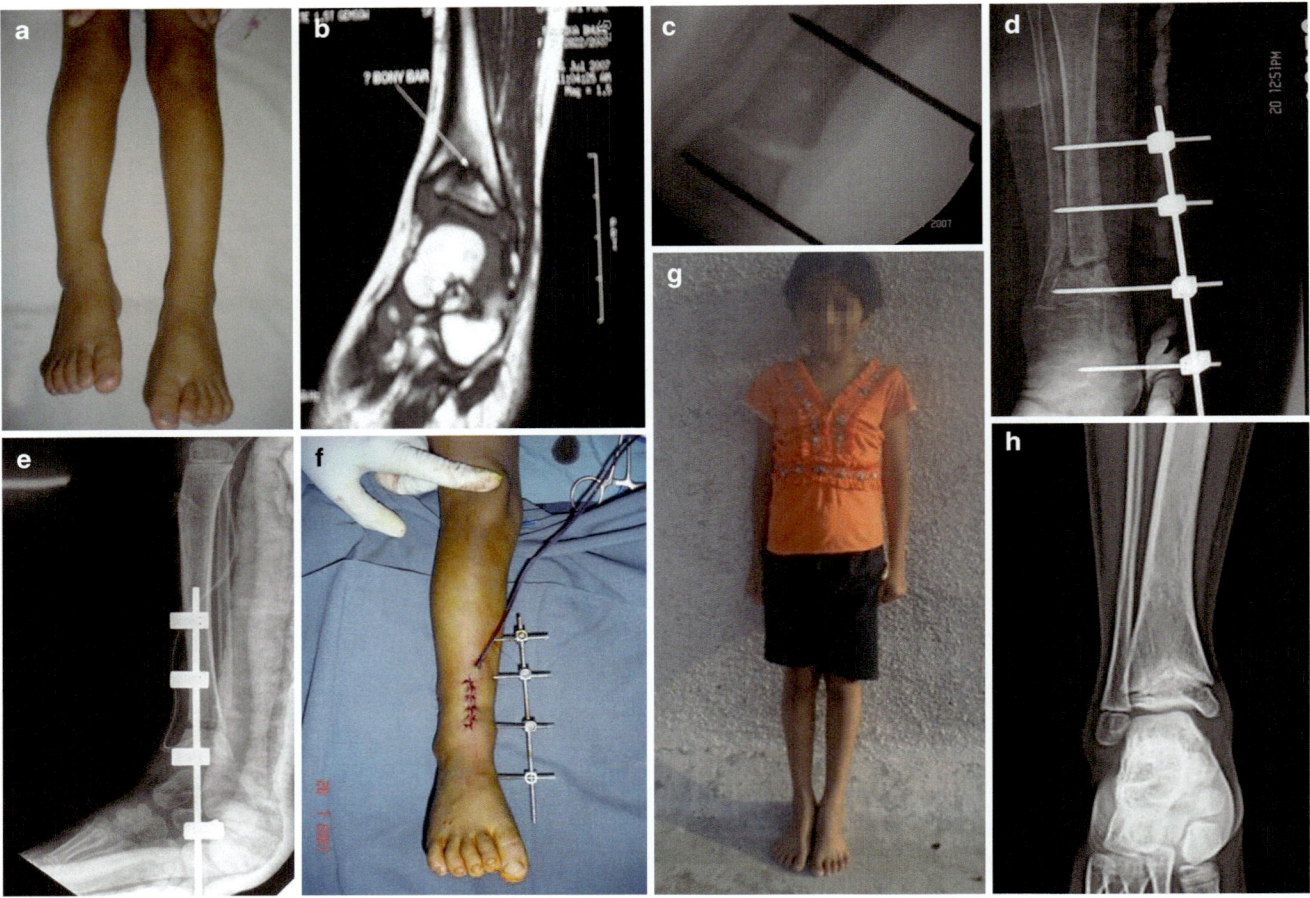

Fig. 37.16 Physeal injury ankle with growth arrest. (**a, b**) After a distal tibial fracture, clinical picture showing deformity and MRI showing physeal central growth arrest with tenting. (**c**) Intraoperative C-arm picture shows osteotomy and central bar excision and fat graft. (**d–f**) Postoperative X-ray showing osteotomy and excision of bar with external fixation. (**g, h**) Five years postoperative, clinical photo and X-rays showing restoration of physeal growth and absence of deformity

Philosophy of Treatment

The treatment was planned with low medial transphyseal osteotomy, and hemiepiphysiodesis of distal tibia to arrest medial growth to achieve correction, with percutaneous physeal drilling for fibular physis.

The patient walks well with full range of ankle motion and no recurrence of deformity at 16 months post surgery.

Soft Tissue Loss with Skeletal Injury

It poses a greater challenge for reconstruction as the management involves restoration of soft tissue cover, muscle length, and skeletal alignment.

This may need soft tissue procedures, use of distraction with external fixation, and osteotomies.

Case Study (Fig. 37.18)

Clinical Summary

A 15-year-old male sustained a runover injury with soft tissue loss and bony injury (distal physeal arrest) to the lower leg 4 years earlier. He was initially treated with skin grafting and external fixation. He presented with a progressive valgus deformity and soft tissue contracture and was walking on the medial aspect of the foot.

Philosophy of Treatment

We did an oblique closed-wedge intraphyseal osteotomy of distal tibia to correct the deformity and stop further progression of deformity. This was combined with fibular resection and application of a simple distractor system for stretching the lateral scarred soft tissues. We were able to achieve plantigrade foot with this strategy.

Fig. 37.17 Twelve-year-old child with posttraumatic ankle valgus. (**a–c**) Clinical picture, X-rays, and MRI 1 year after injury. (**d**) Intraoperative C-arm image after fibular epiphysiodesis and medial lower tibial hemiepiphysiodesis. (**e**) X-rays at 16-month follow-up showing good correction with physeal closure

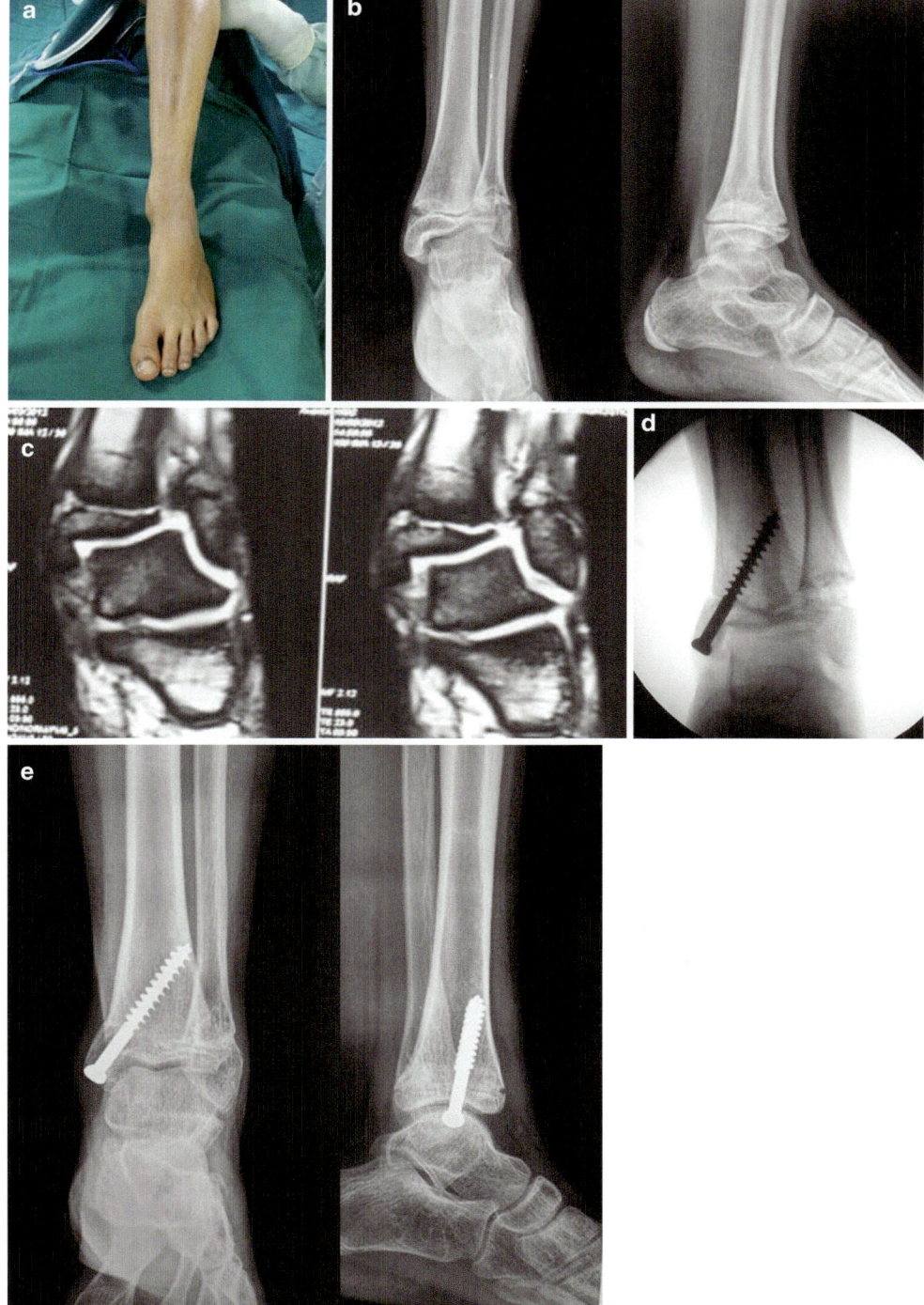

Valgus Deformity at the End of Long Bone Plate

Angular deformity has been reported at the end of long bone plating for fractures of femur and tibia. The exact cause of the deformity is not known but may be related to periosteal stripping leading to growth stimulation.

Case Study (Fig. 37.19)

Clinical Summary

An 8-year-old child with a tibial shaft fracture was treated with plating. The child had uneventful recovery and healing but developed valgus deformity at the proximal end of tibial plate and limb elongation giving rise to limb length discrepancy.

Fig. 37.18 Posttraumatic severe ankle valgus following physeal injury and soft tissue loss in 15-year-old. (**a–c**) Clinical pictures and X-rays at presentation. (**d**) Intraoperative X-ray showing the intraphyseal osteotomy fixed with K wires. (**e**) Intraoperative picture showing mini external fixator. (**f, g**) Postoperative pictures on follow-up after fixator removal showing good correction

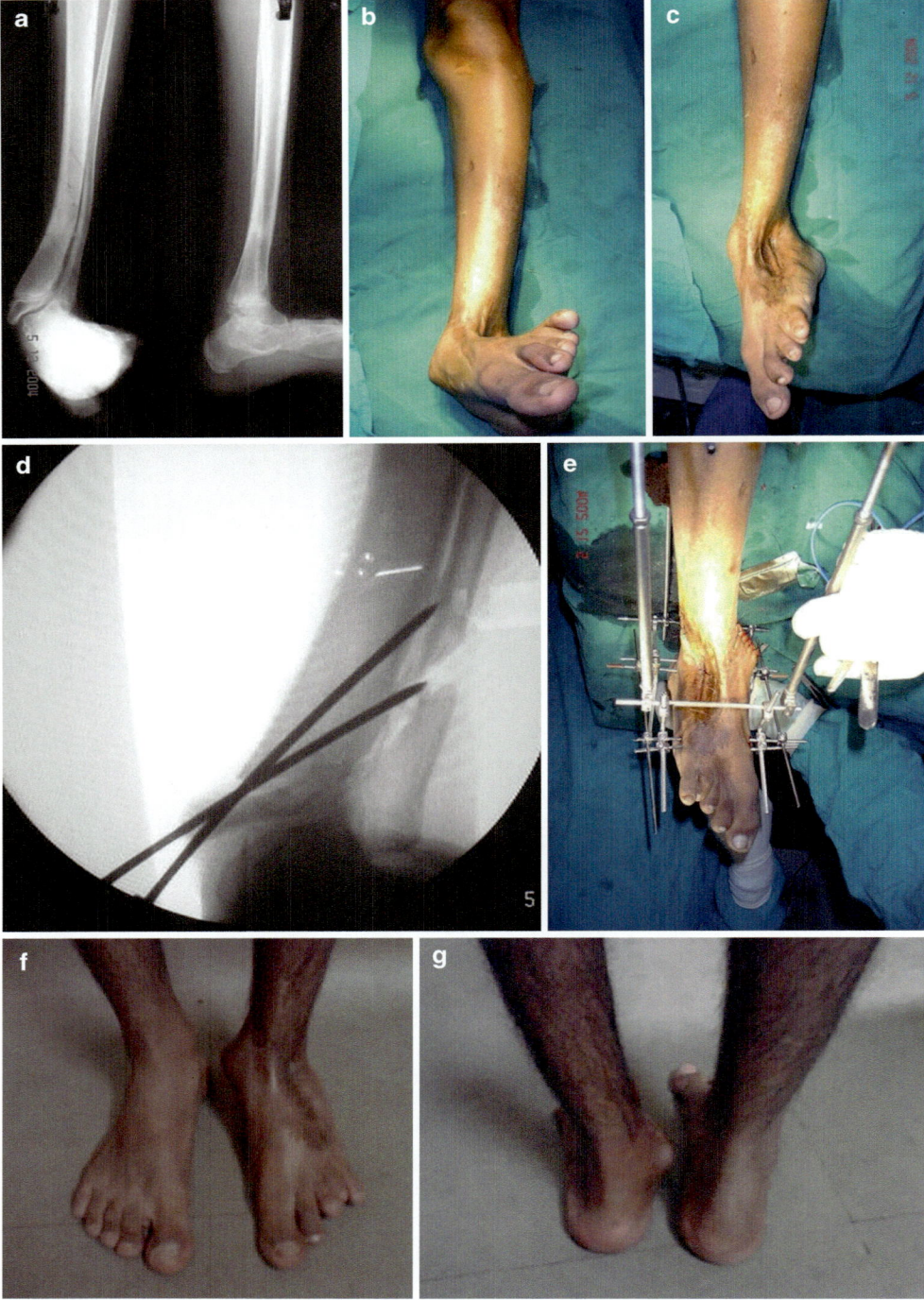

Philosophy of Management

As the deformity and lengthening persisted beyond 2 years post injury, the child was treated with removal of implant with osteotomy to correct the deformity and limb length discrepancy and fixed with external fixation and IM nailing. A repeat plating was avoided to prevent recurrence of the deformity. A metaphyseal or juxta metaphyseal deformity can also be corrected by growth modulation in a skeletally immature child with at least 2 years skeletal growth remaining.

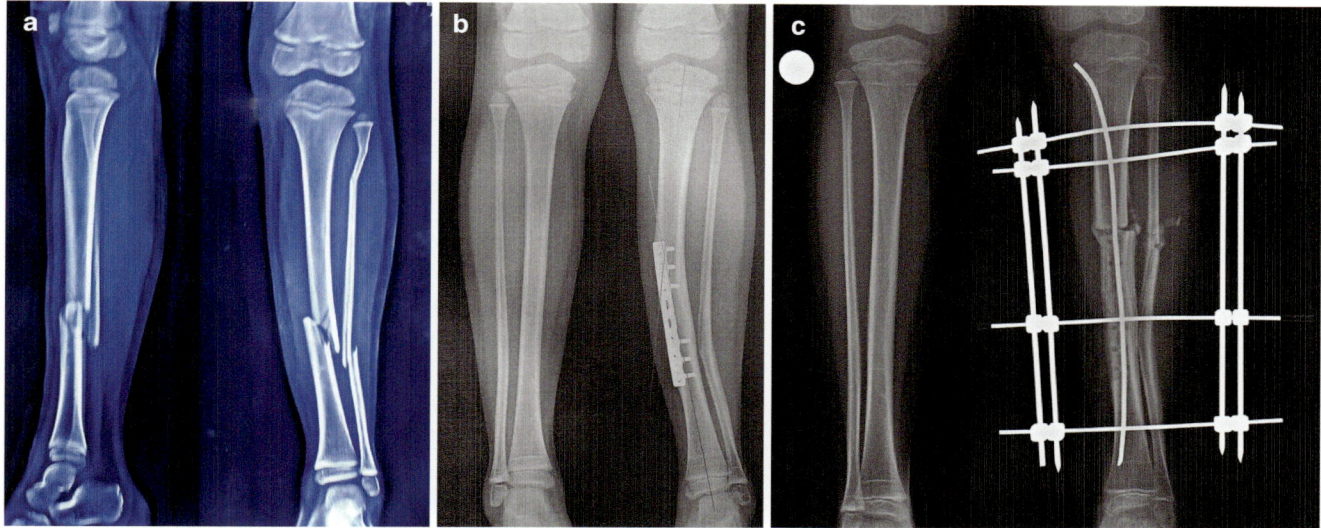

Fig. 37.19 (a) Fracture shaft tibia in 8 years old. (b) Treated with tibial plating with valgus deformity proximal to plate and limb lengthening, noticed 6 months post injury. (c) Treated by tibial osteotomy with shortening and external fixation

Summary

Posttraumatic deformity management requires a comprehensive approach in terms of evaluation and management. Such deformities vary in their complexity from a simple extraarticular joint contracture to the more complex and progressive deformities due to physeal injuries or bone loss. In children, the potential for remodeling has to be kept in mind when developing management strategy. Correction may demand combination of techniques and multispecialty involvement. The aim must be to get an acceptable alignment and limb length by skeletal maturity with adequate function of the extremity.

Acceptability Criteria for Reduction in Lower Limb Fractures

Fracture Neck Femur

Only anatomical reduction is acceptable.

Fracture Shaft Femur
- 0–6 months of age: <1.5 cm of shortening, <30° angulation in varus valgus plane, <30° angulation in AP plane
- 6 months to 6 years: <2 cm of shortening, <15° angulation in varus valgus plane, <20° anterior angulation
- 6–10 years: <1.5 cm shortening, <10° varus valgus angulation, <15° AP angulation
- >10 years: <1 cm shortening, <5° varus valgus angulation, <10° AP angulation.

Fracture: Separation of Distal Physis of Femur

In Salter–Harris Types 1 and 2
- <10 years: <20° anterior or posterior angulation
- >10 years: Only minimal AP angulation
- <5° varus valgus angulation.

In Salter–Harris Types 3 and 4
- Anatomical reduction and ORIF.

Fracture Tibial Tuberosity

Only minimally displaced fractures with possible active extension of knee to 0° can be acceptable. The rest require open reduction and internal fixation.

Fracture Patella
- <3 mm articular step-off
- <3 mm diastasis on X-ray
- Intact extensor mechanism.

Fracture of Tibia and Fibula

Proximal Metaphysis
Closed reduction to anatomic position or slight varus is acceptable.

Diaphysis

	<8 years	>8 years
Varus	<10°	<5°
Valgus	<5°	<5°
Ant. Angulation	<10°	<5°
Post. Angulation	<5°	<0°
Shortening	<10 mm	<5 mm
Rotation	<5°	<5°

Distal Tibial Fractures

Salter–Harris Types 1 and 2
- In patients with at least 2 years of growth remaining: <15° of posterior angulation, <10° of valgus angulation, 0° of varus angulation.
- In patients with less than 2 years of growth remaining angulation in all planes <5°.

Salter–Harris Types 3 and 4
- <2 mm displacement.

Commentary

Commentary to Posttraumatic Deformities in Children

Mark Eidelman
m_eidelman@rambam.health.gov.il

Children suffer traumatic injuries fairly commonly, and despite the progress in fracture treatment, post-traumatic deformities and malunions are quite frequent. The most important difference between adults and children in relation to trauma is the presence of the epiphysis and a growth plate in immature patients. The remodelling potential of post-traumatic deformities in patients with open physes can be quite impressive, though successful remodelling is possible only when the growth plate was not damaged.

When complete growth arrest is present, the result is a shorter limb. Partial growth arrest on the other hand can lead to progressive deformity as well as a shorter affected limb. It is essential to perform closure of the growth plate early after partial growth arrest has been established; otherwise, deformity will inevitably progress.

Correction of post-traumatic deformities in children can be performed in many ways. Age is an important factor in deformity correction planning in children. When the apex of deformity is close to the epiphysis and the growth plate is intact, the easiest and most minimally invasive way to correct malunion is guided growth. However, when the growth plate is involved, or the patient is close to maturity or already mature, the guided growth technique will not work.

Acute correction using an internal fixation device is another method for deformity correction. However, when substantial limb length discrepancy is present, external or internal lengthening should be considered.

External fixation remains the most versatile and useful method for deformity correction and lengthening both in children as well as adolescents. There are many challenges and pitfalls that need to be considered when performing correction for each affected limb.

Posttraumatic Femoral Deformities

Femoral fractures are common. Fractures of the femoral head and neck should be treated as a medical emergency, due to the risk of avascular necrosis to the femoral head. When promptly treated and good fixation achieved, favorable results can be expected (Fig. 37.20).

The majority of diaphyseal femoral fractures in patients younger than 5 years old can be successfully treated by immobilization in a cast. Even in cases with residual deformity and a resultant shorter limb, typically no correction is required, due to the excellent remodeling potential in this age group. Diaphyseal fractures between the ages 5 and 12 years can usually be treated using flexible nails. The ideal candidate for flexible nail fixation is a patient with a transverse diaphyseal fracture. Length unstable and long spiral fractures are less suitable for elastic nail fixation and may require fixation using plates, external fixator or rigid intramedullary nail. Most postoperative troubles in this age group are related to rotational malalignment that was inaccurately judged intraoperatively when the original fracture was fixed.

Fractures of the distal femur that penetrate through the growth plate or fracture epiphysiolysis of the distal femur can occasionally lead to growth arrest (GA). When GA is complete, it results in impaired growth and shorter limb. However, partial growth arrest will cause not only shorter affected bone, but also angular deformity. The bulk of malunions caused by growth arrest will need correction, due to significant malalignment and shorter limb (Fig. 37.21).

External fixation offers almost unlimited options for correction. This is a minimally invasive method, that allows restoration of length, without the need for extensive soft tissue exposure. This is especially important when the skin and muscles were previously injured. Additionally, gradual correction is far more forgiving, compared to acute correction, as it allows "fine tuning" of the correction during the correction process, if required. However, an external fixator is usually somewhat less comfortable for patients. Pins and wires penetrate the skin and muscles causing discomfort. Occurrences of pin site infection are nearly universally following the correction process. Joint contractures are also common.

Therefore, an extended rehabilitation period might be required postoperatively. An alternative gradual correction method had recently been popularized—internal lengthening nails.

Lengthening nails have many advantages over external fixation: no pin site infections, less pain, no bulky frames, and fewer joint contractures. Technically, insertion of the nail is simple, and after a short learning curve, the surgeon can become a "bone lengthening master." Nonetheless, there are several disadvantages. When correction is performed using external fixation, full weight bearing is encouraged immediately after surgery. On the contrary, when internal lengthening is used, patients are required to withhold weight bearing until regenerate consolidation. Another disadvantage is the increased risk of deep intramedullary bone infections, particularly in patients previously treated by external fixation.

The high costs of internal lengthening nails (which in contrast to external fixators cannot be reused) limit their widespread use particularly in low-mid income countries.

In case of significant projected leg length discrepancy not only lengthening of the shorter limb should be considered, but also epiphysiodesis of the long femur and occasionally even contralateral femoral shortening (Fig. 37.21).

Posttraumatic Tibial Deformities

Posttraumatic tibial deformities in children are common and a variety of methods can be used to address those deformities. Most metaphyseal malunions are related to the proximal or the distal physes of the tibia. The proximal tibia grows approximately 6 mm per year and distal tibia approximately 3 mm per year. Consequently, most deformities,

especially in younger patients, also involve some degree of limb length discrepancy as a result of growth impairment. The fibula should also be considered. The tibia-fibular relationship is important, particularly as the distal tibiofibular joint plays a key role in ankle stability. The age of the patient is also a substantial factor to take into account. In younger patients with substantial leg length discrepancy, external fixation with lengthening and gradual correction of deformities is probably the most practical treatment (Fig. 37.22), while in older patients, other options like acute correction might be considered.

Posttraumatic Upper Extremities Deformities

The majority of proximal and diaphyseal humeral deformities in children with open and intact physis have excellent remodeling potential and good prognosis with nonoperative treatment. However, when the physis is injured, the natural history might be development of deformity and a shorter arm. Lengthening of the humerus can be performed by external fixation using either monolateral or circular frames.

Nonetheless, the need for humeral lengthening is exceedingly rare. In contrast to the lower extremities, limb length discrepancy in the upper limb typically does not cause any considerable functional impairment. Consequently, gradual correction of deformities in the upper limbs in not prevalent. The vast majority of upper limb deformities can be corrected using a variety of acute correction techniques. Even so, several specific conditions, like cubitus varus and cubitus valgus, can also be treated by gradual correction.

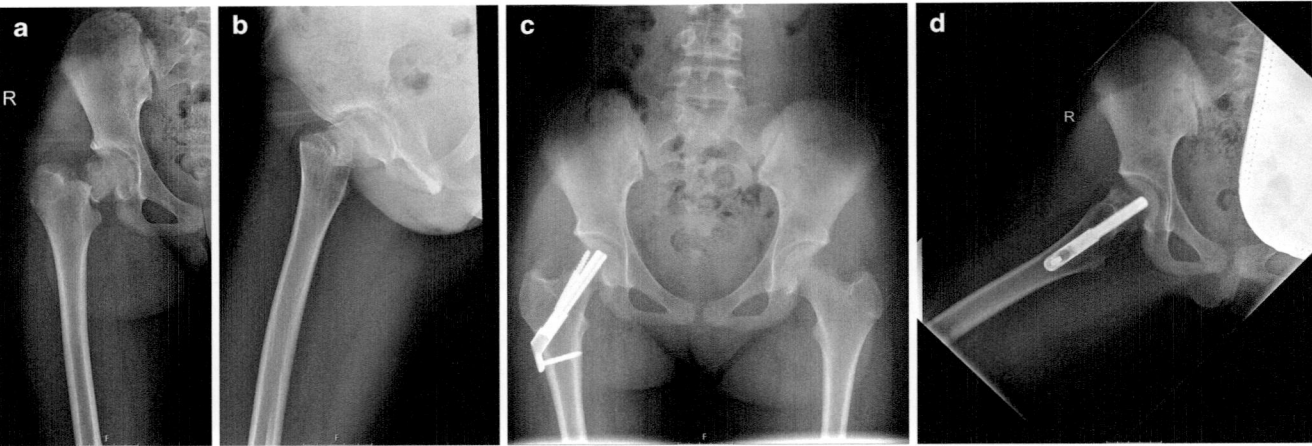

Fig. 37.20 (**a, b**) Displaced transcervical fracture of the femoral head in 14-year-old girl. (**c, d**) One year after open reduction and internal fixation using FNS (femoral neck system, DePuy, Synthes)

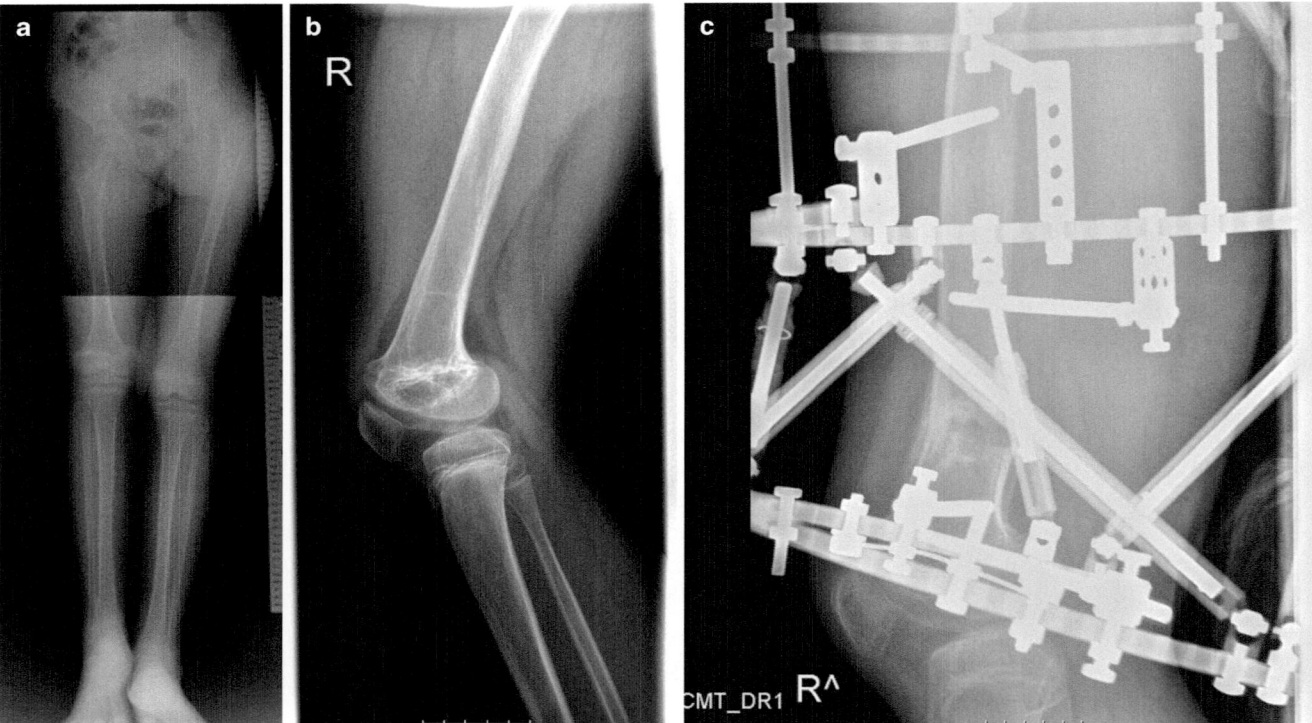

Fig. 37.21 (**a, b**) Nine-year-old girl after severe trauma to the right femur. The X-rays show growth arrest of the distal femur, as well as disturbance of growth of the proximal femur. The patient also had flexion contracture of the right knee and projected leg length discrepancy of more than 10 cm. (**c**) Extension osteotomy of the distal femur using hexapod external fixator. (**d**) Coxa valga and narrow femoral neck that prevent antegrade internal lengthening. (**e**) X-rays after right retrograde femoral lengthening, left distal femoral epiphysiodesis and left proximal femoral shortening using intramedullary nail. (**f**) Clinical photo of the lower limbs after maturity

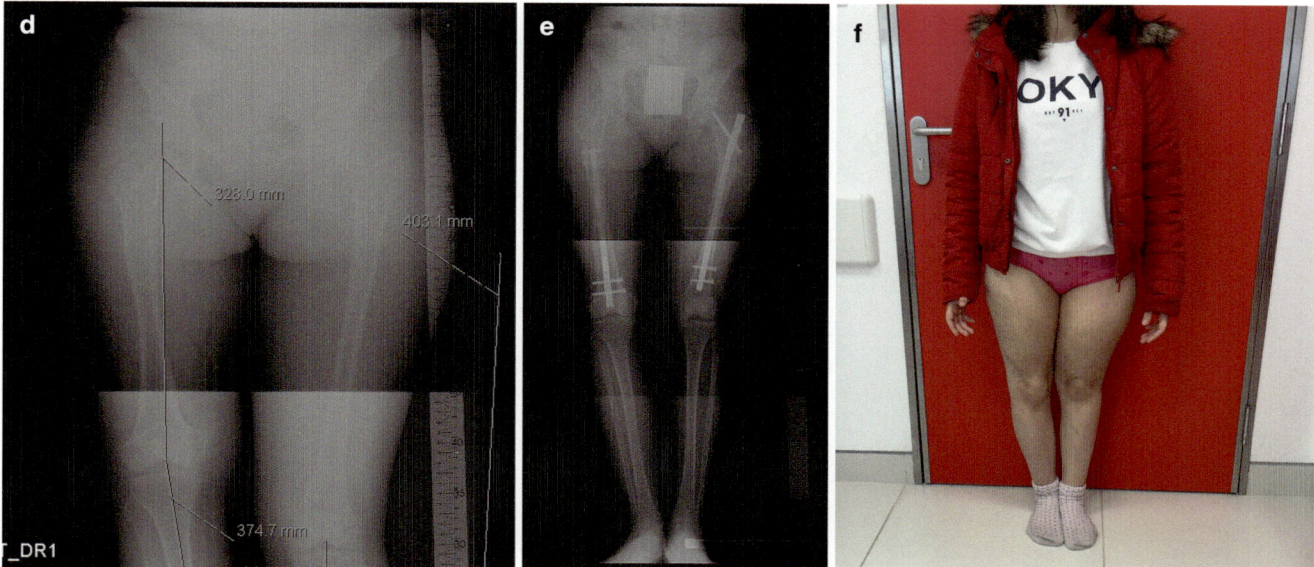

Fig. 37.21 (continued)

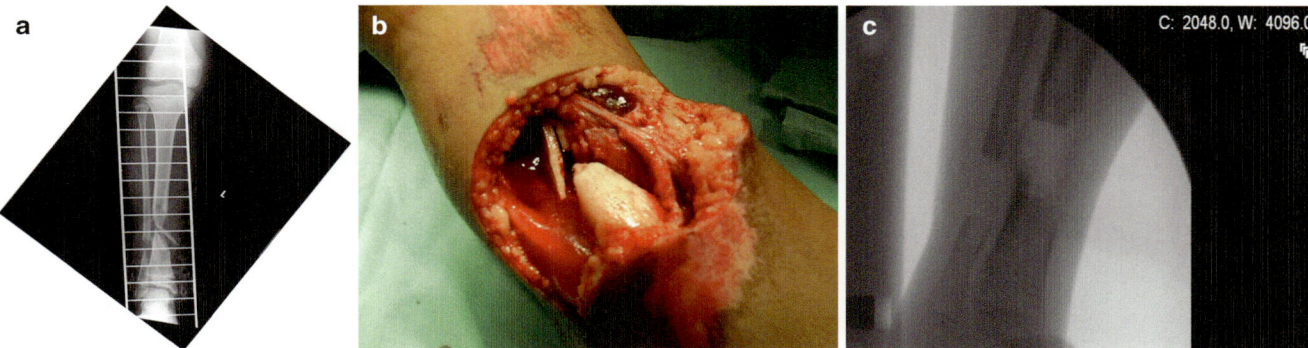

Fig. 37.22 (**a, b**) Eight-year-old boy after motor vehicle accident, with open tibial fracture and bone loss of 4 cm with extensive soft tissue defect. (**c**) Radiological appearance after bone debridement. (**d, e**) X-rays after acute shortening of the tibia and fibula and intentional posterior angulation to achieve wound closure without free skin flap. (**f, g**) Clinical picture demonstrating wound healing and temporary leg deformity. (**h, i**) X-rays after gradual correction and proximal tibial lengthening of 4 cm. (**j, k**) Long leg X-rays at maturity showing anatomic alignment, identical leg length and normal clinical appearance

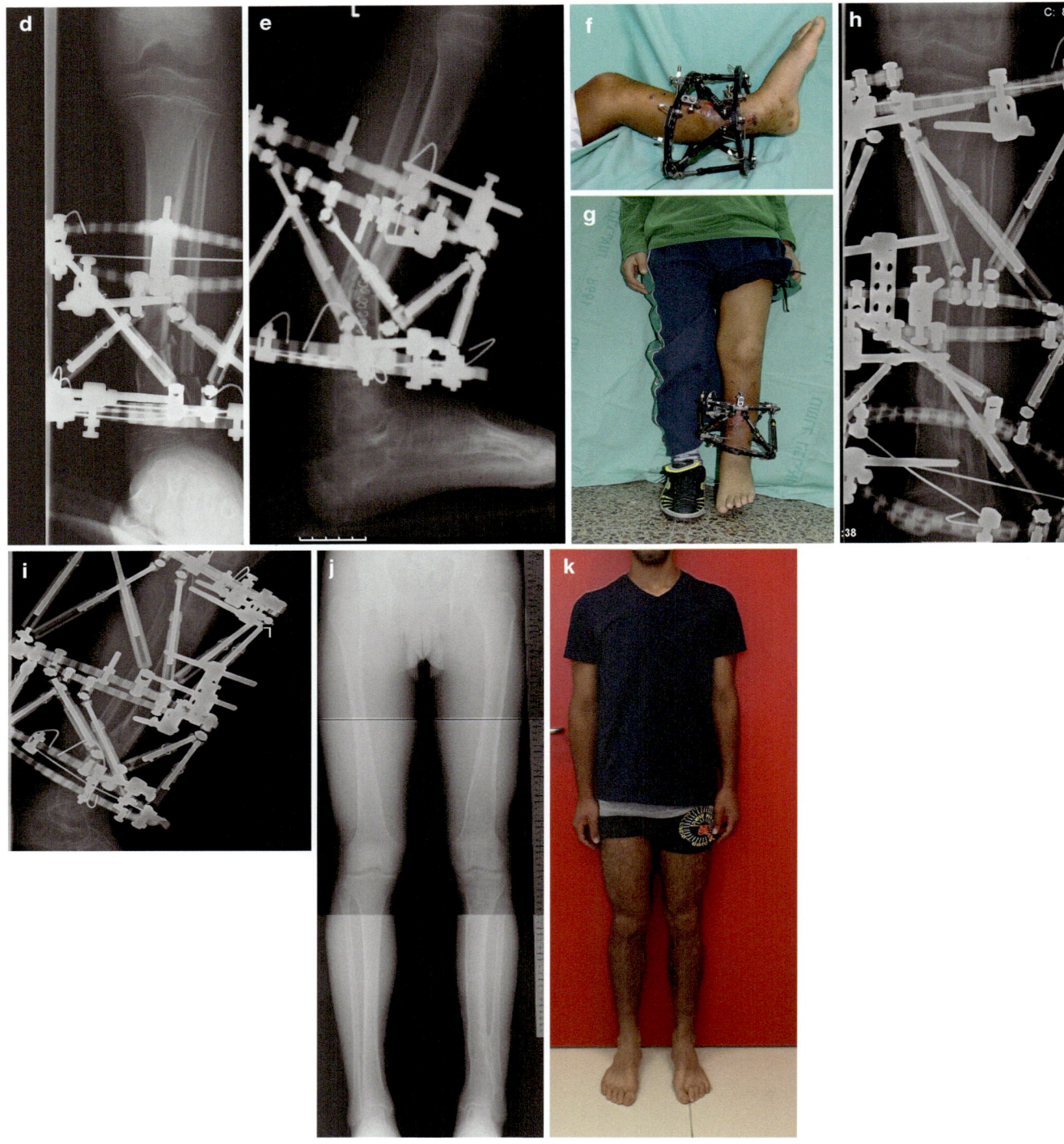

Fig. 37.22 (continued)

References

1. Wilkins KE. Principles of fracture remodeling in children. Injury. 2005;36(Suppl 1):A3–11.
2. Wall EJ, May MM. Growth plate fractures of the distal femur. J Pediatr Orthop. 2012;32(Suppl 1):S40–6.
3. Kalamchi A, MacEwen GD. Avascular necrosis following treatment of congenital dislocation of the hip. J Bone Joint Surg Am. 1980;62-A:876–88.
4. Bucholz RW, Ogden JA. Patterns of ischemic necrosis of the proximal femur in nonoperatively treated congenital hip disease. In: The hip: proceedings of the sixth open scientific meeting of the hip society. St Louis, MO: Mosby; 1978. p. 43–63.
5. Kitakoji T, Hattori T, Ida K, Iwata H. Arthrodiatasis for chondrolysis with hinge abduction: a case report. J Pediatr Orthop B. 2000;9(3):198–200.
6. González-Herranz P. Articulated hip distraction or arthrodiatasis. J Pediatr Orthop B. 2006;15(2):154.
7. Eid AM, Hafez MA. Traumatic injuries of the distal femoral physis. Retrospective study on 151 cases. Injury. 2002;33(3):251–5.
8. Czitrom AA, Salter RB, Willis RB. Fractures involving the distal epiphyseal plate of the femur. Int Orthop. 1981;4(4):269–77.
9. Robert M, Moulies D, Longis B, Laufenburger A, Coville M, Alain JL. Traumatic epiphyseal separation of the lower end of the femur. Rev Chir Orthop Reparatrice Appar Mot. 1988;74(1):69–78.
10. Thomson JD, Stricker SJ, Williams MM. Fractures of the distal femoral epiphyseal plate. J Pediatr Orthop. 1995;15(4):474–8.
11. Basener CJ, Mehlman CT, DiPasquale TG. Growth disturbance after distal femoral growth plate fractures in children: a meta-analysis. J Orthop Trauma. 2009;23(9):663–7.
12. Garrett BR, Hoffman EB, Carrara H. The effect of percutaneous pin fixation in the treatment of distal femoral physeal fractures. J Bone Joint Surg Br. 2011;93(5):689–94.
13. Arkader A, Warner WC Jr, Horn BD, Shaw RN, Wells L. Predicting the outcome of physeal fractures of the distal femur. J Pediatr Orthop. 2007;27(6):703–8.
14. Ilharreborde B, Raquillet C, Morel E, Fitoussi F, Bensahel H, Penneçot GF, Mazda K. Long-term prognosis of Salter-Harris type 2 injuries of the distal femoral physis. J Pediatr Orthop B. 2006;15(6):433–8.
15. Vrettakos AN, Evaggelidis DC, Kyrkos MJ, Tsatsos AV, Nenopoulos A, Beslikas T. Lower limb deformity following proximal tibia physeal injury: long-term follow-up. J Orthop Traumatol. 2012;13(1):7–11.
16. Dorman S, Jariwala A, Campbell D. Cozen's phenomenon: a reminder. Scott Med J. 2013;58(3):e10–3.

Postinfectious Deformities of the Lower Limb

In Ho Choi and Chang Ho Shin

Introduction

There is a diverse range of postinfectious residual deformities of the lower limb depending on the site of infection, patient's age, infecting organism, host resistance, timing and adequacy of initial treatment, and severity of damage to the epiphysis and physis of the affected bone [1–8]. The epiphysis can be damaged extensively, particularly in the neonatal period, by various mechanisms including (a) transphyseal spread of infection from the metaphysis through the physis and into the epiphysis via transphyseal vessels, or (b) following the passage of organisms from the metaphysis to the joint in intracapsular epiphyses such as the hip joint, or (c) from the epiphyses into the adjacent joint following transphyseal spread [9]. As a result, most of the postinfectious juxta-articular and articular deformities are associated with physeal damage and growth disturbance [10].

Proper evaluation based on a thorough musculoskeletal examination and radiographic imaging allows the surgeon to determine an effective treatment plan for deformity correction. A meticulous analysis of the complex deformity of the lower limb by determining the location, magnitude, and direction of the deformity would be the first step in characterizing the deformity. Mechanical axis deviation, mechanical and anatomical alignments, and joint orientation should be accurately determined [11]. In addition, limb length discrepancy (LLD), difference in the knee level, joint laxity, and loss of mobility secondary to soft-tissue contractures and/or juxta-articular skeletal deformity should be evaluated.

The management of severe deformities that occur as a result of fulminant septic arthritis or osteomyelitis is clinically challenging. However, timely and well-performed reconstructive operations can ensure growth and development of the lower limb by restoring the weight-bearing mechanical axis as well as individual joint alignment, and thus providing the best possible joint mechanics at skeletal maturity. This chapter reviews the treatment principles and reconstructive surgical modalities for long-term residual deformities of the lower limb after septic arthritis of the hip, knee, and ankle, and osteomyelitis of the femur and tibia in infancy or early childhood.

Late Sequelae of Infantile Septic Arthritis of the Hip

Residual deformities of infantile septic arthritis of the hip occur due to necrosis of the articular cartilage, ischemic necrosis of the femoral head (FH), premature closure of the triradiate cartilage, acetabular dysplasia, premature or asymmetrical closure of the proximal femoral physis, subluxation, dislocation, pseudarthrosis of the femoral neck, greater trochanteric overriding, and complete destruction of the FH and neck [1–4, 6, 8, 9, 12–15]. The decision to perform either a reconstructive or a salvage procedure should be individualized depending on the type of residual deformity of the hip.

Radiographic Classifications of Late Sequelae of Infantile Septic Arthritis of the Hip

Several radiographic classifications of late sequelae of infantile septic arthritis of the hip have been reported in the literature. In 1982, Hunka et al. [13] first proposed a classification to document the five types of residual deformities of septic arthritis in a logical fashion: Type 1—absent or minimal FH changes; Type II—(A) deformity of the FH, with an intact growth plate and (B) deformity of the FH, with a premature fusion of the growth plate; Type III—pseudarthrosis of the femoral neck; Type IV—(A) complete destruction of the proximal femoral epiphysis, with a stable neck segment and (B) complete destruction of the proximal femoral epiphysis, with a small unstable neck segment; and Type V—complete destruction of the FH and neck to the intertrochanteric line, with dislocation of the hip.

In 1990, Choi et al. devised a radiological classification of residual proximal femoral deformities based on the nature and extent of damage and radiographic appearance at the final follow-up or at maturity, and each of the four major types of residual deformities was further divided into two subtypes (Fig. 38.1) [2]. In 2002, Johari et al. [14, 15] also reported the classification of the sequelae of septic hips. Group 1: loss of capital femoral epiphysis (CFE)/neck,

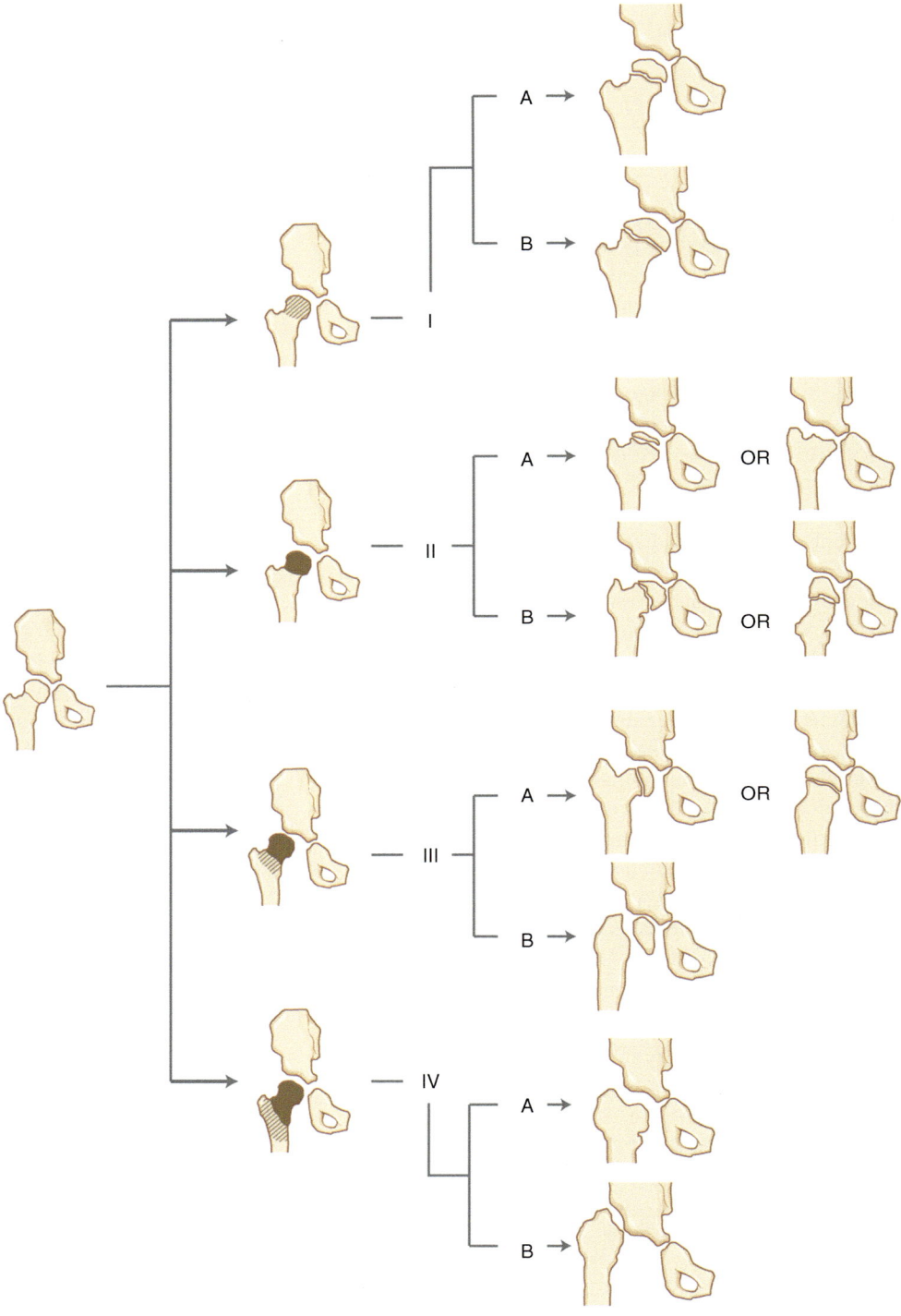

Fig. 38.1 Choi classification [2] of sequelae of infantile septic arthritis of the hip. Type I: No residual deformity (Type IA) or mild coxa magna (Type IB). Type II: Coxa breva with a deformed head (Type IIA) or progressive coxa vara or valga due to asymmetrical, premature physeal closure (Type IIB). Type III: Slipping at the femoral neck, resulting in coxa vara or valga with severe anteversion or retroversion (Type IIIA) or pseudarthrosis of the femoral neck (Type IIIB). Type IV: Destruction of the femoral head (FH) and neck, with a small remnant of the neck (Type IVA) or complete loss of the FH and neck and no articulation of the hip (Type IVB). Adapted from Choi IH, Pizzutillo PD, Bowen JR, Dragann R, Malhis T. Sequelae and reconstruction after septic arthritis of the hip in infants. J Bone Joint Surg Am. 1990;72:1150–65

metaphyseal spike present, stable; Group 2: loss of CFE and neck, unstable; Group 3A: dislocation, CFE present, unstable; Group 3B: subluxation, CFE present, unstable; Group 4: articular incongruity, avascular necrosis, coxa magna, physeal disturbance (coxa breva, coxa vara, coxa valga, and trochanteric overgrowth), stable; Group 5, pseudarthrosis of the femoral neck, stable/unstable. In 2008, Forlin and Milani [12] proposed a relatively simple radiological classification based on the relationship between the femur and the acetabulum, and the severity of the lesion of the proximal femur. Hips with sequelae grade 1 were reduced hips, with the FH preserved (1A) or absent (1B); hips grade 2 were dislocated hips, with the FH preserved (2A) or absent (2B). The category of the presence or absence of dislocation was not included in the original paper by Choi et al. that was reported in 1990 [2]. It was because, in that series, most children had been treated at other medical centers, and were referred to the institute with the hips reduced, at an average of 3 years after the original infection in infancy. We agree that the category of septic hip dislocations with the capital femoral epiphysis present is a distinct entity. Of note, the classification systems proposed by other authors [12–15] do not have a subtype equivalent to the Choi Type IIIA (slipping at the femoral neck, resulting in coxa vara or valga with severe anteversion or retroversion) (Fig. 38.1) [2].

One common drawback of all the aforementioned radiological classifications is that they were mainly devised based on the changes noted on the plain radiographs. Currently, with the help of advanced imaging technologies, e.g., MRI and 3D-CT, deformed osteocartilaginous geometry of the proximal femur can be better visualized in three dimensions, and the dynamics of articular motion between the deformed FH and acetabulum can be better understood. A new, comprehensive three-dimensional radiological classification is anticipated considering the rapid advancement in the imaging technology.

Late Operative Treatment Modalities for Residual Deformities of Septic Arthritis of the Hip

Treatment modalities for the long-term sequelae of infantile septic arthritis of the hip are outlined in Table 38.1. The recommended primary and secondary treatment methods are as varied as the types of deformities. Unfortunately, no definite primary treatment for a severely damaged hip joint makes the affected joint capable of withstanding the forces imposed on it by otherwise healthy children and their long-term physical demands [2]. Thus, any surgical treatment for severe sequelae must be regarded as a measure that temporarily improves the clinical function and delays the more definitive procedures that are reserved for adult patients [2, 3]. The

Table 38.1 Late operative treatment modalities for severe sequelae of infantile septic arthritis of the hip

Purpose	Indications	Procedures
To reduce/contain the hip joint	Subluxation or dislocation	Open reduction; soft-tissue release (adductor-iliopsoas tenotomy)
To optimize joint congruity	Incongruity	Proximal femoral realignment osteotomy (varus or valgus osteotomy with a sagittal or rotational component); redirectional acetabular osteotomy (salter, Pemberton, Dega osteotomy, triple innominate osteotomy, Ganz periacetabular osteotomy)
To improve femoral head coverage	Uncovered femoral head	Redirectional acetabular osteotomy; salvage acetabuloplasty (e.g., Chiari, shelf operation); Ganz femoral head reduction osteotomy
To reduce cam or pincer lesion	Femoroacetabular impingement	Osteochondroplasty via safe surgical hip dislocation or arthroscopy; excision of the femoral head and neck remnant (Choi type IVA or mobile nonunion type of IIIB)
To address intra-articular pathology of the cartilage or labrum	Torn labrum or articular cartilage lesion	Labral debridement or refixation; articular cartilage repair using microfracture technique or osteochondral grafting or chondrocyte transplantation
To correct acetabular dysplasia	Dysplastic acetabulum	Redirectional acetabular osteotomy
To correct abnormal version of the proximal femur and acetabulum	Anteverted or retroverted femur and acetabulum	Proximal femoral rotational/derotational osteotomy; redirectional acetabular osteotomy
To improve abductor muscle function; to correct coxa brevis	Greater trochanteric overriding; short femoral neck	Greater trochanteric advancement; true or relative femoral neck lengthening
To repair pseudarthrosis of the femoral neck	Femoral neck nonunion	Bone grafting, often combined with proximal femoral valgus osteotomy
To reconstruct femoro-pelvic articulation	Destruction of the femoral head and neck	Greater trochanteric arthroplasty; pelvic support osteotomy; Ilizarov hip reconstruction (Choi type IVB or failed type IVA); L'Episcopo, Albee, or Harmon operation, Ilizarov femoral neck lengthening, femoral neck reconstruction using vascularized bone grafting (Choi Type IVA)

(continued)

Table 38.1 (continued)

Purpose	Indications	Procedures
To equalize the lower limb length	Limb length shortening	Lengthening by distraction osteogenesis; contralateral epiphysiodesis or shortening of the femur; Ilizarov hip reconstruction
To manage painful unstable hip as a last resort	Unstable hip with advanced osteoarthritis not amenable to the above-mentioned reconstructive procedures	Hip arthrodesis; total hip replacement arthroplasty; Ilizarov hip reconstruction after excision of the femoral head and neck remnant

Table 38.2 Pearls and pitfalls in the management of late sequelae of infantile septic arthritis of the hip

Assessment	• The surgeon should be familiar with radiological classifications of femoral residual deformities • Use of advanced imaging technologies (MRI, ultrasonography, arthrography, and 3D-CT) to visualize unossified cartilaginous structure of the epiphysis, also to determine osteocartilaginous geometry of the proximal femur, and the dynamics of articular motion between the deformed head and acetabulum • Full-length standing radiograph (teleradiograph) visualizing the entire lower limbs is helpful not only to identify associated sequelae at other sites, if any, but also to determine axial malalignment, joint malorientation, and limb length discrepancy
Treatment	• Femoroacetabular impingement-related symptoms are often encountered in older children and young adults with severe residual deformities • The decision to perform either reconstructive or salvage procedures must be made on an individual basis, after reviewing the clinical findings and imaging studies • Definitive and adjunctive surgical treatment methods can be used alone or in combination (Table 38.1) • Authors' stepwise algorithmic surgical approach to femoroacetabular impingement would be helpful in decision making of treatment for Choi type II and III hips (Fig. 38.2) • Greater trochanteric arthroplasty for reconstruction of femoro-pelvic articulation is a technically demanding procedure with unpredictable outcomes. If performed at younger age, then the transferred greater trochanter can assume a globular shape, but with no or incomplete formation of head-neck offset • Ilizarov hip reconstruction is a highly effective treatment modality for the management of Choi type IVB and IVA hips in which the previous reconstructive surgery has failed, or there is late presentation with a severe abductor lurch and a considerable limb length shortening, particularly in the adolescents and young adults in whom arthrodesis or hip arthroplasty is not suitable

pearls and pitfalls in the management of late sequelae of infantile septic arthritis of the hip are summarized in Table 38.2.

Choi Type II and III Hips Causing Femoroacetabular Impingement and Secondary Hip Dysplasia

Type II and III hips are fundamentally the result of an abnormally shaped, sized, or oriented FH and neck, altered head-neck offset, and acetabular dysplasia. A wide variety of residual deformities of the FH have been observed in Type II and III hips, ranging from deformities similar to those in Perthes disease with coxa vara/valga, coxa plana, coxa breva, coxa magna, coxa irregularis, relative greater trochanteric overriding, sagging rope sign [16], and acetabular dysplasia to the more deformed proximal femur visualized as beard, collared, staghorn, or rugby ball-shaped FH [17, 18].

Children with Type II or III deformities may remain asymptomatic in their younger age, but, in (pre)adolescence, these children often present with clinical problems such as pain, limp, joint instability or contracture, restriction of motion, LLD, pelvic obliquity, lumbar lordosis, and even emotional disturbances. According to the authors' experience, in older children with Type II and III hips, a painful limp is usually associated with femoroacetabular impingement (FAI) with or without damaged acetabular cartilage and/or labrum.

Figure 38.2 depicts a stepwise algorithmic approach to FAI in Perthes-like deformities at the authors' institute. First, the extent of asphericity is assessed; if it is mild and the FH is well contained within the acetabulum, osteochondroplasty of the head and neck junction alone is indicated. Next, the presence or absence of a labral tear is determined. If a labral tear is present, then labral debridement or refixation is necessary. Similarly, the presence of coexisting acetabular dysplasia is assessed. If the hip becomes congruent in abduction, then relative femoral neck lengthening combined with peri-acetabular osteotomy (PAO) or triple innominate osteotomy (TIO) is indicated. In the authors' institute, Bernese PAO is preferred for correction of acetabular dysplasia in adolescents and young adults with closed triradiate cartilage (around 12 years in girls and 14 years in boys) [19], whereas a TIO, in (pre)adolescents with open triradiate cartilage [20]. If the hip becomes congruent in adduction, then proximal femoral valgus osteotomy and PAO or TIO are indicated. The next step is to check whether coxa breva and coxa vara associated with relatively greater trochanteric overriding are severe enough to cause FAI, and if so, a relative or true femoral neck lengthening combined with distal advancement of the greater trochanter (GT) is indicated [21–24]. When the FH asphericity is too severe and the FH is "irreducible," the following procedures should be considered. If the hip becomes congruent in extension and adduction, then femoral valgus-flexion osteotomy plus/minus PAO or TIO should be considered.

If the hip becomes congruent in any rotational position, then transtrochanteric rotational osteotomy with or without a

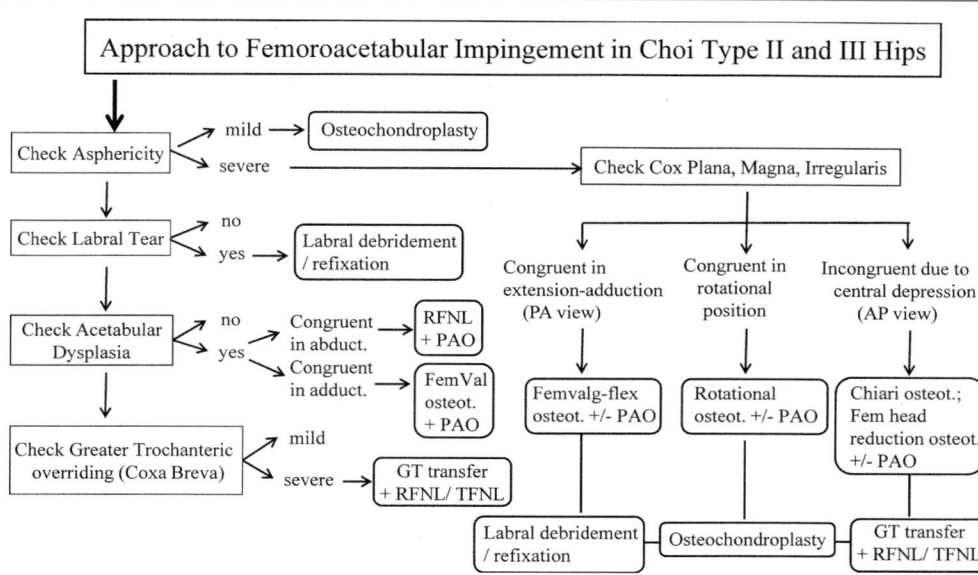

Fig. 38.2 A schema showing the stepwise algorithmic approach to femoroacetabular impingement associated with Choi Type II and III sequelae, which are similar to Perthes(–like) deformities (refer text). *RFNL*, relative femoral neck lengthening; *TFNL*, true femoral neck lengthening; *PAO*, periacetabular osteotomy; *PA*, posteroanterior; *AP*, anteroposterior Note: A triple innominate osteotomy is performed, instead of PAO, in (pre)adolescents with open triradiate cartilage [19]

PAO or TIO may be indicated. If the FH with a central depression is too severely deformed such that the FH cannot be contained within the acetabulum in any position, then a Chiari osteotomy or FH reduction osteotomy [21, 23, 25] with or without a PAO or TIO can be considered. In addition, a combination of osteochondroplasty, labral debridement/refixation, and distal advancement of the greater trochanter should be performed, if necessary.

Late Treatment Options for Choi Type IV Deformity

The available reconstructive procedures for the treatment of Type IV hips are limited, and, in general, have not yielded satisfactory long-term results [2–4, 13, 26–30]. When only a remnant of the FH and neck is present, it is difficult to maintain a stable reduction; and if instability and dislocation persist, the surgeon can either leave the deformity uncorrected or can attempt reconstruction of femoro-pelvic articulation [27]. In young children in whom the FH and neck have been destroyed, as in Type IVA sequelae, a new femoral neck can be fashioned to articulate with the acetabulum by utilizing the L'Episcopo [31], Harmon [32], or Albee [33] reconstruction methods. When a reasonably sized unossified cartilaginous cap persists as a femoral neck remnant, open reduction can be attempted. The repositioning of the femoral remnant into the acetabular socket can be facilitated using a modification of the Harmon technique [32]. An incomplete, spring osteotomy is made at the base of the femoral remnant adjoining the greater trochanter and the resulting opening wedged gap is filled with a block of the cartilage graft taken from the iliac apophysis. This procedure produces a femoral neck-lengthening effect [26]. Dr. Li et al. [33] reported a modified technique of Albee or Harmon arthroplasty; trimming any rough or uneven cartilage surfaces of the acetabulum with a small ball-shaped reamer, detaching the greater trochanter 0.5 cm below the physis, splitting the width of the medial fragment, serving approximately two-thirds of the diameter of the femoral segment as the new FH, and repositioning the greater trochanter with the attached gluteus medius and gluteus minimus distally to the lateral fragment so that muscle tension is restored. Subsequent stability and fulcrum of the hip will depend on the amount the osteochondral tissue assuming a FH and neck produced. They recommended to create a $135° \sim 145°$ between the "new" FH and the proximal part of the femoral shaft. In older children, gradual lengthening of the remnant femoral neck using the Ilizarov technique may be indicated. Nonetheless, the authors believe that open reduction in children older than 6 years of age is not likely to be beneficial because of the high risk of developing stiffness and pain. Therefore, the authors recommend that in children older than 6 years of age, Type IVA hips should be treated in the same manner as hips with Type IVB sequelae [3].

Postponing the treatment of Type IVB hips will result in proximal iliac dislocation with a marked abductor lurch, telescoping, limp, and LLD [6, 28]. Although these patients may remain asymptomatic for a number of years [1, 4, 14], they are at a risk of developing degenerative changes in the lumbosacral spine and hips [27]. Therefore, various treatment modalities for reconstructing a femoro-pelvic articulation in Type IVB hips have been reported: hip reconstruction with vascularized iliac crest grafting [34], arthrodesis, greater trochanteric arthroplasty (GTA) [27, 28, 35–40] with adjunctive or secondary procedures, pelvic support osteotomy (PSO) [41–44], and Ilizarov hip reconstruction (IHR) [41, 45–59]. Of these treatment modalities, the two most commonly performed procedures are GTA and IHR.

Greater Trochanteric Arthroplasty Versus Pelvic Support Osteotomy/Ilizarov Hip Reconstruction

GTA was originally described by Colonna [37] and was popularized by Westin [40] and others [27, 28, 36, 39]. The underlying concept of GTA is based on the following two aspects: first, the GT is viable and therefore retains its growth potential and second, when the hyaline cartilage covering the GT is placed inside the acetabulum, the GT assumes a globular shape, similar to that of an FH [2, 3, 19, 26, 28, 29, 35–41]. The detached abductor muscles must be transferred distally in order to provide hip stability and some degree of abductor function. However, the subsequent progressive subluxation observed in most of the patients necessitates additional procedures, such as femoral varus osteotomy, pelvic osteotomy including Chiari osteotomy, or shelf acetabuloplasty, to improve FH coverage. There are many drawbacks and limitations of GTA for reconstruction of femoro-pelvic articulation due to the uniqueness of the technique. Previous reports have described the potential risk of avascularity of the proximal segment after femoral varus osteotomy, difficulty in osteosynthesis at the varus osteotomy site, gradual straightening of the proximal femur due to remodeling at the osteotomy site, abductor weakness, stiffness, degenerative arthritis, and difficulty during conversion to total hip arthroplasty in adulthood [2, 3, 26–28, 36, 39, 56]. According to the authors' observation, the transferred GT can assume a globular shape with time, but with no or incomplete formation of head-neck offset. For this reason, even those children with satisfactory results at the midterm follow-up often present with FAI-related symptoms (Fig. 38.3).

The two most important factors that determine the success or failure of a procedure after GTA are preoperative abductor weakness and stiffness [3]. Although some authors have reported satisfactory results [27, 28, 35, 37–40], most of the experienced surgeons feel that GTA is a technically demanding procedure with highly unpredictable outcomes.

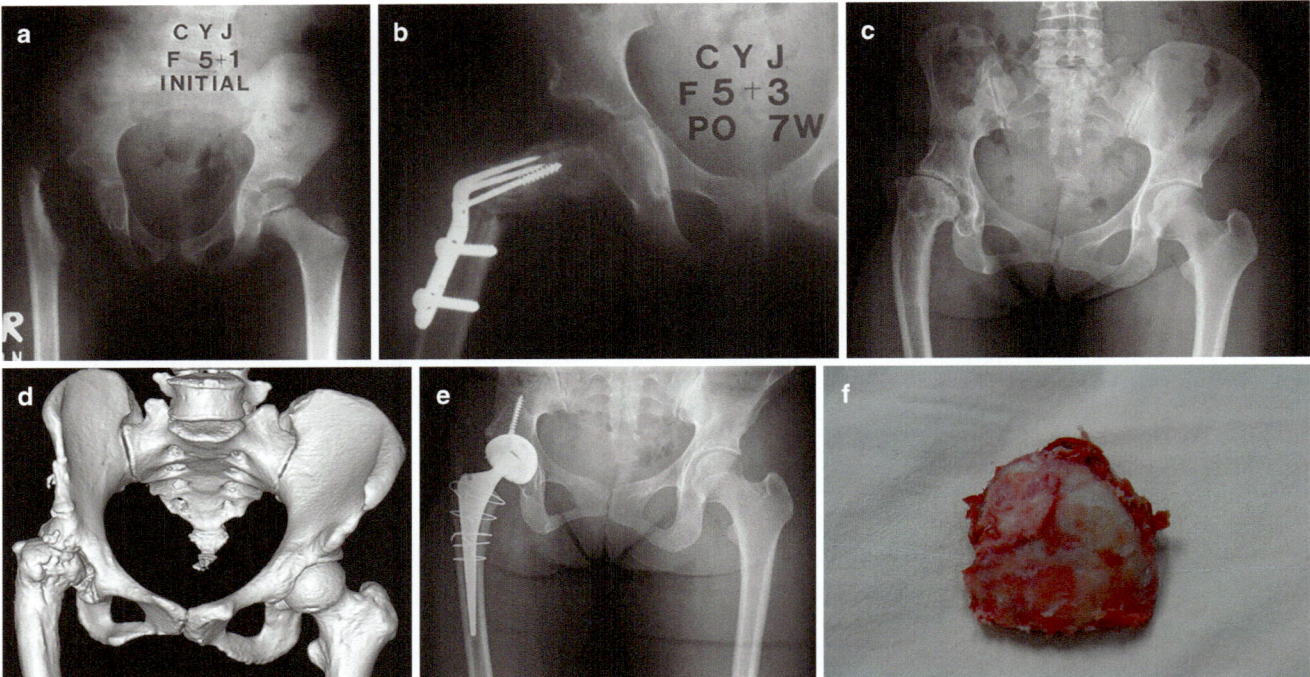

Fig. 38.3 Greater trochanteric arthroplasty in a girl. (**a**) A radiograph in a 5-year—and 1-month-old girl showing Choi Type IVB sequelae in the right hip. (**b**) A radiograph showing trochanteric arthroplasty with adjunctive femoral varus osteotomy. (**c**, **d**) Radiographs taken at 32 years of age showing advanced degenerative arthritis of the right hip joint, despite a well-remodeled greater trochanter which had assumed a globular shape similar to that of a femoral head. Three-dimensional-CT image also shows laterally displaced, remodeled greater trochanter with multiple osteochondral prominences on its margin, suggestive of femoroacetabular impingement. (**e**) A radiograph showing total hip replacement arthroplasty which was performed to treat a painful limp. (**f**) A gross photograph of the remodeled greater trochanter; the articular cartilaginous surface had been markedly degenerated, showing some fibrous adhesions

The authors have noted that the result of GTA may also be correlated with the patient's age at operation. In a retrospective study performed by Choi et al. [26], satisfactory results were obtained only in those children who underwent GTA at less than 6 years of age. This observation may support the opinion that a patient should be old enough to follow the physical therapy instructions, and young enough to allow remodeling of the transferred GT [3].

"Pelvic support osteotomy (PSO)" has a long history in orthopedic surgery. The technique was developed in 1910s and was quite popular until the advent of total hip arthroplasty [41–44, 60]. The basic concept and goal of a PSO is to enhance femoro-pelvic stability by means of a proximal femoral valgus osteotomy and to improve hip biomechanics by displacing the center of gravity medially, resulting in an improvement in the mechanical efficiency of the abductor muscles [41]. However, the clinical application of traditional PSO is limited due to its indigenous shortcomings. It is difficult to achieve the optimal extent of angulation. If the angular correction is too large, then excessive genu valgum, fixed pelvic obliquity, and impingement pain on adduction of the lower limb to neutral position may occur. On the other hand, if the angular correction is too small, the result would lead to an insufficient improvement in hip biomechanics, and most importantly, the issue of persisting LLD cannot be addressed. To overcome the shortcomings of traditional PSO, Ilizarov developed and popularized a modified PSO technique, the so-called IHR, in which a second distal femoral osteotomy is performed in addition to proximal femoral valgus osteotomy for pelvic support to realign the knee joint and to correct the LLD [41, 46–48, 50–53, 55–59]. Furthermore, Ilizarov emphasized the importance of extension of the proximal femoral osteotomy to correct the fixed flexion deformity of the hip and to permit locking of the hip joint [41, 45, 46, 48–53, 55–59].

Evidence has accumulated that IHR is highly effective in eliminating or substantially reducing the Trendelenburg gait and in equalizing the lower limb length while improving the stability and range of motion of the hip joint at the same time [41, 45, 47–50, 52, 56–59]. Hence, the authors currently prefer IHR for the management of Type IVB and IVA hips in which the previous reconstructive surgery has failed, or there is late presentation with a severe abductor lurch and a considerable LLD, particularly in the adolescents and young adults in whom arthrodesis or hip arthroplasty is not suitable [41].

The reported complications of IHR in the literature include knee stiffness, pin tract infection, delayed consolidation, refracture, obturator nerve entrapment, remodeling of the proximal valgus angulation, and persistent Trendelenburg gait. There is a possibility of ischiofemoral impingement if the apex of the proximal femoral valgus angulation site directly abuts the ischium. The literature demonstrates that an average of 30% (range, 0–62.5%) of patients have a persistent positive Trendelenburg sign after IHR, although it is reduced in severity in most of the patients [41].

IHR is not ideal for young children, because in accordance with Wolff's law, gradual straightening of the proximal femur tends to occur at the site of valgus angulation, which may result in loss of pelvic support. The potential for remodeling and subsequent gradual loss of valgus angulation remains important considerations in proximal femoral osteotomy in preadolescence [41, 45, 49, 55–57] (Fig. 38.4). Therefore, if performing IHR at an age before adolescence, then as much as 25°–40° of overcorrection should be empirically added to the valgus correction angle based on the single-leg stance drop angle relative to the horizontal line of the pelvis in the anticipation of remodeling of the proximal femur after IHR [41, 55, 56]. The authors believe that IHR is still indicated even in patients older than 6 years of age, despite the high probability of repeat PSO, because a second femoral lengthening is usually needed at or near skeletal maturity in patients with hip instability associated with marked LLD due to multiple lower limb growth disturbances secondary to neonatal sepsis. Early stabilization of the hip with a newly reconstructed fulcrum of femoral-pelvic articulation can be beneficial for building-up the abductor muscle power, and consequently, leading to an improved gait in emotionally sensitive elementary school children. Another alternative is to perform femoral lengthening without a PSO and insert half pins into the pelvis to prevent proximal migration of the femur at a younger age, and subsequently perform IHR when the patients are near skeletal maturity [41, 57]. Metikata et al. [61] recently proposed a two-stage technique of PSO exclusively using internal devices, avoiding some of the complications of external fixators while facilitating quicker rehabilitation of the ipsilateral hip and knee joints as an alternative to IHR. This technique is composed of stage 1, FH resection and PSO using double plating, and stage II, distal femoral osteotomy avoiding varus followed by the insertion of a retrograde magnetic nail for postoperative lengthening.

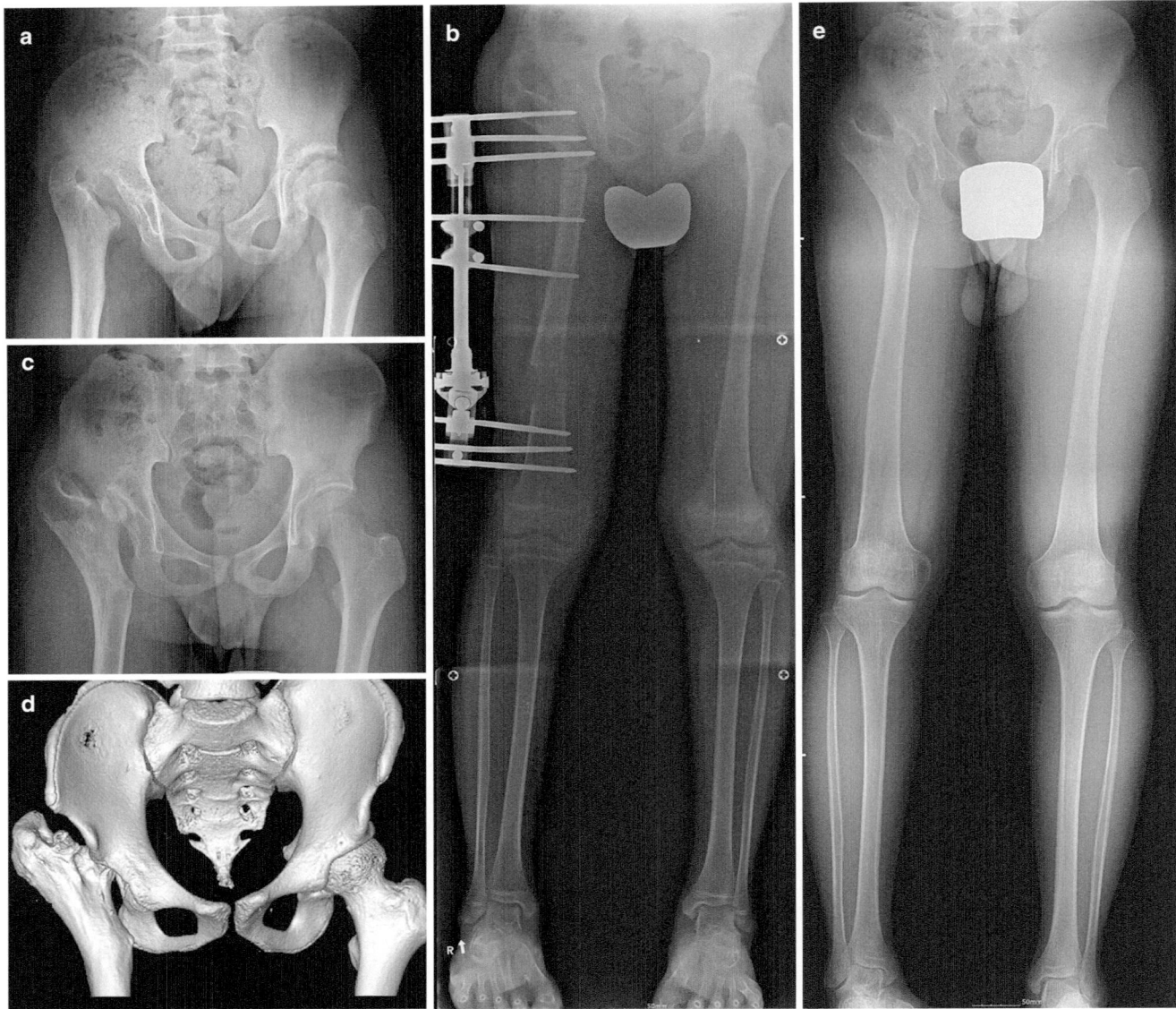

Fig. 38.4 (a) A radiograph in a 12-year—and 4-month-old boy with Choi Type IVB sequelae in the right hip. He had a previous history of Ilizarov hip reconstruction with 40° of proximal valgus osteotomy for pelvic support and 4 cm of distal diaphyseal lengthening for leg length equalization performed at an age of 8 years and 1 month. It is noteworthy to observe a completely remodeled, straightened proximal femur showing no evidence of pelvic support. (b) A teleradiograph showing a repeated Ilizarov hip reconstruction osteotomy. (c, d) A plain radiograph and 3D-CT taken at 17 years of age showing displacement of the lesser trochanter into the acetabulum and proximal femur with valgus angulation near the ischium, which apparently enhances the femoro-pelvic stability and improves abductor mechanics by displacing the center of gravity medially. (e) A teleradiograph taken at 25 years of age showing equalization of the lower limb length after surgery. He had a negative Trendelenburg sign

Late Sequelae After Septic Arthritis and Osteomyelitis Around the Knee and Ankle Joints

The rate of overall unsatisfactory results in terms of residual deformities after infantile or childhood septic arthritis of the knee and ankle joints is less compared to that after septic arthritis of the hip [5, 8], likely because the infection in these more peripheral joints can be diagnosed sooner than that in the hip [9]. Long-term follow-up following a septic arthritis is critical because radiographic improvement in the involved epiphyseal region can occur several months to years after the acute infection. In younger children in whom the secondary ossification center has not yet developed, vascular damage can lead to a marked delay in the formation of the ossific center, but the cartilage model may continue to grow.

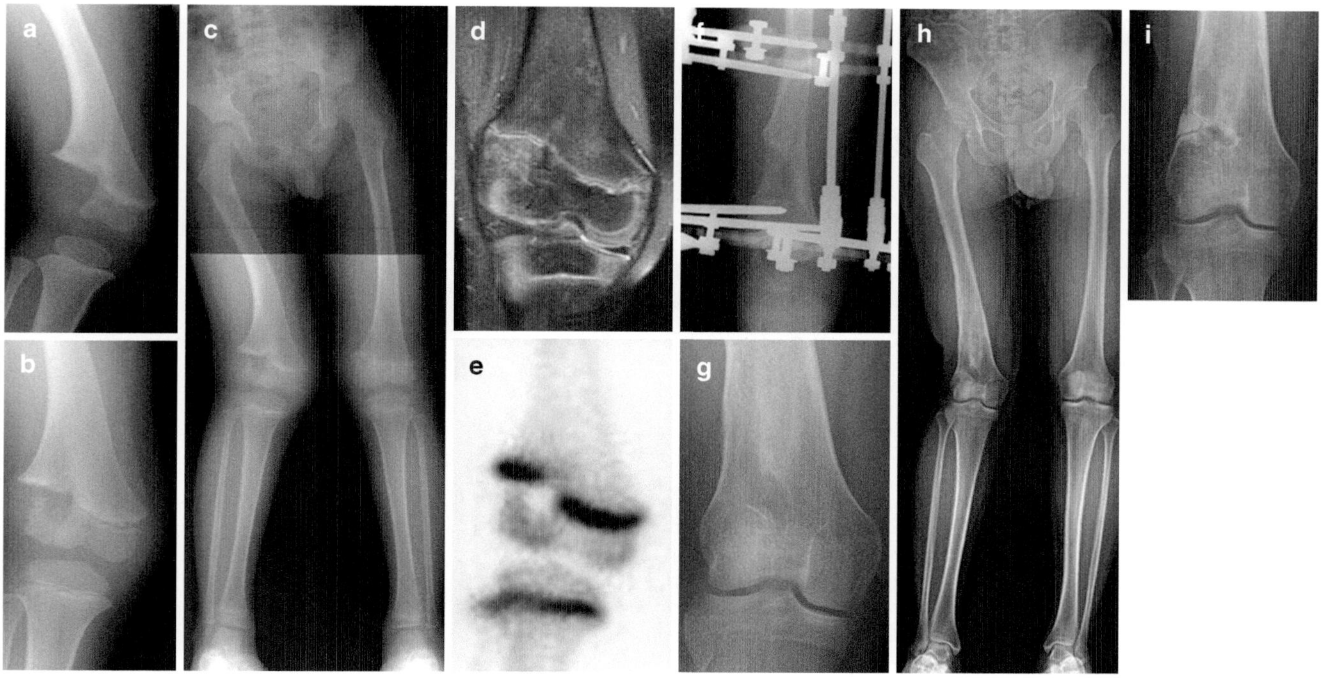

Fig. 38.5 (a) A radiograph showing the deficiency of the lateral half of the distal femoral epiphysis in a 2-year—and 10-month-old boy. (b-e) Radiographic images including plain radiographs, MRI and bone scan, taken at 5 years and 6 months of age at referral, showing almost complete reossification of the lateral epiphysis. (f) A radiograph taken at 3 months after Ilizarov surgery for gradual deformity correction and concomitant lengthening shows nicely formed regenerated bone in the distraction gap. (g, h) However, when he revisited at 19 years of age, recurrent genu valgum, probably due to premature closure of the lateral physis, is seen. (i) Residual genu valgum was corrected by acute opening wedge osteotomy using corticocancellous bone blocks taken from the iliac crest and allograft chips

Therefore, even when bony deficiency is seen on plain radiography, it is necessary to perform advanced imaging studies such as ultrasonography, arthrography, or MRI [9] in order to better visualize the cartilaginous epiphysis (chondroepiphysis) and assess the potential growth of the adjacent physis (Fig. 38.5). When the appropriate treatment is delayed, growth disturbance with a resultant angular deformity, joint incongruity, impingement, and accompanying ligamentous laxity and joint instability may develop gradually. Postinfectious juxta-articular deformity of the knee usually develops as a result of metaphyseal osteomyelitis or primary septic arthritis of the knee, involving the distal femoral physis or the proximal tibial physis, or both. The distal femur is more prone to growth-related sequelae than the proximal tibia. Angular deformities due to partial distal femoral physeal destruction are far more common than complete symmetric growth cessation [9]. The most serious growth sequelae occurs following neonatal sepsis and to a lesser extent within the first 2 years of life [8, 9] (Fig. 38.6). In particular, meningococcemia caused by *Neisseria meningitides* or meningococcus, which is found only in human respiratory secretions, is a devastating illness that primarily affects young children. The disseminated intravascular coagulation and focal infections of the acute phase are primarily responsible for the vascular injuries to the growing chondro-osseous tissues and contiguous soft tissues. Ischemic changes also selectively involve the physeal circulation, which adversely affect the longitudinal and transverse growth of bone. Therefore, children who survive meningococcal septicemia are prone to develop complex deformities of the lower limb due to multiple areas of growth disturbance [54, 62, 63].

The ultimate goal of managing juxta-articular and intra-articular deformity is the prevention of osteoarthritis of the affected joint and the adjacent joint by restoring the weight-bearing mechanical axis and by normalizing the joint orientation as early as possible, because both these factors contribute to abnormal loading of the affected joint, leading to premature osteoarthritis of the affected joint(s) [9, 64, 65]. Juxta-articular realignment and reorientation osteotomy are preferred because of the proximity of such an osteotomy to the adjacent joint that leads to a more anatomic reorientation correction, without iatrogenic translational deformities. The resultant pain reduction and decreased wear rate of the articular cartilage due to redistribution of joint reaction forces increase the longevity of the major weight-bearing joints [64]. The pearls and pitfalls in the management of late sequelae after septic arthritis and osteomyelitis around the knee and ankle joints are summarized in Table 38.3.

To establish an optimal treatment plan for restoring the weight-bearing axis, for stabilizing the unstable joint, and

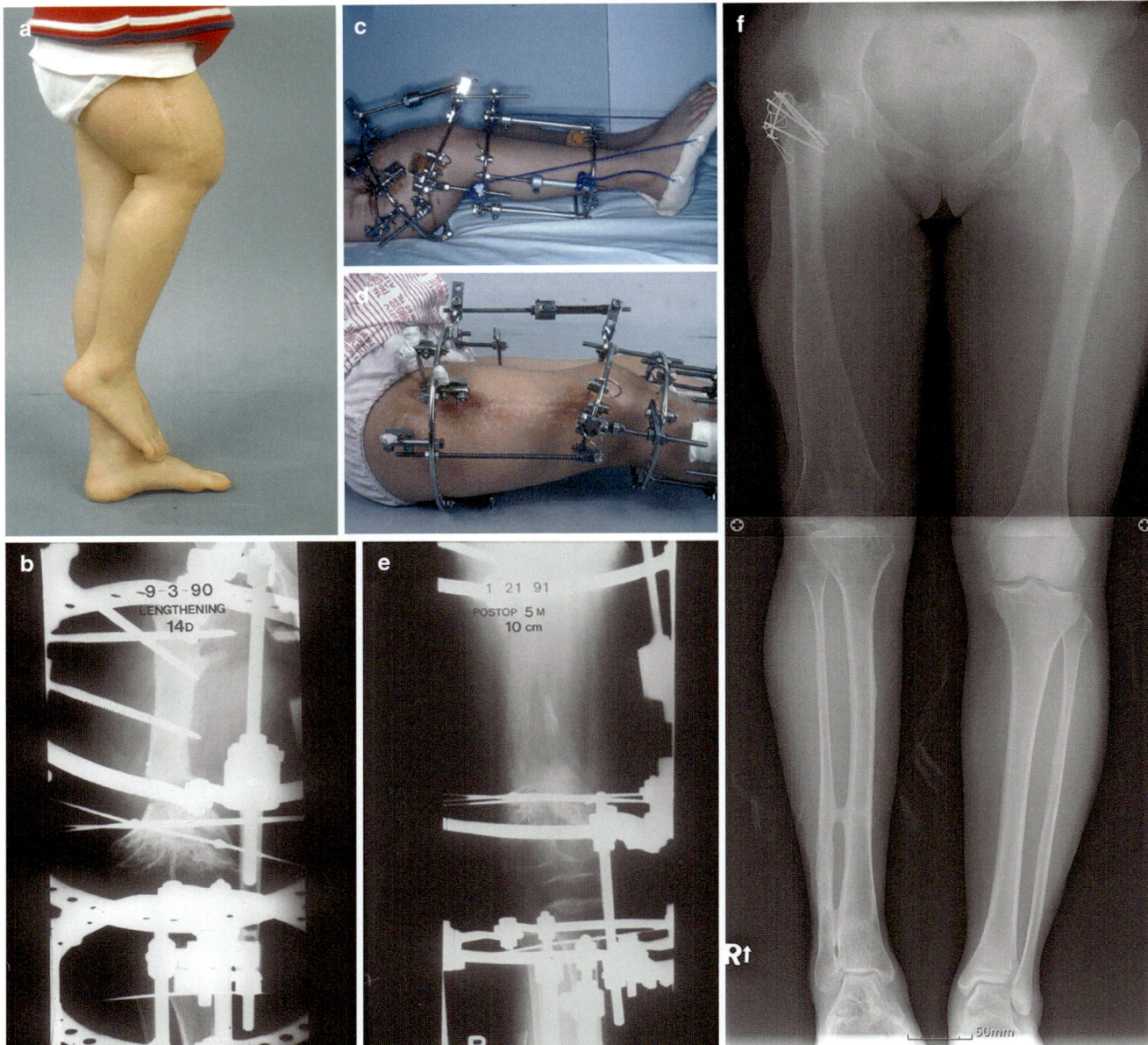

Fig. 38.6 (**a**) A 10-year—and 7-month-old girl presenting with 17.5 cm of shortening of the right femur and a concomitant 30° of flexion contracture of the knee joint after fulminant osteomyelitis of the right femur extending to the hip and knee joints. Further flexion in the knee joint was only marginally limited. (**b, c**) A radiograph and photograph showing the femoral and tibial Ilizarov frames constructed with one proximal full ring and a distal two-third ring for concomitant femoral lengthening and deformity correction at the distal femoral corticotomy site. Tibial frame was applied for the purpose of transarticular fixation during lengthening to prevent potential subluxation of the unstable knee joint apparently caused by deformation of the femoral condyle secondary to central physeal arrest in the distal femur. (**d, e**) A concomitant 10-cm lengthening and deformity correction could be achieved by differential distraction of the anterior and posterior motor rods. Subsequent procedures included right tibial and fibular lengthening followed by left distal femoral epiphysiodesis, concomitant right femoral and tibial lengthening, and right greater trochanteric advancement. (**f**) At the last follow-up at the age of 26 years, her right lower limb function and gait were excellent with equalization of the lower limb length and no knee flexion contracture despite the difference in the knee level

for equalizing the lower limb length, a preoperative three-dimensional assessment of the juxta-articular and intra-articular deformity is essential. The surgeon should recognize that frontal, sagittal, and oblique plane malalignment can result from a variety of sources such as ligamentous laxity, joint subluxation, altered joint line secondary to physeal growth disturbance, and epiphyseal deficiency or deformation. This may be particularly true in children with severe multifocal, angular, and/or rotational deformities, often associated with joint incongruity, joint instability,

Table 38.3 Pearls and pitfalls in the management of late sequelae of septic arthritis and osteomyelitis around the knee and ankle joints

Assessment	• In young children, it is necessary to perform studies assessing the cartilaginous structure of an epiphyseal region to assess the growth potential by using ultrasonography, arthrography, bone scintigraphy, and MRI • Meticulous deformity analysis of the complex deformity by determining the location, magnitude, and direction of the deformity is the first step. Frontal, sagittal, and oblique plane malalignment can also result from ligamentous laxity, joint subluxation, and joint line deformity • It is essential to determine whether a juxta-articular deformity has a compensatory fixed deformity at an adjacent bone and joint. When there exists a compensatory fixed deformity, correction of this deformity must also be included in the treatment plan • Careful assessment of physeal integrity, intra-articular epiphyseal irregularity, joint instability, surrounding soft-tissue condition, and neurovascular condition is essential
Treatment	• The decision whether to perform acute versus gradual deformity correction, and conventional osteotomy versus external fixator-assisted plating or intramedullary nailing, should be made on an individual basis. When a technique of lengthening over an intramedullary nail using external fixation is used, caution is required to prevent deep infection in patients who have a past history of infection, and open trauma • Juxta-articular realignment and reorientation osteotomy are preferred because the closer each osteotomy to the adjacent joint is, the greater the reorientation with angular correction is • When correcting a juxta-articular deformity by conventional metaphyseal osteotomy, the use of the Ilizarov technique with an offset hinge system or external fixation which utilizes the six-axis deformity correction principle is preferred • When correcting severe juxta-articular deformity, adjunctive procedures (e.g., peroneal nerve decompression and compartment release) may be justified to prevent major complications • In the management of juxta-articular ankle deformity, early stabilization of the talocrural joint by leveling the ankle and restoration of the axial alignment and joint orientation are of paramount importance • Intra-articular osteotomy is a very technically demanding procedure and should be selectively performed

LLD, and surrounding soft-tissue scars and contractures. In such children, identification, characterization, and prioritization of each component of the deformity are crucial. The decision and timing of performing multilevel operations either in one stage or in multiple stages must be made on an individual basis.

Patients who have a juxta-articular deformity may also have a compensatory fixed deformity at an adjacent bone and joint, and correction of this deformity must also be included in the treatment plan. Correction of the malunion without addressing the compensatory deformity may result in a straight bone with a maloriented joint, leading to long-term disability due to altered biomechanics. For instance, when distal femoral valgus coexists with compensatory proximal tibia varus or distal femoral varus in the presence of a compensatory proximal tibial valgus deformity, the lower limb may appear aligned with no mechanical axis deviation despite malorientation of the knee joint. However, combinations of femoral valgus and tibial varus would produce shear stress in the knee joint due to increased obliquity of the knee joint to the ground. This deformity can cause lateral subluxation of the proximal tibia associated with progressive degenerative arthritis in late adulthood. In contrast, in the case of distal femoral varus and proximal tibial valgus, patients may tolerate well because obliquity of the joint adds to knee joint stability, buttressing against the lateral subluxation forces [66, 67].

Acute correction of juxta-articular deformity by conventional metaphyseal osteotomy is associated with many challenges, such as fixation stability, geometrical considerations related to the different locations of the osteotomy site and the locus of the deformity, multilevel deformities caused by prior osteotomies, and concurrent LLD. In addition, the disadvantages of acute correction using plate and screw fixation include the requirement of extensive soft-tissue dissection, limitation of early weight bearing and function, and inability to correct a substantial shortening of the involved extremity. It is well known that realignment of the mechanical axis and joint orientation by metaphyseal osteotomy requires a combination of angulation and translation [64, 65]. In this regard, the Ilizarov technique with an offset (juxta-articular) hinge system (true or virtual) is preferred for accurately correcting and restoring the mechanical axis and joint orientation. In recent years, the use of external fixators which utilize the six-axis deformity correction principle using a software program has been advocated due to the convenience and accuracy of such adjuncts in correcting complex juxta-articular deformities of the limb. External fixator assisted acute deformity correction and fixation using a locking compression plate [68–70] is another surgical technique for addressing such deformities. The potential advantages of a fixator-assisted plating include correction of deformities under direct visualization, rigid fixation, and its applicability in various anatomic locations and situations, e.g., open physis, narrow intramedullary canal, and bowing deformity of the femur and tibia. Similarly, external fixator-assisted acute bone realignment and fixation using an intramedullary locking nail or fixator-assisted deformity correction and consecutive lengthening over an intramedullary locking nail can also be performed in certain instances [71–75]. However, while the technique of lengthening over an intramedullary nail using external fixation is used to reduce the time of external fixation, caution is required to prevent deep infection in patients who have a past history of bone and joint infection, or an open trauma [76, 77]. The latest advance is in systems utilizing fully implantable intramedullary nails, e.g., PRECICE™, to accomplish the goal of moderate acute deformity correction and subsequent gradual lengthening [71, 72].

Juxta-articular deformity of the ankle may develop as a result of metaphyseal osteomyelitis of the distal tibia or a primary septic arthritis of the ankle joint, involving the physis. Asymmetric or symmetric premature physeal closure of the distal tibia can be seen along with a normally growing distal fibula (Fig. 38.7), or vice versa. When the length discrepancy between the tibia and fibula is severe, secondary distal tibiofibular dissociation can occur. Similar to the juxta-articular deformity of the knee, the ultimate goal of the treatment for juxta-articular deformity of the ankle is to obtain a painless, stable plantigrade foot with a functional, mobile ankle joint. For this purpose, early stabilization of the talocrural joint by leveling the ankle and restoration of the axial alignment and joint orientation are of paramount importance. Treatment of juxta-articular deformity of the ankle should be individualized after considering the patient's age, relative length discrepancy between the tibia and fibula, physeal integrity, presence or absence of lateral talar subluxation and wedge-shaped epiphysis of the distal tibia, intra-articular epiphyseal irregularity due to epiphyseal deformation, compensatory foot deformity including subtalar joint subluxation/deformation, range of motion, surrounding soft-tissue condition, neurovascular status, LLD, and other factors, in addition to the deformity itself. For instance, the use of internal fixation may not be feasible in patients with a poor soft-tissue envelope and is contraindicated in the presence of an active infection. Circular external fixation is well suited for the management of patients with complex deformities and/or bone loss with a poor soft-tissue envelope and history or presence of infection. The specific advantage of external fixation is that adjustments to achieve the desired alignment can be performed gradually during the postoperative period. In certain complex scenarios, external fixators are utilized in conjunction with internal fixation to provide additional support in order to avoid hardware failure and development of a residual deformity [78].

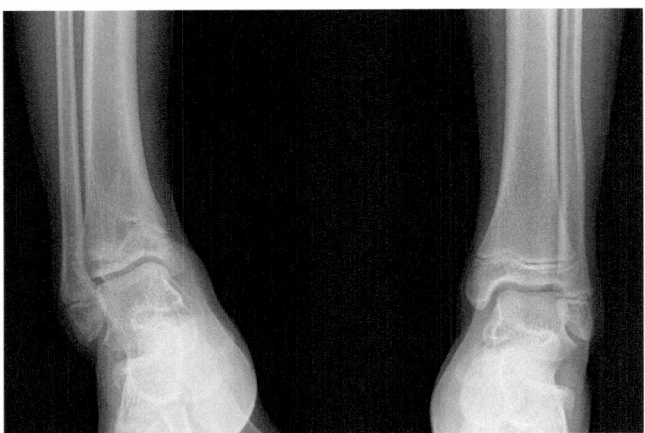

Fig. 38.7 A radiograph showing asymmetrical premature physeal closure of the distal tibia in the presence of normally growing distal fibula in a 13-year—and 8-month-old boy

Figure 38.8 depicts the authors' systematic approach for the assessment of the juxta-articular deformity of the ankle. First, the length of the tibia relative to the fibula is assessed,

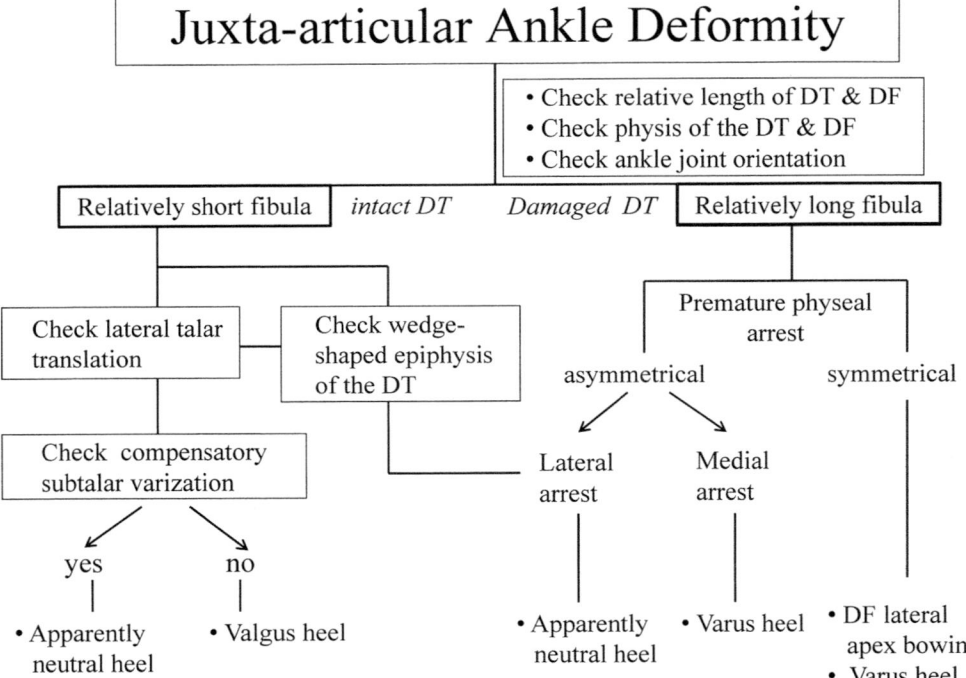

Fig. 38.8 Authors' systematic approach for the assessment of juxta-articular deformity of the ankle (refer text). *DT* distal tibia; *DF* distal fibula

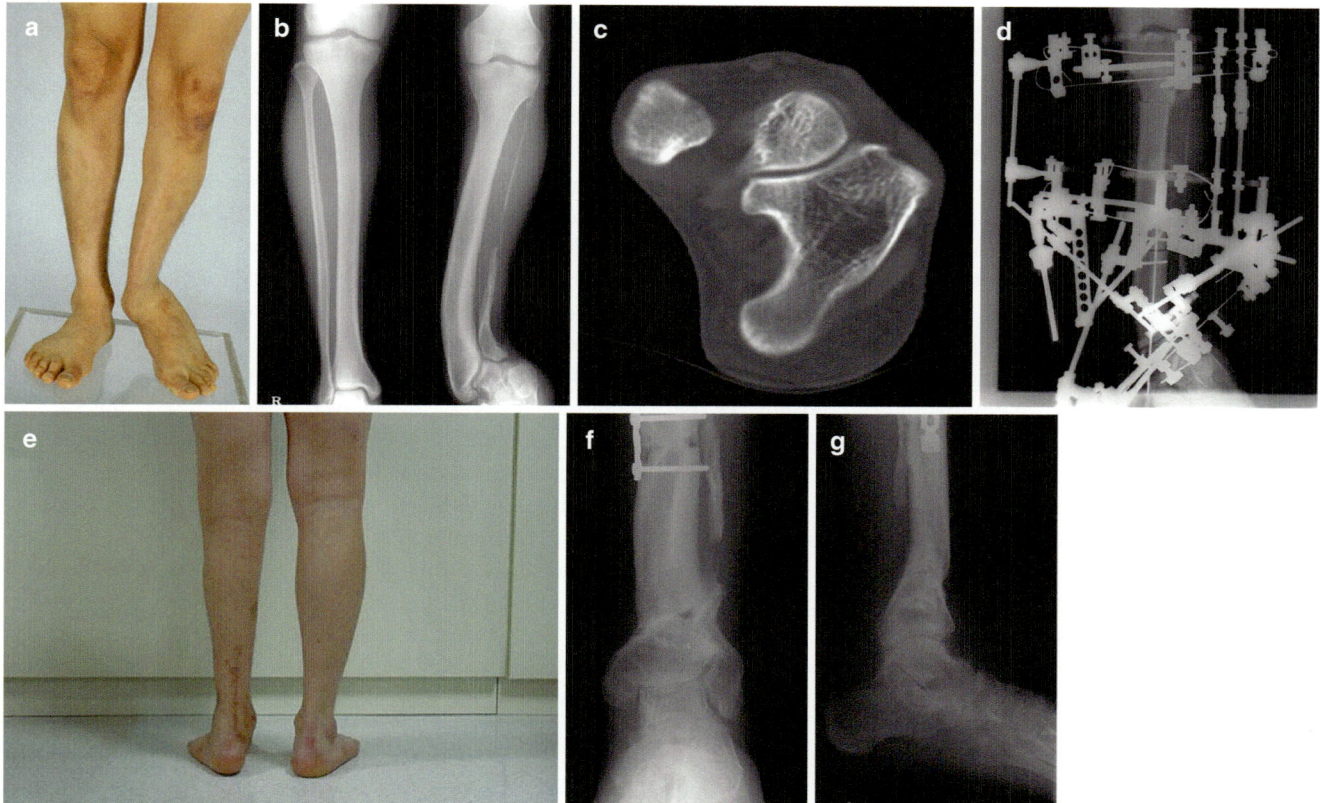

Fig. 38.9 (**a–c**) A 25-year-old man presenting with a severe equinovalgus deformity of the foot. He had a history of undergoing incision and drainage and sequestrectomy for osteomyelitis of the entire fibula at 5 years of age. Compensatory proximal varus and distal anteromedial bowing deformity of the tibia, and a calcaneal varus deformity, is seen on the coronal view of the CT (**c**). (**d**) Tibial osteotomy was made at three levels, for the purpose of acute deformity correction and plate fixation for diaphyseal angulation, and gradual distraction for correction of proximal angular deformity using conventional Ilizarov construct and correction of distal angular deformity at the supramalleolar level using the hexapod system. Lateral calcaneal closing wedge osteotomy was also performed. (**e–g**) At 13 months after removal of the external fixator, which was applied for 9 months, he regained full function of the lower limb with a plantigrade foot and ankle joint motion from neutral to 20° of plantar flexion

physeal integrity of the distal tibia and fibula is checked, and orientation of the ankle joint in the coronal and sagittal planes is assessed. The location and extent of premature physeal closure, angular or joint surface deformities, and secondary osteoarthritis can be determined by using MRI, bone scintigraphy, and CT, together with plain radiographs [79, 80]. Documenting the magnitude of the angular deformity at other site(s) and LLD, if any, is also essential. When a juxta-articular valgus deformity of the ankle, with either a neutral heel or a valgus heel, is associated with a relatively short fibula due to partial deficiency or premature physeal arrest in the presence of intact physis of the distal tibia (Fig. 38.9), it is imperative to determine whether lateral talar subluxation with or without compensatory subtalar varus deformity and wedge-shaped epiphysis of the distal tibia coexist. If possible, acute or gradual reduction of lateral talar subluxation by external fixation should be performed first. Other definitive and adjunctive surgical treatment methods that can be used alone or in combination include fibular lengthening [81, 82], supramalleolar corrective osteotomy [83–85], hemiepiphysiodesis, and occasionally an intra-articular osteotomy [86]. Several techniques of supramalleolar osteotomy for acute deformity correction have been reported, including oblique transphyseal supramalleolar osteotomy [84], transverse supramalleolar osteotomy with translation, Wiltse translational step-cut osteotomy [85], and an arc osteotomy. The oblique medial closing wedge osteotomy allows for correction of the valgus deformity of the ankle and offers the advantage of improved bone healing as minimal periosteal stripping is necessary and the deformity is corrected by hinging the osteotomy at a point along the bisector of the deformity [83]. Hemiepiphysiodesis of the medial aspect of the distal tibia can also be performed by using a transphyseal screw [87, 88], staple, or a tension-band plate [89, 90]. External fixator-assisted acute correction of ankle valgus and fixation using a locking compression plate or multiple screws and gradual correction with external fixation are other viable options.

In contrast, when a juxta-articular varus deformity of the ankle, with an apparently neutral heel or a varus heel, and distal fibular lateral apex bowing, is associated with premature physeal arrest of the distal tibia in the presence of intact physis of the distal fibula, the location and extent of physeal damage of the distal tibia should be checked. In this situation, definitive and adjunctive surgical options that can be used alone or in combination include physeal bar resection, supramalleolar corrective osteotomy [83, 84, 91], distal fibular shortening and/or epiphysiodesis, tibial lengthening and subsequent epiphysiodesis, and occasionally an intraarticular osteotomy. When along with a juxta-articular deformity of the ankle, there is a compensatory deformity of the subtalar joint and/or calcaneus, the correction of this component must also be included in the treatment plan. When a supramalleolar corrective osteotomy is contemplated, the treatment option for acute versus gradual deformity correction should be selected on an individual basis after considering all the aforementioned confounding variables. In patients who have previously undergone surgery for the reorientation of the talocrural joint, a second-stage lengthening of the proximal tibia and fibula may be needed, near or at skeletal maturity for equalizing the lower limb lengths.

Postinfectious Articular Deformity Causing Knee and Ankle Joint Incongruity

The residual deformity of septic arthritis of the knee and ankle joints may include partial epiphyseal destruction with a resultant joint incongruity and accompanying joint instability, subluxation, and impingement that may lead to rapid degenerative arthritis. In this situation, juxtaarticular osteotomy alone cannot solve the problem of joint incongruity. Although intraarticular osteotomy is not a common treatment option for the hip, knee, or ankle, intra-articular osteotomy can be selectively performed to promote joint congruity and stability [86]. Paley [86] demonstrated, through case studies, that intraarticular osteotomy of the FH, the distal femur, or the tibial plafond is technically feasible and can yield successful results when performed for specific indications. When juxta-articular deformity of the ankle is associated with partial epiphyseal deficiency or deformation causing joint incongruity, an intraarticular osteotomy combined with or without juxta-articular osteotomy may be indicated. Theoretically, normalizing the joint articulation between the two adjoining bones is desirable for improving the joint congruency and stability. However, an intra-articular osteotomy is a technically demanding procedure requiring intensive postoperative physiotherapy and should be selectively performed. Furthermore, long-term follow-up results of such intra-articular osteotomies are currently unavailable.

Postinfectious Segmental Long Bone Defects

Fulminant osteomyelitis of the femur or tibia, if not treated properly, can result in segmental long bone defects. The wide array of limb reconstruction options has been described for the management of bone defects depending on the age, anatomical site, size of bone defect, and the status of surrounding soft tissues. The choice of the most appropriate treatment should be based on specific patient requirements after taking all potential risk factors into account. Most of all, in case of poor soft tissue condition, reconstruction of the soft tissues should be preceded by bony reconstruction. Reported treatment modalities for long bone defects include autogenous or mixed autogenous and allogenic bone grafting [92], Masquelet induced membrane technique [93], acute or gradual shortening with or without subsequent gradual lengthening [94], bone transport [95, 96], cross union between the tibia and fibula [97, 98], fibula bypass grafting [99], vascularized fibula grafting [100, 101], and others. Prior studies suggest that when acute shortening is planned, the tibia can be shortened by 10%, and the femur by 20% of its original length without any complications. Femoral and tibial shortening of up to 20 mm without subsequent lengthening is well tolerated [94, 95, 102–104]. Specific limb reconstruction skills are required for the reconstruction of the defect greater than 6 cm in length. Currently, authors' preferred modality for the treatment of massive defect in children is bi—or trifocal bone transport [105] over vascularized fibular grafting, fibular bypass grafting, and induced membrane technique [92]. We think that bone transport is not only cost-effective but also more predictable with fewer surgical interventions. However, greater than 2 cm of residual LLD can be managed by lengthening of the affected limb or contralateral epiphysiodesis of the normal limb in a growing child, or a combination of different options, depending on the severity of residual limb shortening.

In summary, in the last several decades, thanks to the Ilizarov biologic principles and the law of tension-stress, great stride has been made in the field of deformity correction with or without concomitant lengthening. This helped the surgeons upgrade their armamentarium to successfully treat postinfectious juxta-articular deformity and segmental long bone defects of the lower limb. However, when confronted with severe sequelae of septic arthritis of the hip, knee, and ankle showing joint incongruity with or without instability, currently available reconstructive surgical options, e.g., intraarticular osteotomies, are limited, and, in general, they have not yielded satisfactory long-term results. Various techniques of regenerative medicine-based articular cartilage regeneration as a biologic alternative to artificial joint replacement or resurfacing are still under investigation, and yet to achieve the consistency and effectiveness for widespread clinical use [106]. We hope that real progress of cartilage tissue engineering can be expedited, so that we can fight against postinfectious premature osteoarthritis of the joint by incorporating the new advanced technology of articular cartilage tissue engineering in the near future.

Commentary

Janet D. Conway
jconway@lifebridgehealth.org

Dr. Choi has done a remarkable job outlining the complex deformities that occur following septic arthritis and osteomyelitis in the pediatric lower limb. These are some of the most complex deformities in orthopedics because of the high stakes involved in preserving the joint function in these young patients. There are also other considerations in the growing child since with the growth arrest comes a significant limb length discrepancy. The treatment algorithm tables have been carefully laid out and provide practical guidance for evaluating and treating these patients. Spectacular physical therapy postoperatively along with a cooperative child and their parents are essential contributors to successful outcomes. This is essential reading for any pediatric orthopedic surgeon handling these complicated postinfectious deformities.

References

1. Betz RR, Cooperman DR, Wopperer JM, Sutherland RD, White JJ Jr, Schaaf HW, et al. Late sequelae of septic arthritis of the hip in infancy and childhood. J Pediatr Orthop. 1990;10:365–72.
2. Choi IH, Pizzutillo PD, Bowen JR, Dragann R, Malhis T. Sequelae and reconstruction after septic arthritis of the hip in infants. J Bone Joint Surg Am. 1990;72:1150–65.
3. Choi IH, Yoo WJ, Cho TJ, Chung CY. Operative reconstruction for septic arthritis of the hip. Orthop Clin North Am. 2006;37:173–83.
4. Fabry G, Meire E. Septic arthritis of the hip in children: poor results after late and inadequate treatment. J Pediatr Orthop. 1983;3:461–6.
5. Gillespie R. Septic arthritis of childhood. Clin Orthop Relat Res. 1973;96:152–9.
6. Hallel T, Salvati EA. Septic arthritis of the hip in infancy: end result study. Clin Orthop Relat Res. 1978;132:115–28.
7. Shaw BA, Kasser JR. Acute septic arthritis in infancy and childhood. Clin Orthop Relat Res. 1990;257:212–25.
8. Strong M, Lejman T, Michno P, Hayman M. Sequelae from septic arthritis of the knee during the first two years of life. J Pediatr Orthop. 1994;14:745–51.
9. Shapiro F. Pediatric orthopedic deformities. Basic science, diagnosis, and treatment. London: Academic Press; 2001. p. 897–909.
10. Ilharreborde B. Sequelae of pediatric osteoarticular infection. Orthop Traumatol Surg Res. 2015;101(Suppl 1):S129–37.
11. Paley D. Principles of deformity correction. Berlin: Springer Science & Business Media; 2002.
12. Forlin E, Milani C. Sequelae of septic arthritis of the hip in children: a new classification and a review of 41 hips. J Pediatr Orthop. 2008;28:524–8.
13. Hunka L, Said SE, MacKenzie DA, Rogala EJ, Cruess RL. Classification and surgical management of the severe sequelae of septic hips in children. Clin Orthop Relat Res. 1982;171:30–6.
14. Johari AN. Residual Problems in Septic Arthritis of the Hip in Childhood. Thesis submitted for the M. Ch. Ortho., University of Liverpool 1988. In: Current concept: septic arthritis in childhood Trends in paediatric orthopaedics. London: Macmillan (I) Ltd.; 2002. p. 25–32.
15. Johari AN, Dhawale AA, Johari RA. Management of post septic hip dislocations when the capital femoral epiphysis is present. J Pediatr Orthop B. 2011;20:413–21.
16. Kim HT, Eisenhauer E, Wenger DR. The "sagging rope sign" in avascular necrosis in children's hip diseases--confirmation by 3D CT studies. Iowa Orthop J. 1995;15:101–11.
17. El-Tayeby HM. Osteochondroplasty of the femoral head in hip reconstruction for type II late sequelae of septic arthritis: a preliminary report. J Child Orthop. 2008;2:431–41.
18. Shin SJ, Choi IH, Cho TJ, Yoo WJ, Chung CY, Park MS. Unusual osteocartilaginous prominence or bump causing femoroacetabular impingement after septic arthritis of the hip: a report of 2 cases in preadolescence. J Pediatr Orthop. 2009;29:459–62.
19. Ganz R, Klaue K, Vinh TS, Mast JW. A new periacetabular osteotomy for the treatment of hip dysplasias: technique and preliminary results. 1988. Clin Orthop Relat Res. 2004;418:3–8.
20. Wenger DR. Triple innominate osteotomy. In: Flynn JM, Wiesel SW, editors. Operative techniques in pediatric orthopaedics. Philadelphia: Lippincott Williams & Wilkins; 2010. p. 516–26.
21. Ganz R, Huff TW, Leunig M. Extended retinacular soft-tissue flap for intra-articular hip surgery: surgical technique, indications, and results of application. Instr Course Lect. 2009;58:241–55.
22. Hasler CC, Morscher EW. Femoral neck lengthening osteotomy after growth disturbance of the proximal femur. J Pediatr Orthop B. 1999;8:271–5.
23. Leunig M, Ganz R. Relative neck lengthening and intracapital osteotomy for severe Perthes and Perthes-like deformities. Bull NYU Hosp Jt Dis. 2011;69(Suppl 1):S62–7.
24. Standard SC. Treatment of coxa brevis. Orthop Clin North Am. 2011;42:373–87.
25. Paley D. The treatment of femoral head deformity and coxa magna by the Ganz femoral head reduction osteotomy. Orthop Clin North Am. 2011;42:389–99.
26. Choi IH, Shin YW, Chung CY, Cho TJ, Yoo WJ, Lee DY. Surgical treatment of the severe sequelae of infantile septic arthritis of the hip. Clin Orthop Relat Res. 2005;434:102–9.
27. Dobbs MB, Sheridan JJ, Gordon JE, Corley CL, Szymanski DA, Schoenecker PL. Septic arthritis of the hip in infancy: long-term follow-up. J Pediatr Orthop. 2003;23:162–8.
28. Freeland AE, Sullivan DJ, Westin GW. Greater trochanteric hip arthroplasty in children with loss of the femoral head. J Bone Joint Surg Am. 1980;62:1351–61.
29. Wada A, Fujii T, Takamura K, Yanagida H, Urano N, Surijamorn P. Operative reconstruction of the severe sequelae of infantile septic arthritis of the hip. J Pediatr Orthop. 2007;27:910–4.
30. Wopperer JM, White JJ, Gillespie R, Obletz BE. Long-term follow-up of infantile hip sepsis. J Pediatr Orthop. 1988;8:322–5.
31. L'episcopo JB. Stabilization of pathological dislocation of the hip in children. J Bone Joint Surg Am. 1936;18:737–42.

32. Harmon PH. Surgical treatment of the residual deformity from suppurative arthritis of the hip occurring in young children. J Bone Joint Surg Am. 1942;24:576–85.
33. Li XD, Chen B, Fan J, Zheng CY, Liu DX, Wang H, et al. Evaluation of the modified Albee arthroplasty for femoral head loss secondary to septic arthritis in young children. J Bone Joint Surg Am. 2010;92:1370–80.
34. Cheng JC, Aguilar J, Leung PC. Hip reconstruction for femoral head loss from septic arthritis in children. A preliminary report. Clin Orthop Relat Res. 1995;314:214–24.
35. Abrishami S, Karami M, Karimi A, Soufali AP, Aslani HR, Badizadeh K. Greater trochanteric preserving hip arthroplasty in the treatment of infantile septic arthritis: long-term results. J Child Orthop. 2010;4:137–41.
36. Axer A, Aner A. A new technique for greater trochanteric hip arthroplasty. J Bone Joint Surg Br. 1984;66:331–3.
37. Colonna PC. A new type of reconstruction operation for old ununited fracture of the neck of the femur. J Bone Joint Surg Am. 1935;17:110–22.
38. Ferrari D, Libri R, Donzelli O. Trochanteroplasty to treat sequelae of septic arthritis of the hip in infancy. Case series and review of the literature. Hip Int. 2011;21:653–6.
39. Weissman SL. Transplantation of the trochanteric epiphysis into the acetabulum after septic arthritis of the hip: report of a case. J Bone Joint Surg Am. 1967;49:1647–51.
40. Westin GW. The stick femur. Proceedings and reports of university colleges, councils and associations. J Bone Joint Surg Br. 1970;52:778–9.
41. Choi IH, Cho TJ, Yoo WJ, Shin CH. Recurrent dislocations and complete necrosis: the role of pelvic support osteotomy. J Pediatr Orthop. 2013;33(Suppl 1):S45–55.
42. Milch H. The" pelvic support" osteotomy. J Bone Joint Surg Am. 1941;23:581–95.
43. Milch H. The "pelvic support" osteotomy. 1941. Clin Orthop Relat Res. 1989;249:4–11.
44. Peltier LF. The classic. The "pelvic support" osteotomy. Clin Orthop Relat Res. 1989;249:4–11.
45. El-Mowafi H. Outcome of pelvic support osteotomy with the Ilizarov method in the treatment of the unstable hip joint. Acta Orthop Belg. 2005;71:686–91.
46. Ilizarov GA. Treatment of disorders of the hip. In: Green S, editor. Transosseous osteosynthesis. Berlin: Springer; 1992. p. 668–96.
47. Ilizarov GA, Samchukov ML. Ilizarov reconstructive surgery in the treatment of hip osteoarthritis. Ortop Travmatol Profitez. 1988;6:10–3.
48. Ilizarov GA, Samchukov ML, Kurtov VM. Ilizarov restorative reconstruction surgery in the treatment of hip osteoarthritis, congenital and pathological hip dislocation in children and adults. In: Materials of second international symposium on experimental, theoretical, and clinical aspects of Transosseous Osteosynthesis. Kurgan, USSR: Kurgan Scientific Research Institute; 1986. p. 100–2.
49. Inan M, Bomar JD, Küçükkaya M, Harma A. A comparison between the use of a monolateral external fixator and the Ilizarov technique for pelvic support osteotomies. Acta Orthop Traumatol Turc. 2004;38:252–60.
50. Kadykalo OA, Kuftyev LM. Some biomechanical principles of the hip reconstruction with defect on head and neck of the femur by Ilizarov method. In: the value of general biological patterns in regeneration tissue opened by GA Ilizarov. In: Scientific works collection 13th edition, the Ministry of Health, the RSFSR (the Russian soviet federative Socialist Republic). Kurgan All-union scientific center. Rehabilitation Traumatology Orthopedics; 1988. p. 124–9.
51. Kocaoglu M, Eralp L, Sen C, Dincyurek H. The Ilizarov hip reconstruction osteotomy for hip dislocation: outcome after 4-7 years in 14 young patients. Acta Orthop Scand. 2002;73:432–8.
52. Mahran MA, ElGebeily MA, Ghaly NA, Thakeb MF, Hefny HM. Pelvic support osteotomy by Ilizarov's concept: is it a valuable option in managing neglected hip problems in adolescents and young adults? Strategies Trauma Limb Reconstr. 2011;6:13–20.
53. Manzotti A, Rovetta L, Pullen C, Catagni MA. Treatment of the late sequelae of septic arthritis of the hip. Clin Orthop Relat Res. 2003;410:203–12.
54. Nectoux E, Mezel A, Raux S, Fron D, Maillet M, Herbaux B. Meningococcal purpura fulminans in children: I. Initial orthopedic management. J Child Orthop. 2010;4:401–7.
55. Pafilas D, Nayagam S. The pelvic support osteotomy: indications and preoperative planning. Strategies Trauma Limb Reconstr. 2008;3:83–92.
56. Paley D. Hip joint considerations. In: Paley D, editor. Principles of deformity correction. Berlin: Springer Science & Business Media; 2002. p. 647–94.
57. Rozbruch SR, Paley D, Bhave A, Herzenberg JE. Ilizarov hip reconstruction for the late sequelae of infantile hip infection. J Bone Joint Surg Am. 2005;87:1007–18.
58. Samchukov ML, Birch JG. Pelvic support femoral reconstruction using the method of Ilizarov: a case report. Bull Hosp Jt Dis. 1992;52:7–11.
59. Samchukov ML, Ivanova IV, Dolganov DV. Analysis of pelvotrochanteric muscles and weight-bearing after Ilizarov femoral reconstruction in patients with hip osteoarthritis. In: The congress of scientific and technical advances of the young scientists of the Urals. USSR; 1986. p. 86–7.
60. Schiltenwolf M, Carstens C, Bernd L, Lukoschek M. Late results after subtrochanteric angulation osteotomy in young patients. J Pediatr Orthop B. 1996;5:259–67.
61. Metikala S, Kurian BT, Madan SS, Fernandes JA. Pelvic support hip reconstruction with internal devices: an alternative to Ilizarov hip reconstruction. Strategies Trauma Limb Reconstr. 2020;15:34–40.
62. Grogan DP, Love SM, Ogden JA, Millar EA, Johnson LO. Chondro-osseous growth abnormalities after meningococcemia. A clinical and histopathological study. J Bone Joint Surg Am. 1989;71:920–8.
63. Park DH, Bradish CF. The management of the orthopaedic sequelae of meningococcal septicaemia: patients treated to skeletal maturity. J Bone Joint Surg Am. 2011;93:984–9.
64. Nakase T, Yasui N, Kawabata H, Shimizu N, Ohzono K, Hiroshima K, et al. Correction of deformity and shortening due to post traumatic epiphyseal arrest by distraction osteogenesis. Arch Orthop Trauma Surg. 2007;127:659–63.
65. Sakurakichi K, Tsuchiya H, Kabata T, Yamashiro T, Watanabe K, Tomita K. Correction of juxtaarticular deformities in children using the Ilizarov apparatus. J Orthop Sci. 2005;10:360–6.
66. Paley D. Gait considerations. In: Paley D, editor. Principles of deformity correction. Berlin: Springer Science & Business Media; 2002. p. 717–58.
67. Cooke TD, Pichora D, Siu D, Scudamore RA, Bryant JT. Surgical implications of varus deformity of the knee with obliquity of joint surfaces. J Bone Joint Surg Br. 1989;71:560–5.
68. Bar-On E, Becker T, Katz K, Velkes S, Salai M, Weigl DM. Corrective lower limb osteotomies in children using temporary external fixation and percutaneous locking plates. J Child Orthop. 2009;3:137–43.
69. GugenheimJr JJ, Brinker MR. Bone realignment with use of temporary external fixation for distal femoral valgus and varus deformities. J Bone Joint Surg Am. 2003;85:1229–37.
70. Rozbruch SR. Fixator-assisted plating of limb deformities. Oper Tech Orthop. 2011;21:174–9.
71. Hammouda AI, Szymczuk VL, Gesheff MG, Mohamed NS, Conway JD, Standard SC, et al. Acute deformity correction and lengthening using the PRECICE magnetic intramedullary lengthening nail. J Limb Lengthen Reconstr. 2020;6:20.

72. Iobst CA, Rozbruch SR, Nelson S, Fragomen A. Simultaneous acute femoral deformity correction and gradual limb lengthening using a retrograde femoral nail: technique and clinical results. J Am Acad Orthop Surg. 2018;26:241–50.
73. Kocaoglu M, Eralp L, Bilen FE, Balci HI. Fixator-assisted acute femoral deformity correction and consecutive lengthening over an intramedullary nail. J Bone Joint Surg Am. 2009;91:152–9.
74. Rozbruch SR, Birch JG, Dahl MT, Herzenberg JE. Motorized intramedullary nail for management of limb-length discrepancy and deformity. J Am Acad Orthop Surg. 2014;22:403–9.
75. Sabharwal S, Rozbruch SR. What's new in limb lengthening and deformity correction. J Bone Joint Surg Am. 2011;93:2323–32.
76. Simpson AH, Cole AS, Kenwright J. Leg lengthening over an intramedullary nail. J Bone Joint Surg Br. 1999;81:1041–5.
77. Song HR, Oh CW, Mattoo R, Park BC, Kim SJ, Park IH, et al. Femoral lengthening over an intramedullary nail using the external fixator: risk of infection and knee problems in 22 patients with a follow-up of 2 years or more. Acta Orthop. 2005;76:245–52.
78. Cherkashin AM, Samchukov ML, Birch JG, Stapleton JJ, Zgonis T. Stepwise approach to adult and pediatric foot and ankle malunions/nonunions and external fixation. In: Cooper P, Zgonis T, Polyzois V, editors. External fixators of the foot and ankle. Philadelphia: Lippincott Williams & Wilkins; 2012. p. 318.
79. Jaramillo D, Shapiro F, Hoffer FA, Winalski CS, Koskinen MF, Frasso R, et al. Posttraumatic growth-plate abnormalities: MR imaging of bony-bridge formation in rabbits. Radiology. 1990;175:767–73.
80. Thawait SK, Thawait GK, Frassica FJ, Andreisek G, Carrino JA, Chhabra A. A systematic approach to magnetic resonance imaging evaluation of epiphyseal lesions. Magn Reson Imaging. 2013;31:418–31.
81. Weber BG, Simpson LA. Corrective lengthening osteotomy of the fibula. Clin Orthop Relat Res. 1985;199:61–7.
82. Weber D, Friederich NF, Muller W. Lengthening osteotomy of the fibula for post-traumatic malunion. Indications, technique and results. Int Orthop. 1998;22:149–52.
83. Keeler KA, Gordon JE. Distal tibial osteotomy. In: Flynn JM, Wiesel SW, editors. Operative techniques in pediatric orthopaedics. Philadelphia: Lippincott Williams & Wilkins; 2010. p. 251–8.
84. Lubicky JP, Altiok H. Transphyseal osteotomy of the distal tibia for correction of valgus/varus deformities of the ankle. J Pediatr Orthop. 2001;21:80–8.
85. Wiltse LL. Valgus deformity of the ankle: a sequel to acquired or congenital abnormalities of the fibula. J Bone Joint Surg Am. 1972;54:595–606.
86. Paley D. Intra-articular osteotomies of the hip, knee, and ankle. Oper Tech Orthop. 2011;21:184–96.
87. Davids JR, Valadie AL, Ferguson RL, Bray EW, Allen BL. Surgical management of ankle valgus in children: use of a transphyseal medial malleolar screw. J Pediatr Orthop. 1997;17:3–8.
88. Stevens PM, Belle RM. Screw epiphysiodesis for ankle valgus. J Pediatr Orthop. 1997;17:9–12.
89. Saran N, Rathjen KE. Guided growth for the correction of pediatric lower limb angular deformity. J Am Acad Orthop Surg. 2010;18:528–36.
90. Stevens PM, Kennedy JM, Hung M. Guided growth for ankle valgus. J Pediatr Orthop. 2011;31:878–83.
91. Takakura Y, Takaoka T, Tanaka Y, Yajima H, Tamai S. Results of opening-wedge osteotomy for the treatment of a post-traumatic varus deformity of the ankle. J Bone Joint Surg Am. 1998;80:213–8.
92. Ferreira N, Tanwar YS. Systematic approach to the management of post-traumatic segmental diaphyseal long bone defects: treatment algorithm and comprehensive classification system. Strategies Trauma Limb Reconstr. 2020;15:106–16.
93. Masquelet AC, Begue T. The concept of induced membrane for reconstruction of long bone defects. Orthop Clin North Am. 2010;41:27–37.
94. El-Rosasy MA. Acute shortening and re-lengthening in the management of bone and soft-tissue loss in complicated fractures of the tibia. J Bone Joint Surg Br. 2007;89:80–8.
95. Tetsworth K, Paley D, Sen C, Jaffe M, Maar DC, Glatt V, et al. Bone transport versus acute shortening for the management of infected tibial non-unions with bone defects. Injury. 2017;48:2276–84.
96. Wen H, Zhu S, Li C, Xu Y. Bone transport versus acute shortening for the management of infected tibial bone defects: a meta-analysis. BMC Musculoskelet Disord. 2020;21:80.
97. Harmon PH. A simplified surgical approach to the posterior tibia for bone-grafting and fibular transference. J Bone Joint Surg Am. 1945;27:496–8.
98. Foster MJ, O'Toole RV, Manson TT. Treatment of tibial nonunion with posterolateral bone grafting. Injury. 2017;48:2242–7.
99. Weinberg H, Roth VG, Robin GC, Floman Y. Early fibular bypass procedures (tibiofibular synostosis) for massive bone loss in war injuries. J Trauma. 1979;19:177–81.
100. de Boer HH, Wood MB, Hermans J. Reconstruction of large skeletal defects by vascularized fibula transfer. Factors that influenced the outcome of union in 62 cases. Int Orthop. 1990;14:121–8.
101. Bi ZG, Han XG, Fu CJ, Cao Y, Yang CL. Reconstruction of large limb bone defects with a double-barrel free vascularized fibular graft. Chin Med J. 2008;121:2424–8.
102. Salih S, Mills E, McGregor-Riley J, Dennison M, Royston S. Transverse debridement and acute shortening followed by distraction histogenesis in the treatment of open tibial fractures with bone and soft tissue loss. Strategies Trauma Limb Reconstr. 2018;13:129–35.
103. Sigmund IK, Ferguson J, Govaert GAM, Stubbs D, McNally MA. Comparison of Ilizarov bifocal, acute shortening and relengthening with bone transport in the treatment of infected, segmental defects of the tibia. J Clin Med. 2020;9(2):279.
104. Wen H, Zhu S, Li C, Xu Y. Bone transport versus acute shortening for the management of infected tibial bone defects: a meta-analysis. BMC Musculoskelet Disord. 2020;21:1–9.
105. Catagni MA, Azzam W, Guerreschi F, Lovisetti L, Poli P, Khan M, et al. Trifocal versus bifocal bone transport in treatment of long segmental tibial bone defects: a retrospective comparative study. Bone Joint J. 2019;101:162–9.
106. Klein TJ, Malda J, Sah RL, Hutmacher DW. Tissue engineering of articular cartilage with biomimetic zones. Tissue Eng Part B Rev. 2009;15:143–57.

Bone Defects

Abdullah Addar, Reggie C. Hamdy, and Mitchell Bernstein

Definition of Bone Defects

A critical-sized bone defect is best defined as a defect that will not heal spontaneously despite adequate surgical stabilization. Controversy exists in the literature regarding the most accurate manner in determining a critical-sized defect; however, a reliable method is one with a defect greater than 1–2 cm in length and more than 50% of the circumference [1]. Attempts to standardize the quantification of bone defects have been made. A study of patients with post-traumatic bone loss formalized the quantification of bone defects via a measurement termed radiographic apparent bone gap (RABG). The size is obtained by measuring the length of the defect on all four cortices (anterior, posterior, medial, and lateral) and dividing it by 4. It was found that all patients with a RABG $\geq$ 25 mm developed a non-union, whereas those with a RABG <25 mm united with >50% probability [2]. Variables affecting the success of spontaneous healing include whether they occur in skeletally immature patients, the size of the defect, the bone segment affected, the integrity of soft tissues, etiology, and associated comorbidities [3].

The other cause of confusion is the lack of clear differentiation between a bone defect and a non-union. In both bone defects and non-unions there is a lack of a solid bony contact between the bone edges with varying area sizes. However, a bone defect is a circumstance in which there is adequate biological healing potential and mechanical stability but an incapacity to fill in the defect, a non-union, by contrast, is a circumstance in which there is an impaired biological healing potential or mechanical instability, so that once the biological or mechanical issue is resolved the bone will unite. Reports on bone defects involving skeletally immature children do not provide any unique definition that is different from skeletally mature patients [4] [5].

Etiology and Classification

Bone defects occur after trauma, infection, tumour resection, or congenital causes such as congenital pseudoarthrosis of the tibia (CPT). Bone defects in children are uncommon and most frequently occur in the lower extremity (Tibia, femur, fibula) [4] [6]. Generally, the classification should include location within the bone (articular, metaphyseal, and diaphyseal), length of defect, and the amount of circumferential bone loss [3]. Another classification scheme proposed is the Orthopedic Trauma Association Open Fracture Classification System (OTA-OFC) (Fig. 39.1) [7]. In this system, defects are classified into incomplete (cortical discontinuity), subcritical (<2 cm), or critical size defects ($\geq$ 2 cm). This classification has been found to have excellent inter–and intra-

A. Addar (✉)
Department of Orthopaedics, King Saud University, Riyadh, Saudi Arabia
e-mail: aaddar@ksu.edu.sa

R. C. Hamdy
Department of Pediatric Surgery, McGill University Health Center, Montreal, QC, Canada

Shriners Hospital for Children-Canada, Montreal, QC, Canada
e-mail: rhamdy@shriners.mcgill.ca

M. Bernstein
Shriners Hospital for Children-Canada, Montreal, QC, Canada

Department of Surgery and Pediatric Surgery, McGill University, Montreal, QC, Canada

Montreal Children's Hospital, Montreal, QC, Canada

Montreal General Hospital, Montreal, QC, Canada
e-mail: mitchell.bernstein@mcgill.ca

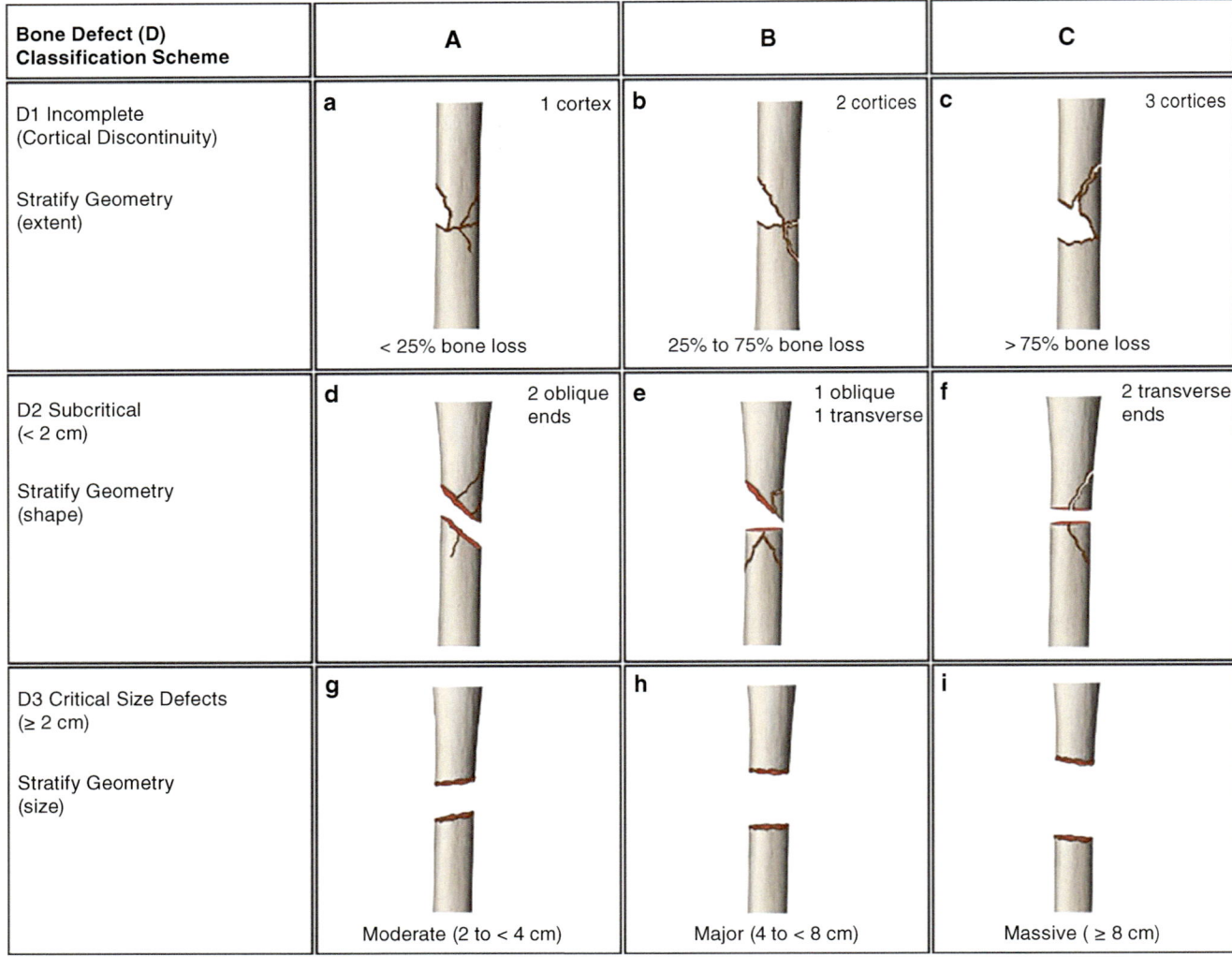

Fig. 39.1 The bone defect classification scheme was described by Tetsworth et al. There are three major categories: D1 (a-c), D2 (d-f), and D3 (g-i). These categories are based upon the size of the defect (incomplete, subcritical, and critical) and the local geometry of the defect. Image adapted with permission from Tetsworth et al. Classification of Bone Defects: An Extension of the Orthopaedic Trauma Association Open Fracture Classification. J Orthop Trauma 2021;35:71–76) DOI: 10.1097/BOT.0000000000001896

observer reliability. However, it still does not provide a guide for treating bone defects, and it is not clear if and how articular defects fit into the scheme.

Evaluation Specific to Bone Defects

Clinical Evaluation

The first issue for the surgeon is the etiology and context in which bone loss occurred. Is this an acute trauma-related bone defect, whether from extrusion of bone or post-debridement? Alternatively, is it chronic osteomyelitis or sarcoma that will need radical excision, resulting in a bone defect? The physical examination is obviously important; the soft tissues' status and the limb's vascular supply are critical to determine as they can shift the treatment pathway considerably. For example, the anterior tibial and peroneal arteries must be intact for vascularized proximal fibula and diaphyseal fibular transfer, respectively [8] [9]. Another aspect is the patient's social support and economic means. This is particularly important in selecting a limb reconstruction plan. Patients with a good social support system and reliable transportation to facilitate regular clinic visits are more amenable to complex treatment strategies, such as bone transport techniques.

Ring external fixators (Ilizarov or hexapod) require strut adjustments, intense physical therapy, clinic appointments for strut changes, and pin site management [10, 11]. In children and adolescents, both first-hand and second-hand smoking must be evaluated and addressed. There is evidence that counselling parents to stop smoking for the benefit of their children might be effective in parental smoking cessation which will help the healing process in bone defects [12]. The economic status and access to healthcare is also a determining factor for bone defect reconstruction; in settings, however patients have limited access to surgical services, single-stage surgery such as primary bone grafting, fibula-pro-tibia, acute shortening, or amputation might be preferable to multiple-stage surgeries. Vitamin D deficiency is an established cause of skeletal pathologies such as rickets, genu varum/valgum, bone pain [13], and fractures [14]; therefore, nutritional status and optimization of vitamin D levels before and throughout the bony reconstruction process are recommended [13]. Another issue is protein malnutrition; currently, there is no precise determination of its prevalence in limb reconstruction; however, it would be prudent to test for protein malnutrition in patients undergoing major limb reconstruction via serum lab levels of albumin and prealbumin [10]. Obesity in children is rising, and its detrimental effects on pediatric bone health are becoming more evident, such as decreased bone mineral density [14].

Identifying if residual infection exists is essential. The success of limb reconstruction will be affected if not treated and cured [15]. How to determine if infection is eradicated is still of debate; however, assessing the clinical picture from soft tissue healing, laboratory markers such as serial C-reactive protein (CRP) measurements, intraoperative inspection, and bone biopsy will aid in making a diagnosis.

Radiographic Evaluation

Orthogonal calibrated plain films of the limb segment are obtained to assess bone defects accurately. It is beneficial to ask the radiology technicians to place the entire bone on one cassette. This can aid in accurately measuring coronal and sagittal malalignment. Additionally, pelvis to floor (hip-to-ankle) weight-bearing films are also valuable to measure coronal limb malalignment and limb length discrepancies. The radiographic assessment might still be spurious due to the apparent geometry of bone defects from displacement. Therefore, the best reduction possible needs to be obtained for a defect to be measured accurately; this is done intraop-

Fig. 39.2 The RABG is a method of standardizing bone defect measurements, it takes into account the size of the defect on all four cortices and then divides it by 4 to get an average of the defect. Adapted with permission from Hainnes et al. Defining the Lower Limit of a "Critical Bone Defect" in Open Diaphyseal Tibial Fractures. J Orthop Trauma 2016;30:e158–e163). DOI: https://doi.org/10.1097/BOT.0000000000000531

Medial Cortex	Lateral Cortex	Anterior Cortex	Posterior Cortex	RABG
20 mm	0 mm	0 mm	0 mm	5 mm

Medial Cortex	Lateral Cortex	Anterior Cortex	Posterior Cortex	RABG
10 mm	0 mm	0 mm	20 mm	7.5 mm

Medial Cortex	Lateral Cortex	Anterior Cortex	Posterior Cortex	RABG
10 mm	10 mm	10 mm	10 mm	10 mm

Medial Cortex	Lateral Cortex	Anterior Cortex	Posterior Cortex	RABG
20 mm	0 mm	20 mm	0 mm	10 mm

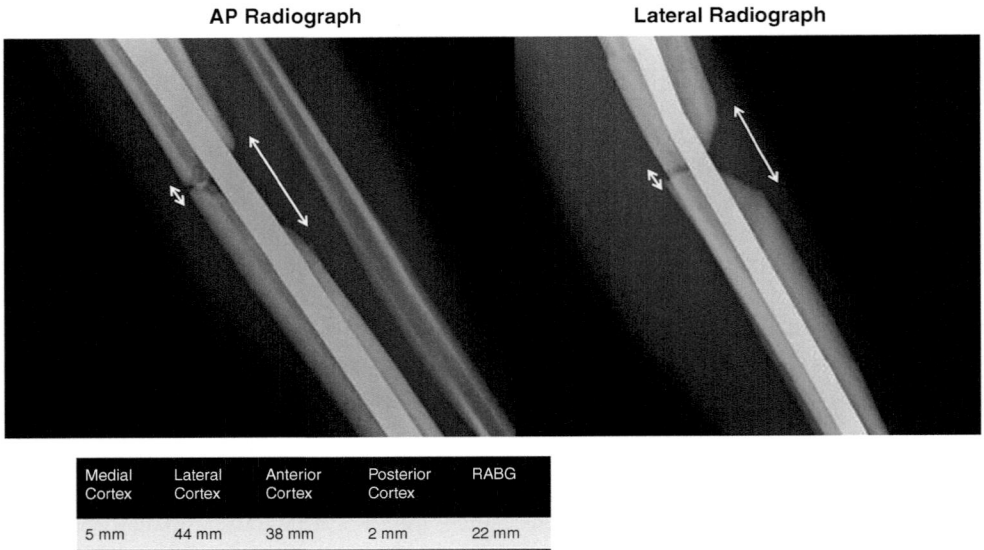

Fig. 39.3 The longitudinal length of the bone defect on all four cortices was measured and divided by 4 to yield an average result. Adapted with permission from Hainnes et al. Defining the Lower Limit of a "Critical Bone Defect" in Open Diaphyseal Tibial Fractures. J Orthop Trauma 2016;30:e158–e163). DOI: https://doi.org/10.1097/BOT.0000000000000531

eratively or after surgery in staged approaches to bone defects [7]. Once accurate films are obtained, a RABG can be measured; this is done as mentioned previously by measuring all four cortices and dividing them by four (Figs. 39.2 and 39.3) [2]. Computed tomography (CT) with three-dimensional (3D) reformatting is helpful in further defining articular bone defects [16].

Treatment of Bone Defects

Goals

In addressing bone defects, the goal is to achieve a bony union that allows patients to use their limbs with minimal morbidity. The "Diamond Concept" is a culmination of four factors contributing equally to bony union: the presence of osteogenic cells, growth factors, an osteoconductive scaffold, and mechanical stability; this concept serves as a guide to treatment [17].

Spontaneous Regeneration

The spontaneous regeneration of bony defects is reported in both skeletally immature and mature patients, may occur in different bones from the cranium to the foot, and in various sizes up to 20 cm [18–20]. This phenomenon can be attributed partially back to the Diamond Concept [17], where osteogenic cells arise from the cambium layer of the periosteum, growth factors are delivered from the ensuing hematoma, and mechanical stability is provided via surgical fixation. Regarding an osteoconductive scaffold, most cases reported did not have any scaffold. This could be due to excellent stabilization combined with favourable patient biology, namely, young with at least partially intact periosteum. Practically speaking, none (except for fibular graft harvest cases) were done intentionally in all reports on spontaneous regeneration; instead, there was a cause to delay definitive bone defect management, from soft tissue coverage and infection, to missing visits. Factors contributing to spontaneous regeneration elucidated include younger age, periosteal preservation, etiology (post-traumatic/post-infectious), traumatic brain injury (TBI), and mechanical stability [20].

Most patients reported were younger on average. Additionally, the time to regeneration in patients ≤ 18 years was almost half those >18 years (2.83 vs. 4.87 months). Periosteal preservation was the case in most patients, but not all. The periosteum's role in providing osteogenic cells and the blood supply is evident. All cases reported had mechanical stability and restored bone length via surgical fixation, with notable exceptions for fibular [21] and cranial bone regeneration [19]. Some of the cases had synthetic factors such as calcium sulphate bone substitute, but the use of these factors was inconsistent. It hence cannot be generalized to be a factor that reliably helps bony regeneration. Factoring spontaneous bone regeneration into the management scheme for bone defects must be further studied, and it cannot be relied upon as the primary treatment plan. However, in some cases in which reconstruction will be delayed, it is worthy of observing. Clear patterns emerging in spontaneous bone regeneration include stabilizing the bone segment mechanically, evaluating positive prognosticators (younger age, periosteal integrity, TBI), serial assessments via imaging and clinically in the cases of reoperation, and having a definitive management plan for the bone defect management in any case.

Considerations for Successful Bone Defect Reconstruction

Developing a treatment plan for a successful bone defect reconstruction entails a complex decision-making process. This process must consider multiple factors, and the weight of each element varies according to the clinical context. Additionally, before selecting and commencing a treatment pathway, the surgeon and patient must define a target goal that determines success. Typically, the first consideration is the etiology of the bone defect. In congenital bone defects, there is a higher likelihood of complications such as soft tissue contractures and non-union. Conversely, in post-traumatic defects, the risk of infection is high. Hence, the primary consideration is to prevent or eradicate infection primarily before undergoing any complex surgical reconstruction. Similarly, in post-tumour cases, the prevention of tumour recurrence is of prime importance. The other consideration is the bone segment involved; tibial defects are more amenable to techniques employing circular fixators, and femoral defects are better managed with intramedullary (IM) nailing techniques when possible. Soft tissue coverage is a primary determinant that imposes a heavy weight in decision-making; if compromised, the options are veered towards acute shortening and re-lengthening (ASRL) or composite free-fibula vascularized transfer (FFVA) (osteomusculocutaneous flap) as these techniques can address both the soft tissue and skeletal defect effectively. Defects that are 5 cm and less are best managed with autogenous bone grafting (ABG), whereas those above 5 cm can employ any of the different techniques other than ABG. The surgeon must also gauge the patient's tolerance with reconstruction, as a patient who cannot tolerate a complex treatment will benefit more from a single-stage procedure if feasible than a multi-stage procedure. Finally, the treating team's resources, from surgeon experience to hospital setting, treatment affordability, and cost-effectiveness, must also be factored in.

Techniques

Bone Grafting

Bone grafting is a process in which bone is transplanted serving as a biological or mechanical function or both, with the goal of achieving a bony union. The biological function is subdivided into osteogenesis (formation of new bone via osteogenic cells), osteoconduction (formation of a scaffold that guides skeletal growth), osteoinduction (growth factors that convert stem cells into osteoblasts and chondroblasts), and in the case of vascularized grafts that provide blood supply. The mechanical function varies from solid mechanical support in cortical grafts to minimal support with cancellous grafts [22].

Autograft vs. Allograft Bone: Autogenous bone graft is superior in the biological function provided as it is osteogenic, osteoconductive, and osteoinductive. Additionally, there is no concern for histocompatibility. The main drawback of autogenous bone graft is donor site morbidity (pain, infection, hematoma, blood loss, and nerve injury) and limited supply, especially in children with notable exceptions that include the Iliac decancellization procedure and vascularized fibula bone graft which provides an excellent amount of bone and excellent biological and mechanical function (refer to section for more details). Allograft bone avoids donor site complications and is abundant but comes with a small risk of transmissible diseases. In most cases, allograft bone is mainly used for mechanical support as it has a poor biological function; therefore, it has limited bone defect management benefits [23]. Exceptions to using allograft for bone defect management include mixing allograft with autograft bone to increase the volume of bone with the induced-membrane technique (IMT) [24], and in the case of an osteoarticular bone defect in which structural support is needed to preserve the geometry and reconstruct articular surfaces [25].

Autograft Specifics: The main indication of non-vascularized bone autograft is in bone defects that are up to 5 cm. Defects above 5 cm and treated with bone grafting undergo significant resorption [26, 27].

Sites to harvest autograft bone include the iliac crest, greater trochanter, proximal tibia, distal tibia, calcaneus distal radius, and IM canal via the reamer-irrigator-aspirator (RIA) device [23, 28]. Iliac crest bone graft (ICBG) is the most used harvest site and provides cancellous and corticocancellous bone graft. The volume of harvest is typically 13 cm^3 for anterior ICBG and 30 cm^3 for posterior ICBG. These volumes can be increased to 90 cm^3 using the acetabular reamer technique. Both anterior and posterior ICBG harvest sites can be done on the same patient, but positioning of the patient must be adjusted to accommodate [23]. The acetabular reamer technique utilizes a low-speed, high-torque reamer, typically 40–42 mm in diameter, and then, the inner or outer ilium is reamed. The harvest via this technique is faster and has proven clinical outcomes in obtaining union. This technique in skeletally immature patients is limited due to the reamer size and risk of apophysis injury [29]. Another technique described by Paley et al. [30] is the iliac decancellization procedure which has been described for skeletally immature patients. This technique involves splitting the iliac crest apophysis and then taking a thin osteotome and splitting the ilium down the middle till it reaches the acetabular dome and triradiate cartilage anteriorly and the sacroiliac joint posteriorly and then curetting the cancellous bone. This technique is reported to provide between 20 and 45 cc of bone graft. Additionally, there is an option to obtain a periosteal graft which can be meshed to increase its volume. Due to a large amount of bone being removed, it is recommended to backfill the harvest area with a bone substitute such as calcium phosphate.

The RIA technique utilizes a unique IM reaming device that allows for irrigation and aspiration; it traps the reamed bone graft via a suction trap mechanism [28]. Volumes harvested have been reported between 30 and 90 cm^3 from the femur and tibia. The quality of the harvest is rich in stem cells and growth factors and might be superior to ICBG and has been proven clinically in obtaining union. Entry into the femoral canal is recommended to be antegrade via the greater trochanter to avoid injury to the femoral neck; the tibia is also entered antegrade similar to IM nailing of the tibia [31]. No studies using RIA are present to date on skeletally immature patients, but this method can be used in mature patients or those nearing skeletal maturity; it is especially indicated in cases of prior ICBG, insufficient volume from other sites, and sites with higher infection risk. The main drawback of RIA is the risk of blood loss from continued aspiration. Other hazards include eccentric reaming, resulting in iatrogenic fractures and incarceration of the reamer [23]. The other sites mentioned (proximal and distal tibia, calcaneus, greater trochanter, and distal radius) are mainly used to obtain cancellous bone graft from the metaphysis when the recipient site is near the harvest site. The metaphysis is accessed with a small bone window which is preferably made circular to limit the risk of a stress-riser and avoid injury to the nearby joint surface or any important neighbouring structures. The main limitation of these sites regarding bone defects is the limited supply of bone ranging from 3 cm^3 to 10 cm^3 [31].

Intraoperative handling of autogenous bone graft: Harvesting autogenous bone graft is done near or immediately before transplantation at the donor site, as open-air might be determinantal to its properties. While waiting for implantation, place the harvested autograft in normal saline, dextrose 5% solution, or wet gauze [23]. Another element to consider is mixing bone grafts with antibiotics. This combination has the theoretical advantage of managing dead space created by bone defects coupled with biological healing potential and local delivery of antibiotics, resulting in superior infection control and bony union. The main concern with mixing antibiotics and bone graft is the possible antibiotic cytotoxic effect, with mixed results reported in the literature depending on the type and dose of antibiotics. Some studies have shown that with appropriate doses, antibiotics mixed with autograft are not harmful to union [32] and, in some cases, even beneficial in preventing infection recurrence [33]. However, the fracture-related infection (FRI) group has reviewed local antibiotic delivery and dead space management for FRI and given the paucity of high-quality studies, it does not recommend mixing antibiotics with autograft as the standard of care [34].

Induced-Membrane Technique (IMT)

The IMT, as described by Masquelet, is suited for bone defects 6 cm and larger. The IMT procedure has been described for both children and adults and for various etiologies [24]. Although not restrictive, IMT in children is mainly reported for post-tumour and congenital pseudoarthrosis reconstruction; in adults, it is used chiefly for post-traumatic or post-infectious reconstruction [6]. The procedure encompasses a 2-stage approach to yield an induced-membrane, which creates a vascularized insulated chamber that protects the bone graft from resorption and is rich in osteoinductive growth factors promoting bony unions such as VEGF, TGF beta, and BMP-2. The first stage involves bony and soft tissue debridement, mechanical stabilization, and cement spacer application. Debridement is done by eliminating all pathological tissues and reaching the healthy bleeding bone. This step is of utmost importance as reports of residual infection in infectious cases have been reported when inadequate debridement was performed leading to further morbidity [6]. The second stage involves removing the cement spacer and applying a morselized cancellous bone autograft (Fig. 39.4).

Mechanical stabilization can be achieved via various means, including using external fixators, plates, IM nails, or elastic nails. An important caveat is that the fixation must be solid, as unstable fixation is a predictor of failure of IMT [35]. Cement preparation and application are also critical parts of the first stage. Poor technique is a risk factor for failure and complications. The poly-methyl-methyl-acrylate (PMMA) cement is typically placed alone; however, it can be mixed with antibiotics in post-infectious reconstruction cases. Proper cement application necessitates that it is done after stabilization, and a material that will act as a mold to contain the cement (i.e., syringe split in half) is placed around the bone defect. When the cement is applied, a helpful technical tip is to make the cement spacer wider than the defect and extending on both ends to cover the bone edges; this will facilitate clear identification of the membrane for the second stage and enable the repair of the membrane. The timing of the second stage is at 6–8 weeks in most instances, as this allows enough time for soft tissue and flap healing [36]. In post-tumour reconstruction cases where chemotherapy courses are needed, delays of 8 months and more have yielded good outcomes, typically 6–8 weeks from the last course of chemotherapy. This delay is necessary to decrease the risk of infection as the patient recovers from any neutropenia and to prevent any cytotoxic effect on osteoblasts that might delay union [37]. In animal studies, it was found that

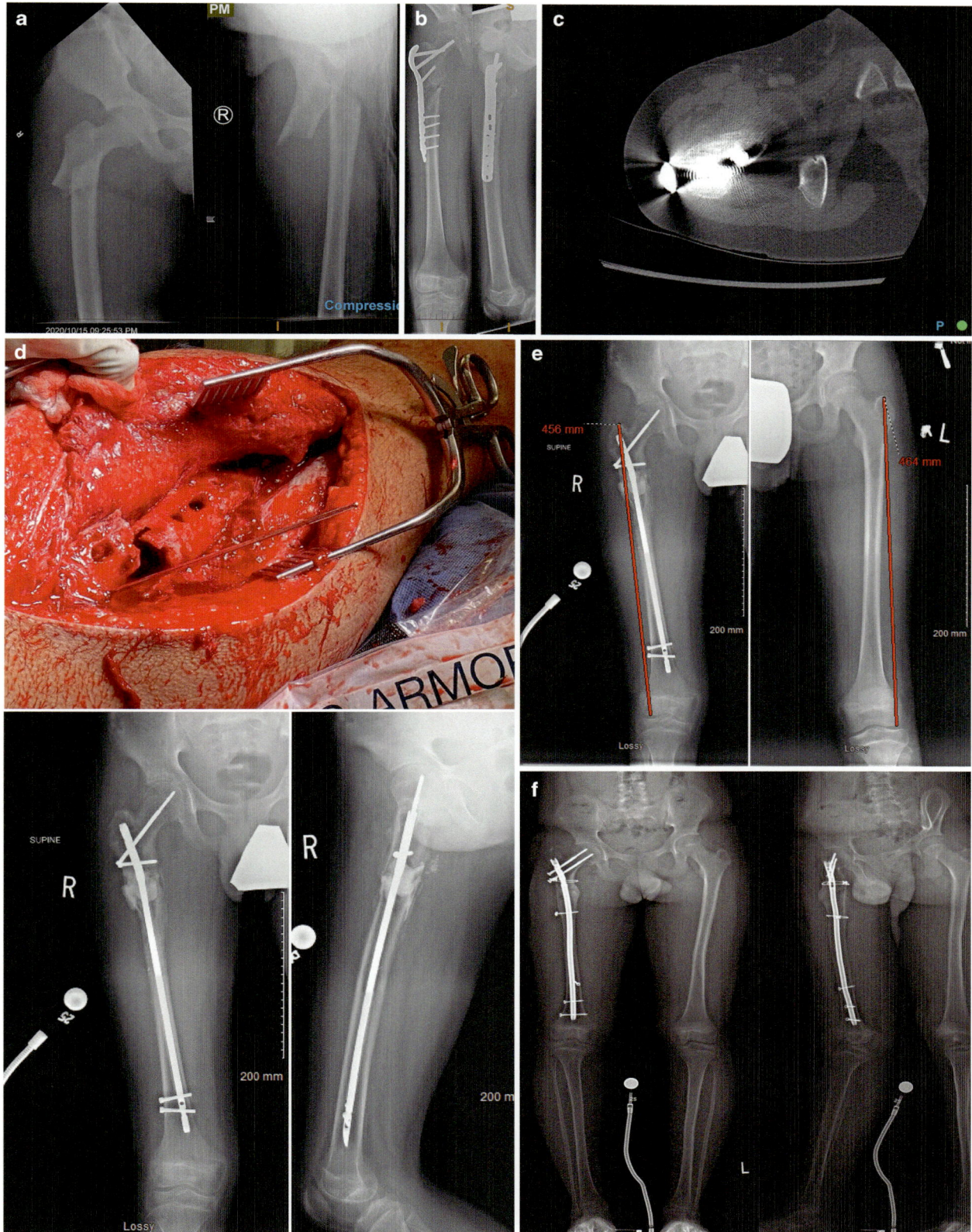

Fig. 39.4 (a) Twelve-year-old male who sustained a left femur subtrochanteric pathological fracture due to solitary fibrous dysplasia. (b) Underwent primary internal fixation with a proximal femur plate. (c) After a period of persistent pain, investigations revealed the development of osteomyelitis with an associated abscess. (d) Treatment included removal of the proximal femoral plate, bony debridement till healthy bleeding bone was encountered and implantation of an antibiotic coated intramedullary nail. The resultant bone defect was filled with cement and treated with the induced membrane technique. (e) Prior to the second stage, a contralateral femur image was obtained, the femoral length discrepancy was 10 mm, and the bone defect was 48 mm; thereby, the final bone defect size was 58 mm. (f) Final orthogonal images at the end of treatment with progressive healing of the bone defect and equalized limb lengths

the maximum amount of growth factors released by the IMT is at 4 weeks [38]; however, this is not practical, as mentioned above. The bone graft used for the second stage is mainly obtained from the iliac crests, the volume of which can be increased by mixing it with allograft in a 3:1 ratio [24]. Growth factors are avoided for pediatric IMT cases as most are post-tumour resection or cases of CPT, where growth factors might promote recurrence risk [6].

Advantages of IMT include low cost, as it consumes material found in most orthopedic settings, and there is no need for advanced microsurgical skills. Additionally, IMT has been described for different bony segments other than the lower extremities, including the clavicle [39], humerus, and forearm bones [6, 40]. The main disadvantages include prolonged union time (37 weeks) and a staged approach that often needs supplementary procedures in 30–40% of cases. Complications of IMT occur in up to 54% of pediatric patients and include fixation failure, fracture, nonunion, mal-union, impaired wound healing, and stiffness [6]. Risk factors of IMT failure have been studied, and it was found that patients were more likely to fail if they were male, had malignancy as an underlying diagnosis, had a femoral bone defect, had a larger area of resection, required delaying the second stage, had autogenous bone mixed with allograft, or had unstable fixation as deemed by the treating surgeon [35]. Unfortunately, at this time, there are no regression analyses or risk ratios that allow the true impact of each of these factors to be determined, but this is an area of active study.

Acute Shortening and re-Lengthening (ASRL)

The advances in distraction osteogenesis (DO) have enabled surgeons more freedom in managing bone defects, with acute shortening and re-lengthening (ASRL) being one option. This technique is versatile as the surgeon can shorten the limb, correct angulation, and even lengthen the limb at a later once the bone defect has healed. Acute shortening alone is well described to manage bone defects in both the upper and lower extremities. Shortening up to 3 cm in the humerus might be well tolerated [41, 42]. In the lower extremities, tolerance for shortening alone is less, given the impact on weight-bearing and the difficulty in obtaining accurate measurements, especially since that in most instances, this procedure is done in the setting of acute trauma. The indications to perform ASRL are in the setting of acute trauma, especially when complicated with soft tissue loss, and in bone defects resulting from the debridement of an infected non-union [43]. In the case of soft tissue loss with acute trauma, ASRL enables DO and distraction histogenesis; this makes ASRL unique in which the orthopedic surgeon can obtain wound closure primarily or with skin graft and regional flaps. In most cases, it spares the need for free tissue transfer with its associated complexity and potential complications [44]. The versatility provided via ASRL is also evident in which angulation can be added to achieve wound closure. Once the injury has healed, angular correction can be performed concurrently with lengthening using the fixator. Another option to correct the angulation is to use guided growth after the lengthening is completed. The amount of bone shortening possible is limited mainly by the limb's vascular supply. In skeletally mature patients, referenced numbers for tibial shortening by El-Rosasy et al. [43] are 3 cm for the upper third of the leg, 3–5 cm for the middle third, and < 6 cm for the lower third. Betz et al. [45] reported that for adult patients with acute traumatic bone loss in addition to neurovascular injury, the limit for ASRL is 15 cm and recommended that amputation be done for defects larger than that. More recent reports have reached amounts of shortening of 8 cm in skeletally immature and mature patients, with no negative consequences on vascularity [5]. In their series, Yokoyama et al. [46] demonstrated that when >25% of the bone is shortened using ASRL for type IIIB tibial fractures, quality-of-life scores are impaired, even after lengthening. Atbasi et al. [47] performed angiography post ASRL for their patients with acute tibial shortening; they found that 4 cm of shortening had no impact on arterial configuration, there was minimal arterial bending with 4–6 cm of shortening, and there was arterial tortuosity with shortening up to 8 cm. There was no arterial kinking in any patient, and the changes were maintained for 2 years. Since ASRL is primarily chosen in a traumatic setting, there is a chance of physeal injury or arrest. Therefore, it is imperative when lengthening to assess the physis viability and to account for any physeal arrest when lengthening, and not simply equalize the current LLD, but account for the potential LLD at skeletal maturity.

Technical tips for tibial ASRL: Examine the limb's vasculature via ultrasound Doppler documenting the patent vessels and their signal intensity (triphasic, biphasic, and monophasic) as well as hallux pulse oximetry before starting [44]. The skin incisions are never longitudinal and should be transverse at the site of the intended union if the shortening will be <5 cm, or Z-shaped if the lengthening is ≥ 5 cm, or the skin is compromised [43]. After preparing the bone edges, the bone is shortened until complete bony contact. Adding angulation can also be done to achieve the best soft tissue closure, but if the angulation is severe, then planning a skin graft or regional flap can be done [48]. Pulses must be checked frequently through the shortening. If the circulation is impaired at any point, then reverse the shortening until restoration of circulation is achieved and plan for gradual shortening of 2–3 mm/day postoperatively until the complete contact is achieved. The fibula must be partially resected (lesser magnitude than tibia) to allow tibial shortening and will overlap after shortening is completed; additionally, the resection should be far from the tibial defect site. If the cause of surgery is non-union, apply bone graft simultaneously. Fixation with a circular fixator is optimal as it allows maximum versatility for lengthening, shortening if needed, and angular correction. Creating a distant tibial corticotomy to allow bone transport is done at the index procedure or delayed as preferred.

A vital link to appreciate is that both bone transport (BT) and ASRL are based upon DO, as described by Gavriil Ilizarov. Comparing BT and ASRL has been studied in comparative studies. Tetsworth et al. [49] studied both techniques for infected tibial non-unions; the authors found that ASRL had 50% fewer complications than BT; however, there was no difference in EFI and clinical outcomes. The authors concluded that ASRL was best for bone defects <3 cm and BT was best for those >10 cm. Sen et al. [50] studied BT and ASRL on bone defects due to femoral non-unions. All the patients had bone defects from 3 cm to 10 cm. They found that ASRL had a shorter EFI by 35%, fewer complications, and less bone grafting of the docking site.

Bone Transport

BT relies on the four phases of DO described by Ilizarov. Phase 1 is performing a low-energy osteotomy, which is ideally in the metaphyseal bone to allow the best regenerate to form. Phase 2 is the latency phase in which the bone segment is undisturbed for 7–10 days in the femur and 10–14 days in tibial cases, to allow the maturation of the hematoma into early callus at the osteoplasty site. Phase 3 is the distraction phase, in which the osteotomy site and the bone segment are transported at a regular rate and rhythm, often starting at 1 mm/day, divided into four 0.25 mm increments. The transport can be done either antegrade or retrograde depending on the integrity of the surrounding soft tissues. Finally, phase 4 is the consolidation phase which in BT comprises both regenerate maturation and docking site union. The docking site frequently needs supplementary bone grafting, and some authors recommend this routinely [51]. The bone segment transported has a leading and trailing edge; the leading edge crosses the defect site gradually and closes it by achieving contact at the docking site; the trailing edge is where the regenerate bone forms. The hallmark feature of BT, which differentiates it from limb lengthening, is that there is no change in overall limb length since the fixation device is applied at the limb's entire length and the BT occurs within the boundaries of the device. In other words, the formation of the regenerated bone will be equal to the bone defect size. Bone transport is advantageous in filling more significant bony defects (>8 cm) with reliable union rates, producing native high-quality bone [52, 53]. The main issues with BT are the length of treatment time and skin complications when using a circular fixator [54]. In most BT cases, a circular fixator guides the transported segment, which is moved along the fixator via either a suspension-wire technique or a central cable bone transport (CBT) system. This entire BT process then can be augmented with fixation using a nail or a plate done during or after the BT process. If sufficient healing is present, the surgeon may choose to forego augmentation. When using a circular fixator for BT, the external fixation index (EFI) is high at about 1.5–2 cm/month for adults [55] and 0.8 cm/month for skeletally immature patients [56]; this is still a significant time for children, especially considering that frequent follow-ups are needed. Skin complications include pin site infections and skin invagination at the docking site. Skin invagination at the docking site is a unique problem with bone transport. Methods to mitigate its development include suspending the skin at the docking site with a suture and tying it to the fixator, or even using Ilizarov wires to suspend the skin. If the invagination develops, some surgeons have simply gone slowly through the invaginated area and prior to docking, they have the flap elevated with the help of a plastic surgeon. It is in the author's experience, although not published, that managing the defect at the docking site proactively with a cement spacer, along with adequate debridement and soft tissue coverage, and once the transported segment has reached the docking site, the cement spacer will be removed and bone graft applied, this technique has resulted in avoiding this complication. Other complications include joint stiffness, axial deviation, residual LLD, delayed union at the docking site, regenerate fracture, and hardware loosening/breakage (Fig. 39.5) [54]. Advancements in techniques of BT enabled shortening of treatment time; these include multifocal BT [57], transport and then nailing (TATN) [58], bone transport over a nail (BTON) [59], bone transport over a plate (BTOP) [60], integrated fixation [61] (CBT and BTON), and all internal BT techniques [62–64]. Union rates with all of these techniques range between 77% and 100%. Multifocal bone transport, usually either bifocal or trifocal, significantly decreases the EFI by about 2.5x, and trifocal transport is 25% less than bifocal. Additionally, there are fewer complications associated with trifocal BT, mainly due to shortened time in the fixator [57]. An important consideration is that multifocal transport does not decrease fixation time proportionate to the number of osteotomies. This is

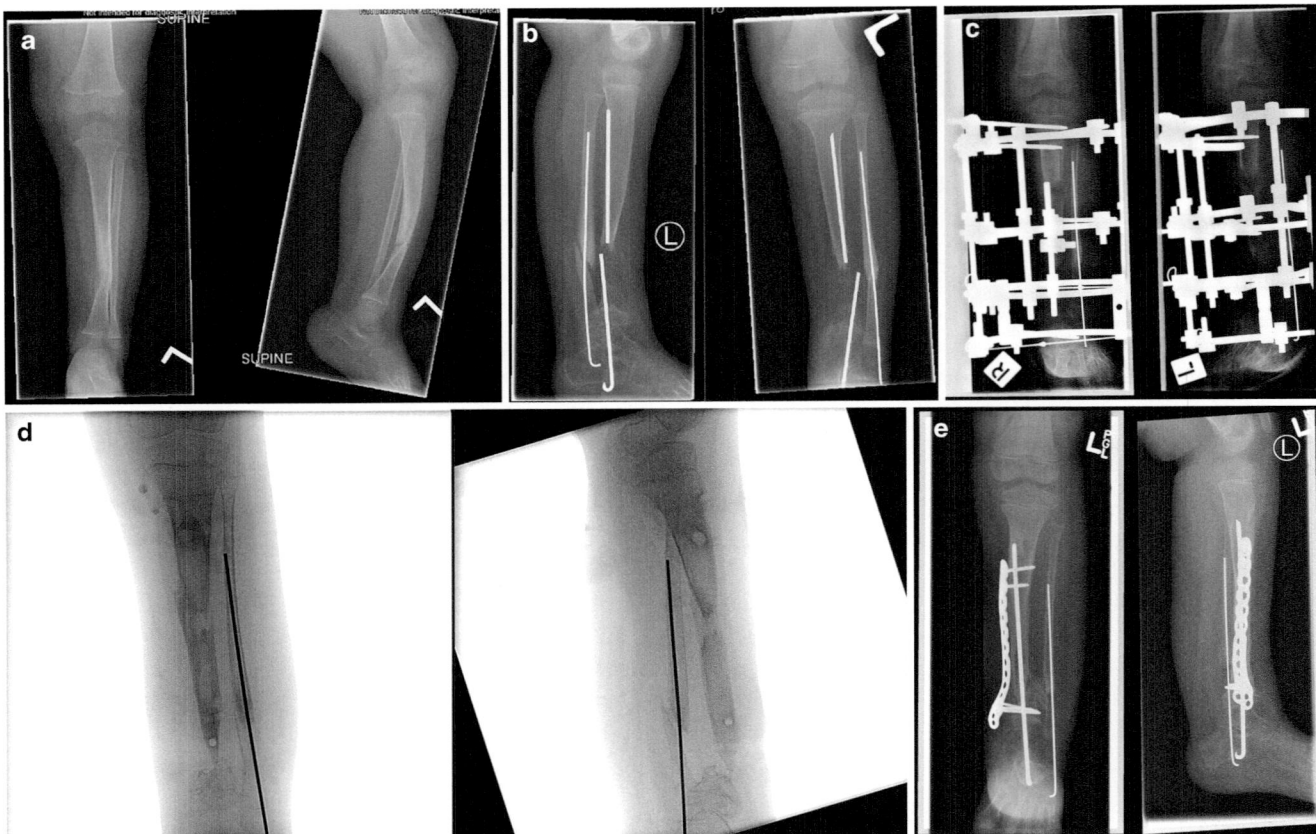

Fig. 39.5 (a) Four-year-old female with Type 1 Neurofibromatosis and congenital pseudoarthrosis of the tibia. (b) Underwent two failed attempts of reconstruction with bone grafting and fixation with a plate once and with Rush rods on the second attempt. (c) Bone transport with an Ilizarov fixator was performed. (d) During follow-ups, docking site non-union was suspected and confirmed on intraoperative imaging. (e) Reconstruction was ultimately successful with autogenous bone grafting and dual intramedullary and extramedullary internal fixation

due to making one of the osteotomies at the diaphysis, which is biologically inferior to the well-vascularized and rapidly healing metaphysis. Also, the distraction rate will need to be reduced, allowing the leading skin pins/wires to heal as they tend to ulcerate with the amount of physiological stress placed on the limb. Internal bone transport (IBT) completely supplants the use of external fixation and all its associated morbidity. Variations of IBT include plate-assisted bone segment transport (PABST) [62] and Cylinder-Kombi-Tube module (CKTST) (Figs. 39.6 and 39.7) [64], also known as MagicTube [63]. In PABST, locking plates fixate the bone segment at the entire length, while a motorized lengthening nail (MLN) is fixed to the segment to be transported, and then, the transport occurs via the MLN. In the case of MagicTube, it is designed as a sleeve that acts as a runway for the MLN. The area of overlap between the MLN and MagicTube is then locked, capturing the segment of transport, the MagicTube, and the MLN. The distal end of the MagicTube is locked distal to the docking site via screws. Oleson et al. [62] described in a series the results of PABST performed on femora and tibiae. The union rate was 78%, and the consolidation index (CI) for the femora was 0.9 mo/cm compared to 1.26 mo/cm for the tibiae. This is less than Ilizarov-type BT which stands at 1.85 mo/cm. Issues to using PABST are implant size limitations and the potential risk of infection, as many patients needing BT are victims of trauma and open fractures. The challenge then becomes in delaying the definitive BT procedure and ensuring eradication of the infection. The MagicTube was reported [64] as a case report on a single 74-year-old male, and hence, more study will be needed to determine its performance.

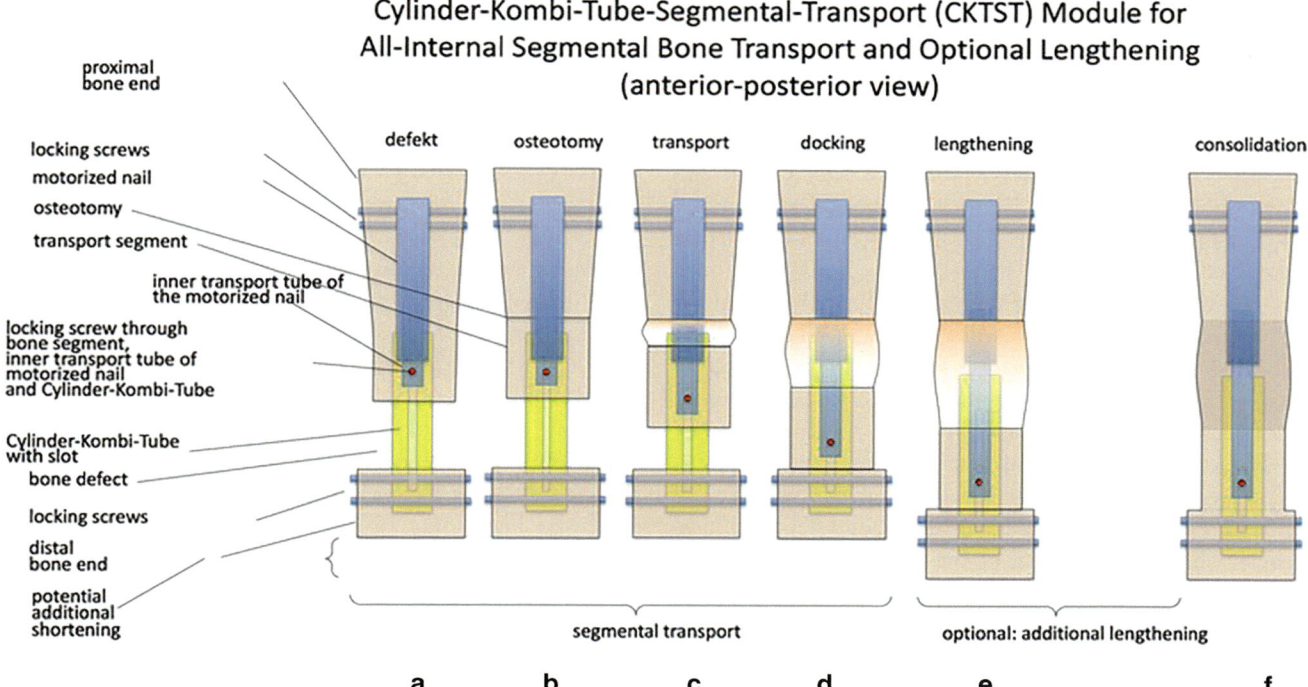

Fig. 39.6 A diagram representation of the CKTST module. (**a**) Example bone defect with motorized nail and CKTST attached. (**b**) Osteotomy for transport performed. (**c**) Bone transport started. (**d**) Transported segment reached docking site. (**e**) Additional lengthening performed. (**f**) Consolidation of the transported segment. Adapted with permission from Krettek et al. All Internal Segmental Bone Transport and Optional Lengthening With a Newly Developed Universal Cylinder-Kombi-Tube Module for Motorized Nails—Description of a Surgical Technique. J Orthop Trauma 2017;31:S39–S41) DOI: 10.1097/BOT.0000000000000986

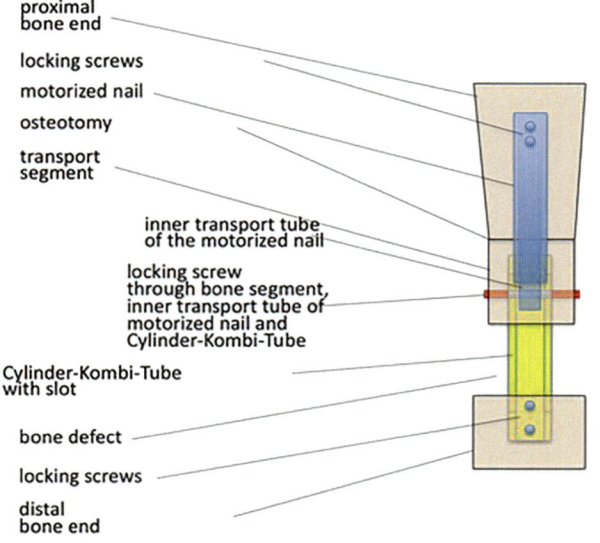

Fig. 39.7 Lateral view of CKTST module, the module is composed of a cylinder that has a holding site for the motorized nail and locking screws to hold both sides of the bone defect. Adapted with permission from Krettek et al. All Internal Segmental Bone Transport and Optional Lengthening With a Newly Developed Universal Cylinder-Kombi-Tube Module for Motorized Nails—Description of a Surgical Technique. J Orthop Trauma 2017;31:S39–S41) DOI: 10.1097/BOT.0000000000000986

Ipsilateral Fibula Transposition

The tibia is the most common location for bone defects [52], and hence, the fibula, whether ipsilateral or contralateral in cases of free fibula transfers, acts as an ideal bone substitute. Ipsilateral fibula transposition (IFT), also known as "Fibula-Pro-Tibia" and the Huntington procedure [65], is a time-tested procedure that is inexpensive and does not require microsurgical skills or advanced implants; it is ideal for tibial bone defects, especially in children [66]. It is also utilized in adults with success [67]. The forearm version of this procedure is termed one-bone-forearm (OBF) [68]. Ipsilateral fibula transposition has been used in post-traumatic, post-infectious, and post-benign or low-grade malignant tumour bone defects. It is preferably avoided in malignant tumour cases due to the risk of contamination. Ipsilateral fibula transfer is considered a semi-vascularized transfer as the fibula is transposed with its periosteal blood supply; although the vascular pedicle is not always identified, every attempt is made to protect it [67].

Technical Tips for IFT: Timing of IFT is critical. It must be after clearance of the active disease process in cases of infection to prevent failure and recurrence. In post-traumatic cases, IFT is done as soon as the surgical bed is clean and healthy; intraoperatively, this is confirmed after debridement by the presence of healthy-appearing and bleeding bone.

Delaying the IFT procedure is a poor prognostic factor likely due to vascular disruption from failed attempts [67]. Practically, IFT is better as a primary treatment for bone defects than it as a revision option. The other consideration is that IFT is done as either a single-stage [67] or two-stage procedure [66]. In the two-stage procedure, only a single end of the fibula (proximal or distal) is transposed to the tibia, this is then left for 6–8 weeks, and then, the other end is transposed; the rationale behind this is that the non-transposed end will have preserved blood supply and allow the other end to vascularize in its new place. Whether a single- or two-staged procedure is selected, the transposition must be mindful of preserving the blood supply; this entails leaving a soft tissue cuff of about 1–2 mm thick surrounding the fibula and avoiding injuring the peroneal artery pedicle. Releasing the fibula to allow free mobilization will need to release it from the interosseus membrane and flexor hallucis muscle, which is a risk to the blood supply. The length of the fibula resection is longer than the tibial defect; this will allow the invagination of the fibula into the tibia, allowing maximal bony contact and increased stability. An important consideration is to place the fibular graft in a well-aligned position, as malalignment is implicated in fibular autograft stress fractures [69, 70]. Another technique for better incorporation is to embed the transposed fibula into a tibial periosteal sleeve if the etiology of defect allows (benign tumour, trauma, or infection) [71]. Fixation of the graft at both ends is done via independent cortical screws and casting, a plate-screw construct, or an external fixator. Applying bone graft (autogenous ICBG) is also recommended when performing IFT in skeletally mature patients as a single-stage procedure. Postoperatively, the patients are instructed to restrict weight-bearing till graft union and hypertrophy.

Outcomes of IFT: Similar to free-fibula transfers, IFT results in hypertrophy of the fibula; this is in response to the load applied weight-bearing [72]. Non-union occurs with IFT in delayed or revision treatment cases, when the non-union/defect is located at the end of the tibia (graft volume inadequate to fill), and not applying bone graft in the single-stage procedure in skeletally mature patients. Other complications with IFT include delayed union, LLD, physeal injury with resultant angular deformity, and stress fractures [67]. Abdelkhalek et al. [73] compared IFT with BT in children; they found that IFT had a shorter union time than BT (3.4 vs. 5.5 months). However, despite this earlier union time, weight-bearing was delayed in IFT until fibular hypertrophy was achieved (about 9 months) in order to prevent graft fractures. The BT group had earlier weight-bearing with circular fixators; however, they also developed the expected fixator-associated issues, from pin site infection, loosened hardware, and stress fractures. Overall, the authors concluded that there is no preferred procedure and that selecting either one is based on considering each technique's unique features tailored to the patient.

Vascularized Autograft

The ability to perform a vascularized autograft transfer provides the surgeon with the versatility to tackle complex bone defect situations [74]. The most common vascularized autograft is the free fibular vascularized autograft (FFVA); this graft has been described in bone defect reconstruction for various etiologies: post-tumour, post-infectious, post-CPT, and post-traumatic [69]. The two basic types of FFVA are an intercalary graft (peroneal artery pedicle) and an epiphyseal transfer (anterior tibial pedicle) [75]. The intercalary FFVA has been described successfully in multiple clinical situations and configurations, including a double-barreled/folded graft [76], a hybrid IM graft with allograft (Capanna technique) [77], a composite soft tissue graft with muscle and skin [78], and an Onlay graft [79]. The epiphyseal FFVA has been reported in reconstructing multiple epiphyseal areas. Although intercalary FFVA is classically indicated in any significant bone defect (>6 cm) [3], it is instrumental in revision or salvage cases where a poor surgical bed, whether due to scarring, radiation, or impaired blood supply, is affected, as the FFVA will come with its circulation and biological healing potential [31, 80]. Bone defects post-tumor resection in children are also a unique situation. Both intercalary and epiphyseal FFVA provides a durable biological reconstruction with growth potential, sparing the patients from endoprosthesis and their complications; the option of lengthening FFVA is also present [81–83]. An advantage of FFVA is performing the treatment in one setting (harvest and transfer), having two teams working simultaneously helps reduce the operative time. Disadvantages include the need for a microvascular surgeon, donor site morbidity (up to 30%), prolonged restricted weight-bearing (6–9 months average till union), and potential complications. Complications of FFVA are divided into early and late. Early complications include wound infection, dehiscence, graft thrombosis, fixation failure, nerve palsy, sensory disturbance, and foot ischemia. Late complications include graft stress fracture, non-union, great-toe contracture, fixation failure, valgus ankle deformity, and LLD [78]. Foot ischemia results when FFVA is performed on a peroneal artery dominant foot; this is not the case in most patients; however, some congenital variants such as peroneal artery hypoplasia (5% of limbs) and in peripheral arterial disease, this might be the case; therefore, preoperative evaluation of the leg's circulation is mandatory [85]. A graft stress fracture is the most common late postoperative complication occurring in 15–52% [69, 84]. Factors to prevent fracture include satisfactory alignment [69], observing graft hypertrophy (defined as a 30% + increase in size) [86], and rigid stabilization. Graft configuration (double-barrel or folded) did not prevent stress fractures [70]. Leg length discrepancy post FFVA is reported successfully to be corrected surgically, whether by epiphysiodesis or leg-lengthening [81–83]. Long-term follow-up studies demonstrate that despite the morbidity and complications associated with FFVA, most patients have a full functional recovery and can lead active lifestyles [78, 84]. Recurrence of underlying diseases such as infection with osteomyelitis and non-union with CPT has been reported. In tumour resection and FFVA reconstruction cases, long-term follow-up series [78, 84] reported no recurrences in any patient, although recurrence is likely due to adequacy of resection and postoperative treatment.

Osteochondral Reconstruction

When encountering an articular-based bone loss in a traumatic setting, the surgeon must attempt to save the piece via replantation, as an osteochondral fragment is precious and there is no excellent alternative; this contrasts with diaphyseal/metaphyseal bone defects [87]. However, replantation is not possible with malignant tumours or resistant infection. Options to manage articular bone loss vary from arthrodesis, arthroplasty, allograft reconstruction, cement and bone grafting, epiphyseal FFVA, and amputation. Arthrodesis works well in the small joints of the hand and feet [88]. Allograft reconstruction is widely described for post-tumour and post-traumatic reconstruction with good results; however, there is a risk of infection, graft failure, early arthritis, and joint instability [25, 89]. Epiphyseal FFVA provides a unique option to reconstruct joint surfaces in the pediatric population. Reconstructed sites reported include the distal radius, proximal humerus, proximal femur, and lateral malleolus [90]. Epiphyseal FFVA is helpful in skeletally immature patients as the transferred physis will provide longitudinal growth and remodelling potential if performed <8 years for the proximal humerus and < 7 years for the distal radius. Epiphyseal FFVA should be avoided if the anterior tibial artery is the main supply to the foot and if the proximal fibula physis is absent or non-functional [91].

Funding Information The authors performed this body of work independently and have no financial disclosures relevant to this work.

Commentary

Commentary from Stephen Quinnan

Stephen M. Quinnan
squinnan@paleyinstitute.org

Treatment of bone loss remains one of the great challenges in orthopaedic surgery. This chapter describes thoroughly the considerations regarding defining and evaluating the problem. It also provides relevant context for the importance of etiology and how this effects the paradigm of treatment. In addition, it describes many of the available techniques to address this challenge. As with many difficult clinical problems, one simple solution that can address all situations does not exist. This is the reason why so many treatment alternatives outlined in the chapter remain relevant.

The above comments are true regarding bone loss in general, but the discussion becomes even more nuanced when addressing bone loss in the pediatric population. The reasons for this are both biological and practical. On the one hand, children have a much greater healing potential than adults. Consequently, they have a much greater potential for spontaneous regeneration and are much more capable of incorporating and hypertrophying vascularized grafts such as a fibula or an osteochondral flap. They also have a greater ability to accommodate and overcome soft tissue stiffness and contractures that can arise during treatment. On the other hand, children with open physes have future growth that must be protected or incorporated into the plan. This restricts the use of some fixation strategies and techniques available to skeletally mature patients or requires addressing of any potential future length discrepancy, especially in the very young patient.

In my experience, the above considerations lead to a general paradigm that helps guide treatment selection. The pediatric upper extremity has such a robust healing potential that almost all bone loss situations can be successfully treated with bone grafting techniques. The various options of autograft, allograft, vascularized grafts, induced membrane techniques, and osteochondral grafts can all be chosen depending on the considerations described well in the chapter.

The lower extremity in younger pediatric patients is also likely to have excellent regenerative potential and can most often also be addressed with similar methods to the upper extremity. In addition, these methods are easier to apply with fixation methods that do not risk damage to the physes. However, bone loss in the lower extremity in older children or select situations in younger children may benefit more from methods that employ DO such as bone transport or shortening and then lengthening. DO allows for a reconstruction that recapitulates the normal biology and anatomy of the bone better than any grafting method and can be applied without donor site morbidity.

Traditionally, the tradeoff for performing reconstruction with DO has been the prolonged treatment time in an external fixator and associated issues like pin site infection. However, newer methods such as balanced cable transport and then nailing and all internal methods such as the Bone Transport Nail or PABST (plate assisted bone segment transport) technique can mitigate or eliminate these concerns and provide an excellent alternative for this patient population. The limitation to these methods is that, at present, they require the option for intramedullary fixation. Fortunately, this often becomes feasible for children starting at around the age of 8 years for trochanteric nailing of the femur and the age of 10 years for tibial nails because the intramedullary canal size becomes large enough to accommodate the fixation and the physis is large enough to allow passage of the implant without limiting the growth potential. Because these limitations are mechanical and based on the size of the bone and physis, evaluation of these aspects is more appropriate than purely age-based decisions. Younger patients who are not amenable to these techniques can still be treated effectively with circular external fixation, but it will require a more prolonged treatment to reach full healing in the external fixator.

While I have found the above considerations to be helpful in my practice, I agree wholeheartedly with the profound importance of individualized decision-making for each patient and circumstance as the authors note in their concluding statement "The surgeon must also gauge the patient's tolerance with reconstruction, as a patient who cannot tolerate a complex treatment will benefit more from a single-stage procedure if feasible than a multi-stage procedure. Finally, the treating team's resources, from surgeon experience to hospital setting, treatment affordability, and cost-effectiveness, must also be factored in."

References

1. Nauth A, Schemitsch E, Norris B, Nollin Z, Watson J. Critical-size bone defects: is there a consensus for diagnosis and treatment? J Orthop Trauma. 2018;32 Suppl 3(3):S7–S11.
2. Haines N, Lack W, Seymour R, Bosse M. Defining the lower limit of a "critical bone defect" in open diaphyseal tibial fractures. J Orthop Trauma. 2016;30(5):e158–63.
3. Keating JF, Simpson AHRW, Robinson CM. The management of fractures with bone loss. Journal of bone and joint surgery. British. 2005;87(2):142–50.
4. Sales de Gauzy J, Fitoussi F, Jouve J, Karger C, Badina A, Masquelet A. Traumatic diaphyseal bone defects in children. Orthop Traumatol Surg Res. 2012;98(2):220–6.
5. Laine J, Cherkashin A, Samchukov M, Birch J, Rathjen K. The Management of Soft Tissue and Bone Loss in type IIIB and IIIC pediatric open tibia fractures. J Pediatr Orthop. 2016;36(5):453–8.
6. Morelli I, Drago L, George D, Romanò D, Romanò C. Managing large bone defects in children: a systematic review of the 'induced membrane technique'. J Pediatric Orthop B. 2018;27(5):443–55.
7. Tetsworth K, Burnand H, Hohmann E, Glatt V. Classification of bone defects: An extension of the Orthopaedic trauma association open fracture classification (OTA-OFC). J Orthop Trauma. 2020;35(2):71–6.
8. Innocenti M, Delcroix L, Manfrini M, Ceruso M, Capanna R. Vascularized proximal fibular epiphyseal transfer for distal radial reconstruction. J Bone Joint Surg Am. 2005;87:237–46.
9. Medda S, King MA, Runyan CM, Frino J. Vascularized Pedicled fibula for pediatric tibia reconstruction. J Orthop Trauma. 2021;35(S 2):S48–9.
10. McClure P, Alrabai H, Conway J. Preoperative evaluation and optimization of reconstruction of segmental bone defects of the tibia. J Orthop Trauma. 2017;31 Suppl 5(5):S16–9.
11. Zura R, Mehta S, Della Rocca GJ, Steen RG. Biological risk factors for nonunion of bone fracture. JBJS Rev. 2016;4(1):1.
12. Rosen LJ, Ben Noach M, Winickoff JP, Hovell MF. Parental smoking cessation to protect young children: a systematic review and meta-analysis. Pediatrics (Evanston). 2012;129(1):141–52.
13. Davies J, Reed J, Blake E, Priesemann M, Jackson AA, Clarke NM. Epidemiology of vitamin D deficiency in children presenting to a pediatric Orthopaedic service in the UK. J Pediatr Orthop. 2011;31(7):798–802.
14. Beck JJ, Mahan ST, Nowicki P, Schreiber VM, Minkowitz B. What is new in pediatric bone health. J Pediatr Orthop. 2021;41(8):e594–9.
15. Morelli I, Drago L, George DA, Gallazzi E, Scarponi S, Romanò CL. Masquelet technique: myth or reality? A systematic review and meta-analysis. Injury. 2016;47:S68–76.
16. Bishop J, Jones G, Rerko M, Donaldson C. 3-D CT is the Most reliable imaging modality when quantifying glenoid bone loss. Clin Orthop Relat Res. 2013;471(4):1251–6.
17. Giannoudis PV, Einhorn TA, Marsh D. Fracture healing: the diamond concept. Injury. 2007;38:S3–6.
18. Cappendijk V, van de Ven K, Madern G, Haverlag R, van Vugt A, Hazebroek aF. Strength of youth: conservative treatment of segmental bone defect in children. J Trauma. 2000;49(6):1123–5.
19. Figueroa-Sanchez JA, Ferrigno AS, Moreno-Cuevas J, Gonzalez-Garza MT, Jamall S, Martinez HR. Spontaneous bone regeneration after large Craniectomy in pediatric patient. World Neurosurg. 2019;127:316–8.
20. Abdulkarim A, Hu SY, Walker BR, Krkovic M. Cambridge experience in spontaneous bone regeneration after traumatic segmental bone defect: a case series and review of literature unusual presentation of more common disease/injury. BMJ Case Rep. 2020;13:e232482.

21. Agarwal A, Kumar A. Fibula regeneration following non-vascularized graft harvest in children. Int Orthop (SICOT). 2016;40(10):2191–7.
22. Khan SN, Cammisa FP Jr, Sandhu HS, Diwan AD, Girardi FP, Lane JM. The biology of bone grafting. J Am Acad Orthop Surg. 2005;13(1):77–86.
23. Myeroff C, Archdeacon M. Autogenous Bone Graft: Donor Sites and Techniques. J Bone Joint Surg Am. 2011;93(23):2227–36.
24. Masquelet AC, Begue T. The concept of induced membrane for reconstruction of long bone defects. Orthop Clin North Am. 2010;41(1):27–37.
25. Borade A, Kempegowda H, Fernandez M, Horwitz DS. Osteoarticular allograft reconstruction of post-traumatic defect of distal femur in a pediatric patient: A case report and literature review. Injury. 2016;47(11):2473–8.
26. Hertel R, Gerber A, Schlegel U, Cordey J, Rüegsegger P, Rahn BA. Cancellous bone graft for skeletal reconstruction. Muscular versus periosteal bed--preliminary report. Injury. 1994;25(Suppl 1):A59–70.
27. Goulet JA, Senunas LE, DeSilva GL, Greenfield ML. Autogenous iliac crest bone graft. Complications and functional assessment. Clin Orthop Relat Res. 1997;339(339):76–81.
28. Yee M, Hundal R, Perdue A, Hake M. Autologous bone graft harvest using the reamer–irrigator–aspirator. J Orthop Trauma. 2018;32 Suppl 1(4):S20–1.
29. Westrich G, Geller D, O'Malley M, Deland J, Helfet D. Anterior iliac crest bone graft harvesting using the Corticocancellous reamer system. J Orthop Trauma. 2001;15(7):500–6.
30. Paley D. Paley cross-union protocol for treatment of congenital Pseudarthrosis of the tibia. Oper Tech Orthop. 2021;31(2):100881.
31. Marecek GS, Little MT, Gardner MJ, Stevanovic M, Lefebvre R, Bernstein M. Management of Critical Bone Defects. Instr Course Lect. 2020;69:417–32.
32. Lindsey RW, Probe R, Miclau T, Alexander JW, Perren SM. The effects of antibiotic-impregnated Autogeneic cancellous bone graft on bone healing. Heidelberg: Springer; 1993.
33. Chan Y, Ueng S, Wang C, Lee S, Chen C, Shin C. Antibiotic-impregnated autogenic cancellous bone grafting is an effective and safe method for the Management of Small Infected Tibial Defects: A comparison study. J Trauma. 2000;48(2):246–55.
34. Metsemakers W, Fragomen A, Moriarty F, Morgenstern M, Egol K, Zalavras C, et al. Evidence-based recommendations for local antimicrobial strategies and dead space Management in Fracture-Related Infection. J Orthop Trauma. 2020;34(1):18–29.
35. Aurégan J, Bégué T, Rigoulot G, Glorion C, Pannier S. Success rate and risk factors of failure of the induced membrane technique in children: a systematic review. Injury. 2016;47:S62–7.
36. Gouron R. Surgical technique and indications of the induced membrane procedure in children. Orthop Traumatol Surg Res. 2015;102(1):S133–9.
37. Fitoussi F, Ilharreborde B. Is the induced-membrane technique successful for limb reconstruction after resecting large bone tumors in children? Clin Orthop Relat Res. 2015;473(6):2067–75.
38. Pelissier P, Masquelet AC, Bareille R, Mathoulin Pelissier S, Amedee J. Induced membranes secrete growth factors including vascular and osteoinductive factors and could stimulate bone regeneration. J Orthop Res. 2004;22(1):73–9.
39. Haddad B, Zribi S, Haraux E, Deroussen F, Gouron R, Klein C. Induced membrane technique for clavicle reconstruction in paediatric patients: report of four cases. Orthop Traumatol Surg Res. 2019;105(4):733–7.
40. Mohseni AA, Boussetta R, Saied W, Zairi M, Msakni A, Bouchoucha S, Nessib MN. Congenital pseudarthrosis of the forearm treated with induced membrane technique: A case report. Int J Surg Case Rep. 2020;77:584–90.
41. Hughes RE, Schneeberger AG, An K, Morrey BF, O'Driscoll SW. Reduction of triceps muscle force after shortening of the distal humerus: A computational model. J Shoulder Elb Surg. 1997;6(5):444–8.
42. Rigal S, Merloz P, Le Nen D, Mathevon H, Masquelet A-. Bone transport techniques in posttraumatic bone defects. Orthop Traumatol Surg Res. 2011;98(1):103–8.
43. El-Rosasy MA, El-Rosasy MA. Acute shortening and re-lengthening in the management of bone and soft-tissue loss in complicated fractures of the tibia. J Bone Joint Surg Br. 2007;89(1):80–8.
44. Pierrie S, Hsu J. Shortening and angulation strategies to address composite bone and soft tissue defects. J Orthop Trauma. 2017;31 Suppl 5(5):S32–5.
45. Betz AM, Stock W, Hierner R, Baumgart R. Primary shortening with secondary limb lengthening in severe injuries of the lower leg: A six year experience. Microsurgery. 1993;14(7):446–53.
46. Yokoyama K, Itoman M, Nakamura K, Uchino M, Tsukamoto T, Suzuki T. Primary shortening with secondary limb lengthening for Gustilo IIIB open Tibial fractures: A report of six cases. J Trauma. 2006;61(1):172–80.
47. Atbasi Z, Demiralp B, Kilic E, Kose O, Kurklu M, Basbozkurt M. Angiographic evaluation of arterial configuration after acute tibial shortening. Eur J Orthop Surg Traumatol. 2014;24(8):1587–95.
48. Pikkel YY, Wilson JJ, Kassis S, Lerner A. Acute shortening and angulation for limb salvage in a paediatric patient with a high-energy blast injury. BMJ Case Rep. 2014;2014:bcr2013203431.
49. Tetsworth K, Paley D, Sen C, Jaffe M, Maar DC, Glatt V, et al. Bone transport versus acute shortening for the management of infected tibial non-unions with bone defects. Injury. 2017;48(10):2276–84.
50. Sen C, Demirel M, Sağlam Y, Balcı HI, Eralp L, Kocaoğlu M. Acute shortening versus bone transport for the treatment of infected femur non-unions with bone defects. Injury. 2019;50(11):2075–83.
51. Tetsworth K, Dlaska C. The art of Tibial bone transport using the Ilizarov fixator: the suspension wire technique. Tech Orthop. 2015;30(3):142–55.
52. Molina CS, Stinner DJ, Obremskey WT. Treatment of traumatic segmental long-bone defects: A critical analysis review. JBJS Rev. 2014;2(4):1.
53. Mauffrey C, Barlow BT, Smith W. Management of segmental bone defects. J Am Acad Orthop Surg. 2015;23(3):143–53.
54. Liu Y, Yushan M, Liu Z, Liu J, Ma C, Yusufu A. Complications of bone transport technique using the Ilizarov method in the lower extremity: a retrospective analysis of 282 consecutive cases over 10 years. BMC Musculoskelet Disord. 2020;21(1):354.
55. Quinnan S. Segmental bone loss reconstruction using ring fixation. J Orthop Trauma. 2017;31 Suppl 5(5):S42–6.
56. Arslan H, Özkul E, Gem M, Alemdar C, Şahin İ, Kişin B. Segmental bone loss in pediatric lower extremity fractures: indications and results of bone transport. J Pediatr Orthop. 2015;35(2):e8–e12.
57. Catagni MA, Azzam W, Guerreschi F, Lovisetti L, Poli P, Khan MS, et al. Trifocal versus bifocal bone transport in treatment of long segmental tibial bone defects. Bone Joint J. 2019;101-B(2):162–9.
58. Quinnan S, Lawrie C. Optimizing bone defect reconstruction—balanced cable transport with circular external fixation. J Orthop Trauma. 2017;31(10):e347–55.
59. Bas A, Daldal F, Eralp L, Kocaoglu M, Uludag S, Sari S. Treatment of Tibial and femoral bone defects with bone transport over an intramedullary nail. J Orthop Trauma. 2020;34(10):e353–9.
60. Park K, Oh C, Kim J, Oh J, Yoon Y, Seo I, et al. Matched case-control comparison of bone transport using external fixator over a nail versus external fixator over a plate for segmental Tibial bone defects. J Orthop Trauma. 2021;35(11):e397–404.
61. Bernstein M, Fragomen A, Sabharwal S, Barclay J, Rozbruch S. Does integrated fixation provide benefit in the reconstruction of posttraumatic Tibial bone defects? Clin Orthop Relat Res. 2015;473(10):3143–53.

62. Olesen UK, Nygaard T, Prince DE, Gardner MP, Singh UM, McNally MA, et al. Plate-assisted bone segment transport with motorized lengthening nails and locking plates: A technique to treat femoral and Tibial bone defects. J Am Acad Orthop Surg Glob Res Rev. 2019;3(8):e064.
63. Krettek C. MagicTube: new possibilities for completely internal bone segmental transport and optional lengthening: new additional module for motorized lengthening nails for treatment of large bone defects. Unfallchirurg. 2018;121(11):884–92.
64. Krettek C, El Naga A. All internal segmental bone transport and optional lengthening with a newly developed universal cylinder-kombi-tube module for motorized nails—description of a surgical technique. J Orthop Trauma. 2017;31 Suppl 5(5):S39–41.
65. Huntington TW. The classic: case of bone transference. Use of a segment of fibula to supply a defect in the tibia. 1905. Clin Orthop Relat Res. 2012;470(10):2651–3.
66. Gupta S, Garg G. The Huntington procedure: still a reasonable option for large tibial defects in paediatric patients. J Child Orthop. 2014;8(5):413–21.
67. Kassab M, Samaha C, Saillant G. Ipsilateral fibular transposition in tibial nonunion using Huntington procedure: a 12-year follow-up study. Injury. 2003;34(10):770.
68. Devendra A, Velmurugesan P, Dheenadhayalan J, Venkatramani H, Sabapathy S, Rajasekaran S. One-bone forearm reconstruction: A salvage solution for the forearm with massive bone loss. J Bone Joint Surg. 2019;0101(15):e74.
69. Minami A, Kasashima T, Iwasaki N, Kato H, Kaneda K. Vascularised fibular grafts: An experience of 102 patients. J Bone Joint Surg Br. 2000;82(7):1022–5.
70. Muramatsu K, Ihara K, Shigetomi M, Kawai S. Femoral reconstruction by single, folded or double free vascularised fibular grafts. Br J Plast Surg. 2004;57(6):550–5.
71. Steiger CN, Journeau P, Lascombes P. The role of the periosteal sleeve in the reconstruction of bone defects using a non-vascularised fibula graft in the pediatric population. Orthop Traumatol Surg Res. 2017;103(7):1115–20.
72. De Meulemeester C, Verdonk R, Bongaerts W. The fibula pro tibia procedure in the treatment of nonunion of the tibia. Acta Orthop Belg. 1992;58(Suppl 1):187–9.
73. Abdelkhalek M, El-Alfy B, Ali A. Ilizarov bone transport versus fibular graft for reconstruction of tibial bone defects in children. J Pediatr Orthop B. 2016;25(6):556–60.
74. Taylor G, Corlett R, Ashton M. The evolution of free vascularized bone transfer: A 40-year experience. Plast Reconstr Surg. 2016;137(4):1292–305.
75. Ghert M, Colterjohn N, Manfrini M. The use of free vascularized fibular grafts in skeletal reconstruction for bone tumors in children. J Am Acad Orthop Surg. 2007;15(10):577–87.
76. Cashin M, Coombs C, Torode I. A-frame free vascularized fibular graft and femoral lengthening for osteosarcoma pediatric patients. J Pediatr Orthop. 2018;38(2):e83–90.
77. Houdek M, Wagner E, Stans A, Shin A, Bishop A, Sim F, et al. What is the outcome of allograft and intramedullary free fibula (Capanna technique) in pediatric and adolescent patients with bone tumors? Clin Orthop Relat Res. 2016;474(3):660–8.
78. McCullough MC, Arkader A, Ariani R, Lightdale-Miric N, Tolo V, Stevanovic M. Surgical outcomes, complications, and long-term functionality for free vascularized fibula grafts in the pediatric population: A 17-year experience and systematic review of the literature. J Reconstr Microsurg. 2020;36(5):386–96.
79. Friedrich JB, Moran SL, Bishop AT, Wood CM, Shin AY. Vascularized fibula flap onlay for salvage of pathologic fracture of the long bones. Plast Reconstr Surg. 2008;121(6):2001–9.
80. Bae D, Waters P, Gebhardt M. Results of free vascularized fibula grafting for allograft nonunion after limb salvage surgery for malignant bone tumors. J Pediatr Orthop. 2006;26(6):809–14.
81. Courvoisier A, Sailhan F, Mary P, Damsin J. Case reports: lengthening of a vascularized free fibular graft. Clin Orthop Relat Res. 2009;467(5):1377–84.
82. Zhang X, Zhang T, Liu T, Li Z, Zhang X. Lengthening of free fibular grafts for reconstruction of the residual leg length discrepancy. BMC Musculoskelet Disord. 2019;20(1):66.
83. Han C, Chung D, Lee J, Jeong B. Lengthening of intercalary allograft combined with free vascularized fibular graft after reconstruction in pediatric osteosarcoma of femur. J Pediatr Orthop B. 2010;19(1):61–5.
84. Sainsbury DCG, Liu EH, Alvarez-Veronesi MC, Ho ES, Hopyan S, Zuker RM, et al. Long-term outcomes following lower extremity sarcoma resection and reconstruction with vascularized fibula flaps in children. Plast Reconstr Surg. 2014;134(4):808–20.
85. Abou-Foul AK, Borumandi F. Anatomical variants of lower limb vasculature and implications for free fibula flap: systematic review and critical analysis. Microsurgery. 2016;36(2):165–72.
86. El-Gammal TA, El-Sayed A, Kotb MM. Hypertrophy after free vascularized fibular transfer to the lower limb. Microsurgery. 2002;22(8):367–70.
87. Toogood P, Miclau T. Critical-sized bone defects: sequence and planning. J Orthop Trauma. 2017;31 Suppl 5(5):S23–6.
88. Schuh R, Trnka H. First metatarsophalangeal arthrodesis for severe bone loss. Foot Ankle Clin. 2011;16(1):13–20.
89. Hornstein S, Moukoko D, Deroussen F, Plancq MC, Collet LM, Gouron R. Successful hemicondylar femoral allograft for traumatic bone loss: A paediatric case study with ten years of follow-up. Knee. 2014;22(1):63–6.
90. Kurlander D, Shue S, Schwarz G, Ghaznavi A. Vascularized fibula epiphysis transfer for pediatric extremity reconstruction: A systematic review and meta-analysis. Ann Plast Surg. 2019;82(3):344–51.
91. Akinbo O, Strauch R. Physeal transfers for skeletal reconstruction. J Hand Surg Am. 2008;33(4):584–90.

Iatrogenic Deformities

40

Austin T. Fragomen and Robert Rozbruch

Introduction

As physicians, we strive to help our patients improve their pain and function. As orthopedic surgeons, we do this through operative or nonoperative intervention. Our treatment choice is based on the standard of care and on our individual training and level of comfort. Despite the best intentions, some patients have deformities after treatments that are unacceptable to them. *Iatrogenic deformity* refers to the circumstance where medical treatment contributed to the limb deformity. It may be that the management of a tibia fracture with casting resulted in a deformity which the patient now complains about as an adult (Fig. 40.1), or, perhaps, an adolescent with Blount's disease whose deformity was overcorrected resulting in a valgus deformity.

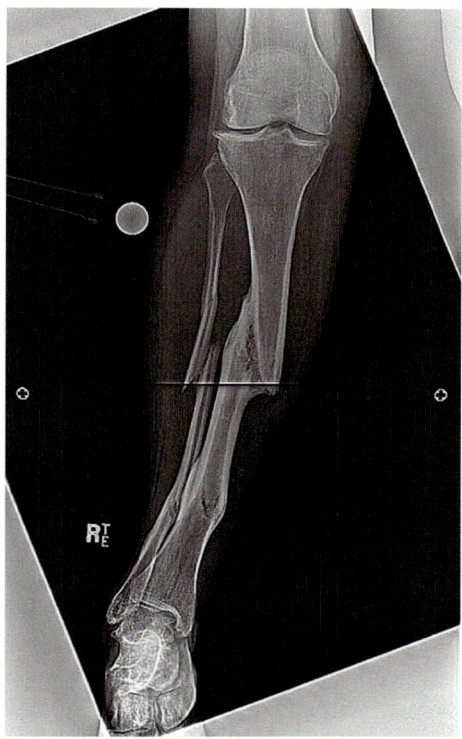

Fig. 40.1 This segmental tibia fracture in an adolescent was treated with casting and went onto malunion. The patient subsequently developed knee and ankle osteoarthritis

A. T. Fragomen (✉)
Department of Orthopedics, Hospital for Special Surgery, New York, NY, USA
e-mail: fragomena@hss.edu

R. Rozbruch
Department of Orthopedics, Hospital for Special Surgery, New York, NY, USA

Weill Cornell Medical College, Cornell University, New York, NY, USA
e-mail: rozbruchsr@hss.edu

What Is Acceptable Alignment?

There has been an evolution in what constitutes acceptable alignment among our peers. Through the 1990's, all focus was on achieving union with the following alignment dogma: less than 10° of angular deformity and less than 2 cm of shortening were well tolerated [1, 2]. Sarmiento stated, "We accept minor losses in length and alignment as small sacrifices in an effort to provide early function and decreased morbidity. [Changes in stress patterns at the tib-

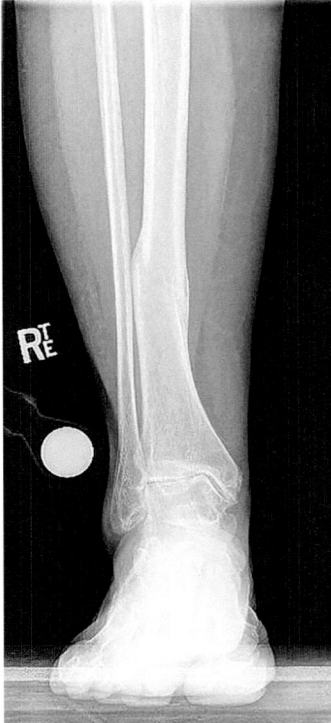

Fig. 40.2 This distal tibial fracture was sustained during adolescence and was treated with casting. The angulation of 10° was accepted and the fracture healed uneventfully. The patient developed ankle arthritis years later with more joint space narrowing seen in the medial aspect of the tibiotalar joint

iotalar joint are not significant with angular deformities less than 10° in any plane. In over 25 years of observation, small amounts of shortening and angulation have not been associated with osteoarthritis or diminished function at a later date and are cosmetically acceptable to the patient]" [3]. Many patients were left with large rotational deformities of the femur and tibia, bone shortening, or angular and translational deformities (Fig. 40.2). Surgeons have moved toward more stringent criteria with less than 5° of angular deformity considered ideal [4–6]. The adoption of intramedullary (IM) nailing and marginalization of casting as a standard of care for adult tibia fractures have given surgeons the ability to obtain more accurate fracture reductions [7]. Similarly, the management of pediatric femur fractures has moved toward surgery making traction and casting less popular [8] (Fig. 40.3).

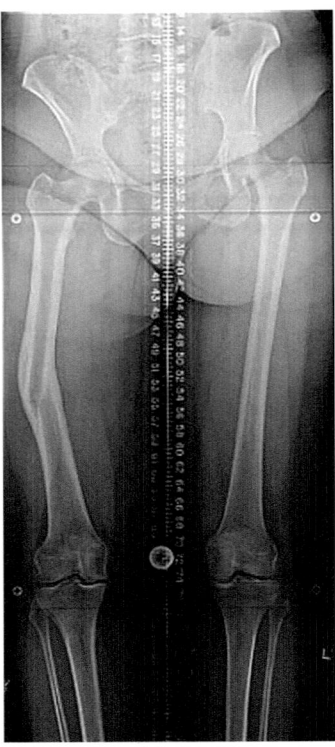

Fig. 40.3 This fracture was treated in adolescence with traction and casting resulting in 16° of varus and 3 cm of shortening

What Are the Consequences of Malalignment?

It is not uncommon to see adult patients with childhood deformities present to the office with knee or ankle arthritis secondary to the long-standing malalignment. This poor alignment places abnormal or asymmetric stress across the adjacent joint(s) leading to premature cartilage breakdown [7–10]. This contention is supported by Vallier et al. who found that a tibial malunion of more than 5° was significantly associated with knee and ankle pain [4]. Palmu found that the treatment of femur fractures in children older than 10 years with traction led to a high incidence of deformities greater than 10° that he later correlated with the development of knee arthritis at a young age [8] (Fig. 40.4). We should strive to reestablish these normal parameters for bone alignment to avoid abnormal limb mechanics. This will help to prevent articular cartilage wear and pelvic and low back

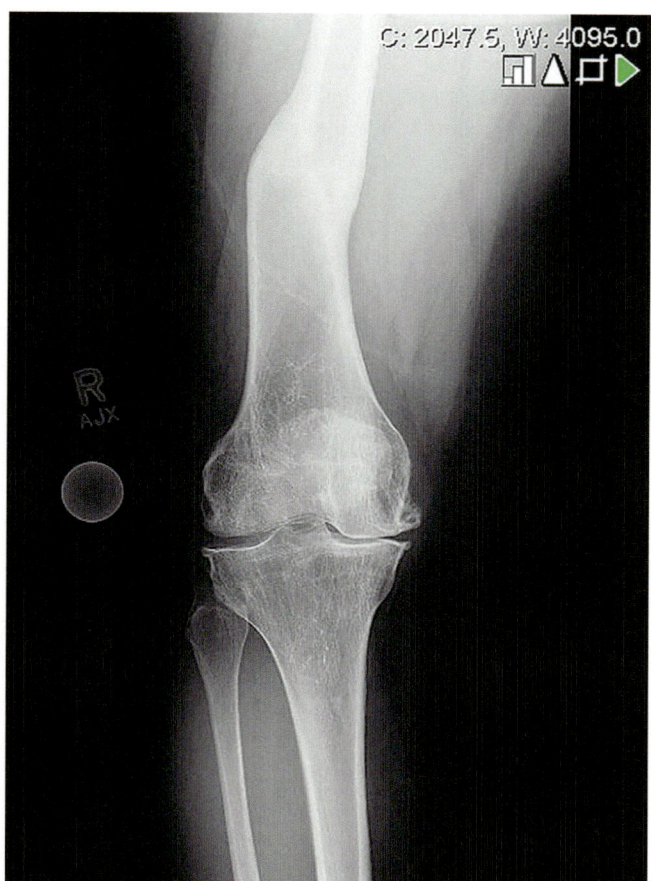

Fig. 40.4 This varus femur malunion resulted in malalignment that developed medial compartment osteoarthritis years after the injury

problems, and facilitate joint replacement, if and when needed. More importantly, if initial treatment results in unacceptable alignment, then we are obligated to consider the long-term implications for this patient and suggest further surgical correction for this patient. If the surgeon is not comfortable performing this "residual correction," then the patient should be referred to a specialized center. Many patients will elect no further treatment or may not be candidates for further intervention, but the malalignment needs to be acknowledged.

What Are the Legal Implications of Iatrogenic Deformities?

Nearly 15% of orthopedic surgeons face a malpractice claim annually [11]. Restricting the criteria for acceptable deformity is analogous to "narrowing the strike zone." This places increased responsibility on the surgeon to have a "perfect" result, thus making our job more difficult. If a malunion is a failure and the criteria for malunion are now broadened, then there are legal implications. Patients are glad to have their concerns about their deformity legitimized, but their next question is why the deformity occurred and whether this was malpractice. Based on our experience, in most cases, the best policy is to concede that the result is not ideal, reassure that every effort was made to provide an optimal result and that there was no medical negligence, and counsel that further surgery to deliver a superior outcome is recommended. The greatest predictor of payment to a plaintiff is the severity of the patient's disability [12]. This implies that the best course of action is to do everything possible to improve their condition and decrease disability. At no time, should the surgeon abandon or blame the patient. A good doctor-patient relationship and better preoperative discussions of known complications will help to calm the impulse to bring legal action against the physician [13, 14]. Contact the hospital legal department and identify this patient as "at risk" for litigation. The hospital will often have patient services mitigate any feelings of discontent or help finance further treatment. When a patient does seek legal action, an angry patient will be less likely to settle the case. So, one must do as much as possible to avoid a hostile relationship with the patient and his or her caretakers. One must keep in mind that we are judged not only by our successes but also by how we handle adversity. These difficult situations are hurdles along the career path of every orthopedic surgeon.

Common Iatrogenic Deformities

Tibia Malunion

The immature skeleton's ability to remodel a "malunion" is determined by the number of years of growth remaining. If the remodeling potential of an angulated bone is limited, then the fracture is considered a malunion and warrants intervention. If a child of advanced age presents with a displaced long bone fracture of the lower extremity that will likely go on to a malunion (impending malunion) if treated with cast immobilization, then the surgeon will often select operative treatment to help ensure acceptable alignment at skeletal maturity. The current criteria for "acceptable" alignment in pediatric fractures fall into two groups. Children aged 8 years old or less often remodel angular deformities of up to 10°. Children older than 8 years and in adolescents, angular deformity of up to 5°, 1 cm of shortening, and less than 10° of rotational deformity is acceptable [15]. Most remodeling occurs within 2 years after fracture healing [15]. Due in part to a robust periosteum and rapid healing, most tibia fractures in children can be treated with casting while still maintaining acceptable alignment, length, and rotation [16]. However, certain fractures are difficult to manage in a cast or are at high risk for displacement and malunion and are often treated surgically: high-energy unstable fractures, open fractures, fractures with soft tissue injury or compartment syndrome, oblique fractures with an intact fibula, floating knee, and fractures in older children [16–19]. The operative management of tibia factures is most commonly performed with elastic titanium IM nails [20]. Circular external fixation has been shown to be superior to monolateral fixation for unstable diaphyseal fractures of the tibia in children and adolescents and is gaining popularity [21]. Circular fixation may also be equivalent to elastic IM nailing in adolescents [22]. External fixation may be superior to casting as it allows for ease of monitoring and management of compartment syndrome, which remains one of the most common complications of pediatric tibia fractures [23, 24]. The use of the programmable, six-axis circular fixator in high-energy pediatric tibia fractures has proved successful affording very accurate alignment and early weight bearing [25, 26]. However, the use of external fixation is associated with a small incidence of refracture and fracture through the pin sites [27].

Case 1

A 12-year-old male presented with a noticeable deformity of the lower leg including varus, external rotation, and shortening. He had sustained a Salter–Harris type II fracture of the distal tibia at the age of 8 years. A metaphyseal osteotomy was performed for deformity correction and was stabilized with a plate and screws. The growth plate became tethered medially driving the epiphysis into varus and slowing the growth of the entire physis (Fig. 40.5a, b). This was recognized by his orthopedist who had been following him yearly after the injury. He was referred for deformity correction and limb lengthening. The sum of these deformities led to significant functional problems with walking and running and put him at increased risk for developing arthritis of the ankle and low back pain. He was noted to have limited ankle dorsiflexion of the injured side compared with the unaffected left ankle. His external rotation deformity of the tibia was 20°. He had a 2.5-cm shortening of the tibia. Surgical planning included calculation of the future shortening that would result from formal closure of the distal tibial physis. Correction with the six-axis circular fixator was considered a good option. This would allow for deformity correction and lengthening. The entire distal tibial growth plate was closed surgically. A distal metaphyseal osteotomy was created with an osteotome to allow for gradual correction of the varus and rotational deformities. Lengthening through the same osteotomy site has two disadvantages: the patient may develop a significant equinus and the time for consolidation of the lengthening regenerate would be lengthy. To address these potential problems, a second more proximal osteotomy was performed for the lengthening (Fig. 40.5c, d). The final result was correction of the deformities including length with a full-functional recovery (Fig. 40.5e–g). He had a contracture of the gastrocnemius that fully resolved with physical therapy 6 months after frame removal. Another option would have been to lengthen the gastrocnemius muscle tendon for a more rapid recovery of ankle motion.

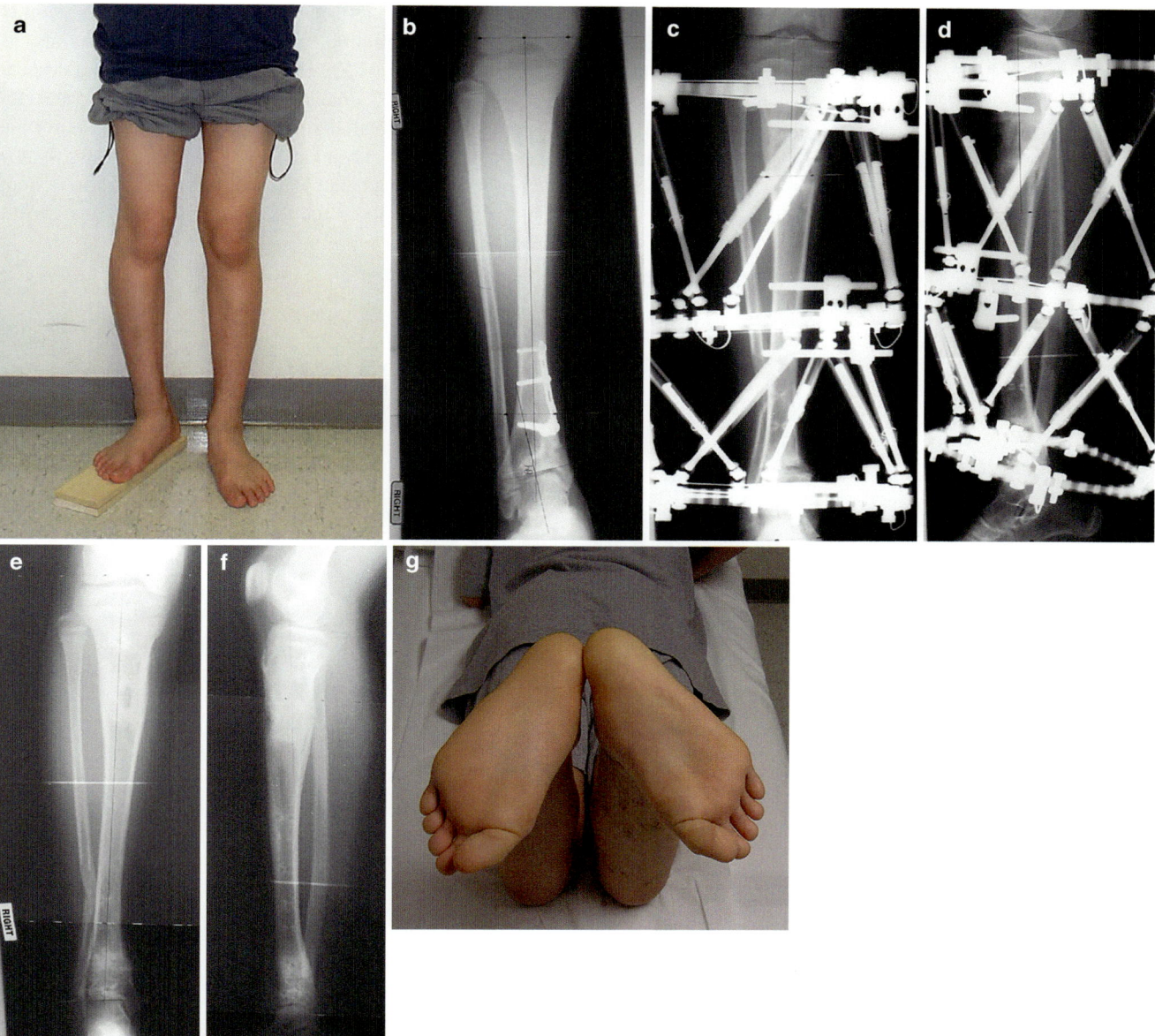

Fig. 40.5 (a) This patient has a malunion with shortening, external rotation, and varus. (b) AP X-ray shows retained hardware, medial physeal tethering, and distal varus deformity. (c, d) AP and lateral radiographs during treatment demonstrating the two-level osteotomy and double-level circular fixation for deformity correction and lengthening. (e, f) These X-rays show healing of both osteotomies with accurate correction of the underlying deformities. (g) Restoration of the axial alignment of the tibia is assessed with the prone exam

Case 2

A high-energy closed tibia fracture in a 13-year-old male was treated with a monolateral pin-to-bar external fixation as the definitive stabilization. The reduction resulted in 2 cm of lateral translation of the distal fragment and 10° of apex anterior angular deformity (Fig. 40.6a, b) The surgeon explained that this was an acceptable alignment and that he was unable to improve it with closed reduction, because the deformity was acceptable and open reduction was not indicated. The family sought a second opinion. This sagittal plane deformity is greater than 5° and will likely not remodel in this adolescent patient. The clinical concern about residual apex anterior deformity of the tibial shaft is that it may create abnormal wear on the knee and ankle joints, increases stress on the anterior cruciate ligament (ACL), and prevents full leg extension. Trepidations about the fixation construct included fur-

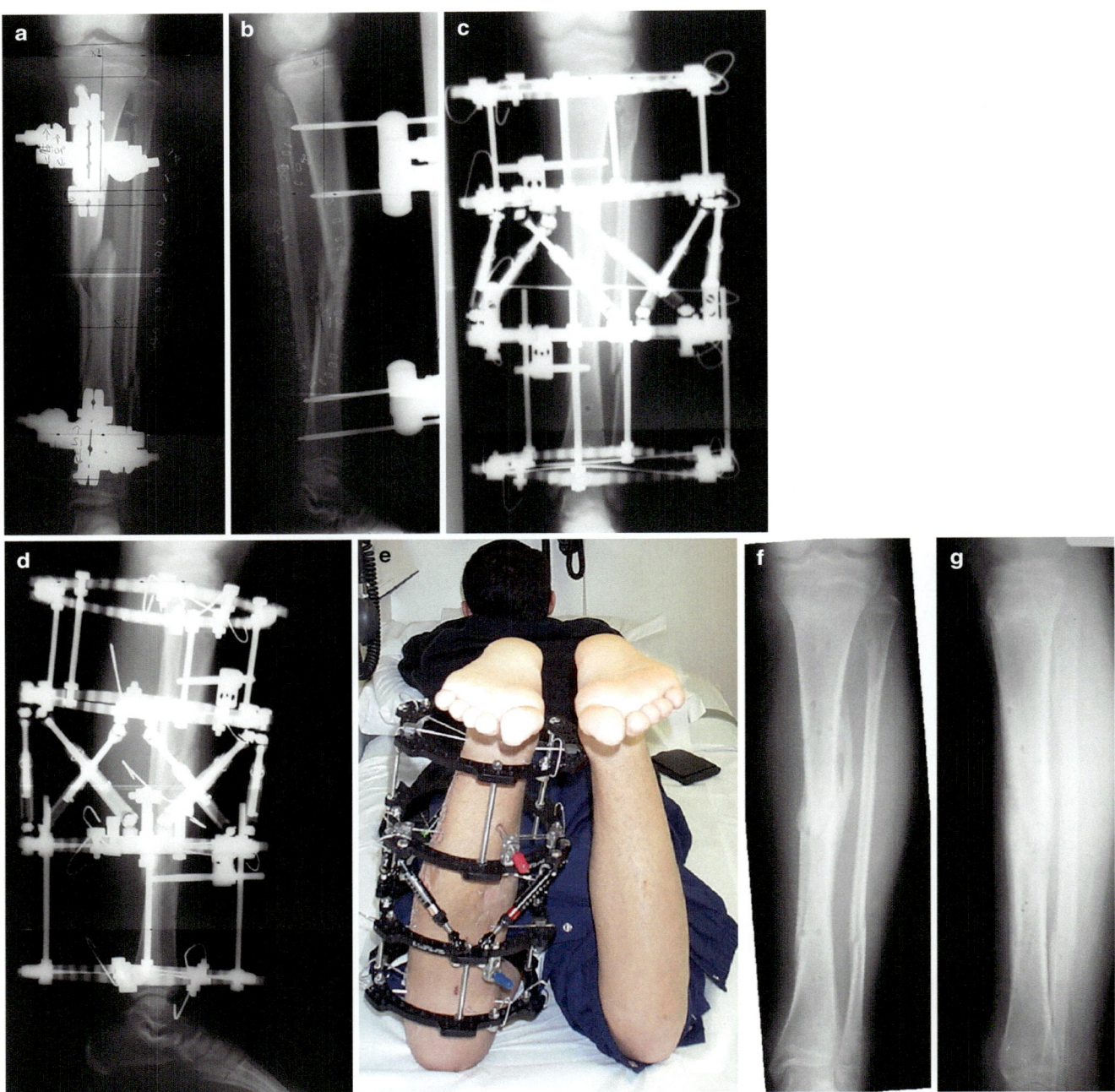

Fig. 40.6 (**a, b**) AP and lateral radiographs show a high-energy tibial fracture treated with temporizing external fixation. Soft-tissue swelling and damage made internal fixation a poor option. (**c, d**) The circular external fixator provided superior stability and allowed for early weight bearing. (**e**) The prone exam is important to confirm that axial alignment has been restored. (**f, g**) The final result is a healed fracture with excellent alignment

ther loss of reduction, impending malunion, and even possible nonunion. Treatment with a six-axis circular fixator using the Taylor Spatial Frame (TSF) (Smith & Nephew, Memphis, TN) was provided. This device allowed for a percutaneous surgery, an accurate and gradual correction of the residual deformity, avoidance of the growth plates, and weight bearing as tolerated ambulation during the entire treatment period (Fig. 40.6c–e). After 3 months of wearing the external fixator, the final result was a near-anatomic bony alignment and no functional impairment was seen (Fig. 40.6f, g).

Fibular Malunion

Fibular fractures in children and adolescents commonly heal without incident. In rare circumstances, growth arrest of the distal fibular physis can occur causing progressive fibular shortening. This leads to valgus orientation of the hindfoot, widening of the syndesmosis, and early ankle joint degeneration [28–33]. Once recognized, this fibular shortening and syndesmotic laxity can be corrected surgically [34–36]. Manoudis et al. reported a case of fibular shortening from physeal arrest corrected by open osteotomy, acute lengthening, grafting with tricortical iliac crest, and internal fixation [37]. An open release of the syndesmosis was necessary to reduce the fibular tip into its proper location. Other authors have reported on the same technique without the need for syndesmotic dissection [29]. Alternatively, a percutaneous technique can be employed to both lengthen the fibula through distraction osteogenesis and utilize distraction histiogenesis to stretch the syndesmotic ligaments and achieve distal migration of the fibular tip.

Case 3

A 13-year-old female presented with a valgus deformity of the hindfoot after premature fibular physeal closure. The patient had previously undergone curettage of a benign distal fibular bone cyst (without apparent physeal involvement) with prophylactic plating to prevent fracture of the distal fibula. The hardware was removed 1 year later without incident. The distal fibular physis closed prematurely postoperatively leading to a shortening deformity of the fibula over time. The etiology of the physeal injury is not clear but an iatrogenic cause could not be excluded. The patient's hindfoot drifted into valgus when compared with the other side. Radiographs revealed a shortened fibula with a distal physeal closure. X-rays of the contralateral ankle were taken to establish the normal fibular length and talocrural angle (Fig. 40.7a, b). This deformity was unacceptable as it would lead to asymmetric wear of the lateral talus and possibly arthritis. Fibular shortening of 1.5 cm was measured. The treatment plan included lengthening of the fibula. The tibia was included in the proximal fibular ring block to protect the proximal tibiofibular joint from subluxation and ensure distal migration and reduction of the fibular tip (Fig. 40.7c, d). The fibula was lengthened with the external fixator. When the correct length was obtained, the patient was brought back to the operating room for insertion of syndesmotic screws and early removal of the frame (Fig. 40.7e). The patient's hindfoot alignment was corrected with no loss of ankle motion (Fig. 40.7f).

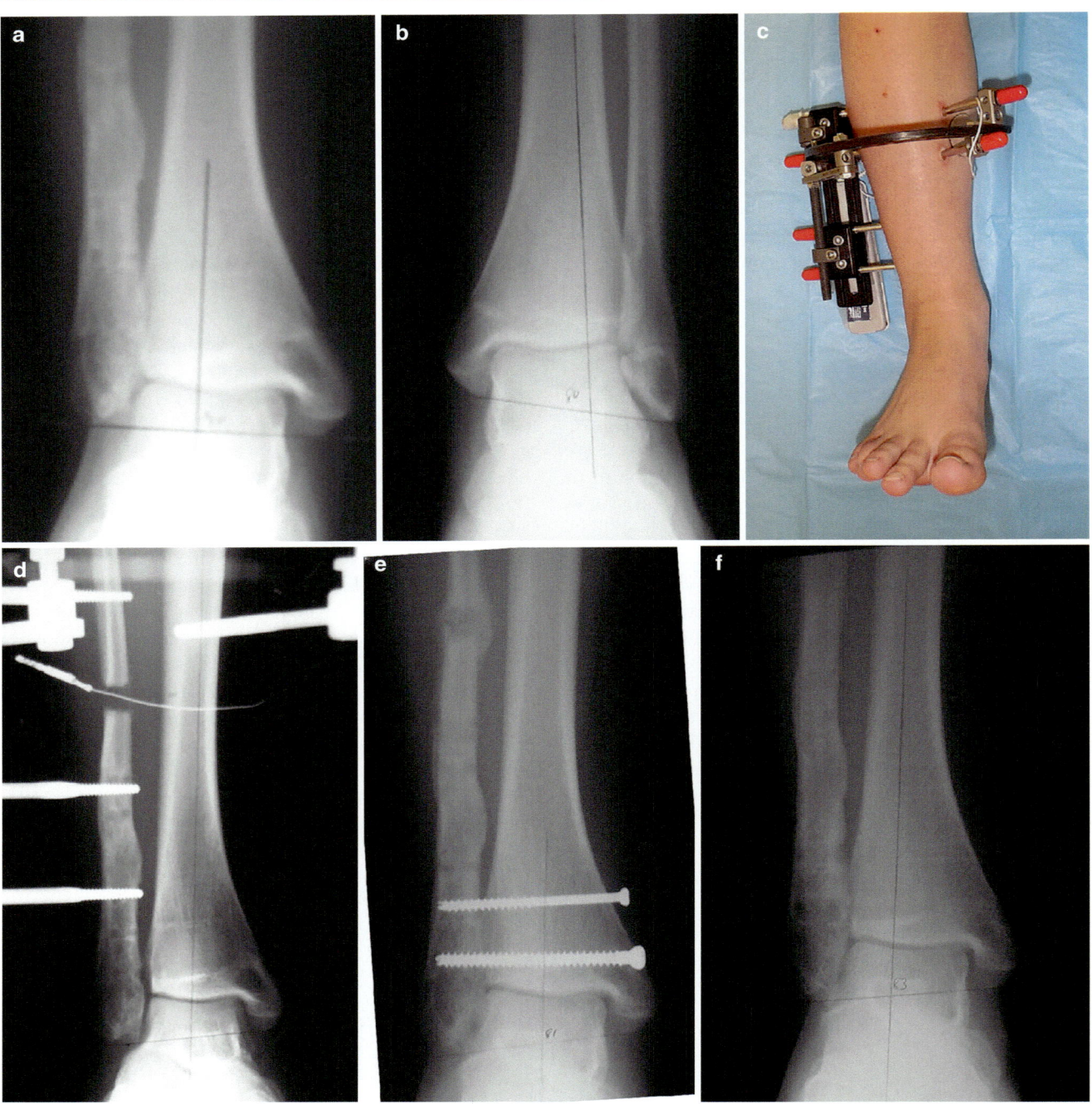

Fig. 40.7 (**a**, **b**) AP radiographs of the shortened right fibula and the normal left fibula. Tibial alignment is within normal. (**c**, **d**) An external fixator was used to lengthen the fibula using half pins. (**e**) At the time of frame removal, the syndesmosis was stabilized with two screws. (**f**) Final radiographs show restoration of the length of the fibula and removal of the screws

Transphyseal ACL Reconstruction Causes Premature Physeal Closure

An option for ACL reconstruction in older children (age 11–14 years) is the transphyseal tunnel technique. Most authors report minimal complications with this method including an average growth plate disturbance risk of 3% [38–44]. Kumar et al. reported on 32 children with an average age of 11.25 years where the transphyseal reconstruction was used with one case of mild valgus and no leg length discrepancy [38]. Similarly, transphyseal surgery in a series of 15 patients, average age of 12.8 years, resulted in one case of valgus malalignment of the knee [39]. Asymmetric growth of the distal femoral physis is the most commonly reported mechanism for the valgus deformity [41]. Other series report no adverse trauma to the physis with this technique, but authors caution to make sure that the graft bone blocks are not in contact with the physis [42–44]. Physeal sparing reconstruction carries minimal risk to the growth plate but may not be as reliable with regard to the maintenance of ligamentous stability of the knee [45]. Although the risk of growth plate disturbance around the knee is small, its occurrence in some cases is undeniable and such iatrogenic angular deformities may require surgical correction.

Case 4

A 15-year-old male presented with a deformity of the proximal tibia including varus, recurvatum, and shortening. At the age of 12 years, he sustained an ACL injury. The ACL was reconstructed using the transphyseal technique in the tibia and an over-the-top technique in the femur. The anterior-medial proximal tibial physis was likely damaged. A progressive angular deformity developed with significant retardation of physeal growth (Fig. 40.8a–c). The radiologic deformities included 15° of varus, 28° of apex posterior (recurvatum), and 4.5 cm of shortening. The clinical deformity included 10° of hyperextension of the knee and normal knee ligamentous stability. Growth remaining discrepancy was calculated to be an additional 1 cm. Treatment was closure of the remainder of the proximal tibial physis to prevent further deformity, proximal tibial osteotomy, and TSF application for deformity correction and lengthening (Fig. 40.8d, e). The latest follow-up at 12-months post-frame removal shows restoration of length and alignment, and a full functional recovery is expected (Fig. 40.8f–h).

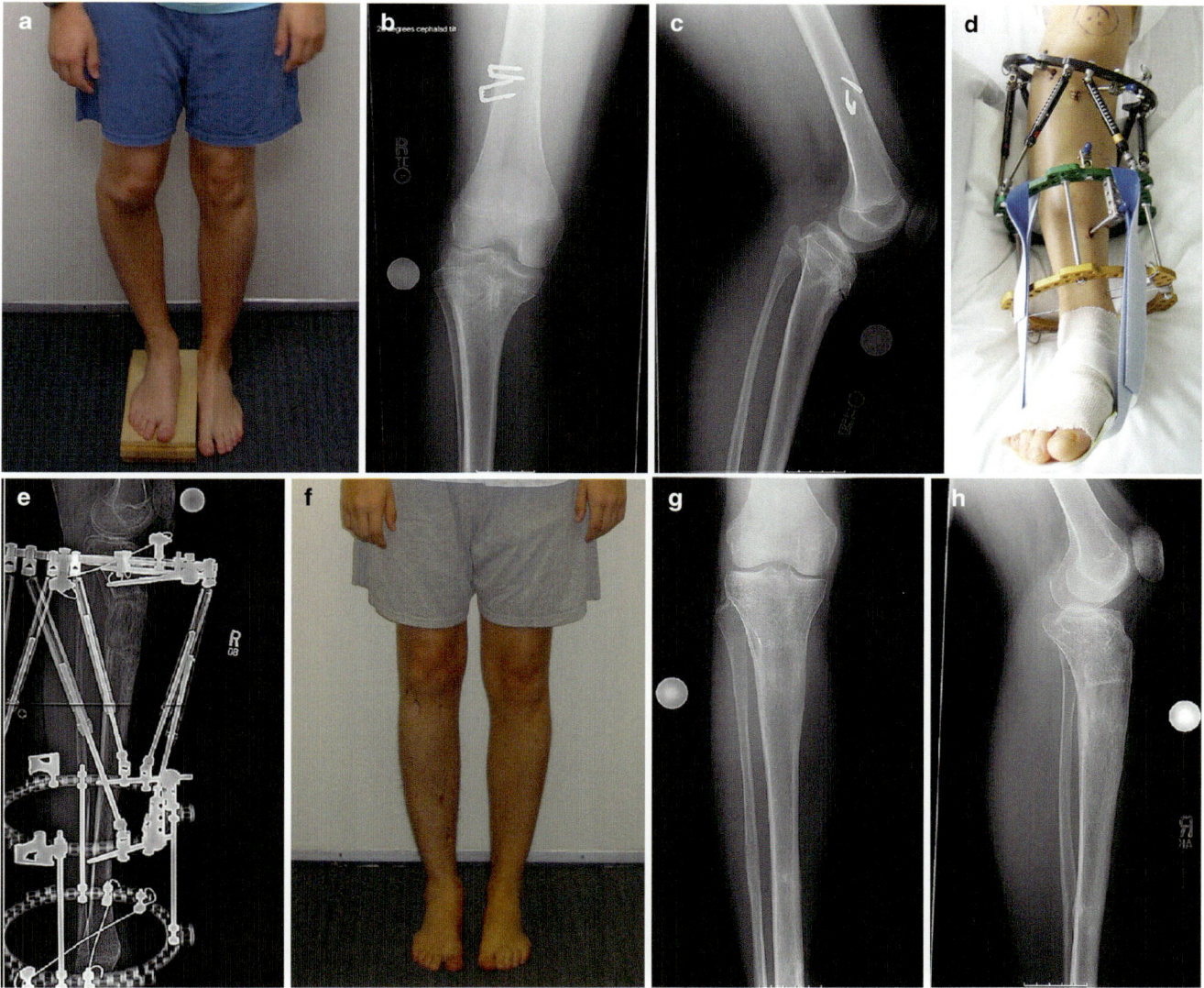

Fig. 40.8 (a) This clinical photo shows a proximal tibial deformity with shortening, varus, and malrotation. (b, c) AP and lateral X-rays show varus and recurvatum angulation with closure of the anteromedial physis. (d, e) This photo shows the early postoperative external fixator mimicking the deformity. The radiograph was taken near the end of the correction showing the proximal tibial lengthening. (f–h) Final clinical photo and radiographs demonstrate full correction of the deformity

Femur Malunion and Growth Disturbance

Distal femur physeal fractures are afflicted by a high rate of physeal arrest and subsequent deformity [46]. Displaced fractures and Salter–Harris II injuries are predictors of a poor outcome with a 40% risk of physeal bar formation [47]. Surgical reduction and fixation are recommended, and smooth Steinman pins crossing the physis do not seem to further increase the already high risk of physeal arrest [46, 48].

Distal femur malunion without growth plate arrest is another complication of pediatric femur fractures. Although the skeletally immature femur has a tremendous remodeling potential, angulation and shortening may not be tolerated as well as many surgeons believe. In children over 10 years of age, varus-valgus angulation of greater than 5° and procurvatum-recurvatum of greater than 10° should not be accepted because such deformities can be associated with premature knee arthritis [8].

Treatment of diaphyseal and distal femoral deformities that occur during childhood and subsequently present in adulthood can be accomplished with various implants including IM nail, plate and screws, and external fixation. The challenge is managing the femoral shortening that is often present in these individuals. External fixation allows for deformity correction and lengthening simultaneously [49]. Integrated fixation techniques provide the best of both devices using external fixation to achieve length and deformity correction and then converting to internal fixation while the immature bone consolidates [50–52]. The newer internal lengthening nails provide an all-internal correction of deformity and bone lengthening solution [53].

Case 5

A 19-year-old male presented with femoral valgus and shortening. He had been struck by a vehicle when he was 11 years old sustaining a distal femur physeal fracture. The fracture was stabilized with internal fixation. It is not known whether the fracture was reduced anatomically or was stabilized with residual valgus angulation. If the initial postoperative alignment was appropriate, then this may not qualify as an iatrogenic deformity. He was an avid soccer player but was having increasing difficulty playing due to the lower limb deformity and knee pain. Partial closure of the lateral distal femoral physis caused a valgus deformity and 3 cm of shortening (Fig. 40.9a, b). The patient was at a risk for knee arthritis, hip, and low back problems. The proposed treatment would address both the valgus deformity and the femur shortening. A distal osteotomy with lengthening is best done with a circular fixator, but the frame would need to be on the leg for a long time and femoral rings are very uncomfortable. The LAP (lengthening and plating) technique was selected. A femoral osteotomy was created and stabilized with a TSF (Fig. 40.9c). The correction was performed gradually with lengthening. Once the acceptable length and alignment were reached, the patient was brought back to surgery for insertion of a plate and screws and removal of the frame (Fig. 40.9d, e). The femur healed and the plate was later removed (Fig. 40.9f, g). He returned to play soccer without any limitations.

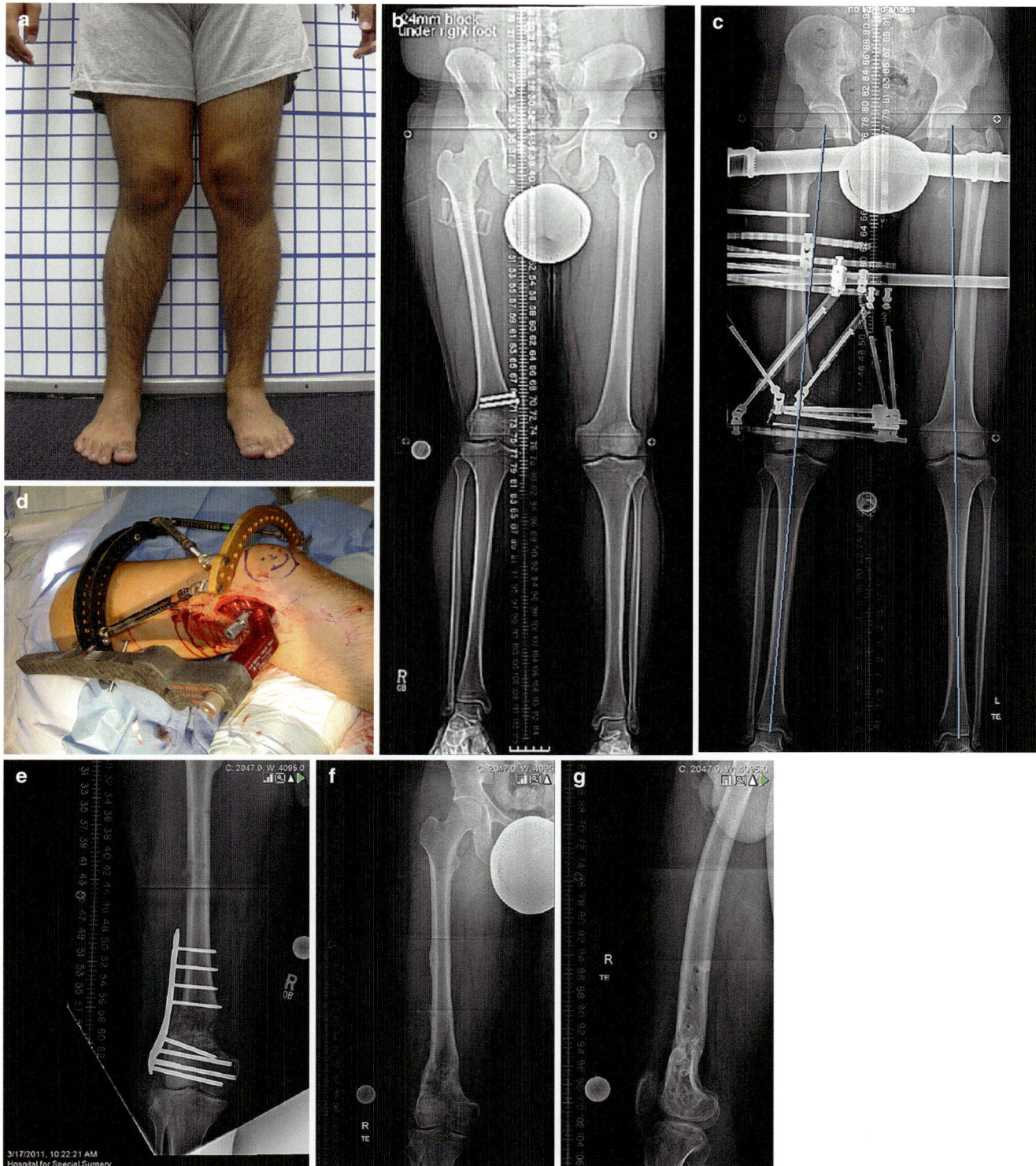

Fig. 40.9 (**a**, **b**) This clinical photo and radiograph show a valgus malunion of the distal femur with shortening. The two medial screws suggest a Salter–Harris 2 fracture with fixation. This X-ray was taken with the patient standing on blocks. (**c**) External fixation was used to distract and angulate the distal femur. (**d**) The external fixator was mounted differently to expose the lateral femur for subsequent plating. Here, the plate is being inserted. (**e**) This radiograph shows the plate spanning the new regenerate bone. (**f**, **g**) Final radiographs show full union of the osteotomy and ideal alignment

Case 6

A 34-year-old female presented with a deformity of the right femur and tibia. She had a femur fracture when she was 11 years old that was treated with skeletal traction followed a few days later by casting. The traction pin was placed into the proximal tibia at that time. She presented with a deformity of the right femur including valgus and shortening, and deformity of the right tibia including recurvatum and shortening. On examination, she had knee hyperextension of 20°, valgus alignment, and lateral knee instability. The radiographs revealed a 20° apex posterior deformity of the proximal tibia with 15-mm shortening and 6° of valgus, relative proximal migration of the proximal fibula, and 5° valgus deformity of the distal femur diaphysis with 20 mm of short-

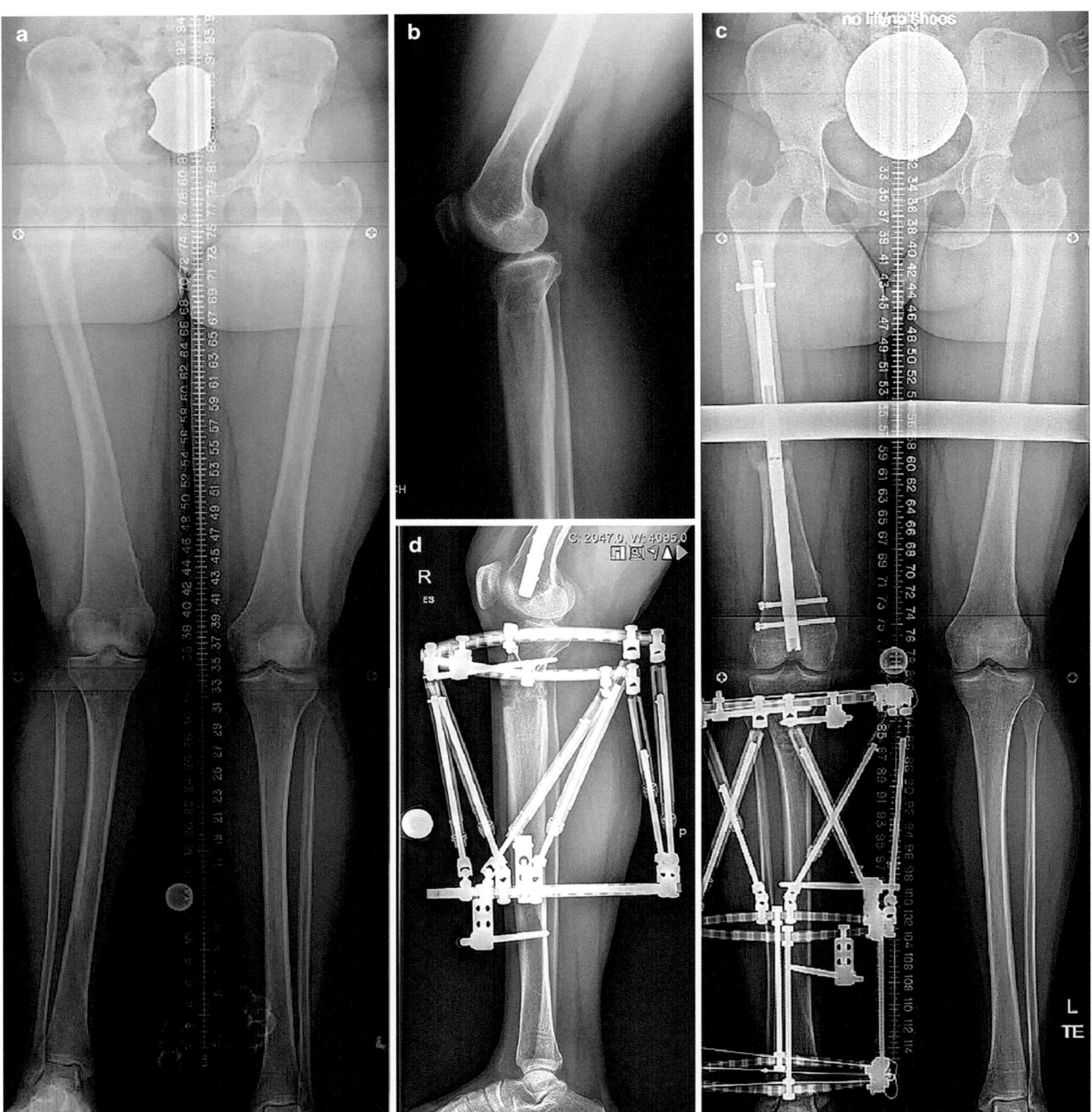

Fig. 40.10 (**a**, **b**) These radiographs show valgus of the distal femur and proximal tibia as well as a 20° recurvatum deformity of the proximal tibia. (**c**, **d**) Correction of the valgus femur malunion and shortening was performed with an internal lengthening nail. The tibia valgus and recurvatum as well as the superior migration of the fibula were all corrected with a tibial osteotomy and external fixation. (**e**–**g**) Final radiographs and a clinical photo show full healing and a successful correction of the deformities

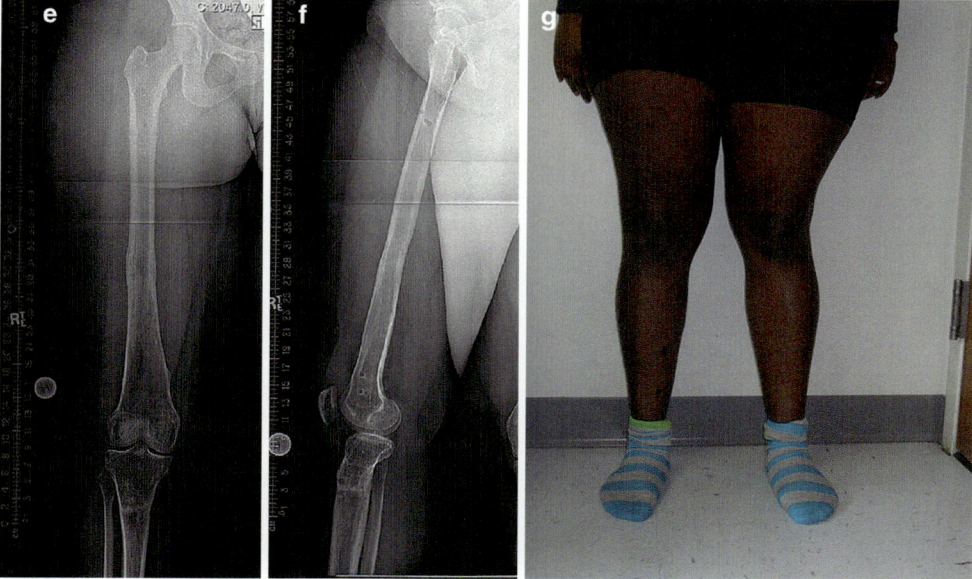

Fig. 40.10 (continued)

ening (Fig. 40.10a, b). The patient has knee instability and pain. She was at a high risk for developing premature knee arthritis and would have likely required living a life of activity modification. The surgical plan included femur surgery to both correct the valgus deformity and lengthen the femur. This was accomplished with a retrograde IM internal lengthening nail. The plan also included a gradual correction of the recurvatum and valgus deformities of the tibia with lengthening. This included translating the intact fibula distally to re-tension the lateral collateral ligament (Fig. 40.10c, d). After removal of the hardware, the patient is recovering well. The deformities have been corrected, and the knee is stable with normal extension (Fig. 40.10e–g).

Vascularized Fibula Graft Nonunion and Valgus Ankle Deformity from the Fibular Donor Site

Reconstruction of the tibia after tumor resection with contralateral vascularized fibular autograft is an effective limb-sparing procedure [54]. The rate of nonunion can be as high as 20% [55]. When the metaphyseal segment is small, achieving stability with internal fixation can be challenging. Circular fixation is especially effective in these situations.

Harvesting of the fibula for reconstruction of a bone defect with a vascularized fibular autograft can be associated with valgus deformity of the donor-side ankle [56–58]. Tibia-fibula syndesmosis synostosis has been recommended to prevent this deformity, but valgus can occur even after this measure [59]. Prevention is also possible and has been successful with stabilization of the fibula to the tibia using a distal syndesmotic screw [58]. Correction of the iatrogenic valgus deformity with external fixation through a supramalleolar osteotomy is effective in the short term but can be complicated by recurrence of the deformity [57]. In this case report, the guided-growth technique is used to restore the distal tibial alignment resulting in normal ankle joint orientation at maturity.

Case 7

A 10-year-old male was referred for the management of a nonunion and deformity at the junction of the proximal tibial metaphysis and a vascularized fibular autograft. The patient had an osteosarcoma excision of the proximal tibia reconstructed with contralateral fibular autograft and flap. The patient did not have recurrence of the tumor and the diaphyseal junction of the graft healed satisfactorily. He had pain, a varus and flexion deformity of the proximal tibia, and difficulty walking despite bracing. Radiographs revealed a nonunion of the proximal graft junction (Fig. 40.11a–c). The treatment plan was to repair the nonunion and correct the deformity with fine-wire fixation. The proximal tibial segment was very small, making it well suited for this technique. A percutaneous repair of the nonunion was performed by making a small incision over the nonunion site and passing a drillbit multiple times and in different planes to stimulate the adjacent bone to bleed. A curette was then passed through the drill holes to scrape the bone surfaces and further stimulate bony bleeding. This approach stimulated a healing response while minimizing trauma to the poor soft tissue envelope (Fig. 40.11d). The minimally invasive wires and pins accomplished the same goals of soft tissue preservation and provided excellent bony fixation. The deformities were corrected with the TSF and the nonunion was compressed (Fig. 40.11e). Weight-bearing ambulation was allowed postoperatively. The patient was also noted to have an iatrogenic deformity of the contralateral ankle. After the fibula was harvested, the ankle had drifted into a valgus deformity. Radiographs showed a valgus deformity of the distal tibia. This was addressed with guided growth using a small extraperiosteal plate and non-locking screws to tether the medial physis and improve the distal tibial valgus (Fig. 40.11f, g). After frame removal of the side with the nonunion, the graft-host junction of the proximal tibia had healed and the deformities were corrected including the contralateral distal tibial alignment. The patient underwent a distal femoral lengthen-

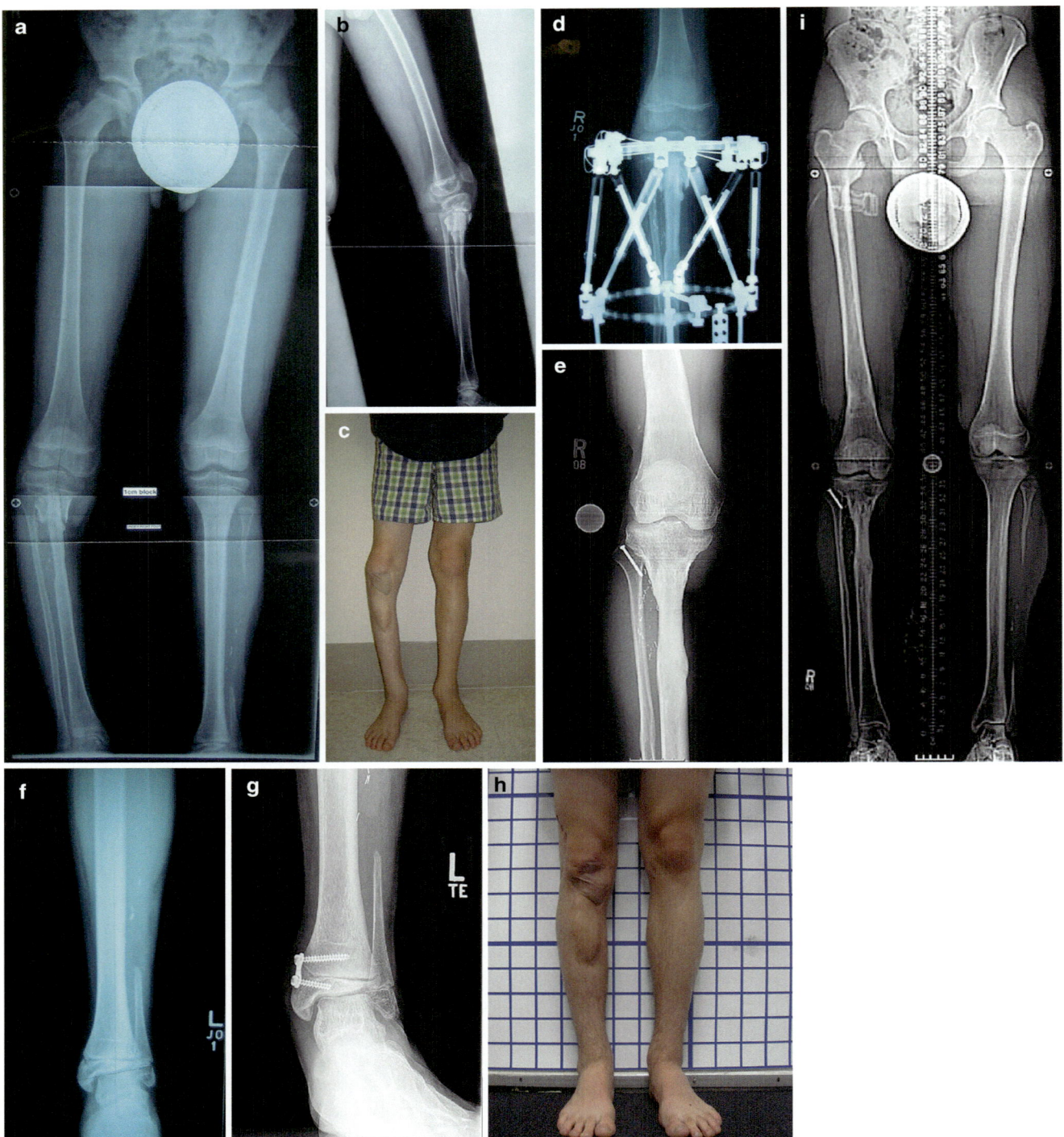

Fig. 40.11 (a–c) The radiographs show tibial shortening and a nonunion with angulation of the proximal graft-host junction. The vascularized fibular graft has hypertrophied but has failed to unite. The patient had a mobile nonunion with bowing and a lateral thrust. (d, e) Fixation with fine wires afforded enough stability for bone healing to progress. (f, g) Valgus deformity was developing at the donor-side ankle, which was treated with guided growth of the physis. (h, i) The final results were correction of the deformity, bony union, and correction of the donor-side ankle valgus

ing of the extremity with the proximal tibial autograft 2 years later to make up for the residual leg length discrepancy. It was felt that the ipsilateral tibia had already suffered enough trauma making a femoral osteotomy a wiser course of action (Fig. 40.11 h, i).

Deformity from Tibial Lengthening

Lengthening of the tibia from congenital or acquired shortening can be accomplished using the methods of Ilizarov. However, there are unbalanced forces from the posterior and lateral muscle groups acting upon the bone that cause predictable deformity: valgus and procurvatum. The challenge of distraction osteogenesis is to create a straight regenerate, thereby avoiding the creation of a tibial deformity. This iatrogenic deformity needs to be anticipated whether using external fixation or an internal lengthening nail. A further problem is bending of the new regenerate bone when the external fixator is removed prematurely. Even if the lengthening is done correctly, the new bone is still at risk for developing angular deformity (Fig. 40.12a, b). Both deformities that occur during lengthening and after lengthening are considered malunions and are considered iatrogenic. The treatment of these malunions is either casting to prevent further angulation, internal fixation with osteotomy to correct the current deformity, or external fixation with osteotomy. If the immature lengthening regenerate bends and is managed early enough, then it can be manually realigned without osteotomy and stabilized with external or internal fixation.

Contracture of the ankle and knee joints is a common complication of tibial lengthening surgery. Tightening of the gastrocnemius muscle and fascia pulls the ankle into equinus and the knee into flexion. A tibial lengthening of greater than 13% of the length of the tibia bone and congenital etiology were risk factors for an equinus contracture. Furthermore, gastro-soleus recession restored preoperative motion in all cases [60]. Acute correction of these contractures should be avoided to prevent undue stretching on the already tight nerves, especially the tibial nerve at the tarsal tunnel. When these contractures occur before the desired tibial length has been achieved, then consideration should be given to stopping or slowing down the lengthening process to allow for improved range of joint motion.

Case 8

A 10-year-old male presented with shortening and deformity of the left tibia. He had no previous trauma, no syndrome, and no femoral involvement. He was felt to have a very mild fibular hemimelia resulting in angular deformity

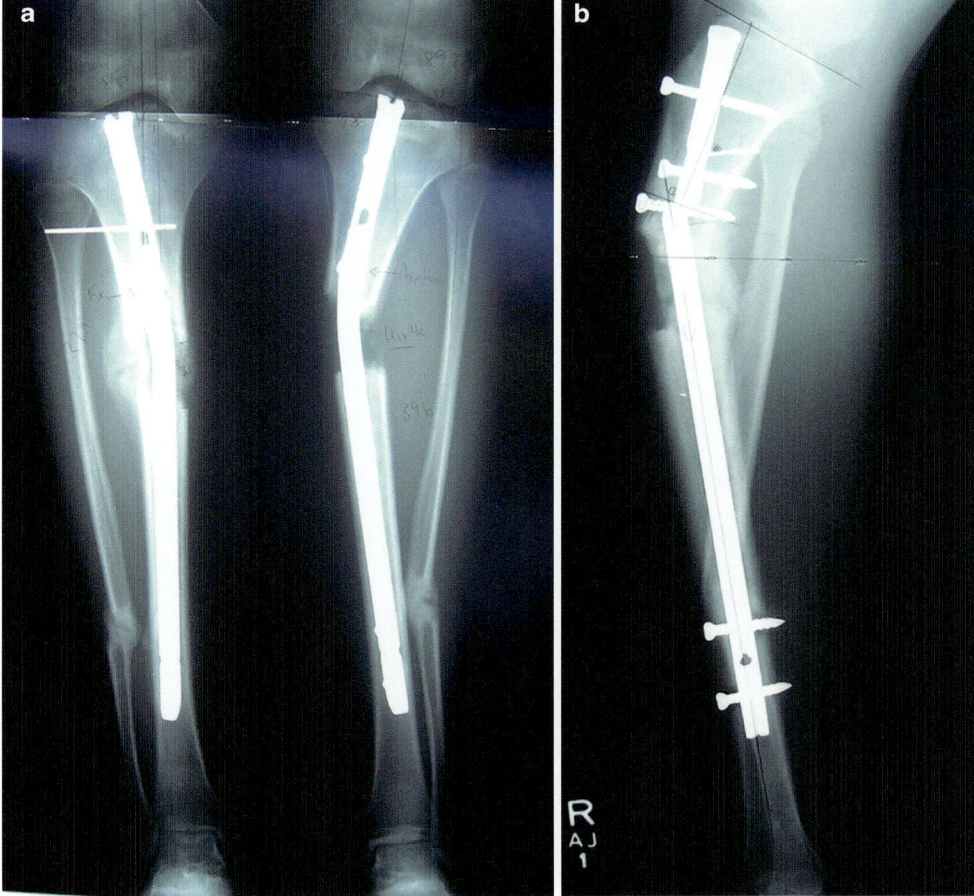

Fig. 40.12 (a, b) A patient underwent bilateral tibial lengthening surgery by lengthening the tibia with an external fixator over an IM nail. Once the desired length was achieved, the fixator was removed and the patient started weight bearing too early. These AP and lateral (respectively) radiographs show collapse and angulation through the tibial lengthening site. The immature bone could not support weight bearing and failed with angulation of the regenerate and fracture of the internal fixation

and shortening of the affected tibia and fibula (Fig. 40.13a–c). He had normal range of motion and stability of both ankle and knee joints. There was 8 cm of shortening with additional shortening expected as growth continued. The goal was to obtain at least 5 cm of shortening, which was an 18% lengthening of the tibia. The patient was treated with double-level tibia osteotomies lengthened at 1.0 mm per day for a total of 2.0 mm per day of limb lengthening (Fig. 40.13d, e). This rate was chosen to prevent premature consolidation at either lengthening site. The result of this rapid lengthening was equinus contracture of the ankle and knee flexion contracture (Fig. 40.13f). The patient and his mother were unable to stretch the contracture despite physical therapy. The patient underwent a gastro-soleus recession at the mid-distal-leg level with attachment of a foot ring and hinges. The ankle joint was distracted acutely 3 mm to prevent articular cartilage compression. The correction of the equinus contracture was performed gradually with the foot ring. A spring-loaded hinged brace was attached to the tibial ring to help correct this knee flexion

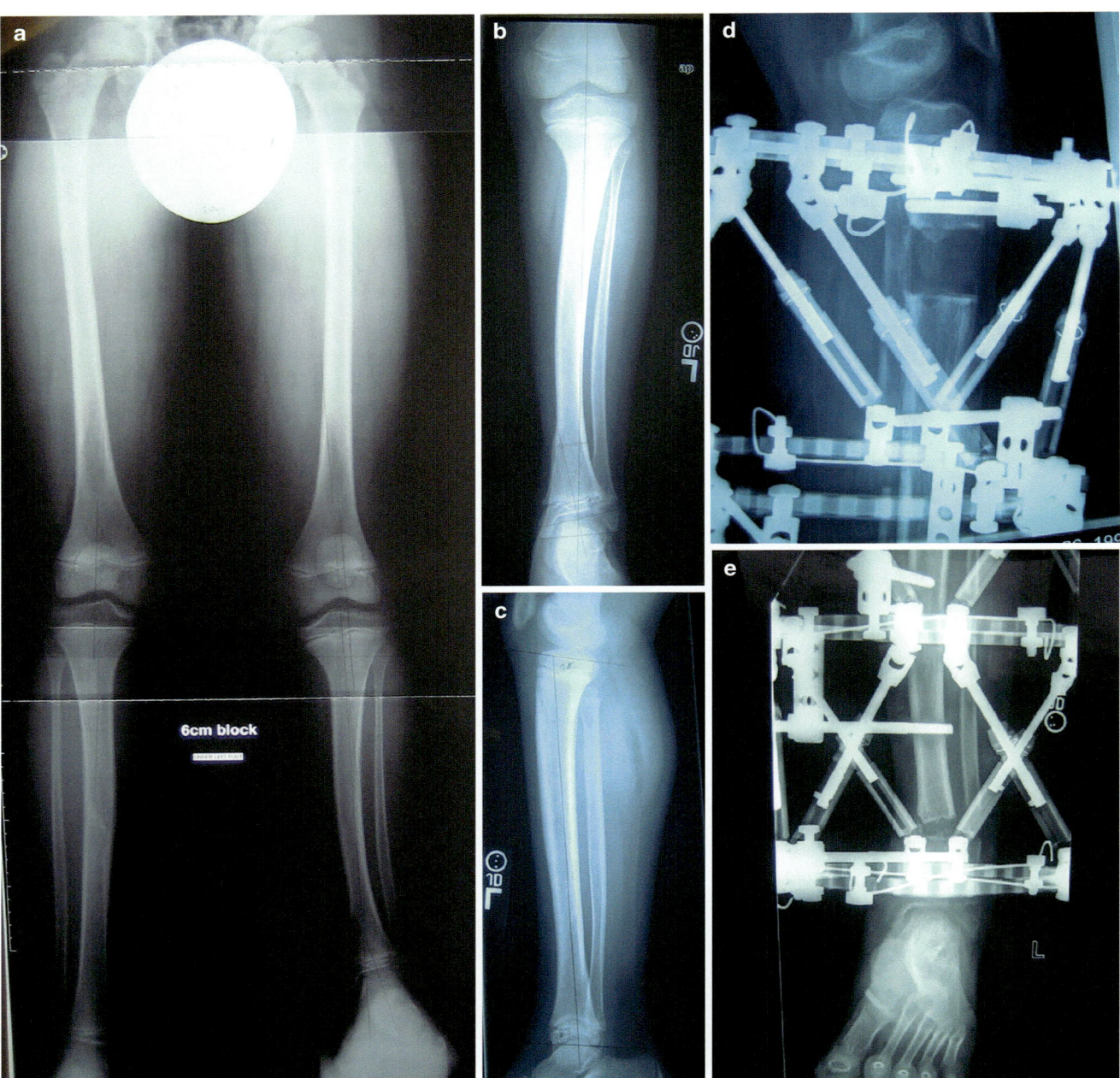

Fig. 40.13 (**a–c**) These radiographs show a two-level, congenital deformity of the left tibia with significant shortening. (**d, e**) The proximal osteotomy allowed for mild deformity correction and lengthening. The distal osteotomy allowed for deformity correction and mild lengthening. (**f**) Ankle and knee contractures are apparent during the lengthening process. (**g**) The foot ring is seen in an overcorrected position to prevent recurrence. The dynamic, spring-loaded brace is seen bolted onto the proximal tibial ring delivering an extension moment. (**h, i**) Final X-rays show full healing, correction of the deformity, and successful attainment of length

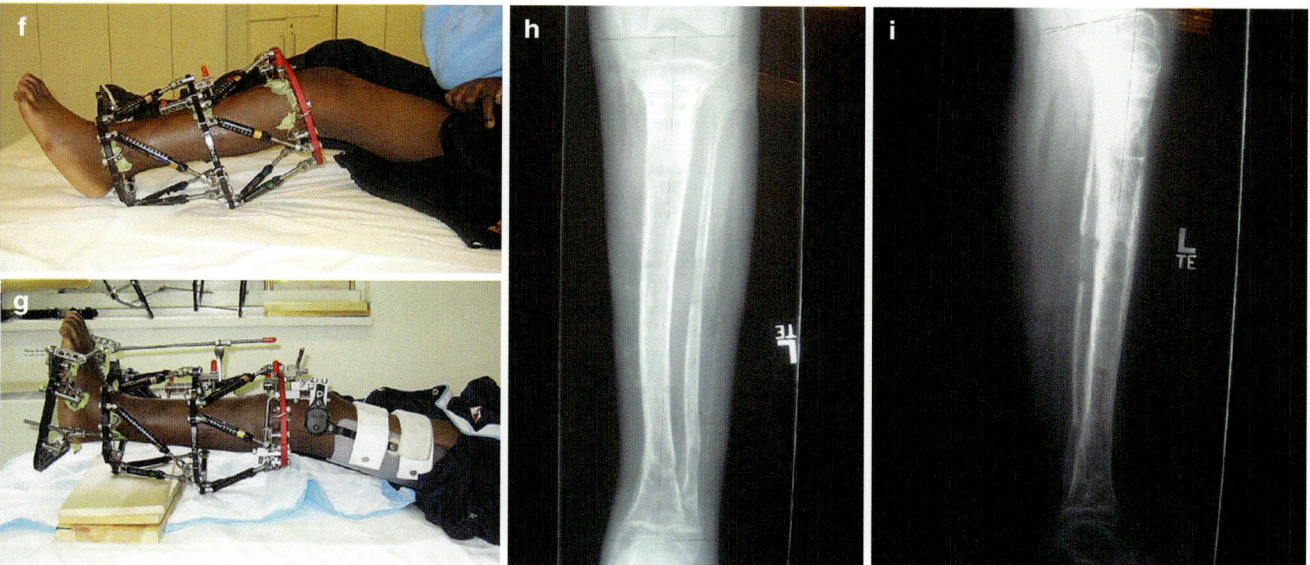

Fig. 40.13 (continued)

deformity (Fig. 40.13g). Further lengthening was stopped. After frame removal, a total of 5 cm of length had been achieved, and ankle and knee range of motion were eventually normal (Fig. 40.13h, i). The patient can undergo further lengthening in the future.

Translational Deformity

Iatrogenic translational deformity can occur when an osteotomy is performed at a location away from the apex of the deformity. These osteotomies require a deliberate translation of the bone fragments to ensure that the joints remain in line with the long axis of the tibia and the mechanical axis of the femur. These intentional translations may look like an accidental iatrogenic deformity when in fact they are planned and desirable. Patients will often need reassurance that the translational "deformity" was intended.

Case 9

A 42-year-old female had a correction of Blount's disease at the age of 10 years. A varus and flexion deformity recurred over time and led to medial compartment arthritis (Fig. 40.14a, b). Preoperative radiographs showed a medial mechanical axis deviation (MAD), 17° of varus, and the apex of the deformity at the knee joint line (Fig. 40.14c, d). The osteotomy performed distal to the tibial tubercle would require a lateral translation of 24 mm (Fig. 40.14e). This would create an iatrogenic deformity of the tibia in order to restore the mechanical axis and the proper joint orientation angles, the medial proximal tibial angle (MPTA). A circular fixator was used to achieve a gradual correction of the deformity and translate the distal fragment laterally (Fig. 40.14f). Final radiographs demonstrate an apparent iatrogenic deformity of the proximal tibia (Fig. 40.14g–j). However, the MAD and MPTA have been restored, and the bone healed without incident. It is likely that this translation, although technically correct, will cause difficulty with conversion to a total knee replacement.

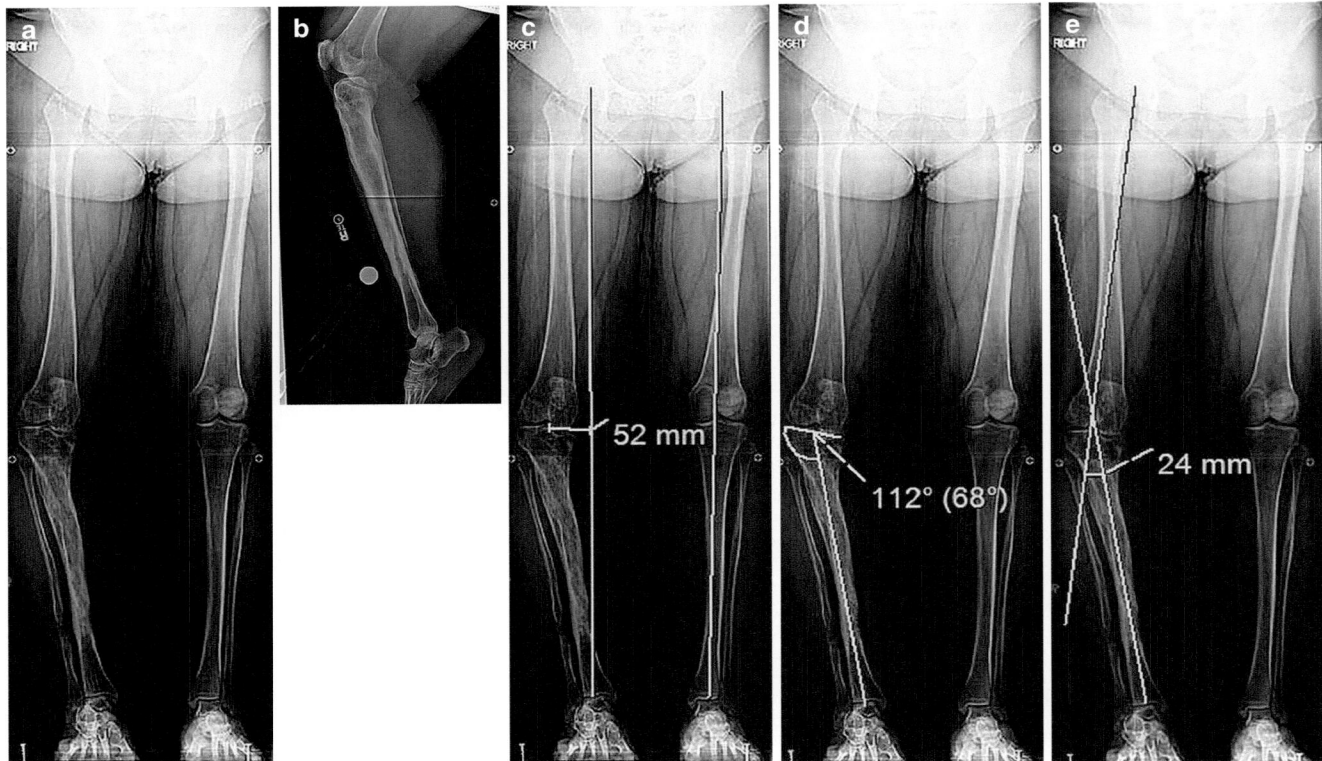

Fig. 40.14 (**a**, **b**) Preoperative radiographs demonstrate varus and flexion deformities of the right proximal tibia. (**c**, **d**) The MAD is 52 mm medial to the midline, and the MPTA is 68°. (**e**) This represents a 17° varus deformity. The CORA is near the knee joint line. The planned osteotomy is below the tibial tubercle. In order to prevent a translational deformity, the distal bone fragment must be translated 24 mm laterally in addition to the angular correction of 17°. (**f**) Circular fixation is ideal for executing angular and translational movements of the bone. (**g**, **h**) Final radiographs after frame removal show what looks like an extreme amount of translation at the osteotomy site. (**i**, **j**) Mechanical axis and joint orientation analysis exhibit a slight lateral MAD and an MPTA of 87°; both were ideal for this patient

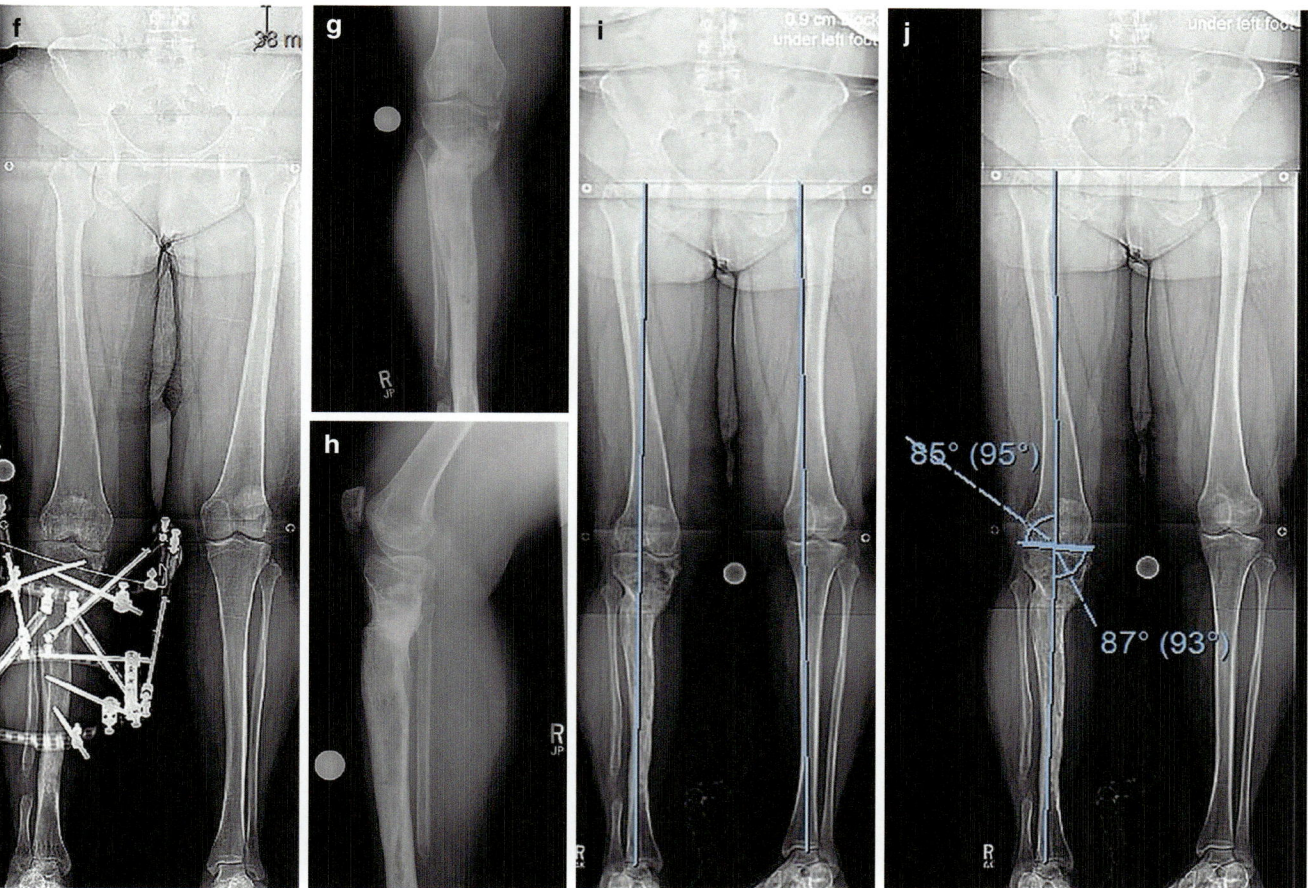

Fig. 40.14 (continued)

Box 40.1 Highlights
- The ability to correct deformity has improved, making anatomic restoration of bone more attainable.
- Posttraumatic malunions are often seen with displaced pediatric tibial shaft fractures and have directed initial treatment in some adolescents toward surgical fixation rather than casting.
- Transphyseal ACL reconstruction can, in rare cases, result in growth disturbance.
- Limb lengthening often creates predictable deformity that the surgeon must be able to anticipate, recognize, and treat.
- Intentional translation after osteotomy for periarticular deformities maintains proper limb alignment, but the bone may appear deformed to the untrained eye.

Summary

Iatrogenic deformity takes many forms (Box 40.1). The surgeon must consider factors such as the location and magnitude of the deformity and the growth remaining when deciding on treatment options. The tools available to repair malunions and restore alignment have improved, and the outcome of surgical reconstruction has become more predictable. Patients with deformity need not suffer for the remainder of their lives or until they are old enough for a joint replacement. Further research will help determine more accurate parameters for acceptable alignment. Advances in technology will continue to make anatomic restoration of deformities and fractures more easily attainable.

Commentary

J. Spence Reid
jreid@pennstatehealth.psu.edu

As sub-specialization in orthopedics continues to evolve, the standard of care continues to rise in each discipline as more surgeons focus their efforts into a narrower range. This has certainly occurred in the field of fracture care for both the adult as well as pediatric population. In addition, there is increasing recognition of the sequela of malalignment. New tools and methods to precisely correct deformity continue to evolve. As the authors point out, this higher bar or "narrowed strike zone" is likely to continue as techniques improve.

Sometimes, patients with a residual deformity after fracture treatment may elect to not undergo additional surgical correction because of practical considerations such as family, educational, or work obligations. As time passes, many of these patients may change their mind and return to either the original treating surgeon or a specialized center.

In the case of litigation, the authors point out that disability not cosmesis per se drives the outcome. Patients need to be educated that not all deformity leads to disability—particularly in the upper extremity where significant deformity can be compatible with normal function.

In the case of an unexpected residual deformity after treatment, the surgeon needs to be both honest with the patient and themselves. If the experience and skill set to correct the problem are not present, it would be best for the treating surgeon to personally find an appropriate referral for the patient and set up the appointment. Given the possibility of litigation, the referred surgeon should be called, and the situation carefully explained (Fig. 40.15a–d).

Fibular malunion: In the adult patient following an ankle fracture, fibular shortening can also occur resulting in a talar tilt and significant risk of future arthritis. This can be corrected with acute lengthening via an oblique osteotomy and use of autologous bone graft from the proximal tibia(Fig. 40.16a–d).

Integrated techniques that employ initial external fixation to allow both slow deformity correction as well as lengthening followed by the use of internal fixation (IM nails or plates) are being increasingly used in deformity correction in both pediatric and adult populations. These techniques allow the "best of both worlds" in that the power of precise deformity correction with hexapod ring fixation is employed, but the extended frame time is avoided. The infection risk associated with the conversion remains a concern, but has been shown to be less of a problem than previously thought. This may be partially due to increased experienced with these techniques and possibly the routine use of hydroxyapatite coated fixator pins which may reduce the incidence of pin site infections. (Saithna A, The influence of hydroxyapatite coating of external fixator pins on pin loosening and pin track infection: a systematic review. Injury. 2010 Feb;41(2):128–32).

Translational deformity as a result of an osteotomy at a distance from the apex of the deformity is not technically iatrogenic since it is simply the geometric result of this technique. But as the authors point out, warning the patient/family of the effect on the overall alignment and radiographic appearance prior to surgery will do much to avoid a surprise as treatment progresses.

Case 1: 25 yo man sustained a bimalleolar ankle fracture, fixed as shown below

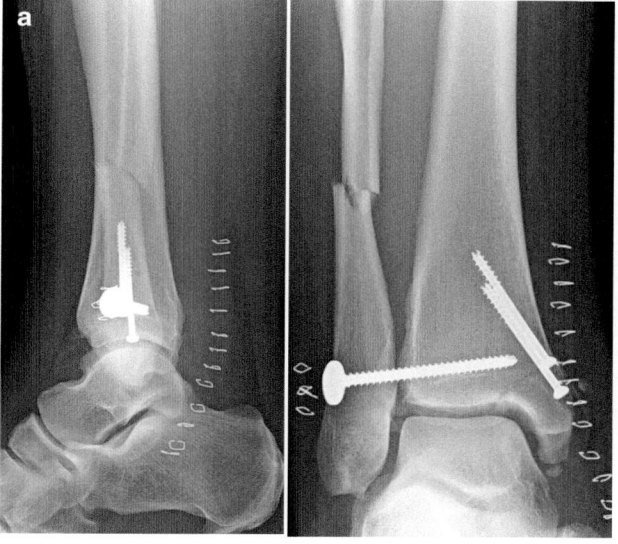

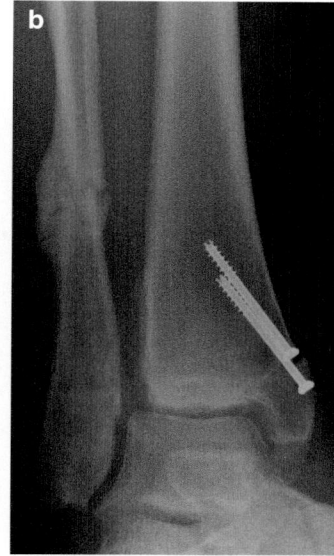

4 months later the patient presented with ankle pain and a talar tilt with fibular shortening and a mal-reduced medial malleolus

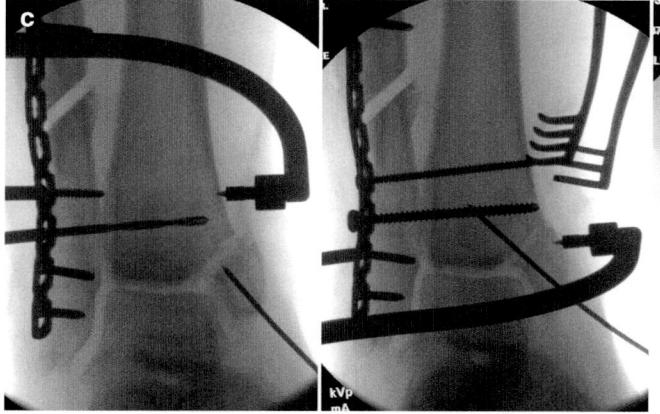

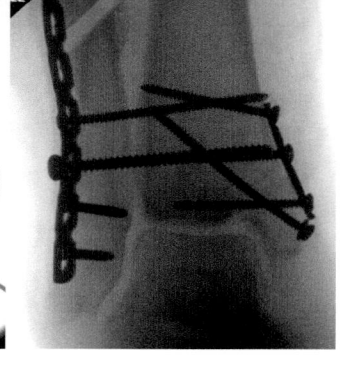

The fibula was acutely lengthened, the syndesmosis, and medial malleolus both open reduced. Autogenous bone from the proximal tibia was placed into the fibular defect.

Fig. 40.15 (**a–d**) This case was incompletely united and still in treatment at the time of the second opinion. In this situation, the surgeon performing the second opinion should specifically ask the family if they are seeking only a second opinion or a possible transfer of care? If care is to be transferred, then a communication (preferably a phone call) should be made to the original treating surgeon to explain the situation and that the care will be transferred. This will create good will and a likely future referral pattern. In addition, it will alleviate a great deal of anxiety on the part of the original treating surgeon

At 6 months post reconstruction, the ankle mortise was well reduced, and patient was pain free.

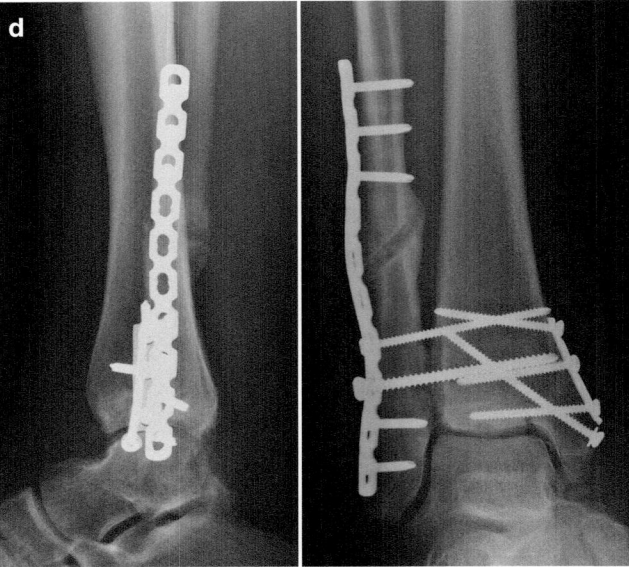

Fig. 40.15 (continued)

Fig. 40.16 (**a–d**) As the authors alluded to, the adult patient with a leg length discrepancy and distal femoral deformity can also be managed with a fixator-assisted retrograde internal lengthening nail using the "reverse planning method" described by Baumgart (Rainer Baumgart; *The reverse planning method for lengthening of the lower limb using a straight intramedullary nail with or without deformity correction. A new method.* Oper Orthop Traumatol. 2009 June 21(2):221–33

Rainer Baumgart; *The reverse planning method for lengthening of the lower limb using a straight intramedullary nail with or without deformity correction. A new method.* Oper OrthopTraumatol. 2009 June 21(2):221-33

Case 2: 36 you woman with fibrous dysplasia in proximal femur.
Presents with a valgus deformity and residual 5 cm LLD. Using the method of Baumgart, a fixator assisted retrograde internal lengthening nail was placed with excellent restoration of length and alignment.

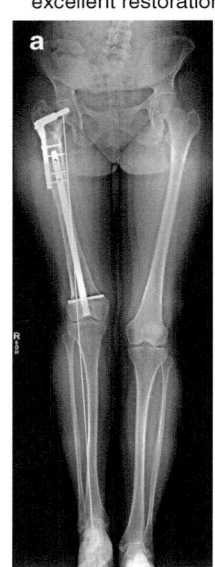 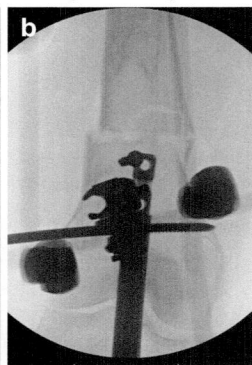 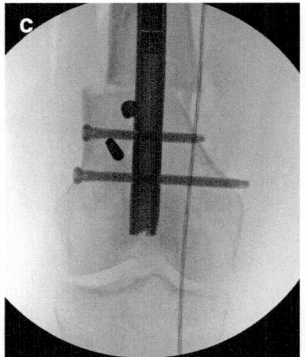 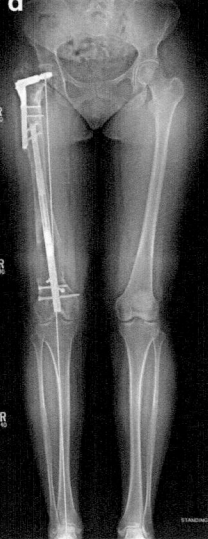

References

1. Sarmiento A. A functional below-knee cast for tibial fractures. J Bone Joint Surg Am. 1967;49-A:855–75.
2. Alho A, Ekeland A, Stromsoe K, Follerås G, Thoresen BO. Locked intramedullary nailing for displaced tibial shaft fractures. J Bone Joint Surg Br. 1990;72-B(5):805–9.
3. Sarmiento A, Gersten L, Sobol P, Shankwiler JA, Vangsness CT. Tibial shaft fractures treated with functional braces. Experience with 780 fractures. J Bone Joint Surg Br. 1989;71(4):602–9.
4. Vallier H, Cureton B, Patterson B. Factors influencing functional outcomes after distal tibia shaft fractures. J Orthop Trauma. 2012;26(3):178–83.
5. Ricci W, O'Boyle M, Borrelli J, Bellabarba C, Sanders R. Fractures of the proximal third of the tibial shaft treated with intramedullary nails and blocking screws. J Orthop Trauma. 2001;15(4):264–70.
6. Russell T, Mir H, Stoneback J, Cohen J, Downs B. Avoidance of malreduction of proximal femoral shaft fractures with the use of a minimally invasive nail insertion technique (MINT). J Orthop Trauma. 2008;22(6):391–8.
7. Valderrabano V, Horisberger M, Russell I, Dougall H, Hintermann B. Etiology of ankle osteoarthritis. Clin Orthop Relat Res. 2009;467(7):1800–6.
8. Palmu S, Lohman M, Paukku R, Peltonen JI, Nietosvaara Y. Childhood femoral fracture can lead to premature knee-joint arthritis. 21-year follow up results: a retrospective study. Acta Orthop. 2013;84(1):71–5.
9. Eckhoff D, Kramer R, Alongi C, VanGerven DP. Femoral anteversion and arthritis of the knee. J Pediatr Orthop. 1994;14:608–10.
10. Mootanah R, Imhauser C, Reisse F, Carpanen D, Walker RW, Koff MF, et al. Development and validation of a computational model oft eh knee for the evaluation of surgical treatments for osteoarthritis. Comput Methods Biomech Biomed Engin. 2014;17(13):1502–17.
11. Jena A, Seabury S, Lakdawalla D, Chandra A. Malpractice risk according to physician specialty. N Engl J Med. 2011;365(7):629–36.
12. Brennan T, Sox C, Burstin H. Relation between negligent adverse events and the outcomes of medical malpractice litigation. N Engl J Med. 1996;335(26):1963–7.
13. Matsen F, Stephens L, Jette J, Warme WJ, Posner KL. Lessons regarding the safety of orthopaedic patient care. An analysis of four hundred and sixty four closed malpractice claims. J Bone Joint Surg Am. 2013;95:e201–8.
14. DeNoble P, Marshall A, Barron O, Catalano LW 3rd, Glickel SZ. Malpractice in distal radius fracture management: an analysis of closed claims. J Hand Surg Am. 2014;39(8):1480–8.
15. Mashru R, Herman M, Pizzutillo P. Tibial shaft fractures in children and adolescents. J Am Acad Orthop Surg. 2005;13(5):345–52.
16. Gordon J, O'Donnell J. Tibia fractures: what should be fixed? J Pediatr Orthop. 2012;32(1):S52–61.
17. Robertson P, Karol L, Rab G. Open fractures of the tibia and femur on children. J Pediatr Orthop. 1996;16:621–6.
18. Bohn W, Durbin R. Ipsilateral fractures of the femur and the tibia in children and adolescents. J Bone Joint Surg Am. 1991;73:429–39.
19. Yang J, Letts R. Isolated fractures of the tibia with intact fibula in children: a review of 95 patients. J Pediatr Orthop. 1997;17:347–51.
20. Kubiak E, Egol K, Scher D, Wasserman B, Feldman D, Koval KJ. Operative treatment of tibial fractures in children: are elastic stable intramedullary nails and improvement over external fixation? J Bone Joint Surg Am. 2005;87:1761–8.
21. Gordon J, Schoenecker P, Oda J, Ortman MR, Szymanski DA, Dobbs MB, et al. A retrospective comparison of monolateral and circular external fixation of unstable diaphyseal tibia fractures in children. J Pediatr Orthop. 2003;12:338–45.
22. Gordon J, Gregush R, Schoenecker P, et al. Complications after titanium elastic nailing of pediatric tibial fractures. J Pediatr Orthop. 2007;27:442–6.
23. Wood D, Hoffer M. Tibial fractures in head injured children. J Trauma. 1987;27:65–8.
24. Paletta C, Dehghan K. Compartment syndrome in children. Ann Plast Surg. 1994;32:141–4.
25. Tafazal S, Madan S, Ali F, Padman M, Swift S, Jones S, et al. Management of paediatric tibial fractures using two types of circular external fixator: Taylor spatial frame and Ilizarov circular fixator. J Child Orthop. 2014;8(3):273–9.
26. Monsell F, Howells N, Lawniczak D, Jeffcote B, Mitchell SR. High energy open tibial fractures in children: treatment with a programmable circular external fixator. J Bone Joint Surg Br. 2012;94(7):989–93.
27. Norman D, Peskin B, Ehrenraich A, Rosenberg N, Bar-Joseph G, Bialik V. The use of external fixators in the immobilization of pediatric fractures. Arch Orthop Trauma Surg. 2002;122:379–82.
28. Al-Aubaidi Z. Valgus deformity after distal fibular fracture. Ugeskr Laeger. 2011;173(42):2656–7.
29. Lui T, Chan K, Ngai W. Premature closure of the fibular growth plate: a case of longitudinal syndesmosis instability. Arch Orthop Trauma Surg. 2008;128(1):45–8.
30. Ramsey P, Hamilton W. Changes in tibio-talar area of contact caused by lateral talar shifts. J Bone Joint Surg Am. 1976;58:356–7.
31. Karrholm J, Hansson L, Selvik G. Changes in tibiofibular relationships due to growth disturbances after ankle fractures in children. J Bone Joint Surg Am. 1984;66:1198–210.
32. Lalonde K, Letts M. Traumatic growth arrest of the distal tibia: a clinical and radiographic review. Can J Surg. 2005;48:143–7.
33. Sharma O, Sharma N, Patond K. Fibular shortening in poliomyelitis. Indian J Pediatr. 1994;61:71–4.
34. Offierski C, Graham J, Hall J. Late revision of fibular malunion in ankle fractures. Clin Orthop Relat Res. 1982;171:145–9.
35. Roberts C, Sherman O, Bauer D. Ankle reconstruction for malunion by fibular osteotomy and lengthening with direct control of the distal fragment: a report of three cases and review of the literature. Foot Ankle. 1992;13:7–13.
36. Weber B, Simpson L. Corrective lengthening osteotomy of the fibula. Clin Orthop Relat Res. 1985;199:61–7.
37. Manoudis G, Kontogeorgakos V, Badras L. Distal fibular lengthening after premature growth arrest: a case report. J Orthop Surg (Hong Kong). 2012;20(3):409–13.
38. Kumar S, Ahearne D, Hunt D. Transphyseal anterior cruciate ligament reconstruction in the skeletally immature: follow up to a minimum of sixteen years of age. J Bone Joint Surg Am. 2013;95(1):e1.
39. Kohl S, Stutz C, Decker S, Ziebarth K, Slongo T, Ahmad SS, et al. Mid term results of transphyseal anterior cruciate ligament reconstruction in children and adolescents. Knee. 2014;21(1):80–5.
40. Lipscomb A, Anderson A. Tears of the anterior cruciate ligament in adolescents. J Bone Joint Surg Am. 1986;68(1):19–28.
41. Lemaitre G, Salle de Chou E, Pineau V, Rochcongar G, Delforge S, Bronfen C, et al. ACL reconstruction in children: a transphyseal technique. Orthop Traumatol Surg Res. 2014;100(4 Suppl):S261–5.
42. Aronowitz E, Ganley T, Goode J, Gregg JR, Meyer JS. Anterior cruciate ligament reconstruction in adolescents with open physes. Am J Sports Med. 2000;28(2):168–75.

43. Cohen M, Ferretti M, Quarteiro M, Marcondes FB, de Hollanda JP, Amaro JT, et al. Transphyseal anterior cruciate ligament reconstruction in patients with open physes. Arthroscopy. 2009;25(8):831–8.
44. Hui C, Roe J, Ferguson D, Waller A, Salmon L, Pinczewski L. Outcome of anatomic transphyseal anterior cruciate ligament reconstruction in Tanner stage 1 and 2 patients with open physes. Am J Sports Med. 2012;40(5):1093–8.
45. Kocher M, Garg S, Micheli L. Physeal sparing reconstruction of the anterior cruciate ligament in skeletally immature prepubescent children and adolescents. J Bone Joint Surg Am. 2005;87(11):2371–9.
46. Garrett B, Hoffman E, Carrara H. The effect of percutaneous pin fixation in the treatment of distal femoral physeal fractures. J Bone Joint Surg Br. 2011;93(5):689–94.
47. Arkader A, Warner W, Horn B, Shaw RN, Wells L. Predicting the outcome of physeal fractures of the distal femur. J Pediatr Orthop. 2007;27(6):703–8.
48. Eid A, Hafez M. Traumatic injuries of the distal femoral physis. Retrospective study on 151 cases. Injury. 2002;33(3):251–5.
49. Palatnik Y, Rozbruch S. Femoral reconstruction using external fixation. Adv Orthop. 2011;2011:967186.
50. Iobst C, Dahl M. Limb lengthening with submuscular plate stabilization: a case series and description of the technique. J Pediatr Orthop. 2007;27(5):504–9.
51. Rozbruch S, Kleinman D, Fragomen A, Ilizarov S. Limb lengthening and then nailing of an intramedullary nail: a case-matched comparison. Clin Orthop Relat Res. 2008;466(12):2923–32.
52. Harbacheuski R, Fragomen A, Rozbruch S. Does lengthening and then plating shorten duration of external fixation? Clin Orthop Relat Res. 2012;470(6):1771–81.
53. Kirane Y, Fragomen A, Rozbruch S. Precision of the precice internal bone lengthening nail. Clin Orthop Relat Res. 2014;472(12):3869–78.
54. Scaglioni M, Arzi R, Gur E, Amotz OB, Barnea Y, Kollender Y, et al. Free fibular reconstruction of distal tibial defects after sarcoma surgery. Ann Plast Surg. 2015;74(6):680–3.
55. Tanaka K, Maehara H, Kanaya F. Vascularized fibular graft of bone defects after wide resection of musculoskeletal tumors. J Orthop Sci. 2012;17(2):156–62.
56. Nathan SS, Athanasian E, Boland PJ, Healey JH. Valgus ankle deformity after vascularized fibular reconstruction for oncologic disease. Ann Surg Oncol. 2009;16(7):1938–45.
57. Kang S, Rhee S, Song S, Chung JW, Kim YC, Suhl KH. Ankle deformity secondary to acquired fibular segmental defect in children. Clin Orthop Surg. 2010;2(3):179–85.
58. Fragniere B, Wicart P, Mascard E, Dubousset J. Prevention of ankle valgus after vascularized fibular grafts in children. Clin Orthop Relat Res. 2003;408:245–51.
59. Kanyata K, Wada T, Kura H, Yamashita T, Usui M, Ishii S. Valgus deformity of the ankle following harvesting of a vascularized fibular graft in children. J Reconstr Microsurg. 2002;18(2):91–6.
60. Rozbruch S, Zonshayn S, Muthusamy S, Borst EW, Fragomen AT, Nguyen JT. What risk factors predict usage of gastrosoleus recession during tibial lengthening? Clin Orthop Relat Res. 2014;472(12):3842–51.

Index

A

Abductor muscle slide, 623
Abnormal growth plate function, 106
Abnormal physis, 106
Accordion maneuver, 865
Accordion technique, 875
Acetabular deformity, 884
Acetabular dysplasia, 673, 884, 886
Acetabular fragment, 891, 892
Acetabular injuries, 933
Acetabular reamer technique, 981
Acetabular version, 27
Acetabuloplasty
   skeletally immature, 887
   techniques, 919
Achilles tenotomy, 716
Achondroplasia, 7, 21, 374, 375, 543–546
Achterman and Kalamchi classification, 716
Achterman and Kalamchi type-II FH, 742
Activated platelets, 868
Acute deformity correction
   acute complications
      compartment syndrome, 143
      iatrogenic fractures, 143
      neurological, 143
      physeal damage, 143–144
      skin and wound problems, 143
      vascular injury, 143
   age considerations, 117–119
   angle stable devices, 137
   angular correction and translation, 122
   angular deformity secondary to physeal insult, 124
   bifocal procedures, 124
   blade plates, 137
   bone void fillers, 138–139
   Cozen's phenomenon, 125–126
   deformity memory effect, 125
   disease-specific indications, 131–132
   external fixation, 138
   fixator-assisted plating, 139
   general considerations, 117
   hardware considerations, 135
   internal lengthening nail, 164
   intramedullary devices, 137–138
   Kirschner (K) wires, 135
   late complications
      acute vs. gradual correction, 145–146
      cast-related complications, 145
      hardware-related complications, 144–145
      joint stiffness, 144
      muscle weakness, 145
      non-union and delayed union, 144
      recurrent deformity, 144
      vascular, 144
   length discrepancy, 130
   limb reconstruction systems, 138
   locked plates, 137
   lower limb alignment, 119
   mango slice effect, 125
   osteotomy
      adjuvant fibular osteotomy, 120
      adjuvant procedures, 130–131
      angular correction and translation, 122–123
      closing wedge osteotomy, 122
      diaphysis, 127
      dome osteotomy, 122
      epiphyseal, 127
      indications, 126
      juxta-apophyseal, 127
      knee, 130
      lengthening osteotomy, 123
      level of, 120
      metaphysis, 126
      oblique osteotomy, 123
      opening wan edge osteotomy, 121
      opening wedge osteotomy, 120–122
      proximal femoral osteotomies, 127, 128
      reorientation of acetabulum, 130
      shortening osteotomy, 123
   planning
      femoral deformity correction, 133, 134
      multiple bony deformities, 134–135
      rules governing osteotomy, 132
      tibial deformity correction, 132–133
   screws, 136
   supracutaneous plate, 142
   technique, 139–141
   tension band wiring, 137
Acute shortening and re-lengthening (ASRL), 981, 984
Adductor releases, 500
Adipose tissue-derived stem cells, 875
Adjunctive treatment, 799
Adjuvant fibular osteotomy, 120
Adolescent Blount's disease, 843, 859
   "classic" deformity, 852
   compressive forces, 852
   growth modulation, 854
   left-sided varus deformity, 855
   microscopic physeal architecture, 852
   morphological characterization/prognostic purposes, 852
   natural history, 846
   radiographic appearance, 844

Adolescent Blount's disease (Cont.)
   treatment
      angular deformity, 852
      angular deformity correction, 853
      ipsilateral deformities of distal femur and distal tibia, 853
      morbid obesity, 853
      obesity in, 852
      surgical treatment, 853, 854
      varus deformity, 853
      weight management program, 853
   "zone of injury" on radiographs, 852
Adolescent tibia vara, 853, 855
Adrenal cell carcinoma, 7
Alkaline phosphatase (ALP), 431
Allogenic bone grafts (allografts), 875
American Academy of Orthopaedic Surgeons (AAOS) Lower Limb Outcomes Questionnaire, 60
Amputation, 757, 799
   CFD
      Gillespie classification, 387, 389, 390, 392
      Hamanishi classification, 387, 388
      Paley classification, 387, 389
   congenital fibular deficiency, 392, 393
   congenital pseudarthrosis of the tibia, 397
   congenital tibial deficiency, 393–396
   fibular hemimelia, 383–385
   Ilizarov approach, 383
   paralympic sports, 383, 384
   patient and family management, 385–387
   trauma, 399, 400
   treatment, 385
   tumor reconstruction, 397–399
   volume changes, 399
Amyoplasia, 526, 531
Anatomic posterior distal femoral angle (APDFA), 31
Androgens, 873
Angiogenesis, 871
Angular deformity, 445
Angular osteotomy, 120–122
Angulatory deformity, 42, 44, 45, 48, 51
Ankle and foot deformity
   assessment tools and indications, 303, 304
   diagnostic matrix, 295
   during normal gait
      ankle dorsiflexion, 297
      clearance and pre-positioning, 298, 299
      ipsilateral initial contact, 296
      lateral column, 296
      medial column, 296
      plantar flexor muscle group, 297
      segments, 295, 296
      shock absorption, 297, 298
   overview, 304, 305
   segmental malalignment, 299–301
   surgical interventions
      clinical decision-making for surgery, 302, 303
      cosmetic improvements, 301
      foot stiffness, 301
      skeletal surgeries, 302
      soft tissue surgeries, 301, 302
Ankle-foot orthosis (AFO), 460, 607, 820
Ankle stabilization, 758
Anterior compartment fasciotomy, 848
Anterior cruciate ligament (ACL), 998
Anterior distal tibial angle (ADTA), 32
Anterior fasciotomy, 801

Anterior inferior iliac spine (AIIS), 815
Anterior muscle placement, 819
Anterior-posterior instability, 597, 631
Anterior superior iliac spine (ASIS), 353, 815
Anticatabolic therapy, 873, 874
Antisense oligonucleotides, 509
Apical ectodermal ridge (AER), 595
Approach-withdrawal technique, 624
Arthrodiatasis, 933
Arthrogryposis, 6, 9, 10
   body, 518, 519
   central nervous system, 519
   child, 520
   classification, 517
   clinical picture, 520, 521
   definition, 517
   etiology, 517
   foot, 521–524
   genetic aspects of, 519
   hip, 528–530
   intellectual skills, 520
   knee, 524–528
   limbs, 518
   lower limb, 521
   management, 521
   orthopedic management
      amyoplasia, 531
      Larsen syndrome, 531
      lower limb deformities, 531
      popliteal pterygium syndrome, 531
      rehabilitation, 532
   prevalence, 517
   prognosis, 521
   scoliosis, 530, 531
   upper limb, 530
Arthrogryposis multiplex congenita, 5
Articular cartilage regeneration, 972
Asymmetrical girth, 8
Asymmetrical premature physeal closure of distal tibia, 970
Autogenous and allogenic bone grafts, 875
Autogenous bone grafting (ABG), 981
   dual intramedullary and extramedullary internal fixation, 986
   intraoperative handling, 982
Autogenous cancellous bone grafting, 673, 875
Autograft specifics, 981
Autologous transplantation of bone marrow concentrate, 867
Avascular necrosis, 445, 919
Axial foot deformities, 24–25
Axial plane deformity, 33

B

Barnhoft questionnaire for hip, 61
Beal's syndrome, 9
Beckwith-Wiedemann syndrome, 8
Berndt and Harty classification, 751
Biceps tendon lengthening, 644
Bifocal procedures, 124
Bilateral ankles, 104
Bilateral infantile Blount's disease, 847
Bioactive scaffolds, in bone bonding, 868
Biological stimulation, 866
   optimal timing, 871
   systemic application, 872, 873
Biologics, 876

Biotechnology on fracture healing, 867
Biplanar/triplanar osteotomy, 899
Birch classification of FH, 718
Bisphosphonate infusion, 673, 801
Bisphosphonates, 459, 460, 462, 799, 873
Blood flow restriction therapy (BFRT), 369
Blount's disease, 11, 12, 19–21, 31, 83, 84, 86, 87, 93, 98, 103, 431, 1009
    acute correction with internal fixation, 855
    acute deformity correction, 858
    acute realignment of the mechanical axis, 857
    adolescent, 843
    bracing/orthosis, 857
    correction with external fixation, 855
    epiphyseal and physeal distortion, 843
    forms, 843
    growth inhibition, 856
    guided growth plate, 857
    infantile form, 843
    intermediate form, 843
    medial hemi-plateau elevation, 858
    postoperative alignment, 857
    progressive varus deformity of left tibia, 845
    recurrence, 857
    slipped proximal tibial epiphysis, 845
    3-stage classification, 843
    unpredictability, 856
Body mass index (BMI), 19, 20
Bone defects
    biological healing potential and mechanical stability, 977
    classification, 977–978
    clinical evaluation, 978–979
    definition, 977
    etiology, 977–978
    laboratory markers, 979
    left femur subtrochanteric pathological fracture, 983
    longitudinal length, 980
    physical examination, 978
    primary internal fixation with proximal femur plate, 983
    radiographic evaluation, 979–980
    reconstruction, 981
    residual infection, 979
    social support system, 978
    spontaneous regeneration, 980
    surgical stabilization, 977
    treatment, 978, 980
Bone formation, 876
Bone grafting, 981
Bone graft substitutes, 876
Bone lengthening with external fixation, 212
Bone marrow aspirate concentrate (BMAC), 867
Bone marrow cells (BMCs), 866
Bone marrow-derived mesenchymal stem cells (MSC), 867
Bone morphogenetic proteins (BMP), 596, 863, 866
Bone morphogenic protein 2 (BMP-2), 626, 764, 782
Bone regeneration, 863, 874, 875
Bone transport (BT), 985
    Ilizarov fixator, 986
    plate/nail assist, 218–220
    procedure, 986
Bone tumors, 6
Bone void fillers, 138–139
Boyd modification, 392
Brittle bone disease, *see* Osteogenesis imperfecta
Brown procedure, 756, 757
Burosumab, 434

C

Calcaneo-cavus deformity, 797
Calcaneo-valgus deformity, 833
Calcaneo-valgus foot deformity, 823, 825, 837
Calcium/phosphate homeostasis, 4
Callotasis, 152, 158
Callus regeneration, 867
Campanacci's disease, *see* Osteofibrous dysplasia
Cancellous bone, 815, 819
Capanna technique, 988
Cartilage tissue engineering, 973
Cat's paw retractor, 622
Center of rotation of angulation (CORA), 120, 122, 125, 127, 128, 132–135, 140, 143, 190, 439
Central bars, 107, 110
Cerebral palsy (CP), 5
    ambulant child, gait, 490–493
    ankle and foot
        gastrocnemius and soleus lengthening, 503, 504
        osteotomies, 504
        SPLATT, 504
        SPOTT, 504
    classification, 479–481
    goals of treatment, 496
    hip
        adductor releases, 500
        femoral derotation and varus derotational osteotomy, 500
        femoral head resection, 501
        iliopsoas lengthening, 500
        periacetabular pelvic osteotomy, 500, 501
    knee and lower leg segment
        anterior hemiepiphyseodesis, 503
        distal femoral extension osteotomy, 501, 502
        distal tibial (supramalleolar) derotational osteotomies, 503
        hamstring lengthening, 501
        PTS, 502
        rectus femoris transfer, 503
    lower extremity
        ankle and foot, 486–488
        knee and lower leg segment, 485, 486
        pelvis and hip, 482–484
    musculoskeletal deformity, 481, 482
    non-ambulant child, 496
    on-table physical examination
        bony alignment, 494, 495
        muscle strength and selective control, 495, 496
        muscle tone and length, 493, 494
    prevalence, 479
    principles of treatment, 497–499
Charcot Maire Tooth disease (CMT), 5, 6
Charcot-Marie-Tooth disease type 1 (CMT type 1A), 507
CHARGE syndrome, 749
Chiari osteotomy, 679, 963
Child Health Questionnaire (CHQ), 59, 62
Childhood Amputee Prosthetics Project- Functional Status Inventory (CAPP-FSI), 60
Childhood Amputee Prosthetics Project-Prosthetics Satisfaction Inventory (CAPP-PSI), 60
Choi classification of sequelae of infantile septic arthritis of the hip, 960
Choi Type II and III hips, femoroacetabular impingement and secondary hip dysplasia, 962, 963
Choi Type IV deformity, 963
Choi Type IVB sequelae in the right hip, 966
Chondro-ectodermal dysplasia, 554–556
Chromosome 17 (17q), 5

Cidex, 410
Circular external fixator, 153
Cleidocranial dysostosis, 10
Closing wedge osteotomy, 122
Clubfeet, 416–420
Clubfoot, 521–524
CO_2 during DO in rabbits, 871
Coleman block test, 507
Compartment syndrome, 135, 138, 143–145
Compensatory foot deformity, 970
Compensatory proximal varus and distal anteromedial bowing deformity of the tibia, 971
Complex hip deformities in older children, 920
Computerized tomography (CT), 603, 605
Congenital bowing of the tibia, 10
Congenital femoral deficiency (CFD), 3, 7–10, 23, 370, 373, 374, 730
    child evaluation
        classification, 606
        CT, 603, 605
        history, 601
        life plan for family, 606
        magnetic resonance imaging (MRI), 603
        non-operative management, 607
        physical examination, 602, 603
        radiographic examination, 603
    classification, 606
    embryology, 595, 596
    epidemiology, 595
    genetics, 596, 597
    Gillespie classification, 387, 389, 390, 392
    Hamanishi classification, 387, 388
    lengthening reconstruction surgery, 608
    ligamentous structures, 597, 599, 600
    limb lengthening surgery, 656, 658, 659
        complications and treatment, 672–675, 678, 679
        epiphysiodesis and hemi-epiphysiodesis, 672
        extramedullary implantable limb lengthening technique, 663, 666
        fixator removal and rodding of femur, 670
        intramedullary implantable limb (IMIL) lengthening technique, 666, 669
        monolateral external fixator technique, 659, 663
        prophylactic rodding of femur at time of external fixator removal, 670
        rehabilitation and follow-up during lengthening, 669, 670
    muscle pathoanatomy, 600
    osseous deformities, 597
    Paley classification, 387, 389
    Paley Type 1
        patellar realignment surgical techniques, 637–639
        posterior capsule release of knee surgical technique, 639, 644, 645
        preparatory surgery of hip, 608, 609
        SUPERhip, 609–612, 623–628
        SUPERknee procedure, 630–632, 635
    Paley Type 2, treatment for, 645
        Femoral Sling Surgical Technique, 646, 648
        pelvic support osteotomy (PSO), 654
        SUPERhip 2 procedure, 648, 649, 654
    Paley Type 3, treatment for, 655
    pathology, 601
    pathophysiology, 596, 597
    prosthetic reconstruction surgery, 679–681, 686, 701, 702, 704
    surgical treatment, 608
    vascular pathoanatomy, 601
Congenital fibular deficiency, 3, 8, 392, 393

Congenital foot deformity
    brachymetatarsia, 317
    calcaneovalgus/oblique talus, 308, 320, 321
    congenital clubfoot
        Achilles tenotomy, 329, 330
        ankle, subtalar and midfoot joints, 325
        anterior tibialis tendon transfer, 330, 331
        atypical clubfoot, 328, 329
        bracing period, 329
        casting, 327
        complex clubfoot, 327, 328
        complications, 332
        fibrous hyperplasia, 325
        overview, 325
        pathogenesis, 325, 326
        physical examination, 326
        posterior medial release, 331, 332
        skewfoot, 332
        surgical management, 329
        treatment, 327
    curly toe
        overview, 309
        parental anxiety, 309, 310
        treatment, 310
    development, 308
    Dobbs method, 319, 320
    etiology, 318, 319
    local factors, 308
    longitudinal epiphyseal bracket, 313, 314
    macrodactyly, 312, 313
    metatarsus adductus, 315–317
    oblique talus, 321, 322
    polydactyly, 310–312
    subungual exostosis, 315
    syndactyly, 312
    systemic factors, 308
    tarsal coalitions
        calcaneonavicular coalition resection, 324–325
        developmental cause, 322
        imaging and diagnostic studies, 323
        physical exam, 322
        prevalence, 322
        talocalcaneal coalition resection, 324
        treatment, 323, 324
    varus fifth toe, 313
    vertical talus, 318
Congenital knee dislocation, 3, 9
Congenital patella dislocation, 3, 10
Congenital posteromedial bowing of the tibia
    deformity
        fibula, 833
        tibia, 832
    demographic features, 831
    etiology, 831
    incidence, 831
    natural history
        evaluation, 836
        rate and pattern of spontaneous remodeling, 834
        residual deformities, shortening, and functional problems, 834, 836
    treatment
        aims of, 837
        calcaneo-valgus foot deformity correction, 837
        decision making, 839, 840
        diagnosis, 840
        indications, 837

limb length inequality correction, 838
muscle imbalance across the ankle correction, 839
sagittal, coronal/torsional deformities of tibia and fibula correction, 837
valgus ankle correction, 837
Congenital pseudarthrosis of the tibia (CPT), 397, 791
classifications of, 791, 792
Paley cross-union protocol surgical technique, 800, 801, 812, 813, 818–821, 823, 824
biomechanical success, 821
4-in-1 osteosynthesis, 820
pathobiology of, 797
pathomechanics of, 797
postoperative considerations
calcaneo-valgus foot deformity, 823, 825
FD rod exchange, 822
FD rod pull out, 822
hemiepiphysiodesis, 822
limb length differences (LLD), 822
pre-CPT, 826
primary vs. secondary changes, 797, 798
treatment, 798–801
Congenital tibial deficiency, 8–9, 393–396
Congenital vertical talus, 522
COnsensus-based Standards for the selection of health Measurement INstruments (COSMIN), 61–64
Consolidation index (CI) for the femora, 986
Construct validity, 62–64
Content validity, 62
Continuous passive motion (CPM) device, 898
Contralateral epiphysiodesis, 838
Controlled compressive, 865
Controlled mechanical stimulation, 865
Cortical allograft, 673
Coventry and Johnson classification, 715
Coxa breva, 883, 884, 902
Coxa magna, 884, 908
deformity, 908
femoral head reduction osteotomy, 909, 911, 912
Coxa valga and narrow femoral neck, 954
Coxa vara, 3, 4, 7, 8, 10, 12, 13, 23, 433, 546
Cozen's phenomenon, 3, 12, 13, 125–126
CPCHILD, 61
Craniofacial bones, 563
Cross-cultural validity, 63, 64
Crouch gait, 490, 492
Cubitus varus, 155, 160
Culture-expanded method, 867
Curettage and bone grafting of fibrous dysplasia, 564
Current procedural terminology (CPT) codes, 77
Custom knee device (CKD), 367, 368
Cutis marmorata telangiectatica congenita, 8
Cylinder-Kombi-Tube module (CKTST), 986, 987

D

Dedifferentiation/reprogramming, 867
Deep posterior compartment fasciotomy, 806
Deformity memory effect, 125
Demineralized bone matrix (DBM), 875
Developmental dysplasia of the hip (DDH), 884
Diamond concept, 980
Diaphyseal and distal femoral deformities, 1002
Diaphyseal-epiphyseal angle, 932
Diaphyseal fractures of the tibia in children and adolescents, 996
Diaphyseal osteotomies, 127

Diastrophic dysplasia, 7, 10, 548–552
Displaced transcervical fracture of the femoral head, 954
Distal arthrogryposes (DA), 518
Distal femoral epiphysis, 967
Distal femoral extension osteotomy, 501, 502
Distal femoral valgus, 740
Distal femur and proximal tibia, 1004
Distal femur diaphysis, 1004
Distal femur physeal fractures, 1002
Distal fibular physis, 999
Distal tibia, 758
epiphysis, 767, 821
fracture, 952, 994
physis, 996
valgus, 853
Distal tibial-fibular syndesmotic ligaments, 731
Distraction osteogenesis (DO), 211, 212, 582–586, 588, 591, 985, 999
autologous and allogenic bone grafting, 863
in vivo tissue engineering, 874
preoperative preparation and planning, 875
Dobbs method, 319, 320
Dome osteotomy, 122
Drill corticotomy, 216
Drill hole technique, 440
Drive Rail, 659, 660
Duchenne's muscular dystrophy (DMD), 508, 509
Dunn procedure, 895
Dwarfing syndromes, 845
Dynamic compression plate (DCP), 136, 139, 141
Dysplasia epiphysealis hemimelica, 573

E

Eccentric ossification of distal tibial epiphysis, 834
Ehlers-Danlos syndrome, 9
Elastic stable intramedullary nails (ESIN), 213
Ellis vanCreveld (EvC) syndrome, 10, 554–556
Ely test, 602
Embryology, 595, 596
Enchondromas, 568
Enchondromatosis, 568, 569
Endogenous retinoids, 597
Endurance limit, 412
Epiphyseal dysplasias, 845
Epiphyseal FFVA, 989
Epiphysiodesis, 672, 724, 848, 849
Epiphysiolysis, 765
Episodic planning, 39, 40
Equinocavovarus deformity, 489
Equinovarus deformities, 486–488, 531, 713
Equinus, 20, 22
Escobar syndrome, 359
Ethylene oxide (EtO), 411
EuroQol-5and Rosenberg self-esteem scale, 60
Exogen™, 673
Extension osteotomy of distal femur, 954
Extensor hallucis longus (EHL), 371
External fixation, 338, 724, 850
External fixation index (EFI), 985
External fixator
intra-operative considerations
bone, 176, 177
half pin/wire coating, 175, 176
pin site dressings, 177, 178
revision of frame, 174, 175
skin preparation and decolonization, 174

External fixator (Cont.)
    soft tissue, 176
    stability principles, 174, 175
    wire and pin design, 175
  pin site infection
    bacteriology and antibiogram properties, 180
    Checketts and Otterburn Classification, 180
    clinical experience, 183
    diagnosis, 180
    dressing variation, 184
    incidence, 184
    pre-tensioning, 183
    proximal and distal tibio-fibular joints, 183
    surgical management, 181, 182
    treatment principles, 180, 181
    wire tension, 184
  postoperative pin site care
    dressing timing, 179
    dressings materials and frequency of changes, 179, 180
    mobilization, 179
    patient and caregiver education, 180
    prophylactic antibiotics, 179
    recovery, 178, 179
  preoperative preparation, 173, 174
  treatment
    half pin removal, 182, 183
    wire removal, 182
Extra-articular ACL reconstruction, 632
Extra-articular PCL reconstruction, 631
Extramedullary implantable limb lengthening technique, 663, 666
Extramedullary internal limb lengthening (EMIL), 659

F
Fassier-Duval telescopic nail, 813
Femoral acetabular impingement (FAI), 895
Femoral deformity, 155–156
    correction, 133, 134
    in fracture shaft femur, 937
Femoral Fassier-Duval (FD) rod technique, 466, 467
Femoral fixator, 659
Femoral fractures, 952
Femoral head fixation, 897, 898
Femoral head reduction osteotomy, 885, 909–912
Femoral length discrepancy, 983
Femoral neck deformity, 899
Femoral neck osteoplasty, 900
Femoral notchplasty, 631
Femoral osteotomy, 1007
Femoral sling surgical technique, 646–648
Femoral version, 23–24
    computerized tomography, 27
    intraoperative assessment, 28
    low dose biplanar radiographs with EOS system, 28
    modified Ogata method, 28, 29
Femoroacetabular impingement associated with Choi Type II and III sequelae, 963
Femoro-fibulo-clacaneal arthrodesis, 755
Femur malunion and growth disturbance, 1002
Fibroblast growth factor (FGF), 595
Fibroblast growth factor-2 (FGF-2), 871
Fibroblast growth factor 23 (FGF 23), 4
Fibrous dysplasia, 3, 6, 10, 12, 562–566
Fibula, 806, 813, 818, 833
Fibula-Pro-Tibia, 987
Fibular centralization, 756, 757
Fibular fractures in children and adolescents, 999
Fibular hemimelia (FH), 374, 601
    classifications, 715–717
    clinical assessment, 719
    Paley classification, 717
    prediction of height and limb length discrepancy, 724
    radiographic assessment, 720, 722
    reduction osteotomy, 963
    surgical outcomes, 742
    surgical techniques
      lengthening for Paley Type 1, 725, 727, 728
      lengthening plus ankle realignment for Paley Type 2, 728, 729
      lengthening plus SUPERankle Reconstruction for Paley Type 3, 729, 732, 735–738
      post-surgical care, 741, 742
    treatment, 724, 725
    typical deformities associated with, 714
    See also Congenital fibular deficiency
Fibular length stabilization screws (FLoSS), 286
Fibular malunion, 1012
Fixator-assisted deformity correction, 141
Fixator-assisted nailing (FAN), 208
    antegrade nailing, 190, 191
    compartment syndrome, 207
    delayed union and nonunion, 207
    external fixation, 190, 191
    fluoroscopy, 190
    focal dome drill guide, 191, 192
    lengthening process, 191
    neurological complication, 206, 207
    peri-implant complications, 207
    postoperative management, 206
    preoperative planning, 190
    recurrence, 207
    retrograde nailing, 190
    soft tissue problem, 207
    technique, 439, 448, 449
    vascular injury, 207
Fixator-assisted plating (FAP), 139, 208, 969
    angular correction, 196
    compartment syndrome, 207
    delayed union and nonunion, 207
    descending geniculate artery, 196
    distal femoral deformities, 196
    distal femur deformity, 197, 201
    indications, 196
    neurological complication, 206, 207
    peri-implant complications, 207
    plate fixation, 196
    postoperative management, 206
    preoperative planning, 190
    proximal tibia deformity, 197, 204
    recurrence, 207
    soft tissue problem, 207
    tibia deformity, 196, 199
    tibia malunion, 196, 197
    vascular injury, 207
Fixed flexion deformity (FFD), 601
Fixed knee flexion deformity (FKFD), 89, 91
Flexion-Valgus osteotomy with bumpectomy and RNL for chronic severe SCFE with closed physis, 924
Foot progression angle, 20, 21, 25
4-in-1 osteosynthesis, 820
Fracture, 678
    distal physis of femur separation, 951
    healing, 931

neck femur, 951
patella, 951
shaft femur, 951
tibial tuberosity, 951
Fracture-Related Infection (FRI) group, 982
Free fibular vascularized autograft (FFVA), 981, 988, 989
Fulminant osteomyelitis of the femur or tibia, 972
Fulminant septic arthritis, 959

G
Gait, 20, 378, 379
  apparent, 490
  crouch, 490, 492
  jump, 490
  observation of, 490
  stiff knee, 492, 493
  true equinus, 490, 491
Gait Outcomes Assessment List (GOAL), 60, 66
Gait Outcomes Assessment List –Lower Limb Differences (GOAL-LD), 60, 66
Galpha-signaling protein, 562
GAlpha-stimulating protein, 562
Ganz osteotome, 890
Gastrocnemius, 503, 504, 996
Genu valgum, 3, 4, 10, 12–14, 84, 85, 433, 447–452, 548, 549
Gigli saw technique, 440
Gillespie classification, 387, 388
Gradual correction
  acute trauma, 348, 349
  adolescent tibia vara, 855
  arthrogryposis, 345
  clubfoot, 340–343
  equino-cavo-varus deformity, 344, 345
  metatarsal lengthening, 349, 350
  osteotomy, 345–348
  soft tissue contracture, 339, 340
  technology update, 339
  tibial lengthening, 348
  weight bearing, 338
Gradual deformity correction, 541, 542
  external fixation
    circular, 152, 153
    femoral deformity, 155–156
    monolateral, 152
    principles of, 153, 155
    tibial osteotomy, 158–159
  foot deformities, 160
  foot extremities, 160
  osteotomy, 159–160
  upper extremities, 160
Graft configuration, 989
Grammont patellar tendon realignment, 630
Grammont procedure, 637, 638
Granulocyte colony-stimulating factor (G-CSF), 873
Greater trochanteric arthroplasty, 964, 965
Gross motor function classification system (GMFCS), 479
Growth differentiation factors (GDFs), *see* Bone morphogenetic proteins
Growth factors, stem cell therapy, 868
Growth hormone (GH), 542, 873
Growth modulation
  angular–frontal
    follow-up, 87
    intermittent guided growth, 89
    pathologic, 85
    physiologic, 85
    technique, 87
    timing, 86, 87, 89
  angular–sagittal/oblique
    knee, 89
    postoperative management, 90
    surgical technique, 89
  ankle/coronal, 90, 92
  ankle/sagittal, 90
  complications, 92, 93
  length-anisomelia
    complications, 98
    pathologic, 93, 94
    physiologic, 93
    timing-< age 10 years, 94–98
    timing-adolescent, 94
    treatment, 98
  lower extremity deformities, 84–85
  management, 93
  rotational guided growth, 98, 99
Growth plate, 927

H
Hall classification, 517
Hamanishi classification, 387, 388
Hamartoma, 806
Hamstring lengthening, 501
Harvesting of the fibula for reconstruction of a bone defect, 1005
Health Inter Network Access to Research Initiative (HINARI), 422
Health-related quality of life (HRQL), 59, 61, 63, 64
Heating, ventilation, and air conditioning (HVAC) systems, 411
Hemaclear tourniquet, 630
Hemiatrophy, 7
Hemiepiphysiodesis, 436, 609, 672, 822, 971
Hemihypertrophy, 3, 7, 8
Hemophilic arthropathy, 7
Hemostat, 356
Hepatoblastoma, 7
Hereditary hypophosphatemic rickets, 432
Hereditary motor sensory neuropathy (HSMN)
  CMT type 1A, 507
  foot deformities, 507, 508
  hip deformities, 508
Herring and Catterall classifications of Perthes, 751
High-energy closed tibia fracture, 998
Higher head-shaft angle (HFA), 483
High tibial osteotomy, 855
  recurrent deformity, 850
  of tibia, 847, 848
Hinged external fixation device, 916
Hip abduction, 494
Hip arthrogram, 623
Hip deformity, 883, 884
Hip distraction treatment for residual femoral head subluxation, 915
Hip distraction with a hinged external fixator, 885
Hip distraction with a hinged external frame, 918
Hip distractor application, 916–917
Hip dysplasia, 505
  diagnosis, 886
  treatment, 885
Hip instability, 483
Hip involvement, 528–530
Hip-knee-ankle angle (HKA), 847
Hip subluxation/dislocation, 673, 674

Hohmann retractor, 625
Host responsibilities, 407
Huntington procedure, 987
Hybrid techniques, 212, 213
Hydroxyapatite tricalcium phosphate calcium silicate scaffold (HASi), 138, 139
Hyperbaric oxygen therapy, 873
Hypertonia, 481
Hyp mice, 435
Hypochondroplasia, 7
Hypophosphatasia, 431, 445, 446
Hypophosphatemic rickets, 4
Hypotheses testing, 63
Hypotrophic regenerate formation, 673

I
Iatrogenic causes, 13
Iatrogenic deformities
  acceptable alignment, 993
  acceptable deformity, 995
  accurate alignment, 996
  "at risk" for litigation, 995
  early function and decreased morbidity, 993
  early weight bearing, 996
  external rotation deformity of tibia, 996
  malalignment, 994
  operative management of tibia factures, 996
  tibia malunion, 995
  varus femur malunion, 995
Iatrogenic translational deformity, 1009
Iatrogenic valgus deformity with external fixation, 1005
Idiopathic genu valgum, 446
Idiopathic osteonecrosis of epiphysis, 901
Iliac apophysis, 815, 818
Iliac bone decancellousization, 819
Iliac crest, 819
Iliac decancellization procedure, 981
Iliac wing osteotomy, 626
Iliopsoas lengthening, 500
Iliotibial band (ITB), 357, 358
Ilizarov external fixation, 435, 798–800
Ilizarov method, 211, 212, 383
Ilizarov technique, 985, 986
Incomplete osteotomy and premature consolidation, 673
Induced-membrane technique (IMT), 981–984
Infantile Blount's disease
  acute deformity correction, 849
  differential diagnosis, 845
  hemi-plateau elevation, 851
  internal tibial torsion and proximal tibial flexion deformities, 847
  medial proximal tibial physeal growth, 848
  radiographic appearance, 848
  "sagging" or "depressed" medial tibial plateau, 851
  treatment of, 847, 851
Infantile/childhood septic arthritis, knee and ankle joints, 966–972
Infantile septic arthritis of the hip
  late operative treatment modalities for severe sequelae, 961–962
  management of late sequelae, 962
  radiographic classifications of late sequelae, 959–961
  residual deformities, 959
Infantile tibia vara, 847
Inflammatory conditions, 6
In-house limb deficiencies questionnaire, 60
Innominate osteotomy (Salter), 886
Instability index, 27

Integrated limb lengthening, 212
Intellectual skills, 520
Intermediate type of Blount's disease, 856
Internal bone transport (IBT), 986
Internal lengthening devices, 376–378
Internal lengthening nail, 164
International Consortium for Health Outcomes Measurement (ICHOM), 61, 62
International Society for Quality of Life Research (ISOQOL), 61–63
Interosseous membrane excision, 806
Intertrochanteric osteotomy, 895
Intra-articular osteotomy, 972
Intra-articular PCL Reconstruction, 635
Intramedullary Fassier-Duval (FD) rod, 820
Intramedullary (IM) nailing, 190, 212, 213, 218, 219
Intramedullary implantable limb (IMIL) lengthening technique, 666, 669
Intramedullary rodding, 798
Intravenous bisphosphonate, 566
In vivo mechanical characterization of the bone callus, 865
Ipsilateral fibula transposition (IFT), 987–988
Ipsilateral iliac crest, 815
Ischial osteotomy for Tönnis Triple Osteotomy, 888

J
Jansen type, 554
Joint contractures
  etiology, 353
  history/examination, 353, 354
  imaging, 354, 355
  non-operative treatment, 356
  operative treatment
    ankle, 360, 361
    hip, 356, 357
    knee, 357–360
  principles of treatment, 356
Joint line congruence angle (JLCA), 30, 31, 42
Joint malorientation, 969
Joint motion/instability, 40
Joint prostheses, 868
Joint stiffness and contracture, 678, 679
Jones classification, 393, 752
Judet quadriceplasty, 360
Juvenile idiopathic arthritis, 6
Juvenile rheumatoid arthritis, 6
Juxta-articular deformity, 967, 969, 970
Juxtaphyseal malignant bone tumor
  distraction osteogenesis, 582–586, 588, 591
  indication, 581
  liquid nitrogen, 583–589, 591
  osteosarcoma, 581

K
Kalamchi classification, 751
Kinematic coupling, 342
Klippel-Trenaunay syndrome, 8
Knee and ankle joint incongruity, postinfectious articular deformity, 972
Knee-ankle-foot orthosis (KAFO), 460
Knee arthrodesis, 390
Knee classification of intercondylar notch, 600
Knee extension mobilization, 375
Knee subluxation/dislocation, 674
Knee thrust, 21

Kniest syndrome, 7
Kujala score for anterior knee pain, 61

L

Langenskiöld classification of infantile Blount's disease, 843
Langenskiöld (Paley) procedure, 630
Langenskiöld radiographic classification of infantile Blount's disease, 844
Langer-Giedion syndrome, 748
Larsen syndrome, 3, 6, 9, 519, 531
Lateral collateral ligament laxity, 21, 31
Lateral distal femur angle (LDFA), 42
Lateral distal tibial angle (LDTA), 32, 87, 90
Legg-Calve-Perthes disease, 372, 373, 548, 901
Leg length discrepancy (LLD), 378, 597, 606, 724, 725, 902
Lengthening and plating (LAP) technique, 1002
Lengthening and screw fixation, 220–222
Lengthening and then nailing (LATN), 215
Lengthening and then plating (LAP), 218
Lengthening osteotomy, 123
Lengthening over nail (LON), 212–215, 438, 439, 727
Ligamentous structures, CFD, 597, 599, 600
Limb deformity
    diagnostic imaging, 25–26
    history, 19
    physical examination, 19, 25
Limb Deformity-Scoliosis Research Society (LD-SRS) score, 59, 60
Limb hypoperfusion, 106
Limb length assessment, 26–27
Limb length differences (LLD), 822
Limb length discrepancy (LLD), 8, 25, 33, 34, 153, 169, 566, 713, 959
Limb lengthening, 271, 758
    achondroplasia, 374, 375
    anatomical axis, 233
    angulation and translation, 278
    antegrade approach, 233
    bifocal oblique osteotomies, 275
    bilateral transfemoral amputations, 275
    blocking screws, 242
    CFD, 373, 374
    challenges, 363
    clinical outcome, 379
    complications
        handling techniques, 366
        joint stiffness, 369
        joint subluxation, 370, 371
        muscle contractures, 366–368
        muscle weakness, 369
        soft tissue dysfunctions, 365, 366
    deformity correction, 59, 65, 243
        after trauma, 243
        anti-rotation pins, 247
        blocking screws, 247
        debridement, 243
        distal osteotomy, 243
        electric vs. magnetic nail, 254, 255
        femur bone position, 243
        follow-up, 243
        functionality, 247
        Gustilo IIIB segmental femoral fracture, 243
        healed osteotomy, 247
        intercondylar notch, 243
        intraoperative draping and position, 247
        intraoperative fluoroscopy, 247
        lateral fluoroscopy, 247
        lengthening gap, 243
        lengthening protocols, 256, 257
        lower limb mechanical axis, 243
        magnet position, 247
        nail removal, 247
        neurovascular structures, 246
        postoperative lengthening, 247
        post-operative period, 255, 256
        postoperative radiograph, 243
        proximal locking screws, 247
        reaming, 246
        retrograde approach, 246, 254
        retrograde Precice™ straight nail, 247
        reverse planning method, 243
        shortening and distal procurvatum, 247
        transverse skin incision, 247
        ventilation holes, 247
    external fixation, 227
    extramedullary lengthening devices, 277
    fibular hemimelia, 374
    Fitbone™ nail, 228
    gait, 378, 379
    history and physical examination
        ankle joint motion, 232
        bone health, 232
        gait/alignment/muscles/shortening/rotation, 230, 231
        hip joint stability, 231, 232
        knee joint stability, 232
        mental health, 232
        social examination, 232
    Ilizarov's elements, 272, 273
    indications, 229, 230
    internal lengthening, 227, 376–378
    intraoperative, 237
        distal locking screws, 241
        nail functionality, 241
        proximal locking screws, 240
        proximal varus deformity, 238
        reaming, 239
        reverse planning method, 236
        rotational markers, 239
        solid nail, 241
        venting holes, 238
    Legg-Calve-Perthes disease, 372, 373
    Length and Deformity Correction Center, 274
    lengthening rate, 278
    mechanical femoral lengthening nail, 227, 228
    neophyte limb lengthening surgeon, 273
    nerve injury, 371
    postoperative follow-up
        clinical examination, 257, 258
        complications, 265–267
        dealing with delayed union/non-union, 267, 268
        dealing with joint complications, 268
        dealing with premature consolidation, 267
        distraction phase, 258, 263
        extramedullary lengthening, 268, 269
        nail removal, 265–267
        physical therapy, 265
        radiographs, 258, 259, 263
        segmental bone defects, 269, 270
        stump lengthening, 269, 270
        weight-bearing protocols, 263, 264
    Precice™ nail, 228, 229
    preoperative assessments, 271
    preoperative planning, 234–236

Limb lengthening (Cont.)
  procedure, 864
  radiographs, 233, 234
  rehabilitation
    consolidation phase, 364, 365
    inpatient phase, 363, 364
    lengthening/correction phase, 364
    post frame removal phase, 365
  retrograde approach, 233
  skeletal dysplasias (see Skeletal dysplasias)
  surgery, 656, 658, 659
    complications and treatment, 672–675, 678, 679
    epiphysiodesis and hemi-epiphysiodesis, 672
    extramedullary implantable limb lengthening technique, 663, 666
    fixator removal and rodding of femur, 670
    IMIL lengthening technique, 666, 669
    monolateral external fixator technique, 659, 663
    prophylactic rodding of femur at time of external fixator removal, 670
    rehabilitation and follow-up during lengthening, 669, 670
    trampoline injury, 278
    weight bearing, 371, 372
Limb Lengthening and Reconstruction Society (LLRS-AIM classification), 59
Limb Lengthening Satisfaction Questionnaire (LLSQ), 60
Limb length equalization, 674, 965
Limb length inequality correction, 838
Limb malalignment, 675
Limb reconstruction surgery, 655, 759
Limb reconstruction team, 71–73
Liquid nitrogen (LN) method, 583–589, 591
Load-sharing intramedullary implants, 565
Locked plates (LCP), 137, 139
Lower extremity, 22
Lower extremity benign bone lesions, 561
  dysplasia epiphysealis hemimelica, 573
  enchondromatosis, 568, 569
  fibrous dysplasia, 562–566
  McCune Albright syndrome, 562–566
  multiple hereditary osteochondromatosis/exostoses (MHE), 570–573
  nonossifying fibroma, 561
  osteofibrous dysplasia, 567, 568
  solitary osteochondromas, 570–573
Lower extremity deformity, 538
  clinical evaluation, 40, 41
  episodic planning, 39, 40
  global planning, 39
  osteotomy
    acute correction, 48–53
    gradual correction, 51–53
  physeal modulation/ablation, 45–48
  problem list, 41
  relative contraindications, 43
  soft tissue modification, 44, 45
  surgical indications, 41, 42
  surgical options, 44
Lower limb alignment, 119
Lower limb deformities, 531
Lower limb fractures, acceptability criteria, 951–952
Lower limb questionnaire, 60
Lower-middle-income countries (LMIC), 78, 79
Low-income countries (LIC), 78
Low-intensity pulsed ultrasound (LIPUS), 865, 866, 875
Low-intensity ultrasound, 865

M
MacFarland fracture, 947
MacIntosh (Paley) extra-articular PCL reconstruction, 630
Maffucci's syndrome, 568
Magnetic resonance imaging (MRI), 603, 722, 723
Malunited fracture left shaft femur with shortening varus and rotational deformity, 936
Malunited shaft femur, 934
Mango slice effect, 125
Manual muscle testing (MMT), 495
Mapi Research Trust, 61
McCune Albright syndrome, 562–566
McKusick type, 554
Mechanical axis deviation (MAD), 30, 959
Mechanical lateral distal femoral angle (mLDFA), 30, 33, 720
Mechanical lateral proximal femoral angle (mLPFA), 31
Mechanical medial proximal tibial angle (mMPTA), 847, 854
Mechanical stabilization, 982
Mechanical stimulation, 865
Medial apophysis, 815
Medial parapatellar tendon arthrotomy, 631
Medial proximal tibial angle (MPTA), 30, 42
Medico-legal issues, 407
Metabolic bone disease, 845
  conditions, 429
  definition, 429
  hypophosphatasia, 445, 446
  idiopathic genu valgum, 446
  pathophysiology, 429–431
  renal osteodystrophy
    angular deformity, 445
    avascular necrosis, 445
    medical treatment, 444
    orthopedic treatment, 444
    prevalence, 444
    SCFE, 445
  rickets
    diagnosis, 431
    laboratory findings, 431
    mineralization, 431
    nutritional rickets, 432
    skeletal symptoms, 431
    XLH (see X-linked hereditary hypophosphatemic rickets (XLH))
Metabolic disorders
  neurofibromatosis, 5
  osteogenesis imperfecta, 4
  renal osteodyrophy, 4
  rickets, 4
Metaphyseal chondrodysplasia, 553, 554
Metaphyseal dysostosis, 10, 845
Metaphyseal dysplasia, 431
Metaphyseal osteotomy, 126
Metatarsophalangeal joint (MTPJ), 349, 350
Metatarsus adductus (MTA), 20, 24, 25
Mild familial genu valgum, 40
Mini-Hohmann retractors, 735
Modified capsulotomy and repair, 923
Modified Dalmonte classification, 742
Modified Dunn procedure, 885, 895, 896, 898, 923

Modified Langenskiöld procedure, 637, 639
Modified Ogata method, 29
Modified Southwick intertrochanteric osteotomy, 885
Modified Southwick osteotomy, 901
Modified triple osteotomy, 895
Monolateral external fixator technique, 152, 659, 663
Morquio syndrome, 550–553
Morscher femoral neck lengthening osteotomy, 885
Morscher osteotomy, 903–905
Motor evoked potentials (MEPs), 540
Motorized internal lengthening nail (MILN)
    blocking screws, 288
    indications, 281, 282, 289
    intra operative execution, 284, 285
    joint contracture, 288
    lengthening rate, 288
    magnet, 287
    outcomes, 287, 290
    post Op recommendations, 287, 289, 290
    pre-operative planning, 282, 284, 289
    reaming and nail insertion, 286, 287, 289
Motorized lengthening nail (MLN), 986
MPS Type 1 (Hurler), 7
MPS Type IV (Morquio), 7
Mucopolysaccharidosis type 4, 550
Multiplanar Ilizarov-type external fixator, 658
Multiple bony deformities, 134–135
Multiple epiphyseal dysplasia (MED), 7, 548, 549
Multiple hereditary exostosis (MHE), 6
Multiple hereditary osteochondromatosis/exostoses (MHE), 6, 570–573
Multiple pterygium syndromes, 519
Multiplier app, 94
Multiplier method, 86
Muscle herniation, 848
Muscle imbalance across, 839
Muscle length testing, 602
Muscle pathoanatomy, 600
Muscular dystrophies, 508, 509
Musculoskeletal deformity, 481, 482
Myelomeningocele
    ankle and foot deformities, 506
    hip dysplasia, 505
    incidence, 505
    knee flexion deformity and tibial torsion, 505, 506

N

Nail patella syndrome, 10
Neoangiogenesis, 871
Neonatal sepsis, 104, 105
Nerve injury, 672
Neurofibromatosis (NF), 5, 10
Neurofibromatosis type 1 (NF1), 5, 8, 10
Neurological disease, 20
Neuromuscular conditions
    arthrogryposis multiplex congenita, 5
    cerebral palsy, 5
    Charcot Maire Tooth disease, 5, 6
    Larsen syndrome, 6
    multiple Pterygium syndrome, 6
    osteochondral dysplasias, 6
Neuromuscular disorder
    cerebral palsy (see Cerebral palsy (CP))
    HSMN
        CMT type 1A, 507
        foot deformities, 507, 508
        hip deformities, 508
    muscular dystrophies, 508, 509
    myelomeningocele (spina bifida), 505, 506
    poliomyelitis, 506, 507
Non-communicating Children's Pain Checklist Postoperative Version for pain in severe intellectual disabilities, 61
Nonossifying fibroma, 561
Non-physeal fractures, 13
Non-weight-bearing phase, 375

O

Obesity in children, 979
Oblique osteotomy, 123
Oblique plane deformity, 35
Olecranization of patella, 782
Ollier's disease, 6, 568
Open epiphysiodesis, 83
Open hemiepiphysiodesis of lateral proximal tibia, 854
Opening wedge osteotomy, 120–122
Open skeletal injuries/iatrogenic issues, 929
Open Vulpius procedure, 726
Osseointegrated Prostheses for the Rehabilitation of Amputees (OPRA), 402
Osseointegration, 401, 402
Osseous deformities, 597
Osteochondral dysplasias, 6
Osteochondral reconstruction, 989
Osteoconduction, 868
Osteofibrous dysplasia, 567, 568
Osteogenesis imperfecta (OI), 3, 4
    classification, 457, 458
    clinical and radiological manifestations, 458, 459
    complications, 473–475
    definition, 457
    diagnosis, 457
    differential diagnosis, 457
    general and anesthesia, 462
    incidence, 457
    medical treatment, 459, 460
    pathogenesis, 458
    preoperative planning, 462, 464, 465
    rehabilitation, 460
    soft tissues, 462, 463
    surgery
        coxa vara correction, 469
        femoral Fassier-Duval rod technique, 466, 467
        guided growth, 465
        osteotomy, 466, 468
        patient positioning, 466
        rodding, 465, 466
        stress and resorbs, 465
        tibial Fassier-Duval rod, 469
        treatment, 460, 461
Osteogenic differentiated progenitor cells, 867
Osteogenic differentiation from bone marrow-derived mesenchymal stem cells, 866
Osteogenic peptides, 871
Osteogenic progenitor stem cell culture techniques, 868
Osteolysis of the tibia, 797
Osteomyelitis, 3, 13, 105, 959, 983
Osteosarcoma, 581

Osteotomy, 110, 663, 666, 735, 889, 890
    acute correction, 48–51
    adjuvant fibular osteotomy, 120
    adjuvant procedures, 130–131
    angular correction and translation, 122–123
    closing wedge osteotomy, 122
    diaphysis, 127
    dome, 122
    epiphyseal, 127
    gradual correction, 51–52
    indications, 126
    juxta-apophyseal, 127
    knee, 130
    lengthening osteotomy, 123
    level of, 120
    metaphysis, 126
    oblique osteotomy, 123
    opening wedge osteotomy, 120–122
    proximal femoral osteotomies, 127, 128
    reorientation of acetabulum, 130
    shortening osteotomy, 123
Overabundant bone formation, 673
Oxford foot and ankle questionnaire, 61

P
"Pagoda" deformity, 48
Paley–Brown rotationplasty, 679, 681, 686, 701
Paley classification, 387, 389, 606, 717, 719, 791, 792
Paley cross-union protocol surgical technique, 800, 801, 818, 821, 823, 824
    anterior fasciotomy, 801
    anterior muscle placement, 819
    backfill the iliac crest, 819
    biomechanical success, 821
    bone end separation, 812
    cancellous bone insertion, 819
    circumferential excision of hamartoma, 806
    deep posterior compartment fascia, 806
    distal locking, 813
    excise hamartoma from fibula, 806
    Fassier-Duval telescopic nail, 813
    female component insertion, 813
    4-in-1 osteosynthesis, 820
    hamartoma incision, 806
    iliac apophysis, 818
    iliac bone decancellousization, 819
    iliac incision closure, 819
    interosseous membrane excision, 806
    intramedullary length measurement, 813
    leg incisions closure, 819
    locking plate, 818
    male component insertion, 813
    periosteal graft harvest and meshing, 819
    periosteal grafting, 819
    periosteum, BMP2 and bone graft preparation, 819
    posterior compartment muscle elevation, 806
    preoperative bisphosphonate infusion, 801
    prep and incision, 801
    proximal tibial reaming, 813
    split iliac bone, 819
    square off tibial bone ends, 812, 813
    syndesmotic ligaments release, 806
Paley modification, 813
Paley periacetabular triple osteotomy (PATO), 620, 625

Paley rotationplasty, 687, 701–703
PaleySUPERhip-Van Nes procedure, 684
Paley type 1b subtrochanteric type surgical technique, SUPERhip 1 for, 627, 628
Paley type 1 CFD
    patellar realignment surgical techniques, 637–639
    posterior capsule release of knee surgical technique, 639, 644, 645
    preparatory surgery of hip, 608, 609
    SUPERhip, 609–612, 623–628
    SUPERknee procedure, 630–632, 635
Paley type 2 CFD, 645
    femoral sling surgical technique, 646, 648
    pelvic support osteotomy (PSO), 654
    SUPERhip 2 procedure, 648, 649, 654
Paley type 3 CFD, 655
Paley unicortical iliac osteotomy, 624
Paley-Weber patellar arthroplasty, 781, 782
Paley-Winkelman rotationplasty, 681
Parathyroid hormone (PTH), 872
Partial prophylactic anterior compartment fasciotomy, 848
Patellar realignment surgical techniques, 637–639
Patellar tendon mobilization, 638
Patellar tendon shortening (PTS), 502
Patelloplasty, 758
Patient –reported outcome measure for lower limb reconstruction (PROLLIT), 59, 60
Patient reported outcome measures (PROMS)
    availability, 63
    in children, 60–61
    clinical practice/implementation science, 64–65
    clinician/researcher and patient burden, 63
    concept of interest, 61
    conceptual and measurement model, 62
    context of use, 61
    guidelines, 63, 64
    ICHOM, 61, 62
    interpretability of scores, 63
    item generation, 64
    item reduction, 64
    limb lengthening and deformity correction, 59
    literacy level, 63
    pilot testing, 63
    PROMIS, 61
    PROQOLID, 61
    psychometric evaluation, 64
    psychometric properties, 62, 63
    Q-portfolio website, 61
    specific context, 61
    validation, 62
Patient-Reported Outcome Measurement Information System (PROMIS), 60, 61
Pediatric femur fractures, 994
Pediatric limb reconstruction
    clinic setting, 73
    hospital commitment, 77
    limb reconstruction team, 71–73
        additional clinic staff, 71
        clinic co-pilot, 71
        limb reconstruction program administrative assistant/office coordinator, 71
        physiatrist, 72
        physical therapists, 71
        psychologist, 72
        radiology team, 72
        social worker, 72

managing expectations, 77
operating room setting, 73–74
patient volume, 74, 75
practice habits, 75–77
    accepting complications, 76
    branding, 76
    conferences, 76
    customer service, 77
    post-operative patient clinic visits, 76
    pre- and post-clinic huddle, 76
    pre-operative planning, 75
    surgical journal, 75
    team meetings, 76
    weekly clinic visits, 76
resource challenged environment, 78–80
    clinic organization, 79
    intraoperative solutions, 79
    personnel, 78
    social media, 79
    training and education, 78
    travel logistics/availability of service, 79
surgeon, 69
    continuing education, 70, 71
    educational foundation, 69, 70
working with industry, 77
Pediatric Outcomes Data Collection Instrument (PODCI), 60, 62
Pediatric Quality of Life Inventory (PedsQL), 59, 60, 63
PedsQL-CP version, 60–61
Pelvic osteotomy, 674, 675, 886
Pelvic support osteotomy (PSO), 654
Pemberton/Dega-type pelvic osteotomy, 920
Percutaneous osteotomy and external fixation, 901
Percutaneous transphyseal screw (PETS) growth modulation methods, 854
Periacetabular triple osteotomy of pelvis, 889, 890
Pericapsular acetabuloplasty (Dega, Pemberton), 886, 887
Periosteal graft cambium layer, 816
Periosteal grafting, 819
Peripheral bars, 107, 110
Peroneal nerve compression, 849
Peroneal nerve issues, 858
Phosphate regulating endopeptidase X linked gene (PHEX), 4, 432
Physeal arrest resection surgery, 849, 850
Physeal bar excision
    abnormal physis, 106
    clinical outcome, 113–114
    computed tomography, 108
    etiology and prognosis, 103–106
    growth plate disturbance, 106
    growth remaining, 109
    infection, 105–106
    interposition material, 113
    magnetic resonance imaging, 108
    neoplasm and tumorlike conditions, 106
    osteotomy, 110
    physeal arrest
        anatomic classification, 107
        extent, 108
        location of, 107
        partial versus complete, 106–107
    plain radiographs, 108
    radiographic markers, 113
    surgical approaches, 110–113
    surgical indications, 109
    surgical technique, 109
    timely identification, 106
    trauma, 104
    vascular insult, 106
Physeal bar resection surgery, 849
Physeal fractures, 12–13
Physeal injury ankle with malunion, 947, 948
Physeal modulation/ablation, 45–48
Physical stimulation, 865, 866
Physical therapy, 679
Physiologic Genu Varum, 10–11
Picture archiving and communication system (PACS), 863–864
Pierre-Robin sequence, 596
Pistol grip deformity, 824
Pixel value ratio (PVR), 863
Plate-assisted bone segment transport (PABST), 986
Plate-assisted lengthening (PAL), 215–218
Platelet-rich plasma (PRP), 863, 867
Poliomyelitis, 506, 507
Poly-methyl-methyl-acrylate (PMMA) cement, 982
Polyostotic diseases, 6
Polyostotic FD, 564
Ponse-Taylor method, 160
Ponseti method, 416, 417, 419, 420, 506
Ponseti technique, 521–523
Poor/failed bone formation, 673
Popliteal pterygium syndrome, 519, 531
Postaxial hypoplasia, 713
Posterior capsule release of knee surgical technique, 639, 644, 645
Posterior proximal tibial angle (PPTA), 31
Posteromedial bowing, 10, 11
Postinfectious articular deformity causing knee and ankle joint incongruity, 972
Postinfectious residual deformities of lower limb
    epiphysis, 959
    intracapsular epiphyses, 959
    musculoskeletal examination and radiographic imaging, 959
    transphyseal spread of infection, metaphysis, 959
Postinfectious segmental long bone defects, 972, 973
Posttraumatic chondrolysis of hip and avascular necrosis, 933, 934
Posttraumatic coxa vara, 934
Posttraumatic deformities
    in children, 927
    lower limb, 933
Posttraumatic femoral deformities, 952, 953
Posttraumatic lower limb deformities, children
    classification, 930
    clinical assessment, 930
    damage to growing area of bone, 929
    deformity correction planning, 952
    etiological factors, 928
    growth, 929
    management and complications, 928
    muscle forces, 928
    neural/vascular injury, 928
    open fracture/ischaemia, 930
    open fracture of tibial tuberosity, 931
    poor skeletal stabilization, 928
    postural or positional, 928
    radiographic imaging, 930
    remodeling, 929–931
    symmetric physeal damage, 929
    types of interventions, 932
Post-traumatic tibia valga, 945
Posttraumatic tibial deformities in children, 953
Posttraumatic upper extremities deformities, 953, 955

Post-tumour reconstruction, 982
PRECICE intramedullary nail, 659
Pressure-sensitive sensory device (PSSD), 672
Pressure specified sensory device (PSSD), 371
"Procurvatum" (flexion deformity) of the proximal tibia, 854
Procurvatum-varus diaphyseal deformity, 797
Progressive deformity, 945
Progressive healing of the bone defect and equalized limb lengths, 983
Progressive proximal tibial varus deformity, 843
Progressive valgus angulation, 13
Prophylactic anterior compartment fasciotomy, 727, 848
PROQOLID, 61
Prosthesis, 400
    developments, 401
    end weight-bearing, 401
    osseointegration, 401, 402
    replacement, 400
    residual limb length, 400
    residual limb overgrowth, 400, 401
Prosthetic reconstruction surgery (PRS), 608
Protein malnutrition, 979
Proteus syndrome, 8
Proximal femoral osteotomies, 127, 128
Proximal femoral plate, 983
Proximal focal femoral deficiency (PFFD), 7–9
Proximal focal fibrocartilaginous dysplasia, 12
Proximal metaphysis, 951
Proximal osteotomy, 654, 858
Proximal tibial autograft, 1007
Proximal tibial epiphysis, 772
Proximal tibial physis, 943–945
Proximal tibial segment, 1005
Pseudarthrosis, 39, 41, 52, 801, 821, 935
Pseudoachondroplasia, 7, 12
Psoas tenotomy, 649
Pulsed electromagnetic field (PEMF), 866

Q

Q-portfolio website, 61
Quadratus femoris, 357
Quality-adjusted life-years (QALYs), 65
Quantitative deformity analysis, 30, 31, 33, 34
Quantitative sensory testing, 672

R

Radiographic apparent bone gap (RABG), 977, 979, 980
Rebound deformity phenomenon, 93
Recombinant homologous growth hormone (GH), 873
Recombinant human growth hormone (rhGH), 434
Rectus femoris transfer, 503
Regeneration of bone defects, 863
Relative neck lengthening (RNL), 921
Relative value units (RVUs), 77
Reliability, 60, 62–64, 66
Renal osteodystrophy, 4
    angular deformity, 445
    avascular necrosis, 445
    medical treatment, 444
    orthopedic treatment, 444
    prevalence, 444
    SCFE, 445
Repercussions, 407
Residual deformity from moderate and severe slipped capital femoral epiphysis, 919
Residual femoral head subluxation or migration, 914, 915
Residual hip deformity, 12, 885, 919
Residual hip dysplasia
    patients after closure of triradiate growth plate, 888, 889
    skeletally immature child, 886, 887
Resource-challenged environments
    clubfeet, 416–420
    cordless power, 413
    educational resources, 422
    globalization, 405
    healthcare expenditures, 406
    income disparity, 405
    indications, 405, 408
    internal vs. external fixation, 412
    operating room set up, 411, 412
    operations in, 412
    partnership
        credentialing and liability, 407, 408
        host responsibilities, 407
        motivation, 407
        program, 406
        repercussions, 407
        volunteers, 406, 407
    perioperative and anesthetic considerations, 408–410
    post-operative care, 413, 414
    re-use of implants and external fixation components, 412, 413
    SIGN Nail, 420, 421
    spica cast, 421, 422
    sterility, 410, 411
    wild, 415, 416
Responsiveness, 62–64, 66
Reverse planning method, 1014
Revolutions per minute (RPMs), 413
Rhythm of distraction, 865
Rickets, 3, 4, 12, 429
    diagnosis, 431
    hereditary hypophosphatemic rickets, 432
    laboratory findings, 431
    mineralization, 431
    nutritional rickets, 432
    skeletal symptoms, 431
    XLH (see X-linked hereditary hypophosphatemic rickets (XLH))
Ring external fixators (Ilizarov or hexapod), 979
Rod migration, 212
Rotational deformity, 33
Rotational profile, 40
Rotationplasty, 679–681, 686, 701
    muscle transfers and closure, 701, 702
    Paley rotationplasty, 701
    Paley–Brown rotationplasty, 686, 701
    postoperative management, 704
    supramalleolar osteotomy/SHORDT for, 702
    surgical technique, 686
Rubinstein-Taybi syndrome, 10
Russel-Silver syndrome, 8

S

Sagittal, coronal, or torsional deformities of tibia and fibula correction, 837
Salter osteotomy, 886
Salter–Harris Types 1 and 2, 952

Index

Salter–Harris Types 3 and 4, 952
Schmid type, 553
Sclerostin antibodies, 434
Scoliosis, 530, 531
Scoliosis Research Society (SRS) outcome instrument, 59
Segmental tibia fracture, 993
Septic arthritis, 13, 105
    of the hip, late operative treatment modalities for residual deformities, 961, 962
    and osteomyelitis around the knee and ankle joints, 969
Severe equinovalgus deformity of the foot, 971
Shepherd's crook deformity, 564, 565
Shortening osteotomy, 123, 128, 130, 131, 142
Shortening Osteotomy Realignment Distal Tibia (SHORDT) procedure, 702, 705, 725, 729, 823
Short Form Health Survey (SF-36), 59, 60
Short leg gait, 20
Silfverskiold test, 360, 494
Single-event multilevel orthopedic surgery (SEMLS), 497
Single level, multi-event surgery (SLMES), 89
Single-stage surgery, 867
Single use devices (SUDs), 413
Skeletal dysplasias, 6, 7
    achondroplasia, 543–546
    anesthesia, 540
    deformity correction
        acute correction, 539, 541
        gradual deformity correction, 541, 542
    diastrophic dysplasia, 548–552
    EvC, 554–556
    genetics of, 537, 538
    imaging, 539, 540
    implant size and design, 540
    lower extremity deformity, 538
    MED, 548, 549
    metaphyseal chondrodysplasia, 553, 554
    morbidity, 537
    Morquio syndrome, 550–553
    planning, 543
    positioning and neuromonitoring, 540
    post-operative considerations, 542
    pre-operative evaluation, 539
    SEDC, 546–548
    stature lengthening, 542
    systemic involvement, 537, 538
Skeletal realignment and stabilization, 934
Skin invagination at the docking site, 985
Slipped capital femoral epiphysis (SCFE), 23, 444, 445, 895, 897
Soft tissue loss, skeletal injury, 948
Soft tissue releases, 916
Soleus lengthening, 503, 504
Solitary osteochondromas, 570–573
Sonic hedgehog (SHH), 595, 748
Southwick osteotomy, 899, 901
Spica cast, 421, 422
Spina bifida
    ankle and foot deformities, 506
    hip dysplasia, 505
    incidence, 505
    knee flexion deformity and tibial torsion, 505, 506
Spine, 19, 20, 22, 30, 32–34
Split iliac apophysis, 357
Split tibialis anterior tendon transfer (SPLATT), 504
Split tibialis posterior tendon transfer (SPOTT), 504
Spondyloepiphyseal dysplasia congenital (SEDC), 7, 546–548
Spondyloepiphyseal dysplasia tarda, 7
Spondylometaphyseal dysplasia, 10
Stanitski classification of FH, 717
Stanmore Limb Reconstruction Score (SLRS), 59, 60
Stem cells, 867
    avascular necrosis of femoral head, 868
    injection, 915
    mixture, 869
    therapy, 868
Stiff knee gait, 492, 493
Structural validity, 63
Subcapital osteotomy versus intertrochanteric osteotomy, 895
Subcutaneous tissue flaps, 623
Submuscular nail placement, 666
Subtrochanteric osteotomy, 624, 924
SUPERankle procedure, 725
SUPERankle reconstruction, 725, 729, 732, 735–738
SUPERankle technique, 729
SUPERhip, 609
SUPERhip 1 surgical technique, Paley type 1 CFD, 612, 623–626
    arthrogram, 623
    blade plate insertion, 624
    bone grafting paley unicortical iliac osteotomy, 625
    bone morphogenic protein (BMP2) insertion, 626
    closure, 626
    distal femur fixation and internal rotation, 625
    external rotation contracture release, 622
    fascia lata release, 612
    femoral shortening, 625
    flap elevation, 612
    iliac wing osteotomy, 626
    incision, 611
    muscle repairs and transfers, 626
    PATO, 625
    Paley unicortical iliac osteotomy, 624
    positioning, prepping, and draping, 611
    post-operative course, 626
    quadriceps, 623
    sub-trochanteric osteotomy, 624
SUPERhip 2 procedure, Paley type 2 CFD, 648, 649, 654
SUPERhip osteotomy, 645
SUPERhip procedure, 639, 684
SUPERhip surgical technique, 611, 612, 626
    evolution of, 610
    guide wire insertion, 623
    hip flexion contracture releases, 619
    Paley type 1b subtrochanteric type surgical technique, 627, 628
    periosteum release, 624
Superior pubic ramus osteotomy, 890
SUPERknee procedure, 612, 619, 631, 632, 635
    extra-articular ACL reconstruction, 632
    extra-articular PCL reconstruction, 631
    femoral notchplasty, 631
    history of, 630
    incision and dissection, 631
    intra-articular PCL reconstruction, 635
    preparation of ligaments, 631
    secure the ends of ligaments, 635
    tibial tunnel, 631
SUPERknee tips and tricks, 645
Supplementary small-diameter solid rod (SLIM), 659, 663, 670
Supracutaneous locked plating, 142
Supramalleolar dome osteotomy, 728, 731
Supramalleolar osteotomy, 159, 702, 838, 971
Supramalleolar reorientation osteotomy, 716

Sural nerve, 735
Surgical Implant Generation Network (SIGN), 420, 421
Symes amputation, 390
Symes procedure, 392
Syndesmotic dissection, 999
Syndesmotic ligaments, 806
Syndromic and idiopathic hemihypertrophy, 7
Systematic Utilitarian Procedure for Extremity Reconstruction (SUPER) procedure, 716

T
Talipes equinovarus, 521
Taylor Spatial Frame (TSF), 153, 999
Telescopic rods, 465, 466, 473
Temporary hemiepiphysiodesis, 847, 857
Temporary reversible epiphysiodesis, 83
Tendo-Achilles lengthening, 503
Tenotomized, 357
Tensor-fascia lata (TFL), 356
Testosterone, 873
TGF-beta signaling pathway, 866
Thigh foot angle (TFA), 24, 495
Third-time repeat height tibial osteotomy, 850
Thrombocytopenia-absent-radius (TAR) syndrome, 845, 846
Tibia, 818, 832
Tibia-fibula syndesmosis synostosis, 1005
Tibia hemimelia, *see* Congenital tibia deficiency
Tibia hemimelia-foot polydactly-tripahlangeal thumb syndrome, 8
Tibia hemimeliala-micromelia-trigonobrachycephaly syndrome, 8
Tibia reconstruction after tumor resection with contralateral vascularized fibular autograft, 1005
Tibia vara, 435, 843
Tibial alignment, 1000
Tibial deformity correction, 132–133
Tibial Fassier-Duval (FD) rod, 469
Tibial hemimelia, 747
    classification system, 750–752
    genetics, 747–749
    pathoanatomy, 749, 750
    treatment
        amputation, 757
        Brown procedure (fibular centralization), 756, 757
        distal tibia and ankle stabilization, 758
        early, 755, 756
        history, 755
        limb lengthening, 758
        limb reconstruction surgery, 759
        olecranization of patella, 782
        Paley Type 1, 759
        Paley Type 2, 760, 762, 764, 767
        Paley Type 3b, 767
        Paley Type 4, 769, 771, 772
        Paley type 5, 773, 783, 784
        Paley-Weber patellar arthroplasty, 781, 782
        tibiofibular synostosis, 757
        Weber Patellar arthroplasty, 758
Tibial hemimelia diplopodia syndrome, 8
Tibial hemimelia–polysyndactyly–triphalangeal thumb syndrome (THPTTS), 748
Tibial hemimelia split hand and foot syndrome, 8
Tibialis anterior muscle, 816
Tibialis posterior tendon lengthening, 504
Tibial lengthening, deformity, 1007–1009
Tibial osteotomy, 158–159, 726, 818
Tibial pilon construct, 607
Tibial plateau osteotomies, 48
Tibial torsion, 24, 28
Tibiofibular diastasis, 767
Tibiofibular synostosis, 757
Tissue engineering, 867, 876
Tönnis triple osteotomy, 888
Total joint arthroplasty (TJA), 543
TP508, 871
Tranexamic acid (TXA), 821
Translation, 119, 122, 137, 141, 144
Translational deformity, 1009, 1012
Translation and cultural adaptation (TCA), 63, 64
Transmalleolar axis (TMA), 24, 495
Transphyseal ACL reconstruction, 1000, 1001
Trendelenburg sign, 21
Trevor's disease, *see* Dysplasia epiphysealis hemimelica
Tricortical iliac crest graft, 944
Triple pelvic osteotomy, 885
Trochanter flip approach, 920
Trochanter flip modified Morscher osteotomy, 922
Trunk, 20–22
2-β-(3-hydroxypropoxy)-1α, 25-dihydroxyvitamin D3 (ED-71), 871
Two-incision Tönnis triple technique, 892, 894
Type 1 neurofibromatosis and congenital pseudoarthrosis of the tibia, 986
Type II tricho-rhino-phalangeal syndrome (TRPS II), 748

U
Uniapical deformity, 41
Upper extremity, 20, 713
Upper limb deformities, 160–164, 530

V
Valgus ankle correction, 837
Valgus ankle deformity, fibular donor site, 1005
Valgus deformity, 572
    at end of long bone plate, 949–951
    and femur shortening, 1002
    of hindfoot, 999
Valgus thrust, 21
Varusings osteotomy with RNL and trochanter distalization for Perthes, 922
Vascularized autograft transfer, 988
Vascularized fibula graft nonunion, 1005
Vascularized fibular grafting, 798, 799
Vascular pathoanatomy, 601
Vastus medialis obliquus (VMO), 549
Venofer (iron) infusion, 821
Verebelyi-Ogston procedure, 522
Vitamin D deficiency, 845, 979
Vitamin D metabolism, 429, 430
Vitamin D-resistent rickets (VDRR), 432, 845, 846
von Recklinghausen disease, 5

W
Warner syndrome, 8
Weber classification, 751
Weber Patellar arthroplasty, 758, 759
Weight-bearing ambulation, 1005

Werner mesomelic syndrome (WMS), 748
Wilm's tumor, 7
Windswept angular deformity, 564

X
X-linked hereditary hypophosphatemic rickets (XLH)
    bilateral femoral varus deformities, 446–448
    clinical features, 432, 433
    CORA, 439
    drill hole technique, 440
    fixator-assisted nailing technique, 439, 440
    follow-up, 444
    genu valgum deformity, 447–450
    genu varum deformity, 447, 450–452
    Gigli saw technique, 440
    guided growth technique, 453
    medical treatment, 434, 435
    non-pharmacological, 435
    orthopedic, 435–439
    patient-centered multidisciplinary care model, 433, 434
    PHEX, 432
    rehabilitation, 435
    surgical technique, 441–444
    varus deformity, 433

Z
Zoledronic acid (ZA), 799, 801
Zone of polarizing activity (ZPA), 595
Z-plasty, 759

Printed by Printforce, the Netherlands